CT and MR Angiography:
Comprehensive Vascular Assessment

CT and MR Angiography:

Comprehensive Vascular Assessment

Geoffrey D. Rubin, MD

Professor of Radiology
Associate Dean for Clinical Affairs
Chief, Section of Cardiovascular Imaging, Department of Radiology
Stanford University School of Medicine
Stanford, California

Neil M. Rofsky, MD

Associate Professor of Radiology
Harvard Medical School
Director, MRI
Beth Israel Deaconess Medical Center
Boston, Massachusetts

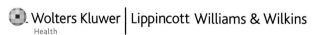
Wolters Kluwer | Lippincott Williams & Wilkins
Health

Philadelphia • Baltimore • New York • London
Buenos Aires • Hong Kong • Sydney • Tokyo

Acquisitions Editor: Lisa McAllister

Managing Editor: Kerry Barrett

Project Manager: Nicole Walz

Manufacturing Coordinator: Kathy Brown

Senior Marketing Manager: Angela Panetta

Design Coordinator: Holly Reid McLaughlin

Cover Designer: Karen Kappe

Production Services: Aptara®

Library of Congress Cataloging-in-Publication Data

Rubin, Geoffrey D.
    CT and MR angiography : comprehensive vascular assessment / Geoffrey
D. Rubin, Neil M. Rofsky.
        p. ; cm.
    Includes bibliographical references and index.
    ISBN-13: 978-0-7817-4525-3
    ISBN-10: 0-7817-4525-X
  1. Blood-vessels—Tomography. 2. Blood-vessels—Magnetic resonance
imaging. I. Rofsky, Neil M. II. Title. III. Title: Computed
tomographic and magnetic resonance angiography.
    [DNLM: 1. Vascular Diseases—diagnosis. 2. Magnetic Resonance
Angiography—methods. 3. Tomography, X-Ray Computed—methods. WG 500
R959c 2008]
    RC691.6.T65R83 2008
    616.1'307548—dc22

                                                2007051427

Care has been taken to confirm the accuracy of the information presented and to describe generally accepted practices. However, the authors, editors, and publisher are not responsible for errors or omissions or for any consequences from application of the information in this book and make no warranty, expressed or implied, with respect to the currency, completeness, or accuracy of the contents of the publication. Application of this information in a particular situation remains the professional responsibility of the practitioner; the clinical treatments described and recommended may not be considered absolute and universal recommendations.

The authors, editors, and publisher have exerted every effort to ensure that drug selection and dosage set forth in this text are in accordance with current recommendations and practice at the time of publication. However, in view of ongoing research, changes in government regulations, and the constant flow of information relating to drug therapy and drug reactions, the reader is urged to check the package insert for each drug for any change in indications and dosage and for added warnings and precautions. This is particularly important when the recommended agent is a new or infrequently employed drug.

Some drugs and medical devices presented in this publication have Food and Drug Administration (FDA) clearance for limited use in restricted research settings. It is the responsibility of health care providers to ascertain the FDA status of each drug or device planned for use in their clinical practice.

The publishers have made every effort to trace copyright holders for borrowed material. If they have inadvertently overlooked any, they will be pleased to make the necessary arrangements at the first opportunity.

To purchase additional copies of this book, call our customer service department at (800) 638-3030 or fax orders to (301) 223-2320. International customers should call (301) 223-2300.

Visit Lippincott Williams & Wilkins on the Internet: http://www.lww.com. Lippincott Williams & Wilkins customer service representatives are available from 8:30 am to 6:00 pm, EST.

10 9 8 7 6 5 4 3 2 1

Dedication

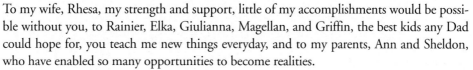

To my wife, Rhesa, my strength and support, little of my accomplishments would be possible without you, to Rainier, Elka, Giulianna, Magellan, and Griffin, the best kids any Dad could hope for, you teach me new things everyday, and to my parents, Ann and Sheldon, who have enabled so many opportunities to become realities.

—GDR

To my wife, Lisa, for empowering and enriching my life, to my children, Anna and Bennett, who make everything worthwhile, and to my parents, Lorraine and David, for showing me that possibilities are infinite.

—NMR

Dedication

Contents

Preface

Cardiovascular diseases represent the leading causes of death in the United States, Europe, and regions of Asia. Conventional angiography has played a dominant role in the diagnosis and characterization of these disorders using high-spatial and temporal resolution for luminal visualization of the cardiovascular system. However, even as a backbone for the evaluation of cardiovascular diseases, its fundamental limitations are noteworthy: each contrast injection typically provides a single perspective of often complex, three-dimensional vascular anatomy; there are geometric constraints that prevent access to many critical imaging perspectives; there is a restricted sensitivity to low contrast details in the anatomy; there is no ability to directly visualize the blood vessel walls and perivascular tissues; and its invasiveness has a substantial impact on both the patient and the cost of performing the diagnostic evaluation.

Due to innovations in hardware, software, and image analysis technology, computed tomography (CT) and magnetic resonance imaging (MR) angiography are now at the forefront of clinical cardiovascular imaging. In fact, these "noninvasive" techniques are replacing conventional angiography and are poised to serve as a new gold standard by providing equivalent or, in many cases, superior characterization of cardiovascular abnormalities. Both CT and MR are three-dimensional imaging tools that are built from thin section acquisitions, yielding volumetric data that can be assessed from innumerable perspectives, both graphical and quantitative. When combined with the advantages of eliminating the need for arterial punctures, a compelling case for the widespread adoption of noninvasive CV imaging with CT and MR emerges.

The rapid and continuous evolution of these tools for cardiovascular evaluations has left medical imaging practitioners in a challenging position. Many physicians with a deep knowledge of cardiovascular anatomy and disease need to master the skills in image acquisition and interpretation required from technologies that are fundamentally different from the traditional skill set required of conventional angiographers. Conversely, many sophisticated users of CT and MR technology may not have the requisite understanding of cardiovascular anatomy, disease, and treatment options. Thus, we intend for this book to fill the respective gaps that now exist and, in so doing, broaden the range of individuals capable of generating terrific images and delivering the key information for effective patient management. Furthermore, referring physicians will be afforded a resource to understand the capability of these modalities to provide the information they may be seeking.

We have been fortunate to have recruited top cardiovascular CT and MR experts to present an integrated approach to the acquisition and analysis of volumetric cardiovascular imaging. We have strived for a balanced and uniform approach supported by ample references. It is our sincere hope that readers find this work to be a staple of cardiovascular imaging and one that will be "well worn" from frequent use in daily practice.

Foreword

When I published the first edition of *Abrams' Angiography* almost a half century ago, the field of vascular imaging had advanced to a point at which a comprehensive reference volume was required. Over the next few decades, a new subspecialty was created based on catheter technologies that were moderately invasive and afforded exquisitely precise selective visualization of many branches of the central and peripheral vascular bed. Just as sophisticated imaging methods have invariably preceded surgical progress in the viscera—the brain, the gastrointestinal tract, the kidneys—so the improvements in vascular radiology underlay much of the progress in vascular surgery and the creation of the entire field of interventional radiology.

During the late 1950s and early 1960s, selective coronary arteriography was introduced and then was evermore widely applied to the study of the coronary circulation. The images were so striking that the arteriogram became the gold standard for confirmation of the presence of disease: the vessels involved, the degree of stenosis, the patency of by-pass grafts, and the congenital anomalies of clinical significance. In this setting, the diagnostic catheter was later converted into a therapeutic instrument, as balloon angioplasty became an important option.

Freeman Dyson, the great physicist at the Institute for Advanced Study (Princeton), has noted that concept-driven science has not always recognized or understood the cataclysmic contributions based on "tool" revolution. Just as the Galileo transformation in astronomy was based on the telescope, so x-ray crystallography radically changed biology. (Rosalind Franklin's images of DNA were the real foundation behind the Watson-Crick formulation of the structure of the DNA molecule.) The huge accumulation of knowledge of cardiovascular physiology and disease that characterized the 20th century was based far less on innovative research ideas than on the application of extraordinarily versatile tools, x-rays first and foremost. Side by side with the electrocardiogram, echocardiography, and the biochemistry laboratory these methods have afforded the clinician with a wealth of information critical to the management of patients with heart disease. Catheter angiography, however, has had its costs, monetary to be sure but also biologic. As an invasive procedure, it has well-known complications as well as contrast media reactions. It also involves exposure to ionizing radiation. Clearly, less-invasive methods would be desirable.

This brings us directly to the rationale behind this impressive volume. In the continuing search for methods that are safer and less consequential to patients, both MRI and multidetector CT have proven to be invaluable approaches to visualizing the heart and vascular bed. At such a point in the history of technologic advance applied to human subjects, an imperative become clear to fine minds in the field. The need becomes pressing to organize the huge amount of pertinent information that has become available. The lessons that have been learned, the variations in technique that have been developed, and the value of the methods in each vascular bed can all be embodied in a single volume to which both newcomers and those already in the field may refer. The challenge is very large, and it can only be surmounted when experience and expertise are coupled with unusual organizational ability, strong motivation, working weekends, and familiarity with the best sources in the field.

Drs. Rubin and Rofsky have risen to the challenge. With the help of their talented colleagues, they have produced a text that is thoroughly documented and profusely illustrated. While its practicality lends a strong "how to" quality to the volume, it responds equally well to the intellectual demands of the large literature which has been analyzed in each chapter.

In line with their hope and desire, *CT and MR Angiography* will be viewed as a seminal text for many years to come.

Herbert L. Abrams, MD
Philip H. Cook Professor of Radiology, Emeritus
Harvard Medical School
Professor of Radiology, Emeritus,
Stanford University School of Medicine

With Special Thanks

Daniel Nóbrega Costa, MD
Editorial Assistance

Nancy Prendergast, MD and Kimberly Battista
Medical Illustrations

Acknowledgments

I am indebted to my mentors for being so giving of their time, their knowledge, and their enthusiasm for medical imaging. They have lead me to a truly rewarding career. As a medical student at UCSD, Skip vanSonnenberg's exuberant spirit helped me appreciate the power of imaging in medical diagnosis and therapeutic guidance and lead me to choose a career in radiology. As a resident, Brooke Jeffrey and Gary Glazer both showed me what it meant to be a CT master. I marveled at their insightful syntheses of keen observation and inference. The foundation for my career in academics and my deep affinity for cardiovascular imaging were created by Michael Dake. Starting a new clinical application as a third year resident was a challenge and without angiographic correlation all I had were pretty pictures. Mike saw to it that anyone in whom he found a stenosis, aneurysm or dissection came to me for CTA. The correlations and Mike's insights were critical; his creativity was an inspiration. Of equal importance to our nascent non-invasive CV imaging program, Sandy Napel exposed me to computer graphics and opened my mind to a wealth of possibility in volumetric image analysis. Our 17-year collaboration (and counting) has been the key to many imaging innovations. It also resulted in the creation of our 3D Laboratory. Lead by Laura Pierce, the tremendously talented staff has been critical to bringing the benefits of 3D applications to tens of thousands of Stanford patients and their physicians. The support, collegiality, and expertise of cardiothoracic and vascular surgeons, Scott Mitchell, Craig Miller, Neal Olcott, and Chris Zarins contributed greatly to the adoption and acceptance of CT angiography at Stanford and brought me opportunities to introduce CTA to a rich worldwide community of cardiovascular specialists.

I am grateful to my many colleagues in the Department of Radiology at Stanford. I wish that I could name you all. Without you I would not be spending my twentieth year in the department. Of equal importance to my contentment has been the energy and enthusiasm of the greatest students, residents, and fellows anywhere. I am particularly indebted to those former Stanford trainees who were invaluable in pulling this book together—Danny Donovan, Tamer El-Helw, Rich Hallett, Amir Pezeshkmehr, Justus Roos, and Pietro Sedati.

Finally a gigantic thank you to Neil Rofsky who has been a tremendous partner in this the most extensive and exhaustive of my academic efforts to date. Thank goodness for those late night jam sessions. What's next, a second edition or a rock opera about writing the first?

—GDR

There are so many individuals that I am indebted to for inspiration, for time and patience, for open mindedness, for intellectual generosity and for posing critical challenges— these gifts and the spirit behind them have allowed me to accomplish much more than I could have imagined possible.

The formative years for my MRA experience at NYU were an era of discovery, productivity, strong collaboration and immeasurable joy. The phenomenal team that included Glynn Johnson, Glenn Krinsky, Vivian Lee and Jeffrey Weinreb ensured our successes. Jeff deserves special recognition since it was his original suggestion that prompted me to pursue MRA, which ultimately changed the course of my professional career. That proposition was initially met with reluctance from me, a radiologist trained in abdominal imaging and fearful of being a fish out of water. But, thanks to the many hours and cases spent with vascular-interventionalist Bob Rosen, and with vascular surgeons, Mark Adelman, Gary Giangola, Pat Lamparello and Tom Riles, a solid foundation was established to launch the new path in my career. I have vivid memories of being the young, upstart radiologist in the NYU vascular surgery conference, always asking "what about MRA?" to which, in the early days, there would be responses of eye-rolling, shoulder shrugging and other physical demonstrations of doubt laced with contempt. This starkly contrasts against a more recent memory, at my very last NYU vascular surgery conference, when one of the vascular surgery attendings was laying into his resident asking, "what about an MRA?", incredulous that this option had not been considered.

Along the way and through a mutual interest in this "new field" I have met many exceptional people. It is with particular gratitude and fondness that I can recognize the gifts of knowledge, nuance and friendship that evolved from lectures, discussions and collaborations with Bob Edelman, Paul Finn, Tom Grist, Gerhard Laub, Chuck Mistretta and Martin Prince, during those early years and to the present day. I continue to learn from the ever growing number of experts in the field, a reflection of the successes and expansion of this important discipline. I am also grateful for the contributions of the technologists who ably implement our developments and the talents of our many students, whose thirst for knowledge insures that the future of our field will be one of boundless opportunity.

Geoff and I have tried our best to credit all those who have been kind enough to share case material—if by chance memory or process has fallen short and you recognize one of your images lacking recognition, please let us know so that we can ascribe the due credit in the (gulp) next edition!

—NMR

Contributors

Juan Gilberto S. Aguinaldo, MD
Research Program Coordinator
Imaging Science Laboratories Departments of Radiology and
    Medicine (Cardiology)
The Zena and Michael A. Wiener Cardiovascular Institute
The Marie-Josée and Henry R. Kravis Cardiovascular Health Center
Mount Sinai School of Medicine
New York, New York

Christoph R. Becker, MD
Associate Professor
Department of Clinical Radiology
Ludwig-Maximilian University
Section Chief CT and PET/CT
Department of Clinical Radiology
Klinikum Grosshadern
Munich, Germany

Michael A. Brooks, MD
Assistant Professor
Section Head of Cardiothoracic Imaging
Department of Radiology
Wake Forest University Health Sciences
Winston-Salem, North Carolina

Patricia E. Burrows, MD
Courtesy Attending
Department of Radiology
Childrens' Hospital
Boston, Massachusetts
Attending Physician, INN
Roosevelt Hospital
New York, New York

J. Jeffrey Carr, MD, MSCE, FAHA, FACC
Professor and Vice Chair for Research
Division of Radiological Sciences
Division of Public Health Sciences
Department of Internal Medicine—Section of Cardiology
Wake Forest University School of Medicine
Winston-Salem, North Carolina

Daniel Nóbrega Costa, MD
Beth Israel Deaconess Medical Center
Hospital Sírio-Libanês
Department of Radiology
São Paulo, Brazil

James P. Earls, MD
Vice President and Medical Director
Fairfax Radiological Consultants
Clifton, Virginia

Zahi A. Fayad, PhD, FAHA, FACC
Professor
Department of Radiology and Medicine (Cardiology)
Mount Sinai School of Medicine
New York, New York

Dominik Fleischmann, MD
Associate Professor
Department of Radiology
Stanford University Medical Center
Stanford, California

W. Dennis Foley, MD
Professor of Radiology
Department of Radiology
Medical College of Wisconsin
Section Head, Digital Imaging
Department of Radiology
Froedtert Hospital
Milwaukee, Wisconsin

Isabela Gosk-Bierska, MD, PhD
Assistant Professor of Medicine
Department of Angiology
Wroclaw Medical University
Wroclaw, Poland

Marc V. Gosselin, MD
Associate Professor of Radiology
Department of Radiology
Oregon Health Science University
Portland, Oregon

Douglas E. Green, MD
Assistant Professor
Department of Radiology
University of Utah
Salt Lake City, Utah

Richard L. Hallett, MD
Chief, Cardiovascular Imaging
Northwest Radiology Network
Indianapolis, Indiana
Adjunct Clinical Assistant Professor of Radiology
Stanford University Medical Center
Stanford, California

Jeffrey C. Hellinger, MD
Assistant Professor of Radiology and Cardiology
Director of Cardiovascular Imaging
Director of CHOP 3D Medical Imaging Laboratory
The Children's Hospital of Philadelphia
University of Pennsylvania School of Medicine
Philadelphia, Pennsylvania

Christoph U. Herborn, MD
Associate Professor of Radiology
Medical Prevention Center Hamburg
University Medical Center Hamburg-Eppendorf
Hamburg, Germany

Nicole M. Hindman, MD
Assistant Professor of Radiology
Body Imaging Section
New York University School of Medicine
New York, New York

Katharine L. Hopkins, MD
Associate Professor
Departments of Radiology and Pediatrics
Chief
Division of Pediatric Radiology
Oregon Health and Science University
Portland, Oregon

R. Brooke Jeffrey, MD
Professor
Department of Radiology
Stanford University School of Medicine
Section Chief, Abdominal Imaging
Department of Radiology
Stanford University Medical Center
Stanford, California

Orhan Konez, MD
Department of Radiology
Vascular and Interventional Radiology
Cleveland Clinic
Cleveland, Ohio

Frank R. Korosec, PhD
Professor
Department of Radiology
University of Wisconsin Hospital and Clinics
Madison, Wisconsin

Roger J. Laham, MD
Associate Professor of Medicine
Department of Cardiology
BIDMC/Harvard Medical School
Boston, Massachusetts

Alexander W. Leber, MD
Imaging Science Laboratories
Departments of Radiology and Medicine (Cardiology)
The Zena and Michael A. Wiener Cardiovascular Institute
The Marie-Josée and Henry R. Kravis Cardiovascular Health Center
New York, New York
Klinikum Grosshadern
Department of Cardiology
Ludwig Maximilians University of Munich

University of Munich, Klinikum
Grosshadern, Medizinische Klinik I
Munich, Germany

Seung Uk Lee, MD
Division of Cardiology
Department of Medicine
Harvard Medical School and
Beth Israel Deaconess Medical Center
Boston, Massachusetts

Tim Leiner, MD, PhD
Assistant Professor
Cardiovascular Research Institute Maastricht (CARIM)
Maastricht University Faculty of Health, Medicine and Life Sciences
Department of Radiology
Maastricht University Hospital
Maastricht, The Netherlands

Jeffrey H. Maki, MD, PhD
Associate Professor
Department of Radiology
University of Washington
Director of Body MRI
Department of Radiology
University of Washington Medical Center
Seattle, Washington

Venkatesh Mani, PhD
Imaging Science Laboratories
Departments of Radiology and Medicine (Cardiology)
The Zena and Michael A. Wiener Cardiovascular Institute
The Marie-Josée and Henry R. Kravis
   Cardiovascular Health Center
Mount Sinai School of Medicine
New York, New York

Warren J. Manning, MD
Professor of Medicine and Radiology
Harvard Medical School
Section Chief, Non-invasive Cardiac Imaging
Beth Israel Deaconess Medical Center
Boston, Massachusetts

James F. M. Meaney, FRCR
Director
Centre for Advanced Medical Imaging
Director, MRI
Department of Radiology
St. James Hospital
Dublin, Ireland

Henrik J. Michaely, MD
Section Chief Vascular and Abdominal MRI
Institute of Clinical Radiology
University Heidelberg–University Hospital Mannheim
Mannheim, Germany

Lee M. Mitsumori, MD
Assistant Professor of Radiology
Department of Radiology
University of Washington
Seattle, Washington

Ivan Pedrosa, MD
Assistant Professor
Department of Radiology
Harvard Medical School
Staff Radiologist
Department of Radiology
Beth Israel Deaconess Medical Center
Boston, Massachusetts

F. Scott Pereles, MD
Director of MRI
Salinas Valley Radiologists and Coastal Valley Imaging
Salinas, California

Mathias Prokop, MD, PhD
Professor of Radiology
Department of Radiology
University Medical Center Utrecht
Utrecht, The Netherlands

Neil M. Rofsky, MD
Associate Professor of Radiology
Harvard Medical School
Director, MRI
Beth Israel Deaconess Medical Center
Boston, Massachusetts

Geoffrey D. Rubin, MD
Professor of Radiology
Associate Dean for Clinical Affairs
Chief, Section of Cardiovascular Imaging, Department of Radiology
Stanford University School of Medicine
Stanford, California

A. Daniel Sasson, MD
Attending
Division of Interventional Neuroradiology
Maimonides Medical Center
Brooklyn, New York
Interventional Neuroradiology
Department of Radiology
The Johns Hopkins Medical Institutions
Baltimore, Maryland

Stefan O. Schoenberg, MD
Oberarzt, Leiter des Funktionsbereichs
Magnetresonanztomographie
Department of Radiology
München, Germany

U. Joseph Schoepf, MD
Associate Professor of Radiology and Medicine
Medical University of South Carolina
Charleston, South Carolina

Pietro Sedati, MD
Resident in Radiology
University of Rome, Rome, Italy

Marilyn J. Siegel, MD
Professor of Radiology and Pediatrics
Mallinckrodt Institute of Radiology
Washington University School of Medicine
St. Louis, Missouri

Daniel Y. Sze, MD, PhD
Associate Professor
Division of Interventional Radiology
Stanford University Medical Center
Stanford, California

Andrzej Szuba, MD, PhD
Assistant Professor of Medicine
Departments of Internal and Occupational Diseases
Wroclaw Medical University
Wroclaw, Poland

Bruce A. Wasserman, MD
Associate Professor of Radiology
Director of Diagnostic Neurovascular Imaging
The Russell H. Morgan Department of Radiology and Radiological
    Sciences
The Johns Hopkins University School of Medicine
The Johns Hopkins Hospital
Baltimore, Maryland

Jesse L. Wei, MD
Instructor in Radiology
Harvard Medical School
Beth Israel Deaconess Medical Center
Boston, Massachusetts

Stephan G. Wetzel, MD
Deputy Head
Department of Diagnostic and Interventional Neruoradiology
University Hospital Basel
Basel, Switzerland

Joanna J. Wykrzykowska, MD
Division of Cardiology
Department of Medicine, Harvard Medical School
Beth Israel Deaconess Medical Center
Boston, Massachusetts

Eric Zeikus, MD
Former Abdominal Imaging Fellow Department of Radiology
Beth Israel Deaconess Medical Center
Harvard Medical School
Boston, Massachusetts

CT and MR Angiography:
Comprehensive Vascular Assessment

IMAGING PRINCIPLES

CHAPTER 1

Principles of Computed Tomographic Angiography

Mathias Prokop

Computed tomographic angiography (CTA) is one of the big success stories in diagnostic radiology. CTA was developed shortly after the introduction of spiral (helical) CT scanning in the early 1990s. Spiral CT had made it possible to cover body regions so rapidly that the transient enhancement of the vascular system following intravenous contrast injection could be captured during one scan. With the introduction of multidetector-row technology, CTA gained a tremendous boost and quickly became an easy-to-perform standard technique for vascular imaging.

Over the years, CTA—together with magnetic resonance angiography—has taken over most diagnostic vascular procedures from invasive catheter angiography, first for the aorta and the pulmonary arteries; later for the carotids, renal, and splanchnic arteries; and recently also for peripheral arteries and the circle of Willis. Most recently, CTA of the coronaries has been developed. While coronary CTA is still technically challenging, it also holds the promise to substitute for part of diagnostic cardiac catheter angiographies.

CTA has the advantage that it can be highly standardized, which makes it a very fast and robust procedure that is the technique of choice in many acute vascular diseases. It provides three-dimensional information with a comparatively high spatial resolution and allows for simultaneous evaluation of the vascular lumen as well as the vessel wall and the surrounding structures. In fact, every arterial phase CT can potentially serve as an arterial CTA, while a portal phase scan can serve as a portal venous CTA.

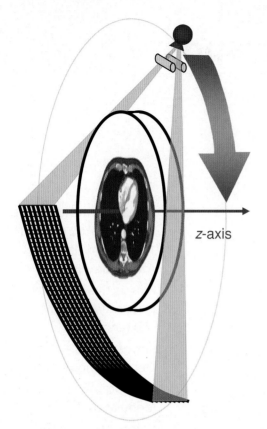

FIGURE 1-1 Principle of current CT scanners: A thin fan-shaped beam rotates around the body and is detected by a synchronously rotating detector array. (From M. Prokop et al. *Spiral and Multislice CT of the Body.* Thieme Medical Publishers 2003, with permission.)

CT technology has seen more rapid improvements than other radiological techniques: over the past decade, scanner performance doubled approximately every two years. While CT technology nowadays is more than sufficient for standard CTA applications, further developments focus on improvement of quality and robustness of coronary CTA as well as CT perfusion imaging.

This chapter will provide the basic understanding of CT technology as it relates to CTA as well as show how to optimize scanner parameter settings, discuss various trade-offs, and suggest solutions to typical problems and pitfalls encountered in clinical practice.

BASIC CONCEPTS OF COMPUTED TOMOGRAPHY

Computed tomography is an x-ray tomographic technique in which an x-ray source rotates around the body and an x-ray beam passes through the patient from various directions (Fig. 1-1). A mathematical image reconstruction (inverse Radon transformation) uses the x-ray attenuation along each of the many paths through the body (the *CT raw data*) to calculate the local attenuation at each point within the acquisition volume. The local attenuation coefficients are normalized to yield *CT numbers* for every point of the image matrix. These *CT image data* are finally converted into shades of gray that are displayed as an image.

The first two generations of CT scanner geometries were already abandoned in the late 1970s and were substituted by third- and fourth-generation scanners. With the advent of multidetector-row CT, only *third-generation geometry* is still available. In these scanners, an x-ray tube and a detector array rotate synchronously around the patient. Parallel collimation is used to shape the x-ray beam to a thin fan, which defines the total thickness of the acquired transaxial volume (Fig. 1-1).

Apart from the first scanner generations in the 1970s, which had two parallel detector arrays, later scanners used a single detector array for measuring the intensity of the attenuated radiation as it emerged from the body. In these *single detector-row scanners*, the thickness of the acquired section could be varied by changing the collimated width of the x-ray beam. For thinner section collimation, only part of the detector array was exposed (Fig. 1-2A). In the early 1990s, one vendor introduced a *dual slice system*, in which the detector array was split in half so that two sections were exposed simultaneously (Fig. 1-2B). In the late 1990s, *multidetector-row scanners* were developed that consisted of multiple parallel arrays that could be combined so that four simultaneous sections could be acquired (Fig. 1-2C). Development went on rapidly, and currently, 128-row scanners are on the market.

In the 1970s and 1980s, the scan volume was covered in a stepwise manner: After acquiring a transaxial section, the table was moved by a certain amount (usually the section thickness) and the next of these *sequential scans* was performed (Fig. 1-3A). This scanning technique was slow and suffered from discontinuities at the border between sections whenever there was motion between consecutive scans.

With the advent of scanners with continuously rotating x-ray tubes, it became possible to acquire a data volume in continuous fashion: Raw data was captured during multiple rotations while the patient table moved through the scan plane (Fig. 1-3B). This technology, which was named *spiral* or *helical CT*, required suitable interpolation techniques to compensate for motion while allowing for reconstruction of a complete three-dimensional data set consisting of overlapping axial images. It became the basis of CT angiography because it avoided step artifacts due to suboptimum registration (for example, as a result of inconsistent depth of inspiration between consecutive sections) and had the advantage that a larger volume could be imaged rapidly and continuously so that transient phases of contrast enhancement could be captured within one scan.

Dynamic scanning is the third scanning technique available in CT: Here, the table remains stationary, and the scanned sections are exposed repeatedly to image dynamic processes such as the enhancement after intravenous contrast

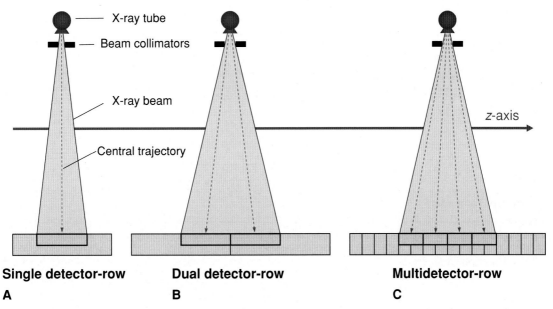

FIGURE 1-2 Comparison of the detector geometry of single detector-row scanners, dual detector-row scanners, and multidetector-row scanners—in this case, with 4 detector rows. (From M. Prokop et al. *Spiral and Multislice CT of the Body*. Thieme Medical Publishers 2003, with permission.)

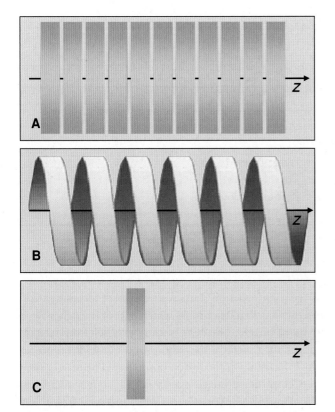

FIGURE 1-3 Principle of sequential scanning **(A)**, spiral or helical scanning **(B)**, and dynamic scanning **(C)**. In sequential scanning, each section is acquired at a constant table position, then the table is moved and the next section is acquired. In spiral scanning, the table is moved during the acquisition process. In dynamic scanning, a particular section is scanned multiple times to evaluate temporal changes.

injection (Fig. 1-3C). Dynamic scanning can be used to find the optimum starting point for a CTA examination and also for evaluating tissue perfusion (CT perfusion imaging, CTP).

Sequential, spiral, or dynamic data acquisition is available with single detector-row as well as with multidetector-row scanners.

SCANNING PARAMETERS

The most important scanning parameters for CT angiography are summarized in Table 1-1.

Acquisition Parameters

The following parameters described in Table 1-1 determine data acquisition:

- Number of active detector rows (N)
- Section collimation (SC)
- Rotation time (RT)
- Table feed per rotation (TF)
- Pitch factor (P): $P = TF/(N \times C)$
- Scan length (L)
- Tube voltage (U), also called the kVp setting
- Tube load (I $\times$ t), also called the mAs setting.

The number of active detector rows or simultaneously acquired sections is one for single detector-row CT, two for dual detector-row CT, and 4 to (presently) 128 for multidetector-row CT. Section collimation is determined by the total width of the acquired volume in the center of the scan field divided by the number of sections. The rotation time is the time it takes for the tube–detector unit to rotate once around the patient.

TABLE 1-1

Overview of the Most Important Scan Parameters for CT Angiography

Acquisition Parameters

N	Number of active detector rows	(1 – 320)
SC	Section collimation (mm)	(nominal section thickness)
TF	Table feed per tube rotation (mm)	(N × SC × P)
P	Pitch	(TF/[N × SC])
RT	Rotation time (s)	(duration of one tube rotation)
L	Scan length (cm)	(T × TS = T × N × SC × P/RT)
SFOV	Scan field of view	(determines area from which data is acquired)

Derivative Parameters

TS	Table speed (mm/s)	(TF/RT)
T	Scan duration (s)	(scan time = L/TS = L × RT/[N × SC × P])

Reconstruction Parameters

M	Matrix size	(usually 512^2; 768^2 or $1,024^2$ also available on some scanners)
FOV	Field of view	(smaller or equal to SFOV)
F	Reconstruction filter	(filter kernel, determines xy-resolution)
SW	Section width (mm)	(effective section thickness, determines z-resolution)
RI	Reconstruction increment (mm)	(reconstruction interval)

Dose Parameters

I × t	Tube load (mAs)	(mAs settings)
U	Tube voltage (kVp)	(kVp setting, usually 80, 90, 100, 120, 130, or 140 kVp)
$CTDI_{vol}$	Volume CT dose index (mGy)	(average dose measured in a 16-cm head or 32-cm body phantom)
E	Effective dose (mSv)	(dose that describes radiation risk)

Table feed per rotation and pitch are parameters that are relevant for spiral scanning: The table feed indicates how much the table moves during the rotation time. The pitch factor provides the relation between table feed and total width of the acquired volume. The maximum pitch depends on the scanner manufacturer and usually varies between 1.5 and 2. For sequential scanning, the table feed between consecutive sections is usually chosen identical to the section collimation, and the resulting pitch is 1.

Scan length depends on the clinical indication. Scan duration can be derived from scan length and table speed, and thus the other parameters as described in Table 1-1.

Tube load, pitch, and tube voltage are main determinants of patient dose. Tube load, also called the mAs setting, is proportional to the radiation dose, while pitch is inversely proportional to it. This has led to the definition of effective tube load (or effective mAs): $mAs_{eff} = mAs/P$. Tube voltage (kVp setting) determines the energy of the x-ray beam: At higher energy, there is more penetrating power. However, the x-ray attenuation of elements with a higher atomic number than water (for example, calcium or iodine) will be relatively higher at lower x-ray energy. At constant mAs, the dose *decreases* if lower kVp settings are chosen.

Reconstruction Parameters

Image reconstruction is influenced by the following parameters (Table 1-1):

- Field of view (FOV)
- Matrix size (M)
- Reconstruction filter (F)
- Raw data interpolation algorithm (for spiral scanning)
- Reconstructed section width (SW), also called section thickness
- Reconstruction increment (RI)

Image reconstruction starts with choice of a reconstruction field of view that determines which part of the data will end up in the images. The FOV is usually chosen from reference images that include the whole body cross sections and allows focusing on the region of interest. The matrix size of the reconstructed image usually is 512^2, but modern scanners allow for other matrices as well (768^2 or $1,024^2$).

The reconstruction filter is required to reconstruct usable images from the projectional raw data. It determines the trade-off between spatial resolution in the imaging plane (*xy*-plane) and the image noise. The raw data interpolation

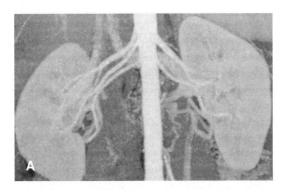
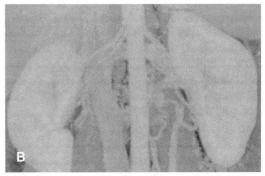

FIGURE 1-4 Contrast-to-noise ratio and image quality. Maximum intensity projection (MIP) of the renal arteries with high CNR in the arterial phase **(A)** and low CNR in the portal venous phase **(B)**. Note that image noise and exposure parameters were similar in both examples, but the contrast enhancement was lower in the portal venous phase. In such a late phase, vessels can no longer be visualized if their enhancement is similar to that of the background tissue.

algorithm is necessary in spiral scanning to compensate for the continuous motion during the scan, but more sophisticated raw data interpolation algorithms are also used to compensate for cone beam effects in multidetector-row CT (p. 20).

Reconstructed section width or section thickness refers to the thickness of the CT sections in the final images. In sequential scanning, section width and section collimation are identical. With spiral scanning, section width is commonly larger than section collimation (p. 13). With multidetector-row CT, section width can be varied almost arbitrarily but is always larger than or equal to the chosen section collimation (p. 14). Section collimation therefore determines the thinnest section width that can be reconstructed.

The reconstruction increment is a parameter for spiral scanning: Here, images can be reconstructed at arbitrary increments that are smaller than the chosen section width or section collimation. In sequential scanning, the reconstruction increment is identical to the table feed between sections.

PERFORMANCE PARAMETERS

In order to be able to optimize image quality for CTA, it is helpful to understand the basic physical parameters that determine performance of a CT scanner or a scanning protocol. The main parameters are contrast-to-noise ratio and spatial resolution, which determine how well a vessel is displayed and how small a detail can be evaluated.

Contrast-to-Noise Ratio

The contrast-to-noise ratio (CNR) determines how well a given vessel can be displayed. At a high CNR, even small vessels can be detected, and vessel contours on 3D displays appear well defined (Fig. 1-4A). At a low CNR, small vessels may no longer be sufficiently visualized to make a diagnosis, and 3D displays of larger vessels may be irregular with insufficiently defined contours (Fig. 1-4B).

CNR is determined by the difference in CT numbers between vessel of interest and surrounding soft tissues in relation to the image noise:

$$CNR = (CT_{vessel} - CT_{soft\ tissue})/Noise$$

Contrast

The contrast in the CNR is determined by the enhancement of the target vessel and the CT number of the surrounding soft tissues. Since a vessel is rarely surrounded by only one type of soft tissue, CNR varies locally and may be difficult to determine in clinical practice. For this reason, water is frequently used as a substitute for soft tissue in the equation above.

To understand how the contrast is influenced by CT numbers, it is useful to have a quick look at CT-number definition: CT numbers are derived from the local x-ray attenuation (μ) by normalizing x-ray attenuation to water: $CT = 1,000 \times (\mu - \mu_{water})/\mu_{water}$. The numbers are set on a scale in which $-1,000$ represents the attenuation of air and 0 is the attenuation of water. Note that there is no upper limit to the scale. In honor of Sir Godfrey N. Hounsfield, the inventor of CT, the unit for CT numbers is called the *Hounsfield unit* (HU). The normalization process reduces the dependence of the CT number on the energy of the radiation as long as the chemical composition of the examined structure is similar to that of water. This holds true for most soft tissues but is not the case for calcium or iodine-containing structures. Optimizing the energy of the x-ray beam therefore can be used to increase the CT numbers of contrast-enhanced vessels.

Enhancement of the target vessel depends on the local intravascular iodine concentration. This local iodine concentration is heavily influenced by the contrast material injection protocol (see Chapter 2) as well as by the timing of the scan. Intravenously injected contrast material first travels through the right heart and pulmonary system; then through the left heart, the aorta, and the arterial system;

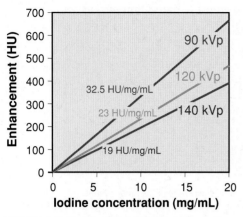

FIGURE 1-5 Vascular enhancement versus iodine concentration for various kVp settings. Note that enhancement per mg iodine is higher at lower kVp settings.

and finally returns back to the right heart via portal and systemic veins. Proper timing, depending on the target vessels, is therefore mandatory.

Enhancement is not only dependent on the local iodine concentration but also on the energy spectrum of the radiation. Within the energy range used for CT examinations, the CT numbers of iodine-containing contrast material increase rapidly as lower tube voltages (kVp settings) are applied (Fig. 1-5). At identical intravascular iodine concentrations, better enhancement and therefore better contrast can be obtained at low kVp settings.

In clinical practice, surrounding tissues may also enhance. This is especially the case for parenchymal organs such as the liver or the kidneys. If such vessels are to be evaluated, the scan must be timed early enough to ensure that there is no substantial tissue enhancement present (compare Fig. 1-4).

Image Noise

Image noise refers to random variations in CT numbers, which cause problems in contour definition and low-contrast resolution (Fig. 1-6). Noise is mainly due to the limited amount of quanta that hit the CT detector array (*quantum noise*), but it is also caused by other sources such as the detector electronics (*electronic noise*). Image noise is usually described by the standard deviation of the CT numbers within a homogenous region of an object. Image noise is determined by the following factors:

- Radiation dose and quantum statistics (in principle, the number of photons that pass through the reconstructed voxel),
- Overall detector efficiency (the ability to detect as many quanta as possible and add as little additional noise from electronic detector components),
- Image interpolation (for example, to correct for motion in the case of spiral scanning), and
- Image reconstruction algorithm (the filter kernel that determines spatial resolution in the scan plane).

High image noise causes similar problems as low contrast: at high noise, small vessels may vanish, and contours are no longer sharply defined (Fig. 1-6).

Windowing

Windowing is a technique used in most imaging systems: It assigns only a small portion (window) on the number scale to actual gray levels that are displayed on a monitor or printed on film. Windowing is used to vary the visual contrast and brightness of a digital image. A window is characterized by its center (also called *level*) and its width.

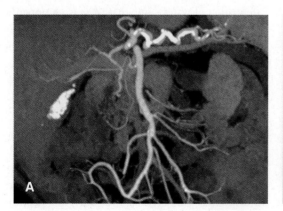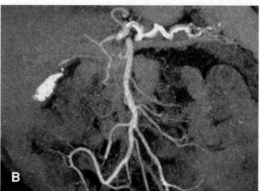

FIGURE 1-6 CTA angiography of a patient with an aberrant right hepatic artery arising from the superior mesenteric artery. The scan was part of an ECG-gated exam with 64 × 0.625 mm collimation acquired with 300 mAs (CTDI$_{vol}$ = 18 mGy). The untagged reconstruction takes advantage of all data and has a low image noise **(A)**, while the gated reconstruction uses only about 15% of the data and therefore suffers from increased image noise **(B)**. The periphery of the hepatic artery can no longer be evaluated in **(B)**. Note that calcified gallstones also are displayed on these maximum intensity projections.

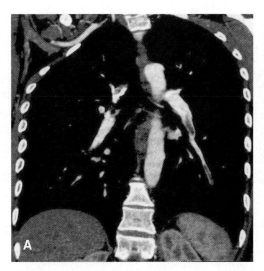 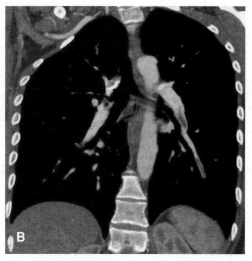

FIGURE 1-7 Effect of windowing. A narrow window enhances contrast and visual noise perception **(A)**, while a wide window reduces contrast and noise perception **(B)**. CNR is not affected. The window has to be wide enough that structures in enhanced lumen can be discerned. It has to be increased in width for vessels with higher enhancement.

Windowing affects visual contrast and noise perception equally. The contrast-to-noise ratio of the image is not affected. A wide window results in low contrast and little noise; a narrow window results in a high contrast but also a high noise (Fig. 1-7).

In practice, the optimum window width for CTA is determined by the intravascular contrast enhancement and, to a lesser degree, by the presence of wall calcifications or differences in tissues around the vessels. High enhancement and the presence of calcifications require a wide window, while insufficient enhancement requires narrower window settings. It is obvious that a high enhancement is desirable because it increases CNR and allows for using wider window settings that suppress image noise.

Spatial Resolution

Spatial resolution determines how small a detail can be evaluated and how sharp a given structure is depicted. Spatial resolution in a CT image depends on matrix size and system resolution. System resolution is determined by the scanner geometry and the chosen acquisition parameters. If the matrix is fine enough (small enough pixels, or picture elements), the spatial resolution in the image equals the system resolution. Commonly, the spatial resolution of an imaging system is described in one of the following three ways.

- The *modulation transfer function* (MTF) describes how much percent of its original contrast a structural detail of a certain size retains in the image (Fig. 1-8). The size of structural details is given in terms of spatial frequencies. The MTF is the most abstract and correct way of describing spatial resolution. The MTF

decreases toward higher spatial frequencies. Vendors usually use a cutoff point around 4% and provide the corresponding spatial frequency (in cycles per centimeter) as the maximum spatial resolution of the imaging system. However, a cutoff point of 4% has little to do with clinical reality. It means that the contrast of the original structure has been reduced by a factor of 25: For a small vessel, that will mean that its original contrast—for example, 500 HU—will have been reduced to 20 HU in the image. A cutoff frequency of 20% is much more realistic, but data at this point are less readily available (Fig. 1-8).

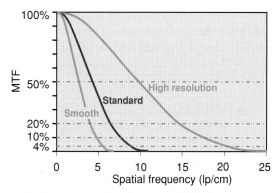

FIGURE 1-8 The modulation transfer function (MTF) describes how the contrast of a detail of a certain size (spatial frequency in line pairs per centimeter) is displayed in an image. In technical reports of scanner systems, spatial resolution is usually described as the spatial frequency at which the MTF reaches 4%. This value is unrealistic for CTA. A cutoff value of 20% or the mean of the cutoff values at 10% and 50% describe the systems better. In this example, MTFs for typical smooth, standard, and high resolution filters are provided. In CTA, only smooth and standard filters are used.

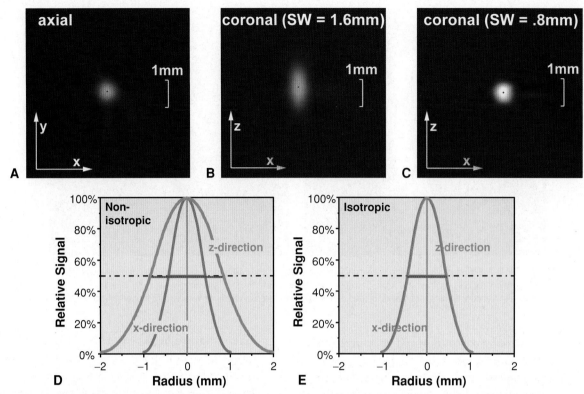

FIGURE 1-9 The point spread function (PSF) describes how a tiny detail is displayed in the image. Compare the images of a tiny gold bead in the axial plane **(A)** and the coronal plane scanned with a section width of 1.6 mm **(B)** and 0.8 mm **(C)**. The CT number profile though the center of the bead corresponds to the PSF. In case of a section width of 1.6 mm, the PSFs in the *x*-direction and *z*-direction will differ **(D)**, while for a section width of 0.8 mm, the PSFs in both directions are equal **(E)**. Note that the width at 50% of the height of the PSF (full width at half maximum) is a good indicator of spatial resolution. (From M. Prokop et al. *Spiral and Multislice CT of the Body*. Thieme Medical Publishers 2003, with permission.)

- The *full width at half maximum* (FWHM) of the point spread function (PSF): The PSF describes how much every detail in an object gets blurred once it is displayed in an image (Fig. 1-9). Hence, the PSF is measured experimentally by imaging a very tiny detail that is substantially below the spatial resolution of the imaging system but that has a very high contrast. In practice, gold spheres or tungsten wires are used for this purpose. The width of the point spread function indicates the spatial resolution of the system: The smaller it is, the better the resolution. It is commonly used in the *z*-direction and is then called *section width* or *effective section thickness* (see also Fig. 1-14). In the *xy*-plane, it is probably the best way of comparing spatial resolution as well, but so far, it is not yet commonly provided by the manufacturers. An approximate relation to the MTF is provided in Table 1-2.

TABLE 1-2

Effect of Reconstruction Filter on Spatial Resolution

Description	Spatial Resolution (4% MTF)	Spatial Resolution (theoretic maximum)	Spatial Resolution (FWHM of PSF)
Smooth	5 cycles/cm	1.00 mm	1.30 mm
Moderately smooth	7 cycles/cm	0.70 mm	1.00 mm
Standard	10 cycles/cm	0.50 mm	0.70 mm
High-resolution	15 cycles/cm	0.33 mm	0.55 mm

Note: Relation between spatial resolution given in line pairs per cm (at 4% MTF) and full width at half maximum (FWHM) of the point spread function (numbers in mm). The relation given here is approximate and varies depending on the actual shape of the MTF curve. The theoretic maximum is directly derived from the 4% value of the MTF but can only be reached for very high contrast structures. Note that the FWHM in the *xy*-plane corresponds to the section width in the *z*-direction.

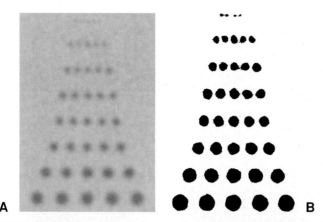

FIGURE 1-10 (A) Spatial resolution as indicated by groups of equidistant drill holes in Plexiglas measured with 64 × 0.625-mm section collimation. **(B)** Note that using a very narrow window setting can influence detail visibility.

- The smallest *size of a group of equidistant lines or holes* (Fig. 1-10): This way of displaying spatial resolution is the one that seems most intuitive, but it is also the one that is most prone to manipulation. By using very high contrast (e.g., air-filled holes or an aluminum grid to create lines) and then using a very narrow window setting (almost black and white), favorable results can be achieved that have little to do with clinical reality.

Matrix Size

Matrix size works as a limiting factor for spatial resolution. Too small a matrix can reduce spatial resolution, but a very large matrix size cannot increase resolution beyond the system resolution (Fig. 1-11). To be more precise, it is not the matrix size in itself but the resulting size of a single picture element (called a *pixel*) that limits spatial resolution. According to the sampling theorem, the pixel size should be at least one half the spatial resolution—as defined by the FWHM of the point spread function. In practice, further improvement in image quality can be seen if pixels are one third of the spatial resolution. Beyond that, the added value of even smaller pixel sizes is very limited.

Pixel size (p) is determined by the field of view (FOV) and the matrix size (M): $p = FOV/M$. In the imaging plane (*xy*-plane), the size of the reconstruction matrix is usually 512^2, but newer scanners allow for 768^2 and $1,024^2$ as well. For a full body cross section in the chest or abdomen, a FOV between 300 and 400 mm is required. The resulting pixel sizes vary from 0.6 to 0.8 mm if a 512 matrix is used.

In a coronal or sagittal plane derived from a 3D-image data set, the pixel size is derived from the pixel size in the *xy*-plane and by the reconstruction increment in the direction of the patient axis (*z*-direction). This reconstruction increment (RI) describes the distance between the centers of consecutive sections that are reconstructed from the CT raw data. In such coronal or sagittal planes, matrix size is no longer square but rectangular: In the *x*- or *y*-direction, it remains 512 (or higher, depending on the chosen reconstruction matrix), but in the *z*-direction, it is defined by the scan length (L) and the reconstruction increment (RI): $M_z = L/RI$. Again, the pixel size in the *z*-direction (i.e., the RI) should be at least one half the spatial resolution in this direction. Spatial resolution in the *z*-direction is defined by the reconstructed section width (SW, see below "*z*-resolution"). For CT angiography, RI should therefore be not larger than SW/2.

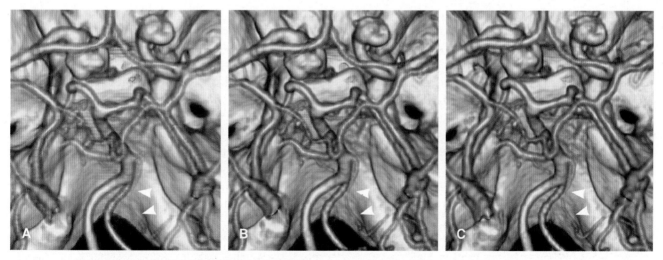

FIGURE 1-11 Effect of field of view (FOV) on spatial resolution. Volume-rendered images of the circle of Willis reconstructed with 40-cm FOV **(A)**, 20-cm FOV **(B)**, and 10-cm FOV **(C)**, each with a 512^2 matrix. The images were enlarged to yield the same details. While too large a FOV reduces quality, excessive reduction of FOV does not further improve it.

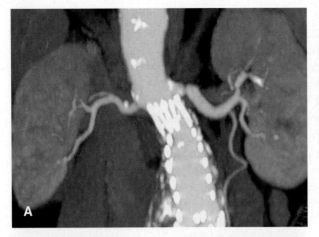

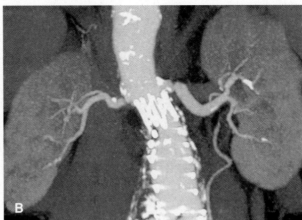

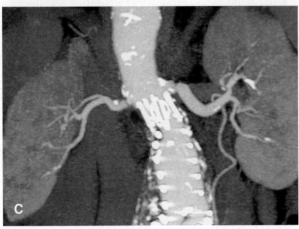

FIGURE 1-12 Comparison of image quality in an anisotropic data set (SW = 3 mm, RI = 1.5 mm) **(A)** and an isotropic reconstruction of the same data set (SW = 0.9 mm, RI = 0.5 mm) **(B)**. Reconstructing even thinner sections leads to no further improvement (SW = 0.67 mm, RI = 0.35 mm) **(C)**.

Taking the concept of pixel from 2D to 3D leads to volume elements (called *voxels*) that are defined by the pixel size in the *xy*-plane and the reconstruction increment in the *z*-direction. In most traditional CT examinations, the voxel has a matchstick shape, that is, the pixel size measured in the *xy*-plane is 5 to 10 times smaller than the reconstruction increment. For CTA, however, the pixel size in the *xy*-plane and the *z*-direction should be adapted to the available spatial resolution. For multidetector-row CT scanners, scan parameters should be chosen so that spatial resolution in the *xy*-plane is similar to resolution in the *z*-direction (*isotropic resolution*), and the voxels should also be isotropic (i.e., have a cubic shape). For this purpose, the reconstruction increment should be chosen similar to the pixel size (Fig. 1-12). With the newest generations of multidetector-row CT scanners, spatial resolution can now be higher in the *z*-direction than in the *xy*-plane, but choosing such parameters makes little sense for most indications (Fig. 1-12C).

xy-Resolution

Spatial resolution in the imaging plane (*xy*-plane) is determined by the reconstruction filter (filter kernel) used for the mathematical process of reconstructing transaxial cross-sectional images from projection data. The filter kernel determines the trade-off between spatial resolution and image noise (Fig. 1-13). The maximum spatial resolution that can be created with such filter kernels depends on the scanner geometry and increases, for example, for smaller detector elements or techniques such as quarter detector offset or flying focal spot. In CT angiography, image noise becomes a limiting factor. Moderately smoothing filter kernels are therefore preferred for most applications.

The *xy*-resolution is commonly given in line pairs per centimeter at the 4% value of the MTF. For practical purposes, however, the width of the point spread function yields numbers that can be better used to optimize scan and reconstruction parameters. Table 1-2 provides an overview of how these numbers relate.

z-Axis Resolution

The *z*-axis resolution is determined by the section width, the thickness of the reconstructed CT section. The section width is defined as the full width at half maximum

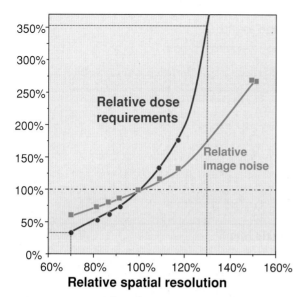

FIGURE 1-13 Spatial resolution versus image noise and dose requirements for constant SNR. Note that reduction in spatial resolution by 30% compared with standard filter kernel requires less than 50% of the dose for identical SNR, while increase in resolution by 30% requires a more than 2.5 times increase in dose. (From M. Prokop et al. *Spiral and Multislice CT of the Body*. Thieme Medical Publishers 2003, with permission.)

(FWHM) of the section sensitivity profile, which shows how much a point in the object contributes to the image as a function of its distance from the center of the section (Fig. 1-14). Speaking in the terms defined earlier, the section profile is nothing other than the point spread function in the *z*-direction, while the section width is the FWHM of this point spread function.

In sequential single detector-row CT scanning, section width and section collimation are identical. In fact, *section collimation* is defined as the FWHM of the section profile in the center of the scan field during a single scan without table movement. Under these conditions, the section profile approaches an "ideal" rectangular shape: Only points within a parallel section in the scanned object contribute to the image. In reality, the finite width of the focal spot of the x-ray tube, the cone shape of the x-ray beam, and other factors contribute to the fact that realistic section profiles are more rounded (Fig. 1-14A–C).

With the introduction of single detector-row spiral scanning, the section profile becomes bell-shaped (Fig. 1-14E). This is due to the interpolation that takes place in order to compensate for the table movement during the scan (p. 21). Depending on the pitch factor and the spiral interpolation algorithm, the section width increases by as much as 30% over the section collimation. Manufacturers differ in how they indicate the section width on their scan interface: Only Philips provides SW, all others provide SC,

from which the user must calculate SW, depending on the pitch.

With multidetector-row CT, the section width becomes independent of the section collimation. The only precondition is that SW is larger than or equal to SC. This means that spatial resolution in the *z*-direction can easily be reduced if thin collimation had been chosen to scan the patient, but choosing too thick a collimation for scanning will not allow for improving *z*-axis resolution after the scan has been acquired. The various manufacturers have taken different approaches to the practical implementation of this principle: Some allow for continuous choice of SW, others allow for multiples of the chosen section width.

Temporal Resolution

Temporal resolution is described by the temporal acquisition window, the time period from which data are sampled to reconstruct an image. If raw data are weighted before reconstruction, the temporal resolution is frequently defined in analogy to spatial resolution as the full width at half maximum of the temporal weighting function.

SCANNER TECHNOLOGY

Detector Technology

Single detector-row scanners use a single detector arc or detector ring that consists of parallel detector elements that are much smaller in the direction of the arc (*xy*-plane) than in the *z*-direction (Fig. 1-2A). In fact, the detector elements are wide enough in the *z*-direction to accommodate the maximum section collimation (usually 10 mm) that is available on such scanners.

Dual detector-row scanners are based on a detector array that is twice as wide as a conventional CT detector and is split in half (Fig. 1-2B). These scanners became available in early 1992, but in 1998, the introduction of 4-detector-row scanners brought a technological breakthrough.

In multidetector-row CT, each element on the detector array is subdivided along the *z*-axis (Fig. 1-2C). These parallel detector rows can be electronically combined to yield between 4 and 128 separate sections per rotation, depending on the type of scanner (1–3). With the exception of most 64- and 128-detector-row scanners, the actual number of detector rows is much larger than the number of active detector rows (channels) in order to accomplish more than one collimation setting. Different collimation settings are achieved by adding the signals of neighboring detector rows.

While there were three distinct types of detector arrays with 4- to 8-detector-row scanners—namely matrix arrays,

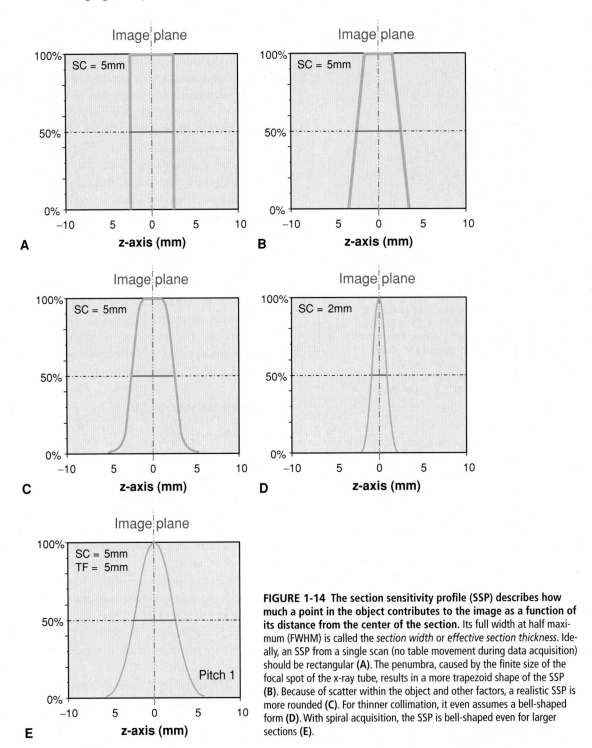

FIGURE 1-14 The section sensitivity profile (SSP) describes how much a point in the object contributes to the image as a function of its distance from the center of the section. Its full width at half maximum (FWHM) is called the *section width* or *effective section thickness*. Ideally, an SSP from a single scan (no table movement during data acquisition) should be rectangular **(A)**. The penumbra, caused by the finite size of the focal spot of the x-ray tube, results in a more trapezoid shape of the SSP **(B)**. Because of scatter within the object and other factors, a realistic SSP is more rounded **(C)**. For thinner collimation, it even assumes a bell-shaped form **(D)**. With spiral acquisition, the SSP is bell-shaped even for larger sections **(E)**.

hybrid arrays, and adaptive arrays (Fig. 1-15)—10- to 16-detector-row scanners use only hybrid arrays, and 32- to 64-detector-row scanners use hybrid or matrix arrays. Matrix arrays consist of detector rows of identical thickness; hybrid arrays have a central group of detector rows whose thickness is half the thickness of the outer detector rows; while adaptive arrays have detector rows that get wider the more peripherally they are located.

All 4- to 16-detector-row scanners provide multiple collimator settings with the maximum number of detector rows (Table 1-3). For hybrid and matrix arrays, the available section collimations are multiples of the thinnest detector width (Fig. 1-16A–B). For adaptive array detectors, the available section collimations are gained by combining signals from one, two, or more parallel rows with appropriate collimator settings (Fig. 1-16C). Most 64- and 128-detector-row scanners, how-

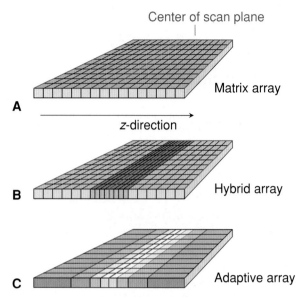

Center of scan plane

A Matrix array

z-direction

B Hybrid array

C Adaptive array

FIGURE 1-15 Detector configurations for multidetector-row CT: matrix array, in which all detector elements are equal **(A)**; hybrid array, in which the innermost detectors are smaller **(B)**; and adaptive array, in which the size detector rows increase with the distance from the center of the scan plane **(C)**. Various section collimations can be created by proper collimation and combination of detector rows.

ever, do no longer provide the maximum number of sections for the largest available collimation (Fig. 1-17A–B). These scanners use matrix detector arrays of between 64 × 0.5 mm (128 × 0.5 mm) and 64 × 0.625 mm width. In these arrays, all 64 to 128 detector rows are read out simultaneously. As a consequence, only half the number of sections are available if the next wider collimation settings are chosen.

The only exception to this rule is a scanner that uses 32 active detector rows and z-flying focal spot technology (Fig. 1-17C). This scanner has a hybrid array that allows for section collimation of 32 × 0.6 mm and 20 × 1.2 mm. While this scanner actually provides a maximum of 32 sections per rotation (in the nonspiral, or sequence, mode), the manufacturer has opted for calling it a 64-slice scanner because the z-flying focal spot technology effectively doubles the data points (and thus the simultaneously acquired slices) along the patient axis without having to increase the number of detector rows.

Flying Focal Spot Technology

Flying focal spot (FFS) technology refers to the position of the focal spot of the x-ray tube. The focal spot varies very rapidly between various positions on the anode, thus creating slightly different views of the object despite an (almost) identical position of the detector. The technology can be used to increase the number of x-ray projections for image reconstruction and, that way, allows for improving the spatial resolution of a scanner without creating "aliasing artifacts." The technology is not new. It has been used for years to increase the number of projections within the imaging plane (xy-plane).

Recently, an additional movement along the z-axis (z-FFS) was introduced that allows for increasing the number of projections also in the z-direction. The idea behind the technology is as follows. For image reconstruction, it is irrelevant whether projections from the tube to the detector or in the opposite direction, from the detector to the tube, are considered. This knowledge has been used for more

TABLE 1-3

Overview of Collimation Settings That are Relevant for CTA with Various Multidetector-row Systems of the Major Vendors

	Manufacturer			
Scanner	GE	Philips	Siemens	Toshiba
4-detector-row	2 × 0.625 mm*	2 × 0.5 mm*	2 × 0.5 mm*	4 × 0.5 mm
	4 × 1.25 mm	4 × 1 mm	4 × 1 mm	4 × 1 mm
	4 × 2.5 mm	4 × 2.5 mm	4 × 2.5 mm	4 × 2 mm
16-detector-row	2 × 0.625 mm	2 × 0.6 mm*	2 × 0.6 mm*	16 × 0.5 mm
	16 × 0.625 mm	16 × 0.75 mm	16 × 0.75 mm	16 × 1 mm
	16 × 1.25 mm	16 × 1.5 mm	16 × 1.5 mm	16 × 2 mm
64-detector-row	2 × 0.5 mm	64 × 0.5 mm		
	64 × 0.625 mm	64 × 0.625 mm	32 × 0.6 mm**	32 × 1 mm
	32 × 1.25 mm	32 × 1.25 mm	20 × 1.2 mm**	16 × 2 mm

*Thinner collimation obtained by collimating the innermost two detector rows.
**Used in combination with a dual z-flying focal spot that doubles data points in the z-direction.

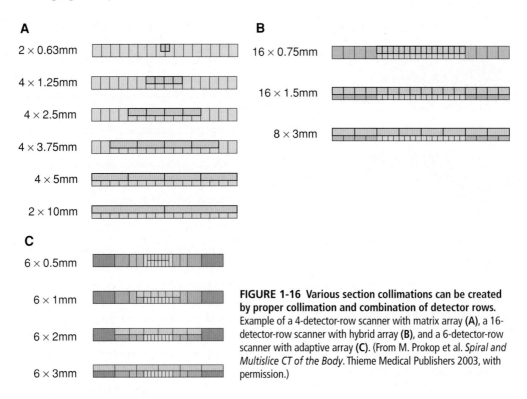

A
2 × 0.63mm
4 × 1.25mm
4 × 2.5mm
4 × 3.75mm
4 × 5mm
2 × 10mm

B
16 × 0.75mm
16 × 1.5mm
8 × 3mm

C
6 × 0.5mm
6 × 1mm
6 × 2mm
6 × 3mm

FIGURE 1-16 Various section collimations can be created by proper collimation and combination of detector rows. Example of a 4-detector-row scanner with matrix array (**A**), a 16-detector-row scanner with hybrid array (**B**), and a 6-detector-row scanner with adaptive array (**C**). (From M. Prokop et al. *Spiral and Multislice CT of the Body.* Thieme Medical Publishers 2003, with permission.)

than a decade for 180-degree interpolation algorithms in spiral CT, in which projection data from a conjugated spiral trajectory (detector to tube) are used for interpolation. Similarly, it can also be used for *z*-flying focal spot techniques (Fig. 1-18A): The linear trajectories from the tube to the centers of adjacent detector elements are identical to the trajectories from a single detector to multiple positions of the focal spot. However, there is a marked difference in the actual regions within the scanned object that are "seen" along each trajectory using these two techniques. In case of separate detector rows, these regions do not overlap, while they markedly overlap in the case of multiple

focal spots (Fig. 1-18B). Currently, *z*-FFS technology is implemented in a way that two overlapping sections are irradiated, which are exactly 50% offset in the scan center. These sections converge (i.e., become identical) toward the detector and diverge (i.e., become separate) toward the tube with its flying focal spot (Fig. 1-18C). One has to keep in mind that despite the fact that the projections overlap in the center of rotation (by 0.3 mm), the thinnest available section width that can be reconstructed with *z*-FFS technology remains identical to the collimation (i.e., 0.6 mm).

Because the *z*-flying focal spot technology provides twice the data points in the *z*-direction over conventional

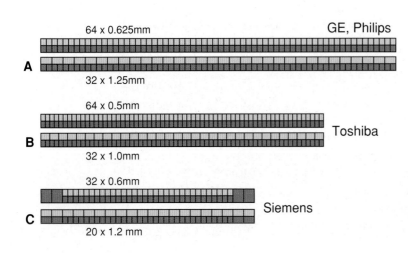

A
64 x 0.625mm
32 x 1.25mm
GE, Philips

B
64 x 0.5mm
32 x 1.0mm
Toshiba

C
32 x 0.6mm
20 x 1.2 mm
Siemens

FIGURE 1-17 Comparison of various 64-slice detector configurations. GE and Philips use the same basic configuration with 64 × 0.625-mm and 32 × 1.25-mm collimation (**A**). Toshiba uses a 64 × 0.5-mm and 32 × 1.0-mm configuration (**B**). Siemens opted for a 32 × 0.6-mm and 20 × 1.2-mm configuration combined with *z*-flying focal spot technology (**C**). (From M. Prokop et al. *Spiral and Multislice CT of the Body.* Thieme Medical Publishers 2003, with permission.)

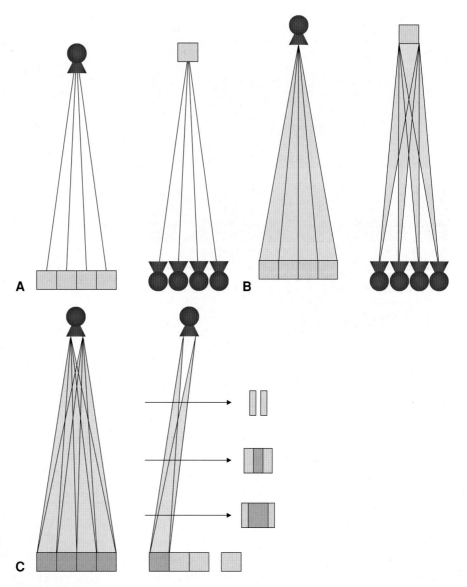

FIGURE 1-18 Principles of *z*-flying focal spot technology (*z*-FFS). The number of projection data can be increased if multiple detector elements or multiple focal spots are used: The central x-ray trajectories from the tube to multiple detector elements are identical to the trajectories from multiple tube positions (or focal spots) to a single-detector element **(A)**. If not only the central line of the trajectory but also the width of the beam is considered, however, it becomes apparent that the sampled data is not identical. While the beams do not overlap in the case of multiple detector rows, the beams overlap to a varying degree in case of multiple focal spots **(B)**. In the center of the scan field, a 50% overlap between beams can be created if only two focal spots are used **(C)**. In the periphery of the scan field, gaps between the two beams occur close to the tube, while there is a higher overlap close to the detector.

technology with a single focal spot, aliasing artifacts in the *z*-direction are markedly reduced, even at higher pitch values (4). This is especially apparent for CTA images of the skull base and posterior fossa. If the number of projections is increased with conventional technology, however, similar artifact suppression can be reached. This requires low pitch factors or increasing the reconstructed section width by at least 30% over the chosen collimation (Fig. 1-19). For this reason, *z*-FFS yields the biggest advantages whenever very thin sections have to be reconstructed or high pitch factors have to be used.

Finally, it has to be noted that the number of focal spots plays no role for the calculation of pitch factors or other crucial scanner characteristics. A scanner with 32 active detector rows and 2 focal spots will therefore behave like a 32-detector-row scanner and not like a 64-detector-

row scanner when it comes to pitch, scanning speed, or even detector width. To mark this difference, it might be useful to distinguish between detector rows on the one hand and slices on the other: A 64-slice scanner that employs two *z*-flying focal spots should therefore correctly be addressed as a 32-detector-row scanner with dual *z*-FFS technology. The technique holds a lot of promise, and in the future, tubes with multiple focal spots can be expected.

Dual Source Technology

Multiple source technology refers to scanners with more than one tube–detector array combination (5). They are primarily being developed for cardiac CT. Presently, dual source scanners are becoming available that have the advantage that the time required to acquire data for one image is

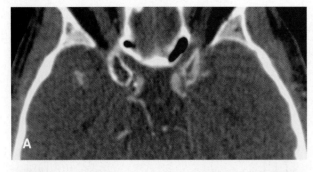

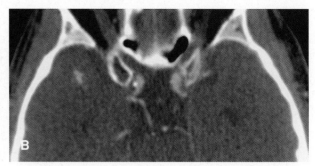

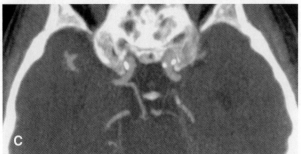

FIGURE 1-19 Aliasing artifacts occur mainly in regions with rapid transitions in x-ray attenuation along the *z*-axis, such as the posterior fossa **(A)**. The artifacts are worse if the thinnest possible section thickness is reconstructed (here, 0.67-mm-thick sections acquired with 64×0.625-mm collimation) but decrease substantially if a >30% wider section thickness (0.9-mm-thick sections reconstructed from the same raw data set) is chosen **(B)**. Using a *z*-flying focal spot, the amount of aliasing at 0.6-mm-thick sections can be expected to be similar to **(B)**. Independent of the aliasing artifacts, however, diagnosis of a hypoplasic posterior communicating artery (*arrow*) can be made from 4-mm-wide thin-slab MIP based on the 0.67-mm-thick image data set **(C)**.

cut in half by the two acquisition systems. Another potential advantage is the availability of a dual energy technique: The two tubes can operate at different kVp settings, and the differences in x-ray absorption at identical projection angles can be used to separately display materials of differing atomic number, such as calcium, iodine, or soft tissues. It remains to be seen whether the ultimate goal of reducing the negative influence of vessel wall calcifications in coronary CTA can be reached.

In dual source scanners, one of the detector arrays has a normal size (in *xy*-direction) to be able to perform standard CT examinations. The second detector array is narrower because it only is used for cardiac examinations (Fig. 1-20). The effective rotation time is reduced from 330 ms for a single source scanner to 165 ms for a dual source scanner. Maximum temporal resolution with these scanners is below 90 ms.

Scanner Performance

The most important factor that determines scanner performance for CTA is the relation between scanning speed and *z*-resolution. This performance parameter can be defined as the ratio between maximum table speed and thinnest section width that can be reconstructed using that table speed. Scanner performance, when defined that way, has been doubling approximately every 2 years since the mid 1980s (Fig. 1-21). As compared to 4-detector-row scanners, performance of 32- to 64-detector-row scanners has increased more than 20 times owing to more detector rows and faster rotation speed.

This increase in performance made it possible to acquire isotropic data and even reduce scan duration with multidetector-row scanners. While spiral CT scanning with single detector-row scanners made it possible to perform thoracic or abdominal CTA during a single breath-hold

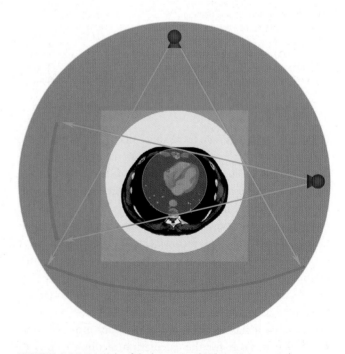

FIGURE 1-20 Principle of dual source technology: Two x-ray tube-detector arrays rotate simultaneously around the body, thus reducing effective rotation time, the time required to acquire a full 360-degrees of projectional data.

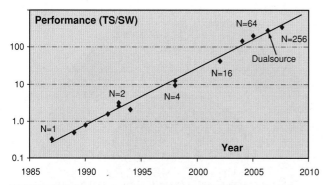

FIGURE 1-21 Increase in scanner performance, defined as the ratio between maximum table speed *(TS)* and thinnest section width *(SW)* that can be reconstructed using that table speed, has approximately doubled every two years over the last decade. (From M. Prokop et al. *Spiral and Multislice CT of the Body*. Thieme Medical Publishers 2003, with permission.)

phase of approximately 30s, the advent of 4-detector-row scanners made it possible to acquire the data in a near isotropic fashion. With 16-detector-row scanners, near-isotropic resolution could be combined with sub-mm resolution and scan durations of between 8 and 15s for chest or abdomen (Table 1-6) (6). With 32- to 128-detector-row scanners, scan duration can always be kept well below 10s, even for submillimeter resolution. However, this decrease in scan duration may not always be advantageous: Especially for large aneurysms or vessel occlusions, it takes longer to completely enhance the vessel of interest, and scanning too early or too fast will lead to suboptimum contrast enhancement (see also Fig. 1-31). For this reason, 16-detector-row units suffice for providing excellent spatial resolution and good handling for the vast majority of CTA examinations.

Further increase in performance is only desirable for the heart or other applications in which electrocardiogram (ECG) synchronization of data acquisition or reconstruction is required. This is where the present advantages of 32- to 128-detector-row scanners lie. Further improvement in effective rotation time and thus, temporal resolution, is especially important for coronary CTA. For CT perfusion imaging, wider detector arrows would be advantageous because whole organ systems could then be imaged within one rotation.

DATA ACQUISITION AND RECONSTRUCTION

Sequential Scanning

In sequential scanning, the table remains stationary during acquisition of a single section. The reconstructed section width is identical to the section collimation. The table feed between sections usually is identical to the section collimation. Sequential scanning is not used for CTA.

In general, data from a 360-degree rotation are sampled to reconstruct an image. However, data from multiple rotations can be combined in order to increase dose, for example, for brain scans. In order to increase temporal resolution, so-called partial scans can be performed, in which the minimum amount of projections are used for reconstructing an image: For each pixel in the final image, a 360-degree circle of evenly spaced projectional rays are required. Since direction of the rays plays no role, projectional data from 180 degrees have to be available. For pixels in the center of the scan field, projections from a 180-degree rotation suffice. Outside the center, more data have to be sampled: This minimum amount of data consists of a rotation that covers 180 degrees plus the fan angle of the x-ray beam or, more precisely, the fan angle that just covers the field of view (Fig. 1-22).

These data or reconstruction techniques are also used for dynamic scanning. The basic principles of data reconstruction, however, also hold true for the spiral data acquisition described below.

Spiral Scanning

Spiral scanning is the basis for CTA. The patient is moved through the scan field during continuous acquisition of raw data. To be able to reconstruct stationary images from such a scan, motion correction is necessary. Basic raw data interpolation techniques are used for single detector-row CT, while more complex algorithms are required for multidetector-row CT. With spiral scanning, a CT image can be generated from any segment within the scanned volume, so the table feed is unrelated to the site of image reconstruction. Sectional images can be produced at arbitrary table positions, and individual images can be overlapped as desired without increasing radiation exposure. The spacing between the reconstructed sections is called the *reconstruction increment, interval,* or *index.*

Cone Beam Effects

Due to the nature of the x-ray beam, which arises from a small focal spot, all CT scanning relies on cone beam geometry. With single detector-row CT, these effects are hardly visible, but they play a major role in multidetector-row scanning because the same structure may be depicted on different detector rows during one revolution of the x-ray tube (Fig. 1-23A). Only in the center of rotation are structures always captured by identical detector rows. The effect becomes more prominent the further a structure is located from the isocenter (rotational axis), the wider the detector rows are, and the more detector rows are used.

Simple raw data interpolation algorithms make the assumption that all beams are parallel, which yields reasonable

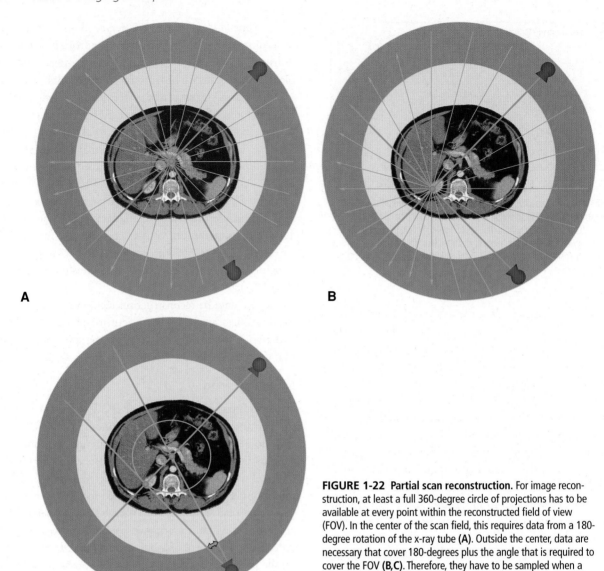

A

B

C

FIGURE 1-22 Partial scan reconstruction. For image reconstruction, at least a full 360-degree circle of projections has to be available at every point within the reconstructed field of view (FOV). In the center of the scan field, this requires data from a 180-degree rotation of the x-ray tube **(A)**. Outside the center, data are necessary that cover 180-degrees plus the angle that is required to cover the FOV **(B,C)**. Therefore, they have to be sampled when a smaller FOV is used for reconstruction and the temporal acquisition window becomes shorter.

results up to six active detector rows but fails with a higher number of rows (Fig. 1-23B). For 8- and 16-detector-row scanners, more sophisticated cone beam algorithms have to be employed for image reconstruction.

Spiral Data Interpolation—Single Detector-row Scanners

The table movement during a scan will produce motion artifacts if the raw data acquired during a 360-degree rotation are used directly for image reconstruction. This is because the first and last projections in the 360-degree rotation sample different data due to the table motion during tube rotation. To avoid these artifacts, interpolation of the raw data before image reconstruction is required. The goal of the interpolation is to obtain a complete set (360 degrees) of projections at the desired z-axis position in the scanned volume. Various interpolation algorithms may be used.

The simplest *linear interpolation* of the projection data is called *360-degree LI* (Fig. 1-24A). At every angular position of a 360-degree rotation, it interpolates between the two projections in the spiral data set that are closest to the chosen z-position and thus produces a complete 360-degree set of projections for this z-position. The 360-degree LI interpolation therefore actually uses data from two rotations, which means that data up to one table feed (TF) away from the chosen z-position contributes to the image. As a consequence, the 360-degree LI interpolation provides the least image noise but substantially broadens the section profile (Fig. 1-24A) (7).

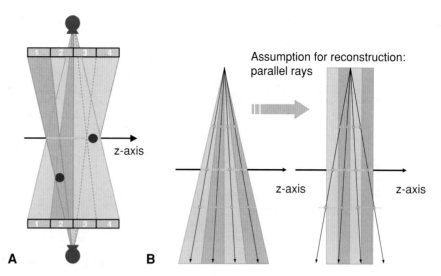

FIGURE 1-23 Cone beam geometry in multidetector-row scanners. Peripheral structures will be seen by different detector rows during one revolution of the x-ray tube **(A)**. Simple raw data interpolation algorithms make the assumption that all beams are parallel as in conventional spiral CT scanning **(B)**. Such algorithms will fail with more than four detector rows. (From M. Prokop et al. *Spiral and Multislice CT of the Body.* Thieme Medical Publishers 2003, with permission.)

More advanced interpolation algorithms exploit the fact that x-ray attenuation is independent of direction, that is, the attenuation along a ray between the tube and detector is equal in both directions. This makes it possible to compute a "virtual" spiral (so-called "conjugate data") for the attenuation values along a ray from the detector to the tube, and to interpolate the projections at corresponding angles between the real and conjugate spiral (7). With this algorithm, called *180-degree LI*, the section profile is substantially narrower (Fig. 1-24B) because the distances between corresponding projections in the real and virtual spirals are less than between corresponding projections in the real spiral alone. The 180-degree LI algorithm, however, results in a larger *image noise* since only half the data are used for interpolation as compared to 360-degree LI. In fact, the noise with 180-degree LI is as high as it would be with a 360-degree LI and half the exposure dose (7).

Higher-order interpolation algorithms use not only two points from adjacent (real or virtual) spirals but instead apply a more complex weighting function (*longitudinal filtration, z-filtering*) to the spiral projection raw data. This z-filter function defines how much each projection contributes to the final image depending on its distance to the chosen z-position. Such algorithms can be optimized to obtain more rectangular section profiles at the cost of more image noise, or they can reduce noise (and thus dose requirements) at the expense of a slightly broadened section.

The width of the section profile (SW) in spiral CT varies with pitch factor. At a pitch of 1, the section width for 180-degree LI is identical to the section collimation. At a pitch of 1, 360-degree LI yields a section width that is approximately 30% (in theory 28%) larger than the section collimation and is identical to the section width with

180-degree LI at a pitch of 2 (Fig. 1-24C). Interpolation artifacts increase with increasing pitch.

Spiral Data Interpolation—4-Detector-row Scanners

With multidetector-row scanners, multiple data channels are available for interpolation at every angular position of a 360-degree rotation. Additional data are available for the projections from the detector to the tube (conjugated data).

In 4-detector-row scanners, cone beam effects can be neglected, and all four projections can be approximated by parallel beams. Under these conditions, the same interpolation techniques can be used as with single detector-row CT. Algorithms that are analogous to 180-degree LI and 360-degree LI from spiral CT are called *180-degree MLI* (*multislice linear interpolation*) and *360-degree MLI* (Fig. 1-25). For each projection angle, they use the projection data from the two detectors that are closest to the scanning plane (360-degree MLI only real trajectories, 180-degree MLI also conjugated trajectories from the detector to the x-ray tube). Section profiles with these algorithms vary between those from conventional 180-degree LI and 360-degree LI spiral CT interpolation, but the dependence on the pitch factor is more complex because of the sampling patterns described below (1,8).

Depending on the pitch factor, the spiral trajectory of the first detector row may overlap with that of the second, third, or fourth row if the table feed per rotation is identical to multiples of the section collimation. For a pitch of 0.5, even the conjugate data from the virtual spiral overlap the real spiral at the isocenter of the scan field (Fig. 1-25C). This makes data sampling particularly inefficient and only allows for an interpolation between data samples that are one section collimation apart. As a consequence, the section width is similar to a 360-degree LI interpolation. Because of varying

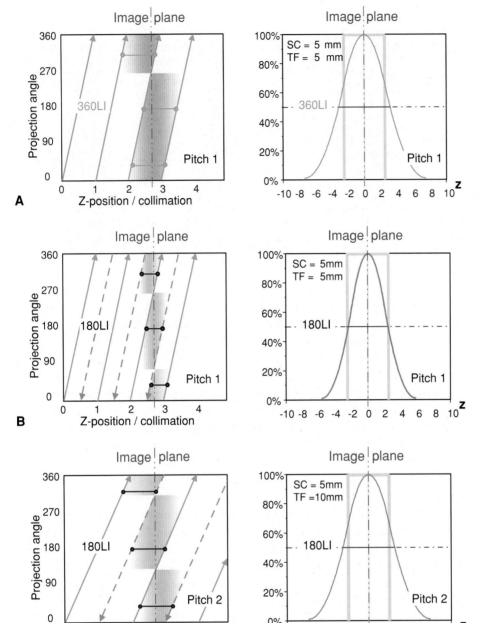

FIGURE 1-24 Principle of raw data interpolation and resulting section sensitivity profiles (SSP). Interpolation between spiral trajectories (tube to detector) with 360-degree LI interpolation at pitch 1 increases section width (SW) by 28% over section collimation (SC) (**A**). Interpolation between spiral trajectories and conjugated trajectories (detector to tube) with 180-degree LI interpolation ensures that SW and SC are identical at pitch 1(**B**). At pitch 2, conjugated trajectories have the same position as spiral trajectories in (**A**), and the resulting SSP with 180-degree LI is identical to the SSP with 360-degree LI and pitch 1 (**C**). (From M. Prokop et al. *Spiral and Multislice CT of the Body*. Thieme Medical Publishers 2003, with permission.)

degrees of overlap with changing pitch factors, the sampling density and thus the section width varies (Fig. 1-26).

Various vendors chose different approaches to tackle this problem. *GE* chose for making only two distinct pitch factors with particularly beneficial properties available (P = 0.75, "high-quality" mode; P = 1.5, "high-speed" mode) (8). In order to simplify the user interface, GE has chosen to let the user reconstruct a section width that is identical to the section collimation for both pitch factors. However, one has to keep in mind that the true section width at pitch 1.5 is some 30% wider than SC. *Toshiba* suggests preferred pitch factors, for

which there is a particularly dense sampling pattern (P = 0.75 and 1.375) but also allows other pitch factors (9). *Siemens* uses a special z-filter to ensure that section width is always some 30% wider than the collimation, independent of the pitch (1). This has the advantage that also image noise and radiation dose (volume CT dose index, $\mathrm{CTDI_{vol}}$) are pitch independent. Only for the thinnest collimation of 4 × 1 mm do they allow for reconstructing sections of 1-mm width if the pitch is less than 1. For this thin collimation, however, there is a noise penalty of some 17% over the theoretical value at 1-mm section width. *Philips* uses a hybrid approach: While the user is

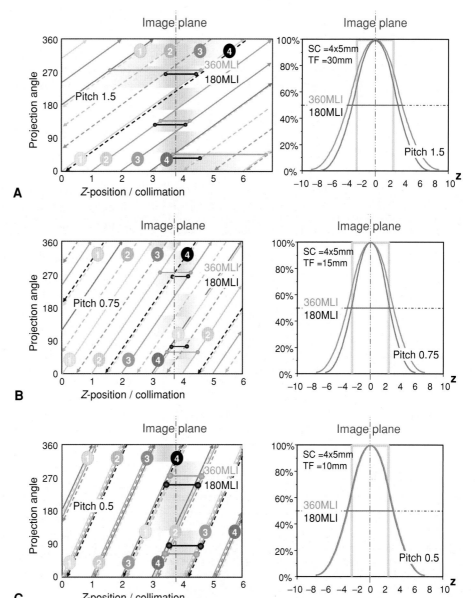

FIGURE 1-25 Multislice linear interpolation is performed in analogy to spiral interpolation in single detector-row scanners. Depending on the pitch factor, various degrees of overlapping data sampling occur when the trajectory of one detector row superimposes on another. Note the effect on section width (*blue line* indicating the full-width-at-half-maximum of the SSP). There is little overlap at a pitch of 1.5 (**A**). More overlap occurs with a pitch of 0.75 (**B**). At a pitch of 0.5, even the conjugate data from the virtual spiral overlap the real spiral trajectory for a pitch of 0.5 (**C**). Note, however, that the cone beam geometry ameliorates this effect, especially for image points farther away from the isocenter. (From M. Prokop et al. *Spiral and Multislice CT of the Body.* Thieme Medical Publishers 2003, with permission.)

allowed to choose any pitch, the system selects (and indicates) a preferred pitch factor that is closest to the user-selected value. With all these approaches, the minimum available section width is identical to the section collimation if the pitch is less than 1 and is approximately 30% wider if pitch is larger than 1.

In order to obtain a section width that is substantially wider than the collimation, a technique called z-*filtering* is used. The z-filter interpolation not only uses the two projections from the detectors that are closest to the scan plane but also adjacent projections (*multipoint interpolation*). These projections are weighted according to their distance from the scan plane. This filter function may even contain negative portions that result in "edge enhancement" along the z-axis. By using a wide filter function, noise is reduced, and the section width becomes larger. As soon as the user chooses a section width

that is some 30% larger than the section collimation, the section width provided on the user interface of a scanner is correct, which means it is identical to the width of the section profile at half maximum (FWHM). Some manufacturers simply combine the data from two or more subsequent rotations and then are limited as to which section widths can be reconstructed. Depending on the manufacturer, various combinations between chosen section collimation and reconstructed section width are available. In principle, the only restraint is that the section width must be larger than the collimation.

Spiral Data Interpolation—Cone Beam Correction

With more than 6 to 8 detector rows, cone beam effects can no longer be neglected without inducing reconstruction

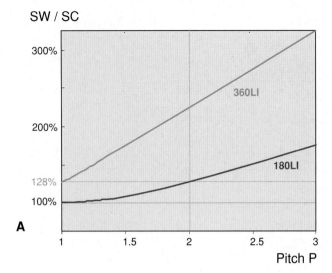

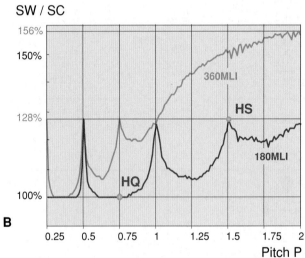

FIGURE 1-26 Effective section thickness (section width) as a function of pitch for 180-degree LI and 360-degree LI with single detector-row CT **(A)** compared with 180-degree MLI and 360-degree MLI with 4-detector-row CT **(B)**. Note that the effects of varying degrees of overlap between sections leads to a more complex curve for multidetector-row CT. (From M. Prokop et al. *Spiral and Multislice CT of the Body*. Thieme Medical Publishers 2003, with permission.)

artifacts (Fig. 1-23). Cone beam corrections require more complex calculations and are constantly refined as detector width increases with new scanner generations (2,4). Variants of 3D back projection (Feldkamp algorithm) should yield the least artifacts and consider only those rays that cross the immediate environment of any voxel that is reconstructed. Other techniques (e.g., advanced single-slice rebinning) shift the plane of interpolation from an axial orientation to an oblique position that better matches the spiral trajectory. The techniques use only partial scan reconstruction for each of these oblique planes to keep the requirement for interpolation low. For each position of the tube, a set of such oblique planes (a "booklet") is created, in which each of the planes corresponds to one detector row (or one particular cone angle). Interpolation between the total number of these oblique planes then creates axial, coronal, or arbitrarily oriented sections of any desired section width without necessarily having to go through a real reconstruction of an orthogonal 3D data set.

Overscanning—Hidden Dose Increase

Overscanning or *over-ranging* refers to the fact that image reconstruction requires approximately one rotation before and one rotation after the planned scan range in order to be able to properly interpolate and reconstruct cross-sectional images from the raw data (10). The amount of overscanning depends on the pitch factor, section collimation, number of detector rows, and the raw data reconstruction technique. If, like theory predicts, one additional rotation at the beginning and at the end of the scan were required, then the range that is exposed is increased by a distance identical to the table feed at either end of the scan range. The scan range indicated on the scanner console usually is defined by the center of the sections, which adds another half collimation at the beginning and end of the scan. Because dose linearly builds up/decreases over these additionally exposed areas, the total dose-length-product is increased by $(TF + SC) \times CTDI_{vol}$.

Overscanning varies with the manufacturer. In general, however, overscanning increases with higher pitch and larger collimation and may cause a substantial "hidden" dose increase of which most users will not be aware. Especially in children or for short scan ranges, overscanning may increase radiation dose by 50% and more (Fig. 1-27). So far, manufacturers have done little to tackle this problem.

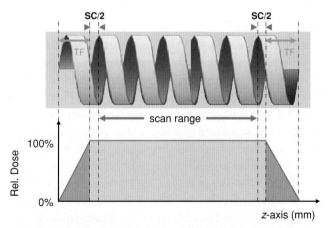

FIGURE 1-27 Overscanning leads to a hidden dose increase because approximately one rotation before and after the beginning of the reconstructed range has to be exposed in order to be able to perform spiral interpolation. The scan range indicated on the scanner console is defined as the distance of the centers of the first and last reconstructed sections.

CHOICE OF SCAN PARAMETERS

CTA relies on thin-section spiral imaging and optimum timing of contrast material injection to ensure proper enhancement of the target territory.

To obtain the best possible spatial resolution along the z-axis, all the spiral scan parameters should be optimized to produce the smallest possible section width in single detector-row CT. While z-axis resolution is a limiting factor with such single detector-row techniques, near isotropic imaging is possible with multidetector-row techniques. Signal-to-noise ratios become a more important limiting factor with multidetector-row scanning because of low detector signals at thin sections. A section width between 1 and 3 mm suffices, depending on the scan length and the size of the patients. Smaller sections may be technically feasible but should be avoided for most body applications because of excessive noise or dose. In general, the scanning technique with multidetector-row CTA becomes more simple and robust. The following paragraphs describe the rationale behind the choice of scan parameters and the most important trade-offs in CTA.

General Aspects

Table 1-4 gives an overview of general aspects for setting up a CTA examination.

Patient Preparation

The patients should refrain from eating a few hours before the examination, but otherwise, no special preparation is needed unless there is known deterioration in renal function or an otherwise increased risk for contrast material application. No positive oral contrast material should be employed. This is especially important to remember if CTA is performed as part of another examination, for example, a biphasic liver CT.

Precontrast Scans

Precontrast scans are not mandatory but may be helpful in patients with suspected hemorrhage, or mural hematoma in suspected aortic dissection (Fig. 1-28). In most cases, however, precontrast scans offer little additional information over contrast-enhanced CT angiograms. Because the abnormalities extend over larger regions, it is usually sufficient to scan in a discontinuous fashion (e.g., 5-mm sections every 20 mm) with single detector row CT or to perform low-dose scans with multidetector row CT that are reconstructed with 7- to 10-mm section width.

Precontrast scans are rarely necessary for determining the scan range. In single detector row CT, however, long scan ranges require the use of thicker collimation and thus reduce spatial resolution, or require increased scan time and

TABLE 1-4

Overview of General Aspects of Setting Up a CTA Examination

Patient preparation	Check for contraindication for contrast material application.
	No positive oral contrast agents.
	Train breath holding.
	Check time it takes the patient to breathe in.
Precontrast scans	Standard in suspected aortic dissection.
	Optional for suspected bleeding.
	Helpful for determining optimum scan range in single detector-row CT.
	Use reduced dose and thicker sections (5 to 10 mm).
Scan length	As short as possible, as long as necessary for solving clinical problem.
Respiratory phase	Normal inspiration (standard).
	Shallow respiration (patients who are unable to hold their breaths).
Window settings	Precontrast CT, W/L = 400/40.
	CT angiography, W/L = 500/150 (adjust as needed).

W/L, window width/window level (HU).

thus need more contrast material and make motion artifacts more probable. For this reason, precontrast scans in the case of, for example, the aorta or the upper abdominal arteries can help to keep the scan range as short as possible.

Scan Length

Scan length is no limiting factor in multidetector-row CT but is critical for spatial resolution in single detector-row CTA. However, keeping the range to a minimum reduces scan time, allowing for thinner collimation and thus better spatial resolution, with reduced motion-related artifacts, contrast material requirements, and patient dose. The cranial and caudal extent of the acquisition can usually be determined on the scanogram.

The scan range may have to be divided into two parts if the scan duration becomes too long, for example, for single detector row examinations of the thoracic and abdominal aorta.

Scan Duration and Breath Holding

CT angiography of the chest and abdomen is performed during an inspirational breath hold. For CTA of the lower abdomen (iliac arteries), breath holding is not mandatory. No breath holding is required for the head and neck and for

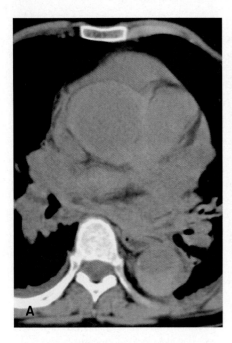
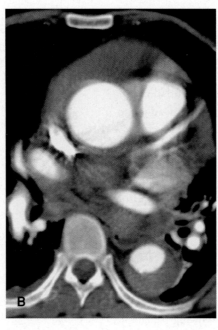

FIGURE 1-28 Precontrast scan in a patient with mural hematoma **(A)** shows a hyperdense rim in the aorta. Such a rim may be more difficult to evaluate if only a CT angiogram is available **(B)**.

the extremities. Scan duration in the chest and abdomen is limited by the breath-holding period in single detector-row CT and to a lesser degree also in 4- and 8-detector-row scanners (see Tables 1-5, 1-6).

In general, most patients will be able to hold their breath for about 30 s if breath holding has been practiced prior to the scan. It is helpful to have the patient hyperventilate briefly (i.e., perform several forced inhalations and exhalations) before each scan. Informing the patient about the procedure and the importance of the breath hold is an important part of a successful CTA examination. In critical patients, the technologists should try the breath-holding maneuver before the actual scan and watch the patient's

abdomen. If it moves during the breath-hold phase, the patient has to be instructed again.

If the patient is not able to hold the breath for sufficient time, the scan duration should be reduced. This is feasible for most emergency examinations but reduces diagnostic evaluation of smaller vessels because of the need to employ a thicker collimation. If this is not possible, no attempt should be made to force a breath-hold examination. In such cases, the patient will continue breathing anyway, resulting in major breathing artifacts. It is better to have the patient hyperventilate before the scan and then breathe shallowly. This is especially important in patients with suspected pulmonary embolism (Fig. 1-29).

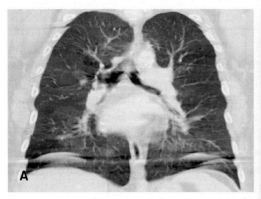
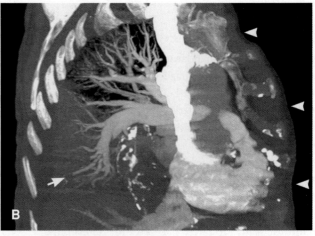

FIGURE 1-29 Comparison of breathing artifacts in dyspneic patients that received a CTA for suspected pulmonary embolism while being asked to hold their breath (and not succeeding) **(A)** and during quiet respiration after a period of prior hyperventilation **(B)**. Note that substantial breathing artifacts commence after the first half of the scan (craniocaudal scanning direction) in **(A)**. There are continuous minor artifacts during shallow continuous breathing (*arrowheads*) that do not interfere with the diagnosis of an occluded peripheral vessel (*arrow*) **(B)**.

In single detector-row CTA, the scan duration can be increased to 40 to 60 seconds by first scanning the part of the imaging volume that is susceptible to respiratory artifacts (e.g., the upper abdomen). After 30 seconds have elapsed, the patient is instructed to resume breathing while the less motion-sensitive part of the volume is imaged. This technique can be used in examinations of the abdominal aorta and renal arteries as a means of reducing the section thickness.

In multidetector-row CTA with more than four detector rows, scan duration can be substantially reduced for many indications. A scan duration of 15 seconds is rarely exceeded with 16 (or more) detector-row scanners (see Table 1-6). Most patients will easily accept a breath-hold duration of 15 seconds. This should not make the technicians less careful in instructing the patients. A sudden breath-hold command in an unprepared patient will often result in substantial breathing artifacts that may spread over the whole scan if scan duration is very short (for example, five seconds for an abdominal exam with a 64-detector-row scanner).

It is also advisable to check how long the patient takes to stop breathing in order to make sure the scan is not started too early. In addition, movement artifacts may occur if the patient relaxes the diaphragm during the breath-hold phase or if there are involuntary diaphragmatic movements toward the end of the scan phase. Again, checking for movement of the abdominal wall during a test breath hold can avoid artifacts later in the scan. In instructing the patient, one should avoid provoking a Valsalva maneuver (Fig. 1-30). In particular, the technician should refrain from asking the patient to take a *deeeep* breath but let the patient breathe in normally.

Since it takes some time to completely fill a vascular bed with contrast-enhanced blood, very short scan durations may not always be beneficial. Scanning too early or too fast may yield suboptimum contrast enhancement, for example, in peripheral arteries or large aortic aneurysms (Fig 1-31). For

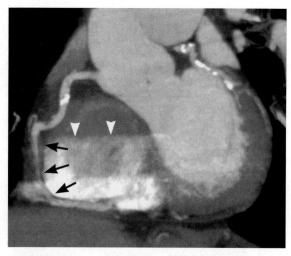

FIGURE 1-30 Effect of ending a Valsalva maneuver in the middle of a coronary CTA scan. The Valsalva maneuver has led to complete obliteration of contrast in the right atrium during the first half of the scan (cranio-caudal scanning direction), which immediately resumes after intrathoracic pressure is relaxed (*arrowheads*). The accompanying slight movement of the diaphragm induces a motion artifact that extends over a larger region in the RCA because of multisector reconstruction of the data (*arrows*).

this reason, 16-detector-row scanners suffice for providing excellent spatial resolution and good handling for the vast majority of CTA examinations. For 64-detector-row scanners, it is advisable either to prolong the start delay (from the arrival of contrast material in the target region to the start of the scan) or to decrease the scan speed to ensure suffice enhancement in the distal portions of the examined vascular territory.

Single Detector-row Computed Tomographic Parameters

Standard parameters can be used in most CTA examinations. The parameters listed in Table 1-5 are for single

TABLE 1-5

Examples of Standard Parameters for Single Detector-row CTA

Region	SC (mm)	TF (mm)	RI (mm)	Scan Direction	Scan Duration
Precontrast CT	7	12	7	↓	20–25s
Circle of Willis*	1	2	1	↑	30s
Carotid arteries	1–2	3	1	↑	30–40s
Pulmonary arteries	3	5	2	↑	30s
Thoracic aorta	3	5	2	↑	30s
Abdominal aorta	3	5	2	↓	40s
Renal arteries	2	3–4	1	↓	30s
Peripheral arteries**	3	5	2	↓	30–40s

↓, cranio-caudal scan direction; ↑, caudo-cranial scan direction; s, seconds.
*Carotid bifurcation.
**Only for local abnormalities, such as aneurysms.

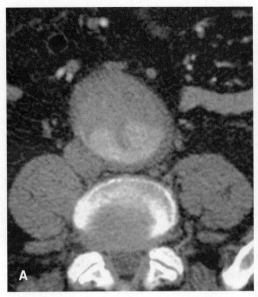
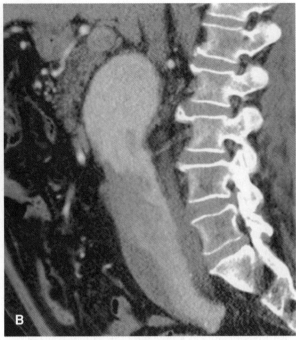

FIGURE 1-31 **Scanning faster than the blood flow may cause inhomogeneous enhancement and is especially common in aneurysms with turbulent flow.** Axial image **(A)** and sagittal reformation **(B)** from a 16-detector-row CTA acquired with 16 × 0.75-mm collimation during a 10-second scan. Despite bolus triggering with a start delay of 8 seconds after reaching a threshold of 100 HU in the aorta, substantial flow artifacts remain.

detector-row scanners with 1-second tube rotation that permit at least a 50-second scan duration. These parameters may have to be adjusted for the available scanner technology because rotation time in particular substantially affects the *z*-axis resolution and the available scan length. In very obese patients in whom the maximum mAs settings do not suffice, the use of a thicker collimation may be necessary to improve the signal-to-noise ratio.

Section Width, Pitch, and Section Collimation

In single detector-row CT, *z*-resolution is the main limiting factor. It is therefore important to obtain the thinnest possible section width while still being able to cover the necessary scan range within the desired scan duration. Section width in single detector-row CT is a parameter that cannot be freely chosen but is a result of the raw data interpolation algorithm, section collimation, and pitch. The main goal for this optimization task is therefore to choose interpolation algorithm, SC, and P so that SW is minimum for a given table feed.

Because of its substantially wider SW, a 360-degree LI algorithm is generally not suited for CTA. With a 180-degree LI algorithm, SW grows by some 30% as pitch is increased from 1 to 2, and SC is kept constant. However, under these conditions, TF also grows by a factor of 2. If SC is reduced at a given TF, pitch (per definition) increases but SW decreases (as much as 35% for a pitch of 2).

For this reason, it is always advisable to use thin collimation and a high pitch factor (1.5 to 2) in order to obtain a small section width (11). A pitch of 3, if available, may be used for selected indications such as scanning of the carotid arteries or the pulmonary arteries with 1-mm collimation and subsecond rotation time (Fig. 1-32). One has to be aware, however, that interpolation artifacts are increased at

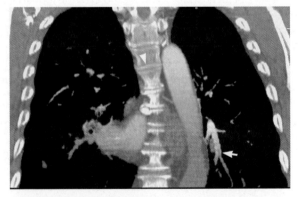

FIGURE 1-32 **For 1-mm collimation, the pitch can be increased to 3 without markedly compromising image quality in single detector-row CTA.** Note the excellent quality of multiplanar reformations with 1-mm collimation and a pitch of 3 for visualization of subsegmental pulmonary emboli (*arrow*). Note that the vertebral end plates are well delineated but suffer from minor horizontal interpolation artifacts (*arrowhead*). (From M. Prokop et al. *Spiral and Multislice CT of the Body*. Thieme Medical Publishers 2003, with permission.)

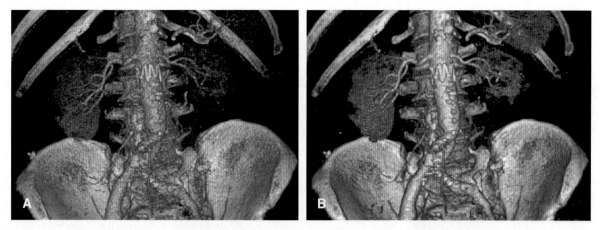

FIGURE 1-33 Comparison of image quality of a volume rendering from a data set reconstructed with a standard filter kernel **(A)** and a smoothing filter kernel **(B)**.

higher pitch factors. In clinical practice, this fact is of less importance than z-resolution.

Image Reconstruction

For optimum results of multiplanar reformations and 3D reconstructions, images should be reconstructed with a high degree of overlap. The reconstruction increment should not be larger than half the section width. Image quality further improves if RI = SW/3. In practice, a reconstruction increment of 1 mm is recommended for short scan ranges and thin SW (≤3mm), while a reconstruction increment of 1.5 to 2 mm is sufficient for larger scan ranges (for example, the aorta or the pulmonary arteries) and SW >3 mm.

In order to reduce image noise and obtain smooth interfaces on 3D reconstruction, a moderately to strongly smoothing filter kernel can be recommended (Fig. 1-33). In general, the more obese the patient, the more smoothing the filter kernel that has to be used.

For optimum display of small detail, it is advisable to reduce the field of view to include only the vascular structures: 12 to 15 cm for the circle of Willis; 25 cm for the aorta or abdominal arteries (Fig. 1-11). This may require reconstructing a second set of images at a full FOV in order to be able to evaluate all nonvascular structures as well.

Multidetector-row Computed Tomographic Parameters

With multidetector-row CT scanning, the number of scanning protocols is substantially reduced (Table 1-6). For small arteries like the circle of Willis, the carotids, the

TABLE 1-6

Examples of Standard Parameters for Multidetector-row CTA

Region	4-row SC	16-row SC	64-row SC	SW/RI	Scan Direction
Precontrast CT	2–2.5	1.25–2	1.2–2	7/5	↓
Circle of Willis*	0.5–0.625	0.5–0.625	0.5–0.625	0.5–0.9/0.4	↑
Carotid arteries	1–1.25	0.5–0.75	0.5–0.625	0.8–1.25/0.5	↑
Pulmonary arteries	1–1.25	0.5–0.75	0.5–0.625	0.8–1.25/0.7	↑
(dyspnoic patients)	2–2.5	1.0–1.5	1–1.25	1.0–3.0/0.7–1.5	↑
Thoracic aorta	2–2.5	1.0–1.5	0.6–1.0	1.0–3.0/0.7–1.5	↑
Abdominal aorta	2–2.5	1.0–1.5	0.6–1.0	1.0–3.0/0.7–1.5	↓
Thoracoabdominal aorta	2–2.5	1.0–1.5	0.6–1.0	1.0–3.0/0.7–1.5	↓
Abdominal arteries	1–1.25	0.625–1	0.5–1.0	0.8–1.25/0.7	↓
Peripheral arteries	2–2.5	0.75–1.25	0.6–1.0	1.0–3.0/0.7–1.5	↓
(distal arteries)**	1–1.25	0.5–0.75	0.5–0.625	0.8–1.25/0.5	↓

SC, section collimation (mm); SW/RI, section width (mm)/reconstruction increment (mm).
↓, cranio-caudal scan direction; ↑, caudo-cranial scan direction.
*May require use of only the two innermost detectors.
**Scan range can be split in two, lower resolution down to knees, highest resolution of lower leg and feet.

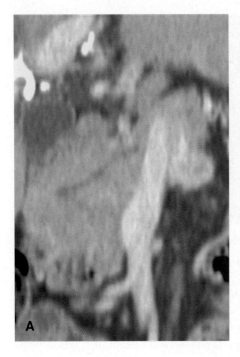
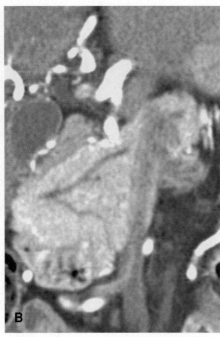

FIGURE 1-34 Comparison of image quality of a coronal reformation from a portal venous data set acquired with 4 × 2.5-mm collimation and a pitch of 0.75 **(A)** and an arterial phase data set acquired with 4 × 1.25-mm collimation and a pitch of 1.5 **(B)**. Note that scan speed is identical for the two acquisitions, but image quality is much better for the thinner sections. (From M. Prokop et al. *Spiral and Multislice CT of the Body.* Thieme Medical Publishers 2003, with permission.)

pulmonary arteries, the abdominal side branches or peripheral arteries, the thinnest collimation is used. For the aorta and venous structures, the next larger collimation may be used, but whenever there is a question about side branches or smaller vessels, the thinner collimation is to be preferred. In 4- to 16-detector-row scanners, the wider collimation may be necessary in dyspneic patients if scanning has to be completed within a very short scan period.

Section Width, Pitch, and Section Collimation

In multidetector-row CT, better z-resolution can be obtained with thinner collimation and high pitch than with wider collimation and low pitch (Fig. 1-34). If the thinnest collimation is already used as a standard, and scan duration is no limiting factor, pitch can be lowered to reduce artifacts. In practice, this means that the pitch in 4-detector-row scanners will be chosen close to 1.5, while it will be reduced to around 1.25 for 16-detector-row scanners and will be chosen around 0.9 for 64-detector-row scanners unless scanning speed is an issue.

Cone beam artifacts are visible at interfaces between structures that are oriented parallel to the scan plane and have substantially different attenuation. Typical examples are the ribs, the intervertebral disks, and the skull base. Such artifacts play a minor role for CTA outside the skull base, but for CTA of the circle of Willis, artifacts may substantially reduce the quality of axial images. These "windmill" artifacts are due to a lack of data points (aliasing) in the z-direction. They can be reduced by reducing the pitch

to between 0.6 and 0.9 (12) or by reconstructing thicker section widths (Fig. 1-19). The z-flying focal spot technology substantially reduces these artifacts even at the thinnest section width.

When it comes to the choice of section width, one should resist the urge to always go for the submillimeter resolution that is available with 16- to 64-detector-row scanners. At a collimation of 0.5 to 0.625 mm, the minimum section width that can be chosen on the scanner interface varies between 0.5 and 0.67 mm, dependent on the manufacturer. One has to keep in mind, though, that the real section width (if measured as the FWHM of the section sensitivity profile) is usually somewhat larger (0.6 to 0.8 mm). Such a submillimeter section width, however, comes at a considerable price: Noise in the resulting images is substantially increased. This holds true not only for the original axial images but also for thicker coronal or sagittal images that are reconstructed from these data sets. In order to compensate for this noise, dose must be increased considerably (p. 31).

For this reason, one should refrain from reconstructing the thinnest available section width unless there is the need for the highest possible spatial resolution (for example, for the circle of Willis or the arteries of the distal extremities). In practice, a section with SW of between 0.9 to 1.25 mm is sufficient for the chest, and a section width of 1.0 to 1.5 mm should be chosen for the abdomen because of its higher attenuation (13–15). Frequently, however, image noise may hamper 3D displays even at these section widths.

Image Reconstruction

In multidetector-row CT, the reconstruction increment should be in the range of SW/2 to SW/3 but need not be chosen smaller than the pixel size within the scan plane (2).

At a field of view of 35 cm—that usually covers the lungs or most of the abdomen—pixel size is 0.7 mm. For CTA with a FOV of 25 cm that is commonly used for aortic exams, pixel size is 0.5 mm. For the hands, feet, or the circle of Willis, the FOV may be reduced to 10 to 15 cm, resulting in a pixel size of 0.2 to 0.3 mm.

Because image noise is such a disturbing factor, smoothing filter kernels are used for reconstruction of thin sections. Such smoothing kernels have a resolution of 5 to 10 line pairs per cm (4% MTF), which translates into a resolution of 0.7 to 1.2 mm in the scan plane (FWHM of the point spread function). This is in the same range as section width, which makes spatial resolution virtually isotropic.

Resolution, Noise, and Dose

Radiation dose is the most important limiting factor for further improvement of spatial resolution in CTA. As thinner and thinner sections are used with the new generations of scanners, detector dose decreases proportionally, and image noise may increase substantially. Image noise, in fact, is influenced by the reconstructed section width (z-axis resolution) and by the filter kernel (xy-resolution).

For identical signal-to-noise ratios, the required radiation dose (D) is inversely proportional to the reconstructed detector-row width SW: $D \sim 1/SW$. For example, when reducing SW from 2.5 mm to 1.25 mm, the required dose will increase by a factor of 2. However, there is an additional noise penalty if the minimum possible SW is chosen (SW $\approx$ section collimation): Noise has been found to increase by an additional 17% over the increase that could be expected when moving to a smaller section width (4). As a result, about 35% more dose is required to compensate for this additional increase in noise. This effect can add substantially to the dose required at thinner sections for identical signal-to-noise ratios (SNR). Let us consider the example of a 64-slice scanner with 0.6 mm collimation: In order to obtain the same SNR as with 0.9-mm-thick sections, the dose for 0.6-mm-thick sections has to be increased by a factor that takes account of the thinner collimation (i.e., 0.9/0.6 = 1.5) and by the additional 35% that stem from the fact that a section width of 0.6 mm is identical with the collimation. As a consequence, radiation dose for 0.6-mm sections would have to be increased by a factor of 2 over 0.9-mm sections to obtain identical image noise. This is in line with the current practice in coronary CTA where—despite a slightly higher noise level with 64-slice CTA—approximately twice the dose is used for 64-slice CTA with 0.6-mm-thick sections as

compared with 16-detector-row CTA with 1.0-mm-thick sections (16,17).

For xy-resolution, the relation is more complex and is influenced by the type of image reconstruction (currently filtered back projection) and geometric considerations. As a rough estimate, the following considerations hold true when comparing the radiation doses required for obtaining the same signal-to-noise as with a standard filter kernel. Reduction of spatial resolution using a smoothing filter kernel will require a dose that is inversely proportional to (spatial resolution)^2. This effect is similar to averaging data in two dimensions. For example, when reducing spatial resolution by 30%, the required dose will decrease to $(100\% - 30\%)^2 = 49\%$. On the other hand, increasing the spatial resolution over that of a standard filter kernel will require a dose that is inversely proportional to (spatial resolution)^3. This old relation (Brook formula) established in the 1970s still holds true today because increasing spatial resolution not only relies on filter kernels but on scanner architecture (detector aperture) as well. For example, if spatial resolution shall be increased by 30%, then the required dose will increase to $(100\% + 30\%)^3 = 220\%$. Doubling the spatial resolution will require a dose that increases to $200\%^3 = 800\%$. Thus, in-plane resolution will become the major limiting factor for CT in the future.

With the new generation of scanners, isotropic imaging is standard. Increasing spatial resolution in all three spatial directions together will require a dose increase that is inversely proportional to (spatial resolution)^4. For the same example of an increase of spatial solution by 30%, but now in all three directions, the required dose will increase to $(100\% + 30\%)^4 = 285\%$. Doubling the spatial resolution will require a dose that increases to $200\%^4 = 1,600\%$.

Unless detector technology, data sampling, image reconstruction techniques, and noise-reducing filters can dramatically decrease image noise, we will not see major improvements of spatial resolution over current values. Even then, the basic trade-offs between spatial resolution and dose requirements will remain valid.

In clinical practice, spatial resolution of current scanners is sufficient for the vast majority of applications. Further improvements may be advantageous for small-vessel CTA, for example, in the brain or for peripheral arteries. A higher spatial resolution, however, is most important for coronary CTA in order to improve evaluation of small coronary arteries, coronary stents, and calcified plaques. Coronary CTA therefore remains the driving force behind efforts to further increase spatial resolution in CT.

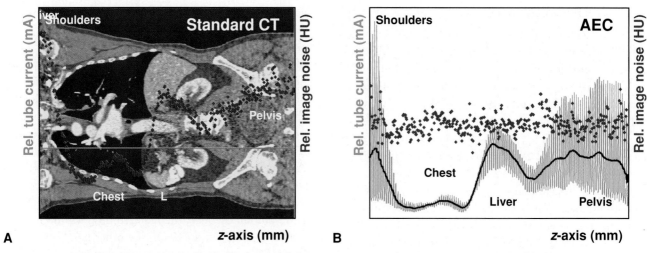

FIGURE 1-35 Dose containment by *xyz*-modulation. At constant mA values, image noise increases in the region of the shoulders and the pelvis and is least for the chest **(A)**. Automated exposure control (AEC) reduces mA values in the sagittal direction (low attenuation) as compared with the lateral direction (high attenuation). In addition, the average mA level per rotation is adapted to the local absorption: higher for the shoulders and the abdomen, and lower for the mid chest **(B)**. As a consequence, image noise remains constant independent of the body region. (Data courtesy of IMP, University of Erlangen, Germany.)

DOSE CONTAINMENT

With increasing pressure on CT to improve spatial resolution, mainly in the area of cardiac CTA, dose containment becomes a major issue. Numerous techniques are being developed, the most important of which fall into the category of dose modulation. All vendors now combine some or all of the following techniques to ensure more constant image quality independent of patient size or body region. The techniques, however, will require further fine-tuning in the future.

xy-Modulation

Dose modulation in the scan plane (*xy*-modulation) varies the tube current as the x-ray tube rotates around the body: In regions with a reduced diameter—for example, the AP direction in the shoulders—the tube current is reduced, while in regions with an increased diameter—for example, the lateral direction in the shoulder region—the tube current is kept constant or increased (Fig. 1-35). The technique reduces streak artifacts and can reduce radiation dose by an average of approximately 20% without affecting signal-to-noise ratios (18). However, most practical implementations are suboptimum: Dose is reduced from a predefined value, which will reduce dose in the shoulders but provide a disproportionably high dose in the mid chest, for example. Better techniques increase the dose in regions with high attenuation and decrease it in regions with low attenuation. However, in general, *xy*-modulation works best if combined with modulation in the *z*-axis as well.

z-Modulation

Dose modulation in the *z*-direction (*z*-modulation) varies the tube current as the scan progresses along the patient axis: In regions with reduced absorption—for example, the neck or the mid chest—tube current is reduced, while in regions with high absorption—for example, the shoulders or the pelvis—tube current is increased (Fig. 1-35). While *xy*-modulation alone cannot be recommended on some scanners, *z*-modulation (if possible combined with *xy*-modulation) should always be used in any clinical patient because it reduces dose where possible, increases dose where necessary, and ensures constant image quality independent of the body region. It can reduce radiation dose by more than 50% in low-absorption areas (19).

Automated Exposure Control

Adaptation of the dose to patient size (automated exposure control) adjusts the general setting of the tube current to the size of the patient. For example, dose in children is substantially reduced as compared to adults. The technique ensures constant image quality independent of patient size (20). The implementation varies between vendors. In one system, the user can choose the desired image noise (noise index) that will be reproduced by the system. In other systems, the user chooses the mA setting for a standard-sized patient, which is then adapted to the current patient. Yet others use a template exam whose quality is then reproduced for the current patient. It is not yet clear, however, which image quality is required in which clinical setting and which of these systems is most easy to use and most reproducible. In particular, it

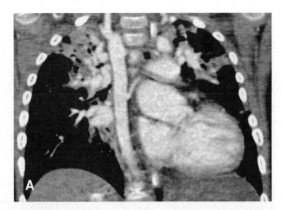
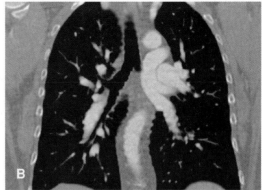

FIGURE 1-36 Comparison of image quality in a child **(A)** and an adult **(B)**: Despite similar image noise (standard deviation of CT numbers), the image of the child appears to be of lower quality. It suffers from less sharply defined contours and a more granular noise pattern. (Figure 1.36 B from M. Prokop et al. *Spiral and Multislice CT of the Body*. Thieme Medical Publishers 2003, with permission.)

appears that less noise can be tolerated in children and slim patients than in obese patients (Fig. 1-36). Whenever possible, such systems should be used if care has to be taken to titrate the noise to the clinical question.

Noise Filters

Image noise can also be reduced by mathematically filtering either the projectional raw data or the image data.

Adaptive filtering of the raw data can reduce streak artifacts and ensures more homogeneous image quality. The technique locally averages raw data for high-absorption and, therefore, high-noise projections, thus substantially improving the signal-to-noise ratio in the resulting image (Fig. 1-37). It

works best in regions with considerable differences in local absorption such as the shoulders or the pelvis (21).

Postprocessing filters work on reconstructed image data and use edge-preserving algorithms to locally reduce image noise without excessively blurring the image (Fig. 1-38) (22).

Low kVp Techniques

While all of the techniques mentioned aim at improving signal-to-noise ratios by reducing the noise component, the SNR can also be improved by increasing the signal. Because CT numbers are normalized to water and air, the CT numbers of most soft tissues remain fairly stable independent of the scan parameters used. The exception is fat that shows a

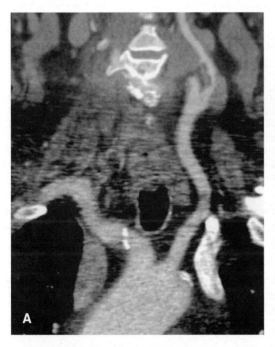
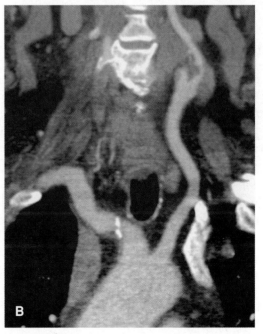

FIGURE 1-37 Comparison of image quality before **(A)** and after adaptive noise filtering **(B)**. The streak artifacts in the region of the shoulders are substantially reduced for carotid CTA.

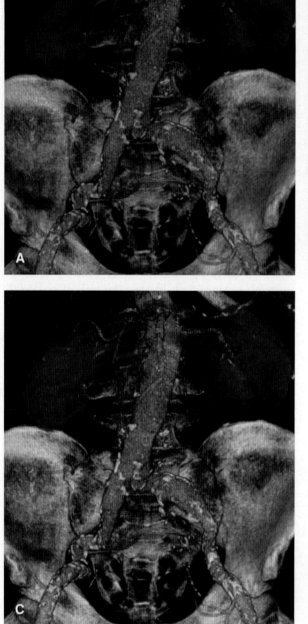

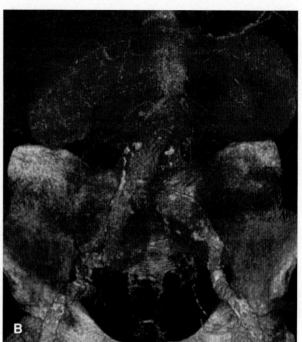

FIGURE 1-38 Effect of edge-preserving postprocessing filters on volume-rendered images. Untagged reconstruction of an ECG-gated CTA of the aorta (ECG information neglected, all projectional raw data used for reconstruction) **(A)**. Gated reconstruction of the same data set (only some 15% of the projectional data and thus, from the total dose, used) **(B)**. Same data set after edge-preserving anisotropic filtering **(C)**.

substantial reduction of CT numbers at low tube voltage settings. Bones and iodinated contrast agents, on the other hand, demonstrate substantially increased CT numbers at low x-ray energies (Fig. 1-5) (23). However, x-ray attenuation also increases at low x-ray energies. For regions with substantial attenuation such as the abdomen or obese patients, low kVp settings would induce a disproportional amount of noise that could no longer be counted by the increased CT number of iodine at such low kVp settings. For contrast-enhanced exams in slim patients or children, or

for the CTA of the pulmonary arteries or the circle of Willis (Fig. 1-39), this kVp dependence of the CT numbers can be used to optimize SNR at constant dose or to reduce dose at constant SNR (23–26). Table 1-7 gives a suggestion for kVp settings depending on patient weight and body region.

Children and Slim Patients

Children are much more radiation sensitive than adults when it comes to the estimated risk of developing radiation-induced cancer. This radiation sensitivity is highest at early age and is

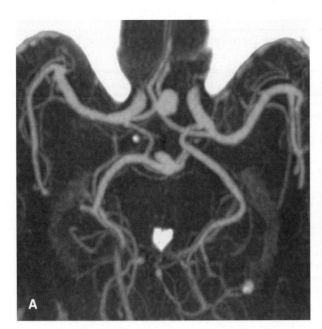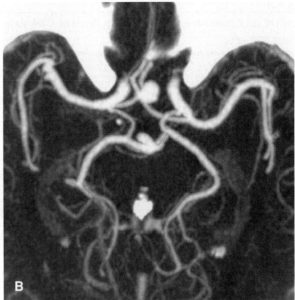

FIGURE 1-39 Comparison of a maximum intensity projection of the circle of Willis obtained at 120 kVp and a $CTDI_{vol}$ of 28.5 mGy **(A)** and 90 kVp and a $CTDI_{vol}$ of 21 mGy **(B)**. Despite a 25% lower dose, the image quality is similar if not better at 90 kVp. (Courtesy of A. Waaijer, Utrecht.)

about twice as high for girls than for boys: A newborn girl has an almost 10 times higher radiation risk than the average population (30-year-old adult). At older age, radiation sensitivity decreases substantially and can be 5 times lower than the population average for a 65-year-old male.

There is another factor that leads to a potential dose increase in children or slim adults: Because there is less radiation attenuation in the body, the local dose is closer to the dose in air. As the attenuation increases (abdomen as opposed to chest or neck, or obese as compared with slim patients), more dose is already absorbed in the outer layers of the body, and the local organ dose is actually reduced. For identical exposure parameters, local organ dose in small individuals will therefore be substantially higher than for large individuals.

The following techniques can be used to reduce radiation dose in children; slim patients; or CTA of the circle of Willis, neck, and chest:

- Keep the scan range as small as possible but as large as necessary.

TABLE 1-7

Suggested kVp Settings for Typical CTA Examinations Depending on Body Region and Patient Weight

Patient Weight	Circle of Willis	Chest	Abdomen
<50 kg	80 kVp	80 kVp	100 kVp
50–80 kg	80 kVp	100 kVp	120 kVp
>80 kg	80 kVp	120 kVp	120 kVp

- Avoid radiation sensitive organs, if possible (for example, the eyes in the case of CTA of the circle of Willis).
- Consider using a maximum of 8 to 16 active detector rows if the scan range is small compared with the total collimation. This reduces the added dose by over-ranging (the additional rotations outside the scan range that are required for image interpolation). This is especially important in small children.
- Use automated exposure control. If not available, use a size-dependent exposure table (Table 1-8).
- As an indicator of exposure dose, do not use mA (or mAs settings), but use the volume CT dose index ($CTDI_{vol}$) indicated on the scanner interface instead. This parameter includes already the effect of kVp setting, scanner type, and section collimation on dose.
- Use *z*-modulation, and combine with *xy*-modulation if possible. If *z*-modulation is not available, refrain from only using *xy*-modulation.
- Use adaptive filtering to reduce noise and artifacts in the shoulder or pelvic regions.
- Consider a moderately (not strongly) smoothing filter kernel because vessels are generally smaller in children or slim patients.
- Reduce kVp setting, depending on size and body region (Table 1-7).
- Optimize contrast enhancement by adapting contrast-injection protocols
- Use a wide window setting to accommodate for the increased vascular contrast (due to adjusted injection

TABLE 1-8

Example of Exposure Settings for Typical CTA Examinations Depending on Body Region and Patient Weight

Region	Suggested CTDI$_{vol}$ Depending on Patient Weight					
	<20 kg	20–50 kg	50–65 kg	65–80 kg	80–100 kg	>100 kg
Circle of Willis*	20	25	30	35	40	40
Carotid arteries**	2.5	4	6	7.5	10	15
Pulmonary arteries	2.5	4	6	7.5	10	15
Thoracic aorta**	2.5	4	6	7.5	10	15
Abdominal aorta	4	6	7.5	10	15	25
Renal arteries	4	6	7.5	10	15	25
Peripheral arteries**	4	6	7.5	10	15	25

Volume CT dose index, CTDI$_{vol}$.
*CTDI for 16-cm head phantom; for other organs, a 32-cm body phantom is used.
**Always combine with *z*-modulation, if available.

parameters and low kVp settings) and in order to make image noise less visually disturbing.

- When reviewing cross-sectional images, interactively increase section width of multiplanar reformations as much as possible without losing vascular detail (1.5 to 3 mm, depending on body size and vascular territory).

Obese Patients

Obese patients pose a different challenge: Here, it is not so much the radiation exposure that is of concern but the image quality that can be very limited. A proper exam contributes to dose containment because otherwise the CTA examination will be wasted and may even have to be repeated.

One also has to keep in mind that the organ dose in obese individuals is substantially lower than for slim individuals if the same exposure parameters are used. The reason is again the fact that the outer layers of the body already attenuate a substantial amount of the radiation. If automated exposure control is used, this translates into a modest increase in organ dose despite a substantial increase in exposure parameters (in particular, CTDI$_{vol}$).

For identical SNR, the exposure parameters may have to be increased considerably since x-ray attenuation increases roughly every 4 to 5 cm of increase in effective body diameter. However, the amount of noise that is clinically acceptable increases in larger patients because most of the contrast-enhanced vessels will be embedded in adipose tissue that serves as a negative contrast agent. For this reason, the required increase in dose is not as high as theoretically expected. Again, automated exposure control can be used to ensure more constant image quality.

The following measures can be used to improve image quality in obese patients:

- Keep the scan range as small as possible but as large as necessary. This will allow for using higher mAs settings (or more precisely, higher CTDI$_{vol}$).
- Use thicker collimation (5 mm on single detector-row scanners, and up to 2.5 mm on multidetector-row scanners) in order to increase detector signal and keep the relative contribution of electronic noise low.
- Try using the full width of the detector to increase geometric dose efficiency.
- When the maximum tube output (mAs setting) is reached for a particular set of scan parameters, further increase is usually possible if pitch is reduced or rotation time is decreased.
- Use 120 kVp, and maximize dose (CTDI$_{vol}$). If more dose is required, switch to 140 kVp (this, however, will reduce intravascular enhancement of iodine).
- Use automated exposure control. If not available, use a size-dependent exposure table (Table 1-8).
- Use *z*-modulation, combine with *xy*-modulation, if possible.
- Use adaptive filtering.
- Consider a strongly smoothing filter kernel to reduce noise.
- Optimize contrast enhancement by adapting contrast injection protocols: Inject larger amounts of iodine with a high injection rate.
- Consider a larger field of view for image reconstruction in order to make image noise less visually disturbing on axial images (Fig. 1-40).
- When reviewing cross-sectional images, interactively increase section width of multiplanar reformations as much as possible without losing vascular detail (3 to 7 mm, depending on body size and vascular territory).

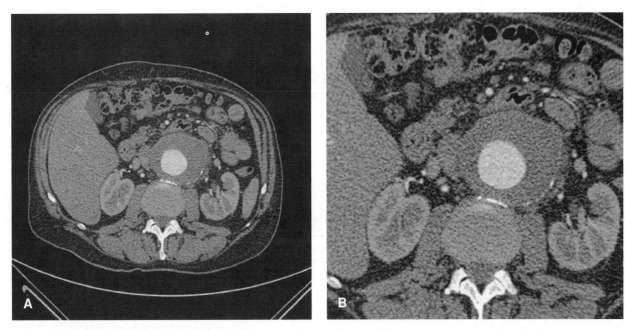

FIGURE 1-40 Effect of field of view (FOV) on noise perception in cross-sectional images: 40-cm FOV in an obese adult **(A)**; 20-cm FOV of the same exam **(B)**. Display of small structures, however, may be adversely affected (Fig. 1-11).

ECG SYNCHRONIZATION AND CARDIAC COMPUTED TOMOGRAPHIC ANGIOGRAPHY

For cardiac imaging but also for reducing or analyzing the effects of vascular pulsatility, ECG synchronization of data acquisition or reconstruction is necessary. Two techniques are available: prospective ECG triggering, in which data is acquired from a predefined interval of the RR cycle, and retrospective gating, in which data is acquired throughout the cardiac cycle but is retrospectively separated into different phases (Figs. 1-41–1-43).

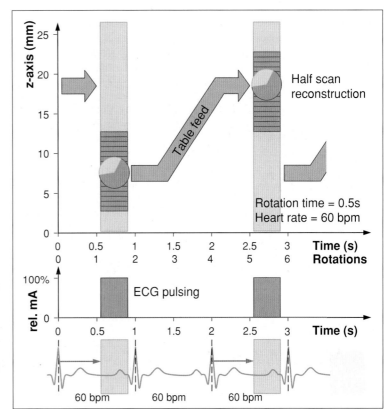

FIGURE 1-41 Principle of prospective ECG triggering. Data acquisition is started at a predefined delay after the R-peak of the ECG. A single section is acquired using a half-scan reconstruction; then, the table is moved to the next position (sequential acquisition). This usually means that data acquisition can only take place every second heartbeat. All radiation dose is used for image generation (ECG pulsing), but the correct temporal window has to be estimated beforehand. If the heart rate changes, data can no longer be acquired during the most optimum phase. (From M. Prokop et al. *Spiral and Multislice CT of the Body.* Thieme Medical Publishers 2003, with permission.)

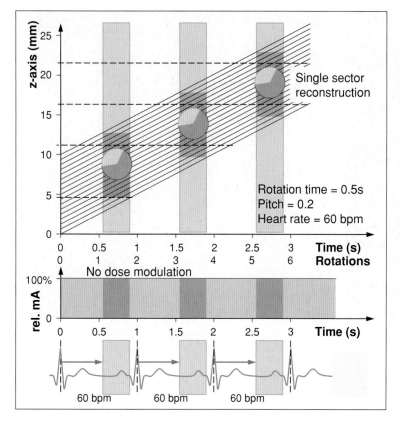

FIGURE 1-42 Principle of retrospective ECG gating using single-sector reconstruction. In this technique, radiation is given continuously during a spiral data acquisition with a low pitch factor (usually 0.2 to 0.3). Only those raw data are retrospectively chosen for half-scan reconstruction that belong to the same motion state of the heart. In single-sector reconstruction, all raw data originate from the same RR interval. The width of the temporal acquisition window is somewhat wider than half the rotation time RF (here, RT = 0.5 seconds). If pitch is low, data could be taken from two consecutive intervals (*gray areas*), but usually only data from the center of one RR interval (*blue*) are used. Because of sharp transitions between RR intervals, step artifacts may occur if cardiac motion is not absolutely identical between consecutive cardiac cycles. The optimum temporal reconstruction window is usually estimated from the RR interval: antegrade from the preceding R-peak, retrograde from the next R-peak, or as a (frequency-adaptive) percentage of the RR interval. Multiple intervals can be chosen to evaluate heart motion. For each interval, only part of all raw data (10% to 30%) contribute to the image, which means that dose efficiency is low (10% to 30%). However, even if the heart rate changes, the phase with the relatively least motion can be retrospectively chosen for reconstruction. (From M. Prokop et al. *Spiral and Multislice CT of the Body.* Thieme Medical Publishers 2003, with permission.)

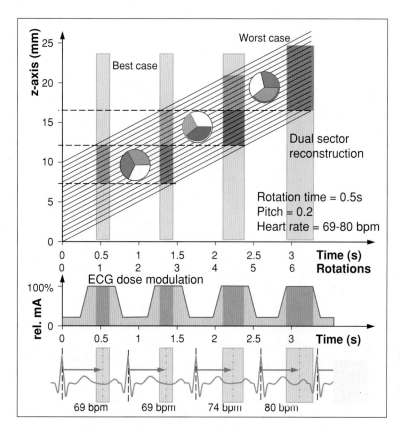

FIGURE 1-43 Principle of retrospective ECG gating using multisector reconstruction. This technique uses the same acquisition as single-sector reconstruction but reduces the width of the temporal acquisition window by filling up the raw data for half-scan reconstruction from two (or more) consecutive RR intervals. In the best case, the width of the temporal acquisition window can be reduced by the number of heart cycles used for reconstruction. At less favorable heart rates, however, data partially overlap, and the temporal acquisition window has to be widened. Motion artifacts are reduced with decreasing width of the temporal acquisition window, but dose efficiency decreases proportionally as well. For this reason, multisector acquisition is frequently combined with ECG dose modulation. ECG dose modulation reduces the mA settings during those phases of the heart cycle that are not used for reconstruction of CTA data sets. However, if heart rate increases during the scan, dose modulation may no longer work optimally.

Prospective Electrocardiogram Triggering

Prospective ECG triggering is used for sequential acquisition of multiple simultaneous sections (equal to the number of active detector rows). Temporal resolution is improved by a partial scan technique. X-ray dose is only switched on during the temporal acquisition window, which is prospectively determined by the user (Fig. 1-41).

A prospective trigger is derived from the ECG to initiate scanning at a user-selectable time after the preceding R-wave or before the next R-peak. This delay is defined to coincide with the end-diastolic phase of the heart cycle. It is usually chosen between 40% and 80% of the RR interval. Due to limitations in scan cycle times (table movement), every other heartbeat is used for data acquisition. The table feed should be identical to the total collimation width or slightly less for overlapping sections.

Standard partial scan techniques require data from half a rotation plus the fan angle of the x-ray beam. With modern short geometries, the fan angle is in the range of 60 degrees. This will result in a temporal resolution that amounts to approximately 65% to 70% of the rotation time. Some manufacturers offer optimized reconstruction by rebinning the fan beam data to parallel beam geometry and using a reduced field of view: At an FOV of 20 cm, the required angle is in the range of 10 degrees, which yields a temporal resolution that is about 53% of the rotation time (Fig. 1-22). As a consequence, the temporal resolution varies between approximately 330 ms for 0.5 second rotation time and traditional partial reconstruction and 175 ms for 0.33 second rotation time and optimized reconstruction. Administration of a beta-blocker is always advisable in order to prolong the diastole as much as possible in order to make sure that no motion occurs within the temporal acquisition window.

Since all data are used for image reconstruction, no increase in radiation dose to the patient is necessary as compared with a conventional CT. At identical noise levels, dose is similar to or smaller than that of electron beam computed tomography.

Retrospective Electrocardiogram Gating

In retrospective cardiac gating, a continuous spiral scan is acquired with simultaneous ECG recording (Fig. 1-42). Images are reconstructed from a temporal acquisition window that can be retrospectively chosen at any arbitrary position within the RR interval. In order to obtain enough projectional data to be able to reconstruct an axial image during this acquisition window, oversampling with a low pitch factor (P = 0.2 to 0.3) is required. At higher heart rates, a higher pitch can be chosen (27,28).

With higher temporal resolution, the temporal acquisition window becomes narrower relative to the RR interval. This means that also a smaller proportion of the total amount of data contributes to any given image. At a heart rate of 80 beats per minute (bpm), for example, the length of the RR interval is 750 ms. If the temporal resolution increases from 150 ms to 75 ms, the percentage of the radiation dose that contributes to the final image decreases from 20% to 10%. In other words, the higher the temporal resolution, the less the temporal dose efficiency of the technique.

The width of the temporal acquisition window is determined by the rotation time and the number of cardiac cycles that are used for data reconstruction. In single-sector reconstruction, only one heart cycle is used for data reconstruction using partial scan techniques (with some sort of interpolation to compensate for table motion) (Fig. 1-42) (27). Single-sector reconstruction results in a temporal resolution that is at best 50% of the rotation time (see Fig. 1-44A). For consistent results, heart rate should be below 60 bpm with most scanners. This requires administration of beta-blockers in the majority of patients.

In multisector reconstruction, multiple heartbeats contribute data to a partial scan reconstruction (Fig. 1-43) (29,30). Under the most favorable condition that each heartbeat contributes a different portion of this data, the temporal resolution with multisector reconstruction can be reduced over single-sector construction by a factor that is identical to the number of sectors used. At a rotation time of 0.4 seconds, for example, single-sector reconstruction will yield at best a temporal resolution of 200 ms, while four-sector reconstruction will yield at best a temporal resolution of 50 ms (Fig. 1-44). However, this effect is heart-rate dependent. If heart motion and tube rotation are synchronized in a way that during each rotation the same tube position coincides with the same position of the heart, then there is no additional information from a new heart cycle, and the temporal acquisition window cannot be reduced conference to that of a single-sector reconstruction (Fig. 1-43). As a consequence of multisector reconstruction, there are favorable and unfavorable heart rates, and temporal resolution varies between the highest values defined by the number of sectors and the lowest values defined by single-sector reconstruction (Fig. 1-44A).

Adaptive multisector reconstruction techniques optimize the number of sectors automatically and always provide the highest temporal resolution at the given heart frequency, pitch factor, and rotation time (29,30). Since the position of unfavorable heart rates varies with rotation time, and better temporal resolution can sometimes be gained if the rotation time is reduced, more sectors are used for reconstruction

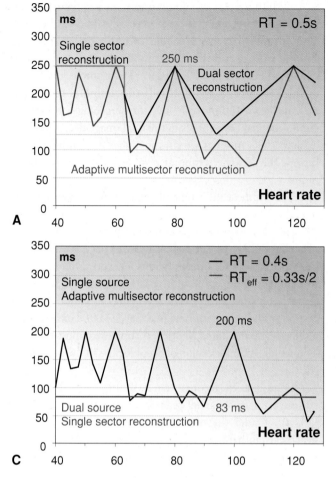

FIGURE 1-44 Comparison of the temporal resolution (width of the temporal acquisition window) for single- and dual-sector reconstruction versus adaptive multisector reconstruction for a rotation time (RT) of 0.5 seconds. Note that multisector reconstruction can improve temporal resolution substantially below 250 ms, but at certain unfavorable heart rates, temporal resolution remains 250 ms (A). Reducing the rotation time can shift the position of these unfavorable heart rates and improves the temporal resolution in the worst case scenario. Note that the heart rates that lower rotation times may provide better temporal resolution (B). Because of the very fast effective rotation time of dual source scanners, temporal resolution is high despite single-sector reconstruction (C). Note that the darker background areas in all graphs indicate a higher probability of motion artifacts. Such artifacts, however, strongly depend on individual patient factors such as cardiac contractility as well. (From M. Prokop et al. *Spiral and Multislice CT of the Body.* Thieme Medical Publishers 2003, with permission.)

(Fig. 1-44B). Most vendors let the user choose the rotation time manually, while some vendors automatically suggest an optimum rotation time depending on the range of hard frequencies recorded during a test inspirational period. Problems occur if the heart frequency deviates substantially from the prescan range and the selected rotation time is no longer optimum. In addition, many problems occur if the position of the heart is not precisely identical during the various heart cycles used for multisector reconstruction.

With dual source systems, in which two tubes rotate with 330 ms, effective rotation time is reduced to 165 ms. At such a speed, single-sector reconstruction is always possible and yields a constant temporal resolution of less than 90 ms independent of the heart rate (Fig. 1-44C). For most patients, that will probably mean that beta-blockers no longer need to be applied. Even with these new systems, the increase in temporal resolution will lead to a substantial reduction in temporal dose efficiency unless dose is reduced during those phases on the cardiac cycle that are not used for creation of images. ECG dose modulation is therefore mandatory for avoiding dose increase with these new scanners.

Electrocardiogram Dose Modulation

ECG dose modulation is a technique that reduces mA settings during predefined phases of the cardiac cycle that are not used for reconstruction of high-quality images (Fig. 1-43) (31,32). Usually the mA setting is reduced to 20% of its original value, which makes it possible to still obtain images of a sufficient quality for gaining functional information from the cardiac chambers. The smaller the portion of the RR interval in which dose is kept high, the better the temporal dose efficiency of the ECG dose modulation. The interval during which dose is kept high should be wide enough to still allow for retrospect adjustment of the reconstruction window to accommodate for interpatient variations or a change in heart rate during the scan. Vendors differ in how they have implemented the technique. In general, however, ECG dose modulation works best for low heart rates because the relatively increased length of the diastole will allow for down-regulating dose during larger portions of the cardiac cycle.

With conventional scanners, low heart rates (usually <60 bpm) are required for effective use of ECG dose modulation. With the constantly high temporal resolution of dual source systems, ECG dose modulation may work even at higher hard frequencies (<80 bpm). At present, a dose reduction of 50% over continuous scanning has been described.

Coronary Computed Tomographic Angiography

Coronary CTA has been gaining a lot of attention because it has the potential to substitute for a substantial part of diagnostic catheter coronary angiographies. Coronary CTA has become feasible with 4-detector-row scanners, but the technique yielded good results mainly in the proximal coronaries and only in a modest amount of patients. With 16-detector-row scanners, coronary CTA has become more stable, and more distal segments can be evaluated. With 64-detector-row scanners, even distal segments can be evaluated in the vast majority of studies, but patient preparation and patient selection still play a major role in the success of the examination. Further improvement can be expected from dual source technology and, ultimately, from wider detectors that are able to cover the heart in one heartbeat.

Patient Preparation

Even with the newest technology, a low and stable heart rate and good patient cooperation are mandatory for a successful exam. For this reason, a well-trained team of CT technologists and doctors are essential for a well-functioning coronary CTA lab. The patient has to experience a relaxed and professional atmosphere to make sure that the heart rate remains as low as possible. In order to keep stress levels down, informed consent for premedication, contrast injection, and potentially also radiation dose should be obtained before the patient enters the exam room, ideally already at the time the patient is scheduled for the exam.

Heart Rhythm

Most institutions will not scan patients with absolute arrhythmia or multiple extrasystolies. While good results can be gained in patients with absolute arrhythmia if the RR interval happens to coincide with those heart rates in which a high temporal resolution is available, the exam may become nondiagnostic when the RR interval is unfavorable and temporal resolution low. As a consequence, scanning patients with absolute arrhythmia is a gamble (Fig. 1-45). Extrasystolies may be corrected by "ECG editing," in which RR intervals with such extrasystolies are removed from the dataset (33). In order to still be able to reconstruct an image, a high data redundancy (low pitch) is required. Paired extrasystolies will make a scan impossible to evaluate

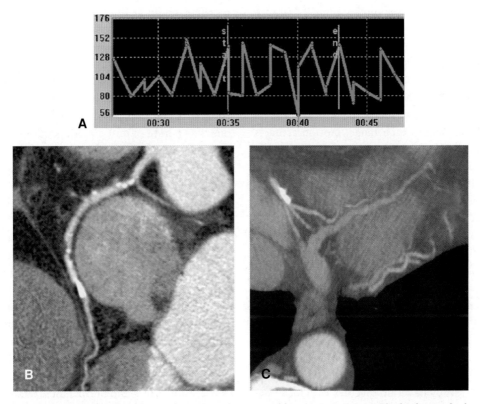

FIGURE 1-45 Image quality of coronary CTA can be acceptable even in patients with absolute arrhythmia if adaptive multisector reconstruction is used. However, the success of this technique is random and depends on the temporal resolution at the specific heart rates encountered during the scan. The faster the scan, the more likely a successful examination. In this 8-second scan performed with 4 × 0.625-mm collimation, heart rate varied from 40 to 140 bpm **(A)**. Note the soft plaques in the right coronary artery **(B)**.

because two consecutive RR intervals will have to be excluded from reconstruction. For this reason, it is not recommended to scan patients with known multiple ventricular extrasystolies or premature beats.

Breathing Instructions

Breathing instructions are an often neglected issue: Since scan durations for CTA of the heart are comparatively longer than in other body regions (because of an up to 5 times lower pitch), the risk of breathing-induced motion is higher than elsewhere. In addition, data from multiple rotations need to be gathered when multisector reconstructions are used. These data must come from identical anatomic locations, so minimum motion is acceptable. Patients should not relax their diaphragm during the breath-hold phase; they should not press or perform a Valsalva maneuver. Such motion will lead to local blurring of the coronaries and slight step artifacts in the contours of the ventricles (Fig. 1-30). Valsalva maneuvers, in addition, can almost completely cut off the venous inflow from the injection veins and can thus ruin the contrast enhancement of an exam. It is therefore important to instruct the patients to *breathe in normally and hold their breath*. The technologist should avoid letting the patient breathe in deeply because this will increase the risk of Valsalva. Explaining too much also may be counterproductive because it increases the stress on patients.

Single-sector reconstruction has an advantage when it comes to motion artifacts: Since data at a specific range of *z*-positions will come from the same RR intervals, motion will often only lead to a step whenever the next RR interval is reconstructed, but within each range, motion artifacts will be minimum. For multisector reconstruction, motion will induce incongruence within the data used for reconstruction and will result in blurring at all *z*-positions that have used the affected RR interval. Single-sector reconstruction, however, has a relatively lower temporal resolution and should be reserved for lower heart rates.

Premedication

In order to keep heart rate low and stable, most institutions will prescribe oral or intravenous beta-blockers before the exam (34). A low heart rate improves image quality and makes efficient dose reduction possible by use of ECG dose modulation. Beta-blockers are usually safe with few side effects, but the approach chosen at each institution should ideally be set up together with local cardiologists. Contraindications are known medication-dependent bronchial asthma, atrioventricular (AV) block, severe hypotension, overt heart failure, or known intolerance to beta-blockers.

Oral beta-blockers have the advantage that they can be administered prior to the exam but may not lead to sufficient reduction of heart rate and may need to be supplemented by intravenous (IV) beta-blockers on the exam table. They are administered at least one hour before the exam (for example, 50 to 100 mg metroprolol tartrate by mouth). Heart rate needs to be checked before the scan. If it is not low enough (ideally less than 60 bpm with most 16- to 64-detector-row scanners), an additional oral dose may be administered, but the patient then has to wait for at least another 30 minutes before the scan can be started. Alternatively, IV beta-blockers may be used to further reduce heart rate, but this should be done under the supervision of a cardiologist.

Intravenous beta-blockers are usually injected while the patient is on the CT table. They have the advantage that patients do not have to wait, but the technique adds another 5 to 10 minutes to the examination time. Usually, the dose is slowly increased (for example, in doses of 5 mg metroprolol tartrate IV up to a maximum dose of 20 mg) until the heart rate is below the desired level.

Even with the injection of beta-blockers, the heart rate cannot always be lowered far enough in every patient. In such a situation, multisector reconstruction can still yield excellent results if the heart rate is stable during the scan (see below). In scanners that only allow for single-sector reconstruction, the patient will need to be rescheduled if heart rate remains too high.

Sublingual application of nitrates has been suggested for vasodilation in order to increase the diameter of the coronaries and improve their evaluation. For this purpose, one to two hubs of nitroglycerin spray have been advocated. In some patients, this will lead to dizziness, but usually it is well tolerated. Again, a general policy should be set up together with local cardiologists.

Scan Range

The scan range should cover the whole heart. On the scanogram, the upper border of the scan range is set slightly caudal to the tracheal bifurcation, while the lower border is estimated from the heart contours. If a noncontrast scan was performed for calcium scoring, the range can be determined directly from appropriate sections. However, an additional centimeter above the highest coronary and below the inferior border of the heart should be included in the scan field to be less sensitive to differences in inspiration between the scanogram or calcium scan and the CTA acquisition.

For evaluation of bypass grafts of the heart including the ascending aorta, the scan range should be extended cranially to 1 cm above the aortic arch. The same holds true for

TABLE 1-9

Suggested Scan Parameters for ECG-gated CTA

Region	4-row SC	16-row SC	64-row SC	SW/RI	Scan Direction
Coronaries	1–2	0.5–0.625	0.5–0.625	0.5–0.9/0.4	↑
Bypass grafts	1–1.25	0.5–0.75	0.5–0.625	0.8–1.25/0.5	↑
Cardiopulmonary workup	2–2.5	1.0–1.5	1–1.25	1.0–3.0/0.7–1.5	↑
Thoracic aorta	2–2.5	1.0–1.5	0.6–1.0	1.0–3.0/0.7–1.5	↑
Thoracoabdominal aorta	2–2.5	1.0–1.5	0.6–1.0	1.0–3.0/0.7–1.5	↓

SC, section collimation (mm); SW/RI, section width (mm)/reconstruction increment (mm).
↓, cranio-caudal scan direction; ↑, caudo-cranial scan direction.
*May require use of only the two innermost detectors.
**Scan range can be split in two, lower resolution down to knees, highest resolution of lower leg and feet.

scans performed for a complete cardiopulmonary workup including the coronaries, aortic dissection, and coronary arteries. For this indication, it is usually not necessary to cover the whole lungs including the posterior recesses and the lung top.

Scan Parameters

For optimum temporal resolution, the shortest available rotation time should be chosen at low heart rates in order to improve the temporal resolution of single-sector reconstruction. At higher heart rates and when adaptive multisector reconstruction is required, it may be advantageous to adapt the rotation time to the heart frequency (Fig. 1-44). Some scanners record the heart frequency during a test breath-holding phase and determine the most optimum rotation time automatically (29).

In order to be able to reconstruct data from only part of the cardiac cycle, sufficient overlap between rotations is required. This means that the pitch factor has to be reduced compared with standard CTA. A lower pitch is required for low heart rates and for multisector reconstruction. In practice, however, more constant pitch factors between 0.2 and 0.25 are used in most instances. Some scanners automatically suggest suitable pitch factors depending on the heart rate that has been recorded during a test breath-holding phase (29).

For optimum spatial resolution, the thinnest possible collimation should be chosen. However, for 4-detector-row scanners, this will mean that the scan time has to be extended to about 40 seconds for covering the whole heart. For this reason, cardiac CTA requires 16 or more detector-row scanners for daily practice (Table 1-9).

Images are reconstructed with 0.9- to 1.25-mm section width, a field of view of approximately 20 cm, and a reconstruction interval of 0.4 to 0.6 mm. A thinner section width of around 0.6 mm could be chosen with 64-detector-row scanners, but it has to be kept in mind that this will substantially increase image noise and will require about twice the dose for identical SNR compared with slightly thicker sections.

For the evaluation of cardiac stents, spatial resolution is critical. For this particular indication, the thinnest possible section width combined with higher resolution filter kernels can improve the display of the stent lumen (Fig. 1-46) (35). However, an additional standard reconstruction with slightly thicker sections can be helpful for the evaluation of the rest of the coronary tree.

For coronary CTA, the acquisition window has been chosen so that motion is minimum. Unfortunately, the phase of the minimum motion varies between patients. Depending on the implementation on the scanner, the position of the acquisition window will be determined relative to the R-wave or as a percentage of the cardiac cycle. For single-sector reconstruction, an acquisition window that starts 350 ms before the R-wave will yield good results in the vast majority of cases. If residual motion artifacts are present, scans should be reconstructed at 300, 400, and 450 ms before the R-wave (16). With multisector construction, good results are usually obtained during mid diastole (70% to 80% of the cardiac cycle) if the heart rate is below 60 bpm (28). For heart rates about 75 bpm, the best results are seen in end systole (30% to 40% of the cardiac cycle) (36). For heart rates between 60 and 75 bpm, images should be reconstructed during mid diastole and end systole (Fig. 1-47). If all images show artifacts, additional phases need to be reconstructed. In the future, however, automatic determination of the most suitable heart phase will become available (37).

Dose

Dose is strongly related to spatial resolution as well as temporal resolution (see above). High temporal resolution (relative to the length of the RR interval) requires more dose if no ECG modulation is used. As a consequence of increasing spatial resolution in the z-axis (thinner

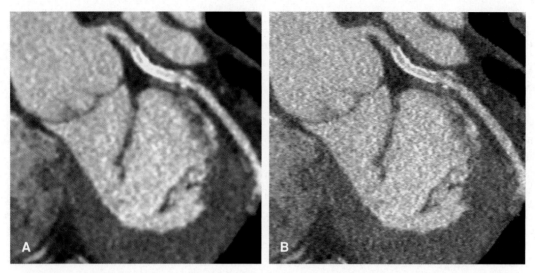

FIGURE 1-46 Higher resolution may be advantageous for coronary stents. Comparison of the quality of curved planar reformations through a stent in the left anterior descending coronary artery reconstructed with a moderately smooth filter and 1.0-mm section thickness **(A)** and a higher resolution filter and 0.6-mm section thickness **(B)**. (Images courtesy of Dominique Sandner-Porkristl, Siemens Medical Solutions, Stanford, California.)

reconstructed sections) or the *xy*-plane (high-resolution filters), image noise will grow (Fig. 1-46). This requires a substantial increase in dose if the advantages of higher resolution shall not be lost due to increased noise. Already, retrospectively ECG-gated coronary CTA scans suffer from either substantially higher noise levels or higher dose requirements.

For optimum quality with 64-detector-row scanners, up to 60 mGy (CTDI$_{vol}$) have been given at some institu-

tions to provide high spatial resolution at reasonable noise levels (17). This dose is approximately twice as high as for coronary CTA using 16-detector-row scanners of the same manufacturer (16,31). This CTDI is about 5 to 10 times higher than for a regular nongated chest CT (31). The effective dose for the patients remains around 10 mSv if only the heart is included in the scan range (31) or larger scan ranges; however, the effective dose will increase proportionally. For example, if the scan range is increased

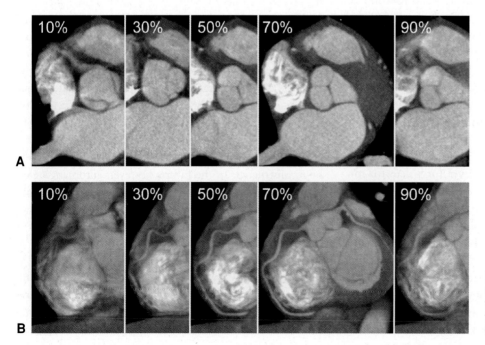

FIGURE 1-47 Image quality of axial sections **(A)** and volume intensity projection **(B)** as a function of the reconstruction window within the RR interval at a heart rate of 65 bpm.

from 12 cm for the heart to 24 cm for the heart including the ascending aorta, the effective dose will double.

Measures for reducing dose in cardiac CT are therefore being developed. ECG dose modulation is most efficient for low heart rates and may reduce patient dose by 50% over standard techniques (32). Dual source technology promises even a further reduced dose by shortening the acquisition window and therefore improving ECG dose modulation. Other measures include narrowing of the fan beam so that only the region of the heart is always within the primary radiation. This will reduce the dose to the outer portions of the chest. Anatomic dose modulation, in which the dose is increased in posterior projections and decreased in anterior projections, may reduce the dose to the breasts.

Lowering the kVp may improve the contrast enhancement of the coronaries, thus allowing for lowering the dose without decreasing SNR. This only is possible for slim patients and may use more artifacts in those stent grafts that have high attenuation on CT.

The most efficient way of keeping dose low is by not exaggerating spatial and temporal resolution and adapting dose to patient size (dose modulation and automated exposure control) (38).

Cardiopulmonary Workup

For a combined workup of cardiopulmonary disease (triple workup: acute coronary disease, aortic dissection, pulmonary embolism), the scan range is increased to include the heart, most of the thoracic aorta, and the pulmonary arteries. For this indication, it is usually not necessary to cover the whole lungs including the posterior recesses and the lung top. Therefore, the scan range extends cranially to 1 cm above the aortic arch and ends approximately 1 cm below the heart. Because of a relatively large scan range, dose would be approximately twice as high as for coronary CTA were the same exposure parameters used.

Since the indication for a complete cardiopulmonary workup might potentially include patients with suspected pulmonary embolism as well as suspected acute myocardial problems, a lot of patients are potentially eligible, but only a small portion will probably demonstrate manifest disease. For this reason, it is important to use a good compromise between image quality and radiation dose.

Such a compromise between image quality and radiation dose can be achieved by reducing the kVp settings in smaller patients (Table 1-7), reconstructing slightly thicker sections (1.2 to 1.5 mm), and reducing mAs settings accordingly (Fig. 1-48). Possible scan parameters are suggested in Table 1-9.

Gated Computed Tomographic Angiography

ECG-gated CTA is a technique that becomes possible with 16-detector-row scanners and is easily performed with 64-detector-row scanners. It uses retrospective ECG gating in very much the same way as cardiac CTA but, in

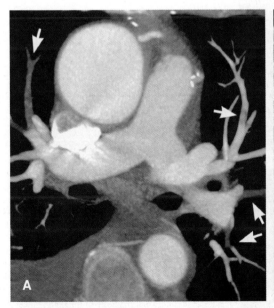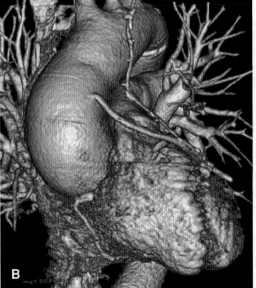

FIGURE 1-48 Cardiopulmonary workup: Example of a patient with constrictive pericarditis and pulmonary embolism after bypass surgery (300 mAs, CTDI$_{vol}$ = 18 mGy). Despite the fact that images were reconstructed with 1.3-mm section thickness, the emboli **(A)** as well as the coronaries **(B)** are depicted sufficiently.

general, with a reduced dose (CTDI$_{vol}$). ECG gating is thereby applied to freeze vessel pulsation, to analyze vessel pulsatility, and to evaluate the heart and—to a lesser degree—the coronaries. Clinical applications include improved visualization of aortic dissection membranes, evaluation of aortic pulsatility before and after stent grafting, analysis of cardiac function, and evaluation of the proximal coronary arteries (39). Unless the coronary arteries are the main focus, application of beta-blockers is not necessary.

The technical challenge is to keep patient dose within reasonable limits: If the same exposure parameters were used as for a typical 64-detector-row cardiac CTA (CTDI$_{vol}$ = 40 to 60 mGy), then the effective patient dose would be in the range of 35 to 50 mSv, which is 2 to 3 times above the dose range usually applied for body CT.

In the chest, this can be done by tweaking the CTA acquisition in a way that keeps the dose as low as possible.

In slim patients, reducing the kVp settings is an obvious option. In addition, section width can be increased to 1.25 to 1.5 mm in order to reduce image noise (see cardiopulmonary workup). However, image quality in the abdomen will suffer despite a substantial radiation exposure. In more obese individuals, quality of ECG-gated CTA will be too low to perform detailed analysis of smaller arteries unless the dose is increased substantially over nongated CTA techniques.

The solution to this dilemma is to reconstruct not only ECG-gated images (that necessarily use only 10% to 20% of the applied dose) but also to reconstruct an image data set that neglects the ECG information and uses all available raw data for image reconstruction. Such untagged or ungated images will have an excellent signal-to-noise ratio but will suffer from blurring of pulsating contours (Fig. 1-49). For most applications, however, blurring of contours will not

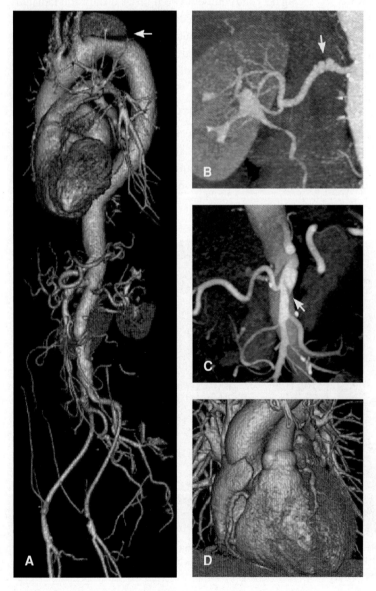

FIGURE 1-49 Gated CTA of a patient with a chronic aortic dissection type B. The untagged reconstruction neglects the ECG information and therefore yields volume-rendered images of excellent quality **(A)**. There is persistent dissection in the proximal descending aorta (*arrow*) but no residual false lumen in the more distal portions of the aorta. However, there is a persistent intimal flap in the superior mesenteric artery (*arrow*) **(B)**, and there are signs of fibromuscular dysplasia of the right renal artery (*arrow*) **(C)**. Gated images reconstructed with 1.4-mm section width to reduce image noise reveal normal coronaries on the volume-rendered display **(D)**.

adversely affect diagnosis. In addition, the ECG-gated data set will freeze motion and allow for precise evaluation of the contours of the aorta or large arteries. Thus, the nongated data can be used for evaluation of small arteries in a fashion similar to conventional CTA, while the gated data can be used for evaluation of vessel pulsation and, to certain extent, the heart and the coronaries. The dose need not be increased much over a standard CTA (Table 1-9). This approach is unfortunately not supported by all vendors.

CT PERFUSION

CT perfusion is firmly established only for the brain (40,41), although applications elsewhere in the body have been suggested for a long time, and commercial software is now available (42–45).

Multiple scans in rapid succession (or even during continuous radiation) are obtained during the injection of a contrast material bolus. The various sections must be registered to obtain the enhancement curve (time-density curve) of each voxel within the organ of interest. For this reason, the organ of interest must be free of motion during data acquisition. The local enhancement curves for each pixel are then used to calculate various perfusion parameters.

Basic Concepts

CT perfusion (CTP) is based on temporal changes in attenuation during the first pass of a bolus of an iodinated contrast agent (time-density curves). Increases of attenuation relative to the precontrast scan are linearly related to the concentration of the contrast agent. Perfusion depends on the velocity and volume of the blood flow through large capacity vessels as well as through the capillary vascular bed. CT perfusion usually applies first-pass evaluation using kinetic models that assume that the contrast material is nondiffusible and neither metabolized nor absorbed by the tissue bed studied.

A simple "slope model," which uses the slope of the enhancement curve to determine regional blood flow (RBF), is most robust. It relies on the Fick principle: Change in enhancement (C) in an ROI is proportional to the blood flow × difference in concentration of contrast material between feeding artery (C_a) and draining vein (C_v):

$$dC(t)/dt = RBF \times [C_a(t) - C_v(t)]$$

This model requires a delta impulse to work best, which means that a sufficient amount of contrast material (e.g., 50 mL) has to be injected within as short a time as possible (i.e., using large bore 14 to 16G venous cannula and a flow rate of 8 to 10 mL/s). Since the absolute concentration of contrast material in the artery is not known, only relative numbers can be obtained for RBF. The time to peak (TTP) is easily established.

Deconvolution models provide both qualitative and quantitative data and allow for slower injection rates (50 mL at 4 to 5 mL/s). They use the time-density curves in a feeding artery and a draining vein (which have to be contained in the imaging volume) as arterial input function (AIF) and venous output function (VOF) to deconvolute the tissue time-density curve to determine RBF, regional blood volume (RBV), mean transit time (MTT), and potentially other parameters such as vascular permeability. In particular, the regional blood volume is calculated as the ratio of the area under the time concentration curve of the first bolus passage through the tissue to the area under the

TABLE 1-10

Suggested Scan Parameters for CT Perfusion Imaging of the Brain

Region	4-row	16-row	64-row
Section collimation (SC)	4 × 5mm	8 × 2.5–3 mm	32 × 1–1.25
Section width (SW)	5–10 mm	5–10 mm	5–10 mm
Tube voltage	80 kVp	80 kVp	80 kVp
CTDI per scan	2 mGy	2 mGy	2 mGy
Cycle time	2s	2s	2s
Number of scans	25	25	25
Contrast volume	40 mL	40 mL	40 mL
Flow rate	5–8 mL/s	5–8 mL/s	5–8 mL/s
Delay	0s	0s	0s

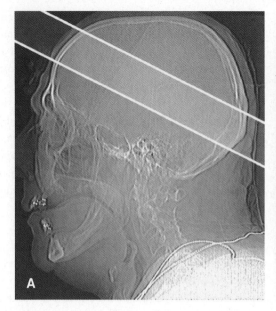

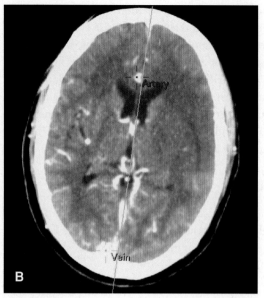

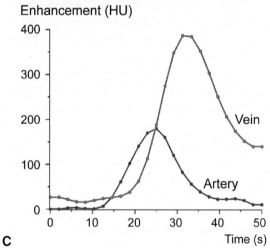

FIGURE 1-50 CT perfusion (CTP) imaging of the brain. The slab for data acquisition is positioned to include the basal ganglia and all major perfusion territories **(A)**. The arterial input function (AIF) is determined automatically from an ROI drawn in the region of the anterior cerebral arteries, while the venous output function (VOF) is determined from an ROI in the region of the sagittal sinus **(B)**. An axis of symmetry can be indicated to facilitate automatic comparison of the two hemispheres. The resulting enhancement curves for AIF and VOF **(C)** are used to calculate tissue perfusion parameters.

curve of the VOF. The MTT, the average time taken by the blood to cross the capillary network, is calculated by a deconvolution operation of the tissue curve with the AIF (41). This can be approximated by the difference between the width of the tissue curve and the width of AIF. According to the central volume principle, RBF can be calculated from RBV and MTT: RBF = RBV/MTT.

Brain Perfusion

CT perfusion imaging is becoming a standard technique in patients with acute stroke. The technique is straightforward (Table 1-10) and can be easily added to any noncontrast scan of the brain. Automated evaluation software is available that performs most of the necessary processing steps automatically.

No special patient preparation is necessary. Because only a small amount of contrast material (40 to 50 ml) is injected, the risk of contrast-induced nephropathy is very low. Patients with manifest renal insufficiency, however, should not be examined. Care has to be taken to place the head symmetrically in the head holder and to fix it as necessary in agitated or uncooperative patients.

For the evaluation of brain perfusion, usually one slab is chosen at the level of the basal ganglia (3 cm above the dorsum sellae) with angulation parallel to the anterior skull base. With single detector-row CT, this slab is 10-mm thick; with multidetector-row, the maximum width of the detector is used (20 to 40 mm, depending on the scanner type), and 5- to 8-mm-thick sections are reconstructed (Fig. 1-50A). Scanning is performed at 80 kVp in order to optimize signal-to-noise ratios and keep radiation exposure low. The CTDI per section is usually chosen to be approximately 2 mGy. Scans are obtained every 2 to 3 seconds. Scanning is started immediately after the beginning

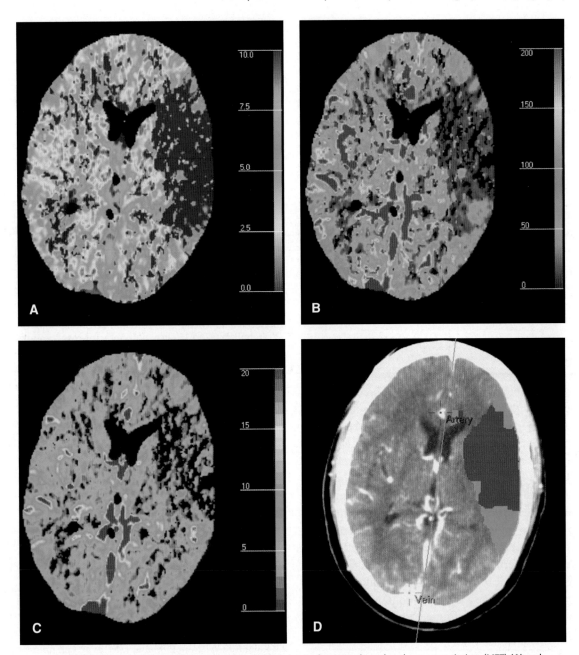

FIGURE 1-51 CTP of the brain in a patient with acute stroke. Note the reduced mean transit time (MTT) **(A)** and cerebral blood flow (CBF) **(B)** in the medial cerebral artery territory. The cerebral blood volume (CBV) is reduced only in the region of the infarct core (*arrow*) **(C)**. By visually displaying those areas with CBF <10mL/s in green and areas with CBV <2 mL/100g tissue in red, one can more easily distinguish areas of penumbra (potentially salvageable tissue) and the (nonsalvageable) infarct core **(D)**. However, one has to be careful not to overinterpret such fixed thresholds because of substantial interindividual variations.

of the contrast injection in order to obtain one to two precontrast scans, which are required for calculating contrast enhancement. Scanning is continued for about 40 to 60 seconds. Ideally, scanning could be performed more rapidly during the phase of contrast arrival (for determining arterial input in venous output) and more slowly during later phases (for determining washout). Most scanners, however, allow only for one fixed interscan delay and cannot increase the interscan delay later during the acquisition.

Once the data are required, the various sections are automatically registered to account for minor motion effects. Sections with gross motion artifacts have to be deleted. The next step is automated noise-filtering requirements to improve signal-to-noise ratios and enhance the gray-white differentiation. In the next step, the user is often to indicate the position of an artery (to determine the arterial input function) and the position of a suitable vein (to determine the venous output function). This can, for example, be done by placing a circular ROI around the vessel of interest (Fig. 1-50B). The computer then automatically finds the position of the vessel and calculates the curves (Fig. 1-50C). The curves are then used to calculate cerebral blood flow, cerebral blood volume, and mean transit time or time to peak (Fig. 1-51A–C). For this purpose, the described techniques are used.

Some programs allow for mirroring the perfusion values from the symptomatic hemisphere on to the asymptomatic hemisphere in order to automatically detect regions with hypoperfusion (penumbra) or manifest infarction (Fig. 1-51D). These regions can also be determined by calculating areas in which cerebral blood flow and cerebral blood volume drop below certain thresholds.

CONCLUSION

While the technology of data acquisition has become more complex with the advent of multidetector-row CT, the actual choice of scanning parameters has become simpler. Patient preparation becomes less important with more modern scanners but remains a critical factor in cardiac CTA. While CTA of all body regions can now be easily performed with 16-detector-row scanners, cardiac CTA will require further technological improvements in order to be easily applicable in any clinical situation at a reasonable radiation dose. Isotropic resolution is available with all modern scanners, but further increase in spatial resolution will be limited by dose requirements. Reduction of image noise and dose containment will become the challenges of the future.

REFERENCES

1. Schaller S, Flohr T, Klingenbeck K, et al. Spiral interpolation algorithm for multislice spiral CT—part I: theory. *IEEE Trans Med Imaging*. 2000;19:822–834.
2. Flohr T, Stierstorfer K, Bruder H, et al. Image reconstruction and image quality evaluation for a 16-slice CT scanner. *Med Phys*. 2003;30:832–845.
3. Mori S, Endo M, Tsunoo T, et al. Physical performance evaluation of a 256-slice CT-scanner for four-dimensional imaging. *Med Phys*. 2004;31:1348–1356.
4. Flohr TG, Stierstorfer K, Ulzheimer S, et al. Image reconstruction and image quality evaluation for a 64-slice CT scanner with z-flying focal spot. *Med Phys*. 2005;32(8):2536–2347.
5. Flohr TG, McCollough CH, Bruder H, et al. First performance evaluation of a dual-source CT (DSCT) system. *Eur Radiol*. 2006 Feb;16(2):256–268.
6. Prokop M. General principles of MDCT. *Eur J Radiol* 2003;45(supp 1):S4–S10.
7. Polacin A, Kalender WA, Marchal G. Evaluation of section sensitivity profiles and image noise in spiral CT. *Radiology*. 1992;185(1):29–35.
8. Hu H, He HD, Foley WD, et al. Four multidetector-row helical CT: image quality and volume coverage speed. *Radiology*. 2000;215:55–62.
9. Taguchi K, Aradate H. Algorithm for image reconstruction in multi-slice helical CT. *Med Phys*. 1998;25:550–553.
10. Tzedakis A, Damilakis J, Perisinakis K, et al. The effect of z overscanning on patient effective dose from multidetector helical computed tomography examinations. *Med Phys*. 2005;32:1621–1629.
11. Rubin GD, Napel S. Increased scan pitch for vascular and thoracic spiral CT (letter). *Radiology*. 1995;197:316–317.
12. van der Schaaf I, van Leeuwen M, Vlassenbroek A, et al. Minimizing clip artifacts in multi CT angiography of clipped patients. *AJNR Am J Neuroradiol*. 2006;27(1):60–66.
13. Remy-Jardin M, Remy J, Baghaie F, et al. Clinical value of thin collimation in the diagnostic workup of pulmonary embolism. *AJR*. 2000;175:407–412.
14. Schertler T, Wildermuth S, Alkadhi H, et al. Sixteen-detector row CT angiography for lower-leg arterial occlusive disease: analysis of section width. *Radiology*. 2005;237:649–656.
15. Heuschmid M, Mann C, Luz O, et al. Detection of pulmonary embolism using 16-slice multidetector-row computed tomography: evaluation of different image reconstruction parameters. *J Comput Assist Tomogr*. 2006;30:77–82.
16. Mollet NR, Cademartiri F, Krestin GP, et al. Improved diagnostic accuracy with 16-row multi-slice computed tomography coronary angiography. *J Am Coll Cardiol*. 2005;45(1):128–132.
17. Mollet NR, Cademartiri F, van Mieghem CA, et al. High-resolution spiral computed tomography coronary angiography in patients referred for diagnostic conventional coronary angiography. *Circulation*. 2005;112(15):2318–2323.
18. Mastora I, Remy-Jardin M, Delannoy V, et al. Multi–detector row spiral CT angiography of the thoracic outlet: dose reduction with anatomically adapted online tube current modulation and preset dose savings. *Radiology*. 2004;230:116–124.
19. Kalra MK, Rizzo S, Maher MM, et al. Chest CT performed with Z-axis modulation: scanning protocol and radiation dose. *Radiology*. 2005;237(1):303–308.
20. Greess H, Lutze J, Nomayr A, et al. Dose reduction in subsecond multislice spiral CT examination of children by online tube current modulation. *Eur Radiol*. 2004;14(6):995–999
21. Kachelriess M, Watzke O, Kalender WA. Generalized multidimensional adaptive filtering for conventional and spiral single-slice, multi-slice, and cone-beam CT. *Med Phys*. 2001;28(4):475–490.
22. Kalra MK, Wittram C, Maher MM, et al. Can noise reduction filters improve low-radiation-dose chest CT images? Pilot study. *Radiology*. 2003;228(1):257–264.
23. Waaijer A, Prokop M, Velthuis BK, et al. Dose reduction and image quality: reducing kVp and increasing mAs settings for CT angiography of the circle of Willis. *Radiology*. 2007;242(3):832–839.
24. Bahner ML, Bengel A, Brix G, et al. Improved vascular opacification in cerebral computed tomography angiography with 80 kVp. *Invest Radiol*. 2005;40(4):229–234.
25. Sigal-Cinqualbre AB, Hennequin R, Abada HT, et al. Low-kilovoltage multi–detector row chest CT in adults: feasibility and effect on image quality and iodine dose. *Radiology*. 2004;231:169–174.
26. Wintersperger BJ, Jakobs T, Herzog P, et al. Aorto-iliac multidetector-row CT angiography with low kV settings: improved vessel enhancement and simultaneous reduction of radiation dose. *Eur Radiol*. 2005;15:334–341.
27. Kachelriess M, Ulzheimer S, Kalender WA. ECG-correlated imaging of the heart with subsecond multislice spiral CT. *IEEE Trans Med Imaging*. 2000;19(9):888–901.

28. Hoffmann MHK, Shi H, Manzke R, et al. Noninvasive coronary angiography with 16–detector row CT: effect of heart rate. *Radiology.* 2005;234:86–97.

29. Lembcke A, Rogalla P, Mews J, et al. Imaging of the coronary arteries by means of multislice helical CT: optimization of image quality with multisegmental reconstruction and variable gantry rotation time [German]. *RöFo Fortschr Röntgenstr.* 2003;175:780–785.

30. Manzke R, Grass M, Nielsen T, et al. Adaptive temporal resolution optimization in helical cardiac cone beam CT reconstruction. *Med Phys.* 2003;30:3072–3080.

31. Hausleiter J, Meyer T, Hadamitzky M, et al. Radiation dose estimates from cardiac multislice computed tomography in daily practice: impact of different scanning protocols on effective dose estimates. *Circulation.* 2006;113:1305–1310.

32. Jakobs TF, Becker CR, Ohnesorge B, et al. Multislice helical CT of the heart with retrospective ECG gating: reduction of radiation exposure by ECG-controlled tube current modulation. *Eur Radiol.* 2002;12:1081–1086.

33. Cademartiri F, Mollet NR, Runza G, et al. Improving diagnostic accuracy of MDCT coronary angiography in patients with mild heart rhythm irregularities using ECG editing. *AJR.* 2006;186:634–638.

34. Shim SS, Kim Y, Lim SM. Improvement of image quality with ß-blocker premedication on ECG-gated 16-MDCT coronary angiography. *AJR.* 2005;184:649–654.

35. Cademartiri F, Mollet N, Lemos PA, et al. Usefulness of multislice computed tomographic coronary angiography to assess in-stent restenosis. *Am J Cardiol.* 2005;96(6):799–802.

36. Sanz J, Rius T, Kuschnir P, et al. The importance of end-systole for optimal reconstruction protocol of coronary angiography with 16-slice multidetector computed tomography. *Invest Radiol.* 2005;40:155–163.

37. Hoffmann MHK, Lessick J, Manzke R, et al. Automatic determination of minimal cardiac motion phases for computed tomography imaging: initial experience. *Eur Radiol.* 2006;16:365–373.

38. Jung B, Mahnken AH, Stargardt A, et al. Individually weight-adapted examination protocol in retrospectively ECG-gated MSCT of the heart. *Eur Radiol.* 2003;13:2560–2566.

39. Roos JE, Willmann JK, Weishaupt D, et al. Thoracic aorta: motion artifact reduction with retrospective and prospective electrocardiography-assisted multi-detector row CT. *Radiology.* 2002;222:271–277.

40. Nabavi DG, Kloska SP, Nam EM, et al. MOSAIC: Multimodal Stroke Assessment using Computed Tomography: novel diagnostic approach for the prediction of infarct size and clinical outcome. *Stroke.* 2002;33:2819–2826.

41. Wintermark M, Smith WS, Ko NU, et al. Dynamic perfusion CT: optimizing the temporal resolution and contrast volume for calculation of perfusion CT parameters in stroke patients. *AJNR.* 2004;25:720–729.

42. Blomley MJ, Coulden R, Bufkin C, et al. Contrast bolus dynamic computed tomography for the measurement of solid organ perfusion. *Invest Radiol.* 1993;28(suppl 5):S72–S77.

43. Harvey C, Dooher A, Morgan J, et al. Imaging of tumour therapy responses by dynamic CT. *Eur J Radiol.* 1999;30(3):221–226.

44. Blomley MJ, McBride A, Mohammedtagi S, et al. Functional renal perfusion imaging with colour mapping: is it a useful adjunct to spiral CT of in the assessment of abdominal aortic aneurysm (AAA)? *Eur J Radiol.* 1999;30(3):214–220.

45. Herzog P, Wildberger JE, Niethammer M, et al. CT perfusion imaging of the lung in pulmonary embolism. *Acad Radiol.* 2003;10:1132–1146.

Principles of Magnetic Resonance Angiography

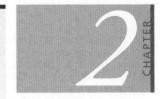

Frank R. Korosec

Magnetic resonance imaging (MRI) is a versatile and useful imaging modality that provides a wealth of diagnostic information. It is able to demonstrate, with striking contrast, differences in signal intensities among different soft tissues. A host of MR imaging parameters can be modified to exploit any one of a number of tissue-specific properties to manipulate image contrast. MRI derives signal using a magnetic field and radiofrequency energy, not ionizing radiation or radioactive materials like other medical imaging systems. Also, MRI is capable of providing tomographic images of any plane without requiring movement of the patient or any of the equipment.

MRI was introduced clinically in the early 1980s, and its applications have grown rapidly and immensely since. A subset of MR techniques, referred to as *magnetic resonance angiography* (MRA) *methods*, is described in this chapter. The chapter begins with an overview of the principles of MRI. This is followed by a description of some phenomena that negatively affect all MRA techniques. Finally, the physical principles, benefits, and limitations of specific MRA techniques are discussed. Additional overviews of MRA techniques may be found in References 1 through 5.

MAGNETIC RESONANCE IMAGING—OVERVIEW

MRI may be used to image nuclei of atoms containing an odd number of protons and/or neutrons. The nucleus of the hydrogen atom on the water molecule satisfies this criterion, as it is composed of a single proton. Because of its abundance in the body, the hydrogen nucleus on the water molecule is imaged in MRI.

The hydrogen nucleus possesses a magnetic dipole moment and will interact with a magnetic field as if it were a tiny bar magnet. The magnetic dipole moment of a hydrogen nucleus can either align or antialign with the strong magnetic field of the MRI scanner. In an ensemble of hydrogen nuclei, the majority will align because it requires less energy than antialigning. The net sum of the magnetic dipole moments from an ensemble of nuclei will yield a bulk magnetization that is aligned with the applied magnetic field. It is this bulk magnetization that is considered in discussions regarding MRI.

In MRI, signal is generated when the bulk magnetization is tipped out of alignment with the applied magnetic field. The maximum signal is generated when the aligned (longitudinal) magnetization is tipped 90 degrees so that it is perpendicular (transverse) to the direction of the applied magnetic field. A pulse of radio frequency (RF) energy is used to tip the longitudinal magnetization transverse. When the magnetization is transverse, it rotates, or precesses, around as shown in Figure 2-1. A receiver coil is placed perpendicular to the direction of the applied magnetic field to detect the oscillating signal that is generated by the precessing bulk magnetization. The precessional rate (and the frequency of the generated signal) is proportional to the strength of the applied magnetic field.

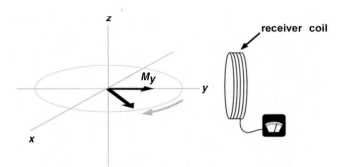

FIGURE 2-1 The bulk magnetization, M, rotates, or precesses, when it is transverse. The receiver coil detects an oscillating signal from the component of magnetization (M_y) that points toward it. The rate of precession and the frequency of the signal are proportional to the strength of the magnetic field. In this diagram, the magnetic field is aligned along the z-axis.

Magnetic field gradients that vary linearly with position are superimposed on the spatially uniform magnetic field during imaging. The resulting spatially varying magnetic fields cause the bulk magnetization at different locations to precess at different rates. Thus, transverse magnetization at different locations will produce signals with different frequencies. During image reconstruction, the detected signals are mapped to the proper positions based on their frequencies. Magnetic field gradients are strategically applied on each of the cartesian axes during imaging to map signal to position in all three dimensions.

Signal intensity in MR depends on a number of factors, and there are a host of parameters in MR imaging protocols that can be modified to accentuate the influence of these factors. One factor that influences signal intensity is the magnitude of the transverse magnetization. The transverse component of magnetization diminishes, or decays, exponentially with time. The rate of decay is characterized by a time constant called T_2. The decay rate depends on the microstructure of the tissue surrounding the magnetic dipole moments that make up the bulk magnetization. Since different tissues have dissimilar microstructures, they have distinct T_2 decay times. So, as time elapses, the transverse magnetization from different tissues decays by different amounts. Tissues with short T_2 decay times lose transverse magnetization quickly, whereas tissues with long T_2 decay times lose it more slowly. Thus, allowing time to elapse between tipping the magnetization transverse and detecting it allows achievement of signal differences from tissues with distinct T_2 decay times. The time from when the magnetization is tipped transverse until the signal is detected is controlled by the MR imaging parameter TE (echo time). Because scans with longer echo times accentuate signal differences based on variations in T_2 decay times, they are referred to as *T_2 weighted*.

Another factor that affects signal intensity in MRI is the amplitude of the longitudinal magnetization. After the bulk magnetization is tipped transverse, the longitudinal component begins to regrow exponentially. This rate of regrowth is characterized by a time constant called T_1. The regrowth rate depends on the microstructure of the tissue surrounding the magnetic dipole moments that make up the bulk magnetization. Since different tissues have dissimilar microstructures, they have distinct T_1 regrowth times. In MR, the longitudinal magnetization must be tipped many times in order to encode enough information to map the signals to the proper locations in the image. If only a short time elapses between application of one tipping pulse and the next, the longitudinal magnetization does not fully regrow. Furthermore, the longitudinal magnetization from short T_1 tissues regrows more than the longitudinal magnetization from long T_1 tissues. Thus, allowing only a short amount of time to elapse between tipping pulses ensures different amounts of magnetization are tipped transverse. This leads to generation of distinct signals from different tissues based on variations in T_1 regrowth times. The time between tipping pulses is controlled by the MR imaging parameter TR (repetition time). Since scans with shorter repetition times accentuate signal differences based on variations in T_1 regrowth times, they are referred to as *T_1 weighted*. In order to minimize T_2 weighting in these scans, the shortest possible echo time is used. In order to minimize T_1 weighting in T_2-weighted scans, a long TR is used.

When a long TR and a short TE are used, the signal is not dependent on T_1 or T_2 differences. In this case, the signal intensity depends on the density of hydrogen nuclei (on the water molecule) in each tissue. Since the hydrogen nucleus consists of a single proton, these scans are referred to as *proton density weighted*.

In addition to being influenced by T_2, T_1, and proton density, the signal in MRI is influenced by diffusion, temperature, magnetic field strength, motion, injection of a T_1-shortening contrast material, and many other factors. MRA techniques achieve contrast by harnessing the effects of motion (phase contrast and time-of-flight MRA) and injection of a T_1-shortening contrast material (contrast-enhanced MRA).

MAGNETIC RESONANCE ANGIOGRAPHY—LIMITATIONS

Shortly after the introduction of MRI, it was realized that this modality could be used to obtain images of the blood vessels. Since then, numerous magnetic resonance angiography methods have been developed for non- or minimally invasive assessment of vascular disease. MRA has many desirable attributes. For example, it can be used to demonstrate vascular information in three dimensions, provide information regarding the velocity and volume flow rate of blood, and produce angiograms without the use of an iodinated contrast material or ionizing radiation. In addition, MR permits soft tissues to be imaged. Therefore, in a single exam, both vascular pathology and its effect on the target tissues may be assessed. In the context of neuroimaging, MR also may be used to gather information regarding diffusion, perfusion (cerebral blood volume, cerebral blood flow, and mean transit time), brain function, and relative metabolite concentration, permitting a comprehensive evaluation using a single modality.

MRA, however, is not without its limitations. All MRA techniques are susceptible to phenomena that cause image degradation. Fortunately, an understanding of these phenomena permits wise selection of imaging parameters and image-enhancing options that lead to minimization of the adverse effects resulting from these phenomena, allowing consistent acquisition of high-quality MR angiograms. Three phenomena that cause image degradation in all MRA techniques are intravoxel dephasing, signal saturation, and signal ghosting. Because they affect all MRA techniques, they are described early in this chapter. The sensitivities of each of the MRA techniques to these phenomena are described later in the chapter.

In MR, the largest signal is produced when the transverse components of the magnetization from all of the nuclei within a voxel are aligned with one another. When they are aligned and rotating in synchronization, all of the signals from the magnetization add constructively to produce a large net signal. If for some reason the transverse components of the magnetization from the nuclei within a voxel start to rotate at different rates, the synchronized condition will decay. The signals from these different nuclei will then begin to destructively interfere with each other, leading to a diminished net signal from that voxel. This phenomenon is referred to as *intravoxel dephasing*, or *phase dispersion*. In MRI, intravoxel dephasing causes signal loss in regions of magnetic field inhomogeneity and at interfaces of tissues having different magnetic susceptibilities.

In MRA, signal loss due to intravoxel dephasing also occurs when nuclei having different velocities are present in the same voxel. This can be explained in the following way. In MRI, nuclei rotate at different rates depending on the magnetic field strength that they experience. If nuclei in a voxel have different velocities, they have traveled different distances to reach that voxel (from the time the magnetization is tipped transverse until the time the signal is detected). This means they have experienced different magnetic field strengths as they traveled to that voxel (due to the application of the spatially varying magnetic field gradients that are used for imaging). This leads to

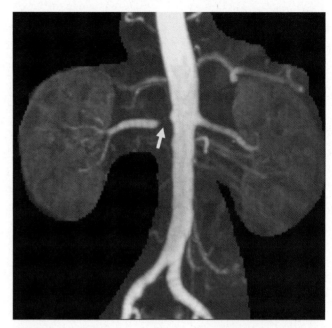

FIGURE 2-2 In regions of complex flow, intravoxel dephasing can lead to complete signal loss as is demonstrated here in this coronal image showing a tight stenosis of the right renal artery (*arrow*).

varied amounts of phase accumulation for the magnetization from the different nuclei, resulting in some element of destructive interference, in turn affecting the signals received from them. To the extent that protons are out of phase at the time of the echo measurement, signal is lost.

Certain types of vascular pathology, including stenoses, generate complex patterns of flow, which causes blood at various locations to travel at different velocities. Thus, blood flowing in the vicinity of stenoses often suffers from signal loss. In the vicinity of very tight or irregularly shaped stenoses, complete signal loss may result, as is shown in Figure 2-2. In these situations, it can be inferred that pathology is present, but details regarding the pathology cannot be determined.

Blood flows at varying velocities as it accelerates around corners; thus, there can be signal loss in regions where vessels turn sharply. These losses in signal can mimic those caused by tight stenoses, which is an important consideration when interpreting images.

Intravascular signal loss can also occur due to susceptibility-induced intravoxel dephasing. In the MR scanner, different amounts of magnetization are induced in tissues with different magnetic susceptibilities. As blood flows past these different tissues, it is influenced by different magnetic fields. High fields cause the magnetization in blood to precess quickly, and lower fields cause magnetization in the blood to precess more slowly. These different precessional rates lead to intravoxel dephasing, which results in signal loss. It is common to observe signal loss in blood vessels as they pass through the skull base due to the magnetic susceptibility differences between bone, extravascular tissues, and intraluminal blood.

The amount of intravoxel dephasing can be reduced by using a short echo time. Using a short TE permits the signal to be detected before the magnetization has had time to dephase. Dephasing only occurs during the TE—from the time the magnetization is tipped into the transverse plane, until the time that the receiver is turned on and the signal is detected. Shortening the TE reduces the amount of time that the magnetization is permitted to dephase. Hence, by employing shorter TEs, these types of signal losses are reduced.

The amount of intravoxel dephasing can also be reduced by using small voxels. This is because magnetization from one voxel is not combined with magnetization from another voxel. Therefore, by using small voxels, the amount of magnetization that is permitted to combine incoherently is reduced, thus limiting signal loss.

Finally, intravoxel dephasing may also be reduced by activating an image-enhancing feature called *flow compensation*. This feature eliminates phase shifts accumulated by blood that is moving at constant velocities. Flow compensation is described more fully later in this chapter.

Another phenomenon that leads to signal loss in MR angiograms is referred to as *signal saturation*. Signal saturation is a diminution of signal caused by rapid and repeated application of radio frequency excitation pulses to an image slice or volume, as shown in Figure 2-3. The rapid and repeated application of these pulses limits the regrowth of longitudinal magnetization of blood. This reduces the magnetization available to generate signal after application of subsequent radio frequency excitation pulses. All MRA methods employ rapid application of radio frequency pulses (short TRs), so saturation of vascular signal is an inherent limitation of all the MRA techniques. The more radio frequency pulses blood experiences, the greater the saturation, until eventually an equilibrium saturation level is reached. Thus, the longer blood stays in an image slice or volume, the more saturated it becomes. Methods to reduce signal saturation have been determined. In general, increasing the TR, reducing the tip angle, decreasing the thickness of the image slice or volume, strategically prescribing the acquisition to ensure that blood spends little time in the slice, and administering a T1-shortening contrast material are all strategies that lead to reduced signal saturation.

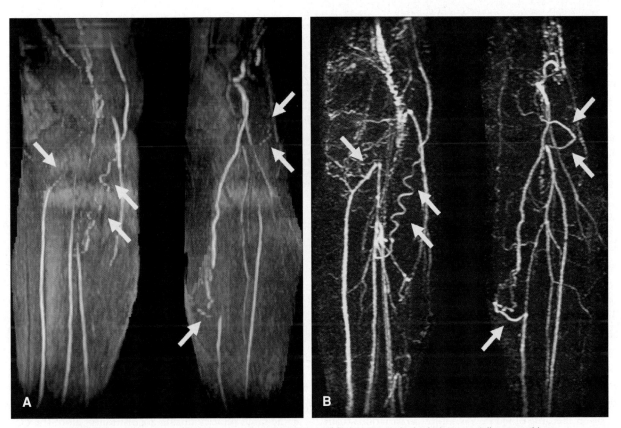

FIGURE 2-3 The image in **(A)** was obtained using a 2D time-of-flight MRA method, which is especially susceptible to signal loss caused by saturation (*arrows*). To produce this angiogram, thin axial slices were imaged, and the data were reprojected. The signal is saturated in regions where blood stays in the axial slices too long. The image in **(B)** was acquired using a contrast-enhanced MRA method, which is less prone to saturation.

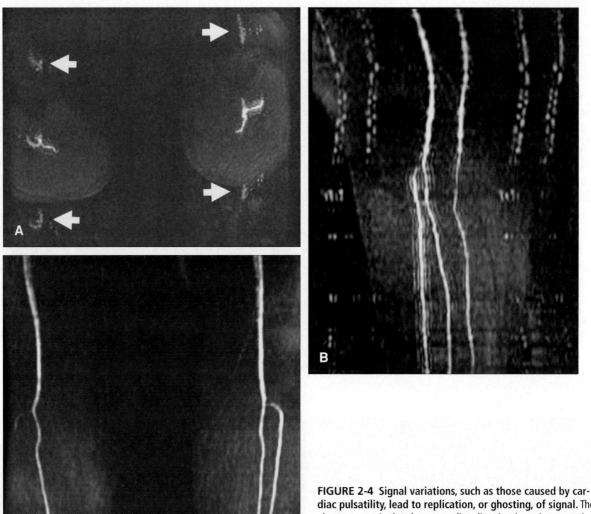

FIGURE 2-4 Signal variations, such as those caused by cardiac pulsatility, lead to replication, or ghosting, of signal. The ghosts appear in the phase-encoding direction (anterior–posterior, in this case) and are apparent here on the **(A)** axial and **(B)** oblique reprojections of the data, but not on **(C)**, the coronal reprojection. The coronal reformation superimposes the ghosts and vessels along the same projection and, therefore, the artifacts are not visualized.

These and other methods used to minimize signal saturation are described in more detail throughout this chapter.

A third phenomenon that affects the quality of MR angiograms is referred to as *signal ghosting*. Ghosting is the replication of signal in an image, resulting in an object appearing at one or more locations where it does not exist, as shown in Figure 2-4. Because replicas appear in locations where the object does not exist, they are referred to as *ghosts*. Signal ghosting originates from several sources. One source of ghosting is variation of signal intensity throughout image acquisition. Because blood flow is subject to variations from the rhythmic beating of the heart, spins in the blood move along the gradients in a varied manner. This motion generates phase gain or loss, resulting in artifacts that appear along the phase-encoding axis. (The position along the

phase-encoding axis is encoded at a specific phase). Mismapped phase information can appear as a varying signal or ghosts of the pulsating vessels in the image. It is the phase shifts of spins flowing along the imaging gradients during the finite time required between phase encoding and signal sampling that produce these ghosts.

Signal ghosts originating from this source can be reduced or eliminated by collecting data for an image always at the same time frame, or phase, within the cardiac cycle. This increases the likelihood that the blood will be flowing at the same velocity during acquisition of all of the data for an image. Elimination of signal variation removes the ghosts.

Like all imaging methods, MR vascular imaging methods have benefits and limitations. The limitations can be minimized and the benefits exploited by understanding the

TABLE 2-1

Benefits and Limitations of Magnetic Resonance Angiography

Benefits

- Safe—no ionizing radiation, no iodinated contrast materials, no intra-arterial injections, and no intra-arterial insertion of catheters.
- Provides information regarding vascular anatomy, hemodynamics, blood velocity, and volume flow rate.
- Can be performed in combination with other MRI acquisitions that provide information regarding the target organ, such as information regarding anatomy, diffusion, perfusion (cerebral blood volume, cerebral blood flow, mean transit time), temperature, and relative metabolite concentrations.
- Three-dimensional methods permit retrospective reformatting and reprojection of the data to evaluate the vascular anatomy from any orientation.
- Vascular signal is not attenuated by bone or other overlying structures.

Limitations

- Susceptible to a variety of artifacts, including signal loss (caused by intravoxel dephasing and saturation) and signal ghosting (caused by patient motion, cardiac pulsatility, and variations in contrast material concentration).
- Appearance of veins in images acquired using some MRA techniques can make image interpretation difficult.
- As with all MR imaging methods, increasing the spatial resolution leads to longer scan times and/or lower SNR.
- The physical principles affecting image quality are quite complex, and a limited understanding of these principles may lead to design of suboptimal imaging protocols.

characteristics of the MRA methods. This understanding is helpful in selecting the appropriate method and scan parameters for the desired application. Some of the more important benefits and limitations of all MRA methods are summarized in Table 2-1.

MAGNETIC RESONANCE ANGIOGRAPHY—SPECIFIC METHODS

The most widely used MRA techniques can be categorized as *phase contrast*, *time-of-flight*, or *contrast-enhanced* MRA techniques. In the remainder of this chapter, an overview of the principles of these techniques is provided, examples of clinical applications are shown, and the benefits and limitations of each of the specific methods are discussed. In addition, two other techniques that can be useful for vascular assessments, dark blood imaging and steady state free precession, will also be discussed.

Phase Contrast Magnetic Resonance Angiography

It is a fundamental MR principle that spins subjected to a magnetic field gradient acquire a shift in their phase of rotation that is proportional to the strength of the field. Moving spins will acquire a phase shift that is related to the distance traveled along the gradient and, therefore, related to the velocity of the spins. Phase contrast MRA capitalizes on this phenomenon such that spin velocities are encoded into a map of the vessels of interest. Thus, those phase contrast techniques that rely exclusively on phase data yield images with complete suppression of stationary tissue (with no velocity, there is no signal). When using PC techniques, stationary tissues that might appear bright by virtue of T1 or T2 characteristics will not be confused with flow.

Phase contrast MRA (6,7) is similar to conventional x-ray angiography in that both methods employ subtraction to eliminate signals from stationary tissues. As a result, only signals from flowing blood are present in the angiogram. Phase contrast MRA differs from conventional x-ray angiography in that no contrast media injection is required with the former method. The mechanism responsible for generating signal in phase contrast MRA is the motion of the blood.

Phase contrast techniques derive contrast between flowing blood and stationary tissues by manipulating the phase of the magnetization, such that the phase of the magnetization is zero for stationary tissues and nonzero for moving tissues (Fig. 2-5). Phase is a measure of how far the magnetization precesses, or rotates, from the time it is tipped into the transverse plane until the time it is detected. The data acquired with phase contrast techniques can be processed to produce magnitude, phase difference, and complex difference images.

In *magnitude* images, the strength of the magnetization at each point in the object is displayed in the appropriate pixel in the image. This is the typical display method employed in general MR imaging. With phase contrast methods, the phase of the magnetization is manipulated, but the strength of the magnetization, or its magnitude, is unaltered. Thus, displaying the magnitude of the magnetization permits simultaneous demonstration of vessels and stationary tissues.

In *phase difference* images, the signal is linearly proportional to the velocity of the blood—the faster the motion of the blood, the larger the signal, and blood moving in one direction is assigned a bright (white) signal, whereas blood moving in the opposite direction is assigned a dark (black) signal (Fig. 2-6). This characteristic of phase difference images permits arteries to be effectively differentiated from veins when they are aligned antiparallel to each other, as is the case with the carotid arteries and jugular veins (Fig. 2-7). Phase difference images also can be used to

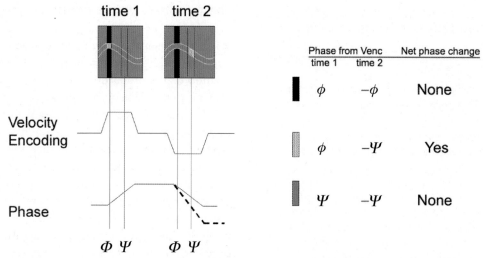

FIGURE 2.5 Schematic of phase contrast angiography. A velocity-encoding gradient pulse pair is added to the sequence. This superimposes a magnetic field to the affected region. The first velocity-encoding gradient is applied at some time (e.g., t_1). Then, an equal but opposite gradient pulse is applied shortly thereafter (e.g., t_2). Stationary spins (*black rectangle, gray rectangle*) experience the same magnetic field magnitude during each pulse but with an opposite polarity; thus, the phase gain acquired at t_1 is returned to its initial state for a net phase change of zero. Moving spins (*stippled box*), having traveled along the gradient, experience a different field (magnetization at t_2 × magnetization at t_1). Thus, the moving spins experience a net phase change (*thick dotted line*). The phase change is proportional to the velocity. (Adapted from Glyn Johnson, Ph.D.)

detect retrograde flow such as in subclavian steal syndrome, where a stenosis or occlusion of the subclavian artery proximal to the vertebral artery causes reversed flow in the latter.

In addition to permitting assessment of vascular anatomy, phase difference images can be used to determine quantitative information regarding speed and direction of blood flow. The signal in each pixel in a phase difference image is linearly proportional to the velocity of the blood or tissue represented by that pixel. So, a cursor or region of interest (ROI) can be placed on the image, and a direct measure of the velocity (mm/sec) of the blood or tissue can be determined. In addition, if the cross section of a vessel is demonstrated in the image, information regarding the volume flow rate of the blood (mL/min) in that vessel can be derived using computer software (8). Flow volumes can be calculated from the equation Q = velocity × area, where Q is flow in mL/min, velocity is determined using the phase map images (cm/sec), and area (cm^2) is defined by a user-generated ROI. By creating a cross-sectional ROI that traces the full lumen of a vessel and is perpendicular to its course, the blood volume (cm/sec × cm^2 = cm^3/sec, or mL/sec) can be calculated. Furthermore, if the acquisition is cardiac gated (9,10), and a series of images is produced demonstrating the cross section of a vessel throughout the cardiac cycle, then the acquired series of images can be

evaluated to determine volume flow rate in that vessel throughout the cardiac cycle (Fig. 2-8). In this case, blood volume across the aorta can be integrated over the cardiac cycle (mL/cardiac cycle), and since the cardiac cycle translates to heart rate, aortic volume flow rate (mL/min) can be calculated.

The physiologic effect of vascular pathology can be evaluated by (a) comparing the volume flow rate on the contralateral side with that on the ipsilateral side, (b) by comparing the volume flow rate before and after a physical or drug-induced challenge, and (c) by comparing the volume flow rate proximal and distal to a stenosis (e.g., coarctation of the aorta).

In *complex difference* images, the signal strength is dependent on the velocity of the blood (as it is in phase difference images), but the dependence is not linear (as it is in phase difference images). Furthermore, the direction of blood flow is not represented, so flow in opposite directions is not represented as bright and dark as it is in phase difference images (Fig. 2-9). Therefore, complex difference images are not used to determine quantitative information regarding blood velocity or volume flow rate, but are used, instead, for demonstrating the anatomy of the vessels.

Phase contrast methods are implemented using two-dimensional or three-dimensional acquisitions (11,12). Two-dimensional acquisitions can be completed rapidly

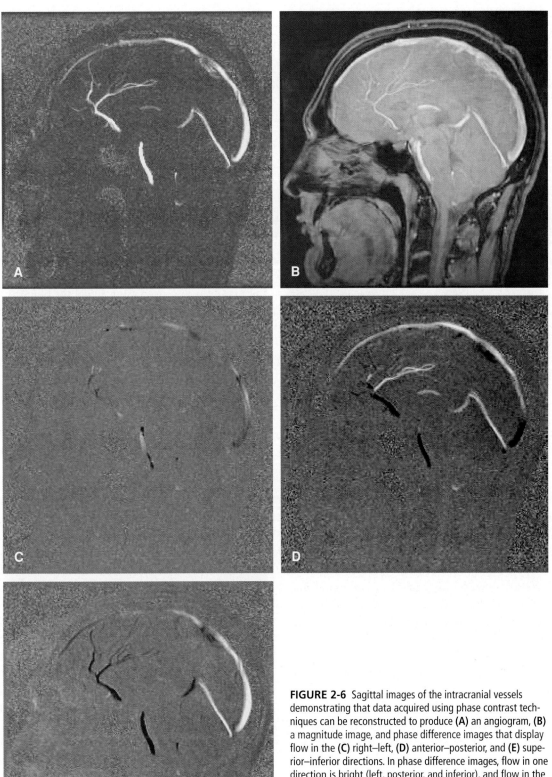

FIGURE 2-6 Sagittal images of the intracranial vessels demonstrating that data acquired using phase contrast techniques can be reconstructed to produce **(A)** an angiogram, **(B)** a magnitude image, and phase difference images that display flow in the **(C)** right–left, **(D)** anterior–posterior, and **(E)** superior–inferior directions. In phase difference images, flow in one direction is bright (left, posterior, and inferior), and flow in the opposite direction is dark (right, anterior, and superior). The intensity of the signal in the images shown in **(C)**, **(D)**, and **(E)** is linearly proportional to the velocity of the blood. The angiogram shown in **(A)** was produced by squaring the signals from the images shown in **(C)**, **(D)**, and **(E)**, summing them and taking the square root of the sum.

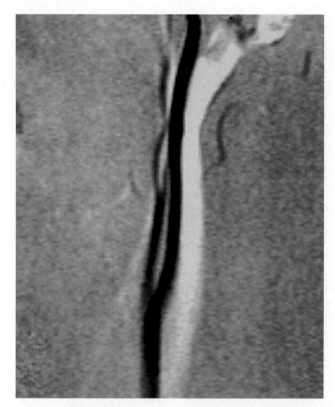

FIGURE 2-7 Phase difference processing of phase contrast data permits differentiation of arterial flow from venous flow as shown here, where flow in the carotid artery is dark, and flow in the jugular vein is bright. Additionally, the signal intensity is linearly proportional to the velocity of the blood.

and are effective for localizing vessels that can then be more thoroughly evaluated using other MRA techniques. In this manner, the 2D PC serves as a vascular scout series. It is also effective for performing cardiac-gated scans as described previously. Three-dimensional acquisitions are more time consuming than two-dimensional acquisitions and thus are used less frequently. Due to the long scan times associated with 3D acquisitions, they are not commonly cardiac gated. Benefits of 3D acquisitions include an inherently high signal-to-noise ratio (SNR) (due to the effective averaging of signal that is acquired throughout the entire scan) and small voxels (due to the encoding method employed). Also, thin section 3D image sets can be retrospectively reprojected or reformatted to permit observation of the vessels from any orientation. When phase difference processing is used, images reformatted perpendicular to a vessel can be used to determine volume flow rate through that vessel.

Phase contrast methods are sensitive to a range of velocities. To specify this range of velocities, the user chooses a velocity-encoding (Venc) value. This range designates the flow velocities to be encompassed within the maximum 360 degrees of phase shift. The Venc is inversely related to the area of the flow-encoding gradients. Hence, for the imaging time to remain unchanged, stronger gradient amplitudes are required to encode smaller velocities.

The Venc is given in centimeters per second. It determines the highest and lowest detectable velocity encoded by a phase contrast sequence. Therefore, $V_{enc} = 100$ cm/sec describes a phase contrast experiment with a measurable range of flow velocities of ±100 cm/sec.

Blood traveling at velocities higher than the Venc value will be misrepresented in the image, so the user must choose this value carefully. This misrepresentation is referred to as *velocity aliasing* and appears differently in phase difference and complex difference images. In phase difference images, aliased signal is easy to identify by an abrupt change from very dark to very bright signal (Fig. 2-10), or vice versa. In complex difference images, velocity aliasing manifests as a decreasing signal for blood traveling at increasing velocities above the Venc value. Blood traveling at some velocities above the Venc value gives rise to no signal at all. Thus, with complex difference processing, selecting a Venc that is too low can yield very misleading results that are not easy to identify. With both phase difference and complex difference processing, choosing a Venc value that is too low should be avoided. Choosing a Venc value that is too high should also be avoided, as it leads to all blood magnetization accumulating only small phase shifts, which results in low SNR, and a small signal range.

To avoid velocity aliasing, some a priori information regarding the anticipated pathology may be helpful in determining the appropriate velocity-encoding value. Often this information is not available, and in such instances, reference velocity values for normal vessels can provide a useful starting point. Alternatively, different velocity-encoding values may be used in different scans to highlight different vessels. For example, arteries and veins in an arteriovenous malformation (AVM) can be displayed in separate images that are sensitive to different velocity ranges (Fig. 2-10).

In order to encode flow in all directions with phase contrast acquisitions, a flow-encoding gradient must be applied on each of the three gradient axes in separate TR intervals. In addition, a fourth nonflow-encoded acquisition must be acquired. This nonflow-encoded acquisition is subtracted from each of the three flow-encoded acquisitions to eliminate signal phase produced from sources other than velocity. Alternatively, the flow-encoding gradients may be strategically applied on more than one axis simultaneously, to improve the SNR of the subtracted images (13,14). These alternative methods still require the acquisition of four scans to acquire velocity information in all three cartesian directions. With all of the phase contrast acquisition methods,

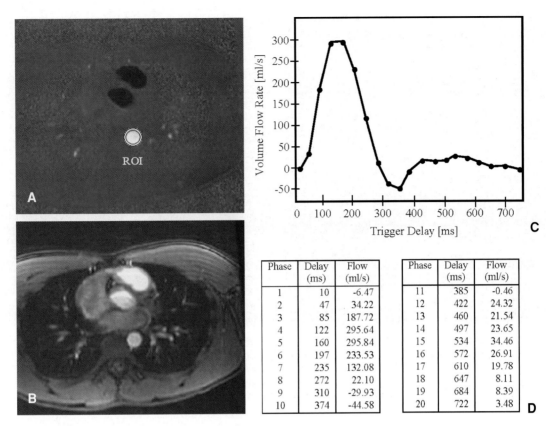

Phase	Delay (ms)	Flow (ml/s)	Phase	Delay (ms)	Flow (ml/s)
1	10	-6.47	11	385	-0.46
2	47	34.22	12	422	24.32
3	85	187.72	13	460	21.54
4	122	295.64	14	497	23.65
5	160	295.84	15	534	34.46
6	197	233.53	16	572	26.91
7	235	132.08	17	610	19.78
8	272	22.10	18	647	8.11
9	310	-29.93	19	684	8.39
10	374	-44.58	20	722	3.48

FIGURE 2-8 Phase difference images can be used to calculate the volume flow rate in a vessel throughout the cardiac cycle. This requires acquisition synchronous with the cardiac cycle, collection of a series of images throughout the cardiac cycle, and demonstration of the vessel cross section in the series of images. **A:** A region-of-interest (*ROI*) is drawn around the cross section of the descending aorta on one of a series of phase difference images acquired throughout the cardiac cycle. Note that flow direction is encoded such that cranial directed flow is represented as black (ascending aorta and pulmonary artery), whereas the caudal directed flow is represented as dark (descending aorta). **B:** The magnitude images can be used as a guide to identify the location and the boundary of the vessel throughout the cardiac cycle. **C:** The volume flow rate of the blood through the vessel as determined from each of the acquired images can be plotted to show the flow waveform as a function of time throughout the cardiac cycle. **D:** The actual values of the volume flow rate at different times within the cardiac cycle can be tabulated.

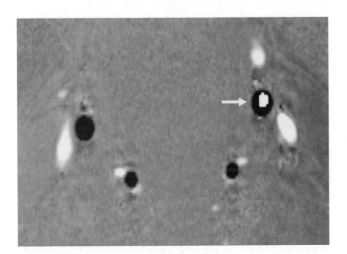

FIGURE 2-9 With phase contrast MRA methods, a velocity-encoding value must be selected. Velocities above this value will be misrepresented, or aliased. In phase difference processed images, such as the one shown here, velocity aliasing is easy to identify as an abrupt change from very dark to very bright signal (*arrow*), or from very bright to very dark signal (not shown).

the subtraction provides high contrast between vessels and stationary tissues, permitting large fields-of-view to be imaged without detrimental effects from saturation, as long as a relatively small tip angle (20 to 30 degrees) is used.

The scan time for encoding flow in all three cartesian directions using 2D acquisitions is $4 \times TR \times NSA \times \#PE$, where TR is the repetition time of the imaging sequence, NSA is the number of signal averages (sometimes referred to as the *number of excitations*, NEX), and #PE is the number of phase-encoding values acquired. If flow is encoded in only a single direction, the factor of four is reduced to a factor of two. With 2D acquisitions, a single thick slab is typically imaged. If multiple slabs are imaged, the scan time is determined by multiplying the above equation by the number of slabs. The scan time for encoding flow in all directions using 3D acquisitions is $4 \times TR \times NSA \times \#PE \times \#SE$, where #SE is the number of slice-encoding values acquired and all other abbreviations are as described previously. If

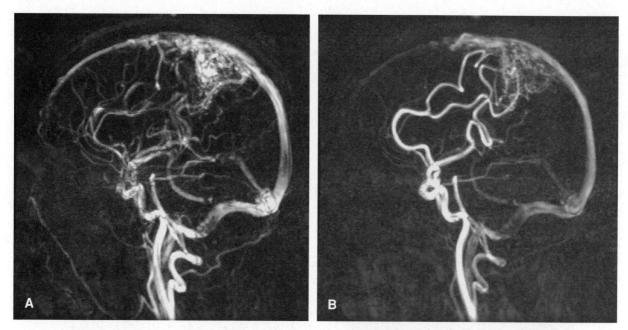

FIGURE 2-10 Phase contrast MRA images can be acquired with different velocity sensitivities (using different Venc values) to highlight vessels containing blood flowing in different velocity ranges. These sagittal complex difference processed phase contrast images of an arteriovenous malformation were acquired with velocity-encoding values of **(A)** 20 cm/sec and **(B)** 80 cm/sec. Note how the slow flow in the nidus of the AVM is better demonstrated in the image shown in **(A)**, whereas the faster flow in the feeding arteries is better demonstrated in the image shown in **(B)**.

flow is encoded in only a single direction, the factor of four is again reduced to a factor of two.

The use of the flow-encoding gradients in phase contrast sequences makes these methods particularly susceptible to signal loss caused by intravoxel dephasing. There are two reasons for this. First, the flow-encoding gradients force an increase in the minimum achievable echo time, which means that there is more time for intravoxel dephasing to occur (from all sources, including susceptibility). Second, the purpose of the flow-encoding gradients is to impart phase to magnetization from moving blood, but this is detrimental when blood at different locations within a voxel is moving at different velocities. In this case, magnetization from blood that is moving at different velocities accumulates different amounts of phase, which leads to intravoxel dephasing (which is exacerbated by the long TE).

The slice-selection and frequency-encoding gradients also cause intravoxel dephasing when blood at different locations within a voxel is moving at different velocities during application of these imaging gradients. *Flow compensation methods* (15,16), also known as *gradient moment nulling methods*, may be employed to reduce intravoxel dephasing caused by the imaging gradients.

Flow compensation methods are designed to eliminate the phase induced by the slice-selection and/or frequency-encoding gradients in the magnetization of all blood that moves at a constant velocity, independent of its velocity. When the phase of the magnetization from all blood (moving at a constant velocity) is nulled, intravoxel dephasing from this source is eliminated. However, the phase induced by the flow-encoding gradients is a necessary part of phase contrast MRA methods, so these phases are intentionally not nulled by the flow compensation methods. As a result, phase contrast MRA methods remain susceptible to signal loss caused by intravoxel dephasing when blood moving at a range of velocities is present in the same voxel. Accelerating blood also causes intravoxel dephasing, so phase contrast methods often exhibit signal loss where blood flows around a corner (centripetal acceleration) or in regions where pathology generates complex flow patterns.

The features of two- and three-dimensional phase contrast MRA methods are summarized in Tables 2-2 and 2-3, respectively, and the benefits and limitations of the two techniques are summarized in Tables 2-4 and 2-5.

Time-of-Flight Magnetic Resonance Imaging

Time-of-flight MRA techniques (17,18) differ from phase contrast techniques in that the former do not employ subtraction, so some signal from stationary tissues remains in the angiograms. In addition, time-of-flight techniques do not provide quantitative information regarding velocity or volume flow rate; thus, these methods are used primarily for assessing vascular anatomy.

TABLE 2-2

Summary of Two-dimensional Phase Contrast Magnetic Resonance Angiography

- A thick or thin slab may be imaged to demonstrate a single vessel or a group of vessels.
- A small tip angle (20 to 30 degrees) is used to reduce saturation of the blood signal.
- A short TR is used to reduce the scan time.
- The velocity-encoding value and the direction of flow sensitization both must be selected by the operator.
- Flow-encoding gradients are applied along the axis or axes of flow sensitization.
- If flow in all directions is to be evaluated, four acquisitions must be performed during a single scan.
- Scan time = $4 \times TR \times NSA \times \#PE$. (TR, repetition time; NSA, number of signal averages; #PE, number of phase-encoding values sampled.)
- A saturation pulse may be applied at the edge of the field-of-view to reduce venous signal, but complete elimination is difficult because the effect of the saturation pulse is diminished as the venous blood penetrates the image volume (see the section on time-of-flight MRA for more details).
- Cardiac gating can be used to reduce ghosting caused by cardiac pulsatility or to reveal flow information throughout the cardiac cycle.
- Data may be processed using complex difference processing to yield qualitative velocity information, or phase difference processing to yield quantitative velocity or volume flow rate information.

TABLE 2-3

Summary of Three-Dimensional Phase Contrast Magnetic Resonance Angiography

- A slab is imaged, and slices are encoded using a technique similar to that used for phase encoding.
- A small tip angle (20 to 30 degrees) is used to reduce the saturation of blood signal.
- A short TR is used to reduce the scan time.
- The velocity-encoding value and the direction of flow sensitization both must be selected by the operator.
- A flow-encoding gradient is applied along the axis or axes of flow sensitization.
- If flow in all directions is to be evaluated, four acquisitions must be performed.
- Scan time = $4 \times TR \times NSA \times \#PE \times \#SE$. May be quite long depending on the number of slices required to achieve adequate coverage. (TR, repetition time; NSA, number of signal averages; #PE, number of phase-encoding values sampled; #SE, number of slice-encoding values sampled.)
- A saturation pulse may be applied at the edge of the field-of-view to reduce venous signal, but complete elimination is difficult because the effect of the saturation pulse is diminished as the venous blood penetrates the image volume (see the section on time-of-flight MRA for more details).
- Data may be processed using complex difference processing to yield qualitative velocity information, or phase difference processing to yield quantitative velocity or volume flow rate information.

Time-of-flight techniques derive contrast between flowing blood and stationary tissues by manipulating the magnitude of the magnetization, such that it is large for moving blood and small for stationary tissues. This leads to a large signal from moving blood and a diminished signal from stationary tissues.

In MR, the signal from tissues decreases with exposure to an increasing number of radio frequency excitation pulses, until an equilibrium saturation value is reached. In time-of-flight imaging, the goal is to subject the flowing blood to at most a very few excitation pulses, and to subject stationary tissues to a large number of excitation pulses, thereby achieving a signal difference between blood and stationary tissues (Fig. 2-11).

This can be accomplished by imaging slices, or thin slabs, oriented perpendicular to the primary direction of flow. When this is done, the moving blood enters the slice fully magnetized, experiences only a few excitation pulses, and then flows out of the slice before it becomes saturated. This ensures that the signal from blood will be relatively large. The stationary tissues, however, remain in the slice, or slab, throughout image acquisition, so they give rise to a diminished signal because the magnetization from them is saturated due to the constant exposure to the excitation pulses.

The number of excitation pulses experienced by moving blood as it traverses the imaging slice depends on a number of factors including the thickness of the slice, the velocity of the blood, the orientation of the vessel relative to the image slice, and the TR of the imaging sequence. In general, thinner slices, faster-flowing blood, vessels oriented perpendicular to the slice, and a longer TR lead to increased vascular signal. A longer TR, however, also leads to increased signal from stationary tissues. Therefore, an intermediate TR must be selected with time-of-flight MRA.

Increasing the tip angle leads to diminished signal from stationary tissues but can also lead to increased saturation of blood that experiences multiple excitation pulses. As a result, an intermediate tip angle also must be selected. These factors and others must be carefully considered when constructing a time-of-flight protocol. Some important parameters and their effect on the signal from blood and stationary tissues are summarized in Table 2-6.

Time-of-flight methods can be implemented using 2D or 3D acquisition. For 2D acquisition (17), data are acquired from multiple slices stacked contiguously along the vessels of interest. Because the image quality is best if the slices remain perpendicular to the direction of flow, 2D time-of-flight

TABLE 2-4

Benefits and Limitations of Two-Dimensional Phase Contrast Magnetic Resonance Angiography

Benefits
- Scan time is short—good for localizing, enhancing different vessels by performing multiple scans with different Venc values, or implementing with cardiac gating to reduce pulsatility artifacts.
- Signal from stationary tissues is eliminated by subtraction, yielding excellent vascular contrast.
- Effects of saturation are minimized by using a small tip angle for imaging and eliminating the signal from stationary tissues via subtraction.
- When phase difference processing is performed, the direction of blood flow is represented in the images, and the velocity and volume flow rate can be calculated (throughout the cardiac cycle if cardiac gating is implemented).

Limitations
- Susceptible to signal loss caused by intravoxel dephasing due to the large voxel depth, the long echo time (TE), and the presence of the flow-encoding gradients.
- Signal loss may result due to phase cancellation of magnetization in overlapping vessels.
- Retrospective image reformatting and reprojection are not possible if only a single slice is imaged.
- Best choice of velocity-encoding value is sometimes unknown.
- Pulsatility causes severe ghosting artifacts if cardiac gating is not employed.
- Veins may appear in the angiogram because the effect of the venous saturation pulse is diminished as the venous blood penetrates the imaging slab.

TABLE 2-5

Benefits and Limitations of Three-Dimensional Phase Contrast Magnetic Resonance Angiography

Benefits
- The voxel size in the slice direction can be small, leading to good spatial resolution and decreased signal loss caused by intravoxel dephasing.
- The SNR is inherently high, being proportional to the square root of the number of slices imaged as a result of the acquisition strategy.
- Data may be retrospectively reformatted and reprojected to demonstrate vascular anatomy at arbitrary angles.
- Signal from stationary tissues is eliminated by subtraction, yielding excellent vascular contrast.
- Effects of saturation are minimized by using a small tip angle for imaging and eliminating the signal from stationary tissues via subtraction.
- When phase difference processing is performed, the direction of blood flow is represented in the images, and velocity and volume flow rate can be calculated.

Limitations
- May be susceptible to signal loss caused by intravoxel dephasing due to the long echo time (TE) and the presence of the flow-encoding gradients.
- Scan time is proportional to the number of slices imaged, so it may be quite long, especially when trying to image a large volume.
- Best choice of velocity-encoding value is sometimes unknown.
- Pulsatility may lead to ghosting artifacts, but less so than in two-dimensional phase contrast acquisitions, due to the averaging effect inherent in three-dimensional acquisitions.
- Veins may appear in the angiogram because the effect of the venous saturation pulse is diminished as the venous blood penetrates the imaging slab.

methods are best suited for imaging vessels that are straight, such as the carotid arteries, or the vessels in the lower extremities (Fig. 2-12). The data from the slices can be retrospectively reprojected or reformatted to demonstrate long segments of the vessels. With 3D acquisition, thin slices are imaged (1 to 3 mm) to increase the likelihood that the blood will experience only a very few radio frequency excitation pulses as it flows through the image slice (18). When thin slices are imaged, a moderately large tip angle (60 degrees) can be used to suppress the signal from the stationary tissues without substantially suppressing the signal from blood that quickly moves through the image plane. Even when the slices are thin, the moderately large tip angle can cause saturation of the signal from slow-moving blood, such as that in the carotid bulb (Fig. 2-13). The degree of saturation can be reduced by decreasing the tip angle and/or increasing the TR of the imaging sequence; however, it must be realized that this also will increase the amount of signal from stationary tissues.

With 2D time-of-flight MRA, a spatial saturation pulse (19–21) can be applied parallel to the image slice at the beginning of each TR to reduce or eliminate unwanted signal from blood flowing into the image slice from a particular direction. For example, applying a saturation pulse superior to an axial image slice is an effective means of eliminating signal from blood in the jugular veins. The signal from the blood in those veins is diminished or eliminated as the blood flows through the region affected by the saturation pulse. The venous blood, therefore, has little signal to give when it flows into the image slice. If blood in the jugular veins were left unsaturated, these vessels would interfere with observation of the carotid arteries (Fig. 2-14A). In this same example, if the saturation pulse is prescribed inferior to the image slice, this mechanism can be used to effectively eliminate the signal from the carotid arter-

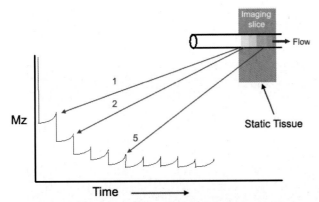

FIGURE 2-11 Schematic of flow-related enhancement. Maximum signal is available at the start of the excitation. With progressive exposure to repeated excitation pulses, the static tissue reaches a steady-state attenuated or saturated signal. However, the blood that emanates from outside the slice has no excitation history until it encounters the slice. As the blood traverses the slice, it may acquire the progressive excitation history of the background tissue and thus become saturated, rendering a decrease in its signal intensity. Thicker slices and slower velocity flow can accentuate this saturation effect.

ies (Fig. 2-14B). If a saturation pulse is not used to image the vessels in the neck, both the carotid arteries and the jugular veins appear in the image, often making interpretation difficult (Fig. 2-14C). An inferior saturation pulse can also be used to image the veins in the head (Fig. 2-15). In general, inferior saturation pulses are used to suppress the signal from arteries above the heart and veins below the heart, whereas superior saturation pulses are used to suppress the signal from veins above the heart and arteries below the heart.

The relatively long acquisition times associated with 2D time-of-flight MRA render the angiograms susceptible to effects of motion resulting from gross patient movement and, in the neck vessels, from swallowing. Because of the way the images are acquired and reprojected, motion during acquisition of one or just a few slices may affect signal in a small section of the vessel, causing a distortion that may mimic a stenosis (Fig. 2-16). Motion can be distinguished from a stenosis because the former typically affects the signal in the entire slice that was being acquired when the motion occurred. Each slice maps to a horizontal line in the reprojected image, so inspecting the information along the horizontal line that runs through the suspicious vascular abnormality can be helpful in identifying motion. Extreme patient motion can cause the vessel to appear to have a dramatically varying diameter similar to that resulting from fibromuscular dysplasia (FMD). Motion of the vessels caused by cardiac pulsatility may result in replication, or ghosting, of the vascular signal. This may be reduced or eliminated by using cardiac gating to synchronize data acquisition with the cardiac cycle. Motion caused by pulsatility may also cause the vessels to blur, which may lead to underestimation of the severity of stenosis.

Because of the large voxels and long echo times inherent to the 2D time-of-flight MRA methods, these techniques often suffer from signal loss in regions of complex flow caused by stenoses. Although these regions of signal loss prevent direct observation of pathology, they are strong indicators of disease. The obvious signal voids produced by complex flow in 2D time-of-flight MRA has led to an effective use of this technique as a screening method for carotid stenosis (22). The 2D time-of-flight screening scan can be immediately followed by a 3D time-of-flight or contrast-enhanced MRA scan to delineate the pathology.

For 3D time-of-flight acquisition (23,24), a slab oriented perpendicular to the vessels of interest is imaged and then encoded into thin slices using an encoding method similar to that used for phase encoding. Because a slab is imaged, a small tip angle (30 degrees) must be used so that the signal from blood remaining in the slab does not become too saturated. The small tip angle, necessary to preserve signal from blood, also leads to an undesirable preservation of some signal from stationary tissues. Therefore, when 3D acquisition is employed, other mechanisms must be implemented in order to reduce the signal from stationary tissues.

One mechanism employed to diminish signal from stationary tissues in 3D time-of-flight is magnetization transfer (25–27). With magnetization transfer, an off-resonance pulse

TABLE 2-6

Summary of Parameters Affecting Signal in Time-of-Flight Magnetic Resonance Imaging

Number of Radiofrequency Pulses Experienced	
Slice thickness	↓ slice thickness, ↓ saturation of blood signal
Blood velocity	↑ blood velocity, ↓ saturation of blood signal
Repetition time (TR)	↑ TR, ↓ saturation of blood and tissue signal
Vessel orientation	↓ in-plane flow, ↓ saturation of blood signal
Tip Angle	
	↑ tip angle, ↑ signal from through-plane blood
	↑ tip angle, ↑ saturation of signal from stationary tissues
	↓ tip angle, ↓ saturation of signal from in-plane blood
T1 of Blood/Stationary Tissues	
	↓ T_1, ↓ saturation of blood and tissue signal

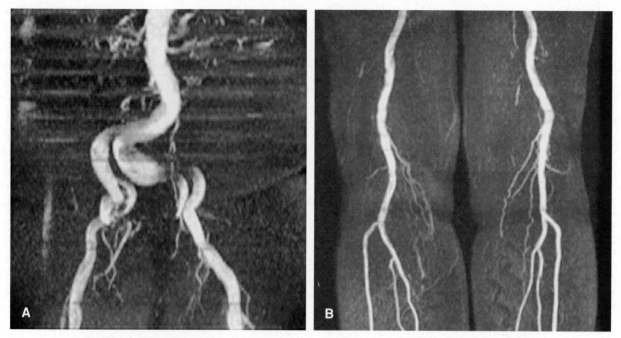

FIGURE 2-12 To produce these 2D time-of-flight angiograms of (A) the lower abdomen and upper legs, and (B) the lower legs, a stack of contiguous thin-section axial slices was imaged, from which these coronal maximum intensity projection images were produced. The images comprise a 3D data set from which projections at any obliquity can retrospectively be constructed. Note the loss of signal uniformity in the tortuous iliac arteries, portions of which course in the plane of acquisition.

is applied at the start of each TR to saturate the magnetization from restricted water molecules. Signal from these molecules does not appear in MR images because the T$_2$ of the signal from them is too short. When the magnetization from these restricted molecules becomes saturated, nearby free water molecules can transfer their magnetization to the restricted molecules, leading to a diminished signal from free water in

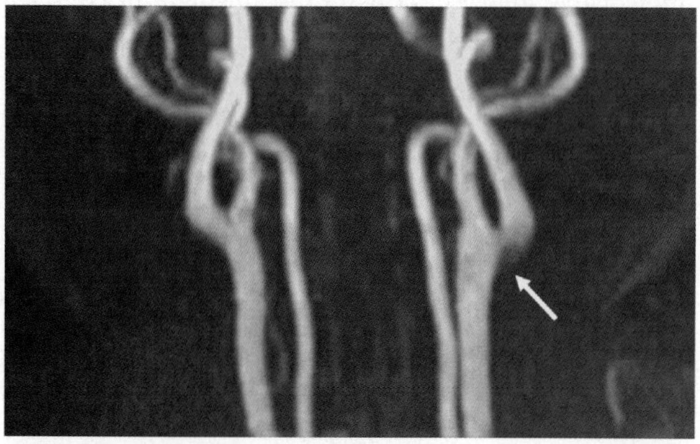

FIGURE 2-13 Relatively large tip angles (60 degrees) and relatively short TR values are used in 2D time-of-flight methods to reduce the signal from stationary tissues. These same parameters diminish the signal from blood that remains in the axial imaging planes for more than a few TR intervals. Signal loss in the carotid bulb due to the slow-flowing blood in these regions is demonstrated here (*arrow*).

tissues that contain restricted molecules. Gray and white brain matter contain restricted molecules, whereas blood does not.

Thus, when applied to cerebral MR angiography, magnetization transfer can be used to diminish the signal from the brain, while leaving the signal from blood virtually unaffected. The resulting increased vessel to background contrast improves the angiograms generated from 3D time-of-flight acquisitions. Because the magnetization transfer pulse is applied in each TR interval, selecting this feature requires that the TR be increased, resulting in a longer scan time. Applying a magnetization transfer radio frequency pulse during each TR also leads to an increase in the deposited energy.

The contrast in 3D time-of-flight angiograms can be further improved by choosing an echo time that leads to the magnetization from fat being 180 degrees out of phase with the magnetization from water at a critical time during signal detection so that their respective signals destructively interfere with each other. Fat and water precess, or rotate, at different rates, so at certain times, the magnetization from them is oriented in opposite directions. At a magnetic field strength of 1.5T, the magnetization from fat is oriented in a direction opposite that of water at echo times of approximately 2.3 m/sec and 6.9 m/sec. Choosing these echo times is an effective means of suppressing signal from tissues that contain both fat and water, leading to an increase in the conspicuity of the signal from blood.

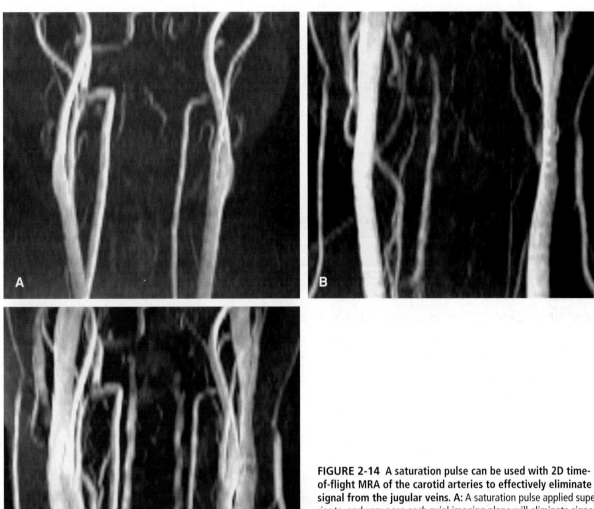

FIGURE 2-14 **A saturation pulse can be used with 2D time-of-flight MRA of the carotid arteries to effectively eliminate signal from the jugular veins. A:** A saturation pulse applied superior to, and very near, each axial imaging plane will eliminate signal from blood in the jugular veins that will flow into each image slice. **B:** A saturation pulse applied inferior to, and very near, each axial imaging plane will eliminate signal from blood in the carotid arteries that will flow into each imaging plane, resulting in production of a venogram. **C:** When no saturation pulse is applied, both arteries and veins appear in the image, making interpretation difficult.

Another mechanism used to achieve higher contrast between flowing blood and stationary tissues in 3D time-of-flight MRA is the use of a ramped tip angle (28). A ramped tip angle is used to diminish the reduction of blood signal as the vessels penetrate farther into the slab. The tip angle is ramped such that a small tip angle is applied where the vessels of interest enter the slab, and a large tip angle is applied where the vessels of interest exit the slab. The tip angle varies linearly between these points. The small tip angle at the entrance of the slab prevents the blood from becoming too saturated as it traverses the slab. The large tip angle at the exit of the slab tips a large component of the magnetization from the almost fully saturated blood into the transverse plane to be sampled just before the blood leaves the slab, providing a larger signal than would be achieved if a small tip angle were used. The large tip angle further saturates the signal from blood, but this is inconsequential, since this blood is exiting the slab and will not be sampled again. The ramped tip angle provides a more uniform signal along the vessels as they traverse the slab, provided they follow a fairly direct path through the slab. A drawback of this imaging feature is that it may cause the signals in vessels that run parallel to the edge of the slab in the region of the large tip angle to become more saturated than they would if a constant tip angle were applied.

Another feature that is used to enhance image quality in 3D time-of-flight MRA is *zero filling* (29,30). This feature, also referred to as *zero interpolation processing* (ZIP), is a reconstruction option that may be used to improve the apparent resolution of images in the phase- and frequency-encoding directions, and, with 3D methods, in the slice

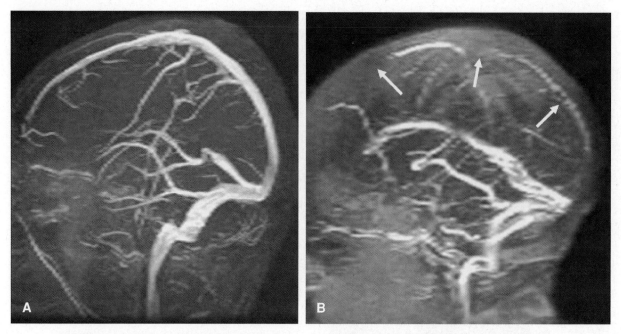

FIGURE 2-15 Intracranial venograms can be produced by acquiring axial or coronal 2D time-of-flight images with a saturation pulse applied at the inferior aspect of each image slice (for axial acquisitions) or FOV (for coronal acquisitions) to eliminate signal from the arteries. The images shown here demonstrate sagittal reprojections of coronal images acquired from **(A)** a healthy adult and **(B)** a child with partial thrombosis of the sagittal sinus (*arrows*).

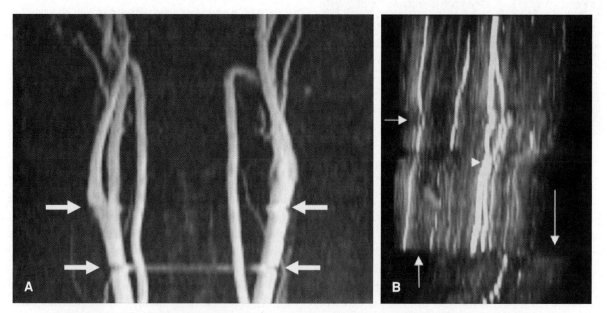

FIGURE 2-16 Effects of motion on TOF MRA. A: A coronal image of the carotid arteries demonstrating that motion of vessels due to gross patient movement or swallowing during 2D time-of-flight imaging results in distortion that may mimic the appearance of a stenosis. In this image, motion can be identified at the locations marked by the *arrows*. Motion affects the signal at multiple points along the horizontal lines indicated by the *arrows*. The motion that occurred during acquisition of the slice identified by the lower pair of *arrows* was in the superior–inferior direction, permitting unsaturated stationary tissues to move into the slice to give rise to a large signal between the vessels. **B:** TOF MRA in the tibial segment of a lower extremity evaluation showing subtle motion (*horizontal arrow*), stair-step artifact (*horizontal arrowhead*), and substantial movement with translation of the leg (*vertical arrows*), the latter rendering the vascular anatomy artifactually discontinuous.

direction as well. Because zero filling is applied during reconstruction, it does not affect the scan time. It does, however, increase the reconstruction time. When this option is selected, zeroes are applied to the edges of data space prior to reconstruction. When zero filling is used in the frequency- or phase-encoding directions, interpolated pixels are inserted between the original pixels. The original pixels are unmodified. The interpolation is nonlinear, meaning that the interpolated values can be greater or less than the average value of the adjacent (original) pixel values. The result is that zero filling makes vessels appear smoother by reducing the stair-step effect (Fig. 2-17A–B) and better representing the data that were acquired. When zero filling is applied in the slice-encoding direction for 3D applications, the original slices remain the same, but interpolated slices are inserted between each pair of adjacent original slices. This results in smoother-appearing vessels in the reformatted and reprojected images (Fig. 2-17C–D).

An awareness of this strategy is essential for resolution considerations. For example, consider a 100-mm slab that is partitioned into 50 slices through traditional slice phase encoding. The true resolution is 100 mm/50 or 2 mm for each slice. In this case, by using an interpolation factor of 2 in the slice dimension, the data would be reconstructed as 2 mm every 1 mm, providing overlap of the slices, hence, the smoother appearance of the maximum intensity projections (MIP). However, some manufacturers report the post-interpolation result, which should not be confused with the true resolution. In the previous example, the slice would be misleadingly reported as 1 mm, whereas the true resolution is 2 mm. A knowledge of the method for reporting resolution is important when creating or modifying protocols or when evaluating results reported in the literature.

Three-dimensional time-of-flight methods are well suited for imaging the intracranial vessels due to the small voxels, short echo times, and inherently high signal-to-

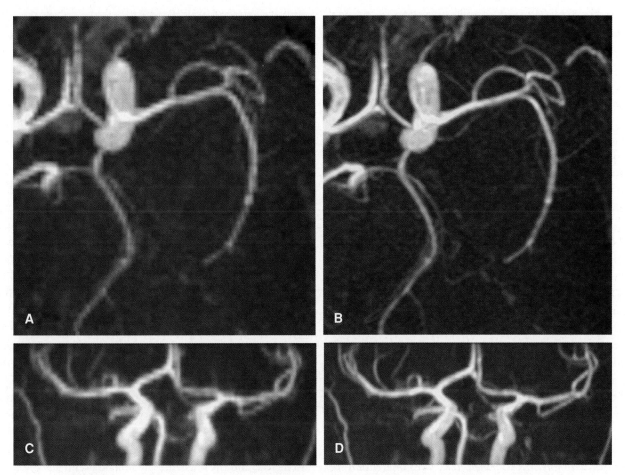

FIGURE 2-17 MIP images produced from 3D time-of-flight image sets. A: Axial MIP with no zero filling. **B:** Axial MIP with zero filling in the phase- and frequency-encoding directions. **C:** Coronal MIP reconstructed with no zero filling. **D:** Coronal MIP reconstructed with zero filling in the slice-encoding (top to bottom) direction. The data used to produce parts A and C is 256 × 256 × 32. The same data set was zero filled to 512 × 512 × 64 to produce the images in figure parts B and D.

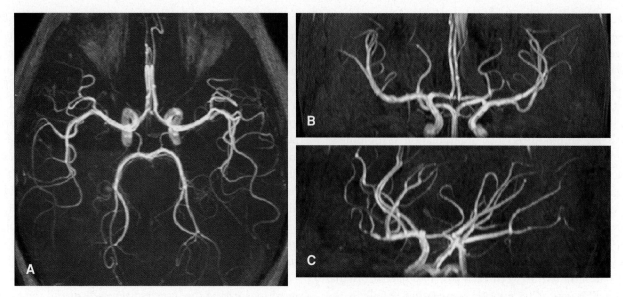

FIGURE 2-18 Shown are (**A**) axial, (**B**) coronal, and (**C**) sagittal reprojections produced from axial images of the intracranial vessels of a healthy adult acquired using a 3D time-of-flight MRA technique.

noise ratios provided by these techniques. The small voxels result in good spatial resolution, and together with the short TEs, they lead to a reduction in the amount of signal loss caused by intravoxel dephasing. The imaging features described earlier can be used collectively with 3D time-of-flight MRA to improve the contrast between the intracranial vessels and the surrounding brain tissue and fat. Images of the intracranial vessels acquired with a 3D time-of-flight imaging sequence are shown in Figure 2-18. Intracranial vascular diseases such as AVMs, aneurysms, and occlusions commonly are evaluated using 3D time-of-flight MRA.

Even with the small voxels and short TEs provided by 3D time-of-flight MRA, these methods are not impervious to signal loss caused by intravoxel dephasing of magnetization. Some types of aneurysm clips and other implanted metal devices can have dramatic effects on the vascular signal, no matter what MRA method is used. The extent of the signal loss is dependent on a number of factors, including the degree to which the metallic device perturbs the magnetic field as well as the velocity of the blood traveling through the affected region. If the extent of the perturbation is large, or if the blood moves a great distance after having its magnetization diminished by passing through the affected region, the extent of the signal loss may be great. *In order to avoid misdiagnosis due to questionable signal in angiograms acquired with any MRA method, the source images and the nonvascular MR images should be inspected for signs of metallic implants that may cause signal loss.*

Even using the imaging features mentioned, contrast between blood and stationary tissues can be small in 3D time-of-flight MRA when thick slabs are used to achieve extended coverage. To achieve greater coverage with reduced saturation effects, 3D time-of-flight data can be acquired from multiple thin slabs (18,31) arranged perpendicular to the vessels of interest in a method called *multiple overlapping thin slab angiography* (MOTSA). The multislab method combines the thin-slice benefits of 2D acquisition (reduced saturation) with the benefits of 3D acquisition (including an inherently high SNR, small voxels, and a short TE) in an effort to provide high-quality images as shown in Figure 2-19.

Even with multiple thin slabs, the signal from slow-flowing blood can become saturated as the blood traverses the slab. This saturation effect causes signal reduction at the distal edge of each slab, and is referred to as the *slab boundary artifact*, or the *venetian blind artifact* (Fig. 2-20A). If this artifact occurs in the slow-flow region of the carotid bulb, it can mimic or mask a stenosis (Fig. 2-20B).

With 3D time-of-flight MRA, a spatial saturation pulse can be applied just outside the slab at the beginning of each TR to eliminate signal from blood that will flow into the imaging slab, as described previously for 2D time-of-flight imaging. With 3D time-of-flight MRA, the saturation pulse is not as effective as with 2D time-of-flight MRA. This is because as the blood that was initially saturated traverses the slab, the longitudinal magnetization from this blood begins to regrow, and the once-saturated blood eventually gives rise to signal. In general, the farther the once-saturated blood penetrates into the slab, the less effective the saturation of the signal because of the increasing amount of time that elapses between saturation and signal detection.

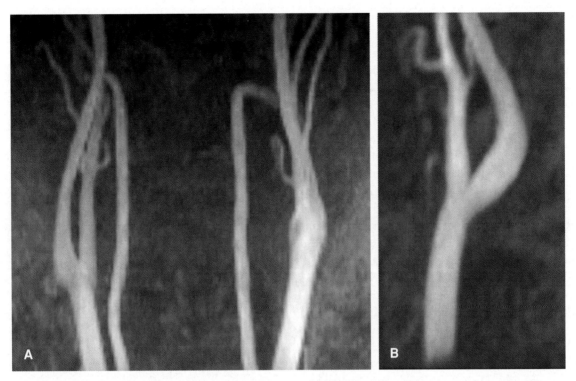

FIGURE 2-19 **MOTSA acquired with a ramped tip angle is widely used for imaging the carotid arteries.** The image in (**A**) shows a coronal projection of the carotid and vertebral arteries, and the image in (**B**) shows a magnified and cropped oblique projection of a single carotid bifurcation.

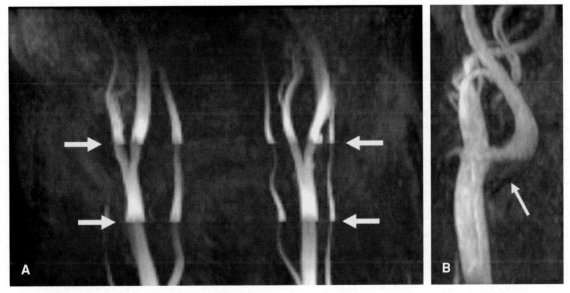

FIGURE 2-20 **A:** A coronal reprojection of the carotid and vertebral arteries produced from axial images acquired using a 3D time-of-flight MOTSA method. This image demonstrates the venetian blind, or slab boundary, artifact that can result when slow-flowing blood at the distal edge of each image slab becomes saturated. This artifact can be reduced by ramping the tip angle, decreasing the tip angle, increasing the TR, or overlapping the slabs by a greater number of slices. **B:** If two slabs of a 3D time-of-flight technique overlap at the carotid bifurcation, the slow-flowing blood in the carotid bulb may become saturated at the distal end of the more inferior slab. The signal loss due to saturation may mimic or mask a stenosis. This effect may sometimes be identified by a straight edge where the saturated signal at the distal edge of the inferior slab meets the strong signal at the proximal edge of the more superior slab. This effect can be avoided by taking care not to place a slab boundary near the carotid bulb.

As demonstrated in this section, both 2D and 3D time-of-flight methods are applicable to imaging the intracranial arteries and veins, and the extracranial carotid and vertebral arteries. Two-dimensional time-of-flight MRA is well suited for imaging the arteries in the neck and lower extremities because these regions contain arteries that are relatively straight and veins that carry blood in an antiparallel direction, which can be well suppressed using a saturation pulse. The use of 2D time-of-flight has also been effective for the peripheral run-off vessels of the lower extremities, particularly for slow flow, distal pedal vessels.

A drawback of 2D time-of-flight is that, due to SNR considerations and the slice-selection process, the imaged slices must be relatively thick (1 to 3 mm) compared with those imaged with 3D time-of-flight MRA. Using thicker slices leads to poorer spatial resolution in the slice direction and results in large voxels that are susceptible to intravoxel dephasing. The effective resolution can be improved by overlapping the slices; however, this does not reduce the size of the voxels. The large voxels and long TEs associated with 2D time-of-flight cause this method to be severely affected by intravoxel dephasing (signal loss) near pathologies that produce complex flow patterns. This sensitivity to complex flow, which manifests as potentially large signal voids, has led to the use of 2D time-of-flight as a screening tool to draw attention to tight stenoses in vessels.

When it is desirable to obtain an accurate depiction of pathology, especially in the carotid arteries (to facilitate quantitative grading of a stenosis, for example), multislab 3D time-of-flight MRA is used. The multislab method, with its high resolution, high SNR, and many contrast-improving features, is also used to assess the intracranial vessels. If the vessels in a small region are being imaged, such as those composing the circle of Willis, the single-slab 3D time-of-flight method is used. If a larger region is being imaged, it is more advantageous to use the multislab technique. The features of 2D and 3D time-of-flight MRA methods are summarized in Tables 2-7 and 2-8, respectively, and the benefits and limitations of the two techniques are summarized in Tables 2-9 and 2-10.

Contrast-enhanced Magnetic Resonance Angiography

Contrast-enhanced MRA techniques are the most recently developed MRA methods (32). They are probably the easiest to understand of the three classes of MRA techniques, and when implemented properly, they provide diagnostic-quality images under very diverse conditions.

TABLE 2-7

Summary of Two-Dimensional Time-of-Flight Magnetic Resonance Imaging

- Thin slices (1.5 to 3.0 mm), oriented perpendicular to the direction of flow, are imaged.
- An intermediate tip angle (45 to 60 degrees) is used so that it is large enough to suppress signal from stationary tissues, but not so large that it suppresses signal from blood that remains in the image plane for an extended amount of time.
- An intermediate TR (30 to 50 m/sec) is used so that it is short enough to suppress signal from stationary tissues, but not so short that it suppresses signal from blood that remains in the image plane for an extended amount of time.
- A saturation pulse that is parallel to and near the image slice may be used to effectively suppress unwanted signal from blood that will flow into the image plane after it is saturated.
- Scan time = TR × NSA × #PE × #slices. (TR, repetition time; NSA, number of signal averages; #PE, number of phase-encoding values; #slices, number of slices imaged to cover the length of the vessels.)
- Cardiac gating may be used to reduce pulsatility artifacts.

TABLE 2-8

Summary of Three-Dimensional Time-of-Flight Magnetic Resonance Imaging

- A slab, oriented perpendicular to the direction of flow, is imaged.
- Multiple, overlapping slabs may be prescribed to prevent saturation when imaging extended coverage.
- A small tip angle (20 to 30 degrees) is used to prevent saturation of blood as it traverses the slab, leading to a less saturated, or brighter, signal from stationary tissues.
- A ramped tip angle may be used to make the vascular signal more uniform throughout the slab or slabs.
- Several image-enhancing features may be used to reduce the signal from stationary tissues, such as magnetization transfer and/or the selection of an echo time that leads to destructive interference of the signals from fat and water.
- A saturation pulse may be applied at the edge of the field of view or the edge of each slab to reduce venous signal, but complete elimination is difficult because the effect of the saturation pulse is diminished as the venous blood penetrates farther into the image slab.
- Scan time = TR × NSA × #PE × #SE × #slabs. (TR, repetition time; NSA, number of signal averages; #PE, number of phase-encoding values; #SE, number of slice-encoding values (slices) per slab; #slabs, number of slabs imaged to cover the length of the vessels.)

TABLE 2-9

Benefits and Limitations of Two-Dimensional Time-of-Flight Magnetic Resonance Imaging

Benefits
- Inflow results in good contrast and uniform signal along the length of the vessels.
- Effective venous suppression may be achieved by using a saturation pulse that stays near and parallel to the image slice.
- Data may be retrospectively reformatted and reprojected to demonstrate vascular anatomy at arbitrary angles.
- May be used effectively as a screening method due to its sensitivity to, and resulting signal loss from, intravoxel dephasing caused by complex flow in regions of pathology.

Limitations
- Scan time may be long depending on the number of slices required to achieve adequate coverage of the vessels of interest.
- The voxel size in the slice direction may be large, leading to poor resolution in the reprojected images and increased signal loss caused by intravoxel dephasing.
- Blood that remains in the image plane due to slow flow or vessel orientation may become saturated.
- Pulsatility and motion can significantly compromise image quality.
- Tissues with short T1 values are not well suppressed.

TABLE 2-10

Benefits and Limitations of Three-Dimensional Time-of-Flight Magnetic Resonance Imaging

Benefits
- The voxel size in the slice direction can be small due to the encoding method used, leading to good spatial resolution in the reprojected images and decreased signal loss caused by intravoxel dephasing.
- The SNR is inherently high due to the characteristics of the 3D acquisition strategy.
- Data may be retrospectively reformatted and reprojected to demonstrate vascular anatomy at arbitrary angles.
- The TE may be made short due to the acquisition strategy, leading to reduced signal loss caused by intravoxel dephasing.

Limitations
- The scan time may be long depending on the number of slices and slabs required to achieve adequate coverage.
- Signal from blood that remains in the imaging slab due to slow flow or vessel orientation may become diminished at the distal regions of the slabs due to saturation. This may lead to slab boundary, or venetian blind, artifacts in the multislab technique.
- Signals from stationary tissues are not well suppressed, especially from those tissues having short T1 values.
- Effective venous suppression may be difficult.

In addition, they suffer from fewer artifacts than phase contrast and time-of-flight MRA techniques. For these and other reasons, contrast-enhanced MRA has quickly gained widespread clinical acceptance and in some institutions has replaced conventional x-ray angiography as the standard method for assessing certain pathologies in various vascular territories.

Contrast-enhanced MRA techniques achieve signal differences between blood and stationary tissues by manipulating the magnitude of the magnetization, such that the magnitude of the magnetization from moving blood is larger than the magnitude of the magnetization from stationary tissues. Manipulating the magnetization to produce signal differences in contrast-enhanced MRA techniques is achieved not only by employing the appropriate sequence parameters (as is the case in time-of-flight techniques), but also by injecting a contrast material intravenously to selectively shorten the T_1 of the blood. By implementing a T_1-weighted imaging sequence during the first pass of the contrast material, images can be acquired that show arteries with striking contrast relative to surrounding stationary tissues and veins (Fig. 2-21).

In order to acquire the majority of the data for the contrast-enhanced angiogram during the first pass of the contrast material (*when the concentration of the contrast material in the arteries is high, and the concentration in the veins and stationary tissues is low*), it is desirable to scan rapidly. To this end, a short TR is used, and a reduced data set is sampled. The TR may be reduced by using a high receiver bandwidth, a fractional echo, and, if available, a scanner with fast gradients. A reduction in the data set may be achieved by employing a fractional field-of-view, a reduced number of phase-encoding values, and a reduced number of slices. To ameliorate the sacrifice in spatial resolution that inevitably results when using a reduced number of phase- and slice-encoding values, the *apparent* spatial resolution both in the plane of the images and in the slice direction (for the reprojected and reformatted images) can be increased by using zero filling as previously described.

Contrast-enhanced methods have been used successfully to image vessels throughout the body, including the carotid and vertebral arteries, the aortic arch and great vessels, the renal and abdominal arteries, and the arteries of the upper and lower extremities. Although less common, veins are also imaged using these methods. Contrast-enhanced methods have been used to image the intracranial arteries (33), but this application has not gained widespread use, mainly because noncontrast-enhanced 3D time-of-flight methods currently provide consistently high-quality images

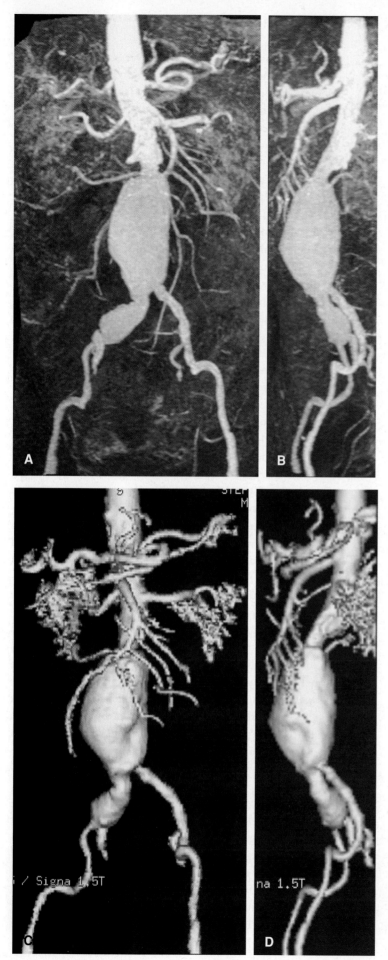

FIGURE 2-21 Shown are **(A)** coronal and **(B)** sagittal MIP images of an abdominal aortic aneurysm acquired using a 3D contrast-enhanced MRA method. The signal difference between the arteries and the surrounding tissues is so great that the signals from stationary tissues can be removed from the data set simply by retaining only signal intensities above a specified threshold value. The remaining bright signals can be used to make volume-rendered images of the vessels, which can demonstrate **(C)** coronal and **(D)** sagittal views of the data used to produce the MIP images in **(A)** and **(B)**.

of these vessels. Also, the presence of the blood–brain barrier and the short transit time from arteries to veins leads to very rapid and intense venous enhancement, leaving little time available for acquisition of a contrast-enhanced intracranial MR angiogram.

Currently, the contrast materials most widely used in MRA are extracellularly distributed gadolinium chelates (Chapter 5). The gadolinium atom has seven unpaired electrons that interact with the hydrogen nuclei on the water molecules (recall that it is these nuclei imaged with MRI). The interaction results in an increased regrowth rate of longitudinal magnetization from these hydrogen nuclei (reduced T_1), so they appear bright in images acquired with T_1-weighted MR acquisition methods.

The gadolinium-based contrast material is typically injected intravenously through an 18- to 22-gauge angiocatheter. The angiocatheter is typically inserted into a large, easily accessible vein, such as one of the veins in the antecubital fossa. However, other injection sites may be selected as well, including the forearm, wrist, or even the back of the hand. Injection into the right arm provides the most direct route to the heart, increasing the likelihood of distributing a tight, highly concentrated bolus of contrast material to the vessels of interest. The size of the angiocatheter selected is dependent on the size of the vessel being injected and the injection rate. Injection rates typically range from 0.5 to 4.0 mL/sec. Injection volumes range from 0.1 to 0.3 millimoles of contrast material per kg of body weight (mmol/kg), with typical values in the range of 20 to 40 mL of contrast material.

Higher volumes usually provide images with higher SNR in which the small vessel detail can be better delineated (Fig. 2-22). Studies are underway to determine the minimum dose necessary to provide diagnostic information. The injection of the contrast material is immediately followed by a flush of normal saline. The injection may be performed manually or by using an MR-compatible, computer-controlled injector. With a computer-controlled injector, the volume and injection rate are precisely programmed to ensure reproducible results. With manual injection, the clinician can better monitor the status of the patient and can more easily detect a misadministration.

Contrast-enhanced imaging methods are less sensitive than phase contrast and time-of-flight MRA methods to artifacts caused by intravoxel dephasing, signal saturation, pulsatility, and motion. The short echo time achievable with contrast-enhanced imaging methods limits the amount of time available for intravoxel dephasing, which leads to less signal loss. The dramatic reduction of the T_1 of blood caused by the intravenous injection of the T_1-shortening contrast material results in rapid regrowth of the

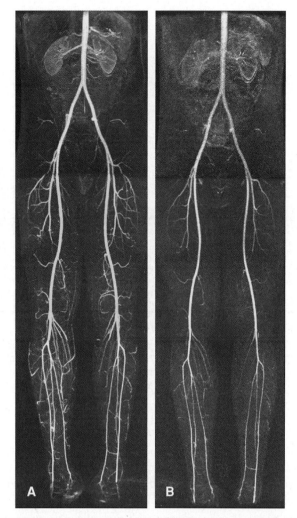

FIGURE 2-22 Images of the blood vessels of the legs of a healthy volunteer acquired using a 3D contrast-enhanced MRA method. The volume of contrast material injected to obtain the images shown in **(A)** was 35 mL (0.22 mmol/kg body weight) and to obtain the images shown in **(B)** was 15 mL (0.09 mmol/kg body weight). Each injection was administered over a 40-second period.

longitudinal magnetization of blood. This limits the amount of signal saturation, even when using a short TR, a large tip angle, and a large image volume.

The 3D acquisition strategy, in effect, averages the signals that are acquired throughout the entire scan, which leads to a reduction of the signal ghosts typically caused by pulsatility of blood and patient motion. Furthermore, the short scan times used with 3D contrast-enhanced MRA methods restricts the amount of motion that occurs during a scan, thus further limiting the appearance of motion-related artifacts in the angiograms. Additionally, the short imaging time allows collection of an entire data set during a single breath-hold interval, permitting acquisition of high-quality angiograms even in areas affected by respiratory motion.

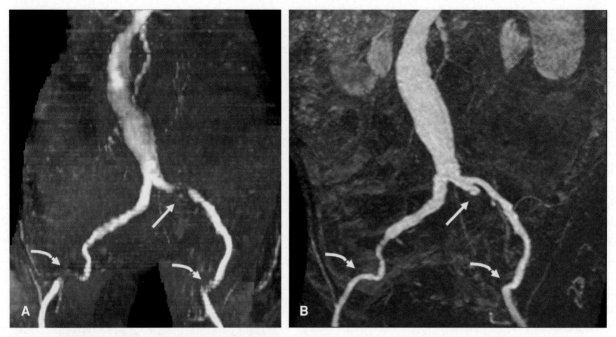

FIGURE 2-23 Images of the abdominal aorta and iliac and femoral arteries acquired from the same patient using **(A)** a 2D time-of-flight MRA method and **(B)** a 3D contrast-enhanced MRA method. The 3D contrast-enhanced method is less sensitive to saturation of in-plane flow (*curved arrows*) and slow or complex flow caused by pathology (*straight arrow*). The slow flow in the abdominal aortic aneurysm is also better demonstrated in the 3D contrast-enhanced method.

Owing to the reduced sensitivity of contrast-enhanced methods to artifacts caused by intravoxel dephasing, signal saturation, pulsatility, and motion, these methods offer improved image quality over 2D and 3D time-of-flight methods, as demonstrated in the images shown in Figures 2-23 and 2-24. As compared with time-of-flight strategies, contrast-enhanced techniques offer better delineation of pathologies with complex flow patterns (tight or irregular stenoses), a better rendition of tortuous vessels as well as those that remain in the acquisition plane, and improved acquisition time efficiency by virtue of the ability to scan parallel to vessels of interest. In addition, the time gained by use of efficient methods when acquiring data in the sagittal or coronal planes offers an opportunity to reinvest in better spatial resolution in the long axis of the main vessels of interest, in turn providing better delineation of the vascular detail (Fig. 2-25). Small tortuous vessels containing slow flow also are well demonstrated with contrast-enhanced methods. Although observation of these small vessels usually is not always necessary for diagnostic purposes, it increases the confidence of the observer in assessing other vessels in the image. The large coverage and excellent delineation of vessels offered by contrast-enhanced methods often permits them to provide information similar to that obtained using digital subtraction angiography (34).

In order to ensure the best possible image quality with contrast-enhanced vascular imaging methods, it is essential to properly synchronize data acquisition with the arrival and passage of the contrast material (Fig. 2-26). If acquisition is completed before the arrival of the contrast material, the blood will not generate enough signal to appear in the angiogram. If the contrast material arrives during the scan—after data acquisition has begun, but before it is completed—the SNR of the arteries may be low, or artifacts may be present in the images (35). The artifacts may manifest as a less intense area in the center of the vessels, ringing or replication of the vessel edges, or demonstration of only the edges of the vessels. The appearance of the artifacts depends on the size of the vessels affected, at what time during the acquisition the contrast material arrives in the vessels being imaged, the order in which the data are acquired, and the rate at which the concentration of the contrast material changes during the scan. If the data are acquired too late, the arterial signal will be diminished, and the veins and stationary tissues will be enhanced.

Several methods have been developed to ensure proper timing of the acquisition relative to the passage of the contrast material. In one method, a small test bolus of contrast material is injected, and then 2D images are rapidly and repeatedly acquired (36). From these images, the arrival time of the contrast material can be determined and used to calculate when to start the acquisition of the 3D angiogram after injecting the full bolus. In other methods, the signal in a volume (37) or an image (38,39) is moni-

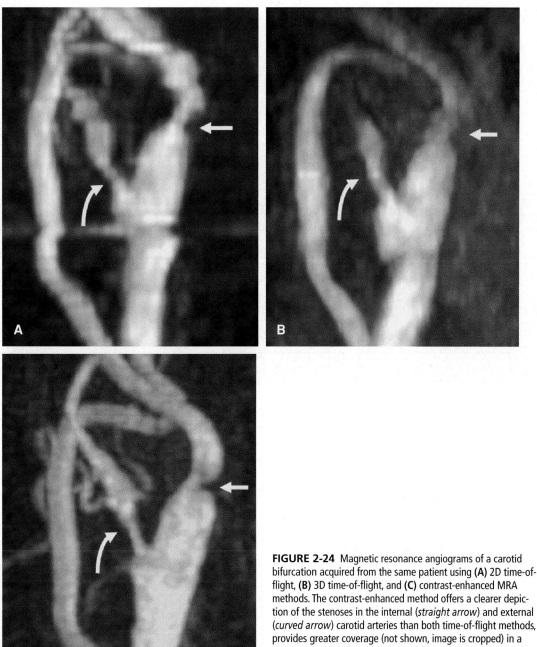

FIGURE 2-24 Magnetic resonance angiograms of a carotid bifurcation acquired from the same patient using **(A)** 2D time-of-flight, **(B)** 3D time-of-flight, and **(C)** contrast-enhanced MRA methods. The contrast-enhanced method offers a clearer depiction of the stenoses in the internal (*straight arrow*) and external (*curved arrow*) carotid arteries than both time-of-flight methods, provides greater coverage (not shown, image is cropped) in a shorter scan time than both time-of-flight methods, is less susceptible to motion than 2D time-of-flight **(A)**, is less sensitive to saturation than 3D time-of-flight **(B)**, and better demonstrates small vessels than either of the time-of-flight methods.

tored, and acquisition of the angiogram begins when it has been determined that the contrast has arrived. Finally, time-resolved methods have been developed that repeatedly acquire 2D (40,41) or 3D (42,43) angiograms continuously during the passage of the contrast material (Fig. 2-27), obviating the need to prospectively determine when the contrast has arrived. In addition to demonstrating the peak arterial frame, time-resolved methods provide some infor-

mation regarding hemodynamics and can provide separate images of both early and late-filling vessels. The dynamic signal intensity changes of the background soft tissue may also provide insights into the disease process, though, at the time of this writing, this feature has not been rigorously evaluated.

A current challenge of contrast-enhanced MR angiography is obtaining high spatial resolution in the

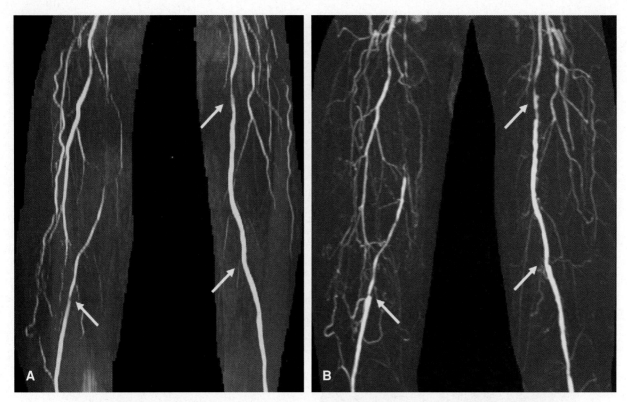

FIGURE 2-25 Images of the vessels in the thighs of a patient acquired using **(A)** a 2D time-of-flight MRA method and **(B)** a 3D contrast-enhanced MRA method. The 3D contrast-enhanced MRA method provides higher spatial resolution, permitting better delineation of the vessels. In this patient, the higher spatial resolution allows a more thorough assessment of the diffuse disease (*arrows*).

short amount of time available between arterial and venous enhancement. To address this issue, a method has been developed in which the data acquisition order is modified to acquire the low spatial frequency data early, during enhancement of the arteries, and the high spatial frequency data later, even after enhancement of the veins and stationary tissues.

This data acquisition order is referred to as *true centric*, or *elliptical centric*, *phase-encoding order* (38). It allows the acquisition time to be extended to increase the spatial resolution of the images without incurring substantial interference from enhancing veins and stationary tissues. In images, low spatial frequencies demonstrate the bulk of the contrast information, whereas high spatial frequencies demonstrate the detail information.

Acquiring the low spatial frequency information (the contrast information) early in the scan, when only the arterial blood is enhanced, minimizes the amount of signal from veins and stationary tissues in the angiogram. If the contrast material reaches the veins and stationary tissues late in the scan, when the high spatial frequencies (the detail information) are being acquired, only the edges of these structures will appear in the images. This

edge information from the veins and stationary tissues usually does not significantly interfere with observation of the arteries.

The signal difference between vessels and stationary tissues can be increased in contrast-enhanced MRA methods by acquiring a precontrast mask image set and subtracting it from the postcontrast image set to produce a subtraction angiogram (Fig. 2-28). This is analogous to digital subtraction angiography in that the signal from stationary tissues (which remains constant between acquisitions) is eliminated by the subtraction, whereas the vascular signal (which is increased after the injection of the contrast material) persists after the subtraction. Disadvantages of subtraction are that it reduces the signal-to-noise ratio of the angiogram (because noise from two images, but signal from only one image, contributes to the angiogram), and it renders the angiograms susceptible to misregistration artifacts that result from motion. For these reasons, mechanisms such as fat saturation are being investigated as alternative means of suppressing the signal from stationary tissues.

Imaging more than one vascular territory, or station, during a single exam session presents challenges for

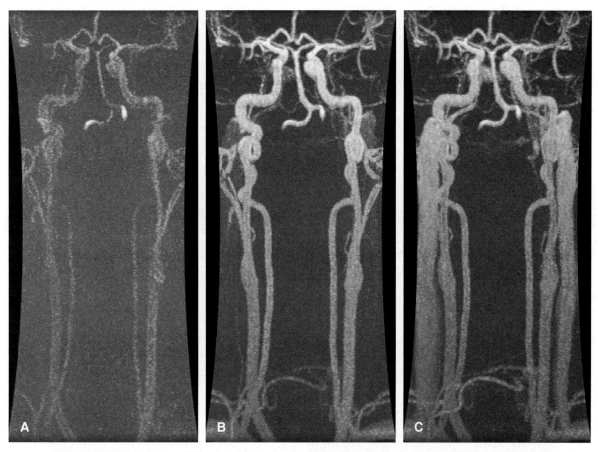

FIGURE 2-26 Three images of the carotid arteries acquired using a contrast-enhanced MRA method. The images demonstrate the effect of acquiring the data **(A)** too early, **(B)** at the appropriate time, and **(C)** too late relative to the passage of the contrast material. When the scan is started too early as in **(A)**, the images suffer from poor SNR and can suffer from other artifacts as described in the text. When the scan is started too late as in **(C)**, veins appear in the image, making it difficult to clearly observe the arteries.

contrast-enhanced MRA methods. Two approaches are currently in use for performing multistation contrast-enhanced MRA. In one approach, a separate injection of contrast material is administered just prior to scanning each territory (44). There are benefits in this multi-injection approach, but the image quality can be adversely affected in two ways. First, the volume of contrast material available for each injection is only a fraction of the maximum allowed because the volume must be split into multiple injections. The reduced volume leads to lower SNR in the angiograms. Second, residual contrast material remaining from the early injections enhances arteries in the mask acquisitions for the later injections. Because the arteries are slightly enhanced in the mask images, subtraction of the mask images leads to a signal reduction in the arteries in the subtracted angiogram. If the mask images from all stations were acquired before the first injection, they could not be used to eliminate venous enhancement in the later images caused by residual contrast material remaining from the ear-

lier injections. One benefit of a multi-injection method over a single-injection method is that more time can be spent imaging each station to achieve high spatial resolution and extended coverage. This is possible because the scan times do not need to be limited in order to chase the bolus of contrast material.

In a second approach utilized for multistation contrast-enhanced MRA, multiple territories are imaged after administration of a single injection of contrast material (45–47). After the administration of the contrast material is initiated in this single-injection approach, an image set is rapidly acquired from the first station, then the table is moved to bring the second station into the sensitive region of the MR scanner, and a scan is performed to image the second station. This table movement and data acquisition cycle is continued until all of the stations are imaged. With this method, it is necessary to scan quickly in order to image all the stations when the arterial signal is enhanced and before the veins and stationary tissues enhance. Scanning

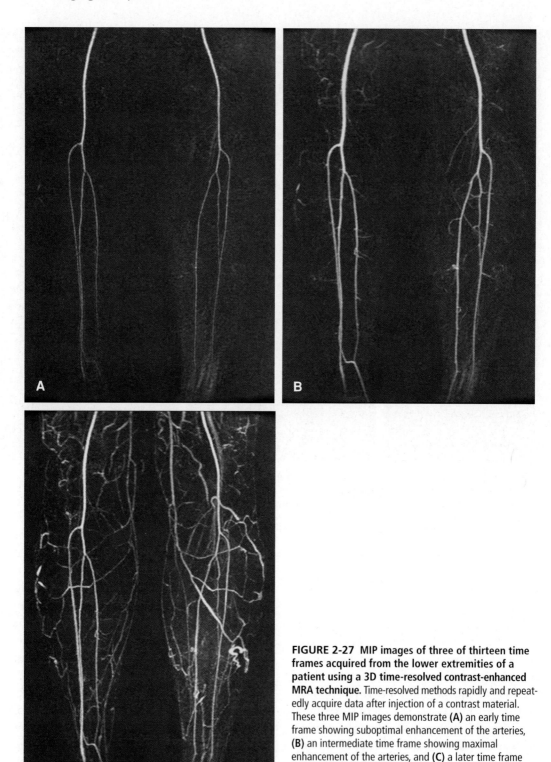

FIGURE 2-27 MIP images of three of thirteen time frames acquired from the lower extremities of a patient using a 3D time-resolved contrast-enhanced MRA technique. Time-resolved methods rapidly and repeatedly acquire data after injection of a contrast material. These three MIP images demonstrate **(A)** an early time frame showing suboptimal enhancement of the arteries, **(B)** an intermediate time frame showing maximal enhancement of the arteries, and **(C)** a later time frame showing diminished enhancement of arteries and interference from enhancing veins.

quickly limits the spatial resolution and coverage that can be achieved at each station.

When the bolus of contrast material advances quicker than the time it takes to acquire and translate the patient, enhancement of veins and stationary tissues may be seen in the later-acquired stations. The images of the vessels of the lower extremities shown in Figure 2-22 were acquired with a single-injection, three-station technique. For this study, acquisition was sufficiently rapid that the images at all three stations were acquired prior to enhancement of

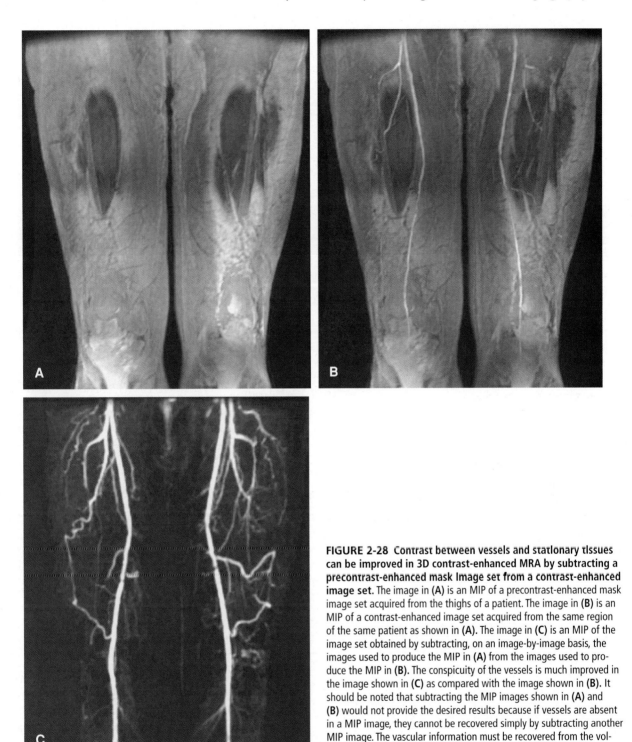

FIGURE 2-28 Contrast between vessels and stationary tissues can be improved in 3D contrast-enhanced MRA by subtracting a precontrast-enhanced mask image set from a contrast-enhanced image set. The image in (A) is an MIP of a precontrast-enhanced mask image set acquired from the thighs of a patient. The image in (B) is an MIP of a contrast-enhanced image set acquired from the same region of the same patient as shown in (A). The image in (C) is an MIP of the image set obtained by subtracting, on an image-by-image basis, the images used to produce the MIP in (A) from the images used to produce the MIP in (B). The conspicuity of the vessels is much improved in the image shown in (C) as compared with the image shown in (B). It should be noted that subtracting the MIP images shown in (A) and (B) would not provide the desired results because if vessels are absent in a MIP image, they cannot be recovered simply by subtracting another MIP image. The vascular information must be recovered from the volume data set.

veins or stationary tissues. When single-injection, multi-station exams are performed, the mask images for all stations are acquired prior to administration of the contrast material to prevent the contrast material from enhancing the vessels in any of the mask images. Finally, the rate of the injection must be reduced (in order to extend the duration of the contrast material administration) to ensure that contrast material is present during imaging of all the stations.

Contrast materials that remain in the blood pool for more than an hour without leaking into the surrounding stationary tissues have been developed and currently are being evaluated (48,49). These so-called intravascular, or blood pool, contrast materials can be used to increase the imaging time in order to achieve greater coverage and higher spatial resolution. The drawback of increased acquisition time is that it results in venous enhancement, which leads to difficulty in evaluating the arteries. Methods are being developed to separate arterial signal from venous signal but are not yet available clinically. An additional benefit of some of the intravascular contrast materials is that they have a higher relaxivity. In other words, they provide greater vascular signal during the first pass of the contrast material by causing a more dramatic decrease in the T1 of blood (per unit volume of contrast material) compared with the currently available extravascular contrast materials.

In summary, 3D contrast-enhanced MRA methods can provide excellent vascular images, and they offer advantages over noncontrast-enhanced MRA methods. The features of 3D contrast-enhanced MRA methods are summarized in Table 2-11, and the benefits and limitations of these techniques are summarized in Table 2-12.

Black Blood Imaging

Flowing blood may appear as low signal on spin echo sequences with high velocity, turbulence, and dephasing. Since the early days of imaging the thoracic aorta, the high velocity of aortic blood provided contrast, yielding the aortic lumen with dark signal. That dark signal can be thought of as the consequence of an outflow phenomenon—excited blood protons flow out of the region of exci-

TABLE 2-11

Summary of Three-Dimensional Contrast-Enhanced Magnetic Resonance Angiography

- A T_1-shortening contrast material is intravenously administered.
- A short TR (<10 m/sec), short TE (<2 m/sec), large tip angle (45 to 60 degrees), T1-weighted 3D gradient echo imaging sequence is used to achieve striking contrast between blood and stationary tissues.
- Data are acquired during the first pass of the contrast material, when the contrast material is most concentrated in the arteries and has not yet reached the veins or stationary tissues.
- A slab, oriented parallel to the vessels of interest, is imaged.
- Scan time = TR $\times$ NSA $\times$ #PE $\times$ #SE. (TR, repetition time; NSA, number of signal averages; #PE, number of phase-encoding values; #SE, number of slice-encoding values.)

TABLE 2-12

Benefits and Limitations of Three-Dimensional Contrast-Enhanced Magnetic Resonance Imaging

Benefits

- The T_1-shortening contrast material reduces the effects of saturation, allowing the entire length of the vessel to be imaged with a large FOV and permitting slow flow to be visualized.
- The effects of intravoxel dephasing are diminished due to the inherently short TE of the imaging sequence, and the high vascular signal made available by the presence of the T_1-shortening contrast material, leading to reduced signal loss in regions affected by complex flow and susceptibility differences.
- A large tip angle (45 to 60 degrees) can be used, leading to a large signal from the short-T_1 blood and a small signal from the longer-T_1 stationary tissues.
- A precontrast image set can be subtracted from the contrast-enhanced image set to improve vessel conspicuity by eliminating signal from stationary tissues.

Limitations

- Image quality is highly dependent on the timing of the acquisition relative to the arrival and passage of the contrast material.
- The modulation of signal caused by changes in the concentration of the contrast material as it passes may lead to artifacts in the image.
- Saturation pulses are ineffective at reducing the signal from T_1-shortened blood and are too time consuming, so suppression of venous signal is achieved by acquiring data prior to the arrival of the contrast material in the veins, which may be difficult in some situations.
- Accumulated contrast material may degrade image quality when multiple sites are imaged with multiple injections.
- Spatial resolution may be limited by the requisite short scan times.

tation prior to the application of a relevant refocusing pulse. For those (flowing) spins unable to undergo both excitation and refocusing pulses, signal cannot be generated. However, depending on the blood velocity and the TR of the sequence, slow-flowing blood may be able to experience both pulses and thus may be able to generate signal. Such flow may be seen in the false channel of an aortic dissection or from an inadvertent sampling of data in diastole.

A more purposeful approach utilizes inversion pulses that can accomplish more uniform dark signal (50) . This strategy is predicated on the application of a double-inversion pulse that is applied to null the signal of blood before the start or the readout. This can be applied to spin echo, echo train, and half-Fourier single-shot readouts. Although termed as *double*

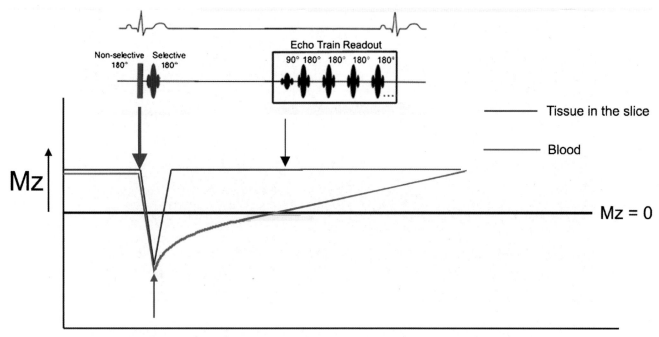

FIGURE 2-29 Pulse sequence schematic for double inversion dark blood imaging. Following the ECG, a nonselective inversion pulse (*purple arrow*) affects the spins within *and beyond* the slice of interest. The next pulse is a slice-selective reversion pulse (*blue arrow*) that restores Mz in the imaging slice, while Mz beyond the slice remains inverted. During a short time interval, blood in the slice exits while blood outside the slice is restoring Mz according to the T_1 of blood. By initiating the echo train pulse sequence at the time where the blood T_1 crosses the null point (*black vertical arrow*), there is no Mz available for registering signal, yielding dark blood in multiple slices.

inversion, this technique can be better understood as an *inversion–reversion technique* (Fig. 2-29).

Following the initial inversion, which is a broad-based nonselective pulse, all protons, including those beyond the slice, are inverted. The next pulse is a selective reversion affecting the slice of interest. Thus, there is no net effect on the protons in the slice of interest, and the readout then follows to capture signal from the tissues in the slice. Meanwhile, the protons outside the slice are recovering magnetization according to their T_1 properties. If the pulse is timed to null the signal of blood, the readout will be initiated when there is no longitudinal magnetization; hence, there will be no signal coming from blood.

This technique is most commonly used in clinical practice when studying the aorta and when evaluating for atherosclerotic plaque (51,52).

Steady-State Free Precession

An approach to MRA that uses a coherent steady-state technique with a fully balanced gradient waveform to recycle transverse magnetization offers rapid image acquisitions with intrinsic high signal in the blood pool. Generically

referred to as *steady-state free precession* (SSFP), this strategy is also known as *TrueFISP, FIESTA,* and *balanced FFE* (fast field echo) as implemented by Siemens Medical Systems, General Electric Healthcare Technologies, and Philips Medical Systems, respectively.

With SSFP, contrast is determined on the basis of the ratio of T_2 to T_1 with some influence of inflow effects, as in spoiled gradient-echo methods. This decreases the sensitivity of SSFP to saturation effects. However, the rendering of the blood signal as bright is not specific and eliminates the ability to use signal intensity as a means to distinguish arteries and veins (Fig. 2-30) (53,54).

Relative to spoiled gradient-echo methods, SSFP is extremely rapid, which allows performance of a cine MR sequence in as little as 5 to 6 seconds. Gated single-phase SSFP images can be acquired in a single heartbeat. This has been used to provide a rapid survey of the thorax in multiple planes in less than 1 minute (53).

RECENT ADVANCES

All MR angiographic methods are benefiting from recent advances in radio frequency coil design and increases in

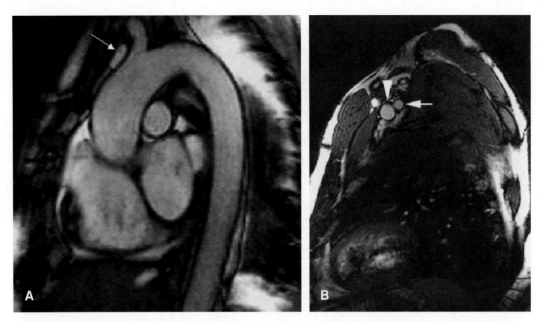

FIGURE 2-30 SSFP images with intrinsic bright blood. A: ECG-triggered, sagittal SSFP (TR = 3.2 m/sec, TE = 1.6 m/sec) image of the normal aorta in a 46-year-old patient. (From Pereles FS, McCarthy RM, Baskaran V, et al. Thoracic aortic dissection and aneurysm: evaluation with nonenhanced true FISP MR angiography in less than 4 minutes. *Radiology.* 2002;223(1):270–274, with permission.) Note that bright signal is visualized in the brachiocephalic vein (*arrow*) and throughout the blood pool. **B:** Sagittal, nontriggered SSFP image (TR = 4.8 m/sec, TE = 2.3 m/sec) along the left mid clavicle shows left subclavian vein (*arrowhead*) has homogeneous hyperintense signal intensity, similar to that of subclavian artery (*arrow*). (Reprinted from Pedrosa I, Morrin M, Oleaga L, et al. Is true FISP imaging reliable in the evaluation of venous thrombosis? *AJR Am J Roentgenol.* 2005;185(6):1632–1640, with permission.)

magnetic field strength of clinically available scanners. There are numerous multielement radio frequency coils available for MRA applications that provide additional spatial coverage and improved SNR. MR vendors are currently providing systems with 16 and 32 receivers, and systems with even greater numbers of receivers are being developed. As the number of system receivers increases, so too can the number of independently active elements per radio frequency coil, thereby permitting even greater increases in coverage and SNR. Additionally, using multi-element coils allows the use of scan-time reduction methods such as SENSE (MR angiography with sensitivity encoding) (55,56) and GRAPPA (generalized autocalibrating partially parallel acquisition) (57). With these methods, the reduction factor is dependent on the number of elements contained in a coil. Therefore, increases in the number of elements will permit even greater reductions in scan time. Higher magnetic fields permit improvements in MRI by providing increased SNRs in the images. Scanners with higher magnetic fields are becoming more prevalent, and MR angiographic methods are being developed for use on these systems (58–62). Initial results demonstrate excellent image quality.

CONCLUSION

Under appropriate conditions, and when properly implemented, all MR angiographic methods can yield diagnostic-quality images. Two-dimensional phase contrast methods offer qualitative and quantitative information regarding blood velocity or volume flow rate. Phase contrast methods are often used to measure these values in the renal arteries, the aorta, the pulmonary vessels, and the intracranial and extracranial arteries. Three-dimensional time-of-flight methods offer small voxels, short echo times, and inherently high signal-to-noise ratios. These methods are often used for imaging the intracranial arteries as well as the extracranial carotid and vertebral arteries. The 2D time-of-flight method is sensitive to signal loss from intravoxel dephasing and is often used as a highly sensitive and specific method for screening for stenoses of the carotid or lower extremity arteries. Two-dimensional time-of-flight may also be used with an inferior saturation pulse to image the intracranial veins. Three-dimensional contrast-enhanced methods can provide high-quality vascular images with less sensitivity to artifacts and shorter scan times as compared with the noncontrast-enhanced MRA methods. Contrast-enhanced MRA is widely used for imaging vessels throughout the body and in some situations is replacing digital subtraction angiography (DSA) as the standard imaging method. Three-dimensional contrast-enhanced methods continue to undergo refinements, making these methods more competitive with DSA.

REFERENCES

1. Anderson CM, Edelman RR, Turski PA. *Clinical Magnetic Resonance Angiography*. New York: Raven Press; 1993.
2. Potchen EJ, Haacke EM, Siebert JE, et al. *Magnetic Resonance Angiography: Concepts and Applications*. St. Louis: Mosby; 1993.
3. Krinsky G. Magnetic resonance imaging clinics of North America. *Body MR Angiography*. 1998;6:2.
4. Keller PJ, Drayer BP, Fram EK. Neuroimaging clinics of North America. *Magn Reson Angiography*. 1992;2:4.
5. Prince MR, Grist TM, Debatin JF. *3D Contrast MR Angiography*. Berlin: Springer; 1999.
6. Moran PR. A flow zeugmatographic interlace for NMR imaging in humans. *Magn Reson Imaging*. 1982;1:197–203.
7. Dumoulin CL, Hart HR. Magnetic resonance angiography. *Radiology*. 1986;161:717–720.
8. Korosec F, Turski P. Velocity and volume flow rate measurements using phase contrast magnetic resonance imaging (review article). *Int J Neuroradiology*. 1997;3:293–318.
9. Nayler GL, Firmin DN, Longmore DB. Blood flow imaging by cine magnetic resonance. *J Comput Assist Tomogr*. 1986;10(5):715–722.
10. Pelc NJ, Herfkens RJ, Shimakawa A, et al. Phase contrast cine magnetic resonance imaging. *Magn Reson Q*. 1991;7: 229–254.
11. Dumoulin C, Souza S, Walker M, et al. Three-dimensional phase contrast angiography. *Magn Reson Med*. 1989;9:139–149.
12. Pernicone JR, Siebert JE, Potchen EJ, et al. Three-dimensional phase-contrast MR angiography in the head and neck: preliminary report. *Am J Roentgenol*. 1990;155: 167–176.
13. Pelc NJ, Bernstein MA, Shimakawa A, et al. Encoding strategies for three-direction phase-contrast MR imaging of flow. *Magn Reson Imaging*. 1991;1:405–413.
14. Hausman R, Lewin JS, Laub G. Phase-contrast MR angiography with reduced acquisition time: new concepts in sequence design. *J Magn Reson*. 1991;1:415–422.
15. Pattany PM, Phillips JJ, Chiu LC, et al. Motion artifact suppression technique (MAST) for MR imaging. *J Comput Assist Tomogr*. 1987;11(3):369–377.
16. Haacke E, Lenz G. Improving MR image quality in the presence of motion by using rephasing gradients. *Am J Roentgenol*. 1987;148:1251–1258.
17. Keller PJ, Drayer BP, Fram EK, et al. MR angiography with two-dimensional acquisition and three-dimensional display: work in progress. *Radiology*. 173:527–532.
18. Parker DL, Yuan C, Blatter DD. MR angiography by multiple thin slab 3D acquisition. *Magn Reson Med*. 17:434–451.
19. Felmlee JP, Ehman RL. Spatial presaturation: a method for suppressing flow artifacts and improving depiction of vascular anatomy in MR imaging. *Radiology*. 1987;164: 559–564.
20. Edelman RR, Atkinson DJ, Silver MS, et al. FRODO pulse sequences: a new means of eliminating motion flow, and wraparound artifacts. *Radiology*. 1988;166:231–236.
21. Ehman RL, Felmlee JP. Flow artifact reduction in MRI: a review of the roles of gradient moment nulling and spatial presaturation. *Magn Reson Med*. 1990;14:293–307.
22. DeMarco JK, Huston J 3rd, Bernstein MA. Evaluation of classic 2D time-of-flight MR angiography in the depiction of severe carotid stenosis. *AJR Am J Roentgenol*. 2004;183(3):787–793.
23. Ruggieri PM, Laub GA, Marsaryk TJ, et al. Intracranial circulation: pulse-sequence considerations in three-dimensional (volume) MR angiography. *Radiology*. 1989;171: 785–791.
24. Schmalbrock P, Yuan C, Chakeres DW, et al. Volume MR angiography: methods to achieve very short echo times. *Radiology*. 1990;175:861–865.
25. Wolff SD, Balaban RS. Magnetization transfer contrast (MTC) and tissue water proton relaxation in vivo. *Magn Reson Med*. 1989;10:135–144.
26. Pike GB, Hu BS, Glover GH, et al. Magnetization transfer time-of-flight magnetic resonance angiography. *Magn Reson Med*. 1992;25:372–379.
27. Edelman RR, Ahn SS, Chien D, et al. Improved time-of-flight MR angiography of the brain with magnetization transfer contrast. *Radiology*. 1992;184(2):395–399.
28. Nagele T, Klose U, Grodd W, et al. The effects of linearly increasing flip angles on 3D inflow MR angiography. *Magn Reson Med*. 1994;31(5):561–566.
29. Du YP, Parker DL, Davis WL, et al. Reduction of partial-volume artifacts with zero-filled interpolation in three-dimensional MR angiography. *J Magn Reson Imaging*. 1994;4(5):733–741.
30. Bernstein MA, Fain SB, Riederer SJ. Effect of windowing and zero-filled reconstruction of MRI data on spatial resolution and acquisition strategy. *J Magn Reson Imaging*. 2001;14(3): 270–280.
31. Blatter DD, Parker DL, Robinson R. Cerebral MR angiography with multiple overlapping thin slab acquisition. *Radiology*. 1991;179:805–811.
32. Prince MR, Yucel EK, Kaufman JA, et al. Dynamic gadolinium-enhanced three-dimensional abdominal MR arteriography. *J Magn Reson Imaging*. 1993;3(6):877–881.
33. Parker DL, Goodrich KC, Alexander AL, et al. Optimized visualization of vessels in contrast enhanced intracranial MR angiography. *Magn Reson Med*. 1998;40:873–882.
34. Huston J, Fain SB, Wald JT, et al. Carotid artery: elliptic centric contrast-enhanced MR angiography compared with conventional angiography. *Radiology*. 2001;218: 138–143.
35. Maki J, Prince M, Londy F, et al. The effects of time varying intravascular signal intensity and k-space acquisition order on three-dimensional MR angiography image quality. *J Magn Reson Imaging*. 1996;6:642–651.
36. Earls J, Rofsky N, DeCorato D, et al. Breath-hold single-dose gadolinium-enhanced three-dimensional MR aortography: usefulness of a timing examination and MR power injector. *Radiology*. 1996;201:705–710.
37. Foo T, Saranathan M, Prince M, et al. Automated detection of bolus arrival and initiation of data acquisition in fast, three-dimensional, gadolinium enhanced MR angiography. *Radiology*. 1997;203:275–280.
38. Wilman A, Riederer S, Huston J, et al. Arterial phase carotid and vertebral artery imaging in 3D contrast-enhanced MR angiography by combining fluoroscopic triggering with an elliptical centric acquisition order. *Magn Reson Med*. 1998;40:24–35.
39. Huston J, Fain S, Riederer S, et al. Carotid arteries: maximizing arterial to venous contrast in fluoroscopically triggered contrast-enhanced MR angiography with elliptical centric view ordering. *Radiology*. 1999;211:265–273.
40. Wang Y, Johnston D, Breen J, et al. Dynamic MR digital subtraction angiography using contrast enhancement, fast data acquisition, and complex subtraction. *Magn Reson Med*. 1996;36:551–556.
41. Hennig J, Scheffler K, Laubenberger J, et al. Time-resolved projection angiography after bolus injection of contrast agent. *Magn Reson Med*. 1997;37:341–345.
42. Korosec F, Frayne R, Grist T, et al. Time-resolved contrast-enhanced 3D MR angiography. *Magn Reson Med*. 1996;36: 345–351.

43. Willig DS, Turski PA, Frayne R, et al. Contrast-enhanced 3D MR DSA of the carotid artery bifurcation: preliminary study of comparison with unenhanced 2D and 3D time-of-flight MR angiography. *Radiology*. 1998;208:447–451.

44. Earls JP, Patel NH, Smith PA, et al. Gadolinium-enhanced three-dimensional MR angiography of the aorta and peripheral arteries: evaluation of a multistation examination using two gadopentetate dimeglumine infusions. *AJR Am J Roentgenol*. 1998;171(3):599–604.

45. Ho KY, Leiner T, de Haan MW, et al. Peripheral vascular tree stenoses: evaluation with moving-bed infusion-tracking MR angiography. *Radiology*. 1998;206(3):683–692.

46. Earls JP, DeSena S, Bluemke DA. Gadolinium-enhanced three-dimensional MR angiography of the entire aorta and iliac arteries with dynamic manual table translation. *Radiology*. 1998;209:844–849.

47. Meaney JF, Ridgway JP, Chakraverty S, et al. Stepping-table gadolinium-enhanced digital subtraction MR angiography of the aorta and lower extremity arteries: preliminary experience. *Radiology*. 1999;211:59–67.

48. Kroft LJ, de Roos A. Blood pool contrast agents for cardiovascular MR imaging. *J Magn Reson Imaging*. 1999;10(3):395–403.

49. Perreault P, Edelman MA, Baum RA, et al. MR angiography with gadofosveset trisodium for peripheral vascular disease: phase II trial. *Radiology*. 2003;229(3):811–820.

50. Simonetti OP, Finn JP, White RD, et al. "Black blood" T_2-weighted inversion-recovery MR imaging of the heart. *Radiology*. 1996;199(1):49–57.

51. Fayad ZA, Fuster V, Fallon JT, et al. Noninvasive in vivo human coronary artery lumen and wall imaging using black-blood magnetic resonance imaging. *Circulation*. 2000;102(5):506–510.

52. Stemerman DH, Krinsky GA, Lee VS, et al. Thoracic aorta: rapid black-blood MR imaging with half-Fourier rapid acquisition with relaxation enhancement with or without electrocardiographic triggering. *Radiology*. 1999;213(1):185–191.

53. Pereles FS, McCarthy RM, Baskaran V, et al. Thoracic aortic dissection and aneurysm: evaluation with nonenhanced true FISP MR angiography in less than 4 minutes. *Radiology*. 2002;223(1):270–274.

54. Pedrosa I, Morrin M, Oleaga L, et al. Is true FISP imaging reliable in the evaluation of venous thrombosis? *AJR Am J Roentgenol*. 2005;185(6):1632–1640.

55. Pruessmann KP, Weiger M, Scheidegger MB, et al. SENSE: sensitivity encoding for fast MRI. *Magn Reson Med*. 1999;42(5):952–962.

56. Weiger M, Pruessmann KP, Kassner A, et al. Contrast-enhanced 3D MRA using SENSE. *J Magn Reson Imaging*. 2000;12(5):671–677.

57. Griswold MA, Jakob PM, Heidemann RM, et al. Generalized autocalibrating partially parallel acquisitions (GRAPPA). *Magn Reson Med*. 2002;47(6):1202–1210.

58. Bernstein MA, Huston J 3rd, Lin C, et al. High-resolution intracranial and cervical MRA at 3.0T: technical considerations and initial experience. *Magn Reson Med*. 2001;46(5):955–962.

59. Thomas SD, Al-Kwifi O, Emery DJ, et al. Application of magnetization transfer at 3.0 T in three-dimensional time-of-flight magnetic resonance angiography of the intracranial arteries. *J Magn Reson Imaging*. 2002;15(4):479–483.

60. Willinek WA, Born M, Simon B, et al. Time-of-flight MR angiography: comparison of 3.0-T imaging and 1.5-T imaging-initial experience. *Radiology*. 2003;229(3):913–920.

61. Leiner T, de Vries M, Hoogeveen R, et al. Contrast-enhanced peripheral MR angiography at 3.0 Tesla: initial experience with a whole-body scanner in healthy volunteers. *J Magn Reson Imaging*. 2003;17(5):609–614.

62. Gibbs GF, Huston J 3rd, Bernstein MA, et al. Improved image quality of intracranial aneurysms: 3.0-T versus 1.5-T time-of-flight MR angiography. *AJNR Am J Neuroradiol*. 2004;25(1):84–87.

Conventional Angiography in the Noninvasive Era

Daniel Y. Sze

Within a few months of Roentgen's publication describing the discovery of x-rays, Haschek and Lindenthal published the first angiogram of an amputated hand (1). While Lord Kelvin was still denouncing x-rays as a "hoax," others already recognized the potential for medical applications of this new phenomenon and the utility of filling hollow structures with a radio-opaque substance to aid in image-based diagnosis. The first seven decades of medical imaging were devoted primarily to the diagnosis of disease.

In 1964, Dotter conceived of angioplasty using sequential introduction of plastic dilators, and the field of angiography and interventional radiology veered away from diagnosis and toward therapy. The previous year, he had predicted that "[t]he angiographic catheter can be more than a tool for passive means for diagnostic observation; used with imagination, it can become an important surgical instrument" (2). This trend was fueled further by the introduction of less invasive diagnostic technologies including ultrasound, computed tomography (CT), and magnetic resonance (MR) imaging. Cross-sectional and volumetric imaging has replaced nearly all of the diagnostic roles previously occupied by angiography. Dotter's prophecy has become completely realized; the tools and techniques of catheter-based therapy have developed into a field that stands as its own "component" in the American College of Radiology (3). Despite this change in function, catheter angiography continues to play a crucial role in vascular medicine.

The current practice of interventional radiology, although highly dependent on miniaturized devices and new pharmacological agents, relies on the generation of anatomical images to pursue its mission of maximum therapeutic yield with minimum risk. To generate these images, tools and techniques currently or formerly used solely for diagnosis were adopted and customized. Aside from facilitating interventions, these customized imaging methods can also provide a few subtle but clinically crucial advantages over noninvasive methods of imaging.

TECHNIQUES

Generation of Images

Early observations that x-ray bombardment of certain substances could cause luminescence, or emission of photons of a wavelength in the visible range, allowed real-time x-ray examination of patients. Unfortunately, the hazards of radiation were not well understood, and many red-spectacled physicians succumbed to the adverse effects of radiation overexposure. Modern fluoroscopy has evolved into a method that reduces physician exposure to acceptable levels yet greatly increases the diagnostic power of the generated images. Standards of practice, including standards of equipment, have been published and are updated periodically (4).

Few modern angiography facilities have retained the capability of producing analog hard-copy photographic film angiograms, sometimes referred to as *cut film*. Film size ranged from 105-mm cinematic roll film, through 14" square rapid sequence film used with a "Puck" film changer, to 51" "long leg" film capable of capturing the entire lower extremities without demagnification. Obtaining subtraction

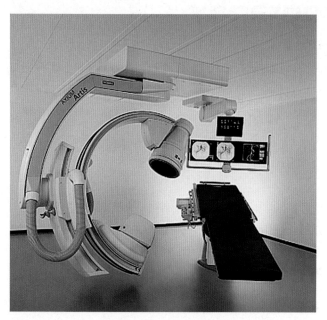

FIGURE 3-1 **A fluoroscopic unit is shown.** Imaging hardware is commercially available in numerous different designs and configurations, including C-arms, U-arms, floor-mounted, ceiling-mounted, biplanar, and the like. This unit is a ceiling-mounted C-arm using an image intensifier. (Courtesy Siemens Medical Solutions USA, Inc., Malvern, PA)

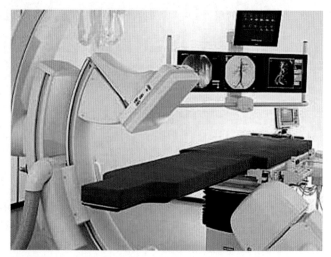

FIGURE 3-2 **This figure shows a flat-panel detector.** In the newest fluoroscopic units, the image intensifier is replaced with a square or rectangular amorphous silicon flat-panel detector, decreasing the effective radiation dose and geometric distortion of the image, and lowering the profile of the instrument. (Courtesy Siemens Medical Solutions USA, Inc., Malvern, PA)

films from these hard-copy films required considerable expertise in a time-consuming process of making a negative of the mask image and reprinting selected images by physically stacking the images onto the negative mask and printing a summating negative. Since the 1970s, digitized images have progressively replaced analog images, and digital subtraction can be performed instantaneously. Even the last bastions of cut-film angiography in mesenteric and pulmonary angiography are yielding to the modernization of digital subtraction angiography (DSA).

The generation of a DSA image starts with generation of x-rays by a tube that usually sits beneath the patient (5) (Fig. 3-1). The thinly collimated x-rays pass upward through the radiolucent table and the patient, and transmitted photons are captured by the detector situated above the patient, coupled to the tube by a C- or U-shaped arm. In the 1950s, fluorescent detectors were replaced by the image intensifier (II). These "cans" contain a vacuum tube photon detector that converts x-ray photons to optical photons. The weak luminescence is converted to photoelectrons, which are then electronically accelerated and focused onto another phosphorescent screen that converts the photoelectrons back to optical photons. These amplified optical photons are then photographed by a video camera and projected in real time onto a high-definition (>1 kilopixel × >1 kilopixel) monitor (6). The newest detectors are flat panel, square or rectangular, and use amorphous silicon to detect photons and convert them directly to electrical signals. Flat-panel detectors

offer the advantages of lower profile than IIs, approximately 30% reduction in radiation due to greater efficiency and much less geometric distortion (Fig. 3-2).

Fluoroscopic images obtained in real time by stepping on a pedal may be archived on videotape or computer memory. Most frequently, though, the real time images are not archived, and only the *runs*, dedicated and prescribed cinematic sequences usually obtained during injection of contrast, are stored electronically. Acquisition parameters that need to be prescribed include the frame rate (up to 30 frames per second) and exposure time per frame, the kilovoltage, and the current or milliamperes. As is true of any other radiography technique, the greater the current (and therefore photons), the higher the signal-to-noise ratio, and the higher the kilovoltage (especially above the k-edges of the penetrated materials), the higher the penetrance.

Images obtained digitally can be displayed as native or subtracted and positive or negative (black bones, white air or white bones, black air). With digital subtraction, the intensity of each pixel in each frame is first converted into logarithmic form and then subtracted from a digital mask image, producing a difference image. If the patient is perfectly still and nothing is injected, the difference image is blank. By blanking out the background, digital subtraction angiography attains sensitivity much greater than in native images. Injected contrast can be seen as black on a blank white background, or vice versa (Fig. 3-3).

Subtraction techniques, though, are subject to a number of artifacts. Perhaps the most frequently encountered

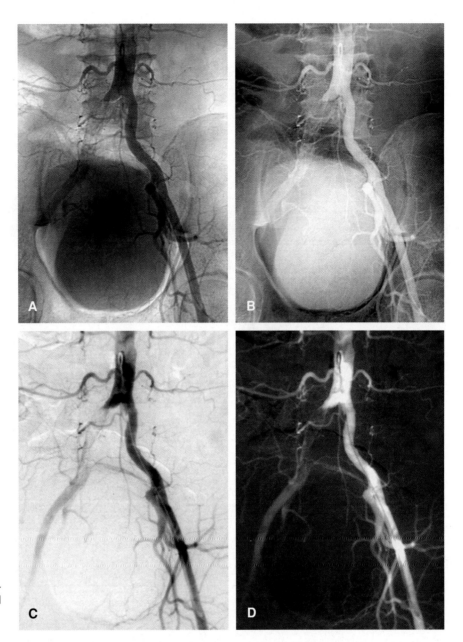

FIGURE 3-3 Shown is a digitally acquired catheter angiogram. The same image can be displayed **(A)** native (unsubtracted), **(B)** inverted native, **(C)** digitally subtracted, or **(D)** subtracted and inverted. Signal-to-noise and contrast-to-noise ratios, and thus diagnostic power, can be greatly enhanced by digital subtraction.

is motion artifact. Motion of a uniform background does not cause artifacts, but the background of the human body is decidedly nonuniform. Any anatomical structures that are fluoroscopically discernable, including bones, bowel gas, lungs, surgical clips, and the like will move as a result of patient respiration, cardiac pulsation, and peristalsis, causing artifacts that can obscure the region of interest. These artifacts can be minimized by apnea (voluntary or otherwise), pharmacological intervention (sedatives, glucagon), and physical restraints. Smaller artifacts can usually be eliminated by optimal choice of which frame to use as a mask, and by reregistration of the mask frame and image frame in a process referred to as *pixel shifting* (Fig. 3-4).

Newer angiography units also feature the capability of *rotational* angiography. In these systems, continuous acquisition is performed while the C-arm rotates and contrast is injected. Preliminary images obtained without contrast allow digital subtraction to be performed. The final product shows the angiogram from a multitude of oblique angles, which when displayed as a loop allows the angiographer to form a three-dimensional (3D) image mentally.

Angiographic Methods

Modern angiography blossomed with the introduction of the Seldinger method of catheter exchange and the introduction of preshaped wires and catheters. Prior to the 1950s, angiography of a vessel required direct puncture of

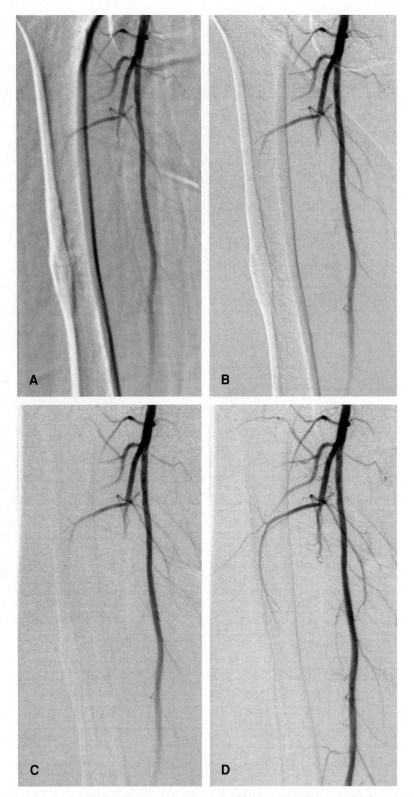

FIGURE 3-4 Optimization of digital subtraction is presented here. A: Digitally acquired catheter angiogram using the default mask for subtraction. **B:** Selection of optimal mask image. **C:** Reregistration of the mask and selected images yields a more diagnostic image. **D:** Multiple frames can be stacked to obtain a maximum opacity image, which can be useful for short or fragmented contrast boluses or for displaying arterial and venous information simultaneously.

that vessel with a needle to inject contrast and obtain images. Building on the techniques of percutaneous access to a vessel and the Forssman technique pioneered in the 1920s of accessing distant structures using a catheter threaded through a vessel, Seldinger published the technique of removing the needle over a guide wire and replacing it with a catheter (1). With rare exception, all modern angiography is performed using the Seldinger technique.

Access to a vessel, arterial or venous, is usually performed with a needle ranging from 18 to 22 gauge (G). Although digital palpation of a pulse combined with knowledge of normal anatomy is usually sufficient to achieve safe access to a vessel, transcutaneous ultrasound can enable success in difficult situations (no palpable pulse, branched or tortuous vessels) and also makes routine access safer. Inadvertent carotid puncture during internal jugular vein access, for instance, has been reported to be as common as 5% to 14% without the use of ultrasound but is now virtually 0% in the hands of the skilled ultrasonographer (7). Other complications, such as pneumothorax and branch vessel injury, can also be minimized using ultrasound guidance. In patients in whom the use of an arterial closure device is anticipated, ultrasound can also optimize access location, avoiding sidewall punctures and punctures near or through bifurcations. Larger needles can accommodate larger wires, so use of an 18G or thin-walled 19G needle may save time by allowing immediate introduction of a 0.035"-diameter wire, but many practitioners now prefer the relative safety of using a smaller needle (21 or 22G) that only accommodates an 0.018" wire. With lower-profile access, a *micropuncture* coaxial dilator must be used to increase the size of the access to accommodate the standard 0.035" wire.

Devices

The default size for diagnostic catheterization is now 5 French (F) (1.67 mm outer diameter), but some practitioners are starting to favor 4F. For patients in whom multiple catheter exchanges are anticipated, a side-arm sheath is usually placed to minimize trauma to the vessel. Sheaths are sized according to inner diameter, so a 5F sheath allows passage of 5 French catheters, but actually measures about 6 to 7F (2.0 to 2.3 mm) on its outer diameter. Catheters are commercially available as thin as about 1.8F (0.6 mm), and the largest devices (used for stent-graft treatment of the thoracic aorta) require a 24F sheath with an outer diameter of 9.5 mm. Diagnostic catheters are available in a large variety of shapes, diameters, and lengths (Fig. 3-5). Most catheters incorporate a radio-opaque substance within the polymer to render them visible on fluoroscopy. In addition, differences in design engineering and manufacturing using materials such as polyethylene (PE), polytetrafluoroethylene (PTFE, Teflon), polyamides (e.g.,

nylon), and aramids (e.g., Kevlar) result in subtle differences in "pushability" or resistance to longitudinal stretching and shortening, "trackability" or conformability to a tortuous course, pliability, torquability, pressure capacity, and surface friction. Similarly, guide wires are available in a large array of designs, varying in diameter, length, stiffness, tip shape and length, torquability, steerability, surface friction, and kink resistance (Fig. 3-6). Different materials including nitinol, stainless steel, and platinum are used in the cores to take advantage of their characteristics such as kink resistance, stiffness, and radio-opacity. Superficially, guide wires may be coated with PTFE or wettable hydrophilic coatings.

Risks and Complications

Some of the reasons for diagnostic catheter angiography being replaced by less invasive methods are (a) greater risk for complications of catheterization and (b) convenience to the patient. For purely diagnostic catheterization procedures, the rate of complications is not alarming, and published guidelines list acceptable rates (8–10) (Table 3-1). The rates of complications increase when therapeutic procedures are performed, due to the larger device profiles, longer duration and greater complexity of manipulation, greater selectivity of catheterization, and the fact that only patients with significant disease require intervention.

Some of the risks of catheter angiography are shared by CT angiography, including exposure to contrast medium and to radiation. The typical diagnostic catheter angiogram uses approximately 100 to 150 mL of contrast medium, no different from CT angiography, so the risks of contrast medium reactions and/or nephrotoxicity are not substantially different. However, in catheter angiography, the contrast is administered in smaller aliquoted boluses, so localized tissue infiltration and necrosis are virtually absent. However, the contrast medium may be injected at rates as high as 25 mL per second and pressure as high as 1700 psi (pounds per square inch, approximately 11.7 kPa) through a multiside-hole nonselective catheter, and approximately half of these parameters through a single endhole selective catheter, so injury to arteries and other vessels is possible. These injuries can include arterial dissection, small vessel rupture, and aneurysmal rupture. These complications should be immediately recognized and rectified by the practitioner. Other risks unique to catheterization include distal embolization of targeted organs or of the accessed extremity, subintimal passage of wires and/or catheters, and access site complications including hematoma, thrombosis, arteriovenous fistula, and pseudoaneurysm.

Radiation dose is highly variable in both conventional and CT angiography, depending on the imaging protocols and body parts imaged. The high frame rates used in

(*text continues on page* 94)

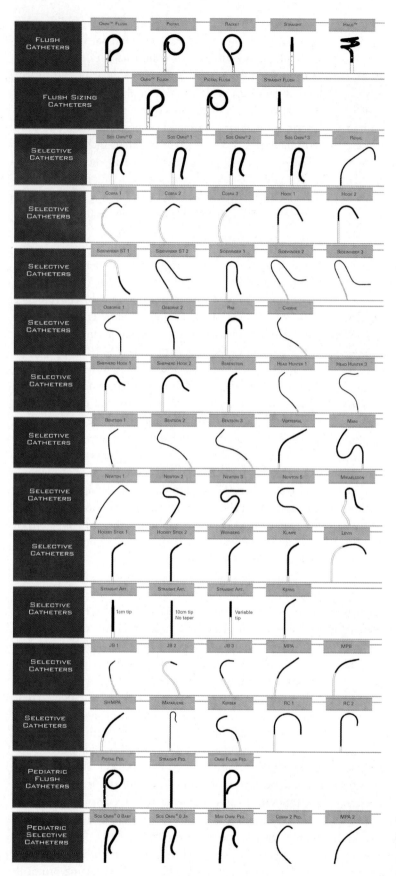

FIGURE 3-5 The standard diagnostic catheter shapes offered by a market-leading company are shown. In addition to differences in shape, catheters are available in different diameters, lengths, and materials. In addition, catheters can be custom shaped commercially or by individual practitioners at the time of angiography. (Courtesy AngioDynamics, Inc., Queensbury, NY)

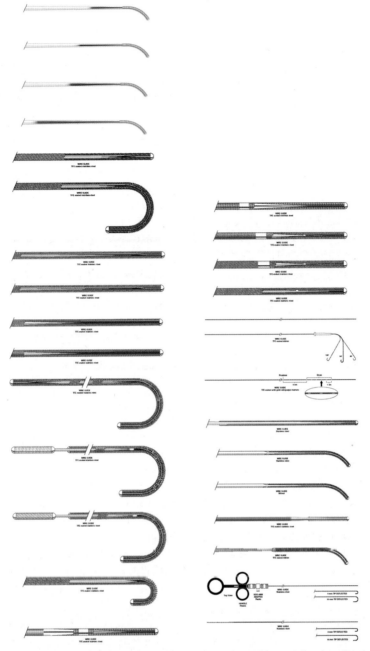

FIGURE 3-6 Standard guide wires (also known as wire guides) are used for peripheral angiography and intervention. The commercial offerings of one market-leading company are listed. These wires range in diameter from 0.014″ to 0.038″ and are available in various lengths from 50 to 300 cm. They differ from each other in core stiffness, steerability, torquability, tip shape and length, kink resistance, and surface treatment. From top to bottom, in order of appearance:

Roadrunner Nimble,
Nimble Floppy,
The Firm,
The Firm LT,
Straight Fixed Core Wire Guides,
Safe-T-J Curved Fixed Core Wire Guides,
Newton Cerebral Wire Guides (LT),
Newton Cerebral Wire Guides (LLT),
Bentson Cerebral Wire Guides,
Bentson Plus Cerebral Wire Guides,
Double Flexible Tipped Wire Guides,
Amplatz Tapered Movable Core Wire Guides,
Tapered Tefcor Movable Core Wire Guides,
Rosen Curved Wire Guides,
Lunderquist Extra Stiff Wire Guides,

Amplatz Ultra Stiff Wire Guides,
Amplatz Extra Stiff Wire Guides,
Amplatz Stiff Wire Guides,
Coon Interventional Wire Guides,
Lunderquist-Ring Torque Wire Guides,
McNamara Renal Exchange Wire Guides,
Graduate Measuring Wire Guides,
Torq-Flex Wire Guides—Australian Modification,
Cope Mandril Wire Guides,
Shorty Wire Guides—TFE Coated,
Roadrunner Extra-Support Wire Guides,
Disposable Reuter Tip Deflecting Wire Guides,
    and Reuter Tip Deflecting Wire Guides
(Courtesy Cook Inc., Bloomington, IN)

TABLE 3-1

Indicators and Thresholds for Complications in Diagnostic Arteriography

Department Indicators	Reported Rates (%)	Major Adverse Event Threshold (%)
Puncture site complications		
Hematoma (requiring transfusion, surgery, or delayed discharge)	0.0–0.68	0.5
Occlusion	0.0–0.76	0.2
Pseudoaneurysm/arteriovenous fistula	0.04–0.2	0.2
Catheter-induced complications (other than puncture site)		
Distal emboli	0.0–0.10	0.5
Arterial dissection/subintimal passage	0.43	0.5
Subintimal injection of contrast	0.0–0.44	0.5
Major contrast reactions	0.0–3.58	0.5
Contrast-media-associated nephrotoxicity	0.2–1.4	0.2

catheter pulmonary angiography result in high radiation dosage of 3.3 to 17.3 (mean 7.1) mSv, substantially higher than that expected with CT angiography of 2.2 to 6.0 (mean 4.2) mSv (14). However, radiation dose reduction remains a challenge in coronary CT angiography, as described in other chapters. For peripheral vessels, measured cumulative dose of a CT angiogram of the abdomen, pelvis, and lower extremities has been reported to be as high as 15 to 20 or as low as 1.6 to 3.9 (mean 2.7) mSv, compared to a dose of 6.4 to 16.0 (mean 11) for catheter angiography (13).

As for convenience to the patient, a diagnostic catheter angiogram is usually completed in less than an hour. However, in preparation for the procedure, most patients undergo laboratory blood tests and receive intravenous sedatives. This means that they need to fast for at least 6 hours before the procedure and may have to pay a preliminary visit or else wait several hours for laboratory test results to be available. After a venous catheterization, only an hour or two of supine recovery is necessary for a common femoral venous access, and even less for internal jugular or brachial. However, after arterial catheterization, most practitioners still recommend a 6-hour recovery with the patient supine and immobile, universally considered by patients to be the worst part of any procedure. With the availability of arterial closure devices, the recovery can be substantially shortened to an hour or so, but these devices carry their own risks for complications, including hemorrhage and hematoma, pseudoaneurysm, stenosis or occlusion, device embolization, and infection (15).

Finally CT and MR angiography, because of their lesser requirement for intensive physician and nursing participation in the acquisition of the images, cost significantly less than diagnostic conventional angiography (16–20).

UTILIZATION

Cross-sectional Imaging as a Preferred Diagnostic Tool

Although complications and convenience are important, the most compelling reason for less invasive cross-sectional imaging to have replaced catheter angiography for diagnostic procedures is the greater diagnostic power (Table 3-2). The specific features of cross-sectional imaging that result in this diagnostic power include 3D rather than projectional imaging of the vessel lumen, better characterization of vessel wall morphology, greater diagnostic characterization of nonvascular structures and tissues, and greater sensitivity to contrast enhancement.

Conventional catheter angiography yields only projectional images with little 3D information. For instance, when assessing vessel lumen diameter in a stenosis, a radially asymmetric lesion could result in gross inaccuracy (Fig. 3-7). Flow dynamics, as described by Poiseuille's law, are a function of

TABLE 3-2

Major Advantages of Cross-sectional Versus Catheter Angiography

1. Lesser risk of complications
2. Convenience to patient
3. Greater diagnostic power
   A. 3D display and analysis
   B. Vessel wall characterization
   C. Portrayal of extravascular structures
   D. Greater sensitivity to contrast enhancement, accumulation
4. Lower cost

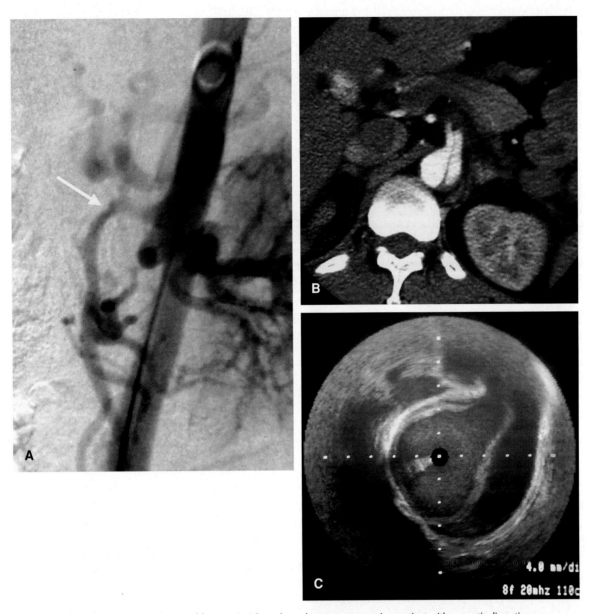

FIGURE 3-7 Asymmetric vessel lumen. A: A lateral true-lumen aortogram in a patient with an aortic dissection shows contrast filling both main renal arteries, the celiac axis, and the superior mesenteric artery (SMA). A mild stenosis of the SMA is seen approximately 2 cm distal to its origin (*arrow*). The diameter of the first 2 cm appears normal, but the contrast column appears attenuated, suggesting effacement of the vessel. CT angiogram **(B)** and intravascular ultrasound (IVUS) **(C)** at the level of the SMA origin shows the aortic dissection flap extending into the SMA. The craniocaudal dimension of the vessel is essentially normal, but the transverse diameter is reduced by about 50%. The false lumen of the SMA is a blind sac without a re-entry tear, containing some thrombus.

the vessel diameter to the fourth power. The traditional guidelines grading severity of stenoses assume that the cross section of the vessel is consistently circular. Deviations from radial symmetry can greatly increase turbulence. Even when catheter angiography is performed with multiple oblique projections, the irregular irregularity of typical atherosclerotic disease and its effect on hemodynamics is probably underestimated.

Another advantage of 3D imaging over projectional imaging is the ability to elongate tortuosity and to untangle overlapping vessels. Redundant, tortuous vessels with focal abnormalities are difficult to image by any modality, but acquiring a 3D data set essentially performs an infinite number of oblique projections simultaneously. Finding the optimal projection to portray an aneurysmal neck, for instance, frequently requires multiple iterative runs during catheter angiography, whereas all of these data are intrinsic to the data set produced by one series of CT or MR angiography (Figs. 3-8–3-10).

(*text continues on page 100*)

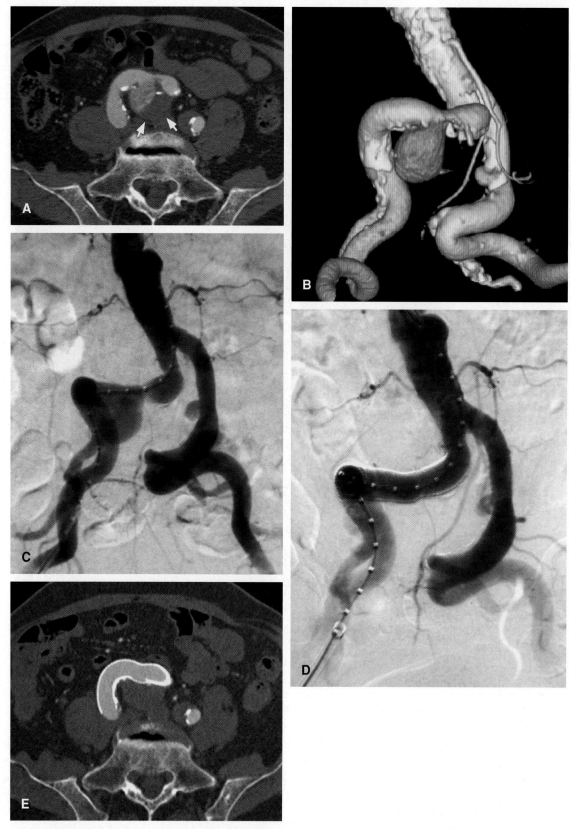

FIGURE 3-8 A three-dimensional depiction of the neck of an aneurysm arising from tortuous vessels. Treatment options for a symptomatic right common iliac artery saccular aneurysm included embolization and stent-graft exclusion. An axial image **(A)** and an oblique volume rendering **(B)** from a CT angiogram revealed a wide neck with adequate length landing areas proximal and distal, and a total aneurysmal diameter of 4.4 cm, including mural thrombus (*arrows*). Anteroposterior catheter angiogram **(C)** using a marker (measuring) catheter confirmed location of aortic and iliac bifurcations and marked tortuosity. However, the neck of the aneurysm is not well depicted, and the total size of the aneurysm is severely underestimated by this lumenogram. Repeat catheter angiogram **(D)** and follow-up CT angiogram **(E)** after stent-graft exclusion.

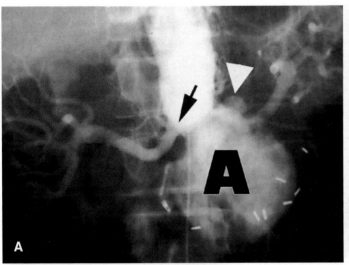

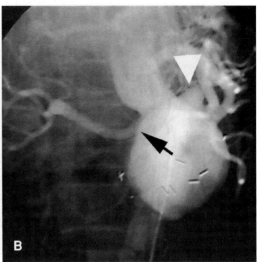

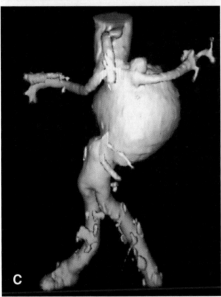

FIGURE 3-9 Overlapping branch arteries over an aortic aneurysm. A: Unsubtracted screen-film anteroposterior catheter angiogram demonstrates an abdominal aortic aneurysm. While unsubtracted screen-film techniques are now obsolete, the challenge of differentiating overlapping structures on projectional images is effectively illustrated. The aneurysm neck projects below the left renal artery origin (*black arrow*), but the locations of the superior mesenteric and right renal arteries are poorly demonstrated. A small saccular aneurysm (*white arrowhead*) originates in the region of the left renal artery origin but is also poorly localized due to the overlap with the aorta and this projection. **B:** Shallow right anterior oblique catheter angiogram results in an ambiguous presentation of the right renal artery origin (*black arrow*), as this projection creates an appearance that suggests that the left renal artery origin is from the wall of the aortic aneurysm. The locations of the superior mesenteric and left renal artery origins as well as the smaller saccular aneurysm (*white arrowhead*) are again ambiguously displayed. Two additional catheter injections obtained with other obliquities (not shown) failed to clarify these key anatomic relationships prior to surgical repair. **C:** Shaded surface display from a single detector-row CT angiogram maps the origins of these overlapping structures. The right renal artery originates above the aneurysm, but the left renal artery originates from the aneurysm wall. The small saccular aneurysm originates at the junction of the posterior wall of the left renal artery with the aortic aneurysm. The superior mesenteric artery origin is well above the aneurysm neck. These findings were confirmed in the operating room, where a cross clamp was placed above the left but below the right renal arteries, and the aortic aneurysm was bypassed with a graft. The proximal aspect of the left renal artery along with the small saccular aneurysm was resected and the remaining renal artery transplanted onto the aortic graft. (Reprinted from Rubin GD. Three-dimensional helical CT angiography. *Radiographics* 1994;14:905–912, with permission.)

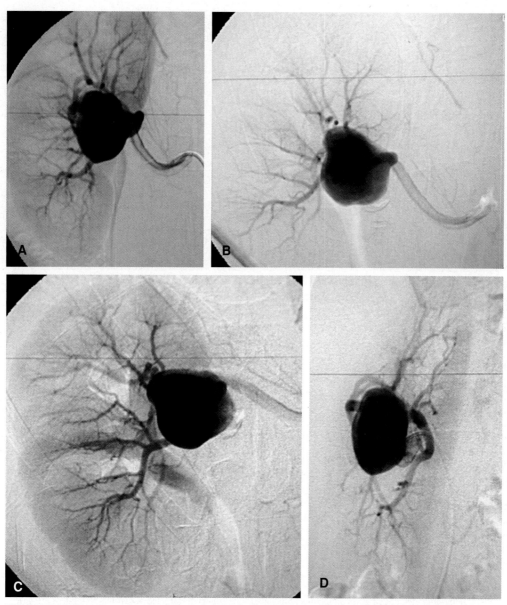

FIGURE 3-10 Treatment planning prior to repair of a renal artery aneurysm. A–D: Four separate catheter injections performed with four different obliquities illustrate a large renal artery aneurysm. Although the aneurysm is clearly demonstrated, it had been previously identified with sonography (not shown). The purpose of the imaging test was to evaluate the number and location of feeding (afferent) and draining (efferent) arteries and their relationship to the aneurysm sac and renal parenchyma for planning repair. Because of the substantial overlap of the afferent and efferent arteries with the aneurysm and renal parenchymal blush, these relationships cannot be ascertained. Cinematic playback and optimization of digital subtraction angiographic runs increases diagnostic power, but limitations in archiving capabilities have historically precluded extensive post-processing of data-intensive catheter angiography. As a result optimal DSA views may not be available in the patient record if they were not created at the time of image capture.

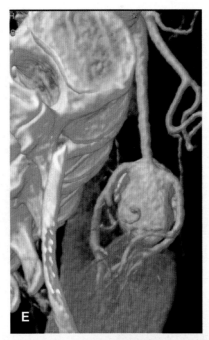

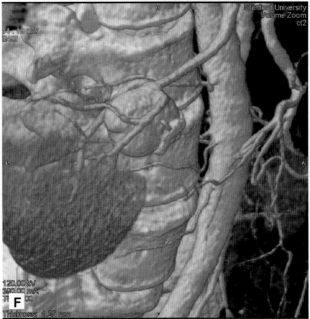

FIGURE 3-10 Continued E, F: Volume renderings created from a single intravenous injection for this 4-row multidetector-row computed tomography (MDCT) angiogram clearly illustrate the single afferent and two efferent arteries originating from the anterior and posterior walls of the medial aspect of the aneurysm. No branches are observed lateral to these primary efferent branches, which supply the anterior and posterior halves of the kidney, respectively. These findings were confirmed in the operating room, where an ex vivo repair of the aneurysm was successfully performed.

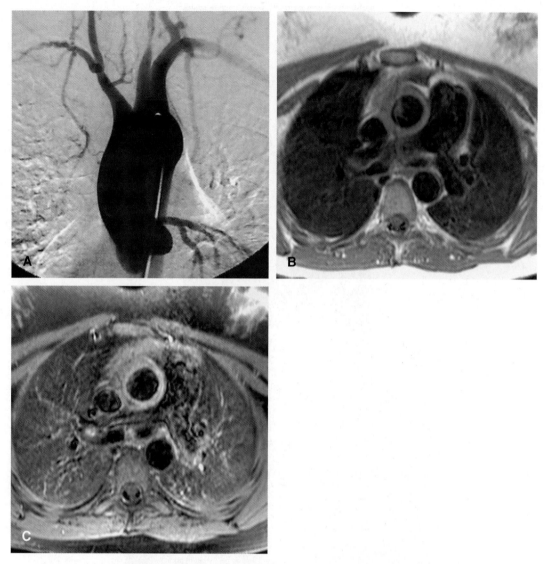

FIGURE 3-11 Imaging of the vessel wall. A: Catheter flush aortogram in the anteroposterior projection in a young female patient showed typical findings of Takayasu arteritis, with severe narrowing of all of the supra-aortic branches. The aorta itself is of normal diameter in this projection. T_1- **(B)** and T_2-weighted **(C)** MR images confirm normal diameter of the aortic lumen but reveal marked wall thickening and edema, representing active vasculitis.

In addition, the imaging of injected contrast yields only a *lumenogram*, yielding limited information about the vessel wall. Although sometimes beyond the limits of spatial resolution, characterization of vessel walls is of particular importance in cases of inflammation, dissection, and intramural hematoma. Frequently, corroborating data can be obtained through laboratory blood tests, physical examination, and obtaining a detailed history including family and travel history. These data can have profound influence on therapeutic decision making, such

as in the patient with a suspected vasculitis (Fig. 3-11), intramural hematoma (Fig. 3-12), or connective tissue disorder (Fig. 3-13).

Aside from vessel wall characterization, cross-sectional imaging also affords analysis of potentially crucial extravascular structures. Some examples include musculoskeletal impingement, such as in arterial or venous thoracic outlet syndrome (Paget-Schrötter syndrome), iliac vein compression (May-Thurner syndrome), popliteal entrapment (Figure 3-14), and shoulder girdle aneurysms in

(text continues on page 105)

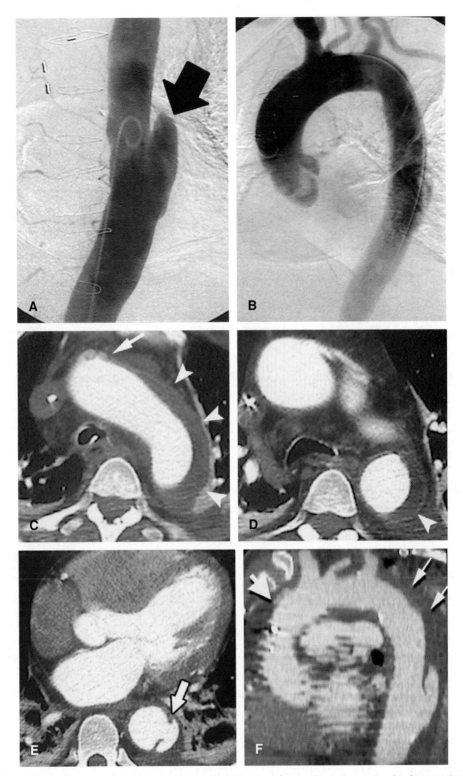

FIGURE 3-12 Imaging of the vessel wall in a 77-year-old patient with acute chest pain. A: Conventional catheter angiogram obtained with contrast medium injection in the descending thoracic aorta demonstrates a contour abnormality (*arrow*), presumed to represent a giant penetrating ulcer. The luminal dimension above the ulcer is smaller than below the ulcer, suggesting luminal compression by an intramural hematoma cephalad to the ulcer. **B:** Conventional catheter angiograms obtained with contrast medium injection in the ascending thoracic aorta in multiple obliquities does not demonstrate evidence for ascending aortic or aortic arch involvement. **C–E:** Transverse CT angiogram sections provide direct demonstration of an intramural hematoma (*arrowheads*) from above the ulcer (*outlined arrow in E*) cephalad to involve the aortic arch. A subtle region of extraluminal contrast medium extravasation is observed in the proximal arch (*thin arrow in C*) to communicate with the intramural hematoma. **F:** Curved planar reformation illustrates the relationship between the ascending aortic intimal discontinuity (*wide arrow*), the intramural hematoma (*thin arrows*), and the descending aortic ulcer. Limitations of projection and low contrast delectability hinder conventional catheter angiography in correctly characterizing the nature and extent of this lesion. (Reprinted from Rubin GD. Helical CT angiography of the thoracic aorta. *J Thorac Imaging* 1997;12:128–149, with permission.)

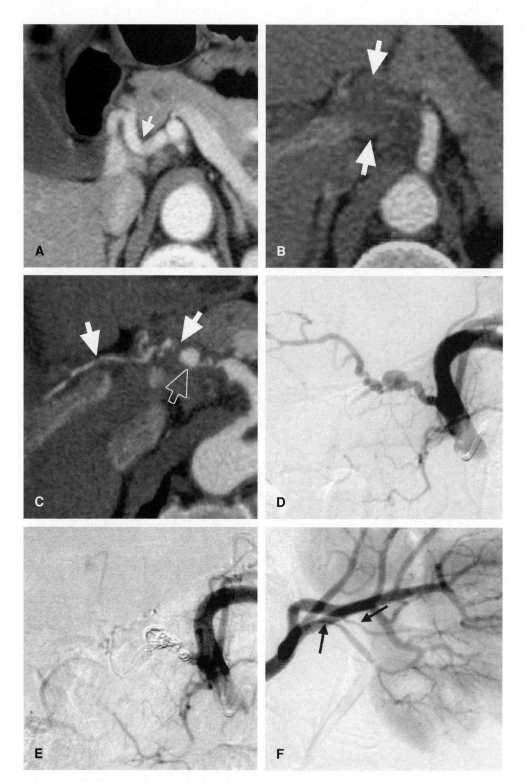

FIGURE 3-13 Imaging of the perivascular space. A: Transverse image from CT scan in a patient with a spontaneous renal infarction showed a normal common hepatic artery (*arrow*). The patient had no history of trauma or illness and had absolutely no laboratory abnormalities (normal white blood cell count, normal erythrocyte sedimentation rate, normal C-reactive protein, normal autoantibody panel, normal blood culture, etc.). **B:** Follow-up two weeks later revealed near occlusion of the hepatic artery and new appearance of low-attenuation material surrounding the artery (*arrows*), interpreted without benefit of the comparison study as a pancreatic neoplasm. **C:** Curved planar reconstruction of a CT angiogram performed 3 weeks after the previous scan demonstrates interval decrease in soft tissue mass, suggesting that it was a hematoma, possibly from a ruptured spontaneous dissection. Note narrowing and discontinuity of the artery (*white arrows*) and development of a small aneurysm (*open arrow*). **D:** Selective celiac arteriogram showed patency but corkscrew tortuosity and aneurysm of the artery, which was coil embolized, preserving the gastroduodenal artery (**E**) for the presumptive diagnosis of segmental arterial mediolysis. **F:** A renal infarction previously identified with CT (not shown) was probably due to other dissections or intramural hematomas within renal arterial branches, seen in the healing phase as long-segment stenoses (*arrows*), which were too subtle for the CT angiograms to resolve.

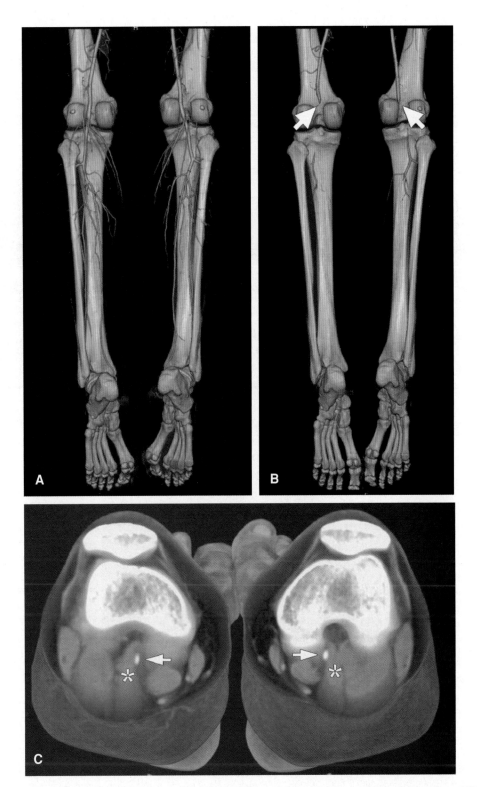

FIGURE 3-14 Popliteal entrapment syndrome in an athlete. A: Posterior volume rendering from a 16-row MDCT angiogram obtained in a 19-year-old collegiate basketball player with calf pain when running the floor demonstrates normal popliteal arteries and run-off to the feet. **B:** Taking advantage of an old catheter angiography technique, a second MDCT angiogram was performed during active dorsiflexion against resistance, demonstrating bilateral popliteal artery occlusions above the knee (*arrows*). **C:** Volume rendering from a position cephalad to the imaging volume demonstrates the aberrant position of the medial head of the gastrocnemius muscles bilaterally (*), displacing the popliteal arteries (*arrows*) medially and occluding them during forced contraction.

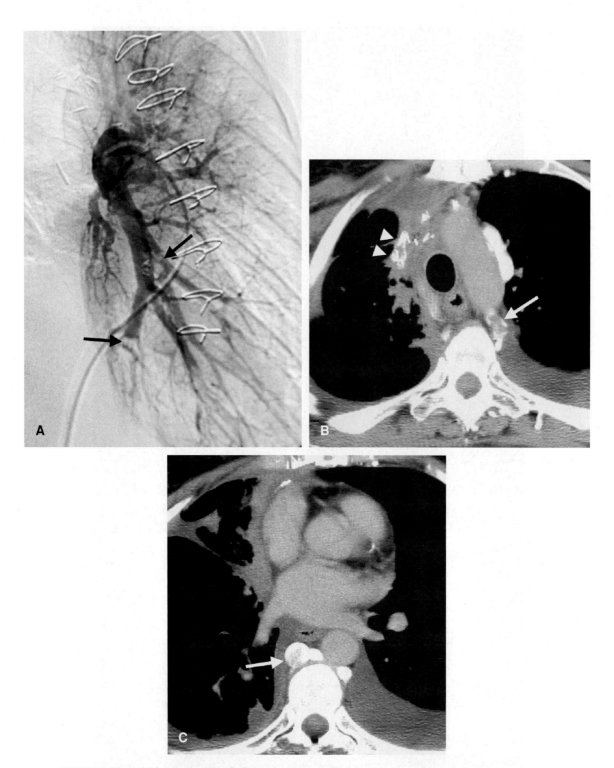

FIGURE 3-15 Multiple corroborative findings in a patient with acute shortness of breath. A: Catheter pulmonary angiogram demonstrated multiple left lower lobe filling defects diagnostic of acute pulmonary embolism (*arrows*). Lower extremity ultrasound examination was unrevealing, but CT scan the same day showed filling defects (*arrows*) in the left superior intercostal (**B**) and azygos veins (**C**) as well as sequelae of a right upper lobe carcinoma (*arrowheads in* **B**), which may have predisposed the patient to hypercoagulability.

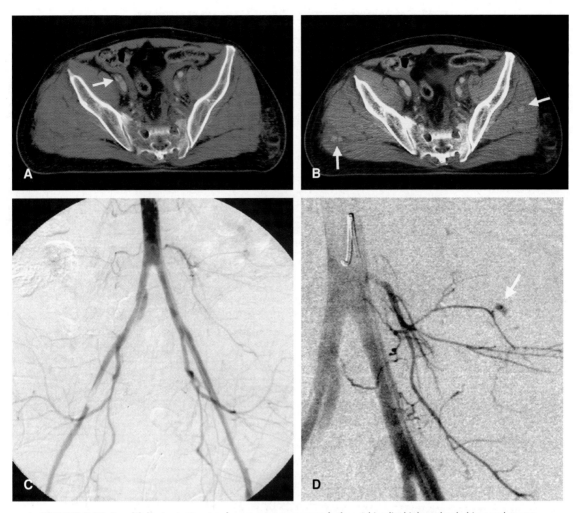

FIGURE 3-16 Sensitivity to contrast enhancement or accumulation. A bicyclist hit by a drunk driver underwent CT scan because of hemodynamic instability and enlarging pelvic hematomas. **A:** Arterial phase image through the pelvis showed dissection of the right external iliac artery without extravasation. **B:** Venous-phase image at same level showed subtle areas of hemorrhage in and around the gluteal muscles (*arrows*). **C:** Catheter angiography confirmed traumatic dissection but revealed no active arterial extravasation except of a branch of the left L4 lumbar artery (*arrow* in **D**), which was embolized with Gelfoam slurry and coils. The internal iliac arteries were also embolized empirically because of the findings on CT scan.

throwing athletes. Other conditions where cross-sectional imaging data influence vascular diagnosis include neoplasm, where direct involvement of vessels can be shown by CT, MRI, and ultrasound. In cases of invasion, as well as in cases of a paraneoplastic hypercoagulable state (Trousseau syndrome), cross-sectional imaging can reveal not only the effect but also the cause (Fig. 3-15).

Both CT angiography and MR angiography also exceed catheter angiography in sensitivity to contrast enhancement and contrast accumulation. This is especially useful for identifying small trickles of blood such as in an endoleak after endovascular repair of an aneurysm (21) or in hemorrhage,

for instance, in a trauma victim or a gastrointestinal bleeder. Nuclear medicine studies may offer even higher sensitivity but can be frustratingly nonspecific for spatial localization. In most cases, a preceding diagnostic cross-sectional study does not preclude catheter angiography and therapy but allows a customized, targeted approach (Fig. 3-16).

Finally, the intravenous delivery of contrast agents for both CT and MR angiography results in near simultaneous and prolonged opacification of all patent arteries in the body. When occluded arteries are reconstituted by collaterals with distant origins, they can be time consuming and potentially risky to locate (Fig. 3-17). Moreover, when

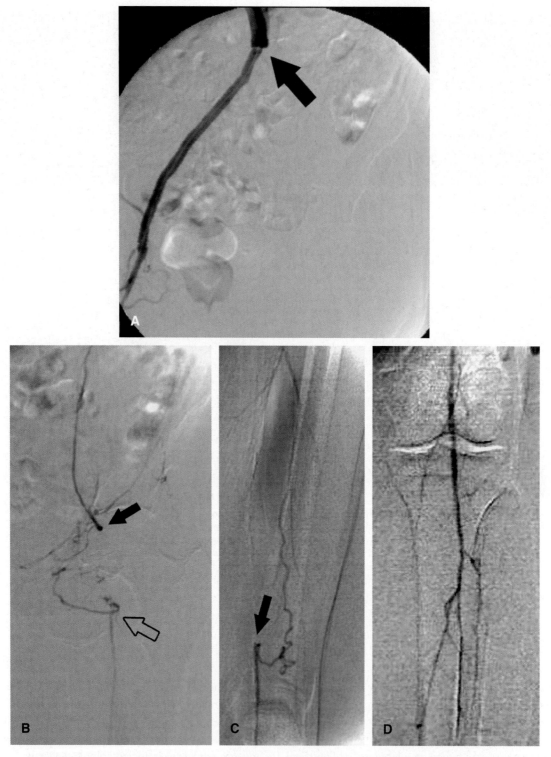

FIGURE 3-17 Opacification of arterial reconstitution—procedural complexity and patient risk. A 78-year-old woman presented with left lower extremity claudication and diminished left femoral pulses several years after aortob-ifemoral bypass graft placement. A conventional catheter angiogram was requested to confirm graft occlusion and to identify the site of distal reconstitution of the left lower extremity arterial system. **A:** Anteroposterior conventional catheter angiogram demonstrates occlusion of the graft at the origin of the left iliac limb (*arrow*). Injections of contrast medium into the distal abdominal aorta failed to opacify the left lower extremity arteries, so the left internal mammary artery was catheterized and injected. Images through the left groin **(B)** demonstrated filling of the left inferior epigas-tric artery with collateral supply to the profunda femoral artery, which in turn reconstitutes the popliteal artery above the knee **(C)** with patency of the proximal aspect of all three crural arteries **(D)**. These images also show the compro-mise of conventional angiographic image quality when optimization of acquisition parameters and of digital subtrac-tion are not carefully performed.

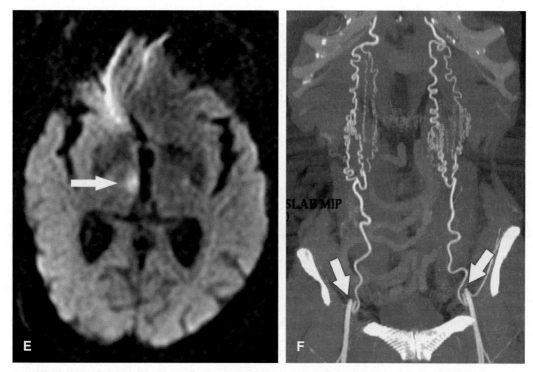

FIGURE 3-17 Continued Following the procedure, the patient experienced left-sided weakness. A diffusion-weighted brain MRI obtained 12 hours after the procedure demonstrated an acute thalamic infarction (*arrow*) **(E)**. This complication could have been avoided if noninvasive imaging were performed with MR or CT. **F:** Frontal maximum intensity projection (MIP) from a CT angiogram in a different patient who had distal abdominal aortic and bilateral iliac arterial occlusions demonstrates internal mammary and inferior epigastric arterial collaterals reconstituting the femoral arteries (*arrows*) without requiring internal mammary arterial catheterization.

reconstitution is by multiple collateral pathways, all sources of reconstitution may be difficult to identify with the multiple selective conventional angiographic injections. The benefit of the prolonged opacification resulting from 20- to 30-second intravenous contrast medium injections for CT or MR angiograms is that arteries distal to occlusions will opacify via collaterals with varying flow rates. During a rapid conventional angiographic injection, these varying flow rates may result in substantial intra-arterial dilution of the contrast medium by unopacified blood, hindering target arterial visualization (Fig. 3-18).

Catheter Angiography as a Preferred Diagnostic Tool

The remaining diagnostic advantages of catheter angiography over less invasive cross-sectional imaging reflect several technical issues (Table 3-3). First, catheter angiography allows real time and cinematic imaging. Second, the spatial resolution of angiography still exceeds that of noninvasive methods. Third, a contrast bolus can be more temporally and spatially defined, allowing dynamic rather than vascular pool imaging. Fourth, the projectional image, although compressed and limited in volumetric resolution, can portray information instantaneously from a large field of tens of liters of tissue.

Fifth, metallic artifacts may be more easily avoided. Sixth, immediate interpretation of acquired images facilitates repetition and modification of technique until optimal results are obtained. In time, many of these advantages will also be equalized by technological advances in noninvasive imaging.

The ability to perform real time and cinematic imaging is the most dramatically exploited advantage in catheter-based vascular imaging. The pace of blood flow is often as important a diagnostic criterion as the morphologic appearance of the vessel. Even direction of flow can be difficult to ascertain from a CT- or MR-derived blood pool study (Fig. 3-19).

TABLE 3-3

Major Advantages of Catheter Versus Cross-sectional Angiography

1. Real-time and/or cinematic imaging; greater temporal resolution
2. Greater spatial resolution
3. Spatially and temporally defined contrast bolus
4. Simultaneous panoramic, summation view of a large volume
5. Usually lesser metallic and beam-hardening artifacts
6. Immediate interpretation of images; repetition, modification for optimization

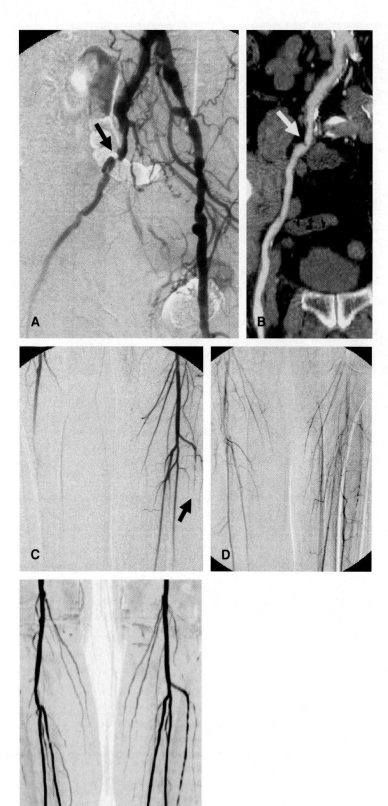

FIGURE 3-18 Asymmetric flow rates in lower extremity arteries. A: Conventional catheter angiogram of the iliac and femoral arteries from a contrast medium injection into the distal abdominal aorta. There is a high-grade stenosis in the proximal right external iliac artery (*arrow*), which slows flow distally, resulting in diminished opacification of the right femoral artery relative to the left. **B:** Curved planar reformation from a 4-row CT angiogram obtained during a 50-second-long intravenous contrast medium injection also shows the right external iliac artery stenosis (*arrow*), but distal opacification is similar to that seen proximal to the stenosis. **C:** Anteroposterior conventional angiogram obtained over the knees from the same contrast medium injection as in **(A)** demonstrates faster contrast medium delivery to the left popliteal and proximal crural arteries than the right, which is minimally opacified proximally and not opacified distally. The left anterior tibial artery appears occluded approximately 4 cm distal to its origin (*arrow*). **D:** Same projection as in **(C)** obtained 13 seconds later and optimized for visualization of the right lower extremity demonstrates the markedly delayed filling of the right crural arteries. The opacification is poor compared with the left, which is due to intra-arterial dilution of the contrast bolus. The right anterior tibial artery appears occluded, but the left anterior tibial artery, while highly diseased, is demonstrated to fill over a greater distance than seen 13 seconds earlier in **(C)**. **E:** MIP of the CTA with an inverted grayscale demonstrates equal opacification of the right and left popliteal and crural arteries due to the use of a prolonged (50-second) intravenous contrast medium injection. The prolonged, generalized delivery of contrast medium reduces the likelihood of intra-arterial dilution. The diseased left anterior tibial artery is opacified greater than on the conventional angiogram. (Reprinted from Rubin GD, Schmidt AJ, Logan LJ, et al. Multi-detector row CT angiography of lower extremity arterial inflow and runoff: initial experience. *Radiology* 2001;221:146–158, with permission.)

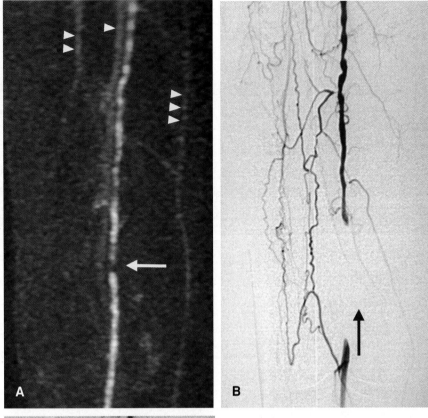

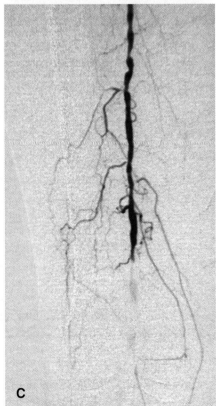

FIGURE 3-19 A 72-year-old diabetic man with a gangrenous right third toe, upper gastrointestinal hemorrhage, and chronic renal failure was evaluated for peripheral arterial occlusive disease. **A:** Gadolinium-enhanced MR angiogram revealed short, focal stenosis of the superficial femoral artery (SFA) near the adductor canal (*arrow*). Superficial femoral (*one arrowhead*), profunda femoral (*two arrowheads*), and greater saphenous (*three arrowheads*) veins are also enhanced. **B:** Selective catheter arteriogram of the SFA with injection into the common femoral artery showed filling of the popliteal artery from profunda femoral collaterals and retrograde flow into the distal SFA (*arrow*). **C:** Selective catheter arteriogram with injection into the SFA confirmed complete occlusion. This was successfully treated by percutaneous atherectomy. Cinematic imaging and higher spatial resolution of catheter angiography allowed correct diagnosis of complete occlusion and determination of direction of flow in each femoral arterial segment.

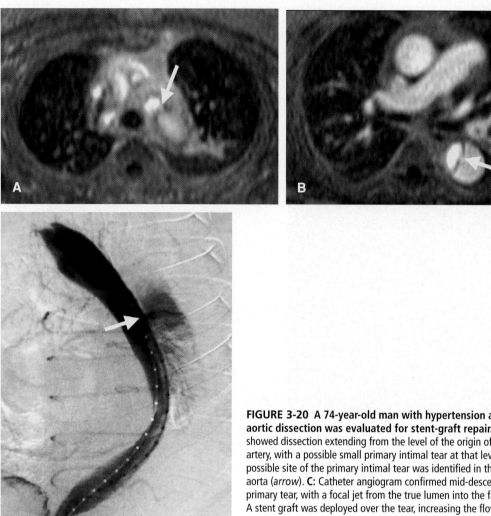

FIGURE 3-20 A 74-year-old man with hypertension and an acute Type B aortic dissection was evaluated for stent-graft repair. A: MR angiogram showed dissection extending from the level of the origin of the left subclavian artery, with a possible small primary intimal tear at that level (*arrow*). **B:** Another possible site of the primary intimal tear was identified in the descending thoracic aorta (*arrow*). **C:** Catheter angiogram confirmed mid-descending thoracic aortic primary tear, with a focal jet from the true lumen into the false lumen (*arrow*). A stent graft was deployed over the tear, increasing the flow into the collapsed true lumen and into compromised visceral branches. Catheter angiography with spatially and temporally defined contrast bolus and rapid sequence cinematic imaging facilitated correct identification and treatment of the primary intimal tear.

Competitive flow in vascular beds with multiple inlets, reversal of flow in collateral vessels, and relative tempos of flow in different vessels can all be assessed by cinematic imaging. Frame rates of modern angiography units can be as fast as 30 images per second, allowing temporal resolution of beating hearts, vessel wall pulsatility and capacitance, dissection flap mobility, and the turbulence of a poststenotic jet (Fig. 3-20). Similarly, the differentiation between arteries and veins is usually trivial, reflecting the continuum of blood flow into and out of the targeted anatomical site (Figs. 3-21–3-23). Real time imaging also serves this patient population particularly well, allowing quick imaging and recognition of clinically pertinent adverse events such as dissections, ruptures, emboli, and thromboses as well as desired outcomes such as resolution of such pathology.

The spatial resolution of projectional angiography still exceeds that of CT and MR (Fig. 3-24). Although submillimeter in-plane resolution is the standard for modern cross-sectional imaging, projectional angiography can resolve up to 4 line pairs per millimeter (Fig. 3-25). Such resolution, although not crucial for macroscopic anatomic structures, can be clinically crucial in small vessels, whereas an angioplasty based on inaccurate measurements can result in insufficient resolution of an obstruction, or worse, injury to a vessel. Measurements using conventional catheter angiography can be accurate when combined with careful techniques to avoid measurement inaccuracies caused by parallax and geometric distortion. Fine spatial resolution is further hampered in CT and MR by heavy calcification, which can be effectively compensated for by digital subtraction during catheter angiography (Fig. 3-26). Nevertheless for some measurements, such as luminal path lengths and arterial curvature, volumetric measurements from CT are superior to

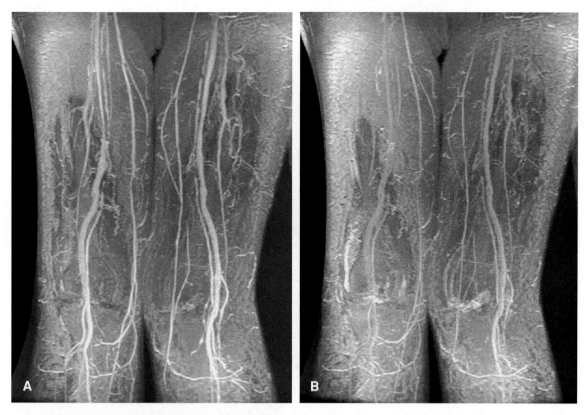

FIGURE 3-21 Venous contamination of MR arteriography images. Early **(A)** and late **(B)** MIP images from a gadolinium-enhanced MR angiogram of the lower extremities showed filling of numerous veins, complicating the interpretation of the arteriogram.

projection-based measurements with conventional angiography (22,23).

The administration of contrast into a peripheral vein for CT or MR angiography, although substantially less invasive and risky than into an artery, also results in a whole-body bolus, which lacks spatial and temporal definition. Although the path of venously administered contrast usually takes a very predictable route to the right heart, lungs, left heart, and peripheral arteries, only a fraction of the administered bolus is in the right place at the right time to be imaged. Selective catheterization allows not only elimination of nontarget contrast administration outside of the field of view, but also minimizes background contrast enhancement within the field of view (Fig. 3-27). Thus, anatomically targeted studies using catheter angiography can usually be performed using less contrast medium than a noninvasive study requiring systemic administration of contrast medium. In case of renal insufficiency or contrast medium allergy, alternative contrast agents including gadolinium chelates and carbon dioxide can be substituted, a technique not as effective in whole-body administrations because of the poorer radio-

opacity of gadolinium agents and the pattern of distribution of injected carbon dioxide. In extreme cases, no nephrotoxic or allergenic contrast media need be administered at all with the exclusive use of carbon dioxide and intravascular ultrasound (Fig. 3-28).

Projectional images can be difficult to interpret, particularly because of the lack of resolution along the axis of the image beam. Nevertheless, panoramic images and images of structures that are not confined to one plane are frequently the most useful when a large field of view and volume of tissue are simultaneously pictured. Guide wires, catheters, drains, stents, bones, and orthopedic and other surgical hardware are examples of structures and devices where projectional images displaying the entire length of the target subject may be preferable to the hundreds of cross-sectional images that need to be compiled to reconstruct the target (Fig. 3-29). Also, because of the relative simplicity of the technique of generating a projectional image, akin to casting a shadow on a wall, the presence of metal hardware is not a great obstacle. Beam hardening and susceptibility artifacts are not issues, and the patient and/or imaging equipment can be positioned to avoid superimposition of the metal and

(*text continues on page 120*)

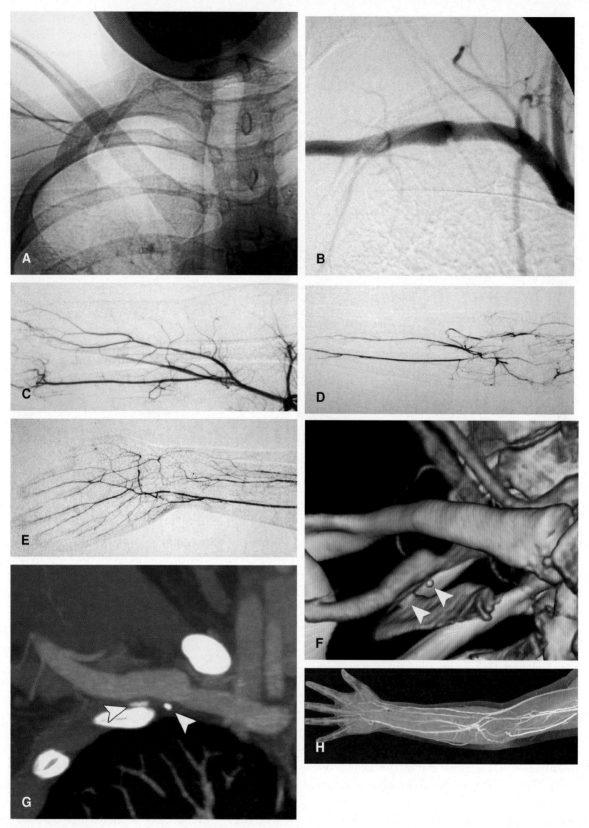

FIGURE 3-22 Venous contamination of CT arteriography images. A 17-year-old high school tennis player suffered ischemic symptoms of her arm, including coolness and fatigue. **A:** Fluoroscopic spot image confirmed cervical rib extending into the region of the thoracic inlet. **B:** Selective subclavian arteriogram showed mild aneurysmal dilatation with luminal irregularity. **C–E:** Run-off showed chronic occlusions of the brachial, distal radial, medial and lateral first digital, and lateral third digital arteries, probably from chronic emboli. Two years following decompression of her thoracic outlet with resection of the cervical rib, she had recurrent symptoms, and a CT angiogram was obtained. A volume rendering projection **(F)** and an MIP **(G)** demonstrate the persistence of the aneurysmal deformity of the proximal right axillary artery. Remnants of the cervical rib remain (*arrowheads*). An overview MIP image of the run-off following removal of the bones **(H)** demonstrates substantial opacification of arteries and veins, particularly around the elbow, challenging the interpretation of arterial disease. The ability of volume rendering to simultaneously display 3D relationships as well as subtle differences in arterial enhancement through color makes it the preferred technique for assessing this portion of the CT scan.

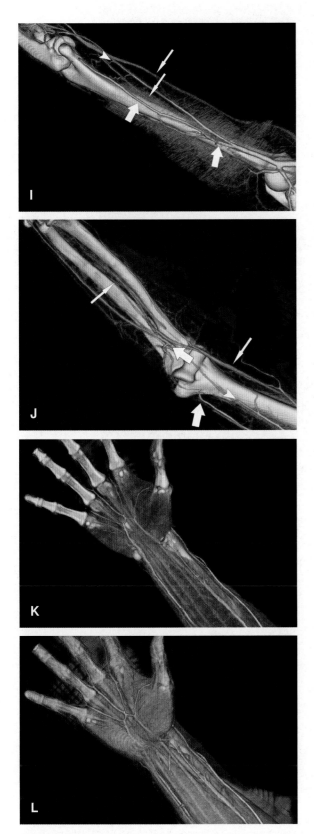

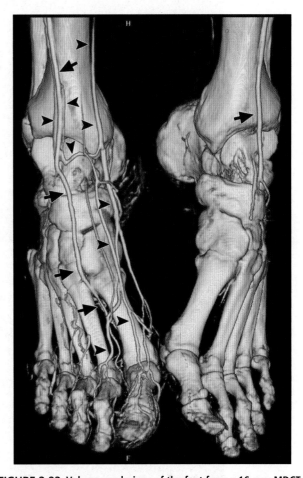

FIGURE 3-23 Volume renderings of the feet from a 16-row MDCT angiogram demonstrate simultaneous opacification of arteries (*arrows*) and veins (*arrowheads*) in the right foot. Arteriovenous shunting, seen in the setting of inflammation and trauma, can complicate separation of arteries and veins. A thorough knowledge of arterial and venous anatomy together with real time manipulation of the 3D data on a workstation helps to overcome this limitation.

FIGURE 3-22 Continued The run-off **(I,J)** demonstrates a diminutive brachial artery terminating proximal to the elbow (*arrowhead*) and a large profunda brachial artery reconstituting the ulnar artery below the elbow (*wide arrows*). Superimposed venous opacification (*narrow arrows*) is substantial and likely secondary to chronic inflammation/ischemia and arteriovenous shunting around the elbow. The use of a proper opacity transfer function and color scale allows the veins to be discriminated from the arteries because the veins are slightly less enhanced and thus rendered with a redder color. **K,L:** Filling of the palmar and digital arteries is demonstrated, but the lower resolution of the CT scan does not allow them to be displayed with the clarity demonstrated on the conventional angiogram **(E)**.

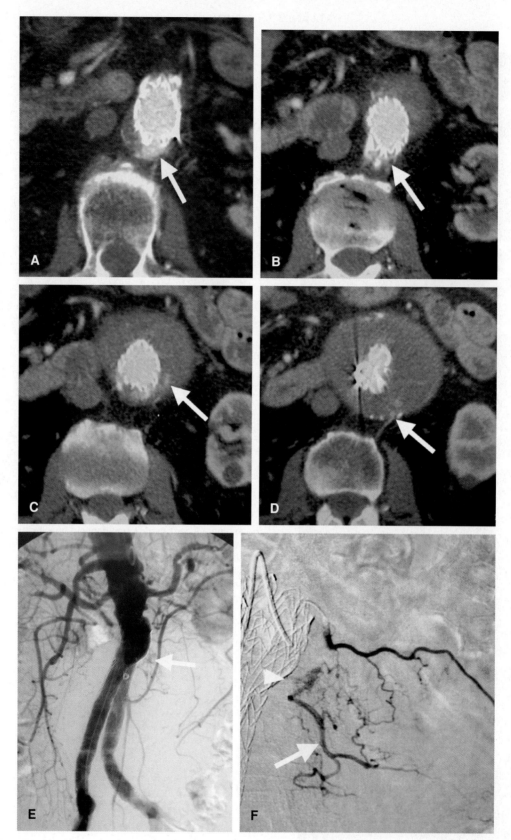

FIGURE 3-24 An 86-year-old man presented with an enlarging abdominal aortic aneurysm despite stent-graft repair two years earlier.
A–D: Transverse CT angiography images suggested a new degenerative ulcer on the posterior wall of the aortic neck, resulting in a Type I endoleak (inadequate seal between device and aortic wall). Flow of blood in the leak was interpreted to be from the infrarenal aorta, around the incomplete seal at the top of the prosthesis, into the aneurysm, and out the lumbar branches (*arrows*). **E:** Catheter flush aortogram confirmed filling of the aneurysm inferior and left of the aortic neck (*arrow*). **F:** Selective catheter angiogram in the ulcer did not demonstrate a Type I leak, but microcatheter selection of the left L2 lumbar artery revealed retrograde filling of the left L3 lumbar artery (*arrow*) and of the aneurysmal sac (*arrowhead*) via microscopic retroperitoneal communications. The tip of the catheter had an outer diameter of 0.8 mm, and the smallest depicted collaterals measured approximately 200 micrometers. This Type II leak was treated with a combination of microcoils and N-butyl-cyanoacrylate glue.

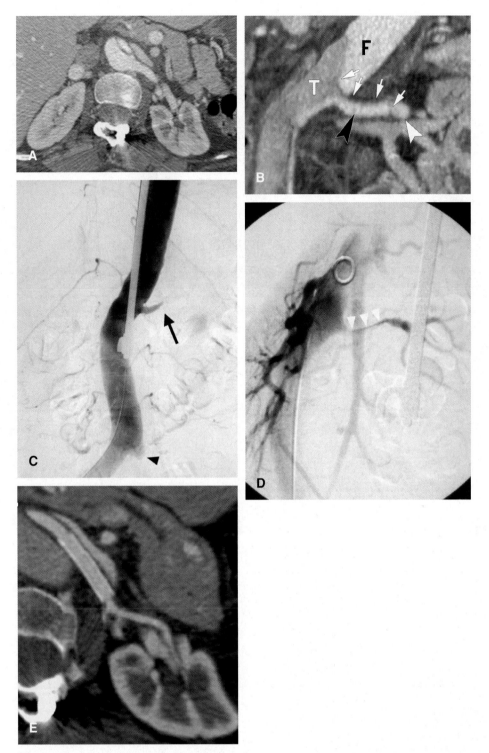

FIGURE 3-25 A 35-year-old woman presented with Marfan syndrome, chronic Type B aortic dissection, and labile hypertension on four antihypertensive medications. A: CT angiogram showed subtle asymmetry in renal parenchymal enhancement, right greater than left. The smaller true lumen fed the right kidney, and the larger false lumen appeared to supply the left kidney. **B:** Coronal curved planar reformation showed false lumen *(F)* supply to the left kidney *(black arrowhead)*. The true lumen *(T)* does not appear to enter the kidney; however, the intimal flap coalesces with the superior margin of the renal artery and terminates in a linear filling defect within the mid renal artery *(white arrows)*. The true lumen is less enhanced than the false lumen at this level because of the relatively delayed nature of this abdominal CT scan, obtained after a cardiac-gated scan of the thoracic aorta was completed. As a result, the peak true luminal enhancement has passed, but the slower flow in the false lumen results in a higher degree of opacification when compared with the true lumen. The distal renal artery *(white arrowhead)* appears to have a similar degree of enhancement as does the false lumen, suggesting that an exit tear might be present at this site with re-entry of flow from the false lumen into the distal renal artery. **C:** False lumen catheter aortogram showed only outflow into the right iliac artery. Extension of dissection into the left renal artery *(arrow)* and left common iliac artery *(arrowhead)* were dead ends with no re-entry tears. **D:** True lumen catheter aortogram in 30-degree left anterior oblique projection showed true lumen supply to the left kidney, with critical narrowing of the left renal artery true lumen *(arrowheads)* by the distended, unopacified false lumen. This was successfully treated with a stent **(E)**. Two factors challenge the CTA interpretation to detect the correct renal arterial physiology—inadequate spatial resolution to resolve the narrow intrarenal arterial true luminal channel and enhancement ambiguities in the distal renal artery caused by slowed delivery of contrast from the true lumen (resulting in a brighter than expected distal renal artery).

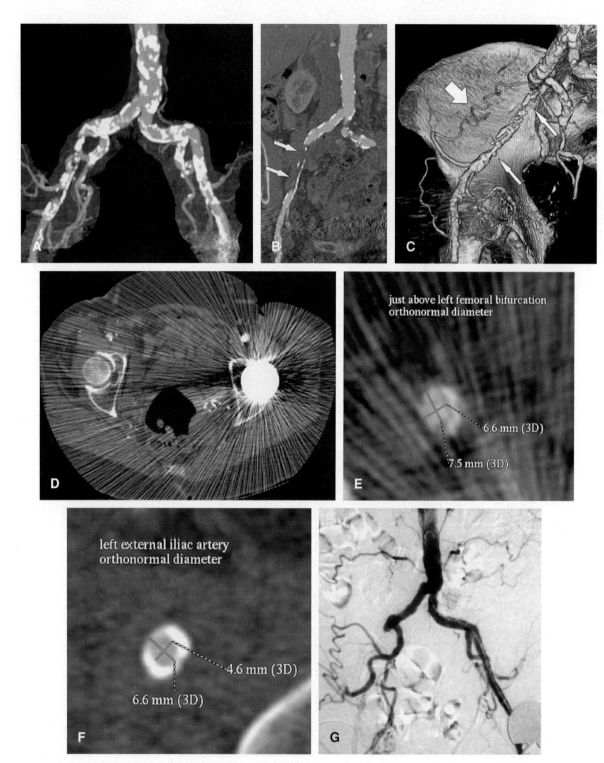

FIGURE 3-26 Beam-hardening artifact from heavy calcification and metallic implant. A: A MIP of CT angiogram performed on a patient with a thoracic aortic aneurysm being evaluated for endovascular repair showed severe calcified atherosclerotic disease in the abdominal aorta and iliac arteries. **B:** A curved planar reformation demonstrates complete occlusion of the proximal right external iliac artery (*arrows*). **C:** A volume rendering displays the external iliac arterial occlusion (*thin arrows*) and a large collateral artery originating from the posterior division of the internal iliac artery and reconstituting the femoral artery (*wide arrow*). **D:** A transverse section through the hip joints reveals a metallic left hip prosthesis, creating substantial spray artifacts throughout the image. **E:** Orthogonal diameter of the common femoral artery was not reliably discernable due to beam-hardening artifact from a hip prosthesis. **F:** Orthogonal diameter of the external iliac artery was measured in a region of maximum calcification. **G:** Catheter angiogram at the time of aneurysm repair effectively subtracted out the calcification. A 24F sheath with an outer diameter of 9.5 mm was passed through the left iliac arteries, although with some difficulty. The overestimation by CT of the dimensions of a dense object such as calcium or a stent strut is sometimes referred to as a *blooming artifact.*

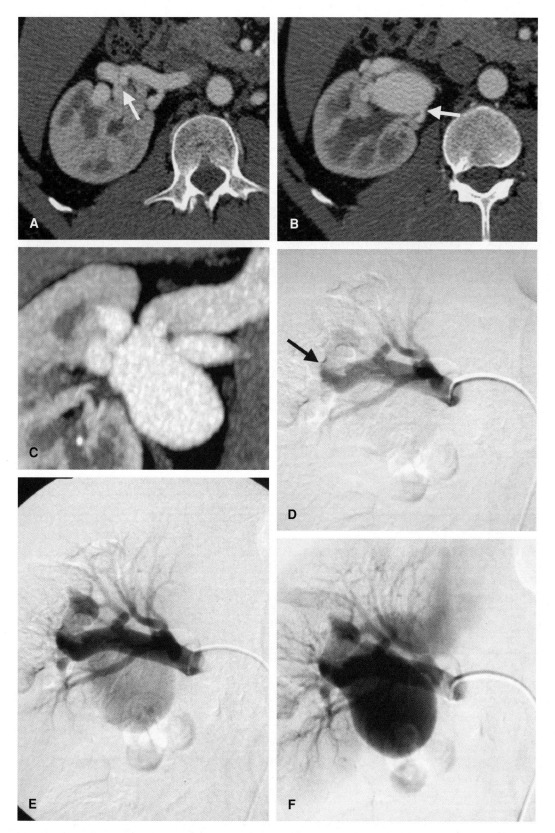

FIGURE 3-27 A 37-year-old man presented with borderline hypertension and a 1-year history of increasing right flank pain. Initial CT scan showed right renal mass. **A,B:** CT angiogram was interpreted as a renal artery aneurysm or fistula, probably fed by anterosuperior **(A)** and inferoposterior **(B)** extrarenal branches of the renal artery. **C:** Numerous reconstructions and reformatted images were inconclusive about identifying the inflow and outflow of the aneurysm, in part because of the rapid and equal opacification of arteries and veins. **D–F:** Selective catheter renal angiogram excluded extrarenal branch supply but instead showed a single, large intrarenal arterial branch supplying a fistula (*arrow*).

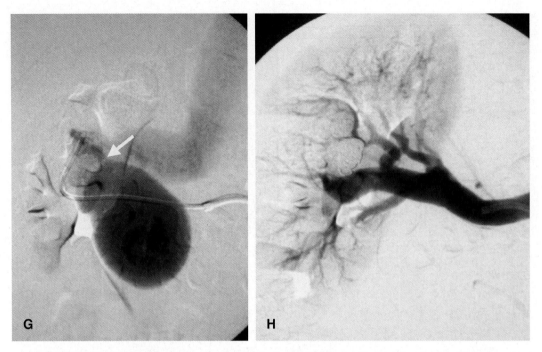

FIGURE 3-27 Continued G: Advancing the catheter through the fistula allowed delineation of a bilobed venous varix with an outflow stenosis (*arrow*), draining into the main renal vein. **H:** The fistula was successfully treated by coil embolization. The sharp temporal definition of the contrast medium bolus and the cinematic imaging of catheter angiography allowed detailed anatomic diagnosis and treatment.

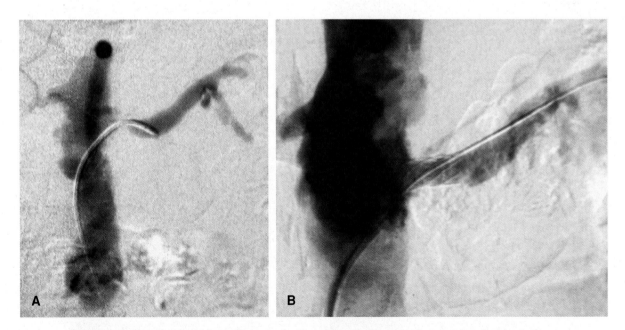

FIGURE 3-28 Renal angiography and intervention in an 82-year-old man with worsening chronic renal insufficiency and MR angiography evidence for a left renal artery stenosis is shown. A: CO_2 selective left renal arteriogram confirmed morphologic stenosis. Hemodynamic measurements revealed a pressure gradient of 72 mmHg systolic, 26 mmHg mean. **B:** Completion angiogram using iodinated contrast showed successful stent deployment. This patient received a total of 12 mL of contrast medium, but in severe cases of renal failure or allergy, iodinated contrast can be avoided completely.

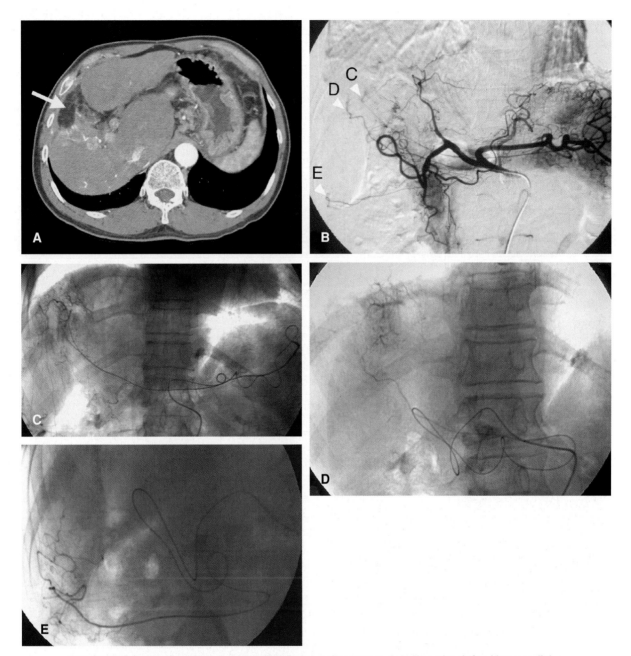

FIGURE 3-29 A 65-year-old man presented with chronic hepatitis C, cirrhosis, and multifocal hepatocellular carcinoma. The patient underwent numerous previous hepatic chemoembolizations and had a recurrent rising serum alpha-fetoprotein. **A:** CT scan showed new hypervascular masses and prominent fatty tissue in the porta hepatis, extending into the fissure for the ligamentum teres (*arrow*). Note hypertrophy of the left and caudate lobes, shifting the fissure for the ligamentum teres laterally. **B:** Selective celiac arteriogram showed hepatic arterial branch occlusions and irregularities, likely secondary to chemical vasculitis from prior chemoembolizations. Numerous parasitized vessels were seen entering the liver (*arrowheads*). With progressive superselectivity, these branches were identified as greater omental branches of the splenic *(C)*, gastroepiploic *(D),* and gastroduodenal *(E)* arteries. Note the long and tortuous courses of these arteries, which could not be traced on the 2.5-mm-slice thickness CT scan, even in retrospect. These were all treated with chemoembolic agents. **C–E:** Images from superselective injections of greater omental branches of the splenic **(C)**, gastroepiploic **(D)**, and gastroduodenal **(E)** arteries are shown.

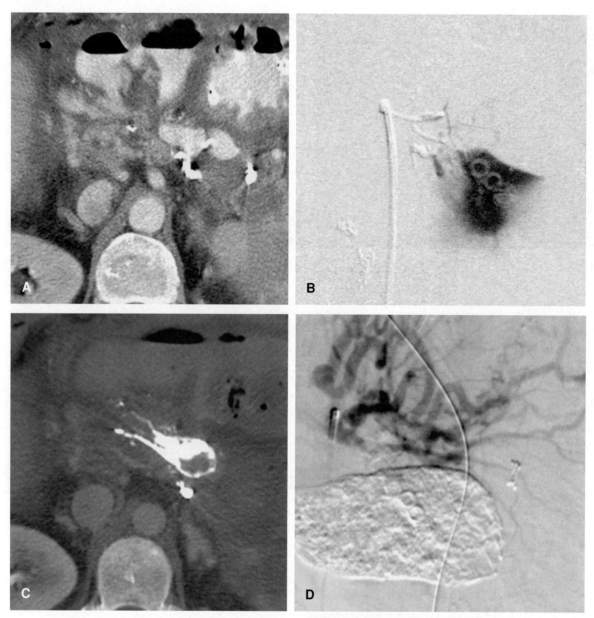

FIGURE 3-30 Beam-hardening artifact from permanent metallic devices. A: Contrast-enhanced CT scan of the abdomen in a patient with a complicated postsurgical course after repair of a perforated gastric ulcer showed embolization coils from previous procedures and contrast-filled structures initially interpreted as bowel. **B:** Because of persistent gastrointestinal hemorrhage, catheter angiography was performed. A superselective microcatheter angiogram of a branch of the left gastric artery revealed a large pseudoaneurysm, which could be seen on the CT in retrospect. This was treated by n-butyl cyanoacrylate and ethiodol glue embolization, which appeared to extravasate into the pseudoaneurysm as well as fill the feeding branch vessel. **C:** The patient remained hemodynamically unstable, but a follow-up CT scan was difficult to interpret because of beam-hardening artifact in the region of embolization. **D:** Repeat left gastric arteriography showed no filling of the feeding vessels and the pseudoaneurysm.

the target tissue (Fig. 3-30). It is important to note that not all metal is a problem for CT and MR scanners. Both the thickness and composition of the metal are key determinants of their impact in CT or MR images (Fig. 3-31).

Even if an angiogram is compromised by an obscuring metallic object or by any imperfection in imaging tech-

nique, the adequacy of the study can be immediately assessed. Inadequate studies can be quickly and easily repeated in an iterative process, usually with only small incremental administrations of contrast medium (Fig. 3-32). In addition, stress views in different positions or before and after administration of vasoactive medications

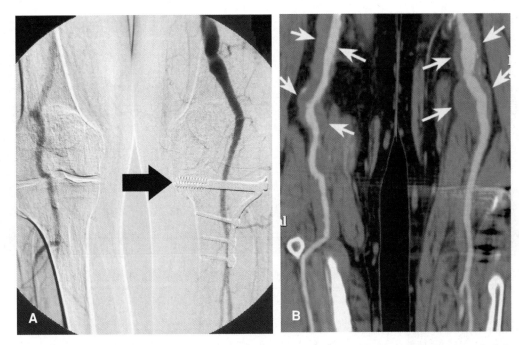

FIGURE 3-31 Bilateral femoropopliteal artery aneurysms post open reduction and internal fixation of a left tibial plateau fracture. A: The metal screws associated with the tibial fixation obscure the underlying popliteal artery on this anteroposterior projection from a catheter arteriogram. **B:** Curved planar reformation from a 4-row MDCT angiogram demonstrates minimal artifact from the metal, allowing visualization of the entire popliteal artery. The true dimensions of the femoropopliteal artery aneurysms are visible because both the mural thrombus and the contrast medium enhanced lumen are visible (*arrows*). Had a lateral or oblique projection been acquired, then the entirety of the lumen of the left popliteal artery and tibioperoneal trunk should have been visible; however, asymmetric intimal abnormalities easily could be missed. (Reprinted from Rubin GD, Schmidt AJ, Logan LJ, et al. Multi-detector row CT angiography of lower extremity arterial inflow and runoff: initial experience. *Radiology* 2001;221:146–158, with permission.)

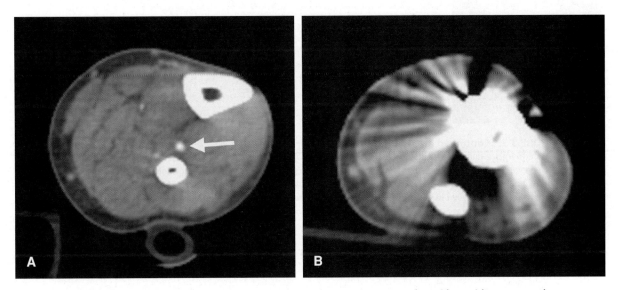

FIGURE 3-32 Images reflect the status of a 48 year-old man post–motorcycle accident with a compound fracture of the left tibia and fibula superior to the site of a previous fracture, which had been fixated with a plate. A: CT angiogram of the extremity showed dominant anterior tibial arterial supply to the mid-calf (*arrow*) and opacification of the distal anterior tibial artery (**C, page 122**), although proof of contiguity was precluded by metallic beam-hardening artifact (**B**).

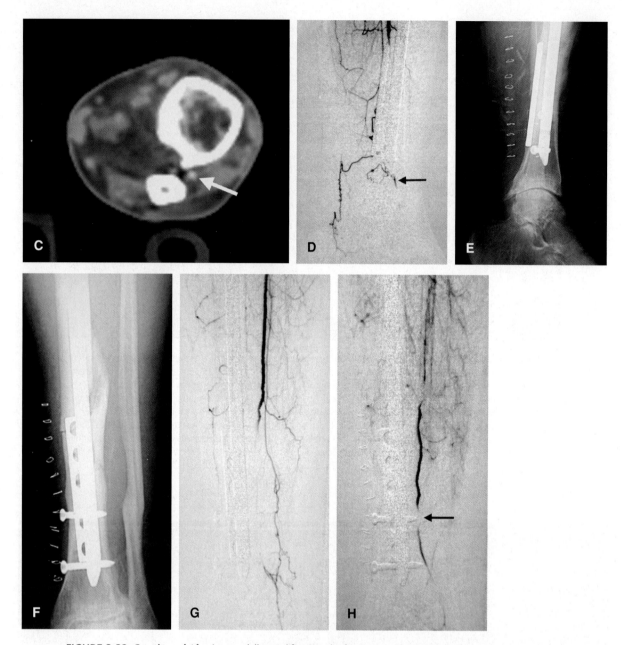

FIGURE 3-32 Continued After intramedullary rod fixation, the foot appeared ischemic, and a catheter angiogram was performed. A lateral view of the ankle **(D)** showed poor flow into the distal anterior tibial artery (*arrow*), but details were obscured by orthopedic hardware **(E)**. In an anteroposterior obliquity **(F)**, sluggish flow was seen in the mid-anterior tibial artery **(G)**, and the dorsalis pedis filled via muscular collateral vessels. **H:** Retrograde flow in the distal anterior tibial artery led to a point of obstruction (*arrows*), which at surgical exploration proved to be a screw or drill injury.

are easily obtained (Fig. 3-33). Noninvasive imaging is usually protocoled using noncontrast scout images and possibly a test injection of a small contrast medium bolus, but repetition of entire studies may be limited by the relatively large bolus necessary to produce a study and by the relatively long time necessary to process and interpret a study.

A final differentiation between cross-sectional and catheter angiography is the level of personnel and clinical care present at the time of the procedure. Catheter angiograms are performed by at least one physician, with real time interpretation of images and of adequacy of the study. The physician is usually aided by a team of technologists, nurses, physician assistants, and/or nurse practitioners. The constant presence of multiple personnel during conventional angiography allows immediate diagnosis and action. Preparation for catheter angiography requires the physician or other qualified member of the team to perform a history and physical examination. In contrast, cross-sectional imaging may be protocoled by a physician but is usually performed without a physician present and is not immediately interpreted. It is not uncommon that a cross-sectional study is later deemed suboptimal because of artifact, contrast medium injection issues, wrong or inadequate pulse sequences, or the wrong body part being scanned.

FUTURE TECHNOLOGICAL DEVELOPMENT

Hybrid Imaging Instruments

The data provided by cross-sectional imaging are frequently complementary to the data provided by catheter angiography. Even when using image guidance for therapeutic procedures, the interventionalist is usually restricted to using one or the other. Modern interventionalists, though, are increasingly comfortable with interpreting cross-sectional images and are interested in using both projectional and cross-sectional images to guide procedures. Perhaps the best-established combination is obtained by the inclusion of ultrasound in the angiography suite. Ultrasound has become the modality of choice to guide percutaneous nephrostomies, cholecystostomies, cholangiograms and biliary drains, simpler biopsies and drainages, and difficult vascular access. As a diagnostic imaging modality, though, ultrasound

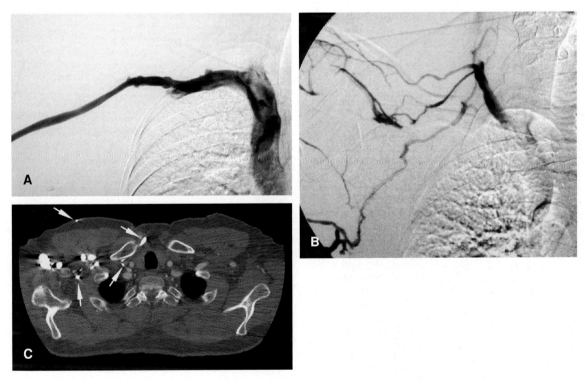

FIGURE 3-33 Iterative procedures for stress views or optimization. A: Catheter venogram of the right upper extremity in a patient with exercise intolerance appeared normal. **B:** Venogram was repeated with a modified Wright maneuver, showing complete obstruction of the subclavian vein at the thoracic inlet, with filling of subscapular, lateral thoracic, and external jugular branches. Numerous sequential evocative maneuvers may be performed on each patient. A contrast medium–filled vessel can also be observed in real time during manipulation of an extremity. **C:** Transverse axial image from a contrast-enhanced CT of the thorax of a different patient, showing filling of numerous collateral veins (*arrows*) when contrast was injected into the abducted right upper extremity. Some iterative optimization is also possible with evocative patient positioning within the gantries and bores of MR and CT scanners.

does not have the power of CT or MR, mostly due to limited tissue penetration and obscuration by gas or bone.

A new class of hybrid instruments is being developed to allow the interventionalist to use both projectional fluoroscopy and either cross-sectional CT or MRI, iteratively in real time during a procedure. For hybrid MRI/x-ray fluoroscopy, at least two designs have been prototyped. One involves the installation of a fixed, solid-state x-ray fluoroscopy system between the superconducting magnets of a double-donut General Electric Signa SP 0.5 Tesla open configuration magnet (Fig. 3-34). Although the patient does not need to be moved to exploit both modalities, the fluoroscopy unit does not allow oblique angulation. In addition, considerable optimization of the hardware and postacquisition image processing is necessary to achieve diagnostic quality images (24). A second prototyped design utilizes a radiolucent and MR-compatible patient table that is mounted on a long track (Fig. 3-35). At one end of the track is a 1.5 Tesla Intera I/T scanner, and at the other end of the track is an Integris C-arm fluoroscopy unit (25). Because both image acquisition systems are essentially standard, state-of-the-art systems, the images produced are also standard and state of the art. However, iteration between the two modalities requires physically moving the patient on a carriage from one room to another, which can result in registration error.

Combining x-ray fluoroscopy with CT may find wider applications than with MRI. Earlier prototypes were engineered similar to the second MRI/x-ray system, where two separate imaging systems were installed in one room and the patient could be physically transported from one room to another in a radiolucent bed on a track, or the CT unit itself could be mounted on a track (Fig. 3-36). Some systems allowed the bed to swivel 90 degrees for a more compact footprint. More recently, the trend of increasing number of detector rows in CT and the advent of rotational x-ray angiography have met in the middle, yielding what amounts to a projectional angiography unit that can also function as a cone beam CT scanner (Fig. 3-36). Although applications of combination cone-beam CT/projectional angiography are still being vetted, three-dimensional vascular imaging has already proven useful in intracranial arteriography at the time of embolization (26) and in abdominal visceral imaging at the time of transjugular intrahepatic portosystemic shunt creation (27) (Fig. 3-37). Other applications, especially in interventional oncology for chemoembolization and radioembolization, are gaining wider acceptance and utilization.

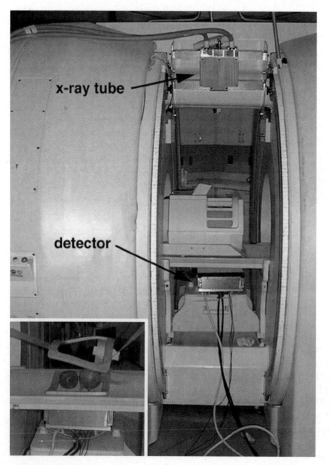

FIGURE 3-34 Hybrid MRI and x-ray fluoroscopy unit (in parallel). A solid state, fixed angle fluoroscopy unit was installed in the gap between the superconducting magnets of a 0.5 Tesla General Electric Signa SP MR scanner. The inset shows the flexible, radiolucent radio frequency coil used to obtain MR images. (Reprinted from Fahrig R, Butts K, Wen Z, et al. Truly hybrid interventional MR/x-ray system: investigation of in vivo applications. *Acad Radiol* 2001:1200–1207, with permission.)

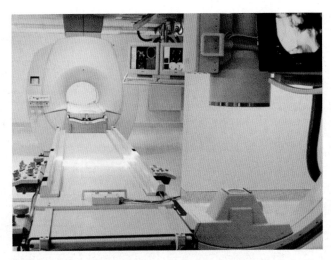

FIGURE 3-35 Hybrid MRI and x-ray fluoroscopy unit (in series). A Philips Integris fluoroscopy unit coupled to a 1.5 Tesla Intera I/T MR scanner allows a patient to be transferred from one to another on a track connecting the two. Reprinted from Martin AJ, Saloner DA, Roberts TP, et al. Carotid stent delivery in an XMR suite: immediate assessment of the physiologic impact of extracranial revascularization. *AJNR Am J Neuroradiol* 2005;26:531–537, with permission.)

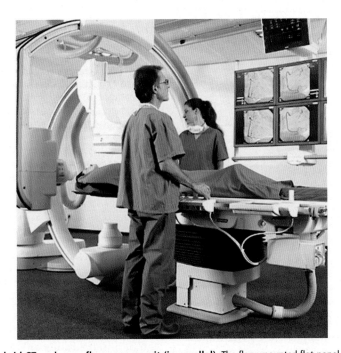

FIGURE 3-36 Hybrid CT and x-ray fluoroscopy unit (in parallel). The floor-mounted flat-panel detector fluoroscopy unit in this biplanar system is capable of rotational angiography as well as cone-beam computed tomography. Although total radiation dose can be decreased, protective aprons are still required for personnel. (Courtesy Siemens Medical Solutions USA, Inc., Malvern, PA)

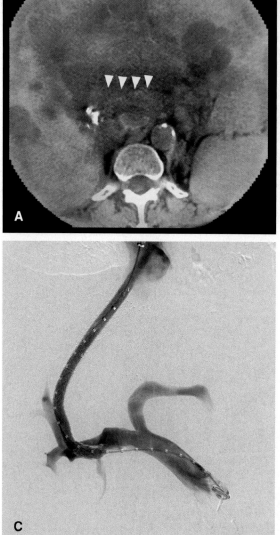

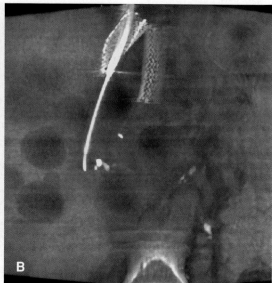

FIGURE 3-37 Transjugular intrahepatic portosystemic shunt (TIPS) creation in a patient with polycystic liver disease. Cone-beam CT axial image without contrast enhancement **(A)** shows the main portal vein (*arrowheads*) and numerous cysts in a markedly enlarged liver. A TIPS needle was passed through a preexisting middle hepatic vein stent, through numerous cysts, and into the main portal vein, as shown in this oblique coronal MIP reconstruction **(B)**. Real-time image guidance of the needle throw, guidewire manipulation, angioplasty, and stent deployment was performed using conventional projectional fluoroscopy, and venography of the portal vein including after creation of the shunt **(C)** was performed using digital subtraction angiography, all using the same imaging hardware. (Reprinted from *J Vasc Interv Radiol* 2006;17:711–715, with permission.)

CONCLUSION

With the tremendous gains in MR and CT technology, noninvasive angiography has supplanted conventional catheter angiography as the preferred diagnostic imaging modality for a majority of vascular abnormalities. Nevertheless, current digital subtraction angiographic technique continues to offer important advantages over noninvasive techniques in selected circumstances. One consistent feature of all three modalities is that they continue to evolve, and even greater capabilities can be expected in the near future.

Catheter-based therapy has evolved into a competitor of traditional open surgical techniques and is winning the competition as the preferred treatment for the majority of vascular diseases. Almost all imaging studies performed by the modern interventional radiologist are not diagnostic in nature but instead are used as maps to guide interventions at the time of intervention. The large majority of interventions are still performed using x-ray fluoroscopy for guidance because of the ability to perform cinematic imaging with high spatial and temporal resolution of the target tissue and of the devices used. It is almost inevitable that future generations of interventionalists will have hybrid projectional/cross-sectional instruments available for both diagnosis and treatment. As these technologies develop, the role of the interventional radiologist will further evolve into one of a surgeon, a primarily therapeutic clinician.

REFERENCES

1. Abrams HL. *Abram's Angiography*. Boston: Little, Brown, and Co.; 1996.
2. Rosch J, Keller FS, Kaufman JA. The birth, early years, and future of interventional radiology. *J Vasc Interv Radiol.* 2003;14:841–853.
3. American College of Radiology Digest of Council Actions 1995–2004; 2001.
4. Cardella JF, Casarella WJ, DeWeese JA, et al. Optimal resources for the examination and endovascular treatment of the peripheral and visceral vascular systems. AHA Intercouncil Report on peripheral and visceral angiographic and interventional laboratories. *J Vasc Interv Radiol.* 2003;14:S517–S530.
5. Hendee WR, Ritenour ER. *Medical Imaging Physics*. New York: Wiley-Liss; 2002.
6. Wang J, Blackburn TJ. X-ray image intensifiers for fluoroscopy. *Radiographics.* 2000;20:1471–1477.
7. Hind D, Calvert N, McWilliams R, et al. Ultrasonic locating devices for central nervous cannulation: meta-analysis. *BMJ.* 2003;327:361.
8. Standards of Practice Committee of the Society of Cardiovascular and Interventional Radiology. Standard for diagnostic arteriography in adults. *J Vasc Interv Radiol.* 1993;4(3): 385–395.
9. Singh H, Cardella JF, Cole PE, et al. Quality improvement guidelines for diagnostic arteriography. *J Vasc Interv Radiol.* 2003;14:S283–S288.
10. American College of Radiology, the American Society of Interventional and Therapeutic Neuroradiology, and the Society of Interventional Radiology. Practice guideline for interventional clinical practice. *J Vasc Interv Radiol.* 2005; 16:149–155.
11. Rubin GD, Schmidt AJ, Logan LJ, et al. Multi-detector row CT angiography of lower extremity arterial inflow and runoff: initial experience. *Radiology.* 2001;221:146–158.
12. Karcaaltincaba M, Foley D. Four- and eight-channel aortoiliac CT angiography: a comparative study. *Cardiovasc Intervent Radiol* 2005;28:169–172.
13. Willmann JK, Baumert B, Schertler T, et al. Aortoiliac and lower extremity arteries assessed with 16-detector row CT angiography: prospective comparison with digital subtraction angiography. *Radiology.* 2005;236(3):1083–1093.
14. Kuiper JW, Geleijns J, Matheijssen NA, et al. Radiation exposure of multi-row detector spiral computed tomography of the pulmonary arteries: comparison with digital subtraction pulmonary angiography. *Eur Radiol.* 2003;13:1496–1500.
15. Hoffer EK, Bloch RD. Percutaneous arterial closure devices. *J Vasc Interv Radiol.* 2003;14:865–885.
16. Swan JS, Langlotz CP. Patient preference for magnetic resonance versus conventional angiography. Assessment methods and implications for cost-effectiveness analysis: an overview. *Invest Radiol.* 1998;33:553–559.
17. Rubin GD, Armerding MD, Dake MD, et al. Cost identification of abdominal aortic aneurysm imaging by using time and motion analyses. *Radiology.* 2000;215:63–70.
18. Visser K, Kock MC, Kuntz KM, et al. Cost-effectiveness targets for multi-detector row CT angiography in the work-up of patients with intermittent claudication. *Radiology.* 2003; 227:647–656.
19. Visser K, Kuntz KM, Donaldson MC, et al. Pretreatment imaging workup for patients with intermittent claudication: a cost-effectiveness analysis. *J Vasc Interv Radiol.* 2003;14:53–62.
20. U-King-Im JM, Hollingworth W, Trivedi RA, et al. Contrast-enhanced MR angiography vs intra-arterial digital subtraction angiography for carotid imaging: activity-based cost analysis. *Eur Radiol.* 2004;14:730–735.
21. Armerding MD, Rubin GD, Beaulieu CF, et al. Aortic aneurysmal disease: assessment of stent-graft treatment-CT versus conventional angiography. *Radiology.* 2000;215: 138–146.
22. Tillich M, Bell RE, Paik DS, et al. Iliac arterial injuries after endovascular repair of abdominal aortic aneurysms: correlation with iliac curvature and diameter. *Radiology.* 2001;219: 129–136.
23. Tillich M, Hill BB, Paik DS, et al. Prediction of aortoiliac stent-graft length: comparison of measurement methods. *Radiology.* 2001;220:475–483.
24. Fahrig R, Butts K, Wen Z, et al. Truly hybrid interventional MR/X-ray system: investigation of in vivo applications. *Acad Radiol.* 2001;8:1200–1207.
25. Wilson MW, Fidelman N, Weber OM, et al. Experimental renal artery embolization in a combined MR imaging/angiographic unit. *J Vasc Interv Radiol.* 2003;14:1169–1175.
26. Heran NS, Song JK, Namba K, et al. The utility of DynaCT in neuroendovascular procedures. *AJNR Am J Neuroradiol* 2006;27:330–332.
27. Sze DY, Strobel N, Fahrig R, et al. Transjugular intrahepatic portosystemic shunt creation in a polycystic liver facilitated by hybrid cross-sectional/angiographic imaging. *J Vasc Interv Radiol* 2006;17:711–715.

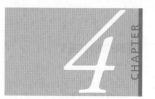

Contrast Medium Administration in Computed Tomographic Angiography

Dominik Fleischmann

Intravenous (IV) contrast medium (CM) administration is one of the essential ingredients of computed tomographic angiography (CTA). Its primary goal is to achieve adequate opacification of the vascular territory of interest synchronized with the CT acquisition. This seemingly simple goal is not always easy to achieve, notably in the light of continuously evolving CT technology, where scan times have become substantially shorter with each new scanner generation. Empirically developed injection protocols designed for the scanning times achievable in the early days of CTA are no longer adequate for current multiple detector-row com-

puted tomography (MDCT) technology. Fast acquisitions require that physiologic constraints of arterial enhancement have to be taken into account when building an integrated scanning and injection protocol for a cardiovascular CT application. The key to any rational design of contrast medium injection protocols is a thorough understanding of the physiologic and pharmacokinetic principles governing arterial enhancement, and knowledge of the effects of user-selectable injection parameters on vascular enhancement.

This chapter first reviews the general properties and safety aspects of iodinated contrast media with particular relevance to CT angiography. The central purpose is, how-ever, to explain the basic principles of arterial enhancement (early contrast medium dynamics) for CT angiography, which are timeless and thus independent of the scanner gen-eration used. Finally, this chapter reviews how the basic prin-ciples and currently available techniques of contrast medium delivery can be assembled into rational injection protocols for state-of-the-art cardiovascular CT.

CONTRAST MEDIA FOR COMPUTED TOMOGRAPHIC ANGIOGRAPHY

Angiographic x-ray CM currently in use are water-soluble derivates of symmetrically iodinated benzene (tri-iodoben-zene). They are either negatively charged ionic (ionic CM) or nonionic (nonionic CM) monomers or dimers, respec-tively (Table 4-1). In addition to ionicity and chemical structure (monomer vs. dimer), CM are also categorized into osmotic classes (high-osmolar, low-osmolar, and iso-osmolar). The diagnostic use of x-ray contrast media is exclusively based on the physical ability of iodine to absorb x-rays, and not on pharmacological effects, which are gener-ally undesired. The desired effect of CM is thus directly related to the iodine concentration of the agent. The increase in CT numbers observed in a given vessel or tissue after con-trast medium administration is directly proportional to the local iodine concentration (1). Other important physico-chemical properties of iodinated contrast agents in the con-text of CT are their osmolality and their viscosity.

Viscosity has been considered a less important factor than osmolality when mechanical power injectors were first introduced (2); however, in the setting of CT angiography where increasing iodine administration rates are desired, viscosity has regained importance. Furthermore, viscosity

may also play a role in CM-induced nephropathy (3), among many other possible factors. The viscosity of a con-trast agent depends mainly on the nature of the active ingre-dient, iodine concentration, and temperature. Viscosity increases exponentially with increasing iodine concentra-tion. Viscosity is reduced by approximately 50% when warmed from room temperature (20°C) to body tempera-ture (37°C) (4). There are distinct differences between non-ionic CM of the same iodine concentration with respect to their viscosity (Fig. 4-1). Dimers are the largest molecules and are generally more viscous than monomers.

The selection of IV contrast medium for CTA is pri-marily governed by safety considerations and the rate of expected adverse reactions. In this context, nonionic CM are generally safer than ionic contrast media, with less idio-syncratic (nondose-dependent, e.g., allergylike) adverse reactions (5–8). Ionic CM also have a greater potential to cause acute nausea and vomiting, and—as a result—motion, when injection rates greater than 2.0 to 2.5 mL/s are used. Furthermore, extravasation of ionic CM is less well tolerated than nonionic CM. Therefore, nonionic CM are preferable in the setting of CTA (9) and are used almost exclusively today.

SAFETY ISSUES OF CONTRAST MEDIA FOR COMPUTED TOMOGRAPHIC ANGIOGRAPHY

While modern nonionic iodinated contrast agents are among the safest medications used worldwide (10), adverse effects occur in approximately 3.13%. An overview of adverse events relevant to CTA is given in Table 4-2. Most reactions to nonionic agents are mild to moderate, but severe reactions do occur in 0.04% (5). Adverse reactions

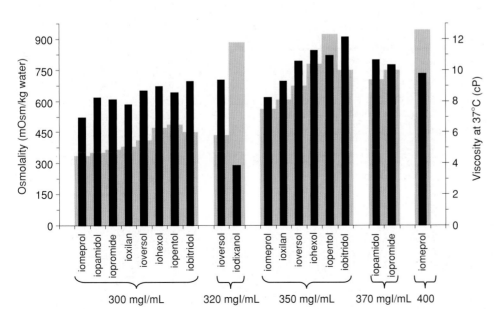

FIGURE 4-1 Physicochemical properties of iodinated contrast media used for CTA. Osmolality (*black bars*) and viscosity (*gray bars*) of low- and iso-osmolar contrast agents are shown in groups of the same iodine concentration.

TABLE 4-1

Physicochemical Properties of Radiographic Contrast Media

Contrast Medium (CM) Type and Agent	Example of Trade Name (Manufacturer)	Molecular Weight (Dalton)	Iodine Concentration (mgI/mL)	Osmolality (mOsm/kg water)	Viscosity at 20°C (cP)	Viscosity at 37°C (cP)
Ionic CM, monomer (High osmolar CM)						
Iothalamate[3]	Conray 60% (Mallinckrodt)	809	282	1,400	6.0[2]	4.0
Ionic CM, dimer (Low osmolar, ionic CM)						
Ioxaglate	Hexabrix (Mallinckrodt, Guerbet)	1,274	320	600	15.7	7.5
Nonionic CM, monomer (Low osmolar CM)						
Iopamidol	Isovue (Bracco)	777	300	616	3.3	4.7
			370	796	20.9	9.4
Iohexol	Omnipaque (GE-HC)	821	300	672	11.8	6.3
			350	844	20.4	10.4
Iopromide	Ultravist (Berlex/Schering)	791	300	607	9.2	4.9
			370	774	22.0	10.0
Ioversol	Optiray (Mallinckrodt/ Guerbet)	807	300	651	8.2[2]	5.5
			320	702	9.9[2]	5.8
			350	792	14.3[2]	9.0
Ioxilan	Oxilan (Guerbet)	791	300	585	9.4	5.1
			350	695	16.3	8.1
Iopentol[1]	Imagopaque (GE-HC)	835	300	640	13.2	6.5
			350	818	26.6	12.0
Iomeprol[1]	Iomeron (Bracco)	777	300	521	8.1	4.5
			350	618	14.5	7.5
			400	726	27.5	12.6
Iobitridol[1]	Xenetix (Guerbet)	835	300	695	11.0	6.0
			350	915	21.0	10.0
Nonionic CM, dimer (iso-osmolar CM)						
Iodixanol	Visipaque (GE-HC)	1,550	270	290	12.7	6.3
			320	290	26.6	11.8

GE-HC, GE Healthcare.

[1]Substance not available in the United States.

[2]Viscosity at 25°C.

[3]Meglumine salt.

TABLE 4-2

Adverse Events of Contrast Media, Risk Factors, and Preventive Measures in the Setting of Computed Tomographic Angiography

Adverse Event, Known (Suspected) Risk Factor	Preventive Measures/Consequences
Idiosyncratic Reactions	
Acute allergylike reaction	
• History of prior moderate or severe CM adverse reaction	Screen for history of prior reactions and drug history.
• History of significant allergy (requiring medical treatment)	Have premedication protocol for patients with increased risk.
• Asthma	Have equipment and guidelines for treatment of acute
• Drugs	CM reactions.
Beta-blockers (increase risk, decrease effect of adrenaline)	
Interleukin-2	
Delayed (cutaneous) reaction	
• History of prior reaction (to specific agent)	Screen for history of prior reactions and drug history.
• Interleukin-2	
• Hydralazine	
Dose-dependent (nonidiosyncratic) Reactions	
Cardiovascular effects	
• It is not excluded that high injection flow rates and volumes can cause cardiopulmonary decompensation in patients with cardiocirculatory compromise.	Avoid large volumes and flow rates in fragile, elderly patients with low body weight.
Contrast medium–induced nephrotoxicity	
• History of renal disease	Screen for history and risk factors of renal disease in outpatients; obtain routine serum creatinine in inpatients.
• Previous kidney surgery (including transplantation)	
• Diabetes	Have protocol for the prevention of CIN.
• Proteinuria	(See also Table 4-4.)
• Hypertension	
• Gout (hyperuricaemia)	
• Multiple myeloma (needs hydration)	
• Documented decrease of renal function (eGFR $<$60 mL/min/1.73 m^2)	
CM Extravasation Injury	
• Increased risk in noncommunicative patients, notably in unconscious and elderly patients.	Manual test injection; Monitor injection site.
	Have policy for treatment and hand-surgery consult.
Drug Interactions	
• Metformin	Obtain thorough drug history; stop metformin and nephrotoxic drugs.
• Nephrotoxic drugs	(See also Table 4-4.)
Aminoglycoside antibiotics	
NSAIDs	
Chemotherapy (cyclosporine, cisplatin)	
• Interleukin-2 (CM precipitates IL-2 toxicity; IL-2 increases risk of CM-induced acute urticarial reaction	
• Beta-blockers (see acute reactions)	
• Hydralazine (may predispose to acute cutaneous vasculitis)	
Interaction with Endocrine Function	
• CM are contradindicated in patients with manifest hyperthyroidism.	Screen for history of thyroid disease.
• Risk of thyrotoxicosis in patients with Graves disease and multinodular goiter with autonomous thyroid tissue, notably in areas of iodine deficiency.	Endocrinology consult and follow-up.
• CM compromises thyroid scintigraphy and radioiodine treatment of thyroid malignancies for 2 months.	

are generally categorized into idiosyncratic (nondose dependent), allergylike reactions and nonidiosyncratic (dose dependent) reactions. The risk of idiosyncratic adverse reactions to intravenously injected contrast medium can be expected to occur in the setting of CTA at the same rate as in any other indication for IV contrast medium use. Acute allergylike reactions are particularly troublesome because of their unpredictability, and also because they may be life threatening. The equipment and expertise to treat acute adverse reactions should be readily available whenever contrast agents are administered. Because serious reactions are infrequent, it is important to review treatment protocols regularly and to check equipment and drugs at regular intervals for expiration and availability. Guidelines for patient screening, premedication, and recognition and management of acute adverse reactions have been published elsewhere (11–13). Delayed cutaneous reactions to contrast agents, presumably immune mediated, may occur 1 to 7 days after administration and are thus rarely recognized by radiologists. However, their incidence is surprisingly high when actively looked for (14). Delayed reactions are clinically important, and they have a tendency to recur with reinjection of the same contrast agent (15), which underscores the importance of accurate documentation of any contrast administration.

Manifest hyperthyroidism is considered an absolute contraindication for iodinated contrast media. Contrast medium–induced thyrotoxicosis is otherwise rare. Patients at risk of developing thyrotoxicosis after contrast medium injection are patients with Graves disease as well as patients with multinodular goiter with thyroid autonomy, especially elderly patients and patients living in areas of iodine deficiency (the United States is not an iodine deficiency area). Routine monitoring of thyroid function tests before contrast medium injection in patients with a normal thyroid is not indicated (16). Patients at high risk should be carefully monitored by endocrinologists after contrast medium examinations. The free iodide load of contrast media interferes with iodide uptake in the thyroid. Contrast media therefore compromise diagnostic thyroid scintigraphy and radio-iodine treatment of thyroid malignancies for 2 months after administration and should be avoided in this setting. Simple guidelines on the CM and thyroid function have recently been published (16).

Because CM delivery for CTA requires comparably large volumes injected at high flow rates with power injectors, it is important not to ignore the potential risks of dose-dependent adverse effects of CM. Based on clinical and experimental evidence for ionic CM, one might naturally assume that rapid injections would be less well tolerated than slower injections (17). However, at least for injection flow rates up to 4 mL/s, no correlation between injection rate and the overall rate of adverse reactions has been found (18). Utilization of noninvasive cardiovascular imaging is increasing (19), however, and there is an increased use of CT particularly in the elderly (20). This patient population is more likely to have cardiovascular disorders and diabetes, and may be more vulnerable than other current and past patient cohorts undergoing CT.

The "classic" dose-dependent adverse reactions in the ionic CM era (particularly with intra-arterial or intracoronary injections) included nausea, vomiting, arrhythmia, pulmonary edema, and cardiovascular collapse. The dose-dependent effects that require specific attention in the setting of CTA are CM extravasation, cardiovascular effects, and CM-induced nephrotoxicity (CIN). Drug interactions are also a concern in this patient population.

Contrast Medium Extravasation

Extravasation is a well-known complication of IV CM administration. The rate of extravasation has been reported to range from 0.2% to 0.6% when mechanical power injectors are used (21). Although injection flow rates of 5 mL/s for CTA were reported as early as 1993, many radiologists were reluctant to inject more than 3 mL/s. Over the years, however, injection flow rates for CTA have increased, and flow rates of 5 or 6 mL/s have become clinically routine at many institutions today. Although there has been concern that these injection flow rates would be associated with a proportionally increased risk of extravasation, no correlation between extravasation frequency and injection rate has been found (18). Ten mL/s are standard for functional imaging studies using CT (22,23). In the era of IV digital subtraction arteriography (DSA), the standard peripheral IV injection rate was 15 mL/s (24) for volumes of 30 to 50 mL, repeated for each view.

Most extravasations of CM involve only small volumes and result in minimal to mild symptoms if nonionic CM is used. When large volumes of CM extravasate, it is usually in noncommunicative patients such as infants and children, the elderly, or unconscious patients. Severe extravasation injuries such as skin necrosis and ulceration, or compartment syndrome, have occasionally been reported even with nonionic agents (21). Thus, a preliminary rapid manual injection of saline with the patient's arm in scanning position (e.g., above the head) is generally recommended to ensure correct and stable cannula position prior to iodinated CM administration. Monitoring of the injection site early during CM administration reduces the risk of significant extravasation but does not eliminate it because extravasation may occur several seconds after the beginning of the injection. The use of a CM extravasation detection device connected to the power injector reduces this risk as well (25).

Conservative management of CM extravasation injury is often adequate, but it is advisable to establish a local policy for management of these injuries together with a plastic or hand surgeon (21,26). Both warm and cold compresses may be beneficial to the treatment of local extravasation. There is no clear consensus on the preferred treatment. Proper documentation of extravasation events is important.

Cardiovascular Effects

Cardiovascular adverse reactions to intra-arterial (notably coronary) but also to intravenous injections of ionic CM are well documented experimentally and clinically, and include arrhythmia, tachycardia, pulmonary edema, and cardiovascular collapse (17,27). With IV administration of nonionic agents, serious cardiovascular adverse events are probably very rare.

Cochran et al. analyzed the trends of adverse events to more than 90,000 CM injections over a period of 15 years (from 1985 to 1999) at their institution (28). As expected, they found decreasing rates of adverse events when the universal use of ionic CM was replaced with selective use of nonionic CM followed by universal use of nonionic contrast agents. Interestingly, the authors found that seven of the ten severe reactions to nonionic CM occurred in patients after CT angiography. The authors also found that severe reactions with nonionic contrast agents were more likely due to cardiopulmonary decompensation than to allergylike reactions in their patients. While the authors could not exclude a statistical glitch and a change in the patient population during the study period (which is not at all unlikely), a potential association between cardiopulmonary decompensation and CT angiography is not excluded.

Because severe reactions to nonionic agents are rare in general, and because it is probably not always easy to differentiate allergylike from cardiopulmonary events retrospectively (and both may coexist), one cannot expect to easily find hard evidence to prove or exclude an increased risk of CTA to cause cardiopulmonary adverse events. For patients with substantial cardiopulmonary compromise, however, it is quite plausible that a rapidly injected volume of CM can result in acute decompensation.

Theoretically, the risk can be reduced when smaller volumes and flow rates are used. In patients with low cardiac output, this will still result in good vascular opacification. Unfortunately, it is unlikely that patients at risk will be easily identifiable beforehand. Individualizing the injection flow rates and volumes to body size is at least one rational technique to avoid excessive CM injections in older persons with small stature.

Contrast Medium–Induced Nephrotoxicity

CIN is commonly defined as an impairment of renal function with an increase of serum creatinine of >25% or 0.5 mg/dL (44 μmol/L) from baseline within three days after CM injection in the absence of alternative etiology (29). The mechanism is incompletely understood and may be due to a combination of several factors, such as a direct toxic effect on renal tubular cells (30), and contrast medium–related changes in renal medullary perfusion subsequent hypoxemia (3). Osmolality and viscosity may both play a role, but at this point, it is quite controversial how and to which extent these factors contribute to CIN (3,31). CIN due to nonionic contrast agents is rare in the general population (less than 2%), but the incidence may be greater than 25% in patients with risk factors (32). The primary risk factors are pre-existing renal impairment, notably if associated with diabetes, volume depletion, and the use of nephrotoxic drugs. While CIN is reversible in the vast majority of cases, it may cause considerable morbidity and mortality. Patients who develop CIN are at significantly higher risk of death, both in the hospital and at 1 year, at least in patients undergoing cardiac catheterization and angiography (33).

There are two practical consequences in the setting of CTA. It is necessary to screen for patients at risk, and once a patient at risk is identified, it is necessary to take measures to reduce the likelihood of CIN. Detailed discussions of this topic and specific guidelines have again been published elsewhere (13,34).

Screening for Patients at Risk

A protocol to identify patients at risk of CIN should be in place in every diagnostic imaging department. The practice of screening these patients in the setting of CTA depends mostly on the clinical setting (outpatients vs. inpatients or emergency room). In an outpatient setting, routine measurement of serum creatinine is not necessary in patients younger than 70 years if a simple questionnaire designed to elicit a history of renal disorders and additional risk factors for CIN suggests normal renal function (35). If the questionnaire indicates a positive history of prior kidney disease, diabetes, kidney surgery (including transplantation), or congestive heart failure (Table 4-2), the serum creatinine should be measured. Recently, a rapid strip-based test has become commercially available that allows bedside determination of serum creatinine and BUN within a few minutes (36), which may be particularly helpful in the outpatient setting. In inpatients, serum creatinine levels should always be known before CM administration.

TABLE 4-3

Serum Creatinine Levels (in mg/dL) Indicating an Estimated Glomerular Filtration Rate of less than 60 mL/min/1.73 m²

Age (years)	20	30	40	50	60	70	80
Men (not African American)	1.57	1.47	1.39	1.34	1.30	1.26	1.23
Women (not African American)	1.21	1.13	1.08	1.03	1.00	0.97	0.95
Men (African American)	1.86	1.73	1.65	1.58	1.53	1.49	1.46
Women (African American)	1.44	1.34	1.27	1.22	1.18	1.15	1.12

MDRD, Modification of Diet in Renal Disease study; S_{cr} = serum creatinine in μmol/L; age is given in years.
Note: Calculations based on 4-parameter MDRD formula:
GFR (mL/min/1.73 m²) = $186(S_{cr} \times 0.011)^{-1.154} \times (age)^{-0.203} \times (1.21$, if African American$) \times (0.742$, if female$)$.
(http://www.kidney.org/kls/professionals/gfr_calculator.cfm.)

Serum creatinine is an imperfect marker of renal dysfunction, and in the setting of CIN, its primary limitation is that a fixed threshold of "normal" creatinine (e.g., 1.3 mg/dL) may not detect even a more than 50% reduction of the glomerular filtration rate and thus miss a significant proportion of patients at risk. It has been suggested that a patient's glomerular filtration rate should be estimated instead of using serum creatinine. This can be done most easily using the 4-variables abbreviated version of the original 6-variable MDRD (modification of diet in renal disease) formula (37–39), which calculates a patient's glomerular filtration rate per body surface area (thus correcting for body size already), based on patient age, sex, race, and serum creatinine. When an estimated glomerular filtration rate equal to or less than 60 mL/min/1.73 m² is used as a threshold to identify patients at risk, one can again simplify the matter and tabulate the creatinine thresholds above which a patient would be considered to have renal insufficiency and thus be at risk for CIN (Table 4-3).

Prevention in Patients at Risk

In patients at high risk for CIN, other imaging modalities such as magnetic resonance imaging (MRI) without contrast medium and Doppler ultrasound should be considered first. If CTA is deemed necessary, the lowest possible dose of a low osmolar or iso-osmolar dose should be used (Table 4-4). With fast scanners, and if only large vessel disease is clinically suspected such as for aortic aneurysm follow-up and evaluation, small volumes and flow rates may suffice, but one should not risk that image quality is nondiagnostic, particularly if acute treatment decisions need to be inferred from a CTA.

Nephrotoxic drugs, such as nonsteroidal anti-inflammatory drugs (NSAID), should be stopped at least 24 hours before CM administration. Volume expansion with IV fluid is known to reduce the risk of CIN. It is not entirely clear if oral hydration would be adequate as well; it certainly does no harm. Studies have shown that it is important to start fluid injection (e.g., 100 mL per hour of normal 0.9% saline) several hours before CM injection and to continue for several hours thereafter (40). A recently published more compact hydration protocol by Merten et al. (41) using bicarbonate seems to be effective and in the setting of CTA has the advantage that it can be started only 1 hour before contrast medium injection (Table 4-4).

There are numerous studies, meta-analysis, and reviews published regarding the pharmacological prevention of CIN using vasodilators (e.g., fenoldopam), receptor antagonists of endogenous vasoactive mediators (e.g., theophyllin), or cytoprotective drugs (e.g., acetylcysteine), all of which do not seem to offer consistent protection against CIN (40). Despite conflicting evidence in the literature, acetylcysteine may still be useful in a pretreatment protocol (together with volume expansion with bicarbonide) in patients with increased risk of CIN because of its low cost, the lack of side effects, and simplicity of use (Solomon R, personal communication).

While it is well recognized that low-osmolar nonionic contrast agents are less nephrotoxic than high-osmolar ionic contrast agents in patients with renal impairment, it is currently unclear if and to what extent iso-osmolar contrast agents (42) further reduce the risk of CIN compared with low-osmolar agents, notably in the setting of IV injections for CTA. More study is required to confirm the reported lower nephrotoxicity of iso-osmolar contrast media. Finally, if patients at risk for CIN undergo a CT angiographic study, it is also important to ensure that serum creatinine levels are being followed-up adequately.

Drug Interactions

Contrast media may interact with the pharmacological action of other drugs. Given the increasing use of CM and

TABLE 4-4

Practical Preventive Measures for Contrast Medium–induced Nephrotoxicity in the Setting of Computed Tomographic Angiography

Outpatients	Routine blood testing not required in all patients; use questionnaire to determine need for blood testing in patients younger than 70 years.
Request serum creatinine	Blood testing required in • Patients older than 70 years • Patients with history of renal disease, renal surgery (including transplantation), diabetes • All inpatients
Estimate risk for CIN	Do not use a single creatinine threshold as an indicator of impaired renal function. Instead, use an estimated GFR <60 mL/min/1.73 m^2 determined by using the MDRD formula or a table (Table 4-3) as an indicator of impaired renal function.
Inpatients at risk for CIN	Consider alternative imaging techniques (MR, ultrasound). Stop potentially nephrotoxic drugs and diuretics for at least 24 hours. Use low or iso-osmolar contrast agents. Use a volume expansion protocol (see below) Acetylcysteine may be beneficial (see below)
Volume expansion protocol	Administer intravenously • 3.50 mL/kg BW per hour for one hour, followed by 1.18 mL/kg BW per hour for 6 hours of the following solution: 3 ampules (150 mEq) of sodium bicarbonate to 1 liter of 5% dextrose (yielding 130-mEq/L concentration of sodium bicarbonate and 4.35% dextrose).
Acetylcysteine	May have a protective effect if given at the dose of 600 to 1,200 mg orally twice daily 24 hours before and continued for 48 hours after CM injection.
Do not forget	Follow up on patients at risk for CIN.

(GFR, glomerular filtration rate; MDRD, Modification of Diet in Renal Disease study.)

the changing patient population, including older patients and patients with multiple medical problems (20), it is important to be aware of these interactions. Knowing a patient's drug history and proper documentation of the CM used are the first of several general guidelines on how to avoid drug interactions with CM (43). In the setting of CTA, the following drugs need special attention.

Metformin may cause lactic acidosis in diabetic patients with renal impairment, notably in diabetic nephropathy, and should be discontinued (44).

Nephrotoxic drugs such as *cyclosporine, cisplatin, aminoglycosides,* and *NSAIDs* and also *loop diuretics* enhance the adverse effects of CM on renal function. A few drugs may enhance allergylike reactions to CM. The most important ones in the context of cardiovascular CT/CTA are *beta-blockers.* Patients on beta-blockers are significantly more likely to have an anaphylactoid reaction than matched controls (45,46). Furthermore, beta-blockers reduce the effectiveness of adrenaline when a life-threatening anaphylaxislike reaction occurs (11). Contrast media may not only precipitate *interleukin-2* (IL-2) toxicity, but patients on IL-2 also have higher rates of immediate urticarial as well as delayed reactions to IV CM. An increased risk may remain for

2 years after the end of treatment. Previous CM reaction in an IL-2 patient should be considered a relative contraindication of further CM (47). Finally, it has been suggested to avoid contrast medium injections in patients treated with *hydralazine* (a compound in some antihypertensive medications), as it may predispose patients to a reaction of acute cutaneous vasculitis (48). Effects of CM on coagulation, fibrinolytic drugs, and interactions with calcium channel blockers are not relevant for intravenous CM administration.

Gadolinium-based Contrast Agents for Computed Tomographic Angiography

Because of the perceived safety of gadolinium-based (Gd) contrast media in the setting of MRI up to a dose of 0.3 mmol/kg, it has been suggested that Gd-based agents could be used in lieu of iodinated agents in patients with significant renal impairment (49). Gadolinium has a higher atomic number (z = 64) than iodine (z = 53), and its k-edge (50 keV) is also more favorable than that of iodine (33 keV) at the kilovoltage settings used in CT, resulting in approximately double the x-ray attenuation. Because Gd-based agents have a substantially lower molar concentration (typically 0.5 mmol Gd/mL, with only one exception) than iodinated agents

(300 mgI/mL = 2.38 mmol I/mL), their x-ray absorption per milliliter is less. In CTA, where arterial opacification is proportional to the quantity of x-ray–attenuating particles administered per unit of time, an injection flow rate of 4 mL/s of Gd-based contrast medium will achieve an arterial enhancement level less than that of an injection rate of 2 mL/s of iodinated (300 mg/mL) CM. So, despite that one would certainly exceed the recommended and approved dose of Gd-based CM, the image quality would still be inferior to that of a typical CTA and not of diagnostic quality when small vessel visualization is desired. Gadolinium-based contrast agents are also nephrotoxic in patients with decreased renal function in doses greater than 0.3 mmol/kg (50). At equivalent x-ray–attenuating doses, Gd-based CM are actually more nephrotoxic than iodinated agents (51). Gd-based agents are therefore not recommended as an alternative to iodinated contrast medium in patients with renal insufficiency undergoing CTA. For a more detailed discussion of gadolinium based contrast agents and nephrogenic systemic fibrosis see Chapter 22. The use of these agents as an alternative may be justified, however, in the setting of prior severe generalized adverse reaction to iodinated contrast medium and in cases of imminent thyroid treatment with radioactive iodine.

PHARMACOKINETICS AND PHYSIOLOGY OF ARTERIAL ENHANCEMENT

All angiographic x-ray contrast media are extracellular fluid markers. After IV administration, they are rapidly distributed between the intravascular and extravascular interstitial spaces (52). Pharmacokinetic studies on CM have tradionally concentrated on the phase of elimination (following CM injection) rather than on the very early phase of CM distribution (during CM administration). For the time frame relevant to CTA, however, it is this particularly complex phase of early contrast medium distribution and redistribution that determines vascular enhancement. Early contrast medium dynamics cannot be studied directly (i.e., measuring the rapid changes of the concentration of CM from blood samples). However, as relative CT attenuation values (ΔHU, ΔHounsfield units), derived by subtracting background attenuation before administration of contrast medium, are linearly related to the concentration of contrast medium (iodine), contrast medium dynamics may be described and expressed in these units (1,52).

It is important to appreciate, at this point, that vascular enhancement (which is the topic of this chapter) and parenchymal organ enhancement are affected by different kinetics. Early vascular enhancement is essentially determined by the relationship between iodine administration per unit of

time (iodine flux [mgI/s]) versus blood flow per unit of time (i.e., cardiac output [L/min]). Parenchymal enhancement, on the other hand, is governed by the relationship of total iodine dose (mgI) versus volume of distribution (extracellular fluid, or as a proxy, body weight [kg]). Thus, the most important injection parameter in CTA is the injection flow rate or—more precisely—the iodine flux, whereas in organ imaging, it is the CM volume or—more precisely—the iodine dose.

Early Arterial Contrast Medium Dynamics

Early contrast medium dynamics have gained substantial interest because of their implications for CTA. Whereas time-attenuation responses to intravenously injected CM may vary between vascular territories and across individuals, the basic pattern is illustrated in the following example.

Figure 4-2 schematically shows the early arterial contrast medium dynamics as observed in the abdominal aorta: When a 16-mL test bolus of CM is injected intravenously at a flow rate of 4 mL/s, it causes an arterial enhancement response in the aorta. The time interval needed for the CM to arrive in the arterial territory of interest is referred to as the *contrast medium transit time* (t_{CMT}). The t_{CMT} is variable between individuals and an important parameter for scan timing (see section titled, Scanning Delay and Automated Bolus Triggering). The first peak in the vascular enhancement response is also referred to as the *first pass effect*. Note that the tail of the arterial enhancement response after the first peak does not return to zero but instead undulates above the baseline attenuation. This is most likely due to broadening of the bolus in the heart and pulmonary circulation, and also due to recirculation of opacified venous blood from highly perfused organs, such as the brain and the kidneys. It is important to realize that within the time frame of CTA, one will not only observe the first pass effect of intravenously injected contrast material but also its bolus-broadening and recirculation effects (generally—though not perfectly correct—referred to as *recirculation*).

For a given individual and vascular territory, the enhancement response is proportional to the iodine administration rate, or iodine flux (mgI/s). Figures 4-2C and 4-2D illustrate the effect of doubling the iodine administration rate (by doubling the injection flow rate) for a given injection duration. The resulting enhancement response is approximately twice as strong. Whereas the proportional effect of the iodine administration rate on arterial enhancement is intuitive, this is not the case for the effect of the injection duration on the degree and the overall shape of the enhancement curve.

A simple additive model, based on the assumption of a time-invariant linear system, may help to explain the effect of prolonged injections on arterial enhancement (53).

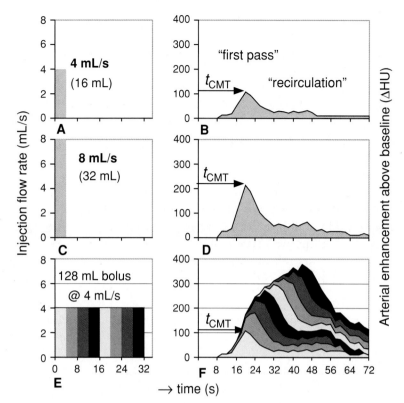

FIGURE 4-2 Simple "additive model" illustrating the effects of injection flow rate and injection duration on arterial enhancement. Intravenous contrast medium (CM) injection **(A)** causes an arterial enhancement response **(B)**, which consists of an early first pass peak and a lower recirculation effect. Doubling the injection flow rate (doubling the iodine administration rate) **(C)** results in approximately twice the arterial enhancement **(D)**. The effect of the injection duration **(E)** can be regarded as the sum (time integral) of several enhancement responses **(F)**. Note that due to the asymmetric shape of the test-enhancement curve as well as the recirculation effects, arterial enhancement following an injection of 128 mL (the "time integral of 8 consecutive 16 ml") increases continuously over time. (Adapted from Fleischmann D. Present and future trends in multiple detector-row CT applications: CT angiography. *Europ Radiol.* 2002;12:S11–S16, with permission.)

As shown in Figures 4-2E and 4-2F, a large (128 mL), prolonged (32 seconds) bolus of CM can be regarded as the sum of 8 subsequent test boluses of 16 mL each. Each of these 8 test boluses has its own effect (first pass and recirculation) on arterial enhancement, respectively. The cumulative enhancement response to the entire 128-mL injection equals the sum (time integral) of enhancement responses to each of the 8 test boluses. Note that the recirculation effects of the earlier test boluses overlap (and thus have to be added) with the first pass effects of later test boluses.

As a result, the general enhancement pattern observed in the arterial system following the IV injection of a prolonged bolus (>10 seconds) of contrast medium can be characterized as follows: After a certain time interval (corresponding to the contrast medium transit time, t_{CMT}), there is a short, steep enhancement increase, which is followed by a more shallow, continuous increase of arterial opacification that is approximately as long as the duration of the CM injection, followed by a rapid decrease of enhancement.

The principles of the early arterial CM dynamics described can be summarized into the first two (of three) key rules of arterial enhancement for cardiovascular CT (Table 4-5):

1. Arterial enhancement is proportional to the iodine flux.
2. Arterial enhancement also increases with longer injection durations.

Physiologic Parameters Affecting Arterial Enhancement

In general, the previously described vascular enhancement response to intravenously injected CM applies to all arterial territories. The specific magnitudes, however, are characteristic for a given vascular territory in a given patient. The exact shape of a time-attenuation curve is determined by an individual's physiology and thus beyond the control of the observer.

The t_{CMT} from the injection site to the vascular territory of interest depends on the anatomic distance between them, but also on the encountered physiologic flow rates between these landmarks. Peripheral IV injection flow rates certainly affect the transit times in the arm veins, but increasing the injection rate only minimally shortens the arterial t_{CMT} because cardiac output is hardly affected by the injected volume. Central venous injections unsurprisingly shorten the t_{CMT} as well (54,55). For systemic arteries, the t_{CMT} is primarily controlled by cardiac output, which also accounts for most of the wide interindividual variability of the t_{CMT}. Low cardiac output prolongs and high cardiac output decreases the t_{CMT}. Obviously, the t_{CMT} can be substantially delayed in patients with venous obstructions downstream from the injection site but also when venous return is temporarily decreased, such as during a forceful Valsalva maneuver by a patient attempting to hold his or her breath.

The *degree of arterial enhancement* following the same IV contrast medium injection is also highly variable between individuals. Even in patients considered to have normal cardiac output, mid aortic enhancement may range from 140 HU to 440 HU (a factor of three) between patients (56). Even if body weight is taken into account, the average aortic enhancement has been shown to range from 92 to 196 HU/mL/kg (a factor of two) in patients with abdominal aortic aneurysms (55). The relationship of arterial enhancement to body weight is illustrated in Figure 4-3. Adjusting the contrast medium volume (and injection rates) to body weight will therefore not eliminate but will reduce interindividual differences of arterial enhancement, notably in patients with extreme deviations from the average. The third key rule of arterial enhancement for cardiovascular CT is thus:

3. Arterial enhancement is highly variable between individuals (Table 4-5).

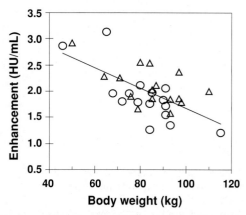

FIGURE 4-3 Arterial enhancement versus body weight. Scatterplot shows significant correlation (rPearson = −0.64, *p* <*0.01*) between arterial enhancement and body weight in 32 patients who underwent abdominal CTA. Patients represented as triangles were injected 120 mL of CM at a flow rate of 4 mL/s. Patients represented as circles received individualized volumes and injection rates. Enhancement is given in Hounsfield Units (HU) per mL of CM injected, correcting for differences in injected volumes in group 2. (Data from Fleischmann D, Rubin GD, Bankier AA, et al. Improved uniformity of aortic enhancement with customized contrast medium injection protocols at CT angiography. *Radiology.* 2000;214:363–371, with permission.)

TABLE 4-5

Key Rules of Early Arterial Contrast Medium Dynamics for Computed Tomographic Angiography and Their Consequences

1. Arterial enhancement is proportional to the iodine flux.
   - Arterial opacification can be increased by increasing the injection flow rate and/or by increasing the iodine concentration of the contrast medium.
   - For example, the iodine flux (and thus arterial enhancement) increases by 46% (from 1.20 to 1.75 g/s) if the flow rate is increased from 4 to 5 mL/s and the iodine concentration is increased from 300 to 350 mgI/mL.

2. Arterial enhancement increases over time in a cumulative fashion.
   - Arterial opacification increases with longer injection durations.
   - A minimum injection duration of approximately 10 seconds is always needed to achieve adequate arterial enhancement.
   - Biphasic (multiphasic) injections result in more uniform enhancement if long scan times and injection durations (>20 seconds) are used.

3. Arterial enhancement is highly variable between individuals.
   - Cardiac output—the main physiologic parameter controlling arterial enhancement—is inversely proportional to arterial opacification (i.e., high cardiac output results in decreased arterial enhancement and vice versa). Cardiac output correlates with body weight.
   - Increasing or decreasing both the injection rate and the injection volumes to body weight, at least for large (>90 kg) and small (<60 kg) individuals, respectively, will reduce the interindividual variability of arterial enhancement and is recommended.

A practical compromise in clinical CTA is therefore to adjust the injection volumes and flow rates at least for patients with body weights differing more than 20% from an average of say 75 kg.

The key physiologic parameters affecting individual arterial enhancement are cardiac output and the central blood volume. *Cardiac output* is inversely related to the degree of arterial enhancement, particularly in first pass dynamics (57): If more blood is ejected per unit of time, the contrast medium injected per unit of time will be more diluted. Hence, arterial enhancement is lower in patients with high cardiac output, but it is stronger in patients with low cardiac output (despite the increased t_{CMT} in the latter). This effect is illustrated in two patients with different physiques (Figure 4-4). Note that the 51-year-old hypertensive man with a body weight (BW) of 88 kg required about 3 times the volume and substantially greater injection flow rates to achieve a similar degree of arterial enhancement when compared with the 67-year-old woman with 59 kg of body weight.

Central blood volume is also inversely related to arterial enhancement—but presumably affects recirculation and tissue enhancement to a greater extent than it affects first pass dynamics (52). Central blood volume correlates with body weight. Very generally speaking, a dose of 1.5 to 2.0 mL/kg of body weight (450 to 600 mgI/kg BW) is a reasonable quantity for arterial CTA.

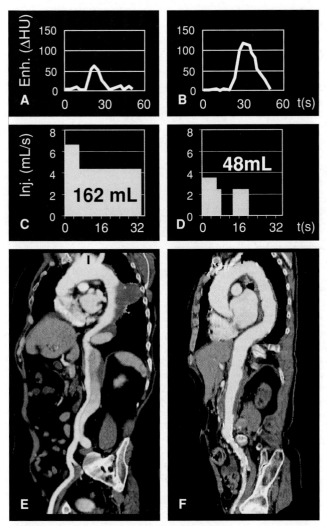

FIGURE 4-4 Variability of arterial enhancement between patients of different physique. The aortic enhancement responses (**A,B**) to a 16-mL test bolus are shown for a 51-year-old hypertensive man with a body weight of 88 kg (**A**), and a 67-year-old woman with 59 kg body weight (**B**). Because of a substantially lower enhancement response to the test bolus, the younger and bigger man required more than 3 times more contrast medium volume (162 mL) than the older and smaller woman (48 mL) (**C,D**) to achieve a similar enhancement in the subsequent CTA of the thoracoabdominal aorta (**E,F**).

User-selectable Parameters Affecting Arterial Enhancement

With key physiologic parameters (such as cardiac output) beyond the control of the observer, it is particularly important to understand the effects of user-selectable injection parameters on arterial enhancement. Traditionally, injection protocols for CTA have been expressed as the volume (mL) and flow rate (mL/s) of contrast medium, likely because those are the parameters that usually can be selected on a power injector. However, volume and injection flow rate poorly reflect underlying physiology. It is more useful and intuitive to express injection protocols for CTA in terms of iodine administration

rate (or its substitute, the injection flow rate, in mL/s) and injection duration (in s). CM volume is a secondary, dependent parameter, derived by simple multiplication, and should not be considered a primary injection parameter.

Iodine administration rate (injection flow rate): The number of iodine molecules administered per unit of time (the *iodine flux*) is proportional to the injection flow rate for a given CM concentration. An iodine flux of 1.0 to 1.2 g/s (3.5 to 4 mL/s) is generally considered a minimum rate for CTA (15 mgI/s/kg BW). The iodine flux or the injection flow rate has a direct, proportional effect on arterial enhancement (Figures 4-2C and 4-2D). For example, a 50% increase of the injection rate (for a given injection duration) will result in a 50% increase of arterial enhancement (at the cost of 50% more contrast medium volume). Similarly, a 30% increase of the iodine concentration will yield a 30% stronger enhancement. Maximum iodine flux can be achieved when both high iodine concentration contrast media (≤350 mgI/mL) and high injection flow rates are combined. Injection flow rates greater than 8 mL/s, however, do not necessarily translate into a proportionally stronger arterial enhancement (58), possibly due to backflow of contrast medium into the inferior vena cava. This physiologic limitation of increasing the flow rate may be even lower in patients with cardiocirculatory disease.

Injection duration: As illustrated in Figure 4-2, arterial enhancement also increases with the injection duration. This effect is not as straightforward and intuitive as the effect of the iodine flux; however, it becomes immediately obvious that very short injection durations—for example, 4 seconds—cannot reach an adequate arterial enhancement level. Therefore, the traditional CTA rule of thumb, where the injection duration equals the scanning duration, is no longer applicable to fast acquisitions. There is a minimum injection duration necessary to raise arterial enhancement to an adequate level of opacification in CTA, which is probably in the order of 10 seconds.

Biphasic or multiphasic injections: As previously noted, the typical arterial enhancement pattern resulting from prolonged (20 to 40 seconds) CM injections is a continuous rise of arterial enhancement. Even with correct scan timing, this will result in lower arterial opacification early during the scan and excessive enhancement later during the data acquisition. For prolonged CT acquisitions (20- to 40-second scan time), a more uniform enhancement can be achieved if the injection rates are varied over time, with high initial flow rates and lower continuing flow rates (59,60). Prolonged acquisitions are encountered with single-slice CTA, with 4-channel MDCT with large volume coverage (e.g., thoracoabdominal CTA), and also with ECG-gated cardiothoracic acquisitions with 16-channel MDCT. There is no benefit of using bi- or multiphasic injections with fast CTA acquisitions (<10 seconds) when the acquisitions are timed correctly.

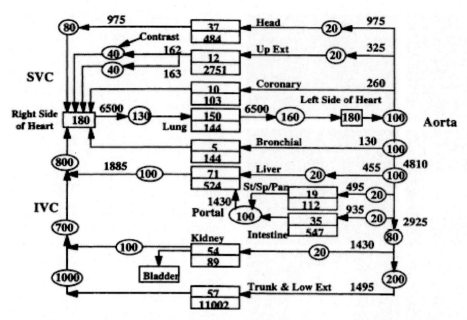

FIGURE 4-5 Global circulation model. Contrast medium (*Contrast*) is introduced into the antecubital site, mixed in the right side of the heart, distributed throughout the body, and excreted by the kidneys according to the glomerular filtration rate. Regional blood flow is expressed according to the magnitude (in milliliters per minute) and direction of the flow. A blood vessel is represented by a circle surrounding a number that represents its volume (in milliliters). Each organ is shown as a box split into two subcompartments: The number in the upper subcompartment denotes capillary volume, and the number in the lower subcompartment denotes ECF volume. (IVC, inferior vena cava; Low Ext, lower extremities; St/Sp/Pan, stomach, spleen, pancreas; SVC, superior vena cava; Up Ext, upper extremities.) (From Bae KT, Heiken JP, Brink JA. Aortic and hepatic contrast medium enhancement at CT. Part I. Prediction with a computer model. *Radiology.* 1998;207:647–655, with permission.)

Mathematical Modeling

Accurate prediction and controlling of time-dependent arterial enhancement is highly desirable for MDCT. Ideally, one wants to predict and control the time course as well as the degree of vascular enhancement in each individual, independent of an individual's underlying physiology. Two mathematical techniques addressing this issue have been developed.

The first is a sophisticated *compartmental model*, which predicts vascular and parenchymal enhancement using a system of more than 100 differential equations to describe the transport of contrast medium between intravascular and interstitial fluid compartments of the body (Fig. 4-5) (61). For CT angiography, this model suggests multiphasic injections to achieve uniform vascular enhancement. The injection flow rate is maximum at the beginning of the injection followed by a continuous, exponential decrease of the injection rate (57). The advantage of this model is that it can predict not only arterial but also parenchymal (e.g., liver) enhancement. The limitation of this approach is, however, that it cannot calculate individualized injections because key physiologic parameters are generally unknown in a given patient. Weight-based estimates are possible, of course, and thus rational injection protocols can be designed.

The second *black-box model* approach is based on the mathematical analysis of a patient's characteristic time-attenuation response to a small test-bolus injection (62). Assuming a time-invariant linear system, one can mathematically extract an individual's contribution ("patient factor") to his or her enhancement response to an intravenously injected test bolus. A subject's patient factor can then be used to individually tailor biphasic injection protocols to achieve uniform, prolonged arterial enhancement at a predefined level (60). The principle of this technique is outlined in Figure 4-6. The method is robust and has been used successfully (Fig. 4-4) and extensively in clinical practice at one institution, but it is not commercially available to a potentially larger group of users.

The greatest practical value of both mathematical models for CTA, however, comes from the gained insights into early contrast medium dynamics, allowing a more rational approach to the design of empiric but routinely applicable injection techniques for current and future CT applications.

INSTRUMENTATION AND TECHNIQUE

Contrast Medium Concentration and Temperature

Vascular enhancement is proportional to the number of iodine molecules administered per unit of time. This *iodine administration rate* (iodine flux) can be increased by

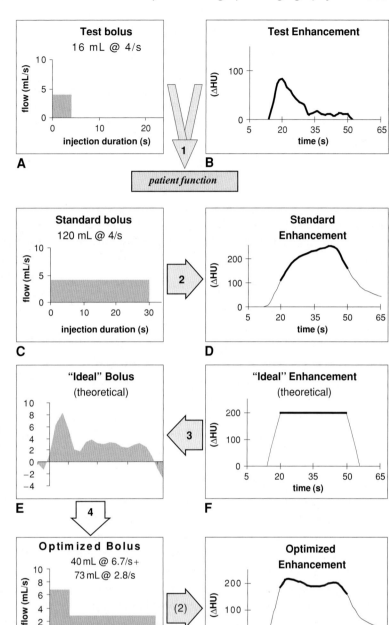

FIGURE 4-6 Mathematical modeling and individualizing of arterial enhancement. Flow chart illustrates the four main steps to characterize, predict, and optimize arterial enhancement in CTA of the aorta using the *black-box* model. The calculation of the optimized biphasic bolus for this 65-year-old patient is based on the selection of an "ideal" enhancement of 200 DHU for 30 s, with slopes of increase and decrease of 200 HU/6 s.

Step 1: The *patient function* is calculated in Fourier space from the relation of a 16-mL test bolus **(A)** to the patient's corresponding aortic time-attenuation response, the test enhancement **(B)**.

Step 2: Once the patient function is known, the standard enhancement **(D)** to an arbitrary bolus, such as a 120-mL standard bolus **(C)** can be predicted.

Step 3: With the use of the patient function, it is also possible to calculate a theoretically ideal bolus **(E)**, which is supposed to achieve an ideal, near-rectangular enhancement **(F)**.

Step 4: As the theoretically ideal bolus **(E)** contains "unreal" components in the time domain, like oscillations, or negative flow rates, a *fitting algorithm* has to be introduced to approximate the ideal flow rates into a practically applicable "optimized" biphasic (Σ, 113 mL) bolus **(G)**. The corresponding optimized enhancement **(H)** can be predicted as described in step 2. Despite the pronounced simplification of the optimized bolus **(G)**, the resulting optimized enhancement **(H)** does not deviate much from the desired form in the scanning period.

(Bolus descriptors are given as: total volume (mL) at flow rate (mL/s); DHU, arterial enhancement over baseline attenuation in Hounsfield units.) (From Fleischmann D, Hittmair K. Mathematical analysis of arterial enhancement and optimization of bolus geometry for CT angiography using the discrete fourier transform. *J Comput Assist Tomogr.* 1999;23:474–484, with permission.)

increasing the injection flow rate and/or by increasing the iodine concentration of the contrast medium used. An iodine administration rate of, say, 1.5 g/s requires a faster injection rate of 5 mL/s with "standard" concentration (300 mgI/mL) CM compared with an injection rate of 4.3 mL/s using a 350 mgI/mL concentration or a flow rate of 3.8 mL/s with the highest concentration (400 mgI/mL) of CM available (the maximum iodine concentration available in the United States is 370 mgI/mL). The obvious advantage of high-concentration agents is that one can achieve a greater iodine flux for a given flow rate—or achieve the same iodine flux at lower injection rates. One potential limitation of high-concentration agents (≥350 mgI/mL) is their disproportionally greater viscosity (Table 4-1). However, with use of power injectors and adequate needle size, this is not a practical limitation. Low-concentration contrast media (<300 mgI/mL), on the other hand, have the advantage that they cause less perivenous artifacts at the level of the brachiocephalic veins and the superior vena cava in thoracic CT, particularly if saline flushing of the veins is not employed (63). Low-concentration agents are also less viscous.

We use 350 mgI/mL and higher contrast agents (370 mgI/mL is the highest iodine concentration available in the U.S., 400 mgI/mL agents are available elsewhere) at our institution. At similar iodine administration rates, the concentration of the agent has probably no effect.

Preheating the contrast agents, using commercially available thermostatically controlled heating cabinets to warm the contrast media to 37°C, significantly reduces the viscosity—approximately 50% compared with the viscosity at room temperature (Table 4-1). Because high injection rates and/or high-concentration (more viscous) contrast agents are often required in the setting of CTA, and the most commonly used cannula is 20G at our institution, we generally preheat our contrast medium.

Intravenous Access

A securely placed peripheral IV cannula in a large cubital or antebrachial vein is the preferred injection site for CTA. There has been a trend to using increasingly higher injection flow rates and high-concentration contrast agents (≥350 mgI/mL) with each new scanner generation. Both high flow rates and high iodine concentration (because of its exponential effect on viscosity) require that an adequate diameter IV cannula be used. There is hardly any data in the literature that could serve as the basis for recommended cannula size. The limitations for flow rates (in mL/min for water!) provided by the manufacturers and the minimum pressure limits an IV cannula must withstand by the ISO (International Organization for Standardization) standard (5 bar [72 PSI]) (4) will almost certainly be exceeded with any CTA injection protocol, but to the best of our knowledge, no specific pressure limits for peripheral IV lines of different size are available for CM injections. The frequency of bursting of an IV cannula is unknown, and so is its relationship to the in-line pressures. The risk to the patient from a ruptured IV line (outside the patient's body) is probably small. The author is currently unaware of any reported cases of the theoretical risk of cannula disintegration and subsequent foreign-body embolism.

At our institution, 20G cannulas (pink ISO color code) are most commonly used by all referring services. We use these 20G cannulas for CTA with our most commonly used injection rate of 5 mL/s, but we also use up to 5.5 or 6 mL/s. As well, we use fairly viscous (Table 4-1) high-concentration monomers (350 mgI/mL or 370 mgI/mL) or an iso-osmolar dimer CM—and therefore routinely preheat the CM—and use a warming cuff on the injector. The pressure limit is set to 300 PSI. In general, larger cannulas 18G (green) are preferable if flow rates equal to or greater than 6 mL/s are anticipated. We have routinely used 17G cannulas (white) for perfusion studies with IV flow rates up to 10 mL/s in the past. A fast manual saline injection with the patient's arms in scanning position (usually above the head for body CTA) before mechanical CM delivery is always performed to assure correct peripheral catheter position. The injection site is monitored at the start of the injection.

Central Venous Catheters and Peripherally Inserted Central Catheter Lines

The safety of using central venous catheters to administer contrast medium using power injectors in patients without sufficient peripheral IV access is not generally established. Even slow injection rates exceed the (probably conservative) pressure limits recommended by the manufacturers (64,65). Sanelli et al. have tested a 7 French (F) triple-lumen central venous catheter used at their institution (Arrow-Howes multilumen catheter) in vitro with flow rates up to 9.9 mL/s. They also tested flow rates between 3.0 and 5.0 mL/s in 104 patients with the pressure limit of the power injector set to 300 PSI. They used a viscous contrast medium (iodixanol at room temperature) injected through proximal and mid 18G ports and the distal 16G port (66) without complications. While it is not possible to generalize these results for all types of central venous lines, this work shows how local guidelines for central venous CM injections can be established successfully. These guidelines do not include only flow rates and pressure limits, but also include measures to clearly identify the catheter tip in the superior vena cava on nonenhanced images before the power injection and a nursing policy for avoiding catheter contamination.

While standard peripherally inserted central venous catheters (PICC lines) do not allow sufficient CM administration rates for CTA (67), the U.S. Food and Drug Administration has recently cleared dedicated high-pressure PICC lines from at least two manufacturers that allow pressure limits of 300 PSI and can thus be used for rapid CM injections (5 mL/s) required for CTA (Powerpick, Bard Access Systems; Turbo-Flo, Cook Inc.).

Power Injectors and Saline Flushing

Mechanical power injectors are indispensable devices for CTA. Power injectors allow for preprogramming the desired CM volume and flow rates, and setting of a pressure limit (usually 300 PSI). Most devices also provide a heating cuff to keep the CM in the syringe of the injector warm. Many power injectors allow more than one injection phase, like biphasic, multiphasic, or even continually decelerating injections, and all major manufacturers have introduced double-barrel systems, which allow one syringe to be filled with CM and the other one to be filled with saline solution, which can be used to flush the arm veins after a CM injection. Some injectors also allow that saline is admixed to CM during the injection to vary the CM concentration.

One manufacturer produces an injector with a CM extravasation detection device, which interrupts the mechanical injection when a skin-impedance change due to fluid extravasation is detected (68). While the reported 100% sensitivity may eliminate significant extravasations (>10 mL) in high-flow-rate CT applications, false positives occur in 2.4% (25).

Several manufacturers of power injectors and CT manufacturers have recently agreed on a generic communication interface between scanner and injector. This will allow the generation of combined scanning and injection protocols that can be automatically loaded and initiated from either the scanner or the injector.

Saline Flushing of the Veins

It is well known from upper extremity venography that a considerable amount (probably about 15 mL, but with wide variation) of contrast medium remains in the arm veins after the end of an injection, from where it is cleared only very slowly. In the setting of CTA, this particular fraction of CM is not utilized because it does not contribute to arterial enhancement. Flushing the venous system with saline immediately after the CM injection pushes the CM column from the arm veins into the circulation, which has two desirable effects. First, saline flushing improves arterial opacification and prolongs the arterial enhancement phase. The best way to intuitively understand the magnitude effect is by asking oneself the question, What is the effect of not using a saline flush? Not using a saline flush has about the same effect as if the last near-15 mL of the CM dose were not injected. So, saline flushing does "save" CM, and this effect has been exploited to reduce the total CM volume in routine thoracic MDCT (69,70). Second, because saline flushing removes CM from the brachiocephalic veins and the superior vena cava, it reduces perivenous streak artifacts (Fig. 4-7). In cardiac and coronary CTA, notably with fast scanners, saline flushing allows the right ventricle to be completely cleared from undiluted CM (the *levocardiogram*. While this avoids artifacts in the right atrioventricular groove portion of the right coronary artery, complete CM voiding of the right ventricle is problematic for functional analysis of the left ventricle because the thickness and motion of the interventricular septum cannot be assessed in this instance. A potential solution for this is not to flush with saline, but to use diluted CM (10% to 20%) instead.

Saline flushing can also be performed by layering saline above contrast in the syringe of a single-barrel power injector. Some mixing cannot be avoided, though, and the technique is more time consuming and less reliable than using double-barrel systems.

Scanning Delay and Automated Bolus Triggering

A fixed, empiric injection-to-scan delay is adequate for many routine nonvascular CT applications. In cardiovascular CT, however, a fixed scanning delay cannot be recommended because the arterial t_{CMT} is prohibitively variable between individual patients. It may range from as short as 8 seconds to as long as 40 seconds in patients with cardiovascular diseases. In CTA, the scanning delay needs to be timed relative to the t_{CMT} of each individual. Transit times can be determined reliably by using either a test-bolus injection or an automatic bolus-triggering technique.

Test bolus: The injection of a small test bolus (15 to 20 mL) while acquiring a series of low-dose dynamic (nonincremental) CT images is the most reliable means to determine the t_{CMT} from the IV injection site to the arterial territory of interest (71). The time-to-peak enhancement interval measured in a region-of-interest (ROI) placed within a reference vessel is generally used as the t_{CMT} for this particular vascular territory of a given individual. The test-bolus technique can also be used when unusual injection sites need to be used (e.g., lower extremity vein), and more than one ROI and t_{CMT} can be obtained from different vessels (e.g., the SVC, the pulmonary artery, and the aorta) (Fig. 4-8). In the era of single-slice CT, the measured t_{CMT} was almost always used directly as the scanning delay for a subsequent CTA. It is important to keep in mind, though, that it is often more favorable not to use the t_{CMT} directly, but to use a slightly longer scanning delay relative to an individual's t_{CMT}. For example, the notion that "scanning delay is $t_{CMT} + 5$ s" means that the CTA acquisition begins 5 seconds after the t_{CMT} (5 seconds after the CM has arrived in the territory of interest).

Bolus triggering: All state-of-the-art MDCT scanners have this feature built into their system. In principle, a circular ROI is placed into the target vessel on a nonenhanced image. While contrast medium is injected, a series of low-dose nonincremental images are obtained, and the attenuation within an ROI is monitored or inspected visually. The CT acquisition is initiated when the desired enhancement threshold (e.g., 100 ΔHU) is reached (Fig. 4-9).

Four specific parameters need to be selected when automated bolus triggering is used. The details as well as the terminology are scanner specific:

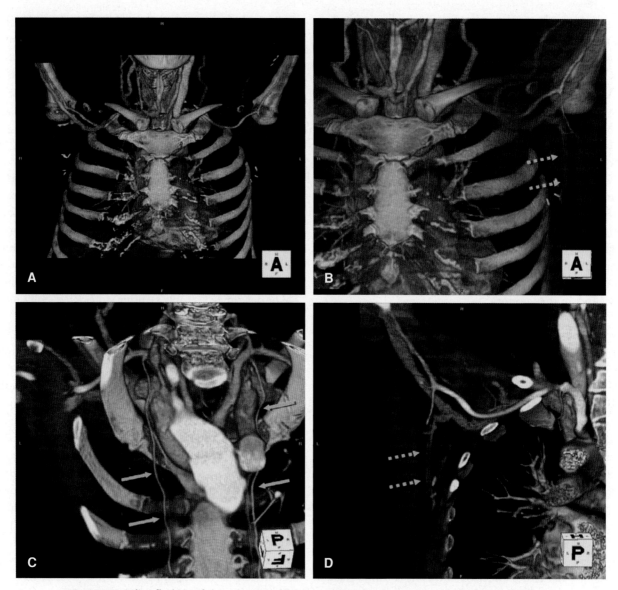

FIGURE 4-7 Saline flushing of the veins. CTA of the chest wall in a 57-year-old woman with a history of bilateral breast cancer, referred to evaluate the size and patency of the bilateral internal mammary and thoracodorsal arteries and veins for possible free flap surgical reconstruction. Injected biphasically were 150 mL of contrast medium over 55 seconds, followed by 40 mL of saline using a double-barrel power injector. A fast caudocranial CTA acquisition (16 × 1.25 mm) was initiated immediately after the CM injection. Volume-rendered images show absence of any streak artifacts at the level of the upper thorax and thoracic inlet **(A)**, allowing the assessment of both internal mammary arteries and veins (*solid arrows* in **C**) and the diminutive thoracodorsal arteries and veins (*dashed arrows* in **B** and **D**).

1. *Monitoring delay* determines when the first monitoring slice is acquired after the beginning of the injection. Usually between 5 and 10 seconds.
2. *Monitoring interval* is the sampling interval for the monitoring slices. While some vendors (e.g., Toshiba) provide continuous monitoring (and low-dose radiation), others acquire the monitoring slices at predefined intervals (1 to 3 seconds).
3. *Trigger threshold* is the enhancement value within the ROI that when reached initiates the CTA acquisition.

Values of 80 to 120 HU (above baseline) are reasonable values in this context.

4. *Trigger delay* ("delay," "diagnostic delay") is the selectable time interval between reaching the trigger threshold (or contrast medium arrival), and the start of the actual CTA data acquisition. The minimum trigger delay depends on the scanner model. The trigger delay can and should be increased with short acquisition times.

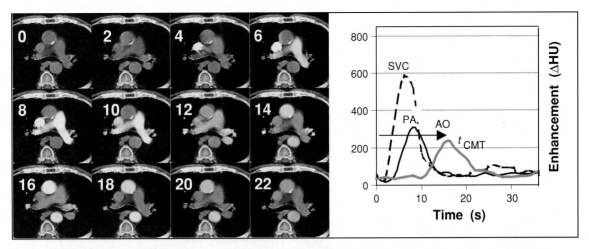

FIGURE 4-8 Time-attenuation curves obtained from a test-bolus injection. Left panel shows 12 nonincremental CT images obtained at the level of the carina in 2-second intervals during IV injection of a small test bolus of CM (16 mL, injected at 4 mL/s). **Right panel** shows time-attenuation curves obtained from the superior vena cava (SVC), the pulmonary artery (*PA*), and the aorta (*AO*). The contrast medium transit time for the aorta (t$_{CMT}$) was 16 seconds in this particular case.

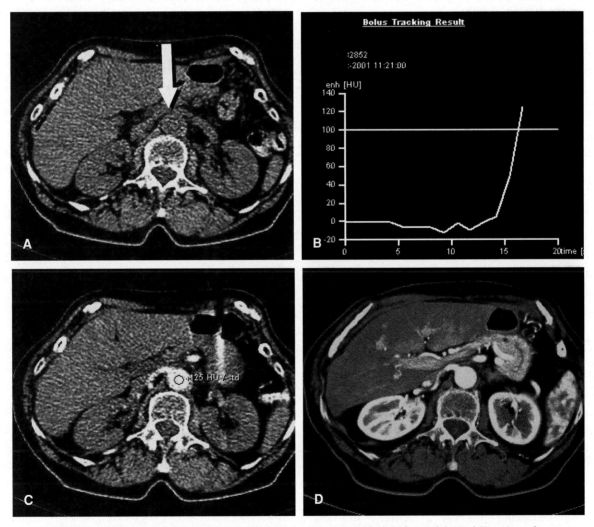

FIGURE 4-9 Automated bolus triggering. The scanning delay is individualized for an abdominal CT angiography by placing a region of interest into the aorta (*arrow* in **A**). Contrast medium is injected, and arterial enhancement is monitored on a time-attenuation curve (**B**) displayed on the scanner console. Once the opacification in the aorta (**C**) exceeds the target enhancement level of 100 HU (*horizontal line* in **B**), the CTA acquisition is initiated after a short interval. Note the bright opacification in the aorta on the first CTA image (**D**).

While bolus triggering is a very effective and robust means for individualizing the scanning delay, it is important to be aware of the fact that it inherently results in longer scanning delays compared with the t_{CMT} obtained with the test-bolus technique. This is because the CT scanner needs a minimum of 1 to 3 seconds to begin data acquisition after the trigger threshold is reached (or more, if the starting position of the scan is not identical to the table position of the monitoring series, but also if the pre-recorded breath-hold command is long). In addition to this, one has to add the time for image reconstruction and the sampling interval of the monitoring images, which may substantially differ between manufacturers as well as between scanner models. Notably, in early models of General Electric MDCT scanners, this image reconstruction time is 3 seconds (what you see is 3 seconds old). In these particular scanners, the actual scan is initiated approximately 8 seconds after the true t_{CMT} (3-s image reconstruction time, 3-s minimum diagnostic delay, 2-s potential sampling error). While this is not necessarily a disadvantage—because arterial enhancement only gets better with a longer scanning delay, and one can accommodate a breath-hold command in this time interval—it has to be accounted for by also increasing the injection duration accordingly. Otherwise, one is at risk to run out of contrast medium opacification at the end of the acquisition.

When the specific details of the bolus-triggering technique of a given scanner are known and taken into account, bolus triggering is a very robust and efficient method for individualizing the scanning delay in all patients undergoing CTA. The primary advantage is that it does not require the additional time and volume of an extra test-bolus injection.

Avoiding the Valsalva Maneuver

Central venous blood flow is subject to intrathoracic pressure changes due to respiration (72). In the setting of CM-enhanced CT, this may be particularly harmful if a patient performs an ambitious Valsalva maneuver during breath holding. During a Valsalva maneuver, the intrathoracic and intra-abdominal pressures increase, which causes a temporary interruption of venous return from the head and upper extremity veins (where CM is usually injected), and a temporary relative increase of (unopacified) venous blood from the inferior vena cava. The effect of this flow alteration is a temporary decrease of vascular opacification in the dependent territories, such as the pulmonary arterial tree, but also later in the arterial system. In some cases (and notably with fast scanners), this may cause nondiagnostic opacification of the entire pulmonary arterial tree (Fig 4-10).

It is thus important that the technologist explains to the patient not to "bear down" during breath holding, and/or advise him or her to keep the mouth open during breath holding, which apparently makes it difficult to perform a Valsalva maneuver.

CLINICAL CONTRAST MEDIUM INJECTION PROTOCOLS FOR COMPUTED TOMOGRAPHIC ANGIOGRAPHY

The common denominator and thus the key parameter for designing rational injection protocols for a given CTA application is the scan time. Scan times vary across scanners and have become substantially shorter with each new scanner generation. Scan times may also differ between applications for different vascular territories of a given scanner model. Acquisition times for CTA may range from more than 30 seconds (e.g., thoracoabdominal CTA with a 4-channel MDCT) or 40 seconds (lower extremity run-off) to as short as 4 seconds (abdominal CTA with a 64-channel MDCT). No single strategy of CM injection for CTA can therefore be applied. The following clinical injection strategies for "slow" and "fast" acquisitions are based on the pharmacokinetics of early contrast dynamics, published clinical and experimental data, mathematical approximations, and practical experience. Most applications with 4-channel MDCT fall into the slow category, while 16-channel applications mostly fall into the fast category, but there is some overlap, depending on the specific application or scanning parameters used. With 64-channel MDCT, however, we have observed a paradigm shift. For the first time, the injection protocols are not designed to match the scan time, but instead, the CT acquisition protocol is designed to match the injection protocol.

Basic Injection Strategy for Slow Acquisitions

The most basic injection strategy for CTA derived from the single-slice CT era, when comparatively long scan times were necessary to image a given volume with thin sections. The rule of thumb was to inject CM for a duration equal to the scan time. So, for a 40-second abdominal CTA acquisition, the injection duration would be 40 seconds as well, which resulted in a quite large CM dose of 160 mL if a typical injection flow rate of 4 mL/s (300 mgI/mL; 1.2 g of iodine/s) was used. Scan timing was done either using a test bolus or bolus tracking, or sometimes even with a fixed scanning delay.

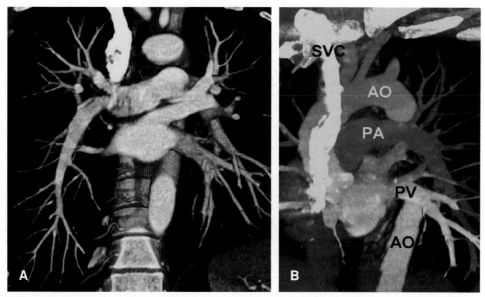

FIGURE 4-10 Detrimental effect of Valsalva maneuver on pulmonary arterial enhancement. Volume-rendered **(left panel)** 64-channel pulmonary CT angiogram obtained in a 40-year-old man with pulmonary hypertension to rule out pulmonary embolism (and deep venous thrombosis). Injected were 150 mL of CM at a flow rate of 5 mL/s, with a scan delay of t_{CMT} + 15 seconds. The patient performed a strong Valsalva maneuver during breath holding for the CT acquisition, which was obtained in the caudocranial direction. Oblique thin-slab MIP image **(right panel)** demonstrates that while CM is still being injected at the end of the acquisition as seen in the superior vena cava (*SVC*), and while there is good opacification of the aorta (*AO*) and pulmonary veins (*PV*), the opacification of the pulmonary arterial (*PA*) tree is nondiagnostic.

This very basic strategy is still useful for many CTA applications. Flow rates should be adapted, though, for shorter acquisitions (up to 5 or even 6 mL/s) and also for patient size. For example, a 20% higher and a 20% lower injection flow rate (and volume) should be used for patients with more than 90 kg or less than 60 kg body weight, respectively. Individual scan timing is crucial for faster acquisitions.

Two widely held misconceptions derived from this initial "injection-duration-equals-scanning-duration" protocol. The first is the intuitive but inaccurate belief that an IV injection at a constant injection rate (e.g., 4 mL/s) results in an equally constant, uniform *enhancement plateau*. From Figure 4-2, it is obvious that such an enhancement plateau does not exist for the time frame of CTA. The second related misconception is the assumption that faster CT acquisitions directly translate into proportionally smaller amounts of CM (Fig. 4-11).

Biphasic and Multiphasic Injections for Slow Acquisitions

Biphasic (or multiphasic) injections are more favorable for prolonged injections (20 to 40 seconds) than uniphasic injections (Table 3-1) because they provide a more uniform enhancement in the vascular territory of interest (60). In general, the injection duration is again chosen equal to the scanning duration. The initial iodine administration rate should be in the order of 1.8 g/s for 5 seconds for an average (75 kg) adult. The second, maintaining injection phase, should be in the order of >1.0 g/s (iodine administration rate). The scanning delay should be short (equal to the t_{CMT} or only slightly longer, up to t_{CMT} + 2 s). Examples of biphasic injections are given in Table 4-6. We have been using biphasic injection routinely for most of our CTA acquisitions with single and 4-channel MDCT, and still use biphasic injections for lower extremity CTA, even with 64-channel MDCT (73). Biphasic injections are less useful for short acquisiton times, because enhancement does not change rapidly after the initial rise during a short CT acquisition.

Rapid Injections for Fast Acquisitions

When scan times became increasingly shorter with MDCT scanners, it became apparent that basic rule of thumb—injection duration equals the scanning duration—is not universally applicable, at least not with injection flow rates unchanged: Let us assume that the same patient who underwent a prior CTA with a slow scanner and a scan time

TABLE 4-6

Biphasic Injection Protocols for Slow Acquisitions

Acquisition Time (s)	Scanning Delay (s)	Iodine		300-mgI/mL CM		350-mgI/mL CM		400-mgI/mL CM	
		Total Dose (g)	Biphasic Iodine Flux (g @g/s)	Total Volume (mL)	Biphasic Injections (mL @ mL/s)	Total Volume (mL)	Biphasic Injections (mL @ mL/s)	Total Volume (mL)	Biphasic Injections (mL @ mL/s)
40	t_{CMT}	42	9 @ 1.8 + 33 @ 0.95	140	30 @ 6 + 110 @ 3.1	120	25 @ 5.1 + 95 @ 2.7	105	23 @ 4.5 + 82 @ 2.4
35	t_{CMT}	39	9 @ 1.8 + 30 @ 1.0	130	30 @ 6 + 100 @ 3.3	110	25 @ 5.1 + 85 @ 2.9	100	23 @ 4.5 + 77 @ 2.5
30	t_{CMT}	36	9 @ 1.8 + 27 @ 1.1	120	30 @ 6 + 90 @ 3.6	105	25 @ 5.1 + 80 @ 3.1	90	23 @ 4.5 + 67 @ 2.7
25	t_{CMT}	33	9 @ 1.8 + 24 @ 1.2	110	30 @ 6 + 80 @ 4.0	95	25 @ 5.170 + @ 3.4	85	23 @ 4.5 + 62 @ 3.0
20	t_{CMT}	30	9 @ 1.8 + 21 @ 1.25	100	30 @ 6 + 70 @ 4.2	85	25 @ 5.1 + 60 @ 3.6	75	23 @ 4.5 + 52 @ 3.1

Note: t_{CMT}, contrast medium transit time, as established individually with a test-bolus or bolus-triggering technique. The total injection duration for the biphasic injections equals the scan time. For the first 5 seconds of the injection, the injection rate always corresponds to 1.8 g of iodine/s; for the remainder of the injection, the flow rates are lower.

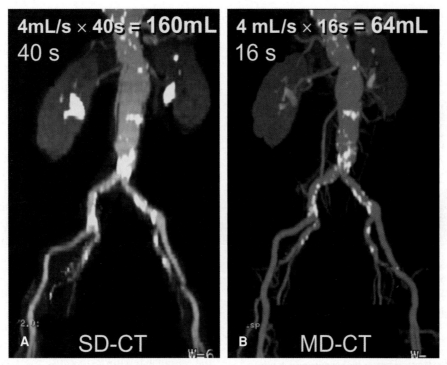

FIGURE 4-11 Arterial enhancement in single (SDCT) versus multiple detector-row CT (MDCT). Comparison of two abdominal CT angiograms in the same patient obtained with a single-slice CT **(left)** and a 4-channel MDCT **(right)** scanner. The image quality with respect to spatial resolution and stair-step artifacts is substantially improved with MDCT. At the same time, it is important to also observe that arterial opacification is actually decreased with MDCT. This is easily explained by the injection protocols that had been used: Both studies were obtained with an injection rate of 4 mL/s, but the injection duration was 40 seconds (equal to the scan time) with single-slice CT and only 16 seconds with MDCT (also equal to the scan time). Hence, there was not enough time to achieve the same degree of enhancement. (From Rubin GD, Shiau MC, Leung AN, et al. Aorta and iliac arteries: single versus multiple detector-row helical CT angiography. *Radiology.* 2000;215:670–676, with permission.)

of 32 seconds (Fig. 4-2F) is rescanned with a new, faster scanner, with half the scan time of 16 seconds (Fig. 4-12). It is readily apparent that if the original injection flow rate of 4 mL/s would have been used for the shorter injection duration of only 16 (vs. 32) seconds, the arterial enhancement with the faster scanner is less than with the slower scanner. To compensate for that, the first and/or the second key rules of early contrast medium dynamics can be applied. First, arterial enhancement can be increased by increasing the iodine flux. Changing the injection flow rate from 4 to 5 mL/s, and using a contrast agent with 350 rather than 300 mgI/mL, the iodine flux and thus arterial enhancement is increased by 45%. Second, arterial enhancement can also be improved by increasing the injection duration and scanning delay (e.g., for 8 seconds, relative to the t_{CMT}), respectively. Of note, the injection duration is no longer equal but is longer than the scan time!

For routine CTA applications with 8- and 16-channel scanners using scan times in the range of 10 to 20 seconds, the following ball park rule can be applied (Table 4-7):

Select an injection rate of 5 mL/s (range: 4 to 6 mL/s) of ≥350 mgI/mL contrast agent (1.75 gI/s). Inject at the selected injection rate for 8 seconds longer than the scan time (e.g., for a 12-second acquisition, inject 5 mL/s for 20 seconds, resulting in 100 mL total volume). Use a test bolus or preferably automated bolus triggering in order to individualize the scanning delay such that the acquisition will start approximately 8 seconds after the t_{CMT} (after the CM arrives in the target vasculature). An example of a 16-channel MDCT angiogram of a patient with visceral artery vasculitis imaged with the above protocol is shown in Figure 4-13.

Strategies for 64-Channel MDCT and Beyond: The Paradigm Shift

What might be the best way to inject CM for a scan time of only 4 seconds—which is easily possible with 64-channel MDCT? Obviously, one cannot inject 4 mL/s for only 4 seconds, as the arterial enhancement effect would be equal to that obtained from injecting a test bolus—certainly not

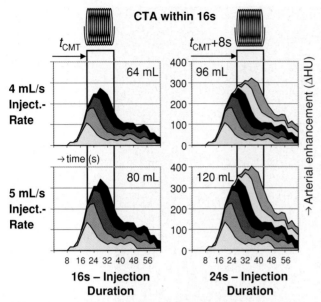

FIGURE 4-12 Strategies to improve arterial enhancement with faster CTA. Two strategies to increase arterial enhancement compared with what can be achieved from a 16-second injection at 4 mL/s **(upper left panel)** can be employed—either alone or in combination: Increasing the injection rate from 4 to 5 mL/s increases the enhancement approximately 20% **(lower left panel)**. Alternatively, one can also increase the injection duration and the scanning delay, taking advantage of the fact that enhancement increases with longer injection durations **(right upper panel)**. Maximum enhancement can be achieved when both the injection rate (and/or the iodine concentration) as well as the injection duration are increased **(right lower panel)** simultaneously. (From Fleischmann D. Contrast-medium administration. In: Catalano C, Passariello R, eds. *Multidetector-row CT Angiography.* New York: Springer; 2005:41–54, with permission.)

greater enhancement. High flow rates are also impractical, and scan timing would become critically important in order to not completely miss a short and high arterial enhancement peak. One solution again would be to increase the iodine flux as well as increase the scanning delay and the injection duration as described earlier.

With 64-channel MDCT, however, one can follow a very different strategy, and for good reasons. First of all, there is no particular advantage of using a 4-s versus a 10-s acquisition for a CT angiographic application. Maximum table speed may even be detrimental because very fast acquisitions may not allow complete and sufficient opacification of a diseased arterial tree. This has been observed in mesenteric CTA, in abdominal or thoracic aortic aneurysms, and most notably in peripheral (lower extremity) CTA (74). Figure 4-14 shows an example of an infrarenal abdominal aortic aneurysm that is incompletely opacified because the scanning speed was chosen too fast. Another general problem with CTA injection protocols is that they are difficult to standardize across different patients and vascular territories because the acquisition times may be quite different, even within the same application. While protocols are usually adjusted for the different scan times, only few attempts have been made to individualize injection protocols at the same time, probably because of the difficulty of intuitively integrating many parameters into an individual injection.

So, our current integrated acquisition and CM injection strategy for 64-channel CTA is to deliberately slow down the CT acquisition and use the same scan time for a given vascular territory for each patient (the pitch thus varies between patients). Automated tube-current modulation is used not only to avoid increasing the radiation dose to the patient but more importantly to control image noise. Automated tube-current modulation allows the user to predetermine the desired (or acceptable)

enough to study small arterial branches at high resolution. Injecting at very high flow rates, for example, 10 mL/s, could work theoretically, but it is known that flow rates greater than 8 mL/s are not linearly transmitted by the circulation and thus do not necessarily lead to a proportionally

TABLE 4-7

Injection Protocols for Fast Acquisitions

Acquisition Time (s)	Scanning Delay (s)	Iodine Dose (g)	Iodine Flux (g/s)	300-mgI/mL CM CM Volume at Injection Rate (mL @ mL/s)	350-mgI/mL CM CM Volume at Injection Rate (mL @ mL/s)	400-mgI/mL CM CM Volume at Injection Rate (mL @ mL/s)
20	t_{CMT} + 8	39	1.35	125 @ 4.5	110 @ 4	95 @ 3.4
15	t_{CMT} + 8	36	1.5	115 @ 5	100 @ 4.5	90 @ 3.8
10	t_{CMT} + 8	33	1.8	110 @ 6	90 @ 5	85 @ 4.5
5	t_{CMT} + 10	27	1.8	90 @ 6	80 @ 5	70 @ 4.5

Note: t_{CMT}, contrast medium transit time, as established individually with a test-bolus or bolus-triggering technique.

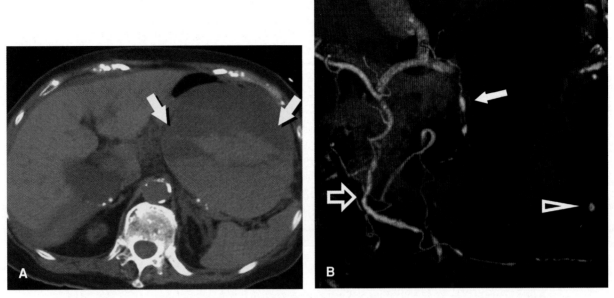

FIGURE 4-13 16-Channel abdominal CT angiography. Abdominal CTA obtained in a 43-year-old woman with a history of spontaneous retroperitoneal hematomas and positive lupus anticoagulant antibodies. Nonenhanced CT image demonstrates large hemorrhage with sedimentation of blood within the lesser sac (*arrows* in A). Volume-rendered image of the celiac vasculature **(B)** shows inflammatory changes with narrowing and beading of the short gastric artery (*arrow*), wall irregularities of the gastroduodenal artery (*open arrow*), and a small aneurysm of the gastroepiploic artery (*arrowhead*). Visualization of small vessels requires bright vessel opacification, which was achieved by an injection flow rate of 5 mL/s, injected for a duration of 20 seconds (100 mL). Scanning delay for this 12-second scan time was set to t_{CMT} + 8 seconds.

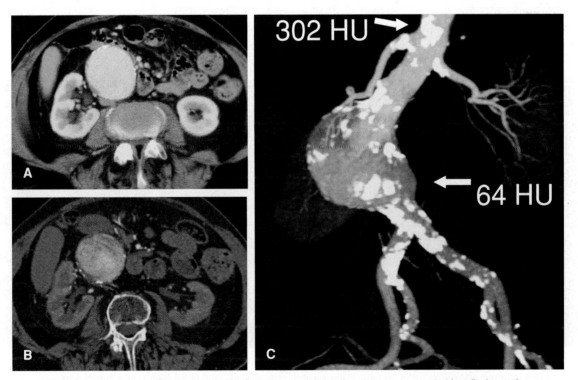

FIGURE 4-14 Poor opacification caused by fast CTA. An abdominal aortic aneurysm was incidentally detected on a routine 5-mm section thickness abdominal CT **(A)**. The patient was referred for a dedicated abdominal CTA **(B,C)** to evaluate his aneurysm. A 64-channel CTA was obtained using automated bolus triggering but inadvertently without an additional delay (t_{CMT} + 0 seconds). Transverse CTA section **(B)** at the same level of **(A)** shows insufficient opacification of the aneurysm sac, which does not allow the differentiation of thrombus from perfused lumen. MIP image **(C)** demonstrates good arterial opacification above the aneurysm (302 HU), but the short time required to scan this territory does not allow adequate opacification of the aneurysm sac (64 HU) and the iliac arteries.

TABLE 4-8

Integrated 64-Channel MDCT in Renal Disease Study Acquisition and Injection Protocol for Abdominal CTA

Acquisition	64 × 0.6 mm (number of channels × channel width); automated tube current modulation (250 quality reference mAs)
Pitch	variable (depends on volume coverage, usually <1.0)
Scan time	FIXED to 10 seconds (in all patients)
Injection duration	FIXED to 18 seconds (in all patients)
Scanning delay	t_{CMT} + 8s (scan starts 8 seconds after CM arrives in the aorta, as established with automated bolus triggering)
Contrast medium	high concentration (370 mgI/mL)
Injection flow rates and volumes	Individualized to body weight

Body weight	CM Flow Rate	CM Volume
<55 kg	4.0 mL/s	72 mL
56–65 kg	4.5 mL/s	81 mL
66–85 kg	5.0 mL/s	90 mL
>85 kg	6.0 mL/s	108 mL

image noise for a given CT application, which will then be constant within and across individuals. When the scan time stays the same for all patients, one can always use the same injection durations as well. The flow rates can then be easily individualized for patient weight in a simple look-up table, an example of which is shown in Table 4-8.

The scan time with 64-channel CTA is therefore no longer chosen as a result of technical trade-offs of spatial resolution versus volume coverage, and it is not chosen by just using the maximum speed available, but it is done so to match the physiologic constraints of arterial CM enhancement. For example, we choose a scan time of 10 seconds for abdominal CTA with an injection duration of

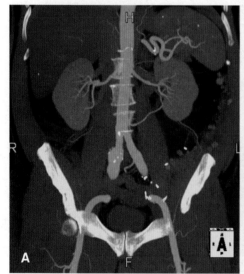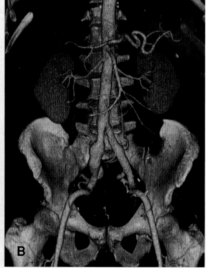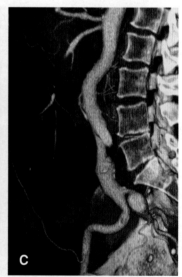

FIGURE 4-15 64-Channel abdominal CT angiography. Abdominal CTA obtained in a 63-year-old obese (95 kg) man for evaluation of right iliac aneurysms, incidentally detected on an MR study of the lumbar spine. Images were acquired within a 10-second scan time. Injection flow rate was 5.5 mL/s, injected for 18 seconds, with a scanning delay of t_{CMT} + 8 seconds (see text). Thin-slab maximum intensity projection image **(A)** nicely demonstrates low image noise throughout the entire scanning range despite the patient's large body habitus. No artifacts or increased noise are seen in pelvis. This image quality is reliably achieved by using a slow acquisition speed (10-second scan time) and automated tube-current modulation. Corresponding frontal **(B)** and sagittal **(C)** volume-rendered images demonstrate the fusiform right common iliac and saccular right hypogastric artery aneurysms.

18 seconds, and a scanning delay of t_{CMT} + 8 seconds determines using bolus triggering. This strategy allows breath holding for virtually all patients, and it results in reliable strong arterial enhancement because of high iodine flux combined with increased scanning delay relative to the t_{CMT} but avoids excessive injection flow rates at the same time. Image quality (noise) is constant within and across individuals by using automated tube-current modulation (Fig. 4-15). Injection volumes and flow rates can easily be adjusted to body weight as well.

CONCLUSION

Contrast medium delivery remains an integral part of cardiovascular MDCT and CTA. While CT technology continues to evolve, the physiologic and pharmacokinetic principles of arterial enhancement will remain unchanged in the foreseeable future. A basic understanding of early contrast medium dynamics thus provides the foundation for the design of current and future CM injection protocols. With these tools at hand, CM utilization can be optimized for various clinical applications of CTA and optimized for each patient. This ensures optimal CM utilization while exploiting the full capabilities of continuously evolving MDCT technology.

REFERENCES

1. Dawson P, Blomley MJ. Contrast media as extracellular fluid space markers: adaptation of the central volume theorem. *Br J Radiol.* 1996;69:717–722.
2. Gries H. Chemistry of x-ray contrast agents. In: Dawson P, ed. *Textbook of Contrast Media.* Oxford: Isis Medical Media; 1999:15–33.
3. Persson PB, Hansell P, Liss P. Pathophysiology of contrast medium-induced nephropathy. *Kidney Int.* 2005;68:14–22.
4. Knopp M, Kauczor HU, Knopp MA, et al. [Effects of viscosity, cannula size and temperature in mechanical contrast media administration in CT and magnetic resonance tomography]. *ROFO.* 1995;163:259–264.
5. Katayama H, Yamaguchi K, Kozuka T, et al. Adverse reactions to ionic and nonionic contrast media. A report from the Japanese Committee on the Safety of Contrast Media. *Radiology* 1990;175:621–628.
6. Palmer FJ. The RACR survey of intravenous contrast media reactions. Final report. *Australas Radiol.* 1988;32:426–428.
7. Wolf GL, Arenson RL, Cross AP. A prospective trial of ionic vs nonionic contrast agents in routine clinical practice: comparison of adverse effects. *AJR Am J Roentgenol.* 1989;152:939–944.
8. Hill JA, Winniford M, Cohen MB, et al. Multicenter trial of ionic versus nonionic contrast media for cardiac angiography. The Iohexol Cooperative Study. Am J Cardiol 1993; 72:770-775.
9. Hopper KD. With helical CT, is nonionic contrast a better choice than ionic contrast for rapid and large IV bolus injections? *AJR Am J Roentgenol.* 1996;166:715.
10. Caro JJ, Trindade E, McGregor M. The risks of death and of severe nonfatal reactions with high- vs low-osmolality contrast media: a meta-analysis. *AJR Am J Roentgenol.* 1991;156:825–832.
11. Thomsen HS, Morcos SK. Management of acute adverse reactions to contrast media. *Eur Radiol.* 2004;14:476–481.
12. Media CiDaC. Manual on Contrast Media, Version 5.0: American College of Radiology, 2004.
13. Thomsen HS, ed. *Contrast Media: Safety Issues and User Guidelines.* New York: Springer; 2005.
14. Webb JA, Stacul F, Thomsen HS, et al. Late adverse reactions to intravascular iodinated contrast media. *Eur Radiol.* 2003;13:181–184.
15. Bettmann MA, Heeren T, Greenfield A, et al. Adverse events with radiographic contrast agents: results of the SCVIR Contrast Agent Registry. *Radiology.* 1997;203:611–620.
16. van der Molen A, Thomsen H, Morcos S; Contrast Media Safety Committee, European Society of Urogenital Radiology (ESUR). Effect of iodinated contrast media on thyroid function in adults. *Eur Radiol.* 2004;14:902–907.
17. Dawson P. Does injection rate affect the tolerance? In: Dawson PH, Clauss W, eds. *Contrast Media in Practice: Questions and Answers.* 2nd ed. New York: Springer Verlag; 1998:135–136.
18. Jacobs JE, Birnbaum BA, Langlotz CP. Contrast media reactions and extravasation: relationship to intravenous injection rates. *Radiology.* 1998;209:411–416.
19. Maitino AJ, Levin DC, Parker L, et al. Practice patterns of radiologists and nonradiologists in utilization of noninvasive diagnostic imaging among the Medicare population 1993–1999. *Radiology.* 2003;228:795–801.
20. Toms A, Cash C, Linton S, et al. Requests for body computed tomography: increasing workload, increasing indications and increasing age. *Eur Radiol.* 2001;11:2633–2637.
21. Bellin MF, Jakobsen JA, Tomassin I, et al. Contrast medium extravasation injury: guidelines for prevention and management. *Eur Radiol.* 2002;12:2807–2812.
22. Blomley MJ, Coulden R, Dawson P, et al. Liver perfusion studied with ultrafast CT. *J Comput Assist Tomogr.* 1995;19:424–433.
23. Bader TR, Herneth AM, Blaicher W, et al. Hepatic perfusion after liver transplantation: noninvasive measurement with dynamic single-section CT. *Radiology.* 1998;209:129–134.
24. Jeans WD. The development and use of digital subtraction angiography. *Br J Radiol.* 1990;63:161–168.
25. Birnbaum BA, Nelson RC, Chezmar JL, et al. Extravasation detection accessory: clinical evaluation in 500 patients. *Radiology.* 1999;212:431–438.
26. Cohan RH, Ellis JH, Garner WL. Extravasation of radiographic contrast material: recognition, prevention, and treatment. *Radiology.* 1996;200:593–604.
27. Rees CR, Palmaz JC, Garcia O, et al. The hemodynamic effects of the administration of ionic and nonionic contrast materials into the pulmonary arteries of a canine model of acute pulmonary hypertension. *Invest Radiol.* 1988;23:184–189.
28. Cochran ST, Bomyea K, Sayre JW. Trends in adverse events after IV administration of contrast media. *AJR Am J Roentgenol.* 2001;176:1385–1388.
29. Morcos SK. Contrast media-induced nephrotoxicity—questions and answers. *Br J Radiol.* 1998;71:357–365.
30. Heinrich MC, Kuhlmann MK, Grgic A, et al. Cytotoxic effects of ionic high-osmolar, nonionic monomeric, and nonionic iso-osmolar dimeric iodinated contrast media on renal tubular cells in vitro. *Radiology.* 2005;235:843–849.
31. Solomon R. The role of osmolality in the incidence of contrast-induced nephropathy: a systematic review of angiographic contrast media in high risk patients. *Kidney Int.* 2005;68:2256–2263.
32. Parfrey PS, Griffiths SM, Barrett BJ, et al. Contrast material-induced renal failure in patients with diabetes mellitus, renal insufficiency, or both. A prospective controlled study. *N Engl J Med.* 1989;320:143–149.
33. Levy EM, Viscoli CM, Horwitz RI. The effect of acute renal failure on mortality. A cohort analysis. *JAMA.* 1996;275:1489–1494.
34. Thomsen HS, ed. *Contrast Media: Safety Issues and User Guidelines.* New York: Springer; 2005.
35. Choyke PL, Cady J, DePollar SL, et al. Determination of serum creatinine prior to iodinated contrast media: is it necessary in all patients? *Tech Urol.* 1998;4:65–69.

36. Namasivayam S, Kalra M, Ritchie J, et al. Role of reagent strip based rapid blood urea nitrogen and creatinine meter (EZ-Chem) in patients undergoing contrast enhanced radiological studies. *RSNA Bulletin.* 2005.

37. Levey AS, Bosch JP, Lewis JB, et al. A more accurate method to estimate glomerular filtration rate from serum creatinine: a new prediction equation. Modification of Diet in Renal Disease Study Group. *Ann Intern Med.* 1999;130:461–470.

38. Levey AS, Greene T, Kusek JW, et al. A simplified equation to predict glomerular filtration rate from serum creatinine. *J Am Soc Nephrol.* 2000;11:155A.

39. Lamb EJ, Webb MC, Simpson DE, et al. Estimation of glomerular filtration rate in older patients with chronic renal insufficiency: is the modification of diet in renal disease formula an improvement? *J Am Geriatr Soc.* 2003;51:1012–1017.

40. Morcos SK. Prevention of contrast media nephrotoxicity—the story so far. *Clin Radiol.* 2004;59:381–389.

41. Merten GJ, Burgess WP, Gray LV, et al. Prevention of contrast-induced nephropathy with sodium bicarbonate: a randomized controlled trial. *JAMA.* 2004;291:2328–2334.

42. Aspelin P, Aubry P, Fransson SG, et al. Nephrotoxic effects in high-risk patients undergoing angiography. *N Engl J Med.* 2003;348:491–499.

43. Morcos SK, Thomsen HS, Exley CM. Contrast media: interactions with other drugs and clinical tests. *Eur Radiol.* 2005;15:1463–1468.

44. Thomsen HS, Morcos SK. Contrast media and metformin: guidelines to diminish the risk of lactic acidosis in non-insulin-dependent diabetics after administration of contrast media. ESUR Contrast Media Safety Committee. *Eur Radiol.* 1999;9:738–740.

45. Lang DM, Alpern MB, Visintainer PF, et al. Increased risk for anaphylactoid reaction from contrast media in patients on beta-adrenergic blockers or with asthma. *Ann Intern Med.* 1991;115:270–276.

46. Lang DM, Alpern MB, Visintainer PF, et al. Elevated risk of anaphylactoid reaction from radiographic contrast media is associated with both beta-blocker exposure and cardiovascular disorders. *Arch Intern Med.* 1993;153:2033–2040.

47. Choyke PL, Miller DL, Lotze MT, et al. Delayed reactions to contrast media after interleukin-2 immunotherapy. *Radiology.* 1992;183:111–114.

48. Reynolds NJ, Wallington TB, Burton JL. Hydralazine predisposes to acute cutaneous vasculitis following urography with iopamidol. *Br J Dermatol.* 1993;129:82–85.

49. Prince MR, Arnoldus C, Frisoli JK. Nephrotoxicity of high-dose gadolinium compared with iodinated contrast. *J Magn Reson Imaging.* 1996;6:162–166.

50. Sam AD 2nd, Morasch MD, Collins J, et al. Safety of gadolinium contrast angiography in patients with chronic renal insufficiency. *J Vasc Surg.* 2003;38:313–318.

51. Thomsen HS, Almen T, Morcos SK. Gadolinium-containing contrast media for radiographic examinations: a position paper. *Eur Radiol.* 2002;12:2600–2605.

52. Dawson P, Blomley MJ. Contrast agent pharmacokinetics revisited: I. Reformulation. *Acad Radiol.* 1996;3[Suppl 2]:S261–S263.

53. Fleischmann D. Present and future trends in multiple detector-row CT applications: CT angiography. *Eur Radiol.* 2002;12:S11–S16.

54. Rubin DL, Burbank FH, Bradley BR, et al. An experimental evaluation of central vs. peripheral injection for intravenous digital subtraction angiography (IV-DSA). *Invest Radiol.* 1984;19:30–35.

55. Hittmair K, Fleischmann D. Accuracy of predicting and controlling time-dependent aortic enhancement from a test bolus injection. *J Comput Assist Tomogr.* 2001;25:287–294.

56. Sheiman RG, Raptopoulos V, Caruso P, et al. Comparison of tailored and empiric scan delays for CT angiography of the abdomen. *AJR Am J Roentgenol.* 1996;167:725–729.

57. Bae KT, Heiken JP, Brink JA. Aortic and hepatic contrast medium enhancement at CT. Part II. Effect of reduced cardiac output in a porcine model. *Radiology.* 1998;207:657–662.

58. Claussen CD, Banzer D, Pfretzschner C, et al. Bolus geometry and dynamics after intravenous contrast-medium injection. *Radiology.* 1984;153:365–368.

59. Bae KT, Tran HQ, Heiken JP. Multiphasic injection method for uniform prolonged vascular enhancement at CT angiography: pharmacokinetic analysis and experimental porcine model. *Radiology.* 2000;216:872–880.

60. Fleischmann D, Rubin GD, Bankier AA, et al. Improved uniformity of aortic enhancement with customized contrast medium injection protocols at CT angiography. *Radiology.* 2000; 214:363–371.

61. Bae KT, Heiken JP, Brink JA. Aortic and hepatic contrast medium enhancement at CT. Part I. Prediction with a computer model. *Radiology.* 1998;207:647–655.

62. Fleischmann D, Hittmair K. Mathematical analysis of arterial enhancement and optimization of bolus geometry for CT angiography using the discrete fourier transform. *J Comput Assist Tomogr.* 1999;23:474–484.

63. Rubin GD, Lane MJ, Bloch DA, et al. Optimization of thoracic spiral CT: effects of iodinated contrast medium concentration. *Radiology.* 1996;201:785–791.

64. Herts BR, O'Malley CM, Wirth SL, et al. Power injection of contrast media using central venous catheters: feasibility, safety, and efficacy. *AJR Am J Roentgenol.* 2001;176: 447–453.

65. Carlson JE, Hedlund LJ, Trenkner SW, et al. Safety considerations in the power injection of contrast media via central venous catheters during computed tomographic examinations. *Invest Radiol.* 1992;27:337–340.

66. Sanelli PC, Deshmukh M, Ougorets I, et al. Safety and feasibility of using a central venous catheter for rapid contrast injection rates. *AJR Am J Roentgenol.* 2004;183:1829–1834.

67. Salis AI, Eclavea A, Johnson MS, et al. Maximal flow rates possible during power injection through currently available PICCs: an in vitro study. *J Vasc Interv Radiol.* 2004;15:275–281.

68. Nelson RC, Anderson FA Jr., Birnbaum BA, et al. Contrast media extravasation during dynamic CT: detection with an extravasation detection accessory. *Radiology.* 1998;209: 837–843.

69. Hopper KD, Mosher TJ, Kasales CJ, et al. Thoracic spiral CT: delivery of contrast material pushed with injectable saline solution in a power injector. *Radiology.* 1997;205:269–271.

70. Haage P, Schmitz-Rode T, Hubner D, et al. Reduction of contrast material dose and artifacts by a saline flush using a double power injector in helical CT of the thorax. *AJR Am J Roentgenol.* 2000;174:1049–1053.

71. Van Hoe L, Marchal G, Baert AL, et al. Determination of scan delay-time in spiral CT-angiography: utility of a test bolus injection. *J Comput Assist Tomogr.* 1995;19:216–220.

72. Gosselin MV, Rassner UA, Thieszen SL, et al. Contrast dynamics during CT pulmonary angiogram: analysis of an inspiration associated artifact. *J Thorac Imaging.* 2004;19:1–7.

73. Fleischmann D, Hallett RL, Rubin GD. CT angiography of peripheral arterial disease. *J Vasc Interv Radiol.* 2006;17:3–26.

74. Fleischmann D, Rubin GD. Quantification of intravenously administered contrast medium transit through the peripheral arteries: implications for CT angiography. *Radiology.* 2005;236:1076–1082.

Contrast Medium Administration in Magnetic Resonance Angiography

Jeffrey H. Maki
Lee M. Mitsumori

The emergence of magnetic resonance angiography (MRA) as an accurate, noninvasive alternative to conventional catheter angiography has been largely due to the marriage of MR technological advances with MR contrast agents. MR angiography began in the mid 1980s (1), using noncontrast techniques such as time-of-flight (TOF) and phase contrast (PC) based on the motion of flowing blood. Formerly, these techniques were the mainstay of MRA and now are largely relegated to studying the central nervous system blood vasculature (2).

In 1988, the approval of the first MR contrast agent for clinical use in the United States (3) set the stage for exciting developments to come in the early 1990s with applications extending to MRA. The first contrast-enhanced MR angiograms (CE-MRA) required a hefty 5-minute-and-10-second acquisition time (4), and although image quality paled in comparison to what can be accomplished today, the results captured the attention of the MR community. Just over a decade later, CE-MRAs of astonishing quality can be produced in seconds, with the same class of MR contrast agent first used in central nervous system (CNS) magnetic resonance imaging (MRI) back in 1988! While MR technology continues to advance at remarkable rates with higher field strength (3 Tesla) clinical machines (5), improved coil technology (6), and parallel imaging acceleration techniques (7), so too does MR contrast development.

This chapter will broadly discuss MR contrast agents in the context of their association with MRA. Newer contrast agents are being developed and while some are already in use in Europe, availability is lagging in the U.S. Decisions regarding the acquisition technique, the choice of contrast media, and method of administration for a given agent will be necessary to optimally perform MRA as one seeks to best answer the clinical question at hand. This chapter attempts to provide tools to assist in such decisions.

First, a review of basic MR physics will enable the understanding of selected principles important for further understanding the mechanism of different classes of contrast agents as they apply to CE-MRA. Next, the physics and efficacy of contrast agents will be discussed in terms of (a) physical properties and mechanism of action for each agent, (b) the pharmacokinetic properties that govern the diagnostic efficacy of an agent at the desired site of action, and (c) the safety issues related to MR contrast agent use. Following this, details of contrast administration, including injection techniques; dosing and timing issues and how they relate to commonly seen CE-MRA artifacts; and specific MRA acquisition techniques will be covered. Finally, some brief comments regarding future direction of MR contrast agents and CE-MRA will be presented.

Before embarking on a comprehensive discussion of contrast agent principles, safety, and administration, it is worth emphasizing that MR contrast agents are considered drugs and as such are regulated by the U.S. Food and Drug Administration (FDA). When a new drug is submitted to the FDA for approval, the manufacturer presents well-controlled investigations supporting its labeling claims. Once that drug is approved, the manufacturer is only permitted to advertise the drug for approved indications and can only do so using the information approved by the FDA for use in labeling (8).

At present, none of the four traditional gadolinium extracellular contrast agents approved by the FDA (Table 5-1) include indications for MRA, and hence, the manufacturers cannot advertise their products in any way for use with MRA. This is in no way a statement about the safety or efficacy of these agents for MRA, but rather is a default position because the manufacturers did not present the FDA with data to specifically support a claim that their agent was evaluated in the context of MRA procedures. Thus, in the United States, administration of an MR contrast agent to perform MRA is considered "off-label" use.

Physicians are permitted by the FDA to lawfully deviate from the conditions for use as approved in the drug package insert as part of the "practice of medicine" (9), and such off-label uses have been upheld by the courts. While the FDA frowns at the marketing of off-label applications, it does permit off-label use provided that use occurs in an independent medical program—meaning a program either not supported by industry or, if partially supported, following specific rules regarding disclosure of commercial sponsors and maintaining control of content and speakers (8). Thus, the radiologist is ultimately responsible for selecting the contrast agent and dose for a particular indication.

BASIC PRINCIPLES

One of the most unique and clinically exploitable properties of MRI is the rich variety of contrast mechanisms available. Indeed, MRI is well known for the rich intrinsic soft tissue contrast found in straightforward acquisitions emphasizing T1 or T2 weighting. The imaging features may be modified by the addition of exogenous contrast agents and how these agents are distributed.

In comparison to CT contrast agents, which function simply through their ability to scatter or absorb x-ray photons, MR contrast agents work indirectly by changing the local magnetic environment of tissue, thereby modifying intrinsic relaxation rates of tissues. In order to more fully understand this process, it is necessary to briefly review the basic principles of how MR signals are generated.

Magnetic Resonance Basics

Nuclear magnetic resonance is a phenomenon exhibited by atoms having odd numbers of nucleons (protons and neutrons) (10). The most clinically relevant of these is the proton (^1H), due to its high abundance given the approximate 70% water (H_2O) content of the human body. Almost all clinical MRI is proton MRI. Other biologically pertinent atoms exhibiting the MR phenomena include ^{13}C, ^{23}Na, and ^{31}P, although these species are much less abundant in the human body and currently are rarely used for clinical imaging.

The hydrogen nucleus, a single proton, can be considered a spinning positive charge, and thus, it generates a magnetic field. This is often described as a *magnetic moment* or *dipole*. When a population of protons is placed into a static magnetic field (called B_0), each proton's magnetic moment aligns either parallel or antiparallel to B_0 (due to two discrete quantum mechanical energy states), with just a slightly greater fraction aligning parallel to B_0 such that there is a small net magnetic moment parallel to B_0.

TABLE 5-1

Physiochemical Properties and Approval Status of All Currently Approved and Selected Experimental MR Contrast Agents

Generic Name	Product Name	Manufacturer	Type	Chemical Abbreviation	Approved?	$R_1{}^a$	$R_2{}^a$	Molarity	Osmolality[b]	Viscosity[c]
Gadopentetate	Magnevist	Berlex	Para–ECF–I	Gd-DTPA	FDA	3.8	—	0.500	1.96	2.90
Gadoversetamide	OptiMARK	Mallinckrodt	Para–ECF–NI	Gd-DTPA-BMEA	FDA	4.7	—	0.500	1.11	2.00
Gadodiamide	Omniscan	Nycomed, Amersham	Para–ECF–NI	Gd-DTPA-BMA	FDA	3.9	—	0.500	0.79	1.40
Gadoteridol	ProHance	Bracco	Para–ECF–NI	Gd-HPDO3A	FDA	3.7	—	0.500	0.63	1.30
Gadoterate	Dotarem	Guerbet	Para–ECF–I	Gd-DOTA	E.U.	3.6	4.8	0.500	1.35	2.00
Gadobenate	MultiHance	Bracco	Para–ECF–I[d]	Gd-BOPTA	FDA	4.4[e] 9.7[f]	5.6	0.500	1.97	5.30
Gadobutrol	Gadovist	Schering	Para–ECF–NI	Gd-DO3A-butrol	E.U.	3.6	—	1.000	1.39	3.70
Mangafodipir	Teslascan	Nycomed, Amersham	Hepatocyte Specific–Para	MN-DPDP	FDA	1.9	2.2	0.010	0.29	0.70
Gadofosveset	Vaosvist	EPIX	Para–Blood Pool[h]	MS-325	Approvable letter from FDA	6.6[e] 44.0[f]	53.0[f]	0.250[g]	—	—
B22956	—	Bracco	Para–Blood Pool[h]	B22956	No	6.5[e] 27.0[f]	—	0.250[i]	—	—
SH L 643A	Gadomer-17	Schering	Para–Blood Pool[j]	Gadomer-17	No	18.7	—	0.500	—	—
P792	P792	Guerbet	Para–Blood Pool[k]	P792	No	39.0[e] 44.5[f]	—	0.035[k]	—	—
Ferumoxide	Ferridex IV Endorem	Berlex, Guerbet	SPIO	AMI-25	FDA E.U.	24.0	107.0	0.200[l]	0.20	0.34
Ferucorbotran	Resovist	Schering	SPIC	SHU555A	E.U.	20.0	190.0	0.500	0.33	1.00
Ferumoxtran	Combidex Sinerem	Cytogen, Guerbet	USP O	AMI-227	No[m]	23.0	51.0	0.360[l]	—	—
NC100150	—	Nycomed, Amersham	USP O	NC100150	No[n]	25.0	41.0	0.360[o]	—	—

All data from Tables 2-1 to 2-3 in Weisskoff et al. MR contrast agent basics. In: Lardo A, Fayad Z, Chronos A, et al., eds. *Cardiovascular Magnetic Resonance*. London: Martin Dunitz; 2003:17–38 unless otherwise stated. (For type: ECF: extracellular fluid; Para, paramagnetic; SPIO, superparamagnetic iron oxide; USPIO, ultrasmall superparamagnetic iron oxide; I, ionic; N, nonionic; FDA, U.S. Food and Drug Administration approval; E.U., European Union approval.) Approval is as of June 2005. Agents in bold print are the four conventional ECF agents approved for human use by the FDA.

[a]@ 0.5T, 37°C, s⁻¹ mM⁻¹, in serum unless otherwise stated.

[b]Osmol/kg.

[c]Centipoise.

[d]Weakly protein binding.

[e]In buffer.

[f]In plasma.

[g]R_1 measured at 0.1 M.

[h]Strongly protein binding.

[i]Data from La Noce A, Stoelben S, Scheffler K, et al. B22956/1, a new intravascular contrast agent for MRI: first administration to humans—preliminary results. *Acad Radiol*. 2002;9 [Suppl 2]:S404–S406, with permission.

[j]Increased size dendritic chelate, 17 kDa. 24 Gd³⁺ complexes per dendrimer.

[k]Increased size, 5kD with some self assembling characteristics. From Weinmann H, Ebert W, Misselwitz B, et al. Tissue-specific MR contrast agents. *Eur J Rad*. 2003;46:33–44, with permission.

[l]Data from Petersein J, Saini S, Weissleder R. Liver. II: Iron oxide-based reticuloendothelial contrast agents for MR imaging. *Magn Reson Imaging Clin N Am*. 1996;4:53–60, with permission.

[m]An "approvable" letter has been received from the FDA.

[n]Development recently discontinued.

[o]Data from Rydland J, Bjørnerud A, Haugen O, et al. New intravascular contrast agent applied to dynamic contrast enhanced MR imaging of human breast cancer. *Acta Radiol*. 2003;44(3):275–283, with permission.

It is this net magnetic moment (sometimes called *proton spin*) that is manipulated to form the MR signal. Of note, the preferential parallel fraction is only 5 per million but does increase as B_0 increases, providing one explanation why increased magnetic fields provide more signal.

The magnetic moment of a proton precesses around B_0 at a frequency called the *Larmor frequency*. The Larmor frequency depends on the strength of the applied magnetic field B, with the angular frequency ω described as $\omega = \gamma B$, where $\gamma/2\pi = 42.57$ MHz/T is called the *gyromagnetic ratio*. MR signal is generated by applying radio frequency (RF) energy at the Larmor frequency (resonance), thereby tipping or "nutating" the magnetic moment away from the axis of B_0. As the proton precesses around B_0, it can be thought of as a magnet rotating within a magnetic field and as such will induce current to flow in a nearby conducting coil (the MR receiver coil) according to the Faraday law of electromagnetic induction (10). Current that is induced in the receiver coil is proportional to the transverse component of magnetization (i.e., the component perpendicular to the axis of B_0). This current oscillates at the Larmor frequency and becomes the basis for creation of an MR image.

The property of how an individual spin "relaxes" to realign with B_0 is described by the *T1 relaxation time*, or *spin-lattice relaxation*. Similarly, the properties of how a collection of spins (we cannot image just one!) precess at slightly different Larmor frequencies and hence lose signal due to phase cancellation is referred to as the *T2*, or *spin-spin relaxation time*. How much signal is lost depends on the echo time (TE), describing the time at which we sample the current induced in our coil.

We further describe a term *T2**, which combines the effects of T2 with local field inhomogeneities and is important when considering gradient echo rather than spin echo imaging. Often, we use the term *relaxivity* (R1, R2) or inverse of T1 or T2 (R1 = 1/T1, R2 = 1/T2) out of convenience when discussing contrast mechanisms. Of note, both R1 and R2 are magnetic field–dependent properties. At 1.5 T, the T1 of blood is 1200 ms, with a T2 of 150 to 200 ms; the T1 and T2 for fat are 300 and 60 ms, respectively (1).

Contrast Media—Relaxation Enhancement

When a contrast agent is administered, the physics of magnetic resonance described earlier do not change. However, the presence of the contrast agent decreases the observed tissue relaxation times T1 and T2, thereby changing the tissue signal intensity. This also can be expressed as increasing the tissue relaxivities R1 and R2 (i.e., observed 1/T1 and 1/T2), and hence, the effect is termed *relaxation*

enhancement. Because the concentration of protons (water) is much greater (55,000 M) than the concentration of contrast agent (perhaps 0.1 to 5.0 mM), individual contrast complexes must exert relaxation effects on extremely large numbers of water molecules. The efficiency of this process can be expressed as the relaxivity of the contrast agent ($R_{contrast}$), which is linearly related to the concentration of the contrast agent and can be written (11):

$$R1_{(observed)} = R1_{(intrinsic)} + c\,R1_{(contrast)} \qquad [1]$$

$$R2_{(observed)} = R2_{(intrinsic)} + c\,R2_{(contrast)} \qquad [2]$$

where c is the concentration of contrast agent. In other words, the observed relaxivities R1,2 can be thought of as the sum of an intrinsic relaxivity (i.e., the true tissue T1 and T2) and a contrast specific relaxivity proportional to the concentration of contrast present. Contrast agents themselves can be classified as paramagnetic or superparamagnetic, as will be described shortly. As stated, both R1 and R2 depend on magnetic field strength. This effect is demonstrated for five different MR contrast agents in Figure 5-1—a nuclear magnetic relaxation dispersion (NMRD) curve, which in this case plots R1 versus field strength.

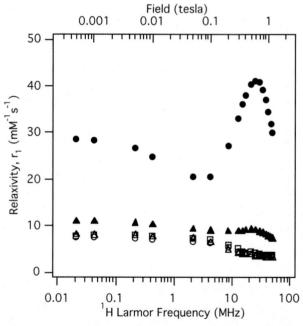

FIGURE 5-1 Relaxivities of contrast agents. Relaxivities (R1) of 0.2 mM contrast agents in 4.5% HSA solution, 358C. Gd-DTPA (Magnevist), open squares; Gd-DTPA-BMA (Omniscan), open circles; Gd-HPDO3A (Prohance), open triangles; Gd-BOPTA (Multihance), filled triangles; MS-325, filled circles, plotted as a function of magnetic field. Reprinted with permission from Weisskoff R, Caravan P. MR contrast agent basics. In: Lardo A, Fayad Z, Chronos A, et al., eds. *Cardiovascular Magnetic Resonance*. London: Martin Dunitz; 2003:17–38.

Contrast Media—Paramagnetic

Examples of paramagnetic agents include molecular oxygen, free radicals, and the metal ions gadolinium (Gd^{3+}), iron (Fe^{2+}), and manganese (Mn^{2+}). All of these agents are characterized by having relatively large numbers of unpaired electrons. These unpaired electrons generate a locally fluctuating magnetic field, which in turn causes an alteration in tissue T1 and T2.

These complex interactions are often broken into two components: inner sphere and outer sphere. *Inner sphere* refers to relaxation enhancement resulting from rapid water exchange of the typically single water molecule intimately associated with the contrast complex, and *outer sphere* refers to the surrounding water solvating the contrast complex (Fig. 5-2) (12).

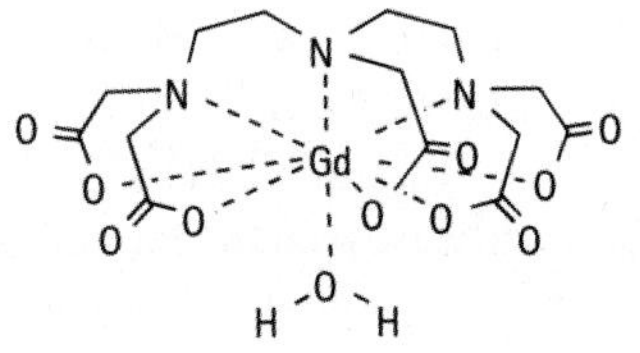

Gd-DTPA (gadopenetate, Magnevist)

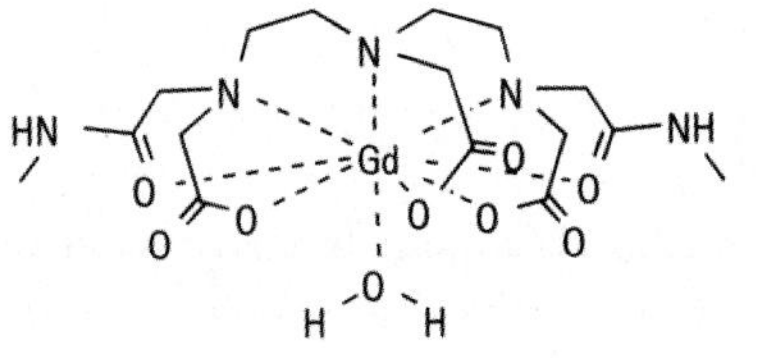

Gd-DTPA-BMA (gadodiamide, Omniscan)

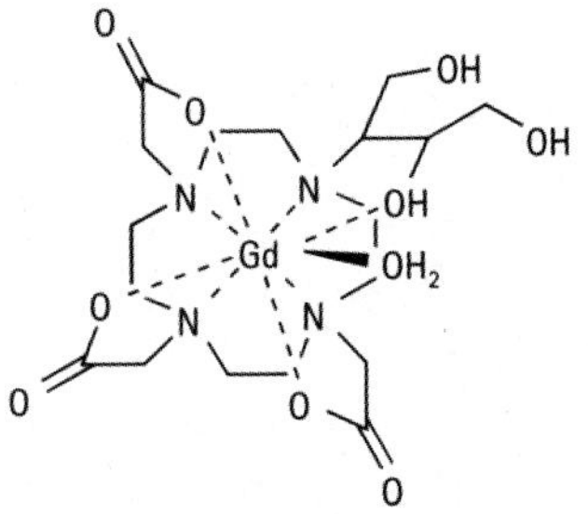

Gd-DO3A-butrol (gadobutrol, Gadovist)

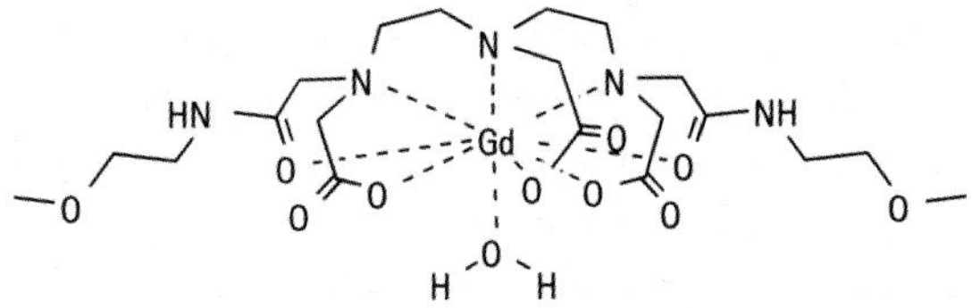

Gd-DTPA-BMEA (gadoversetamide, OptiMARK)

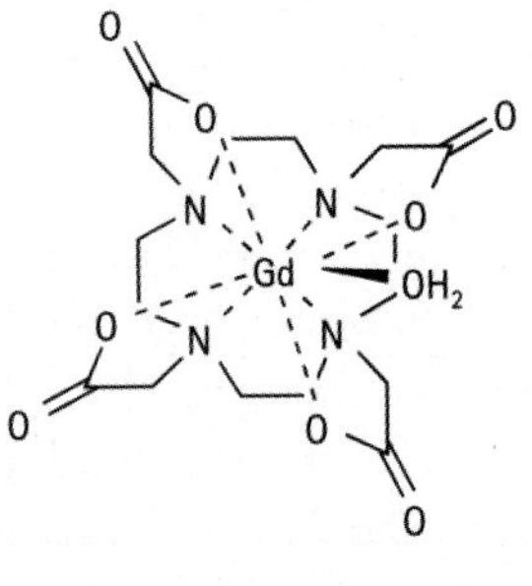

Gd-DOTA (gadoterate, Dotarem)

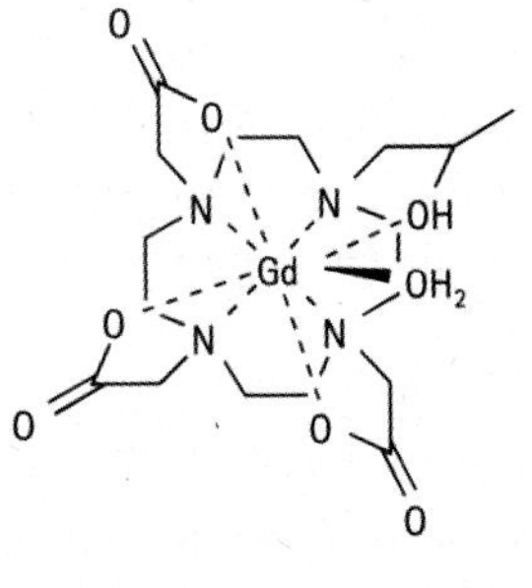

Gd-HPDO3A (gadoteridol, ProHance)

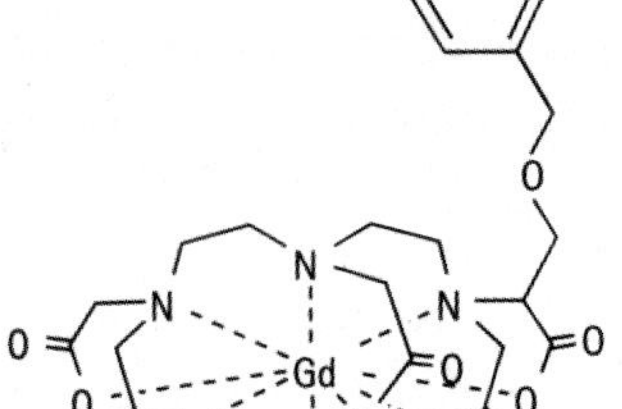

Gd-BOPTA (gadobenate, MultiHance)

FIGURE 5-2 Molecular diagrams comparing structures of various MR contrast agents. Compare the linear-structured gadolinium chelate gadodiamide (Omniscan, Nycomed) with the macrocyclic agent gadoteridol (ProHance, Bracco). Reprinted with permission from Weisskoff R, Caravan P. MR contrast agent basics. In: Lardo A, Fayad Z, Chronos A, et al., eds. *Cardiovascular Magnetic Resonance.* London: Martin Dunitz; 2003:17–38.

Of the two, inner-sphere relaxivity (R1,2^{IS}) is typically the larger term, increasing with the square of the contrast agent magnetic moment μ_{eff}, which is in turn proportional to the number of unpaired electrons. Thus, ions such as Gd^{3+}, Fe^{2+}, and Mn^{2+} (with 7, 5, and 5 unpaired electrons, respectively) make better relaxation agents compared with an ion such as Cu^{2+}, the latter with only 1 unpaired electron. Furthermore, inner-sphere relaxivity falls off as the sixth power of the radius between proton and paramagnetic ion (1/r^6), making it important to formulate contrast agents such that water can gain close proximity to the paramagnetic center.

A third component to inner-sphere relaxivity relates the quantum mechanical probability of contact interaction between the two, which can be described in terms of rotation, electron spin relaxation, and chemical exchange correlation times, respectively (11,13,14).

Outer-sphere relaxivity (R1,2^{OS}) is basically the same as inner sphere, only the correlation times are altered due to the different properties of outer-sphere water; there is a much larger distance between water and the paramagnetic center (1/r^6 dependence); and there exist a vastly greater number of water molecules in that sphere. Nonetheless, the contribution of R1^{OS} can be significant, contributing approximately half the relaxivity for extracellular contrast agents used in medical imaging (12).

Because many metal ions such as Gd^{3+} alone are highly toxic they must be tightly bound to chelates such as DTPA, DOTA, DTPA-BMA, HPDO3A etc. Manganese (Mn^{2+}) is not as toxic, and there is one FDA approved Mn^{2+} compound (Mn-DPDP), from which the Mn^{2+} dissociates in vivo and is taken up by the pancreatic cells and hepatocytes. This compound is typically used for liver and pancreatic imaging.

The prototype gadolinium-based contrast agents, of which there are several (Table 5-1), are termed *extracellular fluid agents* or *ECF agents*, as they quickly equilibrate with the extracellular space and do not associate with proteins. These are the agents typically used for MR angiography. Gadopentetate dimeglumine (Gd-DTPA) was the first agent approved for clinical use, and that initial use was for the evaluation of the CNS, particularly tumors. Clinical trials for Gd-DTPA began in 1983, and the agent was approved for human use in 1988 (3).

All of the traditional ECF agents are quite small (<1,000 Da), and all contain one gadolinium ion, an 8-coordinate ligand binding to Gd^{3+}, and a single water molecule coordination site to the gadolinium (the inner-sphere water). Molecular structures demonstrating these properties are shown for two example ECF compounds in Figure 5-2.

Tight binding of Gd^{3+} to ligands such as DTPA "cages" the gadolinium ion, preventing toxicity, but also reduces the relaxation effect by distancing water molecules from the paramagnetic center (recall the 1/r^6 relationship). The coordinated water molecule, however, undergoes rapid chemical exchange (10^6 exchanges per second) with the solvating outer-sphere water molecules, in effect catalyzing the relaxation process.

The traditional gadolinium ECF agents all have similar relaxivities (Table 5-1), with the R1 and R2 of gadoterate being 3.6 L mmol^{-1} sec^{-1} and 4.8 L mmol^{-1} sec^{-1}, respectively (this and all Table 5-1 relaxivities are measured at 0.5 T— this relates to an artifact of the instrumentation used to measure relaxivities, which only measure up to 20 Mhz, or approximately 0.5 T).

As an example, if gadoterate (0.5 M) were diluted to 1% in the blood (i.e., 5 mmol), we can rewrite Equation [1] for blood as:

$$1/T1_{(observed)} = 1/1{,}200 + c\, R1_{(contrast)} \qquad [3]$$

where (1/1,200 ms^{-1}) is the R1 of nonenhanced blood (i.e., T1 nonenhanced blood = 1,200 ms). Substituting values into [3], 1/T1 would be 1/1,200 + (3.6)(5) = 18 sec^{-1}. This equates to a T1 of 1/18 seconds or 56 milliseconds, a substantial relaxation effect.

Paramagnetic agents are considered to have a relatively balanced effect between R1 and R2, with all medically used contrast agents having R2 greater than R1. Compare this with superparamagnetic relaxation agents, which are less balanced, having a much greater R2 effect and greater R2/R1 ratio (see below). This makes paramagnetic agents ideal for visualizing blood through shortening T1—that is, the lumen becomes bright on T1-weighted imaging. T2 shortening, on the other hand, results in decreased signal intensity.

Another consideration when discussing the relaxivity of paramagnetic agents is the size of the entire gadolinium complex. Water protons move through regions of paramagnetic influence at a very optimal rate for MRA—slowly enough to experience the relaxation effect, yet fast enough to allow other protons the opportunity to relax as well and thereby magnify the effect (15). If, however, a small gadolinium chelate is bound to a large macromolecule (e.g., MW 50,000 to 250,000 Da), the rotation of the entire complex slows down, increasing the probability of contact between the gadolinium complex and the water proton, and thereby further increasing relaxation enhancement. Examples include gadobenate (Gd-BOPTA), which weakly binds the large protein serum albumin (92,000 Da), leading to an approximate doubling of relaxivity at 0.5 T (16). Another example is gadofosveset (MS-325), which tightly binds serum albumin (91% bound fraction), resulting in an approximate eightfold increase in relaxivity (17).

Contrast Media—Superparamagnetic

Superparamagnetic agents develop large magnetic moments when placed into an external magnetic field—much greater than those seen with paramagnetic agents such as gadolinium (18). Once removed from the magnetic field, they retain no net magnetization. In tissues, superparamagnetic agents create strong local magnetic field inhomogeneities. When protons (water) diffuse through these local regions of field inhomogeneity, this induces phase cancellation (phase incoherence) of spins, decreasing the T2 relaxation time (see Magnetic Resonance Basics section, above) and hence, the signal intensity is decreased (15,18). T1 also decreases, but not as dramatically as does T2. Superparamagnetic agents used for MR are iron oxide based, consisting of a biodegradable coating surrounding the iron oxide core.

Two types of compounds are discriminated based on their aggregate size: large ($>$50 nm) particles, referred to as a SPIO (superparamagnetic iron oxide) and small ($<$50 nm) particles, referred to as a USPIO (ultrasmall superparamagnetic iron oxide). Examples of SPIOs include AMI-25 and SHU-555A; USPIOs include AMI-227 and NC100150 (Table 5-1).

Relaxivity of superparamagnetic agents is a function of particle size, with larger particles (SPIOs) having greater relaxivity. More important to consider for vascular MR indications, however, is the ratio of R2 to R1, which tends to be very high for SPIOs (AMI-25: R2/R1 = 160/40 = 4) (18). This means that T2 effects typically dominate T1 effects, and the agents are not appropriate for conventional "bright blood" T1-shortening CE-MRA. Instead, they are used in circumstances where the T2 effect manifesting as signal loss is sought, such as for determining benign from malignant liver lesions and lymph nodes (19–21). USPIOs such as AMI-227 have much more favorable R2/R1 ratios (R2/R1 = 53/23 = 2.3), making them more appropriate as T1-shortening agents but still not as ideal as the paramagnetic agents (22,23).

Contrast Pharmacokinetics and Biologic Factors

In order to properly use MR contrast agents, it is important to understand their formulation, biodistribution, and elimination pathways. Injectable MR contrast agents for MRA use must be formulated at adequate concentration to effectively alter relaxation at achievable blood concentrations and must be either soluble or homogeneously dispersible in blood. Typically, 0.1- to 1.0-M formulations are employed, depending on agent relaxivity (Table 5-1).

Another consideration is viscosity, which must be low enough that bolus injection can be performed through standard-size intravenous (IV) catheters (acceptable range is approximately 0 to 3 centipoise) (11). Warming the contrast agent to body temperature reduces viscosity, which can be useful when injecting high-viscosity agents such as gadopentetate dimeglumine through smaller IVs (24,25).

Osmolality must also be considered, as injection of a sufficient quantity of a hyperosmolar agent can transiently increase serum osmolality (normal serum osmolality is approximately 290 mOsm/kg), which in turn leads to diffusion of extracellular water into the intravascular space. Under extreme circumstances, passage of a high-osmolality contrast bolus can, in theory, disrupt the blood–brain barrier with serious consequences (26). Acceptable contrast agent osmolalities range from 0.3 to 2.0 Osm/kg (11).

The relatively small quantities of MR contrast used (20 to 40 cc) make the issue somewhat less important than is the case of contrast CT, where boluses of 150 to 200 cc are common. The small volumes of MR contrast translate into a low osmotic load (volume $\times$ the osmolality) delivered to the patient, as will be discussed later.

Additionally, injectable compounds must be stable in vivo (or be metabolized to nontoxic products), the compound (as well as any additional MRI-inactive materials added) must be of acceptable toxicity and completely eliminated from the body in a reasonable amount of time, and the compound must have a usefully long shelf life. Finally, when considering gadolinium agents, the toxic gadolinium ion must remain tightly bound to the ligand (see Magnetic Resonance Contrast Safety, below).

The biodistribution of a contrast agent is governed by the kinetics of distribution, clearance, and excretion. Most of the data on MR contrast biodistribution comes from the gadolinium ECF contrast agents gadopentetate (3,27) and gadoterate (28), although the other ECF agents are considered to behave in a relatively similar fashion. In terms of kinetics and imaging behavior, the ECF compounds (Table 5-1) are considered interchangeable, with only slight variations in physical parameters among them (1,12).

The two-compartment model provides the basis for understanding and discussing MR contrast kinetics. In this model, the intravascular space (arteries and veins) makes up one compartment, while the extracellular extravascular space (EES) makes up the other. Contrast agents have varying abilities to diffuse back and forth between the two compartments (ECF agents diffuse rapidly; blood pool agents and SPIOs diffuse slowly). Initially, most of the flux is from the intravascular space into the EES due to the high intravascular concentration after bolus injection. For ECF agents, equilibrium between the two compartments occurs

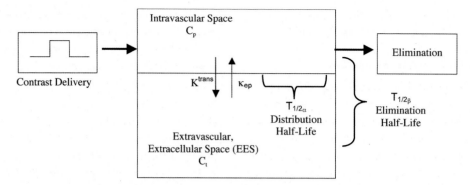

FIGURE 5-3 Two-compartment model depicting the pharmacokinetic parameters that govern the biodistribution of a contrast agent administered intravenously. C_p is the plasma (intravascular) concentration of the contrast agent, and C_t is the contrast concentration in the extravascular, extracellular space (EES). K^{trans} is the volume transfer constant describing contrast transfer between the plasma and EES, and κ_{ep} is the rate constant describing contrast transfer between the EES and intravascular compartment. The distribution half-life $T_{1/2\alpha}$ represents the time required for half of contrast to redistribute from the intravascular space to the EES. The elimination half-life $T_{1/2\beta}$ represents the time required for elimination of one half the total contrast from the body.

quite rapidly (in a matter of minutes), providing one reason why CE-MRA is optimally performed during the "first pass" of contrast. A generalized kinetic model of contrast dynamics can be written (29):

$$dC_t/dt = K^{trans}\, C_p - \kappa_{ep}\, C_t \qquad [4]$$

where C_t is the EES concentration, C_p is the plasma (intravascular) contrast concentration, K^{trans} is the volume transfer constant describing contrast transfer between the plasma and EES, and κ_{ep} is the rate constant describing contrast transfer between the EES and plasma. A simple diagram demonstrating this model is shown in Figure 5-3. This is simply a mathematical way of saying that the rate by which concentration changes in the EES (dC_t/dt) increases proportional to the intravascular contrast concentration (C_p), while at the same time decreases at a rate proportional to the EES contrast concentration (C_t). Of course, C_p also decreases according to how the contrast is eliminated (e.g., renal or hepatic clearance).

Another way to describe contrast kinetics uses a biexponential model of elimination half-lives. This takes into account the two-compartment model in combination with clearance/excretion and is most influenced by physical contrast agent size and the differences in capillary endothelium between different organs. In muscle and connective tissue, the endothelium forms a continuous layer around the capillary, preventing all but the smallest molecules (such as ECF agents) from leaking out. In the kidney, however, the glomerular capillaries have a fenestrated enodothelium with pores measuring 60 to 70 nm in diameter. This allows molecules less than 20,000 Da in weight to pass freely and molecules up to 70,000 Da to pass depending on lipid solubility, polarity, and pH (22).

In this model, two half-lives are defined; the distribution half-life ($T_{1/2\alpha}$), describing the rate by which contrast agent distributes out of the intravascular space, and the elimination half-life ($T_{1/2\beta}$), describing the rate of elimination from the body. These concepts are diagrammed in Figure 5-3. ECF agents are known to rapidly distribute throughout the EES via capillaries (excepting neural tissue due to the blood–brain barrier), as they are all small molecules less than 1,000 Da in size. In fact, it is estimated that 50% of gadopentetate passes from the intravascular space to the EES on the initial pass through the capillaries (30). The half-life values for the ECF agents are well described and relatively similar, with $T_{1/2\alpha}$ ranging from 3.6 to 12 minutes, and $T_{1/2\beta}$ ranging from 1.3 to 1.6 hours (1,28).

In comparison, blood pool agents such as gadofosveset and B22956, which reversibly bind serum albumin, have much longer elimination half-lives (e.g., gadofosveset $T_{1/2\beta}$ estimated at 2 to 3 hours) since the large complex that is formed cannot be filtered through the glomerulus (31). Distribution half-life, however, is very similar to that of the ECF agents ($T_{1/2\alpha}$ 3 minutes for gadofosveset (22)), as the unbound fraction is free to pass through the capillary endothelium.

The macromolecular agents such as Gadomer-17 and P792 have somewhat different pharmacokinetic properties, with a long distribution half-life but a relatively rapid elimination half-life (due to swift glomerular filtration). This means that nearly all the contrast present remains intravascular, but it is rapidly cleared from the bloodstream.

The iron oxides have different properties yet, with the larger SPIOs having quite rapid elimination half-lives (8 to 10 minutes) due to rapid sequestration by liver Kupfer cells (18) and USPIOs having much longer elimination half-lives (90 minutes in the case of NC100150) (32,33).

A third parameter, the steady state distribution volume ($V_{d\ ss}$) can also be calculated using this model, describing the total intra- and extravascular volume over which a contrast agent distributes. Typical distribution volumes range from 171 mL/kg for gadopentetate to 256 mL/kg for gadoterate (28).

Consider again the example in Equation [3], where gadoterate (0.5M) is injected to achieve a 1% arterial phase blood concentration, resulting in a peak T1 of 56 milliseconds. If the total injected volume is 20 cc (into a 75-kg person), and the distribution volume is approximated as 200 mL/kg, the equilibrium concentration (discounting elimination) would be (20 cc $\times$ 500 mmol/L)/(200 mL/kg $\times$ 75 kg) = 0.66 mmol. Putting this value into Equation [3], the equilibrium T1 (EES and intravascular space) is approximately 420 milliseconds, which is much greater than that of fat (270 ms); this example demonstrates that in order for the T1 of blood to be shorter than the T1 background tissue, imaging must be performed in the first-pass arterial phase.

Elimination pathways vary according to the type of contrast agent. The gadolinium ECF agents, small and extremely hydrophilic, are predominately eliminated unmetabolized via a renal route—glomerular filtration, active secretion, or a combination of the two. As stated earlier, elimination half-lives are on the order of 90 minutes. The only exception to pure renal elimination is gadobenate (Gd-BOPTA), which is partially taken up by the hepatocytes and excreted in bile (34). This makes it useful for hepatic imaging in addition to MRA (35).

Gadolinium-based blood pool agents, on the other hand, remain intravascular for a much longer time and are eliminated from the body much more slowly (longer $T_{1/2\beta}$). These agents remain largely intravascular due to one of two mechanisms: (a) a substantial fraction (>80% at any one time [36]) reversibly binds to serum albumin, or (b) the large inherent size (>20,000 Da) of the blood pool agent prevents it from diffusing through the endothelium.

In the first case, because albumin is not eliminated by the healthy kidney, it is only the small unbound (free) fraction of contrast agent that is available for renal excretion (17). In the second case, the macromolecule is large enough to remain intravascular but small enough to be excreted by glomerular filtration (37).

Iron oxide agents (i.e., SPIOs, USPIOs) are metabolized in a completely different fashion from the gadolinium agents. These agents are cleared by the body's reticuloendothelial system (RES), which includes the liver, spleen, bone marrow, and lymph nodes, with the Kupfer cells within the liver being responsible for approximately 80% of the clearance (18). How fast this RES clearance occurs depends on blood half-life, which is in turn dependent on particle size. The larger

SPIOs are cleared rapidly from the blood ($T_{1/2\beta}$ = 8 to 10 minutes), while the smaller USPIOs are not immediately recognized by the RES and have longer elimination half-lives ($T_{1/2\beta}$ = 45 to 200 minutes) (18,32).

While all of the iron oxide aggregates are large enough that they remain predominantly within the intravascular space, only the USPIOs are considered candidates for blood pool MRA. This is not only due to the longer blood half-life of USPIOs, but is also due to their more favorable R_2/R_1 ratio (see Contrast Media—Superparamagnetic, discussed earlier). The SPIOs appear better suited to hepatic and lymph node imaging.

MAGNETIC RESONANCE CONTRAST AGENT SAFETY

Medical imaging contrast agents are considered pharmaceuticals and are therefore regulated by the FDA. As with therapeutic drugs, new imaging contrast agents need to be proven efficacious and safe through a specific and structured process that is overseen by the FDA prior to being approved for human use. In this process, the initial assessment of safety is performed using in vitro and animal studies to establish the toxicity and dose tolerance of the agent (38).

A frequently stated measure of preclinical safety that is established in these tests is the median lethal dose (LD50), which describes the dose of a drug that results in the acute death of approximately half the animals in the study population (39). Though such measures as the LD50 have been correlated with the incidence of idiosyncratic reactions with iodinated contrast media, these types of animal and in vitro measures of toxicity typically do not have well-defined clinical value owing to the significantly lower doses used clinically. These toxicity measures are useful, however, in that they provide a means to compare the theoretical tolerances of different agents (40).

Once the initial safety is established, subsequent studies are performed on humans (Phase I–III trials) to further define the efficacy and tolerance of the agent. On completion of Phase III, the product label is developed, which summarizes the experience with the drug and provides specific guidelines for its use, and the agent is submitted to the FDA for approval. If approved, the drug can then be marketed for its designed application, at which time it enters Phase IV, or the postmarketing stage of development (38).

Currently, there are five widely available FDA-approved gadolinium-based MR contrast agents available in the United States (gadopentetate dimeglumine, gadoteridol, gadodiamide, gadoversetamide, and gadobenate dimeglumine)—the first four representing the conventional extracellular fluid (ECF) gadolinium chelates (41). Though the information describing the safety of these agents obtained from the trials and studies performed during the approval process demonstrate that these agents are exceptionally well tolerated and do not exhibit nephrotoxicity at approved doses, life-threatening reactions can still occur (42–45).

Thus, the MR physician prescribing these pharmaceutical agents must be (a) aware of the potential adverse effects, (b) able to identify patients at increased risk for contrast reactions, and (c) capable of managing a contrast reaction (41,46). As previous sections of this text have presented principles regarding the effectiveness of contrast agents related to their relaxivity and biologic distribution, this section will discuss issues related to contrast agent toxicity and contrast use in special patient populations. Safety-related knowledge should assist the practitioner in understanding subtle differences between the various agents, enabling selection of the most efficacious and safe compounds from a continually growing array of clinically available agents and formulations (46).

Etiology of Contrast Media Reactions

Adverse reactions to contrast media can be classified as anaphylactoid, nonanaphylactoid, or a combination of the two. Anaphylactoid (idiosyncratic) reactions occur unexpectedly, vary in severity, and symptomatically appear similar to anaphylactic reactions. While their precise mechanism is unknown, it is believed to be related to the release of vasoactive substances that subsequently result in systemic vasodilation and/or bronchospasm. The nonanaphylactoid reactions include those that are related to chemotoxic, osmotoxic, and vasovagal mechanisms and do not have the features of an anaphylactoid response. Chemotoxicity refers to the inherent toxicity related to the chemical structure of the compound. Osmotoxicity reflects osmotic effects and the ability to induce water movement across semipermeable membranes. Vasovagal reactions are initiated in the central nervous system and reflect increased vagal tone on the heart and blood vessels (47,48).

Studies into the mechanisms of adverse reactions of iodinated contrast agents hypothesize that the primary pathogenic processes involve cell membrane destabilization and the subsequent release of vasoactive substances or activation of the complement system. What is known from experience with the iodinated contrast media is that the use of low-osmolar, nonionic agents results in nearly a fivefold decrease in the incidence of adverse reactions when compared with ionic agents (47).

Pharmacodynamically, it is postulated that this lower reaction rate with the nonionic compounds is related to the greater number of hydroxyl groups that these agents contain.

The hydroxyl groups attract water, thereby forming a shielding shell of bound water that decreases interactions with hydrophobic segments of proteins and cell membranes (48). Other described nonanaphylactic reactions of iodinated contrast media include chemotoxic renal tubular injury, osmotoxic-induced changes in blood flow and vascular permeability, vasodilation, and the pain that occurs when hyperosmolar agents are administered during arteriography (48,49).

Safety of the Extracellular Fluid Gadolinium Chelates

In comparison to the iodinated contrast media, the gadolinium-based MR agents possess some unique safety issues. The principal chemotoxic concern with gadolinium is that the free ion is extremely toxic (50), with an LD50 in rodents between 0.3 and 0.5 mmol/kg (22). When administered intravenously, the free ion is distributed primarily to the liver, where it forms insoluble colloid particles. Elimination of gadolinium is also extremely slow, with a biologic half-life of several weeks (51).

The unfavorable pharmacologic parameters of the free gadolinium ion are significantly improved by noncovalently linking the gadolinium ion to a chelating molecule such as DTPA, which modifies the biodistribution, elimination, and toxicity of the resulting ion-ligand complex (50). Interestingly, while the four conventional gadolinium chelates approved for use in the United States (gadopentetate dimeglumine, gadoteridol, gadodiamide, and gadoversetamide) differ in the structure of the chelating molecule, they have remarkably similar pharmacokinetics, effectiveness, and safety profiles (41).

These four agents are considered equally efficient as extracellular contrast agents, with no significant difference between their T1 and T2 relaxivities (Table 5-1). They are all labeled as interstitial agents with an apparent volume of distribution ($V_{d\,ss}$) equivalent to the extracellular fluid compartment (200 to 300 mL/kg) (22). Excretion for each compound is primarily by the kidneys, with biologic elimination times being approximately 1.5 hours (51).

Though very similar pharmacokinetically, there are several pharmacologic differences between the four conventional FDA-approved agents that are theoretically important with regards to safety. Given the extreme toxicity of the free gadolinium ion, the agents that are more stable in vivo, and therefore better able to maintain the gadolinium ion-chelating ligand complex, are considered to have a safety advantage (41).

In general, the macrocyclic ring chelate (gadoteridol— see Fig. 5-2) is more stable than the linear agents (gadopentetate, gadodiamide, gadoversetamide), as demonstrated by their thermodynamic stability constants—an in vitro measure of the affinity between the metal ion and the ligand (50) (Table 5-2). The higher stability also reduces the risk of transmetalation, in which other metal ions (e.g., copper and zinc) compete for gadolinium attachment sites, allowing the release of free gadolinium ions. Despite these hypothetical risks, no harmful affects in humans have been reported due to free gadolinium ion deposition resulting from clinical use (41).

The ECF gadolinium chelates also differ in their osmolality and viscosity (Table 5-2). Gadoteridol and gadodiamide have the lowest osmolality and viscosity, in part since they are nonionic. Gadopentetate dimeglumine has the highest osmolality and viscosity. Gadoversetamide is intermediate between the other two groups (41). When comparing these agents with iodinated contrast media, it is important to recognize that the manifestation of osmotoxicity is dependent on the osmotic load that the patient is exposed to rather than the measured in vitro osmolality. This relates to the drug osmolality, volume of drug administered, and the volume of distribution.

For example, the total osmotic load for an injected volume of 14 cc of Gd-DTPA (1960 mOsmol/kg) is 27 mOsmol, which compares with an osmotic load of 104 mOsmol for a 150-cc dose of iohexol (690 mOsmol/kg) (52). Thus, while low osmolality is an important safety parameter for iodinated contrast agents, it is less of a factor with these gadolinium chelates, given the lower volumes and injection rates traditionally employed for MR studies (41). Table 5-3 compares the osmotic loads that result from the administration of some commonly used MR and CT contrast media.

Potential Adverse Events

Multiple variables and numerous differences in study design—such as the phase of development, number of participating sites and their locations, study indications, and selected end points—make it extremely difficult to perform direct comparisons of the overall incidence of adverse reactions derived from various clinical trials performed for each agent (46). For example, the reported incidence of adverse events for gadopentetate in the central nervous system ranges between 6.0 and 19.9%, while it has been reported as high as 44.1% when applied to liver pathology. This is confounded when one includes the finding that the reaction rate with a saline placebo in a different liver study was 44.2% (46).

General comparisons between agents, however, can be made through the use of parallel-group or patient crossover studies that compare agents directly with one another in the same study (53). What these comparative studies have shown is that there are no discernable differences in the incidence of

adverse events between the available ECF gadolinium chelates. As a result, most references to safety are based on the data obtained with gadopentetate dimeglumine, the first agent approved for use in the United States and the one that has been the most extensively studied (53).

Available estimates place the overall incidence rate of adverse events for ECF gadolinium agents at less than 5%, with the incidence of any single adverse event occurring being 1% or less (51). The most frequent reactions that occur with these agents are nausea with or without emesis (25% to 42% of reactions), headache (18%), urticaria (3% to 7%), and taste perversion (<1%) (46,54). Similar to the iodinated agents, numerous other associated reactions from hot flashes to gingivitis have been reported involving every organ system, though at frequencies much less than 1% (51).

Despite that the vast majority of adverse reactions to these MR contrast agents are mild, and reactions requiring any form of treatment are rare (54), severe anaphylactoid reactions can and do occur (41). Reported incidences of severe reactions range from 1 in 10,000 to 1 in 500,000 doses (41,51), which is still low even when compared with the rates quoted for low osmolar iodinated CT contrast media (1.6 in 10,000) (54). The potential for life-threatening reactions necessitates that MR personnel be trained to handle adverse events, and that resuscitation equipment be available whenever these medical imaging agents are administered.

While the exact mechanisms behind these complications are not clearly understood, the similar characteristics of adverse events that occur with both MR and iodinated contrast media has been used to support the use of the empiric therapy employed with iodinated contrast media for treating MR contrast reactions (52,54). Specific treatment protocols are available from the Committee on Drugs and Contrast Media of the American College of Radiology (54).

Safety Considerations with Special Patient Populations

As with the administration of iodinated contrast media, the safe administration of a gadolinium-based MR agent may need to be modified or require preprocedural attention in selected patient populations. These special groups include (a) patients with renal insufficiency/failure, (b) persons who present an increased risk for a reaction due to atopy or prior reaction history, (c) people with sickle cell disease or a hemolytic anemia, (d) patients who are pregnant, (e) women who are breast-feeding, (f) children less than two years of age, and (g) those at risk for contrast extravasation.

Renal Insufficiency/Failure

Patients with decreased renal clearance stand a greater risk of dissociation and toxicity due to the longer half-life and

TABLE 5-2

Summary of the Safety-related Features of the Five FDA-approved Gadolinium Chelates

Generic Name	Product Name	Ligand Structure—(ionic/nonionic)	LD50 in Mice/Rats (mmol/kg)	Thermodynamic Equilibrium Constant (log Keq)	Osmolality (mOsm/kg)	Viscosity at 37°C (cP)	Significant Laboratory Interactions
Gadopentetate dimeglumine	Magnevist	Linear, ionic	6–7[a]	22.2[b]	1960[b]	2.9[b]	
Gadoteridol	Prohance	Macrocyclic, nonionic	12[a]	23.8[b]	630[b]	1.3[b]	
Gadodiamide	Omniscan	Linear, nonionic	30[a]	16.9[b]	783[b]	1.4[b]	spurious hypocalcemia
Gadoversetamide	OptiMARK	Linear, nonionic	25–28[c]	16.6[d]	1110[d]	2.0[d]	spurious hypocalcemia
Gadobenate dimeglumine	MultiHance	Linear, ionic	8–10	22.6	1970	5.3	
Gadoterate meglumine	Dotarem	Cyclic, ionic	10	24.0[b]	1350	2.0	
Gadobutrol	Gadovist	Cyclic, nonionic	23	21.8	1603	5.0	

[a]Data from Oksendal A, Hals P. Biodistribution and toxicity of MR imaging contrast media. *J Magn Reson Imaging.* 1993;3:157–165, with permission.
[b]Data from Runge V. Safety of approved MR contrast media for intravenous injection. *J Magn Reson Imaging.* 2000;12:205–213, with permission.
[c]Data from Wible JJ, Troup C, Hynes M, et al. Toxicological assessment of gadoversetamide injection (OptiMARK), a new contrast-enhancement agent for use in magnetic resonance imaging. *Invest Radiol.* 2001;36(7):401–412, with permission.
[d]Data from Kirchin M, Runge V. Contrast agents for magnetic resonance imaging. *Top Magn Reson Imaging.* 2003;14(5):426–435, with permission.

TABLE 5-3

Osmotic Loads of Magnetic Resonance Imaging Contrast Agents and Computed Tomographic Contrast Agents for a 70-kilogram Patient

Contrast Agent	Osmotic Load (mOsm)
MR (0.1 mmol/kg)	
ProHance	8.8
Omniscan	11.1
Magnevist	27.4
CT	
Iohexol	105.0
Iopamidol	119.0
Diatrizoate	255.0

Adapted from Shellock F, Kanal E. Safety of magnetic resonance imaging contrast agents. *J Magn Reson Imaging.* 1999;10:477–484, with permission.

subsequent longer in vivo exposure to contrast agents. This is related to the concerns regarding nephrogenic systemic fibrosis (NSF), and that entity is discussed more in depth in Chapter 22. With normal renal function, the rapid excretion and high stability of the gadolinium chelates present almost no risk of dissociation. While all four conventional ECF gadolinium chelates are cleared entirely by urinary excretion, none have been found to exhibit nephrotoxicity at approved doses in patients with impaired renal function, when administered intravenously (41,55,56).

For patients undergoing dialysis, contrast clearance depends on the characteristics of the agent and the dialysis equipment. No significant differences in clearance exist between the ECF agents (gadopentetate, gadodiamide, gadoversetamide, and gadoteridol) based on their molecular weight (<1,000 Da), considered the most important factor for dialysis. Although the type of dialysis equipment and the specific hemodialysis membranes in use have not been standardized, the available data demonstrates similar ECF agent elimination, with mean-elimination rates of 98% after three hemodialysis sessions for all of the ECF agents. It had previously been thought that changes in a patient's dialysis schedule were not required after the intravenous administration of an ECF contrast agent (57-59). However, new controversies have arisen regarding this issue based on NSF concerns.

In summary, although there is a theoretical risk associated with lower glomerular filtration rates resulting in a longer cellular exposure to potentially toxic molecules, the ECF gadolinium chelates are felt to be safe for use in patients with an estimated glomerular filtration rate <30 mL/min.

Patients with an Increased Risk for an Adverse Reaction

The risk of an adverse reaction with gadolinium ECF agents, although still low (approximate incidence 1% to 2%) when compared with iodinated media (5% to 12% ionic high osmolar agents, 1% to 3% nonionic media) (54), is increased in several patient populations. Patients with a history of asthma or allergy have an approximate 2 times greater risk (2.6% to 3.7%) than those without an atopic history. The adverse reaction rate is 6.3% in someone with a history of a prior reaction to iodinated contrast and 21.3% for patients who report a prior reaction to a prior MR imaging agent (52,60).

Although at present there are no well-defined policies for patients considered at increased risk for having an adverse reaction, it is generally recommended that those at increased risk be premedicated with corticosteroids. If there has been a prior reaction to an MR contrast agent, then a different agent should be employed in addition to corticosteroid premedication to reduce the risk of a repeat reaction (51,54).

Hemolytic Anemias

While there are still no clinical reports of a sickle crisis or hemolysis being precipitated by the administration of an MR contrast agent, warnings are described for these patients due to two sets of laboratory findings (8,51). The first, an in vitro study of deoxygenated sickled erythrocytes, found that the enhanced magnetic moment induced by MR contrast agents can promote alignment of nearby sickled cells, thereby potentially precipitating vaso-occlusive complications. The second arises from observations of transient elevations in serum iron and bilirubin after administration of early formulations of gadopentetate dimeglumine that were felt to be related to a mild transient hemolysis. Subsequent trials with a reformulated agent, however, have not reproduced these laboratory findings (41). Despite the absence of any reported adverse events, safe use of MR contrast in this group of patients has not yet been confirmed.

Pregnancy

ECF gadolinium chelates cross the placental barrier and appear within the fetal bladder. From there, though unproven, the agents should enter the amniotic fluid and subsequently be swallowed, thereby passing into the fetal gastrointestinal tract and ultimately excreted by the kidneys (51). While there is still no data to suggest that in utero exposure to gadolinium chelates results in chromosomal mutations (11,61) or congenital malformations (41), fetal adverse events such as growth retardation and postimplantation loss do occur in animal studies (41).

Given the lack of adequate controlled MR contrast studies with human pregnancy, a conservative approach is recommended (Pregnancy Category C). MR contrast should only be administered if the clinical benefit justifies the potential risk to the fetus. In the situation where contrast is deemed necessary, it would be appropriate to obtain written, informed consent, specifically stipulating that the risk associated with MR contrast use in pregnancy is unknown (51).

Lactation

The gastrointestinal absorption of orally administered MR contrast is extremely low (99.2% is fecally excreted), thereby reducing the LD50 1,000-fold when compared with parenteral administration. Despite this low absorption, a prudent approach to minimize the amount of contrast agent delivered to a nursing child was initially pursued (51).

It has been shown that less than 0.04% of the intravascular dose given to the mother is excreted into the breast milk in the first 24 hours (62–64). The expected dose of gadolinium contrast agent absorbed by the infant from breast milk is less than 0.0004% of the intravascular dose given to the mother (64).

Taking into consideration the very small amount of contrast media absorbed, the 2005 version of the ACR Manual on Contrast Media states that "the available data suggest that it is safe for the mother and infant to continue breast-feeding after receiving such an agent. . . . If the mother so desires, she may abstain from breast-feeding for 24 hours with active expression and discarding of breast milk from both breasts during that period. In anticipation of this, she may wish to use a breast pump to obtain milk before the contrast study to the infant during the 24-hour period following the examination" (65).

Pediatric Patients

Considered safe for children over 2 years of age, safety of MR contrast administration has not been established by large clinical trials for children under 2 years of age. Nonetheless, there have been no adverse clinical events or significant safety concerns described to date (41,51), and study results are becoming available that should soon document safe use in those patients that are less than 2 years of age (66,67).

Extravasation

Soft tissue injury due to contrast extravasation can result from acute inflammation related to the hyperosmolality of the extravasated fluid, or from mechanical compression produced by a large volume of fluid leading to a compartment syndrome (54,68). Risk factors for extrava-

sation relate to injection technique as well as specific patient features.

Application of ice packs and heating pads as well as elevation are used to alleviate the symptoms associated with extravasation of contrast material. It is theorized that the initial application of heat might facilitate contrast reabsorption.

As is the case for iodinated contrast extravasation, a plastic surgeon should be consulted if the patient experiences an increase in pain over 2 to 4 hours, if skin blistering or ulceration develops, or if circulation or sensation changes at or distal to the level of the extravasation. No specific treatment approach has been documented with unequivocal efficacy; therefore, most extravasation injuries are conservatively treated with supportive measures.

With regard to technique, events occur more frequently with the use of metal needles as opposed to plastic cannulas; with injections made in the hand, wrist, ankle, or feet; with the use of tourniquets or indwelling peripheral catheters; and with power injectors and higher flow rates. Patient risk factors include (a) infants, small children, unconscious patients—those unable to communicate; (b) low muscular mass or atrophic subcutaneous tissue; and (c) abnormal circulation to the particular limb selected for the injection, such as compromised venous or lymphatic drainage due to prior radiation, vein graft harvesting, or node dissection (54,68).

Available estimates on the frequency of extravasation state an incidence between 0.2% to 0.4% in CT cases using a power injector with flow rates of 1 to 2 cc per second (68). While the risk factors are the same for both CT and MR exams, in general, extravasated MR agents are better tolerated due to the smaller volumes injected. It is important to note that tissue injury can occur with the gadolinium chelates. In animal models of gadolinium chelate extravasation, the degree of injury, as with the iodinated agents, was related to the osmolality of the extravasated fluid (69). Thus, in those patients at risk, technical precautions and use of a low osmolar agent might reduce the risk of extravasation and subsequent injury, although firm data to support this have not been reported in patients. General recommendations regarding treatment after extravasation are based on the volume, site, type of agent used (high or low osmolality), and presence of symptoms (54).

Laboratory Interactions

In addition to adverse patient effects, safety evaluations of contrast agents include documentation of changes that occur in laboratory parameters. To date, only a few such laboratory interactions have been discovered. Clinically insignificant and transient elevations in serum iron have been reported in studies of gadopentetate and gadodiamide

(53), and early formulations of gadopentetate were associated with a mild increase in serum bilirubin, which has not been reproduced in subsequent clinical trials after reformulation of the agent with a greater excess of ligand (41).

In comparison to these mild and transient changes, there are reports of altered laboratory measurements that have had an adverse clinical impact. The propensity for gadodiamide and gadoversetamide to interfere with colorimetric assays for serum calcium, resulting in spurious detection of hypocalcemia (pseudohypocalcemia), has been recently described (70). This effect is attributed to the lower thermodynamic stability of these two agents—since it is not seen with gadopentetate or gadoteridol—that allows the colorimetric reagent to competitively displace the Gd^{3+} ion from the chelate. The resulting free imaging agent ligand then binds the calcium in the sample, rendering it unavailable for measurement (71). In one retrospective study, a significant decrease in serum calcium (greater than 2 mg/dL) was observed in 48 of 896 patients, including 18 patients who were actually treated for the spurious hypocalcium (71).

It is important to highlight that these MR contrast agents do not cause hypocalcemia but affect colorimetric assays that then report falsely depressed values. The degree of the fictitious reduction in calcium levels is correlated with the serum concentration of the contrast, a dose dependence that can be prolonged in patients with renal failure (72). This correlation presents special concerns for the MR angiographer due to the large percentage of patients with renal insufficiency who undergo high-dose CE-MRAs and the frequency of laboratory measurements made in these patients (71).

For those who use gadodiamide and gadoversetamide, current recommendations include (a) determining the method of serum calcium measurements used by the clinical laboratory; (b) notifying relevant physicians and allied health professionals of this laboratory interaction; (c) recommending that serum calcium measurements be made either before or more than 24 hours after a CE-MR exam (depending on renal function); and (d) suggesting that alternative means of calcium determination, such as ion-selective electrodes, be used if these measurements must be made soon after the imaging study (72).

Summary—Safety

Currently, noninvasive MR angiography is predominantly performed using widely available, FDA-approved extracellular space gadolinium chelates (gadopentetate, gadodiamide, gadoteridol, and gadoversetamide). These agents have been found to be extremely similar with regards to their diagnostic efficacy and excellent safety profiles. Estimates place the overall incidence of adverse reactions for these agents to be less than 5%, with the vast majority of adverse events being minor complaints of headache, nausea, urticaria, or taste perversion.

Differences in thermodynamic stability and osmolality may provide justification for selecting one agent over another in situations involving potential laboratory interactions and, theoretically, in patients at risk for extravasation. Special considerations are also warranted for those patients at increased risk for a contrast reaction as well as for pregnant or breast-feeding women. While extremely rare, severe life-threatening reactions do occur. Thus, it is important to re-emphasize the need to be aware of potential adverse effects of MR contrast agents, be able to identify higher risk individuals for its administration, and be capable of managing any adverse reaction associated with the use of these agents in a timely manner.

SPECIFIC CONTRAST MEDIA

MRI contrast agents for use in MRA can be grouped into four categories: pure extracellular agents, weakly protein-binding extracellular agents, strong protein-binding or macromolecular blood pool agents, and ultrasmall superparamagnetic iron oxides (USPIOs). Table 5-1 lists the generic names, product names, agent type, and some general characteristics of most of the approved as well as the more promising experimental contrast agents.

Extracellular Fluid Gadolinium Agents

The extracellular agents approved in the United States at the time of this writing (January 2006) are gadopentetate (Magnevist, Berlex), gadodiamide (OmniScan, Nycomed Amersham), gadoversetamide (OptiMARK, Mallinckrodt), and gadoteridol (ProHance, Bracco). Two additional ECF agents are approved in the European Union—gadoterate (Dotarem, Guerbet) and gadobutrol (Gadovist, Schering). These agents are all 0.5 M formulations, with the exception of gadobutrol, which is 1.0 M concentration.

Although there are some differences in the chelating agent (linear vs. macrocyclic, ionic vs. nonionic, high osmolality vs. low osmolality—see section on Magnetic Resonance Contrast Agent Safety and Tables 5-1 and 5-2), these agents, with the exception of gadobutrol, are all considered to be interchangeable in terms of their effectiveness for contrast MRI and MRA. Because of the increased concentration of gadobutrol (1.0 M) as compared with other ECF agents, there are reports suggesting that gadobutrol may be advantageous for MRA (73–75). Other reports find no significant differences with gadobutrol (76), and further investigations will undoubtedly be undertaken.

The first ECF agent to win U.S. FDA approval was gadopentetate dimeglumine. Initially, this and other agents were approved at a dose of 0.1 mmol/kg, with this dose chosen based on safety concerns rather than efficacy (34). Since then, studies have been performed looking at doses of up to 0.3 mmol/kg for efficacy in brain metastasis detection (77). This has led to the FDA approving the use of gadopentetate, gadodiamide, and gadoteridol for CNS indications at 0.3 mmol/kg in a "stepped" fashion, where 0.1 mmol/kg can be followed by an additional 0.2 mmol/kg within 20 minutes ("body" indications remain 0.1 mmol/kg). Although none of these ECF agents has yet been formally "approved" for the specific indication of MRA, it is common practice for radiologists to interpret the FDA dosing guidelines by administering MRA patients up to 0.3 mmol/kg as an off-label indication (8).

Initial studies emphasized the use of 0.2 mmol/kg for MR angiography (4), but subsequent studies have shown the efficacy of lower dose strategies, including 0.1 mmol/kg (78,79) and less (80,81).

Weakly Protein-Binding Gadolinium Agents

The only weakly protein-binding contrast agent approved for human use at present is gadobenate (MultiHance, Bracco), approved for use in the United States in December 2004. Because of weak, reversible binding to serum albumin, this agent exhibits approximately double the R_1 relaxivity as compared with traditional ECF agents (Fig. 5-1). This binding is not, however, strong enough to make gadobenate behave in true "blood pool" fashion, as is the case for gadofosveset (MS-325, EPIX).

Nonetheless, the protein binding and increased relaxivity appear to translate to higher and longer peak vascular enhancement as well as initial reports suggesting improved visualization of smaller vessels when compared with ECF agents (75,82–84). Furthermore, it has recently been shown that gadobenate dimeglumine at a dose of 0.1 mmol/kg was comparable to gadopentetate dimeglumine at 0.2 mmol/kg for CE renal MR angiography (85).

Strongly Protein-Binding and Macromolecular Blood Pool Agents

Both gadofosveset trisodium (Vasovist, Epix) and B22956 (Bracco) are low molecular weight experimental gadolinium-based agents with strong in vivo binding to serum albumin—the most abundant of the serum proteins (in vivo concentration of 600 to 700 μm) (12,17,36,86). Binding is reversible, with bound fractions of 91% and 95% for the two agents, respectively (12).

The association with albumin allows these contrast agents to remain largely intravascular and thereby behave as blood pool agents, as the contrast agent–albumin complex are both too large (albumin, 92,000 Da) to extravasate into the extracellular, extravascular space (EES) and are "protected" from renal and hepatic excretion. In addition, as discussed previously, binding to large proteins such as albumin slows down molecular rotation, leading to substantially increased relaxivity as compared with traditional ECF agents (Table 5-1). The small unbound fraction of contrast agent (<10%) allows for the necessary slow elimination of contrast from the body. At the same time, however, this small fraction behaves like an ECF agent and distributes into the EES, thereby causing some background soft tissue enhancement (87).

In clinical trials, gadofosveset at a dose of 0.03 mmol/kg has been explored for dynamic imaging as well as for delayed blood pool imaging (88,89) and has demonstrated efficacy for dynamic first-pass MRA when used in the same manner as traditional ECF agents (90,91). Furthermore, there is an added capability for collecting blood pool data from multiple vascular territories over a relatively long period, as intravascular half-lives are on the order of 120 minutes or greater (31) (Fig. 5-4). Safety data available from the Phase II trial indicates the percentage of patients with adverse events after gadofosveset administration of 0.03 mmol/kg was identical to that with administration of placebo, and there was no dose-related trend in severe or serious adverse events (88). This agent is approved for use in the European Union at the time of this writing.

As an example of the potency of protein-binding blood pool agents, if a dose of 0.03 mmol/kg of gadofosveset is administered to a 75-kg patient, assuming blood volume of 5 L, equilibrium concentration would be (0.03 mmol/kg × 75 kg)/5 L = 0.45 mM. Using an R_1 of 20 L mmol^{-1} sec^{-1} at 1.5 T (Fig. 5-1) (and making the simplifying assumption that there is no elimination or distribution into the EES, and only the 90% of the agent bound to albumin contributes to relaxation), and then using Equation [3], the equilibrium T1 is approximately 120 milliseconds, well below the approximately 250 milliseconds T1 of fat at 1.5 T (92). This is only a factor of two greater than the T1 of 56 calculated for the arterial phase of an ECF agent in our previous example (see text surrounding Equation [3]), yet as compared to the very short persistence of the arterial phase, this T1 shortening persists for a duration on the order of the half-life.

A second type of blood pool contrast agent, the macromolecular agents, are designed to be inherently large enough to remain intravascular. Early prototypes of this approach included gadolinium ion covalently linked to polylysine, dextran, and modified bovine serum albumin (12,93,94). While these agents had excellent blood pool properties, they exhibited very slow clearance and had

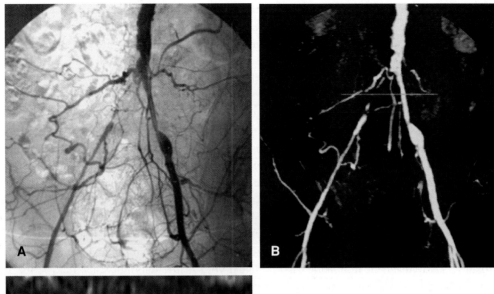

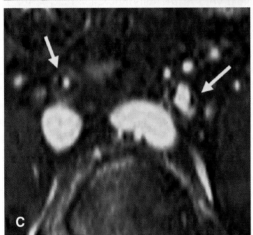

FIGURE 5-4 First-pass and steady-state images using a blood pool agent. A: Coronal projection of a conventional angiogram. **B:** The first pass from gadofosveset-enhanced MR angiography shows excellent correlation with **(A)**. **C:** An axial reconstruction at the level of disease (*white line*) during the steady state of gadofosveset-enhanced MR angiography shows stensoses (*arrows*) in both right and left common iliac arteries and nicely depicts the atherosclerotic plaque. Adapted from Rapp JH, Wolff SD, Quinn SF, et al. Aortoiliac occlusive disease in patients with known or suspected peripheral vascular disease: safety and efficacy of gadofosveset-enhanced MR angiography—multicenter comparative phase III study. *Radiology*. 2005; 236(1):71–78, with permission.

potential adverse immunological responses (12). In response to these problems, compounds have been developed that are sufficiently large to remain intravascular, yet small enough to be eliminated by glomerular filtration.

Two examples of this agent type currently undergoing clinical trials are Gadomer-17 (SH L 643A, Schering) and P792 (Guerbet) (Table 5-1). Gadomer-17 is a large dendrimer with an apparent molecular weight of 30 to 35 kD containing 24 gadolinium ions (37,95,96). A somewhat different approach was taken for P792, a synthetic polymeric Gd-complex based on gadoterate meglumine (Gd-DOTA) with four substituted hydrophilic arms having a total molecular weight of 6.47 kD (97). This agent undergoes some self-assembly and therefore occupies a larger molecular volume (98).

Both of these agents are unique in that the elimination half-lives are relatively rapid, with the elimination half-life of Gadomer-17 (in rabbit) being only 4.4 minutes (97) (approximately the same as standard Gd-DOTA) and the half-life of P792 (in swine) being approximately 20 minutes (99). While rapid elimination shortens the imaging window as compared with more slowly eliminated agents such as gadofosveset, it does give the opportunity to administer additional contrast boluses after only a short delay, eliminating the problem of soft tissue enhancement seen with traditional ECF agents (87,98). In addition, such agents may be well-suited for measurement of blood volume, tissue perfusion, and microvascular permeability (95).

Ultrasmall Superparamagnetic Iron Oxides

The only superparamagnetic agent presently approved for use in the United States is AMI-25 (Feridex, Berlex; Endorem, Guerbet S.A.), although SHU-555A (Resovist, Schering) has been approved in Europe and Japan. Both are SPIOs rather than USPIOs and are mainly used for hepatic and lymphatic imaging (19–21).

A third agent, AMI-227 (Combidex, Cytogen; Sinerem, Guerbet S.A.), a USPIO, is presently under scrutiny by the FDA, with an "approvable" letter having been issued. This agent, mainly developed for lymph node imaging, has potential applications for MRA (23,100). Another USPIO, NC100150 (Clariscan, Nycomed) that was in Stage III clinical trials primarily as a vascular blood pool agent (101,102) recently had development halted by the manufacturer.

Another USPIO, SHU-555C (the small-molecular-size subfraction of SHU-555A) is presently under early investigation as a potential blood pool agent (95,103). This agent has a more favorable R2/R1 ratio (60/24 at 0.47 T) and a longer half-life than its parent, SHU-555A, and hence is a better candidate for a blood pool agent (95).

VSOP-C63 is another small iron oxide in early phases of evaluation as a potential blood pool agent. This agent is of the VSOP (very small superparamagnetic iron oxide particle) class of contrast media and is different from typical USPIOs in that it is coated with monomers rather than polymers (104). At present, protein-binding gadolinium compounds (e.g., gadofosveset) appear much closer to clinical use than do any of the iron oxides.

CONTRAST AGENT ADMINISTRATION

Intravenous Considerations

Location

CE-MRA requires adequate delivery of contrast agent to the vascular region of interest. Contrast is typically administered intravenously either by hand or by using a power injector through a percutaneously placed intravenous catheter (IV), which is ideally placed in a large antecubital or forearm vein. It is important to adequately secure and tighten the connection between the tubing and the hub of the catheter or needle. This minimizes the chances of inadvertently leaking contrast media outside the patient when traction to the IV line occurs during the process of changing patient arm position or moving the table in and out of the magnet.

When possible, it is suggested that the catheter be placed in the right arm, as the right brachiocephalic vein courses more directly into the right atrium, facilitating more rapid and coherent delivery of contrast to the heart. This becomes even more important when performing thoracic or carotid MRA, as contrast in the left brachiocephalic vein has been known to obscure visualization of the arch vessels due to its proximity to these vessels as it crosses left to right, has a greater tendency to reflux up the jugular vein than does a right-sided injection, and can in some circumstances cause frank signal loss in adjacent arch vessels secondary to susceptibility induced signal loss (105). It is the high R2 of undiluted contrast agent during venous injec-

tion that causes this well-known susceptibility artifact that can obscure adjacent arterial structures. Thus, it is recommended that an injection site be designated for the contralateral arm when attempting to image a subclavian artery (Fig. 5-5).

In circumstances where antecubital or forearm placement is not possible, the IV may be placed in the distal forearm or hand, but as these veins are typically smaller and more fragile, injection rates may need to be adjusted downward, and careful monitoring should be performed both before and during the bolus administration. IV placement in the lower extremity is only recommended in times of absolute desperation. While this does work, keep in mind the longer route to the right heart and the high concentration of venous gadolinium that will either opacify or cause a signal void in the femoral veins, iliac veins, and inferior vena cava (depending on concentration).

Injection can be performed into a central line, provided a recent chest radiograph is consulted to verify catheter tip position and a saline test flush is first performed to confirm there is no abnormal resistance (e.g., thrombus on catheter tip) (54). In general, power injection should not be performed into small bore peripheral central access (PICC) lines, as the catheter could break (consult catheter manufacturer specifications). Hand injections are considered safer when this is the only route of administration possible, as pressure can be modulated by the person performing the injection.

Size

It is suggested a 20 to 22G IV be used whenever possible. A 20G catheter allows for injection rates of up to 5 cc per second or greater, which are rarely necessary for MRA. In addition, if injecting by hand, injection will be easier, particularly for the more viscous agents such as gadopentetate dimeglumine. This said, a 22G IV can tolerate up to 5 cc per second as well, but is best reserved for flow rates under 3 cc per second (54). Butterfly type catheters are not recommended, as the sharp tip may lacerate the vein during the extended time the patient is often in the magnet prior to contrast injection.

Injection Considerations

Saline Flush

It is of utmost importance to completely deliver all of the contrast from the venous circulation into the heart in one tight, coherent bolus. This requires "pushing" the contrast through the veins using a saline bolus (flush) to accommodate the high capacitance and variable flow velocity of the venous circulation (106). Without a saline flush, the delivery

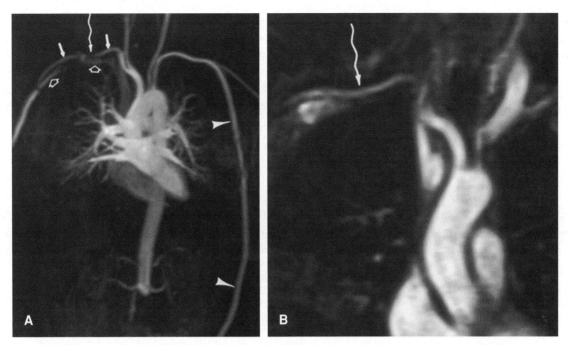

FIGURE 5-5 Pseudostenosis of the right subclavian artery. This 64-year-old man was referred for evaluation of left axillary-femoral bypass graft. **A:** Coronal maximum intensity projection of gadolinium-enhanced MR angiogram, obtained after IV injection of contrast material into right arm, shows contrast material in right axillary and subclavian veins (*open arrows*) and subclavian artery (*solid straight arrows*) with focal signal loss (*wavy arrow*) where the vein passes adjacent to artery. T2* effects of concentrated gadolinium contrast material in the vein cause susceptibility arti-fact affecting adjacent structures such as the subclavian artery. This examination shows patency of the proximal portion of the left axillary-femoral bypass graft (*arrowheads*). **B:** Coronal oblique reconstructed image of delayed three-dimensional acquisition obtained 40 seconds after **(A)** confirms the normal right subclavian artery (*wavy arrow*). Injection into right arm was performed to avoid possible susceptibility artifacts interfering with evaluation of the left axillary-femoral bypass graft anastomosis. Reprinted with permission from Lee V, Martin D, Krinsky G, et al. Gadolinium-enhanced MR angiography: artifacts and pitfalls. *AJR Am J Roentgenol.* 2000;175:197–205.

of contrast into the right heart and subsequently to the arte-rial circulation is unpredictable and vulnerable to being "stretched out" as contrast slowly "trickles" out of the venous circulation into the right heart. This equates to an inefficient use of contrast. All MRA practitioners agree that a saline flush is necessary, although there is no definite agree-ment on the amount. Suggested flush volumes range from 15 to 50 mL, but most authors report using 15 to 20 mL (25,78,107). We suggest using at least a 25-mL saline flush, administered at the same rate as the contrast injec-tion itself. When imaging the subclavian arteries, consider giving extra flush volume to ensure complete washout of the contrast from the subclavian vein to avoid susceptibil-ity artifact.

Methods for Injection

Contrast agents can be administered by hand or by using an automated power injector (multiple vendors offer MR-compatible units). Hand injection is less expensive and less hardware intensive, requiring two syringes (contrast and flush) and an adequate length of IV tubing (dedicated

commercial MRA manual injection tubing sets are avail-able). The addition of a two-way stopcock facilitates rapid transition from contrast to saline flush. Hand injection has the advantages of simplicity and direct caretaker monitor-ing of any immediate problems such as contrast extravasa-tion or leakage. On the down side, manual injection requires medical personnel to be in the magnet room at the time of injection, is imprecise in achieving uniform injec-tion rates (78), has variable switchover time from contrast to saline flush, and can require considerable physical strength depending on IV size, syringe size, and contrast viscosity. In addition, if the person manually injecting con-trast is also responsible for starting the MRA sequence at a precise time and providing breath-hold commands, the sum duties can be burdensome and difficult to successfully achieve.

Power injectors, on the other hand, greatly simplify and standardize contrast injections. Most models are capable of precise infusion of at least two sequential con-trast bolus quantities and rates (biphasic bolus) followed by a saline bolus. The injection can be performed remotely in the control room and initiated with a simple push button action. Thus, the workload is simplified, and full attention can be given to proper timing and patient breath-hold instructions. The negatives for a power injector include increased cost, the possibility of mechanical failures, and the decreased likelihood for monitoring the injection site.

Injection Rate and Dose

Injection Rate

As discussed previously, dynamic CE-MRA can be summarized as acquiring vascular images during a transient period of intravascular T1 shortening caused by the first pass of contrast material. In general, this is performed using a 3D spoiled gradient echo pulse sequence, for which signal intensity (SI) can be written (108):

$$SI \; \alpha \frac{(1 - e^{-TR/T1}) \; \sin(\alpha) \; e^{-TE/T2^*}}{(1 - \cos(\alpha) \; e^{-TR/T1})} \qquad [5]$$

where TR is the repetition time, TE is the echo time, α is the flip angle, T1 is the intravascular T1 relaxation time, and T2* is the combination of intravascular T2 and field homogeneity effects. Examining Equation [5], T1 plays a dominant role—the shorter the T1, the greater the signal intensity. Recall from Equation [3] that $1/T1 = 1/1,200 + c\,R1$, where c is the arterial concentration, and R1 is the relaxivity of the contrast agent. For any significant contrast concentration, the product c R1 overwhelms the scalar term 1/1,200, and we can therefore say:

$$1/T1 \; \alpha \; c\,R1 \qquad [6]$$

(or conversely, $T1 \; \alpha \; 1/c$). Arterial contrast concentration c is a function of how fast the contrast agent enters the arterial circulation. This has been approximated by multiple investigators as (106,109,110):

$$c = IR/CO \qquad [7]$$

where IR is the molar contrast infusion rate, and CO is the cardiac output. This assumes the contrast is pushed into the heart at the prescribed rate (hence, the importance of flush—see earlier) and discounts any recirculation.

Combining Equations [6] and [7] (assuming cardiac output is relatively constant for any given patient), we can say $1/T1 \; \alpha \; IR$, or conversely, $T1 \; \alpha \; 1/IR$. This is a very important point, as it states arterial T1 is inversely proportional to contrast injection rate, not to total contrast dose as might at first be inferred. Thus, for dynamic CE-MRA, contrast injection rate determines how short T1 becomes, and total dose defines how long the arterial concentration remains high—that is, defines the shape or "spread" of the

contrast bolus. Resultant image signal intensity depends on the intravascular T1 at the time the center of k-space is collected, with the shape of the bolus determining subsequent artifacts (see Chapter 2) (111). Proceeding along the lines of Maki et al. (106), we can insert the Ernst angle, or optimum flip angle for a given T1: $\alpha_E = \cos^{-1}(e^{-TR/T1})$, into Equation [5], resulting in:

$$SI \; \alpha \; sqrt(1 - e^{-2TR/T1})e^{-TE/T2^*} \qquad [8]$$

Making the approximation that TR $\ll$ T1 (a reasonable approximation for CE-MRA where a typical TR is 4 to 5 milliseconds, and T1 might be 40 to 50 milliseconds) and writing out Equation [8] as a first-order Taylor series, one arrives at:

$$SI \; \alpha \; sqrt(2 \; TR/T1)e^{-TE/T2^*} \qquad [9]$$

Now substituting in for T1 and then c from Equations [6] and [7], this becomes:

$$SI \; \alpha \; sqrt(TR \; IR \; R1/CO)e^{-TE/T2^*} \qquad [10]$$

This is a useful equation—let us examine it closely. First, it demonstrates that arterial signal intensity is proportional to the square root of TR. This is not unexpected, as MR signal generally scales as the square root of scan time. Second, it tells us that arterial signal intensity also scales as the square root of the infusion rate. This has important implications for CE-MRA. For example, all other things being equal, if one halves the acquisition time by shortening TR by a factor of two, signal decreases by a factor of sqrt(2) (30%). But if one then takes the same volume of contrast material and injects it twice as fast (i.e., double the IR), this increases signal by that same factor of sqrt(2) and in essence "buys back" the signal lost by decreasing scan time. Realize that this occurs without artifacts secondary to shortening the bolus length, as the scan time and bolus duration both decrease to the same degree. This interesting paradox goes against the general trend just stated that MR signal scales as the square root of acquisition time and is a property unique to CE-MRA. This same principle applies when decreasing scan time using other methods such as parallel imaging (112,113). Third, arterial signal intensity scales as the square root of the contrast agent relaxivity R1. This means that an agent such as gadofosveset, with an R1 of 20 at 1.5 T, which is five-fold greater than ECF agents, will in theory give sqrt(5)—more than double the signal for the same molar injection rate. Finally, signal is related to the inverse square root of cardiac output (CO). This means vasculopathic and older patients, who typically have lower cardiac outputs, will actually have greater arterial contrast concentration for a given injection rate.

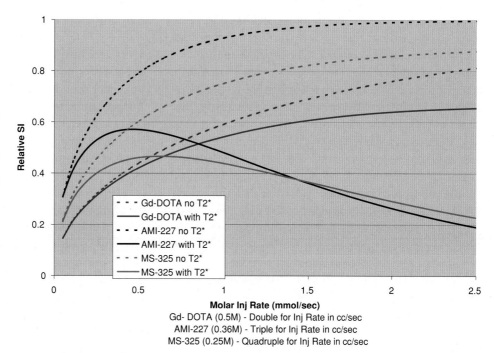

FIGURE 5-6 Predicted signal intensity (SI) versus molar contrast infusion rate using a 3D spoiled gradient CE-MRA sequence with TR = 5 msec and TE = 1.5 msec. The calculations are performed for the ECF agent gadoterate (Gd-DOTA, blue), the USPIO ferumoxtran (AMI-227, black), and the strongly protein-binding blood pool agent gadofosveset (MS-325, red). The calculations are performed both with and without taking into account T2* losses due to the R2 of these compounds in order to demonstrate how profound the R2 losses can be for certain agents at high injection rates. Since injection rate is shown in mmol per second, this can be translated into volume injection rate by dividing the molar injection rate by the contrast concentration.

Based on this discussion, it may appear that injecting contrast at increasingly high flow rates will improve signal (i.e., square root of IR) indefinitely. This is not true for two reasons. The first is that increasing injection rate does not necessarily linearly correlate with achieved arterial contrast rates because of (a) temporal dispersion of the contrast agent as it disperses through the heart and (b) the fact that a given injection rate must be sustained for a long enough duration such that the peak arterial concentration is reached before the bolus ends (110,114). These references are recommended for further clarification of this point. The second reason relates to the $e^{-TE/T2*}$ term at the end of Equation [10]. This term describes the signal loss due to phase cancellation occurring at the echo time (TE) and depends on the arterial T2*, which can be assumed dominated by contrast agent R2 relaxivity when discussing typical dynamic contrast injection rates. By choosing typical TR and TE values of 5.0 and 1.5 ms, we can plot out relative signal level for different contrast agents and molar injection rates (with and without T2* effects included), as shown in Figure 5-6. In this figure, the R2 and R1 values used for gadofosveset differ from those in Table 5-1, as 1.5 T values were used, and gadofosveset has a large dependence on field strength (12) (Fig. 5-1). Note from Figure 5-6 that for the ECF agent gadoterate, with its typical favorable R2/R1 ratio of 1.3, the R2 effects are not extreme but nonetheless indicate that signal intensity flattens for contrast injection rates much more than 1.5 to 2.0 mmol per second (3.0 to 4.0 cc per second).

A very different condition exists for both ferumoxtran (AMI-227) and gadofosveset (MS-325) due to their much more unfavorable R2/R1 ratios of 2.2 and 3.0, respectively. For these agents, the use of low injection rates can yield greater signal compared with extracellular agents. However, at injection rates beyond 0.5 mmol per second (~1.5 cc per second for ferumoxtran and 2.0 cc per second for gadofosveset), there is rapid severe loss in signal due to the T2* factor. Thus, it is important to realize that even though we describe MRA contrast agents as T1 enhancement agents, R2 effects can be extremely important, ultimately limiting achievable signal. As a general rule, investigators typically use injection rates of 1.5 to 2.5 cc per second for most present-day arterial CE-MRA exams using ECF agents (0.75 to 1.25 mmol per second on Fig. 5-6). Specific injection rates for different applications will be discussed in the following chapters.

Injection Dose

Realizing now that contrast injection rate influences arterial signal intensity, we must consider the impact of dose on arterial SI. This impact depends partly on the application. For single-station CE-MRA, the dose must be sustained for long enough that any drop-off in arterial contrast concentration during acquisition does not cause significant artifacts. This is a somewhat complicated issue related to the manner in which the raw data (k-space) is acquired with respect to the arterial enhancement profile (106,111).

Depending on contrast/scan timing and how k-space is collected, it turns out that the arterial concentration need not be maintained at a constant value for the entire acquisition—that is, the IV injection duration can be shorter than the acquisition. When contrast concentration begins to decline (taper off) toward the end of the acquisition, this causes an underrepresentation of the higher spatial frequencies, which in turn causes blurring. This effect, however, has been shown to be relatively mild, with one detailed analysis suggesting that IV bolus durations of approximately 60% of the scan time cause minimal artifact while increasing available signal by allowing a more rapid contrast injection (106).

In fact, there are cases, such as in carotid artery MRA, where very short IV boluses of only 25% to 40% of scan duration have been shown to work well without significant artifact (115,116). In part, this may be related to fast recirculation in the carotid arteries, maintaining a longer "tail" of arterial contrast.

Thus, contrast dose for arterial CE-MRA becomes a choice between how much signal is needed, how much artifact can be tolerated, and how much contrast is available. Moreover, clinical applications for most MRA examinations are performed within the approved ECF agent dose range of 0.1 to 0.3 mmol/kg. Consider the following example. When performing a renal CE-MRA on a 100-kg patient, using 0.1 mmol/kg of contrast media requires 20 cc of a 0.5 M ECF agent. If this amount of contrast is applied for 60% of the scan time for a 17-second acquisition, a 10-second bolus would be required. It follows that an injection of 20 cc of contrast at 2 cc per second yields the 10-second bolus—a reasonable choice for this theoretical patient.

With a faster injection, there will be more signal, but there may also be more blurring artifacts. If you inject more slowly, say at 1 cc per second (20-second bolus), you will not have blurring due to contrast concentration decreasing at the end of the scan, but you will have sqrt(2) less signal and waste the portion of the contrast that arrives in the artery after the acquisition is complete.

When considering dosing for delayed, blood pool, or venous imaging, things are somewhat different. In this case, the early equilibrium or blood pool T1 becomes the relevant signal-determining factor rather than peak arterial T1. This value depends on the pharmacokinetics of the contrast agent—in particular, the distribution volume ($V_{d\,ss}$) as well as the distribution and elimination half-lives ($T_{1/2\alpha}$ and $T_{1/2\beta}$—see previous discussion). ECF agents as well as weakly protein-binding agents can all be considered to have a similar distribution volume reflecting that of the ECF agents—on the order of 200 mL/kg (28).

Macromolecular agents and USPIOs remain nearly entirely intravascular and therefore have distribution vol-

umes on the order of the intravascular volume, which is 70 mL/kg (117). The strongly protein-binding blood pool agents are somewhat more complicated. Although they have distribution half-lives similar to ECF agents due to their small size, it is only the small unbound fraction that rapidly equilibrates with the EES. Because albumin concentration is much greater in the intravascular space than EES space, the net effect is that more agent remains intravascular, and the distribution volume is closer to the intravascular volume.

Having an understanding of the distribution volume as well as the R1 and R2 values for a contrast agent, T1 and signal intensity estimates in delayed phase for any dose and given pulse sequence can be made in a similar fashion to the results presented in Figure 5-6. Of course, elimination and distribution half-lives also need to be considered, but as an approximation, ECF agents have immediate distribution to the EES, and blood pool agents have little or no distribution into the EES.

Elimination half-lives will decrease ECF and macromolecular contrast concentrations within minutes, while strongly protein-binding blood pool agents can be considered not to be eliminated over a period of at least tens of minutes. Examples of how to calculate these values have already been presented for an ECF agent (see Contrast Pharmacokinetics and Biologic Factors section in this chapter) and a blood pool agent (see Specific Contrast Media section in this chapter).

As can be seen from the ECF agent example, where a 10 mmol (20 cc) dose gives an equilibrium T1 greater than 400 ms (i.e., less signal than fat), it is obvious that much larger doses (0.2 to 0.3 mmol/kg) are necessary if high signal-delayed phases are desired. Blood pool agents, on the other hand, with their higher R1 relaxivity, permit delayed imaging (e.g., venous evaluation) at much lower doses (101).

Special Injection Routes

Direct Venous Administration and Imaging

One interesting method of MR venography is to inject dilute contrast agent directly upstream of the target venous system, for example, hand injection for arm MR venography (see Chapter 24) (118,119). This application requires a knowledge of preprocedural contrast agent dilution, as the contrast material will not dilute in the blood as it does when injecting intravenously and waiting to image when contrast arrives in the arteries. Li et al. suggest a 1:20 dilution of ECF agent (119). Assuming gadoterate relaxivities R1 and R2 of 3.6 and 4.8 L mmol^{-1} sec^{-1}, respectively, and using Equation [3], a 1:20 dilution has a T1 of 11 ms, and a T2* on the order of 8 ms. With a further assumption that this dilutes at least another factor of 2 as it mixes with fresh blood, this concentration equates to a molar injection rate of 1.0 mmol per second (2 cc per second) on the Figure 5-6 gadoterate graph—an appropriate place for imaging. Injecting full-strength ECF agent would be disastrous, as the resultant T2* of less than 1 ms would completely eliminate all signal.

Direct Arterial Administration and Imaging

Just as dilute contrast can be administered and imaged directly after injection into the veins, direct intra-arterial injection of dilute contrast material with subsequent MRA imaging has been demonstrated to be feasible, although as of yet primarily in animals (114). This invasive procedure requires an arterial puncture (analogous to conventional angiography) and is being developed for interventional MR, primarily to provide vascular roadmaps during the procedure, but also with potential as a diagnostic tool in these situations (120). As with direct MR venography, ECF contrast agents must be diluted to be effective.

In a dog model, Omary et al. determined that optimum ECF agent dilution factors depended on injection rate, injection duration, vessel flow rate, and imaging parameters (120). He concluded that in a dog aorta, the critical factor is the molar rate of contrast delivery, with optimum molar delivery rates ranging from 0.05 to 0.1 mmol per second. For typical injection rates used in this study, this corresponded to dilution factors of 2% to 14%. Of interest, volume rates of (dilute) intra-arterial contrast injected in this study were on the order of 20 to 30 cc over 3 to 20 seconds—volumes and rates not too dissimilar to conventional angiography using iodinated contrast agents. Exact contrast dilutions and injection protocols remain to be worked out for human imaging.

CONTRAST TIMING AND INFUSION

As can be inferred from much of the preceding discussion, optimum dynamic CE-MRA requires not only proper administration of the most appropriate contrast agent, it also requires precise timing of image data acquisition with respect to the contrast administration. This first requires an understanding of how MR data is collected (121,122). Unlike conventional CT (123), MR imaging does not map spatial data linearly with respect to time. With 3D MR imaging, the entire raw data set—called *Fourier* or *k-space*—is collected before reconstructing individual slices. As such, MR image acquisition is quite unique in that k-space maps spatial frequencies rather than spatial data. Hence, different image "features" are collected at different times within the acquisition time frame (124).

For example, image contrast (i.e., the brightness or darkness of a vessel) corresponds to the low-frequency "center" of k-space, and the fine details (i.e., vessel edge sharpness) corresponds to the high-frequency "periphery" of k-space (111,125). This means certain characteristics of the resultant images can be profoundly influenced by the dynamics or "shape" of the passing contrast bolus and how this relates to the manner in which k-space is collected (view ordering). In particular, the state of the intravascular contrast (concentration in arteries vs. veins) is essentially "captured" at the time the center of k-space is collected—what happens thereafter (or before) relates more to image quality and artifacts (111,124). Proper understanding of these concepts is vital to performing consistent, high-quality MR angiography.

K-space Acquisition Strategies

A 3D CE-MRA data set consists of numerous digitized echoes filling the *x*-dimension, with the *y* and *z* coordinates for each echo being incremented over time by appropriate application of phase-encoding gradients (Fig. 5-7A). How the *y* and *z* phase-encoding gradients are incremented describes what is termed the *k-space acquisition order* or *view order*. Traditionally, MR sequences were implemented using *linear k-space acquisition*, meaning the phase-encoding gradients started at one extreme of k-space (periphery), then incremented through zero (center) and back to the negative extreme (periphery) (Fig. 5-7B). Given that this occurs in two phase-encoding axes (*y* and *z*), there are typically two phase-encoding loops established—for example, start with the maximum *z* phase-encodes value, loop through all *y* phase encodings, then increment *z* and repeat the loop through *y*, and the like.

With linear k-space acquisition, the center of k-space, which determines image contrast (111), is by definition acquired at the midpoint of the scan. While this strategy can work well (126), it presents several limitations for CE-MRA, most notably in instances when real time contrast timing methods are used (see below). When the contrast bolus is detected in the arterial bed of interest in real time, it is necessary to begin the MR data acquisition at or near the center of k-space (127). Failure to do so means that the middle of k-space occurs at some time point after the arrival of arterial contrast, when venous structures may be enhancing (causing venous overlay) or peak arterial contrast concentration may be waning (decreasing arterial signal).

Coincident with the development of real time bolus timing, investigators began modifying the order in which k-space was acquired to better accommodate these new timing techniques. When the center of k-space is obtained at the beginning rather than in the middle of the acquisition,

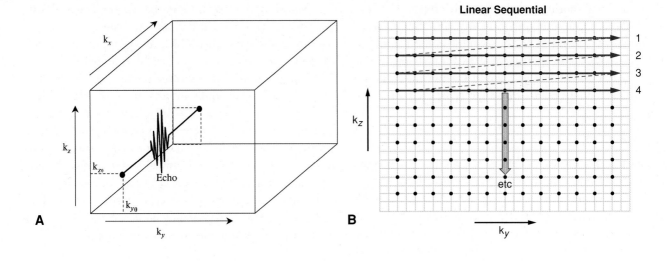

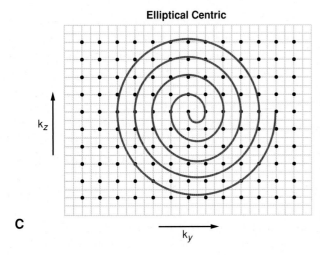

FIGURE 5-7 K-space and filling orders. A: Representation of how a 3D volume of k-space is filled. Each acquired echo (1 per phase encoding) fills out a line (i.e., all values) of k_x space positioned at k_y0, k_z0. Each tiny dot represents the other k_y and k_z values for which subsequent echoes are obtained during a total of $k_y \times k_z$ total phase encoding steps. **B:** Representation of linear k-space acquisition (view ordering). For each successive k_z encoding, the k_y phase encodings are incremented as shown by the *black arrows* (*large dots* represent individual k_z and k_y values—only a subfraction is shown). **C:** Representation of elliptical centric k-space acquisition (view ordering). Sampling begins at $k_z = k_y = 0$. Successive phase encodings are incremented based on their radial distance from the center of k-space (*large dots* represent individual k_z and k_y values—only a subfraction is shown).

this is termed a *centric acquisition* (Fig. 5-7C) (128). In such an acquisition strategy, the y and z phase encodes propagate out from the center of k-space. Most implementations are now termed *elliptical centric*, meaning that y and z phase encodes are ordered based on their true radial distance from the center of k-space, rather than just their numerical ordering (129). Centric view ordering works extremely well and is not only well suited to and often used for CE-MRA (115,127,130), but is also more robust in terms of sensitivity to respiratory motion (131).

With this background of k-space view ordering, timing considerations can now be discussed in greater detail. As k-space reflects the spatial frequency makeup of the anatomic image, different artifacts occur depending on how the arterial contrast concentration (i.e., intravascular T1) changes during the course of k-space acquisition. Artifacts can be considered to come in three varieties—too early, too late, and too peaked (Figs. 5-8 and 5-9).

It is well known that contrast does not arrive in the arteries instantaneously—there is a finite upslope or "rise

time" of contrast concentration, and this depends on injection rate, total contrast volume administered, and patient hemodynamics (110,114). The "too early" artifact occurs when the center of k-space is acquired during the rapid upslope of arterial contrast concentration (Fig. 5-8B) (111). This causes the low (central k-space) spatial frequencies to be under-represented, thus emphasizing the higher spatial frequencies and resulting in an image with overemphasized edges. This then causes a characteristic "ringing" appearance along vessel margins that can at times be quite dramatic (Fig. 5-9B) (111). For this reason, it is paramount not to position the center of k-space too early in the upslope phase of contrast arrival, and experience has taught us that a period of 3 to 5 seconds (depending primarily on cardiac output) must be allowed for the arterial contrast to peak in order to avoid the too early ringing artifact (Fig. 5-8A) (111,124,125,132). Another way of achieving this delay is to slightly recess the absolute center of k-space by a couple of seconds (125,133), which has the added advantage of utilizing at least some of the early contrast arrival

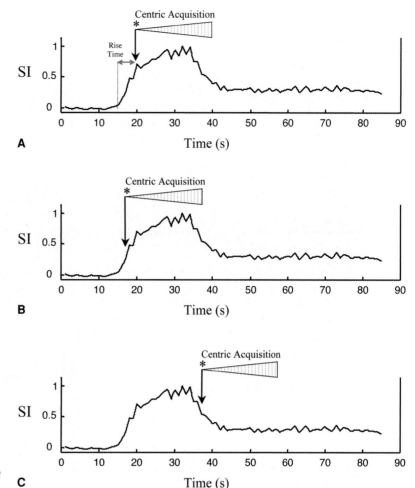

FIGURE 5-8 Aortic response (signal intensity vs. time) to the IV injection of 10 cc ECF contrast agent at 1 cc per second. The "∗" represents the center of k-space. **A:** Perfect timing. Note the rise time from the beginning up-slope to the peak (plateau region) is approximately 5 seconds. **B:** The center of k-space is collected during the arterial contrast upslope. This causes "too early" ringing artifacts. **C:** The center of k-space is collected too late. This causes decreased signal, intensity and (depending on venous contrast arrival time) increased venous signal. This can also cause blurring from under-representation of the high spatial frequencies. Figure 5-9 demonstrates imaging correlates to these aortic response curves.

that might otherwise be wasted. Of interest, the too early ringing artifact is much more pronounced with centric acquisitions than it is for linear acquisitions, likely having to do with the inherent symmetry of a linear acquisition order (111). This makes linear view ordering preferred in cases where no timing is performed (i.e., "best guess") and the relationship between contrast arrival and center of k-space is not known.

On the opposite extreme, when the center of k-space occurs after the arrival of contrast ("too late"—Fig. 5-8C), several things may occur. First, if there is venous enhancement at the time central k-space is collected, the image will have venous overlay. Furthermore, depending on how late central k-space is collected with respect to the arterial enhancement profile, the image can have decreased or no arterial signal as well (Fig. 5-9C). This is particularly problematic with carotid MRA (116), where rapid arteriovenous transit times as short as 5 seconds (134) make accurate timing essential, and with moving-table peripheral MRA

(135,136), where the time required to collect the upper and middle stations often means that the lower station acquisition is well behind the arterial bolus arrival and, unfortunately, sometimes behind venous contrast arrival as well. Second, the bolus can wash out either before the center of k-space is acquired or sometime during the collection of the periphery of k-space. In this instance, which can also occur with a bolus that is properly timed but too compact (114), the decreasing contrast concentration during peripheral k-space acquisition under-represents the high spatial frequencies, resulting in blurring—what we term the *too peaked effect* (Fig. 5-9D). This effect is, however, typically quite minimal, and in examinations such as carotid (115,116) and peripheral (135) MRA, evidence points to recirculation effects prolonging the "tail" of the bolus, moderating this effect. As a general rule for dynamic CE-MRA examinations (nonmoving table), an IV bolus duration of approximately 60% of the planned acquisition time offers a good compromise between artifacts and signal (106,124).

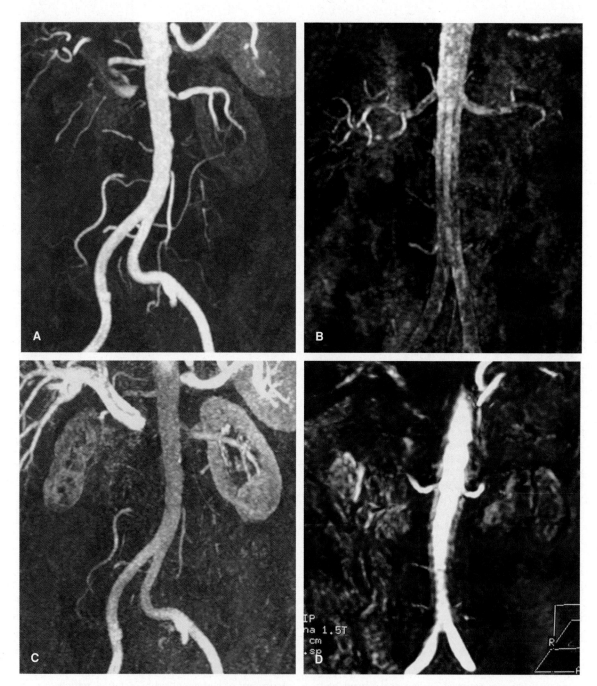

FIGURE 5-9 Renal CE-MRA examinations illustrating contrast timing issues. A: Ideal timing. Good uniform enhancement, no artifacts (s/p right nephrectomy, high grade left renal artery stenosis). **B:** Characteristic "too early" artifact occurring when the center of k-space is acquired during the upslope of contrast arrival. Note the ringing along the vessel edges and poor signal, particularly distally. **C:** The same exam as **(A)**, only 9 seconds later, demonstrating the "too late" effect. Arterial signal is washed out, except distally in the iliac vessels, and venous enhancement predominates. **D:** Examination in which very compact bolus (4 seconds) was used for a 25-second acquisition, causing blurring due to the "too peaked" effect.

The Timing Bolus

Other than a flat-out guess, which is not recommended, performing a timing bolus is the simplest way to determine proper timing (78,134,137). With this technique, 1 to 2 cc of an ECF contrast agent is injected intravenously, followed by adequate saline flush (30 cc suggested). Injection should

be performed at the anticipated rate for the CE-MRA, as arrival time depends on venous injection rate (138).

Coincident with initiating injection, a rapid (0.5 to 1.0 image per second) 2D gradient echo imaging sequence is performed to cover the vascular anatomy of interest, with a duration of at least 50 seconds. This can be either in the plane of or perpendicular to the target vessel. If perpendicular (e.g., axial for the aorta), superior and inferior saturation bands are suggested to suppress inflow effects and improve test-bolus detection. Alternatively, a magnetization-prepared gradient sequence with an inversion time structured to null the signal from nonenhanced blood is very effective and eliminates the need for saturation bands (90).

The time to peak enhancement in a target vessel of interest is determined from examining the images, either manually or by using dedicated software to interpret a specified region of interest. It is important to realize that timing boluses in some hands are limited in accuracy and reproducibility with vulnerability to moment-to-moment changes in venous return and cardiac output (124), and that any alteration in flow rate from the test bolus to the MRA injection can also alter the timing (138). A timing bolus also adds time of approximately 2 to 5 minutes (78) to the overall examination length.

Despite these issues, a timing bolus has been successful for a variety of applications. In addition to providing data about an individual's circulatory physiology, the timing run offers information about IV integrity with 1 to 2 cc of contrast and can lessen the likelihood of a large volume of contrast material extravasating. Finally, the linear order of k-space is less vulnerable to subtle timing nuances compared with centric strategies (94).

Real Time Bolus Detection

The first automated pulse sequence for detecting contrast arrival and then triggering the MRA acquisition was termed *MR SmartPrep* (General Electric Medical Systems, Waukesha, WI) and dates back to 1997 (132,139). To use SmartPrep, the operator first sets up the 3D CE-MRA pulse sequence, then places a monitoring volume (tracker) over the vessel on which to trigger (e.g., aorta or other large artery). The sequence is then started, and baseline tracker signal intensity and standard deviation are computed over a 10- to 20-second period.

Following this, the software instructs the user to inject contrast, meanwhile continuing to monitor the tracker volume. Once contrast arrives, the tracker measures the signal intensity increase. The software is programmed such that a rise beyond a predetermined threshold (e.g., 20% and 2 standard deviations) initiates a user-defined delay of 3 to 5 seconds (allowing contrast to peak and thus avoid the "too early" artifact), and then proceeds with the centric or elliptical centric ordered 3D MRA acquisition. This technique has proven quite successful, but has the disadvantage of not allowing the operator to directly visualize contrast arrival (or lack thereof) and thereby modify the timing "on the fly."

A second real time technique, fluoroscopic triggering, gives the operator much more control over manipulating the timing relationship between bolus arrival and image acquisition (127,140,141). Flouroscopic triggering is available under different labels for all major vendors (BolusTrak, Philips Medical Systems, Best, the Netherlands; Care Bolus, Siemens Solutions, Erlangen, Germany; Flouro Trigger, General Electric Medical Systems, Waukesha, WI). This technique consists of rapid 2D gradient echo images (typically coronal or sagittal) positioned over the vascular territory of interest presented to the operator in real time (1 to 2 frames per second). Some versions employ automated, complex subtraction to increase vessel contrast.

The operator initiates the fluoroscopic sequence, injects the contrast, and visually monitors for the arrival of the contrast bolus in a target vessel of interest. It is often possible to first visualize proximal cardiovascular anatomy (e.g., in the heart or lungs), which provides an indication of an impending arrival along with some insight regarding flow rate. Once the bolus is in the desired location, the operator pushes a button, and the software switches from a monitoring mode to the MRA acquisition mode using a centrically reordered sequence with a user-defined delay (3 to 5 seconds). Fluoroscopic imaging can provide an evaluation of flow dynamics in real time, allowing the operator to make timing adjustments for pooling of contrast in abdominal aneurysms. Without this compensation, such pooling can result in the "too early" phase acquisition and lead to artifacts in the distal aneurysm and iliac vessels as shown in Figure 5-9 (124).

Both automated bolus detection and fluoroscopic triggering share an additional advantage as compared with using a timing bolus. With a timing bolus, a small quantity of contrast is administered several minutes prior to CE-MRA acquisition. This contrast is quickly excreted into the renal collecting systems and sometimes the bladder, where it can potentially complicate interpretation of the MRA images. In addition, it distributes into the extravascular, extracellular space (EES), where it can increase background tissue signal (78), particularly in organs such as the liver and kidneys. While this effect tends to be minimal with small contrast boluses, it becomes much more relevant when discussing second injections, as occur with certain techniques such as multi-injection implementations of peripheral MRA (142).

Time Resolved—No Timing Necessary

In part because achieving proper bolus timing is complex, several authors now advocate time-resolved MRA techniques, where multiple 3D data sets are obtained with a temporal resolution on the order of 2 to 8 seconds. Using this approach, one simply injects the contrast, starts the scan, and then chooses the best temporal data set(s). These time-resolved techniques come in two varieties. The first achieves speed gains through the use of multiple techniques such as ultra-fast TR, reduced matrix size and/or field of view, partial k-space filling, and parallel imaging (76,143–146). Although this approach typically sacrifices spatial resolution and signal to noise (SNR), a side benefit of decreasing scan time to below 10 to 12 seconds is in decreasing motion blurring and providing improved intra-abdominal MRA image quality (147).

The second variety, the so-called *TRICKS* (time-resolved imaging of contrast kinetics) variants synthesize high-resolution data sets from a clever oversampling of central k-space (148–151). In its most basic form, this technique first divides k-space into several blocks. The central k-space block (which provides most of the contrast) is then repeatedly collected in an alternating fashion with the other blocks (more peripheral k-space) such that a unique central block of data is collected every 2 to 8 seconds. Temporal data sets are then "synthesized" by piecing together each unique central k-space block with a linear interpolation of the remaining k-space blocks.

The big advantage of TRICKS over the previously described ultrafast techniques is increased inherent spatial resolution and SNR. Countering this, it may appear at first glance that inherent k-space discontinuities in conjunction with time varying intravascular contrast concentration would cause artifacts. Although this is in fact true, these artifacts have been shown to be relatively mild provided the contrast bolus is not too compact (114,152). Another implementation, time-resolved echo-shared angiographic technique, *TREAT*, combines view sharing with parallel imaging (153). Product versions recently have been released (TRICKS, General Electric Medical Systems, Waukesha, WI; TREAT, Siemens Medical Solutions). Newer TRICKS variants have recently been developed using radial or spiral projections (148,149) and time-resolved echo-shared angiographic technique.

Putting It Together—Choosing the Technique and Timing

The choice of technique—timing bolus versus automated detection versus flouroscopic triggering versus time resolved—depends largely on equipment type, level of proficiency, previous experience and success, and individual preferences. Some general guidelines, however, are in order. For automated detection and fluoroscopic triggering, elliptical centric phase encoding should almost always be used, beginning after a 3- to 5-second delay to allow the bolus to

peak (conveniently also giving time to instruct the patient to breath hold when needed). This is because the MRA acquisition by definition cannot start until the actual bolus arrives. Any view ordering other than centric will displace the center of k-space beyond the arterial arrival, potentially causing venous enhancement. In special circumstances, such as in an ultrafast upper station acquisition in a moving table MRA (154), linear or even reverse centric (middle of k-space at the end of the acquisition) might be beneficial to ensure that the contrast peaks in the distal part of the image in order to avoid the "too early" ringing artifact (Fig. 5-9).

When using a timing bolus, we prefer elliptical centric view ordering, although this is not essential. Some older equipment does not have elliptical centric as an option. However, any machine capable of automated detection or fluoroscopic triggering will have elliptical centric capability. When using elliptical centric view ordering, timing is simply a matter of determining the test-bolus time to peak (t_p), then adding the appropriate rise time (t_R), to allow the imaging bolus to peak (realizing a large bolus requires more time to reach its peak than does a small test bolus (138). We suggest using a rise time of 3 to 4 seconds and adding 1 or 2 seconds to this if there is extremely slow flow or a known aneurysm that will fill slowly. The timing can be summarized as (124):

$$\text{Centric: } T_{start} = t_p + t_R \qquad [11]$$

where t_R is 3 to 6 seconds.

For linear view ordering, the timing is different. Traditionally, the concept has been to position the middle of k-space approximately at the middle of the arterial enhancement profile. This timing can be written as (78):

$$\text{Linear: } T_{start} = t_p - t_s/2 + t_b/2 \qquad [12]$$

where t_s is the scan time, and t_b is the IV bolus duration. The linear view ordering is much less sensitive to the "too early" artifact. The downside to this method is that central k-space is delayed beyond the beginning of arterial enhancement, making venous enhancement more likely. In many cases, such as in renal or aortoiliac MRA, this will be of little consequence. For carotid and pulmonary MRA, venous contamination is more likely.

To decrease chances of venous contamination, Equation [12] can be modified by reducing the calculated T_{start} by a few seconds. The linear view ordering being less sensitive to the "too early" artifact affords the flexibility. Another suggestion for timing when using linear view ordering is to use the same approach taken when using centric view ordering, and to place the center of k-space at the peak of arterial contrast (124). Using the same rise time (t_R) as for centric, this changes Equation [12] to:

$$\text{Linear}_{\text{(alternate)}}: T_{\text{start}} = t_p - t_s/2 + t_R \qquad [13]$$

where t_R is 3 to 6 seconds.

With temporally resolved techniques, no special timing is required, as they are designed to provide at least one temporal data set that demonstrates the desired vascular enhancement. Perhaps the main timing-related consideration concerns abdominal and thoracic examinations, where breath holding is extremely important. Since average contrast transit time from the IV site to the peak arterial enhancement is somewhat lengthy and highly variable, with one investigator reporting 24 +/− 12 seconds (range 10 to 60 seconds) (78), successful breath holding likely cannot begin at the time of injection.

Assuming that injection and acquisition begin simultaneously, operator judgment is required to determine at what point to have the patient initiate a breath hold, keeping in mind that some time-resolved techniques use subtraction and require at least one precontrast-arrival phase for use as a subtraction mask. As operators become more experienced and time-resolved techniques become more refined and available, efficacious and simplified approaches to optimize contrast delivery for MRA will continue to emerge.

CONCLUSION

Successful and reproducible MRA can be achieved by a variety of means. In this chapter, principles and techniques to guide the reader toward high-quality MRA studies have been provided. As the technology evolves, ever simpler strategies to perform will emerge with the capability of easily achieving robust results. With the understanding that CNR is the currency of MRA, combinations of new contrast agents, improved coil designs, and higher field strengths offer continued improvements and expanded capabilities for the MR angiographer.

REFERENCES

1. Potchen E, Haacke E, Siebert J, et al. *Magnetic Resonance Angiography*. 1st ed. St. Louis: Mosby–Year Book; 1993.
2. Al-Kwifi O, Emery D, Wilman A. Vessel contrast at three Tesla in time-of-flight magnetic resonance angiography of the intracranial and carotid arteries. *Magn Reson Imaging*. 2002;20(2):181–187.
3. Weinman H, Brasch R, Press W, et al. Characteristics of gadolinium-DTAP complex: a potential NMR contrast agent. *Am J Roentgenol*. 1984;142:619–624.
4. Prince M, Yucel E, Kaufman J, et al. Dynamic gadolinium-enhanced three-dimensional abdominal MR arterography. *JMRI*. 1993;3:877–881.
5. Leiner T, de Vries M, Hoogeveen R, et al. Contrast-enhanced peripheral MR angiography at 3.0 Tesla: initial experience with a whole-body scanner in healthy volunteers. *J Magn Reson Imaging*. 2003;17(5):609–614.
6. Hayes C, Mathis C, Yuan C. Surface coil phased arrays for high-resolution imaging of the carotid arteries. *J Magn Reson Imaging*. 1996;6(1):109–112.
7. Pruessmann K, Weiger M, Scheidegger M, Boesiger P. SENSE: sensitivity encoding for fast MRI. *Magn Reson Med*. 1999;42:952–962.
8. Runge V, Knopp M. Off-label use and reimbursement of contrast media in MR. *J Magn Reson Imaging*. 1999;10(3):489–495.
9. Torres A. The use of Food and Drug Administration–approved medications for unlabeled (off-label) uses. The legal and ethical implications. *Arch Dermatol*. 1994;130(1):32–36.
10. Roberts T. Basic principles. In: Higgins C, Hricak H, Helms C, eds. *Magnetic Resonance Imaging of the Body*. Philadelphia: Lippencott-Raven; 1997:3–10.
11. Hohenschuh E, Watson A. Theory and mechanisms of contrast-enhancing agents. In: Higgins C, Hricak H, Helms C, eds. *Magnetic Resonance Imaging of the Body*. Philadelphia: Lippencott-Raven; 1997:1439–1464.
12. Weisskoff R, Caravan P. MR Contrast agent basics. In: Lardo A, Fayad Z, Chronos A, et al, eds. *Cardiovascular Magnetic Resonance*. London: Martin Dunitz; 2003:17–38.
13. Solomon I. Relaxation processes in a system of two spins. *Physiol Rev*. 1955;99:559–565.
14. Bloembergen N. Proton relaxation times in paramagnetic solutions. *J Chem Phys*. 1957;27:572–581.
15. Wolf G, Halavaara J. Basic principles of MR contrast agents. *Magn Reson Imaging Clin N Am*. 1996;4:1–10.
16. Cavagna F, Maggioni F, Castelli P, et al. Gadolinium chelates with weak binding to serum proteins. A new class of high-efficiency, general purpose contrast agents for magnetic resonance imaging. *Invest Radiol*. 1997;32:780–796.
17. Lauffer R, Parmelee D, Dunham S, et al. MS-325: albumin-targeted contrast agent for MR angiography. *Radiology*. 1998;207(2):529–538.
18. Petersein J, Saini S, Weissleder R. Liver. II: iron oxide-based reticuloendothelial contrast agents for MR imaging. *Magn Reson Imaging Clin N Am*. 1996;4:53-60.
19. Matsuo M, Kanematsu M, Itoh K, et al. Detection of malignant hepatic tumors: comparison of gadolinium-and ferumoxide-enhanced MR imaging. *AJR*. 2001;177(3):637–643.
20. van Etten B, van der Sijp J, Kruyt R, et al. Ferumoxide-enhanced magnetic resonance imaging techniques in preoperative assessment for colorectal liver metastases. *Eur J Surg Oncol*. 2002;28(6):645–651.
21. Reimer P, Balzer T. Ferucarbotran (Resovist): a new clinically approved RES-specific contrast agent for contrast-enhanced MRI of the liver: properties, clinical development, and applications. *Eur Radiol*. 2003;13(6):1266–1276.
22. Kroft L, de Roos A. Blood pool contrast agents for cardiovascular MR imaging. *J Magn Reson Imaging*. 1999;10(3):395–403.
23. Anzai Y, McLachlan S, Chenevert T, et al. MR angiography with an ultrasmall superparamagnetic iron oxide blood pool agent. *J Magn Reson Imaging*. 1997;7:209–214.
24. Knopp M, Kauczor H, Knopp M, et al. [Effects of viscosity, cannula size and temperature in mechanical contrast media administration in CT and magnetic resonance tomography]. *Rofo Fortschr Geb Rontgenstr Neuen Bildgeb Verfahr*. 1995;163(3):259–264.
25. Prince M, Narasimham D, Stanley J, et al. Breath-hold gadolinium-enhanced MR angiography of the abdominal aorta and its major branches. *Radiology*. 1995;197:785–792.
26. Bhat K, Arroyave C, Crown R. Reaction to radiographic contrast agents: new developments in etiology. *Ann Allergy*. 1976;37:169–173.
27. Weinman H, Laniado M, Mutzel W. Pharmacokinetics of Gd-DTPA/dimeglumine after intravenous injection into

healthy volunteers. *Physiol Chem Phys Med NMR.* 1984;16:167–172.

28. Le Mignon M, Chambon C, Warringon S, et al. Gd-DOTA. Pharmocokinetics and tolerability after intravenous injection into healthy volunteers. *Invest Radiol.* 1990;25:933–937.
29. Tofts P, Brix G, Buckley D, et al. Estimating kinetic parameters from dynamic contrast-enhanced T(1)-weighted MRI of a diffusable tracer: standardized quantities and symbols. *J Magn Reson Imaging.* 1999;10(3):223–232.
30. Schmiedl U, Ogan M, Moseley M, et al. Comparison of the contrast-enhancing properties of albumin-(Gd-DTPA) and Gd-DTPA at 2.0 T: and experimental study in rats. *Am J Roentgenol.* 1986;147(6):1263–1270.
31. Parmelee D, Walovitch R, Ouellet H, et al. Preclinical evaluation of the pharmacokinetics, biodistribution, and elimination of MS-325, a blood pool agent for magnetic resonance imaging. *Invest Radiol.* 1997;32(12):741–747.
32. Krombach G, Wendland M, Higgins C, et al. MR imaging of spatial extent of microvascular injury in reperfused ischemically injured rat myocardium: value of blood pool ultrasmall superparamagnetic particles of iron oxide. *Radiology.* 2002;225(2):479–486.
33. Taylor A, Panting J, Keegan J, et al. Safety and preliminary findings with the intravascular contrast agent NC100150 injection for MR coronary angiography. *J Magn Reson Imaging.* 1999;9(2):220–227.
34. Runge V, Nelson K. Contrast agents. In: Stark D, Bradley W, eds. *Magnetic Resonance Imaging.* St. Louis, MO: Mosby; 1999:257–275.
35. Knopp M, von Tengg-Kobligk H, Floemer F, et al. Contrast agents for MRA: future directions. *J Magn Reson Imaging.* 1999;10(3):314–316.
36. Cavagna F, Lorusso V, Anelli P, et al. Preclinical profile and clinical potential of gadocoletic acid trisodium salt (B22956/1), a new intravascular contrast medium for MRI. *Acta Radiol.* 2002;9[Suppl 2]:S491–S494.
37. Gerber B, Bluemke D, Chin B, et al. Single-vessel coronary artery stenosis: myocardial perfusion imaging with Gadomer-17 first-pass MR imaging in a swine model of comparison with gadopentetate dimeglumine. *Radiology.* 2002;225(1):104–112.
38. Jones J. Radiocontrast media: regulatory aspects. *Invest Radiol.* 1994;29 [Suppl 1]:S54–S58.
39. Hardman J, Limbird L. *The Pharmacological Basis of Therapeutics.* 9th ed. New York: McGraw-Hill; 1996.
40. Speck U. Principles and aims of preclinical testing. *Invest Radiol.* 1994;29 [Suppl 1]:S15–S20.
41. Runge V. Safety of approved MR contrast media for intravenous injection. *J Magn Reson Imaging.* 2000;12:205–213.
42. Murphy KJ, Brunberg JA, Cohan RH. Adverse reactions to gadolinium contrast media: a review of 36 cases. *AJR Am J Roentgenol.* 1996;167(4):847–849.
43. Kirchin MA, Pirovano G, Venetianer C, et al. Safety assessment of gadobenate dimeglumine (MultiHance): extended clinical experience from phase I studies to post-marketing surveillance. *J Magn Reson Imaging.* 2001;14(3):281–294.
44. Runge VM. Safety of magnetic resonance contrast media. *Top Magn Reson Imaging.* 2001;12(4):309–314.
45. Beaudouin E, Kanny G, Blanloeil Y, et al. Anaphylactic shock induced by gadoterate meglumine (DOTAREM). *Allerg Immunol (Paris).* 2003;35(10): 382–385.
46. Kirchin M, Runge V. Contrast agents for magnetic resonance imaging. *Top Magn Reson Imaging.* 2003;14(5):426–435.
47. McClennan B. Adverse reactions to iodinated contrast media: recognition and response. *Invest Radiol.* 1994;29[Suppl 1]:S46–S50.
48. Almen T. The etiology of contrast medium reactions. *Invest Radiol.* 1994;29[Suppl 1]:S37–S45.
49. *Manual on Contrast Media.* 4th ed. American College of Radiology; 1998.
50. Rocklage S, Watson A. Chelates of gadolinium and dysprosium as contrast agents for MR imaging. *J Magn Reson Imaging.* 1993;3:167–178.

51. Shellock F, Kanal E. Safety of magnetic resonance imaging contrast agents. *J Magn Reson Imaging.* 1999;10:477–484.
52. Niendorf H, Alhassan A, Greens V, et al. Safety review of gadopentetate dimeglumine: extended clinical experience after more than five million applications. *Invest Radiol.* 1994;29[Suppl 2]:S179–S182.
53. Brown J, Kristy R, Stevens G, et al. The Optimark Clinical Development Program: summary of safety data. *J Magn Reson Imaging.* 2002;15:446–455.
54. Manual on Contrast Media Version 5.0;2005.
55. Prince M, Arnoldus C, Frisoli J. Nephrotoxicity of high dose gadolinium compared to iodinated contrast. *J Magn Reson Imaging.* 1996;6:162–166.
56. Rofsky N, Weinreb J, Bosniak M, et al. Renal lesion characterization with gadolinium-enhanced MR imaging: efficacy and safety in patients with renal insufficiency. *Radiology.* 1991;180:85–89.
57. Tombach B, Bremer C, Reimer P, et al. Using highly concentrated gadobutrol as an MR contrast agent in patients also requiring hemodialysis: safety and dialysability. *Am J Roentgenol.* 2002;178(1):105–109.
58. Morcos S, Thomsen H, Webb J. Dialysis and contrast media. *Eur Radiol.* 2002;12(12):3026—3030. Epub 2002 Aug 16.
59. Okada S, Katagiri K, Kumazaki T, et al. Safety of gadolinium contrast agent in hemodialysis patients. *Acta Radiologica.* 2001;42(3):339.
60. Nelson K, Gifford L, Lauber-Huber C, et al. Clinical safety of gadopentetate dimeglumine. *Radiology.* 1995;196:439–443.
61. Rofsky N, Pizzarello D, Duhaney M, et al. Effect of magnetic resonance exposure combined with gadopentetate dimeglumine on chromosomes in animal specimens. *Acad Radiol.* 1995;2(6):492–496.
62. Schmiedl U, Maravilla KR, Gerlach R, et al. Excretion of gadopentetate dimeglumine in human breast milk. *AJR Am J Roentgenol.* 1990;154(6):1305–1306.
63. Rofsky NM, Weinreb JC, Litt AW. Quantitative analysis of gadopentetate dimeglumine excreted in breast milk. *J Magn Reson Imaging.* 1993;3(1):131–132.
64. Kubik-Huch RA, Gottstein-Aalame NM, Frenzel T, et al. Gadopentetate dimeglumine excretion into human breast milk during lactation. *Radiology.* 2000;216(2):555–558.
65. Manual on Contrast Media Version 5.0; 2005:45–46.
66. Marti-Bonmati L, Vega T, Benito C, et al. Safety and efficacy of Omniscan (gadodiamide injection) at 0.1 mmol/kg for MRI in infants younger than 6 months of age: phase III open multicenter study. *Invest Radiol.* 2000;35(2):141–147.
67. Eldevik O, Brunberg J. Gadopentetate dimeglumine-enhanced MR of the brain: clinical utility and safety in patients younger than two years of age. *AJNR.* 1994;15(6):1001–1008.
68. Bellin M, Jakobsen J, Tomassin I, et al. Contrast medium extravasation injury: guidelines for prevention and management. *Eur Radiol.* 2002;12(11):2807–2812.
69. Runge V, Dickey K, Williams N, et al. Local tissue toxicity in response to extravascular extravasation of magnetic resonance contrast media. *Invest Radiol.* 2002;37(7):393–398.
70. Doorenbos C, Ozyilmaz A, van Wijnen M. Severe pseudohypocalcemia after gadolinium-enhanced magnetic resonance angiography. *N Engl J Med.* 2003;349:817–818.
71. Prince M, Erel H, Lent R, et al. Gadodiamide administration causes spurious hypocalcemia. *Radiology.* 2003;227(3): 639–646.
72. Hoyke P, Knopp M. Pseudohypocalcemia with MR imaging contrast agents: a cautionary tale. *Radiology.* 2003;227: 627–628.
73. Tombach B, Reimer P, Prumer B, et al. Does a higher concentration of gadolinium chelates improve first-pass cardiac signal changes? *J Magn Reson Imaging.* 1999;10(5):806–812.
74. Goyen M, Lauenstein T, Herborn C, et al. 0.5 M Gd chelate (Magnevist) versus 1.0 M Gd chelate (Gadovist): dose-independent effect on image quality of pelvic three-dimensional MR-angiography. *J Magn Reson Imaging.* 2001;14(5): 602–607.

75. Herborn C, Lauenstein T, Ruehm S, et al. Intraindividual comparison of gadopentetate dimeglumine, gadobenate dimeglumine and gadobutro for pelvic 3D magnetic resonance angiography. *Invest Radiol*. 2003;38:27–33.

76. Fink C, Bock M, Kiessling F, et al. Time-resolved contrast-enhanced three-dimensional pulmonary MR-angiography: 1.0 M gadobutrol vs. 0.5 M gadopentetate dimeglumine. *J Magn Reson Imaging*. 2004;19(2):202–208.

77. Runge V, Wells J, Nelson K, et al. MR imaging detection of cerebral metastases with a single injection of high-dose gadoteridol. *J Magn Reson Imaging*. 1994;4(5):669–673.

78. Earls J, Rofsky N, DeCorato D, et al. Breath-hold single-dose gadolinium-enhanced three-dimensional MR aortography: usefulness of a timing examination and MR power injector. *Radiology*. 1996;(201):705–710.

79. Boos M, Scheffler K, Haselhorst R, et al. Arterial first pass gadolinium-CM dynamics as a function of several intravenous saline flush and Gd volumes. *J Magn Reson Imaging*. 2001;13(4):568–576.

80. Rofsky N, Johnson G, Adelman M, et al. Peripheral vascular disease evaluated with reduced-dose gadolinium-enhanced MR angiography. *Radiology*. 1997;205:163–169.

81. Finn JP, Baskaran V, Carr JC, et al. Thorax: low-dose contrast-enhanced three-dimensional MR angiography with subsecond temporal resolution—initial results. *Radiology*. 2002;224(3):896–904.

82. Knopp M, Giesel F, von Tengg-Kobligk H, et al. Contrast-enhanced MR angiography of the run-off vasculature: intraindividual comparison of gadobenate dimeglumine with gadopentetate dimeglumine. *J Magn Reson Imaging*. 2003;17(6):694–702.

83. Knopp M, Schoenberg S, Rehm C, et al. Assessment of gadobenate dimeglumine (Gd-BOPTA) for MR angiography: phase I studies. *Invest Radiol*. 2002;37:706–715.

84. Wyttenbach R, Gianella S, Alerci M, et al. Prospective blinded evaluation of Gd-DOTA- versus Gd-BOPTA-enhanced peripheral MR angiography, as compared with digital subtraction angiography. *Radiology*. 2003;227(1):261–269.

85. Prokop M, Schneider G, Vanzulli A, et al. Contrast-enhanced MR angiography of the renal arteries: blinded multicenter crossover comparison of gadobenate dimeglumine and gadopentetate dimeglumine. *Radiology*. 2005;234(2):399–408.

86. La Noce A, Stoelben S, Scheffler K, et al. B22956/1, a new intravascular contrast agent for MRI: first administration to humans—preliminary results. *Acad Radiol*. 2002;9(suppl)(2):S404–S406.

87. Corot C, Violas X, Gagneum R, et al. Comparison of different types of blood pool agents (P792, MS325, USPIO) in a rabbit MR angiography-like protocol. *Invest Radiol*. 2003;38(6):311–319.

88. Perreault P, Edelman M, Baum R, et al. MR angiography with gadofosveset trisodium for peripheral vascular disease: phase II trial. *Radiology*. 2003;229(3):811–820.

89. Grist T, Korosec F, Peters D, et al. Steady-state and dynamic MR angiography with MS-325: initial experience in humans. *Radiology*. 1998;207(2):539–544.

90. Goyen M, Edelman M, Perreault P, et al. MR angiography of aortoiliac occlusive disease: a phase III study of the safety and effectiveness of the blood-pool contrast agent MS-325. *Radiology*. 2005;236(3):825–833.

91. Rapp JH, Wolff SD, Quinn SF, et al. Aortoiliac occlusive disease in patients with known or suspected peripheral vascular disease: safety and efficacy of gadofosveset-enhanced MR angiography—multicenter comparative phase III study. *Radiology*. 2005;236(1):71–78.

92. Gold GE, Han E, Stainsby J, et al. Musculoskeletal MRI at 3.0 T: relaxation times and image contrast. *AJR Am J Roentgenol*. 2004;183(2):343–351.

93. Marchal G, Bosman H, Van Hecke P, et al. MR angiography with gadopentetate dimeglumine-polylysine: evaluation in rabbits. *AJR Am J Roentgenol*. 1990;155:407–411.

94. Loubeyre P, Canet E, Zhao S, et al. Carboxymethyl-dextran-gadolinium-DTPA as a blood-pool contrast agent for magnetic resonance angiography. Experimental study in rabbits. *Invest Radiol*. 1996;31(5):288–293.

95. Clarke S, Weinman H, Dai E, et al. Comparison of two blood pool contrast agents of 0.5T MR angiography: experimental study in rabbits. *Radiology*. 2000;214:787–794.

96. Dong Q, Hurst D, Weinmann H, et al. Magnetic resonance angiography with gadomer-17. An animal study original investigation. *Invest Radiol*. 1998;33(9):699–708.

97. Ruehm S, Christina H, Violas X, et al. MR angiography with a new rapid-clearance blood pool agent: initial experience in rabbits. *Magn Reson Med*. 2002;48:844–851.

98. Weinmann H, Ebert W, Misselwitz B, et al. Tissue-specific MR contrast agents. *Eur J Radiol*. 2003;46:33–44.

99. Li D, Zheng J, Weinmann H. Contrast-enhanced MR imaging of coronary arteries: comparison of intra- and extravascular contrast agents in swine. *Radiology*. 2001;218(3):670–678.

100. Mack M, Balzer J, Straub R, et al. Superparamagnetic iron oxide-enhanced MR imaging of head and neck lymph nodes. *Radiology*. 2002;222:239–244.

101. Aschauer M, Deutschmann H, Stollberger R, et al. Value of a blood pool contrast agent in MR venography of the lower extremities and pelvis: preliminary results in 12 patients. *Magn Reson Med*. 2003;50(5):993–1002.

102. Leiner T, Ho K, Ho V, et al. Multicenter phase-II trial of safety and efficacy of NC100150 for steady-state contrast-enhanced peripheral magnetic resonance angiography. *Eur Radiol*. 2003;13(7):1620–1627.

103. Tombach B, Reimer P, Mahler M, et al. First-pass and equilibrium phase MRA following intravenous bolus injection of SH U 555 C: phase I clinical trial in elderly volunteers with risk factors for arterial vascular disease. *Acad Radiol*. 2002;9 [Suppl 2]:S425–S427.

104. Taupitz M, Schnorr J, Abramjuk C, et al. New generation of monomer-stabilized very small superparamagnetic iron oxide particles (VSOP) as contrast medium for MR angiography: preclinical results in rats and rabbits. *J Magn Reson Imaging*. 2000;12(6):905–911.

105. Lee V, Martin D, Krinsky G, et al. Gadolinium-enhanced MR angiography: artifacts and pitfalls. *AJR Am J Roentgenol*. 2000;175:197–205.

106. Maki J, Chenevert T, Prince M. Optimizing three-dimensional gadolinium-enhanced MR angiography. *Invest Radiol*. 1998;33:528–537.

107. Maki J, Chenevert T, Prince M. Contrast-enhanced MR angiography. *Abdom Imaging*. 1998;23:469–484.

108. Hendrick R, Roff U. *Image Contrast and Noise*. Chicago, IL: Mosby–Year Book; 1991.

109. Prince M. Body MR angiography with gadolinium contrast agents. *Magn Reson Imaging Clin N Am*. 1996;4(1):11–24.

110. Verhoeven L. *Digital Subtraction Angiography: The Technique and an Analysis of the Physical Factors Influencing the Image Quality*. Delft: Technische Hogeschule; 1985.

111. Maki J, Prince M, Londy F, et al. The effects of time varying intravascular signal intensity on three-dimensional MR angiography image quality. *J Magn Reson Imaging*. 1996;6:642–651.

112. van den Brink J, Watanabe Y, Kuhl C, et al. Implications of SENSE MR in routine clinical practice. *Eur J Radiol*. 2003;46(1):3–27.

113. Weiger M, Pruessmann K, Kassner A, et al. Contrast-enhanced 3D MRA using SENSE. *J Magn Reson Imaging*. 2000;12:671–677.

114. Frayne R, Grist T, Swan J, et al. 3D MR DSA: effects of injection protocol and image masking. *J Magn Reson Imaging*. 2000;12(3):476–487.

115. Wutke R, Lang W, Fellner C, et al. High-resolution, contrast-enhanced magnetic resonance angiography with elliptical centric k-space ordering of supra-aortic arteries compared with selective x-ray angiography. *Stroke*. 2002;33:1522–1529.

116. Huston J, Fain S, Riederer S, et al. Carotid arteries: maximizing arterial to venous contrast in fluoroscopically triggered contrast-enhanced MR angiography with elliptic centric view ordering. *Radiology*. 1999;211(1):265–273.

117. Karger R, Slonka J, Junck H, et al. Extracorporeal blood volume of donors during automated intermittent-flow plasmapheresis and its relevance to the prevention of circulatory reactions. *Transfusion*. 2003;43(8):1096–1106.

118. Ruehm S, Zimny K, Debatin J. Direct contrast-enhanced 3D MR venography. *Eur Radiol*. 2001;11(1):102–112.

119. Li W, Kaplan D, Edelman R. Three-dimensional low dose gadolinium-enhanced peripheral MR venography. *J Magn Reson Imaging*. 1998;8(3):630–633.

120. Omary R, Henseler K, Unal O, et al. Comparison of intraarterial and IV gadolinium-enhanced MR angiography with digital subtraction angiography for the detection of renal artery stenosis in pigs. *AJR Am J Roentgenol*. 2002;178(1):119–123.

121. Holsinger A, Riederer S. The importance of phase encoding order in ultra-short TR snapshot MR imaging. *Magn Reson Med*. 1990;16:481–488.

122. Jones R, Rinck R. Approach to equilibrium in snapshot imaging. *Magn Reson Med*. 1990;8:797–803.

123. Barnes G, Lakshminarayann A. Conventional and spiral computed tomography. In: Lee J, Sagel S, Stanley R, Heiken J, eds. *Computed Body Tomgraphy with MRI Correlation*. Philadelphia: Lippencott-Raven; 1998:1–20.

124. Maki J, Knopp M, Prince M. Contrast-enhanced MR angiography. *Appl Radiol*. 2003;32(suppl):3–31.

125. Ho V, Foo T, Czum J, et al. Contrast-enhanced magnetic resonance angiography: technical considerations for optimized clinical implementation. *Top Magn Reson Imaging*. 2001;12(4):283–299.

126. Prince M. Gadolinium-enhanced MR aortography. *Radiology*. 1994;191:155–164.

127. Wilman A, Riederer S, King B, et al. Flouroscopically-triggered contrast-enhanced three dimensional MR angiography with elliptical centric view order: application to the renal arteries. *Radiology*. 1997;205(1):137–146.

128. Bampton A, Riederer S, Korin H. Centric phase-encoding order in three-dimensional MP-RAGE sequences: application to abdominal imaging. *J Magn Reson Imaging*. 1992;2:327–334.

129. Wilman A, Riederer S, Breen J, et al. Elliptical spiral phase-encoding order: an optimal, field-of-view-dependent ordering scheme for breath-hold contrast-enhanced 3D MR angiography. *Radiology*. 1996;201(P):328–329.

130. Shetty A, Kostaki G, Vrachliotis T, et al. Contrast-enhanced 3D MRA with centric ordering in k space: a preliminary clinical experience in imaging the abdominal aorta and renal and peripheral arterial vasculature. *J Magn Reson Imaging*. 1998;8(3):603–615.

131. Maki J, Chenevert T, Prince M. The effects of incomplete breath holding on 3D MR image quality. *J Magn Reson Imaging*. 1997;7:1132–1139.

132. Prince M, Chenevert T, Foo T, et al. Contrast-enhanced abdominal MR angiography: optimization of imaging delay time by automating the detection contrast material arrival in the aorta. *Radiology*. 1997;203:109–114.

133. Watts R, Wang Y, B Redd, et al. Recessed elliptical-centric view-ordering for contrast-enhanced 3D MR angiography of the carotid arteries. *Magn Reson Med*. 2002;48(3):419–424.

134. Kim J, Farb R, Wright G. Test bolus examination in the carotid artery at dynamic gadolinium-enhanced MR angiography. *Radiology*. 1998;206:283–289.

135. Maki J, Wilson G, Eubank W, et al. Utilizing SENSE to achieve lower station sub-millimeter isotropic resolution and minimal venous enhancement in peripheral MR angiography. *J Magn Reson Imaging*. 2002;15:484–491.

136. Meaney J, Ridgway J, Chakraverty S, et al. Stepping-table gadolinium-enhanced digital subtraction MR angiography of the aorta and lower extremity arteries: preliminary experience. *Radiology*. 1999;211:59–67.

137. Hany T, McKinnon G, Leung D, et al. Optimization of contrast timing for breath-hold three-dimensional MR angiography. *J Magn Reson Imaging*. 1997;7:551–556.

138. Wilson G, Maki J, Haynor D. Predicting aorta bolus dynamics using a test bolus: theory and validation in human patients. Twelfth scientific meeting of the Magnetic Resonance Angiography Club. Lyon, France; 2000:38.

139. Foo T, Saranathan M, Prince M, et al. Automated detection of bolus arrival and initiation of data acquisition in fast, three-dimensional, gadolinium-enhanced MR angiography. *Radiology*. 1997;203(1):275–280.

140. Fellner F, Fellner C, Wutke R, et al. Fluoroscopically triggered contrast-enhanced 3D MR DSA and 3D time-of-flight turbo MRA of the carotid arteries: first clinical experiences in correlation with ultrasound, x-ray angiography, and endarterectomy findings. *Magn Reson Imaging*. 2000;18(5):575–585.

141. Riederer S, Tasciyan T, Farzaneh F. MR flouroscopy: technical feasibility. *Magn Reson Med*. 1988;8:1–15.

142. Du J, Carroll T, Block W, et al. SNR improvement for multi-injection time-resolved high-resolution CE-MRA of the peripheral vasculature. *Magn Reson Med*. 2003;49(5):909–917.

143. Muthupillai R, Vick GW, Flamm SD, et al. Time-resolved contrast-enhanced magnetic resonance angiography in pediatric patients using sensitivity encoding. *J Magn Reson Imaging*. 2003;17(5):559–564.

144. Goyen M, Laub G, Ladd M, et al. Dynamic 3D MR angiography of the pulmonary arteries in under four seconds. *J Magn Reson Imaging*. 2001;13(3):372–377.

145. Schoenberg S, Bock M, Floemer F, et al. High-resolution pulmonary arterio- and venography using multiple-bolus multiphase 3D-Gd-MRA. *J Magn Reson Imaging*. 1999;10(3):339–346.

146. Levy R, Maki J. Three-dimensional contrast-enhanced MR angiography of the extracranial carotid arteries: two techniques. *AJNR*. 1998;19(4):688–690.

147. Vasbinder G, Maki J, Nijenhuis R, et al. Motion of the distal renal artery during 3D contrast-enhanced breath-hold MRA. *J Magnetic Reson Imaging*. 2002;16:685–696.

148. Barger A, Block W, Toropov Y, et al. Time-resolved contrast-enhanced imaging with isotropic resolution and broad coverage using an undersampled 3D projection trajectory. *Magn Reson Med*. 2002;48(2):297–305.

149. Mazaheri Y, Carroll T, Du J, et al. Combined time-resolved and high-spatial-resolution 3D MRA using an extended adaptive acquisition. *J Magn Reson Imaging*. 2002;15(3):291–301.

150. Turski P, Korosec F, Carroll T, et al. Contrast-enhanced magnetic resonance angiography of the carotid bifurcation using the time-resolved imaging of contrast kinetics (TRICKS) technique. *Top Magn Reson Imaging*. 2001;12(3):175–181.

151. Korosec F, Grist T, Frayne R, et al. Time-resolved contrast-enhanced 3D MR angiography. *Magn Reson Med*. 1996;36:345–351.

152. Mistretta C, Grist T, Frayne R, et al. Contrast and motion artifacts in 4D MR angiography. *Radiology*. 1996;201(P):238.

153. Fink C, Ley S, Kroeker R, et al. Time-resolved contrast-enhanced three-dimensional magnetic resonance angiography of the chest: combination of parallel imaging with view sharing (TREAT). *Invest Radiol*. 2005;40(1):40–48.

154. Maki J, Wilson G, Eubank W, et al. 3D Gd-enhanced peripheral MR angiography using multi-station SENSE (WakiTrak LS) - an update [abstract]. In: Eleventh Scientific Meeting and Exhibition; 2003. Toronto, Canada: International Society of Magnetic Resonance in Medicine; 2003:257.

155. La Noce A, Stoelben S, Scheffler K, et al. B22956/1, a new intravascular contrast agent for MRI: first administration to

humans—preliminary results. *Acad Radiol*. 2002;9 [Suppl 2]: S404–S406.

156. Rydland J, Bjornerud A, Haugen O, et al. New intravascular contrast agent applied to dynamic contrast enhanced MR imaging of human breast cancer. *Acta Radiol*. 2003;44(3):275–283.

157. Oksendal A, Hals P. Biodistribution and toxicity of MR imaging contrast media. *J Magn Reson Imaging*. 1993;3:157–165.

158. Wible JJ, Troup C, Hynes M, et al. Toxicological assessment of gadoversetamide injection (OptiMARK), a new contrast-enhancement agent for use in magnetic resonance imaging. *Invest Radiol*. 2001;36(7):401–412.

Postprocessing and Data Analysis

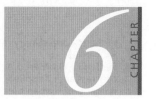

Geoffrey D. Rubin
Pietro Sedati
Jesse L. Wei

Chapters 1 and 2 detail how computed tomographic (CT) and magnetic resonance (MR) angiograms are acquired and images generated. In the case of CT, projection data acquired by the rotating x-ray source and detectors is processed by Fourier transforms to generate transverse reconstructions. Similarly, in MR, the primarily acquired signal is reconstructed to planar images also using Fourier transforms. Although the data acquired during CT scanning are volumetric due to continuous acquisition during table translation, these data are exclusively reconstructed into a stack of transverse sections (1–3). Similarly, although "three-dimensional" (3D) sequences (where an entire volume of anatomy reconstructed is imaged simultaneously) are frequently used in MR angiography, these data are also reconstructed into a stack of planar reformations (4,5).

Although these primary reconstructions when stacked together represent the entire imaged volume, observers have a limited ability to mentally integrate and interpret the many images making up each volume. 3D visualization of volumetric CT and MR data using dedicated image-processing workstations allows different perspectives for visual examination and analysis of these primarily acquired and reconstructed data. Postprocessing of imaging volumes allows visualization of these data in a manner that is most analogous with what is represented in anatomic diagrams as well as what is seen on direct observation in the operating room or in the pathology suite (Fig. 6-1). However, the

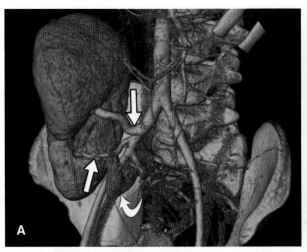 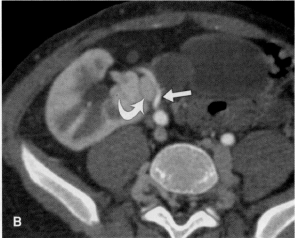

FIGURE 6-1 An intuitive image presentation. CTA following kidney transplantation in the right lower quadrant shows how VR facilitates understanding of complex vascular anatomy. **A:** Oblique 3D VR image shows that the donor's inferior vena cava was transplanted (*curved arrow*), and there are two renal arteries anastomosed to the right common iliac artery (*straight arrows*). **B:** The perspective is less intuitive on a transverse section at the level of one of the renal arteries (*straight arrow*). The donor's inferior vena cava (*curved arrow*) is situated between the renal artery and the kidney parenchyma.

rationale for reformatting and rendering volumetric data extends well beyond simulating direct visualization of anatomic structures. The advantages of postprocessing volumetric CT and MR data fall into four broad categories: alternative visualization, efficiency of interpretation, effective communication, and volumetric quantitation (2–8). Each of these rationales will be discussed in turn.

RATIONALE FOR IMAGE POSTPROCESSING

Alternative Visualization

As mentioned in the preceding paragraph, volumetric rendering techniques of computed tomographic angiography (CTA) and magnetic resonance angiography (MRA) data can display anatomic structures in a manner similar to that experienced on direct visualization. Such techniques emphasize surface representations but have substantial limitations. Many vascular abnormalities are best assessed by using cross-sectional representations through the structures of interest. However, the routine primarily reconstructed cross-sectional images are usually arbitrarily oriented relative to these structures. For example, although the abdominal aorta courses in a cranial to caudal direction nearly parallel to the CT or MR scanner table, it is not truly parallel. Therefore a "transverse," or "axial," primary reconstruction would not be quite perpendicular to the longitudinal axis of the aorta, resulting in oblique cross sections of this structure. Moreover, because even the normal aorta subtly curves with the kyphosis of the thoracic spine and the lordosis of the lumbar spine, a planar reformation perpendicular to the axis of the aorta at one

point when translated cranially and caudally may no longer be perpendicular to the curved centerline axis of the aorta (Fig. 6-2). Because the vascular system is a network of tubes oriented with complex and at times highly variable spatial relationships, and because diagnosis and characterization of vascular diseases necessitate an assessment of a vessel's lumen, wall, and surrounding tissue, a diverse menu of visualization options have been developed to enable physicians to maximize their understanding of the imaged vasculature. The flexibility afforded by volumetric visualization techniques facilitates comparison of changes over time despite subtle shifts in a patient's position between serial examinations. These techniques allow assessment of anatomy by using landmarks and axes that are intrinsically relevant to structures of interest rather than to the orientation of the imaging table (2–8) (Fig. 6-3).

Efficient Interpretation

A single volumetric CT angiogram of the aorta through the lower extremity arterial system can consist of over 2,000 primary reconstructions (Fig. 6-4). Assuming that only 3 seconds are spent examining each image in a CT scan of 2,400 primary transverse reconstructions, an impractical 2 hours would be required for a physician to examine each volumetric data set (3,6,9,10).

A preferable paradigm to consider for the interpretation of such volumetric data arises from ultrasonography. A single sonographic image is a cross-sectional reconstruction similar to a primary planar reconstruction from CTA or MRA; however, the sonographer does not typically save

(*text continues on page 192*)

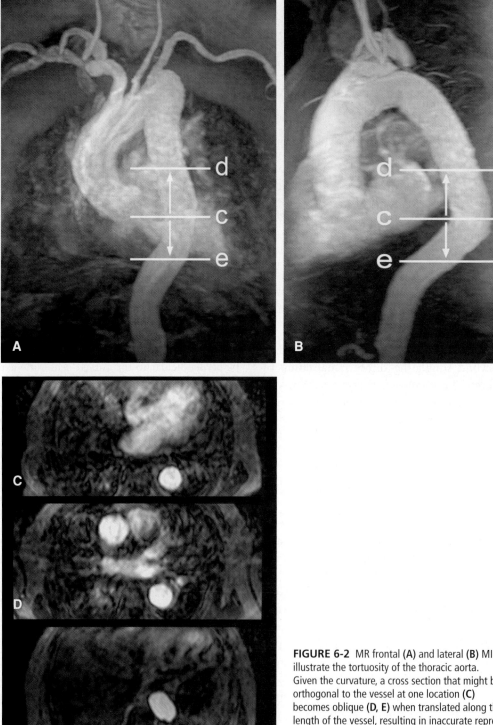

FIGURE 6-2 MR frontal (**A**) and lateral (**B**) MIPs illustrate the tortuosity of the thoracic aorta. Given the curvature, a cross section that might be orthogonal to the vessel at one location (**C**) becomes oblique (**D, E**) when translated along the length of the vessel, resulting in inaccurate representations of the vessel cross section at those locations.

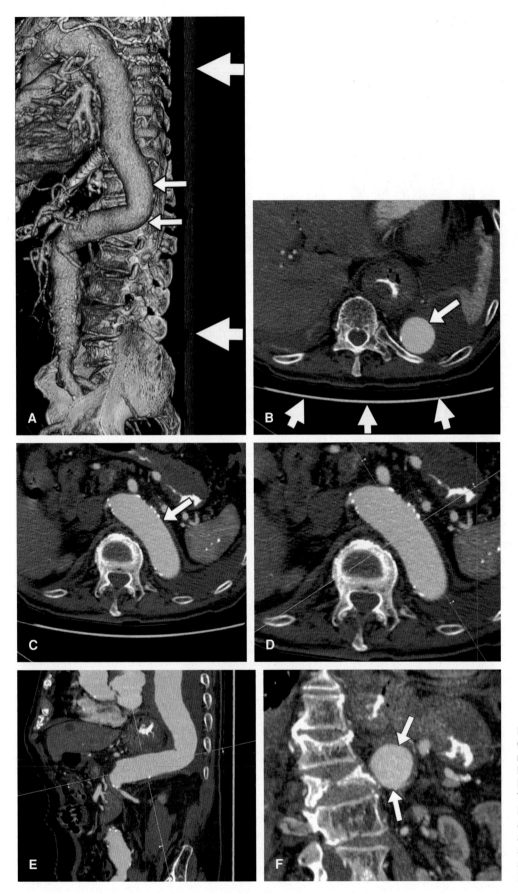

FIGURE 6-3 A: Lateral VR of a CTA shows a tortuous distal thoracic aorta (*small arrows*). The long axis of the aorta is not parallel to the CT table (*big arrows*). The result is that not all transverse images are perpendicular to the aorta but to the table (**B, C**). The axis of the MPR needs to be adjusted (**D, E**) in order to obtain an image perpendicular to the long axis of the vessel (**F**).

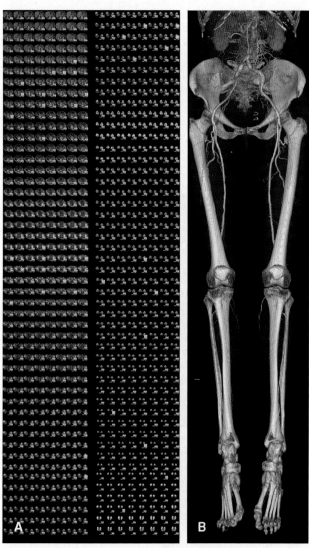

FIGURE 6-4 A: The image shows 864 contiguous transverse sections from a peripheral CTA. Every image needs to be evaluated in order to obtain a diagnosis. **B:** 3D VR image synthesizes all the data in one image.

and interactively explore this volumetric data set both to perform primary interpretation and to record views that are clinically relevant. Using a spectrum of visualization tools in this fashion, the volumetric data can be examined more efficiently than a simple review of individual cross sections.

It should be noted, however, that primary interpretation using interactive volumetric visualization techniques cannot completely replace the routine examination of the primary reconstructions. The pitfalls of each visualization technique utilized should be considered when scanning through the primary reconstructions to assure that all abnormalities have been detected and that volumetric representations are truly representative of the anatomy. Moreover, although the primary goal of vascular imaging is to investigate vascular structures and the organs perfused or drained by those structures, it is incumbent on any interpreter of CTA or MRA data to examine the entirety of the volumetric data set, including structures that are not primarily relevant to the purpose of the examination so that important incidental nonvascular findings may be identified and reported (2–5,7,9–11).

Communication

Individual "screen shots" saved during real-time exploration of volumetric data provide a basis for communication to referring physicians of anatomic findings with complex spatial relationships. The adage that a picture is worth a thousand words is certainly applicable in the case of communicating imaging results (Fig. 6-4). Although a CT or MR angiogram may be composed of thousands of primary reconstructions, key findings can typically be represented in a handful of dedicated views (Fig. 6-5). The advantage of providing this focused output is that it allows the referring clinician to be most efficient in understanding the primary interpretation while reducing the need to wade through piles of film or virtual stacks of cross-sectional images on a computer monitor (3,12). In certain circumstances, the ability for the referring physician to then use those representative images to illustrate the severity and nature of disease to a patient has been shown to alter a patient's treatment choices (e.g., to accept a therapeutic option or undergo lifestyle modifications) (13).

Volumetric Quantitation

The final major rationale for volumetric analysis is the ability to quantify the complex geometric relationships and features of the vasculature. Length, area, and volume measurements of vascular disease serve as objective metrics for evaluating disease severity as well as change over time. In an era where percutaneous delivery of stents, stent grafts, and

entire stacks of cross sections for interpretation while sweeping the transducer from top to bottom of the imaging volume. Rather, the sonographer watches the image display changing in real time as the transducer is swept over the surface of the patient. Based on knowledge of normal and abnormal anatomy, only relevant and representative images in standard planes are captured for further review and archive. Primary diagnosis is made based on direct real-time observation by the sonographer; the saved static images serve primarily to document clinically relevant information in familiar organ-specific planes.

CTA and MRA data can be explored in an analogous fashion. If one considers the volumetric data as a virtual patient lying on a gurncy in the ultrasound suite and conceptualizes the workstation as a virtual sonographic transducer, the interpreter of such examinations can rapidly scan through other therapeutic devices has significantly reduced the direct visualization and measurement afforded by an open procedure, vascular quantitation based on imaging has become a critical process both for triaging patients to appropriate therapeutic options as well as for determining the appropriate size and type of medical devices to be used when intervention is planned (14).

VISUALIZATION TECHNIQUES

Primary Planar Reconstructions

While many sophisticated visualization techniques critical to interpretation of cardiovascular imaging are the focus of this chapter, the importance of review of primary planar reconstructions both with CTA and MRA cannot be understated.

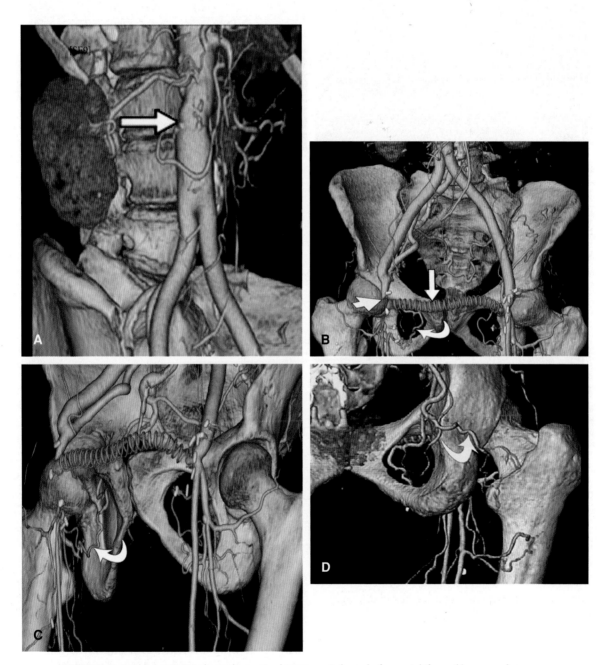

FIGURE 6-5 A: Oblique VR CTA shows the proximal anastomosis (*arrow*) of an aortobifemoral bypass graft. **B:** Frontal 3D VR shows an occlusion at the origin of right superficial femoral artery (*short arrow*) and the presence of an occluded femorofemoral bypass graft (*long arrow*). A large collateral artery emerges from the right obturator foramen (*curved arrow*), bringing arterial blood to the medial circumflex femoral artery, which in turn supplies the profunda femoris (**C**). **D:** Posterior VR shows an enlarged superior gluteal artery (*arrow*), which also serves to reconstitute the femoral arterial system.

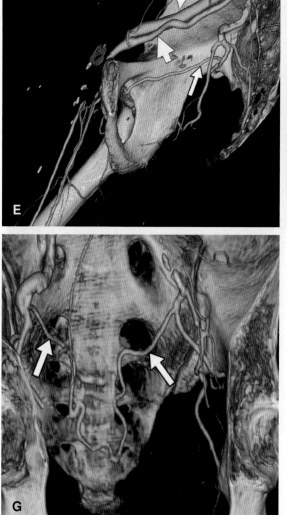

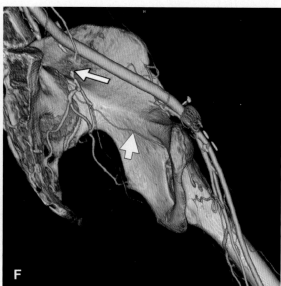

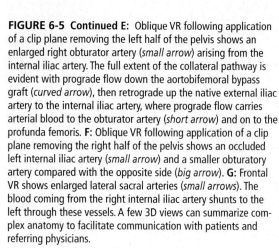

FIGURE 6-5 Continued E: Oblique VR following application of a clip plane removing the left half of the pelvis shows an enlarged right obturator artery (*small arrow*) arising from the internal iliac artery. The full extent of the collateral pathway is evident with prograde flow down the aortobifemoral bypass graft (*curved arrow*), then retrograde up the native external iliac artery to the internal iliac artery, where prograde flow carries arterial blood to the obturator artery (*short arrow*) and on to the profunda femoris. **F:** Oblique VR following application of a clip plane removing the right half of the pelvis shows an occluded left internal iliac artery (*small arrow*) and a smaller obturatory artery compared with the opposite side (*big arrow*). **G:** Frontal VR shows enlarged lateral sacral arteries (*small arrows*). The blood coming from the right internal iliac artery shunts to the left through these vessels. A few 3D views can summarize complex anatomy to facilitate communication with patients and referring physicians.

The "source data" provide the highest spatial resolution and the lowest likelihood of motion-related misregistration and off-axis artifacts.

Artifacts related to beam hardening in CT and magnetic susceptibility in MR are easiest to recognize on the primary image reconstructions. These effects frequently result from metallic clips and prostheses and can cause vascular pseudo-lesions due to localized loss of detail in affected regions. A similar effect can occur where the high concentration of intravenous contrast medium along the course of venous access results in x-ray beam hardening or magnetic suscepti-bility. While 3D volume-rendered images may deceivingly suggest stenosis or occlusion due to susceptibility, review of the primary reconstructions show affected regions as signal voids that cross normal anatomic boundaries (Fig. 6-6).

A critical consideration in the visualization process lies in the setting of the grayscale window and level for image review. When performing cardiovascular imaging, the ves-sel lumen should never be rendered with the highest gray values (white). If the lumen is rendered at these highest gray values, then the grayscale is truncated, which can mis-represent vessel dimensions. This consideration is particu-larly critical for visualization of arterial wall calcifications or metallic stents and stent grafts in CTAs—truncation may render mural calcifications and metal indistinguish-able from the lumen (Fig. 6-7). In fact, in the presence of mural calcification in an image, the window and level should be adjusted so that the calcification is not trun-cated. If the calcium is allowed to be represented as white, its dimensions may be overrepresented and arterial lumina

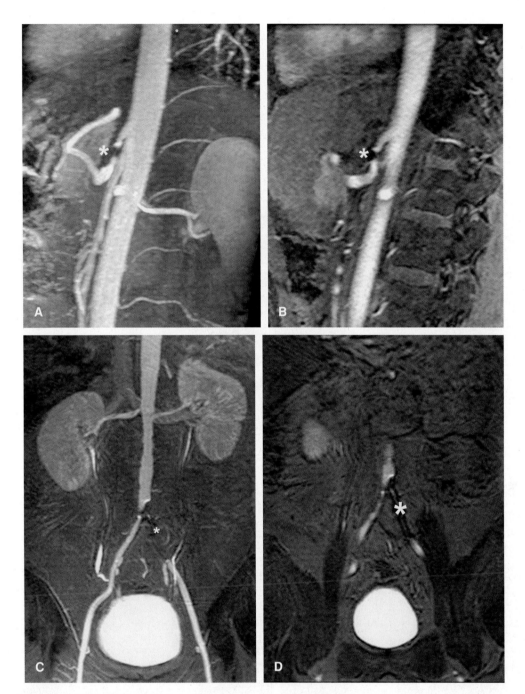

FIGURE 6-6 Susceptibility artifacts in MRA. MIPs may suggest stenosis in regions of focal magnetic susceptibility. However, planar images such as MPRs or CPRs demonstrate signal voids extending beyond normal anatomic borders, which implies that a focus of susceptibility is to blame for the pseudostenosis (∗). *Celiac axis:* MIP **(A)** and MPR **(B)** show pseudo-lesion in the celiac axis from surgical staple. *Common iliac artery:* MIP **(C)** and MPR **(D)** show pseudo-lesion of the left common iliac artery extending to the iliac bifurcation caused by an endovascular stent.

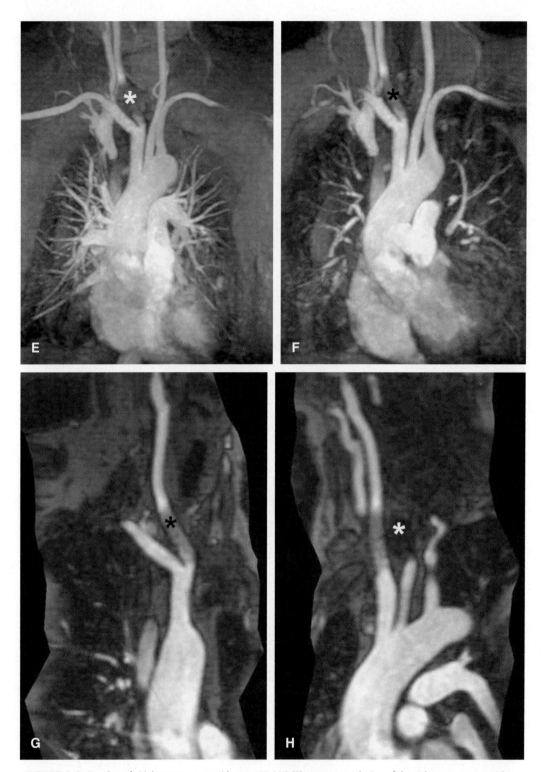

FIGURE 6-6 Continued *Right common carotid artery:* 3D MIP **(E)** suggests occlusion of the right common carotid artery. A 1-cm thick-slab MIP **(F)** and two CPRs **(G, H)** show that the vessel is attenuated in signal but not narrowed or occluded. This appearance is due to the presence of a metallic stent within the vessel and the associated susceptibility.

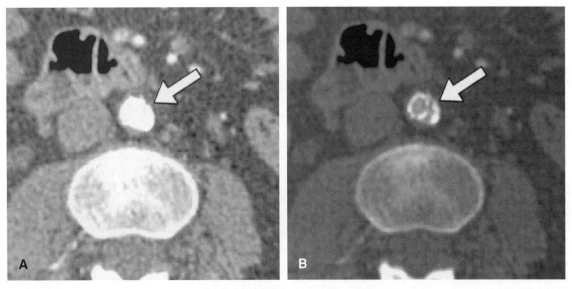

FIGURE 6-7 A transverse CT section through the abdominal aorta (*arrow*) is visualized with inappropriate window settings (**A**). It is impossible to correctly evaluate the vessel lumen and wall. If this is adjusted, it is possible to visualize the endoluminal stent graft and mural calcium (**B**).

adjacent to calcifications underrepresented, suggesting higher grades of stenosis than are actually present (Fig. 6-8). Similarly, when the lumina of metallic stents or stent-grafts need to be assessed, a window and level should be selected to avoid rendering the metallic components of the stents or stent grafts as bright white (Fig. 6-9). These principles for selecting grayscale window and level are equally applicable and clinically important when assessing multiplanar reformations and maximum intensity projections (5,7,10).

Multiplanar Reformations

Multiplanar reformations (MPR) refer to planar cross sections that are oriented through planes other than those of the primary reconstructions. If the primary reconstruction is transverse, then simple sagittal or coronal MPRs orthogonal to these transverse images may be created; however, just as primary transverse reconstructions that are perpendicular to the MR or CT table are generally oriented arbitrarily to human anatomic structures, coronal and sagittal MPRs suffer from the same limitation. MPRs become most valuable when obliqued

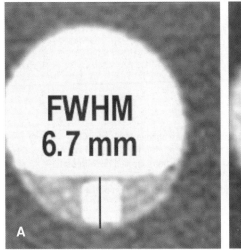 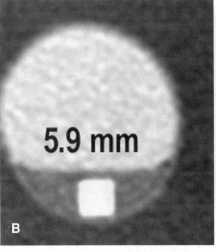 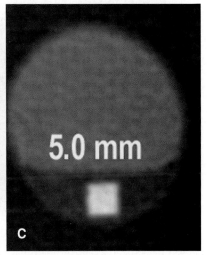

FIGURE 6-8 A–C: A correct window setting is mandatory in order not to overestimate vessel wall calcification dimension. In this example, a 5-mm cube of calcium is shown with different window centers and widths of 40/400, 150/500, and 500/2000, respectively. The measurement values were determined by creating a line density profile through the calcified cubes and measuring the full width at half maximum (FWHM). Only when the calcium is visualized at a gray level below white is the measurement accurate (**C**).

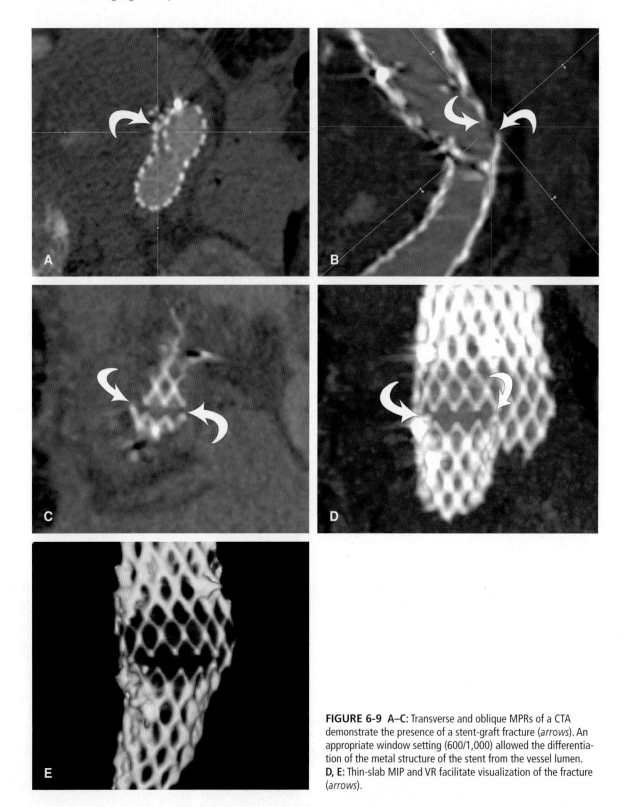

FIGURE 6-9 A–C: Transverse and oblique MPRs of a CTA demonstrate the presence of a stent-graft fracture (*arrows*). An appropriate window setting (600/1,000) allowed the differentiation of the metal structure of the stent from the vessel lumen. **D, E:** Thin-slab MIP and VR facilitate visualization of the fracture (*arrows*).

parallel or perpendicular to the primary axes of a structure to be examined (Fig. 6-10), again in a manner analogous to the cross-sectional images or drawings typically shown in anatomic diagrams. Because blood vessels have a curved course, MPRs are rarely the best means of summarizing vascu-

lar anatomy. Nonetheless, MPRs can be useful for examining the cross-sectional characteristics of short segments of targeted vasculature, particularly in the vessel wall (5,7,10) (Fig. 6-11).

An important limitation of evaluating planar CT or MR images (whether primary reconstructions or MPRs)

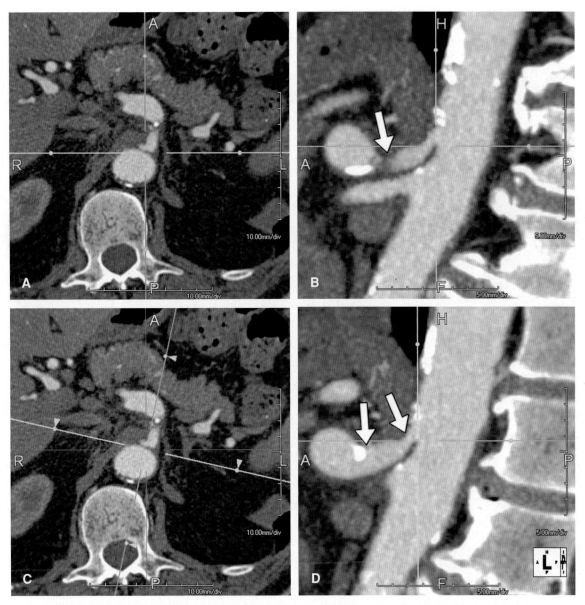

FIGURE 6-10 Transverse CT section **(A)** demonstrates celiac axis dilatation. Sagittal MPR **(B)** shows the origin of the celiac trunk from the aorta but not the entire length of the vessel prior to the dilatation (*arrow*). Reorienting the plane for the MPR on image A **(C)**, it is possible to illustrate the entire course of the vessel (*arrows* in **D**).

occurs because most structures are only partially represented within a single image. When examining blood vessels, planar images must be evaluated in a stacked cine mode rather than in a tiled presentation as would traditionally be represented on photographic film. In this manner, cine paging is performed on a workstation to progressively scroll through a stack of planar images. By dynamically paging through the stack, the interpreting clinician can develop a much better understanding of the spatial relationships of imaged structures than when the stack of images are spatially dissociated by the tiled format (5,7,10).

Curved Planar Reformations

Unlike MPRs, where planes are created via the propagation of a straight line through the imaging volume, curved planar reformations (CPR) are created via the propagation of a curved line through the imaging volume. The curved line typically represents a trace through the centerline of a

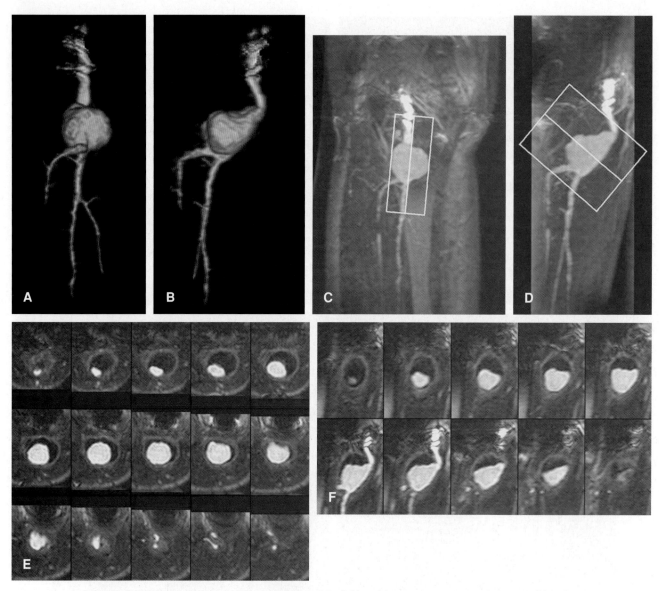

FIGURE 6-11 Popliteal artery aneurysm. Because minimal changes in curvature occur over shorter vessel lengths, short segments of vasculature frequently are easily and accurately assessed by using multiplanar reformatted images. VR **(A, B)** and MIP **(C, D)** MR images provide an overview of the luminal morphology; however, cross-sectional **(E)** and longitudinal **(F)** MPRs through the aneurysm allow visualization of mural thrombus.

blood vessel or other curvilinear structures such as the pancreatic duct or biliary tree, which is then extruded through the volume. Intuitive representations of curved planar reformations, illustrated in Figure 6-12, have been euphemistically referred to as "magic-carpet views," but are not standard in clinical practice. Instead, CPRs are represented on a flat plane as if the folds of the magic carpet have been laid out on a flat surface. This powerful form of display provides the best overview for evaluating wall irregularities along the longitudinal course of blood vessels (Fig. 6-13). It can also be very useful for evaluating the

relationship of filling defects such as thrombi or intimal flaps to the vessel wall and the origins of vessel branches (Fig. 6-14). CPRs in CTA are particularly useful for assessing the luminae of arteries with high attenuation material in or along the arterial wall, such as calcifications or metal stents (Fig. 6-15). One might wonder why CPRs are not more widely used in the assessment of vascular structures, given these capabilities (5,7,10,15).

While CPRs are routinely utilized at the Stanford University 3D Laboratory, many practices eschew this technique for several reasons. Until recently, curved planar

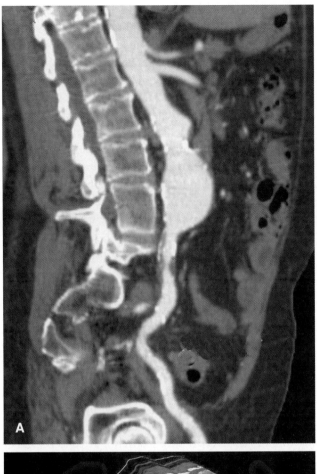

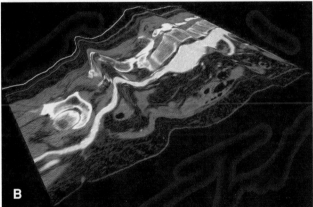

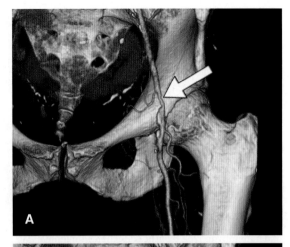

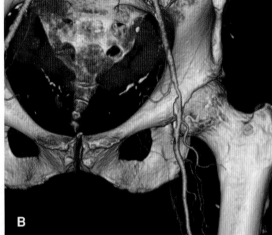

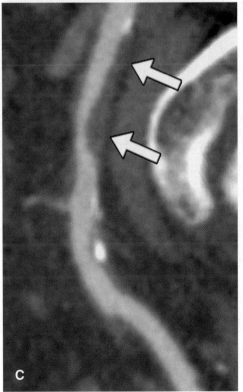

FIGURE 6-12 **A:** CPRs are MPRs that follow a curved path through the imaging volume. **B:** The nature of the curved plane is best represented in the "magic-carpet view," which shows the deviation of the plane through the lateral axis of the imaging volume when progressing from superior to inferior.

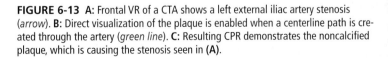

FIGURE 6-13 **A:** Frontal VR of a CTA shows a left external iliac artery stenosis (*arrow*). **B:** Direct visualization of the plaque is enabled when a centerline path is created through the artery (*green line*). **C:** Resulting CPR demonstrates the noncalcified plaque, which is causing the stenosis seen in **(A)**.

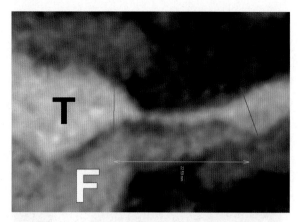

FIGURE 6-14 CPR of the left renal artery origin from a CTA of a patient with type B aortic dissection with intimal flap extending into the left renal artery. Treatment planning is facilitated by quantitative measurement of the length of intimal flap extension into the renal artery (shown in *yellow*) along the median centerline that was used to create the CPR. The true (*T*) and false (*F*) lumina are indicated.

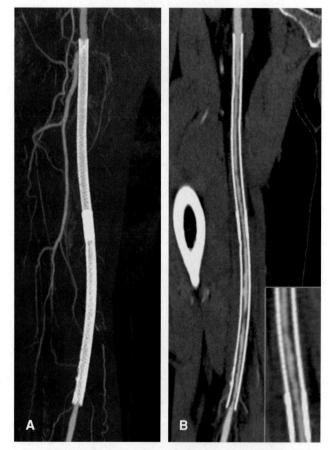

FIGURE 6-15 A: MIP CTA of a right superficial femoral artery with multiple stents placed to treat occlusive lesions. The arterial lumen within the stent is not visible. **B:** A CPR displays the arterial lumen and demonstrates extensive neointimal hyperplasia within the stent.

reformations could only be achieved through manual tracing of a vessel centerline (Fig. 6-16). This labor-intensive process is both time consuming and operator dependent, with potential for substantial variability in the quality of the CPR. Over the past several years, software algorithms to automatically extract the median centerline of blood vessels have resulted in the introduction of automated techniques for creating CPRs (Fig. 6-17). Such automation eliminates both the time-consuming aspects of tracing the curve as well as the operator dependence associated with creating the curve. The interpreter must be cautioned, however, that different implementations of centerline algorithms have varying degrees of effectiveness in finding the true median path, and thus, the interpretation of a CPR should always be made in association with the review of the centerline trace. Another limitation of CPRs is that to the unfamiliar eye, they can present bizarre spatial representations of structures outside the vessels of interest. Particularly when blood vessels course in one direction and then double back on themselves, unusual artifacts called "loop artifacts" can be created (Fig. 6-18). As long as the observer focuses on the primary structure through which the curve is created (while ignoring unusual appearances of other structures), mistakes in interpretation can be avoided. Just as we typically think of MPRs as a collection of parallel planes stacked through the imaging volume, CPRs are more effectively created as a series of radially oriented planes through the curved centerline. By rotating through a series of CPRs created at regular intervals (e.g., 5 degrees) around the centerline, eccentric manifestations of mural thickening or disease deposition are readily demonstrated (Fig. 6-19) and provide greater analytical efficiency when compared with planar reformation translated through a cartesian axis (15).

An important adjunct to CPRs is stacks of cross sections oriented orthogonal or perpendicular to the median centerline of a vessel. The creation of a stack of cross sections in this fashion results in planes that are not parallel to one another but that maintain a perpendicular relationship to the median axis of the vessel as these images propagate along the length of the vessel (Fig. 6-20). This allows for a true assessment of variations in cross-sectional area (CSA) or cross-sectional wall thickening and forms the basis for many quantification techniques described later in this chapter. The stacked review of these orthogonal cross sections has been referred to as a "slice-through" display (15).

Volume Rendering and Ray Casting

Although the current connotation of "volume rendering" (VR) in medical imaging implies a specific 3D visualization technique that uses sophisticated algorithms to represent MR signal or CT attenuation characteristics, volume

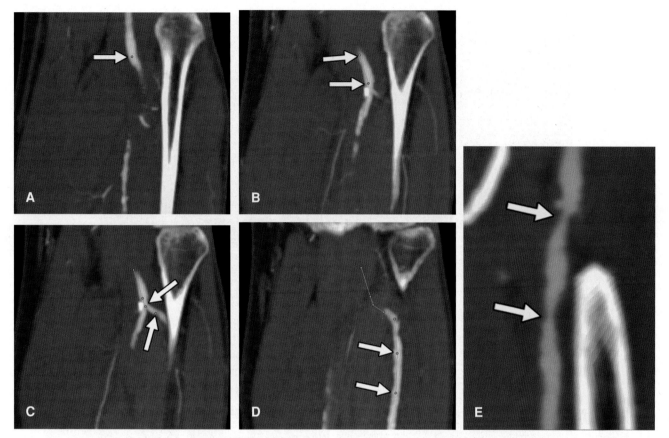

FIGURE 6-16 Manual tracing of vessel centerline in a CTA. In order to create a CPR, the operator needs to deposit points (*arrows* in **A** and **B**) within the vessel lumen, moving through the displayed to track the target vessel—in this case, the distal popliteal and anterior tibial arteries. Once drawn, the curve connecting the deposited points needs to be carefully examined to assure that it remains within the vessel lumen along its entire path (*arrows* in **C** and **D**). The resulting CPR demonstrates the presence of two regions of anterior tibial arterial narrowing (*arrows* in **E**).

rendering also more broadly refers to a family of visualization techniques generally linked by "ray casting," a process which creates 2D images derived from the information in 3D volumetric data sets. Ray casting is a process where the computer projects rays along a specified viewing direction through a volume or subvolume of the CT or MR data and uses characteristics of voxels encountered along each of these rays to compute pixel characteristics that compose an output image. By doing so, ray casting produces 2D images that represent projections from 3D volumes. Commonly seen ray casting techniques include maximum- and minimum-intensity projection (MIP and MinIP, respectively), ray sum, shaded-surface display (SSD), and VR (2–8,10,12,15–17).

Maximum-intensity Projections

MIPs were introduced in the 1980s for MRA. They remain a mainstay of MRA visualization and have also found an important niche in CTA visualization.

As an example of ray casting, the value of the highest intensity voxel encountered by each ray becomes encoded in the output image (Fig. 6-21). Because pulse sequences for MR angiographic acquisitions are designed so that vascular lumina are the highest intensity structures, MIPs are a logical means to flatten 3D MR imaging volumes into 2D representations. This technique is perhaps the most commonly used VR technique for 3D MR angiographic data because it is operator independent, free of intensity thresholding, and easy to perform. Although MIPs seem tailor-made for MRA, there are important limitations to the MIP technique that must be understood (10,16,17).

First, when a ray encounters multiple blood vessels along its path through the imaging volume, only the brightest (maximum intensity) voxel encountered will be encoded on the final MIP image. As a result, in regions of vessel overlap, only the voxels from the brightest vessel will contribute to the pixels of the output image. Unlike conventional angiography, however, there is no summation of

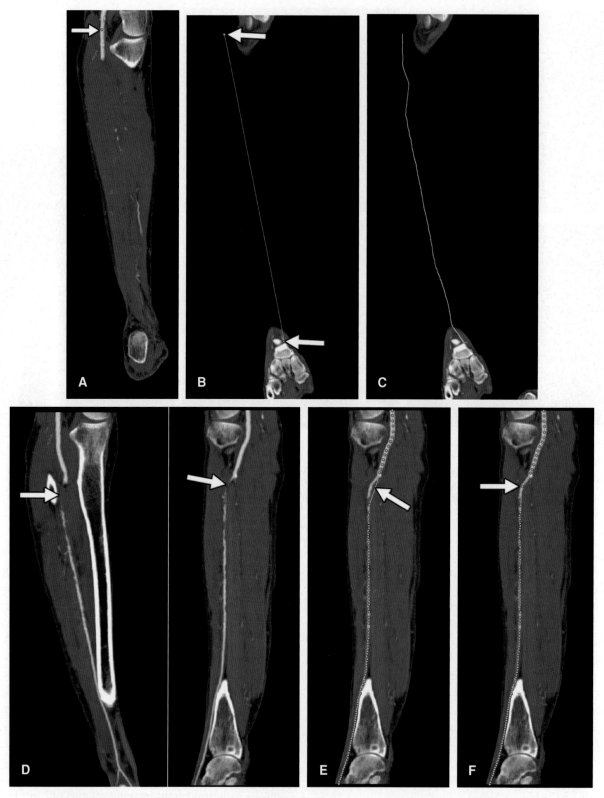

FIGURE 6-17 An automatic tracing of vessel centerline using CT. A seed is placed on a coronal MPR at the top of the vessel segment to be processed (*arrow* in **A**). Another seed is placed at the bottom of the vessel segment (*arrow* in **B**). A centerline along the vessel is automatically extracted (**C**). The extracted centerline is projected over a coronal section. Note that the curved path follows the vessel on multiple cross sections. **D:** When an abnormality is revealed, such as the apparent occlusion (*arrow,* **D**) of the anterior tibial artery, the path must be reviewed and corrected, if necessary, to assure that the path follows the vessel lumen (*arrows*). The correction requires manual repositioning of one of the vertices of the extracted path. Uncorrected and corrected paths are shown in (**E**) and (**F**), respectively.

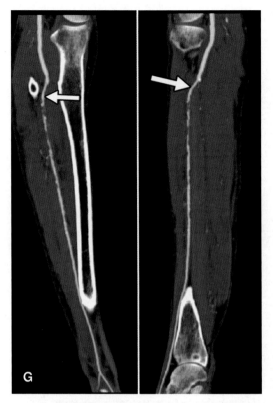

FIGURE 6-17 Continued After the correction, the anterior tibial artery is correctly displayed (**G**).

structures in these regions of overlap to help separate the overlapping vessels. From a practical standpoint, this means that in areas of complex vascular branching or overlap, it can become impossible to decipher the specific path of individual arterial branches (Fig. 6-22). More importantly, while the assessment of arterial ostia and proximal portions of arteries originating from the aorta is critical to the evaluation of many vascular disease processes, these portions of branch vessels could be obscured if an MIP view is created with overlap of an aortic branch ostium and the aorta itself (Fig. 6-23).

Another important limitation of the MIP technique is its tendency to overgrade vessel stenoses. Stenosis overgrading is a well-recognized phenomenon with MIP (Fig. 6-24). This occurs as a consequence of an undesirable side effect of MIP where background intensity values are increased by the MIP process. As rays are cast through the background, noise in the background data will be present, and therefore the rays will encounter a variety of voxel values. Because only the brightest voxel (defined as the one having the maximum value) encountered by any ray will be encoded on the output image, greater degrees of noise will result in a greater variation of background voxel values and, consequently, higher maximum values encountered by the ray tracing.

(*text continues on page 209*)

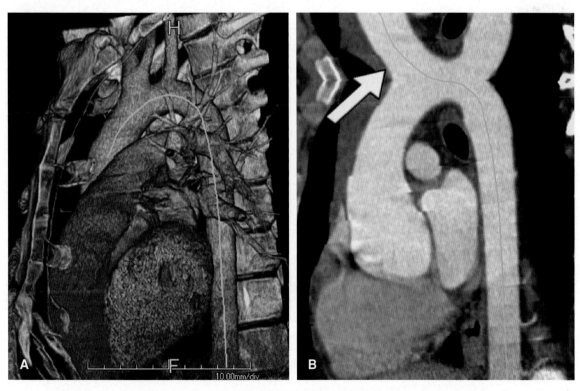

FIGURE 6-18 Loop artifact. A: VR of a CTA through the thoracic aorta with the green centerline path coursing through the ascending aorta, through the arch, and down the descending aorta. **B:** Resulting CPR presents a confusing image termed *loop artifact* (*arrow*) as the curved path intersects the same cross sections at two points.

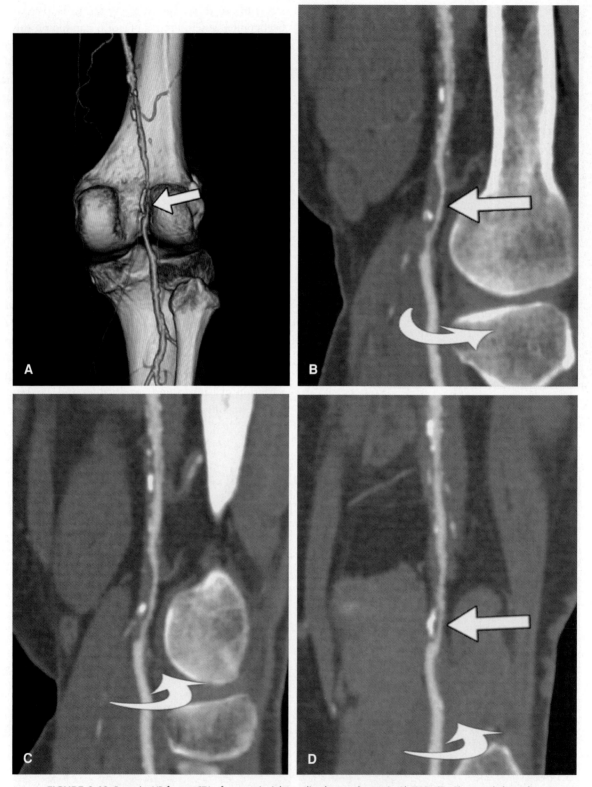

FIGURE 6-19 Posterior VR from a CTA of a stenotic right popliteal artery (*arrow* in **A**). CPRs **(B–G)** rotated about the median centerline through 180 degrees of the popliteal artery allow for a complete assessment of the mixed calcified and noncalcified plaque and the resulting eccentric popliteal artery stenosis (*straight arrows*).

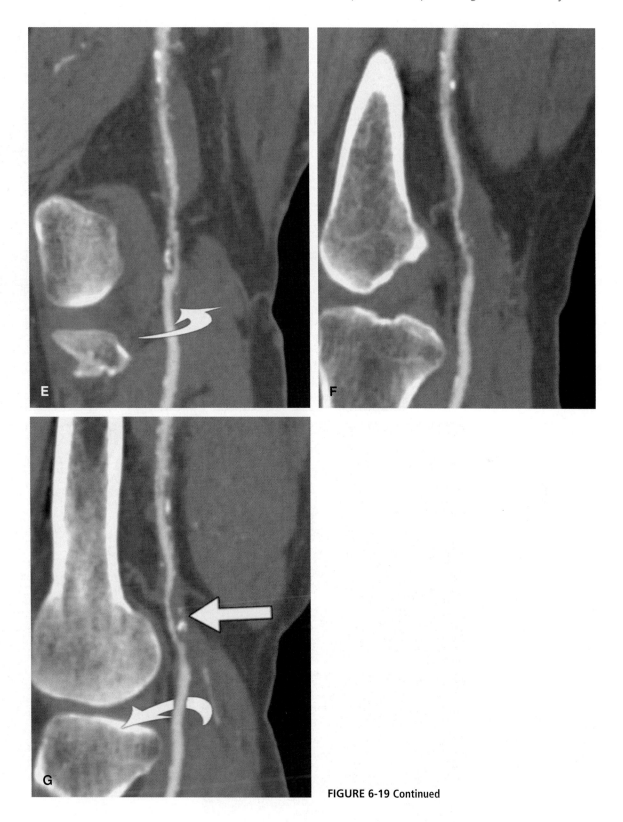

FIGURE 6-19 Continued

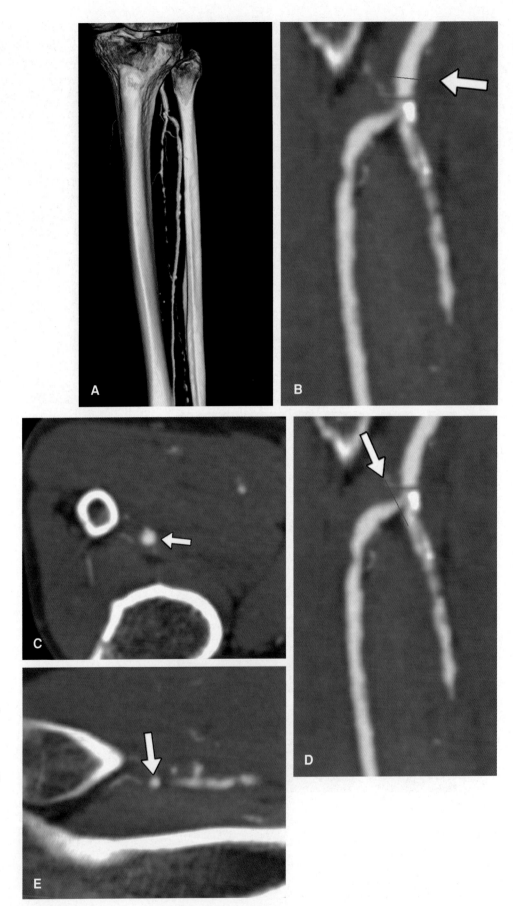

FIGURE 6-20 Orthogonal cross-section assessment of vessel lumina by using CPR. A: VR of a CTA through the distal popliteal and anterior tibial arteries illustrates the extracted centerline path in green. The resulting CPR serves as a guide for the selection of points along the path for automated creation of MPRs that are perpendicular to the path (*arrows* in **B** and **D**), allowing automated creation of true axial MPRs regardless of the orientation of the artery within the imaging volume (**C, E**).

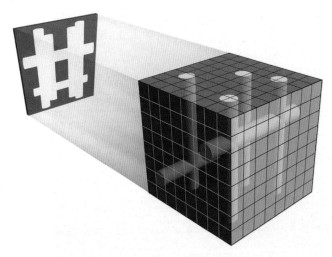

FIGURE 6-21 Schematic diagram illustrating the principle of MIP. Ray casting through the volume encodes the maximum voxel value encountered onto the output image. Because only one of the rods is represented at any particular location, when there are overlapping rods or blood vessels, they cannot be discriminated on the output image and relative depth information within the volume is lost. (Adapted with permission from Fishman EK, Ney DR, Heath DG, et al. Volume rendering versus maximum intensity projection in CT angiography: what works best, when, and why. *Radiographics*. 2006;26:905–922.)

Thus, background signal increases proportional to increasing noise in the data (Fig. 6-25).

Because vessel visualization is directly dependent on the contrast between the vessel lumen and background, there are two consequences of this phenomenon. First, small or less enhancing vessels can disappear in an MIP as background signal increases. Of greater practical importance, however, is that the ability to discriminate the outermost margins of narrowed blood vessels decreases and the degree of apparent narrowing increases as background noise increases (Figs. 6-25, 6-26). This occurs because voxels at the boundary of a vessel's lumen have decreased signal due to volume averaging with unenhanced tissues and can blend into the background as the background noise increases. When vessels with narrower lumina (including segments of stenosis) are evaluated, the proportion of the luminal diameter with significant intravascular enhancement tends to decrease relative to the proportion of the vessel's diameter composed of these boundary pixels that may be obscured by higher background signal levels.

Therefore, while MIP images conveniently provide a gross overview of vascular anatomy that tend to be easy to understand and are generally analogous to conventional angiographic images, there are also limitations to this technique. These limitations can be overcome when used in conjunction with curved planar reformatted images, which should provide the most accurate representation of vessel dimensions or in conjunction with planar images such as the primary reconstructions or MPRs.

When considering the use of MIP with CTA data, all of the aforementioned attributes of using MIP with MRA exist but with an additional important limitation. Because contrast-enhanced vascular lumina are frequently not the highest attenuation structures encountered within a CT volume, they may be obscured by overlying nonvascular structures with high density from mineralization or metal. The most common sources of mineralization are bones and arterial wall calcifications. However, other causes of mineralization (renal calculi, gallstones, myositis ossificans, calcified graft material, oral radiopaque contrast material) as well as metallic structures (wires, clips, joint prostheses, osseous fixation hardware, cardiac pacemakers) and associated streak artifact may also obscure vessel lumina on MIPs (Fig. 6-27). The elimination of nonvascular high-attenuation structures may be accomplished through a variety of segmentation processes that create subvolumes of data free of these high-attenuation structures. Currently, arterial wall calcification cannot be eliminated easily for the purpose of the creation of MIPs. Although some investigators have suggested that applying a threshold to the CT data can eliminate the calcification for the purpose of MIP creation, this approach is fraught with error. The arbitrary selection of the threshold assumes that the transition between luminal attenuation and mural calcium is constant, which is usually not the case. Without a dedicated method to analyze regional attenuation variations at interfaces between calcium and arterial lumina, or until availability of prospective methods for discriminating calcium from iodine such as dual energy approaches, automated removal of calcium from MIPs will remain a highly suspect pursuit.

It is important to note, however, that although arterial wall calcification obscures the arterial lumen on MIPs, the same MIPs can be a very effective means of conveying anatomic distribution of vascular calcifications. This qualitative calcium map can facilitate the selection of optimal locations for graft anastomoses and cross-clamp placement when performing arterial bypass procedures (Fig. 6-28). In the presence of moderate to extensive arterial wall calcification, luminal assessment is best performed with MPRs and CPRs rather than with MIPs.

Minimum-intensity Projections

MinIPs can be considered the opposite of MIPs. Specifically, ray casting results in encoding of the lowest (minimum intensity) encountered voxel value into the output image rather than the highest voxel value (as used in MIPs). While there is currently no widespread use for MinIPs in CTA or MRA, MinIPs can play a limited role to

(text continues on page 213)

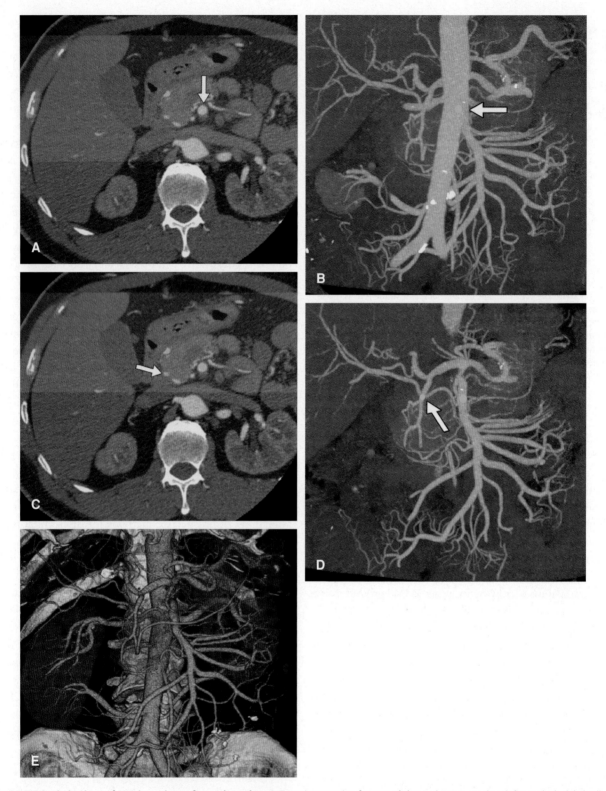

FIGURE 6-22 Limitations of MIP in regions of vessel overlap. A: Transverse section from an abdominal CTA is used to define a thick slab (*yellow shading*) for the purpose of MIP creation. This slab, while excluding the spine as well as the distal portions of the renal arteries, includes the majority of the arteries of the abdomen, including the aorta. *Green dots* positioned in the middle of the abdominal aorta and on the gastroduodenal artery are referenced in subsequent figure parts. **B:** MIP through the thick slab defined in **(A)** does not allow delineation of the superior mesenteric artery at the level identified by the *arrow* in **(A)**. Because the aorta has slightly higher attenuation than the SMA, its attenuation value contributes to the pixel value on the MIP at the expected location of the SMA (*green dot*). **C:** Restriction of the slab to exclude the aorta (*yellow shading*) should allow visualization of the SMA (*green dot*). However, the gastroduodenal artery (*smaller green dot*) is directly in line with the dorsal pancreatic artery (*arrow*). **D:** MIP through the slab defined in **(C)** allows visualization of the proximal SMA (*larger green dot*); however, ambiguity of the visualization is seen at the point of overlap between the gastroduodenal artery and the dorsal pancreatic artery (*arrow*). **E:** VR of the entire volume, including the spine, avoids the pitfalls of MIP by allowing delineation of crossing branches.

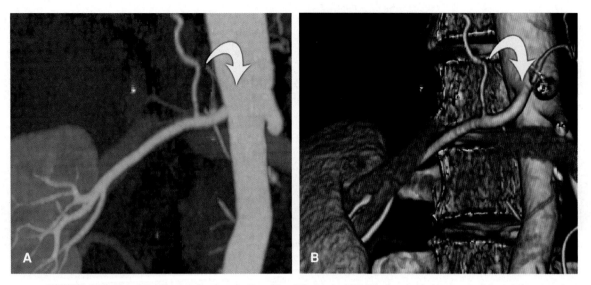

FIGURE 6-23 Normal right renal artery depicted by CTA. On the MIP **(A)**, the proximal segment of the renal artery (*curved arrows*) is obscured due to overlap between this vessel and the aorta. The vessel origin is precisely localized on the VR **(B)**.

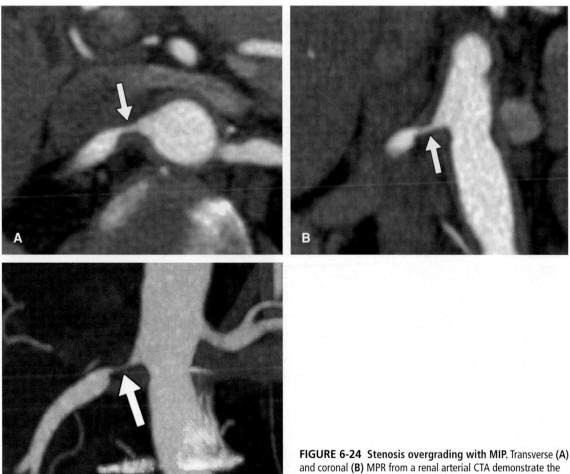

FIGURE 6-24 Stenosis overgrading with MIP. Transverse **(A)** and coronal **(B)** MPR from a renal arterial CTA demonstrate the presence of a right renal artery stenosis (*arrows*). The degree of luminal narrowing shown by MIP **(C)** is overrepresented relative to the cross-sectional views.

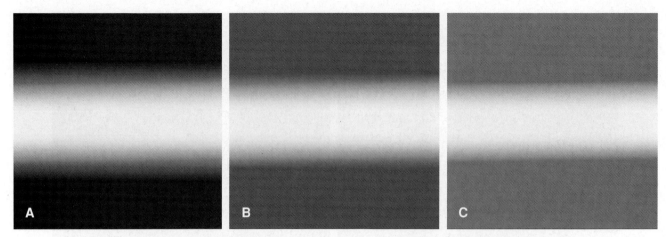

FIGURE 6-25 Apparent narrowing increases as background signal increases. The first image (**A**) shows the simulated appearance of a vessel when using MIP rendering. Assuming that the brightness of this "vessel" remains unchanged, the apparent diameter of the vessel decreases as the background becomes brighter (**B, C**).

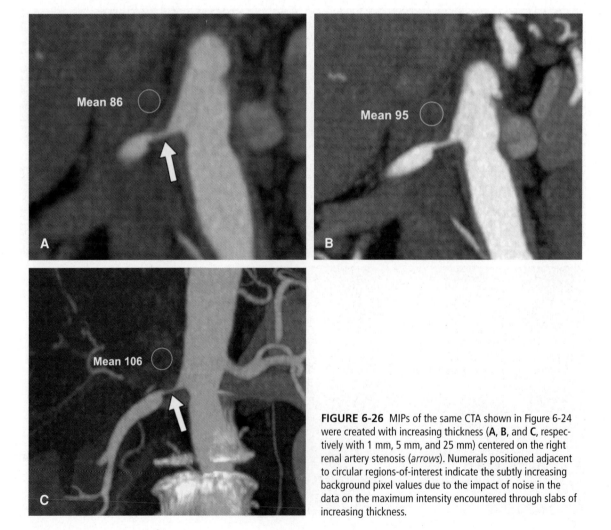

FIGURE 6-26 MIPs of the same CTA shown in Figure 6-24 were created with increasing thickness (**A, B,** and **C,** respectively with 1 mm, 5 mm, and 25 mm) centered on the right renal artery stenosis (*arrows*). Numerals positioned adjacent to circular regions-of-interest indicate the subtly increasing background pixel values due to the impact of noise in the data on the maximum intensity encountered through slabs of increasing thickness.

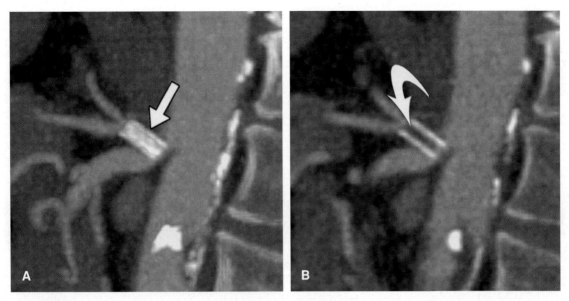

FIGURE 6-27 Sagittal 5-mm-thick MIP of a CTA **(A)** demonstrates the presence of a stent in the celiac axis (*arrow*) in a patient with a common celiomesenteric trunk. The lumen of the stent is obscured by the surrounding stent metal structure. Sagittal MPR image **(B)** shows neointimal hyperplasia (*curved arrow*) resulting in an in-stent occlusion not visible on the MIP. Opacification of the hepatic and left gastric arteries was by pancreaticoduodenal collaterals (not shown).

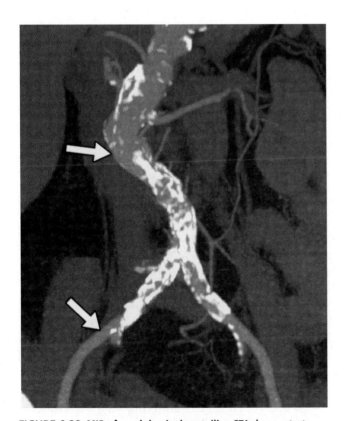

FIGURE 6-28 MIP of an abdominal aortoiliac CTA demonstrates diffuse arterial wall calcifications. This image provides a map that may facilitate the selection of optimal locations for graft anastomoses and cross-clamp placement when performing arterial bypass procedures (*arrows*).

define and accentuate intraluminal filling defects, particularly aortic and mitral valve leaflets. Because valve leaflets are thin and in motion, volume averaging and motion blurring can limit their visualization even on primary cross sections. By selecting a 5- to 20-mm thick slab subvolume that is perpendicular to the aortic root, application of a MinIP can substantially improve visualization of valve leaflets (Fig. 6-29).

Ray Sum

The ray sum, or average-intensity projection, is yet another ray casting technique available on most clinical workstations. Its creation is directly analogous to MIP and MinIP, except the averaged voxel value (rather than the maximum- or minimum-intensity voxel value) encountered along the ray's path is encoded on the output image. In the setting of CT data, these ray sum images may appear very similar to conventional radiographs or "scout images" of the projected slab. Ray sum projections traditionally have little utility in CTA and MRA. These projections are typically created through a slab with thicknesses up to 20 mm. Within this context, they are analogous to obtaining a thick primary reconstruction from a CT or MR acquisition. The use of ray sum projections essentially volume average along the slab direction and consequently reduce edge detail and the ability to delineate fine structures. Unlike MIP and MinIP, noise is reduced in a ray sum projection due to the averaging

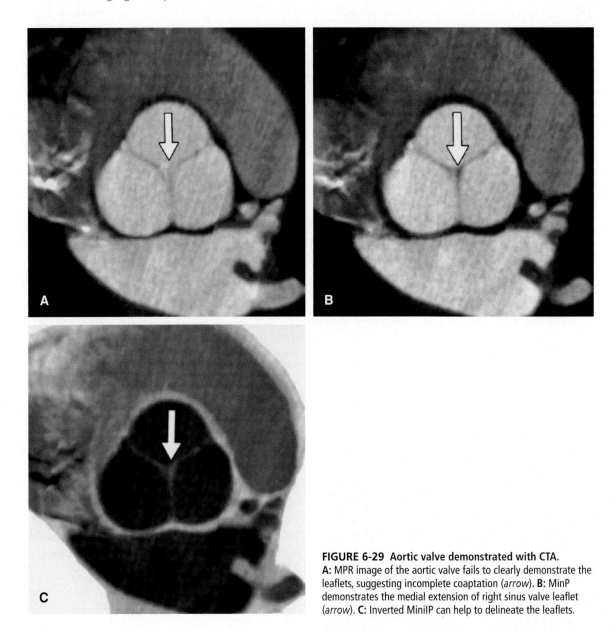

FIGURE 6-29 Aortic valve demonstrated with CTA.
A: MPR image of the aortic valve fails to clearly demonstrate the leaflets, suggesting incomplete coaptation (*arrow*). **B:** MinP demonstrates the medial extension of right sinus valve leaflet (*arrow*). **C:** Inverted MiniIP can help to delineate the leaflets.

that occurs along the ray's path. As a result, in occasional circumstances where noise levels are unacceptable for image interpretation, a ray sum projection can reduce the noise of a primary reconstruction at the expense of an increase in partial volume effects (18) (Fig. 6-30).

Shaded-Surface Displays

For routine clinical CTA and MRA, SSDs are of historical interest only. Although SSDs maintain a role in biomechanical applications where luminal surface extraction facilitates modeling of complex blood flow phenomena, SSDs have been supplanted clinically by VR for purposes of visualization and diagnostic analysis. Nevertheless, SSDs were key to the initial development of CTA in the early 1990s when standard medical postprocessing workstations were insufficiently powered to support the complexity of contemporary VR. Many early scientific publications establishing the clinical utility of CTA utilized SSDs. Like other volume techniques described previously, SSDs are also applicable to MRA data; however, the widespread application of SSDs for MRA data never occurred due to the adoption of MIP and the subsequent direct transition to VR.

In brief, SSDs are created by applying a threshold to the CTA or MRA data resulting in a binary classification of every voxel within the volume as being either above or below the threshold. The interface between voxels above and those below the threshold define a surface that is

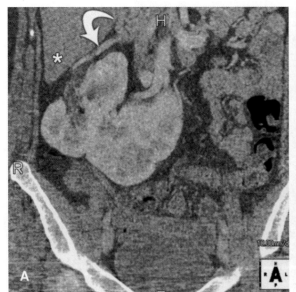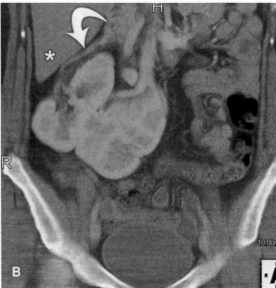

FIGURE 6-30 Low radiation dose CTA in a patient with cross-fused renal ectopia. The coronal MPR **(A)** demonstrates high noise levels. The 10-mm-thick ray sum projection **(B)** reduces the noise at the expense of an increase in partial volume effect. Compare the definition of the liver parenchyma (∗) and the renal vein (*curved arrow*) in both images.

rendered with a polygonal mesh. An imaginary source of illumination is created by the SSD algorithm and directed toward the surface mesh; the reflected light off of the surface back to a viewpoint is calculated to represent the surface shading, which simulates visualization of this surface under real light conditions.

While SSDs overcome many of the aforementioned limitations of MIPs by delineating vessel ostia and allowing clear separation of overlapping blood vessels, their greatest limitation is the requirement for application of a single threshold value. This threshold typically is selected arbitrarily. Even when based on principled image analysis, the assumption in selecting the threshold is that a single value can serve to define the interface between the enhancing vessel lumen and the vessel wall. Due to variations in enhancement relative to vessel position within the imaging volume, the effects of partial volume averaging, or a multitude of other technical factors, it is as a practical matter impossible to represent this interface as a single threshold value (Fig. 6-31). The net result is that vessel dimensions and most notably the portrayed degrees of arterial stenosis vary highly depending on the selection of the threshold value (7,19–21).

Volume Rendering

As previously discussed, VR in the image-processing field is broadly defined to include many algorithms that project 3D volumetric data onto 2D images. However, this same term has in recent years come to connote a more specific type of visualization. Currently, the most computationally intensive visualization method, VRs are created by assigning varying levels of transparency to voxels based on individual voxel values. The opacity transfer function defines the degree of opacity from 0% (completely transparent) to 100% (completely opaque) for each possible voxel value. Thus, when an individual ray is cast, multiple voxels along that ray can contribute to the output image, provided that the cumulative voxel opacity does not exceed 100%. Once the ray has traversed sufficient voxels whose contributions to opacity sum to 100%, subsequent voxels encountered along the ray's path will not contribute to the output image (2,10,12,15–17).

From a practical standpoint, most VR of CTA and MRA data uses these opacity transfer functions in an attempt to isolate contrast-enhanced vessel lumina from adjacent unenhanced tissues. This goal is typically accomplished by creating an opacity ramp with three distinct zones: transparent zone, transitional zone, and plateau (Figs. 6-32 and 6-33). Increases in the steepness of the transition zone tend to accentuate edges; the extreme where the transition zone is vertical results in images that mimic the SSDs described previously.

Another application for VR in cardiovascular imaging is the creation of endoluminal views. The opacity transfer function for this type of application is essentially a mirror image of the aforementioned transfer function with the luminal voxels being rendered transparent and the "vessel wall" or perivascular tissues being rendered opaque (3,12) (Fig. 6-34).

(*text continues on page 218*)

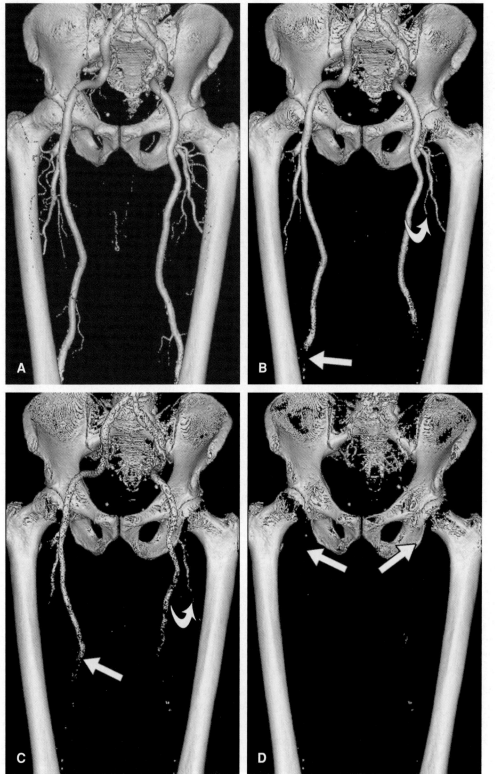

FIGURE 6-31 **A:** Frontal SSD of the iliac and femoral arteries. The threshold is fixed at 250 HU (Hounsfield units). All the voxels with CT numbers below this threshold are not represented. **B:** Increasing the threshold to 280 HU results in the loss of distal and smaller arteries due to a lesser degree of enhancement or volume averaging, respectively (*arrows*). **C, D:** Increasing the threshold to 300 and 350 HU, respectively, the iodine-filled arterial lumen is lost, and only calcified structures remain.

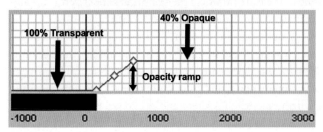

FIGURE 6-32 Example of linear opacity ramp used to create VR images defines three distinct zones—0% opacity (100% transparency), the linear transition zone, and the opacity plateau at 40% opacity.

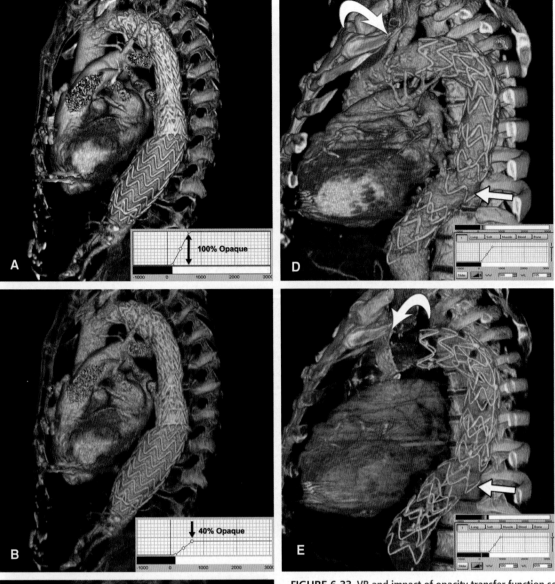

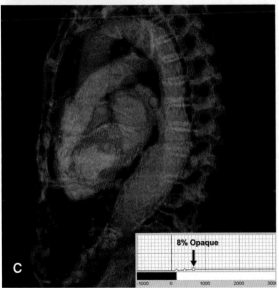

FIGURE 6-33 VR and impact of opacity transfer function selection. A: Lateral VR of a thoracic aortic CTA created with the corresponding opacity transfer function demonstrated at the **lower right**. This transfer function is characterized by 0% opacity (100% transparency) below 120 HU and 100% opacity (0% transparency) above 550 HU. The transition zone between these two plateaus is a linear ramp. **B:** When the peak opacity above 550 HU is limited to 40% opacity, large structures remain opaque due to their thickness, allowing a summation of voxel opacity values achieving 100% as rays are cast through the volume. In contrast, smaller branches such as the apical posterior segmental branches of the left upper lobe pulmonary artery and the branches of the celiac axis are partially transparent. **C:** Clamping peak opacity to 8% results in relatively thick structures, such as the descending thoracic aorta, are rendered with sufficient transparency that the other structures, such as the spine, can be seen through them. Thinner structures, even those with relatively high attenuation such as the metallic elements of the descending thoracic aortic stent graft, are poorly visualized due to the low level of opacity with which they are rendered using this opacity transfer function. **D:** Opacity transfer functions can be modified in innumerable ways. This VR obtained with the opacity transfer function shown at the **lower right** renders the metallic elements of the stent graft (*straight arrow*) and the descending thoracic aortic lumen adjacent to it as completely opaque. The left common carotid artery (*curved arrow*) is also completely opaque obscuring visualization of the superior vena cava deep to it. **E:** Shifting the entire opacity transfer function 300 HU higher results in the iodinated contrast opacified lumina being rendered nearly completely transparent. Only attenuation values over 900 HU are rendered with high opacity (80%), such as the metallic elements of the descending thoracic aortic stent graft (*straight arrow*) and the undiluted iodinated contrast within the superior vena cava (*curved arrow*), which is now visible through the ascending aorta.

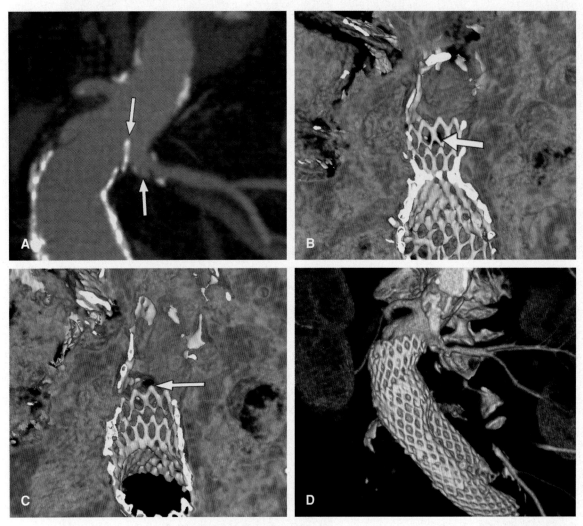

FIGURE 6-34 CTA following stent-graft placement. The oblique MPR **(A)** shows the relationship between the proximal stent graft and the ostium of the left renal artery (*arrows*), which is partially covered but still patent. Endoluminal VRs are more effective at conveying these relationships in 3D (*arrows* in **B, C**) when compared with traditional external VRs **(D)**.

There are many other nuances to the effective creation of opacity transfer functions; however, a detailed discussion of these approaches is beyond the scope of this book. Subtle differences in the characteristics of opacity transfer functions represent the true artistry and complexity of VR, with virtually every vendor of 3D visualization software using a unique VR algorithm. Each of these algorithms has its own idiosyncrasies, and thus while generalities can be drawn, nuanced control requires familiarity with each algorithm and its accompanying user interface.

If VR were based exclusively on opacity transfer functions, then it would bear little resemblance to the 3D representations that we have come to know. Lighting effects play an important role in conveying 3D spatial relationships. Similar to the method described for SSDs, an imaginary source or sources of illumination can be created by using computer algorithms. Because a discrete surface is not calculated in VR, lighting effects are generated relative to the spatial gradient of neighboring voxel values. That is, where adjacent voxels are similar, minimal lighting effects are applied; however, where differences are great such as at the edge of the vessel lumen, lighting effects are applied more strongly. In this way, surfaces appear to be created in regions of high spatial gradient (Fig. 6-35). The encoding of the lighting effects is performed with grayscale shading based on calculated reflections of light in these areas of high spatial gradient. The typical model for lighting VRs is with an imaginary source of illumination originating from the same position as the viewpoint. However, the light source can be decoupled from the viewpoint in order to accentuate surface irregularities (Fig. 6-36). The controls for lighting effects can also be labeled with varying names such as "brightness," "contrast," or "ambient light" (6,7,14,17) (Fig. 6-37).

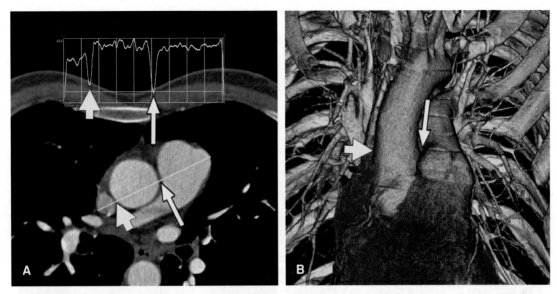

FIGURE 6-35 Lighting effects result in shading at regions of high spatial gradient. A: A line-density profile through the ascending aorta (*yellow line*) illustrates two regions of high spatial gradient at the surface of the aorta (*arrows*), visualized in the plot as regions of high slope at the edges of the luminal plateau. **B:** VR with lighting effects conveys surface features by applying shading in the areas of high spatial gradient (*arrows*).

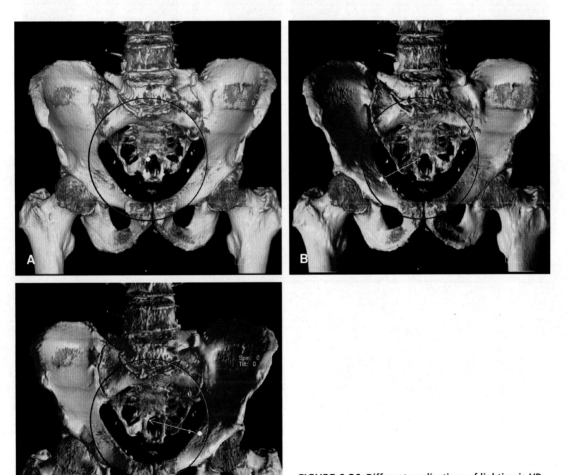

FIGURE 6-36 Different applications of lighting in VR. A: An imaginary source of illumination originates from the same position as the viewpoint. **B, C:** Alternative lighting directions from upper left and lower left, respectively emphasize different surface features.

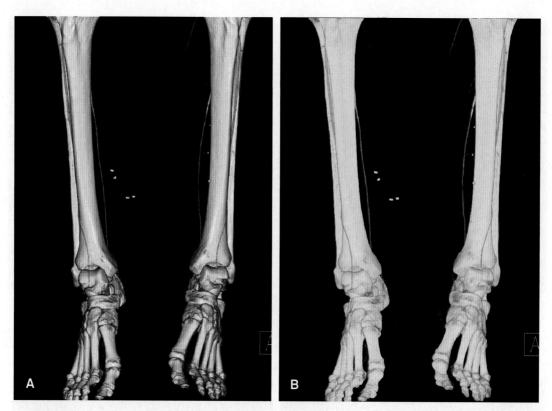

FIGURE 6-37 Lighting effects. A: Standard VR with a combination of ambient and directional lighting originating from the viewpoint. **B:** With ambient lighting only, features appear flat and surface relationships are not conveyed.

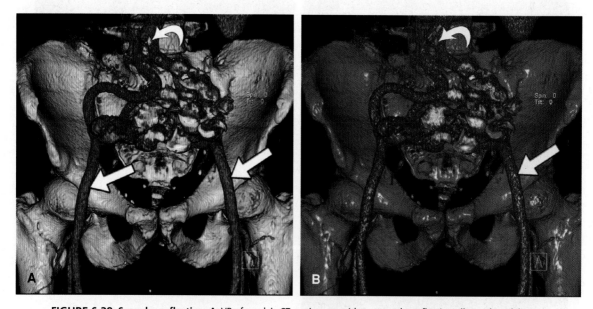

FIGURE 6-38 Specular reflection. A: VR of a pelvic CT angiogram without specular reflection allows clear delineation of mural calcium (*curved arrow*) and contrast-enhanced femoral arterial lumen (*arrows*), because a color scale has been established to map the calcified plaque as white and the lesser attenuation of the contrast-enhanced lumen as red. **B:** The same VR as in **(A)** with a high degree of specular reflection creates a glistening surface; however, ambiguity is created in zones rendered white. White may represent calcification (*curved arrow*) or regions of high specular reflection (*straight arrow*). The ability to confidently discriminate mural calcium from noncalcified arteries is lost when specular reflection is applied.

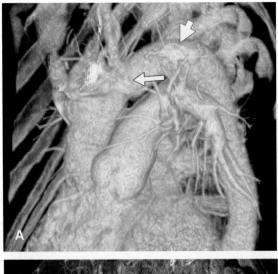

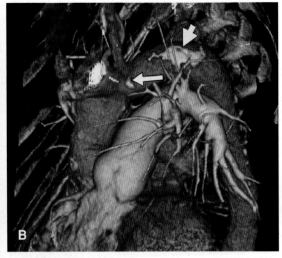

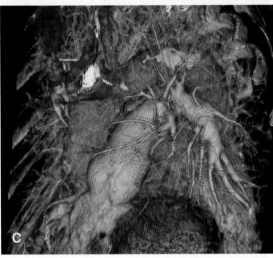

FIGURE 6-39 **A:** VR of the aortic arch and left pulmonary artery using grayscale does not allow effective separation of differing regions of attenuation. The varying shades of gray primarily map shading at the margins of structures. Two regions of calcified plaque in the aortic arch (*arrows*) are barely discriminated from the remainder of the aorta. **B:** The addition of a color scale where red is mapped to attenuation values of 150 HU and transitioned to white at 500 HU renders the 300 HU attenuation within the aortic arch as orange and the 400 HU attenuation within the left pulmonary artery as beige. Calcification (700 HU) is rendered white and is easily discriminated from the adjacent aortic arch lumen (*arrows*). **C:** An additional triangular opacity transfer function with peak attenuation at −300 HU is rendered blue and allows visualization of small pulmonary vessels superimposed on the anatomy shown in (**B**).

Another variable found in many VR interfaces is the degree of "specular reflection" associated with high spatial gradient regions. As specular reflection is raised to higher values, rendered "surfaces" appear to be wet and can also help to accentuate subtle surface variations (Fig. 6-38). The application of specular reflection can be disconcerting and provide ambiguous information relating to voxel values; thus, its use is generally not recommended (1).

Although VR does not need to incorporate color, the use of only grayscale to encode varying voxel values and lighting effects as well as specular reflectiveness can create images that are difficult to interpret. An effective means of creating images that are easier to interpret is the application of a color scale based on voxel value. When chosen and applied effectively, color in VR can result in almost photorealistic representations of anatomic structures. Particularly for CTA, color can be an important element of VR to allow

instant visual differentiation of regions of mural calcium, metallic structures such as stents or stent grafts, contrast-enhancing lumen, and mural thrombus (Fig. 6-39). Because VRs may appear nearly photorealistic, it is important to remind both referring physicians as well as patients who are not familiar with VR that many features potentially seen on direct inspection may not be represented in these renderings.

The majority of VR utilizes orthographic perspective, where individual rays are cast parallel to one another and perpendicular to the plane of display. The resultant image is free of the perspective with which humans visually perceive the world, where objects closer to the viewer appear larger than those farther away. Consequently, with orthographic rendering the relative size of objects are rendered independent of their distance from the viewpoint (Fig. 6-40). In certain circumstances, VR with perspective is

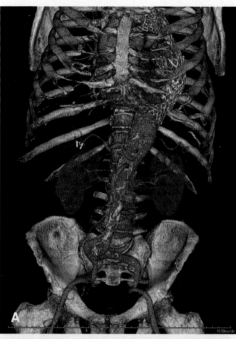

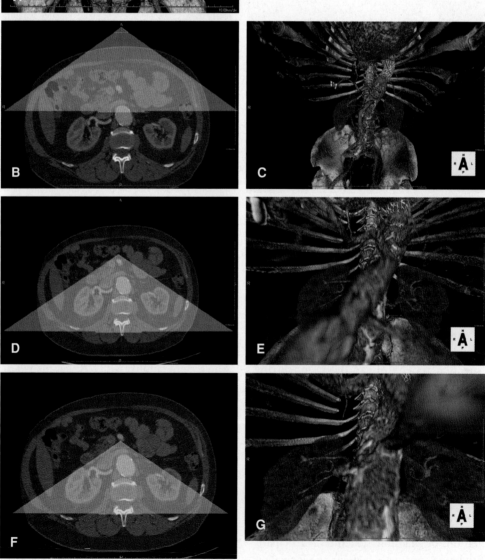

FIGURE 6-40 Perspective VR. **A:** Standard orthographic projection of an abdominal aortic CTA is rendered without perspective. **B:** Transverse CT section illustrates a 110-degree viewing frustum (*yellow triangle*) with a vertex positioned 3 cm anterior to the skin surface. **C:** The resulting perspective VR is rendered and shows that structures closer to the viewpoint, such as the rib ends, appear larger when compared with more distant structures such as the aorta. **D:** Entering the data set (immersive visualization) the vertex of the viewing frustum is positioned immediately anterior to the superior mesenteric artery, resulting in the VR in **(E)**. **E:** The SMA now appears substantially larger than in **(C)** and dominates the visualization, obscuring the underlying aorta. **F:** Advancement of the viewing frustum an additional centimeter eliminates the SMA and allows direct visualization of the aortic surface without segmentation of the data set **(G)**.

desired and is accomplished by using divergent ray casting from a single point. The degree of divergence defines the viewing frustum or field of view (Fig. 6-41). Practical viewing frusta for clinical VR may vary from a low of 30 degrees to as high as 90 degrees. Higher viewing frusta that might provide greater "peripheral vision" are limited by substantial distortions and are rarely useful in vascular imaging (1).

While perspective VRs is may be applied from viewpoints external to the imaging volume, their value is particularly pronounced for immersive visualization, such as in the endoluminal views previously described. With the viewpoint for the VRs created from within the imaging volume, virtual angiography can be performed by using a scripted flight path along the lumen of a vessel. Although this visualization method has limited clinical applicability, it is occasionally useful for demonstrating arterial ostia and in particular establishing the relationship of metallic stents and stent grafts relative to aortic branches (Fig. 6-42) or the intimal flaps of aortic dissections.

WHICH VISUALIZATION METHOD IS BEST?

Many articles have been published comparing the aforementioned visualization methods with one another in an attempt to identify a superior method for assessing a given clinical condition. Unfortunately, due to the substantial variability in the implementation of the different visualization algorithms and in the experiences and approaches of the individual users, these comparisons rarely produce conclusive or generalizable results. Based on our experience, the most powerful and effective means of analyzing cardiovascular imaging data is to work within a visualization environment that allows rapid switching between the various visualization methods, allowing for interactive exploration of the data. A formal assessment of the underlying anatomy and pathology is thus made through a composite assessment by using the various available visualization techniques. Although as a general rule there may be no single visualization method that is best for a specific clinical assessment, each visualization technique has strengths and weaknesses (17) (Table 6-1).

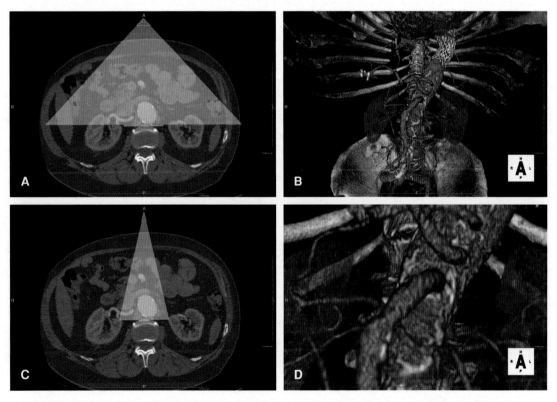

FIGURE 6-41 A: A 90° viewing frustum 5 cm anterior to the abdominal wall results in the VR shown in **(B)**, where there is moderate distortion of spatial relationships with proximal structures such as the heart and rib ends appearing substantially larger than distant structures such as the aorta and kidneys. **C:** Narrowing of the viewing frustum to 15° provides a visualization that more closely represents standard orthographic visualization **(D)**. Perspective is still detectable, as the SMA appears substantially larger than the right renal artery, which is only 1 mm narrower when viewed on the transverse section in **(C)**. In general, smaller viewing frusta, while limiting the field of view, provide less distortion and serve as an effective middle ground between orthographic projection and perspective VR with a wide viewing frustum.

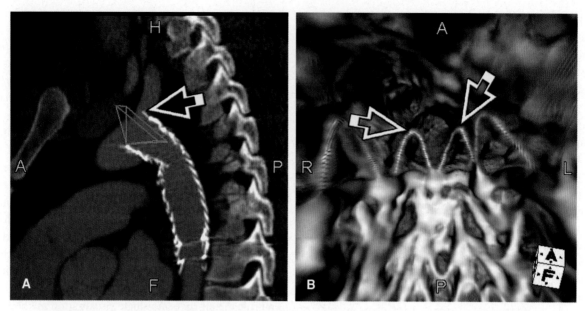

FIGURE 6-42 Practical application of perspective VR. A: Sagittal oblique MPR from a CTA with a thoracic aortic stent graft projecting over the origin of the left subclavian artery (*arrow*). The proximal end of the stent graft appears to overlie over 50% of the left subclavian arterial ostium, raising concerns for hemodynamically significant obstruction (*arrow*). A 90° 3D viewing frustum represented by *red* and *blue lines* illustrates the viewpoint for the perspective VR shown in (**B**). **B:** Perspective VR clearly displays the serrated edge of the proximal stent graft (*arrows*) with the ostium of the left subclavian artery visualized deep to the stent graft. The majority of the left subclavian artery ostium is preserved because of the proximal serration. This feature is not appreciable on the MPR and is visible with this perspective VR that results from an opacity transfer function that renders the lumen of the aorta as transparent.

TABLE 6-1

Visualization Techniques

	Display	Major Uses	Advantages	Disadvantages
MIP	3D	• Angiographic overview providing context with adjacent structures	• Depicts course of small caliber vessels • Depicts poorly enhancing vessels	• Vessel, bone, visceral overlap • Limited stent lumen evaluation • Limited by heavy calcium • Cannot measure vessel dimensions
VR	3D	• Angiographic overview providing context with adjacent structures	• Structural overview • Best display of complex spatial relationships	• Opacity-transfer function dependent rendering • Cannot measure vessel dimensions
MPR	2D	• Flow lumen and vessel wall analysis	• Best display of stenoses, occlusions, calcification, stents	• Limited display of spatial relationships • Limited display of the vessel of interest when the vessel follows a curved path
CPR	2D	• Flow lumen and vessel wall analysis	• Best display of stenoses, occlusions, calcification, stents	• Dependent on accuracy of centerline drawing or extraction • Distortion of extravascular structures

MIP, maximum-intensity projection; VR, volume rendering; MPR, multiplanar reformation; CPR, curved planar reformation; 2D, two dimensional; 3D, three dimensional.

SEGMENTATION

Segmentation is the process through which regions of interest, or regions of extraneous data, are isolated from an imaging volume. Within the context of cardiovascular imaging, segmentation may remove structures that are not relevant to the visualization such as bones, prostheses, and extraneous soft tissue of overlying vasculature. Alternatively, structures to be analyzed such as the arterial wall, arterial lumen, and heart may be retained with the remainder of the background removed. The purpose of segmentation is twofold—to improve visualization by removing extraneous structures or to facilitate quantitation. The precision required when segmentation is applied for the purpose of visualization is usually less critical than when it is used to provide measurements of luminal dimensions, vessel length, or tissue volumes.

It is rarely advantageous when visualizing MR or CT data to render the entirety of the imaging volume by using volumetric display techniques. In general, eliminating extravascular and overlapping structures from the volume improves the visualization of the remaining blood vessels (Fig. 6-43). Because detailed vessel extraction can be a complicated and time-consuming process and complete vessel extraction is often not necessary to achieve a diagnosis, simpler although less complete methods of segmentation may be very effective (1,3).

The simplest segmentation tools available on workstations are clip or cut planes. These planes default to the edges of the imaging volume. The six standard cut planes (anterior, posterior, superior, inferior, right, and left) can be individually advanced into the volume to create cuboid subvolumes. This simple tool can be useful for removing the table from the imaging volume in a CT acquisition (Fig. 6-44); it is also useful in MR imaging for removing superficial tissues that frequently appear brighter than deeper structures because of increased receiver coil sensitivity to surface structures and intentional or unintentional phase wrap as well as the high intrinsic signal of subcutaneous fat.

An extension of this technique is the use of oblique cut planes that can be rotated arbitrarily through the volume. These oblique planes can be used to define a thick-slab region of interest or can be used to intentionally exclude structures on either side of the oblique plane. Multiple oblique planes can be used to carve away extraneous tissues in order to isolate a structure of interest; however, because of the curved and often tortuous course of blood vessels through the body, cut planes are frequently only partially effective at isolating arteries and veins for visualization (Fig. 6-45).

The next level of manual segmentation is region-of-interest drawing. The user creates a trace over a projection or cross section of the imaging volume that defines a region to be included in or excluded from this volume. The trace can be applied to a single cross section, extended over several contiguous cross sections, or extruded through the entire imaging volume (Fig. 6-46). Region-of-interest drawing can be used effectively to "sculpt" the volume. The user can begin with a VR and roughly trace around structures to be included or excluded and then repeatedly rotate the volume and draw additional regions of interest to further

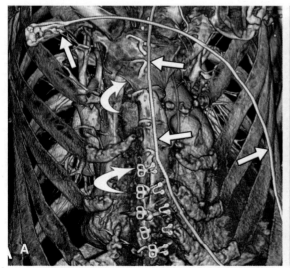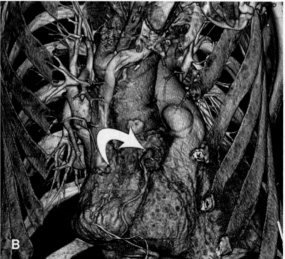

FIGURE 6-43 Chest CTA displayed with VR **(A)**. Vascular visualization is improved after eliminating electrodes (*straight arrows*), metallic clips (*curved arrows*), and the sternum **(B)**.

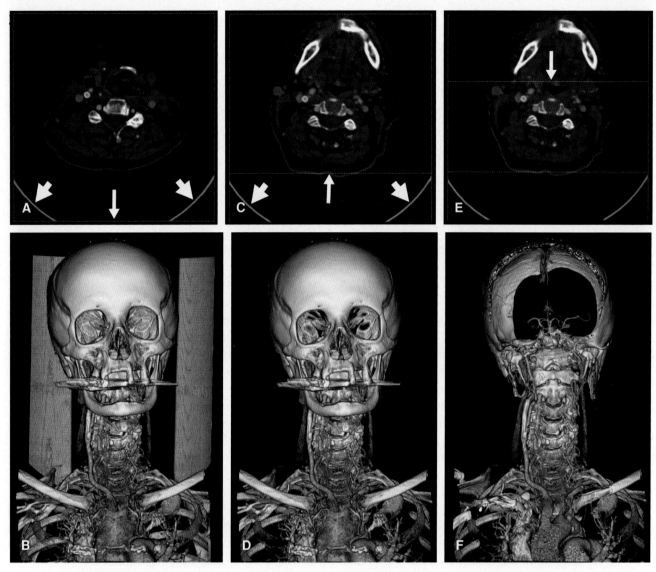

FIGURE 6-44 CT table removal using clip or cut planes. The table is usually seen as a concave structure in transverse images (*wide arrows* in **A** and **C**) and interferes with the visualization of 3D reformats (**B**). After moving the posterior clip plane anteriorly (*thin arrow*), the table is removed from the visualization (**D**). An anterior clip plane (*arrow* in **E**) unmasks the cerebral arteries (**F**).

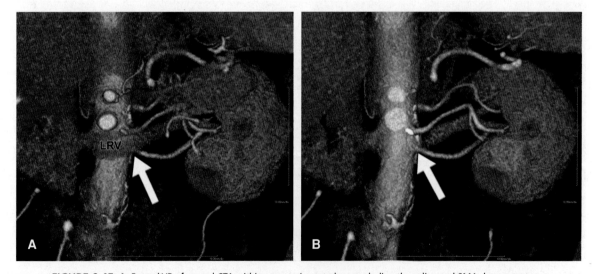

FIGURE 6-45 A: Frontal VR of a renal CTA within an anterior cut plane excluding the celiac and SMA demonstrates the left renal vein (LRV) obscuring the origin of one of three left renal arteries (*arrow*). **B:** Advancement of an oblique cut plane oriented parallel to the LRV successfully excludes only a portion of the LRV, sufficient to expose the origin of the inferior-most left renal artery.

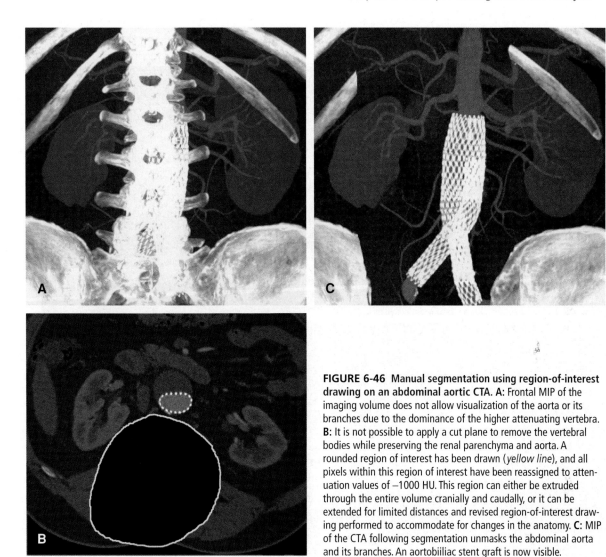

FIGURE 6-46 Manual segmentation using region-of-interest drawing on an abdominal aortic CTA. A: Frontal MIP of the imaging volume does not allow visualization of the aorta or its branches due to the dominance of the higher attenuating vertebra. **B:** It is not possible to apply a cut plane to remove the vertebral bodies while preserving the renal parenchyma and aorta. A rounded region of interest has been drawn (*yellow line*), and all pixels within this region of interest have been reassigned to attenuation values of −1000 HU. This region can either be extruded through the entire volume cranially and caudally, or it can be extended for limited distances and revised region-of-interest drawing performed to accommodate for changes in the anatomy. **C:** MIP of the CTA following segmentation unmasks the abdominal aorta and its branches. An aortobiiliac stent graft is now visible.

refine the volume (Fig. 6-47). The advantage of this technique when compared with cut planes is that the region-of-interest drawing can follow complex curved paths that closely follow the contours of vessels of interest and are not constrained to a flat plane. Some workstations allow the user to draw several regions of interest at key points through the imaging volume between which the computer interpolates the intervening regions. For example, this method can be applied to every 10 or 15 cross sections and then interpolated to include the intervening sections to remove the lumbar spine and pelvis from an abdominal CT angiogram (1,3).

A final manual segmentation method employs "region-growing." Region-growing occurs when the user deposits a seed point within a structure to be retained or to

be removed. The user provides an upper and a lower boundary for the growth of the segmentation into contiguous voxels. In the case of CT, an upper and lower attenuation value is defined; in the case of magnetic resonance imaging (MRI), an upper and lower signal value is defined. The region-growing will occur into all connected voxels within the threshold range. Once identified in this fashion, these voxels can either be selected for retention within the imaging volume or for deletion from the volume (1,3) (Fig. 6-48).

Region-growing can be a very effective means for removing complex geometries such as pelvic bones from CT data. A challenge occurs when enhanced arterial lumina and skeletal structures lie next to one another, allowing the segmentation of osseous structures to "bleed"

(*text continues on page 230*)

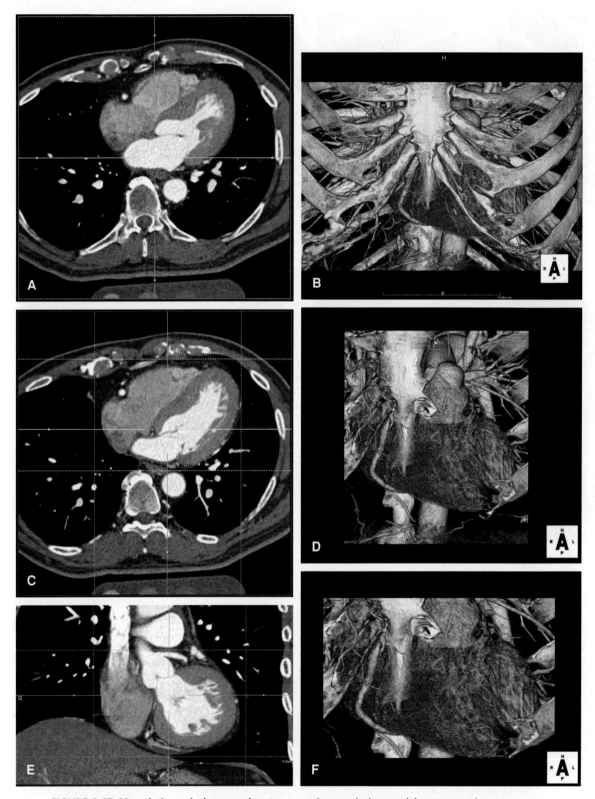

FIGURE 6-47 3D sculpting to isolate complex structures. Because the heart and the accompanying coronary arteries lie in close proximity to other high attenuation structures such as the chest wall, pulmonary vessels, diaphragm and abdominal contents, and great vessels, greater intervention is required to sufficiently segment the heart for coronary artery visualization on VR. **A:** Transverse section through the midventricular level and **(B)** accompanying VR demonstrate the inability to visualize the coronary arteries without segmentation. **C:** Initial application of cut planes (*dashed blue and green lines*) results in a VR **(D)** that is free of some portions of the chest wall; however, substantial regions of the sternum and anterior ribs remain. **E:** Superior and inferior cut planes can be applied (*red dashed lines*) to eliminate the majority of the abdominal contents and great vessels **(F)**.

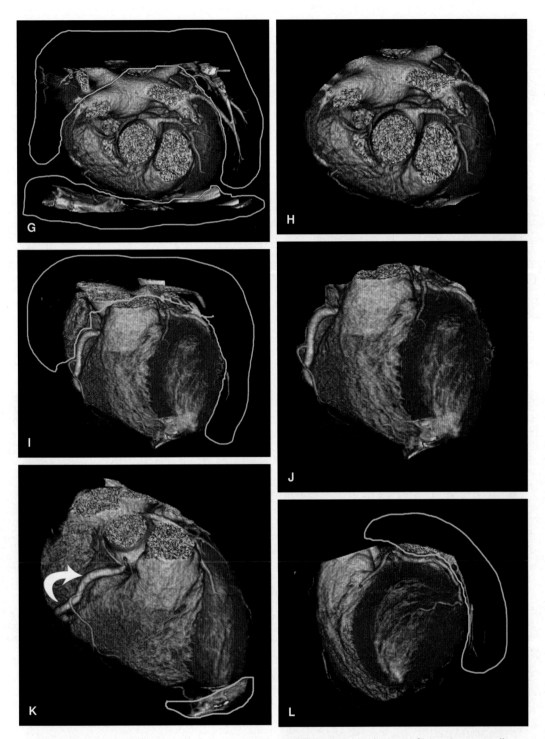

FIGURE 6-47 Continued G: The VR is then reoriented to a cranial projection, and regions of interest are manually drawn (*green*) around the remaining anterior chest wall and portions of the left atrium, posterior diaphragm, and left posterior pulmonary vessels. Critical to the effectiveness of this approach is the identification of a projection that allows display of a cleavage plane between the heart and the anterior chest wall, for example, that allows drawing of a region of interest between the two structures. **H:** VR following extrusion of these regions of interest perpendicularly through the volume and subsequent elimination of these voxels isolated in **(G)** from the rendering. **I:** Rotation of the VR identifies additional cardiac regions to eliminate in order to improve visualization of the left main and right coronary arteries. An additional region of interest (*green*) is drawn. Elimination of these voxels extruded through the volume results in the VR shown in **(J)**. **K:** A small region of the anterior chest wall remains and is isolated with an additional small green region-of-interest drawing. The right coronary artery (*curved arrow*) is now fully exposed. **L:** Pulmonary venous branches in close proximity to the circumflex coronary artery are excluded with a final region-of-interest drawing. (*continues on next page*)

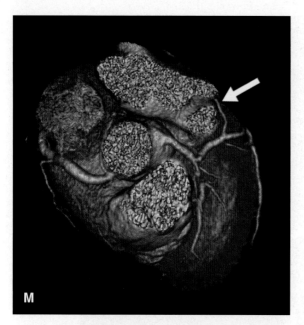

FIGURE 6-47 Continued M: Rotation of the VR allows unencumbered view of a left atrial branch (*straight arrow*) coursing posteriorly from the left circumflex coronary artery.

or "grow" contiguously into the adjacent blood vessels. Typical points of contact within the abdomen and pelvis include lumbar arteries and the superior gluteal arteries as they pass through the sciatic notch. Using preliminary region-of-interest drawing, it is possible to identify and separate these small connection points and allow the seeded region-growing to then proceed exclusively in the bones or blood vessels (Fig. 6-49). Another strategy that can be effective for disconnecting these "bridges" between bones and opacified blood vessels includes the application of erosion procedures that remove a user-selected number of voxels from the surface of the segmentation. Yet another approach involves the use of algorithms that are designed to identify thin bridges of a user-defined width (1 to 3 voxels) and remove those connection points prior to finalizing the segmentation.

In order to use region-growing for identifying structures that will remain or be removed, a fixed threshold value for the segmentation must be selected despite the presence of volume averaging at the periphery of structures

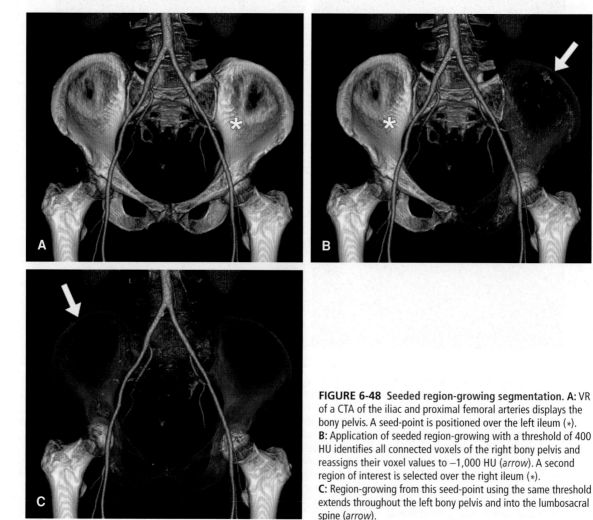

FIGURE 6-48 Seeded region-growing segmentation. A: VR of a CTA of the iliac and proximal femoral arteries displays the bony pelvis. A seed-point is positioned over the left ileum (∗).
B: Application of seeded region-growing with a threshold of 400 HU identifies all connected voxels of the right bony pelvis and reassigns their voxel values to −1,000 HU (*arrow*). A second region of interest is selected over the right ileum (∗).
C: Region-growing from this seed-point using the same threshold extends throughout the left bony pelvis and into the lumbosacral spine (*arrow*).

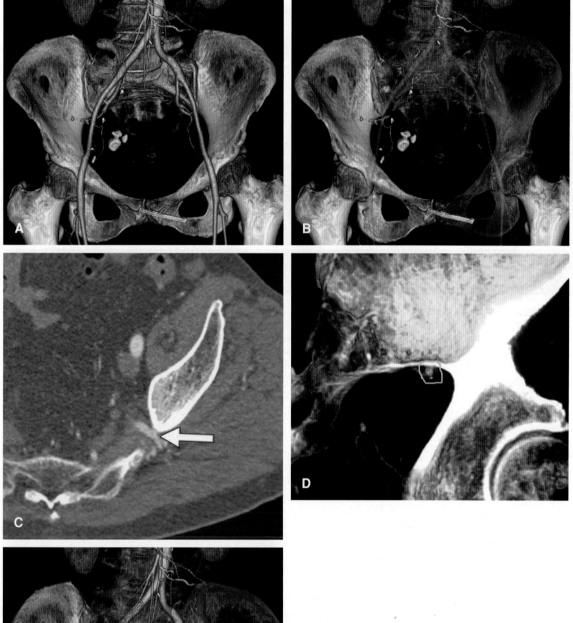

FIGURE 6-49 Controlling region-growing to prevent leakage into vascular structures. A: VR of a CTA of the iliac arteries and bony pelvis. **B:** Region-growing applied to the left hemipelvis results in simultaneous elimination of the arterial system. This occurs when enhanced arterial luminal voxels are in contiguity with skeletal voxels above the threshold desired for region-growing. **C:** A common culprit for this phenomenon within the pelvis is the superior gluteal artery as it passes underneath the sacrum (*arrow*). **D:** A small region of interest can be drawn to exclude a portion of the superior gluteal artery and thus disconnect the arterial system from the bony pelvis. **E:** Subsequent application of region-growing to the left hemipelvis allows preservation of the arterial system while excluding the bony structures.

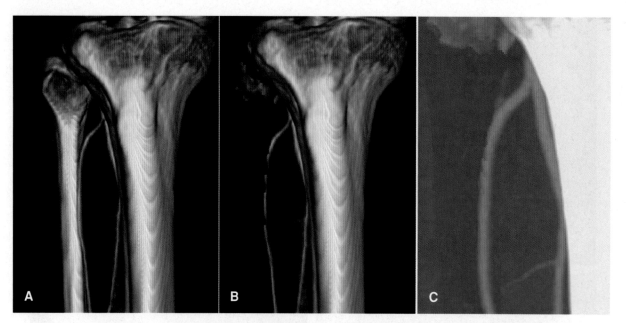

FIGURE 6-50 A: Frontal VR of CTA of the proximal right leg. **B:** Region-growing applied to the right fibula excludes the majority of the fibula; however, the close proximity of the anterior tibial artery to the surface of the fibula has resulted in discontinuity, mimicking stenoses, in the proximal anterior tibial artery. **C:** Regional dilation of the segmentation around the proximal anterior tibial artery recruits voxels back into the imaging volume and allows a normal anterior tibial artery to be visualized on this frontal MIP.

that results in a transition zone between any object and its background. Segmentation using threshold values may not remove these peripheral transition voxels. After removing skeletal structures from a volume, for example, the "ghost" edges of bones can obscure visualization of the target blood vessels. If on the other hand segmented arteries isolated from a volume are selected for display, the absence of the transition voxels of vascular lumina results in an unrealistic visualization that diminishes the caliber of the blood vessel and can create artifactual stenoses. The solution to both of these limitations is the application of a dilation procedure where voxels are recruited onto the surface of the selected segmentation, allowing the inclusion of the edge voxels prior to deleting the segmentation in the case of skeletal removal or prior to deleting the background in the case of vessel isolation (Fig. 6-50).

Automated, single-click algorithms have recently been introduced on commercial workstations for a number of specific tasks. These include but are not limited to bone removal, chest wall removal, cardiac extraction, and coronary arterial extraction. The implementation of these algorithms varies substantially by vendors and tends to be proprietary. In general, when these algorithms work properly, they can quickly and effectively complete their targeted task and can greatly facilitate image interpretation. However,

none of these algorithms works on all cases, and when applying these algorithms, the data should be scrutinized carefully to recognize unintended removal of key structures or artificial creation of pseudo-lesions (Fig. 6-51).

MASK SUBTRACTION

Mask subtraction is a method of increasing the signal-to-background ratio currently used in MRI. By using identical imaging parameters to obtain unenhanced "mask" images followed immediately by postcontrast (timed for optimal vascular enhancement) images, enhancement images with very little background contamination can be obtained by subtracting the mask from the contrast-enhanced images. This principle is similar to that in digital subtraction angiography (DSA), although like DSA, such subtraction images can be rendered misrepresentative or virtually useless if the patient moves between the mask and the contrast-enhanced acquisition (11,16,22).

Subtraction of pre- and postcontrast 3D MRA data sets can be performed in two ways. The process can be performed by subtracting the complex numbers composing the two corresponding raw data sets and then generating a magnitude data set from the result or by first reconstructing the magnitude data of the pre- and postcontrast acquisitions and then subtracting these magnitude values (16).

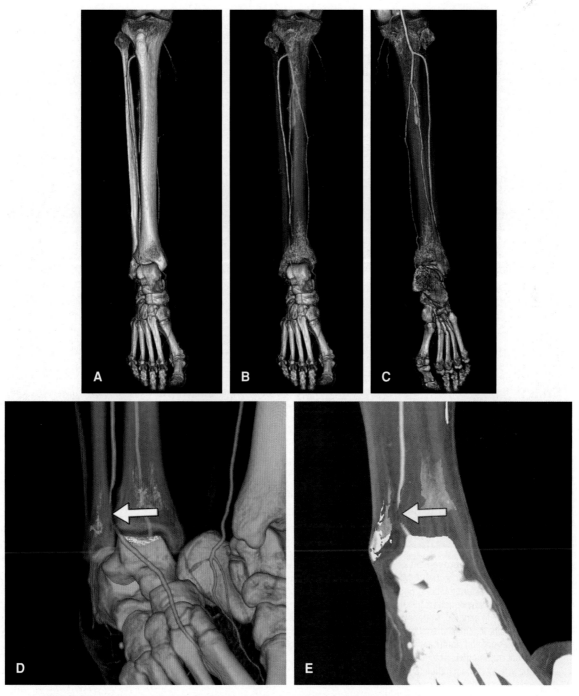

FIGURE 6-51 Automated tibial and fibular bone removal. A: VR of CTA of the right leg prior to segmentation allows minimal visualization of the arterial system. **B:** Automated extraction of tibia and fibula unmasks the majority of the infrapopliteal arteries as viewed anteriorly and **(C)** posteriorly. **D:** Careful examination of the distal anterior tibial artery reveals spurious removal of a portion of the vessel during the segmentation process (*arrow*). **E:** The irregular/jagged edge of the segmentation (*arrow*) is best seen on an MIP and a telltale sign that the abnormality is artifactual rather than evidence for disease.

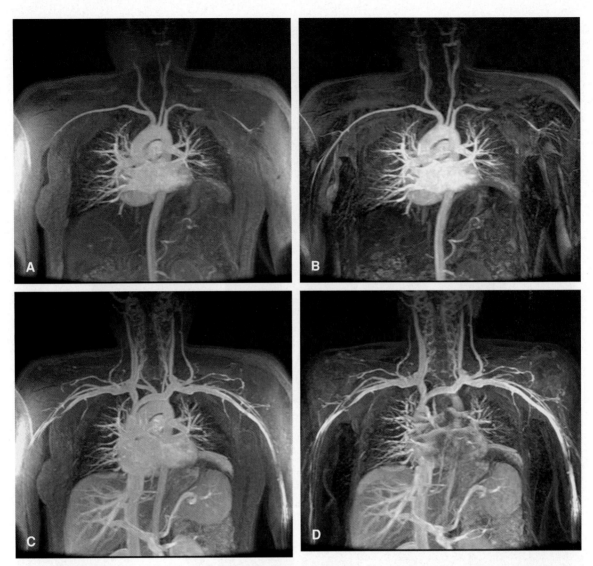

FIGURE 6-52 Improvement of MIP MR images using subtraction on chest MRA/magnetic resonance venography (MRV). This chest MRA/MRV was performed with an otherwise identical set of images obtained before contrast (mask), at peak arterial bolus of gadolinium contrast, and in a venous delayed phase. From a technical standpoint, the examination was optimal. MIPs from primary reconstructions of both the arterial phase **(A)** and the delayed phase **(C)** are shown. In addition, MIPs of the peak arterial subtraction **(B;** arterial phase minus mask) and venous subtraction **(D;** delayed phase minus arterial phase) are shown. In this case, the decreased background levels of the arterial subtraction MIP does not add significant value to interpretation based on the primary arterial reconstructions. However, subtracting arterial contributions of enhancement **(A)** from the delayed acquisition **(C)** yields images of venous enhancement with little arterial contamination **(D)**.

Most commonly, magnitude images reconstructed by the scanner are used for subtraction, as this represents the simplest and least time-consuming approach. However, complex subtraction has an advantage in that it may overcome partial volume effects related to the phase difference between flowing and stationary spins in a voxel. Complex subtraction is especially beneficial for time-resolved thick-slab 2D imaging and to improve conspicuity of small vessels and edges of vessels (11,16).

Subtraction data can make the images created by using the ray casting techniques of VR, including MIP, MinIP, and

ray sum, easier to understand and more aesthetically pleasing, providing arterial or venous enhancement images (Fig. 6-52). Even more important than for VR as a whole, it is imperative to examine the nonsubtracted primarily reconstructed source images to ensure that misregistration of mask and postcontrast images do not artificially obscure real lesions or create pseudo-lesions (Fig. 6-53).

While there is no technical reason that subtraction could not be utilized in CTA, the additional radiation dose required for a mask acquisition makes this endeavor less practical than in MRA.

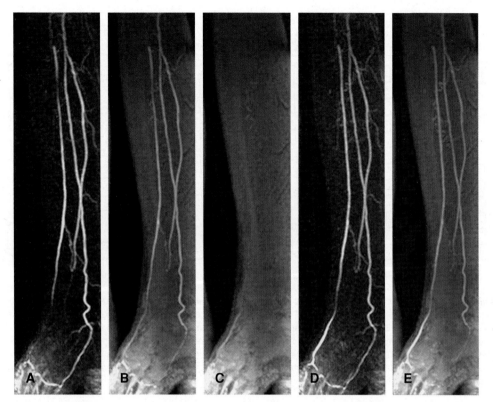

FIGURE 6-53 Identification of pseudo-lesions from subtraction. When utilizing subtraction images for 3D image processing, it is essential to review the original, nonsubtracted images in conjunction with the subtracted images. In this MRA, MIPs of the arterial phase subtraction series suggest occlusion of the distal dorsalis pedis artery of the right foot **(A)**. However, review of MIPs from the prospective, nonsubtracted images show an enhancing dorsalis pedis artery **(B)**. MIP from the preinjection mask series **(C)** shows residual gadolinium in the dorsalis pedis from a prior injection of contrast; this vessel is slow to fill and drain. Because of the high background signal in the mask **(A)**, the low level of enhancement in the early postgadolinium images **(B)**, and the high background levels from the MIP process, this vessel was obscured. On MIP images from both a more delayed series **(D)** as well as the corresponding subtraction series **(E)**, this vessel clearly fills as expected.

IMAGE QUALITY AND THREE-DIMENSIONAL VISUALIZATION AND ANALYSIS

It is an undeniable feature of 3D analysis that the quality of the visualization is directly related to the quality of the input data. The imaging strategies discussed in Chapters 1 and 2 create a critical foundation for effective 3D visualization and analysis. The adage "garbage in, garbage out," certainly applies to image analysis. Effective 3D analysis is ideally achieved by using isotropic voxels (voxels of equal size on all three dimensions), preferably with less than 1 mm^3 dimensions (Fig. 6-54). While as a generalization optimal 3D imaging requires isotropic voxels, isotropy is an impractical goal in MRI since the acquisition time penalty for increasing resolution in the frequency encode direction is significantly less than an equivalent increase in resolution in either the slice or phase directions. As a result, MRA volumes are frequently acquired with appreciably anisotropic voxels, with the greatest voxel dimension in the slice-encode direction but also with variability of in-plane voxel dimensions depending on the phase and frequency encode steps of the imaging matrix. In MRI, the imaging volume should be set up such that the directions of spatial encoding resulting in the smallest voxel dimensions can be prescribed to correspond with the axes of imaging that require the finest spatial detail.

Of equal importance to the spatial resolution is the contrast-to-noise ratio. This ratio can be adversely impacted both by a reduction in the numerator (contrast) and an increase in the denominator (noise). Key vascular structures can disappear into the background from inadequate blood pool contrast due to insufficient or poorly timed delivery of a contrast agent, or especially in the case of MR, from inappropriate acquisition parameters that result in either excessive background signal or insufficient blood pool signal. Minimizing image noise requires an appropriate balance between patient-specific factors such as patient size and movement and acquisition-specific parameters as discussed

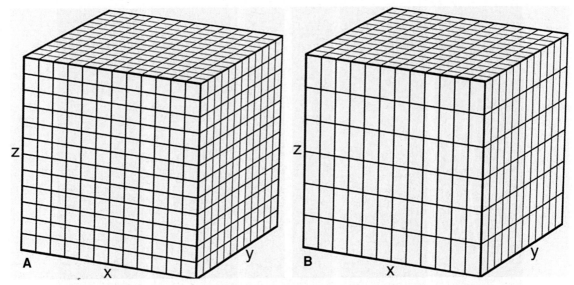

FIGURE 6-54 Isotropic versus nonisotropic voxels. Isotropic voxels refer to imaging voxels where the dimensions and resolution of the voxels are equivalent in all three planes **(A)**, shaped like a cube. The advantage of acquiring data by using isotropic voxels is that reformatted images have the same spatial resolution as the primarily reconstructed ones. In contrast, when voxels are not isotropic, the spatial resolution of the output image depends on the axis of measurement. **B:** The *z*-axis has half the spatial resolution of the other two dimensions. Assuming that the primary reconstructions are in the *xy* plane, any reformatted images will have a spatial resolution that is poorer than the resolution in the primary reconstruction.

in Chapters 1 and 2. Once data acquisition is complete, it may be possible to improve the contrast-to-noise ratio by using noise reduction filters; however, the application of these filters comes at the expense of spatial resolution. Typical with CT, these filters may involve the retrospective reconstruction of a data set by using a "soft" or "low-resolution" reconstruction algorithm in order to minimize noise. Although the diminished spatial resolution reduces the quality of the source reconstructions, it can be an effective option for creating key visualizations of larger structures such as aortic aneurysms in difficult patients for whom their CT acquisition has an inherently low contrast-to-noise ratio.

An additional challenge for 3D visualization specific to MRI results from signal heterogeneity within the imaging volume typically related to the use of surface coils. This limitation has diminished in recent years with the effective use of phased array coils, surface intensity correction algorithms, and parallel imaging techniques. As described previously, segmentation can also reduce the impact of such signal heterogeneities on VR images (1,3,5,9,14,22).

Vessel Quantification

While 3D and 4D visualization are key enablers for maximizing the diagnostic potential of CT and MR angiographic data sets, quantitative treatment planning necessitates the measurement of a variety of vascular and lesion characteristics. Although open surgical repair of vascular

lesions may allow for direct fitting and adjustment of vascular prostheses based on intraoperative measurements, the trend toward transluminal therapy for many vascular lesions requires that accurate measurements be made based on imaging alone. Although some arterial quantification is possible by using projectional angiographic techniques immediately prior to endovascular device deployment, limitations of projection such as parallax and magnification can limit the effectiveness of measurements obtained by using projectional angiography (23).

The two most important measurements for characterizing vascular lesions, both occlusive and aneurysmal, are measurements of vessel cross section by using images orthogonal to the vessel lumen/wall and measurements of vessel length by using images parallel to the lumen (1,9,14,24).

Orthogonal Dimensions

When assessing arterial occlusive disease, luminal dimensions are used to quantify the severity of arterial stenoses. While measurement of the outer wall dimension will provide an opportunity to assess for the presence of positive or negative remodeling and may at some point have an important bearing on the method chosen for revascularization, at the present time quantification of outer wall dimensions has no routine clinical application in the setting of occlusive disease.

In contrast, when assessing arterial aneurysms, both luminal and outer wall dimensions are relevant for planning

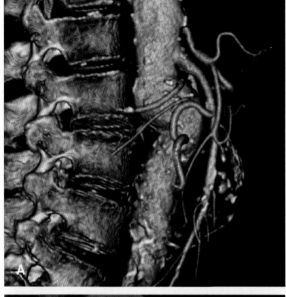

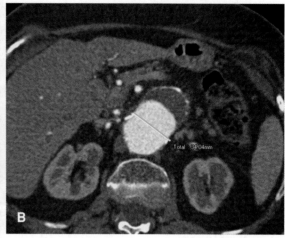

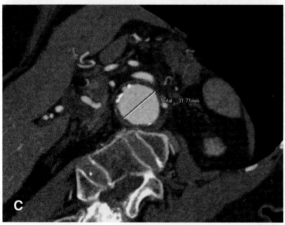

FIGURE 6-55 Importance of double oblique cross sections for measuring vessel dimensions. A: Lateral VR of an abdominal aortic CTA demonstrates tortuosity of the suprarenal neck of an abdominal aortic aneurysm. **B:** Transverse section through the neck of the aneurysm with measurement of the shortest cross-sectional diameter provides a measurement of the luminal dimension of 34 mm. Reorientation of the axes to the aortic flow lumen results in a double oblique cross section at this level **(C)** that provides a minimum luminal dimension of 32 mm. Measurement variation of as little as 2 mm can impact the sizing of endovascular devices.

therapy. In general, luminal dimensions impact the delivery of endoluminal devices, while the dimensions of the outer wall define the origin and terminus of the aneurysm and help to establish landmarks for the fixation of the endoluminal devices. Greater detail of the planning for endoluminal device deployment is provided in subsequent chapters.

Varying degrees of rigor can be brought to bear on the measurement of orthogonal vessel dimensions. It first should be stated that accurate cross-sectional dimensions of a blood vessel should only be made from a cross section that is perpendicular (orthogonal) to the median axis of the blood vessel. The median axis for a given segment of artery may be different depending on whether measurement of the lumen or of the outer wall is desired. While it is convenient to measure arterial dimensions from a primary reconstruction, this measurement may not be accurate even when the shortest dimension is used to quantify vascular size. This is particularly true when cross-sectional vessel dimen-

sions are not circular as is frequently the case in the setting of atheroma, which may be both irregular and eccentrically positioned within the vessel lumen (23) (Fig. 6-55).

Orthogonal cross sections of a vessel can be manually created using a 3D workstation by rotating orientation crosshairs to be perpendicular in all reference planes to the vessel wall or lumen at the measurement point (Fig. 6-56). Automatic methods are also available to extract the median centerline for the purpose of cross-sectional dimensional measurement and are discussed subsequently (1,9,14,24).

Diameter Measurement

Once an orthogonal cross section is available, there are a variety of methods to measure the lumen or outer wall. The simplest method is to manually position measurement cursors on opposite walls of the blood vessel. While these "digital calipers" should provide an accurate indication of the defined distance, the arbitrary nature of the positioning of

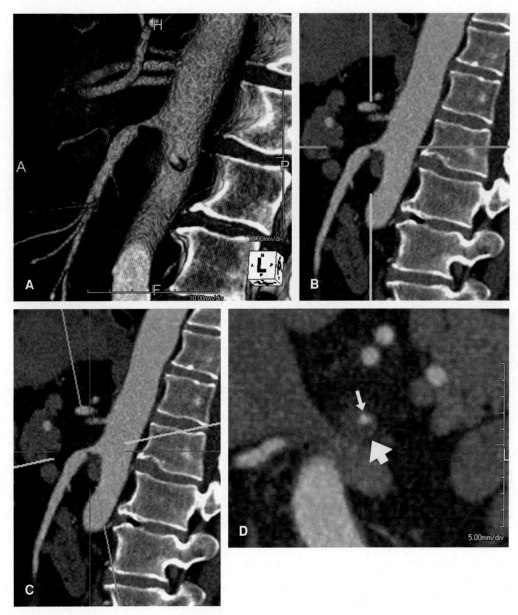

FIGURE 6-56 Cross-sectional area characterization of arterial stenoses, manual method. A: Lateral VR and **(B)** sagittal MPR of an abdominal CTA demonstrate stenosis in the proximal superior mesenteric artery. **C:** Orientation of the cross hairs perpendicular to the region of stenosis (*green line*) allows a cross section perpendicular to the stenosis axis (*red line*) to be created **(D)**. Both the lumen and outer wall of the SMA with direct visualization of mural atheroma (*wide arrow*) and the lumen (*small arrow*) results. Both regions are now available for measurement.

the origin and terminus of the calipers can introduce variability in the measurement (Fig. 6-57). A more consistent means for measuring luminal dimension is to utilize a line density profile through the vessel cross section and quantify the luminal dimension by identifying the half maximum value between the lumen and the wall or between the outer wall and the periarterial tissues (Fig. 6-58). The availability and ease of use of this method varies depending on the workstation available; however, this technique should provide more consistent measurements of vessel

dimension when compared with visual deposition of digital cursors (23).

Cross-sectional Area Measurement

Although the measurement of a single cross-sectional dimension or possibly maximum and minimal dimensions have become the convention for quantifying arterial cross sections, volumetric data acquired by using CT and MR provide the opportunity for quantification of the cross-sectional area (CSA) of the artery. Because CSA length and

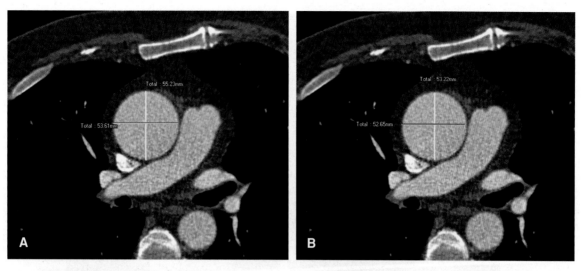

FIGURE 6-57 Variability of manual measurements made by using digital calipers. A, B: Two sets of manual measurements of the ascending aorta on a transverse CT section result in dimensions of 54 × 55 mm and 53 × 53 mm. When examining the red and yellow traces of the measurements, both sets of measurements seem valid.

shape dictate the hemodynamic impact of occlusive lesions, there are theoretic advantages to characterizing arterial stenoses based on measurements of CSA and irregularity. Nevertheless, drawing on years of collective experience quantifying arteries from projectional angiographic data, vir-

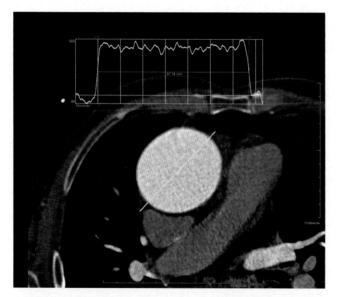

FIGURE 6-58 Automated determination of vessel dimension. A line density profile is plotted above the transverse CT section of the ascending aorta. The aortic lumen is represented as the central plateau, and the mediastinal fat is represented as the lower plateaus at the extremes of the curve. The transition between these plateaus corresponds to the aortic wall, burred by in-plane volume averaging. The dimension of the ascending aorta can be reproducibly measured by calculating the full width at half maximum of the line density profile, indicated by the horizontal *yellow line* between the two vertical *red lines*. The length of the resulting line segment, 67 mm, is automatically determined.

tually all published literature and vascular device deployment guidelines are based on diameter measurements. This fact should not hinder the imager from using tools to quantify CSA as a means of providing a mean cross-sectional diameter of the blood vessel. The mean diameter (D_m) of the blood vessel can be calculated as $D_m = \frac{2}{\pi} \sqrt{CSA}$.

Workstation-based tools for quantifying CSA rely on accurate edge detection between the lumen and the vessel wall. While seemingly a simple task, accurate vessel lumen segmentation must be adaptable to varying degrees of luminal enhancement both between different patients as well as within the arterial tree of a single patient examination, where depending on the timing of the contrast medium bolus, substantial variations in intraluminal density/signal can occur as one proceeds proximally to distally along the arterial tree (Fig. 6-59). Another challenge specific to CT scanning is the need for segmentation algorithms to accurately discriminate the interfaces between luminal opacification and both the adjacent higher attenuation mural calcifications or metal as well as the lower attenuation noncalcified vessel wall. Again, it is critical for the imager to directly visualize the segmentation created by the workstation prior to accepting any automated quantification of CSA area or D_m (Fig. 6-60). It is not uncommon for segmentation algorithms to inappropriately include mural calcium with the arterial lumen, leading to spurious measurements (Fig. 6-60)(23).

One final point relating to the accuracy of CSA and diameter measurements is that measurement accuracy becomes harder to define with greater voxel anisotropy. With appropriate MDCT acquisitions, near-isotropic

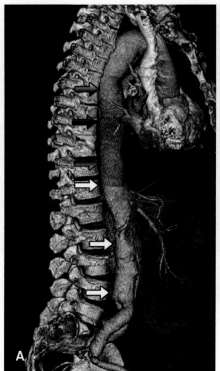

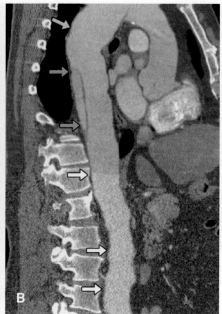

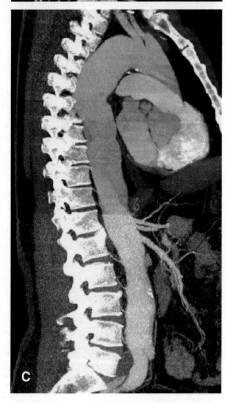

FIGURE 6-59 Variations in contrast enhancement within the aorta. A–C: Volume rendering, curved planar reformation, and MIP, respectively, following acquisition of a gated CTA of the thoracic aorta, 5 seconds elapsed before a nongated helical acquisition of the abdominal aorta commenced. This delay resulted in greater time for the opacification for the aorta to develop and thus a discrete transition zone between the lesser enhancing thoracic aorta (*gray arrows*) and the more enhanced abdominal aorta (*white arrows*). Threshold-based segmentation of the lumen will not provide accurate aortic measurements unless the threshold value adapts to the aortic attenuation at the point of measurement.

resolution is routine. The voxel anisotropy frequently seen in MRI acquisitions causes the measurement accuracy to vary depending on the axes and planes of measurement, making accurate quantification of arterial cross sections more difficult (Fig. 6-61).

Vessel Length

The length of an arterial stenosis determines both the type of therapy (transluminal vs. open bypass) and the length of the stent, when indicated. Additionally, the location of a stenosis or aneurysm relative to arterial branch points can be a critical

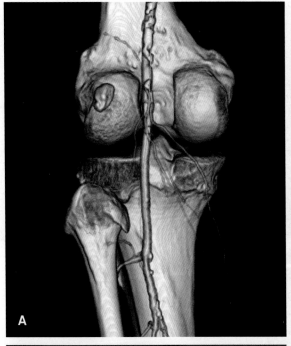

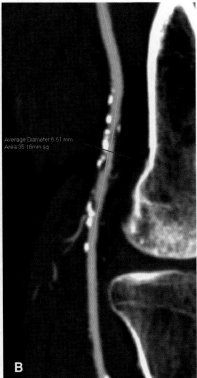

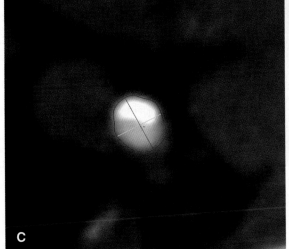

FIGURE 6-60 Automated quantification of a calcified artery. A: The automatically extracted median centerline (*green*) appears to track the lumen of the popliteal artery on this CTA. **B:** Careful examination of the centerline on the resulting CPR demonstrates that the centerline is biased toward the mural calcium, suggesting that the luminal margin detection algorithm is spuriously including the mural calcium. The *blue line* segment is selected for cross-sectional analysis. **C:** The orthogonal MPR resulting from the blue line segment in **(B)** shows the automated segmentation of the vessel as a blue line, confirming the spurious inclusion of calcium and overestimation of luminal dimension.

determinant in device selection and treatment method. For the majority of applications, vessel length as measured by the length of the median centerline of the blood vessel provides the most relevant arterial dimension. This length can be manually extracted by summing multiple line segments positioned through the median axis of the artery from the origin to the terminus of the length measurement, or it can be automatically determined through the use of algorithms that extract the median centerline (Fig. 6-62). Segmentation algorithms that might inappropriately include calcifications in the vessel lumen may result not only in inaccurate cross-sectional dimensional measurements but also in incorrect vessel length measurements if the path of the centerline deviates toward regions of calcifications (Fig. 6-63). Analogous

to the confirmation of cross-sectional luminal segmentation for D_m measurement, visual confirmation of the position of the automatically extracted median centerline should be performed by the imager prior to relying on such a path for length measurements (23).

One notable circumstance where the median centerline may not be the preferred measurement for determining appropriate endovascular therapy occurs in the setting of arterial aneurysms. When the aneurysms are large and eccentrically positioned relative to the proximal and distal necks, the median centerline through the aneurysm can deviate substantially from the ultimate path of a stent graft deployed within the lumen. With respect to aortic stent grafts, the stiffness of current generation devices tends to

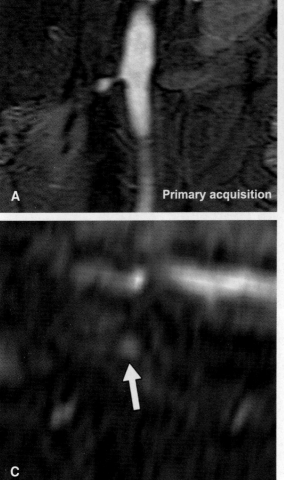

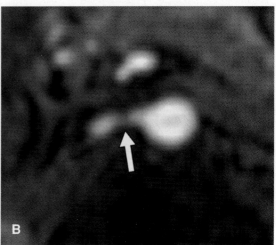

FIGURE 6-61 **Voxel anisotropy in MRA. A:** Primary coronal reconstruction from a gadolinium-enhanced 3D MRA from a 320-mm field-of-view acquisition with 512 frequency and 256 phase-encoding steps, resulting in pixel dimensions of 0.6 mm (superoinferior) × 1.25 mm (right to left). There is a stenosis at the origin of the right renal artery. **B:** Transverse MPR through the stenosis (*arrow*) has pixel dimensions of 1.25 mm (right to left) × 2 mm (anteroposterior). The greater pixel dimensions result in a blurrier image than that shown in **(A)**. **C:** The position of maximal stenosis (*arrow*) is presented on this orthogonal MPR. Differential blurring as a result of varying pixel dimensions will result in varying degrees of measurement accuracy, depending on the orientation of the measurement.

dictate that they follow the shortest distance through an aortic aneurysm between the proximal and distal necks. In planning stent-graft deployment into aortic aneurysms that have large luminal CSA dimensions, modification of the median centerline toward a method that identifies a shorter path through the aneurysm may result in more accurate planning (23,25) (Fig. 6-64).

Arterial Tortuosity

Arterial tortuosity can be highly variable from patient to patient and across arterial beds. The degree of tortuosity can have an important impact on endoluminal therapy, as stiff devices are more apt to injure the vessel wall at sites of greater local curvature (26). Throughout the era of projectional angiography, vessel tortuosity has been poorly characterized due to the inability of the 2D projections to indicate true vessel curvature in three dimensions (Fig. 6-65A, B). As a result, there is a paucity of literature describing meth-

ods for quantifying vessel tortuosity and applying those measurements to clinical decision making. However, volumetric data provided by CT and MR are readily amenable to tortuosity quantification (25,27). This quantification is predominately performed by calculating median centerline curvature, which is the inverse of the radius of curvature as defined by a circle fit to a region of the arterial centerline. The length of arterial centerline selected for circle fitting can impact local curvature measurements. In general, noise along the centerline can result in widely variable curvature measurements if too short of a segment of the centerline is considered for local curvature measurement. For most applications within the aortoiliac system, 5- to 10-mm vessel lengths produce the most useful characterization of arterial curvature. A plot of arterial curvature relative to vessel length thus can be created by incrementing at regular intervals the location of circle fits to the arterial centerline (Fig. 6-65C).

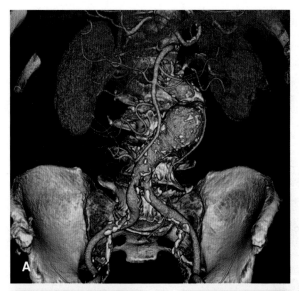

FIGURE 6-62 Manual versus automated centerline extraction. A: VR of a CTA with an abdominal aortic aneurysm. Accurate centerline extraction is required prior to measuring the aneurysm length. **B:** Manual centerline drawn over eight selected transverse sections. Linear interpolation between the manually selected vertices results in the red curve. The insufficient selection of centerline points results in several long, straight segments that do not pass through the center of lumen, evident by the smaller than expected width of the aneurysm. **C:** Automatically extracted centerline (*green*) is smoother than the manual centerline but tends to bias to the inner curve of the aneurysm neck and is not perfectly positioned in the center of the aneurysm. Neither technique is perfect, and manual adjustment of the automated centerline is typically required for a precise measurement.

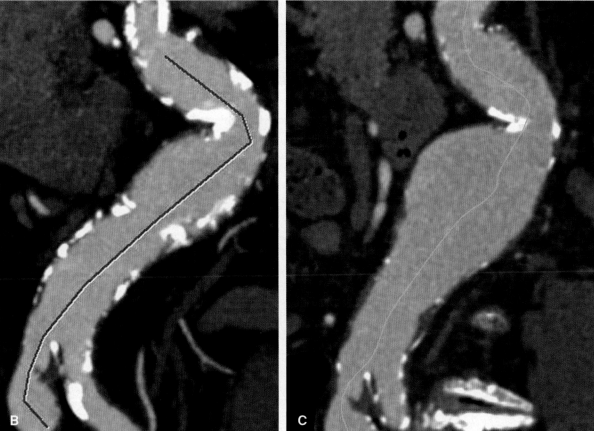

Arterial Branch and Aneurysm Neck Angle Measurements

Although the literature is replete with recommendations on how to perform arterial angle measurements, rarely is a specific method for angle measurement articulated to allow for reproducible results. While it is intuitive to conceptualize the measurement of particular arterial branch angles or to define an angle between the supra-aneurysmal aortic neck and the aneurysm body, the variability and arbitrary nature with which the vertices of the angles are selected can result in widely disparate angle measurements. For characterizing an aneurysm neck, curvature measurements are likely

(*text continues on page 246*)

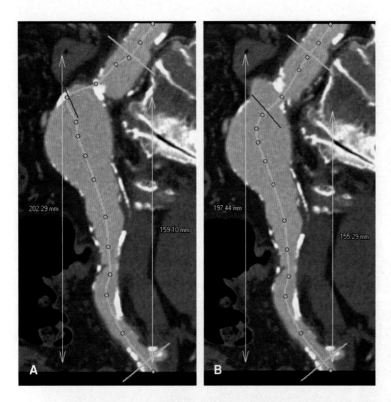

FIGURE 6-63 Inaccurate automated centerline biased by mural calcium. A: Automatically extracted centerline (*green*) with control points (*green dots*) demonstrates an erroneous control point within anterior calcification in the proximal aneurysm (*blue line*). The length of the centerline segment defined by the *green line* segments is 202 mm. **B:** Following correction of the erroneous control point, the centerline segment length measures 197 mm.

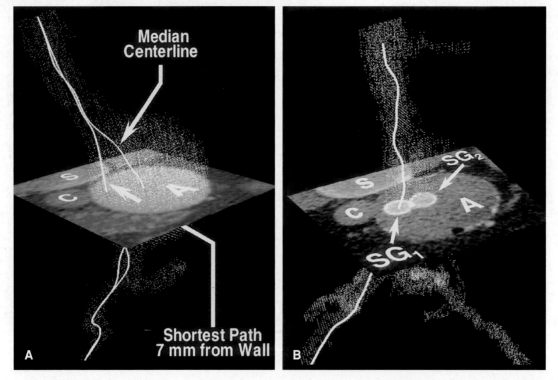

FIGURE 6-64 Prediction of stent-graft path for accurate length measurement for stent-graft sizing. A: Automated extraction of the median centerline and the shortest path through an abdominal aortic aneurysm that maintains a 7-mm distance (equal to the radius of the stent graft to be placed) from the wall. The shortest path measures 36 mm less than the median centerline. (A, aneurysm; C, inferior vena cava; S, spine.) **B:** CTA of the same patient as in **(A)** 1 day after deployment of a stent graft. The aneurysm around the stent graft has thrombosed. The primary stent-graft limb (SG_1) and the secondarily positioned contralateral limb (SG_2) also are indicated. The median centerline of SG_1 is indicated by the *white line*. Note the similarity between the position of this path and that of the shortest path calculated predeployment in **(A)**. The length of this path was 139 mm long, 2 mm more than the predeployment shortest path length measurement and 34 mm less than the predeployment median centerline length. (Reprinted from Tillich M, Hill BB, Paik DS, et al. Prediction of aortoiliac stent-graft length: comparison of measurement methods. *Radiology.* 2001;220:475–483.)

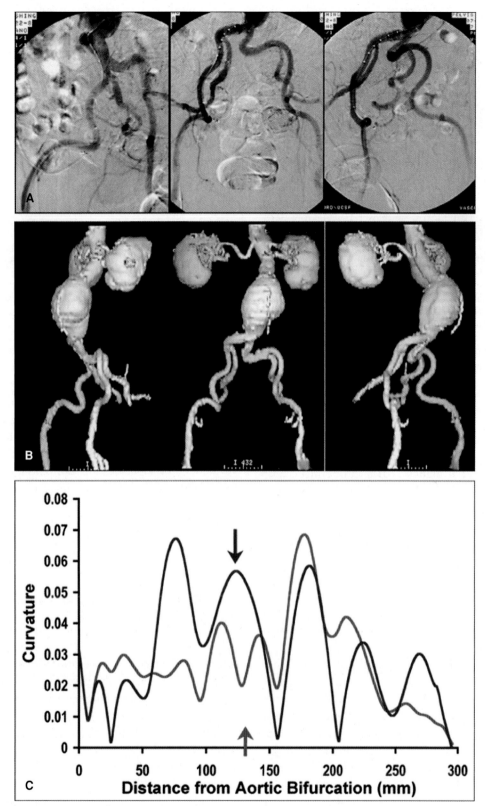

FIGURE 6-65 Arterial tortuosity quantified as median centerline curvature. A: Three views (**left to right**: 45-degree right posterior oblique, anteroposterior, and 45-degree left posterior oblique) from a conventional iliac arteriogram demonstrates tortuosity of the iliac arteries bilaterally. The appearance of the local arterial curvature varies depending on the projection. Because curvature can be both over and underrepresented on projectional views, it is unlikely that any of these standard projections accurately represents the local curvature at all points along the iliac arteries. B: Three SSDs from a CTA in the same patient provide somewhat better assessment of curvature owing to the representation of surface shading, but the basic limitations of the conventional angiograms persist. C: Plot of arterial curvature for the left (*blue*) and right (*red*) iliac arteries from the aortic bifurcation to the femoral arteries. The *blue* and *red arrows* indicate the bifurcations of the common iliac arteries, respectively. Curvature is quantified as the inverse of the radius of a circle fit to a 5-mm long arc incremented every millimeter along the lengths of the iliac arteries. This quantitative output does not suffer from the limitations of the image-based analysis, as curvature values are absolute and independent of projection.

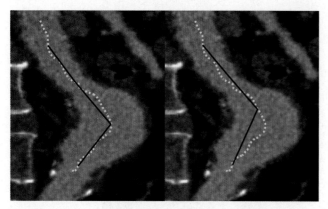

FIGURE 6-66 Measurement of proximal aneurysm neck angulation. Two CPRs of an abdominal aortic aneurysm demonstrate differing approaches to measuring proximal neck angulation. *Yellow points* denote the median centerline of the lumen. The *black line* denotes the angle measured. Without strict rules for establishing measurement landmarks, substantial angle measurement variability can result. Although there are an innumerable number of potential selectable points for determining the proximal neck angulation, the curvature of the centerline at any point along the aorta is defined and could be a more reliable means for quantifying "angulation."

to provide a more reproducible and principled means for determining thresholds for treatment (Fig. 6-66). The calculation of arterial branch angles can be made more reproducible, particularly when using median centerlines, provided that specific rules are established for identifying the vertex of the angle as well as the distance into each branch that defines the endpoint of the line segments forming the angle (27,28).

Vessel Volume

Because aneurysms have complex 3D shapes, it has been hypothesized that the determination of aneurysm growth or shrinkage based on maximum cross-sectional measurements would not be as sensitive to aneurysm change as would be a measurement of aneurysm volume (29,30). Although the clinical relevance and applicability of tracking aneurysm volume is controversial, such volume determination is readily performed by using a 3D workstation. Because aneurysm volume measurement necessitates accurate segmentation of the outer wall of the aneurysm from perianeurysmal tissues and because those perianeurysmal tissues frequently have similar CT attenuation or MR signal characteristics as thrombus, the task of segmentation is challenging. To date, a robust automated solution has not been created for the complete segmentation of the outer wall of aneurysms. Structures that present particular challenge include the diaphragmatic crura, the inferior vena cava, the left renal vein and lumbar veins, the third portion of the duodenum, and retroperitoneal lymph nodes. Thus, pub-

lished data relating to aneurysm volumes are the result of manual or semiautomated segmentation typically performed by skilled technologists. This method of segmentation, where region-of-interest drawing is applied over individual cross sections or stacks of cross sections, and possibly combined with seeded region-growing and other higher order segmentation procedures, tends to be labor intensive and time consuming.

Arterial Quantification Software Packages

While all of the aforementioned measurement methods can be applied within the context of general tools available on 3D visualization workstations, most workstation designers have developed dedicated software routines for the purpose of quantifying vessel dimensions, particularly for planning aortic aneurysm stent-graft deployment. The spectrum of these packages spans the gamut from a collection of dedicated tools that facilitate clinically relevant measurements to a system that employs a highly scripted "wizard" that leads the user to graphically localize key anatomical landmarks so that the software algorithm can generate a battery of measurements that are then automatically populated into a graphical and/or tablature format (Fig. 6-67). Regardless of the level of sophistication and polish apparent in these remarkable applications, the imager remains ultimately responsible for the accuracy of these measurements. Therefore, the use of these software systems should always be performed in a manner that allows the imager to confirm the legitimacy of the final reported measurements.

IMAGE PROCESSING WORKSTATIONS

Until recently, all image processing workstations were stand-alone, closed-system desktop computers, and the majority of image analysis workstations in use today still follow this model. In the past, stand-alone workstations used computer systems that ran Unix-based operating systems; virtually all stand-alone workstations today operate under Microsoft Windows or Linux operating workstations. Within these systems are a variable number of central processing units (CPUs) and frequently specialized graphics processing units (GPUs) that might represent commercially available products or might be proprietary and specially designed for the workstation. Imaged volumes are transferred in their entirety onto the hard drive of the image processing workstation either by a scripted DICOM push procedure from the CT or MR scanner or through a user-initiated query (pull) at the imaging workstation of volume data either from a PACS database or directly from the scanner.

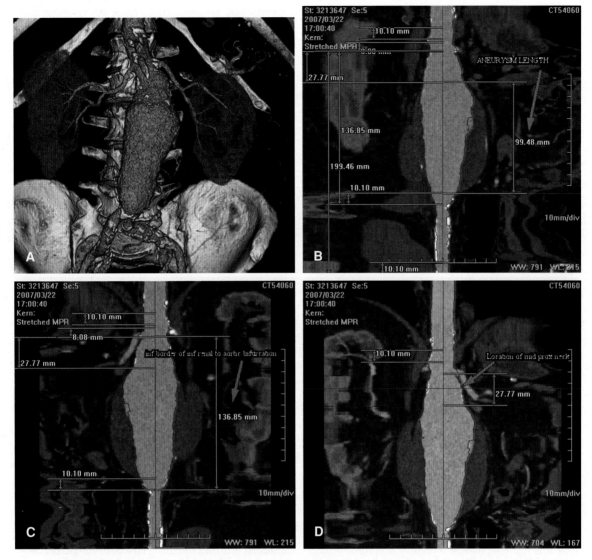

FIGURE 6-67 Automated quantification of aortic dimensions. A: VR of a CTA obtained for planning transluminal abdominal aortic aneurysm repair. Following median centerline extraction, a "stretched MPR" is generated from which key measurements are derived, including the aneurysm length (**B**), the distance from the inferior-most renal artery to the aortic bifurcation (**C**), and the length of the infrarenal neck (**D**).

Because a closed-system workstation prevents users from installing or launching software other than the image analysis software and supporting programs, the workstation can operate at its peak efficiency within the limits of the hardware configuration, software design, and size of the data set.

An alternative model for 3D analysis workstations is a purely software-based model, where the user purchases the 3D analytical software to load onto an open computer system either purchased specifically to run the software or possibly one that is already in use for other purposes (such as PACS). The software vendor typically specifies minimum configuration requirements of the CPU, GPU, random access memory (RAM), and hard drive needed for the software to perform

effectively. When purchasing software for 3D analysis, there is typically an option to purchase concurrent-use licenses, which then allow the user to install the software on an unlimited number of computers. In order to launch and use the software, however, the system may ensure that no more computers are simultaneously running the software than the license allows. This can be achieved by querying the network for other computers where the software is being run, by requiring that a specific hardware key is inserted into a universal serial bus (USB) port, or by utilizing a network license server that meters and regulates concurrent software use. Because this model offers substantially greater flexibility in the hardware that may be used, it provides an opportunity to deploy many image analysis workstations within a medical facility without the expense of purchasing new hardware where satisfactory hardware already exists. However, the performance of the software-based image processing workstations may not be as robust as with the stand-alone systems. Moreover, to date, stand-alone workstations tend to offer more features and specialized processing applications than do the software solutions.

A third model for providing image analysis is the "client-server model," also referred to as a "thin-client" solution. Client-server systems rely on a single server or multiple computer servers, each with many CPUs or GPUs to allow simultaneous processing of multiple volumetric data sets. The server hardware is typically placed in a computer room with a robust high-speed network connection, such that all image processing computations occur within the server. Client computers that run small, noncomputationally or graphically intensive programs communicate with the server by using a network connection to inform the server what manipulations are desired by the user and to receive and display images based on those manipulations. The communications between the client computer and the server occurs over a network, and thus the perceived performance of the thin-client system is dependent both on the server's computational performance as well as the available bandwidth on the network. With sufficient network bandwidth and server capacity, the performance of the client computer for directing and receiving 3D analysis can seem as effective and seamless as a stand-alone workstation. A substantial advantage of a system of this type is that with the purchase and configuration of a single server, an innumerable number of clients can exist within a medical center or even multiple medical centers linked by a common network to the server. The client computers can be typical desktop and laptop configurations; recent mainstream computers deployed for productivity applications and web browsing would be expected to have sufficient hardware resources to adequately function as clients. The client-server model can be a cost-effective solution that allows an institution to deploy 3D analytical capabilities well beyond the traditional locations of image interpretation reading rooms and into clinics, operating rooms, conference rooms, and physician offices. There is generally no added cost or limit to the number of clients that are created; however, licensing and the configuration of the server dictates the number of clients that can concurrently connect to the server or the number of imaging volumes that can be simultaneously loaded and analyzed. Because many physicians desiring access to 3D visualization may wish to manipulate a data set only sporadically, this configuration can easily support hundreds of clients. However, for a larger radiology department with increasing 3D image processing needs, additional servers may be required to meet the ongoing demands of the enterprise.

The primary limitation of the client-server model is insufficient network bandwidth, which is most often due to inadequacy of network cabling and switches but occasionally may be due to competing high-bandwidth network traffic, including data streams traveling from scanners to PACS or traveling from PACS to workstations. Another limitation of client-server systems is that current software releases do not include some of the more advanced processing tasks and features offered on stand-alone workstations such as complex segmentation and quantization tools. This limitation likely results from the relatively recent introduction of these systems and would be expected to diminish as these systems mature.

Workstation Features

While an image analysis workstation should be capable of creating MPRs, MIPs, VRs, and CPRs, there are many additional aspects of workstation design that impact the efficiency and ergonomy with which the workstation is to be used.

The method and ease with which data are transferred to the workstation or to the server for analysis should be flexible and rapid. Whenever possible, prefetching or pushing should be implemented so that the data are available when analysis and manipulation are desired. In some cases, 3D image processing workstations can be integrated with PACS workstations to maximize user convenience, although PACS vendors that offer this option usually only support pairing of 3D software packages from select partner vendors, limiting the user's choice of integrated 3D software packages. An effective independent workstation should be capable of managing data from multiple imaging modalities and generated by the full spectrum of imaging equipment vendors.

The interface between the user and the workstation should be intuitive, customizable, and easily mastered. While a common thread for all clinical workstations today is the use of a keyboard with a computer mouse or trackball, the integration of keyboard shortcuts and the effective application of the three-button mouse is heterogeneously applied across workstations. If possible, a cluttered screen with deeply embedded menu options and an interface that necessitates moving the cursor to various corners and edges of the display in order to activate tools should be avoided. Ultimately, the user's preference for certain types of interfaces and tools is a personal choice, but prior to purchasing a workstation, a thorough investigation of the features and user interface of the workstation represents a critical step in choosing an optimal solution (Fig. 6-68).

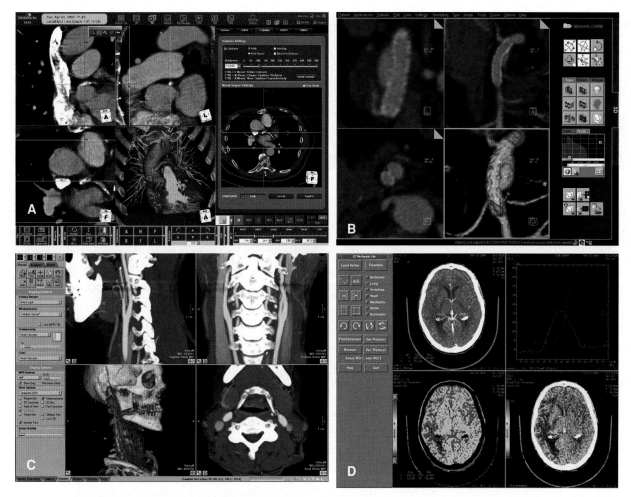

FIGURE 6-68 The spectrum of workstation interfaces currently available is a testament to the adage that one size does not fit all. What is an intuitive interface to one may be opaque and complex to another. Because all commercially available workstations accept DICOM data from all CT and MR scanners, the imager should feel free to investigate all available options before choosing the best solution for their postprocessing needs.

An important function of an image analysis workstation that is often overlooked is the ability to load, view, and compare multiple data sets representing follow-up examinations performed at different time points during the course of a patient's disease. Workstations that are most effective at allowing an understanding of disease variation over time will facilitate analysis by providing the means for linking the imaging volumes so that manipulation of one imaging volume will be reflected in the other linked examinations (Fig. 6-69).

Once 3D visualizations and analyses are created, the workstation should offer a range of methods for saving visualizations and transferring them to databases and referring physicians. While the DICOM format is a key export format for the PACS, the ability to save images as JPEG files facilitates transfer to referring physicians. Additionally, an intuitive interface for the creation of video files (AVI, MPEG, or Quicktime) allows portrayals to referring physi-

cians of intuitive visualizations of either time-varying data or using scripted navigations through complex anatomy. Once the output images are created, a range of output choices should be available, including direct export to PACS, hardcopy printing, creation of portable document format (PDF) files, e-mail, HTML forms for posting on secure web sites, and transfer to media such as drives, CDs, or DVDs.

PHYSICIAN-DIRECTED VERSUS TECHNOLOGIST-DIRECTED VISUALIZATION

Volumetric analyses of CTA and MRA data can be performed both by physicians and by technologists. While it may be tempting to select one of these two models for the delivery of all analytical services within an imaging practice, a combination of the two methods has optimized the delivery of volumetric imaging services at Stanford University over the past 10 years.

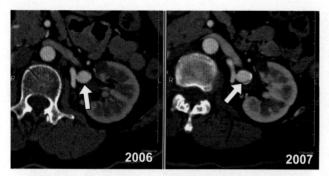

FIGURE 6-69 Follow-up CT in a patient with a renal artery aneurysm (*arrows*), stable in size during the 1-year interval and developing a discrete mural thrombus (*arrow* in the **right** image). The possibility of loading and comparing different exams side by side is of great importance, allowing more accurate comparison and saving time.

In 1996, the Stanford Radiology 3D Laboratory was established with a single technologist processing 20 CT angiograms per month. In late 2006, the laboratory had six full-time 3D technologists processing over 800 examinations per month. When the lab originally opened, analytical workstations were in a primitive state that precluded their routine use by physicians due to the time-consuming nature of the image processing. Although substantial improvements in workstation design have made physician-directed visualization practical, the role of the 3D laboratory remains important at Stanford University. Visualization driven by dedicated technologists assures a level of consistency and reliability in the analyses and visualizations that are not possible with physician-directed visualization. Protocols for specific visualizations and analyses are written for a broad spectrum of clinical applications. 3D technologists are experts at creating these visualizations and reliably measuring key anatomic landmarks for planning therapy.

Because the task of image creation, measurement, and transfer of results to the PACS is the primary responsibility of the technologist in the 3D lab, physicians are freed to use the workstation as a means for exploring the volumetric data for primary interpretation. Although volumetric CT and MR data sets emerge from the scanner as a stack of primary cross sections, many disease processes cannot be efficiently assessed without interaction on a workstation. The availability of the workstation in the reading room with convenient access for the physician, or even 3D workstation capabilities integrated into PACS workstations, provides the opportunity for a comprehensive data assessment. Directed analyses and visualizations can be created and saved to convey complex anatomy. Physician-directed visualizations allow for the creation of nonstandard views that best depict complex anatomy and can augment the scripted visualizations created by the 3D laboratory.

As previously described, this partnership model between technologists and physicians in analysis of volumetric data sets and in creating 3D imaging is very similar to the partnership widely accepted in sonography: The sonographer first creates the scripted visualizations for the physician to review, and if necessary, the physician reinterrogates the patient, exploring and creating dedicated views that clarify the images captured by the sonographer.

OUTSOURCING THREE-DIMENSIONAL VISUALIZATIONS

There are expanding opportunities for medical practices to transfer their imaging data to independent companies or laboratories for the purpose of creating 3D visualizations. It should not be surprising that the quality of analysis and visualization is highly variable among these options. The decision to outsource 3D visualizations does not eliminate the interpreting physician's responsibility to confirm that the visualizations are an accurate representation of the underlying data. Careful examination of 3D images must be performed to verify segmentation and validate conclusions implied by these images, lest an incorrect diagnosis result. It is important to remember that although a 3D laboratory—whether within the home institution, at another medical institution, at an image processing company, or halfway around the world—can facilitate the analysis of CT and MR angiographic data, it is ultimately up to the interpreting physician to provide an accurate interpretation by ensuring that these visualizations are concordant with and accurately depict conclusions that would have been reached during review of the original source data.

CONCLUSION

Volumetric analysis by using image processing workstations is a key element of interpretation in CTA and MRA. A thorough understanding of the spectrum of visualization and measurement techniques as well as a willingness of the imager to interactively explore volumetric imaging data is essential for fully realizing the wealth of clinically important information contained within 3D data sets.

REFERENCES

1. Rubin GD. 3-D imaging with MDCT. *Eur J Radiol.* 2003;45: S37–S41.
2. Rubin GD. Techniques for performing multidetector-row computed tomographic angiography. *Tech Vasc Interv Radiol.* 2001;4:2–14.

3. Cody DD. AAPM/RSNA physics tutorial for residents: topics in CT. Image processing in CT. *Radiographics.* 2002;22:1255–1268.
4. Price RR, Creasy JL, Lorenz CH, et al. Magnetic resonance angiography techniques. *Invest Radiol.* 1992;27:S27–S32.
5. Vannier MW. Digital imaging, image processing, and three-dimensional computer graphics for radiology. *Curr Opin Radiol.* 1992;4:1–10.
6. Sirineni GK, Kalra MK, Pottala KM, et al. Visualization techniques in computed tomographic coronary angiography. *Curr Probl Diagn Radiol.* 2006;35:245–257.
7. Salgado R, Mulkens T, Ozsarlak O, et al. CT angiography: basic principles and post-processing applications. *JBR-BTR.* 2003;86:336–340.
8. Rubin GD, Dake MD, Napel S, et al. Spiral CT of renal artery stenosis: comparison of three-dimensional rendering techniques. *Radiology.* 1994;190:181–189.
9. Prokop M. Multislice CT: technical principles and future trends. *Eur Radiol.* 2003;13:M3–M13.
10. Fishman EK, Lawler LP. CT angiography: principles, techniques and study optimization using 16-slice multidetector CT with isotropic datasets and 3D volume visualization. *Crit Rev Comput Tomogr.* 2004;45:355–388.
11. Wang Y, Johnston DL, Breen JF, et al. Dynamic MR digital subtraction angiography using contrast enhancement, fast data acquisition, and complex subtraction. *Magn Reson Med.* 1996;36:551–556.
12. Davis CP, Hany TF, Wildermuth S, et al. Postprocessing techniques for gadolinium-enhanced three-dimensional MR angiography. *Radiographics.* 1997;17:1061–1077.
13. Wong ND, Detrano RC, Diamond G, et al. Does coronary artery screening by electron beam computed tomography motivate potentially beneficial lifestyle behaviors? *Am J Cardiol.* 1996;78:1220–1223.
14. Lell MM, Anders K, Uder M, et al. New techniques in CT angiography. *Radiographics.* 2006;26:S45–S62.
15. Raman R, Napel S, Beaulieu CF, et al. Automated generation of curved planar reformations from volume data: method and evaluation. *Radiology.* 2002;223:275–280.
16. Huang Y, Webster CA, Wright GA. Analysis of subtraction methods in three-dimensional contrast-enhanced peripheral MR angiography. *J Magn Reson Imaging.* 2002;15:541–550.
17. Fishman EK, Ney DR, Heath DG, et al. Volume rendering versus maximum intensity projection in CT angiography: what works best, when, and why. *Radiographics.* 2006; 26:905–922.
18. Philipp MO, Kubin K, Mang T, et al. Three-dimensional volume rendering of multidetector-row CT data: applicable for emergency radiology. *Eur J Radiol.* 2003;48:33–38.
19. Sato Y, Shiraga N, Nakajima S, et al. Local maximum intensity projection (LMIP): a new rendering method for vascular visualization. *J Comput Assist Tomogr.* 1998;22:912–917.
20. Pelizzari CA. Image processing in stereotactic planning: volume visualization and image registration. *Med Dosim.* 1998;23:137–145.
21. Prokop M, Shin HO, Schanz A, et al. Use of maximum intensity projections in CT angiography: a basic review. *Radiographics.* 1997;17:433–451.
22. Frayne R, Grist TM, Korosec FR, et al. MR angiography with three-dimensional MR digital subtraction angiography. *Top Magn Reson Imaging.* 1996;8:366–388.
23. Ota H, Takase K, Rikimaru H, et al. Quantitative vascular measurements in arterial occlusive disease. *Radiographics.* 2005;25:1141–1158.
24. Kelekis NL, Semelka RC, Worawattanakul S, et al. Magnetic resonance imaging of the abdominal aorta and iliac vessels using combined 3-D gadolinium-enhanced MRA and gadolinium-enhanced fat-suppressed spoiled gradient echo sequences. *Magn Reson Imaging.* 1999;17:641–651.
25. Tillich M, Hill BB, Paik DS, et al. Prediction of aortoiliac stent-graft length: comparison of measurement methods. *Radiology.* 2001;220:475–483.
26. Tillich M, Bell RE, Paik DS, et al. Iliac arterial injuries after endovascular repair of abdominal aortic aneurysms: correlation with iliac curvature and diameter. *Radiology.* 2001;219: 129–136.
27. Rubin GD, Paik DS, Johnston PC, et al. Measurement of the aorta and its branches with helical CT. *Radiology.* 1998;206: 823–829.
28. Raman B, Raman R, Baek DN, et al. Automated measurement of aortoaortic and aortoiliac angulation for CT angiography (CTA) of abdominal aortic aneurysms (AAA) prior to endograft repair. *Radiology.* 2002;225(P):452.
29. Wolf YG, Tillich M, Lee WA, et al. Changes in aneurysm volume after endovascular repair of abdominal aortic aneurysm. *J Vasc Surg.* 202;36:305–309.
30. Giannoglou G, Giannakoulas G, Soulis J, et al. Predicting the risk of rupture of abdominal aortic aneurysms by utilizing various geometrical parameters: revisiting the diameter criterion. *Angiology.* 2006;57:487–494.

ESSENTIALS OF VASCULAR DISEASE

Atherosclerosis: Epidemiology and Pathophysiology

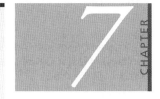

CHAPTER 7

Seung Uk Lee
Joanna J. Wykrzykowska
Roger J. Laham

Atherosclerosis, a progressive disease characterized by the accumulation of lipids and fibrous elements in the large arteries, is the leading cause of death and disability in the United States and other industrialized nations (1). Cardiovascular atherosclerotic disease with its resultant ischemic heart disease, stroke, and peripheral vascular disease is responsible for approximately 50% of all deaths in the United States (2,3). The clinical manifestations of atherosclerotic disease are myriad often coexisting conditions. These include chronic conditions such as stable angina pectoris, peripheral vascular disease, and aneurysmal dilation as well as acute life-threatening conditions such as stroke, myocardial infarction, limb-threatening ischemia, and aneurysm rupture. However, the prevalence of atherosclerotic disease far exceeds the incidence of its adverse events. This raises a concern that with the aging population, atherosclerotic disease will become more manifest.

Significant improvements in the treatment of atherosclerotic heart, cerebral, and peripheral vascular disease have been made. These have included risk factor modifications, antiplatelet and anticoagulant, lipid-lowering agents ("statins"), and antihypertensive medications as well as procedures and devices (such as percutaneous and surgical revascularization). Despite this, the prevalence of atherosclerotic disease continues to rise, and its resultant events continue to burden the health care system. This is partly due to the pro-

gressive nature of this disorder, improved survival with treatment, increasing age of the population, and an incomplete understanding of the underlying biology.

Recent advances in our understanding of the fundamental cellular and molecular pathways involved have established an essential role for inflammation, vessel wall injury, and angiogenesis in the various stages of atherosclerosis.

The inflammatory processes result from the interaction between modified lipoprotein, macrophages, and T-cells, among others. This mechanism provides a more direct link between the known risk factors and the pathogenesis of the disease.

Thus, atherosclerosis, formerly considered a degenerative lipid storage disease, is currently viewed as a form of chronic inflammation that can result in acute plaque rupture, thrombosis, and embolization (4,5). This chapter will focus mainly on the epidemiology, biology, and clinical manifestations of atherosclerosis, with a special emphasis on the emerging dominant role for inflammation in this disease.

ATHEROSCLEROSIS STATISTICS

In 2002, the estimated prevalence of total cardiovascular disease (CVD), coronary heart disease (CHD), and congestive heart failure (CHF) in the U.S. population was 70 million, 13 million, and 4.9 million, respectively. The estimated prevalence of myocardial infarction and stroke, the

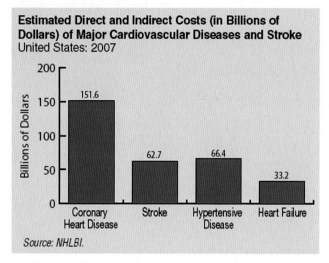

FIGURE 7-1 Estimated direct and indirect costs (in billions of dollars) of cardiovascular diseases and stroke in the United States in 2007. (Reprinted from Heart Disease and Stroke Statistics—2007 Update, American Heart Association.)

TABLE 7-1

Risk Factors Associated with Atherosclerosis

Factors with a Significant Genetic Component

Elevated levels of LDL and VLDL
Low levels of HDL
Elevated lipoprotein(a)
Elevated blood pressure
Elevated levels of homocysteine
Male gender
Metabolic syndrome
Elevated levels of hemostatic factors
Obesity
Diabetes mellitus
Systemic inflammation
Depression and other behavioral traits
Family history

Environmental Factors

High-fat diet
Smoking
Lack of exercise
Infectious agents
Low antioxidant levels

most serious acute complication of atherosclerotic disease, was 7.1 and 5.4 million, respectively. CVD accounted for 38% of all deaths, or 1 of every 2.6 deaths, in 2002. CHD caused 494,382 deaths, or 1 of every 5 deaths, in the United States. Despite marked improvement in therapeutic options and a significant decline in the death rate of CVD from 1992 to 2002, the actual number of deaths increased 0.8%. According to current statistics and estimates, 865,000 new and recurrent myocardial infarctions and 700,000 new and recurrent stroke attacks are expected annually.

Furthermore, the economic impact of atherosclerotic disease is staggering. In the United States, costs related to stroke are expected to reach an estimated $62.7 billion in 2007; CHD is projected to cost an estimated $151.6 billion in direct and indirect costs in 2007 (Fig. 7-1).

RISK FACTORS FOR ATHEROSCLEROSIS

Epidemiological studies (both experimental and observational) over the last 50 years have identified several risk factors for the development of atherosclerosis. These can be grouped into factors with an important genetic component and factors with a largely environmental component (Table 7-1). It is important to emphasize that the factors reported are the ones that were investigated, and it is likely that new risk factors will be identified with a better understanding of the biology of atherosclerosis. Large, prospective, community-based observational studies confirmed

suspected links between suggested factors and cardiovascular risk. A variety of factors, often acting in concert, have been shown to be associated with an increased risk of atherosclerotic plaques in coronary arteries and other arterial beds (1,6,7).

As portrayed in the Framingham Heart Study, which has been ongoing for decades, the different coronary risk factors have an additive effect on the likelihood of developing coronary heart disease (8). The major risk factors and predisposing conditions include dyslipidemia, tobacco use, diabetes mellitus, hypertension, and genetic factors (family history). Metabolic conditions, infectious agents, and psychiatric conditions can each contribute to the risk of developing atherosclerosis.

Dyslipidemia

Elevated levels of serum cholesterol are important in the development of atherosclerosis in humans and experimental animals even in the absence of other known risk factors. High-fat, high-cholesterol diets are usually required for the development of atherosclerosis in experimental animals (9). Epidemiologic studies have demonstrated a continuous, graded relationship between total serum cholesterol and coronary atherosclerotic risk (10). There are five major groups of lipoproteins that may be separated by ultracentrifugation: the chylomicrons, very-low-density lipoproteins (VLDL), low-density lipoproteins (LDL), intermediate-density lipoprotens (IDL), and high-density lipoproteins (HDL).

The major plasma lipids are not water soluble, and they do not circulate in a free form in the blood. Instead, they are complexed and bound to a specific group of protein carriers called *apolipoproteins*, which are found on the surface of the lipoproteins.

Much of the progress in understanding atherosclerosis over the past several decades has depended on the lipid hypothesis, which links cholesterol with heart disease and atherosclerosis. LDL cholesterol undoubtedly contributes to atherosclerosis in many cases and may indeed constitute a permissive factor for atherogenesis.

Reduction of LDL cholesterol by differing modalities, such as diet, several kinds of lipid-lowering agents, ilial bypass, and LDL apheresis, are associated with a reduction in atherosclerosis progression (11–15). It is clear that serum cholesterol, in particular LDL, may initiate the pathological processes of atherosclerosis.

Lipid-lowering strategies, particularly using the statin class of drugs (3-hydroxy-3-methylglutaryl coenzyme A reductase inhibitors, an enzyme essential in cholesterol synthetic pathway), promote features of experimental atheroma associated with plaque stability. These features include a reduction in macrophage number, a decrease in expression of matrix metalloproteinases (MMP), proinflammatory cytokines, leukocyte adhesion molecules, and decrease in production of reactive oxygen molecules. All of these steps are essential for progression of atherosclerosis. Statins also increase interstitial collagen content and smooth muscle maturation (16,17). They have been shown to reduce cardiovascular mortality and may stabilize the plaque (18–27).

Several large, randomized, controlled trials have established the effect of cholesterol-lowering therapy on the risk of death and cardiovascular events across a wide range of cholesterol levels (with or without history of CHD) (21–26). Patients with an acute coronary syndrome benefit from an intensive lipid-lowering (statin) regimen that in turn helps stop the progression of atherosclerosis (27,28). Several statin trials have shown that reduction in LDL cholesterol is associated with a reduced incidence of stroke (29–32). Therefore, dyslipidemias are an important contributor to the pathophysiology of atherosclerosis.

However, most patients with proven coronary artery disease have "average" levels of cholesterol (33), and statins slow but do not stop the progression of atherosclerosis, suggesting that additional risk factors may be as important.

Tobacco Use

Smoking is strongly associated with atherosclerosis (34–39). Between 1995 and 1999, an average of 442,398 Americans died yearly of smoking-related illnesses, with 33.5% of these deaths being cardiovascular. Approximately 90% of peripheral vascular disease in the nondiabetic population can be attributed to cigarette smoking, as can 50% of aortic aneurysms.

Smoking is also a powerful risk factor for CHD (40,41). The global INTERHEART study showed that smoking was a major contributor to 36% of first myocardial infarction (42). The risk of recurrent infarction in a study of smokers fell by 50% within 1 year of smoking cessation and normalized to that of nonsmokers within 2 years (9,43). Moreover, current smoking is a powerful independent predictor of sudden cardiac death in patients with CHD (43).

Cigarette smoking increases inflammatory markers, endothelial dysfunction (ED), platelet aggregation, leukocyte recruitments, and thrombosis in the atheromatous plaque (34,35,38,39). The risk of smoking is amplified by other risk factors, such as diabetes, hypertension, and elevated serum lipid levels (44). The benefits of smoking cessation are evident regardless of how long or how much the patient has previously smoked and should be emphasized in every patient.

Diabetes Mellitus

Diabetes mellitus affects 150 million people worldwide, and the number of diabetics in the United States approaches 20 million. The prevalence of diabetes among adults in the United States has increased by 40% in the past decade and is expected to increase by 165% between 2000 and 2050 (45–47). Mortality from myocardial infarction in patients with diabetes is markedly higher than in nondiabetic patients (48,49). Patients with diabetes but without previous myocardial infarction carry the same level of risk for subsequent acute coronary events as nondiabetic patients with previous myocardial infarction. Diabetes worsens early and late outcomes in acute coronary syndromes and long-term prognosis after myocardial infarction (50–56). Thus, the Adult Treatment Panel III of the National Cholesterol Education Program mandates aggressive antiatherosclerotic therapy in all diabetics (50).

Patients with diabetes have a two- to fourfold increase in the rate of peripheral artery disease (57). Diabetes is associated with arterial bruits, loss of pulse, arterial occlusion, amputation risk, and intermittent claudication (57–63).

Diabetes also adversely affects the cerebral circulation, with more extracranial atherosclerosis and a fivefold increase in the prevalence of calcified carotid atheroma (64,65). The risk of stroke is increased 150% to 400% with diabetes and is directly related to worsening glycemic control (66–69). In the Multiple Risk Factor Intervention Trial (MRFIT), subjects taking medications for diabetes were three times more likely to develop a stroke (70).

Diabetes also affects the risk of stroke among younger patients (71,72) and affects stroke outcomes. There is a threefold increase in the risk of stroke-related dementia, the risk of recurrence is doubled, and there is an increase in total and stroke-related mortality (73–75). The abnormal metabolic state in diabetes causes vascular dysfunction and atherosclerosis through several mechanisms, including chronic hyperglycemia, dyslipidemia, and insulin resistance. Diabetes mellitus alters the function of multiple cell types, including endothelial cells, smooth muscle cells, and platelets (76). Hyperglycemia impairs endothelial function, augments vasoconstriction, increases inflammation, and promotes thrombosis. By decreasing nitric oxide (NO) and increasing endothelin-1 and angiotensin II concentrations, hyperglycemia increases vascular tone and vascular smooth muscle cell proliferation and migration (77–79).

Increase in vascular tone in hyperglycemia is mediated by activation of protein kinase-C and nuclear factor [kappa] B in vascular smooth muscle cells and endothelial cells. This leads in turn to increased production of O^{2-} and contributes to the oxidant-rich milieu (80). Arterial vascular smooth muscle cells cultured from patients with type 2 diabetes demonstrate enhanced migration (81). LDL that has undergone nonenzymatic glycation induces vascular smooth muscle cell migration in vitro, while oxidized glycated LDL can induce apoptosis of vascular smooth muscle cells (82). Thus, diabetes alters vascular smooth muscle function in multiple ways that promote atherosclerotic lesion formation, plaque instability, and clinical events.

Impaired platelet function and increased blood coagulability are also involved in atherogenesis, progression of atheromatous plaque, plaque disruption, and thrombotic occlusion in diabetic patients (83–90).

As the prevalence of diabetes among CHD patients increases (91) and other risk factors such as smoking and hypercholesterolemia are better controlled, diabetes is likely to become the predominant risk factor for atherosclerosis.

Hypertension

Systemic hypertension is well established as a major risk factor for cardiovascular mortality and morbidity in the general population, being more common than cigarette smoking dyslipidemia, and diabetes (92,93). Hypertension is not only a well-established cardiovascular risk factor for the development of atherosclerosis but also appears to increase the risk of atherosclerosis (94–96). The INTERHEART study showed that hypertension accounted for 18% risk of a first myocardial infarction (26).

Increased blood pressure may damage the vessel wall directly and serve as a stimulus for inflammation (97). Indeed, impaired fibrinolysis in patients with hypertension may play an important role in the pathogenesis of cardiovascular disease in hypertensive patients (98).

There is increasing evidence that hypertension, through the vasoactive peptides angiotensin and endothelin-1, promotes and accelerates the atherosclerotic process via inflammatory mechanisms. Angiotensin II does decrease NO bioavailability by promoting oxidative stress (99) and may induce intimal inflammation and elicit the production of superoxide anion, a reactive oxygen species, from endothelial cells (100–102). It can also increase expression of proinflammatory cytokines and leukocyte adhesion molecules.

Indeed, angiotensin II–induced hypertension accelerates the development of atherosclerosis in ApoE-deficient mice (103). Therapeutic blockade of angiotensin II using angiotensin-converting enzyme inhibitors or angiotensin II receptor blockers in experimental studies and in clinical trials has been shown to correct ED and to retard the progression of atherosclerosis, in part related to the decreased expression of inflammatory mediators and improved endothelial function (104–106).

Endothelin-1 is another important mediator of chronic inflammation in the vascular wall. It is capable of inducing NFkB expression and increasing the expression on CD40L. It also mediates vasoconstriction and is expressed at high levels in carotid plaques. Chronic inhibition of endothelin reduces fatty streaks and plaque burden, and restores NO-responsiveness of the endothelium.

Like atherosclerosis, inflammation may contribute to the hypertensive state and may provide a pathophysiological link between these two diseases (107,108).

Other Risk Factors

Obesity not only predisposes to insulin resistance and diabetes, but also contributes to atherogenic dyslipidemia. The resulting elevation in VLDL from visceral fat can lower HDL cholesterol by augmenting exchange from HDL to VLDL by cholesteryl ester transfer protein. Adipose tissue itself can give rise to cytokines that worsen insulin sensitivity and provide a systemic proinflammatory stimulus (109).

Although not yet truly identified as risk factor, morbid obesity and the resultant *metabolic syndrome*, a current worldwide epidemic, are setting the stage for type 2 diabetes, its microvascular complications, and acceleration of macrovascular disease. Insulin resistance, hyperglycemia, dyslipidemia, hypertension, and thrombotic disorders as well as adiposity define the metabolic syndrome and contribute to ED and atherosclerosis.

In the metabolic syndrome, LDL particles may have qualitative alterations reducing their size and their vulnerability to oxidation. The low levels of HDL and elevated levels of triglyceride may blunt other endogenous anti-inflammatory mechanisms (110,111).

Nontraditional, emerging risk factors include lipoprotein(a); homocysteine; infectious agents such as *Chlamydia pneumoniae*, cytomegalovirus, and herpesvirus; and oxidant stress evoked by angiotensin II.

Elevated homocysteine levels appear to injure endothelial cells and stimulate proliferation of vascular smooth muscle cells (SMC) (112).

Infection by cytomegalovirus has been linked to atherosclerosis and arterial restenosis (113). Infection with *C. pneumoniae* is the most widely studied and may contribute to formation and progression of atherosclerotic lesions (114–129). The obligate intracellular bacterium has been detected in atherosclerotic lesions by immunohistochemistry, polymerase chain reaction, and electron microscopy and has also been cultured from atheromatous plaques (115–119). SMCs and macrophages in the intima have been found to be infected by *C. pneumoniae* (120,121). If the inflammatory response does not effectively neutralize or remove the offending agents, it can continue indefinitely, resulting in progression (122). Treatment with antibiotics such as azithromycin, however, has not been consistently shown to reduce the number of cardiovascular events of atherosclerosis progression.

Psychiatric manifestations, such as depression, hostile behaviors, and anger expression, can affect clinical outcome and may play a role in atherosclerotic progression (130–134).

Family history of CHD is a major risk factor, particularly when it involves an immediate relative with premature coronary disease (135).

Exercise is considered an antiatherogenic factor, thus lack of activity and a sedentary lifestyle may be permissive for atheroma formation (136).

PATHOGENESIS

It is now clear that systemic and local inflammatory events mediate plaque formation, progression, and degeneration:

Atherosclerosis is a chronic inflammatory disease (33,122, 137–143). No longer regarded as a bland, simple, and degenerative process, plaque evolution is best illustrated as a continuous tug of war between proinflammatory and anti-inflammatory cellular and molecular pathways.

Animal models have enabled a better understanding of the pathways involved. Targeted disruption of the apolipoprotein E (Apo E) or LDL receptor genes or overexpression of the human apolipoprotein B (Apo B) gene in mice resulted in marked increases in plasma cholesterol levels and development of advanced atherosclerotic lesions (144,145). While providing great insights into pathogenesis of atherosclerosis, the animal models currently available have important limitations in their applicability to the human disease.

In virtually all animal models, atherosclerosis is driven by extreme elevations in circulating cholesterol levels over a time scale of weeks to months. In contrast, atherosclerosis in humans is developed over decades. In autopsy studies, men and women, aged 15 to 34 years, had aortic fatty streaks with the more advanced lesions occurring with increasing age (146–148), and inflammation was at the center of it all. In fact, there is increasing evidence that the classically imagined "response-to-injury" is truly an inflammatory reaction (141,142).

Histologic Classification of Atherosclerotic Plaque

Atherosclerotic disease has been classified as a six-stage stepwise process of cross-sectional morphologic and histologic change (148–150) (Fig. 7-2). A normal artery evolves into types I and II initial lesions of atherosclerosis. These lesions have a characteristic architecture of fatty streaks and appear even in childhood at injury-prone areas such as bifurcations (151). The histologic features of atherosclerotic stages are

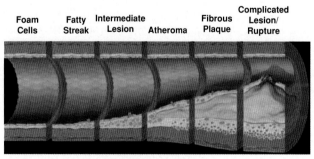

FIGURE 7-2 Evolution of atherosclerosis from earliest fatty streaks to plaque rupture and myocardial infarction. Adapted from Pepine CJ. *Am J Cardiol.* 1998.

shown in Table 7-2; a host of complex interactions occur in atherogenesis.

Fatty streaks are considered the first phase in atherosclerotic plaque development. Histologically, it presents as focal thickening of the intima with an increase in leukocytes, SMCs, and extracellular matrix (152). The fatty streaks also consist of macrophages with a variable number of T lymphocytes and lipid accumulation. Apoptosis of SMC within the fatty streak is associated with further macrophage infiltration and cytoplasmic remnants that contribute to the transformation of fatty streaks into atherosclerotic plaques (153).

Subsequently, fatty streaks progress into fibrous plaques via accumulation of connective tissue with an increased number of smooth muscle cells and lipid-laden macrophages. More advanced lesions often contain a necrotic lipid-rich core and receive vascular supply from both the luminal and medial sides.

A spectrum of possible advanced lesions can result, ranging from the chronic stable type IV atheroma of adulthood to the complicated type VI plaque of acute coronary syndromes. Furthermore, long-standing repetitive inflammatory injury can be the primary factor stimulating the transformation of stable mature type IV lesions into type V fibroatheromas prone to symptomatic luminal stenosis or degenerated type VI plaques vulnerable to acute rupture, hemorrhage, ulceration, thrombosis, or embolization (137,154).

Initiation of Atherosclerosis and Inflammation

Endothelial Dysfunction

The endothelium is not an inert, single-cell lining covering the intima of arteries, but in fact plays an essential role in regulating vascular tone and structure. It also functions as a selective permeability barrier between blood and tissues and can produce various molecules essential for regulation of thrombosis, inflammation, and vascular remodeling. In atherogenesis, ED is the earliest measurable functional abnormality of the vessel wall. It is a consequence of the harmful effects of the risk factors of atherosclerosis on the vessel wall.

Under healthy circumstances, the endothelial monolayer resists firm adhesion of platelets and leukocytes and maintains a balance of profibrinolytic and prothrombotic activity (33). Removal of the endothelium results in platelet adhesion and in a burst of SMC migration and proliferation, the latter subsiding when the endothelium regenerates (155).

Common factors predisposing to atherosclerosis such as hypercholesterolemia and diabetes are associated with ED, which might be the initial step in atherogenesis. Both local and systemic factors such as mechanical denudation

TABLE 7-2

Criteria for American Heart Association Lesion Classification System and Correspondence with Classification of Gross Arterial Specimens

AHA Grade	Criteria	Comments and Corresponding Gross Classification
0	Normal artery with or without adaptive intimal thickening; no hold	Normal tissue
1	Isolated MFCs containing lipid; no extracellular lipid; variable adaptive intimal thickening grossly with lipid staining	Initial atherosclerotic lesion, sometimes visible grossly with lipid staining
2	Numerous MFCs, often in layers, with fine particles of extracellular lipid; variable adaptive intimal thickening	Fatty streak, visible grossly with lipid staining
3	Numerous MFCs with 2 pools of extracellular lipid; no well-defined core of extracellular lipid	Fatty plaque, raised fatty streak, intermediate lesion, or transitional lesion
4	Numerous MFCs plus well-defined core of extracellular lipid, but with luminal surface covered by relatively normal intima	Atheroma, fibrous plaque, or raised lesion
5	Numerous MFCs, well-defined core or multiple cores of extracellular lipid plus reactive fibrotic cap, vascularization, or calcium	Fibroartheroma, fibrous plaque, or raised lesion
6	All of the above plus surface defect, hematoma, hemorrhage, or thrombosis	Complicated lesion

MFC, macrophage foam cell; AHA, American Heart Association.

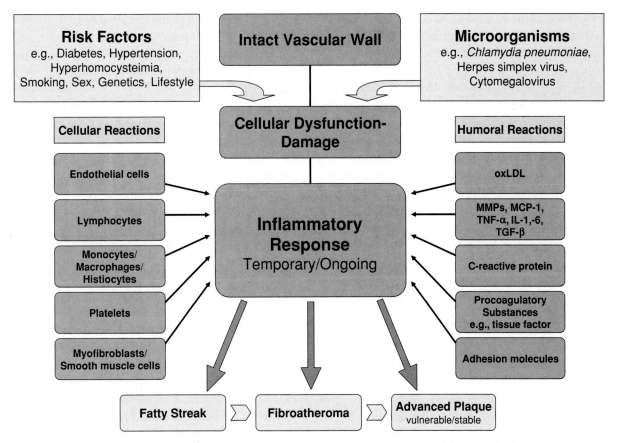

FIGURE 7-3 Schematic construction of the interrelationship between cellular and humoral factors involved in the inflammatory response of atherogenesis.

(angioplasty), advanced glycation end products, infectious agents, uremia, cigarette toxins, oxidative stress, genetic variability, radiation injury, homocysteinemia, chronic autoimmune conditions, and shear stress are associated with ED (156–163).

Endothelial cells in regions of arterial branching with turbulent blood flow have polygonal shape and no particular direction, while in areas with uniform flow, endothelial cells are ellipsoid in shape and aligned in the direction of flow. An absence of laminar flow may reduce local production of endothelium-derived nitric oxide (142).

ED is also associated with increased oxidative stress, an important promoter of the inflammatory processes. Oxidative stress is a harmful condition that occurs when there is an excess of free radicals, a decrease in antioxidant levels, or both.

NO is a potent oxidant and chemical mediator with multiple anti-atherogenic properties, including vasodilatory and anti-inflammatory properties. Its production is impaired in ED.

Experimental studies have demonstrated that leukocyte adhesion and infiltration into the intima, an essential step in atherosclerotic lesion formation, is regulated by leukocyte adhesion molecules and chemokines (164–166).

Pharmacologic inhibition of endothelium-derived NO production results in marked increase in endothelial adhesiveness for monocytes (167,168), an effect attenuated by dietary L-arginine, the substrate of endothelial NO synthase (eNOS).

At the molecular level, inhibition of eNOS results in increased expression of leukocyte adhesion molecules and critical chemokines, which are thought to be responsible for the migration of monocytes into the intima at sites of atherosclerotic lesion formation (169).

In contrast, NO synthase gene therapy dramatically reduces hypercholesterolemia-induced leukocyte adhesion molecule expression and inhibits monocyte infiltration into the arterial wall in a hypercholesterolemic rabbit model (170). Accelerated atherosclerotic lesion formation in the aorta has been demonstrated in eNOS knockout mice (171). Thus, NO serves as a protective moiety. ED with impaired NO production makes the affected intima more vulnerable.

Following a variety of injuries, including shear stress, the endothelial cells respond with an expression of adhesion molecules, increase their permeability, undergo further endothelial cell proliferation, and initiate thrombosis (137).

When the physiologic properties of endothelial cells are altered, several endothelium-derived adhesion molecules are expressed, leading to attachment and accumulation of monocytes, macrophages, T lymphocytes, and platelets on the arterial wall.

Both endothelial and attached cells become activated and release proinflammatory cytokines, membrane receptors, and enzymes. By-products of this cell activation include expression of interleukins (IL) 1, 2, 6, 7, 8, and 18; tumor necrosis factor-α(TNF-α); interferon-γ (IFN-γ); monocyte chemotactic protein (MCP-1); MCP-4; CD40 ligand (CD40L); parathyroid hormone-related protein (PTHrP); osteopontin; cyclo-oxygenase-2 (COX-2); and MMPs (172–174) (Table 7-3).

Then, proinflammatory positive feedback loops are activated, as these mediators recruit additional cells, release more cytokines, and promote LDL receptor expression. This results in aggregation of oxidized LDL particles on the endothelial surface and promotes the release of hepatic acute-phase reactants with attendant activation of the systemic inflammatory cascade (137).

The endothelial layer also increases its permeability. Endothelial penetration of adherent oxidized LDL and circulating macrophages results in formation of lipid-laden "foam cell" macrophage. Furthermore, activated dysfunctional endothelium proliferates and synthesizes several growth factors such as platelet-derived growth factor (PDGF). PDGF promotes platelet and inflammatory cell recruitment, thereby maintaining the inflammatory cascade, which may become self-sustaining.

Dysfunctional endothelial cells also lose their intrinsic anticoagulant properties. Platelet activation, blunted NO release, increased phospholipase A_2, and release of vasoactive agents such as thromboxanes, serotonin, and endothelin-1 all create a thrombogenic milieu (175–178). This may result in occlusive thrombus or embolization, responsible for feared complications such as myocardial infarction, stroke, and critical limb ischemia.

Low-density Lipoprotein Modification

Accumulation of LDL in the subendothelial matrix is an initiating event in atherosclerosis. When levels of circulating LDL are raised, subendothelial accumulation is greater,

and both the transport and retention of LDL are increased (138). LDL diffuses passively through endothelial cell junctions. LDL retention in the arterial wall seems to promote interactions between the LDL constituent apo B and matrix proteoglycans (179).

Native LDL is not taken up by macrophages rapidly enough to induce atherosclerosis, so it has been suggested that LDL is modified in the arterial wall (180). Trapped LDL undergoes modification including oxidation, lipolysis, proteolysis, and aggregation.

Lipid oxidation, a result of exposure to the oxidative waste of vascular cells, is the most important modification for the earliest histologic lesion, the so called *fatty streak formation*, a lesion that has been found in human fetal arteries. The recruitment of macrophages and their subsequent uptake of LDL-derived cholesterol comprise the major cellular events inducing fatty streak formation (181). However, oxidative modification of LDL in lipid and apo B components promotes the initial formation of fatty streaks and can precede the presence of macrophages (182–184).

While minimally oxidized LDL can be recognized by LDL receptors, extensive oxidative LDL particles are not bound by LDL receptors, but rather by several scavenger receptors expressed on macrophages and SMCs (181,184–185).

Accumulation of minimally oxidized LDL is a triggering event for recruitment of monocytes and lymphocytes to the arterial wall. Oxidized LDL stimulates the endothelial cells to produce a number of proinflammatory molecules and growth factors and can also inhibit the production of NO (138).

LDL becomes susceptible to enzymatic and nonenzymatic modifications when retained by extracellular matrix proteins in the arterial wall (186,187). A number of potential oxidant-generating systems including myeloperoxidase, nitric oxide synthase, and 15-lipoxygenase (15-LO) have been studied and implicated as being directly or indirectly responsible for LDL oxidation (144,148, 188–190).

Although there is substantial evidence that LDL oxidation initiates the atherosclerotic process, antioxidant therapy in humans is still controversial and unproven. However, numerous studies have shown that antioxidant treatment with various agents reduces the development of atherosclerosis in hypercholesterolemic animal models (184). Moreover, epidemiologic study in humans has demonstrated that antioxidant supplementation has a protective role (191).

Despite these results, recent prospective clinical trials with antioxidant vitamins such as vitamin E failed to show a significant beneficial effect on atherosclerotic events

TABLE 7-3

Molecular and Cellular Inflammatory Elements of Endothelial Dysfunction

Endothelial Dysfunction	Mediators After Vascular Injury	Cellular Elements	Inflammatory Response	Biologic Effect
Adhesiveness —	ICAM VCAM-1 PECAM-1 Integrins L, E, and selectins	Monocytes Macrophages T lymphocytes Platelets	Cytokines Receptor expression IL-1, -2, -6, -7, -8, -18 TNF-α IFN-γ MCP-1 CD40L PTHrP Osteopontin COX-2 MMP	Recruit additional cellular elements Promote LDL receptor expression Aggregation of ox-LDL Release of hepatic acute phase reactants Activate inflammatory cascade
Permeability	ox-LDL	Macrophages Monocytes T lymphocytes Mast cells	MCP-1 MCP-4 RANTES	Macrophage foam cells Sequestration, modification, and phagocytosis of lipid antigens Activation of complement VSMC proliferation Cytokine and chemokine release
Proliferation	PDGF IDGF-1 FGF TGF-β IL-1 TNF-α	VSMC	VSMC proliferation VSMC migration Collagen synthesis Matrix deposition Fibrous cap production	Transformation of early lesion to mature plaque
Thrombogenesis	Phospholipase A$_2$ PAI-1 Cigarette toxins Thromboxanes Leukotrienes Serotonin Endothelin-1 Angiotensin II Tissue factor MMP	Platelets Endothelial cells	Thrombogenic environment	Hemorrhage Plaque rupture Thrombosis Embolization Occlusion

(CD40L, CD-40 ligand; COX, cyclo-oxygenase; FGF, fibroblast growth factor; ICAM, intracellular adhesion molecule; IDGF, insulin-derived growth factor; IFN, interferon; IL, interleukin; ox-LDL, oxidized low-density lipoprotein; MCP, monocyte chemotactic protein; MMP, matrix metalloproteinase; PAI, platelet activator inhibitor; PDGF, platelet-derived growth factor; PECAM, platelet-endothelial cell adhesion molecule; PTHrP, parathyroid hormone–related protein; RANTES, regulated on activation, normally T-cell expressed and secreted; TGF, transforming growth factor; TNF, tumor necrosis factor; VCAM, vascular cell adhesion molecule; VSMC, vascular smooth muscle cell.)

(192–195). So, defining the most suitable patient population and more investigation of molecular mechanisms responsible for LDL oxidation are necessary to establish a therapeutic strategy.

Leukocyte Recruitment

Leukocyte recruitment is an essential step in the progression of atherosclerosis. Under normal circumstances, adhesion of leukocytes is inhibited by the endothelial monolayer. Although the recruitment of monocytes to the arterial wall and their subsequent differentiation into macrophages initially serve a protective action including removal of cytotoxic and proinflammatory oxidized LDL particles, progressive accumulation of macrophages leads to the development of atherosclerosis (181).

The recruitment of monocytes to lesion-prone sites of large arteries is regulated by chemotactic factors and leukocyte adhesion molecules that are expressed on the surface of endothelial cells in response to ED, oxidized LDL, various inflammatory stimuli, and flow patterns (196) (Fig. 7-4).

These molecules include vascular cell adhesion molecule-I (VCAM-I); intracellular adhesion molecule-I (ICAM-I); integrins; platelet-endothelial cell adhesion molecule-I (PECAM-I); and L, E, and P selectins. Neutrophils, normally involved in most inflammatory responses, are notably absent in atherosclerotic lesions. After cultured endothelial cells are exposed to oxidized LDL, they will attach monocytes and T lymphocytes but not neutrophils.

VCAM-I plays a major role in atherosclerosis initiation. VCAM-I binds monocytes and T lymphocytes found in nascent atheroma, and VCAM-I expression on endothelial cells over lesion-prone areas is increased in response to cholesterol feeding (197). In addition, VCAM-1 rises

before leukocyte recruitment begins in both hypercholesterolemic mouse and rabbit models (198).

Although targeted deletion of VCAM-1 in mice results in early embryonic lethality, dominant negative variants of VCAM-1 confer resistance to atherogenesis and show decreased lesion formation (199). Among constituents of modified lipoprotein particles, certain oxidized phospholipids and short-chain aldehydes arising from lipoprotein oxidation can induce transcriptional activation of the VCAM-1 gene mediated in part by nuclear factor kappa-B (200).

A number of proinflammatory cytokines induce VCAM-1 expression in endothelial cells by this pathway. Since human atherosclerotic lesions contain theses cytokines, proinflammatory cytokines may link hyperlipidemia to VCAM-1 expression.

In addition to VCAM-1, E selectin and P selectin, which bind to carbohydrate ligands on leukocytes, also appeared to contribute to monocyte recruitment in atherosclerotic-susceptible mice (201,202). Similarly, targeted ICAM-1 gene deletion resulted in small but significant reduction in monocyte recruitment to atherosclerotic lesions in apo E–deficient mice (203).

Another adhesion molecule, integrin VLA-4, on monocytes and T cells can mediate recruitment of these cells to the endothelium by interaction with both VCAM-1 on the endothelium and the connecting segment 1 (CS-1) domain of fibronectin (204). Various adhesion molecules and their features are summarized in Table 7-4.

Morphologic studies have established that once adherent to the endothelium, the leukocytes penetrate into the intima. This migration can induce the expression of chemotactic molecules by endothelial cells, such as monocyte chemotactic protein 1 (MCP-1) (183). Monocyte expression of CCR2, the receptor for MCP-1, is stimulated by hypercholesterolemia, and monocytes derived from hypercholesterolemic patients exhibit increased chemotactic responses to MCP-1 (205).

Mice deficient in MCP-1 or CCR2 have less atherosclerosis, mononuclear phagocyte accumulation, and local lipid levels, suggesting that MCP/CCR2 interaction plays a key role in monocyte recruitment in atherosclerosis (164,169,206,207).

IL-8 may have a similar role as a leukocyte chemoattractant during atherogenesis (208). Other chemokines such as CC chemokine and a trio of CXC chemokines are responsible for chemoattraction of leukocytes (209,210). Recent studies revealed that osteopontin, IL-7, and IL-18 are also related to inflammation seen in atherogenesis (173,174,211,212).

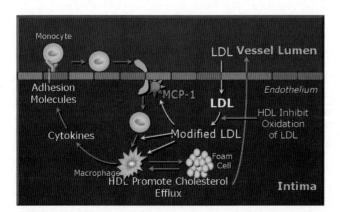

FIGURE 7-4 Schematic presentation of some of the cellular and molecular mechanisms involved in atherogenesis and plaque progression. Adapted from http://www.pbrc.edu/huec7004/slides/Lefevre05.ppt#91

TABLE 7-4

Characteristics of Adhesion Molecules

Adhesion Molecule	CD	Distribution	Function
Selectins			
L-selectin	CD62L	Leukocytes	Rolling
P-selectin	CD62P	Platelets, endothelium	Rolling, β_2-integrin upregulation
E-selectin	CD62E	Endothelium	Rolling
β_2-Integrins			
LFA-1	CD11a/CD18	Leukocytes	Adhesion, emigration
Mac-1	CD11b/CD18	Leukocytes	Adhesion, emigration
P150/95	CD11c/CD18	Dendritic cells, macrophages	Monocyte adhesion
Supergene Immunoglobulins			
ICAM-1	CD54	Endothelium, leukocytes	Adhesion, emigration
ICAM-2	CD102	Endothelium, leukocytes, platelets	Adhesion, emigration
VCAM-1	CD106	Endothelium	Adhesion
PECAM-1	CD31	Endothelium, leukocytes, platelets	Adhesion, emigration

LFA, lymphocyte function associated antigen-1. Other abbreviations are as defined in text.

Foam Cell Formation

Once resident in the arterial intima, monocytes acquire the morphologic characteristics of macrophages. The subsequent development of lipid-laden macrophages, known as *foam cells*, characterizes the early atherosclerotic lesion.

Once within the arterial intima, the monocytes increase expression of scavenger receptors such as the scavenger receptor A (SRA) and CD36 and then internalize modified lipoprotein. These two scavenger receptors appear to be of primary importance, and mice lacking either receptor develop significantly less atherosclerosis (213,214). The expression of scavenger receptors is regulated by peroxisome proliferator-activated receptor-γ and cytokines such as TNF-α and INF-γ (215).

LDL must be extensively modified before it can be taken up by macrophages to form foam cells. Several enzymes are thought to be involved in this modification, including myeloperoxidase, sphingomyelinase, and a secretory phospholipase.

Myeloperoxidase generates myeloperoxidase-modified LDL, which binds to macrophage scavenger receptors (216). Sphingomyelinase may induce lipoprotein aggregation, resulting in increased retention and enhanced uptake by macrophages (217).

A secretory phospholipase can also promote LDL oxidation. Transgenic mice overexpressing this enzyme show increased atherosclerosis (218). Cholesterol accumulation in these cells is thought to be mediated primarily by uptake of extensively modified LDL via scavenger receptors (219).

Macrophages phagocytose and internalize accumulating modified lipoproteins, such that cholesterol esters accumulate in cytoplasmic droplets (33,220). Although resultant lipid-laden foam cell formation is protective in nature, it can effect a disproportionate recruitment of additional monocytes, macrophages, T lymphocytes, and mast cells with attendant cytokine and chemokine release (221). Macrophages within the lesion also secrete a number of growth factors involved in disease progression, and they can replicate within the arterial intima.

Some studies have identified macrophage colony stimulating factor (M-CSF) as a candidate activator, promoting the transition of the monocyte to the lipid-laden macrophage. M-CSF stimulates SRA expression, increases production of cytokines and growth factors by macrophages, and serves as a comitogenic stimulus (222–225).

Targeted disruption of M-CSF gene results in delayed and markedly reduced macrophage accumulation (224–226). Granulocyte macrophage colony stimulating factor (GM-CSF) may have a role in promoting inflammation in atherosclerosis. GM-CSF supports the survival of a population of mononuclear phagocytes that contain myeloperoxidase, one of the potential sources of oxidative stress and inflammation in human plaque (227).

Free cholesterol in the macrophage has a number of potential metabolic fates, including esterification by acyl Co-A: cholesterol acyltransferase-1 (ACAT-1) and storage in the lipid droplets that characterize foam cells. Cholesterol esters within lipid droplets can be hydrolyzed, generating free cholesterol for transport out of the cell. This mechanism is important for maintenance of cholesterol homeostasis in the macrophage.

Disruption of ACAT-1 results in marked systemic abnormalities in lipid homeostasis and extensive deposition of free cholesterol in the skin and brain (228). Interestingly, in one study, ACAT deficiency did not prevent development of atherosclerosis, but it reduced the lipid and macrophage content of lesions (229).

ApoE secreted by macrophages may promote cholesterol efflux to HDL, inhibiting the transformation of macrophages to foam cells (230). Thus, the macrophage has the ability to dispose of excess cholesterol by enzymatic and molecular mechanism.

Since HDL is the primary extracellular acceptor, HDL is thought to be critical for physiologic "reverse cholesterol transport" and to at least partially explain why risk of atherosclerosis is inversely correlated with HDL cholesterol levels (231).

From the adherence to VCAM-1 and LDL modification to the chemoattractant response to MCP-1, inflammatory processes not only promote initiation but also contribute decisively to maintaining and participating development of the initial step of atherosclerosis.

Atheroma Progression and Fibrous Plaque

After formation of the fatty streak, the nascent atheroma typically evolves into a more complex lesion, fibrous plaque, which eventually leads to clinical manifestations. According to the traditional notion, the transition from the relatively simple fatty streak to fibrous plaque is characterized by a growing mass of extracellular lipid, mostly cholesterol and its esters, and by accumulation of SMCs and SMC-derived extracellular matrix from the medial layer of the artery.

Intimal SMCs may also proliferate and take up modified lipoproteins, contributing to foam cell formation and development of a fibrous cap (122). Cytokines and growth factors secreted by macrophages and T cells are important for SMC migration and proliferation as well as extracellular matrix production.

Lymphocytes do not appear to be required for the development of atherosclerosis. Once the early lesions develop, immune responses modulate progression. Immune response appears to have both atherogenic and antiatherogenic effects.

For example, INF-γ stimulates macrophage production of proinflammatory cytokines and reduces scavenger receptor expression on macrophages (140). Some studies have shown that immune activation is ongoing in atherosclerotic lesions (232,233).

Macrophages are thought to generate a variety of autoantibodies in response to oxidative lipids and proteins elaborated with progression of atherosclerosis. There are many proofs in mice and humans of a strong correlation between autoantibody titers to epitopes of oxidative LDL and extent of atherosclerosis. Intravenous (IV) administration of polyspecific immunoglobulin decreased lesion formation, as did hyperimmunization of hypercholesterolemic rabbit and murine models with homologous oxidative LDL (234). These observations suggest that it might be possible to modulate the development of atherosclerosis by immunization or other immunologic techniques.

Thus, this phase of fibrous plaque in atherosclerosis is continuously influenced by interactions between monocytes/macrophages and T cells, resulting in a wide range of cellular, hormonal, and immunologic responses and possession of many features of a chronic inflammatory state. Many growth factors from macrophages in the arterial intima stimulate SMC replication, which is responsible for lesion growth.

Plaque Disruption

Plaque destabilization, the detrimental process that results in clinical events, is caused by a multitude of inflammatory effects that involve cellular plaque components and various proinflammatory mediators, such as cytokines and chemokines (139,235). According to the classical notion, advanced atherosclerotic lesions can lead to progressive narrowing of the vessel lumen, and atherosclerotic processes occur in an inevitable and progressive fashion.

However, data from serial angiographic studies suggest that many coronary arterial lesions in humans develop stenoses discontinuously. Those studies revealed that smooth progression of the lesions proved the exception rather than the rule (236,237).

Similarly, acute cardiovascular events are generally thought to result from plaque rupture and thrombosis (238,239). The "bursts" of atheroma can be explained by microscopic evaluation of atherosclerotic plaque and inflammatory processes. It is suggested that physical disruption of plaques may trigger thrombosis and thus promote sudden expansion of atheromatous lesions (240). Three types of physical disruption may occur (241).

First, superficial erosion, or microscopic denudation of endothelium, occurs frequently. Such areas of limited endothelial denudation can form the nidus of a platelet thrombus. The binding of platelets to exposed regions of the subendothelial matrix is mediated by specific adhesion glycoproteins expressed on platelets. These glycoproteins bind to ligands embedded in the matrix, such as von Willebrand factor and collagen, which in turn promote platelet adhesion and activation (242). Although common and most often asymptomatic, such superficial erosion may be responsible for approximately one quarter of fatal coronary thromboses.

As a hallmark of superficial erosion of atherosclerotic plaque, loss of endothelium is an important and critical process in progression of atherosclerosis. Two inflammatory mechanisms may partake in endothelial desquamation (33).

The first is programmed endothelial cell death, and the second is disruption of the microvessels in atherosclerotic plaques.

Programmed endothelial cell death results from local production of inflammatory mediators or cytolytic attack by activated killer T cells. Additionally, expression and activation of MMPs that specialize in degrading components of the subendothelial basement membrane can be stimulated by inflammatory mediators and oxidized lipoproteins (243).

Inflammatory stimulation may promote the production of enzymes that degrade the extracellular matrix, to which endothelial cells adhere under normal circumstances. The role of MMPs in intimal thickening and atherosclerotic plaque rupture is increasingly acknowledged (244). MMPs are deeply involved in SMC migration, cell-mediated collagen organization, arterial remodeling, and plaque growth (245–250).

There is evidence that platelets can also bind to the surface of activated endothelial cells and to leukocytes that are already adherent to the intima (251–255). These adhesive interactions between platelets and endothelial cells can be mediated by a variety of glycoproteins that are expressed on activated platelets, including P-selectin, von Willebrand factor, and glycoprotein IIb/IIIa. In fact, the binding of activated platelets to endothelial cells and leukocytes can influence the strength of and inflammatory response through the release of different bioactive compounds (256).

Platelets can release a variety of inflammatory molecules that can promote endothelial cell and neutrophil interaction (257–259). Activated platelets also induce chemokine secretion in endothelial and SMCs (260). Recent studies in mice show that platelets adhere to the endothelium before the development of atherosclerotic lesions, and that prolonged blockade of platelet adhesion reduces leukocyte recruitment into the arterial wall and attenuates atherosclerotic lesion formation (261,262).

It is also known that activated platelets trigger an inflammatory response and enhance migration of aortic SMCs and macrophages (263). Activated platelets secrete transforming growth factor beta (TGF-β), the most powerful stimulus for interstitial collagen synthesis by SMCs. In conclusion, platelets are not only involved in hemostasis and thrombosis but also can modulate acute and chronic inflammatory responses in atherogenesis and thereby promote disease progression.

The second scenario for sudden plaque progression is disruption of the microvessels in atherosclerotic plaques (264). Inflammatory cells in the plaque produce mediators such as fibroblast growth factor and vascular endothelial growth factor (VEGF) (265,266).

This intraplaque neovascularization may lead to further enhanced influx of macrophages into the plaque (267). Like microvessels in diabetic retina, the new blood vessels in the plaque are particularly fragile and prone to intraplaque hemorrhage (268). Intraplaque deposition of fibrin, fibrin-split products, and hemosiderin provides evidence for intraplaque hemorrhage (33).

Microvessels in the plaque have the capacity to regulate their own tone independently of the host vessel and may therefore also develop ED independently (235). They may not only serve as a site for hemorrhage and thrombosis but may also perform a nutritive function inducing plaque growth. Indeed, experimental and human pathology studies have shown that the number of intraplaque capillaries increases with plaque progression (269,270). In animal studies, inhibitors of angiogenesis can retard lesion evolution in atherosclerosis (263,271). So, it is clear that plaque microvasculature promotes plaque evolution in atherosclerosis.

There is much evidence to support the role of thrombosis during human atherogenesis. Fibrin is an abundant protein in the arterial vessel wall but is not confined to atherosclerotic lesions (272,273). It is suggested that some fibrin deposition in the vessel wall is the result of inflammatory influences.

In the intima, fibrin can be polymerized by enzymes other than thrombin (274). Fibrin stimulates proliferation of SMCs, while split products inhibit this process. Fibrin cleavage products, degradation products, and D-dimer fragments modulate endothelial function, chemotaxis of SMCs and monocytes, and induction of IL-6 (272,275,276).

Thrombin is another link between coagulation and inflammation. When thrombin binds to its receptor on endothelial cells, such as protease-activated receptor-1, it induces the expression of P-selectin, E-selectin, VCAM-1, and ICAM-1 (277). Thrombin can stimulate SMC migration and proliferation by the release of PDGF from platelets (278). A silent microvascular hemorrhage within the atherosclerotic intima could give rise to a growth spurt in the evolution of the plaque. This growth usually is a result of an interaction between thrombotic and inflammatory processes in the arterial wall.

The third mechanism of plaque disruption, most common and best understood, is a fracture of the plaque's fibrous cap or plaque rupture (279). Although advanced atherosclerotic lesions can lead to ischemic symptoms as a result of progressive narrowing of the vessel lumen, acute cardiovascular events that result in myocardial infarction and stroke are generally thought to result from this plaque rupture and thrombosis (238,239).

Plaque rupture exposes lipid core and tissue factor to blood components, initiating the coagulation cascade, platelet adherence, and thrombosis (33,280). It results in repetitive cycles of microhemorrhage, thrombosis, and inflammation. The fibrous cap protects the thrombogenic lipid-rich core of the atheroma from the bloodstream.

Like the other forms of plaque disruption, most events of plaque rupture probably cause no clinical symptoms. Three quarters of acute myocardial infarctions, however, are caused by a ruptured fibrous cap (280). The likely explanation for these statistics is that when the fibrinolytic pathways outweigh the procoagulant pathways, a limited mural thrombus can be formed rather than an occlusive blood clot, and the event is clinically silent.

Interstitial collagen molecules confer most of the tensile strength to the fibrous cap (239). The level of collagen amount is crucial for stability of the fibrous cap, and its deposition is a tightly controlled process. SMCs are the principal source of extracellular matrix in the arterial wall.

Collagen production by SMCs is also controlled by proinflammatory cytokines. For example, IFN-γ can inhibit collagen production by SMCs. Interstitial collagen fibrils usually resist proteolytic degradation.

Overexpression of all three human interstitial collagenases, MMP-1, -8, and -13, have been found in atheromatous plaques (281–283). MMPs secreted by macrophages also have been detected in regions of plaque rupture and may influence plaque stability by degrading extracellular matrix proteins (284). After the early small proteolytic cleavage by the action of interstitial collagenases, gelatinases, MMP-2, and MMP-9 continue collagen catabolism (281).

Although arteries express the endogenous antagonist of MMPs, the tissue inhibitors of metalloproteinases (TIMPs), there is evidence for collagenolysis, which indicates excess activity of interstitial collagenase over TIMPs in human atherosclerotic plaques (282).

A number of studies have shown that inflammatory mediators, such as IL-1β, TNF-α, and CD40 ligand (CD 154) augment MMP expression in mononuclear phagocytes, endothelial cells, SMCs, and mast cells. All of these

cells within the lesion may in turn release the MMP-induced TNF-α and serine proteinases. The latter can stimulate latent MMP proenzymes (285–287). CD40 and CD154 result in production of inflammatory cytokines, MMPs, and adhesion molecules, contributing to the development of advanced lesions (288).

Recently, multiple lines of evidence have established that expression of MMPs is augmented by several transcription factors, NO, mechanical stretch, and oxidized LDL (289–294). Interestingly, expression and secretion of MMPs are inhibited by doxycycline and statins (295,296). Overexpression of MMP-9 and tissue factor in unstable plaques is associated with chlamydial infection, inflammation, and apoptosis (297).

Dynamic regulation of collagen levels in the fibrous cap is essential for maintenance of stable plaque. Indeed, MMP and TIMP gene transcription is differentially regulated in isolated vascular cells in culture (244). However, when collagen degradation increases due to overexpression of active MMPs, dissolution of the collagenous matrix of the fibrous cap leads to friability. In the clinical arena, the so-called vulnerable plaques are considered to be a predictive factor of acute coronary syndrome (298,299).

Thus, inflammation occupies a central position in the pathophysiology of atherosclerosis. There are many interactions between various injuries as triggers for inflammation and cellular, immunologic, and hormonal responses resulting in the progression of atherosclerosis.

Inflammatory Markers

In addition to measurement of lipid profile, based on the evidence supporting a role for inflammation in the pathogenesis of atherosclerosis, serum markers of inflammation have acquired considerable interest as markers of atherosclerotic risk (Table 7-5).

Among these, high-sensitivity C-reactive protein (CRP) has emerged as a key marker. Plasma CRP is an acute phase reactant produced primarily by the liver in response to inflammatory cytokines such as IL-6. CRP is a powerful independent predictor of myocardial infarction, stroke, and vascular death in a variety of settings and appears to be a better prognostic marker of cardiovascular events than LDL cholesterol (300–302).

Recent studies have suggested that CRP is not only a predictor but is also a mediator of atherosclerosis (303–318). It contributes to the pathogenesis of lesion formation, plaque rupture, and coronary thrombosis by interacting with and altering the endothelial cell phenotype (319).

CRP has also been demonstrated to promote the release of plasminogen inhibitor-1 from endothelial cells,

TABLE 7-5

Circulating Inflammatory Markers

Putative Marker	
hs-CRP	PTHrP
ox-LDL	MMP-9
Phospholipase A$_2$	MCP-1, -4
PAI-1	Endothelin-1
Homocysteine	Angiotensin II
IL-1, -2, -6, -7, -8, -18	Fibrinogen
Myeloperoxidase	Serum amyloid-A
TNF-α	TGF-β
D-dimer	ICAM
IFN-α	Lipoprotein(a)
MCP-1	Leukotrienes
CD40L	Peroxisome proliferator-activated receptors

(CRP, C-reactive protein; CD40L, CD-40 ligand; COX, cyclo-oxygenase; IFN, interferon; IL, interleukin; ICAM, intracellular adhesion molecule; MCP, monocyte chemotactic protein; MMP, matrix metalloproteinase; ox-LDL, oxidized low-density lipoprotein; PAI, platelet activator inhibitor; PDGF, platelet-derived growth factor; ox-LDL, oxidized low-density lipoprotein cholesterol; PTHrP, parathyroid hormone–related protein; TGF, transforming growth factor; TNF, tumor necrosis factor.)

up-regulate angiotensin-mediated neointimal formation, and alter endothelial progenitor cell survival and differentiation (303–305). Elevated blood CRP levels may also promote accumulation of monocytes in the atherogenic arterial wall by increasing chemotactic activities of monocytes in response to MCP-1 (320).

In addition to CRP, many inflammatory markers currently are being investigated as predictors or risk factors for atherosclerosis (321,322). These include lipoprotein-associated A$_2$, fibrinogen, cytokines, and soluble adhesion molecules, and all have been shown to have prognostic values (323–331).

All of these data have altered our perception of atherosclerosis as a degenerative condition. It is now considered to be a chronic inflammatory process susceptible to treatment strategies that may prevent, cause regression, or control this devastating disease.

REFERENCES

1. Braunwald E. Shattuck lecture—cardiovascular medicine at the turn of the millennium: triumphs, concerns, and opportunities. *N Engl J Med.* 1997;337:1360–1369.
2. Ross R. The pathogenesis of atherosclerosis: a perspective for the 1990s. *Nature.* 1993;362:801–809.
3. Faxon DP, Fuster V, Libby P, et al. Atherosclerotic vascular disease conference: writing group III: pathophysiology. *Circulation.* 2004;109:2617–2625.
4. Navab M, Berliner JA, Watson AD, et al. The yin and yang of oxidation in the development of the fatty streak. *Arterioscler Thrombo Vasc Biol.* 1996;16:831–842.
5. Steinberg D, Parthasarathy S, Darew, TE, et al. Modifications of low-density lipoprotein that increase its atherogenicity. *N Engl J Med.* 1989;320:915–924.
6. Wilson PW, D'Agostino RB, Levy D. Prediction of coronary heart disease using risk factor categories. *Circulation.* 1998;97(18)(May 12):1837–1847.
7. Libby P. Changing concepts of atherogenesis. *J Intern Med.* 1999;247:349–358.
8. Kannel WB. Framingham Study insights into hypertensive risk of cardiovascular disease. *Hypertens Res.* 1995;18:181–196.
9. Assmann G, Cullen P, Jossa F, et al. Coronary heart disease: reducing the risk. *Arterioscler Thrombo Vasc Biol.* 1999;19:1819–1824.
10. Stamler J, Wentworth D, Neaton JD, et al. Is relationship between serum cholesterol and risk of premature death from coronary heart disease continuous and graded? Findings in 356,222 primary screenees of the Multiple Risk Factor Intervention Trial (MRFIT). *JAMA.* 1986;256(20)(Nov 28):2823–2828.
11. Watts GF, Lewis B, Brunt JN, et al. Effects on coronary artery disease of lipid-lowering diet, or diet plus cholestyramine, in the St Thomas' Atherosclerosis Regression Study (STARS). *Lancet.* 1992;339:563–569.
12. Brown G, Albers JJ, Fisher LD, et al. Regression of coronary artery disease as a result of intensive lipid-lowering therapy in men with high levels of apolipoprotein B. *N Engl J Med.* 1990;323:1289–1298.
13. Jukema JW, Bruschke AV, van Boven AJ, et al. Effects of lipid lowering by pravastatin on progression and regression of coronary artery disease in symptomatic men with normal to moderately elevated serum cholesterol levels. The Regression Growth Evaluation Statin Study (REGRESS). *Circulation.* 1995;91:2528–2540.
14. Hahmann HW, Bunte T, Hellwig N, et al. Progression and regression of minor coronary arterial narrowings by quantitative angiography after fenofibrate therapy. *Am J Cardiol.* 1991;67:957–961.
15. Buchwald H, Moore RB, Rucker RD Jr., et al. Clinical angiographic regression of atherosclerosis after partial ileal bypass. *Atherosclerosis.* 1983;46:117–128.
16. Peter L. Current concepts of the pathogenesis of the acute coronary syndromes. *Circulation.* 2001;104:365–372.
17. Kausik KR, Christopher PC. Pathological changes in acute coronary syndromes: the role of statin therapy in modulation of inflammation, endothelial function and coagulation. *J Thromb Thrombolysis.* 2004;18:89–101.
18. Goldsten JL, Brown MS. The low-density lipoprotein pathway and its relation to atherosclerosis. *Ann Review Biochem.* 1977;46:897–930.
19. Gould LA, Rossouw JE, Santanello NC, et al. Cholesterol reduction yields clinical benefit: impact of statin trials. *Circulation.* 1988;97:946–952.
20. Davies MJ. Going from immutable to mutable atherosclerotic plaques. *Am J Cardiol.* 2001;88:2F–9F.
21. Scandinavian Simvastatin Survival Study Group. Randomised trial of cholesterol lowering in 4,444 patients with coronary heart disease: the Scandinavian Simvastatin Survival Study (4S). *Lancet.* 1994;344:1383–1389.
22. Sacks RM, Pfeffer MA, Moye LA, et al. The effect of pravastatin on coronary events after myocardial infarction in patients with average cholesterol levels. *N Engl J Med.* 1996;335:1001–1009.
23. The Long-Term Intervention with Pravastatin in Ischaemic Disease (LIPID) Study Group. Prevention of cardiovascular events and death with pravastatin in patients with coronary heart disease and a broad range of initial cholesterol levels. *N Engl J Med.* 1998;339:1349–1357.
24. Heart Protection Study Collaborative Group. MRC/BHF Heart Protection Study of cholesterol lowering with

simvastatin in 20,536 high-risk individuals: a randomised placebo-controlled trial. *Lancet*. 2002;360:7–22.

25. Shepard J, Cobbe SM, Ford I, et al. Prevention of coronary heart disease with pravastatin in men with hypercholesterolemia. *N Engl J Med*. 1995;333:1301–1307.

26. Downs JR, Clearfield M, Weis S, et al. Primary prevention of acute coronary events with lovastatin in men and women with average cholesterol levels: results of AFCAPS/TexCAPS: Air Force/Texas Coronary Atherosclerosis Prevention Study. *JAMA*. 1998;279:1615–1622.

27. Cannon CP, Braunwald E, McCabe CH, et al. Intensive versus moderate lipid lowering with statins after acute coronary syndromes. *N Engl J Med*. 2004;350:1495–1504.

28. Nissen SE, Tuzcu EM, Schoenhagen P. Statin therapy, LDL cholesterol, C reactive protein, and coronary artery disease. *N Engl J Med*. 2005;452:29–38.

29. White HD, Simes RJ, Anderson NE, et al. Pravastatin therapy and the risk of stroke. *N Engl J Med*. 2000;343:317–326.

30. Plehn JF, Davis BR, Sacks FM, et al. Reduction of stroke incidence after myocardial infarction with pravastatin: the Cholesterol and Recurrent Events (CARE) Study. *Circulation*. 1999;99:216–223.

31. Shepherd J, Blauw GJ, Murphy MB, et al. Pravastatin in elderly individuals at risk of vascular disease (PROSPER): a randomised controlled trial. *Lancet*. 2002;360: 1623–1630.

32. The ALLHAT officers and coordinators for the ALLHAT Collaborative Research Group. Major outcomes in moderately hypercholesterolemic, hypertensive patient care vs. randomized to pravastatin vs. usual care: the Antihypertensive and Lipid-Lowering Treatment to prevent Heart Attack Trial (ALLHAT-LLT). *JAMA*. 2002;288:2998–3007.

33. Libby P. Inflammation in atherosclerosis. *Nature*. 2002;420: 868–874.

34. Kangavari S, Matetzky S, Shah PK, et al. Smoking increases inflammation and metalloproteinase expression in human carotid atherosclerotic plaques. *Cardiovasc Pharmacol Ther*. 2004;9:291–298.

35. Matetzky S, Tani S, Kangavari S, et al. Smoking increases tissue factor expression in atherosclerotic plaques: implications for plaque thrombogenicity. *Circulation*. 2000;102: 602–604.

36. Ockene IS, Miller NH. Cigarette smoking, cardiovascular disease, and stroke: a statement for healthcare professionals from the American Heart Association. *Circulation*. 1997;96: 3243–3247.

37. Miller GJ, Bauer KA, Cooper JA, et al. Activation of the coagulant pathway in cigarette smokers. *Thromb Haemost*. 1998;79:549–553.

38. Hautamaki RD, Kobayashi DK, Senior RM, et al. Requirement for macrophage elastase for cigarette-smoke-induced emphysema in mice. *Science*. 1997;277:2002–2004.

39. Shen Y, Rattan V, Sultana C, et al. Cigarette smoke condensate-induced adhesion molecule expression and transendothelial migration of monocytes. *Am J Physiol*. 1996;270:H1624–H1633.

40. Njolstad I, Arnesen E, Lund-Larsen PG. Smoking, serum lipids, blood pressure, and sex differences in myocardial infarction. A 12-year follow-up of the Finnmark Study. *Circulation*. 1996;93(Feb 1):450–456.

41. Prescott E, Hippe M, Schnohr P, et al. Smoking and risk of myocardial infarction in women and men: longitudinal population study. *BMJ*. 1998;316(Apr 4):1043–1047.

42. Yusuf S, Hawken S, Ounpuu S, et al. Effect of potentially modifiable risk factors associated with myocardial infarction in 52 countries (the INTERHEART study): case-control study. *Lancet*. 2004;364(Sept 11):937–952.

43. Wilhelmsson C, Vedin JA, Elmfeldt D, et al. Smoking and myocardial infarction. *Lancet*. 1975;1(Feb 22):415–420.

44. Karim R, Buchanan TA, Hodis HN, et al. The association of smoking and subclinical atherosclerosis in Type 2 diabetes: modification by duration of diabetes. *Diabet Med*. 2005;22(1)(Jan):81–87.

45. Pedro RM, Valentin F. New aspects in the pathogenesis of diabetic atherothrombosis. *J Am Coll Cardiol*. 2004;44: 2293–2300.

46. Mokdad AH, Ford ES, Bowman BA, et al. Diabetes trends in the U.S.: 1990–1998. *Diabetes Care*. 1998;23:1278–1283.

47. Mokdad AH, Bowman BA, Ford ES, et al. The continuing epidemics of obesity and diabetes in the United States. *JAMA*. 2001;286:1195–1200.

48. Otter W, Kleybrink S, Doering W, et al. Hospital outcome of acute myocardial infarction in patients with and without diabetes mellitus. *Diabet Med*. 2004;21: 183–187.

49. Norhammar A, Malmberg K, Diderholm E, et al. Diabetes mellitus: the major risk factor in unstable coronary artery disease even after consideration of the extent of coronary artery disease and benefits of revascularization. *J Am Coll Cardiol*. 2004;43:585–591.

50. Executive summary of the third report of the National Cholesterol Education Program (NCEP) Expert Panel on Detection, Evaluation, and Treatment of High Blood Cholesterol in Adults (Adult Treatment Panel III). *JAMA*. 2001;285: 2486–2497.

51. Kjaergaard SC, Hansen HH, Fog L, et al. In-hospital outcome for diabetic patients with acute myocardial infarction in the thrombolytic era. *Scand Cardiovasc J*. 1999;33: 166–170.

52. Malmberg K, Yusuf S, Gerstein HC, et al. Impact of diabetes on long-term prognosis in patients with unstable angina and non-Q-wave myocardial infarction: results of the OASIS (Organization to Assess Strategies for Ischemic Syndromes) Registry. *Circulation*. 2000;102:1014–1019.

53. Zuanetti G, Latini R, Maggioni AP, et al. Influence of diabetes on mortality in acute myocardial infarction. *J Am Coll Cardiol*. 1993;22:1788–1794.

54. Shindler DM, Palmeri ST, Antonelli TA, et al. Diabetes mellitus in cardiogenic shock complicating acute myocardial infarction. *J Am Coll Cardiol*. 2000;36:1097–1103.

55. Miettinen H, Lehto S, Salomaa V, et al. Impact of diabetes on mortality after the first myocardial infarction. *Diabetes Care*. 1998;21:69–75.

56. Herlitz J, Karlson BW, Lindqvist J, et al. Rate and mode of death during five years of follow-up among patients with acute chest pain with and without a history of diabetes mellitus. *Diabet Med*. 1998;15:308–314.

57. Newman AB, Siscovick DS, Manolio TA, et al. Ankle-arm index as a marker of atherosclerosis in the Cardiovascular Health Study. *Circulation*. 1993;88:837–845.

58. Meijer WT, Hoes AW, Rutgers D, et al. Peripheral arterial disease in the elderly: the Rotterdam Study. *Arterioscler Thromb Vasc Biol*. 1998;18:185–192.

59. Jude EB, Oyibo SO, Chalmers N, et al. Peripheral arterial disease in diabetic and nondiabetic patients. *Diabetes Care*. 2001;24:1433–1437.

60. Beks PJ, Mackaay AJ, de Neeling JN, et al. Peripheral arterial disease in relation to glycaemic level in an elderly Caucasian population: the Hoorn study. *Diabetologia*. 1995;38:86–96.

61. Uusitupa MI, Niskanen LK, Siitonen O, et al. 5-Year incidence of atherosclerotic vascular disease in relation to general risk factors, insulin level, and abnormalities in lipoprotein composition in non-insulin-dependent diabetic and nondiabetic subjects. *Circulation*. 1990;82: 27–36.

62. Kannel WB, McGee DL. Update on some epidemiologic features of intermittent claudication: the Framingham Study. *J Am Geriatr Soc*. 1985;33:13–18.

63. Diabetes-related amputations of lower extremities in the Medicare population—Minnesota, 1993–1995. *MMWR Morb Mortal Wkly Rep*. 1998;47:649–652.

64. Fabris F, Zanocchi M, Bo M, et al. Carotid plaque, aging, and risk factors. *Stroke*. 1994;25:1133–1140.

65. Friedlander AH, Maeder LA. The prevalence of calcified carotid artery atheromas on the panoramic radiographs of

patients with type 2 diabetes mellitus. *Oral Surg Oral Med Oral Pathol Oral Radiol Endod.* 2000;89:420–424.

66. Himmelmann A, Hansson L, Svensson A, et al. Predictors of stroke in the elderly. *Acta Med Scand.* 1988;224:439–443.

67. Jamrozik K, Broadhurst RJ, Forbes S, et al. Predictors of death and vascular events in the elderly. *Stroke.* 2000;31:863–868.

68. Folsom AR, Rasmussen ML, Chambless LE, et al. Prospective associations of fasting insulin, body fat distribution, and diabetes with risk of ischemic stroke. *Diabetes Care.* 1999;22:1077–1083.

69. Kuusisto J, Mykkanen L, Pyorala K, Laakso M. Non-insulin-dependent diabetes and its metabolic control are important predictors of stroke in elderly subjects. *Stroke.* 1994;25:1157–1164.

70. Stamler J, Vaccaro O, Neaton JD, et al. Diabetes, other risk factors, and 12-yr cardiovascular mortality for men screened in the Multiple Risk Factor Intervention Trial. *Diabetes Care.* 1993;16:434–444.

71. Jorgensen H, Nakayama H, Raaschou HO, et al. Stroke in patients with diabetes: the Copenhagen Stroke Study. *Stroke.* 1994;25:1977–1984.

72. You RX, McNeil JJ, O'Malley HM, et al. Risk factors for stroke due to cerebral infarction in young adults. *Stroke.* 1997;28:1913–1918.

73. Luchsinger JA, Tang MX, Stern Y, et al. Diabetes mellitus and risk of Alzheimer's disease and dementia with stroke in a multiethnic cohort. *Am J Epidemiol.* 2001;154: 635–641.

74. Hankey GJ, Jamrozik K, Broadhurst RJ, et al. Long-term risk of first recurrent stroke in the Perth Community Stroke Study. *Stroke.* 1998;29:2491–2500.

75. Tuomilehto J, Rastenyte D, Jousilahti P, et al. Diabetes mellitus as a risk factor for death from stroke. *Stroke.* 1996;27: 210–215.

76. Neckman JA, Creager MA, Libby P. Diabetes and atherosclerosis: epidemiology, pathophysiology, and management. *JAMA.* 2002;287:2570–2581.

77. Williams SB, Cusco JA, Roddy MA, et al. Impaired nitric oxide-mediated vasodilation in patients with non-insulin-dependent diabetes mellitus. *J Am Coll Cardiol.* 1996;27:567–574.

78. Johnstone MT, Creager SJ, Scales KM, et al. Impaired endothelium-dependent vasodilation in patients with insulin-dependent diabetes mellitus. *Circulation.* 1993;88: 2510–2516.

79. De Vriese AS, Verbeuren TJ, Van de Voorde J, et al. Endothelial dysfunction in diabetes. *Br J Pharmacol.* 2000;130:963–974.

80. Inoguchi T, Li P, Umeda F, et al. High glucose level and free fatty acid stimulate reactive oxygen species production through protein kinase C–dependent activation of NAD(P)H oxidase in cultured vascular cells. *Diabetes.* 2000;49:1939–1945.

81. Suzuki LA, Poot M, Gerrity RG, et al. Diabetes accelerates smooth muscle accumulation in lesions of atherosclerosis. *Diabetes.* 2001;50:851–860.

82. Taguchi S, Oinuma T, Yamada T. A comparative study of cultured smooth muscle cell proliferation and injury, utilizing glycated low density lipoproteins with slight oxidation, auto-oxidation, or extensive oxidation. *J Atheroscler Thromb.* 2000;7:132–137

83. Vinik AI, Erbas T, Park TS, et al. Platelet dysfunction in type 2 diabetes. *Diabetes Care.* 2001;24:1476–1485.

84. Assert R, Scherk G, Bumbure A, et al. Regulation of protein kinase C by short term hyperglycaemia in human platelets in vivo and in vitro. *Diabetologia.* 2001;44: 188–195.

85. Li Y, Woo V, Bose R. Platelet hyperactivity and abnormal Ca(2+) homeostasis in diabetes mellitus. *Am J Physiol Heart Circ Physiol.* 2001;280:H1480–H1489.

86. Carr ME. Diabetes mellitus: a hypercoagulable state. *J Diabetes Complications.* 2001;15:44–54.

87. Ceriello A, Giugliano D, Quatraro A, et al. Blood glucose may condition factor VII levels in diabetic and normal subjects. *Diabetologia.* 1988;31:889–891.

88. Ceriello A, Giugliano D, Quatraro A, et al. Evidence for a hyperglycaemia-dependent decrease of antithrombin III-thrombin complex formation in humans. *Diabetologia.* 1990;33:163–167.

89. Ceriello A, Giacomello R, Stel G, et al. Hyperglycemia-induced thrombin formation in diabetes. *Diabetes.* 1995;44:924–928.

90. Nordt TK, Bode C. Impaired endogenous fibrinolysis in diabetes mellitus. *Semin Thromb Hemost.* 2000;26: 495–501.

91. Takaishi H, Taniguchi T, Fujioka Y, et al. Impact of increasing diabetes on coronary artery disease in the past decade. *J Atheroscler Thromb.* 2004;11:271–277.

92. Wilson PW. Established risk factors and coronary artery disease: the Framingham Study. *Am J Hypertens.* 1994;7(7 Pt 2): 7S–12S.

93. Aram VC, George LB, Henry RB, et al. Seventh Report of the Joint National Committee on Prevention, Detection, Evaluation, and Treatment of High Blood Pressure. *Hypertension.* 2003;42(Dec):1206–1252.

94. Stamler J, Neaton JD, Wentworth DN. Blood pressure (systolic and diastolic) and risk of fatal coronary heart disease. *Hypertension.* 1989;13[Suppl 1]:I-2–I-12.

95. Kannel WB, Neaton JD, Wentworth D, et al. Overall and coronary heart disease mortality rates in relation to major risk factors in 325,348 men screened for the MRFIT: Multiple Risk Factor Intervention Trial. *Am Heart J.* 1986;112: 825–836.

96. Alexander RW. Hypertension and the pathogenesis of atherosclerosis oxidative stress and the mediation of arterial inflammatory response: a new perspective. *Hypertension.* 1995;25:155–161.

97. Claudia UC, Richard TL, Nader R, et al. Blood pressure and inflammation in apparently healthy men. *Hypertension.* 2001;38:399.

98. Kim AP, Geoffrey HT, Martin GL, et al. Association of blood pressure with fibrinolytic potential in the Framingham offspring population. *Circulation.* 2000;101:264.

99. Ivonne HS, Ming SZ, Leopoldo R. Nitric oxide, angiotensin II, and reactive oxygen species in hypertension and atherogenesis. *Curr Hyper Rep.* 2005 7:61–67.

100. Berliner J, Leitinger N, Watson A, et al. Oxidized lipids in atherogenesis: formation, destruction and action. *Thromb Haemost.* 1997;78:195–199.

101. Williams KJ, Tabas I. The response-to-retention hypothesis of atherogenesis reinforced. *Curr Opin Lipidol.* 1998;9:471–474.

102. Witztum JL, Berliner JA. Oxidized phospholipids and isoprostanes in atherosclerosis. *Curr Opin Lipidol.* 1998;9:441–448.

103. Weiss D, Kools JJ, Taylor R. Angiotensin II-induced hypertension accelerates the development of atherosclerosis in ApoE-deficient mice. *Circulation.* 2001;103:448–454.

104. Ernesto LS. (CIHR) Multidisciplinary Research Group on Hypertension. Beyond blood pressure: the endothelium and atherosclerosis progression. *Am J Hypertens.* 2002;15: s115–s122.

105. Yusuf S, Sleight P, Pogue J, et al. Effects of an angiotensin-converting-enzyme inhibitor, ramipril, on cardiovascular events in high-risk patients. *N Engl J Med.* 2000;342: 145–153.

106. Dahlöf RB, Devereux SE, Kjeldsen S, et al. Cardiovascular morbidity and mortality in the Losartan Intervention For Endpoint reduction in hypertension study (LIFE): a randomised trial against atenolol. *Lancet.* 2002;359: 995–1003.

107. Li JJ, Chen JL. Inflammation may be a bridge connecting hypertension and atherosclerosis. *Med Hypotheses.* 2005; 64:925–929.

108. Virdis A, Schiffrin EL. Vascular inflammation: a role in vascular disease in hypertension? *Curr Opin Nephrol Hypertens.* 2003;12(2)(Mar):181–187.
109. Yudkin JS, Stehouwer CD, Emeis JJ, et al. C-reactive protein in healthy subjects: associations with obesity, insulin resistance, and endothelial dysfunction: a potential role for cytokines originating from adipose tissue? *Arterioscler Thromb Vasc Biol.* 1999;19:972–978.
110. Navab M, Hama SY, Hough GP, et al. High density associated enzymes: their role in vascular biology. *Curr Opin Lipidol.* 1998;9:449–456.
111. Caglayan E, Blaschke F, Takata Y, et al. Metabolic syndrome-interdependence of the cardiovascular and metabolic pathways. *Curr Opin Pharmacol.* 2005;5:135–142.
112. Gerhard GT, Duell PB. Homocysteine and atherosclerosis. *Curr Opin Lipidol.* 1999;10:417–429.
113. Gupta S, Pablo AM, Jiang X, et al. IFN-γ potentiates atherosclerosis in apoE knock-out mice. *J Clin Invest.* 1997;99:2752–2761.
114. Ngeh J, Anand V, Gupta S. Chlamydia pneumoniae and atherosclerosis—what we know and what we don't. *Clin Microbiol Infect.* 2002;8:2–13.
115. Campbell LA, O'Brien ER, Cappuccio AL, et al. Detection of Chlamydia pneumoniae TWAR in human coronary atherectomy tissues. *J Infect Dis.* 1995;172:585–588.
116. Kuo C, Grayston JT, Campbell LA, et al. Chlamydia pneumoniae (TWAR) in coronary arteries of young adults (15–34 years old). *PNAS.* 1995;92:6911–6914.
117. Maass M, Krause E, Engel PM, et al. Endovascular presence of Chlamydia pneumoniae in patients with hemodynamically effective carotid artery stenosis. *Angiology.* 1997;48:699–706.
118. Ramirez JA. Isolation of Chlamydia pneumoniae from the coronary artery of a patient with coronary atherosclerosis. The Chlamydia pneumoniae/Atherosclerosis Study Group. *Ann Intern Med.* 1996;125:979–982.
119. Gieffers J, Solbach W, Maass M. In vitro susceptibilities of Chlamydia pneumoniae strains recovered from atherosclerotic coronary arteries. *Antimicrob Agents Chemother.* 1998;42:2762–2764.
120. Shor A, Phillips JI. Histological and ultrastructural findings suggesting an initiating role for Chlamydia pneumoniae in the pathogenesis of atherosclerosis. *Cardiovasc J S Afr.* 2000;11:16–23.
121. Hammerschlag MR. The intracellular life of chlamydiae. *Semin Pediatr Infect Dis.* 2002;13:239–248.
122. Ross R. Atherosclerosis—an inflammatory disease. *N Engl J Med.* 1999;340:115–126.
123. Fischer SF, Hacker G. Characterization of antiapoptotic activities of Chlamydia pneumoniae in infected cells. *Ann NY Acad Sci.* 2003;1010:565–567.
124. Fischer SF, Harlander T, Vier J, et al. Protection against CD95-induced apoptosis by chlamydial infection at a mitochondrial step. *Infect Immun.* 2004;72:1107–1115.
125. Wahl C, Maier S, Marre R, et al. Chlamydia pneumoniae induces the expression of inhibitor of apoptosis 2 (c-IAP2) in human monocytic cell line by an NF-kappaB-dependent pathway. *Int J Med Microbiol.* 2003;293:377–381.
126. Greene W, Xiao Y, Huang Y, et al. Chlamydia infected cells continue to undergo mitosis and resist induction of apoptosis. *Infect Immun.* 2004;72:451–460.
127. Bonanomi A, Dohm N, Rickenbach Z, et al. Monitoring intracellular replication of Chlamydophila (Chlamydia) pneumoniae in cell cultures and comparing clinical samples by real-time PCR. *Diagn Microbiol Infect Dis.* 2003;46:39–47.
128. Perfettini JL, Ojcius DM, Andrews CWJ, et al. Role of proapoptotic BAX in propagation of Chlamydia muridarum (the mouse pneumonitis strain of Chlamydia trachomatis) and the host inflammatory response. *J Biol Chem.* 2003;278:9496–9502.
129. Claudia D, Christine FM, Daniel G, et al. *Chlamydia pneumoniae* induces aponecrosis in human aortic smooth muscle cells. *BMC Microbiology.* 2005;5:2.
130. Rozanski A, Blumenthal JA, Kaplan J. Impact of psychological factors on the pathogenesis of cardiovascular disease and implications for therapy. *Circulation.* 1999;99:2192–2217.
131. Lesperance F, Frasure-Smith N, Talajic M, et al. Five-year risk of cardiac mortality in relation to initial severity and one-year changes in depression symptoms after myocardial infarction. *Circulation.* 2002;105:1049–1053.
132. Rugulies R. Depression as a predictor for coronary heart disease. A review and meta-analysis. *Am J Prev Med.* 2002;23:51–61.
133. Matthews KA, Gump BB, Harris KF, et al. Hostile behaviors predict cardiovascular mortality among men enrolled in the Multiple Risk Factor Intervention Trial. *Circulation.* 2004;109:66–70.
134. Alan R, James AB, Karina W, et al. The epidemiology, pathophysiology, and management of psychosocial risk factors in cardiac practice. *J Am Coll Cardiol.* 2005;45:637–651.
135. Watt G, McConnachie A, Upton M, et al. How accurately do adult sons and daughters report and perceive parental deaths from coronary disease? *J Epidemiol Community Health.* 2000;11:859–863.
136. Anne Marie WP, Bente KP. The anti-inflammatory effect of exercise. *J Appl Physiol.* 2005;98:1154–1162.
137. Philip SM, Charles AA, Benjamin WS. Atherosclerosis as inflammation. *Ann Vasc Surg.* 2005;19:130–138.
138. Aldons JL. Atherosclerosis. *Nature.* 2000;407:233–241.
139. Peter L, Paul MR, Attilio M. Inflammation and atherosclerosis. *Circulation.* 2002;105:1135–1143.
140. Christopher KG, Joseph LW. Atherosclerosis: the road ahead. *Cell.* 2001;104:503–516.
141. Ross R, Glomset JA. Atherosclerosis and the arterial smooth muscle cell: proliferation of smooth muscle is a key event in the genesis of the lesions of atherosclerosis. *Science.* 1953;180:1332–1339.
142. Ross R, Glomset JA. The pathogenesis of atherosclerosis. *N Engl J Med.* 1976;295:369–377,420.
143. Mullenix PS, Andersen CA, Starnes BW. Atherosclerosis as inflammation. *Ann Vasc Surg.* 2005;19:130–138.
144. Breslow JL. Mouse models of atherosclerosis. *Science.* 1996;272:685–688.
145. Tamminen M, Mottino G, Qiao JH, et al. Ultrastructure of early lipid accumulation in apoE-deficient mice. *Arterioscl Thromb Vasc Biol.* 1999;19:847–853.
146. Strong JP, Malcom GT, McMahan CA, et al. Prevalence and extent of atherosclerosis in adolescents and young adults. Implications for prevention from the pathobiological determinants of atherosclerosis in youth study. *JAMA.* 1999;281:727–735.
147. McGill HC, McMahon A, Zieske AW, et al. Association of coronary heart disease risk factors with microscopic qualities of atherosclerosis in youth. *Circulation.* 2000;102:374–379.
148. Stary HC, Chandler AB, Dinsmore RE, et al. Definition of advanced types of atherosclerotic lesions in a histological classification of atherosclerosis: a report from the Committee on Vascular Lesions of the Council on Arteriosclerosis, American Heart Association. *Circulation.* 1995;92:1355–1374.
149. Stary HC, Chandler AB, Glagov S, et al. A definition of intimal fatty streak, and intermediate lesions of atherosclerosis. *Circulation.* 1994;89:2462–2478.
150. Sidawy AN. Basic considerations of the arterial wall in health and disease. In: Rutherford RB, ed. *Vascular Surgery.* 5th ed. Philadelphia: W. B. Saunders; 2000:60–72.
151. Ross R. Cell biology of atherosclerosis. *Annu Rev Physiol.* 1995;57:791–804.
152. Davies MJ, Woolf N, Rowles PM, et al. Morphology of the endothelium over atherosclerotic plaques in human coronary arteries. *Br Heart J.* 1988;60(6):459–464.
153. Kockx MM, De Meyer GR, Muhring J, et al. Apoptosis and related proteins in different stages of human atherosclerotic plaques. *Circulation.* 1998;97:2307–2315.

154. Stary HC. The histological classification of atherosclerotic lesions in human coronary arteries In: Fuster V, Ross R, Topol EJ, et al. *Atherosclerosis and Coronary Artery Disease.* Vol. 1. Philadelphia: Lippincott-Raven; 1996: 463–474.
155. Gimbrone MA Jr. Vascular endothelium, hemodynamic forces, and atherogenesis. *Am J Pathol.* 1999;155:1–5.
156. Gonzales MA, Selwyn AP. Endothelial function, inflammation, and prognosis in cardiovascular disease. *Am J Med.* 2003;115 [Suppl 8A]:99S–106S.
157. Keller TT, Mairuhu AT, de Kruif MD, et al. Infections and endothelial cells. *Cardiovasc Res.* 2003;60:40–48.
158. Steele SR, Martin MJ, Mullenix PS, et al. Carotid artery stenosis following radiation therapy for head and neck cancer—should we be more aggressive in focused high-risk population screening? *Am J Surg.* 2004;187:594–598.
159. Al Aly Z, Edwards JC. Vascular biology in uremia: insights into novel mechanisms of vascular injury. *Adv Chronic Kidney Dis.* 2004;11:310–318.
160. Basta G, Schmidt AM, De Caterina R. Advanced glycation end products and vascular inflammation: implications for accelerated atherosclerosis in diabetes. *Cardiovasc Res.* 2004;63:582–592.
161. Asanuma Y, Oeser A, Shintani AK, et al. Premature coronary-artery atherosclerosis in systemic lupus erythematosus. *N Engl J Med.* 2003;349:2407–2415.
162. Libby P, Egan D, Skarlatos S. Roles of infectious agents in atherosclerosis and restenosis: an assessment of the evidence and need for future research. *Circulation.* 997;96:4095–4103.
163. Albert MA, Ridker PM. Inflammatory biomarkers in African Americans: a potential link to accelerated atherosclerosis. *Rev Cardiovasc Med.* 2004;5[Suppl 3]:S22–S27.
164. Boring L, Gosling J, Cleary M, et al. Decreased lesion formation in CCR2$^{-/-}$ mice reveals a role for chemokines in the initiation of atherosclerosis. *Nature.* 1998;394:894–897.
165. Cybulsky MI, Iiyama K, Li H, et al. A major role for VC18AM-1, but not ICAM-1, in early atherosclerosis. *J Clin Invest.* 2001;107:1255–1262.
166. Rosenfeld ME. Leukocyte recruitment into developing atherosclerotic lesions: the complex interaction between multiple molecules keeps getting more complex. *Arterioscler Thromb Vasc Biol.* 2002;22:361–363.
167. Taso PS, Mcevoy LM, Drexler H, et al. Enhanced endothelial adhesiveness in hypercholesterolemia is attenuated by L-arginine. *Circulation.* 1994;89:2716–2182.
168. De Caterina R, Libby P, Peng HB, et al. Nitric oxide decreases cytokine induced endothelial expression of adhesion molecules and proinflammatory cytokines. *J Clin Invest.* 1995;96:60–68.
169. Gu L, Okada Y, Clinton SK, et al. Absence of monocyte chemoattractant protein-I reduces atherosclerosis in low-density lipoprotein receptor-deficient mice. *Mol Cell.* 1998;2:275–281.
170. Qian H, Neplioueva V, Shetty GA, et al. Nitric oxide synthase gene therapy rapidly reduces adhesion molecule expression and inflammatory cell infiltration in carotid arteries of cholesterol-fed rabbits. *Circulation.* 1999;99: 2979–2982.
171. Kuhlencordt PF, Gyurko R, Han F, et al. Accelerated atherosclerosis, aortic aneurysm formation, and ischemic heart disease in apolipoprotein E/endothelial nitric oxide synthase double-knockout mice. *Circulation.* 2001;104: 448–454.
172. Jonasson L, Holm J, Skalli O, et al. Regional accumulations of T cells, macrophages, and smooth muscle cells in the human atherosclerotic plaque. *Arteriosclerosis.* 1986;6:131–138.
173. Ito T, Ikeda U. Inflammatory cytokines and cardiovascular disease. *Curr Drug Targets Inflamm Allergy.* 2003;2:257–265.
174. Strom A, Franzen A, Wangnerud C, et al. Altered vascular remodeling in osteopontin-deficient atherosclerotic mice. *J Vasc Res.* 2004;41:314–322.
175. De Caterina, Zampoli A. From asthma to atherosclerosis—5-lipoxygenase, leukotrienes, and inflammation. *N Engl J Med.* 2004;350:4–7.
176. Cracowski JL. Isoprostanes: an emerging role in vascular physiology and disease? *Chem Phys Lipids.* 2004;128:75–83.
177. Mawatari K, Kakui S, Harada N, et al. Endothelin-1(1-31) levels are increased in atherosclerotic lesions of the thoracic aorta of hypercholesterolemic hamsters. *Atherosclerosis.* 2004;175:203–212.
178. Hamsten A, Wiman B, de Faire U, et al. Increased plasma levels of a rapid inhibitor of tissue plasminogen activator in young survivors of myocardial infarction. *N Engl J Med.* 1985;313:1557–1563.
179. Boren J, Olin K, Lee I, et al. Identification of the principal proteoglycan-binding site in LDL. A single-point mutation in apo-B100 severely affects proteoglycan interaction without affecting LDL receptor binding. *J Clin Invest.* 1998;101:2658–2664.
180. Goldstein JL, Ho YK, Basu SK, et al. Binding sites on macrophages that mediate uptake and degradation of acetylated low density lipoprotein, producing massive cholesterol deposition. *Proc Natl Acad Sci USA.* 1979;76:333–337.
181. Christopher KG, Joseph LW. Atherosclerosis: the road ahead. *Cell.* 2001;104:503–516.
182. Napoil C, D'Armiento FP, Mancini FP, et al. Fatty streak formation occurs in human fetal aortas and is greatly enhanced by maternal hypercholesterolemia. Intimal accumulation of low density lipoprotein and its oxidation precede monocyte recruitment into early atherosclerotic lesions. *J Clin Invest.* 1997;100:2680–2690.
183. Navab M, Berliner JA, Watson AD, et al. The yin and yang of oxidation in the development of the fatty streak. *Arterioscler Thromb Vasc Biol.* 1996;16:831–842.
184. Steinberg D, Witztum JL. *Lipoproteins, Lipoprotein Oxidation, and Atherogenesis.* In: Chien KR, ed. Philadelphia: W. B. Saunders Co.; 1999.
185. Navab M, Berliner JA, Watson AD, et al. The yin and yang of oxidation in the development of the fatty streak. *Arterioscler Thromb Vasc Biol.* 1996;16:831–842.
186. Schwenke DC, Carew TE. Initiation of atherosclerotic lesions in cholesterol-fed rabbits. I. Focal increases in arterial LDL concentration precede development of fatty streak lesions. *Arteriosclerosis.* 1989;9:895–907.
187. Williams KJ, Tabas I. The response-to-retention hypothesis of atherogenesis reinforced. *Curr Opin Lipidol.* 1998;9: 471–474.
188. Heinecke JW. Oxidants and antioxidants in the pathogenesis of atherosclerosis: implications for the oxidized low density lipoprotein hypothesis. *Atherosclerosis.* 1998;141:1–15.
189. Cyrus T, Witztum JL, Rader DJ, et al. Disruption of the 12/15-lipoxygenase gene diminishes atherosclerosis in apo E-deficient mice. *J Clin Invest.* 1999;103:1597–1604.
190. Harats D, Shaish A, George J, et al. Overexpression of 15-lipoxygenase in vascular endothelium accelerates early atherosclerosis in LDL receptor-deficient mice. *Arterioscler Thromb Vasc Biol.* 2000;20:2100–2105.
191. Jha P, Flather M, Lonn E, et al. The antioxidant vitamins and cardiovascular disease. A critical review of epidemiologic and clinical trial data. *Ann Intern Med.* 1995;123: 860–872.
192. Yusuf S, Dagenais G, Pogue J, et al. Vitamin E supplementation and cardiovascular events in high-risk patients. The Heart Outcomes Prevention Evalulation Study Investigators. *N Engl J Med.* 2000;342:154–160.
193. Lonn E, Yusuf S, Dzavik V, et al. Effects of ramipril and vitamin E on atherosclerosis: the study to evaluate carotid ultrasound changes in patients treated with ramipril and vitamin E (SECURE). *Circulation.* 2002;103:919–925.
194. GISSI-Prevenzione Investigators (Gruppo Italiano per lo Studio della Sopravvivenza nell'Infarto miocardico). Dietary supplementation with n-3 polyunsaturated fatty acids and vitamin E after myocardial infarction: results of the GISSI-Prevenzione trial. *Lancet.* 1999;354:447–455.

195. The Heart Outcomes Prevention Evaluation Study Investigators. Vitamin E supplementation and cardiovascular events in high-risk patients. *N Engl J Med.* 2000;342:154–160.

196. Nagel T, Resnick N, Atkinson WJ, et al. Shear stress selectively upregulates intercellular adhesion molecule-I expression in cultured human vascular endothelial cells. *J Clin Invest.* 1994;94:885–891.

197. Cybulsky MI, Gimbrone MA Jr. Endothelial expression of a mononuclear leukocyte adhesion molecule during atherogenesis. *Science.* 1991;251:788–791.

198. Li H, Cybulsky MI, Gimbrone MA Jr., et al. An atherogenic diet rapidly induces VCAM-1, a cytokine regulatable mononuclear leukocyte adhesion molecule, in rabbit endothelium. *Arterioscler Thromb.* 1993;13:197–204.

199. Cybulsky MI, Iiyama K, Li H, et al. A major role for VCAM-1, but not ICAM-1, in early atherosclerosis. *J Clin Invest.* 2001;107:1255–1262.

200. Collins T, Cybulsky MI. NF-κB: pivotal mediator or innocent bystander in atherogenesis? *J Clin Invest.* 2001;107:255–264.

201. Johnson RC, Chapman SM, Dong ZM, et al. Absence of P-selectin delays fatty streak formation in mice. *J Clin Invest.* 1997;99:1037–1043.

202. Dong ZM, Chapman SM, Brown AA, et al. The combined role of P- and E-selectins in atherosclerosis. *J Clin Invest.* 1998;102:145–152.

203. Collins RG, Velji R, Guevara NV, et al. P-selectin or intercellular adhesion molecule (ICAM)-1 deficiency substantially protects against atherosclerosis in apolipoprotein E–deficient mice. *J Exp Med.* 2000;191:189–194.

204. Shih PT, Brennan ML, Vora DK, et al. Blocking very late antigen-4 integrin decreases leukocyte entry and fatty streak formation in mice fed an atherogenic diet. *Circ Res.* 1998;84:345–351.

205. Han KH, Han KO, Green SR, et al. Expression of the monocyte chemoattractant protein-1 receptor CCR2 is increased in hypercholesterolemia: differential effects of plasma lipoproteins on monocyte function. *J Lipid Res.* 1999;40;1053–1063.

206. Gosling J, Slaymaker S, Gu L, Tseng S, et al. MCP-1 deficiency reduces susceptibility to atherosclerosis in mice that overexpress human apolipoprotein B. *J Clin Invest.* 1999;103:773–778.

207. Sheikine Y, Hansson GK. Chemokines and atherosclerosis. *Ann Med.* 2004;36:98–118.

208. Boisvert WA, Santiago R, Curtiss LK, et al. A leukocyte homologue of the IL-8 receptor CXCR-2 mediates the accumulation of macrophages in atherosclerotic lesions of LDL receptor-deficient mice. *J Clin Invest.* 1998;101:353–363.

209. Haley KJ, Lilly CM, Yang JH, et al. Overexpression of eotaxin and the CCR3 receptor in human atherosclerosis: using genomic technology to identify a potential novel pathway of vascular. *Circulation.* 2000;102:2185–2189.

210. Mach F, Sauty A, Iarossi AS, et al. Differential expression of three T lymphocyte-activating CXC chemokines by human atheroma-associated cells. *J Clin Invest.* 1999;104:1041–1050.

211. Damas JK, Waehre T, Yndestad A, et al. Interleukin-7-mediated inflammation in unstable angina: possible role of chemokines and platelets. *Circulation.* 2003;107:2670–2676.

212. Yamaoka-Tojo M, Tojo T, Masuda T, et al. C-reactive protein-induced production of interleukin-18 in human endothelial cells: a mechanism of orchestrating cytokine cascade in acute coronary syndrome. *Heart Vessels.* 2003; 18:183–187.

213. Suzuki H, Kurihara Y, Takeya M, et al. A role for macrophage scavenger receptors in atherosclerosis and susceptibility to infection. *Nature.* 1997;386:292–296.

214. Febbraio M, Podrez EA, Smith JD, et al. Targeted disruption of the class B scavenger receptor CD36 protects against atherosclerosis lesion development in mice. *J Clin Invest.* 2000;105:1049–1056.

215. Tontonoz P, Nagy L, Alvarez JL, et al. PPAR gamma promotes monocyte/macrophage differentiation and uptake of oxidized LDL. *Cell.* 1998;93:241–252.

216. Podrez EA, Febbraio M, Sheibani N, et al. Macrophage scavenger receptor CD36 is the major receptor for LDL modified by monocyte-generated reactive nitrogen species. *J Clin Invest.* 2000;105:1095–1108.

217. Marathe S, Kuriakose G, Williams KJ, et al. Sphingomyelinase, an enzyme implicated in atherogenesis, is present in atherosclerotic lesions and binds to specific components of the subendothelial extracellular matrix. *Arterioscl Thromb Vasc Biol.* 1999;19:2648–2658.

218. Ivandic B, Castellani LW, Wang XP, et al. Role of group II secretory phospholipase A$_2$ in atherosclerosis I. Increased atherogenesis and altered lipoproteins in transgenic mice expressing group IIa phospholipase A$_2$. *Arterioscl Thromb Vasc Biol.* 1999;19:1284–1290.

219. Yamada Y, Doi T, Hamakubo T, et al. Scavenger receptor family proteins: roles for atherosclerosis, host defense and disorders of the central nervous system. *Cell Mol Life Sci.* 1998;54:628–640.

220. Linton MF, Fazio S. Macrophages, inflammation, and atherosclerosis. *Int J Obes Relat Metab Disord.* 2003;21[Suppl 3]:S35–S40.

221. Jeziorska M, McCollum C, Wooley DE. Mast cell distribution, activation, and phenotype in atherosclerotic lesions of human carotid arteries. *J Pathol.* 1997;183:248.

222. Clinton S, Underwood R, Sherman M, et al. Macrophage colony-stimulating factor gene expression in vascular cells and in experimental and human atherosclerosis. *Am J Pathol.* 1992;140:301–316.

223. Rosenfeld ME, Yla-Herttuala S, Lipton BA, et al. Macrophage colony-stimulating factor mRNA and protein in atherosclerotic lesions of rabbits and humans. *Am J Pathol.* 1992;140:291–300.

224. Smith JD, Trogan E, Ginsberg M, et al. Decreased atherosclerosis in mice deficient in both macrophage colony-stimulating factor (op) and apolipoprotein E. *Proc Natl Acad Sci USA.* 1995;92:8264–8268.

225. Rajavashisth T, Qiao JH, Tripathi S, et al. Heterozygous osteopetrotic (op) mutation reduces atherosclerosis in LDL receptor-deficient mice. *J Clin Invest.* 1998;101:2702–2710.

226. Qiao JH, Tripathi J, Mishra NK, et al. Role of macrophage colony-stimulating factor in atherosclerosis: studies of osteopetrotic mice. *Am J Pathol.* 1997;150:1687–1699.

227. Sugiyama S, Okada Y, Sukhova GK, et al. Macrophage myeloperoxidase regulation by granulocyte macrophage colony-stimulating factor in human atherosclerosis and implications in acute coronary syndromes. *Am J Pathol.* 2001;158:879–891.

228. Yagu H, Kitamine T, Osuga J, et al. Absence of ACAT-1 attenuates atherosclerosis but causes dry eye and cutaneous xanthomatosis in mice with congenital hyperlipidemia. *J Biol Chem.* 2000;275:21324–21330.

229. Accad M, Smith SJ, Newland DL, et al. Massive xanthomatosis and altered composition of atherosclerotic lesions in hyperlipidemic mice lacking acyl CoA:cholesterol acyltransferase 1. *J Clin Invest.* 2000;105:711–719.

230. Fazio S, Babaev VR, Murray AB, et al. Increased atherogenesis in mice reconstituted with apolipoprotein E null macrophages. *Proc Natl Acad Sci USA.* 1997;94:4647–4652.

231. Tall AR, Jiang X, Lou Y, et al. George Lyman Duff memorial lecture: lipid transfer proteins, HDL metabolism and atherogenesis. *Arterioscler Thromb Vasc Biol.* 2000;20:1185–1188.

232. Mallat Z, Besnard S, Duriez M, et al. Protective role of interleukin-10 in atherosclerosis. *Circ Res.* 1999;85:17–24.

233. Pinderski L, Hedrick C, Olvera T, et al. Interleukin-10 blocks atherosclerotic events in vitro and in vivo. *Arterioscler Thromb Vasc Biol.* 1999;19:2847–2853.

234. Horkko S, Binder CJ, Shaw PX, et al. Immunological responses to oxidized LDL. *Free Radic Biol Med.* 2000;28:1771–1779.

235. Lerman A, Zeiher AM. Endothelial function. *Circulation.* 2005;111:363–368.

236. Bruschke AV, Kramer JR Jr., Bal ET, et al. The dynamics of progression of coronary atherosclerosis studied in 168

medically treated patients who underwent coronary arteriography three times. *Am Heart J.* 1989;117:296–305.

237. Yokoya K, Takatsu H, Suzuki T, et al. Process of progression of coronary artery lesions from mild or moderate stenosis to moderate or severe stenosis: a study based on four serial coronary arteriograms per year. *Circulation.* 1999;100:903–909.

238. Davies MJ, Richardson PD, Woolf N. Risk of thrombosis in human atherosclerotic plaques: role of extracellular lipid, macrophage, and smooth muscle cell content. *Br Heart J.* 1993;69:377–381.

239. Lee RT, Libby P. The unstable atheroma. *Aterioscler Thromb Vasc Biol.* 1997;17:1859–1867.

240. Davies MJ. Stability and instability: the two faces of coronary atherosclerosis. The Paul Dudley White Lecture, 1995. *Circulation.* 1996;94:2013–2020.

241. Virmani R, Burke AP, Farb A, et al. Pathology of the unstable plaque. *Prog Cardiovasc Dis.* 2002;44:349–356.

242. Massberg S, Enders G, Leiderer R, et al. Platelet-endothelial cell interactions during ischemia/reperfusion: the role of P-selectin. *Blood.* 1998;92:507–512.

243. Rajavashisth TB, Liao JK, Galis ZS, et al. Inflammatory cytokines and oxidized low density lipoproteins increase endothelial cell expression of membrane type 1-matrix metalloproteinase. *J Biol Chem.* 1999;274:11924–11929.

244. Andrew CN. Dual role of matrix metalloproteinases (matrixins) in intimal thickening and atherosclerotic plaque rupture. *Physiol Rev.* 2005;85:1–31.

245. Chase AJ, Newby AC. Regulation of matrix metalloproteinase (matrixin) genes in blood vessels: a multi-step recruitment model for pathological remodelling. *J Vasc Res.* 2003;40:329–343.

246. Cho A, Reidy MA. Matrix metalloproteinase-9 is necessary for the regulation of smooth muscle cell replication and migration after arterial injury. *Circ Res.* 2002;91:845–851.

247. Galis ZS, Johnson C, Godin D, et al. Targeted disruption of the matrix metalloproteinase-9 gene impairs smooth muscle cell migration and geometrical arterial remodeling. *Circ Res.* 2002;91:852–859.

248. Johnson C, Galis ZS. Matrix metalloproteinase-2 and -9 differentially regulate smooth muscle cell migration and cell-mediated collagen organization. *Arterioscler Thromb Vasc Biol.* 2004;24:54–60.

249. Luttun A, Lutgens E, Manderveld A, et al. Loss of matrix metalloproteinase-9 or matrix metalloproteinase-12 protects apolipoprotein E-deficient mice against atherosclerotic media destruction but differentially affects plaque growth. *Circulation.* 2004;109:1408–1414.

250. Rotmans JI, Velema E, Verhagen HJM, et al. Matrix metalloproteinase inhibition reduces intimal hyperplasia in a porcine arteriovenous-graft model. *J Vasc Surg.* 2004;39:432–439.

251. Massberg S, Enders G, Matos FC, et al. Fibrinogen deposition at the postischemic vessel wall promotes platelet adhesion during ischemia-reperfusion in vivo. *Blood.* 1999;94:3829–3838.

252. Kirton CM, Nash GB. Activated platelets adherent to an intact endothelial cell monolayer bind flowing neutrophils and enable them to transfer to the endothelial surface. *J Lab Clin Med.* 2000;136:303–313.

253. Russell J, Cooper D, Tailor A, et al. Low venular shear rates promote leukocyte-dependent recruitment of adherent platelets. *Am J Physiol Gastrointest Liver Physiol.* 2003;284:G123–G129.

254. Granger DN, Vowinkel T, Petnehazy T. Modulation of the inflammatory response in cardiovascular disease. *Hypertension.* 2004;43:924.

255. Mannaioni PF, DiBello MG, Masini E. Platelets and inflammation: role of platelet-derived growth factor, adhesion molecules and histamine. *Inflammation Res.* 1997;46:4–18.

256. Bazzoni G, Dejana E, Del Maschio A. Platelet-neutrophil interactions, possible relevance in the pathogenesis of thrombosis and inflammation. *Haematologica.* 1991;76:491–499.

257. Lindemann S, Tolley ND, Dixon DA, et al. Activated platelets mediate inflammatory signaling by regulated interleukin 1β synthesis. *J Cell Biol.* 2001;154:485–490.

258. Christian W. Platelets and chemokines in atherosclerosis. *Circ Res.* 2005;96:612–616.

259. Huo Y, Schober A, Forlow SB, et al. Circulating activated platelets exacerbate atherosclerosis in mice deficient in apolipoprotein E. *Nat Med.* 2003;9:61–67.

260. Massberg S, Brand K, Gruener S, et al. A critical role of platelet adhesion in the initiation of atherosclerotic lesion formation. *J Exp Med.* 2002;196:887–896.

261. Steffen M, Felix V, Timm D, et al. Activated platelets trigger an inflammatory response and enhance migration of aortic smooth muscle cells. *Thromb Res.* 2003;110: 187–194.

262. de Boer OJ, van der Wal AC, Teeling P, et al. Leucocyte recruitment in rupture prone regions of lipid-rich plaques: a prominent role for neovascularization? *Cardiovasc Res.* 1999;41:443–449.

263. Moulton KS, Vakili K, Zurakowski D, et al. Inhibition of plaque neovascularization reduces macrophage accumulation and progression of advanced atherosclerosis. *Proc Natl Acad Sci USA.* 2003;100:4736–4741.

264. Kolodgie FD, Gold HK, Burke AP, et al. Intraplaque hemorrhage and progression of coronary atheroma. *N Engl J Med.* 2003;349:2316–2325.

265. Brogi E, Winkles JA, Underwood R, et al. Distinct patterns of expression of fibroblast growth factors and their receptors in human atheroma and non-atherosclerotic arteries: association of acidic FGF with plaque microvessels and macrophages. *J Clin Invest.* 1993;92:2408–2418.

266. Ramos MA, Kuzuya M, Esaki T, et al. Induction of macrophage VEGF in response to oxidized LDL and VEGF accumulation in human atherosclerotic lesions. *Arterioscler Thromb Vasc Biol.* 1998;18:1188–1196.

267. Moulton KS, Vakili K, Zurakowski D, et al. Inhibition of plaque neovascularization reduces macrophage accumulation and progression of advanced atherosclerosis. *Proc Natl Acad Sci USA.* 2003;100:4736–4741.

268. Kolodgie FD, Gold HK, Burke AP, et al. Intraplaque hemorrhage and progression of coronary atheroma. *N Engl J Med.* 2003;349:2316–2325.

269. Kwon H, Sangiorgi G, Ritman E, et al. Enhanced coronary vasa vasorum neovascularization in experimental hypercholesterolemia. *J Clin Invest.* 1998;101:1551–1556.

270. Wilson S, Herrmann J, Lerman L, et al. Simvastatin preserves the structure of coronary adventitial vasa vasorum in experimental hypercholesterolemia independent of lipid lowering. *Circulation.* 2002;105:415–418.

271. Moulton KS, Heller E, Konerding MA, et al. Angiogenesis inhibitors endostatin or TNP-470 reduce intimal neovascularization and plaque growth in apolipoprotein E-deficient mice. *Circulation.* 1999;99:1726–1732.

272. Khrenov AV, Ananyeva NM, Griffin JH, et al. Coagulation pathways in atherothrombosis. *Trends Cardiovasc Med.* 2002;12:317–324.

273. Tanaka K, Sueishi K. The coagulation and fibrinolysis systems and atherosclerosis. *Lab Invest.* 1993;69:5–18.

274. Valenzuela R, Shainoff JR, DiBello PM, et al. Immunoelectrophoretic and immunohistochemical characterizations of fibrinogen derivatives in atherosclerotic aortic intimas and vascular prosthesis pseudo-intimas. *Am J Pathol.* 1992;141:861–880.

275. Koenig W. Fibrin(ogen) in cardiovascular disease: an update. *Thromb Haemost.* 2003;89:601–609.

276. Robson SC, Shephard EG, Kirsch RE. Fibrin degradation product D-dimer induces the synthesis and release of biologically active IL-1 beta, IL-6 and plasminogen activator inhibitors from monocytes in vitro. *Br J Haematol.* 1994;86: 322–326.

277. Strukova SM. Thrombin as a regulator of inflammation and reparative processes in tissues. *Biochemistry (Mosc).* 2001;66:8–18.

278. Spronk HMH, van der Voort D, ten Cate H. Blood coagulation and the risk of atherothrombosis: a complex relationship. *Thromb J*. 2004;2:12.

279. Libby P. The molecular bases of the acute coronary syndromes. *Circulation*. 1995;91:2844–2850.

280. Davies MJ, Thomas AC. Plaque fissuring: the cause of acute myocardial infarction, sudden ischaemic death and crescendo angina. *Br Heart J*. 1985;53:363–373.

281. Galis Z, Sukhova G, Lark M, et al. Increased expression of matrix metalloproteinases and matrix degrading activity in vulnerable regions of human atherosclerotic plaques. *J Clin Invest*. 1994;94:2493–2503.

282. Sukhova GK, Schonbeck U, Rabkin E, et al. Evidence for increased collagenolysis by interstitial collagenases-1 and -3 in vulnerable human atheromatous plaques. *Circulation*. 1999;99:2503–2509.

283. Herman MP, Sukhova GK, Libby P, et al. Expression of neutrophil collagenase (matrix metalloproteinase-8) in human atheroma: a novel collagenolytic pathway suggested by transcriptional profiling. *Circulation*. 2001;104:1899–1904.

284. Cameliet P. Proteins in cardiovascular aneurysm and rupture: targets for therapy? *J Clin Invest*. 2000;105:1519–1520.

285. Saren P, Welgus HG, Kovanen PT. TNF-α and IL-1β selectively induce expression of 92-kDa gelatinase by human macrophages. *J Immunol*. 1996;157:4159–4165.

286. Kovanen PT, Kaartinen M, Paavonen T. Infiltrates of activated mast cells at the site of coronary atheromatous erosion or rupture in myocardial infarction. *Circulation*. 1995; 92:1084–1088.

287. Leskinen MJ, Kovanen PT, Lindstedt KA. Regulation of smooth muscle cell growth, function and death by activated mast cells—a potential mechanism for the weakening and rupture of atherosclerotic plaques. *Biochem Pharmaeol*. 2003;66:1493–1498.

288. Schönbeck U, Sukhova GK, Shimizu K, et al. Inhibition of CD40 signaling limits evolution of established atherosclerosis in mice. *Proc Natl Acad Sci USA*. 2000;97:7458–7463.

289. Blankenberg S, Rupprecht HJ, Poirier O, et al. Plasma concentrations and genetic variation of matrix metalloproteinase 9 and prognosis of patients with cardiovascular disease. *Circulation*. 2003;107:1579–1585.

290. Bond M, Chase AJ, Baker AH, et al. Inhibition of transcription factor NF-_B reduces matrix metalloproteinase-1, -3 and -9 production by vascular smooth muscle cells. *Cardiovasc Res*. 2001;50:556–565.

291. Chase AJ, Bond M, Crook MF, et al. Role of nuclear factor-kappa B activation in metalloproteinase-1, -3 and -9 secretion by human macrophages in vitro and rabbit foam cells produced in vivo. *Arterioscler Thromb Vasc Biol*. 2002;22:(5)765–771.

292. Chen HH, Wang DL. Nitric oxide inhibits matrix metalloproteinase-2 expression via the induction of activating transcription factor 3 in endothelial cells. *Mol Pharmacol*. 2004;65:1130–1140.

293. Grote K, Flach I, Luchtefeld M, et al. Mechanical stretch enhances mRNA expression and proenzyme release of matrix metalloproteinase-2 (MMP-2) via NAD(P)H oxidase-derived reactive oxygen species. *Circ Res*. 2003;92:80e–86e.

294. Li D, Liu L, Chen H, et al. Lox-1 mediates oxidized low-density lipoprotein-induced expression of matrix metalloproteinases in human coronary artery endothelial cells. *Circulation*. 2003;107:612–617.

295. Liu J, Xiong WF, Baca-Regen L, et al. Mechanism of inhibition of matrix metalloproteinase-2 expression by doxycycline in human aortic smooth muscle cells. *J Vasc Surg*. 2003;38:1376–1383.

296. Luan Z, Chase AJ, Newby AC. Statins inhibit secretion of metalloproteinases-1, -2, -3, and -9 from vascular smooth muscle cells and macrophages. *Arterioscler Thromb Vasc Biol*. 2003;23:769–775.

297. Sebastian S, Peter H, Letterio B, et al. Overexpression of MMP9 and tissue factor in unstable carotid plaques associated with *Chlamydia pneumoniae*, inflammation, and apoptosis. *Ann Vasc Surg*. 2005;19:1–10.

298. Naghavi M, Libby P, Falk E, et al. From vulnerable plaque to vulnerable patient: a call for new definitions and risk assessment strategies, I. *Circulation*. 2003;108:1664–1672.

299. Naghavi M, Libby P, Falk E, et al. From vulnerable plaque to vulnerable patient: a call for new definitions and risk assessment strategies, II. *Circulation*. 2003;108:1772–1778.

300. Ridker PM, Rifai N, Rose L, et al. Comparison of C-reactive protein and low-density lipoprotein cholesterol levels in the prediction of first cardiovascular events. *N Engl J Med*. 2002;347:1557–1565.

301. Ridker PM, Hennekens CH, Buring JE, et al. C-reactive protein and other markers of inflammation in the prediction of cardiovascular disease in women. *N Engl J Med*. 2000;342:836–843.

302. Ridker PM. Clinical application of C-reactive protein for cardiovascular disease detection and prevention. *Circulation*. 2003;107:363–369.

303. Verma S, Li SH, Badiwala MV, et al. Endothelin antagonism and interleukin-6 inhibition attenuate the proatherogenic effects of C-reactive protein. *Circulation*. 2002;105: 1890–1896.

304. Verma S, Wang CH, Li SH, et al. A self-fulfilling prophecy: C-reactive protein attenuates nitric oxide production and inhibits angiogenesis. *Circulation*. 2002;106:913–919.

305. Pasceri V, Chang J, Willerson JT, et al. Modulation of C-reactive protein-mediated monocyte chemoattractant protein-1 induction in human endothelial cells by anti-atherosclerosis drugs. *Circulation*. 2001;103:2531–2534.

306. Pasceri V, Willerson JT, Yeh ET. Direct proinflammatory effect of C-reactive protein on human endothelial cells. *Circulation*. 2000;102:2165–2168.

307. Zwaka TP, Hombach V, Torzewski J. C-reactive protein-mediated low-density lipoprotein uptake by macrophages: implications for atherosclerosis. *Circulation*. 2001;103: 1194–1197.

308. Wang CH, Li SH, Weisel RD, et al. C-reactive protein upregulates angiotensin type 1 receptors in vascular smooth muscle. *Circulation*. 2003;107:1783–1790.

309. Verma S, Li SH, Wang CH, et al. Hyperglycemia potentiates the proatherogenic effects of C-reactive protein: reversal with rosiglitazone. *J Mol Cell Cardiol*. 2003;35: 417–419.

310. Verma S, Kuliszewski MA, Mickle DAG, et al. C-reactive protein attenuates endothelial progenitor cell survival and differentiation. *Can J Cardiol*. 2002;18[Suppl B]:325.

311. Yeh ET, Willerson JT. Coming of age of C-reactive protein: using inflammation markers in cardiology. *Circulation*. 2003;107:370–371.

312. Venugopal SK, Devaraj S, Yuhanna I, et al. Demonstration that C-reactive protein decreases eNOS expression and bioactivity in human aortic endothelial cells. *Circulation*. 2002;106:1439–1441.

313. Devaraj S, Xu DY, Jialal I. C-reactive protein increases plasminogen activator inhibitor-1 expression and activity in human aortic endothelial cells: implications for the metabolic syndrome and atherothrombosis. *Circulation*. 2003;107:398–404.

314. Mazer SP, Rabbani LE. Evidence for C-reactive protein's (CRP) role in vascular disease: atherothrombosis, immunoregulation and CRP. *J Thromb Thrombolysis*. 2004;17:95–105.

315. Zimmerman MA, Selzman CH, Cothren C, et al. Diagnostic implications of C-reactive protein. *Arch Surg*. 2003;138: 220–224.

316. Mullenix PS, Steele SR, Martin MJ, et al. Comparison of C-reactive protein and low-density lipoprotein cholesterol levels in the prediction of carotid stenosis. *J Am Coll Surg*. 2004;194(3S).

317. Alvarez Garcia B, Ruiz C, et al. High-sensitivity C-reactive protein in high-grade carotid stenosis: risk marker for unstable carotid plaque. *J Vasc Surg*. 2003;38:1018–1024.

318. Mullenix PS, Steele SR, Martin MJ, et al. C-reactive protein and traditional vascular risk factors in the prediction of

carotid stenosis. Presented at the 19th Annual Meeting of the Western Vascular Society, Victoria, BC; September 2004.

319. Subodh V, Michael RB, Todd JA. Endothelial function testing as a biomarker of vascular disease. *Circulation.* 2003;108:2054–2059.

320. Han KH, Hong KH, Park JH, et al. C-reactive protein promotes monocyte chemoattractant protein-1—mediated chemotaxis through upregulating CC chemokine receptor 2 expression in human monocytes. *Circulation.* 2004;109: 2566–2571.

321. Pearson TA, Mensah GA, Alexander RW, et al. Markers of inflammation and cardiovascular disease—application to clinical and public health practice. *Circulation.* 2003;107: 499–511.

322. Mosca L. C-reactive protein: to screen or not to screen? *N Engl J Med.* 2002;347:1615–1617.

323. Zalewski A, Macphee C. Role of lipoprotein-associated phospholipase A2 in atherosclerosis. Biology, epidemiology, and possible therapeutic target. *Arterioscler Thromb Vasc Biol.* 2005;25:1–9.

324. Gaines Das RE, Poole S. The international standard for interleukin-6: evaluation in an international collaborative study. *J Immunol Methods.* 1993;160:147–153.

325. Whitton CM, Sands D, Hubbard AR, et al. A collaborative study to establish the 2nd International Standard for Fibrinogen, Plasma. *Thromb Haemost.* 2000;84:258–262.

326. Poole S, Walker D, Gaines Das RE, et al. The first international standard for serum amyloid A protein (SAA): evaluation in an international collaborative study. *J Immunol Methods.* 1998;214:1–10.

327. Whicher JT. BCR/IRMM reference material for plasma proteins (CRM470). *Clin Biochem.* 1998;31:459–465.

328. Mosca L. C-reactive protein: to screen or not to screen? *N Engl J Med.* 2002;347:1615–1617.

329. Ford ES, Giles WH. Serum C-reactive protein and fibrinogen concentrations and self-reported angina pectoris and myocardial infarction: findings from National Health and Nutrition Examination Survey III. *J Clin Epidemiol.* 2000;53: 95–102.

330. Yano K, Grove JS, Chen R, et al. Plasma fibrinogen as a predictor of total and cause-specific mortality in elderly Japanese-American men. *Arterioscler Thromb Vasc Biol.* 2001;21: 1065–1070.

331. Gronholdt ML, Sillesen H, Wiebe BM, et al. Increased acute phase reactants are associated with levels of lipoproteins and increased carotid plaque volume. *Eur J Vasc Endovasc Surg.* 2001;21:227–234.

Atherosclerosis: In Vivo Characterization

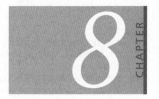

Alexander W. Leber

Venkatesh Mani

Juan Gilberto S. Aguinaldo

Zahi A. Fayad

Atherosclerosis is a chronic inflammatory disease that affects essentially all arterial beds of the human vascular system. It is the main cause of death in the Western Hemisphere, due to cardiovascular syndromes such as myocardial infarction (MI), heart failure, and cerebrovascular accidents. It derives from a complex interaction between genetic and environmental factors with inflammatory stimuli altering the structure of the arterial wall. An improved understanding of the disease process along with the emerging capability to noninvasively assess this process may facilitate preventative strategies for atherosclerosis or the identification of patients at risk for acute events.

CORONARY ATHEROSCLEROSIS IMAGING

Despite advances in our understanding of the pathogenesis of atherosclerosis, coronary heart disease is still the leading cause of death in Western societies. Approximately 50% of all MIs occur in patients with no prior symptoms. It is well established that the risk for plaque rupture is predicated by plaque burden and plaque composition (1). Reliable and accurate assessment of the composition of coronary atherosclerosis currently can be achieved mainly by invasive methods like intracoronary ultrasound or angioscopy (2). Since these are invasive procedures, they are not suitable for preventive investigations in asymptomatic patients.

Electron beam computed tomography (EBCT) and multidetector computed tomography (MDCT) enable an accurate noninvasive identification and quantification of calcified coronary plaques (3). Although calcified plaques reflect only a small proportion of the entire plaque burden and the proportion of lesions containing calcium reveals a broad variability among humans, it is suggested that the extent of coronary calcium is a surrogate marker for total plaque burden. It has been demonstrated that future coronary events may be predicted on the basis of the calcium score derived by various CT modalities (4,5).

However, MI is initiated by rupture or superficial erosion of vulnerable coronary plaques, and these plaques are not necessarily calcified, as calcium is considered to be a frequent feature of stable lesions (1). Further, there are several potential morphologic features such as lipid cores that constitute potential targets for noninvasive imaging in particular for multislice CT and magnetic resonance imaging (MRI). Hence, for risk stratification and guidance of antiatherosclerotic therapies, a noninvasive tool that can identify both calcified and noncalcified plaques would be of great interest.

CLINICAL VALUE OF CORONARY ATHEROSCLEROSIS IMAGING

Coronary atherosclerosis starts very early in life, and early stages of atherosclerotic lesions are already present in young adults under 20 years of age. In general, the disease remains clinically silent for years—50% of acute MIs occur in previously asymptomatic patients as the first clinical manifestation of coronary artery disease (CAD).

In other patients, the first clinical sign of CAD is typically stable angina pectoris, which is due to myocardial ischemia from a high-grade coronary lumen obstruction. The reason for the late development of clinical symptoms is that plaque accumulation within the vessel wall leads to compensatory diameter expansion, a process called *coronary vessel remodeling* (6). Therefore diagnostic tests targeting the detection of myocardial ischemia due to high-grade coronary stenosis identify only the late development stage of coronary atherosclerosis.

Currently, catheter-based invasive modalities like intravascular ultrasound (IVUS) and angioscopy are almost exclusively used for identification of coronary atherosclerosis in a preclinical stage. IVUS has been shown to allow an accurate determination of coronary plaque burden and plaque composition (compared with histology).

From postmortem histopathologic studies investigating the coronaries of victims of MI, it is known that the responsible culprit lesion in most cases reveals typical characteris-

tics: It is an eccentric plaque containing a large lipid core that is covered by a very thin fibrous cap with an abundance of inflammatory cells (macrophages) on its shoulders. Calcium is not necessarily present (7).

In accordance to these histologic criteria, IVUS has shown that plaque rupture initiating MI occurred most frequently in plaques with a large plaque volume with hypoechoic tissue revealing echolucent zones and presenting extensive compensatory vessel remodeling (8). Interestingly, most of these plaques caused no significant luminal obstruction on initial angiograms.

Evidence from recent investigations suggests that plaque rupture is a systemic coronary process rather than a focal event. In a multivessel IVUS study of patients with MI, Riofoul et al. (9) identified multiple silent plaque ruptures in vessels distinct from the culprit lesion. Similar observations were made by angioscopy, where multiple yellow (lipid-rich) lesions were found in patients with acute coronary syndromes, whereas in patients with stable coronary artery disease, the predominant plaque type was a white (fibrotic, calcified) plaque (10).

Goldstein et al. reported the presence of multiple complex lesions in patients with acute MI (11). In accordance, Leber et al. found significantly more noncalcified and less calcified lesions by multislice CT in patients with acute MI as compared with patients with stable coronary artery disease (12). Those studies indicate that it may not be sufficient to identify the one vulnerable plaque that will cause MI in the future because patients at risk have several of them. Moreover, it is necessary to identify the vulnerable patient on the basis of the "pan-coronary" morphology of atherosclerosis.

The reasons for the sudden rupture of multiple plaques are not fully understood at the present time. It is suggested that systemic inflammatory factors play a key role in the development of vulnerable plaques and their progression to rupture. Therefore, a combined approach of determining plaque burden and plaque composition in conjunction with the determination of biomarkers like CRP or s-CD40 ligand will play an important role for risk stratification in the future.

COMPUTED TOMOGRAPHIC IMAGING OF CORONARY PLAQUE—TECHNICAL ASPECTS

The rapid motion of the beating heart presents a challenge to acquiring high-quality motion and artifact free images. In the past, CT failed to generate diagnostic-quality images because of its restricted temporal resolution. Former spiral CT technology needed at least 500 ms to obtain one tomographic slice. With the introduction of electron beam CT (EBCT) and its fast acquisition time of 100 ms, the first motionfree images of the coronaries were obtained. Albeit, the excellent temporal resolution motion artifacts can only be avoided in a certain phase of the heart cycle during diastole. Thus, irrespective of the heart rate, it is mandatory to generate images at identical time points of the R-R interval, which is achieved by using an electrocardiogram (ECG) trigger.

With the introduction of MDCT, a temporal resolution of 83 to 250 ms is now available. In addition to the faster gantry rotation, the major advantage of this technology compared with conventional mechanical spiral CT scanners is that it consists of 4 to 32 detector rows, which allow generation of 4 to 64 slices simultaneously. For coronary applications, the whole volume of the heart is covered in the spiral technique with simultaneous digital registration of the ECG signal. Using this approach, images can be reconstructed after data acquisition retrospectively at every time point of the ECG cycle. The net result is a robustness against extra systoles and arrhythmias. Furthermore, different trigger points can be tailored to each coronary vessel.

CT scanners using 16- and 64-slice technology offer a very high spatial resolution and generate very thin slices, allowing the acquisition of isotropic voxels. This has already led to a major advance in noninvasive coronary angiography. For visualizing noncalcified plaques (unlike calcium scoring), a contrast agent has to be administered intravenously, and specific protocols for coronary computed tomography angiography (CTA) are applied.

To obtain diagnostic image quality with MDCT, it is essential to reduce heart rates below 65 beats per minute (bpm), generally accomplished by administering oral or intravenous beta-blockers. However, slowing the heart rate sufficiently can be a challenge, highlighted by the results in a recent study where 15% of patients failed to achieve a sufficient reduction in heart rate despite beta-blockade (13). Furthermore, patients with renal insufficiency or those allergic to contrast agent cannot be investigated by MDCT. Therefore, CTA is not suitable for a considerable number of patients.

COMPUTED TOMOGRAPHIC IMAGING OF NONCALCIFIED CORONARY PLAQUE

Plaque Composition

The recent advances in CT technology allow for the detection and classification of many atherosclerotic lesions affecting the coronary arteries. The CT attenuation of plaque components correlates well with the echogenicity of ultrasound and even histopathologic criteria. However, only limited data concerning CT imaging specific to the coronary plaque exists.

A recent ex vivo study by Becker et al. showed that advanced stages of coronary plaques in heart specimens can be detected by MDCT (Fig. 8-1) (14). In their comparison with the histologic Stary classification (Fig. 8-1A), they found that CT could visualize type III to type VI plaque, whereas early stages (types I and II) were not detectable.

In a 4-slice CT study, Schroeder et al. found a good correlation between the CT attenuation measured within coronary plaques and the echogenicity of plaques on IVUS (15). In another recent study, Leber et al., using a 16-slice CT, demonstrated that noncalcified lesions could be detected with a reasonable sensitivity of 78% (Table 8-1).

TABLE 8-1

Sensitivity of Multidetector Computed Tomography in the Detection of Different Coronary Plaques in Vessels (58/68) and Specificity to Exclude Coronary Lesions

	Soft (sensitivity)	Fibrous (sensitivity)	Calcified (sensitivity)	Total (specificity)
RCA	(12/16) 75% (48%–92%)	(27/34) 79% (62%–91%)	(49/49) 100% —	(94/102) 92% (85%–97%)
LAD	(44/54) 81% (69%–91%)	(47/62) 76% (63%–86%)	(76/83) 92% (83%–97%)	(294/315) 93% (90%–96%)
RCX	(6/10) 60% (26%–88%)	(13/16) 82% (54%–95%)	(25/26) 96% (80%–99%)	(96/108) 89% (81%–94%)
Total	(62/80) 78% (67%–86%)	(87/112) 78% (69%–85%)	(150/158) 95% (90%–98%)	(484/525) 92% (89%–94%)

Values are (n), %, (95% confidence interval).

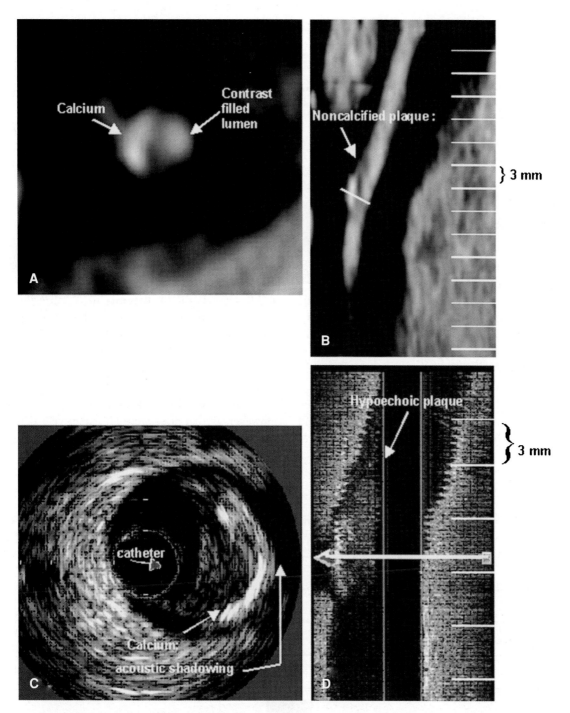

FIGURE 8-1 For analysis of IVUS and MDCT data, the coronary arteries were divided into 3-mm sections. *White lines* indicate 3-mm intervals of the RCA in the longitudinal view of IVUS **(D)** and MDCT **(B)**. **A:** Axial MDCT view of a calcified plaque. **B:** Longitudinal MDCT view of the RCA containing a partly calcified and noncalcified plaque; the level of image **(A)** is indicated by the *white line*. **C:** Corresponding axial IVUS view. **D:** Longitudinal IVUS view of the RCA; the level of the axial image **(C)** is indicated by the *arrow*.

However, they found that the ability of 16-slice CT to identify noncalcified plaques is restricted to larger, more advanced lesions (with a plaque diameter of at least 1.5 mm) that are located in proximal and middle coronary segments, limitations related to temporal resolution (13).

Quantitative characteristics of MDCT detected versus nondetected coronary plaques are shown in Table 8-2. Similar results were also reported by Achenbach et al. (16).

In accordance with previously reported results, Leber et al. also found a good correlation between CT density

TABLE 8-2

Quantitative Characteristics of Multidetector Computed Tomography Detected vs. Nondetected Coronary Plaques

	Detected	Nondetected
Plaque thickness	1.5 mm ± 0.3	0.9 mm ± 0.3
Vessel size (EEM CSA)	4.5 mm ± 1.2	3.6 mm ± 1.1
% Plaque cross-sectional area	42% ± 16%	22 ± 5%

p-values <0.05 for all categories.

measurements within plaques and echogenicity on IVUS. Hypoechoic plaques on IVUS that represented lipid-rich plaques had a significantly lower density than fibrotic plaques. Corresponding longitudinal and axial IVUS and MDCT images are shown in Figure 8-2. However, as in ex vivo studies, they also observed a wide overlap of density values among fibrous and soft plaques, making the differentiation of these lesions very difficult.

There are several reasons for this observation: (a) Even by IVUS analysis, the separation between lipid-rich and fibrous tissue is difficult, as the echogenicity differences between these plaques are relatively small. (b) Density values measured within plaques vary depending on the CT-attenuation within the lumen. The optimal luminal contrast enhancement for plaque differentiation has been found to be within 200 and 250 HU. This value however cannot be consistently achieved in clinical practice. (c) Coronary plaques are rarely composed only from fibrous, calcified, or lipid-rich tissue. In the majority of cases, all kinds of tissue can be observed. CT density values for hypoechoic, hyperechoic, and calcified plaques are shown in Figure 8-3.

Vessel Remodeling

As mentioned previously, positive coronary vessel remodeling is supposed to be a characteristic feature of vulnerable plaques. Schoenhagen et al. have demonstrated that MDCT offers the opportunity to visualize this compensatory diameter expansion (17). Achenbach et al. have also demonstrated that in highly selected patients, the 16-slice CT can determine positive and negative vessel remodeling, and it is feasible to accurately determine plaque areas (18).

The limitation of all these quantitative CT analyses, however, is that they were all exclusively performed in patients with high CT-image quality. This high quality

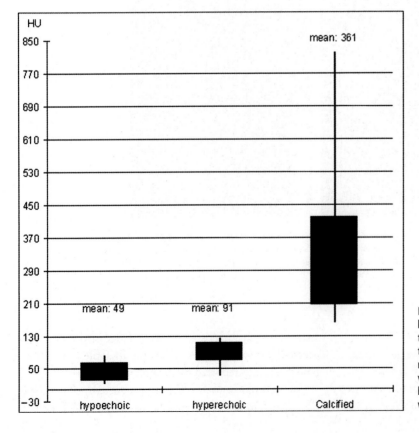

FIGURE 8-2 CT density values for hypoechoic, hyperechoic, and calcified plaques. Each box describes the distribution of density values within 1 standard deviation, the whiskers above and below each box describe the range between the lowest and highest observed density value. The differences of the mean CT density values between hypoechoic, hyperechoic, and calcified plaques were significant, with a *p* value <0.02.

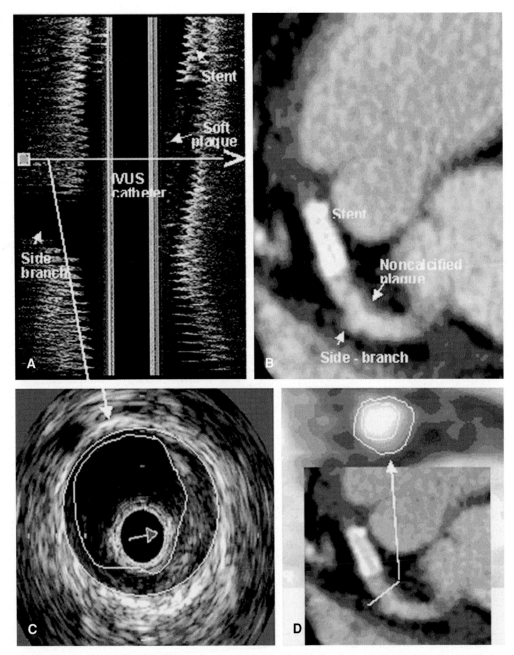

FIGURE 8-3 Corresponding longitudinal and axial IVUS and MDCT images. A: IVUS of a LAD in longitudinal direction containing a hypoechoic plaque adjacent to a stent. **B:** Corresponding MDCT reconstruction using maximum-intensity projection. **C:** Axial tomographic view of the hypoechoic plaque on the level of the arrow in image **(A)**. **D:** Same plaque in axial view using multiplanar reformatted MDCT data.

could only be achieved in approximately 75% of patients. Nevertheless, these study results indicate that MDCT provides a unique opportunity to identify several morphologic features associated with plaque vulnerability like plaque composition, plaque volume, and positive vessel remodeling. Although the prognostic impact of these features is unknown so far and the first follow-up studies are just under way, evidence from first clinical studies underline the predictive potential of MDCT.

In a clinical study, MDCT-derived plaque morphology of patients with acute myocardial infarction (AMI) and stable angina pectoris was compared. In this population, patients with stable angina had significantly more calcified and less noncalcified lesions than patients with MI.

As a consequence, total plaque burden of patients with MI would have been significantly underestimated by calcium scoring alone. Moreover, in 10% of patients with AMI, only noncalcified lesions were present. These observations imply that noncalcified lesions may be involved in the process leading to unstable coronary disease.

Schroeder et al. have demonstrated that the prevalence of noncalcified lesions is inhomogeneous even among a patient selection with a similar high-risk profile, which might reflect different prognostic outcomes. They observed in 14% of patients only noncalcified lesions, in 50% calcified and noncalcified lesions, and in 36% of patients only calcified lesions. However, future prospective studies comparing these populations are needed to assess the relative risk for developing adverse coronary events.

FUTURE DEVELOPMENTS IN COMPUTED TOMOGRAPHIC IMAGING

Due to a rapid improvement of the new generation submillimeter multislice CT technology, noninvasive tomographic imaging of the coronary vessel wall has now become a reality. The early clinical studies have shown the ability of 16-slice CT to determine plaque burden, plaque composition, and compensatory vessel wall remodeling. These novel findings already constitute an important step forward in assessing coronary atherosclerosis noninvasively in a detailed manner that opens promising new opportunities for a better understanding and risk stratification of coronary atherosclerosis. Current limitations, mainly the insufficient accuracy to detect small lesions in distal coronary segments, might be overcome by improved spatial and temporal resolution of the next generation of CT scanners operating with 64 and more detectors.

MAGNETIC RESONANCE IMAGING OF CORONARY PLAQUE—TECHNICAL ASPECTS

Compared with CT, MRI has several advantages when it comes to atherosclerosis plaque imaging. First, MRI does not use ionizing radiation for imaging. Second, MRI does not require the use of a nephrotoxic contrast agent.

High-resolution MRI has been used extensively for noninvasive evaluation of the arterial walls (19–21). With improvements in imaging technology, the ability of magnetic resonance (MR) to delineate these vessels has significantly improved (22–26). Over time, a diverse array of black blood MRI techniques (27,28) have developed into practical tools for the arterial imaging and evaluation of atherosclerosis. Dedicated coils and pulse sequences have

become more readily available for time-efficient multislice imaging (24,25,29,30). Black blood MRI has now become the preferred method for arterial vessel wall imaging. With this strategy, the signal from the blood is nulled, allowing for a clear depiction of the arterial wall. Most MR plaque imaging is currently being performed on a whole-body 1.5 T MR system.

The innate difference in relaxation times among various tissues can generate strong contrast on the image without the use of exogenous contrast media. To take advantage of this phenomenon, black blood multicontrast MRI can be employed with different excitation times, repetition time (TR), and echo time (TE) (21,31,32). For example, T1-weighted sequences will produce a brighter signal from tissues with short longitudinal magnetization recovery times (i.e., fat). T2-weighted sequences will produce a brighter signal from tissues with long transverse magnetization decay times (i.e., dense fibrous tissue). Proton density (PD)-weighted sequences, being a mixture of both T1 and T2 contrasts, will produce brighter signal with tissues with greater free-water content. To delineate the lumen of vessel walls, a bright blood technique such as time-of-flight (TOF) imaging is typically used.

In black blood MR, images are commonly acquired using a turbo spin echo (TSE) sequence with double inversion recovery (DIR) pulses (28) to provide good contrast between the lumen and vessel wall. DIR modules consist of two 180-degree radio frequency (RF) pulses. Magnetization in the whole volume is inverted by the first nonselective RF pulse, while magnetization in the slab of interest is subsequently restored by the second selective RF pulse (Chapter 2). The application of these two preparatory RF pulses causes spins outside the slab of interest to be inverted, with no effect on spins within the slab. Image acquisition begins following a time delay (TI) necessary for magnetization of inverted blood flowing into the imaging slice to reach null point (28). DIR techniques can be used to acquire multiple imaging slices simultaneously (25,26).

Two-dimensional (2D) and three-dimensional (3D) black blood (25,28,33) multicontrast techniques are commonly used in MR to visualize the vessel wall. To enhance the visualization of atherosclerotic plaque, intravenously administered contrast agents are used in conjunction with MR imaging (34–36). Integration of these modalities yields identification of plaque components. Multicontrast MRI has been used for classification of atherosclerotic plaque components (37–39). Shinnar et al. (32) have used multicontrast MRI to identify fibrocellular tissue, calcium, and lipid core with the help of semiautomated algorithms. Qualitative assessment of plaque composition using pattern recognition was performed on

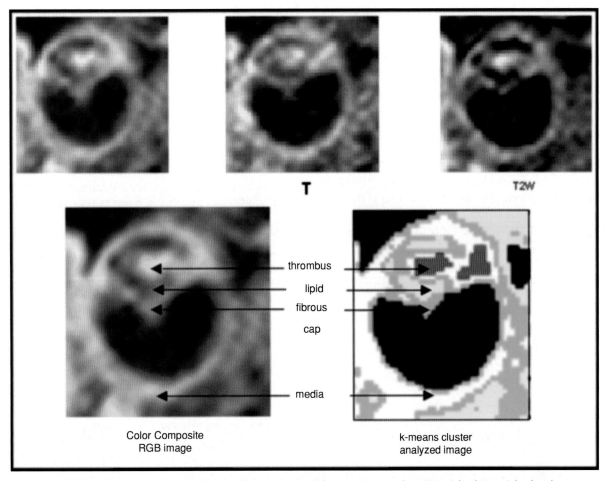

FIGURE 8-4 Multicontrast MR images of an in vivo carotid artery. Top row shows T1-weighted, PD-weighted, and T2-weighted images of the same plaque. The **bottom left panel** shows the RGB color composite image obtained by mapping the T1-weighted image to the red, the PD-weighted image to the green, and the T2-weighted image to the red channel, respectively. The **bottom right panel** shows the plaque segmented automatically into its various components using an automated k-means cluster analysis algorithm. Thrombus, lipid, media, and the fibrous cap can be clearly differentiated.

human aortas using T1-, T2-, and PD-weighted MR images. Normal wall (media), lipid-rich plaques, and fibrous plaques can be differentiated with a clustering algorithm (40). 3D fast time-of-flight imaging can be used in assessing fibrous cap thickness and morphologic "integrity" of the carotid artery plaques (41). This sequence is a bright blood technique in which the signal from flowing blood, and a mixture of T2 contrast weighting and PD contrast weighting highlights the fibrous cap (42). An example of multicontrast MRI showing different plaque components and automatic segmentation of these plaques with a k-means cluster algorithm is shown in Figure 8-4.

MAGNETIC RESONANCE PLAQUE BURDEN

Evidence from several studies show that MR is an excellent technique for quantitative measurement of total plaque volume and disease burden in vivo. MR is also a very accurate technique for plaque measurement. It has been shown that error in vessel wall area measurement was 2.6% for aortic and 3.5% for carotid plaques (43). Similar low measurement errors in plaque area and volume (4% to 6%) were reported by others, proving that plaque area and volume can be accurately assessed (44,45). Therefore, we estimate that changes in plaque size $>5.2\%$ or 9 mm^2 (for aortic lesions) and $>7\%$ or 3 mm^2 (for carotid lesions) are likely to be correctly detected by MR. This has clear benefits for study design, since only a relatively small number of subjects is needed to show a statistically significant change in vessel area by MR. For example, to measure a 6% true change in vessel wall area compared with baseline measurements, with a power of 0.8 and alpha of 0.05, 29 subjects would be required. Similarly, a 3% true change would require 108 subjects, and for a 12% true change, 15 subjects would be required.

MAGNETIC RESONANCE CAROTID ARTERY PLAQUE ASSESSMENT

The carotid arteries are located very superficially and do not move substantially during the cardiac cycle and therefore are ideal candidates for MR plaque imaging. Some of the MR studies of carotid arterial plaques include imaging and characterization of atherosclerotic plaques (46,47), quantification of plaque size (48), and detection of fibrous cap "integrity" (42).

Black blood cross-sectional images of the carotids of a 59-year-old patient with extensive atherosclerotic disease and a corresponding longitudinal section is shown in Figure 8-5.

Yuan et al. (46) have showed that in vivo multicontrast MR of human carotid arteries had a sensitivity of 85% and a specificity of 92% for identifying lipid cores and acute intraplaque hemorrhage. Cai et al. (47) have demonstrated a good agreement between the American Heart Association classifications of plaque and those obtained by MR. That study also demonstrated the feasibility of multicontrast MR for in vivo classification of the human carotid atherosclerotic plaques.

A strong association has been shown between fibrous cap thinning or rupture, as determined by MR imaging, and the history of recent transient ischemic attack (TIA) or stroke (49). Compared with patients with thick fibrous caps, patients with ruptured caps were 23 times more likely to have had a recent TIA or stroke (95% CI = 3,210). This study indicated that MR identification of a ruptured fibrous cap was highly associated with a recent history of TIA or stroke. There was also a strong and statistically significant trend showing a higher percentage of symptomatic patients for ruptured caps (70%) compared with patients with a thick cap (9%) ($p = 0.001$, Mann-Whitney test for cap status vs. symptoms).

MAGNETIC RESONANCE AORTIC PLAQUE ASSESSMENT

Wall thickness of the ascending aorta measured by MR is increased in patients with homozygous familial hypercholesterolemia (50). Thoracic aortic plaque composition and size were compared with matched MR and transesophageal echocardiography (TEE) cross-sectional aortic segments,

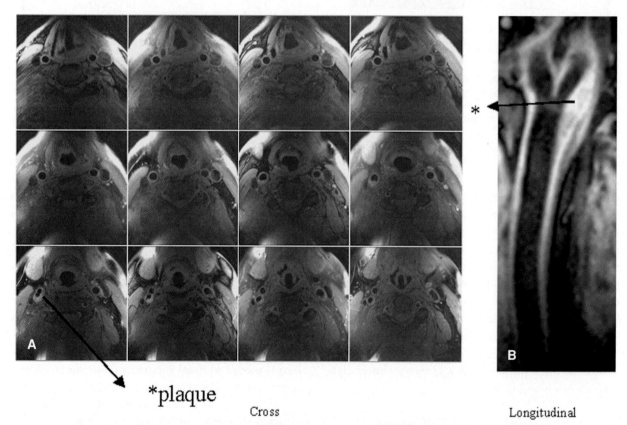

*plaque

Cross

Longitudinal

FIGURE 8-5 A: Axial MR images of carotid arteries in a 59-year-old patient with a history of coronary artery disease. The 12 consecutive axial slices are acquired using the 2D rapid extended coverage (REX) black blood sequence. **B:** The corresponding longitudinal section of the carotid artery. The PD–weighted images obtained show complex atherosclerotic plaque in the carotid wall. The *arrows* indicate plaque.

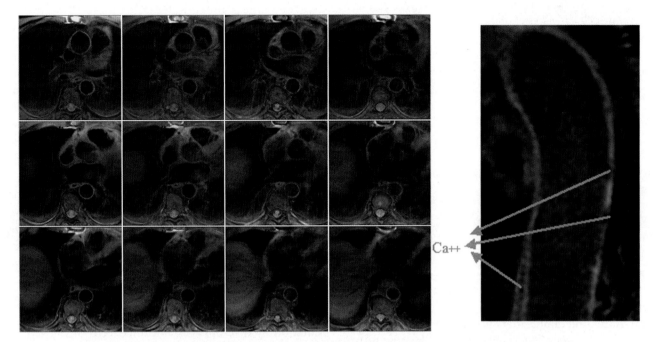

FIGURE 8-6 **Twelve axial images of the thoracic aorta of a 68-year-old patient with a history of coronary artery disease showing atherosclerotic plaque in the vessel wall.** PD–weighted images obtained using the REX sequence are shown. The corresponding candy cane (longitudinal section) image of the aorta shows areas of calcification in the aortic wall.

and there was a strong correlation for plaque composition and mean maximum plaque thickness. Black blood cross-sectional images and a corresponding longitudinal section of the aorta of a patient with atherosclerotic disease are shown in Figure 8-6.

In a subset of patients from the Multiethnic Study of Atherosclerosis (MESA), 196 participants 45 to 84 years old (99 black, 97 white; 98 men, 98 women) without clinical cardiovascular disease were recruited from six study centers across the United States. It was found that blacks had greater mean maximal wall thickness than whites. It was also observed that the maximal and average wall thickness as measured by MRI increased with the age of the patient. Additionally, men were found to have had greater maximal and mean wall thickness than women. This study demonstrates the feasibility of MR as a reliable method to measure aortic wall thickness with high interobserver agreement.

An MR imaging investigation of asymptomatic subjects from the Framingham Heart Study (FHS) showed that aortic atherosclerosis prevalence and burden (i.e., plaque volume/aortic volume) increased significantly with age and was higher in the abdominal aorta as compared with the thoracic aorta (51). It was also found that long-term measures of risk factors and FHS coronary risk score were strongly correlated with asymptomatic aortic atherosclerosis (51).

CORRELATIONS OF MAGNETIC RESONANCE–BASED ATHEROSCLEROTIC ASSESSMENT WITH CARDIOVASCULAR RISK FACTORS

One of the fundamental components of atherosclerosis is inflammation. A recent study was done showing associations of risk factors and plasma inflammatory markers with plaques in both the thoracic and abdominal aortas in 102 patients undergoing coronary angiography (52). C-reactive protein (CRP) has become a primary inflammatory marker. The inflammatory markers, fibrinogen and C-reactive protein levels, correlated with total plaque extent in the aortas.

The patient's age and systolic blood pressure correlated well with the extent of the plaque components in both the abdominal and thoracic aorta. Other risk plaques in the thoracic region were independently associated with CAD. The thoracic and abdominal aortas may have different susceptibilities to risk factors. However, the plasma inflammatory markers appear to reflect the total extent of aortic atherosclerosis.

A study by Weiss et al. (53) in 52 subjects, 40 to 79 years of age, showed that 22 (42%) of patients had increased wall thickness on T2W signal and/or on gadolinium contrast-enhanced MR in the carotid arteries and aorta with elevated serum levels of the inflammatory markers interleukin-6,

CRP, intercellular adhesion molecule-1 (ICAM-1), and vascular cell adhesion molecule-1 (VCAM-1).

MRI can assist in determining the risk of future cardiovascular events by measuring the serum markers of inflammation, and aggressive therapies can be instituted to reduce vascular inflammation factors such as LDL cholesterol and smoking, which are characteristically associated with plaques in the thoracic and abdominal aortas, respectively.

ASSESSMENT OF MAGNETIC RESONANCE TREATMENT EFFECTS

With continued improvements in MRI as a diagnostic tool, more studies are focusing on evaluation of treatments by MR. In one study, we have shown that MR can be used to measure the effects of lipid-lowering therapy (statins) on plaque regression in asymptomatic, untreated, hypercholesterolemic patients with carotid and aortic atherosclerosis (43). Aortic and carotid artery plaques were evaluated in 51 patients at baseline. This pioneering work was the first to demonstrate that maintaining lipid-lowering therapy with simvastatin is associated with significant regression of established human atherosclerotic lesions.

A case-controlled study demonstrated substantially reduced carotid plaque lipid content (with no substantial overall plaque area reduction) in patients treated for 10 years with an aggressive lipid-lowering regimen compared with untreated controls (54).

Recently, in an experimental rabbit study, Corti et al. demonstrated the beneficial effects of statins on atherosclerosis followed by MRI and compared it with the additional antiatherogenic benefits of combining a PPAR-gamma agonist with simvastatin (55). Finally, MRI has shown that lipid-lowering treatment with a statin may have different effects on different segments of the aorta, with a greater effect on atherosclerotic plaque in the thoracic aorta than in the abdominal aorta (56). Treatment with atorvastatin 20 mg for 12 months resulted in marked LDL cholesterol reduction and significant plaque regression in the thoracic aorta but only slowed plaque progression in the abdominal aorta. In patients treated with just 5 mg of atorvastatin, investigators also noted a significant progression of atherosclerotic plaque in the abdominal aorta, whereas vessel wall thickness and vessel wall area in the thoracic aorta increased slightly, but not significantly.

TARGETED MAGNETIC RESONANCE IMAGING OF MOLECULAR COMPONENTS IN ATHEROSCLEROTIC PLAQUE

One emerging technology in MR molecular imaging is its ability to detect unique biochemical activities for the in vivo diagnosis of pathological processes. The ability to target specific molecules of plaques may greatly enhance detection and characterization of atherosclerotic and atherothrombotic lesions using MRI (57). Atherosclerotic plaque components may be differentiated by introduction of plaque-specific contrast agents related to molecular signatures involved in the disease process. Another strategy is to link the contrast agents to antibodies (58–61) or peptides (62,63) that target specific plaque components or molecules that localize to specific regions of atherosclerotic plaques (64–67).

Cellular targeting of mononuclear cells such as monocytes, macrophages, and foam cells is an attractive means of identifying atherosclerosis, as these cells have been shown to play a pivotal role in the progression of atherosclerosis (68,69). At present, macrophages have only been imaged with iron oxide compounds (ultrasmall paramagnetic iron oxides [USPIO] and superparamagnetic iron oxides [SPIO]) that are removed from the circulation by macrophages and other cells of the reticuloendothelial system (65–67). In a study by Kooi et al. on 11 symptomatic patients scheduled for carotid endarterectomy, 75% of ruptured or rupture-prone lesions demonstrated uptake of USPIOs compared with only 7% of stable lesions and a decrease in signal intensity of 24% on T2* (66).

Research to determine the uptake of target macrophages with gadolinium-based contrast agents linked in the form of immunomicelles (micelles containing an antibody) that target the macrophage scavenger receptor in vitro showed a 79% increase in signal intensity in the aortas incubated with immunomicelles compared to a 34% increase in the control (70). The accuracy and validity of this approach were corroborated using fluorescently labeled immunomicelles (70,71). These are the first studies to target macrophages with paramagnetic immunomicelles. This biological activity imaging approach may ultimately become useful in vivo to detect the high macrophage density characteristic of the high-risk.

Neovascularization has been shown to play an important role in atherosclerosis, and the integrin $\alpha_v\beta_3$ has been targeted to identify regions in the vessel wall undergoing neovascularization (59–61). In a rabbit model of atherosclerosis, Winter et al. recently demonstrated that regions of neovascularization in plaque had a 47% increase in signal intensity following treatment with $\alpha_v\beta_3$-targeted nanoparticles (61).

Potential targets of interest for imaging atherosclerotic plaque with molecular-specific MR contrast agents include oxidized low-density lipoprotein (oxLDL), tissue factor, endothelial integrins, matrix metalloproteinases, and extracellular matrix proteins and were discussed

TABLE 8-3

Molecular Magnetic Resonance Imaging

Target	Ligand	Agent	Disease/ Process	Model	Field Strength*	Maximum Spatial Resolution**
ICAM-1	Anti-ICAM-1 antibody	Antibody-conjugated paramagnetic liposome (ACPL)	Encephalitis	Mouse brain ex vivo	9.4	0.04 × 0.04 × 0.04
E-selectin	Sialyl Lewis mimetic	Gd-DTPA-B(sLEx)	Multiple sclerosis	Rat brain in vivo	7	0.23 × 0.23 × 2
$\alpha_v\beta_3$ integrin	DM 101 antibody	Gd-perfluorocarbon nanoparticles	Corneal angiogenesis	Rabbit in vivo	4.7	0.2 × 0.1 × 2
$\alpha_v\beta_3$ integrin	RGD peptide vitronectin antagonist	Peptide-conjugated LEFPC	Atherosclerosis	Rabbit aorta in vivo	1.5	0.25 × 0.23 × 5
Ib^3	RGD cyclic peptide	RGD-USPIO	Platelet thrombus	Pig vein in vivo	1.5	0.3 × 0.3 × 1
Fibrin	Antifibrin monoclonal antibody	Paramagnetic nanoparticles	Thrombus	Human thrombus ex vivo	4.7	0.05 × 0.05 × 0.5
Fibrin	Antifibrin F(ab)	F(ab) monoclonal LEPFC	Venous thrombus	Dog in vivo	1.5	0.9 × 0.7 (in plane)

*Measured in Tesla.
**Resolution given in mm^3.
DTPA, diethylene triamine pentaacetic acid; F(ab), antigen-binding fragment; Gd, gadolinium; ICAM-1, intercellular adhesion molecule-1; LEPFC, lipid-encapsulated perfluorocarbon; USPIO, ultrasmall superparamagnetic particles of iron oxide.

extensively in a recent paper by Choudhury et al. (72) and listed in Table 8-3. While targeted nuclear imaging through the use of antibodies specific to oxLDL has demonstrated promise in detecting atherosclerosis (73), estimating plaque volume (74), and following progression/regression of atherosclerosis (75), we are unaware of any studies evaluating oxLDL as a target for molecular MRI of atherosclerosis.

Additionally, molecules such as tissue factor (76) and endothelial integrins (76–78) such as E-selectin, P-selectin, ICAM-1, or VCAM-1 have been targeted with antibodies linked to echogenic contrast agents for sonographic enhancement. While these agents utilize echocardiography or nuclear imaging, the echogenic or nuclear contrast agents could easily be replaced by linking an MR contrast agent to the monoclonal antibody to target the molecule of interest. Ultimately, the identification of molecules found only in atherosclerotic plaque will enable improved detection of atherosclerotic plaque, assuming that the target is expressed in adequate quantity for detection by molecular MRI.

The ability to identify components of thrombus with molecular MRI may enable enhanced detection and characterization of both luminal thrombus and components of an organized thrombus in an old atherothrombotic lesion.

Therefore, selection of targets in the coagulation cascade, such as fibrin, factor XIII, integrins on the surface of platelets, and tissue factor, is vital for identifying the areas of active or old thrombus formation. Monoclonal antibodies or peptide ligands with MR contrast agents that specifically bind to components of thrombus have been performed in animal models (63,79–81) and humans (82,83).

Additionally, thrombus resulting from plaque rupture has been identified using fibrin-specific MR contrast agents in a rabbit carotid crush injury model (62,84). In the 25 arterial thrombi induced by carotid crush injury, Botnar et al. demonstrated a sensitivity and specificity of 100% for in vivo thrombus detection using MRI (62). Sirol et al. (84) recently investigated a similar fibrin-specific MR contrast agent in 12 guinea pigs, demonstrating that thrombus signal intensity was increased more than 4-fold after intravascular delivery of contrast agent, and thrombus was detected in 100% of animals postcontrast compared with 42% identification of thrombus precontrast (84).

A new class of contrast agents, called Gadofluorines, achieves plaque enhancement. This macrocyclic, lipophilic gadolinium chelate complex (1,528 Da) with perfluorinated side chains forms micelles in aqueous solution. The driving force of binding and accumulation is the hydrophobic moiety of the molecules interacting with hydrophobic

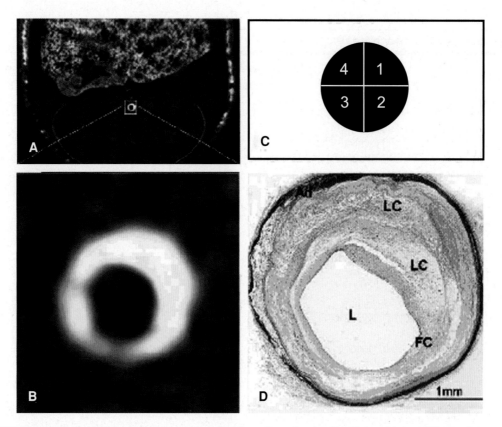

FIGURE 8-7 In vivo T1-weighted MR transverse image of an atherosclerotic rabbit abdominal aorta 24 hours after gadofluorine injection with the use of IR-DIFF-TFL **(A)**. The magnified panel **(B)** shows plaque enhancement after injection. Corresponding histopathological section is shown in **(D)**. The combined Masson trichrome elastin staining allows characterization of different plaque components. MR images and histopathological sections were divided into four quadrants for further analysis **(C)**. The appearance of the MR image correlates closely with the matched histopathological section shown in **(D)**. (Ad, adventitia; FC, fibrous cap; L, lumen; and LC, lipid core.)

plaque materials. Thus Gadofluorine M accumulates within the fibrous plaque or in the fibrous cap of a plaque containing high amounts of extracellular matrix components, but not in the lipid-rich areas (85).

Studies on rabbits showed enhancement in atherosclerotic plaque following gadofluorine administration, although results for determining the uptake of the agent on a particular plaque component have been limited. Sirol et al. (64) and others (86) demonstrated that Gadofluorine M enhanced aortic wall imaging in New Zealand White (NZW) rabbits but did not enhance the aorta of control rabbits. Gadofluorine M increased signal intensity by 164% at 1 hour postcontrast and increased signal intensity by 207% at 24 hours postcontrast (64). A strong correlation was found between the lipid-rich areas in histologic sections and signal intensity in corresponding MR images (64), which suggests a high affinity of gadofluorine M for lipid-rich plaques (Fig. 8-7). Further studies of the ApoE knockout mice showed it to be

colocalized in the extracellular matrix in the atherosclerotic plaque (Fig. 8-8).

Another novel imaging agent that is being developed uses a recombinant high-density lipoprotein (rHDL) molecule that incorporates gadolinium-DTPA phospholipids (87). High-density lipoproteins present in the plasma play a key role in reverse cholesterol transport by removing excess cellular cholesterol from the peripheral tissues. This imaging agent has several advantages; it has a diameter of 7 to 12 nm, is endogenous, does not trigger an immune reaction, and is easy to reconstitute (87). This agent was tested in vivo in apolipoprotein E (ApoE) knockout mice and demonstrated a 35% mean normalized enhancement ratio in the atherosclerotic plaque 24 hours following intravascular injection as well as a significant uptake of fluorescently labeled rHDL, as imaged by confocal microscopy (87). Figure 8-9 demonstrates the enhancement of plaque with rHDL and provides an illustration of the contrast agent.

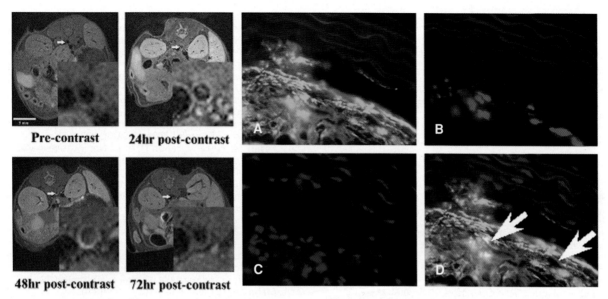

FIGURE 8-8 Left: MR images obtained pre- and at three post-contrast time points on the same ApoE knockout mouse. The lower right inserts of these images denote remagnified views of the abdominal aorta (*arrow*). **Right:** Immunofluorescence of ApoE knockout mouse at 24 hours post injection showing co-localization of Gadofluorine M within the extracelluar matrix. **(A)** Fluorescently labeled antibody to tenascin for extracelluar matrix; **(B)** Carbocyanin labeled Gadofluorine M; **(C)** DAPI staining for cell nuclei; and **(D)** Resultant image from the combination of A, B, and C.

FUTURE DEVELOPMENTS IN MAGNETIC RESONANCE IMAGING

Further improvements in MR coronary plaque imaging (88) are on the horizon and if successful could solidify the simultaneous multivessel (aorta, coronary arteries, carotid arteries, and other peripheral arteries) assessment of atherosclerosis. Future work will be geared toward 3.0 T or higher whole-body MR systems. New black blood techniques have recently been introduced for the simultaneous acquisition of multiple slices and have been shown to greatly reduce total examination time (26,89). Prospective studies are needed to determine the predictive value of fibrous cap characteristics of atherosclerosis, as visualized by MR, for risk of subsequent ischemic events (49).

MR use for serial monitoring of atherosclerotic plaque progression and regression in the carotid arteries and aorta is clearly growing rapidly and may be the noninvasive imaging

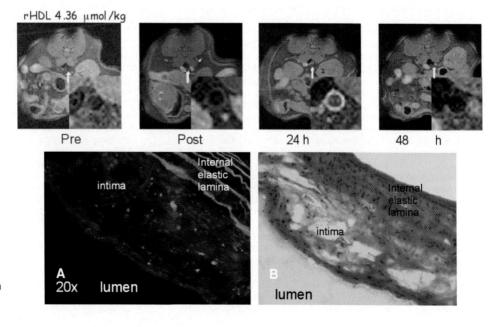

FIGURE 8-9 Above: In vivo MRI at different time points (pre- and postinjection of contrast agent at 24 and 48 hours, with the dosage of gadolinium as determined by plasma mass spectrometry (ICP-MS) measurement. *White arrows* point to the abdominal aorta; the **insets** denote a magnified aorta. **Below:** Confocal fluorescence microscopy of an atherosclerotic plaque **(A)**. *Blue* denotes nuclei (DAPI staining), and *green* denotes rHDL NBD labeled. Histopathological section stained with hematoxylin and eosin (H&E) **(B)**.

technology of choice for this purpose in the future, given the high image quality and the sensitivity to small changes in plaque size and possible characterization.

Combining different imaging modalities and adding new biomarkers of disease, such as MR molecular targeting that can be detected noninvasively, may be necessary to grasp the full picture of the disease; aid in its diagnosis, risk stratification, and management; and may help to predict future cardiovascular events.

REFERENCES

1. Naghavi M, Libby P, Falk E, et al. From vulnerable plaque to vulnerable patient: a call for new definitions and risk assessment strategies: Part II. *Circulation* 2003;108(15):1772–1778.
2. Schoenhagen P, White RD, Nissen SE, et al. Coronary imaging: angiography shows the stenosis, but IVUS, CT, and MRI show the plaque. *Cleve Clin J Med.* 2003;70(8):713–719.
3. Agatston AS, Janowitz WR, Hildner FJ, et al. Quantification of coronary artery calcium using ultrafast computed tomography. *J Am Coll Cardiol.* 1990;15(4):827–832.
4. Arad Y, Spadaro LA, Goodman K, et al. Prediction of coronary events with electron beam computed tomography. *J Am Coll Cardiol.* 2000;36(4):1253–1260.
5. Shaw LJ, Raggi P, Schisterman E, et al. Prognostic value of cardiac risk factors and coronary artery calcium screening for all-cause mortality. *Radiology.* 2003;228(3):826–833.
6. Glagov S, Weisenberg E, Zarins CK, et al. Compensatory enlargement of human atherosclerotic coronary arteries. *N Engl J Med.* 1987;316(22):1371–1375.
7. Virmani R, Burke AP, Farb A, et al. Pathology of the unstable plaque. *Prog Cardiovasc Dis.* 2002;44(5):349–356.
8. Yamagishi M, Terashima M, Awano K, et al. Morphology of vulnerable coronary plaque: insights from follow-up of patients examined by intravascular ultrasound before an acute coronary syndrome. *J Am Coll Cardiol.* 2000;35(1):106–111.
9. Rioufol G, Finet G, Ginon I, et al. Multiple atherosclerotic plaque rupture in acute coronary syndrome: a three-vessel intravascular ultrasound study. *Circulation.* 2002;106(7):804–808.
10. Asakura Y, Furukawa Y, Ishikawa S, et al. Successful predilation of a resistant, heavily calcified lesion with cutting balloon for coronary stenting: a case report. *Cathet Cardiovasc Diagn.* 1998;44(4):420–422.
11. Goldstein JA, Demetriou D, Grines CL, et al. Multiple complex coronary plaques in patients with acute myocardial infarction. *N Engl J Med.* 2000;343(13):915–922.
12. Leber AW, Knez A, White CW, et al. Composition of coronary atherosclerotic plaques in patients with acute myocardial infarction and stable angina pectoris determined by contrast-enhanced multislice computed tomography. *Am J Cardiol.* 2003;91(6):714–718.
13. Leber AW, Knez A, Becker A, et al. Accuracy of multidetector spiral computed tomography in identifying and differentiating the composition of coronary atherosclerotic plaques: a comparative study with intracoronary ultrasound. *J Am Coll Cardiol.* 2004;43(7):1241–1247.
14. Becker CR, Nikolaou K, Muders M, et al. Ex vivo coronary atherosclerotic plaque characterization with multi-detector-row CT. *Eur Radiol.* 2003;13(9):2094–2098.
15. Schroeder S, Flohr T, Kopp AF, et al. Accuracy of density measurements within plaques located in artificial coronary arteries by X-ray multislice CT: results of a phantom study. *J Comput Assist Tomogr.* 2001;25(6):900–906.
16. Achenbach S, Moselewski F, Ropers D, et al. Detection of calcified and noncalcified coronary atherosclerotic plaque by contrast-enhanced, submillimeter multidetector spiral com-

puted tomography: a segment-based comparison with intravascular ultrasound. *Circulation.* 2004;109(1):14–17.
17. Schoenhagen P, Tuzcu EM, Stillman AE, et al. Non-invasive assessment of plaque morphology and remodeling in mildly stenotic coronary segments: comparison of 16-slice computed tomography and intravascular ultrasound. *Coron Artery Dis.* 2003;14(6):459–462.
18. Achenbach S, Ropers D, Hoffmann U, et al. Assessment of coronary remodeling in stenotic and nonstenotic coronary atherosclerotic lesions by multidetector spiral computed tomography. *J Am Coll Cardiol.* 2004;43(5)(Mr):842–847.
19. Fayad ZA, Fuster V, Fallon JT, et al. Noninvasive in vivo human coronary artery lumen and wall imaging using black-blood magnetic resonance imaging. *Circulation.* 2000;102(5):506–510.
20. Worthley SG, Helft G, Fuster V, et al. Serial in vivo MRI documents arterial remodeling in experimental atherosclerosis. *Circulation.* 2000;101(6):586–589.
21. Yuan C, Mitsumori LM, Beach KW, et al. Carotid atherosclerotic plaque: noninvasive MR characterization and identification of vulnerable lesions. *Radiology.* 2001;221(2):285–299.
22. Griswold MA, Jakob PM, Heidemann RM, et al. Generalized autocalibrating partially parallel acquisitions (GRAPPA). *Magn Reson Med.* 2002;47(6):1202–1210.
23. Vignaux OB, Augui J, Coste J, et al. Comparison of single-shot fast spin-echo and conventional spin-echo sequences for MR imaging of the heart: initial experience. *Radiology.* 2001;219(2):545–550.
24. Yarnykh VL, Yuan C. Multislice double inversion-recovery black-blood imaging with simultaneous slice reinversion. *J Magn Reson Imaging.* 2003;17(4):478–483.
25. Mani V, Itskovich VV, Szimtenings M, et al. Rapid extended coverage simultaneous multisection black-blood vessel wall MR imaging. *Radiology.* 2004;232(1):281–288.
26. Itskovich VV, Mani V, Mizsei G, et al. Parallel and nonparallel simultaneous multislice black-blood double inversion recovery techniques for vessel wall imaging. *J Magn Reson Imaging.* 2004;19(4):459–467.
27. Nishimura DG, Macovski A, Pauly JM. Considerations of magnetic resonance angiography by selective inversion recovery. *Magn Reson Med.* 1988;7(4):472–484.
28. Simonetti OP, Finn JP, White RD, et al. "Black blood" T2-weighted inversion-recovery MR imaging of the heart. *Radiology.* 1996;199(1):49–57.
29. Song HK, Wright AC, Wolf RL, et al. Multislice double inversion pulse sequence for efficient black-blood MRI. *Magn Reson Med.* 2002;47(3):616–620.
30. Parker DL, Goodrich KC, Masiker M, et al. Improved efficiency in double-inversion fast spin-echo imaging. *Magn Reson Med.* 2002;47(5):1017–1021.
31. Cai JM, Hatsukami TS, Ferguson MS, et al. Classification of human carotid atherosclerotic lesions with in vivo multicontrast magnetic resonance imaging. *Circulation.* 2002;106(11):1368–1373.
32. Shinnar M, Fallon JT, Wehrli S, et al. The diagnostic accuracy of ex vivo MRI for human atherosclerotic plaque characterization. *Arterioscler Thromb Vasc Biol.* 1999;19(11): 2756–2761.
33. Edelman RR, Chien D, Kim D. Fast selective black blood MR imaging. *Radiology.* 1991;181(3):655–660.
34. Bedaux WL, Hofman MB, Wielopolski PA, et al. Three-dimensional magnetic resonance coronary angiography using a new blood pool contrast agent: initial experience. *J Cardiovasc Magn Reson.* 2002;4(2):273–282.
35. Goyen M, Debatin JF. Gadopentetate dimeglumine-enhanced three-dimensional MR-angiography: dosing, safety, and efficacy. *J Magn Reson Imaging.* 2004;19(3):261–273.
36. Regenfus M, Ropers D, Achenbach S, et al. Noninvasive detection of coronary artery stenosis using contrast-enhanced three-dimensional breath-hold magnetic resonance coronary angiography. *J Am Coll Cardiol.* 2000;36(1):44–50.
37. Corti R, Osende JI, Fayad ZA, et al. In vivo noninvasive detection and age definition of arterial thrombus by MRI. *J Am Coll Cardiol.* 2002;39(8):1366–1373.

38. Toussaint JF, LaMuraglia GM, Southern JF, et al. Magnetic resonance images lipid, fibrous, calcified, hemorrhagic, and thrombotic components of human atherosclerosis in vivo. *Circulation.* 1996;94(5):932–938.

39. Yuan C, Mitsumori LM, Ferguson MS, et al. In vivo accuracy of multispectral magnetic resonance imaging for identifying lipid-rich necrotic cores and intraplaque hemorrhage in advanced human carotid plaques. *Circulation.* 2001;104(17): 2051–2056.

40. Itskovich VV, Samber DD, Mani V, et al. Quantification of human atherosclerotic plaques using spatially enhanced cluster analysis of multicontrast-weighted magnetic resonance images. *Magn Reson Med.* 2004;52(3):515–523.

41. Yuan C, Zhang SX, Polissar NL, et al. Identification of fibrous cap rupture with magnetic resonance imaging is highly associated with recent transient ischemic attack or stroke. *Circulation.* 2002;105(2):181–185.

42. Hatsukami TS, Ross R, Polissar NL, et al. Visualization of fibrous cap thickness and rupture in human atherosclerotic carotid plaque in vivo with high-resolution magnetic resonance imaging. *Circulation.* 2000;102(9):959–964.

43. Corti R, Fayad ZA, Fuster V, et al. Effects of lipid-lowering by simvastatin on human atherosclerotic lesions: a longitudinal study by high-resolution, noninvasive magnetic resonance imaging. *Circulation.* 2001;104(3):249–252.

44. Kang X, Polissar NL, Han C, et al. Analysis of the measurement precision of arterial lumen and wall areas using high-resolution MRI. *Magn Reson Med.* 2000;44(6):968–972.

45. Chan SK, Jaffer FA, Botnar RM, et al. Scan reproducibility of magnetic resonance imaging assessment of aortic atherosclerosis burden. *J Cardiovasc Magn Reson.* 2001;3(4): 331–338.

46. Yuan C, Mitsumori LM, Ferguson MS, et al. In vivo accuracy of multispectral magnetic resonance imaging for identifying lipid-rich necrotic cores and intraplaque hemorrhage in advanced human carotid plaques. *Circulation.* 2001;104(17): 2051–2056.

47. Cai JM, Hatsukami TS, Ferguson MS, et al. Classification of human carotid atherosclerotic lesions with in vivo multicontrast magnetic resonance imaging. *Circulation.* 2002;106(11): 1368–1373.

48. Yuan C, Beach KW, Smith LH Jr., et al. Measurement of atherosclerotic carotid plaque size in vivo using high resolution magnetic resonance imaging. *Circulation.* 1998;98(24): 2666–2671.

49. Yuan C, Zhang SH, Polissar NL, et al. Identification of fibrous cap rupture with magnetic resonance imaging is highly associated with recent transient ischemic attack or stroke. *Circulation.* 2002;105(2):181–185.

50. Summers RM, Andrasko-Bourgeois J, Feuerstein IM, et al. Evaluation of the aortic root by MRI: insights from patients with homozygous familial hypercholesterolemia. *Circulation.* 1998;98(6):509–518.

51. Jaffer FA, O'Donnell CJ, Larson MG, et al. Age and sex distribution of subclinical aortic atherosclerosis: a magnetic resonance imaging examination of the Framingham Heart Study. *Arterioscler Thromb Vasc Biol.* 2002;22(5):849–854.

52. Taniguchi H, Momiyama Y, Fayad ZA, et al. In vivo magnetic resonance evaluation of associations between aortic atherosclerosis and both risk factors and coronary artery disease in patients referred for coronary angiography. *Am Heart J.* 2004;148(1):137–143.

53. Weiss CR, Arai AE, Bui MN, et al. Arterial wall MRI characteristics are associated with elevated serum markers of inflammation in humans. *J Magn Reson Imaging.* 2001;14:698–704.

54. Zhao XQ, Yuan C, Hatsukami TS, et al. Effects of prolonged intensive lipid-lowering therapy on the characteristics of carotid atherosclerotic plaques in vivo by MRI: a case-control study. *Arterioscler Thromb Vasc Biol.* 2001;21(10):1623–1629.

55. Corti R, Osende JI, Fallon JT, et al. The selective peroxisomal proliferator-activated receptor-gamma agonist has an additive effect on plaque regression in combination with simvastatin in experimental atherosclerosis: in vivo study by high-

resolution magnetic resonance imaging. *J Am Coll Cardiol.* 2004;43(3):464–473.

56. Yonemura A, Momiyama Y, Fayad ZA, et al. Effect of lipid-lowering therapy with atorvastatin on atherosclerotic aortic plaques detected by noninvasive magnetic resonance imaging. *J Am Coll Cardiol.* 2005;45(5):733–742.

57. Lipinski MJ, Fuster V, Fisher EA, et al. Targeting of biological molecules for evaluation of high-risk atherosclerotic plaques with magnetic resonance imaging. *Nat Clin Pract Cardiovasc Med.* 2004;1(1):48–55.

58. Kang HW, Josephson L, Petrovsky A, et al. Magnetic resonance imaging of inducible E-selectin expression in human endothelial cell culture. *Bioconjug Chem.* 2002;13(1): 122–127.

59. Kerwin W, Hooker A, Spilker M, et al. Quantitative magnetic resonance imaging analysis of neovasculature volume in carotid atherosclerotic plaque. *Circulation.* 2003;107(6): 851–856.

60. Anderson SA, Rader RK, Westlin WF, et al. Magnetic resonance contrast enhancement of neovasculature with alpha(v)beta(3)-targeted nanoparticles. *Magn Reson Med.* 2000;44(3):433–439.

61. Winter PM, Morawski AM, Caruthers SD, et al. Molecular imaging of angiogenesis in early-stage atherosclerosis with alpha(v)beta3-integrin-targeted nanoparticles. *Circulation.* 2003;108(18):2270–2274.

62. Botnar RM, Perez AS, Witte S, et al. In vivo molecular imaging of acute and subacute thrombosis using a fibrin-binding magnetic resonance imaging contrast agent. *Circulation.* 2004;109(16):2023–2029.

63. Johansson LO, Bjornerud A, Ahlstrom HK, et al. A targeted contrast agent for magnetic resonance imaging of thrombus: implications of spatial resolution. *J Magn Reson Imaging.* 2001;13(4):615–618.

64. Sirol M, Itskovich VV, Mani V, et al. Lipid-rich atherosclerotic plaques detected by gadofluorine-enhanced in vivo magnetic resonance imaging. *Circulation.* 2004;109(23): 2890–2896.

65. Ruehm SG, Corot C, Vogt P, et al. Magnetic resonance imaging of atherosclerotic plaque with ultrasmall superparamagnetic particles of iron oxide in hyperlipidemic rabbits. *Circulation.* 2001;103(3)(Jan 23):415–422.

66. Kooi ME, Cappendijk VC, Cleutjens KB, et al. Accumulation of ultrasmall superparamagnetic particles of iron oxide in human atherosclerotic plaques can be detected by in vivo magnetic resonance imaging. *Circulation.* 2003;107(19): 2453–2458.

67. Trivedi RA, JM UK-I, Graves MJ, et al. In vivo detection of macrophages in human carotid atheroma: temporal dependence of ultrasmall superparamagnetic particles of iron oxide-enhanced MRI. *Stroke.* 2004;35(7):1631–1635.

68. Falk E. Plaque rupture with severe pre-existing stenosis precipitating coronary thrombosis. Characteristics of coronary atherosclerotic plaques underlying fatal occlusive thrombi. *Br Heart J.* 1983;50(2):127–134.

69. Ross R. Atherosclerosis—an inflammatory disease. *N Engl J Med.* 1999;340(2):115–126.

70. Amirbekian V. Lipinski MJ, Briley-Saebo KC, et al. Detecting and assessing macrophages in vivo to evaluate atherosclerosis noninvasively using molecular MRI. *Proc Natl Acad Sci USA.* 2007;104(3):961–966.

71. Lipinski MJ, Amirbekian V, Frias JC, et al. MRI to detect atherosclerosis with gadolinium-containing immunomicelles targeting the macrophage scavenger receptor. *Magn Reson Med.* 2006;56(3):601–610.

72. Choudhury RP, Fuster V, Fayad ZA. Molecular, cellular and functional imaging of atherothrombosis. *Nat Rev Drug Discov.* 2004;3(11):913–925.

73. Tsimikas S, Palinski W, Halpern SE, et al. Radiolabeled MDA2, an oxidation-specific, monoclonal antibody, identifies native atherosclerotic lesions in vivo. *J Nucl Cardiol.* 1999;6(1 Pt 1): 41–53.

74. Tsimikas S. Noninvasive imaging of oxidized low-density lipoprotein in atherosclerotic plaques with tagged oxidation-specific antibodies. *Am J Cardiol.* 2002;90(10C):22L–27L.

75. Tsimikas S, Shortal BP, Witztum JL, et al. In vivo uptake of radiolabeled MDA2, an oxidation-specific monoclonal antibody, provides an accurate measure of atherosclerotic lesions rich in oxidized LDL and is highly sensitive to their regression. *Arterioscler Thromb Vasc Biol.* 2000;20(3):689–697.

76. Hamilton AJ, Huang SL, Warnick D, et al. Intravascular ultrasound molecular imaging of atheroma components in vivo. *J Am Coll Cardiol.* 2004;43(3):453–460.

77. Villanueva FS, Jankowski RJ, Klibanov S, et al. Microbubbles targeted to intercellular adhesion molecule-1 bind to activated coronary artery endothelial cells. *Circulation.* 1998;98(1):1–5.

78. Lindner JR, Song J, Christiansen J, et al. Ultrasound assessment of inflammation and renal tissue injury with microbubbles targeted to P-selectin. *Circulation.* 2001;104(17):2107–2112.

79. Schmitz SA, Winterhalter S, Schiffler S, et al. USPIO-enhanced direct MR imaging of thrombus: preclinical evaluation in rabbits. *Radiology.* 2001;221(1):237–243.

80. Johnstone MT, Botnar RM, Perez AS, et al. In vivo magnetic resonance imaging of experimental thrombosis in a rabbit model. *Arterioscler Thromb Vasc Biol.* 2001;21(9):1556–1560.

81. Flacke S, Fischer S, Scott MJ, et al. Novel MRI contrast agent for molecular imaging of fibrin: implications for detecting vulnerable plaques. *Circulation.* 2001;104(11):1280–1285.

82. Yu X, Song SK, Chen J, et al. High-resolution MRI characterization of human thrombus using a novel fibrin-targeted paramagnetic nanoparticle contrast agent. *Magn Reson Med.* 2000;44(6):867–872.

83. Winter PM, Caruthers SD, Yu X, et al. Improved molecular imaging contrast agent for detection of human thrombus. *Magn Reson Med.* 2003;50(2):411–416.

84. Sirol M, Aguinaldo JG, Graham PB, et al. Fibrin-targeted contrast agent for improvement of in vivo acute thrombus detection with magnetic resonance imaging. *Atherosclerosis.* 2005;182(1):79–85.

85. Meding J, Urich M, Licha K, et al. Magnetic resonance imaging of atherosclerosis by targeting extracellular matrix deposition with Gadofluorine M. *Contrast Media Mol Imaging.* 2007;2(3):120–129.

86. Barkhausen J, Ebert W, Heyer C, et al. Detection of atherosclerotic plaque with Gadofluorine-enhanced magnetic resonance imaging. *Circulation.* 2003;108(5):605–609.

87. Frias JC, Williams KJ, Fisher EA, et al. Recombinant HDL-like nanoparticles: a specific contrast agent for MRI of atherosclerotic plaques. *J Am Chem Soc.* 2004;126(50)(Dec 22):16316–16317.

88. Fayad ZA, Fuster V, Fallon JT, et al. Noninvasive in vivo human coronary artery lumen and wall imaging using black-blood magnetic resonance imaging. *Circulation.* 2000;102(5):506–510.

89. Mani V, Itskovich VV, Szimtenings M, et al. Rapid extended coverage simultaneous multisection black-blood vessel wall MR imaging. *Radiology.* 2004;232(1):281–288.

Thromboembolism

Andrzej Szuba
Izabela Gosk-Bierska
Richard L. Hallett

VENOUS THROMBOEMBOLISM

Deep vein thrombosis (DVT) and its primary complication—pulmonary embolism (PE)—are the two elements of venous thromboembolism (VTE), and epidemiological considerations regarding VTE always, to a greater or lesser extent, apply to both diseases.

Incidence

The incidence of VTE in the United States may be more than 100 per 100,000 patients; encompassing about 2 million new cases annually (1,2). About 30% of new VTE patients die within 30 days from the diagnosis, and 20% suffer sudden death due to PE (3). Long-term consequences of VTE include recurrent VTE, development of postthrombotic syndrome, and pulmonary hypertension.

Frequency estimates of fatal PE are much less reliable than of DVT, as diagnosis of PE is difficult, and postmortem studies are selective. Only one third of PEs are recognized antemortem (4). VTE, therefore, remains a serious socioeconomic problem (5).

Rudolf Virchow described three main factors responsible for activation of coagulation process and formation of blood clot: changes in the vessel wall, changes in the blood

TABLE 9-1

Prothrombotic Risk Factors

General
Thrombophilia, hereditary and acquired
Age
Immobilization
Obesity
Smoking
Pregnancy
Risk Factors Related to Other Diseases
Previous venous thromboembolism
Malignancy
Infection (HIV, herpes, sepsis)
Major trauma
Congestive heart failure
Stroke with associated paralysis
Nephrotic syndrome
Inflammatory bowel diseases
Hematological hyperviscosity syndromes (polycythemia vera, macroglobulinemia, plasmacytoma, essential thrombocytosis, etc.)
Iatrogenic Risk Factors
Major surgery
Intravenous catheters
Hormone replacement therapy and hormonal contraception

components, and venous stasis, later called *Virchow's triad*. After more than 100 years, all identified prothrombotic risk factors still fall into one of the original Virchow categories (Table 9-1):

Vessel wall factors: trauma (iatrogenic, accidents), surgery, sepsis, varicose veins, post-thrombotic syndrome

Blood component abnormalities: inherited and acquired thrombophilia (Fig. 9-1), hyperviscosity syndromes, surgery and the postoperative period, pregnancy, use of oral contraceptives, cancer, nephrotic syndrome, trauma, burns, infections

Venous stasis: due to immobilization (critically ill patients, surgery), congestive heart failure, chronic venous insufficiency, obesity, hyperviscosity syndromes, and the postpartum period and pregnancy

Any disturbance in the fine balance between coagulation and fibrinolysis will result in either a procoagulant state or a bleeding diathesis.

Inherited Thrombophilia

Inherited Thrombophilic States

Hereditary predisposition to vascular thrombosis due to genetic alterations appears to be quite common. In a study of New York newborns, mutations of four genes related to thrombophilia were found in 17.5% of tested newborns (6). Inherited risk factors for thromboembolism (antithrombin III deficiency, protein C deficiency, protein S deficiency, factor V Leiden, prothrombin 20210A) were found in 40% of patients with spontaneous lower extremity DVT before the age of 45 and in 33% of all other patients with leg DVT (7).

Antithrombin III Deficiency

Antithrombin III (AT III) is a member of the serpin family of proteins, which inactivates serine proteases. AT III inactivates thrombin, active factors III, IX, X, XI, and factor VIIa/TF complex.

Multiple genetic defects can lead to quantitative (type I) or qualitative (type II) AT III deficiency. Homozygous AT III deficiency leads to thromboembolic complications early in childhood (8) and is rarely described. Most patients with AT III deficiency have the heterozygous form. AT III deficient patients (heterozygous) of both the quantitative and qualitative types have AT III activity usually at about 40% to 60% of the normal value. The risk of VTE in these people with AT III deficiency was increased eightfold in one comparative study (9).

AT III deficiency is detected in 1.9% of unselected patients with VTE (10) but might be less common in the black population (11).

Protein C Deficiency

Protein C is activated by a thrombin-thrombomodulin complex. Active protein C is a potent coagulation inhibitor and inactivates factors Va and VIIIa on the platelet surface.

Multiple mutations causing type I or type II protein C deficiency have been found. The risk ratio of VTE in protein C deficient patients was reported as 7.3 (9).

Protein C deficiency is found in 2.3% of unselected patients with VTE (10).

Protein S Deficiency

Protein S is a protein C cofactor. Both quantitative and qualitative hereditary protein S deficiencies have been reported. Protein S deficiency increases risk of venous thrombosis five- to eightfold (9,12). Protein S deficiency is present in 2.3% of unselected patients with VTE (10).

Factor V Leiden

Factor V Leiden (FVL) is a hereditary defect that is caused by a single point mutation Arg506→Gln of factor V. This renders activated FVL resistant to hydrolysis by activated protein C, thus prolonging its thrombogenic effect.

It is the most common known cause of hereditary hypercoagulability in Caucasians and is present in almost 5% of

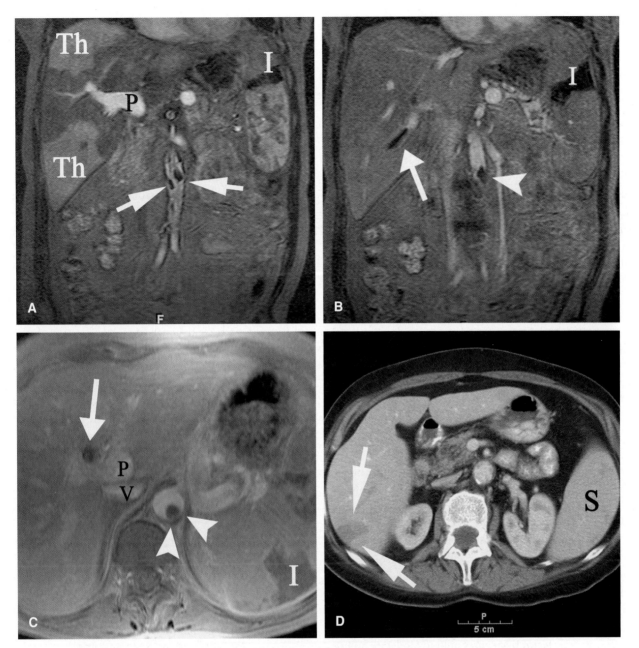

FIGURE 9-1 Thrombotic complications in a patient with essential thrombocytosis. Essential thrombocytosis is a chronic myeloproliferative disorder characterized by overproduction of platelets and subsequent thrombotic and hemorrhagic disorders. **A:** Coronal MRA (arterial phase). There is evidence of significant transient hepatic perfusion abnormality *(Th)* secondary to thromboembolic disease. There are clots hanging in the aorta *(arrows)*, which shows a lack of significant atherosclerotic disease. There is a splenic infarct *(I)*. Portal vein *(P)* is patent. **B:** Coronal MRA (hepatic venous phase). There is low-signal thrombus in a branch of the right hepatic artery *(arrow)*. The splenic infarct is also again seen *(I)*. Thrombus in the aorta is also depicted *(arrowhead)*. **C:** Axial gradient echo T2–weighted image after administration of gadolinium. There is a low-signal thrombus in the distal hepatic artery near the origin of the left hepatic artery *(arrow)*. There is prominent thrombus in the aorta *(arrowheads)* that could result in embolic material. The splenic infarct is again seen *(I)*. (P, portal vein; V, inferior vena cava.) **D:** Axial contrast-enhanced CT image, hepatic venous phase. There is a focal wedge-shaped hepatic lesion *(arrows)* compatible with a small hepatic infarct. The included portion of the spleen *(S)* is unremarkable.

people of European descent (13). In unselected patients with VTE, FVL is found in 18.8% of Caucasians (13) but only in 1.4% in blacks (11). Relative risk for VTE was found to be 7 in heterozygotes and 40 to 80 in homozygotes (14).

Prothrombin G20210A

The G20210A mutation of the prothrombin gene results in higher gene expression without a change in protein structure (15). The G20210A prothrombin gene allele is present in 2% of healthy Caucasian individuals and in 4% to 8% of patients with VTE (10,16). The risk of VTE in heterozygotes is 1.3 to 3-fold higher than in controls (17,18). This defect was not found in samples of the Indian population (19).

The G20210A mutation is found more frequently in children with central nervous system (CNS) thrombosis and arterial thrombosis (20).

Hyperhomocysteinemia

Elevated serum homocysteine may be caused by genetic and environmental factors.

Homocystinuria occurs in homozygotes for the genetic deficiency of cystathionine β-synthase (CBS). It is a recessively inherited disorder with a reported incidence of 1:650,000 to 1:344,000 (21). Patients with homozygotic CBS deficiency have very high levels of plasma homocysteine (>100 μmol/L) and carry an increased risk of vascular complications (22,23). Heterozygotes for CBS deficiency have a mild elevation of plasma homocysteine but a comparable risk to the normal control group (24). However, some authors suggest an increased risk (25).

Mild to moderate hyperhomocysteinemia may increase risk of DVT (26–28) and stroke (29); however, some studies show only a weak effect or no effect at all to elevated homocysteine in reference to the risk of VTE (30). The relationship between hyperhomocysteinemia and arterial occlusive disease is much better documented (31).

One genetic factor that causes mild to moderate homocysteinuria is thermolabile methylenetetrahydrofolate reductase (MTHFR)—a C677T polymorphism of the MTHFR gene (32).

The MTHFR C677T gene polymorphism is found in 13.7% of Caucasians (33). Recent studies on MTHFR gene polymorphism did not prove an increased incidence of venous and arterial thromboembolic disease (30,34). One recent study showed an increased risk of small artery occlusive disease in subjects with C677T MTHFR polymorphism (35).

Lipoprotein(a)

Lipoprotein(a) [Lp(a)] inhibits fibrinolysis by binding to fibrin and other plasminogen substrates (36). Elevated plasma Lp(a) is a well-established risk factor of atherosclerosis

(37,38). Lp(a) may also increase the risk of venous and arterial thrombosis; however, the results of published studies are conflicting (39–42).

Other Risk Factors for Inherited Thrombophilia

Multiple other abnormalities of genetic or undefined origin are postulated to cause thrombophilia. These include elevated plasma levels of coagulation factor VIII (43), especially prevalent in black patients with VTE (11); elevated levels of factors IX, X, XI (44); activated protein C (APC) resistance not related to factor V Leiden (45); heparin cofactor II deficiency (46); histidine-rich glycoprotein elevation (47); TAFI gene polymorphism (48); dysfibrinogenemia (49); dysplasminogenemia (50,51); PAI-1 gene polymorphism (52); and hyperprolactinemia (53).

Multifactor Genetic Thrombophilia

Coexistence of two or more genetic risk factors is not uncommon and significantly increases the risk of venous and arterial thrombosis (54,55).

In pooled analysis of eight studies, double heterozygotes for factor V Leiden and prothrombin G20210A were found in 2.2% of patients with VTE and none in the control group. The odds ratio for VTE in the double heterozygotes was 20.0 in comparison with 4.9 for FVL or 3.8 for prothrombin G20210A only (56).

An increased risk of thromboembolic complications was reported also for double heterozygotes for FVL and protein C deficiency (57), FVL and HR2 haplotype of factor V (54), FVL and homocysteinuria (58), FVL and MTHFR polymorphism, prothrombin G20210A and MTHFR polymorphism (55).

Acquired Thrombophilia
Acquired Prothrombotic States

Acquired thrombophilia may result from antiphospholipid syndrome (APS), the use of oral contraceptives, acquired deficiencies of natural anticoagulants, hyperfibrinogenemia, or acquired hyperhomocysteinemia. Other acquired risk factors for thrombosis include age, malignancy, immobilization, previous VTE, major surgery, trauma, intravenous (IV) catheters, congestive heart failure (CHF), nephrotic syndrome, diabetes mellitus, vasculitis, hematological hyperviscosity syndromes, inflammatory bowel diseases, infection (HIV, herpes, sepsis), obesity, and pregnancy.

Antiphospholipid Syndrome

APS, being probably the most common autoimmune disorder, is characterized by venous and/or arterial vascular thrombotic complications (including miscarriages) and the presence of autoantibodies against membrane phospholipids (antiphospholipid antibodies or APAs) in blood. APAs are responsible for the prolongation of clotting time in patients with systemic lupus erythematosus (SLE) and were named *lupus anticoagulant*. However, the presence of APA was found to predispose to thrombotic complications rather than to bleeding (59).

APAs occur in 1% to 5% of the population and increase with age (50% of patients older than 80 years have APAs) (60). These antibodies can be detected in 12% to 30% of patients with SLE (61). They are also detected in syphilis, tuberculosis, viral infections (HIV, hepatitis C virus), mycoplasma, and other infections (62,63); however, APAs associated with infections usually do not predispose to thrombotic complications (63). APAs may be present more frequently in patients with cancer and severe alcoholic intoxication (64). Familial occurrence of APA is also reported (65).

APAs form a heterogeneous group of antibodies against complexes of phospholipids and their protein cofactors (66), especially beta2-glycoprotein-I (67,68) and prothrombin (69). The mechanism of the prothrombotic action of APA is not fully elucidated and may include endothelial damage, impairment of fibrinolysis, platelet activation, interference with natural anticoagulants, and possibly other mechanisms (70–72).

Preliminary diagnostic criteria were proposed in 1998 in Sapporo, Japan, and published in 1999 (73). The APS diagnosis can be made in presence of one clinical and one laboratory criterion (Table 9-2).

The clinical presentation of antiphospholipid syndrome includes venous thromboembolic disease, arterial thrombosis (often cerebrovascular), mild thrombocytopenia, and recurrent fetal loss.

Secondary APS most often is recognized in patients diagnosed with SLE, while primary APS is diagnosed when no primary associated disease is recognized.

Catastrophic antiphospholipid syndrome (CAS) is a rare, dramatic worsening of APS with symptoms of multiorgan failure caused by widespread thrombosis of the microvascular bed.

CAS mortality rate approaches 50%. Of survivors, 26% develop APS-related thrombotic complications (74).

Antiphospholipid Syndrome Treatment. Although recognized as an autoimmune disorder, APS does not respond to immunosuppression. Typical treatment is limited to oral anticoagulants, sometimes with low doses of acetylsalicylic acid.

Patients with APS and venous or arterial thrombosis require lifelong oral anticoagulation with an international normalized ratio (INR) for blood clotting time between 3 and 4; however, there is no consensus on this issue

---

TABLE 9-2

Antiphospholipid Syndrome—Diagnosis and Clinical Presentation

Clinical Criteria
1. Vascular thrombosis. One or more clinical episodes of arterial, venous, or small vessel thrombosis occurring in any tissue or organ.
2. Complications of pregnancy. One or more unexplained deaths of morphologically normal fetuses at or after the 10th week of gestation; or one or more premature births of morphologically normal neonates at or before the 34th week of gestation; or three or more unexplained consecutive spontaneous abortions before the 10th week of gestation.

Laboratory Criteria
1. Anticardiolipin antibodies. IgG or IgM antibodies present in moderate or high levels in the blood on two or more occasions at least 6 weeks apart.
2. Lupus anticoagulant antibodies. Lupus anticoagulant antibodies detected in the blood on two or more occasions at least 6 weeks apart, according to the guidelines of the International Society on Thrombosis and Hemostasis.

Reprinted with permission from Wilson WA, Gharavi AE, Koike T. International consensus statement on preliminary classification criteria for definite antiphospholipid syndrome: report of an international workshop. *Arthritis Rheum.* 1999;42(7):1309–1311.

(61,75,76). Pregnant women with APS and a history of miscarriages will require anticoagulation with heparin and low-dose acetylsalicylic acid (77,78).

There are no data on the benefits of prophylactic anticoagulation therapy in patients with high titers of anticardiolipin antibodies without a previous history of thrombosis (61).

Risk Factors

Age

Age is an independent risk factor for VTE (3,79). Risk of VTE increases with a hazard ratio of approximately 1.7 per decade of life (80), and at an age >80 years, the incidence of VTE may be as high as 500 per 100,000 (1).

Immobilization

Immobility, regardless of the reason, increases the risk of VTE as a result of venous stasis. It is an important and easily recognizable risk factor and an indication for VTE prophylaxis in hospital patients (81,82). Immobility due to nonmedical conditions like prolonged air travel predisposes to calf DVT and PE. Asymptomatic DVT may occur in up to 10% of passengers on long flights (83,84); however, only passengers with preexisting thrombophilia may have an increased risk of VTE (85).

Obesity

Obesity increases the risk of VTE (80,86). Decreased fibrinolytic activity and increased levels of procoagulant factors (87) as well as lower level of physical activity may contribute to increased incidence of VTE in overweight and obese individuals.

Smoking

Smoking results in injury to the vessel wall (88) and increases the risk of arterial cardiovascular events. Smoking is a well-known risk factor for cardiovascular arterial thrombotic events, including myocardial infarction (MI) and ischemic stroke, but also might predispose to VTE (89). The risk is probably small and was not found in other studies (80). Smoking increases the risk of arterial and venous thrombosis in women who take oral contraceptives (90–92).

Pregnancy and Puerperium

Pregnant women are at a six times higher risk of VTE than nonpregnant women. VTE remains a major cause of morbidity and mortality in pregnancy (93), and the risk of VTE is even higher in the postpartum period (94). Risk of VTE is further increased with obesity, age >35 years, emergency cesarean section, preeclampsia, previous VTE, or the presence of acquired or inherited thrombophilia (94–97).

Arterial thromboembolism in pregnancy is rare and is related to thrombophilia, vasculitis, and arterial dissection (98).

Previous Venous Thromboembolism

Patients with a history of VTE are at higher risk of recurrent VTE. The increased risk may result from preexisting thrombophilia as well as injury to the vessel wall.

After the first episode of VTE, 7% to 10% of patients develop recurrent thrombosis within 6 months despite anticoagulation (1,99) and up to 30% after anticoagulation is stopped (99,100). The risk of recurrence is higher in subjects who present with other risk factors (99).

Malignancy

Patients with malignancy are at a higher risk for venous and arterial thrombosis. Vascular thrombosis is a major cause of morbidity and mortality in cancer patients (101–103). Breast, colorectal, and lung cancer are frequently associated with vascular thrombosis (Fig. 9-2); the malignancies with the highest risk of thrombotic complications are pancreatic cancer, brain tumors, liver cancer, ovarian and uterine cancer, prostate cancer, and Hodgkin lymphoma (104–108). Increased risk of thrombosis is multifactorial, related to hypercoagulability, vascular injury, and hemodynamic

changes in cancer patients. Identified mechanisms of thrombophilia in malignancy include expression of tissue factor and cancer procoagulant on cancer cells (109) and hyperviscosity related to polycythemia vera and/or thrombocytosis (110,111). Cancer infiltration of blood vessels may result in vascular stenosis or occlusion (Fig. 9-3). Cancer therapy may also trigger vascular thrombosis (long-term IV catheters, endothelial injury caused by chemotherapy, radiation injury to the vascular wall) (112–115).

Idiopathic VTE can be a first symptom of occult malignancy (116,117). Up to 12% of patients with idiopathic VTE may have occult cancer (105).

Infections

Infections may trigger formation of venous or arterial thrombosis, due to systemic activation of the coagulation cascade (118–120) or through local injury to the vessel wall per continuitatem from an adjacent infected organ (121–124).

Certain infectious agents like Chlamydia pneumoniae and HIV are suspected to predispose to VTE; however, the association is yet to be confirmed in larger studies (125–127).

Septic arterial embolization may complicate infectious endocarditis (128,129) or aortitis (130,131).

Major Trauma

Patients with major trauma are at higher risk of thromboembolic complications (132). The frequency of VTE varies depending on the type of trauma and the evaluation method. The average incidence of DVT in trauma patients was found to be around 11% and 1.5% for PE (133).

Other Diseases

Multiple medical conditions are associated with an increased incidence of venous and/or arterial thrombosis. Up to 12% of patients with CHF had evidence of PE in autopsy studies (134). Risk of VTE is higher in patients with a low ejection fraction (135). Also, patients with paralysis caused by stroke or spinal cord injury (136) are at risk of thromboembolic complications. Children and adults with nephrotic syndrome suffer more frequently from venous and arterial thromboembolic events secondary to dysproteinemia (low AT III, high fibrinogen) (137,138). Inflammatory bowel diseases are associated with thrombophilia and increased incidence of VTE (139).

Major Surgery

Surgical procedures are considered a risk factor for VTE. However, recent analysis suggests that the frequency of VTE in hospitalized nonsurgical and surgical patients is similar (136). A large retrospective analysis of over 1.6 million surgical

(*text continues on page 303*)

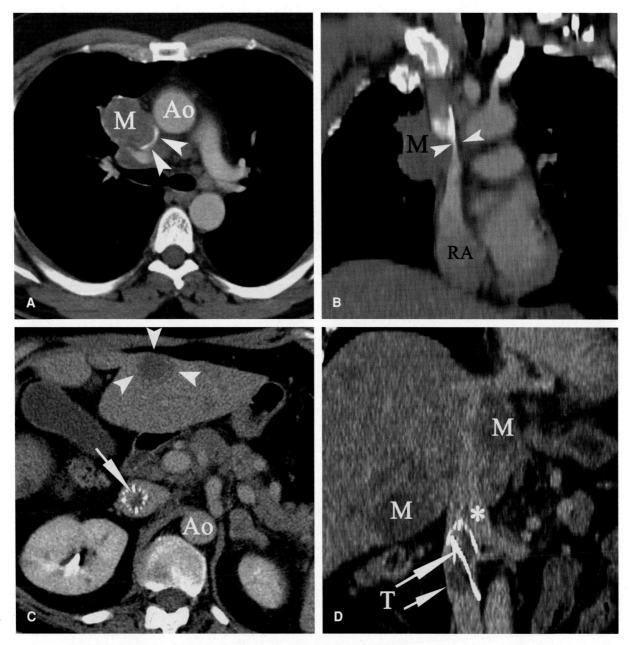

FIGURE 9-2 A 55-year-old nonsmoker with bronchogenic carcinoma. A: Axial image from contrast-enhanced chest CT shows significant mass effect on the superior vena cava (*arrowheads*) from a large pulmonary mass *(M)*, which proved to be adenocarcinoma on biopsy. (Ao, aorta.) **B:** Coronal reformatted image from chest CT shows narrowing of the SVC (*arrowheads*) by the mass *(M)*. Note caudal portions of the SVC are patent, emptying into the right atrium *(RA)*. **C:** Axial image from routine abdominal CT. The same patient 1 month later, after placement of IVC filter for symptomatic DVT and PE. There is thrombus visualized within the interstices of the filter (*arrow*). Note also the mass in the lateral segment left lobe of the liver (*arrowheads*), consistent with a metastasis. (Ao, aorta.) **D:** Coronal reformatted image from the same exam, showing thrombus *(T)* collecting in the IVC filter struts. Additional metastatic liver lesions are demonstrated *(M)*. Note also a second IVC filter (*) placed above the first, secondary to incomplete opening of the first filter and lack of complete coverage of the IVC. Clot is seen in this more cephalad filter as well.

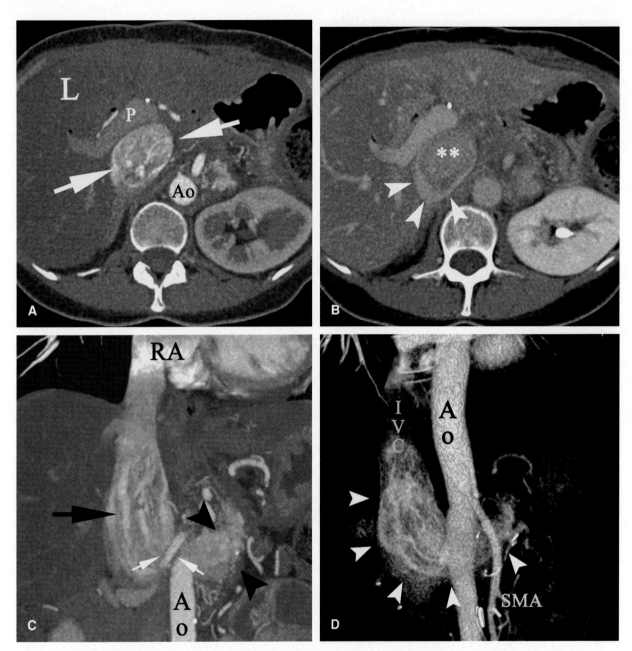

FIGURE 9-3 Invasion and obstruction of inferior vena cava secondary to islet cell tumor of pancreas. A: Axial arterial-phase image from dual-phase abdominal CT. There is a hypervascular mass (*arrows*) in the inferior vena cava. Some lower attenuation regions within the lesion also reflect thrombus. (L, liver; P, portal vein; Ao, aorta.) **B:** Axial venous-phase image at same level shows narrowing of the flow lumen in the IVC (*arrowheads*). The mass and clot (**) are now more homogeneous in density secondary to washout of arterial phase contrast. **C:** Coronal reformatted arterial-phase image shows the pancreatic mass (*arrowheads*) with extension of mass into the IVC (*black arrow*) but not into the right atrium (*RA*). The superior mesenteric artery (*white arrows*) provides blood flow to the hypervascular mass. (Ao, aorta.) **D:** Volume-rendered bone segmented image shows mass extending into IVC (*arrowheads*). The relation of the mass to the superior mesenteric artery (*SMA*) is well displayed without evidence of narrowing or occlusion. (IVC, inferior vena cava; Ao, aorta.)

patients revealed an overall frequency of VTE within 3 months after surgery of 0.8%. Increased risk of VTE was associated with age, Latino and Asian/Pacific Islander ethnicity, malignancy, and a history of previous VTE. Higher incidence of symptomatic VTE (2% to 3%) were associated with invasive neurosurgery, total hip arthroplasty, major vascular surgery, and radical cystectomy (140). Forty percent to 50% of VTE incidents occurred after discharge from the hospital (140,141), which supports the need for longer anticoagulant prophylaxis after surgery (142).

The incidence of asymptomatic VTE was examined in many trials and is much more frequent, exceeding 50% of patients undergoing elective knee or hip surgery (143,144).

Intravenous Catheters

Central venous catheters pose an important risk of venous thrombosis, especially in cancer patients (112,145). Central venous catheters in children with lymphoblastic leukemia have been associated with venous thrombosis in 34% of patients (146).

Oral Contraceptives and Hormone Replacement Therapy

Use of oral contraceptives (OC) increases the risk of VTE. The overall risk of VTE is about three times higher than in nonusers (147). The risk of VTE increases with the dose of estrogen and might be higher with third-generation progestins as compared with second-generation progestins (147,148); however, these differences were not found in some studies (149). The risk of VTE in women taking OC increases dramatically (17-fold) in clinical situations that predispose to VTE (150). Hormone replacement therapy also carries two- to fourfold increased risk of VTE and MI (151–153). The risk of venous and arterial thrombosis is further increased in patients with primary or secondary thrombophilia (154–156).

LOWER AND UPPER EXTREMITY DEEP VEIN THROMBOSIS

DVT is a common and frequently underdiagnosed disorder, characterized by formation of a thrombus within the lumen of the vein. Venous thrombi are composed mainly from erythrocytes and are dark red in appearance. Usually, they originate in the valve pocket of the deep vein and extend to fill the whole vessel lumen. They are loosely attached to the venous endothelium and can be easily fragmented and cause pulmonary embolization.

The deep venous system of the lower extremities is the most common location of DVT, and the deep calf veins are the most common site in the lower extremity (143,157,158).

Lower Extremity Deep Vein Thrombosis

Lower extremity DVT is difficult to diagnose by means of clinical symptoms only. So-called "typical" symptoms are frequently absent or falsely positive; however, a combination of clinical symptoms and risk factors can often lead to proper diagnosis (159). The majority of lower extremity DVT is asymptomatic (1,160,161) and resolve spontaneously. Frequently, an episode of PE is the first sign of DVT.

Classic local clinical symptoms of lower extremity DVT include unilateral increased calf circumference and/or "pitting" edema of the distal part of extremity, calf pain, and Homan sign (calf pain during passive dorsiflexion of the foot), calf and thigh tenderness, skin discoloration (cyanosis), and erythema. Those symptoms are notoriously nonspecific and have low value for clinicians (162). Therefore, multiple clinical score systems are used since combinations of symptoms have better diagnostic value (163–165).

Natural History of Lower Extremity Deep Vein Thrombosis

The deep veins of the calf are the most common location of lower extremity DVT (143,158). Without therapy, up to 25% of calf DVT progresses to the popliteal and femoral veins (166). Spontaneous resolution occurs more frequently in DVT that is limited to the calf (143,166). In patients with isolated calf DVT, Meissner found 50% thrombus load reduction in one month and 100% after 1 year (167). Kim, studying patients with venography after knee arthroplasty, documented thrombus resolution in all patients within 6 months (143).

Patients with proximal DVT are more likely to have PE, which occurs in about 50% of patients (166) (Fig. 9-4). Proximal DVT is also more likely to cause chronic venous occlusion (168). Post-thrombotic syndrome (PTS) features chronic pain, edema, hyperpigmentation, and skin ulceration and is a frequent late sequel of DVT. Its incidence varies in different studies from 82% (169) to 11% in patients after hip arthroplasty complicated by DVT (170). Risk factors of PTS after DVT included multilevel DVT, calf DVT, recurrence of ipsilateral DVT, and insufficient oral anticoagulation (169).

Phlegmasia cerulea dolens is an uncommon presentation of severe multilevel lower extremity DVT, usually in patients with malignancy or other causes of thrombophilia. Almost complete obstruction of the venous outflow results in rapidly progressive leg edema with compromise of arterial perfusion and distal gangrene (171). The high mortality rate is the result of hypovolemic shock and preexisting medical conditions (172).

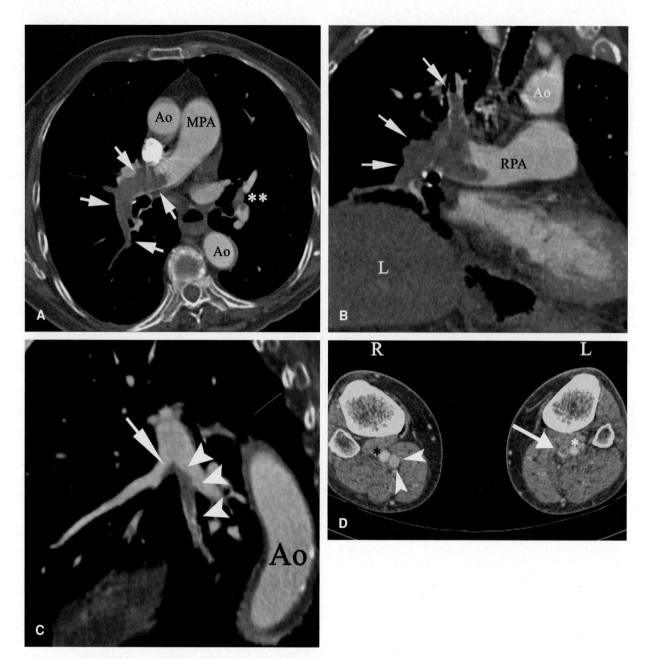

FIGURE 9-4 Acute pulmonary embolus in a 58-year-old woman with chest pain and shortness of breath, status post hip replacement. A: Axial image from pulmonary CTA shows large clot-burden PE involving the distal right main pulmonary artery and lobar branches (*arrows*). Contralateral emboli are also noted (**). (MPA, main pulmonary artery; Ao, aorta.) **B:** Coronal reformatted image from CTA shows extension of clot into the right upper and lower lobe lobar and segmental arteries (*arrows*). (RPA, right pulmonary artery; L, liver; Ao, aorta.) **C:** Sagittal reformatted image from CTA shows emboli assuming a "saddle" configuration (*arrow*) in the left lower segmental pulmonary arteries (*arrowheads*). It is typical for emboli to lodge at and near arterial bifurcations. **D:** Axial image from indirect CT venography obtained 180 seconds after injection of contrast shows filling defect in the left popliteal vein (*arrow*), consistent with DVT. The right popliteal vein is normal (*arrowheads*). (*, normal popliteal arteries.)

Upper Extremity Deep Vein Thrombosis

DVT in the upper extremities is less common, frequently of iatrogenic origin associated with IV catheters (173) and pacemaker electrodes (174) (Figs. 9-5, 9-6). Other risk factors for upper extremity DVT include malignancy, thrombophilia, previous DVT, IV drug abuse, and thoracic outlet syndromes including effort thrombosis in athletes (175–177).

Typical symptoms include upper extremity swelling, skin discoloration, and arm and shoulder pain, although

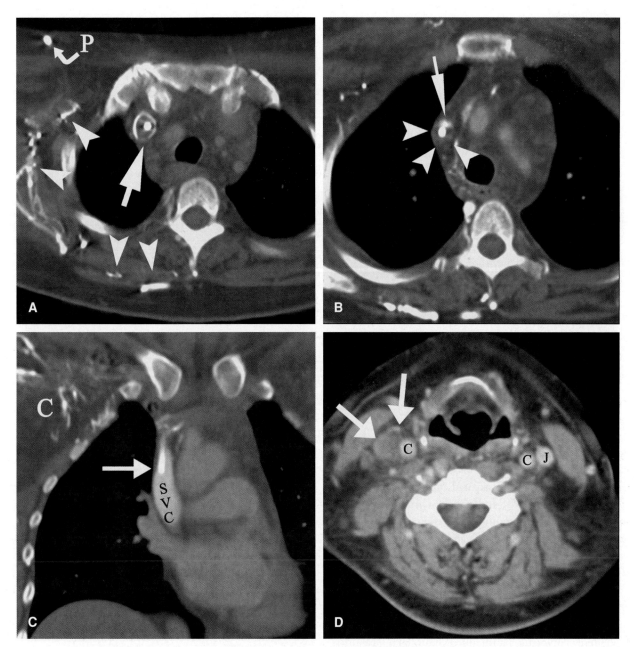

FIGURE 9-5 Thrombus around implantable port catheter. A 53-year-old patient with implantable port for chemotherapy. **A:** Axial image during routine chest CT with injection from the right arm shows thrombus surrounding the intravascular portion of an implantable port (*arrow*). There is evidence of venous collateral filling from the right antecubital injection (*arrowheads*). A portion of the subcutaneous tubing is also seen *(P)*. **B:** Axial image caudal to **(A)** shows narrowing of the SVC lumen (*arrow*), accounting for the collateral vein flow seen on the right. Thrombus (*arrowheads*) is again seen around the catheter. **C:** Coronal reconstruction shows tip of the port to be free of thrombus (*arrow*). The caudal aspects of the superior vena cava *(SVC)* are also patent. **D:** Axial image through the neck shows thrombus in the right internal jugular vein (*arrows*). The left jugular system *(J)* is patent. (C, internal carotid arteries.)

like lower extremity DVT, upper extremity DVT is frequently asymptomatic (178,179).

PE is not an unusual complication of upper extremity DVT and may be detected in 36% of patients (175), especially in those with malignancy and IV catheters (180). Adequate anticoagulation lowers the risk of PE (173).

Diagnosis of Extremity Deep Vein Thrombosis

Contrast venography has long been considered the gold standard for the diagnosis of extremity DVT. However, ultrasound examination correlates remarkably well with venographic findings (181) and became widely adopted as the initial screening tool for patients with suspected DVT

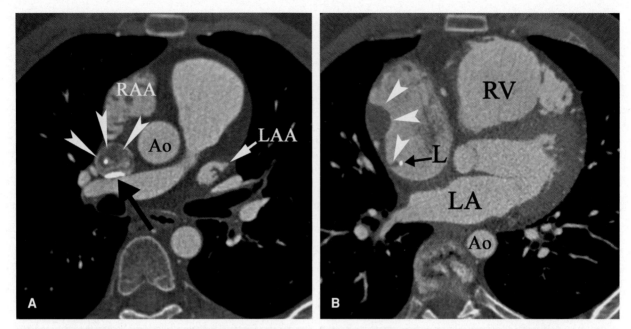

FIGURE 9-6 Thrombus formation around pacer lead. A 27-year-old man with previous pacer/implantable cardiac defibrillator *(ICD)* placement for arrhythmia. **A:** Axial image at the level of the right and left atrial appendages *(RAA, LAA)*. There is subocclusive thrombus formation *(arrowheads)* around the indwelling ICD lead. The flow lumen of the SVC is compressed *(arrow)*. (Ao, aorta.) **B:** Axial image through the right atrium shows the ICD lead *(L)*, with thrombus extending from the lead to the lateral wall of the right atrium *(arrowheads)*. (RV, right ventricle; LA, left atrium; Ao, aorta.)

in general clinical practice as well as in clinical trials (182). Limitations of ultrasound examination include poor visualization of pelvic vein DVT, isolated calf vein DVT, proximal subclavian vein DVT, and poor visualization of other veins in the presence of significant leg edema. Despite limitations, ultrasound examination can be safely used to make therapeutic clinical decisions in patients with suspected DVT (183,184).

The differential diagnosis of lower extremity DVT includes muscle cramps, aggravated chronic venous insufficiency, superficial thrombophlebitis, Baker's cyst, cellulitis, lymphedema, myositis, panniculitis, neuralgia, vasculitis, calf hematoma, arthritis, and leg injury.

Treatment of Extremity Deep Vein Thrombosis

The cornerstone of extremity DVT therapy is anticoagulation. Initial therapy includes IV heparin or low-molecular-weight heparin (LMWH) administered subcutaneously (SC) or IV. A significant advantage of LMWH is the ability to carry on therapy on an outpatient basis, resulting in significant cost savings.

Thrombolytic therapy is indicated in patients with severe iliofemoral DVT and phlegmasia (185,186).

Oral anticoagulation with warfarin should be continued after an initial DVT event. The INR should be maintained between 2 and 3. The duration of anticoagulation

therapy must be determined individually, depending on the clinical condition and presence of risk factors.

Inferior vena cava filters (IVCF) are used for prevention of PE in patients with DVT. Many different devices, both permanent and retrievable, are available currently for percutaneous delivery; routes for access include the femoral, jugular, and antecubital veins. Indications for caval filter placement include contraindications to anticoagulation therapy and recurrent PE despite adequate anticoagulation.

VISCERAL VEIN THROMBOSIS

Portal and Mesenteric Venous Thrombosis

Thrombosis of the veins of the splanchnic system may involve intrahepatic veins (Budd-Chiari syndrome) and the extrahepatic portal vein and its tributaries: the splenic vein and mesenteric veins. The development of new imaging techniques with computed tomography (CT) and magnetic resonance imaging (MRI) has greatly improved our ability to visualize visceral veins and diagnose visceral venous thrombosis (187).

Portal Vein Thrombosis

Thrombosis in the portal venous system (PVT) is associated with liver cirrhosis regardless of the etiology in about 30% of patients. In one series of patients with liver cirrhosis who were undergoing a portocaval shunt operation, PVT was found in 6.5% of cases (188). Other causes of PVT include primary and metastatic liver malignancy (189,190), thrombophilia (191,192), myeloproliferative disorders (193), splenectomy (194,195), liver transplantation (196), abdominal surgery, abdominal trauma, pancreatitis (197,198), pylephlebitis (199), inflammatory bowel diseases (200), and congenital abnormalities of visceral veins. In 50% to 65% of patients, the etiology cannot be determined (201,202).

Thrombosis of the portal vein leads to increased pressure in the portal venous system and development of collateral venous circulation if the process is slow or visceral congestion with bowel necrosis in acute thrombosis (Fig. 9-7).

Patients with acute PVT present with sudden onset of abdominal pain, bloody diarrhea, hematemesis, ileus, and the development of peritonitis due to bowel necrosis (203). Reported mortality in acute PVT varies from 0% to 74% (204).

Subacute disease with partial occlusion of the portal vein may be less dramatic with development of splenomegaly, quickly progressive ascites, and more frequent gastrointestinal (GI) bleeding.

Chronic PVT in patients who have liver cirrhosis is associated with more severe liver disease, GI bleeding, and severe ascites (188,205). PVT is often an accidental finding in patients with liver/pancreatic pathology.

Reported 5-year survival for patients with PVT varies between 47% (197) and 61% (190). Lack of underlying malignancy, liver cirrhosis, and mesenteric vein thrombosis (MVT) is associated with better prognosis and 5-year survival of 89% (190).

Portal Vein Thrombosis Treatment

Choice of therapy depends on clinical presentation and underlying pathology. Surgery is necessary in cases of peritonitis and bowel necrosis (204). Endoscopic sclerotherapy of esophageal varices is a treatment of choice in cases of upper GI bleeding (206).

In cases of acute or subacute PVT, pharmacological or mechanical thrombolysis should be implemented (207–209). Thrombolysis should be followed by chronic anticoagulation. Anticoagulant therapy alone results in recanalization in the majority of patients who have PVT without underlying liver cirrhosis or malignant disease (210).

In patients with chronic portal vein occlusion, symptomatic therapy includes portosystemic shunt operations (202) and sclerotherapy for variceal bleeding.

In cases of chronic portal hypertension related to extrahepatic PVT in children, mesenterico-left portal vein bypass caused a normalization of coagulation parameters (211).

Mesenteric Vein Thrombosis

MVT may occur in association with portal vein thrombosis or alone. Isolated MVT has a distinct clinical presentation and is sometimes recognized as a separate clinical entity (212).

The presence of MVT worsens the clinical presentation and prognosis in patients with PVT (190).

Isolated MVT is more difficult to diagnose and more often causes intestinal necrosis that requires surgery. Clinical presentation of acute MVT in a small, published series included abdominal pain in 96%, symptoms of ileus in 35%, fever in 26%, diarrhea in 17%, and GI bleeding in 13% of patients (203). Isolated MVT was more frequently detected in patients without liver cirrhosis or malignancy as compared with MVT accompanying PVT (212) and, therefore, has a better prognosis, with a reported 2-year survival of 76.9% (213).

Mesenteric Vein Thrombosis Treatment

Peritonitis, bowel necrosis, and ileus are definite indications for surgery. However, in patients without intestinal wall infarction, anticoagulation with or without initial thrombolysis might be sufficient (213,214). Initial pharmacological or mechanical thrombolysis is warranted in cases with acute MVT without bowel necrosis. Anticoagulation should be continued indefinitely in those patients (215).

Budd-Chiari Syndrome

Budd-Chiari syndrome (BCS) can develop in multiple clinical situations as the result of hepatic vein thrombosis, or hepatic veins or inferior vena cava (IVC) obstruction causing post hepatic venous occlusion. The most common causes are myeloproliferative disorders, liver neoplasms, paroxysmal nocturnal hemoglobinuria, sickle cell disease, hereditary and acquired thrombophilia, pregnancy, and membranous obstruction of the IVC. Hematological myeloproliferative disorders account for 25% of BCS. In Asia, membranous obstruction of the IVC is identified in 40% of BCS cases. Factors predisposing to PVT can also predispose to hepatic vein thrombosis. In many cases, the etiology of BCS cannot be identified (216,217).

Veno-occlusive Disease

Veno-occlusive disease (VOD) is a separate disorder resembling BCS.

VOD is caused by fibrosis of hepatic veins and secondary thrombosis of terminal hepatic veins and sinusoids. It was first described in Jamaica and is related to ingestion of pyrrolizidine alkaloids from certain plants (Senecio, Crotalaria, Heliotropium). VOD was also described in Africa, Asia, and South America in tribes drinking "bush tea."

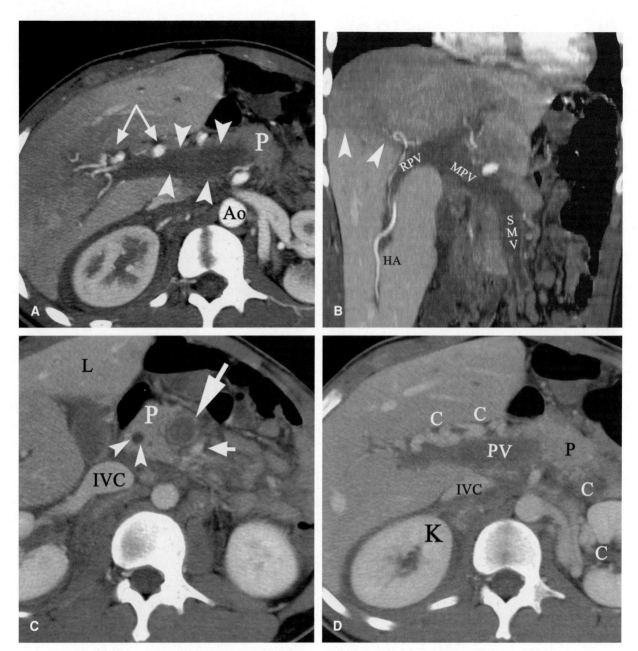

FIGURE 9-7 Portal venous thrombosis in a 32-year-old man with history of hepatitis and portal hypertension. A: Axial image from arterial phase of dual-phase contrast-enhanced abdominal CT shows low-attenuation thrombus (*arrowheads*) in the extrahepatic portal vein, extending into the liver hilum. Periportal collaterals are seen (*arrows*), consistent with long-standing (nonacute) PVT. (P, pancreas; Ao, aorta.) **B:** Coronal reformatted arterial-phase image shows thrombus in the right portal vein *(RPV)*, main portal vein *(MPV)*, and superior mesenteric vein *(SMV)*. Hepatic arteries *(HA)* are dilated, as they are now the sole blood supply to the liver. Note the alteration in enhancement of the left lobe (*arrowheads*), most consistent with THAD (transient hepatic attenuation difference), which is not uncommonly seen in the setting of PVT. **C:** Axial delayed-phase image demonstrates distension of the superior mesenteric vein by thrombus (*large arrow*). The adjacent superior mesenteric artery is patent (*small arrow*). A normal common bile duct (*arrowheads*) is seen coursing through the pancreatic head *(P)*. (L, liver; IVC, inferior vena cava.) **D:** Axial delayed-phase image shows multiple collaterals *(C)*, both periportal and renal. Thrombus in the portal vein *(PV)* is again seen. (IVC, inferior vena cava; P, pancreas; K, right kidney.) Note the THAD-like enhancement seen in **(B)** has resolved.

Other causes of VOD include SLE, bone marrow transplantation, and chemo- and radiation therapy (218). Clinical presentation is similar to BCS (217).

Clinical Presentation

BCS usually develops as a result of chronic or subacute obstruction; acute thrombosis is less common and may present as fulminant liver failure with progressive jaundice, ascites, encephalopathy, and coma. Fulminant BCS is seen in pregnancy-related hepatic vein thrombosis and hematological cases (217,219,220).

Symptoms of chronic BCS are similar to liver cirrhosis with hepatomegaly, ascites, progressive liver insufficiency, and lower extremity edema (216,217).

Budd-Chiari Syndrome Treatment

Fulminant BCS usually requires liver transplantation and is frequently fatal. Thrombolysis and anticoagulant therapy is used in patients with early diagnosis of thrombosis.

Portacaval shunts are performed in patients with progressive portal hypertension. Currently, the transjugular intrahepatic caval shunt (TIPS) procedure is recommended for those patients (221).

Many patients with progressive liver failure require liver transplantation. Orloff published observation of 60 patients with BCS. Thirty-two patients with hepatic vein occlusion had portacaval shunts with excellent long-term results; 8 patients with concomitant IVC occlusion were treated with mesoatrial shunt unsuccessfully (5 patients died); and 10 patients with concomitant IVC occlusion had portacaval shunts inserted and a cavoatrial anastomosis with good results. Ten patients with progressive liver failure underwent orthotopic liver transplantation with a 5-year survival rate of 30% (222).

Orthotopic liver transplantation should be considered in patients who have a fulminant form of BCS with encephalopathy and laboratory evidence of liver failure, chronic BCS with decompensated cirrhosis and encephalopathy, and no effect to previous portosystemic shunt procedures (217,223,224).

Diagnosis

Computed tomography angiography (CTA) and contrast-enhanced MRI and MR angiography (MRA) are the diagnostic tools of choice in detection of visceral venous and arterial pathology, including thrombosis and bowel ischemia (187,225–228). Three-dimensional (3D) MR was found to be very accurate diagnosis of BCS (229).

Ultrasound imaging is helpful in diagnosis of PVT and liver architecture (230) and is a valuable diagnostic procedure, replacing catheterization of the IVC or percuta-

neous transhepatic hepatovenography in the diagnosis of BCS. The typical ultrasonographic features of BCS include the inability to visualize normal hepatic venous connections to the vena cava, comma-shaped intrahepatic collateral vessels, and the absence of Doppler waveform in the hepatic veins. MRI and CT also can distinguish specific parenchymal and vascular abnormalities in the liver and are becoming indispensable in more complex diagnostic cases (231) and prior to liver transplantation (232). Liver biopsy is frequently necessary for differential diagnosis of hepatic malignancy.

Renal Vein Thrombosis

Renal vein thrombosis (RVT) is a rare disorder that is more commonly described in children, although it may occur at any age. Risk factors for RVT include hereditary and acquired thrombophilia (233–236), nephrotic syndrome (237,238) (Fig. 9-8), renal cancer (239), abdominal trauma (240), Behçet disease (241), and kidney transplantation (242).

An abdominal mass, hematuria, proteinuria, and thrombocytopenia all belong to the classic presentation. In acute RVT, patients complain of flank pain; in bilateral RVT, progressive renal failure is observed. Usually, only a few of these symptoms are present in patients with RVT (235).

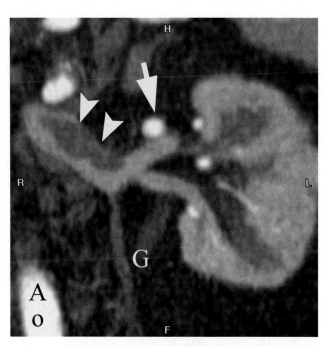

FIGURE 9-8 A 27-year-old man with nephrotic syndrome. Coronal reformatted image from CTA exam shows filling defects in the left main renal vein (*arrowheads*), consistent with thrombus. The entering left gonadal vein (*G*) is also seen, as is a patent left renal artery (*arrow*). (Ao, aorta.)

VENA CAVA THROMBOSIS

Thrombosis of the superior or IVC occurs in patients with malignancy (243,244), primary and secondary thrombophilia, and congenital abnormalities of the vena cava.

Thrombosis of the IVC usually develops as an extension of common iliac vein thrombosis, RVT, or hepatic vein thrombosis. It may also occur as a consequence of tumor invasion (243,245) (Fig. 9-3), IVC compression, or IVC instrumentation (246).

Symptoms depend on the level of IVC occlusion. In distal IVC thrombosis, lower extremity and groin edema develops. In IVC thrombosis at the level of renal veins, accompanied by bilateral RVT, symptoms of venous stasis are accompanied by pain in the lumbar area, hematuria, proteinuria, and renal insufficiency. Thrombosis of the hepatic portion of IVC presents as a BCS with development of portal hypertension (247).

Initial diagnosis can be made with Doppler ultrasound examination (248); however, venography remains the gold standard. CT and MR venography can also be helpful and can often make the diagnosis noninvasively.

Treatment depends on clinical presentation and etiology. Acute thrombosis requires anticoagulation with or without initial thrombolysis. Chronic occlusion can be treated with endovascular recanalization and stenting (249). Development of BCS may require appropriate surgery. Occlusion secondary to malignancy may require surgical resection and replacement with a vascular graft (246).

Superior vena cava (SVC) thrombosis develops as a result of local compression, invasion by malignant (Fig. 9-1) or benign tumors (250), or SVC instrumentation [central IV lines (251), pacemaker electrodes (252), and dialysis catheters (253)] (Figs. 9-5, 9-6). Other causes such as thrombophilia or vasculitis are rare.

Clinical symptoms of SVC syndrome are consequences of venous congestion in the upper part of the body and include arm and head edema, bluish discoloration of skin and mucous membranes, distended jugular veins, and presence of distended superficial veins in the upper chest (Fig. 9-9).

Diagnosis is usually confirmed by contrast-enhanced chest CT, CTA, or MRI.

Therapy includes thrombolysis with subsequent anticoagulation and endovascular procedures (venous angioplasty with or without stenting) (254,255).

CEREBRAL VEIN THROMBOSIS

Cerebral venous and sinus thrombosis (CVST) is a rare but alarming disease that usually begins with headache. Sinus thrombosis may lead to cerebral venous infarction, which is frequently hemorrhagic and may cause focal neurological deficits, seizures, or death. Infection, trauma, tumors, autoimmune disease, and prothrombotic states (e.g., APAs, protein C or S deficiency, factor V Leiden mutation, pregnancy, puerperium, OCs, and malignancy) are all regarded as risk factors, but in many cases, the cause remains unknown (256). A recent retrospective study of 130 patients revealed that the most common causes of CVST were OC use (15%), vascular malformation (11%), infection (10%), and malignancy (9%). In 29% of patients, no etiological factor was identified (257).

Diagnosis of a thrombosed dural sinus, although frequently suspected on CT scan, is often made by MRI. Diagnosis by MR is based on an increased signal in both T1-weighted and T2-weighted MRI and lack of flow by MR venography (MRV). Conventional angiography is rarely needed when MRI is available (258). Diffusion-weighted imaging is also performed to demonstrate areas of infarction (259–262). CTA is also utilized with the diagnosis of CVST (263).

Based on the results of randomized trials and observational studies, both unfractionated and low-molecular-weight heparin are safe and probably effective in CVST (258, 264,265). Bousser recommends heparin as a first-line treatment, even in patients with hemorrhagic venous infarcts, followed by oral anticoagulation for a period of 3 to 6 months (266). In patients who demonstrate progressive neurological deterioration despite adequate anticoagulation, other options such as local intrathrombotic infusion of a thrombolytic agent together with IV heparin are under investigation (258,267).

A recent retrospective series showed that patients with CVT may have a less favorable outcome than previously reported with mortality in about 14%, cognitive impairment in 35%, and lifestyle limitations in 40% (268). Clinical features signifying a poor prognosis are rapidity of onset, early reduced Glasgow coma score (GCS), focal neurological signs, seizures, and concomitant infection (269).

PULMONARY EMBOLISM

PE is a serious and notoriously underdiagnosed medical condition, remaining a significant cause of overall mortality and morbidity.

True incidence of PE can only be estimated, and in the United States, the incidence is thought to be 100 per 100,000 persons per year. Recent analysis of death certificates in the Multiple-Cause Mortality Files revealed that in the United States, PE accounted for almost 25,000 deaths in 1998, showing significant reduction from over 35,000 in 1979 (270). It should be remembered, however, that in autopsy studies, only one third of PEs were diagnosed antemortem (271).

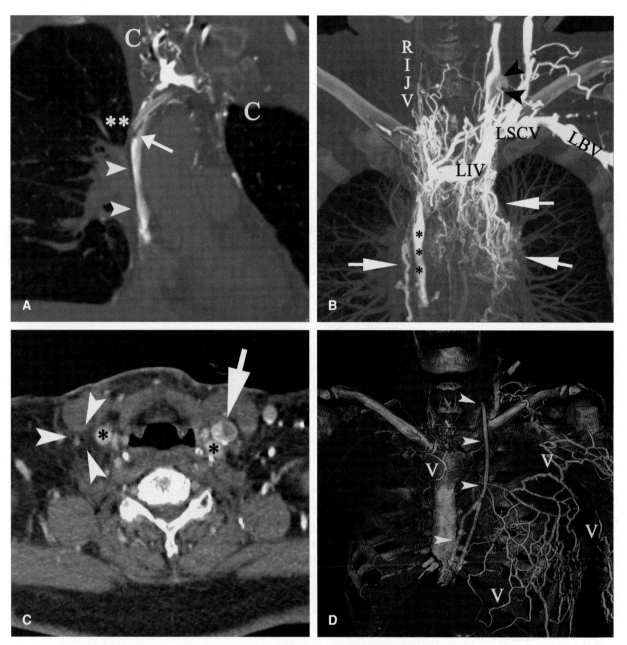

FIGURE 9-9 Superior vena cava syndrome in a 55-year-old man with history of long-term hemodialysis with multiple previous catheters. Patient now presents with dysfunctional tunneled venous catheter and worsening facial and neck swelling. **A:** Coronal thin-slab MIP from CT venography shows the dialysis catheter (∗∗) at the cephalad aspect of the SVC. There is adjacent thrombus around the end of the catheter (*arrow*), which traverses and occludes an area of high grade SVC/left innominate venous stenosis. Neck collaterals *(C)* are seen. Caudal aspects of the SVC are patent (*arrowheads*). The position of the catheter can predispose to inadequate dialysis flow rates and venous stenosis; optimally, the tips should be positioned (depending on catheter) at the SVC/right atrial junction or in the right atrium. **B:** Coronal thick-slab MIP image shows extensive mediastinal, paracardiac, and external jugular collateral veins (*arrows*). Caudal aspects of the SVC are also opacified (∗). Filling defect in the left internal jugular vein is subocclusive thrombus (*arrowheads*). The right IJV *(RIJV)* is chronically occluded from previous tunneled venous catheter accesses. (LIV, left innominate vein; LSCV, left subclavian vein; LBV, left brachial vein.) **C:** Axial image from delayed CTV phase shows the subocclusive LIJV thrombus (*arrow*). The chronic occlusion of the RIJV is also shown (*arrowheads*). (∗, common carotid arteries.) **D:** Volume-rendered coronal image with opacity transfer settings to accentuate superficial soft tissues. There are extensive superficial venous collaterals *(V)*, which communicate to the central veins via mammary, intercostals, and external jugular pathways. The indwelling LIJV tunneled dialysis catheter is also visualized (*arrowheads*).

PE results from fragmentation and migration of thrombi from peripheral veins into pulmonary arteries, leading to arterial occlusion. It is often difficult to prove coexistence of DVT and PE in patients. Evidence of DVT by using lower extremity ultrasound was found in less than one third of patients with PE (272). On the other hand, in patients with proximal lower extremity DVT, a high probability of PE was found in 40% of asymptomatic patients when imaged by scintigraphy (273).

In symptomatic cases, clinical presentation is usually not specific. Most common symptoms include dyspnea (81%), chest pain (72%), apprehension (59%), cough (54%), tachycardia >100 bpm (44%), fever (42%), hemoptysis (34%), diaphoresis (34%), cyanosis (18%), and syncope (14%) (274). Death occurred within 2.5 hours in 10% of cases (275).

Pulmonary angiography remains the gold standard for diagnosis of PE, although combinations of noninvasive tests (D-dimer, pulmonary scintigraphy, CTA, and MRA) can exclude or confirm the diagnosis of PE in the vast majority of patients without the need to perform pulmonary angiography (276). D-dimer testing was reported to have high negative predictive value for VTE, but this seems to be true only for some specific tests (277,278) and for selected patient populations (279). Combined pulmonary CTA and indirect CT venography (Fig. 9-4) offers the unique ability to study pulmonary arteries, right ventricle dilatation, and peripheral veins during the same short examination (280), which could improve our ability to diagnose VTE. Another promising technique is that of direct thrombus imaging with MR, which allows better visualization of the clot and is highly sensitive in detection of DVT and PE (281).

Treatment of PE depends on severity of presentation. Thrombolytic therapy should be considered in patients with massive pulmonary embolism (282,283), and it remains controversial in submassive PE (284,285). Anticoagulation with heparin should be started in all patients with suspected PE. LMWH is preferred and should be followed with oral anticoagulants. The length of anticoagulant therapy should be determined individually for each patient (286). When anticoagulation is contraindicated, vena cava filters should be considered.

Venous Thromboembolism Prophylaxis

Prophylactic strategies for VTE include pharmacological and nonpharmacological means. Pharmacological prophylaxis relies on use of anticoagulants—mainly heparins and warfarin (also, newer agents such as pentasaccharide and ximelagatran are currently under investigation). Nonpharmacological methods include compression stockings and intermittent compression pumps.

Current guidelines of the American College of Chest Physicians for VTE prophylaxis are available at http://www.chestjournal.org/content/vol126/3_suppl/.

Generally, in all hospitalized patients, risk of VTE should be assessed and appropriate measures should be undertaken.

Failure of prophylaxis in VTE prevention is caused by nonadherence to current guidelines resulting in lack of prophylaxis or insufficient prophylaxis (287,288).

Current guidelines may also need to be modified in selected patient populations (144).

ARTERIAL THROMBOEMBOLISM

Arterial Embolism

Arterial embolization occurs when an artery is partially or completely blocked by material flowing with the blood current. The most common emboli are blood clots, while less common emboli include fragmented atherosclerotic plaques and cholesterol crystals, bacterial vegetations, fatty tissue, neoplastic tissue, air, and amniotic fluid. Occasionally, blood clots from the deep venous system can cross over to the arterial circulation, causing arterial embolization.

Arterial embolism (AE) is a prevalent cause of acute ischemia, accounting for 50% to 80% of patients presenting with acute limb ischemia (289–291).

The heart is the source of arterial emboli in over 50% of cases (292–294) (Fig. 9-10). Conditions that are most frequently associated with peripheral embolization are atrial fibrillation (AF) in 70% to 90% of heart emboli, ischemic heart disease (myocardial infarction, left ventricle aneurysm), rheumatic valvular disease (mitral stenosis), and implanted mechanical valves. AE also occurs in congestive heart failure, cardiomyopathy, endocarditis, and atrial myxoma.

AF in patients without valvular disease and age <65 years is associated with the lowest risk of AE—<1 in 100 patients per year (295). Presence of valvular heart disease, age >65 years, and/or other risk factors of AE increases the incidence of arterial embolization to 14 in 100 patients per year (296).

Anticoagulation therapy with warfarin is associated with 50% to 70% risk reduction of AE as compared with lack of anticoagulation therapy (297,298). Aspirin can be used as the sole prophylactic agent in AF patients who are <65 years of age without other prothrombotic risk factors (299).

Arterioarterial Embolism

Arterial emboli can originate from the aorta and large arteries (arterioarterial embolism).

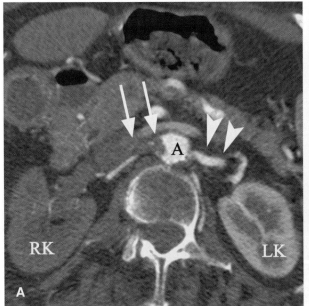

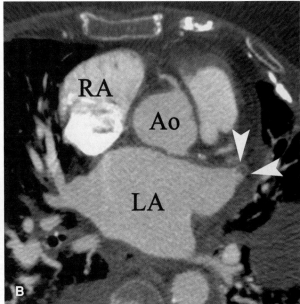

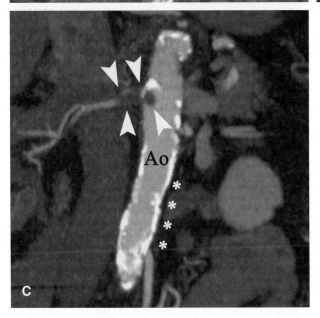

FIGURE 9-10 Cardiogenic embolus to right renal artery with acute renal ischemia in a 48-year-old man with atrial fibrillation. A: Axial image from abdominal CTA shows a large clot (*arrows*) filling the proximal right renal artery and protruding into the aorta *(A)*. The right kidney *(RK)* shows lack of enhancement consistent with acute ischemia. The left kidney *(LK)* and left renal artery (*arrowheads*) are normal. **B:** Axial image at the level of the left atrium from same study. There is dilatation of the left atrium *(LA)*. There is a small thrombus remaining in the left atrial appendage (*arrowheads*). (RA, right atrium; Ao, aorta.) **C:** Coronal reformatted image from CTA shows extent of thrombus (*arrowheads*) in proximal right renal artery, dangling into the aorta *(Ao)*. There is a background of extensive calcific aortic atherosclerotic disease (∗∗∗∗).

Aneurysms (294,300), surgical grafts (301), stent grafts (301), hemodialysis grafts (302), atherosclerotic lesions (294) (Fig. 9-11), and arterial injury may be the sources of peripheral arterial embolization.

Carotid stenosis is a frequent cause of emboli to the cerebrovascular circulation. Risk of stroke is closely related to the severity of stenosis and the type of plaque (303–305). For internal carotid stenosis >75%, the combined risk for transient ischemic attack (TIA) and stroke was 10.5% per year (306), and for symptomatic patients with 90% to 94% stenosis, the incidence increased to 35% per year (305). Risk of stroke is much lower for asymptomatic patients, even in those with high-grade stenosis (307).

Antiplatelet therapy is recommended to reduce rate of stroke and cardiovascular events in patients with symptomatic carotid artery stenosis (308,309).

Arterial Thrombosis

Arterial thrombosis resulting in the occlusion of an artery often develops in atherosclerotic arteries. Plaque rupture and slow blood flow at the site of arterial stenosis are predisposing factors (310). Aneurysms, especially saccular aneurysms, can be complicated by thrombosis and acute occlusion of the artery (e.g., popliteal artery aneurysm) (311).

Arterial compression in thoracic outlet syndromes (300), popliteal artery entrapment (312) (Fig. 9-1), adventitial

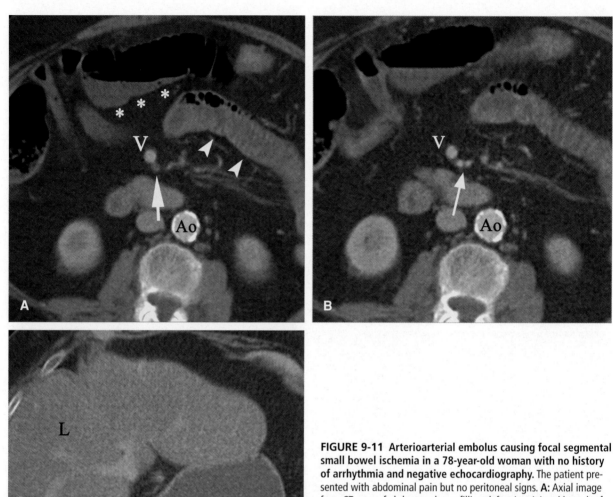

FIGURE 9-11 Arterioarterial embolus causing focal segmental small bowel ischemia in a 78-year-old woman with no history of arrhythmia and negative echocardiography. The patient presented with abdominal pain but no peritoneal signs. **A:** Axial image from CT scan of abdomen shows filling defect in a jejunal branch of superior mesenteric artery (*arrow*). The adjacent mesenteric vein branch *(V)* is patent. Note the lack of enhancement of a segment of small bowel (∗∗∗) relative to adjacent loops (*arrowheads*). (Ao, aorta.) **B:** Axial image immediately cephalad to **(A)** shows normal enhancement of the more proximal jejunal branch (*arrow*). (Ao, aorta; V, patent mesenteric venous branch.) **C:** Axial image at level of diaphragm shows irregular, excavated plaque in the aorta at the thoracoabdominal junction (*arrowheads*). At surgery, early ischemic changes of a segment of jejunum were resected, and the small arterioarterial embolus was removed. (L, liver; S, spleen; St, stomach.)

cyst of the popliteal artery (313) (Fig. 9-12), or compression by external masses (314) can result in local thrombosis and occlusion. Arterial injury, both acute and chronic, like hypothenar hammer syndrome (315), can cause thrombosis. Iatrogenic arterial thrombosis may develop at the site of arterial angioplasty, stent placement (316–319), or arterial injury during surgical procedure (320,321). Arterial instrumentation can be complicated by arterial thrombosis (322). Finally, inherited or acquired thrombophilic states can be complicated by arterial thrombosis (323–327) (Fig. 9-1).

Clinical Presentation

Clinical presentation of embolic/thrombotic arterial occlusion depends primarily on the extent of collateral circulation. Lack of well-developed collateral circulation will result in acute ischemia of the area supplied by the occluded artery with corresponding clinical symptoms. If sufficient collateral circulation exists, occlusion might be asymptomatic or present with fewer symptoms.

Coexisting conditions that limit peripheral perfusion, especially congestive heart failure, diabetes, dehydration,

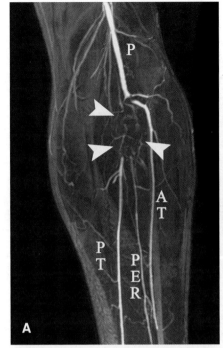

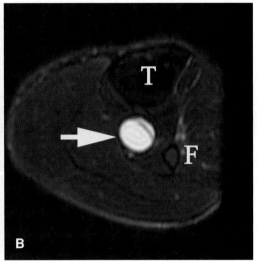

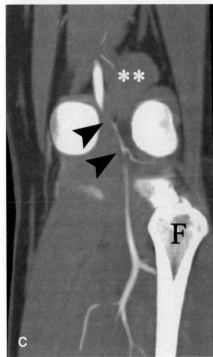

FIGURE 9-12 Compressive lesions that can lead to arterial thrombosis. A, B: Adventitial cystic disease in a 37-year-old software engineer who presents with left calf claudication. **A:** Coronal thick-slab MIP image from MRA. There is occlusion of the tibioperoneal trunk and proximal anterior tibial artery (*arrowheads*) secondary to a mass lesion. There is distal reconstitution of a three-vessel runoff. (AT, anterior tibial artery; PER, peroneal artery; PT, posterior tibial artery.) **B:** Axial fat-suppressed fast spin echo T2-weighted image in proximal left calf. The mass represents a large cystic lesion (*arrow*) that at surgery was found to be intimately associated with the distal left popliteal artery and proximal tibioperoneal trunk. Pathology was consistent with adventitial cystic disease. (F, fibula; T, tibia.) **C:** Popliteal entrapment syndrome in a 20-year-old female intercollegiate athlete with calf claudication. Coronal MIP image from CTA with provocative maneuver (forced plantar-flexion) shows near-complete occlusion of the popliteal artery (*arrowheads*) secondary to an anomalous (accessory) head of the medial gastrocnemius (∗∗), which originates laterally and crosses the popliteal artery in the region of narrowing. (F, fibula.)

and hyperviscosity syndromes, worsen the symptoms and the prognosis of acute arterial obstruction.

Asymptomatic arterial thrombosis often occurs at the site of chronic arterial stenosis, where slow progression of narrowing allows sufficient development of collateral circulation. This situation is frequently found in peripheral arterial disease patients with occlusion of the superficial femoral artery.

Acute Limb Ischemia

The manifestations of acute limb ischemia are often described with five Ps: Pain, Pulselessness, Pallor, Paresthesia, and Paralysis. Sudden onset of limb pain with pallor and lack of peripheral pulse are followed within hours by paresthesia and paralysis. Sudden onset with quick progression of symptoms is characteristic for AE. Pains in the limb, usually severe, together with disappearance of pulses are the first symptoms, followed by a drop in skin temperature. The limb becomes pale, and superficial veins collapse due to limited inflow. Skin cyanosis frequently develops. Sensory loss and motor paralysis occur within hours of the onset of acute ischemia and usually are the signs of nonreversible damage. Arterial thrombosis is characterized frequently by gradual worsening of symptoms. It usually develops in atherosclerotic arteries at the site of a previously existing arterial narrowing, where collateral circulation has already developed (Fig. 9-13).

Clinical history of risk factors for AE (e.g., AF) or peripheral arterial disease (claudication) helps with diagnosis.

Atheroembolism

Small emboli from atherosclerotic sites in the aorta or large arteries can cause distal microembolization of the skin arteries presenting as *livedo reticularis*, or blue toe syndrome. Embolic materials include cholesterol crystals, debris, and small thrombi from ulcerated plaques. Atheroembolism is seen in patients with advanced atheromatosis of the aorta and large arteries. It occurs spontaneously (328) or in connection with endovascular procedures (329). Symptoms vary from benign skin discoloration to limb gangrene, renal insufficiency, and death (330).

Differential Diagnosis of Acute Limb Ischemia

The diagnostic process in acute ischemia should rule out conditions not related to ischemia (e.g., neuropathy, hypoperfusion); identification of the cause of arterial occlusion such as embolus, thrombosis, trauma (e.g., arterial dissection, compression syndromes, vasculitis, thromboangiitis obliterans, vasospasm, vascular procedures); and underlying condition (e.g., atherosclerosis, AF, connective tissue disease, thrombophilic states).

Evaluation of the Patient with Acute Limb Ischemia

Patients who have suspected ALI should be quickly evaluated and diagnosed. Diagnosis of ALI can be made on the

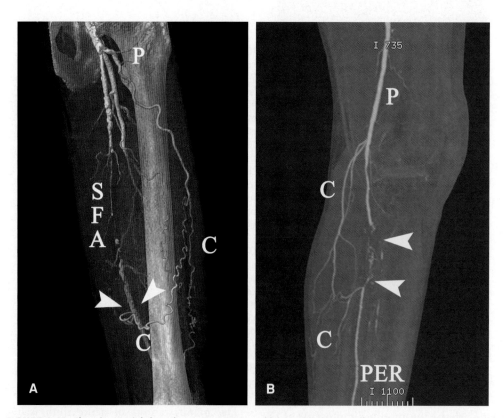

FIGURE 9-13 Chronic arterial thromboses. A: A 65-year-old man with chronic calf claudication. Volume-rendered image from CTA runoff study shows long-segment occlusion of the superficial femoral artery *(SFA)*, with abundant collateral vessels *(C)* from the profunda femoris artery *(P)*. There is reconstitution of the distal SFA *(arrowheads)*. **B:** Chronic popliteal artery and tibioperoneal trunk occlusion in a 73-year-old woman. MIP image with bone segmentation from CTA runoff study is viewed from lateral. There is segmental occlusion of the tibioperoneal trunk *(arrowheads)*. The patient did not have an acutely ischemic foot or leg but presented with calf and foot claudication. There is reconstitution of the peroneal artery *(PER)* via sural and geniculate collaterals *(C)*. (P, popliteal artery.)

TABLE 9-3

Clinical Categories of Acute Limb Ischemia

	Category	Rest Pain	Capillary Circulation	Neurological Deficit DPA	Doppler Assessment	Clinical
I	Viable	(−)	(+)	(−)	(+)	no immediate threat
IIa	Marginally threatened	(−)	delayed capillary refill	(+/−) toes only	(+/−)	marginal threat
IIb	Immediately threatened	(+)	weak/ not detectable	(+) sensory or motor	(−/+)	immediate threat
III	Irreversible ischemia	(+)	no	paralysis	(−)	not viable

Modified from *Management of peripheral arterial disease (PAD)*. TransAtlantic Inter-Society Consensus (TASC). Section C: acute limb ischaemia. *Eur J Vasc Endovasc Surg.* 2000;19[Suppl A]:S115–S143.

basis of history (e.g., sudden onset of limb pain, history of AF) and physical exam (five Ps). Doppler evaluation of peripheral flow should be performed to detect peripheral pulses and to measure the ankle-brachial index (ABI) (Table 9-3). Diagnosis might be more difficult in patients with diabetes, leg paralysis, sensory neuropathy, and severe leg edema. Medial sclerosis in diabetics causes stiffening of arteries and, therefore, falsely elevated arterial pressures and ABI with Doppler examination (332). Sensory neuropathy may alleviate or abolish sensation of pain. Severe edema may cause difficulties in detection of peripheral pulses. Further imaging studies like color Doppler ultrasound or CT/MR angiography are increasingly helpful to delineate vascular anatomy and diagnose underlying conditions.

The main reason for imaging the arteries supplying ischemic legs is to define the responsible arterial lesion(s) and to determine the most appropriate intervention, whether endovascular or surgical. The current options are catheter angiography, duplex scanning, and CT or MR angiography.

Contrast angiography remains the gold standard for ALI patients. It provides the anatomical information necessary to undertake decision on intervention. In certain situations, it can be immediately followed by appropriate endovascular therapy (e.g., thrombolysis or/and mechanical clot disruption, angioplasty, stenting, etc.).

Color duplex imaging has been proposed as an attractive alternative to angiography because it is safe, much less expensive, and can provide essential anatomic and some functional information. However, US is time consuming and significantly dependent on the skill of the operator. CTA and MRA offer the additional advantages of detailed anatomical information not limited to arteries and relative freedom of operator dependency. These modalities can help therapeutic decision making, especially in complex medical patients (e.g., multiorgan trauma, coexisting malignancy, arterial aneurysms, etc.).

Treatment for Acute Limb Ischemia

Limb salvage depends on efficient, accurate diagnosis of the cause of acute ischemia and prompt restoration of adequate blood flow. Initial IV heparin reduces morbidity and mortality compared with no anticoagulant use. If not contraindicated, full anticoagulation with heparin should be initiated at the time of diagnosis (331,333).

Therapeutic options include the following:

Endovascular procedures: thrombolysis, angioplasty with or without stenting, percutaneous aspiration thrombectomy (PAT), percutaneous mechanical thrombectomy (PMT), catheter embolectomy

Surgery: embolectomy, thrombectomy, surgical revascularization

Nonlimb Peripheral Arterial Occlusions: Acute Mesenteric Ischemia and Stroke

The development of arterial thrombosis is frequently related to vascular wall injury; therefore, it is a common complication of atherosclerosis. Thrombosis of noncardiac arteries may occur in patients with atherosclerosis, vasculitis, and a variety of thrombophilic states. It may also complicate the course of arterial trauma, aneurysm, or malignancy that is invading or compressing the artery.

Clinical symptoms, being the consequence of regional ischemia, are similar in arterial thrombosis and embolism.

Risk factors for arterial thrombosis are then the same as established risk factors for atherosclerosis: hypertension, obesity, diabetes mellitus and impaired glucose tolerance (IGT), dyslipidemia, smoking, and lack of physical activity. Newer atherosclerosis risk factors include left ventricular hypertrophy, hyperhomocysteinemia, and elevated Lp(a). Hyperfibrinogenemia, low plasma fibrinolytic activity, and other hereditary and acquired hypercoagulopathies are also recognized cardiovascular risk factors.

Acute Mesenteric Ischemia

Acute mesenteric ischemia (AMI) most frequently results from arterial thromboembolic phenomena or can be a sequel of MVT, as described earlier. Occasionally, vasculitis or aortic dissection can cause AMI.

In one prospective study from Sweden, the incidence of AMI was 5.3 in 100,000 inhabitants per year. Embolic events were the cause of ischemia in 83% (95% of these patients had AF) (334). In another 10-year hospital series, embolism accounted for 42% of patients, while 58% had mesenteric thrombosis (335). The majority of patients presented with signs of peritonitis, and one third had hypotension.

Intestinal necrosis in this series was present in 81% of patients. Reported perioperative mortality can be very high—62%; it was highest in patients with peritonitis and bowel necrosis (335).

Diagnosis

Clinical presentation is often not characteristic. Sudden onset of abdominal pain is followed by peritonitis and hypotension (334). Sudden onset of abdominal pain in patients with AF suggests mesenteric embolism. A history of chronic abdominal angina suggests mesenteric thrombosis.

Mesenteric arteriography is currently the gold standard, but it should be avoided in patients with peritonitis. Therefore, the diagnosis of bowel ischemia and necrosis is sometimes made during surgery (336).

CTA can easily delineate mesenteric artery anatomy and diagnose AMI before bowel necrosis occurs and can change the course of treatment (226,337) (Fig. 9-11). Also, 3D MRA can be applied to study visceral arterial anatomy (338).

Treatment

The majority of patients present with an acute abdomen, and a therapeutic decision is made during laparotomy. In the case of mesenteric embolism, surgical embolectomy should be performed. In patients with mesenteric thrombosis, after thrombectomy, surgical revascularization is necessary. After the flow in the mesenteric artery is restored,

resection of nonviable intestine is often required. Perioperative mortality is very high, especially in cases of mesenteric thrombosis, usually due to coexisting morbidities (339).

Thrombolytic treatment of AMI is rarely reported (340,341). It should be attempted only when there is no doubt regarding intestinal viability. However, even in carefully selected patients, late complications (e.g., intestinal stricture) may develop (339).

Acute Thromboembolism of Cerebral Arteries—Stroke

Thromboembolism of the cerebral arteries is the major cause of ischemic stroke.

Stroke is a major cause of morbidity and mortality. It is estimated that over 760,000 patients in the United States suffer from symptomatic ischemic stroke. However, the number of silent strokes might be much higher, reaching perhaps 11 million patients annually (342).

Etiology

Major causes of acute cerebral ischemia are atherosclerosis of cerebral arteries, lipohyalinosis of small cerebral arteries, cardiogenic emboli, atheroembolism from the carotid arteries and aorta, arterial thrombosis, vasculitis of cerebral arteries, arterial dissection, and others (344) (Fig. 9-14).

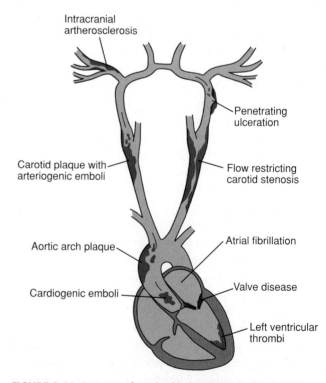

FIGURE 9-14 Anatomy of cerebral ischemic stroke. [Modified from Sherman DG, Dyken ML Jr, Gent M, et al. Antithrombotic therapy for cerebrovascular disorders. An update. *Chest.* 1995;108(4)(suppl):444S–456S.]

Major risk factors for ischemic stroke are hypertension, smoking, hypercholesterolemia, diabetes, alcohol abuse, and AF. In a retrospective autopsy study of 100 fatal ischemic strokes, 28% were thrombotic, 26% were cardioembolic, 12% were atheromatous, and 11% were undetermined (343). In another large study of the Japanese population, followed for 32 years, a high prevalence of lacunar infarction (56%) was found, followed by atherothrombotic (20%), cardioembolic (18%), and undetermined (4%).

Types of Ischemic Infarct

Lacunar infarcts are usually caused by the thrombosis of intracranial arterioles, already narrowed due to the proliferative processes of lipohyalinization (also called *small vessel disease*). This occurs primarily in hypertension and diabetes. Lacunar infarcts are most frequently localized in the internal capsule, thalamus, and basal ganglia. Infarction resolves, leaving behind a small "lacune." Lacunar infarcts are frequently asymptomatic. Symptomatic lacunar strokes present with neurological deficit that can be either motor or sensory.

Atherothrombotic stroke is usually a complication of atherosclerotic lesions in extracranial arteries. Internal carotid artery stenosis may be a source of artery to artery embolization or may cause stroke through carotid artery thrombosis and subsequent hypoperfusion (Fig. 9-15).

Primary intracranial artery thrombosis is a rather infrequent cause of stroke and may happen in patients with thrombophilia (344,345).

Carotid artery stenosis is responsible for over 20% of ischemic strokes (346). The severity of carotid stenosis (347) and increased heterogeneity of the carotid plaque correlate with the incidence of ischemic stroke (303).

Annual incidence of stroke in patients with carotid artery stenosis was found to be 1.3% in patients with stenosis <75% diameter reduction and 3.4% in stenosis >75% (306). In a recent retrospective study, the 10-year risk of ischemic stroke was 5.7% for asymptomatic carotid stenosis <75% and 9.3% in asymptomatic stenosis >75% (307). The number of silent strokes is probably higher according to CT data (304).

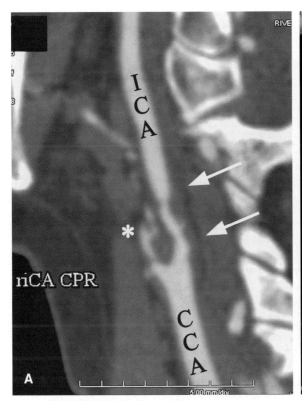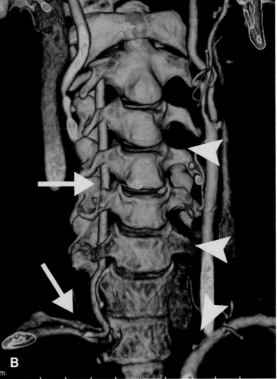

FIGURE 9-15 Internal carotid artery atherosclerotic stenosis in a 77-year-old woman with transient ischemic attack. **A:** Curved planar reconstruction of right internal carotid artery *(RICA)* from CTA exam. There is extensive soft plaque *(arrows)* in the proximal riCA, which causes hemodynamically significant (75% diameter reduction) stenosis. The internal and common carotid arteries are labeled. (∗, external carotid artery origin.) **B:** Subvolume slab volume-rendered image of same patient shows occlusion of the left vertebral artery *(arrowheads)* immediately after the origin from the left subclavian artery. The right vertebral artery *(arrows)* is normal.

Cardioembolic Stroke

Embolic materials migrate from the heart and lodge in cerebral arteries. The majority of infarcts occur in the territory of the middle cerebral artery and its branches, and about one fifth occur in posterior cerebral circulation (348).

AF is the most common heart condition associated with cerebral infarcts. Advanced age and valvular heart disease significantly increase the risk of stroke in patients with AF (296). Other causes of cardiac embolism include MI, endocarditis, rheumatic heart disease, artificial valves, myxoma of left atrium, and cardiomyopathy. Right-to-left cardiac shunts (patent foramen ovale, interventricular septal defect, and pulmonary arteriovenous fistula) predispose to paradoxical embolization.

Clinical Presentation

Recent imaging studies suggest that the vast majority of acute ischemic events are silent (342). Symptoms of ischemic stroke depend on the location and size of the ischemic territory. A sudden onset of neurological sensory and motor symptoms suggest cerebral embolism, while a slower progression of stroke symptoms suggests arterial thrombosis. Neurological symptoms that resolve within 24 hours are characteristic for TIA; resolution within 48 hours is classified as reversible ischemic neurological deficit (RIND).

History and physical examination should identify the type and the extent of neurological deficit and diagnose any underlying/coexisting conditions (e.g., arrhythmia, hypertension, diabetes, autoimmune disorders, history of cancer).

Differential diagnosis should include hemorrhagic stroke, brain tumors, and cerebral abscess.

Imaging

Differentiation between ischemic and hemorrhagic stroke is critical and requires a rapid diagnostic process. Noncontrast brain CT can quickly rule out hemorrhagic stroke, but in the early hours of stroke, it cannot detect brain ischemia. Diffusion-weighted MR and CT angiography with CT perfusion imaging are more sensitive in the detection of an early infarct (349).

Angiography of cerebral arteries is performed when endovascular intervention such as intracranial thrombolysis is planned.

Results of thrombolysis can be monitored with MR (350,351).

Doppler ultrasound of extracranial arteries is mandatory in all cases of acute cerebral ischemia to assess carotid and vertebral arteries. Evaluation of the heart with echocardiography should be done when a cardioembolism is suspected. CTA is

TABLE 9-4

Stroke Prevention

Prophylaxis of Stroke Recurrence
1. Antiplatelet therapy: Aspirin 150–325 mg/day or clopidogrel
2. Anticoagulation in patients with cardioembolic stroke: high risk, Coumadin INR 2–3; low risk, aspirin 150–325 mg/day
3. Surgical endarterectomy in patients with carotid stenosis >75%

Primary Prevention of Stroke
1. Adequate therapy of hypertension
2. Effective control of glycaemia in diabetes
3. Statins for hypercholesterolemia
4. Cessation of smoking
5. Antiplatelet therapy for patients with diabetes, carotid stenosis, and peripheral artery disease
6. Anticoagulation for patients at risk of cardioembolic stroke

useful when further evaluation of abnormal carotid Doppler and exclusion of cardiogenic source is required; these territories can be imaged during the same examination.

Treatment

Management of acute ischemic stroke requires concomitant therapy of coexisting conditions like hypertensive crisis, acute MI, cardiac arrhythmia, hypo- or hyperglycemia, and the like.

Patients presenting within 3 hours of the onset of symptoms can be treated with thrombolytic therapy with rt-PA (352). Unfortunately, the majority of patients present to the emergency room later.

In patients immobilized by stroke, DVT prophylaxis with LMWH should be considered if no contraindications exist (353). Aspirin 150 to 300 mg by mouth (PO) within 48 hours should be given to reduce stroke mortality and morbidity (353) (Table 9-4).

Dexamethasone, IV mannitol 10%, and glycerol are given in patients with increased intracranial pressure and who are in danger of acute herniation.

REFERENCES

1. White RH. The epidemiology of venous thromboembolism. *Circulation.* 2003;107(23)[Suppl 1]I4–I8.
2. Haines ST. Venous thromboembolism: pathophysiology and clinical presentation. *Am J Health Syst Pharm.* 2003;60(22)[Suppl 7]:S3–S5.
3. Heit JA, Silverstein MD, Mohr DN, et al. The epidemiology of venous thromboembolism in the community. *Thromb Haemost.* 2001;86(1):452–463.
4. Kroegel C, Reissig A. Principle mechanisms underlying venous thromboembolism: epidemiology, risk factors, pathophysiology and pathogenesis. *Respiration.* 2003;70(1):7–30.

5. Ollendorf DA, Vera-Llonch M, Oster G. Cost of venous thromboembolism following major orthopedic surgery in hospitalized patients. *Am J Health Syst Pharm.* 2002;59(18):1750–1754.
6. Conroy JM, Trivedi GT, Sovd T, et al. The allele frequency of mutations in four genes that confer enhanced susceptibility to venous thromboembolism in an unselected group of New York State newborns. *Thromb Res.* 2000;99(4):317–324.
7. De Stefano V, Rossi E, Paciaroni K, et al. Screening for inherited thrombophilia: indications and therapeutic implications. *Haematologica.* 2002;87(10):1095–1108.
8. Kuhle S, Lane DA, Jochmanns K, et al. Homozygous antithrombin deficiency type II (99 Leu to Phe mutation) and childhood thromboembolism. *Thromb Haemost.* 2001;86(4):1007–1011.
9. Martinelli, I, Mannucci PM, De Stefano V, et al. Different risks of thrombosis in four coagulation defects associated with inherited thrombophilia: a study of 150 families. *Blood.* 1998;92(7):2353–2358.
10. Seligsohn U, Lubetsky A. Genetic susceptibility to venous thrombosis. *N Engl J Med.* 2001;344(16):1222–1231.
11. Patel RK, Ford E, Thumpston J, et al. Risk factors for venous thrombosis in the black population. *Thromb Haemost.* 2003;90(5):835–838.
12. Makris M, Leach M, Beauchamp NJ. et al. Genetic analysis, phenotypic diagnosis, and risk of venous thrombosis in families with inherited deficiencies of protein S. *Blood.* 2000;95(6):1935–1941.
13. De Stefano V, Chiusolo P, Paciaroni K, et al. Epidemiology of factor V Leiden: clinical implications. *Semin Thromb Hemost.* 1998;24(4):367–379.
14. Rosendaal FR, Koster T, Vandenbroucke JP, et al. High risk of thrombosis in patients homozygous for factor V Leiden (activated protein C resistance). *Blood.* 1995;85(6):1504–1508.
15. Simioni P, Tormene D, Manfrin D, et al. Prothrombin antigen levels in symptomatic and asymptomatic carriers of the 20210A prothrombin variant. *Br J Haematol.* 1998;103(4):1045–1050.
16. Coen D, Zadro R, Honovic L, et al. Prevalence and association of the factor V Leiden and prothrombin G20210A in healthy subjects and patients with venous thromboembolism. *Croat Med J.* 2001;42(4):488–492.
17. Tosetto A, Missiaglia E, Frezzato M, et al. The VITA project: prothrombin G20210A mutation and venous thromboembolism in the general population. *Thromb Haemost.* 1999;82(5):1395–1398.
18. Martinelli I, Bucciarelli P, Margaglione M, et al. The risk of venous thromboembolism in family members with mutations in the genes of factor V or prothrombin or both. *Br J Haematol.* 2000;111(4):1223–1229.
19. Ghosh K, Shetty S, Madkaikar M, et al. Venous thromboembolism in young patients from western India: a study. *Clin Appl Thromb Hemost.* 2001;7(2):158–165.
20. Young G, Manco-Johnson M, Gill JC, et al. Clinical manifestations of the prothrombin G20210A mutation in children: a pediatric coagulation consortium study. *J Thromb Haemost.* 2003;1(5):958–962.
21. Yap S. Classical homocystinuria: vascular risk and its prevention. *J Inherit Metab Dis.* 2003;26(2–3):259–265.
22. Mudd SH, Skovby F, Levy HL, et al. The natural history of homocystinuria due to cystathionine beta-synthase deficiency. *Am J Hum Genet.* 1985;37(1):1–31.
23. Simorre B, Quéré I, Berrut G, et al. [Vascular complications of homocystinuria: a retrospective multicenter study.] *Rev Med Interne.* 2002;23(3):267–272.
24. Mudd SH, Havlik R, Levy HL, et al. A study of cardiovascular risk in heterozygotes for homocystinuria. *Am J Hum Genet.* 1981;33(6):883–893.
25. Kelly PJ, Furie KL, Kistler JP, et al. Stroke in young patients with hyperhomocysteinemia due to cystathionine beta-synthase deficiency. *Neurology.* 2003;60(2):275–279.
26. Ray JG. Meta-analysis of hyperhomocysteinemia as a risk factor for venous thromboembolic disease. *Arch Intern Med.* 1998;158(19):2101–2106.
27. Langman LJ, Ray JG, Evrovski J, et al. Hyperhomocyst(e)inemia and the increased risk of venous thromboembolism: more evidence from a case-control study. *Arch Intern Med.* 2000;160(7):961–964.
28. Hainaut P, Jaumotte C, Verhelst D, et al. Hyperhomocysteinemia and venous thromboembolism: a risk factor more prevalent in the elderly and in idiopathic cases. *Thromb Res.* 2002;106(2):121–125.
29. Kelly PJ, Rosand J, Kistler JP, et al. Homocysteine, MTHFR 677C—>T polymorphism, and risk of ischemic stroke: results of a meta-analysis. *Neurology.* 2002;59(4):529–536.
30. Tsai AW, Cushman M, Tsai MY, et al. Serum homocysteine, thermolabile variant of methylene tetrahydrofolate reductase (MTHFR), and venous thromboembolism: longitudinal investigation of thromboembolism etiology (LITE). *Am J Hematol.* 2003;72(3):192–200.
31. Cattaneo M. Hyperhomocysteinaemia and atherothrombosis. *Ann Med.* 2000;32[Suppl 1]: 46–52.
32. Kang SS, Zhou J, Wong PW, et al. Intermediate homocysteinemia: a thermolabile variant of methylenetetrahydrofolate reductase. *Am J Hum Genet.* 1988;43(4):414–421.
33. De Stefano V, Casorelli I, Rossi E, et al. Interaction between hyperhomocysteinemia and inherited thrombophilic factors in venous thromboembolism. *Semin Thromb Hemost.* 2000;26(3):305–311.
34. Ray JG, Shmorgun D, Chan WS. Common C677T polymorphism of the methylenetetrahydrofolate reductase gene and the risk of venous thromboembolism: meta-analysis of 31 studies. *Pathophysiol Haemost Thromb.* 2002;32(2):51–58.
35. Choi BO, Kim NK, Kim SH, et al. Homozygous C677T mutation in the MTHFR gene as an independent risk factor for multiple small-artery occlusions. *Thromb Res.* 2003;111(1–2):39–44.
36. Boonmark NW, Lawn RM. The lysine-binding function of Lp(a). *Clin Genet.* 1997;52(5):355–360.
37. Price JF, Lee AJ, Rumley A, et al. Lipoprotein(a) and development of intermittent claudication and major cardiovascular events in men and women: the Edinburgh Artery Study. *Atherosclerosis.* 2001;157(1):241–249.
38. Matsumoto Y, Daida H, Watanabe Y, et al. High level of lipoprotein(a) is a strong predictor for progression of coronary artery disease. *J Atheroscler Thromb.* 1998;5(2): 47–53.
39. von Depka M, Nowak-Gottl U, Eisert R, et al. Increased lipoprotein(a) levels as an independent risk factor for venous thromboembolism. *Blood.* 2000;96(10):3364–3368.
40. Lippi G, Bassi A, Brocco G, et al. Lipoprotein(a) concentration is not associated with venous thromboembolism in a case control study. *Haematologica.* 1999;84(8):726–729.
41. Nowak-Gottl U, Junker R, Hartmeier M, et al. Increased lipoprotein(a) is an important risk factor for venous thromboembolism in childhood. *Circulation.* 1999;100(7):743–748.
42. Revel-Vilk S, Chan A, Bauman M, et al. Prothrombotic conditions in an unselected cohort of children with venous thromboembolic disease. *J Thromb Haemost.* 2003;1(5):915–921.
43. Tsai AW, Cushman M, Rosamond WD, et al. Coagulation factors, inflammation markers, and venous thromboembolism: the longitudinal investigation of thromboembolism etiology (LITE). *Am J Med.* 2002;113(8):636–642.
44. Robetorye RS, Rodgers GM. Update on selected inherited venous thrombotic disorders. *Am J Hematol.* 2001;68(4):256–268.
45. Alhenc-Gelas M, Nicaud V, Gandrille S, et al. The factor V gene A4070G mutation and the risk of venous thrombosis. *Thromb Haemost.* 1999;81(2):193–197.
46. Lopaciuk S, Bykowska K, Kopec M. Prevalence of heparin cofactor II deficiency in patients with a history of venous thrombosis. *Pol J Pharmacol.* 1996;48(1):109–111.

47. Ehrenforth S, Junker R, Koch HG, et al. Multicentre evaluation of combined prothrombotic defects associated with thrombophilia in childhood. Childhood Thrombophilia Study Group. *Eur J Pediatr*. 1999;158[Suppl 3]:S97–S104.
48. Kostka H, Kuhlisch E, Schellong S, et al. Polymorphisms in the TAFI gene and the risk of venous thrombosis. *Clin Lab*. 2003;49(11–12):645–647.
49. Mosesson MW. Dysfibrinogenemia and thrombosis. *Semin Thromb Hemost*. 1999;25(3):311–319.
50. Song KS, Lee Sm, Choi JR. Detection of an Ala601Thr mutation of plasminogen gene in 3 out of 36 Korean patients with deep vein thrombosis. *J Korean Med Sci*. 2003;18(2):167–170.
51. Robbins KC. Classification of abnormal plasminogens: dysplasminogenemias. *Semin Thromb Hemost*. 1990;16(3):217–220.
52. Sartori MT, Danesin C, Saggiorato G, et al. The PAI-1 gene 4G/5G polymorphism and deep vein thrombosis in patients with inherited thrombophilia. *Clin Appl Thromb Hemost*. 2003;9(4):299–307.
53. Wallaschofski H, Kobsar A, Koksch M, et al. Prolactin receptor signaling during platelet activation. *Horm Metab Res*. 2003;35(4):228–235.
54. Folsom AR, Cushman M, Tsai M, et al. A prospective study of venous thromboembolism in relation to factor V Leiden and related factors. *Blood*. 2002;99(8):2720–2725.
55. Salomon O, Steinberg DM, Zivelin A, et al. Single and combined prothrombotic factors in patients with idiopathic venous thromboembolism: prevalence and risk assessment. *Arterioscler Thromb Vasc Biol*. 1999;19(3):511–518.
56. Emmerich J, Rosendaal FR, Cattaneo M, et al. Combined effect of factor V Leiden and prothrombin 20210A on the risk of venous thromboembolism—pooled analysis of 8 case-control studies including 2310 cases and 3204 controls. Study Group for Pooled-Analysis in Venous Thromboembolism. *Thromb Haemost*. 2001;86(3):809–816.
57. Brenner B, Zivelin A, Lanir N, et al. Venous thromboembolism associated with double heterozygosity for R506Q mutation of factor V and for T298M mutation of protein C in a large family of a previously described homozygous protein C-deficient newborn with massive thrombosis. *Blood*. 1996;88(3):877–880.
58. Mandel H, Brenner B, Berant M, et al. Coexistence of hereditary homocystinuria and factor V Leiden—effect on thrombosis. *N Engl J Med*. 1996;334(12):763–768.
59. Vogel JJ, Reber G, de Moerloose P. Laboratory and clinical features in systemic lupus erythematosus patients with or without anticardiolipin antibodies. *Thromb Res*. 1991;62(5):545–556.
60. Manoussakis MN, Tzioufas AG, Silis MP, et al. High prevalence of anticardiolipin and other autoantibodies in a healthy elderly population. *Clin Exp Immunol*. 1987;68:557–565.
61. Gezer S. Antiphospholipid syndrome. *Dis Mon*. 2003;49(12):696–741.
62. Nahass GT. Antiphospholipid antibodies and the antiphospholipid antibody syndrome. *J Am Acad Dermatol*. 1997;36(2 Pt 1):149–168; quiz 169–172.
63. Dalekos GN, Zachou K, Liaskos C. The antiphospholipid syndrome and infection. *Curr Rheumatol Rep*. 2001;3(4):277–285.
64. Schved JF, Dupuy-Fons C, Biron C, et al. A prospective epidemiological study on the occurrence of antiphospholipid antibody: the Montpelier Antiphospholipid (MAP) Study. *Haemostasis*. 1994;24(3):175–182.
65. Goel N, Ortel TL, Bali D, et al. Familial antiphospholipid antibody syndrome: criteria for disease and evidence for autosomal dominant inheritance. *Arthritis Rheum*. 1999;42(2):318–327.
66. Triplett DA. Antiphospholipid antibodies. *Arch Pathol Lab Med*. 2002;126(11):1424–1429.
67. Shoenfeld Y, Krause I, Kvapil F, et al. Prevalence and clinical correlations of antibodies against six beta2-glycoprotein-I-related peptides in the antiphospholipid syndrome. *J Clin Immunol*. 2003;23(5):377–383.
68. Neville C, Rauch J, Kassis J, et al. Thromboembolic risk in patients with high titre anticardiolipin and multiple antiphospholipid antibodies. *Thromb Haemost*. 2003;90(1):108–115.
69. Galli M, Barbui T. Antiphospholipid antibodies and thrombosis: strength of association. *Hematol J*. 2003;4(3):180–186.
70. Field SL, Brighton TA, McNeil HP, et al. Recent insights into antiphospholipid antibody-mediated thrombosis. *Baillieres Best Pract Res Clin Haematol*. 1999;12(3):407–422.
71. Rand JH. The pathogenic role of annexin-V in the antiphospholipid syndrome. *Curr Rheumatol Rep*. 2000;2(3):246–251.
72. Forastiero RR, Martinuzzo ME, Lu L, et al. Autoimmune antiphospholipid antibodies impair the inhibition of activated factor X by protein Z/protein Z-dependent protease inhibitor. *J Thromb Haemost*. 2003;1(8):1764–1770.
73. Wilson WA, Gharavi AE, Koike T. International consensus statement on preliminary classification criteria for definite antiphospholipid syndrome: report of an international workshop. *Arthritis Rheum*. 1999;42(7):1309–1311.
74. Erkan D, Asherson RA, Espinosa G, et al. Long term outcome of catastrophic antiphospholipid syndrome survivors. *Ann Rheum Dis*. 2003;62(6):530–533.
75. Petri M. Management of thrombosis in antiphospholipid antibody syndrome. *Rheum Dis Clin North Am*. 2001;27(3):633–642, viii.
76. Meroni PL, Moia M, Derksen RH, et al. Venous thromboembolism in the antiphospholipid syndrome: management guidelines for secondary prophylaxis. *Lupus*. 2003;12(7):504–507.
77. Heilmann L, von Tempelhoff GF, Pollow K. Antiphospholipid syndrome in obstetrics. *Clin Appl Thromb Hemost*. 2003;9(2):143–150.
78. Galli M, Barbui T. Antiphospholipid antibodies and pregnancy. *Best Pract Res Clin Haematol*. 2003;16(2):211–225.
79. Abbate R, Prisco D, Rostagno C, et al. Age-related changes in the hemostatic system. *Int J Clin Lab Res*. 1993;23(1):1–3.
80. Tsai AW, Cushman M, Rosamond WD, et al. Cardiovascular risk factors and venous thromboembolism incidence: the longitudinal investigation of thromboembolism etiology. *Arch Intern Med*. 2002;162(10):1182–1189.
81. Harenberg J. Risk assessment of venous thromboembolism in medical patients. *Semin Hematol*. 2000;37(3 Suppl 5):3–6.
82. Arnold DM, Kahn SR, Shrier I. Missed opportunities for prevention of venous thromboembolism: an evaluation of the use of thromboprophylaxis guidelines. *Chest*. 2001;120(6):1964–1971.
83. Scurr JH, Machin SJ, Bailey-King S, et al. Frequency and prevention of symptomless deep-vein thrombosis in long-haul flights: a randomised trial. *Lancet*. 2001;357(9267):1485–1489.
84. Jacobson BF, Munster M, Smith A, et al. The BEST study—a prospective study to compare business class versus economy class air travel as a cause of thrombosis. *S Afr Med J*. 2003;93(7):522–528.
85. Arya R, Barnes JA, Hossain U, et al. Long-haul flights and deep vein thrombosis: a significant risk only when additional factors are also present. *Br J Haematol*. 2002;116(3):653–654.
86. Kim V, Spandorfer J. Epidemiology of venous thromboembolic disease. *Emerg Med Clin North Am*. 2001;19(4):839–859.
87. Bowles LK, Cooper JA, Howarth DJ, et al. Associations of haemostatic variables with body mass index: a community-based study. *Blood Coagul Fibrinolysis*. 2003;14(6):569–573.
88. Powell JT. Vascular damage from smoking: disease mechanisms at the arterial wall. *Vasc Med*. 1998;3(1):21–28.

89. Tosetto A, Frezzato M, Rodeghiero F. Prevalence and risk factors of non-fatal venous thromboembolism in the active population of the VITA Project. *J Thromb Haemost.* 2003;1(8):1724–1729.

90. Nightingale AL, Lawrenson RA, Simpson EL, et al. The effects of age, body mass index, smoking and general health on the risk of venous thromboembolism in users of combined oral contraceptives. *Eur J Contracept Reprod Health Care.* 2000;5(4):265–274.

91. Roy S. Effects of smoking on prostacyclin formation and platelet aggregation in users of oral contraceptives. *Am J Obstet Gynecol.* 1999;180(6)[Pt 2]:S364–S368.

92. Farley TM, Meirik O, Chang CL, et al. Combined oral contraceptives, smoking, and cardiovascular risk. *J Epidemiol Community Health.* 1998;52(12):775–785.

93. Eldor A. Thrombophilia, thrombosis and pregnancy. *Thromb Haemost.* 2001;86(1):104–111.

94. Pabinger I, Grafenhofer H. Thrombosis during pregnancy: risk factors, diagnosis and treatment. *Pathophysiol Haemost Thromb.* 2002;(5–6):322–324.

95. Hague WM, Dekker GA. Risk factors for thrombosis in pregnancy. *Best Pract Res Clin Haematol.* 2003;16(2): 197–210.

96. Greer IA. Prevention of venous thromboembolism in pregnancy. *Best Pract Res Clin Haematol.* 2003;16(2):261–278.

97. Tan JY. Thrombophilia in pregnancy. *Ann Acad Med Singapore.* 2002;31(3):328–334.

98. Walker ID. Arterial thromboembolism in pregnancy. *Best Pract Res Clin Haematol.* 2003;16(2):297–310.

99. Heit JA, Mohr DN, Silverstein MD, et al. Predictors of recurrence after deep vein thrombosis and pulmonary embolism: a population-based cohort study. *Arch Intern Med.* 2000;160(6):761–768.

100. Kyrle PA, Eichinger S. The risk of recurrent venous thromboembolism: the Austrian Study on Recurrent Venous Thromboembolism. *Wien Klin Wochenschr.* 2003; 115(13–14):471–474.

101. Cook N, Thomas DM. Retrospective survey of unselected hospital patients with and without cancer comparing outcomes following venous thromboembolism. *Intern Med J.* 2002;32(9–10):437–444.

102. Lin JT. Thromboembolic events in the cancer patient. *J Womens Health (Larchmt).* 2003;12(6):541–551.

103. Sorensen HT, Johnsen SP, Norgard B, et al. Cancer and venous thromboembolism: a multidisciplinary approach. *Clin Lab.* 2003;49(11–12):615–623.

104. Baron JA, Gridley G, Weiderpass E, et al. Venous thromboembolism and cancer. *Lancet.* 1998;351(9109): 1077–1080.

105. Monreal M, Fernandez-Llamazares J, Perandreu J, et al. Occult cancer in patients with venous thromboembolism: which patients, which cancers. *Thromb Haemost.* 1997; 78(5):1316–1318.

106. Lee AY. Epidemiology and management of venous thromboembolism in patients with cancer. *Thromb Res.* 2003;110(4):167–172.

107. Goldschmidt N, Linetsky E, Shalom E, et al. High incidence of thromboembolism in patients with central nervous system lymphoma. *Cancer.* 2003;98(6):1239–1242.

108. Marras LC, Geerts WH, Perry JR. The risk of venous thromboembolism is increased throughout the course of malignant glioma: an evidence-based review. *Cancer.* 2000;89(3):640–646.

109. Hillen HF. Thrombosis in cancer patients. *Ann Oncol.* 2000;11[Suppl 3]:273–276.

110. Randi ML, Fabris F, Cella G, et al. Cerebral vascular accidents in young patients with essential thrombocythemia: relation with other known cardiovascular risk factors. *Angiology.* 1998;49(6):477–481.

111. Schwarcz TH, Hogan LA, Endean ED, et al. Thromboembolic complications of polycythemia: polycythemia vera versus smokers' polycythemia. *J Vasc Surg.* 1993;17(3): 518–522; discussion 522–523.

112. Verso M, Agnelli G. Venous thromboembolism associated with long-term use of central venous catheters in cancer patients. *J Clin Oncol.* 2003;21(19):3665–3675.

113. Shlebak AA, Smith DB. Incidence of objectively diagnosed thromboembolic disease in cancer patients undergoing cytotoxic chemotherapy and/or hormonal therapy. *Cancer Chemother Pharmacol.* 1997;39(5):462–466.

114. Prandoni P. Cancer and thromboembolic disease: how important is the risk of thrombosis? *Cancer Treat Rev.* 2002;28(3):133–136.

115. Holm T, Singnomklao MS, Rutqvist L-E, et al. Adjuvant preoperative radiotherapy in patients with rectal carcinoma. Adverse effects during long term follow-up of two randomized trials. *Cancer.* 1996;78(5):968–976.

116. Rickles FR, Levine MN. Epidemiology of thrombosis in cancer. *Acta Haematol.* 2001;106(1–2):6–12.

117. Otten HM, Prins MH. Venous thromboembolism and occult malignancy. *Thromb Res.* 2001;102(6):V187–V194.

118. Valtonen V, Kuikka A, Syrjanen J. Thrombo-embolic complications in bacteraemic infections. *Eur Heart J.* 1993;14[Suppl K]:20–23.

119. Herzberg MC, Weyer MW. Dental plaque, platelets, and cardiovascular diseases. *Ann Periodontol.* 1998;3(1): 151–160.

120. Ben Hamouda-M'Rad IA, Mrabet A, Ben Hamida M. [Cerebral venous thrombosis and arterial infarction in pregnancy and puerperium. A series of 60 cases.] *Rev Neurol (Paris).* 1995;151(10):563–568.

121. Bhatia K, Jones NS. Septic cavernous sinus thrombosis secondary to sinusitis: are anticoagulants indicated? A review of the literature. *J Laryngol Otol.* 2002;116(9):667–676.

122. Bradley DT, Hashisaki GT, Mason JC. Otogenic sigmoid sinus thrombosis: what is the role of anticoagulation? *Laryngoscope.* 2002;112(10):1726–1729.

123. Gallagher RM, Gross CW, Phillips CD. Suppurative intracranial complications of sinusitis. *Laryngoscope.* 1998;108 [11 Pt 1]:1635–1642.

124. Sanchez TG, Cahali MB, Murakami MS, et al. Septic thrombosis of orbital vessels due to cutaneous nasal infection. *Am J Rhinol.* 1997;11(6):429–433.

125. Lozinguez O, Arnaud E, Belec L, et al. Demonstration of an association between Chlamydia pneumoniae infection and venous thromboembolic disease. *Thromb Haemost.* 2000;83(6):887–891.

126. Emmerich J. Infection and venous thrombosis. *Pathophysiol Haemost Thromb.* 2002;32(5–6):346–348.

127. Copur AS, Smith PR, Gomez V, et al. HIV infection is a risk factor for venous thromboembolism. *AIDS Patient Care STDS.* 2002;16(5):205–209.

128. Horstkotte D. Endocarditis: epidemiology, diagnosis and treatment. *Z Kardiol.* 2000;89[Suppl 4]:IV2–IV11.

129. Tunkel AR, Kaye D. Neurologic complications of infective endocarditis. *Neurol Clin.* 1993;11(2):419–440.

130. Maclennan AC, Doyle DL, Sacks SL. Infectious aortitis due to penicillin-resistant Streptococcus pneumoniae. *Ann Vasc Surg.* 1997;11(5):533–535.

131. Cherri J, Freitas MA, Llorach-Velludo MA, et al. Paracoccidioidomycotic aortitis with embolization to the lower limbs. Report of a case and review of the literature. *J Cardiovasc Surg (Torino).* 1998;39(5):573–576.

132. Yoo HH, De Paiva SA, Silveira LV, et al. Logistic regression analysis of potential prognostic factors for pulmonary thromboembolism. *Chest.* 2003;123(3):813–821.

133. Velmahos GC, Kern J, Chan LS, et al. Prevention of venous thromboembolism after injury: an evidence-based report—part I: analysis of risk factors and evaluation of the role of vena caval filters. *J Trauma.* 2000;49(1):132–138; discussion 139.

134. Morpurgo M, Schmid C, Mandelli V. Factors influencing the clinical diagnosis of pulmonary embolism: analysis of 229 postmortem cases. *Int J Cardiol.* 1998;65[Suppl 1]:S79–S82.

135. Howell MD, Geraci JM, Knowlton AA. Congestive heart failure and outpatient risk of venous thromboembolism: a

retrospective, case-control study. *J Clin Epidemiol.* 2001;54(8):810–816.

136. Anderson FA Jr, Spencer FA. Risk factors for venous thromboembolism. *Circulation.* 2003;107(23)[Suppl 1]:I9–I16.

137. Citak A, Emre S, Sairin A, et al. Hemostatic problems and thromboembolic complications in nephrotic children. *Pediatr Nephrol.* 2000;14(2):138–142.

138. Lee C-H, Chen K-S, Tsai F-C, et al. Concurrent thrombosis of cerebral and femoral arteries in a patient with nephrotic syndrome. *Am J Nephrol.* 2000;20(6):483–486.

139. Solem CA, Loftus EV Jr, Tremaine WJ, et al. Venous thromboembolism in inflammatory bowel disease. *Am J Gastroenterol.* 2004;99(1):97–101.

140. White RH, Zhou H, Romano PS. Incidence of symptomatic venous thromboembolism after different elective or urgent surgical procedures. *Thromb Haemost.* 2003;90(3): 446–455.

141. Khushal A, Quinlan D, Alikhan R, et al. Thromboembolic disease in surgery for malignancy-rationale for prolonged thromboprophylaxis. *Semin Thromb Hemost.* 2002;28(6):569–576.

142. Rasmussen MS. Does prolonged thromboprophylaxis improve outcome in patients undergoing surgery? *Cancer Treat Rev.* 2003;29[Suppl 2]:15–17.

143. Kim YH, Oh SH, Kim JS. Incidence and natural history of deep-vein thrombosis after total hip arthroplasty. A prospective and randomised clinical study. *J Bone Joint Surg Br.* 2003;85(5):661–665.

144. White RH, Henderson MC. Risk factors for venous thromboembolism after total hip and knee replacement surgery. *Curr Opin Pulm Med.* 2002;8(5):365–371.

145. Behrendt CE, Ruiz RB. Venous thromboembolism among patients with advanced lung cancer randomized to prinomastat or placebo, plus chemotherapy. *Thromb Haemost.* 2003;90(4):734–737.

146. Male C, Chait P, Andrew M, et al. Central venous line-related thrombosis in children: association with central venous line location and insertion technique. *Blood.* 2003;101(11):4273–4278.

147. Lidegaard O, Edstrom B, Kreiner S. Oral contraceptives and venous thromboembolism: a five-year national case-control study. *Contraception.* 2002;65(3):187–196.

148. Hennessy S, Berlin JA, Kinman JL, et al. Risk of venous thromboembolism from oral contraceptives containing gestodene and desogestrel versus levonorgestrel: a meta-analysis and formal sensitivity analysis. *Contraception.* 2001;64(2):125–133.

149. Todd J, Lawrenson R, Farmer RD, et al. Venous thromboembolic disease and combined oral contraceptives: a re-analysis of the MediPlus database. *Hum Reprod.* 1999;14(6): 1500–1505.

150. Black C, Kaye JA, Jick H. Clinical risk factors for venous thromboembolus in users of the combined oral contraceptive pill. *Br J Clin Pharmacol.* 2002;53(6):637–640.

151. Hoibraaten E, Qvigstad E, Arnensen H, et al. Increased risk of recurrent venous thromboembolism during hormone replacement therapy: results of the randomised, double-blind, placebo-controlled estrogen in venous thromboembolism trial (EVTET). *Thromb Haemost.* 2000;84(6):961–967.

152. Mannucci PM. Venous thromboembolism and hormone replacement therapy. 2001;12(6):478–483.

153. Lowe GD. Hormone replacement therapy: prothrombotic vs. protective effects. *Pathophysiol Haemost Thromb.* 2002;32(5–6):329–332.

154. Peverill RE. Hormone therapy and venous thromboembolism. *Best Pract Res Clin Endocrinol Metab.* 2003;17(1):149–164.

155. Herrington DM, Vittinghoff E, Howard T, et al. Factor V Leiden, hormone replacement therapy, and risk of venous thromboembolic events in women with coronary disease. *Arterioscler Thromb Vasc Biol.* 2002;22(6):1012–1017.

156. Hoibraaten E, Qvigstad E, Andersen TO, et al. The effects of hormone replacement therapy (HRT) on hemostatic variables

in women with previous venous thromboembolism—results from a randomized, double-blind, clinical trial. *Thromb Haemost.* 2001;85(5):775–781.

157. Navarro F, Bartholomew JR. Deep vein thrombosis. In: Young JR, Olin JW, Bartholomew JR, eds. *Peripheral Vascular Diseases.* St. Louis: Mosby-Year Book, Inc., 451–467.

158. Kearon C. Natural history of venous thromboembolism. *Circulation.* 2003:107(23)[Suppl 1]:I22–I30.

159. Criado E, Burnham CB. Predictive value of clinical criteria for the diagnosis of deep vein thrombosis. *Surgery.* 1997;122(3):578–583.

160. de Thomasson E, Strauss C, Girard P, et al. [Detection of asymptomatic venous thrombosis after lower limb prosthetic surgery. Retrospective evaluation of a systematic approach using Doppler ultrasonography: 400 cases.]. *Presse Med.* 2000;29(7):351–356.

161. Ascani A, Radicchia S, Parise P, et al. Distribution and occlusiveness of thrombi in patients with surveillance detected deep vein thrombosis after hip surgery. *Thromb Haemost.* 1996;75(2):239–241.

162. Giannoukas AD, Tsetis D, Kostas T, et al. Suspected acute deep vein thrombosis of the lower limb in outpatients: considerations for optimal diagnostic approach. *World J Surg.* 2003;27(5):554–557.

163. Lennox AF, Delis KT, Serunkuma S, et al. Combination of a clinical risk assessment score and rapid whole blood D-dimer testing in the diagnosis of deep vein thrombosis in symptomatic patients. *J Vasc Surg.* 1999;30(5): 794–803.

164. Kelly J, Hunt BJ. The utility of pretest probability assessment in patients with clinically suspected venous thromboembolism. *J Thromb Haemost.* 2003;1(9):1888–1896.

165. Constans J, Boutinet C, Salmi LR, et al. Comparison of four clinical prediction scores for the diagnosis of lower limb deep venous thrombosis in outpatients. *Am J Med.* 2003;115(6):436–440.

166. Dalen JE. Pulmonary embolism: what have we learned since Virchow? Natural history, pathophysiology, and diagnosis. *Chest.* 2002;122(4):1440–1456.

167. Meissner MH, Caps MT, Bergelin RO, et al. Early outcome after isolated calf vein thrombosis. *J Vasc Surg.* 1997;26(5):749–756.

168. O'Shaughnessy AM, Fitzgerald DE. Natural history of proximal deep vein thrombosis assessed by duplex ultrasound. *Int Angiol.* 1997;16(1):45–49.

169. Ziegler S, Schillinger M, Maca TH, et al. Post-thrombotic syndrome after primary event of deep venous thrombosis 10 to 20 years ago. *Thromb Res.* 2001;101(2):23–33.

170. Warwick D, Perez J, Vickery C, et al. Does total hip arthroplasty predispose to chronic venous insufficiency? *J Arthroplasty.* 1996;11(5):529–533.

171. Szuba A, Cooke JP, Rockson SG. Images in vascular medicine. Phlegmasia coerulea dolens—venous gangrene. *Vasc Med.* 1998;3(1):29–31.

172. Perkins JM, Magee TR, Galland RB. Phlegmasia caerulea dolens and venous gangrene. *Br J Surg.* 1996;83(1):19–23.

173. Mustafa S, Stein PD, Patel KC, et al. Upper extremity deep venous thrombosis. *Chest.* 2003;123(6):1953–1956.

174. Da Costa SS, Scalabrini NA, Costa R, et al. Incidence and risk factors of upper extremity deep vein lesions after permanent transvenous pacemaker implant: a 6–month follow-up prospective study. *Pacing Clin Electrophysiol.* 2002;25(9):1301–1306.

175. Prandoni P, Polistena P, Bernardi E, et al. Upper-extremity deep vein thrombosis. Risk factors, diagnosis, and complications. *Arch Intern Med.* 1997;157(1):57–62.

176. Lindblad B, Tengborn L, Bergqvist D. Deep vein thrombosis of the axillary-subclavian veins: epidemiologic data, effects of different types of treatment and late sequelae. *Eur J Vasc Surg.* 1988;2(3):161–165.

177. DiFelice GS, Paletta GA, Phillips BB, et al. Effort thrombosis in the elite throwing athlete. *Am J Sports Med.* 2002;30(5): 708–712.

178. Kommareddy A, Zaroukian MH, Hassouna HI. Upper extremity deep venous thrombosis. *Semin Thromb Hemost.* 2002;28(1):89–99.

179. Oginosawa Y, Abe H, Nakashima Y. The incidence and risk factors for venous obstruction after implantation of transvenous pacing leads. *Pacing Clin Electrophysiol.* 2002;25(11):1605–1611.

180. Monreal M, Raventos A, Lerma R, et al. Pulmonary embolism in patients with upper extremity DVT associated to venous central lines—a prospective study. *Thromb Haemost.* 1994;72(4):548–550.

181. Theodorou SJ, Theodorou DJ, Kakitsubata Y. Sonography and venography of the lower extremities for diagnosing deep vein thrombosis in symptomatic patients. *Clin Imaging.* 2003;27(3):180–183.

182. Leizorovicz A, Kassai B, Becker F, et al. The assessment of deep vein thromboses for therapeutic trials. *Angiology.* 2003;54(1):19–24.

183. Noren A, Ottosson E, Rosfors S. Is it safe to withhold anticoagulation based on a single negative color duplex examination in patients with suspected deep venous thrombosis? A prospective 3–month follow-up study. *Angiology.* 2002;53(5):521–527.

184. Elias A, Mallard L, Elias M, et al. A single complete ultrasound investigation of the venous network for the diagnostic management of patients with a clinically suspected first episode of deep venous thrombosis of the lower limbs. *Thromb Haemost.* 2003;89(2):221–227.

185. Semba CP, Dake MD. Catheter-directed thrombolysis for iliofemoral venous thrombosis. *Semin Vasc Surg.* 1996;9(1):26–33.

186. Sharafuddin MJ, Sun S, Hoballah JJ, et al. Endovascular management of venous thrombotic and occlusive diseases of the lower extremities. *J Vasc Interv Radiol.* 2003;14(4): 405–423.

187. Bradbury MS, Kavanagh PV, Bechtold RE, et al. Mesenteric venous thrombosis: diagnosis and noninvasive imaging. *Radiographics.* 2002;22(3):527–541.

188. Orloff MJ, Orloff MS, Orloff SL, et al. Portal vein thrombosis in cirrhosis with variceal hemorrhage. *J Gastrointest Surg.* 1997;1(2):123–131.

189. Rabe C, Pilz T, Klostermann C, et al. Clinical characteristics and outcome of a cohort of 101 patients with hepatocellular carcinoma. *World J Gastroenterol.* 2001;7(2):208–215.

190. Janssen HL, Wijnhoud A, Haagsma EB, et al. Extrahepatic portal vein thrombosis: aetiology and determinants of survival. *Gut.* 2001;49(5):720–724.

191. Amitrano L, Brancaccio V, Guardascione MA, et al. Inherited coagulation disorders in cirrhotic patients with portal vein thrombosis. *Hepatology.* 2000;31(2):345–348.

192. Higa M, Kojima M, Ohnuma S, et al. Portal and mesenteric vein and inferior vena cava thrombosis associated with antiphospholipid syndrome. *Intern Med.* 2001;40(12): 1245–1249.

193. McNamara C, Juneja S, Wolf M, et al. Portal or hepatic vein thrombosis as the first presentation of a myeloproliferative disorder in patients with normal peripheral blood counts. *Clin Lab Haematol.* 2002;24(4):239–242.

194. Franciosi C, Romano F, Caprotti R, et al. Splenoportal thrombosis as a complication after laparoscopic splenectomy. *J Laparoendosc Adv Surg Tech A.* 2002;12(4): 273–276.

195. Fujita F, Lyass S, Otsuka K, et al. Portal vein thrombosis following splenectomy: identification of risk factors. *Am Surg.* 2003;69(11):951–956.

196. Marroquin CE, Tuttle-Newhall JE, Collins BH, et al. Emergencies after liver transplantation. *Semin Gastrointest Dis.* 2003;14(2):101–110.

197. Berney T, Morales M, Broquet PE, et al. Risk factors influencing the outcome of portal and mesenteric vein thrombosis. *Hepatogastroenterology.* 1998;45(24):2275–2281.

198. Condat B, Valla D. [Portal vein thrombosis.) *Presse Med.* 2003;32(31):1460–1465.

199. Shin DH, Park JH, Yoon KW, et al. Clostridium perfringens septicemia with thrombophlebitis of the portal vein. *J Infect.* 2003;46(4):253–255.

200. Hagimoto T, Seo M, Okada M, et al. Portal vein thrombosis successfully treated with a colectomy in active ulcerative colitis: report of a case. *Dis Colon Rectum.* 2001;44(4):587–590.

201. Di Cataldo A, Lanteri R, Dell'Arte M, et al. Portal vein thrombosis. A multifactorial clinical entity. *Chir Ital.* 2003;55(3):435–439.

202. Orloff MJ, Orloff MS, Girard B, et al. Bleeding esophagogastric varices from extrahepatic portal hypertension: 40 years' experience with portal-systemic shunt. *J Am Coll Surg.* 2002;194(6):717–728; discussion 728–730.

203. Rieu V, Ruivard M, Abergel A, et al. [Mesenteric venous thrombosis. A retrospective study of 23 cases.] *Ann Med Interne (Paris).* 2003;154(3):133–138.

204. Gertsch P, Matthews J, Lerut J, et al. Acute thrombosis of the splanchnic veins. *Arch Surg.* 1993;128(3):341–345.

205. Tanaka H, Horie Y, Idobe Y, et al. Refractory ascites due to portal vein thrombosis in liver cirrhosis—report of two cases. *Hepatogastroenterology.* 1998;45(23):1777–1780.

206. Janssen HL. Changing perspectives in portal vein thrombosis. *Scand J Gastroenterol Suppl.* 2000;(232):69–73.

207. Uflacker R. Applications of percutaneous mechanical thrombectomy in transjugular intrahepatic portosystemic shunt and portal vein thrombosis. *Tech Vasc Interv Radiol.* 2003;6(1):59–69.

208. Baccarani U, Gasparini D, Risaliti A, et al. Percutaneous mechanical fragmentation and stent placement for the treatment of early posttransplantation portal vein thrombosis. *Transplantation.* 2001;72(9):1572–1582.

209. Guckelberger O, Bechstein WO, Langrehr JM, et al. Successful recanalization of late portal vein thrombosis after liver transplantation using systemic low-dose recombinant tissue plasminogen activator. *Transpl Int.* 1999;12(4):273–277.

210. Condat B, Pessione F, Denninger MH, et al. Recent portal or mesenteric venous thrombosis: increased recognition and frequent recanalization on anticoagulant therapy. *Hepatology.* 2000;32(3):466–470.

211. Mack CL, Superina RA, Whitington PF. Surgical restoration of portal flow corrects procoagulant and anticoagulant deficiencies associated with extrahepatic portal vein thrombosis. *J Pediatr.* 2003;14(2):197–199.

212. Kumar S, Kamath PS. Acute superior mesenteric venous thrombosis: one disease or two? *Am J Gastroenterol.* 2003;98(6):1299–1304.

213. Brunaud L, Antunes L, Adler SC, et al. Acute mesenteric venous thrombosis: case for nonoperative management. *J Vasc Surg.* 2001;34(4):673–679.

214. Tateishi A, Mitsui H, Oki T, et al. Extensive mesenteric vein and portal vein thrombosis successfully treated by thrombolysis and anticoagulation. *J Gastroenterol Hepatol.* 2001;16(12):1429–1433.

215. Rhee RY, Gloviczki P. Mesenteric venous thrombosis. *Surg Clin North Am.* 1997;77(2):327–338.

216. Singh V, Sinha SK, Nain CK, et al. Budd-Chiari syndrome: our experience of 71 patients. *J Gastroenterol Hepatol.* 2000;15(5):550–554.

217. Shafer DF, Sorrell MF. Vascular diseases of the liver. In: Feldman M, Friedman LS, Sleisenger MH, eds. *Sleisenger & Fordtrans Gastrointestinal and Liver Disease.* 7th edition. Philadelphia, Saunders, 2002.

218. Poreddy V, DeLeve LD. Hepatic circulatory diseases associated with chronic myeloid disorders. *Clin Liver Dis.* 2002; 6(4):909–931.

219. Karti SS, Yilmaz M, Kosucu P, et al. Early medical treatment is life saving in acute Budd-Chiari due to polycythemia vera. *Hepatogastroenterology.* 2003;50(50):512–514.

220. Nezakatgoo N, Shokouh-Amiri MH, Gaber AO, et al. Liver transplantation for acute Budd-Chiari syndrome in identical twin sisters with Factor V leiden mutation. *Transplantation.* 2003;76(1):195–198.

221. Perello A, Garcia-Pagan JC, Gilabert R, et al. TIPS is a useful long-term derivative therapy for patients with Budd-Chiari syndrome uncontrolled by medical therapy. *Hepatology.* 2002;35(1):132–139.

222. Orloff MJ, Daily PO, Orloff SL, et al. A 27–year experience with surgical treatment of Budd-Chiari syndrome. *Ann Surg.* 2000;232(3):340–352.

223. Malkowski P, Michalowicz B, Pawlak J, et al. Surgical and interventional radiological treatment of Budd-Chiari syndrome: report of nine cases. *Hepatogastroenterology.* 2003;50(54):2049–2051.

224. Srinivasan P, Rela M, Prachalias A, et al. Liver transplantation for Budd-Chiari syndrome. *Transplantation.* 2002;73(6):973–977.

225. Kaushik S, Federle MP, Schur PH, et al. Abdominal thrombotic and ischemic manifestations of the antiphospholipid antibody syndrome: CT findings in 42 patients. *Radiology.* 2001;218(3):768–771.

226. Fleischmann D. Multiple detector-row CT angiography of the renal and mesenteric vessels. *Eur J Radiol.* 2003;45 [Suppl 1]:S79–S87.

227. Rha SE, Ha HK, Lee S-H, et al. CT and MR imaging findings of bowel ischemia from various primary causes. *Radiographics.* 2000;20(1):29–42.

228. Laissy JP, Trillaud H, Douek P. MR angiography: noninvasive vascular imaging of the abdomen. *Abdom Imaging.* 2002;27(5):488–506.

229. Lin J, Chen XH, Zhou KR, et al. Budd-Chiari syndrome: diagnosis with three-dimensional contrast-enhanced magnetic resonance angiography. *World J Gastroenterol.* 2003;9(10):2317–2321.

230. Vogt W. [Abdominal ultrasound diagnosis.] *Schweiz Rundsch Med Prax.* 2000;89(24):1061–1066.

231. Morrin MM, Pedrosa I, Rofsky NM. Magnetic resonance imaging for disorders of liver vasculature. *Top Magn Reson Imaging.* 2002;13(3):177–190.

232. Smith PA, Klein AS, Heath DG, et al. Dual-phase spiral CT angiography with volumetric 3D rendering for preoperative liver transplant evaluation: preliminary observations. *J Comput Assist Tomogr.* 1998;22(6):868–874.

233. Chan HH, Douketis JD, Nowaczyk MJ. Acute renal vein thrombosis, oral contraceptive use, and hyperhomocysteinemia. *Mayo Clin Proc.* 2001;76(2):212–214.

234. Giordano P, Laforgia N, Di Guilio G, et al. Renal vein thrombosis in a newborn with prothrombotic genetic risk factors. *J Perinat Med.* 2001;29(2):163–166.

235. Zigman A, Yazbeck S, Emil S, et al. Renal vein thrombosis: a 10-year review. *J Pediatr Surg.* 2000;35(11):1540–1542.

236. Amigo MC, Garcia-Torres R. Morphology of vascular, renal, and heart lesions in the antiphospholipid syndrome: relationship to pathogenesis. *Curr Rheumatol Rep.* 2000; 2(3):262–270.

237. Louis CU, Morgenstern BZ, Butani L. Thrombotic complications in childhood-onset idiopathic membranous nephropathy. *Pediatr Nephrol.* 2003;18(12):1298–1300.

238. Stella N, Rolli A, Catalano A, et al. [Simultaneous urokinase perfusion in renal artery and vein in a case of renal vein thrombosis.] *Minerva Cardioangiol.* 2001;49(4):273–278.

239. Laissy JP, Menegazzo D, Debray MP, et al. Renal carcinoma: diagnosis of venous invasion with Gd-enhanced MR venography. *Eur Radiol.* 2000;10(7):1138–1143.

240. Berkovich GY, Ramchandani P, Preate DL Jr, et al. Renal vein thrombosis after martial arts trauma. *J Trauma.* 2001;50(1):144–145.

241. Akpolat T, Akkoyunlu M, Akpolat I, et al. Renal Behçet's disease: a cumulative analysis. *Semin Arthritis Rheum.* 2002;31(5):317–337.

242. Giustacchini P, Pisanti F, Citterio F, et al. Renal vein thrombosis after renal transplantation: an important cause of graft loss. *Transplant Proc.* 2002;34(6):2126–2127.

243. Manavis Alexiadis G, Deftereos S, et al. Testicular tumors manifested as inferior vena cava thromboses. Case reports. *Acta Radiol.* 2003;44(1).24–27.

244. Bissada NK, Yakout HH, Babanouri A, et al. Long-term experience with management of renal cell carcinoma involving the inferior vena cava. *Urology.* 2003;61(1): 89–92.

245. Kaplan S, Ekici S, Dogan R, et al. Surgical management of renal cell carcinoma with inferior vena cava tumor thrombus. *Am J Surg.* 2002;183(3):292–299.

246. Bower TC, Cherry KJ Jr, Toomey BJ, et al. Replacement of the inferior vena cava for malignancy: an update. *J Vasc Surg.* 2000;31(2):270–281.

247. Okuda K. Inferior vena cava thrombosis at its hepatic portion (obliterative hepatocavopathy). *Semin Liver Dis.* 2002;22(1):15–26.

248. Kazmers A, Groehn H, Meeker C. Duplex examination of the inferior vena cava. *Am Surg.* 2000;66(10):986–989.

249. Razavi MK, Hansch EC, Kee ST, et al. Chronically occluded inferior venae cavae: endovascular treatment. *Radiology.* 2000;214(1):133–138.

250. Chen CH, Sheu JC, Huang GT, et al. Recurrent hepatocellular carcinoma presenting with superior vena cava syndrome. *Hepatogastroenterology.* 2000;47(34):1117–1119.

251. Salonvaara M, Riikonen P, Kokomäki R, et al. Clinically symptomatic central venous catheter-related deep venous thrombosis in newborns. *Acta Paediatr.* 1999;88(6): 642–646.

252. Fernandez Vazquez E, Ortega Antelo M, Merlos Navarro S, et al. [Superior vena cava syndrome secondary to intracavitary implantation of a pacemaker.] *Arch Bronconeumol.* 2002;38(7):336–338.

253. Madan AK, Allmon JC, Harding M, et al. Dialysis access-induced superior vena cava syndrome. *Am Surg.* 2002; 68(10):904–906.

254. Kee ST, Kinoshita L, Razavi MK. Superior vena cava syndrome: treatment with catheter-directed thrombolysis and endovascular stent placement. *Radiology.* 1998;206(1): 187–193.

255. Sharafuddin MJ, Sun S, Hoballa JJ. Endovascular management of venous thrombotic diseases of the upper torso and extremities. *J Vasc Interv Radiol.* 2002;13(10):975–990.

256. Bousser MG, Chiras J, Bories J, et al. Cerebral venous thrombosis—a review of 38 cases. *Stroke.* 1985;16(2): 199–213.

257. Gosk-Bierska I, Wysokinski WE, Brown RD, et al. Cerebral venous sinus thrombosis. Incidence of venous thrombosis recurrence and survival. *Neurology.* 2006;67 (5):814–819.

258. Bousser MG. Cerebral venous thrombosis: nothing, heparin, or local thrombolysis? *Stroke.* 1999;30(3):481–483.

259. Fink JN, McAuley DL. Cerebral venous sinus thrombosis: a diagnostic challenge. *Intern Med J.* 2001;31(7):384–390.

260. Wasay M, Bakshi R, Bobustuc G, et al. Diffusion-weighted magnetic resonance imaging in superior sagittal sinus thrombosis. *J Neuroimaging.* 2002;12(3):267–269.

261. Gaudino S, Vadala R, Valenti V, et al. Combined diagnostic and therapeutic imaging in the diagnosis of venous sinus thrombosis in postpartum patients. *Rays.* 2003;28(2): 147–156.

262. Connor SE, Jarosz JM. Magnetic resonance imaging of cerebral venous sinus thrombosis. *Clin Radiol.* 2002;57(6): 449–461.

263. Klingebiel R, Busch M, Bohner G, et al. Multi-slice CT angiography in the evaluation of patients with acute cerebrovascular disease—a promising new diagnostic tool. *J Neurol.* 2002;249(1):43–49.

264. de Bruijn SF, Stam J. Randomized, placebo-controlled trial of anticoagulant treatment with low-molecular-weight heparin for cerebral sinus thrombosis. *Stroke.* 1999;30(3): 484–488.

265. Stam J, De Bruijn SF, DeVeber G. Anticoagulation for cerebral sinus thrombosis. *Cochrane Database Syst Rev.* 2002(4):CD002005.

266. Bousser MG. Cerebral venous thrombosis: diagnosis and management. *J Neurol.* 2000;247(4):252–258.

267. Frey JL, Muro GJ, McDougall CG, et al. Cerebral venous thrombosis: combined intrathrombus rtPA and intravenous heparin. *Stroke*. 1999;30(3):489–494.

268. de Bruijn SF, Budde M, Teunisse S, de Haan RJ, et al. Long-term outcome of cognition and functional health after cerebral venous sinus thrombosis. *Neurology*. 2000;54(8):1687–1689.

269. Preter M, Tzourio C, Ameri A, et al. Long-term prognosis in cerebral venous thrombosis. Follow-up of 77 patients. *Stroke*. 1996;27(2):243–246.

270. Horlander KT, Mannino DM, Leeper KV. Pulmonary embolism mortality in the United States, 1979–1998: an analysis using multiple-cause mortality data. *Arch Intern Med*. 2003;163(14):1711–1717.

271. Morpurgo M, Schmid C. The spectrum of pulmonary embolism. Clinicopathologic correlations. *Chest*. 1995;107[Suppl 1]:18S–20S.

272. Turkstra F, Kuijer PM, van Beek EJ, et al. Diagnostic utility of ultrasonography of leg veins in patients suspected of having pulmonary embolism. *Ann Intern Med*. 1997;126(10):775–781.

273. Moser KM, Fedullo PF, LittleJohn JK, et al. Frequent asymptomatic pulmonary embolism in patients with deep venous thrombosis. *JAMA*. 1994;271(3):223–225.

274. Sasahara AA, Sharma GVRK, McIntyre KM. Pulmonary embolism. In: Young JR, Olin JW, Bartholomew JR, eds. *Peripheral Vascular Diseases*. St. Louis: Mosby-Year Book; 1996:468–490.

275. Stein PD, Henry JW. Prevalence of acute pulmonary embolism among patients in a general hospital and at autopsy. *Chest*. 1995;108(4):978–981.

276. Kruip MJ, Leclercq MG, van der Heul C, et al. Diagnostic strategies for excluding pulmonary embolism in clinical outcome studies. A systematic review. *Ann Intern Med*. 2003;138(12):941–951.

277. Frost SD, Brotman DJ, Michota FA. Rational use of D-dimer measurement to exclude acute venous thromboembolic disease. *Mayo Clin Proc*. 2003;78(11):1385–1391.

278. Eichinger S, Minar E, Biolonczyk C, et al. D-dimer levels and risk of recurrent venous thromboembolism. *JAMA*. 2003;290(8):1071–1074.

279. Brotman DJ, Segal JB, Jani JT, et al. Limitations of D-dimer testing in unselected inpatients with suspected venous thromboembolism. *Am J Med*. 2003;114(4):276–282.

280. Greco F, Zanolini A, Bova C, et al. [Combined diagnostic approach to venous thromboembolism with multidetector computed tomography.] *Ital Heart J*. 2003;4(3)(suppl): 226–231.

281. Kelly J, Hunt BJ, Moody A. Magnetic resonance direct thrombus imaging: a novel technique for imaging venous thromboemboli. *Thromb Haemost*. 2003;89(5):773–782.

282. Goldhaber SZ. Thrombolysis in pulmonary embolism: a debatable indication. *Thromb Haemost*. 2001;86(1):444–451.

283. De Gregorio MA, Gimeno MJ, Mainar A, et al. Mechanical and enzymatic thrombolysis for massive pulmonary embolism. *J Vasc Interv Radiol*. 2002;13(2 Pt 1):163–169.

284. Dalen JE. Pulmonary embolism: what have we learned since Virchow?: treatment and prevention. *Chest*. 2002;122(5):1801–1817.

285. Dalen JE. Thrombolytic therapy in patients with submassive pulmonary embolism. *N Engl J Med*. 2003;348(4):357–359; author reply 357–359.

286. Prandoni P, Simini P, Pagnan A. [Treatment guidelines of acute venous thromboembolism. Current status and future perspectives.] *Minerva Cardioangiol*. 2003;51(4):361–371.

287. Stratton MA, Anderson FA, Bussey HI, et al. Prevention of venous thromboembolism: adherence to the 1995 American College of Chest Physicians consensus guidelines for surgical patients. *Arch Intern Med*. 2000;160(3): 334–340.

288. Goldhaber SZ, Dunn K, MacDougall RC. New onset of venous thromboembolism among hospitalized patients at Brigham and Women's Hospital is caused more often by

prophylaxis failure than by withholding treatment. *Chest*. 2000;118(6):1680–1684.

289. Cambria RP, Abbott WM. Acute arterial thrombosis of the lower extremity. Its natural history contrasted with arterial embolism. *Arch Surg*. 1984;119(7):784–787.

290. Pentti J, Salenius JP, Kuukasjarvi P, et al. Outcome of surgical treatment in acute upper limb ischaemia. *Ann Chir Gynaecol*. 1995;84(1):25–28.

291. Illuminati G, Bertagni A, Calio FG, et al. [Acute ischemia of the lower limbs.] *Riv Eur Sci Med Farmacol*. 1996; 18(1):19–27.

292. Becquemin JP, Kovarsky S. Arterial emboli of the lower limbs: analysis of risk factors for mortality and amputation. Association Universitaire de Recherche en Chirurgie. *Ann Vasc Surg*. 1995;9(suppl):S32–S38.

293. Pereira Barretto AC, Nobre MR, Mansur AJ, et al. Peripheral arterial embolism. Report of hospitalized cases. *Arq Bras Cardiol*. 2000;74(4):324–328.

294. Reber PU, Patel AG, Stauffer E, et al. Mural aortic thrombi: an important cause of peripheral embolization. *J Vasc Surg*. 1999;30(6):1084–1089.

295. Matchar DB, McCrory DC, Barnett HJM, et al. Medical treatment for stroke prevention. *Ann Intern Med*. 1994;121(1):41–53.

296. Aronow WS, Ahn C, Kronzon I et al. Risk factors for new thromboembolic stroke in patients > or = 62 years of age with chronic atrial fibrillation. *Am J Cardiol*. 1998; 82(1):119–121.

297. Go AS, Hylek EM, Chang Y, et al. Anticoagulation therapy for stroke prevention in atrial fibrillation: how well do randomized trials translate into clinical practice? *JAMA*. 2003;290(20):2685–2692.

298. Risk factors for stroke and efficacy of antithrombotic therapy in atrial fibrillation. Analysis of pooled data from five randomized controlled trials. *Arch Intern Med*. 1994;154(13):1449–1457.

299. Hart RG, Halperin JL, Pearce LA, et al. Lessons from the Stroke Prevention in Atrial Fibrillation trials. *Ann Intern Med*. 2003;138(10):831–838.

300. Davidovic LB, Kostic DM, Jakovljevic NS, et al. Vascular thoracic outlet syndrome. *World J Surg*. 2003;27(5): 545–550.

301. Christenson JT, Al-Huneidi W, Saleh RA. Distal embolisation from the surface of PTFE grafts in vivo and the effect of low molecular weight dextran. *Eur J Vasc Surg*. 1988;2(2): 121–125.

302. Valji K, Hye RJ, Roberts AC, et al. Hand ischemia in patients with hemodialysis access grafts: angiographic diagnosis and treatment. *Radiology*. 1995;196(3):697–701.

303. AbuRahma AF, Wulu JT Jr, Crotty B. Carotid plaque ultrasonic heterogeneity and severity of stenosis. *Stroke*. 2002;33(7):1772–1775.

304. Norris JW, Zhu CZ. Silent stroke and carotid stenosis. *Stroke*. 1992;23(4):483–485.

305. Morgenstern LB, Fox AJ, Sharpe BL, et al. The risks and benefits of carotid endarterectomy in patients with near occlusion of the carotid artery. North American Symptomatic Carotid Endarterectomy Trial (NASCET) Group. *Neurology*. 1997;48(4):911–915.

306. Norris JW, Zhu CZ, Bornstein NM, et al. Vascular risks of asymptomatic carotid stenosis. *Stroke*. 1991;22(12): 1485–1490.

307. Nadareishvili ZG, Rothwell PM, Beletsky V, et al. Long-term risk of stroke and other vascular events in patients with asymptomatic carotid artery stenosis. *Arch Neurol*. 2002;59(7):1162–1166.

308. Goertler M, Blaer T, Krueger S, et al. Acetylsalicylic acid and microembolic events detected by transcranial Doppler in symptomatic arterial stenoses. *Cerebrovasc Dis*. 2001;11(4):324–329.

309. De Fabritiis A, Conti E, Coccheri S. Management of patients with carotid stenosis. *Pathophysiol Haemost Thromb*. 2002;32(5–6):381–385.

310. Rauch U, Osende JI, Fuster V, et al. Thrombus formation on atherosclerotic plaques: pathogenesis and clinical consequences. *Ann Intern Med*. 2001;134(3):224–238.

311. Gouny P, Bertrand P, Duedal V, et al. Limb salvage and popliteal aneurysms: advantages of preventive surgery. *Eur J Vasc Endovasc Surg*. 2000;19(5):496–500.

312. Ring DH Jr, Haines GA, Miller DL. Popliteal artery entrapment syndrome: arteriographic findings and thrombolytic therapy. *J Vasc Interv Radiol*. 1999;10(6):713–721.

313. Samson RH, Willis PD. Popliteal artery occlusion caused by cystic adventitial disease: successful treatment by urokinase followed by nonresectional cystotomy. *J Vasc Surg*. 1990; 12(5):591–593.

314. Kwolek CJ, Matthews MR, Hartford JM, et al. Endovascular repair of external iliac artery occlusion after hip prosthesis migration. *J Endovasc Ther*. 2003;10(3):668–671.

315. Wong GB, Whetzel TP. Hypothenar hammer syndrome—review and case report. *Vasc Surg*. 2001;35(2):163–166.

316. Wolosker N, Nakano L, Morales Anacleto MM, et al. Primary utilization of stents in angioplasty of superficial femoral artery. *Vasc Endovascular Surg*. 2003;37(4):271–277.

317. Dougherty MJ, Young LP, Calligaro KD. One hundred twenty-five concomitant endovascular and open procedures for lower extremity arterial disease. *J Vasc Surg*. 2003;37(2):316–322.

318. Ferreira AC, Eton D, de Marchena E. Late clinical presentation of femoral artery occlusion after deployment of the angio-seal closure device. *J Invasive Cardiol*. 2002;14(11): 689–691.

319. Kitchens C, Jordan W, Wirthlin D, et al. Vascular complications arising from maldeployed stents. *Vasc Endovascular Surg*. 2002;36(2):145–154.

320. Wu RW, Hsu CC, Wang CJ. Acute popliteal artery occlusion after arthroscopic posterior cruciate ligament reconstruction. *Arthroscopy*. 2003;19(8):889–893.

321. Wilson JS, Miranda A, Johnson BL, et al. Vascular injuries associated with elective orthopedic procedures. *Ann Vasc Surg*. 2003;17(6):641–644.

322. Nanas JN, Gougoulakis A, Kanakais J. Acute coronary and peripheral arterial thrombosis following percutaneous coronary intervention in a patient with previously undiagnosed inherited thrombophilia. *Can J Cardiol*. 2003;19(9): 1063–1065.

323. Kottke-Marchant K. Genetic polymorphisms associated with venous and arterial thrombosis: an overview. *Arch Pathol Lab Med*. 2002;126(3):295–304.

324. Harrington DJ, Malefora A, Schmeleva V, et al. Genetic variations observed in arterial and venous thromboembolism—relevance for therapy, risk prevention and prognosis. *Clin Chem Lab Med*. 2003;41(4):496–500.

325. Bohm G, Al-Khaffaf H. Thrombophilia and arterial disease. An up-to-date review of the literature for the vascular surgeon. *Int Angiol*. 2003;22(2):116–124.

326. Van Cott EM, Laposata M, Prins MH. Laboratory evaluation of hypercoagulability with venous or arterial thrombosis. *Arch Pathol Lab Med*. 2002;126(11):1281–1295.

327. Rigdon EE. Trousseau's syndrome and acute arterial thrombosis. *Cardiovasc Surg*. 2000;8(3):214–218.

328. Katz SG, Kohl RD. Spontaneous peripheral arterial microembolization. *Ann Vasc Surg*. 1992;6(4):334–337.

329. Nasser TK, Mohler ER, Wilensky RL, et al. Peripheral vascular complications following coronary interventional procedures. *Clin Cardiol*. 1995;18(11):609–614.

330. Theriault J, Agharazi M, Dumont M, et al. Atheroembolic renal failure requiring dialysis: potential for renal recovery? A review of 43 cases. *Nephron Clin Pract*. 2003;94(1):c11–c18.

331. Management of peripheral arterial disease (PAD). TransAtlantic Inter-Society Consensus (TASC). Section C: acute limb ischaemia. *Eur J Vasc Endovasc Surg*. 2000;19[Suppl A]: S115–S143.

332. Quigley FG, Faris IB, Duncan HJ. A comparison of Doppler ankle pressures and skin perfusion pressure in subjects with and without diabetes. *Clin Physiol*. 1991;11(1):21–25.

333. Eliason JL, Wainess RM, Proctor MC, et al. A national and single institutional experience in the contemporary treatment of acute lower extremity ischemia. *Ann Surg*. 2003;238(3):382–389; discussion 389–390.

334. Acosta S, Bjorck M. Acute thrombo-embolic occlusion of the superior mesenteric artery: a prospective study in a well defined population. *Eur J Vasc Endovasc Surg*. 2003;26(2):179–183.

335. Edwards MS, Cherr GS, Craven TE, et al. Acute occlusive mesenteric ischemia: surgical management and outcomes. *Ann Vasc Surg*. 2003;17(1):72–79.

336. Luther B, Moussazadeh K, Muller BT, et al. [The acute mesenteric ischemia—not understood or incurable?] *Zentralbl Chir*. 2002;127(8):674–684.

337. Kirkpatrick ID, Kroeker MA, Greenberg HM. Biphasic CT with mesenteric CT angiography in the evaluation of acute mesenteric ischemia: initial experience. *Radiology*. 2003;229(1):91–98.

338. Vosshenrich R, Fischer U. Contrast-enhanced MR angiography of abdominal vessels: is there still a role for angiography? *Eur Radiol*. 2002;12(1):218–230.

339. Chitwood RW, Ernst CB. Visceral ischemic syndromes. In: Young JR, Olin JW, Bartholomew JR, eds. *Peripheral Vascular Diseases*. St Louis: Mosby-Year Book; 305–320.

340. Calin GA, Calin S, Ionescu R, et al. Successful local fibrinolytic treatment and balloon angioplasty in superior mesenteric arterial embolism: a case report and literature review. *Hepatogastroenterology*. 2003;50(51): 732–734.

341. Savassi-Rocha PR, Veloso LF. Treatment of superior mesenteric artery embolism with a fibrinolytic agent: case report and literature review. *Hepatogastroenterology*. 2002;49(47):1307–1310.

342. Leary MC, Saver JL. Annual incidence of first silent stroke in the United States: a preliminary estimate. *Cerebrovasc Dis*. 2003;16(3):280–285.

343. MacKenzie JM. Are all cardio-embolic strokes embolic? An autopsy study of 100 consecutive acute ischaemic strokes. *Cerebrovasc Dis*. 2000;10(4):289–292.

344. Sherman DG, Dyken ML Jr, Gent M, et al. Antithrombotic therapy for cerebrovascular disorders. An update. *Chest*. 1995;108(4)(suppl):444S–456S.

345. Kahn MJ. Hypercoagulability as a cause of stroke in adults. *South Med J*. 2003;96(4):350–353.

346. Simioni P, De Ronde H, Prandoni P, et al. Ischemic stroke in young patients with activated protein C resistance. A report of three cases belonging to three different kindreds. *Stroke*. 1995;26(5):885–890.

347. Aronow WS. Extracranial carotid arterial disease. *Compr Ther*. 1994;20(3):192–197.

348. Caplan LR. Brain embolism, revisited. *Neurology*. 1993;43(7):1281–1287.

349. Schramm P, Schellinger PD, Fiebach JB, et al. Comparison of CT and CT angiography source images with diffusion-weighted imaging in patients with acute stroke within 6 hours after onset. *Stroke*. 2002;33(10):2426–2432.

350. Uno M, Harada M, Yoneda K, et al. Can diffusion- and perfusion-weighted magnetic resonance imaging evaluate the efficacy of acute thrombolysis in patients with internal carotid artery or middle cerebral artery occlusion? *Neurosurgery*. 2002;50(1):28–34; discussion 34–35.

351. Pillekamp F, Grune M, Brinker G, et al. Magnetic resonance prediction of outcome after thrombolytic treatment. *Magn Reson Imaging*. 2001;19(2):143–152.

352. Devuyst G, Bogousslavsky J. Recent progress in drug treatment for acute ischemic stroke. *Cerebrovasc Dis*. 2001; 11[Suppl 1]:71–79.

353. Coull BM, Williams LS, Goldstein LB, et al. Anticoagulants and antiplatelet agents in acute ischemic stroke: report of the Joint Stroke Guideline Development Committee of the American Academy of Neurology and the American Stroke Association (a division of the American Heart Association). *Stroke*. 2002;33(7):1934–1942.

Vasculitides and Connective Tissue Disorders

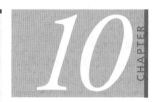

Andrzej Szuba
Izabela Gosk-Bierska
Richard L. Hallett

VASCULITIDES

The clinical and pathological features of vasculitis are variable and depend on the site and type of blood vessels that are affected. Diseases in which vasculitis is a primary process are called *primary systemic vasculitides*. Different classifications will be described, but the final description will be based on the Chapel Hill 1994 Consensus Conference classification. Vasculitis may also occur as a secondary feature in other diseases, such as systemic lupus erythematosus and rheumatoid arthritis (1,2).

Systemic vasculitides form a heterogeneous group of vascular inflammatory diseases that can be subgrouped

TABLE 10-1

Classification of Vasculitides, Chapel Hill Consensus Conference, 1994

I. Affecting Predominantly Large Vessels
Giant cell arteritis/temporal arteritis
Takayasu arteritis
Isolated CNS vasculitis
Cogan's syndrome

II. Affecting Predominantly Medium Blood Vessels
Polyarteritis nodosa
Kawasaki disease

III. Affecting Predominantly Small Blood Vessels
Wegener's granulomatosis
Microscopic polyangiitis
Churg-Strauss syndrome
Henoch-Schönlein purpura (HSP)
Essential mixed cryoglobulinemia
Cutaneous leukocytoclastic angiitis
Behçet disease
Buerger's disease
Hypocomplementemic urticarial vasculitis
Degos' syndrome
Serum sickness

From Jennette JC, Falk RJ, Andrassy K, et al. Nomenclature of systemic vasculitides. Proposal of an international consensus conference. *Arthritis Rheum.* 1994;37(2):187–192. ©1994 Wiley-Liss, Inc. Reprinted with permission of Wiley-Liss, Inc., a subsidiary of John Wiley & Sons, Inc.

based on the underlying histopathology and the size of the vessels involved as well as the target organs involved. The resultant clinical picture is illustrated in Table 10-1 (3).

LARGE VESSELS VASCULITIS

Takayasu Arteritis

Takayasu arteritis (TA), also known as pulseless disease, occlusive thromboaortopathy, and Martorell syndrome is a chronic inflammatory arteritis affecting large vessels (4). It is typically characterized by granulomatous inflammation of the aorta and its major branches, usually occurring in patients younger than 50 years of age. Vessel inflammation leads to wall thickening, fibrosis, stenosis, thrombus formation, and visceral ischemia. Acute inflammation can destroy the arterial media and can lead to aneurysm formation (5).

TA is most commonly seen in Japan, Southeast Asia, India, and South America. In a Japanese population autopsy study, evidences of TA were found in 0.033% of all individuals. Female-to-male ratio was 4.5:1 (6). A study of North American patients by Hall et al. found the incidence to be 2.6 per million per year (7).

Pathogenesis of TA is unknown. Infectious factors including viruses and Mycobacterium are proposed to play a role (5,8,9).

Clinical Manifestation

Manifestations range from asymptomatic disease to catastrophic vascular and neurological complications. TA is usually diagnosed in the second or third decade of life; however, it can occur even in young children. In a large published cohort (n = 107), 80% of patients were between 11 and 30 years, 77% had disease onset between the ages of 10 and 20 years, with time from onset of symptoms to diagnosis of 2 to 11 years in 78% (8). The clinical features of TA in young patients appear to be similar to those of adults (10).

Diagnostic criteria for TA developed by American College of Radiology (ACR) require that at least three of the six criteria are met (11):

1. Development of symptoms or findings related to TA at age <40 years.
2. Claudication of extremity: development and worsening of fatigue and discomfort in muscles of one or more extremity while in use, especially the upper extremities.
3. Decreased pulsation of one or both brachial arteries.
4. Difference of >10 mmHg in systolic blood pressure between arms.
5. Bruit audible on auscultation over one or both subclavian arteries or abdominal aorta.
6. Arteriographic narrowing or occlusion of the entire aorta, its primary branches, or large arteries in the proximal upper or lower extremities not caused by arteriosclerosis, fibromuscular dysplasia (FMD), or similar causes; changes usually focal or segmental.

It should be remembered that sensitivity and specificity of ACR (as well as other) criteria to detect TA and other vasculitides varies (71.0% to 95.3% for sensitivity and 78.7% to 99.7% for specificity) in published studies (12,13) and should be used with caution when applied to an individual patient.

Characteristic clinical features of TA (present in over 80% of patients) include:

- Diminished or absent pulse, limb claudication, and/or blood pressure discrepancies
- Vascular bruits, particularly in carotid, subclavian, and abdominal vessels

Symptoms occurring less frequently are hypertension, aortic root dilatation with aortic regurgitation, chronic heart failure, neurological symptoms (dizziness, visual disturbances, cerebrovascular accident), pulmonary artery involvement, abdominal angina, and myocardial ischemia. Carotidynia and erythema nodosum may occur. Systemic symptoms associated with TA include fever, dyspnea, night sweats, weight loss, arthralgias, and myalgia (7,8,14–19).

It should be noted that significant differences in clinical patterns of TA exist between different populations. Aortic root involvement with aortic regurgitation is the most common presentation of TA in the Japanese population, while involvement of abdominal aorta and renal arteries is most frequently found in Indian patients (17).

Diagnosis and Differential Diagnosis

Various sets of criteria may assist in diagnosis of TA. Adequate vascular imaging studies are necessary for assessment of vascular anatomy. Conventional angiography of the aorta and other large arteries has been the gold standard in diagnosis of TA. However, it is being rapidly replaced by computed tomographic (CT) and magnetic resonance (MR) angiography, techniques that are less invasive and allow detailed visualization of arterial anatomy in conjunction with characterization of the arterial wall (20) (Table 10-2) (Figs. 10-1–10-3). Assessment of arterial wall thickness and inflammatory process can help with diagnosis, monitoring of disease activity, and response to therapy (21,22). The

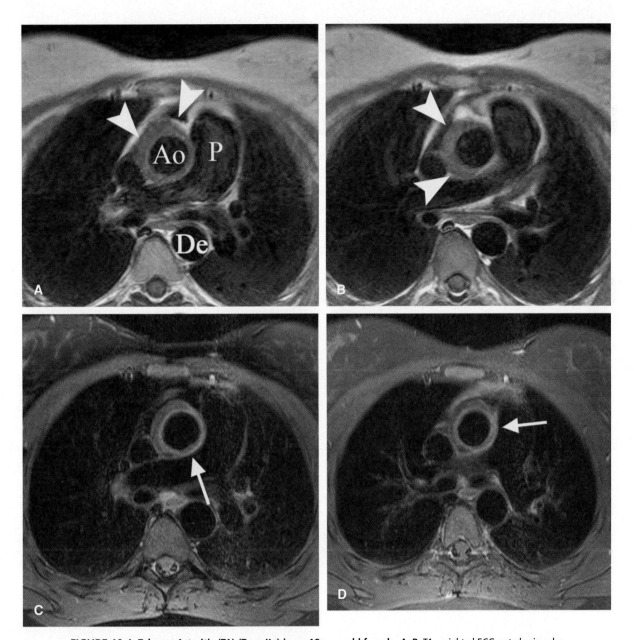

FIGURE 10-1 **Takaysu Arteritis (TA) (Type IIa) in an 18-year-old female. A, B:** T1-weighted ECG-gated spin echo images show circumferential mural thickening (*arrowheads*) involving the ascending thoracic aorta (*Ao*). Descending aorta (*De*) is not involved. (P, main pulmonary artery.) **C, D:** T1-weighted fat-suppressed postgadolinium images at similar levels to (**A, B**) demonstrate ringlike enhancement of portions of the mural thickening (*arrows*). The presence of mural enhancement is thought to correlate with clinically active disease. (*Figure 10-1 continues*)

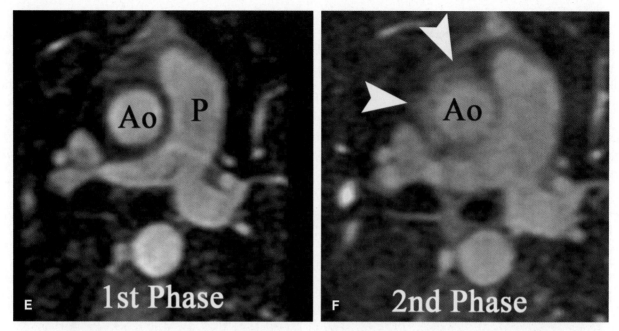

FIGURE 10-1 Continued E, F: Axial multiplanar reconstruction (MPR) images from MR angiography (MRA) study in the initial arterial (**E**) and second equilibrium (**F**) phases in same patient. Note the brisk wall enhancement again noted in the ascending thoracic aorta (*Ao*) on the equilibrium phase (*arrowheads*). This is analogous to the enhancement seen in (**C, D**) and is reflective of clinically active disease site. (P, pulmonary artery.) (Courtesy of Richard L. Hallett, M.D., and Geoffrey D. Rubin, M.D.)

latter, however, needs to be further assessed. As the disease progresses, arterial wall inflammation is replaced by arterial strictures and occlusions (Fig. 10-4).

Doppler ultrasound is a useful noninvasive procedure for the assessment of vascular anatomy and vessel wall inflammation. Histopathological changes are characteristic for TA; however, the specimens are obtained usually during surgery.

Laboratory Evaluation

No biochemical marker specific to TA exists; neither is there a good surrogate marker of disease activity. Erythrocyte sedimentation rate (ESR) and C-reactive protein (CRP) were proposed but proved to correlate poorly with disease activity

TABLE 10-2

Angiographic Classification of Takayasu Arteritis, Takayasu Conference 1994

Type	Vessel Involvement
Type I	Branches from the aortic arch
Type IIa	Ascending aorta, aortic arch and its branches
Type IIb	Ascending aorta, aortic arch and its branches, thoracic descending aorta
Type III	Thoracic descending aorta and/or renal arteries
Type IV	Abdominal aorta and/or renal arteries
Type V	Combined features of types IIb and IV

Note: According to this classification system, involvement of the coronary or pulmonary arteries should be designated as C (+) or P (+).

From Moriwaki R, Noda M, Yajima M, et al., Clinical manifestations of Takayasu arteritis in India and Japan—new classification of angiographic findings. *Angiology.* 1997;48(5):369–379.

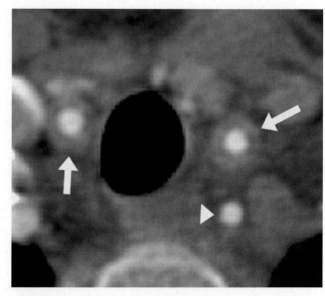

FIGURE 10-2 A 25-year-old woman with TA demonstrates marked wall thickening in the common carotid arteries bilaterally (*arrows*) without narrowing of the lumina. In contrast, the wall of the left vertebral artery (*arrowhead*) is normal. (Courtesy of Richard L. Hallett, M.D., and Geoffrey D. Rubin, M.D.)

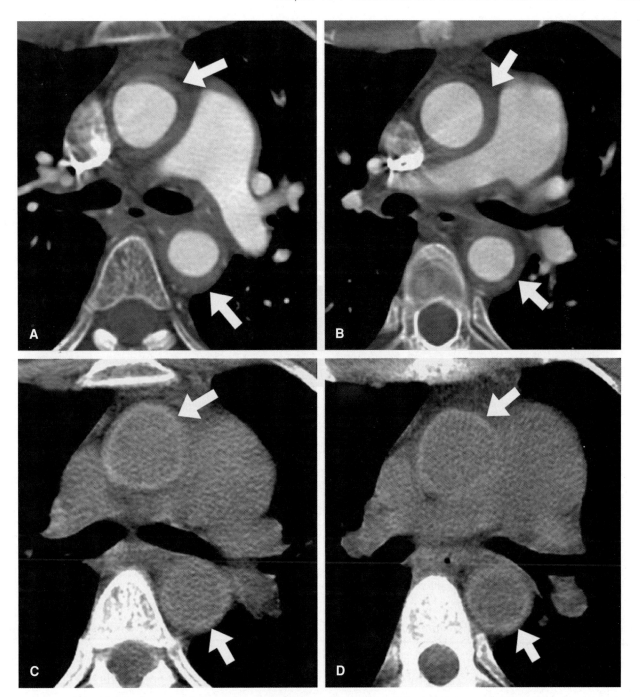

FIGURE 10-3 Mural hemorrhage from active TA. Transverse CT sections following administration of intravenous iodinated contrast material **(A, B)** demonstrates 5–7 mm wall thickening about the ascending and descending aorta. The luminal dimensions of the aorta are normal. Unenhanced CT sections **(C, D)** obtained prior to the administration of iodinated contrast material at the same levels as **(A)** and **(B)**, respectively, demonstrate high attenuation within the wall of the ascending and descending aorta (*arrows*). This finding is suggestive of hemorrhage in the aortic wall secondary to the active inflammatory process of the TA. (Courtesy of Geoffrey D. Rubin, M.D.)

(23–25). More recently, IL-6 and RANTES (26) and plasma matrix metalloproteinases (27) have been proposed as surrogate markers for TA activity.

Histopathology

In the acute phase: vasoritis in adventitia, infiltration by lymphocytes and giant cells with neovascularization in the media, smooth muscle cells, mucopolysaccharides, fibroblasts, and thickening of the intima. In the chronic phase: fibrosis with destruction of elastic tissue is seen.

The differential diagnoses include inflammatory aortitis (syphilis, tuberculosis, Cogan's syndrome [CS], rheumatoid arthritis, giant cell arteritis [GCA], Behçet disease [BD], Kawasaki disease [KD]), coarctation of the aorta,

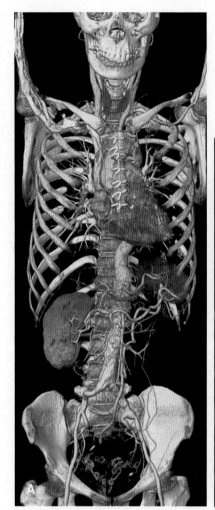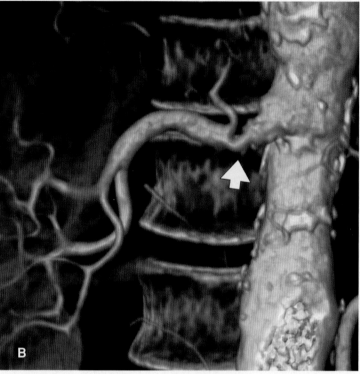

FIGURE 10-4 A 36-year-old woman with Takayasu Arteritis (TA) in advanced stage. The imaging findings of active inflammation and wall thickening have been replaced with multiple regions of arterial stricture and occlusion. **A:** A single 15-second MDCT scan acquired with 16 × 1.25 mm section thickness allows all relevant arterial territory (carotid through femoral arteries) to be evaluated. **B:** A focal 50% stenosis is present in the proximal right renal artery (*arrow*) and is demonstrated with volume rendering. (*Figure10-4 continues*)

Ehlers-Danlos syndrome, Marfan syndrome (MFS), FMD, and neurofibromatosis.

Treatment

Some patients (about 20%) do not require therapy because of a mild, self-limiting course of the disease. Active disease should be treated with steroids (prednisone 1 mg/kg/d), and in 50% of patients it will result in remission. Cyclophosphamid and/or methotrexate should be added if steroids alone do not control disease. This may result in remission in an additional 40% of steroid-resistant patients (24). Hypertension is frequently observed in TA patients. Treatment of hypertension is critical to prevent cardiovascular complications. However, the diagnosis of hypertension in TA may be delayed in patients with subclavian artery stenosis (24). Surgery or angioplasty may be required for treatment of stenoses once active inflammation has been controlled (28).

Giant Cell Arteritis (Temporal Arteritis)

GCA (temporal arteritis, Horton's disease, Horton's giant cell arteritis, giant cell arteritis of elderly) is a granulomatous arteritis of large vessels frequently affecting the temporal artery.

Etiology of GCA is unknown; association with HLA-DR4 and HLA-DRB1 has been reported (29,30). GCA is the most common type of primary systemic vasculitis with an incidence of 200 per million population per year. It usually occurs in patients older than 50 years and is prevalent in women. Sixty-five percent of GCA patients are women >70 years old. Caucasian patients seem to be affected more frequently than Asian and Hispanic patients (31–33).

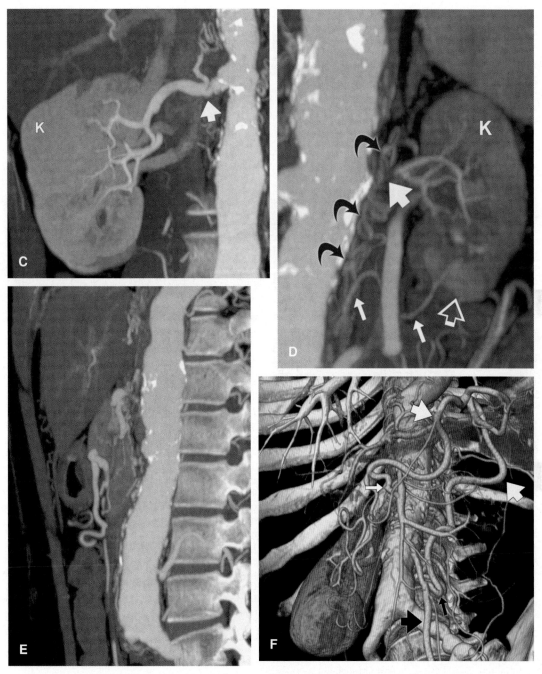

FIGURE 10-4 Continued C: Although on this maximum intensity projection a slight variation in obliquity partially obscures the stenosis (*arrow*), the renal parenchyma is demonstrated to be of normal size and enhancement (*K*). **D:** The left main renal artery (*large arrow*) is completely occluded. The kidney parenchyma (*K*) is poorly enhancing, and the kidney is substantially atrophied compared to the right, measuring 6 cm longitudinally. A blush of greater parenchymal opacification in the lower pole (*open arrow*) indicates slightly better perfusion to this small renal segment supplied by an accessory renal artery (*small white arrows*). Although the origins of the accessory renal artery and the main renal artery are not patent, numerous tortuous retroperitoneal collaterals (*curved black arrows*) provide some blood flow to the kidney, preventing complete infarction. **E:** Lateral maximum intensity projection through the entire width of the aorta demonstrates that the celiac, superior mesenteric, and inferior mesenteric arteries are all occluded at their origins. No branches are observed to originate from the anterior surface of the abdominal aorta, which is mildly aneurysmal. **F:** This patient did not suffer from symptoms of mesenteric ischemia despite the occluded mesenteric arterial branch origins. This volume rendering demonstrates a large meandering artery (*large white arrows*) connecting the superior mesenteric artery and the inferior mesenteric artery (*large black arrow*) via the middle colic artery (*small white arrow*) and the left colic artery (*small black arrow*). Although flow directionality cannot be directly observed, retrograde flow within the inferior mesenteric artery and the meandering artery to perfuse the superior mesenteric artery can be inferred by the pattern of arterial occlusions. (*Figure10-4 continues*)

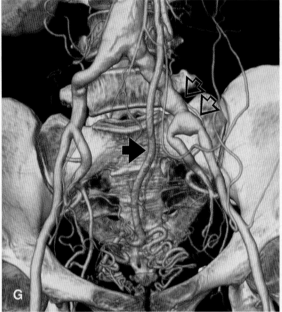
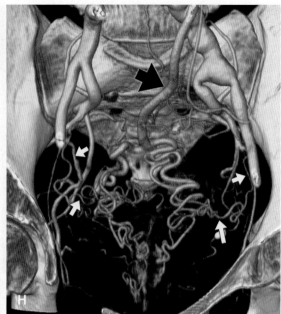
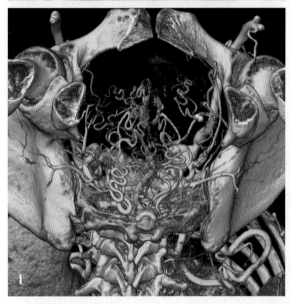

FIGURE 10-4 Continued G: Within the pelvis, the large inferior mesenteric artery (*black arrow*) is seen overlying the sacrum and terminating in numerous serpentine vessels deep within the pelvis. Aneurysms within the left common iliac artery are also observed (*open arrows*). **H:** Anteriorly angulated view through the pelvic inlet demonstrates the termination of the inferior mesenteric artery (*large black arrow*) into paired serpentine superior hemorrhoidal arteries. Direct communication between branches of the internal iliac arteries and the superior hemorrhoidal branches are demonstrated (*small white arrows*). This collateral pathway from the internal iliac arteries to the superior hemorrhoidal arteries is the key pathway for blood to reach the small and large bowel. **I:** The flexibility of volumetric CT data allows depiction of these complex arterial pathways from a variety of perspectives, including this pelvic outlet view. (Courtesy of Geoffrey D. Rubin, M.D.)

GCA is a granulomatous arteritis of the aorta (Fig. 10-5) and its major branches, especially extracranial branches of the carotid artery. Extracranial artery involvement is present in 15% of GCA patients (34). In a review of 75 patients with extracranial GCA, 25% had asymptomatic temporal arteritis. GCA of the ascending aorta and arch occurred in 39%, the subclavian and axillary artery in 26%, and the femoropopliteal artery in 18% of those patients (34). The risk of development of a thoracic aortic aneurysm is 17 times higher in GCA patients (35). Some authors suggest, however, that GCA of the cranial arteries (classic temporal arteritis) and GCA affecting the subclavian/axillary/brachial arteries are two separate pathological entities (36). Rarely, GCA may present as a breast, ovarian, or other type of tumor (37).

Major clinical signs and symptoms are (33,38–40):

- Persistent headache (often unilateral) associated with fever, myalgias, weight loss
- Temporal artery changes: swollen and tender to palpation, pulseless
- Ischemic manifestations: necrosis of the tongue, multiple cranial nerve palsies, dysphagia, hearing loss, and ischemic stroke
- Visual manifestations: partial or complete visual loss may be sudden and painless, diplopia may also occur
- Jaw claudication
- Frequent association with polymyalgia rheumatica (40% to 62%)

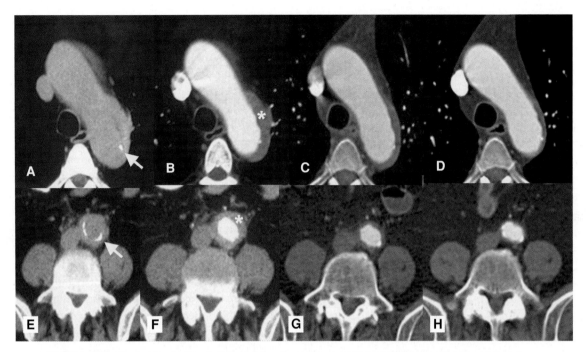

FIGURE 10-5 Giant cell arteritis. A, B: Pre- and postcontrast axial CT images before treatment depict irregular wall thickening (*asterisk* in **B**) with tiny calcifications (*arrow* in **A**) involving the posterior aspect of the aortic arch. **C, D:** Images obtained following treatment for 2 and 5 months, respectively, show significant and progressive regression of the abnormal findings. **E, F:** Pre- and postcontrast axial CT images reveal similar involvement of the distal abdominal aorta. **G, H:** Regression of these findings is progressively observed in the follow-up examinations after treatment for 2 and 5 months, similar to that observed in the thoracic aorta.

Diagnosis is made on characteristic clinical presentation and markedly elevated ESR (>50, frequently >100). In doubtful cases, biopsy of the temporal artery is the gold standard to confirm the diagnosis of GCA. Arterial biopsy reveals granulomatous inflammatory reaction with destruction and calcification of internal elastic lamina, cellular infiltrates of lymphocytes, macrophages, and giant cells. Areas of fibrosis and neovascularization might be also present (41). Temporal artery biopsy is frequently negative in GCA involving the subclavian/axillary/brachial artery (36). Vascular imaging studies (CT, MR, or catheter angiography) should be performed in patients with visual disturbance, limb claudication, suspected involvement of aorta, or other large arteries (42).

Treatment with corticosteroids (prednisone 60 mg to 80 mg/d) should be started as soon as the diagnosis is suspected to avoid visual loss (43). After 6 weeks, the prednisone dose may be slowly tapered to a minimal maintenance dose of 5 to 10 mg/d. Mean duration of therapy is 1 to 2 years; however, some patients require 4 to 6 years of treatment (24). GCA arterial aneurysms may require surgery (44).

Cogan's Syndrome

CS (45) is a rare disorder of children and young people of unknown etiology. Autoimmune mechanisms are suspected. It is characterized by inflammatory eye disease (interstitial keratitis, uveitis, scleritis, optic neuritis) and audiovestibular symptoms resembling Meniere's attacks. CS is associated with vasculitis and aortitis. The onset is usually rapid with ocular symptoms followed within a year by tinnitus, vertigo, nausea and vomiting, and hearing loss. The majority of untreated patients will become deaf, and 5% will become blind (46). Systemic manifestations may be present in half of the patients and include fever, musculoskeletal pains, fatigue, and weight loss. Splenomegaly and lymphadenopathy might also be detected. Aortitis with aortic insufficiency develops in 10% to 15% of patients. Aneurysms of the thoracic and abdominal aorta are also reported. Other vessels including the coronary, renal, extremity, and cerebrovascular arteries may be involved (46–51).

Laboratory evaluation reveals elevated sedimentation rate, anemia, thrombocytosis, and leukocytosis (48). Histological findings in aortitis show involvement of intima and media with cellular infiltrates of neutrophils, mononuclear cells and giant cells, disruption of the internal elastic lamina, and scarring (52). Diagnosis can be suspected in patients with interstitial keratitis and audiovestibular symptoms after infectious etiology (syphilis) is ruled out.

Treatment includes systemic and topical steroids. Aortic valve replacement might be needed in patients with aortic insufficiency, and cochlear implants in patients with deafness.

Prognosis is good in patients without symptoms of aortitis. Early steroid therapy may prevent deafness (48,51,53).

Isolated Vasculitis of the Central Nervous System

Isolated vasculitis of the central nervous system (IVCNS) or primary angiitis of the CNS is a vascular inflammatory disease of the CNS involving mainly small and medium-sized leptomeningeal and parenchymal arteries. It is a rare disease that may present with a variety of neurological symptoms. Headache, focal neurological deficits, stroke, seizures, memory loss, personality changes, and loss of consciousness may appear. Patterns of progressive encephalopathy, space occupying lesions, or multiple sclerosis-like disease have been described (54).

Diagnosis is usually suspected after cerebrovascular angiography. Multifocal segmental or diffuse narrowing of arteries is seen; arterial dilatation and aneurysms are less common (55). Angiographic presentation is not specific for IVCNS and occasionally may be normal (56). MR and CT angiography can be helpful in visualization of vascular and parenchymal CNS changes (57,58).

Brain biopsy is usually necessary to confirm diagnosis of IVCNS (55,59). The histological picture is heterogeneous and may reveal granulomatous, necrotizing, or lymphocytic vasculitis often coexisting in the same patient. Vascular thrombosis may be present (55).

Aggressive immunosuppressive treatment with systemic steroids and cytotoxic agents improved the outcome of IVCNS (59).

MEDIUM VESSELS VASCULITIS

Inflammation affecting predominantly visceral arteries is classified as medium vessels vasculitis. This group includes two vasculitis syndromes: polyarteritis nodosa (PAN) and Kawasaki disease (KD).

Polyarteritis Nodosa

PAN (classic polyarteritis nodosa, periarteritis nodosa) is a rare systemic necrotizing vasculitis of medium and small arteries frequently associated with hepatitis B virus (HBV) infection (7% to 30% of patients have HBs antigen) (60). The majority of affected people are in the fourth to fifth decade of life; men are more frequently affected than women (M:F ratio is 2–3:1). Arterial inflammation leads to formation of aneurysms and thrombosis of affected arteries with ischemia or infarction of supplied organs and/or rupture of an aneurysm.

Etiology of PAN is unknown. Association with HBV infection can be documented only in a minority of patients (7%) (60); however, the rate of latent HBV infection may

be higher (61). Other viruses (cytomegalovirus, parvovirus B-19, human T-cell lymphotropic virus [HTLV-1], and hepatitis C virus [HCV]) are also occasionally implicated in PAN etiology (62–64).

Pathology

Arterial lesions affect segments of medium-sized arteries and frequently are localized at the branching points. Necrosis and inflammatory infiltrates of mononuclear cells are found in the adventitia and media with disruption of the internal elastic lamina. Weakened arterial walls lead to the formation of aneurysms. Intimal proliferation and arterial thrombosis may occur.

Laboratory Finding

Elevated ESR, white blood count, CRP, and normochromic anemia are seen frequently. HBs antigen is present in 7% to 30% (60). No specific laboratory test exists for PAN. Antinuclear cytoplasmic antibodies (ANCA) are usually not found (24,65).

Clinical Presentation

Constitutional symptoms include weakness, myalgias, arthralgias, fever, and weight loss frequently >4 kg. Symptomatology of PAN depends on presence and severity of organ involvement. Kidneys, gastrointestinal system, muscles, and the central and peripheral nervous system are often affected. Involvement of lungs is rare. Kidneys are affected in up to 60% of patients (Fig. 10-6) (cortical infarcts, renal vasculitis, rupture of renal artery aneurysm) (66,67)—glomerulonephritis is absent in PAN by definition. Neurological symptoms related to CNS disease are present in 10% to 25% of PAN patients (68). Cerebral artery occlusion may result in stroke, seizures, amaurosis, and cognitive impairment. Peripheral neurological involvement is present in up to 50% of patients and include polineuropathy, Guillain-Barré syndrome, and mononeuritis multiplex (24,69,70).

Gastrointestinal symptoms are present in more than half of patients. Symptoms are related to bowel ischemia (abdominal angina, ischemic colitis, acute abdomen due to intestinal necrosis and/or perforation) (71,72); occasionally, acute pancreatitis, appendicitis, or cholecystitis may develop (24,72,73).

Cardiovascular involvement is common and includes arterial aneurysms and stenoses/occlusions in peripheral arteries (74), including renal (67), cerebral (75), mesenteric (76), and coronary arteries (77,78). Congestive heart failure may develop. Involvement of the limb arteries is also frequent (74).

Musculoskeletal manifestations of PAN include polymyositis (in up to 40%) (79), arthralgia, and occasionally polyarthritis (24).

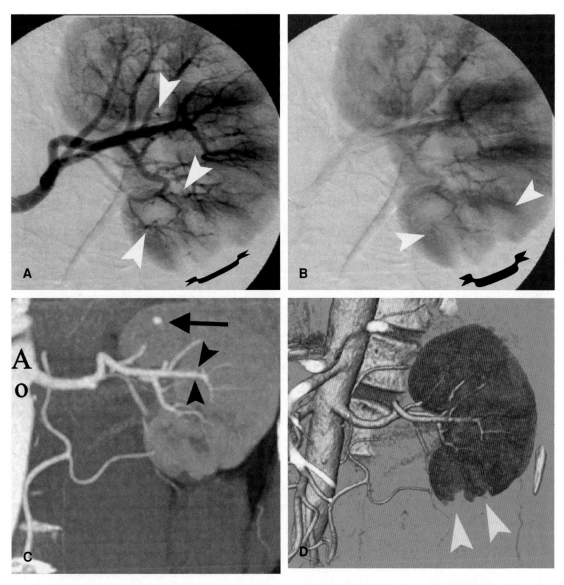

FIGURE 10-6 Polyarteritis nodosa. A: Arterial-phase image from digital subtraction angiography (DSA) of the left kidney shows focal areas of medium-vessel irregularity and tiny microaneurysms (*arrowheads*). Note a zone of hypoperfusion in the lower pole (*bracket*). **B:** Later-phase image from same DSA run shows again the hypoperfusion in the lower pole of the left kidney (*bracket*), in the area served by the diseased vessels (*arrowheads*). **C:** Coronal thick-slab maximum intensity projection (MIP) image from CT angiogram shows a microaneurysm (*arrow*) in the upper pole of the left kidney. The medium-vessel vasculitic changes seen on DSA are less well visualized on the CTA (*arrowheads*), as these vessels approach the spatial resolution limits of CTA. (Ao, aorta.) **D:** Volume-rendered image from CTA again corroborates the lack of perfusion in the lower pole (*arrowheads*).

Skin lesions are less frequent and include subcutaneous palpable purpura, painful inflammatory nodules, and livedo reticularis. Orchitis with testicular pain and tenderness may be found in 10% to 15% of male patients (24).

Diagnosis of PAN may be difficult because of the variety of clinical presentations and infrequent occurrence. It should be suspected in any case of unexplained systemic diseases with multiorgan involvement.

Biopsy of affected tissue can confirm the diagnosis. Biopsy of affected skin or muscles can document presence of necrotizing vasculitis. Sural nerve biopsy may reveal necrotizing vasculitis of epineural arteries in the presence of conduction abnormalities, even in the absence of clinical symptoms of neuropathy (24,80,81).

Angiography can help in the diagnosis of PAN. Evidence of multiple microaneurysms and arterial ectasia, especially in visceral arteries, is thought to be specific for PAN and is found in 40% to 75% of patients (67,74,82). The majority of PAN patients have evidence of arterial occlusions in visceral vessels (74).

Treatment

PAN therapy should be tailored to the severity of presentation. In milder cases (without renal, CNS or cardiac involvement), only steroids (prednisone 1 mg/kg/d) are recommended. Cyclophosphamide 500 to 1,000 mg intravenously (IV) once every 2 weeks (six rounds) should be added in more severe cases. The duration of therapy should last 12 months (83).

Treatment of PAN associated with HBV additionally requires an antiviral drug such as interferon or/and lamivudine in combination with plasmapheresis (84). Aggressive immunosuppression should be limited to life-threatening complications (85,86). Low-dose aspirin is recommended for thrombocytosis. Surgical intervention is necessary in acute abdominal catastrophies (e.g., bowel perforation or hemorrhage).

Prognosis depends on severity of presentation. Five-year mortality varies from 12% to 46%, depending on initial presentation and organ involvement (83).

Kawasaki Disease

KD (mucocutaneous lymph node syndrome) is an acute febrile illness of childhood first described by Kawasaki in 1967. KD affects children usually under the age of 12 years with the peak incidence in children 18 to 24 months old. In Japan, the incidence exceeds 100 to 150/100,000 children <5 years but is 4 to 15/100,000 in this age group in the United States (87).

Diagnosis

KD is an arteritis affecting large, medium, and small arteries and is associated with mucocutaneous lymph node syndrome. It is probably the most common vasculitis in children. Diagnosis is based on clinical criteria: at least 5 days of fever and four or five signs of mucocutaneous inflammation rather than angiographic findings or biopsy. Features of mucocutaneous lymph node syndrome include:

- Fever for >5 days
- Bilateral nonpurulent conjunctivitis
- Polymorphous exanthem, macular polymorphous rash on trunk
- Characteristic oral mucosal changes of lips and oral cavity: dry, red, fissured lips, "strawberry tongue"
- Acute nonsuppurative cervical lymphadenopathy
- Typical extremity changes: red palms and soles, indurative edema, desquamation of fingertips during convalescence
- Other symptoms: abdominal pain, aseptic meningitis, encephalopathy

The most serious feature of KD is coronary arteritis, leading to coronary artery aneurysms and/or occlusions in 25% of untreated patients. Cardiac involvement is usually asymptomatic; however, it may lead to coronary incidents including sudden death in children and young adults. In a review of 74 cases, mean age of presentation of KD cardiac sequelae was 24.7 ±8.4 years. The most common presentation was chest pain (60%); arrhythmia occurred in 10% of cases. Sudden death was a first presentation in 16% of cases. In a majority of cases, symptoms were triggered by exercise. Two thirds of patients had coronary occlusions on angiography. Coronary aneurysms were found in all autopsy cases (88). Aneurysms and thromboses of peripheral arteries leading to limb gangrene are uncommon (89–93).

Laboratory and Other Diagnostic Methods

Laboratory abnormalities include elevated ESR, CRP, leukocytosis, thrombocytosis, proteinuria, and abnormal liver function tests. Early echocardiogram with follow-up study after 4 to 6 weeks is recommended to detect cardiac involvement (94). Electrocardiogram frequently reveals various conduction abnormalities. Evidence of myocardial ischemia and myocardial infarction (MI) may also be present (95,96).

Treatment

Standard therapy with IV immunoglobulin (IVIG; 400 mg/kg/d IV for 4 days) and aspirin (80–100 mg/kg/d by mouth [PO] for 2 weeks) given within the first 10 days of illness greatly reduces this risk of coronary artery aneurysms (CAA). Unfortunately, approximately 5% of children still develop CAA after KD, and a larger number demonstrate coronary artery ectasia (2). Corticosteroid treatment has been controversial since a report by Kato (97) that patients treated with steroids alone had a higher incidence of CAA. A recent study indicated beneficial effects of steroids in patients with severe KD who did not respond to IVIG (98).

SMALL VESSELS VASCULITIS ASSOCIATED WITH ANTINEUTROPHIL CYTOPLASMIC ANTIBODY (ANCA+)

Small vessels vasculitis primarily affects vessels other than arteries, especially capillaries and venules. Depending on the anatomic sites of involvement, patients with small vessels vasculitis may present with purpura, glomerulonephritis, or pulmonary capillaritis.

Wegener's Granulomatosis

Wegener's granulomatosis (WG) is a necrotizing granulomatous vasculitis affecting small- to medium-sized vessels. The upper and lower respiratory tracts and kidneys are most frequently involved. Estimated annual incidence in Europe is 5 to 20 per million (99–102), being highest in Great Britain and Norway. WG affects individuals in their fourth to sixth decade of life, equally among men and women.

Pathology

Necrotizing vasculitis of small- and medium-sized arteries and chronic granulomatous inflammation are the two pathological hallmarks of Wegener's disease. Granulomas contain macrophages, giant cells, epithelioid cells, foci of tissue necrosis, and fibrosis. Granulomas in the lung may coalesce into larger masses that cavitate (Fig. 10-7). The vasculitis affects capillaries particularly in the lung, causing lung hemorrhages. Kidney biopsy frequently demonstrates glomerulonephritis that may be segmental, global, focal, or diffuse with capillary thrombosis. Affected arteries or arterioles show an inflammatory infiltrate and fibrinoid necrosis with destruction of the internal elastic lamina. There is no or little deposition of immune complexes within the kidney or vessel walls (1,24).

Clinical Findings

The classic triad of WG symptoms includes involvement of the upper airways, lungs, and kidneys. Disease may begin acutely with systemic presentation or may be limited to one organ, with years of delay before the next area of the body is affected. The onset of WG may be acute or insidious. The course may be fulminant with multiorgan involvement quickly leading to death or chronic, lasting years before the diagnosis is made (103).

Ninety percent of patients present with symptoms from upper respiratory tracts: perforation of the nasal sep-

tum, bleeding, obstruction and collapse of the nasal bridge, tracheal stenosis, and chronic sinusitis, occasionally with otitis media, hearing loss, and vertigo.

Lungs are affected in 70% to 80% of patients. Symptoms of pneumonia, occasionally with massive hemoptysis from alveolar hemorrhage, are frequently present. Kidneys are involved in 48% to 80% of WG patients (proteinuria, hematuria, erythrocyte casts). Arthralgias and arthritis are frequent. Cutaneous lesions include palpable purpura, and skin ulcerations resembling pyoderma gangrenosum are present in half of patients. Other symptoms include ocular involvement (frequent) with conjunctival hemorrhages, scleritis, uveitis, keratitis, proptosis, ocular muscle paralysis, central and peripheral nervous system granulomas with cranial nerve palsies, sensory neuropathy, and mononeuritis multiplex. Cardiovascular involvement is not frequent but includes coronary arteritis that may lead to MI, pericarditis, cardiomyopathy, aortitis, and aneurysm formation (104). Gastrointestinal vasculitis is uncommon but may cause bowel perforation, fatal hemorrhage, and bloody diarrhea. WG may also present as a tumor (e.g., breast tumor) (1,24,105,106). Constitutional symptoms of WG include fever, malaise, fatigue, and weight loss.

Diagnosis

Diagnosis is based on clinical presentation, histopathological assessment, and serological evidence. The ACR criteria include (107):

• Abnormal urinary sediment (red cell casts or microhematuria)

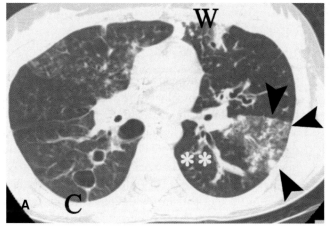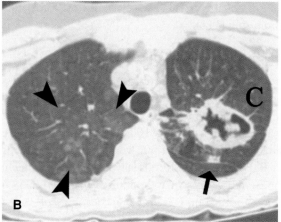

FIGURE 10-7 Wegener's granulomatosis (WG). Evaluation of patient with WG using high resolution computed tomography (HRCT). **A:** Axial CT image shows a constellation of CT findings in WG, including ground glass opacities and nodules (*arrowheads*), wedge-shaped lesion abutting the pleura (*W*), cystic changes from previous cavitary lesions (*C*), and bronchiectasis with mucous plugging (∗∗). **B:** Axial image obtained cephalad to **(A)** shows additional manifestations of WG, including ground glass opacities (*arrowheads*), solid pulmonary mass (*arrow*), and cavitary lesion (*C*). (Courtesy of Richard L. Hallett, M.D., and Geoffrey D. Rubin, M.D.)

- Abnormal chest x-ray (nodules, cavities, or fixed infiltrates)
- Oral ulcers or nasal discharge
- Granulomatous inflammation on biopsy

The presence of two or more of these four criteria is associated with a sensitivity of 88.2% and a specificity of 92.0%.

Biopsy material is usually acquired from lung or upper airways lesions. Serological evidence of antineutrophil cytoplasmic antibodies (ANCA) strongly supports the diagnosis. c-ANCA is almost always present in patients with WG. Other laboratory findings include elevated ESR, CRP, leukocytosis, and anemia (24).

Imaging studies are also helpful in assessment of vascular involvement in WG.

Treatment

Previously, untreated WG usually had a fatal course with median survival of 6 months from diagnosis. However, current therapy has greatly improved the prognosis for WG patients. Early diagnosis is crucial. Cyclophosphamid 1–2 mg/kg/d PO (or 800–1,000 mg IV once every 2–4 weeks during 3–6 months) with a low dose of prednisone should be continued for 1 year, then tapered and discontinued after 18 to 24 months. This regimen led to improvement in 91% of WG patients and caused remission of WG in 75% of WG patients (108). In nonresponders methotrexate and prednisone are the alternative therapy, inducing remission in over 70% of patients (109). Trimethoprim-sulfamethoxazole was found to be useful in control of the upper respiratory tract lesions. Currently, etanercept, a TNF-alpha antagonist, is undergoing evaluation for efficacy in WG patients (110). Early results in WG patients are promising (111).

Microscopic Polyangiitis/arteritis

Microscopic polyangiitis/arteritis (MPA) is a small vessel nongranulomatous necrotizing systemic vasculitis with focal segmental glomerulonephritis. Prevalence of MPA is estimated on 1 to 2 cases per 100,000. The onset of MPA is usually around the age of 50; women are less frequently affected. Patients with MPA usually have glomerulonephritis, and rarely, disease may be limited to the kidney. No granuloma formation is seen. Cutaneous, musculoskeletal, neurological, pulmonary, and gastrointestinal involvement is frequent.

Clinical Presentation

Patients usually present with symptoms of systemic disease and quickly deteriorating renal function due to rapidly progressive glomerulonephritis. Lung involvement is common, and alveolar hemorrhage occurs in 12% to 29% of patients. Otherwise, clinical presentation may resemble PAN. Myalgias, arthralgias, and arthritis are present in 65% to 72% of the patients. Cutaneous vasculitis (palpable purpura, livedo reticularis, digital gangrene) is found in 44% to 58% of the patients. Gastrointestinal (GI) symptoms of abdominal pain are found in 32% to 58% and GI bleeding in 29%; peripheral neuropathy occurs in 14% to 36% of cases. Cardiovascular system involvement is manifested by hypertension (34%), congestive heart failure (17%), pericarditis (10%), and MI (2%). Ocular manifestations and ear, nose, and throat lesions are commonly seen (112,113).

Laboratory Findings

ANCA are found in 75% to 90% of MPA patients; p-ANCA (perinuclear) are more prevalent than c-ANCA (114,115). ANCA testing is used both for the diagnosis and monitoring disease activity (116). Other laboratory studies usually reveal elevated ESR, leukocytosis, normocytic anemia, elevated creatinine, and blood urea nitrogen (BUN). Urinalysis shows proteinuria, leukocyturia, and hematuria with erythrocyte casts.

Diagnosis

Diagnosis is usually based on clinical presentation, presence of ANCA, and histopathological findings from biopsy. Biopsy can be taken from affected lung, skin lesions, kidney, or sural nerve.

Histologically, vascular lesions are identical to PAN but are present in arterioles, capillaries, and venules (in PAN small- and medium-size arteries are affected).

Imaging studies can help to delineate organ involvement. Visceral angiography usually does not show the microaneurysms, however.

Treatment

Choice of therapy depends on the severity of clinical presentation. Therapy usually begins with oral or IV steroids. Use of cyclophosphamide, methotrexate, and other cytotoxic agents should be limited to the most severe cases not responding to steroids (117,118). Patients with lung involvement and capillary hemorrhage may require concomitant plasmapheresis (114). Improvement with therapy is seen in 90% of patients, with 75% entering remission. Relapse occurs in 30% of patients (114,119).

Churg-Strauss Syndrome

Churg-Strauss syndrome (CSS) (allergic granulomatous angiitis) is a rare systemic granulomatous necrotizing vasculitis originally described by Churg and Strauss in 1951.

Estimated incidence is 2.4 per 100,000 people per year (120). Men are affected more frequently than women; M:F ratio is around 2:1. Peak age of onset is typically in the fourth to fifth decade of life.

CSS is associated with an atopic tendency, usually asthma, and characterized by pulmonary and systemic necrotizing vasculitis, extravascular granulomas, and eosinophilia.

Clinical Presentation

Adult onset asthma usually develops 2 to 3 years before symptoms of vasculitis occur. Patients present commonly with asthma that is frequently severe, and with symptoms of systemic disease.

In a series of 96 patients with CSS, asthma was the most common presentation (97%) followed by mononeuritis multiplex in 77%, sinusitis (61%), and skin lesions (palpable purpura, urtricaria, skin nodules, digital gangrene) in almost half of patients. Pulmonary infiltrates (Loeffler's syndrome, pneumonia) and/or hemoptysis were found in over one third of patients. Gastrointestinal involvement (GI bleeding, perforation, abdominal pain, pancreatitis) were present in 30% of cases. Kidney involvement was common with focal segmental or crescentic glomerulonephritis, but symptoms were usually mild and rarely progressed to renal failure. Cardiovascular manifestations included coronary vasculitis, MI, pericarditis, myocarditis and congestive heart failure; occasionally, coronary aneurysms and dissections were reported. Cardiovascular complications were the major cause of death in CSS patients. The CNS was infrequently affected; however, cerebral infarct and fatal cerebral hemorrhages were reported (121,122). Hypercoagulopathy with formation of intracardiac thrombus and peripheral thromboembolism has also been reported in CSS patients (123,124). Constitutional symptoms include fever, fatigue, myalgias, and weight loss.

Classic presentation of CSS may be less frequent today thanks to routine use of inhaled steroids in therapy of asthma. Low-dose steroids may modify the presentation of CSS, making the diagnosis more challenging (125).

Laboratory findings include eosinophilia >10% of white blood cells (WBC), anemia, and elevated ESR and CRP. ANCA are detected in half of patients. p-ANCA are prevalent in CSS (121). Other findings include elevated serum immunoglobulin E (IgE), eosinophilic cationic protein, thrombomodulin, and soluble interleukin-2 receptor. Eosinophilia in bronchoalveolar lavage fluid is found in one third of patients.

Diagnosis of CSS is made on the presence of classic clinical symptoms and laboratory/ histopathologic findings. Six criteria were proposed by the ACR for CSS classification:

(1) asthma, (2) eosinophilia (>10% of WBC), (3) paranasal sinusitis, (4) transient pulmonary infiltrates, (5) histologic evidence of vasculitis with extravascular eosinophils, and (6) mononeuritis multiplex or polyneuropathy. The presence of four or more findings is associated with a sensitivity of 85% and a specificity of 99.7% (126).

Biopsy of skin, lung, kidney, or muscles may help the diagnosis. Histologic findings in CSS include the presence of segmental necrotizing vasculitis with eosinophilic perivascular infiltrates and small necrotizing granulomas with central eosinophilic core (usually found in lungs) (122).

Treatment

Corticosteroids (prednisone 0.5–1 mg/kg/d orally) are sufficient therapy in the majority of CSS patients. IV methylprednisolone may be necessary in severe cases. Steroid therapy is continued until symptoms resolve, then slowly tapered. Twelve months of steroid therapy is usually sufficient (117).

In patients who are nonresponsive to steroids, cyclophosphamide can be added. Remission can be achieved in over 90% of patients treated with steroids or steroids/cyclophosphamide (121).

Prognosis

Ninety percent of treated patients survive 1 year, and the 5-year survival rate is 62%. Overall prognosis correlates with the initial disease severity (127).

SMALL VESSELS VASCULITIS NOT ASSOCIATED WITH ANTINEUTROPHIL CYTOPLASMIC ANTIBODY (ANCA–)

Henoch-Schönlein Purpura

Henoch-Schönlein purpura (HSP) is most commonly observed in children aged 4 to 11 years but can occur at any age. It is the most common vasculitis in children.

HSP is a systemic vasculitis with immunoglobulin A (IgA)–dominant immune deposits affecting small vessels (capillaries, venules, or arterioles). Skin, gut, and glomeruli are typically affected. Arthralgias or arthritis are usually present.

Clinical features include nonthrombocytopenic palpable purpura predominant in dependent areas, lower limbs, and buttocks. Fever, arthritis, and arthralgia are present in over 70% of cases.

GI symptoms include abdominal pain and bloody diarrhea, which are found in 68% of patients.

Kidneys are affected in half of HSP patients (hematuria, proteinuria). Kidney biopsy reveals IgA-associated glomerulonephritis (128).

Laboratory investigations reveal elevated ESR and leucocytosis and elevated serum IgA levels in one third of patients. Biopsy of the skin or kidneys documents IgA immune deposits, which are found in vascular walls; sometimes, deposits of IgG and C3 are also found.

HSP is an idiopathic leukocytoclastic vasculitis and should be distinguished from vasculitis related to infections, which especially can follow bacterial infections (group A beta-hemolytic streptococcus). Recently, however, HSP has been linked with Bartonella henselae infection (129).

Long-term prognosis of HSP is determined by renal involvement. Patients with nephrotic syndrome, decreased factor XIII activity, hypertension, and renal failure at onset have an increased risk of developing chronic renal failure (130).

Treatment

The disease is usually self-limiting, and only supportive treatment is required. Corticosteroids and immunosuppression are indicated for vasculitic glomerulonephritis (131) or serious GI or pulmonary hemorrhage (132).

Buerger's Disease—Thromboangiitis Obliterans

Thromboangiitis obliterans (TAO) is a non-necrotizing vasculitis of small- and medium-sized arteries and veins. TAO is called *Buerger's disease*, after Leo Buerger, who gave a detailed description of a series of patients with TAO in 1908.

This inflammatory vascular disease mainly affects young male smokers; however, incidence in women seems to have risen from the previously reported 1% to 20% (133,134). TAO is encountered throughout the world but is more prevalent in Asia and Eastern Europe. The incidence of Buerger's disease is declining in the world for unexplained reasons and is only partially related to a decline in smoking. According to the Mayo Clinic, the incidence of TAO has fallen from 104.3 in 100,000 people in 1947 to 12.6 in 100,000 people in 1986 (135). Similar trends have been reported from other countries (136,137).

Etiopathogenesis of TAO is not fully understood; however, there is striking relation to tobacco smoking. Virtually all TAO patients are tobacco smokers, and the activity of the disease is closely related to smoking patterns (138). Hypersensitivity to tobacco antigens, autoimmune mechanisms, and genetic predisposition may play a role in TAO development (139). The histopathological picture of affected vessels is characteristic and diagnostic. However, biopsy is not frequently utilized in clinical practice because of reluctance to biopsy ischemic tissue and because of the typical clinical presentation. Specimens for histopathological diagnosis usually are obtained from an

amputated limb. Histopathological examination of affected vessels in TAO reveals non-necrotizing panvasculitis with occlusive thrombus infiltrated with macrophages (pseudoabscess) (139).

Classic clinical features are tobacco smoker (100%), age of onset <45 (90%), male gender (80% to 90%), distal ischemic ulcer/gangrene (50% to 90%), rest pain (50% to 90%), migratory superficial thrombophlebitis (40% to 60%), involvement of upper extremities (up to 90%), and Raynaud's phenomenon (16% to 44%) (139). The majority of patients present with advanced disease and a relatively short history of foot/calf claudication, with quick progression to rest pain and gangrene. Physical examination reveals a lack of peripheral pulses, also frequently found on asymptomatic limbs, and a lack of proximal arterial bruits (otherwise atherosclerosis is suspected); active or resolved superficial thrombophlebitis, distal cyanosis, and toe/finger gangrene. Nonlimb arteries rarely are involved. Occlusions of visceral, coronary, and cerebral arteries are occasionally reported in TAO patients (140–142).

Differential diagnosis should include premature atherosclerosis, vasculitis, arterial embolism, and thrombophilia with arterial thrombosis.

Laboratory tests in TAO are usually normal. The diagnostic panel in TAO should include complete blood count, ESR, antinuclear antibodies, antiphospholipid antibodies, hepatitis serology, and screening for hereditary thrombophilia.

Angiography confirms arterial occlusion and may reveal characteristic vascular abnormalities. Angiographic findings in TAO are characteristic but not specific. Typical angiographic signs in TAO include (Fig. 10-8): multiple arterial occlusions ("skip lesions") with normal, smooth nonaffected arteries; abrupt arterial occlusions; corkscrew collaterals; "direct" collaterals (Martorell sign); and "tree root" collaterals (139,143,144).

Prognosis in TAO is strictly related to tobacco abstinence. Progression of TAO is halted in patients who abstain from smoking, and TAO recurs in patients who continue to smoke (138).

It is difficult for TAO patients to quit cigarette smoking. Tobacco cessation programs are indicated for a majority of TAO patients.

Pharmacological therapy should improve peripheral circulation and alleviate pain. Only prostanoid therapy was found to improve peripheral circulation and cause remission in patients with Buerger's disease (145).

Bypass surgery is available for selected patients (146), with patency rates up to 88% after 10 years (147,148). Thrombolytic therapy can be successful in cases of recent thrombosis (149).

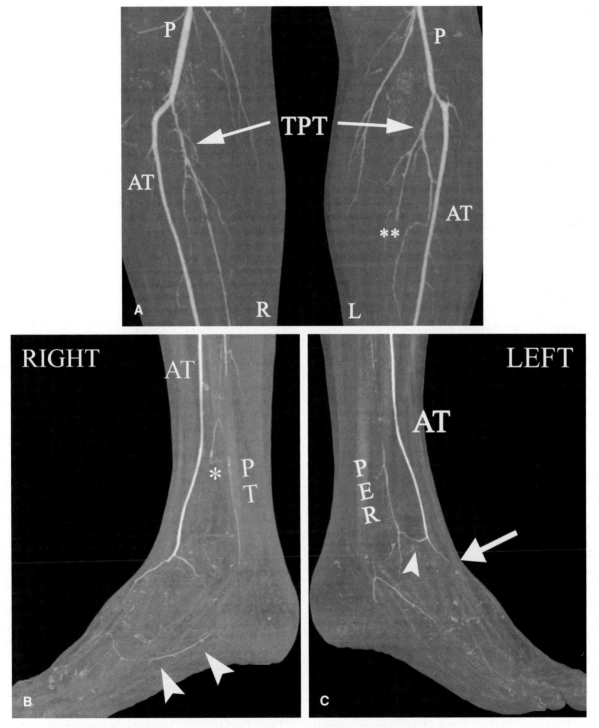

FIGURE 10-8 Lower extremity Buerger's disease in a 26-year-old smoker. The patient is status post right femoropopliteal bypass graft and continues to smoke. He presents with bilateral rest pain and tissue loss in the feet. **A:** Coronal MIP image with bone segmentation from CT angiogram shows fairly symmetric disease involving the tibioperoneal trunk (*TPT*) bilaterally, with disease extending into the posterior tibial and peroneal vessels. There is occlusion of the left posterior tibial artery (**). The anterior tibial artery (*AT*) is the dominant runoff bilaterally and is relatively unaffected. Note the absence of calcified atherosclerotic disease. **B, C:** Coronal MIP images with bone segmentation from CTA of both feet. There are patent anterior tibial arteries bilaterally (*AT*), but the dorsalis pedis and dorsal arch are diminutive. There is collateral (*arrowhead* in **C**) from the left AT to the distal peroneal artery (*PER*). On the right, there is a highly diseased right peroneal artery, which gives a collateral (*) to the previously occluded right posterior tibial artery (*PT*). There is a small amount of flow to the plantar arch (*arrowheads* in **B**). Note the lack of more distal mid- and forefoot arteries in this patient with digital gangrene.

Behçet Disease

Behçet disease (BD) is a chronic inflammatory systemic disease occurring throughout the world, with the highest prevalence in the Mediterranean basin, Middle East, and Central and Eastern Asia (or along the Silk Road). It is a chronic disease with a relapsing and remitting course and multiorgan involvement. BD is significantly more common in males (approximately 10-20:1). BD onset may occur at any age but is most common in young patients, typically in the third decade of life.

Clinical Presentation

The hallmarks of the disease are recurrent oral and/or genital ulcerations (up to 100%). Cutaneous lesions (50% to 85%) (150), arthritis (7% to 60%) (150), ocular involvement (23% to 80%) (150,151), CNS involvement (3.5% to 40%) (150,152), GI disease (3% to 16%) (150,153,154), and cardiac disease (155) are also present. Cutaneous lesions beside genital ulcerations include erythema, papulopustular lesions, neurodermatitis, and pyoderma gangrenosum-like lesions (150,156,157). Ocular involvement (uveitis, marginal keratitis, iridocyclitis, retinal vasculitis) is common and may lead to blindness (151). Arthritis is common in BD and may present as monoarthritis, palindromic rheumatism, and seronegative rheumatoid arthritis (150,158,159). GI involvement BD includes colitis and ileocolitis (160), Budd-Chiari syndrome, mesenteric thrombosis, and involvement of the liver and pancreas. Patients may have chronic symptoms or present with acute abdomen or GI hemorrhage (150,153,154,161). Neurological presentation may include vasculitis with ischemic or hemorrhagic stroke (152,162), meningoencephalitis (163), encephalitis (164), cerebral sinus thrombosis (165–167), or a multiple sclerosis-like syndrome (168). Vascular involvement of veins and/or arteries was reported in 2% to 46% of patients with BD (150,169,170). Venous involvement was twice as common as arterial and included deep vein thrombosis, superficial thrombophlebitis, and superior and inferior vena caval thrombosis (169). Arterial involvement is less common, diagnosed in 1% to 11% of patients (169,171). Arterial lesions include aneurysms and pseudoaneurysms of large- and medium-sized arteries and arterial thrombosis occasionally mimicking Buerger's disease (171–175).

Pulmonary involvement is not uncommon in patients with BD and is reported in 3% of cases (171). Pulmonary artery aneurysms and venous thromboembolism are the most common presentations (176,177). Cardiac involvement may include aortic valve insufficiency (178) and aneurysm of the sinus of Valsalva (179).

Diagnosis

The diagnosis is made mainly on the clinical presentation, because no specific diagnostic laboratory test exists. Diagnostic criteria proposed by International Study Group for Behçet's Disease (180) are:

1. Presence of oral ulceration *and*
2. Minimum *two* of the following:
   a. Genital ulceration
   b. Typical eye lesions
   c. Typical skin lesions
   d. Positive pathergy test[1] (181)

Differential diagnosis depends on the clinical presentation and should include other vasculitis syndromes, hereditary and acquired thrombophilia, and infections including HIV, herpesvirus, and HCV.

CT and MR are useful in characterization of multiorgan involvement in BD (182–185). In cases with vascular involvement, CT and MR angiography are extremely helpful to delineate vascular lesions (174,186) (Fig. 10-9).

Etiopathogenesis

The etiology of BD is unknown. Autoimmune mechanisms and genetic factors are suggested. An association with HLA B51 and MICA gene polymorphism suggests a genetic predisposition (187–189). Recently, autoimmunity to alpha-tropomyosin was described in patients with BD (190).

In pathological specimens, panvasculitis and vasculitis of vasa vasorum has been observed (175,188). Vascular thrombosis is common in BD, but its pathophysiology of thrombophilia is unclear (191–193).

Treatment

Colchicine, nonsteroidal anti-inflammatory drugs (NSAIDs), steroids, pentoxifilline, sulfasalazine, and cyclosporine A have been used in therapy of BD. In severe cases of vasculitis, steroids with cyclophosamide, methotrexate, and other cystostatics are proposed. More recently, thalidomide, interferon-alpha (IFN-α), and infliximab—a chimeric monoclonal antibody to tumor necrosis factor-alpha (TNF-α)—have been employed with varying degrees of success (150,194–197).

Prognosis

BD is a significant cause of morbidity and mortality. Blindness may affect 25% of patients with ocular involvement (151). Neurological and vascular/cardiac involvement is associated with higher mortality (150,156,178).

Degos Disease

This rare disease is also called *malignant atrophic papulosis* or Köhlmeier-Degos' disease. Degos disease (DD) is a

---

[1]Pathergy test: intradermal prick with a 21-gauge needle under sterile condition; formation of a papule or pustule after 48 hours is considered a positive test.

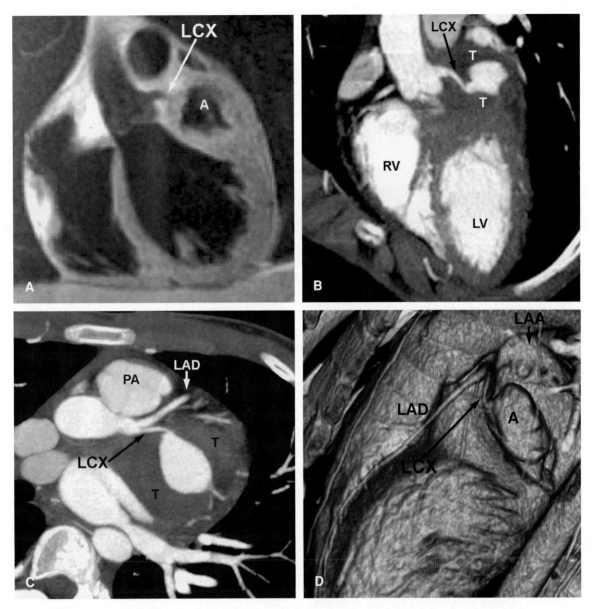

FIGURE 10-9 A 14-year-old patient with recurrent chest pain and a cardiac mass from Behçet disease.
A: Coronal double inversion-recovery fast spin echo (DIRFSE), MRI image demonstrates a low signal mass (*A*) adjacent to the left circumflex coronary artery (*LCX*). **B, C:** Multiplanar reformatted and **(D)** volume-rendered images from an ECG-gated MDCT angiogram demonstrate a large aneurysm (*A*) of the proximal left circumflex artery (*LCX*), causing mass effect on the left atrium and left atrial appendage (*LAA*). The aneurysm has circumferential mural thrombus (*T*). (LV, left ventricle; RV, right ventricle; PA, pulmonary artery; LAD, left anterior descending coronary artery.) (Courtesy of Tamer El-Helw and Geoffrey D. Rubin.)

systemic disorder mainly affecting skin, the GI tract (50% to 60%), and the CNS (20%) (198,199).

Etiopathogenesis is unknown; vasculitis, mucinosis, and/or hypercoagulopathy are proposed. Some authors regard DD as a distinct expression of lupus erythematosus rather than a unique disease (200).

The most characteristic lesion is a dome-shaped skin papula with central porcelain white atrophy. This is the presentation of a skin infarct resulting from thrombosed skin arteriole.

Small vessel infarction may occur in the GI tract, causing perforation, and in the CNS, causing a variety of neurological symptoms (201).

Histopathological examination reveals obliteration of skin arterioles, lymphocytic vasculitis, and deposition of mucin (202–204).

Diagnosis is based on clinical presentation with characteristic skin changes and on the histopathological examination of skin biopsy.

There is no specific therapy for DD. Antiplatelet therapy with aspirin and dipyridamole is occasionally effective alone or with pentoxyfylline (205–207) (Vicktor, 2001 #8143) in treatment of skin lesions (208).

Patients with disease limited to the skin have a good prognosis. Involvement of GI and CNS systems may result in significant morbidity and mortality (201,204,205,209).

Essential Mixed Cryoglobulinemia

Essential mixed cryoglobulinemia (EMC) is a systemic autoimmune vasculitis of small- and medium-sized vessels caused by vascular deposition of circulating immune complexes and presence of cryoglobulins. EMC is a subset of mixed cryoglobulinemias where no underlying disease is detected. Cryoglobulins are serum immunoglobulins that precipitate at a temperature less than 37°C and resolubilize after warming.

Classification of cryoglobulinemia is based on the type of immunoglobulin and presence of rheumatoid factor (RF) activity (210,211):

> *Type I:* Monoclonal immunoglobulin without RF activity (lymphoma, Waldenström's macroglobulinemia, and multiple myeloma)
>
> *Type II:* Mixed mono and polyclonal immunoglobulin with monoclonal RF (frequently EMC, HCV infection, myeloproliferative disorders)
>
> *Type III:* Polyclonal immunoglobulin with polyclonal RF (autoimmune CTD, EMC, chronic infections, myeloproliferative disorders, malignancy)

Clinical presentation is different in type I and types II and III.

In the majority of cases, MC is associated with HCV infection. HCV is thought to be a causative factor of both liver damage and cryoglobulinemia (211–214). MC is found in 40% to 50% of patients with HCV infection (215,216). HBV (215), HIV(217,218), mycoplasma (219), and leprosy (220) can also be associated with MC.

EMC is a rare disorder. A retrospective study of 179 patients with cryoglobulins found only 49 patients with symptoms related to cryoglobulinemia. The majority of them (33) had HCV infection, while systemic autoimmune disease was present in 20 patients; HIV and HBV infection were present in one patient each. In this series, only six patients had no evidence of an underlying disorder and were diagnosed with EMC (3.3% of asymptomatic and 12% of symptomatic patients) (221).

The MC associated with HCV infection has the same clinical pattern as EMC (221). It is possible that it is the same disease, and patients with EMC may have an occult HCV infection (222).

The classic clinical presentation of EMC includes a triad of symptoms (Meltzer's triad): purpura, arthralgia, and

weakness. Peripheral nerves, liver, and kidneys are also frequently involved (223–225). Occasionally, CNS symptoms (stroke, encephalopathy) may develop (226,227). Involvement of the GI tract may resemble Crohn disease (228). Skin purpura and Raynaud's phenomenon may occur spontaneously or after exposure to cold (229,230). In one series of 40 patients, recurrent palpable purpura was present in 100% of patients, arthralgias in 72%, liver involvement in 79%, and renal disease in 55%. Renal involvement was associated with worse prognosis (225).

Symptoms in type I cryoglobulinemia (not EMC) are often related to hyperviscosity and cold-induced small vessel occlusions. Severe Raynaud's phenomenon with acral gangrene, leg ulcerations, brain hemorrhage, peripheral neuropathy, and glomerulonephritis have been reported (231–237).

Histological examination of skin or organ biopsy in EMC reveals leukocytoclastic vasculitis (212) and in the kidneys, membranoproliferative glomerulonephritis (238).

Laboratory evaluation reveals elevated ESR, mild anemia, positive RF, C4 hypocomplementemia, and presence of cryoglobulins (239).

Treatment

Choice of therapy depends on severity of symptoms and underlying condition. In mild cases, antinflammatory therapy with NSAIDs might be sufficient (240). In severe cases associated with HCV, antiviral therapy is often sufficient to alleviate symptoms of cryoglobulinemia (241–243).

Interferon-alpha with or without steroids (244), colchicines (245), cryofiltration (246), immunoadsorbtion apheresis (247), and, recently rituximab (248,249) have been used with good short-term results. Plasma exchange may also be used to quickly remove circulating cryoglobulins (250). In cryoglobulinemic glomerulonephritis, fludarabine was effective (251).

Hypocomplementemic Urticarial Vasculitis

Recurrent urticaria, polyarthralgia, and a low-grade fever in a young person are characteristic for hypocomplementemic urticarial vasculitis (HUV). Other symptoms may include angioneurotic edema in the face and intestines and glomerulonephritis (252–254). Complement activation with low levels of plasma C1-C3 accompanies clinical symptoms. Laboratory findings include elevated sedimentation rate and positive, low-titer antinuclear antibodies. Skin biopsy reveals leucocytoclastic vasculitis. The etiology of HUV is unknown. A similar syndrome may be associated with systemic lupus, HBV, and other immune-complex disorders (255–257). HUV is a rare syndrome, with 70 cases reported in the literature (258).

Diagnosis can be made in patients with characteristic clinical symptoms after exclusion of other autoimmune disorders.

Initial treatment may include combinations of antihistamines, dapsone, colchicine, hydroxychloroquine, or indomethacin. In resistant or severe cases, corticosteroids and immunosupression might be necessary (255).

SECONDARY VASCULITIS

There are five types of secondary vasculitis: drug-induced vasculitis (DIV), infection-related vasculitis, malignancy-related vasculitis, vasculitis secondary to connective tissue diseases (CTDs), and inflammatory bowel disease (IBD)–associated vasculitis.

Drug-induced Vasculitis

Multiple chemicals (insecticides, pesticides, petroleum products, silica [259]), including drugs, can induce systemic vasculitis (Fig. 10-10). Small vessel leukocytoclastic vasculitides including HSP are probably the most common, but other specific vasculitides like WG, CSS, PAN, and MPA have also been reported (260–262).

Humoral and cell-mediated immune response are involved, but mechanisms of DIV are not fully understood.

Drugs frequently reported to induce vasculitis are propylthiouracil, hydralazine, colony-stimulating factors, allopurinol, cefaclor, minocycline, D-penicillamine, phenytoin, isotretinoin, and methotrexate (261). Published reports on DIV cover drugs from all pharmacological groups (e.g., penicillins, sulfonamides, iodides, tetracyclines, and phenothiazines; also, quinidine, aspirin, propylothiouracil, phenylbutazone, methyldopa, cimetidine, thioridazine, glyburide, phenylpropanolamine, and others).

Symptoms of vasculitis may occur hours to years after initial exposure to the offending drug. Symptomatology varies from a mild cutaneous eruption to severe systemic disease with multiorgan failure. In a recent review, 10% of reported DIV resulted in death (261).

Clinical presentation, histopathological exams, and laboratory findings are almost identical in DIV and idiopathic vasculitic syndromes (262). ANCA are usually present in DIV (263). The type and pattern of ANCA may help to distinguish DIV from idiopathic syndromes (264).

Treatment

Symptoms frequently resolve after discontinuation of the offending agent. In more severe cases, steroids, plasmapheresis, and cytotoxic agents have been necessary (260).

Infection-related Vasculitis

Viral, bacterial, and fungal agents can cause inflammation of the vessel wall by direct invasion, autoimmune reaction

with formation of immune complexes, or by acting as superantigens (see an excellent review by Naides) (265).

Bacterial arteritis includes chronic infections like syphilitic arteritis, tuberculous arteritis, and acute/subacute arteritis caused by other bacteria.

Syphilitic Arteritis

Arteritis occurs in the late phase of syphilis, 15 to 20 years after the onset of infection. Syphilitic arteritis, once uncommon, may be on the rise due to the increasing incidence of syphilis in immunocompromised patients (266).

Syphilitic vasculitis usually affects the ascending aorta and frequently involves coronary arteries. Destruction of the aortic wall leads to aneurysmal dilatation of the ascending aorta. Aortic insufficiency frequently develops (267). Ostial stenosis of coronary arteries is common (268). Involvement of peripheral arteries is rare, but arteritis with formation of aneurysms or arterial occlusions can occur in all large- and medium-sized arteries (269).

Histological examination reveals vasculitis of vasa vasorum and inflammation of the outer media with mononuclear cell infiltrates. Destruction of internal elastic fibers, occasionally with foci of necrosis and scarring, is present in the media and intima (270).

Syphilitic aortitis is often asymptomatic until vascular complications (aortic insufficiency, angina, ruptured aneurysm, claudication) develop.

Positive syphilis serology and polymerase chain reaction (PCR) for *Treponema pallidum* may help in diagnosis (271).

Vasculitis Related to Tuberculosis

Tuberculosis may affect the arterial wall by direct spread from infected structures (lymph nodes, kidneys, lungs); blood-borne tuberculous vasculitis was also described in the setting of milliary tuberculosis (270). Leukocytoclastic cutaneous vasculitis associated with tuberculosis has also been reported (272,273).

Mycobacterial aortitis causes destruction of the aortic wall with formation of aneurysms, pseudoaneurysms, and/or aortic rupture (274). Mycobacterial vasculitis involving multiple arteries may occur in HIV patients (275).

Diagnosis can be suspected in patients with pulmonary tuberculosis. Histological evaluation is necessary to confirm tuberculous etiology.

Bacterial Arteritis

Staphylococcus, Salmonella, Pseudomonas, Klebsiella, and other bacteria were identified to cause bacterial arteritis. Predisposing factors are IV drug abuse, endocarditis (12%), immunocompromise, and postoperative cardiac surgery

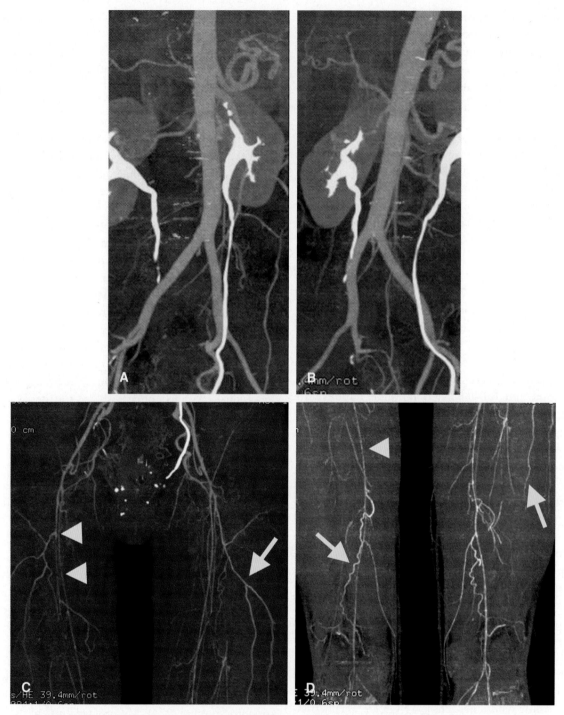

FIGURE 10-10 Ritonavir-induced vasospasm mimicking vasculitis. CTA **(A, B)** reveals unremarkable aortoiliac segments but high grade long-segment stenoses in the superficial femoral (*arrowheads*) and popliteal arteries bilaterally with extensive collateralization (*arrows*) **(C, D)**. In a follow-up exam 5 days after a steroid trial, the abnormalities had resolved. (Courtesy of Dennis Foley, M.D., Medical College of Wisconsin.)

patients (276–278). Infection of the arterial wall usually occurs as a result of embolization with infected material (e.g., embolization of vasa vasorum). Infection and inflammation cause destruction of the arterial wall with rapid formation of an aneurysm and/or arterial rupture.

Rapid enlargement of an aneurysm, fever, pain, and sepsis with positive blood cultures may suggest infectious (mycotic) aneurysm (279,280).

Infectious (mycotic) aneurysms occur most frequently in the aorta, followed by visceral, cerebral, and extremity arteries. Infectious aneurysms are usually saccular. If not treated aggressively, they can lead to arterial rupture with life-threatening hemorrhage and death.

CTA and MRA will delineate the lesion and reveal the presence of arterial wall inflammation. FDG-PET was recently advocated to confirm inflammation of the aortic wall (281).

Surgical resection with an extra-anatomical bypass and aggressive antibiotic therapy may improve the prognosis in this highly lethal condition (276,282,283). In patients with endocarditis, simultaneous valve replacement surgery might be necessary (284).

Human Immunodificiency Virus–associated Vasculitis

In HIV patients, vasculitis may result from autoimmune mechanisms (285) or be related to opportunistic infections (275). Several vasculitis syndromes have been described in association with HIV infection, including a Kawasaki-like syndrome, PAN, MPA, primary angiitis of the CNS, peripheral arterial occlusions, and vasculitic aortic aneurysms (62,286). Opportunistic infections associated with vasculitis in HIV patients include varicella-zoster virus (287), cytomegalovirus, tuberculosis, syphilis, and fungi (288).

Diagnosis of vasculitis in HIV-positive patients is challenging because systemic symptoms of vasculitis-like fever, fatigue, arthralgia, and mononeuropathy are frequently found in these patients. A special effort should be made, including imaging studies (CTA, MRA), while searching for opportunistic infections in suspected cases to uncover the diagnosis of vasculitis and to institute appropriate therapy (62).

Hepatitis B and C Viruses

HBV and HCV infections are associated with immune complex vasculitides. HBV-associated PAN may have worse prognosis than PAN without HBV infection. Specific antiviral therapy may improve the outcome and occasionally is sufficient to induce remission of vasculitis (85,289); aggressive immunosuppression should be used sparingly (see PAN treatment, above).

HCV infection is a frequent cause of mixed cryoglobulinemia (MC) and systemic vasculitis. In a majority of patients, MC is asymptomatic and does not require additional therapy. Antiviral treatment is necessary in HCV-associated vasculitis (see EMC treatment, above).

Malignancy-related Vasculitis

Vasculitis can be associated with malignancy; however, this is rather infrequent. It may precede the diagnosis of malignant disease (290) or appear later. In a retrospective study from the Cleveland Clinic, a documented diagnosis of vas-

culitis was found in 0.1% of 69,000 cancer patients. Only in 12 patients (0.02%) was a temporal association (both diagnoses within 12 months) found. Half of the patients had solid tumors, and half had myeloproliferative disorders. Cutaneous leukocytoclastic vasculitis was most common (7); GCA, PAN, and WG occurred in two patients, two patients, and one patient, respectively. In the majority of patients, symptoms of vasculitis paralleled the neoplasm's response to therapy (291). In a series of 303 adults and children with cutaneous vasculitis, all but one child had primary cutaneous vasculitis; however, in adults, an underlying malignancy was found in four cases (2.3%) (292).

In some cases, vasculitis is a paraneoplastic condition; therefore, a search for underlying malignancy in adults with idiopathic vasculitis is warranted, especially when a poor response to standard therapy is observed.

Vasculitis Secondary to Connective Tissue Diseases

Vasculitis may be associated with autoimmune connective tissue disorders, including systemic lupus erythematosus (SLE), rheumatoid arthritis, scleroderma, and Sjogren's. The pathogenesis is related to the deposition of immune complexes. Cutaneous leukocytoclastic vasculitis is probably the most common presentation; however, other types may be present, and vessels of all sizes can be affected. Occasionally, vascular ectasia and aneurysms may occur (293,294) (Fig. 10-11).

Clinical symptoms found in patients with various CTDs were secondary to vasculitis of the digital arteries with finger gangrene (295,296), peripheral vascular disease of extremities (297–299), intestinal ischemia (300,301), pulmonary and renal vasculitis (302), and vasculitic ischemic neuropathy (303,304). In one study of patients with various CTDs, an association of anti-SM antibodies and immune-complex mediated vasculitis were found (305).

Treatment is focused on the underlying condition, unless the severity of symptoms requires a more aggressive approach.

Inflammatory Bowel Disease–associated Vasculitis

Vasculitis is rare and probably coincidental in patients with IBD. In a large series of 7,199 patients with IBD, various manifestations of vasculitis were found in 21 patients (0.3%) (306), while thromboembolic complications were more common.

CONNECTIVE TISSUE DISORDERS WITH VASCULAR INVOLVEMENT AND NONCLASSIFIED VASCULAR DISEASES

Fibromuscular Dysplasia

FMD is a nonatherosclerotic vascular disease (also see review in [307]) affecting mainly young Caucasian women.

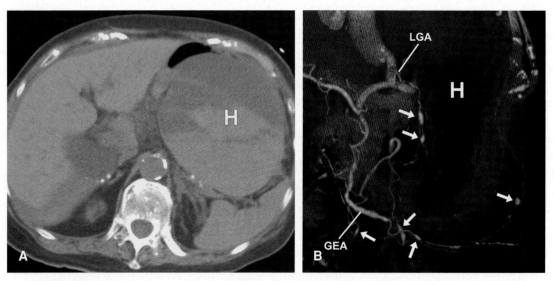

FIGURE 10-11 Acute abdominal pain in a patient with systemic lupus erythematosus. A: Transverse unenhanced CT section demonstrates a large hematoma (*H*) in the lesser peritoneal sac. **B:** Volume-rendered CT angiogram with isolation of the celiac artery reveals multiple aneurysms (*arrows*) from the left gastric artery (*LGA*) and multiple aneurysms (*arrows*) of the right and left gastroepiploic arteries (*GEA*). The central black zone within the left upper quadrant corresponds to the unenhanced hematoma (*H*). (Courtesy of Richard L. Hallett, M.D., Dominik Fleischmann, M.D., and Geoffrey D. Rubin, M.D.)

It usually affects medium- and large-sized arteries, although venous FMD has also been reported (308–310). FMD most commonly affects renal arteries but may affect extracranial, visceral, and extremity arteries as well (Table 10-3).

FMD encompasses a group of most likely congenital vascular abnormalities affecting one or more layers of the vascular wall. Arterial narrowing, aneurysms, and dissection may be present. A histopathological classification of renal artery FMD distinguishes three types of the disease (311):

intimal fibroplasia, medial fibromuscular dysplasia, and periadventitial fibrosis. Histopathological types correspond with radiological presentation.

Intimal Fibroplasia

Intimal fibroplasia occurs in 1% to 10% of all lesions. Angiography reveals smooth focal stenosis in the middle portion of the artery, long tubular stenosis, or corkscrew stenosis. Arterial dissection may complicate the course of intimal fibroplasia. Histological examination reveals fibrous

TABLE 10-3

Features of Extrarenal Fibromuscular Dysplasia

Artery Involved	Predominant Fibromuscular Dysplasia Subtype	Site of Involvement	Associated Lesions	Imaging Appearance
Internal carotid	Intimal and medial fibroplasia	Segment adjacent to C1-2	Intracranial aneurysms Renal FMD	String of beads, tubular stenoses, dissection
Vertebral	Medial fibroplasia	Segment adjacent to C5	Carotid FMD	String of beads
Mesenteric and celiac	Intimal fibroplasia	Midvessel segment beyond orifice	Renal FMD, visceral aneurysms	Focal stenosis, long tubular stenoses
Upper extremity (subclavian, axillary)	Intimal fibroplasia	Middle or distal segments of vessel	Renal FMD	Long tubular stenoses
Lower extremity (external iliac, femoral, tibial)	Medial fibroplasia	Proximal segment of external iliac	Carotid FMD Renal FMD	String of beads

Reprinted with permission from Gray BH, Young JR, Olin JW. Miscellaneous arterial diseases. In: Young JR, Olin JW, Bartholomew JR, eds. *Peripheral Vascular Diseases.* 2nd ed. St. Louis: Mosby–Year Book; 1996:432.

intimal thickening. The internal elastic lamina, media, and adventitia are usually not affected. Without treatment, progression of stenosis with distal organ ischemia occurs.

Medial Fibromuscular Dysplasia

Medial fibromuscular dysplasia is the most common type of FMD. It occurs in 70% to 80% of renal FMD. *Medial fibroplasia* is the most common subtype of medial FMD. The internal elastic lamina is thinned or is simply lacking in certain parts of the vessel, while the medial muscular layer is focally thickened with collagen deposits. The arterial wall may be thinned in some places with thinned or missing media and the formation of saccular aneurysms. Angiography reveals the characteristic *string of beads* picture, where stenotic areas interchange with aneurysmal dilatations (Figs. 10-10, 10-11). The degree of stenosis may be difficult to assess because of the frequent presence of thin membranous stenoses.

Perimedial fibroplasia is considered a second subtype of medial fibromuscular dysplasia. It is characterized by a circumferential accumulation of fibrotic tissue within the outer media, with resulting compression of the arterial lumen. Angiography shows a series of severely stenotic areas (beading) without intervening dilatations. Histology reveals deposits of collagen in the external layer of the media, occasionally with neovascularization.

Fibromusclar hyperplasia of the media is rare. Smooth focal or tubular stenosis frequently progresses and may lead to occlusion of the renal artery. Histological examination reveals thickening of media with proliferation of smooth muscle cells. The angiographic picture resembles intimal fibroplasia.

Periadventitial Fibrosis

In periadventitial fibrosis, the artery is compressed by fibrosis of the adventitia, which may also involve perivascular tissue (308,312–315).

Specific Vascular Distributions— Regional Considerations

Renal Artery Fibromuscular Dysplasia

Renal artery FMD (Fig. 10-12) is found to be the cause of pathologic changes in 40% of renovascular hypertension cases (311). It is a major cause of hypertension in patients <30 years old, including children (316). The natural history depends on the histological type. The most common, medial fibroplasia, rarely progresses to total occlusion of the renal artery. The other types (intimal and perimedial fibroplasia and fibromuscular hyperplasia) may progress to vascular obstruction (308). The clinical presentation and the complications of renal artery FMD include renovascular hypertension, renal

artery thrombosis and dissection, renal artery embolism, renal artery dissection, and renal artery aneurysm (317).

Renal artery FMD may be accompanied by FMD in other arteries. In one series of 92 patients with FMD, 89% had renal artery involvement, 26% had cerebrovascular involvement, 9% had visceral arteries involved, 9% had subclavian arteries involved, 5% had iliac artery involvement, 2% had aortic involvement, and 2% had coronary arteries affected by FMD. In this series, 26% of patients had more than one artery involved, and half of the patients with bilateral renal artery disease had other arteries affected (318).

Treatment of renal artery FMD depends on the presentation. In isolated renal artery stenosis, angioplasty is a safe and effective procedure (319) with durable results (320,321). In a recently published small series of 19 patients, the 8-year re-stenosis rate was 25% (319). Renal artery aneurysms require endovascular obliteration/exclusion or surgical repair (317,322,323).

Cerebrovascular Fibromuscular Dysplasia

The internal carotid artery is the second most common site of FMD (90% of all cerebrovascular FMD), whereas vertebral artery and intracranial FMD is less common (307,324). As in other areas, FMD may be asymptomatic or cause symptoms related to severity and localization of the stenosis, arterial dissection, distal embolization, aneurysm formation and rupture, or arterial thrombosis. Internal carotid artery FMD usually affects its proximal extracranial portion (325,326) (Fig. 10-13) and is frequently bilateral. Angiography may reveal a string of beads appearance, tubular or focal stenosis with elongation of the artery, carotid aneurysm, and dissections (327).

Extracranial carotid artery FMD is not associated with an increased incidence of cerebral aneurysm, which was suggested earlier (328). Clinical symptoms include transient ischemic attack (TIA), ischemic stroke, and subarachnoid hemorrhage (324,329,330).

Diagnosis can be made with Duplex Ultrasound examination; however, due to a proximal localization, the diagnosis can be missed. CT and MR angiography can be helpful (331,332).

Treatment varies from antiplatelet therapy to endovascular angioplasty and stenting to surgical repair (327,333–335).

Visceral and Extremity Artery Fibromuscular Dysplasia

FMD may affect arteries at any location; however, usually involvement of a limb and/or of visceral arteries accompanies renal and/or carotid FMD. Mesenteric, celiac, gastric, hepatic, splenic, pulmonary, and coronary artery involvement has been reported. Visceral FMD may be associated with aortic coarctation at different levels. An angiographic

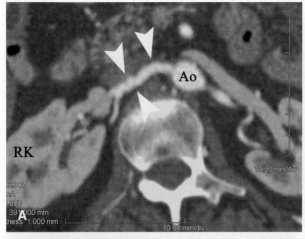

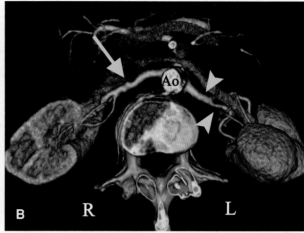

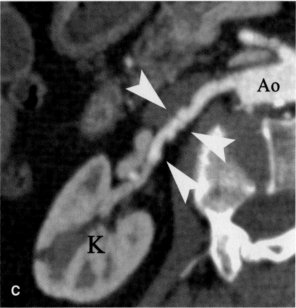

FIGURE 10-12 Renal FMD in a 41-year-old hypertensive female. A: Oblique axial image from a CTA study shows typical "string of beads" appearance (*arrowheads*) of the most common subtype of renal FMD—medial fibroplasia. Note the lack of calcified plaque and postostial location—other factors that distinguish this entity from atherosclerotic renal artery stenosis. (Ao, aorta.) **B:** Volume-rendered image of both renal arteries viewed from below shows the typical beading the right main renal artery (*arrow*). There is also subtle irregularity of the mid-distal left main renal artery (*arrowheads*), suggesting contralateral FMD as well. The findings were subsequently proven by catheter angiography; the patient underwent angioplasty with normalization of blood pressure. (Ao, aorta.) **C:** Curved planar reconstruction through the right renal artery shows alternating areas of stenosis and aneurysmal dilatation (*arrowheads*). Note should be made that given the fine nature of stenoses that may be present in medial FMD, correlation with pressure measurements by catheter may be required to determine the hemodynamic significance of an individual lesion. (Ao, aorta, K, right kidney.) (Courtesy of Richard L. Hallett, M.D., and Geoffrey D. Rubin, M.D.)

presentation may reveal tubular narrowing more frequently than the string of beads presentation; saccular aneurysms are also common (315,336–341). Limb arteries affected by FMD include iliac, superficial and deep femoral, popliteal, subclavian, axillary, brachial, radial, and ulnar arteries.

The clinical presentation includes claudication, limb hypoplasia, distal embolization with Raynaud's phenomenon and/or gangrene, or acute limb ischemia (309,342–351). Interestingly, hypothenar hammer syndrome might be related to underlying FMD of the ulnar artery (352). Diagnosis is usually made with angiography; however, it should be confirmed with histopathological examination. The differential diagnosis should include vasculitis, arterial trauma, thromboangiitis obliterans, vasospastic disorders, and atherosclerosis. Atherosclerotic lesions may develop in arteries affected by FMD in older patients, making the diagnosis more challenging.

Treatment depends on clinical symptoms and location and the type of lesion and may vary from surgical repair or endovascular treatment to medical therapy only.

Medial Degeneration

Nonatherosclerotic degeneration of media is a common underlying cause of aortic aneurysms and dissection and the most common cause of ascending aortic aneurysm (353). In the literature, various types have been described, and various terms are used (Gsell and Erdmann medionecrosis, medionecrosis aortae, cystic medial necrosis, mucoid medionecrosis, mediolytic arteriopathy, mucoid degeneration of the media, and others). Some pathologists distinguish two or more pathological types (354,355), and it is possible that different pathological processes can lead to medial degeneration (MD) or that these are different stages of the same process. MD of aorta is characteristic for

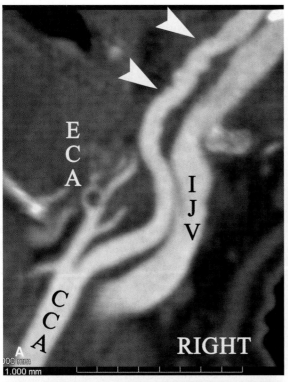

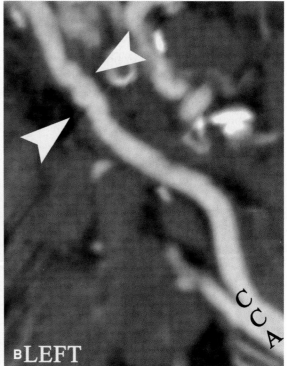

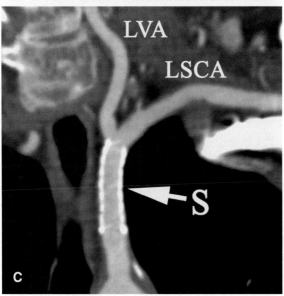

FIGURE 10-13 Cerebrovascular FMD in a 51-year-old female with history of renal and subclavian FMD, now presenting with TIA. A: Curved planar reconstruction (CPR) of right carotid system from a CTA study of neck. There is irregular "beading" of the right internal carotid artery in its midcervical course (*arrowheads*), consistent with FMD. Note the lack of associated plaque and normal distal common carotid (CCA) and external carotid (*ECA*) vessels. (IJV, right internal jugular vein.) **B:** CPR of the left carotid system from same study shows symmetric internal carotid artery (ICA) disease (*arrowheads*). (CCA, common carotid artery.) **C:** CPR of left subclavian segment shows patency of previously placed subclavian stent (*S*), without significant intimal hyperplasia. Note the normal adjacent left vertebral artery (*LVA*) and distal left subclavian segment (*LSCA*).

Marfan disease and may be different from the idiopathic form (355), but according to other authors, it is indistinguishable (356). MD with thoracic aortic aneurysms and dissections (TAAD) may occur in families in an autosomal dominant pattern of inheritance (357).

Classic histological findings include fragmentation and degeneration of elastic fibers and cystic accumulation of mucopolysaccharides within the media.

Pomerance, in a series of 63 thoracic aneurysms, found MD in majority of cases (71.3%) (356); however, MD was less common in extra-aortic aneurysms (358). MD can probably occur in all medium- and large-sized arteries in different age groups, although this is less common than its occurrence in the aorta (359–361).

Segmental Arterial Mediolysis

Segmental arterial mediolysis (SAM), formerly known as segmental mediolytic arteriopathy, is a rare disorder that involves splanchnic arteries in the elderly and coronary arteries in the young. SAM occurs when the arterial smooth muscle cytoplasm is transformed into heterogeneously distributed fluid-filled vacuoles. When the vacuoles rupture, the smooth muscle cells are disrupted, completing the mediolytic process. Mediolysis is accompanied by fibrin deposition and hemorrhages at the adventitiomedial junction and within the media. Inflammation can be observed but typically is limited to periadventitial tissues. Transmural mediolysis leads to formation of arterial wall defects bridged by a serofibrinous layer, leading to regions of aneurysm formation. Focal intimal dissection and intramural hematomas are other common features of SAM. Dissection frequently occurs adjacent to gaps in the arterial wall at sites of total mediolysis or as a result of capillary hemorrhages in areas of partial mediolysis. Lumen occlusion, either by thrombi or dissection, can result in sequela of ischemic bowel, renal infarction, splenic infarction, or intra-abdominal hemorrhage due to aneurysm rupture. While the pathogenesis of these lesions is unknown, it has been hypothesized that SAM is due to vasospasm.

The hallmark of the disorder is the involvement of multiple abdominal splanchnic arteries (Fig. 10-14). The absence of aortic dissection helps to exclude other CTDs such as MFS, Ehlers-Danlos syndrome type IV, or homocystinuria. Uncomplicated SAM lesions can resemble FMD both on imaging as well as at histologic examination. In rare instances, SAM has been reported to coexist with cystic medial necrosis of the aorta.

Adventitial Cystic Disease

Adventitial cystic disease (ACD) (adventitial cystic degeneration, cystic mucoid degeneration) is an uncommon disorder usually affecting the popliteal artery. Only a little over 300 cases of ACD were reported in the literature, the majority of them affecting the popliteal artery. It is found in about 1 of every 1,000 to 1,200 claudicants (362). Other locations are rare and may include both arteries and veins. Iliofemoral axis vessels other than the popliteal artery were the second most common locations of ACD. Other vessels adjacent to large joints (knee, ankle, shoulder, elbow, wrist) were occasionally reported (363–365).

One or multiple mucoid-filled cysts develop in the outer media and adventitia of the affected vessel. Growing cysts compress the affected artery with resulting stenosis and occasionally occlusion (366). Sometimes, communication between an adventitial cyst and the knee joint is found (366).

Etiology of ACD is unclear; developmental abnormalities are proposed (367). ACD affects predominantly younger men; however, it was reported in both sexes and in all age categories.

A typical patient presents with a new (over a period of a few months) onset of calf claudication. Usually, no other symptoms of atherosclerotic disease are present. Ultrasound

examination reveals the presence of a cyst or cysts within the arterial wall with compression of the lumen. CT and MR angiography provide an adequate image of the lesion and suggest the correct diagnosis (368) (Fig. 10-15). Contrast angiography reveals signs of external compression of lumen, but this can occasionally be mistaken for atherosclerotic stenosis (369).

Therapy may begin with a simple needle aspiration of the cyst in qualified cases (370,371). However, recurrent or complicated, multilocular cysts should be managed surgically (368,371). Angioplasty has been occasionally attempted without success (372).

Pseudoxanthoma Elasticum

Pseudoxanthoma elasticum (PXE) (Gronblad-Strandberg syndrome, Gronblad-Strandberg-Touraine syndrome, systemic elastorrhexis) is a rare genetic disorder characterized by the degradation and calcification of elastic fibers.

The prevalence of PXE is estimated to be around 1:70,000–100,000 people. Both autosomal dominant and recessive inheritance patterns have been reported, the latter being more frequent (373). PXE is twice as common in women as it is in men. The underlying genetic defect is probably a mutation of the ABCC6 gene (374,375).

PXE is a systemic disorder with cutaneous, ocular, and vascular manifestations. Clinical symptoms are infrequently seen in children, and the disease is often not diagnosed until the third or fourth decade of life. There is a significant phenotypic variability in PXE patients, even between members of the same family (376,377).

The characteristic clinical presentation includes formation of yellowish skin papules (pseudoxanthomas) on the lateral aspects of the neck and on the skin of joint flexures in about 70% to 85% of cases (377). Skin lesions are symmetric and may coalesce to involve larger areas. Affected skin is thick with an "orange peel" or cobblestone appearance. Increased skin laxity may in some patients lead to the formation of excessive redundant skin folds, requiring surgical removal (378,379). Other clinical symptoms include visual disturbances (occasionally leading to blindness), angina pectoris, claudication, abdominal angina, TIA and/or stroke, and recurrent GI or genitourinary bleeding.

Vascular abnormalities are described in 40% to 50% of PXE patients and include aneurysms as well as arterial stenoses and occlusions of small- and medium-sized arteries, which may occur separately or coexist in the same patient. Involvement of the heart, aorta, and large arteries is less common (380). Recurrent GI and uterine bleeding is frequent, due to the weakened and fragile walls of small arteries (381,382). Vascular abnormalities described in PXE patients include aortic dilatation (377), aortic and coronary

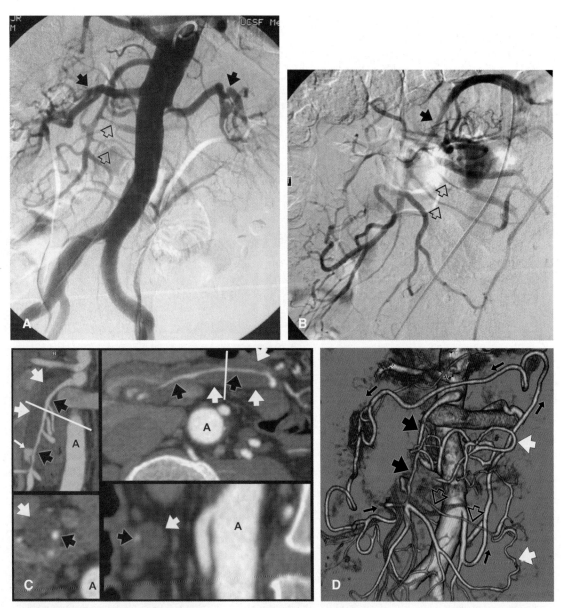

FIGURE 10-14 Segmental arterial mediolysis in a 55-year-old man with a 2-year history of intermittent abdominal pain and GI bleeding. Although arterial abnormalities were noted on three separate conventional arteriograms during this 2-year period, the diagnosis of segmental arterial mediolysis was made only after the acquisition of a 16 × 1.25 mm MDCT angiogram. **A:** Abdominal aortogram demonstrates narrowed branches of the superior mesenteric artery (SMA) (*open arrows*), regions of apparent aneurysmal dilation in second-order branches of the left renal artery (*black arrow*). No abnormalities were identified within the right renal artery, where a dual lumen appearance (*black arrow*) was felt to represent overlapping branches. **B:** Selective superior mesenteric arterial angiogram demonstrates narrowing of the mid SMA as well as confirming narrowing of at least two jejunal branches (*open arrows*). **C:** A longitudinal oblique MPR through the SMA **(upper left)** and transverse section through the SMA at the level of the line segment drawn on the longitudinal view **(lower left)** demonstrates the narrowed SMA lumen (*black arrows*) and the markedly dilated thrombosed false lumen (*large white arrows*). Communication between the true and false lumen is observed approximately 10 cm distal to the SMA origin (*small white arrow*). The SMA measures approximately 15 mm in diameter. Transverse CT section in the mid abdomen **(upper right)** demonstrates the lumen of one of the narrowed jejunal branches seen in **(B)** (*black arrows*) as well as the markedly dilated arterial wall with associated false luminal thrombus (*white arrows*). An oblique MPR orthogonal to this jejunal branch is displayed in the **lower right** and similarly illustrates the small residual lumen (*black arrow*) and the dilated, thrombosed false lumen (*white arrow*). The (*A*) in all four portions of this figure part indicates the aorta. **D:** Volume rendering of the CT angiogram does not allow visualization of the outer wall of the SMA and its branches, neither does it show the thrombus within the false lumen. The strength of the volume rendering is the mapping of the extensive collateral network that maintains adequate perfusion to the small bowel despite the substantial occlusive disease proximally in the SMA (*black arrows*) as well as the proximal jejunal branches (*open black arrows*). A primary collateral pathway visualized in this patient is the meandering artery bridging the left colic artery, which was the first branch of the unaffected inferior mesenteric artery, to the middle colic artery, which enters the SMA distal to the occlusive lesions. The direction of flow in this collateral pathway is indicated by *small black arrows*. Additional intramesenteric collateral pathways are evident bridging regions of stenosis (*white arrows*). (*Figure 10-14 continues*)

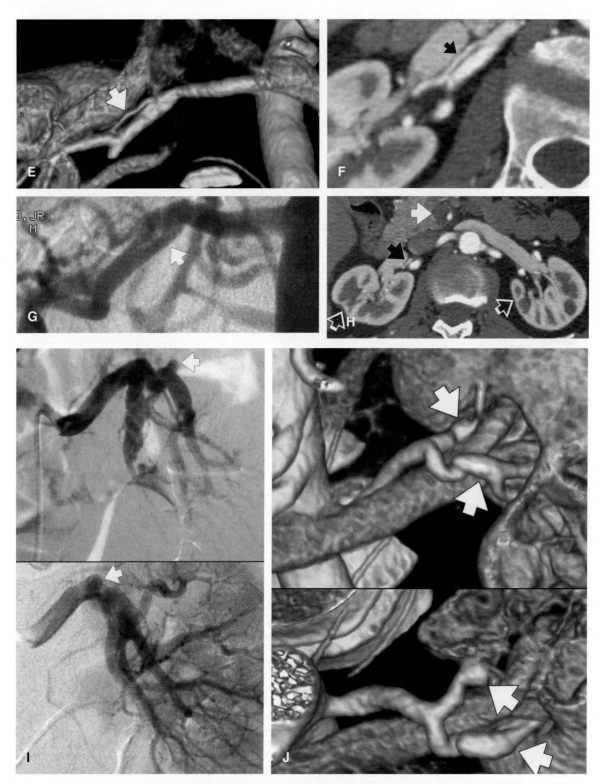

FIGURE 10-14 Continued Volume rendering (**E**) and oblique MPR (**F**) demonstrate that the dual-channel appearance reported in **A** within the right renal artery and better visualized on the magnified right renal arteriogram (**G**) corresponds to a 2 cm long intimal dissection (*arrows*). The limitations of projectional angiography hinder the correct recognition of the dissection clearly evident on the CT scan both with volume rendering and MPR. **H:** Transverse CT section through the mid abdomen demonstrates cortical thinning in both kidneys (*open white arrows*) indicating regional ischemia likely due to occlusion of intrarenal branches. The short dissection of the right renal artery is evident (*black arrows*), as is the dissection of the SMA (*white arrow*). **I:** Two views from a selective left renal arteriogram illustrate irregularity of the renal artery in the renal hilum (*arrows*) without documentation of dissection. **J:** Volume renderings from the CT scan document the presence of two separate aneurysmal abnormalities in anterior and posterior branches of the left renal artery (*arrows*). (*Figure 10-14 continues*)

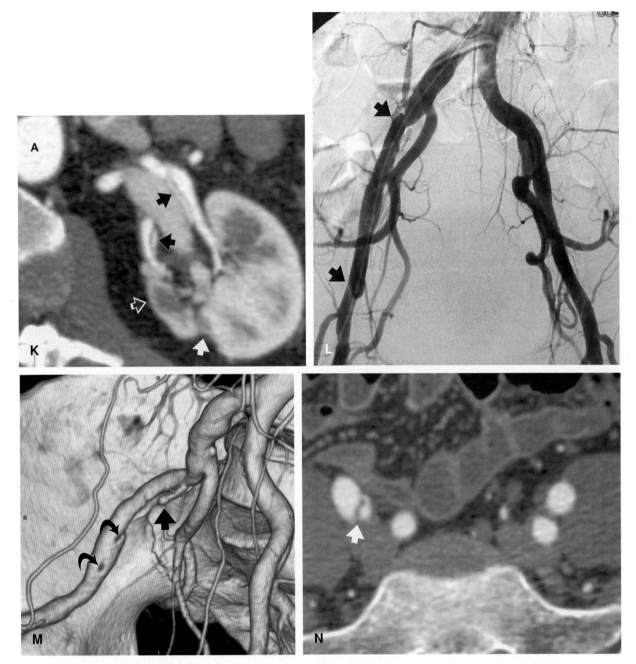

FIGURE 10-14 Continued K: Oblique MPR through the left renal hilum documents focal dissections in both the anterior and posterior renal arterial branches (*black arrows*). A scar (*white arrow*) in the renal parenchyma is associated with complete loss of renal cortex due to chronic renal infarction. The more medially located zone of diminished enhancement and cortical thinning (*open arrow*) is indicative of ongoing ischemia. (A, aorta.) **L:** Conventional angiography of the iliac arteries illustrates ectasia of the right external iliac artery without demonstration of dissection. **M:** Volume rendering obtained with substantial cranial angulation unmasks false luminal opacification (*black arrow*) as well as filling defects (*curved arrows*) corresponding to intimal dissection. **N:** Transverse section allows direct visualization of the intimal flap in the proximal right external iliac artery (*white arrow*). (*Figure 10-14 continues*)

aneurysms (383), visceral artery aneurysms and occlusions (384,385), premature coronary artery disease (386), renovascular hypertension (387,388), peripheral arterial occlusive disease (389,390), carotid stenosis with stroke (391), and cerebral artery involvement with central retinal artery occlusion (392). Classic ocular lesions present in the major-ity of patients and are characterized by retinal angioid streaks, occasionally causing visual loss (385).

Diagnosis

Variability in the clinical presentation, even within the same family, can make the diagnosis difficult. The presence of skin

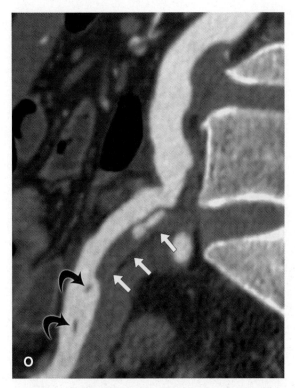

FIGURE 10-14 Continued O: Oblique longitudinal MPR through the right common and external iliac artery allows direct visualization of the partially thrombosed false lumen (*white arrows*) as well as the residual regions of intimal flap (*curved black arrows*). (Courtesy of Geoffrey D. Rubin, M.D.)

lesions and skin biopsy can establish the diagnosis. Genetic analysis is also possible (376). Vascular imaging studies including CTA and MRA can be very helpful in delineating the extent of vascular involvement in patients with PXE.

Histology

The histopathological picture is diagnostic for PXE. Skin biopsy reveals disruption and derangement of elastic fibers with microcalcifications. Degeneration of collagen fibers is also visible. The vascular wall in muscular arteries shows fragmentation of elastic fibers in the elastic laminae with calcification of media identical with Mönckeberg sclerosis. Intimal thickening of intrarenal arteries was also observed (380).

Differential diagnosis in suspected cases should include beta-thalassemia major, which is frequently associated with pseudoxanthomalike lesions (393), and other hereditary CTDs like MFS and Ehlers-Danlos syndrome.

Treatment

No specific therapy exists for PXE. Prophylactic measures include cardiovascular risk factor reduction (smoking cessation, cholesterol-lowering techniques) and avoidance of anticoagulation and antiplatelet drugs because of the high

risk of bleeding complications. Vigorous exercise is also contraindicated. Ophthalmological treatment may prevent visual loss (394).

Surgical revascularization and vascular repair (383,390) including thromboendarterectomy (389) is necessary in patients with severe vascular complications. In patients with excessive redundant skin, skin excision can be performed (379).

Neurofibromatosis Type I

Neurofibromatosis type I (NFI) (von Recklinghausen disease, von Recklinghausen neurofibromatosis) is one of the most common neurological genetic disorders. The prevalence of NFI is estimated to be 1:3,000 newborns in the United States. The disease is caused by a mutation of the neurofibromin gene on chromosome 17. NFI has an autosomal dominant type of inheritance; however, 30% to 50% of cases arise from new spontaneous mutations. Affected individuals develop peripheral schwannomas and neurofibromas, CNS tumors, and cardiovascular abnormalities.

Clinical presentation includes characteristic skin changes with multiple brownish discolored spots of various shapes and sizes (café au lait) and multiple skin tumors of different sizes from very small to large, representing peripheral nerve tumors. Bony abnormalities may also be present.

The prevalence of cardiovascular malformations in 2,322 NFI patients registered by the National Neurofibromatosis Foundation International Database was 2.3%. Peripheral vascular abnormalities were noted in 0.8% of patients and pulmonary stenosis in 1.1% (395).

Aneurysms and stenoses are seen in the aorta and large arteries, while dysplastic features are found in smaller vessels (396–398). Vascular abnormalities arise from the proliferation of Schwann cells within the arterial wall, with subsequent fibrosis. Mesodermal dysplasia affects small arteries (399).

Vascular symptoms in NFI include renovascular hypertension (400), cerebrovascular disease (401,402), visceral ischemia (403), limb artery involvement (404,405), aortic coarctation, and pulmonary hypertension (406). Aneurysms may also occur in coronary arteries (407). The rupture of peripheral aneurysms may occur with formation of a pseudoaneurysm or hemorrhage (408–410). Renal artery stenosis leading to renovascular hypertension was found in 5% of children with NFI (411), and NFI accounted for 15% to 58% of renovascular hypertension in children (316,412).

Although not very common, vascular involvement is a significant problem for patients with NFI. According to recent U.S. study, young individuals <30 years old with NFI are two to three times more likely to die due to cardiovascular problems than their peers of the same age (413).

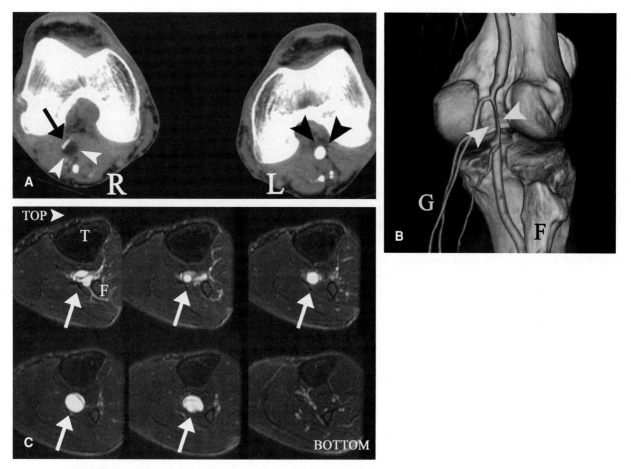

FIGURE 10-15 Adventitial cystic disease. A: Axial image from extremity CTA study of a middle-aged, nonsmoking male with right calf claudication. There is an eccentric, fluid-density lesion (*white arrowheads*) compressing the right popliteal artery (*arrow*). Note the adjacent, normal left popliteal artery (*black arrowheads*). The lesion was fluid echotexture when visualized by ultrasound. **B:** Posterior view volume-rendered image from CTA shows the degree of compression of the popliteal artery (*arrowheads*). There are prominent geniculate arteries (*G*), which attempt to provide collateral blood flow to the calf. The lesion was drained by ultrasound guidance but recurred, necessitating surgical excision of the cyst. (F, fibula.) **C:** Series of axial fat-suppressed fast spin echo T2-weighted images in a different patient (37-year-old male) with ACD and calf claudication. Note the multilobulated cystic lesions (*arrows*) surrounding the popliteal artery and tibioperoneal trunk region. (T, tibia; F, fibula.) (Courtesy of Richard L. Hallett, M.D., Dominik Fleischmann, M.D., and Geoffrey D. Rubin, M.D.)

Diagnosis of NFI is based on the clinical presentation in patients who meet two or more of the following criteria:

- Neurofibromas (two or more, or one plexiform neurofibroma)
- Café-au-lait macules (six or more measuring 1.5 cm in their greatest dimension)
- Freckling (in the axillary or inguinal areas)
- Optic glioma
- Iris hamartomas (known as Lisch nodules; two or more)
- Sphenoid dysplasia or thinning of the cortex of the long bones
- Affected first-degree relative

No specific treatment exists for NFI-associated vasculopathy. Renovascular hypertension and arterial stenoses are treated by angioplasty and stenting (400,414). Aneurysms and other arterial anomalies may require surgical or endovascular repair (415,416).

Williams Syndrome

Williams syndrome (WS) (Beuren syndrome, early hypercalcemia syndrome with elfin facies, elfin facies with hypercalcemia, hypercalcemia-supravalvar aortic stenosis, Williams-Beuren syndrome) is a hereditary disorder caused by 7q11.23 chromosomal deletion—what results in deletion of multiple genes including the elastin gene (417).

Individuals affected with WS syndrome may present with a variety of findings: cardiovascular abnormalities (supravalvular aortic stenosis in 75% of patients, thoracic and abdominal aortic stenosis, and stenosis involving any visceral and peripheral artery); characteristic facial features (elfin facies) with broad brow, short nose, wide mouth, small jaw, and prominent earlobes; connective tissue abnormalities including soft, lax skin; and/or some degree of mental retardation, although some have average intelligence and a unique cognitive profile. Additional endocrinological findings include idiopathic hypercalcemia (15%), hypercalciuria (30%), hypothyroidism (10%), early (but not precocious) puberty (50%), and failure to thrive in infancy (70%) (418).

Arterial elastopathy in WS is characterized by an increased arterial distensibility, arterial wall hypertrophy with abnormal elastic fibers, and a thickened internal elastic lamina (419). Reduced deposition of elastin in WS individuals may lead to increased proliferation of SMC and thickening of media, in some cases leading to arterial occlusion (420).

Vascular abnormalities include supravalvular aortic stenosis found in 75% of patients, stenosis of the pulmonary artery and its branches in 50%, and aortic branch stenosis (20%) (421). Occasionally, cerebral artery stenoses (422), coronary artery stenosis (423), and portal hypertension (424) have been reported. In a series of 112 patients diagnosed with WS, 25 were studied with arteriography. In 19 patients, segmental narrowing of the thoracic or abdominal aorta was present. Eleven patients had renal artery stenosis; 10 of them were associated with aortic hypoplasia. Seventeen patients had arterial hypertension (425). Caution should be used, however, when arterial blood pressure is measured, because arterial wall thickening may cause falsely elevated blood pressure recordings (426). Arterial lesions can initially be mild but may progress over time (421). Long-term follow-up with ultrasound suggests that the more mild aortic stenoses did not change or tended to normalize (427).

Diagnosis in clinically suspected individuals should be confirmed by genetic analysis. The cardiovascular system should be thoroughly examined. MRA or CTA are often the initial diagnostic procedures of choice to detect asymptomatic and potentially dangerous lesions. Close follow-up of arterial stenoses is necessary because of the tendency to progression in some patients. Severe arterial lesions may require surgical repair (421,428). Angioplasty and stenting have also been succesfully utilized (429,430); however, restenosis after endovascular and surgical procedures may be more frequent (427,431).

Marfan Syndrome

MFS is a genetic disorder caused by mutations of the fibrillin gene (FBN1). These fibrillin mutations affect the development of connective tissue in affected individuals and are manifest by predominantly skeletal, ocular, and cardiovascular symptoms. Over 200 mutations of the fibrillin gene were identified in individuals with MFS. The estimated population prevalence of MFS is 1:4,000 (432).

Clinical manifestations vary greatly. Affected individuals can be almost asymptomatic, or symptoms in multiple body systems might be present. Ectopia lentis is present in 60% of MFS patients. Skeletal manifestations of MFS include elongation of the extremities, joint hypermobility (thumb and wrist signs), rib cage abnormalities (pectus excavatum or carinatum), lumbosacral dural ectasia scoliosis, and high-arched palate (Fig. 10-16).

Progressive dilatation of the ascending aorta and spontaneous aortic dissections represent typical cardiovascular involvement in MFS. Mitral valve prolapse with mitral insufficency, aortic insufficiency, and pulmonary artery enlargement are also observed (Fig. 10-17). Aortic disease is the major cause of morbidity and mortality in MFS, leading to death, if untreated, in the third decade of life. Optimal clinical care with surgical therapy of aneurysmal and valvular disease can increase the lifespan of MFS patients to the population average (433).

In a series of 52 children with MFS, followed for nearly 8 years, mitral valve prolapse occurred in 46 patients, mitral regurgitation in 25 patients, aortic dilatation in 43, and aortic regurgitation in 13 (434). The majority of adults with MFS have cardiovascular involvement (435).

Diagnosis is based on the presence of clinical findings and a family history of MFS. Diagnosis of MFS requires clinical evidence of involvement of cardiovascular system (ascending aortic dilatation or dissection), eye (ectopia lentis), lumbosacral dural ectasia, and typical skeletal abnormalities (436). Genetic testing for the FBN1 mutation is available.

Differential diagnosis should include Ehlers-Danlos type IV, familial thoracic aortic aneurysm and dissection (TAAD) syndrome, homocystinuria, congenital contractural arachnodactyly, and other genetic disorders related to FBN1 mutations (e.g., mitral valve prolapse syndrome, MASS phenotype [**M**yopia, **m**itral valve prolapse, borderline and nonprogressive **a**ortic enlargement, and nonspecific **s**kin and **s**keletal features], isolated thoracic aortic aneurysm, ectopia lentis, or skeletal abnormalities) (437).

Management of MFS patients requires a multidisciplinary approach with close cardiovascular monitoring. Progressive enlargement of the aorta requires surgical repair. Criteria for surgical repair may vary slightly between different centers. Elective surgery is recommended before the aortic root diameter reaches 5.0 to 6.0 cm. Replacement of

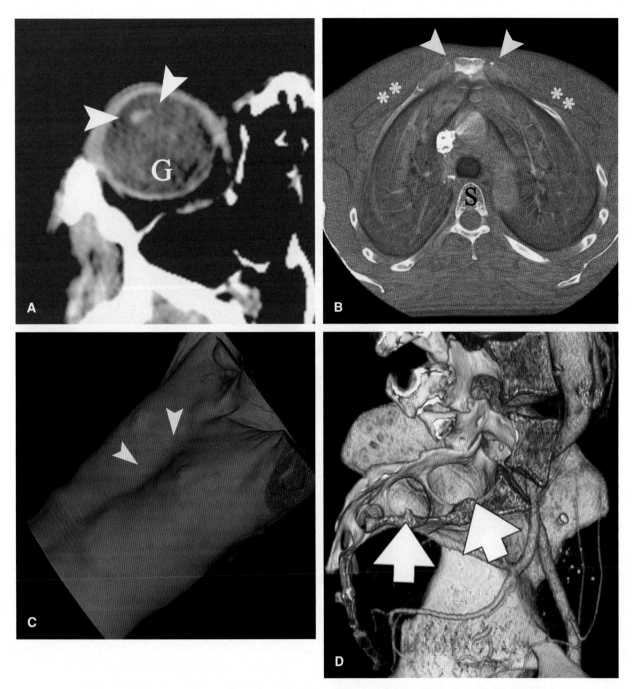

FIGURE 10-16 Extravascular manifestations of MFS. A: Axial image from head CT in a patient with MFS shows ectopia lentis, with displacement of the lens of the right eye (*arrowheads*). This finding can be seen in up to 60% of patients with MFS. (G, globe.) **B:** Subvolume volume-rendered CT image of the chest viewed from below shows prominent convex outward bowing of the sternum consistent with pectus carinatum. Note the anterior orientation of the ribs (******). (S, spine.) **C:** Volume-rendered image viewed tangentially in another patient with MFS shows severe pectus excavatum, with inward depression of the sternum (*arrowheads*) and narrowing in the anteroposterior diameter of the chest. **D:** Volume rendering of the sacrum and pelvis with a sagittal cut-plane demonstrates the expanded sacral spinal canal (*arrows*) due to dural ectasia. (*Figure 10-16 continues*)

the aortic root with a composite graft is a life-saving operation with low perioperative mortality and an excellent long-term prognosis (438–440). Reoperation of the aorta was necessary in 26% of patients during a 20-year follow-up (440).

Recent reports suggest that in closely monitored and adequately treated MFS, patient death is rarely due to ruptured aortic aneurysm or dissection and might be caused by ventricular arrythmias secondary to left ventricle dilation (435).

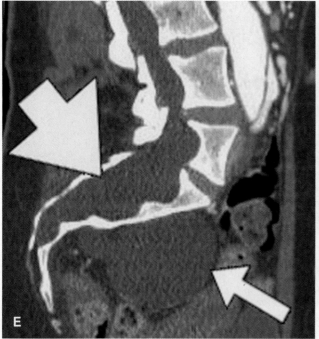

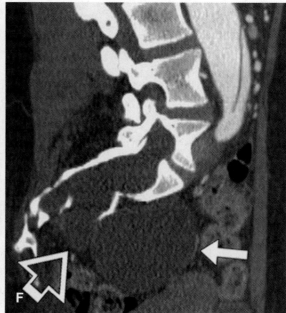

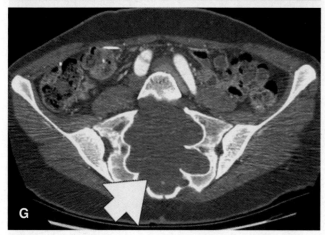

FIGURE 10-16 Continued E–G: Sagittal and parasagittal multiplanar reformations and a transverse section provide direct visualization of the dural ectasia (*large arrow*) and a large anterior meningocele (*small arrow*), which directly communicates with the dural sac through the left S3 neural foramen (*open arrow*). Note intimal flap of aortic dissection in the aorta and right common iliac artery. (Courtesy of Richard L. Hallett, M.D., and Geoffrey D. Rubin, M.D.)

Ehlers-Danlos Syndrome, Vascular Type

Ehlers-Danlos syndrome, vascular type (EDS-IV) (acrogeria; EDS type IV; Ehlers-Danlos syndrome type IV; Ehlers-Danlos syndrome, arterial-ecchymotic type; Sack-Barabas syndrome) is an autosomal dominant disorder linked to a mutation of the gene encoding procollagen type III. About 50% of new cases arise from spontaneous mutations. Estimated prevalence of EDS-IV is 1 in 50,000 to 100,000 people.

Clinical Presentation

Affected individuals have thin, translucent, fragile, easily bruising skin and a characteristic face with large eyes, small chin, thin lips, and nose and joint hypermobility. This connective tissue defect results in a propensity for the spontaneous rupture of arteries, intestines, uterus, pleura (with resulting pneumothorax), tendons, and muscles. Individu-

als with EDS-IV may suffer from chronic joint subluxations and varicose veins at an early age. Vascular and GI complications or organ rupture are the initial presenting events in 70% of adults with EDS-IV (441–445).

A review of over 400 EDS-IV patients revealed high morbidity and mortality. By the age of 20, 25% of patients had one complication, and by the age of 40, up to 80% had one or more complications. The calculated median lifespan of EDS-V individuals was 48 years. Arterial rupture was the major cause of death. Almost 15% of pregnant women died. Bowel rupture accounted for 25% of the complications but rarely resulted in death (442).

Vascular complications (Fig. 10-18) include spontaneous arterial rupture with or without preceding aneurysm, arterial dissection, and the formation of arteriovenous fistulas. Arterial rupture may affect any artery but

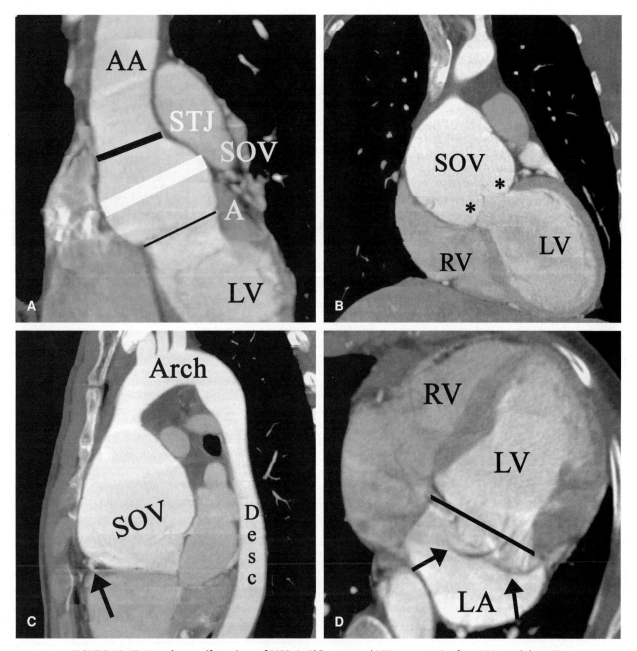

FIGURE 10-17 Vascular manifestations of MFS. A: Oblique coronal MIP reconstruction from ECG-gated chest CTA shows dilated annulus (*A, thin black line*) and sinuses of Valsalva (*SOV, white line*), measuring 33 and 47 mm, respectively. There is a normal-sized sinotubular junction (*STJ, thick black line*), measuring 29 mm. **B:** Marked root dilatation in another patient with MFS. The sinuses of Valsalva (*SOV*) measured 89 mm, with annulus measuring 37 mm. There is incomplete coaptation of the aortic valve leaflets (∗), leading to aortic regurgitation and dilatation of the left ventricle (*LV*). (*RV*, right ventricle.) **C:** Sagittal reconstruction of the aorta of the patient in (**B**) shows the "green onion" appearance of the preferential annuloaortic dilatation. (SOV, sinuses of Valsalva; Arch, thoracic aortic arch; Desc, descending thoracic aorta.) **D:** Four-chamber view from ECG-gated chest CTA shows prolapse of the mitral valve leaflets (*arrows*) into the left atrium (*LA*) when the mitral valve is closed, consistent with mitral valve prolapse. The *black line* indicates the level of the mitral valve annulus. (LV, left ventricle; RV, right ventricle.) (*Figure 10-17 continues*)

is most prevalent within the thorax and abdomen (444, 446,447).

Diagnosis is based on the clinical presentation and a positive family history. Specific clinical diagnostic criteria have been developed (444). In suspected cases, diagnosis should be confirmed by biochemical tests. Genetic testing is available for patients with positive biochemical tests (444).

Catastrophic events in EDS-IV patients require emergency procedures. Surgery for intestinal perforation is usually successful and lifesaving. Arterial rupture is

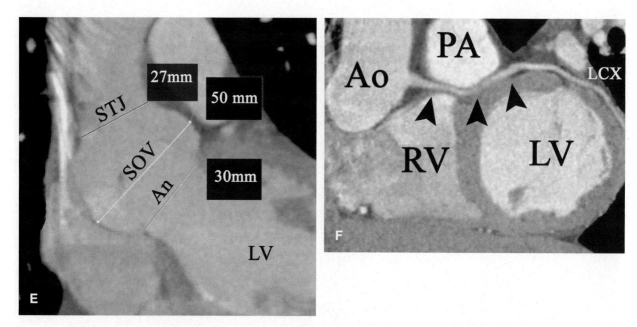

FIGURE 10-17 Continued E: Oblique coronal MIP reconstruction of a 35-year-old physician with MFS, evaluated by ECG-gated chest CTA to exclude dissection. There was evidence of annuloaortic ectasia, with annulus (*An*) measuring 30 mm, sinuses of Valsalva (*SOV*) measuring 50 mm, and sinotubular junction (*STJ*) measuring 27mm. There is no dissection. **F:** Curved-planar reconstruction of left coronary system in the same patient as **(E)** shows existence of an anomalous left main coronary artery originating from the right coronary cusp. The aberrant vessel (*arrowheads*) then courses between the aorta (*Ao*) and the right ventricular outflow tract (*RV*) and pulmonary trunk (*PA*) before giving off the left anterior descending (LAD) and circumflex (*LCX*) branches. This variant can predispose to sudden cardiac death. (LV, left ventricle.) (Courtesy of Richard L. Hallett, M.D., and Geoffrey D. Rubin, M.D.)

frequently fatal (448), and surgical repair is difficult due to the fragility of arteries (449). Occasionally, an endovascular approach may be helpful (450,451).

A conservative approach is recommended, if possible, in EDS-IV patients. In nonurgent patient evaluations, invasive studies should be avoided. Noninvasive imaging is preferred because needle puncture for catheterization can result in arterial laceration and dissection or rupture. CT and MR angiography offer a minimally invasive method for diagnosis and therapy planning, and yield much valuable information for the requesting surgeon or interventionalist. The value of screening EDS-IV patients for aneurysm is doubtful, since arterial rupture frequently happens in nondilated arteries (444).

Hypereosinophilic Syndrome

The idiopathic hypereosinophilic syndrome (HES) is a good example of a condition in which vasculitis is not a prominent feature, but may occur and result in significant morbidity and mortality (Figure 10-19). This condition has heterogeneous clinical manifestations with the common features of prolonged eosinophilia of an undetectable cause and organ system dysfunction. It

affects predominantly men (male-to-female ratio is 9:1) and can occur at any age, but 70% of the patients have onset of disease between 20 and 50 years of age (452,453).

Initial presentation usually consists of nonspecific symptoms, and eosinophilia is sometimes discovered incidentally during routine laboratory tests. Virtually any organ can be affected, but cardiovascular involvement is the major source of morbidity and mortality. Empiric criteria based on clinical (a wide spectrum of signs and symptoms and lack of evidence of recognized causes of eosinophilia) and laboratory findings (persistent eosinophilia of 1,500 eosinophils/mm^3 for at least 6 months) are used to establish the diagnosis (452).

Postmortem specimens have shown injury to the endothelial cells of the endocardium and microvasculature thought to be secondary to eosinophilia (although the precise mechanism whereby eosinophils exert their tissue damaging effects is poorly understood). This results in endocardial fibrosis, restrictive endomyocardiopathy, and thrombosis. Heart failure may be relentlessly progressive—its course varying from days to years. Reported prognosis is variable in the literature, but studies have consistently shown high

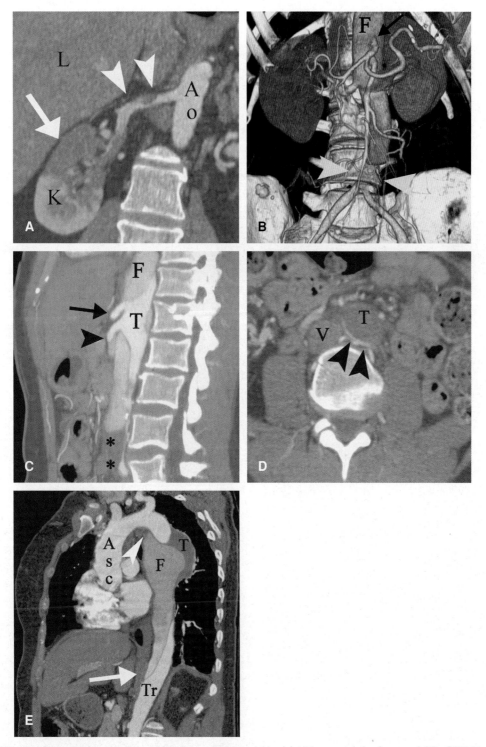

FIGURE 10-18 EDS-IV: vascular complications. A: Coronal thin-slab MIP reconstruction from renal CTA of EDS-IV patient. There is a dissection (*arrowheads*) extending from the right main renal artery to the renal hilum and upper pole branches. There are ischemic hypoperfusion changes in the upper pole (*arrow*) of the right kidney (*K*). (L, liver; Ao, aorta.) **B–D:** Windsock abdominal aortic dissection in another patient with EDS-IV. **B:** Volume-rendered coronal image shows termination of the contrast column in the distal abdominal aorta (*arrowheads*). The celiac axis (*arrow*) and SMA arise from the true lumen, evidenced by their increased opacity (with these opacity transfer settings) compared with the false lumen (*F*). **C:** Sagittal MIP image demonstrates fenestration of the false lumen by the celiac (*arrow*) and SMA (*arrowhead*) as well as thrombus (**) in the windsock portion of the distal abdominal aorta, which has invaginated upon itself. **D:** Axial image at aortic bifurcation demonstrates thrombus (*T*) filling the invaginated portion of the aorta, with marked compression of the flow (true) lumen (*arrowheads*). (V, inferior vena cava.) **E:** Sagittal reconstruction of chest CTA in another patient with EDS-IV demonstrates a Stanford type B dissection, which originates along the undersurface of the arch (*arrowhead*) and extends to the supraceliac abdominal aorta (*arrow*). The dissection does not involve the ascending thoracic aorta (*Asc*). There is aneurysmal enlargement of the false lumen (*F*), which also contains thrombus (*T*). (Tr, true lumen.) (Courtesy of Richard L. Hallett, M.D., and Geoffrey D. Rubin, M.D.)

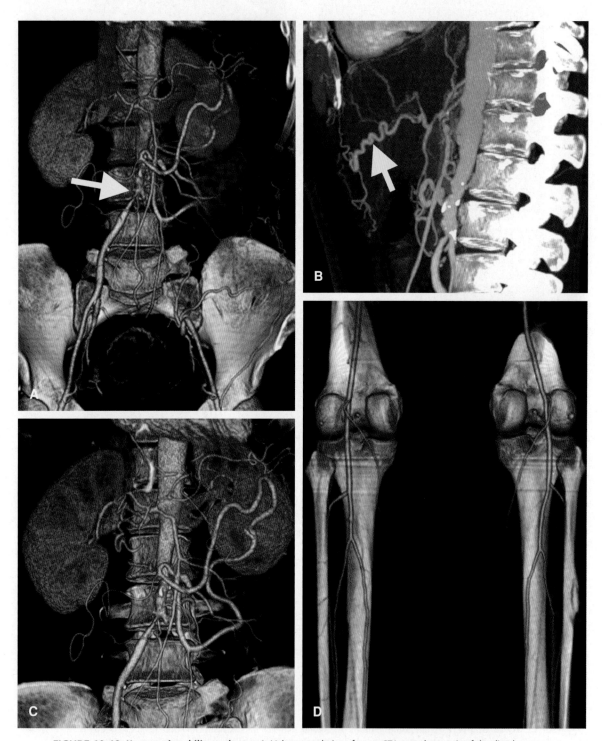

FIGURE 10-19 Hypereosinophilic syndrome. A: Volume renderings from a CTA reveal stenosis of the distal aorta and the proximal right common iliac artery (*arrow*). The left common iliac artery is occluded with the left external iliac artery reconstituted by collaterals from the left internal iliac artery. **B:** A lateral MIP reveals that the celiac, superior mesenteric artery (SMA) and inferior mesenteric artery (IMA) origins are occluded and supplied by abdominal and pelvic sidewall collaterals (*arrow*). **C:** A large, meandering artery provides collateral flow between the SMA and IMA. **D:** Arteries in both lower limbs are unremarkable. (Courtesy of Carlo Catalano, M.D., University of Rome.)

mortality, including an average survival of 9 months and a 3-year survival of 12% in a review of 57 patients. Therapy consists of corticosteroids titrated to control the progression of the disease, sometimes combined with chemotherapeutic agents such as hydroxyurea. Surgical intervention is also warranted in patients with cardiovascular complications. Of note, organ system dysfunction may be seen in some patients with eosinophilia of a known cause, such as those secondary to drug reactions and parasitic diseases (452,453).

REFERENCES

1. Savage COS, Harper L, Cockwell P, et al. ABC of arterial and vascular disease: vasculitis. BMJ. 2000;320(7245):1325–1328.
2. Yalcindag A, Sundel R. Vasculitis in childhood. *Curr Opin Rheumatol.* 2000;13(5):422–427.
3. Jennette JC, et al. Nomenclature of systemic vasculitides. Proposal of an international consensus conference. *Arthritis Rheum.* 1994;37(2):187–192.
4. Johnston SL, Lock RJ, Gompels MM. Takayasu arteritis: a review. *J Clin Pathol.* 2002;55(7):481–486.
5. Numano F, et al. Takayasu's arteritis. *Lancet.* 2000;356(9234):1023–1025.
6. Hotchi M., Pathological studies on Takayasu arteritis. *Heart Vessels Suppl.* 1992;7:11–17.
7. Hall S, Barr W, Lie JT, et al. Takayasu's arteritis. A study of 32 North American patients. *Medicine (Baltimore).* 1985;64(2):89–99.
8. Lupi-Herrera E., et al. Takayasu's arteritis. Clinical study of 107 cases. *Am Heart J.* 1977;93(1):94–103.
9. Robles M, Reyes PA. Takayasu's arteritis in Mexico: a clinical review of 44 consecutive cases. *Clin Exp Rheumatol.* 1994;12(4):381–388.
10. Jain S, et al. Takayasu arteritis in children and young Indians. *Int J Cardiol.* 2000;75[Suppl 1]:S153–S157.
11. Arend WP, et al. The American College of Rheumatology 1990 criteria for the classification of Takayasu arteritis. *Arthritis Rheum.* 1990;33(8):1129–1134.
12. Sharma BK, et al. Diagnostic criteria for Takayasu arteritis. *Int J Cardiol.* 1996;54(suppl):S141–S147.
13. Watts RA, Scott DG. Classification and epidemiology of the vasculitides. *Baillieres Clin Rheumatol.* 1997;11(2):191–217.
14. Sato EI, et al. Takayasu arteritis. Treatment and prognosis in a university center in Brazil. *Int J Cardiol.* 2000;75[Suppl 1]:S163–S166.
15. Sharma S, et al. The association between aneurysm formation and systemic hypertension in Takayasu's arteritis. *Clin Radiol.* 1990;42(3):182–187.
16. Numano F. Differences in clinical presentation and outcome in different countries for Takayasu's arteritis. *Curr Opin Rheumatol.* 1997;9(1):12–15.
17. Moriwaki R, et al. Clinical manifestations of Takayasu arteritis in India and Japan—new classification of angiographic findings. *Angiology.* 1997;48(5):369–379.
18. Subramanyan R, Joy J, Balakrishnan KG. Natural history of aortoarteritis (Takayasu's disease). *Circulation.* 1989;80(3):429–437.
19. Ishikawa K. Natural history and classification of occlusive thromboaortopathy (Takayasu's disease). *Circulation.* 1978;57(1):27–35.
20. Fraga A, Medina F. Takayasu's arteritis. *Curr Rheumatol Rep.* 2002;4(1):30–38.
21. Matsunaga N, et al. Takayasu arteritis: MR manifestations and diagnosis of acute and chronic phase. *J Magn Reson Imaging.* 1998;8(2):406–414.
22. Atalay MK, Bluemke DA. Magnetic resonance imaging of large vessel vasculitis. *Curr Opin Rheumatol.* 2001;13(1):41–47.
23. Sharma BK, Jain S, Radotra BD. An autopsy study of Takayasu arteritis in India. *Int J Cardiol.* 1998;66[Suppl 1]:S85–S90; discussion S91.
24. Calabrese LH, Hoffman GS, Clough JD. Systemic vasculitis. In: Young JR, Olin JW, Bartholomew LE, eds. *Peripheral Vascular Diseases.* St. Louis: Mosby–Year Book; 1996:380–406.
25. Hoffman GS, Ahmed AE. Surrogate markers of disease activity in patients with Takayasu arteritis. A preliminary report from the International Network for the Study of the Systemic Vasculitides (INSSYS). *Int J Cardiol.* 1998;66[Suppl 1]:S191–S194; discussion S195.
26. Noris M, et al. Interleukin-6 and RANTES in Takayasu arteritis: a guide for therapeutic decisions? *Circulation.* 1999;100(1):55–60.
27. Matsuyama A, et al. Matrix metalloproteinases as novel disease markers in Takayasu arteritis. *Circulation.* 2003;108(12):1469–1473.
28. Hoffman GS. Treatment of resistant Takayasu's arteritis. *Rheum Dis Clin North Am.* 1995;21(1):73–-80.
29. Wernick R, Davey M, Bonafede P. Familial giant cell arteritis: report of an HLA-typed sibling pair and a review of the literature. *Clin Exp Rheumatol.* 1994;12(1):63–66.
30. Weyand CM, Goronzy JJ. Molecular approaches toward pathologic mechanisms in giant cell arteritis and Takayasu's arteritis. *Curr Opin Rheumatol.* 1995;7(1):30–36.
31. Liu NH, et al. The epidemiology of giant cell arteritis: a 12-year retrospective study. *Ophthalmology.* 2001;108(6):1145–1149.
32. Emmerich J, Fiessinger JN. [Epidemiology and etiological factors in giant cell arteritis (Horton's disease and Takayasu's disease).] *Ann Med Interne (Paris).* 1998;149(7):425–432.
33. Gonzalez EB, et al. Giant-cell arteritis in the southern United States. An 11-year retrospective study from the Texas Gulf Coast. *Arch Intern Med.* 1989;149(7):1561–1565.
34. Lie JT. Aortic and extracranial large vessel giant cell arteritis: a review of 72 cases with histopathologic documentation. *Semin Arthritis Rheum.* 1995;24(6):422–431.
35. Levine SM, Hellmann DB. Giant cell arteritis. *Curr Opin Rheumatol.* 2002;14(1):3–10.
36. Brack A, et al. Disease pattern in cranial and large-vessel giant cell arteritis. *Arthritis Rheum.* 1999;42(2):311–317.
37. Kariv R, Sidid Y, Gur H. Systemic vasculitis presenting as a tumorlike lesion. Four case reports and an analysis of 79 reported cases. *Medicine (Baltimore).* 2000;79(6):349–359.
38. Procter CD Sr, Hollier LH, Trosclair CM. Temporal arteritis. Clinical implications for the vascular surgeon. *J Cardiovasc Surg (Torino).* 1992;33(5):599–603.
39. Chmelewski WL, et al. Presenting features and outcomes in patients undergoing temporal artery biopsy. A review of 98 patients. *Arch Intern Med.* 1992;152(8):1690–1695.
40. Hellmann DB. Temporal arteritis: a cough, toothache, and tongue infarction. *JAMA.* 2002;287(22):2996–3000.
41. Nordborg C, Nordborg E, Petursdottir V. The pathogenesis of giant cell arteritis: morphological aspects. *Clin Exp Rheumatol.* 2000; 18[4 Suppl 20]:S18–S21.
42. Stanson AW. Imaging findings in extracranial (giant cell) temporal arteritis. *Clin Exp Rheumatol.* 2000;18[4 Suppl 20]:S43–S48.
43. Birkhead NC, Wagener HP, Shick RM. Treatment of temporal arteritis with adrenal corticosteroids; results in fifty-five cases in which lesion was proved at biopsy. *J Am Med Assoc.* 1957;163(10):821–827.
44. Hamano K, et al. An ascending aortic aneurysm caused by giant cell arteritis: report of a case. *Surg Today.* 1999;29(9):957–959.
45. Cogan DG. Ophthalmic manifestations of systemic vascular disease. *Major Probl Intern Med.* 1974;3(0):1–187.
46. Oldenski R. Cogan syndrome: autoimmune-mediated audiovestibular symptoms and ocular inflammation. *J Am Board Fam Pract.* 1993;6(6):577–581.

47. Haynes BF, et al. Cogan syndrome: studies in thirteen patients, long-term follow-up, and a review of the literature. *Medicine (Baltimore)*. 1980;59(6):426–441.

48. Vollertsen RS, et al. Cogan's syndrome: 18 cases and a review of the literature. *Mayo Clin Proc*. 1986;61(5): 344–361.

49. Tseng JF, et al. Thoracoabdominal aortic aneurysm in Cogan's syndrome. *J Vasc Surg*. 1999;30(3):565–568.

50. Ferrari E, et al. [Cardiovascular manifestations of Cogan syndrome. Apropos of a case.] *Arch Mal Coeur Vaiss*. 1992;85(6):913–916.

51. Gaubitz M, et al. Cogan's syndrome: organ-specific autoimmune disease or systemic vasculitis? A report of two cases and review of the literature. *Clin Exp Rheumatol*. 2001; 19(4):463–469.

52. Cheson BD, Bluming AZ, Alroy J. Cogan's syndrome: a systemic vasculitis. *Am J Med*. 1976;60(4):549–555.

53. St. Clair EW, McCallum RM. Cogan's syndrome. *Curr Opin Rheumatol*. 1999;11(1):47–52.

54. Scolding NJ, et al. Cerebral vasculitis—recognition, diagnosis and management. *QJM*. 1997;90(1):61–73.

55. Lie JT. Primary (granulomatous) angiitis of the central nervous system: a clinicopathologic analysis of 15 new cases and a review of the literature. *Hum Pathol*. 1992;23(2); 164–171.

56. Panda KM, et al. Primary angiitis of CNS: neuropathological study of three autopsied cases with brief review of literature. *Neurol India*. 2000;48(2):149–154.

57. Reuter M, et al. [Radiology of the primary systemic vasculitides.] *Rofo Fortschr Geb Rontgenstr Neuen Bildgeb Verfahr*. 2003;175(9):1184–1192.

58. Wynne PJ, et al. Radiographic features of central nervous system vasculitis. *Neurol Clin*. 1997;15(4):779–804.

59. West SG. Central nervous system vasculitis. *Curr Rheumatol Rep*. 2003;5(2):116–127.

60. Trepo C, Guillevin L. Polyarteritis nodosa and extrahepatic manifestations of HBV infection: the case against autoimmune intervention in pathogenesis. *J Autoimmun*. 2001;16(3):269–274.

61. Marcellin P, et al. Latent hepatitis B virus (HBV) infection in systemic necrotizing vasculitis. *Clin Exp Rheumatol*. 1991;9(1):23–28.

62. Johnson RM, Barbarini G, Barbaro G. Kawasaki-like syndromes and other vasculitic syndromes in HIV-infected patients. *Aids*. 2003;17[Suppl 1]:S77–S82.

63. Meyer MF, et al. Cytomegalovirus infection in systemic necrotizing vasculitis: causative agent or opportunistic infection? *Rheumatol Int*. 2000;20(1):35–38.

64. Gaches F, et al. [Periarteritis nodosa and parvovirus B19 infection.] *Rev Med Interne*. 1993;14(5):323–325.

65. Lhote F, Cohen P, Guillevin L. Polyarteritis nodosa, microscopic polyangiitis and Churg-Strauss syndrome. *Lupus*. 1998;7(4):238–258.

66. Uyama H, et al. [A case of polyarteritis nodosa presenting with multiple intrarenal aneurysms and accelerated hypertension.] *Nippon Jinzo Gakkai Shi*. 1995;37(1):57–61.

67. Brogan PA, et al. Renal angiography in children with polyarteritis nodosa. *Pediatr Nephrol*. 2002;17(4):277–283.

68. Provenzale JM, Allen NB. Neuroradiologic findings in polyarteritis nodosa. *AJNR Am J Neuroradiol*. 1996;17(6): 1119–1126.

69. Folwaczny C, et al. [Recurrent abdominal colic, myalgia and mononeuritis multiplex.] *Z Gastroenterol*. 1998;36(9):839–845.

70. Daoud MS, Hutton KP, Gibson LE. Cutaneous periarteritis nodosa: a clinicopathological study of 79 cases. *Br J Dermatol*. 1997;136(5):706–713.

71. Levine SM, Hellmann DB, Stone JH. Gastrointestinal involvement in polyarteritis nodosa (1986-2000): presentation and outcomes in 24 patients. *Am J Med*. 2002;112(5):386–391.

72. Cacoub P, et al. [Causes of death in systemic vasculitis of polyarteritis nodosa. Analysis of a series of 165 patients.] *Ann Med Interne (Paris)*. 1988;139(6):381–390.

73. Ozcay N, et al. Polyarteritis nodosa presenting with necrotising appendicitis and hepatic aneurysm rupture. *Turk J Gastroenterol*. 2003;14(1):68–70.

74. Stanson AW, et al. Polyarteritis nodosa: spectrum of angiographic findings. Radiographics. 2001;21(1):151–159.

75. Munn EJ, et al. Polyarteritis with symptomatic intracerebral aneurysms at initial presentation. *J Rheumatol*. 1998; 25(10):2022–2025.

76. Harada M, et al. Polyarthritis nodosa with mesenteric aneurysms demonstrated by angiography: report of a case and successful treatment of the patient with prednisolone and cyclophosphamide. *J Gastroenterol*. 1999;34(6):702–705.

77. Kastner D, Gaffney M, Tak T. Polyarteritis nodosa and myocardial infarction. *Can J Cardiol*. 2000;16(4):515–518.

78. Chu KH, et al. Polyarteritis nodosa presenting as acute myocardial infarction with coronary dissection. *Cathet Cardiovasc Diagn*. 1998;44(3):320–324.

79. Plumley SG, et al. Polyarteritis nodosa presenting as polymyositis. *Semin Arthritis Rheum*. 2002;31(6):377–383.

80. Ohkoshi N, et al. Sural nerve biopsy in vasculitic neuropathies: morphometric analysis of the caliber of involved vessels. *J Med*. 1996;27(3–4):153–170.

81. Hawke SH, et al. Vasculitic neuropathy. A clinical and pathological study. *Brain*. 1991;114(Pt 5):2175–2190.

82. Travers RL, et al. Polyarteritis nodosa: a clinical and angiographic analysis of 17 cases. *Semin Arthritis Rheum*. 1979;8(3):184–199.

83. Guillevin L. Treatment of classic polyarteritis nodosa in 1999. *Nephrol Dial Transplant*. 1999;14(9):2077–2079.

84. Erhardt A, et al. Successful treatment of hepatitis B virus associated polyarteritis nodosa with a combination of prednisolone, alpha-interferon and lamivudine. *J Hepatol*. 2000;33(4):677–683.

85. Filer A, et al. Successful treatment of hepatitis B-associated vasculitis using lamivudine as the sole therapeutic agent. *Rheumatology (Oxford)*. 2001;40(9):1064–1065.

86. Deleaval P, et al. Life-threatening complications of hepatitis B virus-related polyarteritis nodosa developing despite interferon-alpha2b therapy: successful treatment with a combination of interferon, lamivudine, plasma exchanges and steroids. *Clin Rheumatol*. 2001;20(4):290–292.

87. Burns JC, et al. Kawasaki disease: a brief history. *Pediatrics*. 2000;106(2):E27.

88. Burns JC, et al. Sequelae of Kawasaki disease in adolescents and young adults. *J Am Coll Cardiol*. 1996;28(1): 253–257.

89. Kuijpers TW, et al. Longstanding obliterative panarteritis in Kawasaki disease: lack of cyclosporin A effect. *Pediatrics*. 2003;112(4):986–992.

90. Chang JS, et al. Kawasaki disease complicated by peripheral gangrene. *Pediatr Cardiol*. 1999;20(2):139–142.

91. Tomita S, et al. Peripheral gangrene associated with Kawasaki disease. *Clin Infect Dis*. 1992;14(1):121–126.

92. Brenner JL, et al. Severe Kawasaki disease in infants: two fatal cases. *Can J Cardiol*. 2000;16(8):1017–1023.

93. Bradway MW, Drezner AD. Popliteal aneurysm presenting as acute thrombosis and ischemia in a middle-aged man with a history of Kawasaki disease. *J Vasc Surg*. 1997;26(5):884–887.

94. Scottt JS, Ettedgui JA, Neches WH. Cost-effective use of echocardiography in children with Kawasaki disease. *Pediatrics*. 1999;104(5):e57.

95. Peduzzi TL, Pitetti RD. Myocardial infarction and atypical Kawasaki disease in a 3-month-old infant. *Pediatr Emerg Care*. 2002;18(5):E16–E19.

96. Kitamura S. The role of coronary bypass operation on children with Kawasaki disease. *Coron Artery Dis*. 2002;13(8): 437–447.

97. Kato H, Koike S, Yokoyama T. Kawasaki disease: effect of treatment on coronary artery involvement. *Pediatrics*. 1979;63(2):175–179.

98. Dale RC, et al. Treatment of severe complicated Kawasaki disease with oral prednisolone and aspirin. *J Pediatr*. 2000;137(5):723–726.

99. Takwoingi YM, Dempster JH. Wegener's granulomatosis: an analysis of 33 patients seen over a 10-year period. *Clin Otolaryngol*. 2003;28(3):187–194.
100. Reinhold-Keller E, et al. No difference in the incidences of vasculitides between north and south Germany: first results of the German vasculitis register. *Rheumatology (Oxford)*. 2002;41(5):540–549.
101. Koldingsnes W, Nossent H. Epidemiology of Wegener's granulomatosis in northern Norway. *Arthritis Rheum*. 2000;43(11):2481–2487.
102. Watts RA, et al. Epidemiology of systemic vasculitis: a ten-year study in the United Kingdom. *Arthritis Rheum*. 2000;43(2):414–419.
103. Gross WL. [Wegener's granulomatosis: immunologic aspects of diagnosis, etiology and therapy.] *Immun Infekt*. 1987;15(1):15–25.
104. Shitrit D, et al. Large vessel aneurysms in Wegener's granulomatosis. *J Vasc Surg*. 2002;36(4):856–858.
105. Jordan JM, Rowe WT, Allen NB. Wegener's granulomatosis involving the breast. Report of three cases and review of the literature. *Am J Med*. 1987;83(1):159–164.
106. Lie JT. Wegener's granulomatosis: histological documentation of common and uncommon manifestations in 216 patients. *VASA*. 1997;26(4):261–270.
107. Leavitt RY, et al. The American College of Rheumatology 1990 criteria for the classification of Wegener's granulomatosis. *Arthritis Rheum*. 1990;33(8):1101–1107.
108. Hoffman GS, et al. Wegener granulomatosis: an analysis of 158 patients. *Ann Intern Med*. 1992;116(6):488–498.
109. Sneller MC, et al. An analysis of forty-two Wegener's granulomatosis patients treated with methotrexate and prednisone. *Arthritis Rheum*. 1995;38(5):608–613.
110. Design of the Wegener's Granulomatosis Etanercept Trial (WGET). *Control Clin Trials*. 2002;23(4):450–468.
111. Gause A, Arbach O, Lamprecht P. [Treatment of primary systemic vasculitis with TNF alpha-antagonists.] *Z Rheumatol*. 2003;62(3):228–234.
112. Lhote F, et al. Microscopic polyangiitis: clinical aspects and treatment. *Ann Med Interne (Paris)*. 1996;147(3):165–177.
113. Lauque D, Pourrat J. [Microscopic polyangiitis.] *Rev Prat*. 2000;50(3):268–270.
114. Lauque D, et al. Microscopic polyangiitis with alveolar hemorrhage. A study of 29 cases and review of the literature. Groupe d'Etudes et de Recherche sur les Maladies "Orphelines" Pulmonaires (GERM"O"P). *Medicine (Baltimore)*. 2000;79(4):222–233.
115. Hagen EC, et al. Diagnostic value of standardized assays for anti-neutrophil cytoplasmic antibodies in idiopathic systemic vasculitis. EC/BCR Project for ANCA Assay Standardization. *Kidney Int*. 1998;53(3):743–753.
116. Savige J, et al. Addendum to the International Consensus Statement on testing and reporting of antineutrophil cytoplasmic antibodies. Quality control guidelines, comments, and recommendations for testing in other autoimmune diseases. *Am J Clin Pathol*. 2003;120(3):312–318.
117. Guillevin L, Pagnoux C. When should immunosuppressants be prescribed to treat systemic vasculitides? *Intern Med*. 2003;42(4):313–317.
118. Guillevin L, et al. Treatment of polyarteritis nodosa and microscopic polyangiitis with poor prognosis factors: a prospective trial comparing glucocorticoids and six or twelve cyclophosphamide pulses in sixty-five patients. *Arthritis Rheum*. 2003;49(1):93–100.
119. Venetz JP, Rossert J. [Microscopic polyangiitis.] *Ann Med Interne (Paris)*. 2000;151(3):193–198.
120. Watts RA, Carruthers DM, Scott DG. Epidemiology of systemic vasculitis: changing incidence or definition? *Semin Arthritis Rheum*. 1995;25(1):28–34.
121. Guillevin L, et al. Churg-Strauss syndrome. Clinical study and long-term follow-up of 96 patients. *Medicine (Baltimore)*. 1999;78(1):26–37.
122. Lanham JG, et al. Systemic vasculitis with asthma and eosinophilia: a clinical approach to the Churg-Strauss syndrome. *Medicine (Baltimore)*. 1984;63(2):65–81.
123. Leon-Ruiz L, et al. Churg-Strauss syndrome complicated by endomyocardial fibrosis and intraventricular thrombus. Importance of the echocardiography for the diagnosis of asymptomatic phases of potentially severe cardiac complications. *Lupus*. 2002;11(11):765–767.
124. Ames PR, et al. Thrombosis in Churg-Strauss syndrome. Beyond vasculitis? *Br J Rheumatol*. 1996;35(11):1181–1183.
125. Churg A. Recent advances in the diagnosis of Churg-Strauss syndrome. *Mod Pathol*. 2001;14(12):1284–1293.
126. Masi AT, et al. The American College of Rheumatology 1990 criteria for the classification of Churg-Strauss syndrome (allergic granulomatosis and angiitis). *Arthritis Rheum*. 1990;33(8):1094–1100.
127. Guillevin L, et al. Prognostic factors in polyarteritis nodosa and Churg-Strauss syndrome. A prospective study in 342 patients. *Medicine (Baltimore)*. 1996;75(1):17–28.
128. Lee HS, et al. Henoch-Schoenlein nephritis in adults: a clinical and morphological study. *Clin Nephrol*. 1986;26(3):125–130.
129. Ayoub EM, et al. Role of Bartonella henselae in the etiology of Henoch-Schonlein purpura. *Pediatr Infect Dis J*. 2002;21(1):28–31.
130. Kawasaki Y, et al. Clinical and pathological features of children with Henoch-Schoenlein purpura nephritis: risk factors associated with poor prognosis. *Clin Nephrol*. 2003;60(3):153–160.
131. Worth DP. Immunosuppression in rapidly progressive Henoch-Schoenlein nephritis. *Clin Nephrol*. 1996;45(2):135–136.
132. Paller AS, Kelly K, Sethi R. Pulmonary hemorrhage: an often fatal complication of Henoch-Schoenlein purpura. *Pediatr Dermatol*. 1997;14(4):299–302.
133. Aqel MB, Olin JW. Thromboangiitis obliterans (Buerger's disease). *Vasc Med*. 1997;2(1):61–66.
134. Lie JT. The rise and fall and resurgence of thromboangiitis obliterans (Buerger's disease). *Acta Pathol Jpn*. 1989;39(3):153–158.
135. Lie JT. Thromboangiitis obliterans (Buerger's disease) revisited. *Pathol Annu*. 1988;23(Pt 2):257–291.
136. Mishima Y. [Japanese clinical statistical data of patients with Buerger's disease.] *Nippon Rinsho*. 1992;50(suppl):361–367.
137. Matsushita M, et al. Decrease in prevalence of Buerger's disease in Japan. *Surgery*. 1998;124(3):498–502.
138. Matsushita M, Shionoya S, Matsumoto T. Urinary cotinine measurement in patients with Buerger's disease—effects of active and passive smoking on the disease process. *J Vasc Surg*. 1991;14(1):53–58.
139. Szuba A, Cooke JP. Thromboangiitis obliterans. An update on Buerger's disease. *West J Med*. 1998;168(4):255–260.
140. Lie JT. Visceral intestinal Buerger's disease. *Int J Cardiol*. 1998;66[Suppl 1]:S249–S256.
141. Campello Morer I, et al. [Thromboangiitis obliterans with cerebral involvement.] *Neurologia*. 1995;10(9):384–386.
142. Kim KS, et al. Acute myocardial infarction in a patient with Buerger's disease. A case report and a review of the literature. *Korean J Intern Med*. 1987;2(2):278–281.
143. Hagen B, Lohse S. Clinical and radiologic aspects of Buerger's disease. *Cardiovasc Intervent Radiol*. 1984;7(6):283–293.
144. Suzuki S, et al. Buerger's disease (thromboangiitis obliterans): an analysis of the arteriograms of 119 cases. *Clin Radiol*. 1982;33(2):235–240.
145. Fiessinger JN, Shafer M. Trial of iloprost versus aspirin treatment for critical limb ischaemia of thromboangiitis obliterans. The TAO Study. *Lancet*. 1990;335(8689):555–557.
146. Shindo S, et al. Arterial reconstruction in Buerger's disease: by-pass to disease-free collaterals. *Int Angiol*. 2002;21(3):228–232.
147. Shionoya S. Buerger's disease: diagnosis and management. *Cardiovasc Surg*. 1993;1(3):207–214.
148. Ohta T, Shionoya S. Fate of the ischaemic limb in Buerger's disease. *Br J Surg*. 1988;75(3):259–262.

149. Hodgson TJ, Gaines PA, Beard JD. Thrombolysis and angioplasty for acute lower limb ischemia in Buerger's disease. *Cardiovasc Intervent Radiol.* 1994;17(6):333–335.

150. Chang HK, Kim JW. The clinical features of Behçet's disease in Yongdong districts: analysis of a cohort followed from 1997 to 2001. *J Korean Med Sci.* 2002;17(6):784–789.

151. el Belhadji M, et al. [Ophthalmological involvement in Behçet disease. Apropos of 520 cases.] *J Fr Ophtalmol.* 1997; 20(8):592–598.

152. Martinez-Yelamos A, et al. [The involvement of the parenchyma of the central nervous system in Behçet disease.] *Rev Neurol.* 1998;27(156):223–225.

153. Kram MT, et al. Behçet's ileocolitis: successful treatment with tumor necrosis factor-alpha antibody (infliximab) therapy: report of a case. *Dis Colon Rectum.* 2003;46(1):118–121.

154. Houman MH, et al. Esophageal involvement in Behçet's disease. *Yonsei Med J.* 2002;43(4):457–460.

155. Song JK, et al. Echocardiographic and clinical characteristics of aortic regurgitation because of systemic vasculitis. *J Am Soc Echocardiogr.* 2003;16(8):850–857.

156. Lee LA. Behçet disease. *Semin Cutan Med Surg.* 2001;20(1):53–57.

157. Rakover Y, et al. Behçet disease: long-term follow-up of three children and review of the literature. *Pediatrics.* 1989;83(6):986–992.

158. Park JH. Clinical analysis of Behçet disease: arthritic manifestations in Behçet disease may present as seronegative rheumatoid arthritis or palindromic rheumatism. *Korean J Intern Med.* 1999;14(1):66–72.

159. Kchir MM, et al. [Destructive polyarthritis in Behçet's disease. Apropos of a case and review of the literature.] *Rev Med Interne.* 1992;13(3):211–214.

160. Kim JS, et al. Prediction of the clinical course of Behçet's colitis according to macroscopic classification by colonoscopy. *Endoscopy.* 2000;32(8):635–640.

161. Bayraktar Y, Ozaslan E, Van Thiel DH. Gastrointestinal manifestations of Behçet's disease. *J Clin Gastroenterol.* 2000;30(2):144–154.

162. Hasegawa Y, Okada H, Okamoto S. [Neuro-Behçet disease with bilateral cheiro-oral syndrome following simultaneous multiple brain hemorrhage.] *Rinsho Shinkeigaku.* 1991;31(7):754–759.

163. Meusser S, et al. [Manifestation of neuro-Behçet disease in cyclosporin A therapy.] *Z Rheumatol.* 1997;56(1):31–39.

164. Canhao P, Ferro JM, Freitas JP. [Neurologic manifestations of Behçet disease. Review of the caseload of the Neurology and Dermatology services at the Santa Maria Hospital.] *Acta Med Port.* 1992;5(7):369–371.

165. Chaloupka K, et al. [Cerebral sinus thrombosis in Behçet disease: case report and review of the literature.] *Klin Monatsbl Augenheilkd.* 2003;220(3):186–188.

166. Hata T, et al. [Behçet disease with superior sagittal sinus and inferior vena caval thrombosis.] *Rinsho Shinkeigaku.* 1988;28(10):1217–1224.

167. Proebstle TM, et al. [Behçet disease with primary involvement of the cerebral vessels.] *Dtsch Med Wochenschr.* 1996;121(1–2):16–20.

168. Ashjazadeh N, et al. Neuro-Behçet's disease: a masquerader of multiple sclerosis. A prospective study of neurologic manifestations of Behçet's disease in 96 Iranian patients. *Exp Mol Pathol.* 2003;74(1):17–22.

169. Sagdic K, et al. Venous lesions in Behçet's disease. *Eur J Vasc Endovasc Surg.* 1996;11(4):437–440.

170. Grana Gil J, et al. [Vascular manifestations in 30 cases of Behçet's disease.] *Rev Clin Esp.* 1992;191(7):375–379.

171. Barlas S. Behçet's disease. An insight from a vascular surgeon's point of view. *Acta Chir Belg.* 1999;99(6):274–281.

172. Nonaka K, et al. [Pseudo-aneurysm of aortic arch and rupture into pericardium, a case report of successful surgical management.] *Jpn J Thorac Cardiovasc Surg.* 1998;46(8): 772–776.

173. Bensaid Y, et al. [Arterial complications of Behçet's disease. Report of 13 cases.] *J Mal Vasc.* 1997;22(1):24–28.

174. Berkmen T. MR angiography of aneurysms in Behçet disease: a report of four cases. *J Comput Assist Tomogr.* 1998;22(2):202–206.

175. Amahzoune B, et al. [Arterial manifestations of Behçet's disease. A report of five operated cases.] *Arch Mal Coeur Vaiss.* 2002;95(2):109–16.

176. Yassine N, et al. [Aneurysms of the pulmonary artery in Behçet disease. Apropos of 5 new cases.] *Rev Pneumol Clin.* 1997;53(1):42–48.

177. Tunaci A, Berkmen YM, Gokmen E. Thoracic involvement in Behçet's disease: pathologic, clinical, and imaging features. *AJR Am J Roentgenol.* 1995;164(1):51–56.

178. Lee CW, et al. Aortic valve involvement in Behçet's disease. A clinical study of 9 patients. *Korean J Intern Med.* 2002;17(1):51–56.

179. Kusuyama T, et al. Unruptured aneurysm of the sinus of valsalva with Behçet's disease. *Circ J.* 2002;66(1):107–108.

180. Criteria for diagnosis of Behçet's disease. International Study Group for Behçet's Disease. *Lancet.* 1990;335(8697): 1078–1080.

181. Chang HK, Cheon KS. The clinical significance of a pathergy reaction in patients with Behçet's disease. *J Korean Med Sci.* 2002;17(3):371–374.

182. Cakirer S. Isolated spinal neurobehcet disease. MR imaging findings. *Acta Radiol.* 2003;44(5):558–560.

183. Sener RN. Neuro-Behçet's disease: diffusion MR imaging and proton MR spectroscopy. *AJNR Am J Neuroradiol.* 2003;24(8):1612–1614.

184. Kunimatsu A, et al. Neuro-Behçet's disease: analysis of apparent diffusion coefficients. *Neuroradiology.* 2003;45(8):524–527.

185. Choi JA, et al. Arthropathy in Behçet disease: MR imaging findings in two cases. *Radiology.* 2003;226(2):387–389.

186. Niimi H, et al. [CT & MRI findings of refractory vasculitis.] *Nippon Rinsho.* 1994;52(8):2047–2053.

187. Picco P, et al. MICA gene polymorphisms in an Italian paediatric series of juvenile Behçet disease. *Int J Mol Med.* 2002;10(5):575–578.

188. Yazici H, Yurdakul S, Hamuryudan V. Behçet disease. *Curr Opin Rheumatol.* 2001;13(1):18–22.

189. Tohme A, el-Khoury I, Ghayad E. [Behçet disease. Genetic factors, immunologic aspects and new therapeutic methods.] *Presse Med.* 1999;28(20):1080–1084.

190. Mor F, Weinberger A, Cohen IR. Identification of alpha-tropomyosin as a target self-antigen in Behçet's syndrome. *Eur J Immunol.* 2002;32(2):356–365.

191. Kiraz S, et al. Pathological haemostasis and "prothrombotic state" in Behçet's disease. *Thromb Res.* 2002; 105(2):125–133.

192. Espinosa G, et al. Vascular involvement in Behçet's disease: relation with thrombophilic factors, coagulation activation, and thrombomodulin. *Am J Med.* 2002;112(1):37–43.

193. Yazici H. Behçet's syndrome: an update. *Curr Rheumatol Rep.* 2003;5(3):195–199.

194. Kari JA, Shah V, Dillon MJ. Behçet's disease in UK children: clinical features and treatment including thalidomide. *Rheumatology (Oxford).* 2001;40(8):933–938.

195. Hassard PV, et al. Anti-tumor necrosis factor monoclonal antibody therapy for gastrointestinal Behçet's disease: a case report. *Gastroenterology.* 2001;120(4):995–999.

196. Sakane T, Takeno M. Novel approaches to Behçet's disease. *Expert Opin Investig Drugs.* 2000;9(9):1993–2005.

197. Kaklamani VG, Kaklamanis PG. Treatment of Behçet's disease—an update. *Semin Arthritis Rheum.* 2001;30(5):299–312.

198. Degos R. Malignant atrophic papulosis. *Br J Dermatol.* 1979;100(1):21–35.

199. Bogenrieder T, et al. Benign Degos' disease developing during pregnancy and followed for 10 years. *Acta Derm Venereol.* 2002;82(4):284–287.

200. Ball E, Newburger A, Ackerman AB. Degos' disease: a distinctive pattern of disease, chiefly of lupus erythematosus, and not a specific disease per se. *Am J Dermatopathol.* 2003;25(4):308–320.

201. Sugai F, et al. [An autopsy case of Degos' disease with ascending thoracic myelopathy.] *Rinsho Shinkeigaku*. 1998;38(12):1049–1053.

202. Vicktor C, Schultz U. [Malignant atrophic papulosis (Kohlmeier-Degos): diagnosis, therapy and course.] *Hautarzt*. 2001;52(8):734–737.

203. Harvell JD, Williford PL, White WL. Benign cutaneous Degos' disease: a case report with emphasis on histopathology as papules chronologically evolve. *Am J Dermatopathol*. 2001;23(2):116–123.

204. Burg G, et al. [Malignant atrophic papulosis (Kohlmeier-Degos disease).] *Hautarzt*. 1989;40(8):480–485.

205. Ojeda Cuchillero RM, Sanchez Regana M, Umbert Millet P. Benign cutaneous Degos' disease. *Clin Exp Dermatol*. 2003;28(2):145–147.

206. Torrelo A, et al. Malignant atrophic papulosis in an infant. *Br J Dermatol*. 2002;146(5):916–918.

207. Farrell AM, et al. Benign cutaneous Degos' disease. *Br J Dermatol*. 1998;139(4):708–712.

208. Melnik B, et al. [Malignant atrophic papulosis (Kohlmeier-Degos disease). Failure to respond to interferon alpha-2a, pentoxifylline and aspirin.] *Hautarzt*. 2002;53(9):618–621.

209. Gonzalez Valverde FM, et al. Presentation of Degos syndrome as acute small-bowel perforation. *Arch Surg*. 2003;138(1):57–58.

210. Ramos-Casals M, et al. Mixed cryoglobulinemia: new concepts. *Lupus*. 2000;9(2):83–91.

211. Cacoub P, et al. Cryoglobulinemia vasculitis. *Curr Opin Rheumatol*. 2002;14(1):29–35.

212. Ferri C, Zignego AL, Pileri SA. Cryoglobulins. *J Clin Pathol*. 2002;55(1):4–13.

213. Schott P, Hartmann H, Ramadori G. Hepatitis C virus-associated mixed cryoglobulinemia. Clinical manifestations, histopathological changes, mechanisms of cryoprecipitation and options of treatment. *Histol Histopathol*. 2001;16(4):1275–1285.

214. Lunel F, Musset L. Mixed cryoglobulinemia and hepatitis C virus infection. *Minerva Med*. 2001;92(1):35–42.

215. Christodoulou DK, et al. Cryoglobulinemia due to chronic viral hepatitis infections is not a major problem in clinical practice. 2001;12(5):435–441.

216. Kerr GS, et al. Prevalence of hepatitis C virus associated cryoglobulinemia at a veterans hospital. *J Rheumatol*. 1997;24(11):2134–2138.

217. Fabris P, et al. Prevalence and clinical significance of circulating cryoglobulins in HIV-positive patients with and without co-infection with hepatitis C virus. *J Med Virol*. 2003;69(3):339–343.

218. Dimitrakopoulos AN, et al. Mixed cryoglobulinemia in HIV-1 infection: the role of HIV-1. *Ann Intern Med*. 1999;130(3):226–230.

219. Janney FA, Lee LT, Howe C. Cold hemagglutinin cross-reactivity with Mycoplasma pneumoniae. *Infect Immun*. 1978;22(1):29–33.

220. Thappa DM, et al. Leg ulcers in active lepromatous leprosy associated with cryoglobulinaemia. *Clin Exp Dermatol*. 2002;27(6):451–453.

221. Rieu V, et al. Characteristics and outcome of 49 patients with symptomatic cryoglobulinaemia. *Rheumatology (Oxford)*. 2002;41(3):290–300.

222. Casato M, et al. Occult hepatitis C virus infection in type II mixed cryoglobulinaemia. *J Viral Hepat*. 2003;10(6):455–459.

223. Caniatti LM, et al. Cryoglobulinemic neuropathy related to hepatitis C virus infection. Clinical, laboratory and neurophysiological study. *J Peripher Nerv Syst*. 1996;1(2):131–138.

224. Gemignani F, et al. Cryoglobulinaemic neuropathy manifesting with restless legs syndrome. *J Neurol Sci*. 1997;152(2):218–223.

225. Gorevic PD, et al. Mixed cryoglobulinemia: clinical aspects and long-term follow-up of 40 patients. *Am J Med*. 1980;69(2):287–308.

226. Khella SL, Souayah N. Hepatitis C: a review of its neurologic complications. *Neurolog*. 2002;8(2):101–106.

227. Filippini D, et al. [Central nervous system involvement in patients with HCV-related cryoglobulinemia: literature review and a case report.] *Reumatismo*. 2002;54(2):150–155.

228. Baxter R, et al. Gastrointestinal manifestations of essential mixed cryoglobulinemia. *Gastrointest Radiol*. 1988;13(2):160–162.

229. Schirren CA, et al. A role for chronic hepatitis C virus infection in a patient with cutaneous vasculitis, cryoglobulinemia, and chronic liver disease. Effective therapy with interferon-alpha. *Dig Dis Sci*. 1995;40(6):1221–1225.

230. Bollinger A, Butti P. [Primary and secondary Raynaud's syndrome.] *Schweiz Med Wochenschr*. 1976;106(12):415–421.

231. Mazzola L, et al. Brain hemorrhage as a complication of type I cryoglobulinemia vasculopathy. *J Neurol*. 2003;250(11):1376–1378.

232. Gray Y, et al. Type I cryoglobulinemia presenting as hemorrhagic crusted leg ulcers. *Cutis*. 2002;70(6):319–323.

233. Kawabata K, et al. [A case of mononeuritis multiplex associated with type I (monoclonal) IgG kappa cryoglobulinemia.] *Rinsho Shinkeigaku*. 2001;41(2–3):117–120.

234. Karras A, et al. Renal involvement in monoclonal (type I) cryoglobulinemia: two cases associated with IgG3 kappa cryoglobulin. *Am J Kidney Dis*. 2002;40(5):1091–1096.

235. Sanmugarajah J, et al. Monoclonal cryoglobulinemia with extensive gangrene of all four extremities—a case report. *Angiology*. 2000;51(5):431–434.

236. Hoffkes HG, et al. [Type I cryoglobulinemia.] *Dtsch Med Wochenschr*. 1995;120(28–29):990–995.

237. Woltjen HH, Hansmann E, Bremer K. [Pseudoleukocytosis in cryoglobulinemia type I.] *Dtsch Med Wochenschr*. 1993;118(8):260–264.

238. Bridoux F, et al. [Renal damage during type II cryoglobulinemia.] *Presse Med*. 2003;32(12):563–569.

239. Daoud MS, et al. Chronic hepatitis C, cryoglobulinemia, and cutaneous necrotizing vasculitis. Clinical, pathologic, and immunopathologic study of twelve patients. *J Am Acad Dermatol*. 1996;34(2 Pt 1):219–223.

240. Friedman ES, LaNatra N, Stiller MJ. NSAIDs in dermatologic therapy: review and preview. *J Cutan Med Surg*. 2002;6(5):449–459.

241. Laganovic M, et al. Complete remission of cryoglobulinemic glomerulonephritis (HCV-positive) after high dose interferon therapy. *Wien Klin Wochenschr*. 2000;112(13):596–600.

242. Mazzaro C, et al. Interferon plus ribavirin in patients with hepatitis C virus positive mixed cryoglobulinemia resistant to interferon. *J Rheumatol*. 2003;30(8):1775–1781.

243. Willson RA. The benefit of long-term interferon alfa therapy for symptomatic mixed cryoglobulinemia (cutaneous vasculitis/membranoproliferative glomerulonephritis) associated with chronic hepatitis C infection. *J Clin Gastroenterol*. 2001;33(2):137–140.

244. Laura VM, De Sangro MA. Long-term results regarding the use of recombinant interferon alpha-2b in the treatment of II type mixed essential cryoglobulinemia. *Med Oncol*. 1995;12(4):223–230.

245. Monti G, et al. Colchicine in the treatment of mixed cryoglobulinemia. *Clin Exp Rheumatol*. 1995;13[Suppl 13]:S197–S199.

246. Mori Y, et al. Cryofiltration and oral corticosteroids provide successful treatment for an elderly patient with cryoglobulinemic glomerulonephritis associated with hepatitis C virus infection. *Intern Med*. 2000;39(7):564–569.

247. Stefanutti C, et al. Immunoadsorption apheresis (Selesorb) in the treatment of chronic hepatitis C virus-related type 2 mixed cryoglobulinemia. *Transfus Apheresis Sci*. 2003;28(3):207–214.

248. Zaja F, et al. Efficacy and safety of rituximab in type II mixed cryoglobulinemia. *Blood*. 2003;101(10):3827–3834.

249. Sansonno D, et al. Monoclonal antibody treatment of mixed cryoglobulinemia resistant to interferon alpha with an anti-CD20. *Blood*. 2003;101(10):3818–3826.

250. Dominguez JH, Sha E. Apheresis in cryoglobulinemia complicating hepatitis C and in other renal diseases. *Ther Apher*. 2002;6(1):69–76.

251. Rosenstock JL, et al. Fludarabine treatment of cryoglobulinemic glomerulonephritis. *Am J Kidney Dis*. 2002;40(3):644–648.

252. Meyrier A, et al. [Hypocomplementemic urticarial vasculitis with glomerulopathy and renal venulitis.] *Nephrologie*. 1984;5(1):1–7.

253. Iannello S, et al. [Urticarial vasculitis syndrome. A case report and review of the literature.] *Minerva Med*. 1997;88(11):459–467.

254. el Maghraoui A, et al. [McDuffie hypocomplementemic urticarial vasculitis. Two cases and review of the literature.] *Rev Med Interne*. 2001;22(1):70–74.

255. Venzor J, Lee WL, Huston DP. Urticarial vasculitis. *Clin Rev Allergy Immunol*. 2002;23(2):201–216.

256. Gammon WR, Wheeler CE Jr. Urticarial vasculitis: report of a case and review of the literature. *Arch Dermatol*. 1979;115(1):76–80.

257. Wisnieski JJ. Urticarial vasculitis. *Curr Opin Rheumatol*. 2000;12(1):24–31.

258. Houser SL, et al. Valvular heart disease in patients with hypocomplementemic urticarial vasculitis syndrome associated with Jaccoud's arthropathy. *Cardiovasc Pathol*. 2002;11(4):210–216.

259. Tervaert JW, Stegeman CA, Kallenberg CG. Silicon exposure and vasculitis. *Curr Opin Rheumatol*. 1998;10(1):12–17.

260. Doyle MK, Cuellar ML. Drug-induced vasculitis. *Expert Opin Drug Saf*. 2003;2(4):401–409.

261. ten Holder SM, Joy MS, Falk RJ. Cutaneous and systemic manifestations of drug-induced vasculitis. *Ann Pharmacother*. 2002;36(1):130–147.

262. Cuellar ML. Drug-induced vasculitis. *Curr Rheumatol Rep*. 2002;4(1):55–59.

263. Mansi IA, Opran A, Rosner F. ANCA-associated small-vessel vasculitis. *Am Fam Physician*. 2002;65(8):1615–1620.

264. Wiik A. Laboratory diagnostics in vasculitis patients. *Isr Med Assoc J*. 2001;3(4):275–277.

265. Naides SJ. Known causes of vasculitis in man. *Cleve Clin J Med*. 2002;69[Suppl 2]:SII15–SII19.

266. Internet use and early syphilis infection among men who have sex with men—San Francisco, California, 1999–2003. *MMWR Morb Mortal Wkly Rep*. 2003;52(50):1229–1232.

267. Sugiura M, Matushita S, Ueda K. A clinicopathological study on valvular diseases in 3,000 consecutive autopsies of the aged. *Jpn Circ J*. 1982;46(4):337–345.

268. Cohen MG, et al. Syphilitic aortitis. *Catheter Cardiovasc Interv*. 2001;52(2):237–239.

269. Aupy M, et al. [Neurosyphilitic arteritis. Clinical, paraclinical and therapeutic data. A review of six cases (author's transl).] *Sem Hop*. 1982;58(18):1101–1106.

270. Lewicki Z, Szczawinski A. Arteritis. In: Rykowski H, ed. *Vascular Diseases*. Warszawa: PZWL; 1981:251–296.

271. O'Regan AW, et al. Barking up the wrong tree? Use of polymerase chain reaction to diagnose syphilitic aortitis. *Thorax*. 2002;57(10):917–918.

272. Sais G, et al. Tuberculous lymphadenitis presenting with cutaneous leucocytoclastic vasculitis. *Clin Exp Dermatol*. 1996;21(1):65–66.

273. Lee A, Jang J, Lee K. Two cases of leukocytoclastic vasculitis with tuberculosis. *Clin Exp Dermatol*. 1998;23(5):225–226.

274. Allins AD, et al. Tuberculous infection of the descending thoracic and abdominal aorta: case report and literature review. *Ann Vasc Surg*. 1999;13(4):439–444.

275. Chetty R. Vasculitides associated with HIV infection. *J Clin Pathol*. 2001;54(4):275–278.

276. Soravia-Dunand VA, Loo VG, Salit IE. Aortitis due to Salmonella: report of 10 cases and comprehensive review of the literature. *Clin Infect Dis*. 1999;29(4):862–868.

277. Sawamura Y, et al. Successful surgical management of patients with infective endocarditis associated with acute neurologic deficits. *Jpn J Thorac Cardiovasc Surg*. 2002;50(5):220–223.

278. Inoue T, et al. Mycotic aneurysm of the palmar artery associated with infective endocarditis. Case report and review of the literature. *Minerva Cardioangiol*. 2001;49(1):87–90.

279. Carreras M, et al. Evolution of salmonella aortitis towards the formation of abdominal aneurysm. *Eur Radiol*. 1997;7(1):54–56.

280. Ewart JM, Burke ML, Bunt TJ. Spontaneous abdominal aortic infections. Essentials of diagnosis and management. *Am Surg*. 1983;49(1):37–50.

281. Hoogendoorn EH, et al. Pneumococcal aortitis, report of a case with emphasis on the contribution to diagnosis of positron emission tomography using fluorinated deoxyglucose. *Clin Microbiol Infect*. 2003;9(1):73–76.

282. Katz SG, Andros G, Kohl RD. Salmonella infections of the abdominal aorta. *Surg Gynecol Obstet*. 1992;175(2):102–106.

283. Safar HA, Cina CS. Ruptured mycotic aneurysm of the popliteal artery. A case report and review of the literature. *J Cardiovasc Surg (Torino)*. 2001;42(2):237–240.

284. Shinonaga M, et al. Simultaneous mitral valve replacement and bypass grafting for mycotic aneurysm of the femoral artery during the active phase of infective endocarditis: a case report. *Ann Thorac Cardiovasc Surg*. 2001;7(6):381–383.

285. Zandman-Goddard G, Shoenfeld Y. HIV and autoimmunity. *Autoimmun Rev*. 2002;1(6):329–337.

286. Nair R, et al. Occlusive arterial disease in HIV-infected patients: a preliminary report. *Eur J Vasc Endovasc Surg*. 2000;20(4):353–357.

287. Kleinschmidt-DeMasters BK, Gilden DH. Varicella-Zoster virus infections of the nervous system: clinical and pathologic correlates. *Arch Pathol Lab Med*. 2001;125(6):770–780.

288. Brannagan TH 3rd. Retroviral-associated vasculitis of the nervous system. *Neurol Clin*. 1997;15(4):927–944.

289. Bedani PL, et al. HBV-related cutaneous periarteritis nodosa in a patient 16 years after renal transplantation: efficacy of lamivudine. *J Nephrol*. 2001;14(5):428–430.

290. Naschitz JE, et al. Vascular disorders preceding diagnosis of cancer: distinguishing the causal relationship based on Bradford-Hill guidelines. *Angiology*. 2003;54(1):11–17.

291. Hutson TE, Hoffman GS. Temporal concurrence of vasculitis and cancer: a report of 12 cases. *Arthritis Care Res*. 2000;13(6):417–423.

292. Blanco R, et al. Cutaneous vasculitis in children and adults. Associated diseases and etiologic factors in 303 patients. *Medicine (Baltimore)*. 1998;77(6):403–418.

293. Haug ES, et al. Inflammatory aortic aneurysm is associated with increased incidence of autoimmune disease. *J Vasc Surg*. 2003;38(3):492–497.

294. Ohara N, et al. Aortic aneurysm in patients with autoimmune diseases treated with corticosteroids. *Int Angiol*. 2000;19(3):270–275.

295. Herrick AL, et al. Vasculitis in patients with systemic sclerosis and severe digital ischaemia requiring amputation. *Ann Rheum Dis*. 1994;53(5):323–326.

296. Truckenbrodt H, Hafner R. Vasculitis and calcinosis in juvenile dermatomyositis. *Acta Univ Carol [Med] (Praha)*. 1991;37(1–2):8–15.

297. Wheatley MJ, Hennein HA, Greenfield LJ. Lower extremity arterial disease in systemic lupus erythematosus. *Arch Surg*. 1991;126(1):109–110.

298. Youssef P, et al. Limited scleroderma is associated with increased prevalence of macrovascular disease. *J Rheumatol*. 1995;22(3):469–472.

299. Dorevitch MI, Clemens LE, Webb JB. Lower limb amputation secondary to large vessel involvement in scleroderma. *Br J Rheumatol*. 1988;27(5):403–406.

300. Ho MS, Tech LB, Goh HS. Ischaemic colitis in systemic lupus erythematosus—report of a case and review of the literature. *Ann Acad Med Singapore*. 1987;16(3):501–503.

301. Ebert EC, Ruggiero FM, Seibold JR. Intestinal perforation. A common complication of scleroderma. *Dig Dis Sci*. 1997;42(3):549–553.

302. Cossio M, et al. Life-threatening complications of systemic sclerosis. *Crit Care Clin*. 2002;18(4):819–839.

303. Yoshikawa Y, Mizutani H, Shimizu M. Systemic lupus erythematosus with ischemic peripheral neuropathy and

lupus anticoagulant: response to intravenous prostaglandin E1. *Cutis.* 1996;58(6):393–396.

304. Matsui N, et al. Dermatomyositis with peripheral nervous system involvement: activation of vascular endothelial growth factor (VEGF) and VEGF receptor (VEGFR) in vasculitic lesions. *Intern Med.* 2003;42(12):1233–1239.

305. Singh RR, et al. Clinical significance of anti-Sm antibody in systemic lupus erythematosus & related disorders. *Indian J Med Res.* 1991;94:206–210.

306. Talbot RW, et al. Vascular complications of inflammatory bowel disease. *Mayo Clin Proc.* 1986;61(2):140–145.

307. Begelman SM, Olin JW. Fibromuscular dysplasia. *Curr Opin Rheumatol.* 2000;12(1):41–47.

308. Olin JW, Novick A. Renovascular disease. In: Young JR, Olin JW, Bartholomew LE, eds. *Peripheral Vascular Diseases.* St. Louis: Mosby–Year Book, Inc.; 1996:321–342.

309. Guzman R, et al. Arterial fibrodysplasia causing occlusive vascular disease simulating primary vasculitis. *Rev Invest Clin.* 1994;46(1):67–71.

310. Iwai T, et al. Fibromuscular dysplasia in the extremities. *J Cardiovasc Surg (Torino).* 1985;26(5):496–501.

311. Harrison EG Jr, McCormack LJ. Pathologic classification of renal arterial disease in renovascular hypertension. *Mayo Clin Proc.* 1971;46(3):161–167.

312. Harrison LH Jr, Flye MW, Seigler HF. Incidence of anatomical variants in renal vasculature in the presence of normal renal function. *Ann Surg.* 1978;188(1):83–89.

313. Luscher TF, et al. Arterial fibromuscular. *Mayo Clin Proc.* 1987;62(10):931–952.

314. Virmani R, Darcy T, Robinowitz M. Congenital malformations of the vasculature. In: Loscalzo J, Creager MA, Dzau VJ, eds. *Vascular Medicine.* Boston/Toronto/London: Little, Brown and Company; 1992.

315. Gray BH, Young JR. Miscellaneous arterial diseases. In: Young JR, Olin JW, Bartholomew LE, eds. *Peripheral Vascular Diseases.* St. Louis: Mosby–Year Book, Inc.; 1996: 425–440.

316. Estepa R, et al. Renovascular hypertension in children. *Scand J Urol Nephrol.* 2001;35(5):388–392.

317. Pfeiffer T, et al. Reconstruction for renal artery aneurysm: operative techniques and long-term results. *J Vasc Surg.* 2003;37(2):293–300.

318. Luscher TF, et al. Fibromuscular hyperplasia: extension of the disease and therapeutic outcome. Results of the University Hospital Zurich Cooperative Study on Fibromuscular Hyperplasia. *Nephron.* 1986;44[Suppl 1]:109–114.

319. Surowiec SM, Sivamurthy N, Rhodes JM, et al. Percutaneous therapy for renal artery fibromuscular dysplasia. *Ann Vasc Surg.* 2003;17(6):650–655.

320. Birrer M, et al. Treatment of renal artery fibromuscular dysplasia with balloon angioplasty: a prospective follow-up study. *Eur J Vasc Endovasc Surg.* 2002;23(2):146–152.

321. Mounier-Vehier C, et al. Renal atrophy outcome after revascularization in fibromuscular dysplasia disease. *J Endovasc Ther.* 2002;9(5):605–613.

322. Lupattelli T, et al. Embolization of a renal artery aneurysm using ethylene vinyl alcohol copolymer (Onyx). *J Endovasc Ther.* 2003;10(2):366–370.

323. Bisschops RH, Popma JJ, Meyerovitz MF. Treatment of fibromuscular dysplasia and renal artery aneurysm with use of a stent-graft. *J Vasc Interv Radiol.* 2001;12(6): 757–760.

324. DiFazio M, et al. Intracranial fibromuscular dysplasia in a six-year-old child: a rare cause of childhood stroke. *J Child Neurol.* 2000;15(8):559–562.

325. Schievink WI, Bjornsson J. Fibromuscular dysplasia of the internal carotid artery: a clinicopathological study. *Clin Neuropathol.* 1996;15(1):2–6.

326. Tan AK, et al. Ischaemic stroke from cerebral embolism in cephalic fibromuscular dysplasia. *Ann Acad Med Singapore.* 1995;24(6):891–894.

327. Moreau P, Albat B, Thevenet A. Fibromuscular dysplasia of the internal carotid artery: long-term surgical results. *J Cardiovasc Surg (Torino).* 1993;34(6):465–472.

328. Cloft HJ, et al. Prevalence of cerebral aneurysms in patients with fibromuscular dysplasia: a reassessment. *J Neurosurg.* 1998;88(3):436–440.

329. Camacho A, et al. Vertebral artery fibromuscular dysplasia: an unusual cause of stroke in a 3-year-old child. *Dev Med Child Neurol.* 2003;45(10):709–711.

330. Nomura S, et al. Childhood subarachnoid hemorrhage associated with fibromuscular dysplasia. *Childs Nerv Syst.* 2001;17(7):419–422.

331. Zuccoli G, et al. Carotid and vertebral artery dissection: magnetic resonance findings in 15 cases. *Radiol Med (Torino).* 2002;104(5–6):466–471.

332. Clifton AG. MR angiography. *Br Med Bull.* 2000;56(2): 367–377.

333. Finsterer J, et al. Bilateral stenting of symptomatic and asymptomatic internal carotid artery stenosis due to fibromuscular dysplasia. *J Neurol Neurosurg Psychiatry.* 2000;69(5):683–686.

334. Takigami M, Baba T, Saitou K. [Percutaneous transluminal angioplasty in fibromuscular dysplasia of the internal carotid artery: case report.] *No Shinkei Geka.* 2002;30(3):301–306.

335. Kubaska SM 3rd, et al. Internal carotid artery pseudoaneurysms: treatment with the Wallgraft endoprosthesis. *J Endovasc Ther.* 2003;10(2):182–189.

336. Horie T, et al. Unusual petal-like fibromuscular dysplasia as a cause of acute abdomen and circulatory shock. *Jpn Heart J.* 2002;43(3):301–305.

337. Sandmann W, Schulte KM. Multivisceral fibromuscular dysplasia in childhood: case report and review of the literature. *Ann Vasc Surg.* 2000;14(5):496–502.

338. Ebaugh JL, et al. Staged embolization and operative treatment of multiple visceral aneurysms in a patient with fibromuscular dysplasia—a case report. *Vasc Surg.* 2001;35(2):145–148.

339. Kojima A, et al. Successful surgical treatment of a patient with multiple visceral artery aneurysms due to fibromuscular dysplasia. *Cardiovasc Surg.* 2002;10(2):157–160.

340. Abbas MA, et al. Hepatic artery aneurysm: factors that predict complications. *J Vasc Surg.* 2003;38(1):41–45.

341. Campman SC, et al. Pulmonary arterial fibromuscular dysplasia: a rare cause of fulminant lung hemorrhage. *Am J Forensic Med Pathol.* 2000;21(1):69–73.

342. Flowers MJ, et al. Unilateral lower limb hypoplasia in arterial fibromuscular dysplasia. *Clin Orthop.* 1996(324): 217–221.

343. Khatri VP, Gaulin JC, Amin AK. Fibromuscular dysplasia of distal radial and ulnar arteries: uncommon cause of digital ischemia. *Ann Plast Surg.* 1994;33(6):652–655.

344. Lin WW, et al. Fibromuscular dysplasia of the brachial artery: a case report and review of the literature. *J Vasc Surg.* 1992;16(1):66–70.

345. Reilly JM, McGraw DJ, Sicard GA. Bilateral brachial artery fibromuscular dysplasia. *Ann Vasc Surg.* 1993;7(5):483–487.

346. Yoshida T, et al. Fibromuscular disease of the brachial artery with digital emboli treated effectively by transluminal angioplasty. *Cardiovasc Intervent Radiol.* 1994;17(2):99–101.

347. Verhelst H, Lauwers G, Schroe H. Fibromuscular dysplasia of the external iliac artery. *Acta Chir Belg.* 1999;99(4): 171–173.

348. Schneider PA, et al. Isolated thigh claudication as a result of fibromuscular dysplasia of the deep femoral artery. *J Vasc Surg.* 1992;15(4):657–660.

349. Sauer L, et al. Clinical spectrum of symptomatic external iliac fibromuscular dysplasia. *J Vasc Surg.* 1990;12(4):488–495; discussion 495–496.

350. Esfahani F, et al. Arterial fibrodysplasia: a regional cause of peripheral occlusive vascular disease. *Angiology.* 1989;40(2):108–113.

351. Edwards JM, Antonius JI, Porter JM. Critical hand ischemia caused by forearm fibromuscular dysplasia. *J Vasc Surg.* 1985;2(3):459–463.

352. Ferris BL, et al. Hypothenar hammer syndrome: proposed etiology. *J Vasc Surg.* 2000;31(1 Pt 1):104–113.

353. Leu HJ, Julke M. [Thoracic aortic aneurysm. Pathologico-anatomical analysis of 111 cases.] *Schweiz Med Wochenschr.* 1984;114(45):1593–1595.

354. Leu HJ. [Erdheim-Gsell medial necrosis and mucoid degeneration of the media as a cause of aorto-arterial aneurysm. Pathologico-anatomical analysis of 150 excised vessels.] *Schweiz Med Wochenschr.* 1988;118(18):687–691.

355. Trotter SE, Olsen EG. Marfan's disease and Erdheim's cystic medionecrosis. A study of their pathology. *Eur Heart J.* 1991;12(1):83–87.

356. Pomerance A, Yacoub MH, Gula G. The surgical pathology of thoracic aortic aneurysms. *Histopathology.* 1977;1(4):257–276.

357. Milewicz DM, Urban Z, Boyd C. Genetic disorders of the elastic fiber system. *Matrix Biol.* 2000;19(6):471–480.

358. Julke M, Leu HJ. [Extra-aortic aneurysms. Analysis of 163 aneurysms in 142 patients.] *Schweiz Med Wochenschr.* 1985;115(1):10–13.

359. Gibson WG, Reimer KA. Multiple coronary artery dissections in old age. A unique case. *Arch Pathol Lab Med.* 1980;104(8):419–421.

360. Segal GH, Ratliff NB, Cosgrove DM. Cystic medionecrosis of the coronary arteries and fatal coronary vasospasm. *Ann Thorac Surg.* 1990;50(4):653–655.

361. Slavin RE, Cafferty L, Cartwright J Jr. Segmental mediolytic arteritis. A clinicopathologic and ultrastructural study of two cases. *Am J Surg Pathol.* 1989;13(7):558–568.

362. Wali MA, et al. Mucoid degeneration of the brachial artery: case report and a review of literature. *J R Coll Surg Edinb.* 1999;44(2):126–129.

363. Chakfe N, et al. [Extra-popliteal localizations of adventitial cysts. Review of the literature.] *J Mal Vasc.* 1997;22(2):79–85.

364. Flanigan DP, et al. Summary of cases of adventitial cystic disease of the popliteal artery. *Ann Surg.* 1979;189(2):165–175.

365. Elster EA, et al. Adventitial cystic disease of the axillary artery. *Ann Vasc Surg.* 2002;16(1):134–137.

366. Unno N, et al. Cystic adventitial disease of the popliteal artery: elongation into the media of the popliteal artery and communication with the knee joint capsule: report of a case. *Surg Today.* 2000;30(11):1026–1029.

367. Levien LJ, Benn CA. Adventitial cystic disease: a unifying hypothesis. *J Vasc Surg.* 1998;28(2):193–205.

368. Miller A, et al. Noninvasive vascular imaging in the diagnosis and treatment of adventitial cystic disease of the popliteal artery. *J Vasc Surg.* 1997;26(4):715–720.

369. Ishikawa K. Cystic adventitial disease of the popliteal artery and of other stem vessels in the extremities. *Jpn J Surg.* 1987;17(4):221–229.

370. Do DD, et al. Adventitial cystic disease of the popliteal artery: percutaneous US-guided aspiration. *Radiology.* 1997;203(3):743–746.

371. Colombier D, et al. [Cystic adventitial disease: importance of computed tomography in the diagnostic and therapeutic management.] *J Mal Vasc.* 1997;22(3):181–186.

372. Fox RL, et al. Adventitial cystic disease of the popliteal artery: failure of percutaneous transluminal angioplasty as a therapeutic modality. *J Vasc Surg.* 1985;2(3):464–467.

373. Struk B, et al. Mapping of both autosomal recessive and dominant variants of pseudoxanthoma elasticum to chromosome 16p13.1. *Hum Mol Genet.* 1997;6(11):1823–1828.

374. Pulkkinen L, et al. Identification of ABCC6 pseudogenes on human chromosome 16p: implications for mutation detection in pseudoxanthoma elasticum. *Hum Genet.* 2001;109(3):356–365.

375. Hu X, et al. Pseudoxanthoma elasticum: a clinical, histopathological, and molecular update. *Surv Ophthalmol.* 2003;48(4):424–438.

376. Uitto J, Pulkkinen L, Ringpfeil F. Molecular genetics of pseudoxanthoma elasticum: a metabolic disorder at the environment-genome interface? *Trends Mol Med.* 2001;7(1):13–17.

377. Aissaoui R, et al. [Pseudoxanthoma elasticum, 5 case reports.] *Presse Med.* 2003;32(34):1595–1598.

378. Kaplan EN, Henjyoji EY. Pseudoxanthoma elasticum: a dermal elastosis with surgical implications. *Plast Reconstr Surg.* 1976;58(5):595–600.

379. Chen TH, Wei FC. Pseudoxanthoma elasticum. Case report. *Scand J Plast Reconstr Surg Hand Surg.* 1998;32(4):421–424.

380. Mendelsohn G, Bulkley BH, Hutchins GM. Cardiovascular manifestations of Pseudoxanthoma elasticum. *Arch Pathol Lab Med.* 1978;102(6):298–302.

381. Keim HJ, et al. [Massive upper gastrointestinal bleeding as first clinical manifestation of pseudoxanthoma elasticum (author's transl).] *Z Gastroenterol.* 1980;18(1):20–29.

382. Kundrotas L, et al. Gastric bleeding in pseudoxanthoma elasticum. *Am J Gastroenterol.* 1988;83(8):868–872.

383. Heno P, et al. [Aorto-coronary dysplasia and pseudoxanthoma elastica.] *Arch Mal Coeur Vaiss.* 1998;91(4):415–418.

384. Belli A, Cawthorne S. Visceral angiographic findings in pseudoxanthoma elasticum. *Br J Radiol.* 1988;61(725):368–371.

385. Yap EY, Gleaton MS, Buettner H. Visual loss associated with pseudoxanthoma elasticum. *Retina.* 1992;12(4):315–319.

386. Kevorkian JP, et al. New report of severe coronary artery disease in an eighteen-year-old girl with pseudoxanthoma elasticum. Case report and review of the literature. *Angiology.* 1997;48(8):735–741.

387. Dymock RB. Pseudoxanthoma elasticum: report of a case with reno-vascular hypertension. *Australas J Dermatol.* 1979;20(2):82–84.

388. Ekim M, et al. Pseudoxanthoma elasticum: a rare cause of hypertension in children. *Pediatr Nephrol.* 1998;12(3):183–185.

389. Ruhlmann C, et al. [Gronblad-Strandberg syndrome from the angiological viewpoint.] *Dtsch Med Wochenschr.* 1998;123(11):312–317.

390. Rodriguez-Camarero SJ, et al. [Acute arterial thrombosis of the extremity in pseudoxanthoma elasticum.] *Angiologia.* 1992;44(2):58–61.

391. Galle G, et al. [Stenoses of the cerebral arteries in pseudoxanthoma elasticum (author's transl).] *Arch Psychiatr Nervenkr.* 1981;231(1):61–70.

392. Takeshita T, Ozaki M. Central retinal artery occlusion in a patient with pseudoxanthoma elasticum. *Hiroshima J Med Sci.* 2003;52(2):33–34.

393. Tsomi K, et al. Arterial elastorrhexis: manifestation of a generalized elastic tissue disorder in beta-thalassaemia major. *Eur J Haematol.* 1999;63(5):287–294.

394. Meislik J, et al. Laser treatment in maculopathy of pseudoxanthoma elasticum. *Can J Ophthalmol.* 1978;13(3):210–212.

395. Lin AE, et al. Cardiovascular malformations and other cardiovascular abnormalities in neurofibromatosis 1. *Am J Med Genet.* 2000;95(2):108–117.

396. Pezzetta E, et al. Spontaneous hemothorax associated with von Recklinghausen's disease. *Eur J Cardiothorac Surg.* 2003;23(6):1062–1064.

397. Wertelecki W, et al. Angiomas and von Recklinghausen neurofibromatosis. *Neurofibromatosis.* 1988;1(3):137–145.

398. Karadimas P, Hatzispasou E, Bouzas EA. Retinal vascular abnormalities in neurofibromatosis type 1. *J Neuroophthalmol.* 2003;23(4):274–275.

399. Huffman JL, et al. Neurofibromatosis and arterial aneurysms. *Am Surg.* 1996;62(4):311–314.

400. Fossali E, et al. Renovascular disease and hypertension in children with neurofibromatosis. *Pediatr Nephrol.* 2000;14(8–9):806–810.

401. Muhonen MG, Godersky JC, VanGilder JC. Cerebral aneurysms associated with neurofibromatosis. *Surg Neurol.* 1991;36(6):470–475.

402. Sasaki J, et al. [Neurofibromatosis associated with multiple intracranial vascular lesions: stenosis of the internal carotid artery and peripheral aneurysm of the Heubner's artery; report of a case.] *No Shinkei Geka.* 1995;23(9):813–817.

403. Breul P, Zierz S. [Vascular involvement in neurofibromatosis 1.] *Nervenarzt.* 1991;62(8):490–492.

404. Singh S, et al. Radial artery aneurysm in a case of neurofibromatosis. *Br J Plast Surg.* 1998;51(7):564–565.

405. Ilgit ET, et al. Peripheral arterial involvement in neurofi-bromatosis type 1—a case report. *Angiology*. 1999; 50(11):955–958.
406. Samuels N, et al. Pulmonary hypertension secondary to neurofibromatosis: intimal fibrosis versus thromboem-bolism. *Thorax*. 1999;54(9):858–859.
407. Ruggieri M, et al. Multiple coronary artery aneurysms in a child with neurofibromatosis type 1. *Eur J Pediatr*. 2000; 159(7):477–480.
408. Mullan FJ, Herron BM, Curry RC. Fatal haemorrhage associ-ated with neurofibromatosis. *Eur J Vasc Surg*. 1994;8(3):366–368.
409. Shimizu Y, et al. [A case report of spontaneous rupture of bilateral lumbar artery in a patient with von Reckling-hausen disease.] *Nippon Geka Gakkai Zasshi*. 1993;94(4):420–423.
410. Kunz J, Maxeiner H. [Neurofibromatosis type 1 associated arteriopathy. Case report and literature review.] *Pathologe*. 1997;18(6):480–483.
411. O'Regan S, Mongeau JG. Renovascular hypertension in pediatric patients with neurofibromatosis. *Int J Pediatr Nephrol*. 1983;4(2):109–112.
412. McTaggart SJ, et al. Evaluation and long-term outcome of pediatric renovascular hypertension. *Pediatr Nephrol*. 2000;14(10–11):1022–1029.
413. Rasmussen SA, Yang Q, Friedman JM. Mortality in neurofi-bromatosis 1: an analysis using U.S. death certificates. *Am J Hum Genet*. 2001;68(5):1110–1118.
414. Booth C, et al. Management of renal vascular disease in neurofibromatosis type 1 and the role of percutaneous transluminal angioplasty. *Nephrol Dial Transplant*. 2002;17(7):1235–1240.
415. Criado E, et al. Abdominal aortic coarctation, renovascular, hypertension, and neurofibromatosis. *Ann Vasc Surg*. 2002;16(3):363–367.
416. Smith BL, et al. Ruptured internal carotid aneurysm result-ing from neurofibromatosis: treatment with intraluminal stent graft. *J Vasc Surg*. 2000;32(4):824–828.
417. Perez Jurado AL. Williams-Beuren syndrome: a model of recurrent genomic mutation. *Horm Res*. 2003;59[Suppl 1]:106–113.
418. Morris CA. Williams syndrome. In: *GeneReviews at GeneTests*. Seattle: University of Washington; 2003.
419. Lacolley P, et al. Disruption of the elastin gene in adult Williams syndrome is accompanied by a paradoxical reduc-tion in arterial stiffness. *Clin Sci (Lond)*. 2002;103(1):21–29.
420. Urban Z, et al. Connection between elastin haploinsuffi-ciency and increased cell proliferation in patients with supravalvular aortic stenosis and Williams-Beuren syn-drome. *Am J Hum Genet*. 2002;71(1):30–44.
421. Vernant P, et al. [120 cases of the Williams and Beuren syn-drome.] *Arch Mal Coeur Vaiss*. 1980;73(6):661–666.
422. Kaplan P, Levinson M, Kaplan BS. Cerebral artery stenoses in Williams syndrome cause strokes in childhood. *J Pediatr*. 1995;126(6):943–945.
423. Bonnet D, et al. Progressive left main coronary artery obstruction leading to myocardial infarction in a child with Williams syndrome. *Eur J Pediatr*. 1997;156(10):751–753.
424. Casanelles Mdel C, et al. Portal hypertension in Williams syndrome: report of two patients. *Am J Med Genet*. 2003;118A(4):372–376.
425. Rose C, et al. Anomalies of the abdominal aorta in Williams-Beuren syndrome—another cause of arterial hypertension. *Eur J Pediatr*. 2001;160(11):655–658.
426. Narasimhan C, Alexander T, Krishnaswami S. Pseudohyper-tension in a child with Williams syndrome. *Pediatr Cardiol*. 1993;14(2):124–126.
427. Wessel A, et al. Three decades of follow-up of aortic and pulmonary vascular lesions in the Williams-Beuren syn-drome. *Am J Med Genet*. 1994;52(3):297–301.
428. O'Connor WN, et al. Supravalvular aortic stenosis. Clinical and pathologic observations in six patients. *Arch Pathol Lab Med*. 1985;109(2):179–185.
429. Siwik ES, Perry SB, Lock JE. Endovascular stent implanta-tion in patients with stenotic aortoarteriopathies: early and medium-term results. *Catheter Cardiovasc Interv*. 2003;59(3):380–386.
430. Courtel JV, et al. Percutaneous transluminal angioplasty of renal artery stenosis in children. *Pediatr Radiol*. 1998;28(1):59–63.
431. Apostolopoulou SC, et al. Restenosis and pseudoaneurysm formation after stent placement for aortic coarctation in Williams syndrome. *J Vasc Interv Radiol*. 2002;13(5): 547–548.
432. Wilcken DE. Overview of inherited metabolic disorders causing cardiovascular disease. *J Inherit Metab Dis*. 2003;26(2–3):245–257.
433. Nienaber CA, Von Kodolitsch Y. Therapeutic management of patients with Marfan syndrome: focus on cardiovascular involvement. *Cardiol Rev*. 1999;7(6):332–341.
434. van Karnebeek CD, et al. Natural history of cardiovascular manifestations in Marfan syndrome. *Arch Dis Child*. 2001;84(2):129–137.
435. Yetman AT, Bornemeier RA, McCrindle BW. Long-term out-come in patients with Marfan syndrome: is aortic dissec-tion the only cause of sudden death? *J Am Coll Cardiol*. 2003;41(2):329–332.
436. De Paepe A, et al. Revised diagnostic criteria for the Mar-fan syndrome. *Am J Med Genet*. 1996;62(4):417–426.
437. Dietz HC. Marfan syndrome. In: *GeneReviews at GeneTests*. Seattle: University of Washington; 2003.
438. Gott VL, et al. Replacement of the aortic root in patients with Marfan's syndrome. *N Engl J Med*. 1999;340(17): 1307–1313.
439. Tambeur L, et al. Results of surgery for aortic root aneurysm in patients with the Marfan syndrome. *Eur J Car-diothorac Surg*. 2000;17(4):415–419.
440. Gott VL, et al. Aortic root replacement in 271 Marfan patients: a 24-year experience. *Ann Thorac Surg*. 2002;73(2):438–443.
441. de Wazieres B, et al. [Vascular and/or cardiac manifesta-tions of type IV Ehlers-Danlos syndrome. 9 cases.] *Presse Med*. 1995;24(30):1381–1385.
442. Pepin M, et al. Clinical and genetic features of Ehlers-Danlos syndrome type IV, the vascular type. *N Engl J Med*. 2000;342(10):673–680.
443. Ayres JG, et al. Abnormalities of the lungs and thoracic cage in the Ehlers-Danlos syndrome. *Thorax*. 1985;40(4):300–305.
444. Pepin MG, Byers PH. Ehlers-Danlos syndrome, vascular type. In: *GeneReviews at GeneTests*. Seattle: University of Washington; 2003.
445. Cikrit DF, et al. The Ehlers-Danlos specter revisited. *Vasc Endovascular Surg*. 2002;36(3):213–217.
446. Lauwers G, et al. Ehlers-Danlos syndrome type IV: a hetero-geneous disease. *Ann Vasc Surg*. 1997;11(2):178–182.
447. Mattar SG, Kumar AG, Lumsden AB. Vascular complications in Ehlers-Danlos syndrome. *Am Surg*. 1994;60(11):827–831.
448. Karkos CD, et al. Rupture of the abdominal aorta in patients with Ehlers-Danlos syndrome. *Ann Vasc Surg*. 2000;14(3):274–277.
449. Zheng Y, et al. Ehlers-Danlos syndrome: case and pedigree report and review. *Zhonghua Yu Fang Yi Xue Za Zhi*. 2002;36(7):491–494.
450. Sugawara Y, et al. Successful coil embolization for sponta-neous arterial rupture in association with Ehlers-Danlos syn-drome type IV: report of a case. *Surg Today*. 2003;34(1):94–96.
451. Sultan S, et al. Operative and endovascular management of extracranial vertebral artery aneurysm in Ehlers-Danlos syndrome: a clinical dilemma—case report and literature review. *Vasc Endovascular Surg*. 2002;36(5):389–392.
452. Fauci AS, et al. The idiopathic hypereosinophilic syn-drome—clinical, pathophysiologic and therapeutic consid-erations. *Ann Intern Med*. 1982;97:78–92.
453. Weller PF, et al. The idiopathic hypereosinophilic syn-drome. *Blood*. 1994;83(1):2759–2779.

VASCULAR ANATOMY AND PATHOLOGY

11 CHAPTER

Cerebral Arteries and Veins

Stephan G. Wetzel

In 1927, about 30 years after Conrad Wilhelm Roentgen's detection of x-rays, Egas Moniz of Portugal performed the first cerebral arteriogram in a human by direct puncture of the carotid artery. Since then, conventional angiographic technique has been continuously refined to reduce the risk of the procedure and to increase the diagnostic yield. Major technical developments along the way included a technique to facilitate percutaneous access, the Seldinger technique in 1953, the development of digital subtraction angiography (DSA) by C. A. Mistretta in 1973, improvements of contrast agents and catheters, and more recently, the introduction of rotational acquisitions that have made three-dimensional (3D) DSA imaging possible. For half a century, conventional angiography was *the* method for imaging of the cerebral vasculature.

In the early 1970s, Godfrey N. Hounsfield introduced "computer tomography" (CT), and Paul Lauterbur laid the foundation for magnetic resonance imaging (MRI). These cross-sectional imaging techniques revolutionized diagnostic strategies in clinical neurology and neurosurgery. Refinements in the technique soon allowed not only detection of parenchymal brain disease (e.g., tumors) or sequela of vascular disease (e.g., bleedings and infarcts) but dedicated assessment of the cerebral vasculature as well.

The non- or minimally invasive nature of these techniques, combined with the ability to obtain information about the brain parenchyma within the same examination, represent clear advantages of CT angiography (CTA) and MR angiography (MRA) compared with all other imaging techniques. Continuing developments in the field of CT (e.g., advanced multidetector techniques) as well as MR (e.g., parallel imaging techniques and high field imaging) steadily enable improved assessment of the cerebral arteries and veins. The trend toward greater diagnostic accuracy of these techniques has led to expanded clinical indications. CTA, for example, is beginning to challenge the role of DSA for search of aneurysms in patients presenting with subarachnoid hemorrhage.

Based on these encouraging developments, one would assume that CTA and MRA, by replacing established imaging techniques such as conventional angiography, would lead to a decline in the use of these modalities. Interestingly, an analysis of trends in neuroimaging based on U.S. nationwide Medicare data revealed that the use of conventional angiography increased by almost 25% between 1993 and 1998 (1). While a thorough discussion about the merits, pitfalls, and implications of these data is beyond the scope of this text, it is plausible to consider that a limited understanding of the techniques and advantages inherent to CTA and MRA may substantially contribute. Supporting this assumption is the fact that conventional angiography has had the highest geographic variation in the use of *all* diagnostic neuroimaging procedures, and MRA has had the highest of the noninvasive cross-sectional techniques.

For CTA and MRA of the cerebral vasculature to replace DSA, the essential information to make a diagnosis and to establish a treatment plan must be obtainable in a reliable and reproducible manner. Apart from clinical and technical knowledge, dedication to analyzing the images is required to achieve this goal. Despite advances in postprocessing, a rigorous and sometimes tedious analysis of source images or of tailored targeted views is often necessary to provide the diagnostic information. An analysis of CTA images in the search for an aneurysm is often more time consuming than the analysis of the images from conventional angiography.

Because CTA and MRA should be considered as methods that can replace conventional angiography for many indications, knowledge of the specific imaging properties of DSA is required. This and the indications and limitations of ultrasonography, the other important noninvasive imaging technique, are outlined here.

DSA is still considered to be the standard of reference for the depiction of the cerebral vasculature and for most vascular pathology. The main advantages of the technique compared with CTA and MRA are the unsurpassed spatial and temporal resolution, and the ability to selectively view vessels.

The spatial resolution with matrix sizes of 1024 × 1024 available on most modern DSA units allows an excellent assessment of the morphological changes of the small intracranial vessels and an anatomic display of arteries that cannot be visualized with even the most advanced CTA or MRA techniques. An example of the latter is the perforating arteries, which are crucial to visualize in the treatment planning of some aneurysms.

The high temporal resolution of DSA together with selective injections into the cervical or cerebral vessels provides the possibility to qualitatively assess cerebral hemodynamics. Such a capacity is used to characterize high-flow arteriovenous malformations with great detail and enables the demonstration of collateralization patterns in steno-occlusive disease (Fig. 11-1).

On the other hand, DSA has definite limitations in that it is time consuming, expensive, and requires exposure to radiation. Moreover, DSA is associated with definable risks. Transient neurological complications occur with selective catheter angiography in approximately 1% of patients, and the risk for permanent neurological deficit is about 0.3%. These complication risks are higher for the subgroup of patients with transient ischemic attacks or stroke, demonstrating transit deficits in 3% and permanent deficits in 0.7% when used as a purely diagnostic tool (2).

As a 2D projectional technique, the DSA assessment is restricted to the intraluminal part of the vessel, which is a further disadvantage of the technique. With DSA, unlike CTA

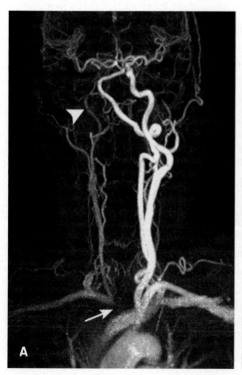 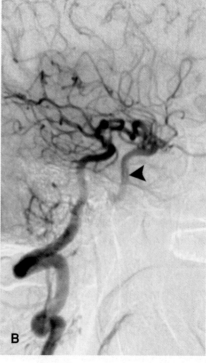

FIGURE 11-1 A: CE MRA MIP image of the cervicocranial vessels. Occlusion of the brachiocephalic trunk (*arrow*), the right ICA is poorly delineated (*arrowhead*), the left VA is enlarged. **B:** DSA, injection into the left VA shows cross flow via the PCoA into the distal ICA (*arrowhead*).

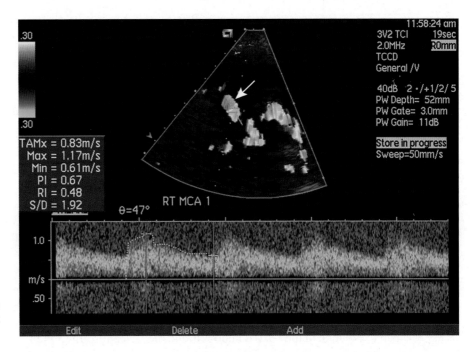

FIGURE 11-2 TCD of the right MCA. The Doppler probe (*arrow*) reveals a poststenotic flow pattern.

or MRA, vessel wall pathology, such as mural pathology or thrombus formation, cannot be directly assessed. As well, numerous views with repeated injections of contrast material from different angles are often necessary to obtain the desired display of the vessels. This has been overcome on modern DSA units with the use of rotational acquisitions and 3D reconstructions.

Finally, forced arterial injections are required with DSA to obtain the angiographic effect, thus altering hemodynamics. In contrast, flow dynamics visualized with MRA techniques are based on innate flow effects.

Ultrasonographic techniques provide information on hemodynamics and structural changes of the intracranial vessels. Transcranial Doppler sonography (TCD), introduced in the early 1980s (3), depicts hemodynamic information by measuring the difference in frequency between two successive echos—the Doppler shift—thus indicating the velocity and direction of the moving blood cells. The differentiation between individual vessels can be difficult, however, since this method has no imaging component, and the signal obtained is assigned to a specific vessel on the basis of indirect parameters (depth of the sample volume, position of the transducer, direction of the blood flow).

With transcranial color-coded duplex sonography, a frequency-based 2D color-coded depiction of the anatomical course of cerebral vessels became possible, which enabled a more exact, angle-corrected measurement of blood flow velocities (Fig. 11-2). The subsequent development of ultrasonographic techniques include power Doppler that depicts the integrated intensity of moving particles and contrast-enhanced (CE) sonographic techniques.

A major advantage of sonography is the ability to detect flow alterations of the major cerebral vessels, including cross-flow patterns through the circle of Willis, with a relatively inexpensive bedside examination. A unique feature of TCD is the ability to detect embolic material traveling within the arteries (4), which seems to be a promising tool to assess pathophysiological factors of cerebral ischemia, and to assess, for example, the effectiveness of antiplatelet agents in the prevention of stroke. Furthermore, the technique can be used to detect cardiac and extracardiac right-to-left shunts by monitoring for intravenously injected microbubbles that normally do not survive the pulmonary passage, thus providing information in the workup of patients with stroke.

The main disadvantages of sonography include poor morphological information compared with other neurovascular imaging techniques, operator dependence, and the limited field of view of the insonation window.

The main clinical indications for transcranial ultrasonographic studies are the evaluation of patients with suspected steno-occlusive disease of the cerebral arteries, in particular of the MCA, and the evaluation and follow-up of patients with vasospasm after subarachnoid hemorrhage.

COMPUTED TOMOGRAPHIC AND MAGNETIC RESONANCE ANGIOGRAPHY OF CEREBRAL ARTERIES AND VEINS: TECHNICAL CONSIDERATIONS

A basic understanding of some key principles of CT and MR physics is necessary for optimizing protocols and for maximizing the diagnostic yield of the obtained information (Chapters 1 and 2). In this section, a clinician's view on the essential technical considerations for CTA and MRA of the cerebral vasculature is provided.

Computed Tomographic Angiography

Until the late 1980s, CT scanners acquired data in discrete slices of patient anatomy, a method often called *axial scanning*. The advent of slip-ring technology and new reconstruction techniques provided a gateway to the data acquisition currently in use, spiral or helical CT, and multislice spiral or multidetector/multirow CT (MDCT) data acquisition systems, that, in turn, have paved the way toward the high-quality dedicated CTA examinations of the cerebral vessels currently obtainable.

In spiral or helical CT, the patient translates through the gantry while the x-ray tube rotates around the patient. Compared with conventional or axial CT a *volume* of data is collected, the spatial resolution in the z-axis is improved, and the scan time is reduced. These features are the prerequisites for optimized CT angiography and an enhanced capacity to generate meaningful multiplanar (MPR) or 3D renderings.

Key parameters for spiral tomography are section collimation, the table feed per rotation, and the pitch (table feed per rotation/section collimation). By extending the pitch factor (e.g., from 1 to 1.5) for a given scan length, the patient dose can be reduced (in this example by 33%) as well as the acquisition time. The accompanying trade-off is a slight broadening of the slice sensitivity profile (effective axial slice thickness). Recent implementations of faster gantry rotations can further speed up acquisitions or be used to obtain higher z-axis resolution.

The development of spiral CTs with multiple-row detectors, MDCT, has allowed a more efficient use of the x-rays produced by the tube while improving z-axis resolution. Owing to the faster acquisition of a long scanning range, MDCT is particularly useful for the evaluation of the thoracoabdominal region, where large organs can be scanned during a single breath hold.

As applied to neurovascular imaging, MDCT yields near isotropic submillimeter resolution scanning. A depiction of the circle of Willis in the arterial phase without venous contamination is now readily obtainable, in particular if MDCTs capable of acquiring greater than four sections per rotation are used.

As in spiral CT, section collimation and the table feed per rotation are the most important acquisition parameters. Unfortunately, different definitions of the pitch factor are used with multislice CT scanners, depending on whether the *total collimation* (number of active arrays × section collimation) or a *section* of the detector array is chosen as a reference. In the first case, the pitch is termed *beam pitch* or *volume pitch* and often is denoted with P [table feed per rotation/(number of active arrays × section collimation)] consistent with the notion of pitch used in single-row detector helical CT. The detector pitch, denoted P*, used by most vendors, indicates the width of a single active detector channel (table feed per rotation/section collimation). The relation between the two definitions of pitch is:

$$P = P^*/n.$$

Protocols

Optimized patient preparation is a prerequisite for any neurovascular CTA examination. In those patients who are confused, irritable, or uncooperative, strategies to reduce motion artifacts such as immobilization of the head by using an adhesive tape or the administration of a short-acting sedative should be considered.

To achieve a reasonably homogenous vascular opacification, the use of a power injector is mandatory, and an injection rate of 3 to 5 mL per second should be chosen. For all neurovascular applications, 80 to 100 mL of iodinated contrast material is usually sufficient. With MDCT, the dosage might be reduced especially if a small volume of anatomy (e.g., the circle of Willis) is scanned with a high acquisition speed (e.g., ≥16-slice CT). To assure that the contrast material is pushed forward through the venous system past the end of the actual contrast injection, a saline chaser bolus (e.g., 40 mL, injection rate of 3 to 5 mL per second, identical to that used for the contrast media) should be injected immediately after contrast administration.

Scanning should only take place during the plateau phase of vessel enhancement. Due to known large variation of circulation times of patients (5), the synchronization of the start of the scan with the arrival of the contrast material in the arteries of the brain should be planned on a per patient basis (Fig. 11-3). The synchronization is important to ensure maximal contrast within the vessels if single slice CT is used but becomes crucial if fast MDCT for arterial imaging with little or no venous overlay is desired, given the short arteriovenous transit time within the brain of about 6 to 8 seconds.

For synchronization, two methods are available. With the first method, the test-bolus injection, a small amount of contrast (15 to 20 mL) is injected. Following an empiric 10-second delay, a low-dose dynamic, nonincremental CT scan at the midcervical level or at the level of the frontal sinus (e.g., 15 slices at a rate of 1 image per second) is performed to determine the arrival time of the small test-dose bolus. Based on the test-bolus arrival time, the CTA examination can be adequately planned and based on the physiology of the individual. Thus, with the test bolus, two separate injections are necessary—one for the arrival time assessment followed by a diagnostic run with a full dose of contrast media.

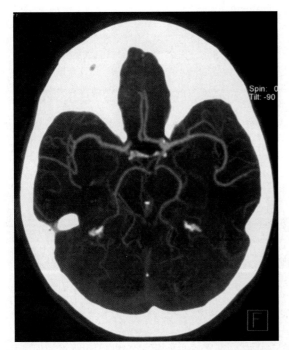

FIGURE 11-3 CTA MIP image of the intracranial arteries obtained with a 16-slice scanner using the test bolus injection. The opacification of the veins and sinuses is minimal.

ner model—in the order of 2 to 8 seconds, which might be too long to image within the arterial phase.

For imaging of the venous system, an individual timing of the contrast administration is not necessary from our experience. In this scenario, we usually start scanning 30 seconds after contrast administration, which ensures a good opacification of the cerebral veins and sinuses.

The coverage of the investigation volume depends on the clinical demand. For cerebral arterial imaging, our standard protocol covers the distance from the anterior arch of C1 to the top of the frontal sinus. Depending on the clinical question, it is restricted to the central section (e.g., for imaging of a middle cerebral artery stenosis) or expanded to include the cervical vessels as well. For venous imaging, the entire head is scanned.

Protocols for performing dedicated CTA examinations depend in detail on the equipment being used. Detailed imaging protocols depend on the type of CT scanner used. Table 11-1 gives the protocols we found useful for a 4-slice, a 16-slice, and a 64-slice scanner (Siemens, Erlangen, Germany).

Visualization Techniques

Image acquisition with thin collimation is a prerequisite to obtain secondary reconstructions with a high spatial resolution. Four main visualization techniques are currently in use to evaluate the volumetric data sets—multiplanar reformations (MPR), maximum-intensity projections (MIP), shaded surface display (SSD), and volume rendering (VR). On most commercially available 3D workstations, it is possible to display images in three planes simultaneously to allow for cross referencing and to change the display mode on the fly (Fig. 11-4).

MPR images that are single voxel tomograms are usually the primary mode of evaluation. They are particularly

To avoid these separate injections, many CT scanners have a bolus-triggering feature built into their system. With this approach, online monitoring of a region-of-interest (e.g., carotid or cerebral arteries) is carried out using low-dose, nonincremental scans during the injection of contrast medium. Then, the diagnostic CTA acquisition is initiated on achieving a predefined enhancement threshold (e.g., 100 HU). However, a drawback of this method is a delay time in the start of the actual acquisition—depending on the scan-

TABLE 11-1

Imaging Parameters for Computed Tomographic Angiography of the Intracranial Arteries*

	4-Slice MDCT	16-Slice MDCT	64-Slice MDCT
Collimation (mm)	4 × 1	16 × 0.75	64 × 0.6
Table feed (mm)	5	13.5	46.1
Gantry rotation (s)	0.5	0.5	0.5
Pitch (P/P*)	1.25/5	1.125/18	1.2/77
kV	120	120	100
Eff. mAs	130	130	160
Contrast volume (mL)	100	80	80
Delay	Test bolus or auto triggered		
Reconstruction/increment (mm)	1.25/0.6	0.75/0.4	0.6/0.5

*Volume Zoom Sensation 4, Somatom Sensation 16 and 64 scanner; Siemens, Erlangen, Germany.

Note: The scanning range extends from the top of the circle of Willis to the anterior arch of C1. For scanning of the venous system, the scanning range extends from the vertex to the anterior arch of C1, with a fixed scan delay of 30 seconds (eff. mAs 120).

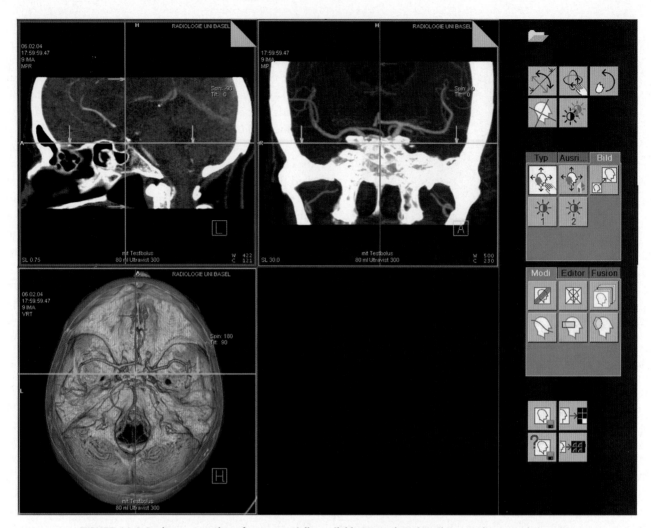

FIGURE 11-4 Desktop screenshot of a commercially available 3D workstation. Three visualization techniques are displayed. **Top left:** MPR image in sagittal plane. **Top right:** 30-mm MIP slab in coronal plane, centered around the green line as displayed on the image top left (cross referencing). **Bottom left:** VR image.

useful when evaluating intraluminal pathologies and for the visualization of brain parenchyma or osseous structures in conjunction with the vessels. Because the course of most vessels does not lie within a single plane, however, the entirety of a vessel can rarely be depicted. To overcome this problem, curved planar reformats can be reconstructed. These images are created from a line that connects points that were manually positioned over a vessel as viewed on standard MPR, MIP, SSD, or VR. Depending on the software, these reconstructions can be rotated, and sections perpendicular to the central pathline can be obtained, allowing for precise assessment of vessel cross section and degree of stenosis.

MIPs are created when a specific projection is selected (e.g., anteroposterior), and then rays are cast perpendicular to the view through the volume data, with the maximum value encountered by each ray encoded on a 2D output image. As a result, the entire volume is collapsed, with only the brightest structures being visible. In contrast to MPR, vascular structures that do not lie in a single plane in their entirety can be visualized. MIP images preserve the "attenuation" information (which allows distinguishing between contrast-material–filled vessels and calcifications); however, the "depth" information (which allows distinguishing "closer" from "farther away" anatomic structures) is lost.

A practical limitation to this technique is the obscuration of contrast-enhanced blood vessels by structures that are more attentuative than the vessels—a particular problem in the display of the cerebral vessels due to the close relation between the vessels and the bone. Editing of the data set to obtain images of, for example, the circle of Willis is time consuming; therefore, slab MIPs (targeted MIPs) are an excellent alternative for image display. Slab MIPs are created when a plane through the data is defined

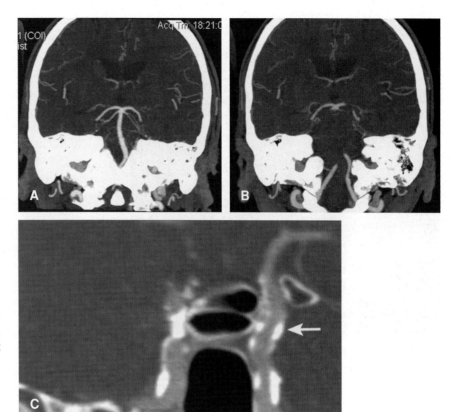

FIGURE 11-5 CTA MIP slab images of cerebral arteries. A, B: Two thin slices in paracoronal orientation already give a good overview about the anatomy of the vertebrobasilar circulation. **C:** For evaluation of the intracranial ICA that follows a complex course, curved MIP images (here, 2-mm thickness) can be helpful. Note vessel calcifications on both sides (*arrow*) that can be well differentiated from the contrast-filled vessel lumen.

and then "thickened" to the desired width. By selecting a slab thickness and slab orientation that does not include high attenuation structures, an increased display of the vessel throughout its course is available while preserving delineation (Fig. 11-5).

SSD is an efficient modality that usually requires no prior editing to obtain 3D views for the demonstration of complex 3D vascular anatomy. With this technique, the user defines a range of Hounsfield values to select the tissue to be rendered. Rays are passed through the entire volume that "stop" at the point the threshold range is reached for the first time. Only the surface is displayed in this method, and the "depth" information is preserved. Shading the voxels enhances the effect so that the volume appears to be illuminated by a light source.

However, with SSD, the "attenuation" information is lost. The major disadvantage of SSD is the limited accuracy of the 3D images as the display depends on the selected threshold values (Fig. 11-6). Thus, arteries will appear to vary in caliber depending on the thresholds that are selected, unsuitable threshold values may simulate occlusion or stenosis of vessels, and calcified plaque that accompany a stenosis that fall within the same threshold range as the blood vessel lumen result in the appearance of a local dilatation, rather than a stenosis (6).

The VR technique is the most complex rendering method that allows the integration of all available information from a volumetric data set with control of the opacity or translucency of selected tissue types (Fig. 11-7) (7).

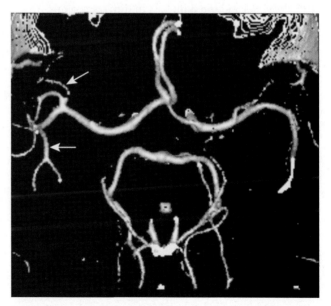

FIGURE 11-6 SSD of the cerebral arteries. Smaller arteries are rendered irregular or with gaps (*arrows*).

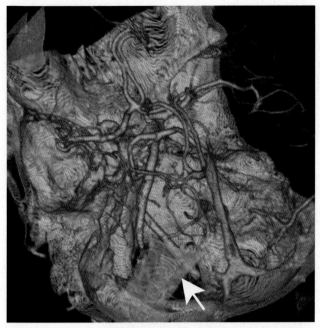

FIGURE 11-7 VR image of the cerebral vessels. The vessels here can be well differentiated from the bony structures. Due to differences in opacity levels, it is possible to look "through" the bone (*arrow*).

There are many different versions of volume rendering, but in general, the user defines the opacity values for various HUs. In a second step, rays are passed through the volume that accumulate values along the way. Groups of voxels within defined attenuation thresholds are assigned a color and an opacity level that can be varied from total transparency to total opacity. With this technique, it is possible to demonstrate, for example, a vessel calcification together with the vessel and the skull base in different colors.

For image presentation, some standardized slab MIPs are usually sufficient. However, these images are not sufficient for a reliable image interpretation! The actual analysis of the complex anatomy of the cerebral vessels requires a free-form interrogation of the source data set on the 3D workstation and should include as many types of image display as required to understand the geometry and pathology.

Magnetic Resonance Angiography

MRA was introduced into clinical practice about 15 years ago and has rapidly become a mainstay in the evaluation of neurovascular disease. Compared with CTA, there is no ionizing radiation and no need for nephrotoxic contrast media. Flow-dependent acquisition techniques, phase contrast MRA (PC MRA), and in particular, the time-of-flight MRA (TOF MRA) have predominated for the evaluation of the cerebral vessels.

These techniques are highly versatile and, in addition to the morphological assessment of the neurovascular anatomy, allow the user to determine blood flow direction or the quantification of blood flow. The main drawbacks are the relative long acquisition times and the vulnerability to artifacts—for example, signal loss due to saturation effects or turbulent flow (Chapter 2).

With flow-independent, contrast-enhanced MR angiography (CE MRA) techniques, the hyperintense signal intensities in the vessels result from the T1 shortening of blood in response to an injection of a gadolinium chelate. This approach offers an image that emphasizes morphological features of the vessel lumen rather than the physiological features of blood vessel flow. However, CE MRA requires trade-offs between imaging speed, volume coverage, and resolution in order to obtain satisfactory venousfree images.

At the current time, no single technique for optimal visualization of all intracranial vessels exists. However, for both the flow-dependent and the flow-independent acquisition modalities, numerous technical variations exist for evaluation of the cerebral vessels that are chosen in dependence of the clinical question.

Time-of-flight Magnetic Resonance Angiography

In general, the robust, flow-dependent TOF MRA technique is primarily used for imaging of the cerebral vessels (Fig. 11-8). TOF MRA is based on the differences in saturation between the extravascular and intravascular (moving blood) constituents. The signal intensity of static tissue (extravascular)

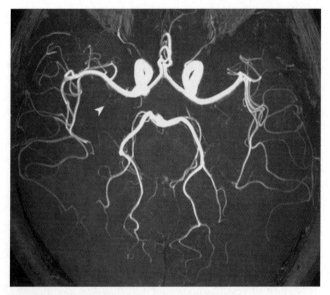

FIGURE 11-8 3D TOF at 3T with a voxel size of 0.13 mm3 (TE 3.4, TR 26, 832 3 1024 matrix). Small lenticulostriate arteries can be visualized (*arrowhead*). Courtesy of W. Willineck, University Hospital Bonn, Bonn, Germany.

is progressively suppressed by repetitive radio frequency pulses, and the inflow enhancement in the investigated vessel produces the angiographic effect.

The most important drawbacks of TOF MRA are the saturation effect and (poststenotic) signal voids, the latter caused by intravoxel incoherence in regions with turbulent flow. Numerous variations of the technique to reduce these shortcomings and methods to improve the inflow-related enhancement have been introduced.

In 3D TOF, one single volume (slab) is excited and segmented into small slices by a second-phase encoding gradient, while in 2D TOF, multiple single slices are acquired sequentially. Both methods have specific advantages and disadvantages as well as resulting different applications.

A major benefit of 3D TOF acquisition is the optimized resolution in all directions. With 3D techniques, slice thickness can be reduced to below 1 mm. In 2D techniques, slice thickness usually varies between 2 and 3 mm, which makes this technique more prone to dephasing effects as the number of different possible phases within the voxel increase. On the other hand, compared with the 3D technique, the 2D method shows an improved sensitivity for inflowing magnetization based on minimized flow saturation effects: In sequential acquisitions, each slice of the data set represents an "entry" slice with the strongest possible intravascular signal. This enables the use of a slightly higher flip angle and as a consequence an overall improvement in signal-to-noise ratio (SNR). Therefore, this technique is well suited for the detection of slow laminar flow conditions.

Based on these properties, 3D TOF MRA is mainly used for the depiction of the relatively small cerebral arteries, while 2D TOF MRA is used for the depiction of the slower flowing cerebral veins. For both techniques, optimized inflow conditions are achieved by orientating the imaging plane perpendicular to the predominant vascular flow direction—for imaging of the cerebral arteries, the preferred imaging plane is therefore axial; for imaging of cerebral veins, the coronal plane is preferred.

To reduce saturation effects in 3D TOF MRA, titled optimized nonsaturating excitation (TONE) radio frequency pulses are frequently used. These pulses provide flip angles that are variable along the slice selection direction. Typically, low flip angles are applied at the entrance side of the arteries in the volume of interest to delay saturation. The flip angle is then steadily increased in cranial direction; the increasing flip angles offer maximal signal recovery from that which remains in the flowing blood, deeper in the slab. The gradient of the TONE pulse (or ramped flip angle) depends on the velocity and the slab thickness (e.g., for imaging of the intracranial arteries 10 degrees at the entrance side and 30 degrees near the top of the volume).

Another method to improve the inflow-related enhancement in 3D acquisitions represents the multiple overlapping thin slice acquisitions (MOTSA) technique. Instead of one thick slab, multiple, consecutively acquired 3D data sets are combined to yield a single reconstruction of the final volume (Fig. 11-9). Because the slab excitation profiles in the slice selection direction are never ideal, these 3D acquisitions have to be mutually overlapping in order to portray the vessels in a smooth and continuous manner.

Incorrect matching of the separate volumes due to gross patient motion might occur as well as visible transitions between the different slabs, leading to a slab boundary or "venetian blind" called *artifact* on the MRA MIP image. The latter artifact can be reduced by increasing the slab overlap and reducing the number of partitions.

A common way to cope with saturation of the intracranial arteries using 3D TOF MRA is to suppress the stationary tissue using a magnetization transfer prepulse. A strong, off-resonance radio frequency pulse saturates the spins of large molecules (macromolecules) that contain protons or are associated with water molecules bound to them. This bound proton pool is able to exchange energy with the free proton pool (water).

The saturated macromolecular spins with zero magnetization will exchange for water spins having magnetization of one. Thus, when the magnetization of the water spins is subsequently measured, it will be found to be less than one.

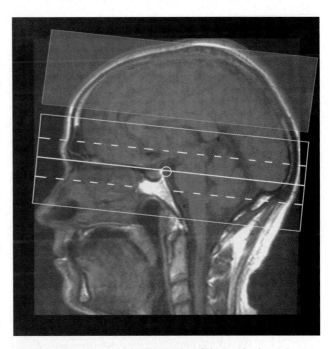

FIGURE 11-9 Planning of 3D TOF MRA of the cerebral arteries with MOTSA. Three separate volumes are acquired; a saturation pulse is applied cranially to suppress venous structures.

As a result, the signal of brain tissue decreases, whereas the signal of flowing blood is unaffected.

Finally, in standard TOF sequences, a presaturation pulse is implemented into the sequence, nulling the cephalocaudad (venous) flow. This saturation pulse is placed parallel and directly superior to the imaging plane (Fig. 11-9).

The image quality of the long-established TOF technique can be considerably improved by two recently introduced MR technologies that have become widely available: high-field imaging and parallel imaging. With 1.5T imaging, the spatial resolution of 3D TOF MRA is limited, and attempts to pursue 1024 spatial resolution would be associated with lower SNR with reasonable scan times. Apart from an increased SNR, 3T high-field-strength MR imaging provides an improved vessel-to-tissue contrast due to the shortening of the T1 relaxation (8,9).

In a study comparing standard resolution 3D TOF MRA (true voxel volume 0.92 mm^3) at 1.5T and 3T with high resolution MRA (true voxel volume, 0.13 mm^3), the high-spatial-resolution 3T examination was found to provide a superior image quality and a significantly better depiction of small vessels segments and vascular disease (9).

Parallel MR imaging techniques, for example, sensitivity encoding (SENSE), facilitate imaging by partially shifting the burden of spatial encoding from magnetic field gradients to receive coils (10). This allows faster imaging, or, alternatively, with an equivalent acquisition time, images with increased spatial resolution can be obtained. However, especially in high spatial resolution examinations at 1.5T where the SNR is already borderline, the relative loss of SNR that scales with the square root of the SENSE reduction factor can be a drawback.

Willinek et al. recently combined the advantages of 3T imaging (high signal-to-noise) with that of SENSE (speed) and found this technique compared with the technique without SENSE promising, as it allowed a substantially reduced measurement time while maintaining the image quality of the 3D TOF MRA examination without SENSE (11).

Phase-contrast Magnetic Resonance Angiography

PC MRA is based on the application of a bipolar gradient pulse pair producing a phase shift depending on the velocity component along the gradient (Fig. 11-10). The technique is very flow sensitive and provides full background suppression but requires a relatively long acquisition time if flow is encoded in all three spatial directions (3D PC MRA).

A velocity-encoding gradient (VENC) of 15 to 20 cm per second for imaging of the venous system and of 60 to 80 cm per second for display of the arteries is usually recommended. However, a variety of velocities can occur in cerebral arterial disease, complicating the correct selection of the VENC. Thus, the method is not as widely used for depiction of the cerebral vessels as is the TOF technique.

Projective 2D PC MRA images on the other hand can be acquired fast (1 min) and easily. This technique is often used to determine the topographic location of the craniocervical

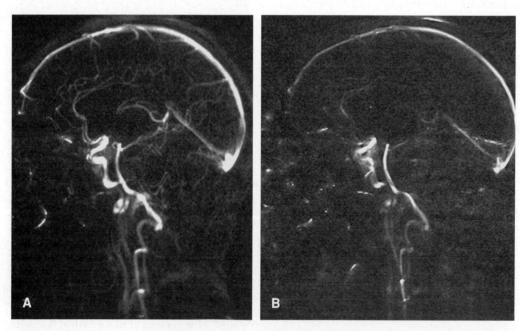

FIGURE 11-10 Single-slice 2D PC MRA obtained in sagittal orientation. With **(A)** a VENC of 15 cm per second, the venous structures are considerably better visualized compared with image acquisition with **(B)** a VENC of 60 cm per second.

arteries in coronal direction, enabling an adequate volume to be investigated by contrast-enhanced MRA methods. It can also provide a good depiction of flow in the major cerebral veins.

The unique capability for PC MRA to measure the flow velocity offers information unobtainable by other MRA strategies. In neurovascular applications, MR flow quantification techniques have most often been applied to evaluate the carotid arteries, intracranial arteries, and venous sinuses (12,13).

Recent technical advances allow for acquisitions of flow-sensitive time-resolved 3D MR based on ECG synchronized 3D phase contrast MRI. This enables a visual assessment and in vivo evaluation of local cerebral blood flow patterns with high temporal and spatial resolution (Fig. 11-11).

The typically long measurement times associated with MR flow quantification have hindered its widespread use in routine clinical practice. The feasibility of a technique to measure flow velocities of the carotid arteries and the cerebral sinuses in real time without the need for cardiac gating was recently described (14). For that purpose, a real time MR phase contrast technique was applied that uses a 2D selective radio frequency pulse followed by flow-sensitizing gradients with echoplanar readout. With this technique, the flow velocities are displayed as time-velocity curves, closely resembling Doppler flow-velocity distribution plots; hence, the technique was termed *duplex MR*. By controlling scan position and orientation interactively, flow signal is optimized (Fig. 11-12).

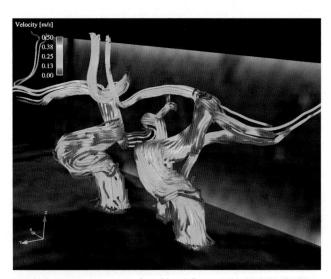

FIGURE 11-11 Overview of 3D blood-flow patterns and velocities of the circle of Willis. The image is based on an ECG-synchronized 3D phase-contrast MRI technique with advanced postprocessing strategies. The complex flow patterns and segmental changes in absolute blood flow velocities are color coded.

Contrast-enhanced Magnetic Resonance Angiography

Unlike TOF or PC MRA methods, CE MRA does not rely on the natural flow effects, but on the shortening of the T1 relaxation time of blood after intravenous injection of a paramagnetic contrast agent bolus. While for TOF techniques an acquisition perpendicular to the vessel is recommended to reduce saturation effects, CE MRA can be generated in any

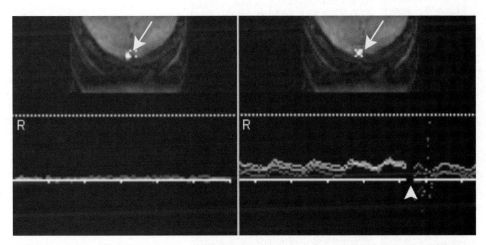

FIGURE 11-12 Duplex MR imaging of the SSS. At **top,** the anatomic image is displayed. The region of interest, representing four voxels, is indicated by four white circles (*arrows*). No flow signal is observed if the region of interest is placed outside the sinus **(left).** When all voxels are placed over the sinus **(right),** a slow uniform pulsatile flow can be observed, with craniocaudally directed flow displayed above the baseline **(bottom).** The distance from the baseline to the measured line represents the velocity (here, 35 cm per second), depending on the VENC (here, 100 cm per second). The baseline tick interval is 1 second; the gap on the baseline indicates the current point of measurement (*arrowhead*).

desired orientation, including acquisitions in the plane of the vessels of interest. The considerably shorter measurement times minimize the vulnerability to motion artifacts.

There are two principle techniques of CE MRA that have been applied for imaging of the cerebral vasculature that differ in acquisition time and pharmacodynamic distribution of contrast material during image acquisition: It can either be performed during the *steady state* after intravenous injection of the contrast medium or during the *initial transit* of the contrast bolus.

CE MRA during the steady state is technically less demanding, and a high resolution can be obtained (Fig. 11-13). These sequences can be helpful in differentiating true stenosis of large arteries from artifactual narrowing, to visualize distal intracranial arteries, and to image vascular pathologies that can contain areas of slow flow (e.g., large aneurysms, arteriovenous malformations) (15–17). For steady state arterial imaging, 3D TOF techniques are typically used with slightly increased flip angles to optimize vessel signal intensities (15).

Jung et al. found a small dose of 5 to 10 mL of gadopentetate dimeglumine to be optimal, as a larger dose of 20 mL limited the interpretation of the small and large arteries due to venous overlap—*the* shortcoming of CE steady state MRA (18). On the other hand, the dedicated assessment of the venous system is usually not hampered by the arteries.

Steady state MRA with 3D T1-weighted gradient-echo sequences was found to be an effective way to demonstrate the venous system with high resolution (Fig. 11-14). However, due to the long acquisition time—in the order of minutes—a chronic thrombus might enhance and be obscured if a steady state MRA technique is used. This pitfall is important to know in the work up of patients suspected to have a venous sinus thrombosis (see subsequent discussion) (19–21).

First-pass CE MRA is the more recent of the two CE MRA techniques (22). For clinical routine neuroradiological examinations, this technique has been mainly applied for assessment of the extracranial carotid arteries (23–25). Given the short transit time of 5 to 6 seconds between the middle cerebral artery and the straight or transverse sinus, the demanding part of this technique is obtaining images of the cerebral arteries without venous overlay. Therefore, to obtain an acceptable resolution, fast sequences that require high-performance gradients with fast rise times and high gradient strength are mandatory.

In general, two methods of first-pass CE MRA can be distinguished (26). In the first, dynamic, or time-resolved CE MRA, a 3D sequence with a measurement time in the order of 5 to 6 seconds is started simultaneously to the contrast injection and sequentially is repeated. This allows to distinguish arterial, early arteriovenous, late arteriovenous, and washout arteriovenous phases. However, due to the

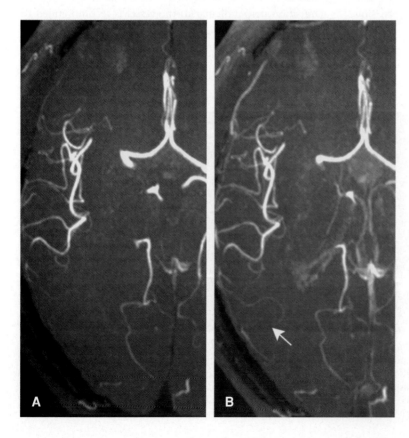

FIGURE 11-13 A: 3D TOF MRA MIP slab before and **(B)** after administration of 10 mL of gadopentetate dimeglumine. Smaller peripheral vessel branches are better visualized; however, there is overlap of the cerebral veins.

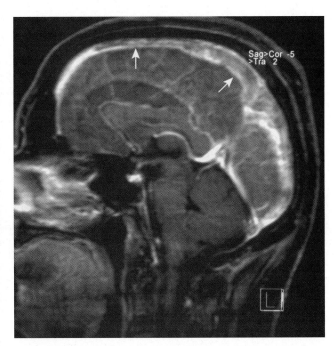

FIGURE 11-14 MIP slab in sagittal orientation of CE MRA in the steady state showing an extensive cerebral venous thrombosis in the SSS (*arrows*) (compare with Fig. 11-52A–D).

short acquisition time, the spatial resolution and hence the usefulness for arterial imaging is limited. For imaging of the cerebral veins, this fast imaging can be of use (27).

An alternative and effective way to visualize the dynamic transit of a contrast bolus from the arterial to the venous phase represents dynamic 2D MR projection angiography, also termed *magnetic resonance digital subtraction angiography* (28,29). This technique employs a modified gradient-echo sequence that is combined with a subtraction technique to maximize vessel-to-background contrast and allows 2D projection angiograms to be obtained of the entire cerebral circulation at a subsecond temporal frame rate with a high *in-plane* resolution (e.g., 1 mm^2). In practice, the sequence is simultaneously started to the injection of the contrast bolus, and the first images before arrival of the contrast are used to form a mask image. All further images are then calculated by complex subtraction of the mask from the subsequent images.

The technique can be extremely valuable for the detection of vascular pathologies that are characterized by fast arteriovenous transit times, parenchymal arteriovenous malformations, and foremost in the detection of dural arteriovenous fistulas (30,31). The lack of volumetric information with these 2D images, however, represents a limitation. More recently, the advantages of parallel imaging were exploited to obtain whole-brain 3D CE MRA images with high temporal resolution (<2 seconds per image). Although the spatial resolution is still limited (voxel size 2 mm^2), the information can be likewise of value for numerous pathologies that are characterized by fast arteriovenous transit times (Fig. 11-15).

To obtain first-pass CE MRA volumetric data sets with high spatial resolution that allow for detailed visualization

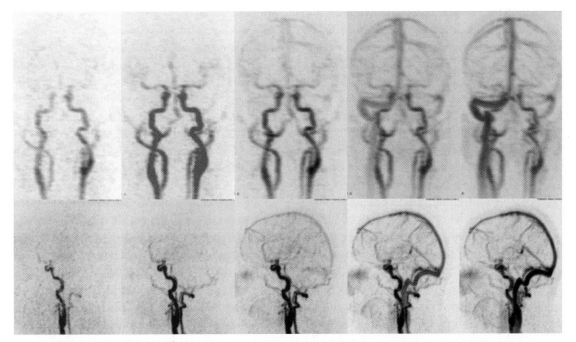

FIGURE 11-15 Time-resolved whole-brain 3D contrast-enhanced MRA with parallel imaging. Subsequently acquired data sets are displayed as MIP images in coronal and sagittal orientation (gray values inverted). The temporal resolution of 1.5 seconds allows visualizing of the dynamics of the contrast bolus passage through the brain (voxel size 2 mm^2).

of smaller intracranial arteries, longer measurement times are necessary. For venous contamination to be minimized, the data acquisition must be synchronized with the arrival of the contrast bolus such that the filling of central k-space lines (where the key determinants of image contrast are established) coincides with the maximal arterial signal prior to the arrival of contrast media in the veins. In the central part of k-space, the low frequencies are sampled, whereas at the periphery of k-space, the higher frequencies are sampled. At the periphery of k-space, the key determinants of image resolution are established.

In a linear phase-encoding table (symmetrical sampling), the low frequencies are sampled in the middle of the measurement time. If the bolus arrival time is determined with a small test bolus of contrast agent (1 to 2 mL) by a rapid and repetitive acquisition of 2D images, an exact timing of the bolus and the sequence becomes possible, and images with little or, ideally, no venous overlay can be generated. As in the case for the fast time-resolved techniques, a precontrast image set is usually subtracted from a postcontrast image set to maximize vessel-to-background contrast.

When this approach is compared with 3D TOF technique, the resolution is limited. However, CE MRA can be valuable, for example, for the detection and characterization of intracranial aneurysms by boosting intravascular contrast, minimizing vulnerability to slow flow signal loss, and the lack of a T1 contamination artifact from blood clot (16,32).

The use of fluoroscopic triggering in CE MRA overcomes the need for the separate test bolus. The arrival of the contrast agent bolus is displayed on-line with the 2D sequence. When the arteries in the monitoring image enhance, the operator starts the angiographic 3D sequence without delay. The contrast determining parts of k-space must be sampled early because the bolus maximum has arrived at the time the 3D MRA sequence begins.

This requires a specific order for k-space sampling in which the central portions of k-space are obtained at the beginning of the data acquisition. Referred to as *centric view ordering*, or *elliptical centric view ordering* if it is centric in both phase-encoding directions, this technique has been shown to be feasible for arterial imaging (33). Since the image contrast is established early in the acquisition, a much longer sampling time can be pursued with less chance of venous contamination.

Farb et al. used the centric-ordered technique with a long measurement time of about two minutes (34). In that study of arteriovenous malformations, pure arterial imaging was thus not possible, but images with a high resolution were created that were valuable for the evaluation of arteriovenous malformations (34).

INTRACRANIAL VASCULAR ANATOMY

A thorough understanding of the brain vascular anatomy is fundamental to making accurate interpretations in neuroimaging. Numerous excellent neuroradiological textbooks and atlas provide an exhaustive anatomic description of the normal vessels, the embryology of vessel formation, and anatomic variations (35–37). This is beyond the scope of this text. Rather, this chapter intends to give a description of the major cerebral vessels that are of importance for the assessment of CTA and MRA. Moreover, common variants and anatomic structures that are of special importance in certain clinical contexts are highlighted as well as some limitations in the anatomic display of the noninvasive techniques compared with DSA.

Arterial Anatomy

Neurovascular Extracranial Arteries

The right and left common carotid arteries (CCA) arise from the brachiocephalic trunk and the aortic arch, respectively. The CCAs typically divide at the C3 to C5 level into the external and internal carotid arteries (ECA and ICA). The first segments of the ICA are extracranial: (a) the carotid bulb, a dilatation at the origin of the ICA; and (b) the cervical segment of the ICA that terminates where the artery enters the temporal bone (petrous segment).

The ECA supplies most extracranial structures of the head and neck. The major branches are the superior thyroid, ascending pharyngeal, lingual, facial, occipital, posterior auricular, internal maxillary, and superficial temporal arteries.

The right and left vertebral arteries (VA) typically arise from the subclavian arteries. They normally ascend through the transverse foramen from C6 to C1. After looping posteriorly above the posterior part of the atlas, they pass through the foramen magnum and unite intradurally to form the basilar artery (BA). Small extracranial branches of the VA supply the spine and muscles; the posterior meningeal artery supplies the falx cerebelli and a part of the dura of the occipital bone.

Variants and clinical remarks. It is evident that the anatomic evaluation of the supra-aortic arteries is essential for a thorough analysis of numerous cerebrovascular disorders, foremost in the evaluation of patients with stroke. The major locations for atherosclerotic plaque formation that might lead to embolic infarcts or a critical hypoperfusion are the carotid bifurcation and the origin of the vertebral arteries. Dissections that may also result in cerebral infarcts are likewise more commonly extracranial in location: (a) at the ICA about two centimeters distal to the bifurcation; and (b) at the VA between the distal cervical segment and skull base.

Anastomoses between the extracranial and intracranial vasculature exist that can provide collateral flow in cases of

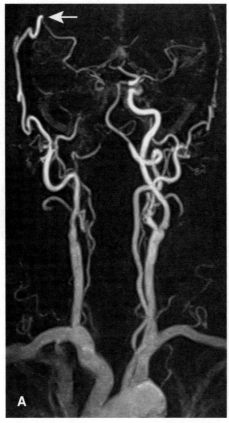

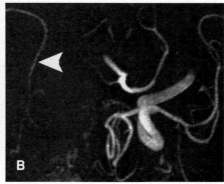

FIGURE 11-16 A: CE MRA of the cervico-cranial vessels showing a bypass between the right superficial temporal artery and the MCA (*arrow*). **B:** On 3D TOF MRA, flow is depicted in the periphery of the MCA (*arrowhead*), but not in the proximal part due to saturation effects.

vessel stenosis or occlusion (e.g., between the angular branch of the facial artery and the ICA). A surgical bypass ("iatrogenic bypass") between the extra- and intracranial vasculature is most commonly formed between the superficial temporal and the middle cerebral artery (Fig. 11-16).

Numerous variants on the origin of the great vessels from the aortic arch have been described. In order from proximal to distal, the most common are described: (a) right subclavian artery arising as the last instead of the first brachiocephalic vessel (aberrant right subclavian artery); (b) right CCA arising directly from the aortic arch; (c) left CCA as common origin or arising from the brachiocephalic trunk; and (d) left ICA, ECA, and left VA with direct origin from the aortic arch. The anatomy of the ECA branches and the hemodynamic balance between adjacent branches are highly variable.

Intracranial Arteries

The Circle of Willis

The circle of Willis is an arterial polygon surrounding the ventral surface of the diencephalon. The following vessels comprise the circle of Willis (Figs. 11-17, 11-18): (a) the two ICAs; (b) the first segment (A1) of both anterior cerebral arteries (ACAs); (c) the basilar artery (BA); (d) the first segment (P1) of both posterior cerebral arteries (PCA); (e) the anterior communicating artery (ACoA); and (f) the two posterior communicating arteries (PCoAs). This polygon that surrounds the ventral surface of the diencephalon is the principal source of collateral flow in cases of an occlusion or severe stenosis of a major cerebral artery. A complete circle of Willis with no absent or hypoplastic segment is seen only in about 25% of cases.

The ICAs usually supply the territory of the ACAs and the middle cerebral arteries (MCAs), often termed the *anterior circulation*. The *posterior circulation* refers to the vascular territory supplied by the VA and BA, including the PCA.

The parenchymal vascular supply of the cerebral arteries is depicted in Figure 11-19, although individual vascular territories have considerable variability (38).

The Anterior Circulation

The Internal Carotid Artery. Numerous anatomic classification schemes exist for the ICA, and this can be a source of confusion. A simple anatomic description is to divide the artery into five segments, in ascending order: (a) the extracranially located carotid bulb; (b) the extracranially located cervical segment; (c) the intraosseous petrous segment; (d) the cavernous segment; and (e) the intracranial segment.

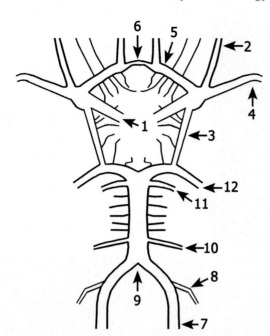

FIGURE 11-17 Schematic drawing of the circle of Willis. Branches of the ICA (1) are the ophthalmic artery (2) and the posterior communicating artery (3). The artery divides into the MCA (4) and the ACA (5) that is connected via the ACoA (6) to the contralateral side. The VA (7) gives rise to the PICA (8) and unites to form the BA (9). The basilar gives rise to the AICAs (10), the SCAs (11), and divides into the PCAs (12) that are connected via the posterior communicating artery (3) to the anterior circulation.

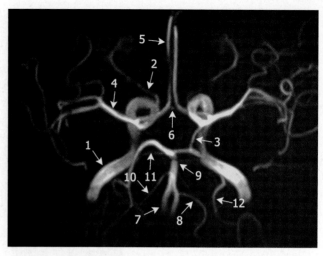

FIGURE 11-18 3D TOF MRA MIP image of the circle of Willis. The left PCoA (3), the right AICA (10), and the left PICA (8) are well displayed, but not their counterparts on the contralateral side. Note the ICA (1), the ophthalmic artery (2), the MCA (4), the ACA (5), the ACoA (6), the VA (7), the BA (9), and the SCAs (11), with numbering as in Fig. 11-17.

A more detailed classification proposed by Bouthillier et al. in 1996 separates the artery into seven segments according to the adjacent structures and the compartments transversed (39). The segments are C1, cervical; C2, petrous; C3, lacerum; C4, cavernous; C5, clinoid; C6, ophthalmic; and C7, communicating. This classification system takes modern anatomic and clinical considerations into account and utilizes a logical scale in the direction of blood flow (Fig. 11-20; Table 11-2).

However, the classification system by Fischer published in 1938 that is based on the *angiographic course* of the intracranial ICA rather than its arterial branches or anatomic compartments is still widely used. With this classification system, the segments are numbered *opposite* to the direction of blood flow, and the extracranial ICA is excluded (40).

Numerous branches arise from the ICA. The ophthalmic artery, arising from the anterosuperior ICA (C6) and passing through the optic canal, and the PCoA, arising from the posterior aspect of the intradural ICA (C7), are usually visible on CTA and MRA (41). However, small but important branches—foremost the anterior choroidal artery (AChA) that arises a short distance above the PCoA and supplies crucial anatomic structures including the posterior limb of the internal capsule—are not visible unless pathologically enlarged (e.g., in the presence of arteriovenous malformations).

Variants and clinical remarks. In patients with an occlusion of an ICA, a small (<1 mm) or absent PCoA is a risk factor for ischemic cerebral infarction, which indicates the importance of the collateral pathways provided by this artery (42). Aneurysms at the origin of the PCoA are common, and as the artery courses posterolaterly over the oculomotor nerve, a third nerve palsy can result. This is a classic example of cranial neuropathies caused by aneurysmal compression.

Distinguishing aneurysms of the cavernous segment of the ICA from those that involve the proximal intradural portion of the artery is of importance for determining treatment options. Intradural aneurysms are at risk for subarachnoid hemorrhage and are usually treated with endovascular or surgical obliteration. In contrast, extradural aneurysms involving the cavernous segment of the ICA pose little or no risk of hemorrhage and are commonly monitored unless they enlarge and produce symptoms related to compression of cavernous sinus structures.

The ophthalmic artery has traditionally served as a landmark in distinguishing extradural (below the ophthalmic artery) from intradural (at or above the ophthalmic artery) aneurysms (43). This origin is variable, however, and may be extradural in 10% of cases.

According to first results from a recent study by Gonzalez et al., the inferior border of the *optic strut* as identified on CTA might be a more reliable anatomic location to discriminate between intradural and extradural aneurysms (Fig. 11-21) (44). This structure is the inferior root that connects the anterior clinoid process with the lesser wing of the sphenoid bone and separates the optic canal from the

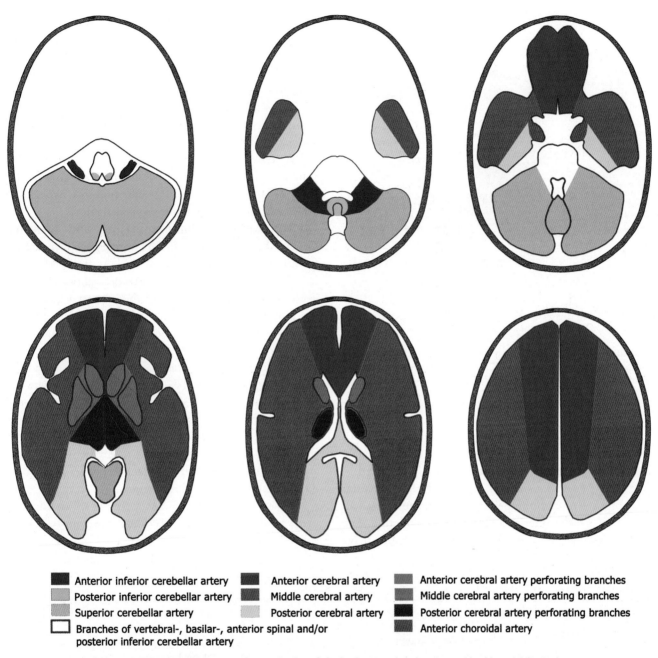

Anterior inferior cerebellar artery
Posterior inferior cerebellar artery
Superior cerebellar artery
Branches of vertebral-, basilar-, anterior spinal and/or posterior inferior cerebellar artery

Anterior cerebral artery
Middle cerebral artery
Posterior cerebral artery

Anterior cerebral artery perforating branches
Middle cerebral artery perforating branches
Posterior cerebral artery perforating branches
Anterior choroidal artery

FIGURE 11-19 Approximate vascular territories of the brain. Note that there is considerable variability in the borders and size of the territories. Adapted and modified from Osborne A. *Diagnostic Neuroradiology.* St. Louis: Mosby; 1994, and Kretschmann H, Weinrich W. *Cranial Neuroimaging and Clinical Neuroanatomy. Atlas of MR Imaging and Computed Tomography.* 3rd ed., revised and expanded ed. New York: Georg Thieme Verlag; 2003, with permission.

superior orbital fissure. Aneurysms that arose distal (with respect to the blood flow) to the optic strut were located intradurally. Conversely, aneurysms that arose proximal to the optic strut were located within the cavernous sinus. Aneurysms at the optic strut were located within the clinoid segment or the interdural space.

The intrapetrous ICA can take an aberrant posterolateral course traversing the hypotympanum. The differentiation of this anomaly from a glomus tympanicum paraganglioma is essential. A rare persistent stapedial artery originating from the petrous ICA is, in the majority of the cases, reported to be enclosed within a bony canal on the cochlear promontory. The artery becomes the middle meningeal artery, and an absent foramen spinosum indicates this anomaly. A possible course of the artery through the footplate of the stapes complicates prosthetic surgery for impaired hearing.

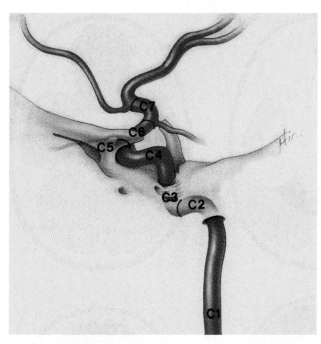

FIGURE 11-20 Classification of segments of the ICA. Reprinted from Bouthillier A, van Loveren HR, Keller JT. Segments of the internal carotid artery: a new classification. *Neurosurgery.* 1996;38:425–432; discussion 432–433, with permission.

The absence of an ICA is rare. When trans-sphenoidal surgery is planned, the intrasellar intercarotid communicating arteries typically seen with this anomaly must be identified.

More common anomalies are carotid-vertebrobasilar anastomoses resembling persisting embryonic connections between the anterior and posterior circulation. The most common anastomosis is the persistent primitive trigeminal artery—present in up to 1%—that arises where the ICA exits the carotid canal (Fig. 11-22). It has two types, the lateral and the medial. The *medial type*, also termed *intrasellar* or *transhypophyseal artery* courses posteromedially, compresses the pituitary gland, penetrates the dorsum sellae, and anastomoses with the BA. This artery must be recognized if trans-sphenoidal surgery is planned (45).

A persistent otic artery arising from the petrous ICA is extremely rare. A little more common are the connections that arise from the cervical ICA: the primitive hypoglossal artery and the proatlantal intersegmental artery.

The Anterior Communicating and Anterior Cerebral Artery. From the A1 segment, which extends from the ICA bifurcation to the ACoA, arise perforating branches, the medial lenticulostriate arteries that pass cephalad to supply the head of the caudate nucleus and the anterior limb of the internal capsule (Fig. 11-23). These are not visible under normal conditions on CTA or MRA, nor are the branches of the ACoA that supply, for example, the superior surface of the optic chiasm and the anterior hypothalamus. The segment of the ACA between the junction of the ACoA and its bifurcation into the main terminal branches, the pericallosal and callosomarginal arteries, is termed *A2*. It curves around the genu of the corpus callosum. The largest medial lenticulostriate artery, the recurrent artery of Heubner, arises most commonly from the proximal A2 segment (less common from the A1 segment). Cortical branches of the A2 and A3 segment supply the anterior two thirds of the medial hemispheric surface.

TABLE 11-2

Classification of Segments of the Internal Carotid Artery*

Segment	Termination Point	Remark
C1—Cervical	Petrous bone entry	Divided into carotid bulb and ascending segment
C2—Petrous	End of petrous carotid canal	Divided into vertical and horizontal segment
C3—Lacerum	Petrolingual ligament	Petrolingual ligament: continuation of periosteum of carotid canal
C4—Cavernous	Proximal dural ring	Extradural; divided into ascending portion, posterior genu, horizontal portion, ascending genu
C5—Clinoid	Distal dural ring	Interdural
C6—Ophthalmic	Proximal to PCoA	Intradural; ophthalmic artery usually visible on CTA or MRA
C7—Communicating	ICA bifurcation	Posterior communicating artery usually visible on CTA or MRA

*According to Bouthillier A, van Loveren HR, Keller JT. Segments of the internal carotid artery: a new classification. *Neurosurgery.* 1996;38:425–432; discussion 432–433.

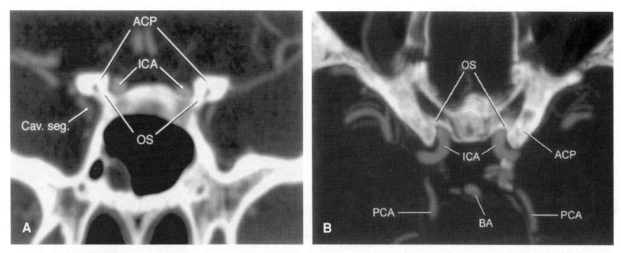

FIGURE 11-21 A: Coronal reconstructed CTA showing the optic strut and its relationship to the cavernous and intradural ICA. **B:** Axial reconstructed CTA showing the position of the intradural ICA and the relationships of the optic strut and the anterior clinoid process. (OS, optic strut; ACP, anterior clinoid process; Cav. seg., cavernous segment.) Reprinted from Gonzalez LF, Walker MT, Zabramski JM, et al. Distinction between paraclinoid and cavernous sinus aneurysms with computed tomographic angiography. *Neurosurgery.* 2003;52:1131–1137; discussion 1138–1139, with permission.

Variants and clinical remarks. The most common variant is a hypoplastic, very rarely absent A1 segment. If a single trunk arises from the confluence of the A1 segments, instead of the paired A2 segments, it is termed *azygous ACA*, present in about 0.25% to 4%. A bihemispheric ACA is more common: In this entity, two ACAs exist, but the more dominant ACA sends branches to the contralateral hemisphere.

The Middle Cerebral Artery. The MCA can be divided into four major segments (Fig. 11-23). First is the M1 segment, which is orientated horizontally and laterally, extending from the origin at the ICA bifurcation to the point where the MCA begins to curve posterosuperiorly over the insula, and includes the bifurcation or trifurcation

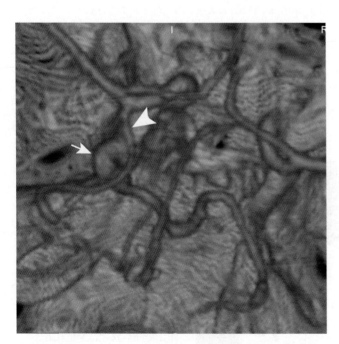

FIGURE 11-22 CTA VR image of a persistent trigeminal artery (*arrow*). The large anomalous artery arises from the precavernous segment of the ICA. The PCoA is present on the side of the persistent trigeminal artery (*arrowhead*); the distal BA is not visible.

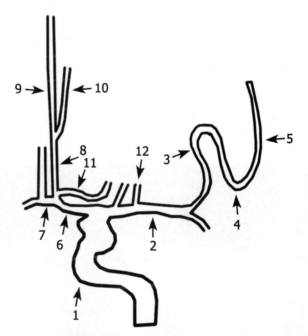

FIGURE 11-23 Schematic drawing of the ICA branches as viewed in a coronal projection. ICA (1); MCA (M1) (2); MCA (M2) (3); MCA (M3) (4); MCA (M4) (5); ACA (A1) (6); ACoA (7); ACA (A2) (8); pericallosal artery (9); callosomarginal artery (10); recurrent artery of Heubner (11); perforating arteries of the MCA (12).

at the sylvian fissure. Deep perforating branches arise from this segment—the lateral lenticulostriate arteries—which supply the lentiform nucleus, parts of the internal capsula, and the caudate nucleus. The insular M2 segments extend from the genu to the top of the sylvian fissure and loop over the insula. The opercular M3 segments extend laterally through the sylvian fissure. The cortical M4 segments curve over the frontal, temporal, and parietal operculae, supplying large parts of the cerebral cortex and white matter.

Variants and clinical remarks. Variants are rare and include fenestration, duplication, single trunk, and accessory arteries.

The Posterior Circulation

The Arteries of the Posterior Fossa. The VAs pass through the foramen magnum and unite anteriorly to the medulla oblongata to form the BA (Fig. 11-24). The left VA is commonly the larger, dominant vessel. Important intracranial branches are the anterior spinal artery and the posterior inferior cerebellar artery (PICA).

After its origin from the distal parts of the vertebral arteries of both sites, the anterior spinal artery courses caudally in the anteromedial sulcus of the cervical cord. The PICA likewise originates from the distal VA, courses caudally along the medulla and the cerebellar tonsils, and with its cortical branches provides blood supply to the posteroinferior surface of the cerebellar hemispheres. Furthermore, the artery supplies the posterolateral medulla, the cerebellar tonsils, and parts of the vermis.

The BA runs cephalad in front of the pons and divides in front of the pons into the PCAs. Major branches are the anterior inferior cerebellar artery (AICA), the superior cerebellar artery (SCA), and perforating vessels. The AICA has a posterolaterally orientated course within the cerebellopontine angle cistern, directed toward the internal auditory canal, and supplies the anterolateral surface of the cerebellar hemisphere and parts of the brain stem. The SCA arises near the tip of the basilar artery and curves posterolaterally around the pons and mesencephalon to supply the parts of the vermis and the cerebellar hemispheres. The perforating branches that arise along the entire BA supply the ventral pons and rostral brain stem.

Variants and clinical remarks. Occasionally, a hypoplastic VA does not have a connection to the BA and terminates in the PICA. A shared AICA/PICA trunk is relatively common. Rarely, the origin of the PICA might be extradural. The BA may be hypoplastic if the PCA has a fetal origin (see next section) or if rare persistent fetal anastomoses exist. Duplications or fenestrations of the vertebral or basilar arteries have been described.

The Posterior Cerebral Artery. The PCAs originate usually from the BA (Figs. 11-17, 11-24). The first segment, P1, is termed the *precommunicating segment* and extends laterally to the junction with the PCoA. Important branches, the posterior thalamoperforating that supply large parts of the thalamus and the midbrain arise from this segment—and from the basilar bifurcation—and are not recognizable on CTA or MRA.

The ambient or P2 segment courses posteriorly around the midbrain. Major branches are the medial and lateral posterior choroidal arteries, and the thalamogeniculate artery. These branches supply the tectal plate; parts of the midbrain, thalamus, and crus cerebri; the pineal gland; and the choroid plexus of the third and the lateral ventricular choroids plexus.

The P3 segment runs behind the midbrain in the quadrigeminal plate cistern. Branches supply the undersurface of the temporal lobe, the posterior third of the interhemispheric surface, the splenium of the corpus callosum, and the occipital pole including the visual cortex (calcarine artery).

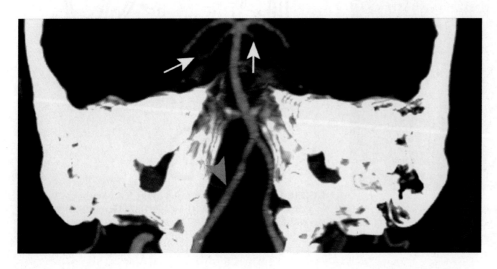

FIGURE 11-24 CTA MIP slab image in paracoronal orientation. The SCA is well delineated on both sides (*arrows*) as well as the right PICA (*arrowhead*).

Variants and clinical remarks. An origin of the PCA from the ICA, termed *fetal origin of the PCA*, is a commonly (20%) seen variant. This is by far the most frequently observed form of carotid-basilar anastomoses. If this anomaly is present, emboli from the carotid circulation might cause symptoms that are classically seen in pathologies of the vertebral or basilar arteries—for example, hemianopsia.

Venous Anatomy

Dural Sinuses

The superior sagittal sinus (SSS), located between the skull and the leaves of the falx cerebri, extends from the crista galli anteriorly and extends posteriorly to its confluence with the straight and lateral sinus (Fig. 11-25). The inferior sagittal sinus is located along the inferior free margin of the falx cerebri and, with the vein of Galen, forms the straight sinus. The straight sinus is enclosed by the dura of the falx cerebri and tentorium cerebelli, and drains into the superior sagittal sinus at the confluens sinuum. Near the confluence, multiple tentorial sinuses that drain the adjacent hemispheres and the cerebellum join the neighboring sinuses. The confluens sinuum divides into the transverse sinuses (TS), which course laterally around the tentorial attachment. At the posterolateral wall of the petrous bone, the transverse sinuses turn inferiorly to form the sigmoid sinus, which continues to the jugular bulb at the jugular foramen.

The cavernous sinuses are paired, septated venous structures located on either side of the sella turcica. The carotid artery, oculomotor nerves (third, fourth, and sixth cranial nerves), and the ophthalmic branch of the fifth nerve are contained within its lateral wall or traverse (sixth nerve) the sinus. The sinuses receive venous tributaries from the orbital veins and drain into the superior and inferior petrosal sinuses. They communicate with each other via intercavernous sinuses and posteriorly with the periclival venous plexus. The superior petrosal sinus connects the cavernous with the TS, and the inferior petrosal sinus connects the cavernous sinus with the jugular bulb.

Variants and clinical remarks. Common variants that are important to know when searching for cerebral venous thrombosis include a hypoplastic or atretic rostral SSS (in this case, prominent superior cortical veins are present) that should not be mistaken for a venous thrombosis; direct termination of the SSS in a TS (usually the right one; in this case, the straight sinus drains into the left— usually hypoplastic TS); "high-splitting" SSS; asymmetry of the TS (the right TS is usually dominant); or agenesis of the TS (in this case, an occipital sinus is prominent). In the majority of patients, arachnoid villi (pacchionian granulations) are visible on CTA or CE MRA techniques and can usually be differentiated easily by their smooth contour from pathological filling defects, as seen in venous thrombosis.

Cerebral Veins

The cerebral veins are often divided into superficial cortical veins and deep veins (Figs. 11-25, 11-26). The superficial cortical veins are highly variable. Three prominent veins can

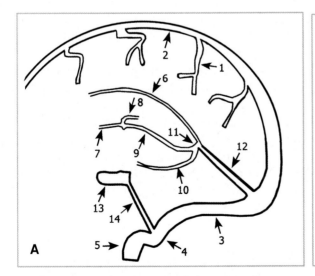
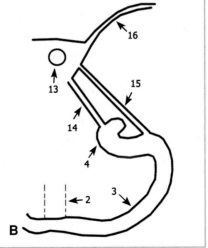

FIGURE 11-25 Schematic drawing of the cerebral veins in **(A)** sagittal and **(B)** axial orientation. Cortical veins (1); SSS (2); TS (3); sigmoid sinus (4); jugular vein (5); inferior sagittal sinus (6); septal veins (7); thalamostriate veins (8); internal cerebral veins (9); basal vein of Rosenthal (10); vein of Galen (11); straight sinus (12); cavernous sinus (13); inferior petrosal sinus (14); superior petrosal sinus (15); sphenoparietal sinus (16).

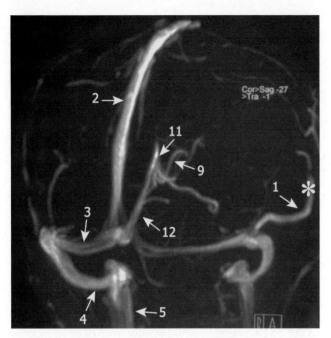

FIGURE 11-26 2D TOF MRA of the cerebral veins. The numbers refer to Figure 11-25. Cortical veins (1); SSS (2); TS (3); sigmoid sinus (4); jugular vein (5); inferior sagittal sinus; internal cerebral veins (9); vein of Galen (11); straight sinus (12). The ISS is not visualized. The prominent cortical vein is the vein of Labbé (∗).

be often recognized, however: (a) the vein of Labbé, which extends from the sylvian fissure posterolaterally to the TS; (b) the vein of Trolard, which runs from the sylvian fissure to the SSS; and (c) the superficial middle cerebral veins, which run along the sylvian fissure.

The deep cerebral veins include the medullary veins, which drain the white matter and course centrally toward the subependymal veins that surround the ventricles. Prominent subependymal veins are the septal veins that run posteriorly from the frontal horn along the septum pellucidum and join near the foramen of Monro with the thalamostriate veins, which course over the caudate nuclei, to form the internal cerebral veins.

The internal cerebral veins course above the roof of the third ventricle and drain into the (unpaired) vein of Galen, which curves under the splenium of the corpus callosum and joins with the inferior sagittal sinus to form the straight sinus. The basal veins of Rosenthal run along the midbrain and drain either into the internal cerebral veins or the vein of Galen. In the posterior fossa, the anterior pontomesencephalic vein lies along the surface of the pons and mesencephalon. The large cerebellar veins are the precentral cerebellar vein and the superior and inferior vermian vein.

Variants and clinical remarks. Although the drainage pattern of the superficial cortical veins and deep veins is highly variable, true anomalies are uncommon.

CLINICAL APPLICATIONS OF COMPUTED TOMOGRAPHIC AND MAGNETIC RESONANCE ANGIOGRAPHY

Stroke and Atherosclerotic Disease

Clinical Background

Stroke is the third most common cause of death worldwide after myocardial infarction and cancer, and the most common cause for permanent disability in developed countries. The term *stroke* is commonly used but imprecise. According to the World Health Organization (WHO) definition, stroke describes the rapid onset of a cerebral deficit, which lasts 24 hours or leads to death, with no apparent cause other than vascular. Ischemic stroke is the most common cause, accounting for approximately 80% of all events. Primary intraparenchymal and subarachnoid hemorrhage account for approximately 15% and 5%, respectively. The remainder are due to a miscellany of much rarer causes (e.g., vasculitis, dissection, venous thrombosis) (46).

Numerous classification schemes describing subtypes of ischemic stroke have been proposed. A classification system based on the patient's neurologic signs, the results of brain imaging, and the findings of ancillary diagnostic tests is widely used. It distinguishes based on etiology large artery or atherosclerotic infarctions, cardioembolic infarctions, and small vessel or lacunar infarctions.

Clinical studies refer to this as the TOAST classification, as it was adopted for the evaluation of patients participating in a trial of low molecular weight heparinoid, the Trial of Org 10172 in Acute Stroke Treatment (47). It should be recognized, however, that it may be difficult in certain clinical settings to determine the clinical subtype, and that many strokes are reported to be of undetermined etiology (48).

The relative frequencies of the stroke subtypes vary from study to study, with incidences of 15% to 40% for large artery or atherosclerotic infarction, 15% to 30% for cardioembolic stroke, and 15% to 30% for lacunar infarctions (46,49).

Atherosclerotic infarctions result from thrombosis directly at the site of atherosclerotic plaque formation or from emboli originating from a plaque that then lodges downstream, causing artery-to-artery embolism. The most common site for atherosclerotic plaque formation is the extracranial circulation, specifically the carotid bifurcation. Another common site of extracranial plaque formation is at the origin of the supra-aortic vessels, including the subclavian and VAs. Common intracranial locations include the carotid siphon, the proximal MCAs and ACAs, the most distal aspects of the VAs, and the BA.

Identification of atherosclerotic stenosis of the major intracranial arteries is important in the workup of a patient with stroke. It is assumed that intracranial arterial stenosis accounts for approximately 10% of ischemic strokes (50). The visualization of a stenosis does not establish the etiology of stroke, however. For example, it had been shown that almost half of the strokes that occur in the territory of a symptomatic carotid appear to be cardioembolic or small artery strokes (51).

Apart from atherosclerosis, numerous other etiologies can lead to large artery thromboembolic stroke. Although these are far less common, they include arterial dissection, vasculitis, and moyamoya disease (discussed in subsequent sections). Hematological disorders that cause hyperviscosity or lead to hypercoagulable state and vasculopathies may also account for large artery territory infarction.

Cardioembolic strokes can be caused by mural thrombus formation in settings of relative stasis (e.g., myocardial infarction or atrial fibrillation or flutter), by valvular heart disease (e.g., development of valvular vegetations, prosthetic valves), or may occur in congenital heart disease.

Lacunar infarctions are caused by occlusion of small perforating arteries and are generally not larger than 1.5 cm. The perforating arteries in the anterior circulation are the lenticulostriate arteries. In the posterior circulation, the thalamoperforating arteries and the small perforating arteries from the main stem of the BA serve as end vessels. Patients with hypertension and diabetes mellitus are predisposed to lacunar infarctions; however, small vessel infarction can also be a manifestation of nonatherosclerotic etiologies (e.g., collagen-vascular disease and vasculitis).

In the radiological community, the terms *territorial infarcts* and *borderzone infarctions* are commonly applied to describe infarct patterns as visualized on CT or MR (Fig. 11-27). Territorial infarctions are confined to the perfusion territory of a cerebral artery. Borderzone infarctions are ischemic lesions situated between two neighboring vascular territories (e.g., between the MCA and PCA territories) (52,53).

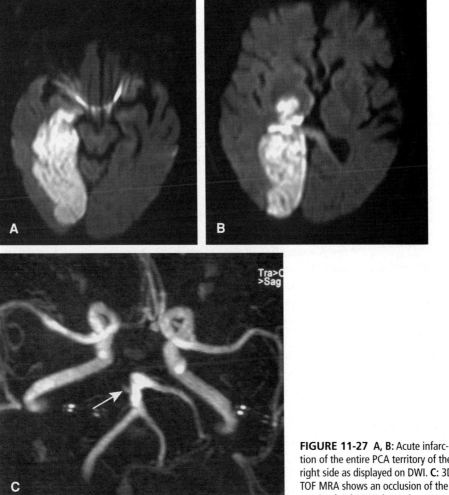

FIGURE 11-27 A, B: Acute infarction of the entire PCA territory of the right side as displayed on DWI. **C:** 3D TOF MRA shows an occlusion of the proximal right PCA (*arrow*).

Early work suggested that territorial infarctions would likely be embolic from a cardiac source or a carotid plaque, and that lesions restricted to border zones would more likely represent hypotensive events of the most vulnerable tissue in the presence of severe large vessel disease. Continuing research has shown that this concept might be an oversimplification.

In particular, it has been shown by van der Zwan et al. (38,54) that the territorial supply area of the cerebral arteries, and therefore the location of borderzone areas, is individually highly variable. Infarctions formerly classified, based on classical textbook templates, as borderzone infarctions might actually lay entirely within a cerebral territory (55).

The concept of borderzone infarctions was furthermore challenged by the observation that (a) there was no significant difference in the incidence of *cortical* borderzone infarctions in patients with and without hemodynamic compromise; that (b) borderzone infarctions were rarely the initial manifestation of carotid occlusion, as might be expected for acute low-flow states; and that (c) postmortem examinations revealed emboli as a possible cause of borderzone infarctions (56–58).

Only so-called *deep* borderzone infarctions, small lesions arranged in a linear fashion parallel to the lateral ventricle in the corona radiate or centrum semiovale, seem to correlate with hemodynamic compromise and were seen with a high specificity in patients with carotid occlusion and an increased cerebral oxygen extraction fraction (59).

Stroke treatment has undergone a rapid evolution in the last decade. The most important development has been the recognition of stroke as an acute emergency and the application of acute-phase therapies to improve outcome. This is summed up with the clinical catchphrase "time is brain."

Of the various therapeutic options available, the administration of intravenous (IV) recombinant tissue plasminogen activator (tPA) *within the first 3 hours* after stroke is the only thrombolytic therapy approved by the U.S. Food and Drug Administration (60). The approval was based on the results from randomized study of IV tPA versus placebo in the American National Institute of Neurological Disorders and Stroke trial (NINDS) (61).

Patients randomized to IV tPA had, depending on the clinical outcome parameter applied, an 11% to 13% increase in the rate of minimal or no disability compared with those who had received placebo. Despite the higher rate of symptomatic intracranial hemorrhage in the tPA group (6%) versus the placebo group (0.6%), there was no significant difference in mortality between the groups.

Three additional trials, the European Cooperative Acute Stroke Studies (ECASS I and II) and the Acute Non-interventional Therapy in Ischemic Stroke (ATLANTIS), evaluated the use of IV tPA in extended time windows of up to six hours (62–64). All had negative results, with no substantial benefit to IV tPA therapy demonstrated beyond three hours of stroke onset using the predetermined primary endpoints of the study.

The debate about tPA treatment of patients remains a matter of intense discussion, however. On the one hand, it has been pointed out that many patients with symptoms of acute ischemic stroke may not have occlusive thromboembolism (65). Thus, many patients might receive a potentially dangerous drug although they do not have the disease for which the drug is intended. On the other hand, given the three-hour window, more than 95% of all patients presenting with symptoms of acute stroke will not be eligible for tPA treatment (66).

Intra-arterial (IA) thrombolysis, as compared with IV therapy, has the advantage that during cerebral angiography, clot lysis can be directly assessed. Since the first report in 1983 (67), numerous case series have been published, with minimal or no neurologic deficit reported in 15% to 75% (68). The rate of complete or partial recanalization was on average 40% and 35%, respectively, and higher than those of IV thrombolysis.

The Prolyse in Acute Cerebral Thromboembolism (PROACT II) showed a benefit of IA thrombolysis up to six hours after ischemic stroke onset (69). The trial randomized patients with MCA thromboembolic occlusion into two arms: (a) IA thrombolytic therapy with prourokinase and low-dose IV heparin, and (b) low-dose IV heparin alone. Despite a higher rate of symptomatic intracranial hemorrhage, treatment with the IA thrombolytic therapy improved the clinical outcome.

Moreover, additional therapeutic protocols for thrombolytic therapy, such as combination of IV and IA therapy, are being evaluated (70). Other therapeutic tools, such as mechanical recanalization of vessels or the administration of neuroprotective drugs to reduce the volume of infarcted tissue, are under investigation.

Apart from efforts to evaluate and optimize the treatment of acute stroke, large efforts are undertaken as well to improve the *secondary prevention* of stroke. These include optimization of treatment plans for patients presenting with the thromboembolic risk factor of an extracranial or intracranial atherosclerotic vascular lesion. Large multicenter trials have established the efficacy to treat *extracranial* carotid atherosclerosis with endarterectomy, and current trials compare surgical approaches with endovascular treatment utilizing stents (71,72).

In an effort to reduce the rate of stroke in symptomatic patients with *intracranial* stenosis of over 50%, the

Warfarin-Aspirin Symptomatic Intracranial Disease (WASID) trial examines the effects of aspirin versus warfarin (50). This study aims to identify patients whose rate of stroke on the best medical therapy is sufficiently high to warrant intracranial angioplasty/stenting.

Imaging Strategies

Acute stroke must be regarded as a medical emergency. The diagnosis of stroke by specialists is reasonably accurate on clinical grounds alone, but in general medical and emergency settings, up to 20% of patients with suspected stroke turn out to have another diagnosis (46,73). As infarction cannot be reliably distinguished from these additional diagnoses, brain imaging plays a pivotal role in the initial workup. The exclusion of hemorrhagic stroke and of lesions that can clinically mimic ischemic stroke (e.g., subdural hematoma, cerebritis, or tumor) remains a major contribution of the radiologist in the setting of acute stroke.

CT is the imaging modality of choice at most institutions for the evaluation of patients in the initial hours of acute stroke because of its widespread availability, rapid acquisitions, capacity to evaluate often uncooperative patients, and the ease of excluding intracranial hemorrhage.

In most cases, a normal unenhanced CT scan is observed within the first 2 to 3 hours; however, some early signs may allude to underlying vascular pathology (Fig. 11-28). These include obscuration of the lentiform nucleus, the insular ribbon sign, and the "hyperdense" media sign or "dot sign." The lentiform nucleus is supplied by the lenticulostriate branches of the MCA, which are end vessels, and are therefore prone to early irreversible damage after proximal MCA occlusion. The *insular ribbon sign* refers to relative hypoattenuation of

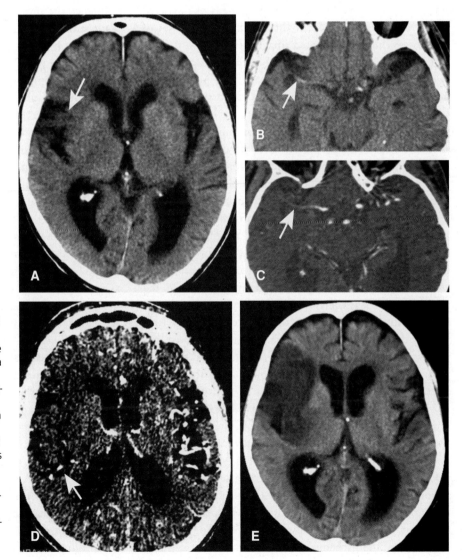

FIGURE 11-28 Three hours after the clinical onset of a right hemispheric stroke, unenhanced CT shows **(A)** a hypoattenuation of the insular cortex (*arrow*) and **(B)** a positive media sign (*arrow*). On **(C)**, an axial CTA source image, the MCA is not opacified in the M2 segment (*arrow*). A source image **(D)** with a narrow window setting depicts a hypoattenuation of a large area of the MCA territory. Pial vessels are only visualized on the posterior aspect of the area (*arrow*). Unenhanced CTA five days later **(E)** reveals a large infarct in the anterior part of the MCA territory. The territory of the perforating vessels that arise from the M1 segment of the MCA have been spared from infarction. The posterior aspect of the MCA territory was most likely supplied by collateral supply via cortical branches of the PCA.

the insular cortex. The insula is distal to potential collateral supply from the PCAs in the early stage of MCA occlusion and thus is susceptible to early damage. If the MCA is occluded by a fresh thrombus, it may appear as hyperintense relative to the normal contralateral MCA, hence the *hyperdense media sign*. This sign has a high specificity but a sensitivity of only about 30%. Thrombosis of more distal branches might also be visible as hyperattenuating dots, termed the *dot sign* (74).

Conventional MR images are more sensitive and specific than CT for acute cerebral ischemia. Findings include hyperintense signal on T2-weighted images, mass effect in the area of infarction, loss of arterial flow voids, and stasis of contrast material within vessels in affected territories following contrast material administration. As with CT, within the first hours, false negative studies might be seen with MR.

The introduction of diffusion-weighted imaging (DWI), however, revolutionized imaging of patients with (hyper)-acute stroke by demonstrating areas of restricted water movement that occur during the initial onset of ischemia, while T2-weighted images still show a normal appearance (Fig. 11-27) (75). MRI furthermore allows the exclusion of intracranial hemorrhage and possibly the definitive diagnosis of subarachnoid hemorrhage as well (76–78).

The large randomized studies of thrombolysis in stroke as mentioned earlier have been based on unenhanced CT findings exclusively. However, the state-of-the-art CT and MR methods can provide more than information on morphological aspects of the brain parenchyma or indirect signs of vessel occlusion. They can now provide information about the perfusion of the brain parenchyma—the microvasculature—and can give detailed information on the larger arteries of the brain—the macrovasculature.

For a comprehensive CT imaging of acute stroke, the unenhanced CT is therefore followed by a perfusion CT examination, which permits the differentiation of irreversibly damaged brain tissue from reversibly impaired "tissue at risk" by assessing changes of cerebral blood flow and volume, and by the CTA examination to assess the cerebral arteries (79,80).

With MR, the combination of DWI with perfusion imaging was found to be of considerable interest in identifying the ischemic yet viable and not fully infarcted areas of the brain surrounding an infarct core (81). For example, it is assumed that in cases where the area of the diffusion abnormality is smaller than the area of reduced perfusion, the area with normal diffusion but decreased perfusion may represent the potentially salvageable tissue, or tissue at risk—that is, the "ischemic penumbra" (82,83).

Several studies have demonstrated the feasibility and the practicality of performing these advanced imaging methods in clinical settings and the use of information obtained to triage patients before therapy (81,84,85). The driving force behind the application of these advanced imaging techniques is to optimize and tailor treatment to the needs of the individual patient in the acute stroke setting. A longer time window of up to 6 hours or even 24 hours might be safe if the decision to treat a patient is not based solely on findings of unenhanced CT, but rather incorporates the additional input from CTA or MRA to assess vessel occlusion and the information about tissue perfusion (86–88).

Computed Tomographic and Magnetic Resonance Angiography in Atherosclerotic Disease

In most institutions, findings from CTA and MRA are already integrated in the workup of patients with stroke and influence the process of therapeutic decision making. In acute stroke, the most important task of CTA is to provide information about possible vessel thrombosis or vessel occlusion. In practice, a comprehensive assessment of the cerebral circulation should include the cervical vessels. This is of particular value if IA thrombolysis is considered a therapeutic option, as the subsequent intervention can be guided by the findings from CTA (Fig. 11-29). The postprocessing procedures should be performed quickly.

Occlusion of the ICA can be detected immediately by surveying the source images; however, the diagnosis of stenosis or occlusion of the smaller branches (e.g., the MCA) might be difficult solely on the basis of source images. Here, MPRs in conjunction with MIP slabs provide for rapid assessment while VR and SSD reconstructions should be mainly reserved for demonstration purposes after analysis of the MPRs and MIP slabs.

CTA has been demonstrated to be highly reliable for the detection or exclusion of thrombotic occlusion of large intracranial vessels—ICA, MCA trunk up to the M2 segment, and the BA (87,89–92). The proper interpretation of CTA images requires special attention to vessel wall calcification, particularly circumferential calcification to analyze for the presence or absence of luminal enhancement, and hence vessel patency.

An analysis of MPR images at varied window settings is required to detect or exclude flow within the vessel when surrounded by calcium. This display technique should likewise be applied for evaluation of the cavernous carotid arteries if the cavernous sinus is hyperattenuated. Venous contamination may be minimized by taking advantage of the imaging speed of multidetector CTs, careful timing of

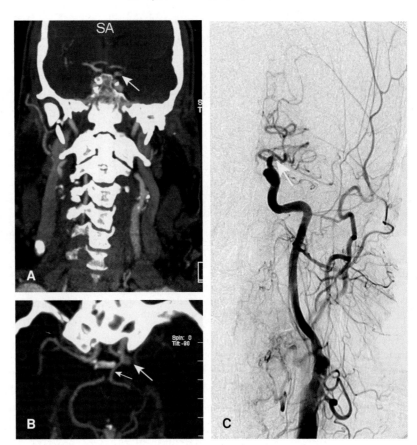

FIGURE 11-29 CTA MIP slab in **(A)** coronal and in **(B)** axial orientation shows an occlusion of the ICA bifurcation (*arrows*), the so-called "carotid T occlusion" that extends from the supraclinoid portion of the ICA into the proximal segments of MCA and ACA (PCoA, *small arrow*). Below the occlusion side, the ICA, and in particular the ICA bifurcation, was displayed without underlying pathologies. DSA **(C)** confirmed the site of occlusion (*arrow*), and IA thrombolysis was successfully performed.

the contrast bolus, or the use of an automatic contrast triggering system, as outlined in the technical section.

Besides the detection of an underlying vascular occlusion, the possibility to assess the extent of hypoperfused brain tissue has to be emphasized (89,93). For that purpose, the CTA source images (CTA SI) that emphasize the contrast of perfused and malperfused brain areas and render information about collateral circulation should be inspected (Fig. 11-28). A comparison of CT, CTA, and CTA SI findings with diffusion-weighted MRI and MRA in 20 patients, 16 with vessel occlusions, revealed a close to equal accuracy of infarct volumes according to CTA SI and DWI, and it was furthermore shown that patients with poor collaterals surrounding the lesion side were prone to experience infarct growth (94).

The most commonly used MRA technique for the assessment of patients with stroke is the unenhanced 3D TOF technique. MRA has a very high sensitivity and specificity to detect occlusions of the major cerebral arteries (95,96). Interpretation of MR images requires more experience, however, as artifacts can cause intraluminal loss of signal intensity and decreased vessel depiction.

Large differences in the magnetic susceptibility between air in the sphenoid sinus and the surrounding

tissue can cause artifactual narrowing of the adjacent intracranial carotid artery. Intravoxel dephasing caused by turbulent flow conditions might contribute to artifactual narrowing at the carotid siphon and at vessel bifurcations (95,97,98); severely stenotic vessels might show a post-stenotic flow void and apparent discontinuity in a vessel.

Even with short echo times, small voxel sizes, and flow compensation applied in new MR sequences, the problem of signal loss cannot always be overcome. In contradistinction, artifacts might also lead to the false diagnosis of vessel *patency*. This occurs in cases where a flow gap within an artery is regarded as artifactual but in reality, the distal branches of the occluded artery are filled by collaterals (99). Problems might also occur if larger arteries below the volume of investigation are occluded (Fig. 11-30).

The correct *grading* of intracranial stenosis is more demanding than the demonstration of a vessel occlusion (Fig. 11-31). The investigators of the WASID trial explicitly demanded DSA to be performed on patients with stenosis of the large intracranial arteries, as there were concerns about false positive tests with noninvasive tests (50). In an unselected population of patients, the sensitivity and specificity for the detection of substantial vessel stenosis with 3D TOF MRA was below 90% (95). In another study that was

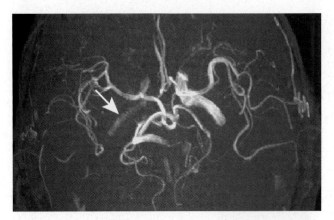

FIGURE 11-30 3D TOF MRA of the intracranial vessels shows the right ICA narrowed and with low signal. This display pattern can be observed in the presence of a high-grade ICA stenosis proximal to investigation volume, foremost at the level of the ICA bifurcation. In this case, however, the ICA was perfused in a retrograde fashion and was mainly supplied by the prominent left VA. CE MRA of the cervical vessels revealed an occlusion of the brachiocephalic trunk (compare with Fig. 11-1, same patient).

focused on the degree of stenosis of the vertebrobasilar system, overestimations were observed in 63% of patients (100).

In a recent study by Hirai et al. (101), the sensitivity, specificity, and accuracy of identifying intracranial stenosis of more than 50% was 92%, 91%, and 91% for 3D TOF MRA compared with DSA. Grades of stenoses at MRA agreed with those obtained from DSA only in 81% of cases, and 8% of normal vessels were interpreted as having moderate or severe stenosis.

However, when CTA was combined with MRA, overestimation decreased substantially, and complete agreement with DSA was observed in 97%. At the current stage of technology, using modern multidetector CTs with voxel

sizes well below 1 mm^3 and optimized postprocessing tools, CTA is superior for grading of intracranial stenosis compared with the 3D TOF MRA technique. The exact depiction of intracranial atherosclerotic lesions is of particular importance for treatment planning of intracranial stenting (Fig. 11-32). Several reports have shown the feasibility, effectiveness, and safety of the procedure in selected patients, and it is likely that this procedure will be more widely applied in the future (102–104).

CTA has the advantage over both MRA and DSA that mural calcifications in relation to the stenosis can be visualized. Furthermore, with high resolution CTA examinations, measurements on the vessel diameters adjacent to the stenosis can be compared with measurements from rotational angiography to optimize the choice of the optimal stent diameter.

A major problem of angioplasty with stent placement is the occurrence of in-stent neointimal growth, which might lead to a hemodynamically relevant restenosis or occlusion of the stented vessel segment. With the current materials used for stenting of intracranial atherosclerotic lesions, MR shows a signal loss at the level of the stent, and patency of the vessel can only be assumed by the flow signal distal to the stent. CTA has some capacity to assess the vessel lumen; however, artificial luminal narrowing, depending on the stent model and the size of the stent, impairs the evaluation, as shown in an in vivo study by Hahnel et al. (105). For a detailed assessment, DSA therefore remains the method of choice for the detection of restenosis.

MR techniques have the advantage over CT that hemodynamic alterations in patients with intracranial steno-occlusive disease can be detected. Selective MRA of the

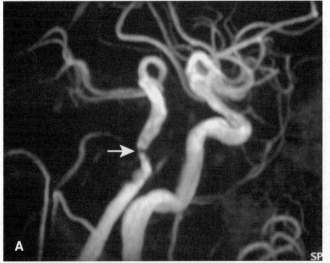
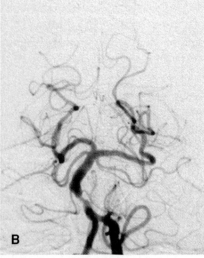

FIGURE 11-31 **A:** 3D TOF MRA MIP reconstruction of the circle of Willis reveals a stenosis at the level of the proximal BA with complete signal cancellation (*arrow*). Compared with (**B**) DSA, the degree of stenosis was overestimated.

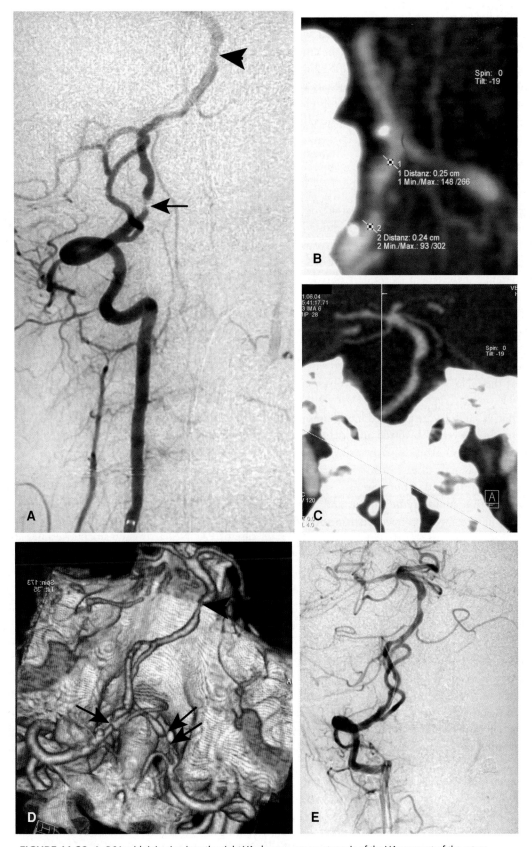

FIGURE 11-32 **A:** DSA with injection into the right VA shows a severe stenosis of the V4 segment of the artery (*arrow*) and a second stenosis of the BA (*arrowhead*). For treatment planning, CTA images (**B, C**) were used to visualize the stenosis to assess calcifications of the vessel wall and to perform measurements of the artery in order to choose the correct stent diameter. **D:** CTA displayed with VR shows a third stenosis of the left VA (*double arrow*). **E:** DSA control after stenting of the right VA stenosis shows an improved flow.

carotid or vertebrobasilar territory by means of presaturation of brain-supplying arteries, or the use of PC MR, allows the detection of intracranial collateral circulation via the anterior and posterior communicating arteries (106–110). However, up to now, these advanced angiographic techniques, as well as velocity measurements with MR, are mainly used for research purposes and are not integrated into the routine clinical workup of patients with stroke.

Cerebral Vasculitis

Clinical Background

Vasculitis refers to a spectrum of disorders that are defined by inflammation of the blood vessel with or without vessel wall necrosis. In primary angiitis of the central nervous system (PACNS), the vasculitis is restricted to the CNS with no apparent systemic involvement. Secondary nervous system vasculitic syndromes occur in the setting of a known systemic vasculitis or other disorders associated with inflammatory vasculopathy such as systemic infections, drug-induced forms, connective tissue disorders, and Behçet's disease. These disorders may present initially with vasculitic involvement of the CNS, without similar involvement at other sites (111).

The systemic vasculitides are classified most commonly based on the size of the vessels involved and include giant cell arteritis and Takayasu arteritis (large arteries), polyarteritis nodosa and Kawasaki disease (medium vessels), and Wegener granulomatosis and Churg-Strauss syndrome (small vessels). Systemic lupus erythematosus and Sjögren syndrome are the most common connective tissue disorders associated with nervous system vasculopathies.

Vasculitis clinically restricted to the CNS is a rare disorder, which is clinically more frequent in secondary forms. The incidence of the idiopathic form, PACNS, is probably less than 1:2,000,000 (112). Overall, vasculitis has been reported to be responsible for 3% to 5% of strokes occurring at young age (<50 years) (113).

Both primary and secondary CNS vasculitides can present with a broad variety of CNS involvement patterns. Clinically, headache, focal neurological dysfunction, and altered cognition or consciousnesses are most common. The diagnosis can be extremely difficult and often needs to be based on careful evaluation of the clinical signs, laboratory/serologic and CSF studies, findings of radiological studies, and exclusion of other causes. A histological diagnosis remains the gold standard and resembles one of the criteria to be fulfilled for establishing the diagnosis of PACNS (114).

Imaging Strategies

In approaching patients with possible CNS vasculitis, MR imaging is usually the first imaging procedure requested by the clinician. MRI is highly sensitive (approaching a sensitivity of 100%) and typically reveals multifocal white- and gray-matter lesions caused by ischemia or infarction. MRI has been rarely reported to remain normal in cases of CNS vasculitis (115). CSF findings are abnormal in the vast majority of cases of PACNS. The combination of normal MRI and CSF is regarded as a very powerful negative predictor to exclude the possibility of CNS vasculitis in many patients (111).

MRI, however, is not specific. Although multiple subcortical infarctions are consistent with the typical appearance of CNS vasculitis on MR images, in a recent study, substantial variations in number and location of lesions were reported with a nearly equal distribution between cortical, subcortical, and deep gray-matter structures (116). Similar findings might occur in patients with multiple sclerosis, low-grade gliomas, mitochondrial disorders, substance abuse, and other conditions.

To date, DSA is considered the imaging reference standard in the diagnostic workup of patients with suspected vasculitis. The typical findings are multiple segmental narrowings and dilations of cerebral arteries. As with MRI, the findings are not specific. Findings consistent with vasculitis are known to occur in numerous disorders, including intracranial atherosclerotic disease, vasospasm, and hypertensive vasculopathy.

The sensitivies of DSA reported in different studies vary widely and have to be regarded with care. In many case series, patients without histological proof of the diagnosis were reported. The sensitivity may be especially low in the case of PACNS, as usually small arterioles and venules of less than 300 μm in diameter are affected, below the resolution of conventional DSA equipment.

In a recent study of 38 patients who were suspected to suffer from PACNS, and who had undergone both DSA and biopsy (parenchymal and leptomeningeal), 14 patients had findings suggestive of vasculitis on DSA, but biopsy failed to confirm the diagnosis. In 2 of the remaining 24 patients, PACNS was found at biopsy (117). Although these results might be limited to a certain extent by the retrospective nature of the analysis (i.e., bias in patient selection), it certainly underscores the diagnostic difficulties in imaging cerebral vasculitis.

Computed Tomographic and Magnetic Resonance Angiography in Vasculitis

CTA and MRA have been used to show the characteristic findings of large artery vasculitis, in particular, stenosis of the aorta and its branches in Takayasu arteritis (118). The ability to assess the vessel wall and the mural inflammation with MRA provides information that cannot be derived from DSA. High-resolution MRI techniques have been recently employed for wall imaging in giant cell arteritis as well (119). Given the considerable lower spatial resolution of MRA compared with DSA, and due to the typical fine vascular abnormalities in PACNS and most secondary forms of CNS vasculitis, the impact of MRA remains rather limited.

A 3D TOF MRA along with the standard MRI examination of the brain that should include FLAIR and diffusion-weighted images gives an overview about the cerebral arteries and can exclude stenosis of the larger vessels. If a stenosis is present, it can evidently be caused by a variety of pathological entities (atherosclerotic changes in particular). The decision to perform a further workup of the patient (DSA or brain biopsy) after the MR examination is then discussed with the neurologists, rheumatologists, and neurosurgeons.

Demaerel et al. recently reviewed findings from 14 patients with suspected cerebral vasculitis who had been investigated with DSA and 3D TOF (120). They concluded that DSA did not add a significant diagnostic contribution in a patient with suspected vasculitis if more than two stenoses in at least two separate vascular distributions were depicted on MRA, and that DSA remains necessary when MRA is normal or less than three stenoses were seen. These interesting conclusions, however, have to be interpreted with care, as the number of patients was small, and information about biopsies was not elaborated in this report.

Moyamoya Disease

Clinical Background

Moyamoya disease is a rare cerebrovascular disease that features progressive stenosis and occlusion starting at the terminal portion of the bilateral ICAs. The term *moyamoya* is derived from a Japanese word meaning "a puff of smoke" and refers to the angiographic appearance of collateral blood vessels around the circle of Willis distal to the ICA occlusion (121). The origin of the disease is still unknown.

Histologically, the vessels show intimal fibrous thickening and thinning of the media. Infection in the head and neck regions may be related to moyamoya disease, although a certain infectious pathogen has not been determined (122). Some genetic factors may also play an important role in pathogenesis of moyamoya disease. The hypothesis is based on reports of familial occurrence, the higher incidence of moyamoya disease in Far Eastern as compared with that in Western countries, and on chromosomal studies (123,124).

Moyamoya disease can occur at any age, although it is most commonly found in children and young adults. Patients may be asymptomatic or present with severe neuro-

logical deficits. As the ICAs continue to narrow, the collateral vessels are unable to supply the brain sufficiently, and ischemic injuries result. Children often present with strokes, seizures, and recurrent headaches. Adults, on the other hand, may suffer from intraventricular hemorrhage and subarachnoid hemorrhage. Patients with unilateral disease may progress over time from unilateral to bilateral disease.

Treatment is symptomatic and supportive. Patients experiencing TIAs and stroke may be given medical therapy to reduce the risk of future attacks. In some cases, revascularization surgery, direct (EC-IC bypass) or indirect bypass (encephaloduroarteriosynangiosis) may be performed.

The term *moyamoya syndrome* was frequently used to describe a phenomenon caused by an olegemic state similar in presentation as moyamoya disease but caused by acquired or systemic disorders (e.g., atherosclerotic disease, irradiation, infections, neurofibromatosis, and Down syndrome). Recently, this terminology has been questioned, and it was proposed to use the term *angiographic moyamoya* for this group of patients (125). A unilateral involvement without any known cause should be called *probable moyamoya* (126).

Imaging Strategies

Classically, DSA is the standard of reference for diagnosis of moyamoya disease. The diagnostic criteria include (a) a stenosis or occlusion at the terminal portion of the ICA and/or at the proximal portions of the ACA and/or MCA, (b) abnormal vascular networks in the vicinity of the stenotic or occlusive lesions, and (c) these findings should be bilateral (127). Apart from abnormal networks through adjacent small perforating and leptomeningeal vessels, cerebral blood supply might be derived from transdural leptomeningeal collaterals arising from ECA branches and from branches of the ophthalmic artery.

According to a staging scheme proposed by Suzuki and Takaku, the angiographic pattern was graded in severity with intensification of the moyamoya in the early stages and disappearance in the late stages. In these late stages, branches from the ICA disappear, and the collateralization is seen from branches of the ECA (121).

CT may be useful to depict hemorrhage and low-density areas suggestive of infarctions in the acute stage. For the workup of patients with suspected moyamoya disease, MRI imaging is the noninvasive imaging procedure of choice (Fig. 11-33). On standard sequences, the moyamoya vessels might be visible as multiple flow voids extending from the suprasellar cisterns to the basal ganglia and accompanying parenchymal injuries might be found. Various methods including perfusion-weighted MR imaging have

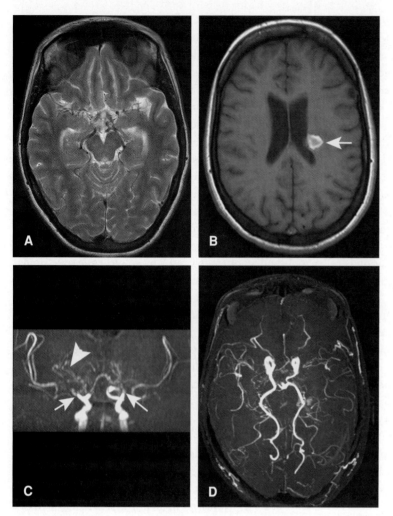

FIGURE 11-33 **Adult, young, female patient with moyamoya disease. A:** On T2-weighted images, the MCAs appear small on both sides. **B:** On the T1-weighted image, a subacute bleeding adjacent to the lateral ventricle is depicted (*arrow*). **C:** 3D TOF MTR MIP slab in coronal orientation and **D:** In the axial orientation shows bilateral occlusion of the supraclinoid ICAs (*arrows*), prominent PCoAs, and, clearly, the collateral vessels (*arrowhead*).

been used to study cerebral blood flow alterations in moyamoya disease, which might become useful as a marker of disease severity (128,129).

Computed Tomographic and Magnetic Resonance Angiography in Moyamoya

The depiction of moyamoya disease with CTA, and in particular with MRA, has been investigated in numerous studies (130–132). Using state-of-the-art 3D TOF MRA, Yamada et al. recently reported on 46 patients who underwent MRI, MRA, and DSA (133). The well-known pitfall of TOF MRA, the overestimation of stenotic arteries as occluded, was the major shortcoming of the technique (18 out of 107 stenotic vessels were rated as occluded on MRA). However, the accuracy for detecting *steno-occlusive* lesions was excellent with MRA (100%) as well as the detection of basal cerebral, leptomeningeal, and transdural collateral vessels. On a patient-to-patient basis, the sensitivity and specificity for diagnosis of moyamoya disease were 98% and 100%, respectively.

According to recent guidelines, DSA is not considered mandatory for the diagnosis of moyamoya disease in children if MRI and MRA clearly show the characteristic criteria (127). MRA was found useful as well to study the postoperative changes after bypass surgery. For example, a reciprocal relation between neovascularization artificially induced by combined bypass surgery and moyamoya vessels was found in a longitudinal study performed by Houkin et al. (134). DSA is thus, in the majority of cases, reserved for equivocal cases, for the preoperative workup, and for the investigation of adults in whom secondary disorders might be underlying.

The typical findings of moyamoya disease might be likewise depicted with CTA, and CTA can be valuable to depict the patency of a bypass after surgery (135,136). If the CT shows an intracranial hemorrhage, CTA might allow the diagnosis of an underlying moyamoya disease at the time of clinical presentation (137). However, larger prospective studies on the role of CTA in this disease are not available.

Aneurysms

Clinical Background

Subarachnoid hemorrhage (SAH) as a consequence of rupture of an intracranial aneurysm has a high mortality and morbidity. It accounts for about one fourth of cerebrovascular deaths, and the case fatality despite improvements in the management of patients with SAH is still between 25% and 50% (138); one half of the survivors will be left disabled and dependent on others in activities of daily living (139,140). CTA and MRA play an increasingly important role for the workup of patients with ruptured or suspected aneurysms as well as in the follow-up of patients treated by surgical or endovascular procedures.

Classification and Pathology of Aneurysms

Aneurysms are localized dilatations of the vessel wall and are traditionally classified based on their morphology or etiology. Based on their morphology, the more common saccular and fusiform aneurysms can be distinguished. The etiologies include vessel degeneration from hemodynamic factors, a presumed congenital disorder that affects the vessel wall, atherosclerosis, dissection, infection (mycotic aneurysms), vascular disease, trauma, and neoplastic invasion.

Saccular Aneurysms. Saccular aneurysms that occur without any underlying predisposing factor (hereditary predisposition, collagen-vascular disease, or arteriovenous malformation) present the vast majority of aneurysms. On histological examination, the aneurysmal sac is usually composed of intima and adventitia only, while the media and the elastic membrane end at the ostium of the aneurysm.

In the past, the development of aneurysms was thought to result from congenital focal defects in the media that were weakened over years under arterial pressure. However, no clear evidence of congenital, developmental, or inherited weakness has been found (141).

A current focus of research is the investigation of hemodynamic stress on aneurysm formation, growth, thrombosis, and rupture. For example, it had been shown that the site of maximal increased wall shear stress is located at the apex of vessel bifurcations (142), which presumably leads to continuing damage of the intima progressing to the initiation and progression of most aneurysms.

Clinically, most aneurysms are found to arise at vessel bifurcations, typically on the convexity of a curve in the parent vessel wall. The relation between the aneurysm and its parent artery is a principal factor that determines the intra-aneurysmal flow pattern (Fig. 11-34). For example, computer simulations of lateral aneurysms have shown shear stress and pressure to be maximal at the downstream site of the ostium (143). These lateral aneurysms project nearly perpendicular from the side of the parent artery and are often localized at the ICA. Blood typically enters these aneurysms at the distal site of the ostium, and it exits at its proximal aspect, producing a slow-flow vortex in the central part of the aneurysm (144). Especially in giant aneurysms (larger than 25 mm), stagnant flow is an important factor for thrombus formation. In contradistinction, the intra-aneurysmal flow is typically rapid in smaller aneurysms that arise at the origin of a branching vessel or terminal bifurcation, and vortex formation is rare. These flow patterns are not only important for the progression of aneurysms but have as well important implications on the imaging display with MR and may influence the selection and placement of endovascular treatment devices in the future (144–147).

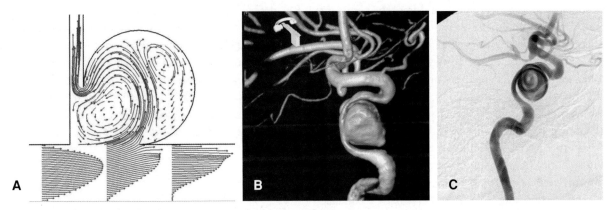

FIGURE 11-34 A: Computer simulation (finite element modeling) of flow velocities in a 2D aneurysmal model located at a vessel bifurcation at the systolic peak. The length of the *arrows* represents the velocity. Note the complex flow pattern with a small recirculating vortex near the dome of the aneurysm and the great variability of flow velocities. Courtesy of P. Dantan, Université Paris7, Paris, France. **B:** Rotational DSA shows a side wall aneurysm located at the cavernous segment of the ICA. **C:** On a single lateral frame, a complex flow pattern within the aneurysm can be observed.

Numerous conditions or diseases are known to be associated with an increased incidence of aneurysms. The frequency of aneurysms with arteriovenous malformations has been reported in the range from 3% to 30%. These aneurysms can be located at the feeding arteries or within the nidus itself and are probably related to increased hemodynamic stress (148). Congenital anomalies of the intracranial vessels, like persistent carotid-basilar anastomoses, also have an increased risk for aneurysm formation, perhaps due to altered hemodynamics. Hereditary conditions associated with intracranial aneurysms include adult polycystic kidney disease (~10% of those affected) and type IV Ehlers-Danlos syndrome.

The risk of aneurysm formation is furthermore increased in families who have a history of aneurysmal SAH—the relative risk is especially elevated in patients with two or more first- or second-degree relatives who suffered from aneurysmal SAH (prevalence of aneurysms: 9.8%) (149). In patients with substance abuse, especially with cocaine, various vascular complications have been described, including SAH and aneurysms.

About 85% of aneurysms are located in the anterior circulation, and of these, more than 80% arise at one of the following locations: the junction of the ACA and the ACoA, the ICA at the origin of the PCoA, the bifurcation of the MCA, and the bifurcation of the ICA. Aneurysms of the posterior fossa account for about 15% of all aneurysms and arise in approximately 50% from the basilar bifurcation; less common locations are the junction of the VAs with the PICA or the SCAs (150).

Aneurysms of the ICA can arise from the extradural or intradural location. If in an intradural location and proximal to the origin of the PCoA, they are termed, depending on their location, as *ophthalmic* or *paraclinoid segment aneurysms*. Aneurysms arising from more peripheral cerebral vessels are less common and should raise the suspicion of an inflammatory, traumatic, or tumoral etiology.

About 20% of aneurysms are multiple. With aneurysms at the ICA or MCA, there is a tendency for either symmetrical aneurysms or a second aneurysm on the same vessel.

Giant aneurysms, those with a diameter of at least 25 mm, represent about 5% of all saccular aneurysms. They are most commonly located at the ICA within the cavernous sinus, at the MCA, or at the apex of the BA.

The majority of all aneurysms are asymptomatic until they rupture. However, some aneurysms may cause neuropathies. A classic example is a third nerve palsy secondary to a PCoA aneurysm. Evidently, clinical signs indicative of a mass lesion are more common with giant aneurysms. Compressive symptoms depend on the location of the aneurysm and include retro-orbital pain, diplopia, impaired visual acuity, and visual field defects for a location at the intracranial carotid arteries; seizures and hemiparesis for the MCA; and signs of brain stem compression and cranial nerve dysfunction at a vertebrobasilar location (151).

Fusiform Aneurysms. Especially in older patients, exaggerated arterial ectasias and elongations that often extend over a considerable length might be found, termed *fusiform aneurysms*. These aneurysms are regarded as a severe and unusual form of atherosclerosis and are most commonly seen at the vertebrobasilar system. Symptoms usually result from thrombosis within the aneurysm, producing brain stem infarction, or from mass effect on the adjacent brain or cranial nerves (35).

Dissecting Aneurysms. In a dissecting aneurysm, the plane of dissection is localized between the internal elastic lamina and the tunica media, which extends transmurally if SAH occurs (152,153). Most cases of dissecting aneurysms that cause bleedings involve the posterior circulation (for a more detailed discussion: see section on dissection) (Fig. 11-35).

Traumatic Aneurysms. Aneurysms caused by a trauma in an intracranial location are relatively rare. These are often called *false saccular aneurysms* or *pseudoaneurysms*, as they are cavitated, paravascular hematomas, typically within blood clots, that lack any components of vessel walls. Mainly caused by penetrating trauma, there are also aneurysms resulting from nonpenetrating trauma, the latter typically localized in vessels near the skull base or at peripheral intracranial vessels. For example, shearing forces between the inferior free margin of the falx and the artery resulting from frontolateral impacts might cause traumatic pericallosal aneurysms.

Mycotic Aneurysms. The term mycotic aneurysm was introduced by Osler in 1885 to describe infective aneurysm formation complicating bacterial endocarditis in a single case. The nomenclature has been subsequently used to describe all types of infective aneurysms. These aneurysms are rare, occur with greater frequency in children, are often found on vessels distal to the circle of Willis, and are most likely caused by infected embolic material that reaches the adventitia through the vasa vasorum. In addition to bacterial endocarditis, meningitis, skull base osteomyelitis, sinusitis, and cavernous infections are known as causative factors (35,154,155).

Screening for Asymptomatic Aneurysms with Computed Tomographic and Magnetic Resonance Angiography

Compared with the management of ruptured aneurysms, surgery for an unruptured aneurysm carries with it a comparably low risk of stroke and death. Based on this clinical consideration and the possibility of using CTA and MRA to

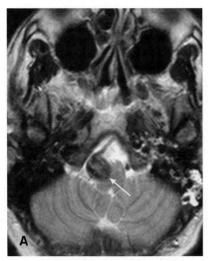 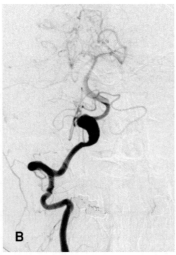 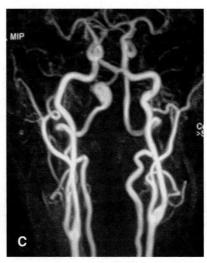

FIGURE 11-35 A middle-aged patient with a minor car accident in his history with developing headache and neck pain. A: T2-weighted image shows a right-sided aneurysm with mixed but predominantly low signal intensity (*arrow*). **B:** CE first-pass MRA and **C:** DSA shows the aneurysm as a fusiform dilatation of the right V4 segment of the VA, proximal to the origin of the PICA. Treatment with parent vessel occlusion.

avoid the costs and risks of DSA, the possibility of a screening role for imaging in aneurysmal detection is receiving attention. Insights into the natural history of asymptomatic aneurysms and the risks associated with their repair are needed in order to approach this complex and controversial subject. Related issues to be clarified include the identification of subgroups of patients at high risk and a selection of the best methods to screen these individuals (149,156).

It is estimated that about 3% to 6% of the population harbor an aneurysm (149). Important data on the natural history and on the risks of repair of asymptomatic aneurysms was derived from two recently published reports, including a total of 2,621 and 4,060 patients, respectively, conducted by the International Study of Unruptured Intracranial Aneurysms Investigators (ISUIA) group (157,158).

The natural history was assessed in the first study, on retrospective data obtained from 1,449 patients with 1,937 unruptured aneurysms. The key results in that study indicated, compared with previous estimates, a tiny rupture risk of 0.05% per year for small aneurysms (<10 mm in diameter) in patients who have not had an SAH previously, and a risk of about 0.5% per year for patients who had a history of previous aneurysm rupture and subsequent repair in another location. For aneurysms larger than 10 mm and giant aneurysms, the rupture rate was less than 1%, and 6%. Despite the size, the location of the aneurysms was the only significant predictor of rupture, with an increased relative risk for aneurysm in the posterior circulation.

The second study included a prospective assessment of patients followed-up, and data was derived from 1,692

patients with a total of 2,686 unruptured aneurysms (6,544 years of follow-up) that did not have aneurysmal repair. Compared with the retrospective study, the rupture rate for patients with an aneurysm of at least 7 mm in diameter was found to be higher, but for aneurysms below 7 mm, the rupture rate was found again to be low. Apart from size, the location was found to have a significant role in determining the risk of future rupture, and as noted in the findings from the retrospective study, aneurysms located at the posterior circulation artery were associated with an increased risk for rupture. For patients without a history of subarachnoid hemorrhage from an aneurysm at another location, the 5-year cumulative rupture rates for aneurysms located at the ICA, ACoA, ACA, or MCA was 0% (aneurysm smaller than 7 mm), 2.6% (7 to 12 mm), 14.5% (13 to 24 mm), and 40% (25 mm or greater), respectively, compared with rates of 2.5%, 14.5%, 18.4%, and 50%, respectively, for the same size categories involving posterior circulation and posterior communicating artery aneurysms.

In the second study, treatment was followed prospectively in a second cohort that included 1,917 patients who had undergone open surgical repair or in 451 patients who had undergone endovascular repair. The combined morbidity and mortality at 1 year for patients without a prior SAH was 12.6% and 9.8% for open surgical repair and endovascular treatment, respectively. For both treatment options, predictors of poor outcome were a large diameter; a location of the aneurysm at the posterior circulation; and for the open surgical group, among other factors as well, an older age. The authors concluded from these results that many factors are involved in the decision about management of patients with unruptured aneurysms; that according to the rupture rate of small aneurysms (<7 mm), it would be difficult to improve on the natural history of these lesions; and that overall, the natural rupture rates for the different sizes of aneurysms were often equaled or exceeded by the risks with surgical or endovascular repair.

In an excellent review based on studies that focused on risk factors for aneurysm formation and rupture, Wardlaw and White recommended that patients who are at the greatest risk of having an aneurysm that subsequently ruptures—females over 30 years from families with two or more first- or second-degree relatives affected by SAH and autosomal dominant polycystic kidney disease patients—should be assessed on an individual basis (149). These authors were wary of introducing a "screening" program that might lead to the detection and treatment of cases that would never have caused clinical disease and that equally might miss cases, including those arising de novo, after screening (149).

Given that the surgical risk is relatively high in comparison to the risk of aneurysm rupture, a lack of data demonstrating cost effectiveness for screening, and the lack of clear information about how often or how long to screen an individual, screening for the asymptomatic patient cannot be fully endorsed at this time. Clearly, more data are required, and continued research is ongoing.

Imaging Strategies

The imaging strategy for the detection or depiction of cerebral aneurysms depends on the clinical setting. Basically, four scenarios can be distinguished: (a) the search for aneurysms in patients presenting with an SAH; (b) the search for aneurysms that might cause a mass effect; (c) the evaluation of asymptomatic patients with increased risk of aneurysms; and (d) the post-treatment imaging of aneurysms.

DSA is still considered the mainstay for the diagnosis of cerebral aneurysms (159), and the recent introduction of rotational angiography with 3D reconstructed images furthermore has increased the sensitivity and accuracy for detection of aneurysms. The precise assessment of the aneurysm neck, incorporated branch segments, and the relationships with the parent vessel has made 3D DSA extremely valuable for treatment planning, especially in complex cases (160). However, like biplane DSA, only the interior of an arterial lumen is depicted, and the nonluminal information, such as the extent and location of mural calcifications and intra-aneurysmal thrombus, is limited or not available.

CTA and MRA are challenging the role of DSA in the clinical workup of patients with known or suspected aneurysm not only because of their technical improvements in imaging quality mimicking the display of DSA, but also as these techniques provide unique information that cannot be derived from DSA.

A noncontrast CT examination is usually the first step in the imaging workup in patients with suspected SAH. This examination can provide important information on an aneurysm location, as some bleeding patterns have been associated with particular aneurysms. For example, a hemorrhage located predominantly within the interhemispheric fissure is common with anterior communicating aneurysms and within the sylvian fissure with MCA aneurysms. On unenhanced scans, larger nonthrombosed aneurysms might already be visualized as a well delineated isodense to slightly hyperdense mass (161). Thrombosed aneurysms, especially the larger ones, often have a thickened, partially calcified wall (Fig. 11-36).

The usefulness of MR in the diagnosis of acute SAH has been a subject of considerable interest. However, despite promising results of gradient-echo T2* and FLAIR images to detect these bleedings (162), no convincing data is available to indicate the role of MR in this clinical setting. Given the limited ability to investigate uncooperative, severely sick patients with MR contributes to the fact that MR is only applied in a few institutions for evaluating acute SAH. MR imaging of aneurysms is most commonly used for the follow-up of treated patients and for screening purposes in those practices pursuing such a program.

On conventional MR scans, the appearance of aneurysms is highly variable and depends on the sequence employed as well as on the flow properties and the presence of clot, fibrosis, and calcification within the aneurysms. The typical patent aneurysm lumen with rapid flow shows flow void on T1- and T2-weighted images; however, signal heterogeneity may be seen if turbulent flow within the aneurysm is present (Fig. 11-35).

Partially thrombosed large aneurysms often show concentric layers of a multilaminated clot with variable signal intensities around the patent lumen and a signal loss at the fibrous capsule. Completely thrombosed aneurysms also have variable MR findings; subacute thrombus is predominately hyperintense on T1- and T2-weighted studies, but isointensity with the brain parenchyma in acute thrombus might occur.

While both conventional CT and MR might already give important diagnostic clues for the detection of aneurysms, it is the addition of CTA and MRA that detects smaller aneurysms and provides an ability to characterize larger aneurysms. The qualities and limitations inherent to each of these angiographic techniques largely influence

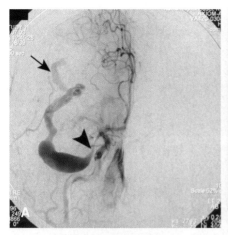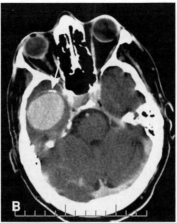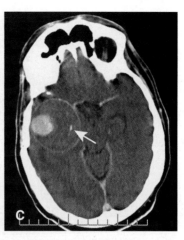

FIGURE 11-36 Giant aneurysm of the right MCA in a patient who had undergone repeated clipping and wrapping operations over the last 25 years. A: During the arterial phase of DSA, a tubular structure pointing in the superior direction is depicted (*arrow*). The aneurysmal dilation begins at the M1 segment (*arrowhead*). **B, C:** CTA source images show that large parts of the aneurysm are thrombosed. Small calcifications can be visualized at **(B)** the wall of the aneurysm (*arrow*)—the wall shows some enhancement—and **(C)** within the aneurysm (*arrow*). The tubular structure as shown on DSA resembled only the small perfused part in the upper part of the aneurysm.

the choice between CT and MR for the different clinical settings.

Computed Tomographic and Magnetic Resonance Angiography in Imaging of Cerebral Aneurysms

Detection of Aneurysms. Over the last two decades, a number of studies were performed comparing the reliability of CTA and/or MRA in comparison with DSA as the standard of reference in depicting cerebral aneurysms. In a meta-analysis of the literature on the diagnostic accuracy of noninvasive imaging methods with that of DSA, White et al. (163) identified and analyzed 38 out of 103 studies that fulfilled their primary inclusion criterion of achieving a sufficiently high quality according to their scoring system.

Similar accuracies for CTA and MRA (89% and 90%, respectively) were demonstrated on a per aneurysm basis. CT showed a greater sensitivity for detection of aneurysms with values of 96% and 61% for CTA and MRA, respectively, in those aneurysms larger than 3 mm and values of 94% and 38%, respectively, for those smaller than 3 mm.

As these authors remarked, the results of direct comparison between CTA and MRA had to be interpreted with caution, as few patients underwent both of the noninvasive examinations. Further caution is required if the results of this meta-analysis are extrapolated to the circumstance of screening for aneurysms, as most studies were performed in populations with a high aneurysm prevalence—many focused on patients with known aneurysms or recent SAH, which might bias the results.

In a prospective study, the same group compared CTA *and* MRA in 142 patients who also underwent DSA to detect aneurysms (164). A similar accuracy was found for CTA and MRA; however, for both modalities, it was slightly lower compared with the meta-analysis results. In accordance to the results of the meta-analysis, the sensitivity for small aneurysms (<5 mm) was lower and reached only a sensitivity of 57% for CTA and of 35% for MRA (164). Based on these results, the authors concluded that CTA and MRA *cannot* safely replace intra-arterial DSA in the diagnostic workup of patients with acute SAH. They did suggest that CTA and MRA can help to exclude aneurysms larger than 5 mm (e.g., those large enough to possibly cause compressive symptoms).

Further improvements in technology and experience, particularly with CTA, will continue to challenge the role of DSA as the method of choice not only for the diagnosis but as well for the triage and treatment planning of aneurysms.

Computed Tomographic Angiography. For all CTA examinations, an optimized patient preparation, as stated previously, is essential to generate high-quality angiograms. This is of special importance in uncooperative patients presenting with SAH, where the smallest vascular abnormalities have to be detected (Fig. 11-37). Overlapping of venous structures can potentially obscure the arterial vessel of interest, which might especially pose problems for the detection of aneurysms at the origin of the PCoA (obscuration by the vein of Rosenthal) and for those at the level of the cavernous segment. A bolus-timing examination is therefore recommended.

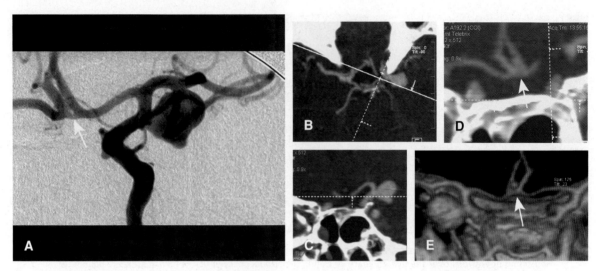

FIGURE 11-37 A: DSA, injection into left ICA, shows a large aneurysm at the communicating segment of the ICA pointing in the lateral direction. A second small ACoA aneurysm (*arrow*) can hardly be visualized in this view. **B–D:** Thin-slab MIP images that are planned with the help of the cross-referencing tool allow display of the large aneurysm with great detail and in relation to the osseous structures and as well to visualize the small ACoA pointing in the superior direction (*arrow*). As shown in **(E),** this small aneurysm was better detected with the VR technique (*arrow*).

A scan volume that covers the distance from the anterior arch of C1—to encompass the PICA—to the third and fourth order sylvian branches, or the top of the frontal sinus, includes 99% of all berry aneurysm sites (5,165). The actual scan parameters should be optimized for resolution (see technical section).

A free-form interrogation of the image data set is recommended, and both 2D and 3D image displays are required. MPR images and sliding thin-slab MIPs should be evaluated using cross-referencing tools in three planes, a crucial step in confirming or excluding a suspected aneurysm.

For the detection of mural calcification and of an intraluminal thrombus, appropriate window settings is important. Bone (1,800 to 4,000 HU) can be easily diffentiated from contrast-opacified blood (150 to 450 HU), and the contrast-opacified arteries (220 to 350 HU) are readily distinguished from SAH (65 to 85 HU).

The free-form interrogation of the image data set should be used to determine the dimensions of the aneurysmal sac, neck, and parent artery. Curved planar reformatted images can be especially useful for the evaluation of aneurysms at the carotid siphon (166). For a further assessment of the anatomical spatial relationships, the VR technique has been advocated as the 3D method of choice (167,168).

With the VR technique, a clearer visualization of vascular relationships and other tissues with different compositions becomes possible. A recent study of Villablanca et al. (169) underlined the importance of this technique. Approximately 10% of the aneurysms were identified initially on 3D images and only retrospectively detected on 2D images.

Using these advanced image acquisition and evaluation techniques, the results of recent studies were more favorable than most of the older studies. For example, Wintermark et al. found a very high sensitivity, specificity, and accuracy (94.8%, 95.2%, 94.9%) in comparison with DSA for the detection of aneurysms using an MDCT technique. Using the VR display technique in conjunction with 2D images, Villablanca et al. found CTA in several studies equal to DSA in the detection of aneurysms and superior to DSA and MRA in the characterization of brain aneurysms (5,168,169).

Given these encouraging results, the question arises if CTA could replace DSA as a tool to diagnose and appropriately manage aneurysmal SAH. Recently, Dehdashti et al. and Matsumoto et al. found CTA sufficient in the vast majority of cases (170,171). In fact, Dehdashti et al. required DSA in only 11 out of 100 patients when the CTA characteristics of the ruptured aneurysm was found to be unsatisfactory (170).

The most important limitation of CTA is the inability to visualize very small vessels, including the anterior choroidal and lenticulostriate arteries, and the perforating arteries at the ACoA and the apex BA. If visualization of these small vessels (<0.5 mm in diameter) would influence the therapeutic approach, DSA should be performed. The inability to visualize collateral flow patterns can be considered a second disadvantage for treatment planning. On the other hand, the identification of calcium in the wall of an aneurysm and the visualization of the relationship of thrombus is best provided by CTA and has shown to be of considerable importance for treatment planning (168).

In light of these results and our experience, we agree with the conclusion by Chappel et al. who stated: "clinicians treating patients with possible aneurysmal SAH might consider following the diagnostic CT scans with CTA. If insufficient experience with or confidence in the technology raises concerns in cases in which an aneurysm is not identified or clearly delineated, despite a high level of suspicion, then DSA can also be used until more confidence and experience are gained. Most patients can be easily and comfortably treated without DSA" (159).

Magnetic Resonance Angiography. For evaluation of patients, using the 3D TOF MRA technique predominates and has been shown to be more effective than the 3D PC MR technique (172). As with CTA, a free-form interrogation of the image data set using both the 2D and 3D image display modalities (MPR images, MIPs, and SSD) is recommended to optimize the detection of aneurysms.

Compared with modern multislice CTA, the image resolution of MRA is generally slightly lower, and saturation of slow-flow and intravoxel phase dispersion in the presence of turbulent flow can lead to incomplete delineation on 3D TOF MRA images (Fig. 11-38). Moreover, diagnostic difficulties might arise from high signal artifact (methemoglobin) caused by intraluminal thrombus or a hematoma surrounding a recently ruptured aneurysm, which can mimic flow signal (173,174). These factors contribute to lower aneurysm detection rates with MRA compared with DSA and state-of-the-art CTA examinations, particularly with small (<3 mm) aneurysms, and to a less accurate quantification and characterization of the lesions (175–177). However, new imaging strategies using CE MRA, as well as sequence and hardware improvements, showed promising results.

The use of CE MRA in search of or to characterize aneurysms was applied both as a fast first-pass dynamic technique and as a steady state technique using a 3D TOF sequence. These techniques were not shown to be useful to distinguish thrombus from patent lumen in large aneurysms but did show promising results for the detection of smaller aneurysms (16,32). Based on initial results at 3T, further improvements in aneurysm detection can be expected capitalizing on the higher signal-to-noise and resolution. When used in combination with parallel imaging techniques, such as sensitivity encoding (SENSE), new synergies are possible (11).

Post-treatment Imaging of Aneurysms

Open surgical clipping and endovascular techniques—coiling, stent implantation, embolization with liquid agents, and parent vessel occlusion—are applied for the treatment of intracranial aneurysms. For post-treatment assessments of all therapies, DSA is the gold standard, but noninvasive CTA and MRA are increasingly being considered for that task. Both imaging modalities, however, in particular CTA, have limitations for the follow-up of these patients. The optimal noninvasive imaging technique depends on the type of treatment that has been applied.

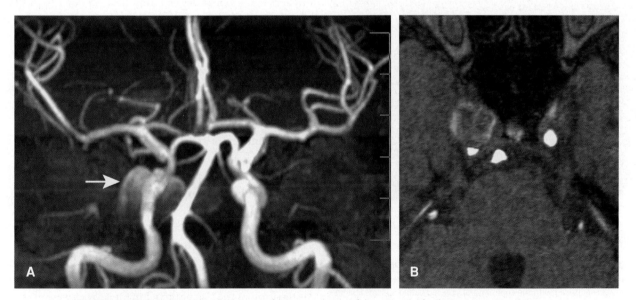

FIGURE 11-38 A: 3D TOF MRA MIP image and **(B)** source image of the patient with a large aneurysm at the cavernous segment of the ICA (same patient as in Fig. 11-1). The aneurysm can be detected (*arrow*), but the turbulent flow leads to an incomplete delineation of the aneurysm, in particular, in the inferior part of the aneurysm.

Clipping. Cerebral angiography performed after aneurysm surgery can identify potential causes of morbidity and mortality, such as an aneurysm remnant or vessel occlusion. This evaluation should be strongly considered for patients with large aneurysms or cerebrovascular atherosclerosis and for those who develop new postoperative neurological deficits (179).

In the long term, follow-up exclusion of an aneurysm from the circulation by clipping appears to be reliable: Tsutsumi et al. (180) observed in their series of 112 patients with 140 aneurysms a 0.26% annual risk of regrowth of completely clipped aneurysms. This rate was far less than the rate of de novo aneurysm formation (0.89%) reported at that time. Based on their results, the authors concluded that long-term follow-up angiography might be indicated about 10 years after surgery: The task of imaging focuses on the treated aneurysm as well as an evaluation of the rest of the cerebral vasculature.

Both CT and MR give important information about the brain parenchyma in patients who have undergone clipping, with CTA and MRA providing information about the patency of vessels distant to the clip. However, both imaging modalities are vulnerable to artifacts, especially in close proximity to clips. DSA remains necessary if the clinical question is for regrowth and reperfusion of the *treated* aneurysm (Fig. 11-39).

If patients with clips undergo a CTA examination, it should be kept in mind that image degradation is less if titanium clips have been placed and in general if a thin

collimation is used. There are techniques to reduce the artifacts on the (a) image acquisition level—tilting the head along the axis of the clip during image acquisition—and (b) postprocessing level have been described. These techniques do not eliminate the artifacts entirely and are rather complicated to use in the daily routine (181–183).

MR imaging of patients with successfully clipped aneurysms is, in general, safe. However, it is necessary to ensure that nonferromagnetic clips, available for many years, have been placed; otherwise, there is a risk of deflection and dislocation of the clip. Evidently, safety of the clip does not imply good image quality.

Coiling. Selective endovascular treatment with Guglielmi detachable coils (GDCs; Boston Scientific/Target Therapeutics, Boston, MA) and other coils is increasingly being used in the management of intracranial aneurysms, especially in light of the first encouraging results from the International Subarachnoid Aneurysm Trial (ISAT) (184).

In the ISAT trial, the outcome of patients treated with coils in terms of survival free of disability at 1 year was significantly better than with clipping. However, the long-term occlusion rates of coiled aneurysms and the most useful duration and frequency for follow-up after coiling have not been established. Moreover, some aneurysms cannot be completely packed with coils, and residual filling within the interstices of the coil mass or a residual aneurysm neck may remain after treatment. Two recent studies made clear that the stability of aneurysm occlusion after coiling must be regularly evaluated, even in cases of initial total occlusion (185,186).

As in the evaluation of patients treated with clips, CTA images are severely degraded by beam-hardening artifacts from the implant material, and these may hinder the detection of a residual flow in the aneurysm. MR artifacts together with some heat production and ferromagnetism of GDCs have been reported. However, compared with CT, these artifacts are minimal, and an obscuration of approximately 2 to 3 mm of surrounding brain parenchyma has been observed (Fig. 11-40) (187).

A number of studies have attempted to evaluate the role of MRA in the follow-up of patients treated with GDCs. In the majority of these studies, 3D TOF MRA with or without gadolinium was compared with findings from DSA (188–192). The sensitivity of 3D TOF MRA without contrast material in revealing residual flow within the aneurysm ranged from about 70% to 90%, with specificity in the range of 90% to 100%. In general, missed remnants were small (<3 mm). Both exaggerations and underestimation of the size of the remnant cavities were observed.

False negative examinations were explained by saturation effects as a result of slow flow in the aneurysm, or by

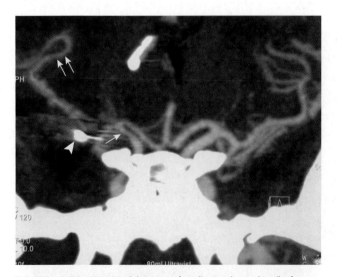

FIGURE 11-39 CTA MIP slab image after clipping (*arrowhead*) of a right sided MCA aneurysm. Note the communicating segment of the ICA is narrowed compared with the contralateral side, indicating spasms (*single arrow*). Severe artifacts adjacent to the clip impair the visualization of the vessel adjacent to the clip. Distal branches, however, are well visualized (*double arrows*).

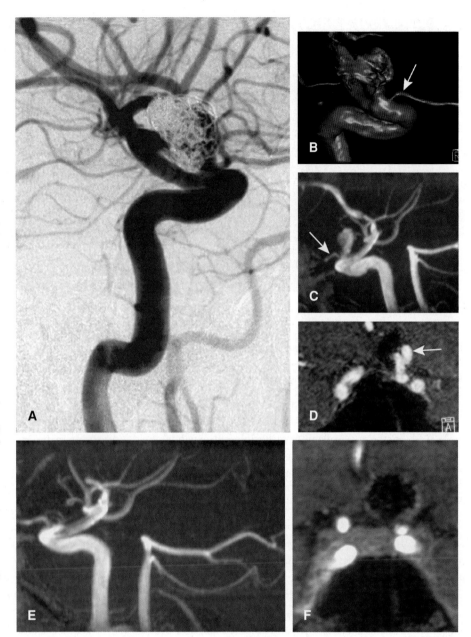

FIGURE 11-40 Patient with partial recanalization of a coiled aneurysm at the ophthalmic segment of the ICA as depicted with **(A)** DSA in lateral oblique view and **(B)** rotational angiography (*arrow* indicates ophthalmic artery). **C:** 3D TOF MRA MIP image without contrast shows the aneurysm and the relation to the ophthalmic artery (*arrow*). **D:** On a thin MIP image in coronal view, the reperfused lateral part of the aneurysm (*arrow*) can be distinguished from the coiled part, the latter being hypointense (*arrowheads*). **E:** Recoiling of the aneurysm resulted in an exclusion of the aneurysm as shown on 3D TOF MRA without contrast and **(F)** after a low-dose contrast injection (thin MIP slab in the coronal orientation).

susceptibility artifact of the coil mass; false positive results, by the presence of intraluminal blood clot interpreted as flow. Cottier et al., who performed a direct comparison of unenhanced and enhanced 3D TOF MRA for the follow-up of GDC-treated aneurysms, observed no benefit with contrast material to depict residual or recurrent aneurysms, but did observe a better delineation of a residual sac in a giant aneurysm. Further technical improvements will facilitate the evaluation of aneurysms treated with coils. For example, it has already been shown that 3D TOF MRA sequences with a short TE, minimizing intravoxel spin-dephasing artifacts, reduce the signal intensity dropout induced by GDCs (193). Coil artifacts were found as well to be reduced by the use of a first-pass CE MRA, probably related to the shorter TE employed (194). MRA may have the potential to replace DSA for follow-up of GDC-treated aneurysms entirely. At the present time, MRA imaging should be regarded as an adjunct to DSA, replacing the invasive technique at certain intervals of follow-up.

Stent Implantation. In the first case reports and case series, stents were mainly used in combination with coils to treat aneurysms in difficult-to-access areas such as the proximal intracranial segments of the ICA or VA, or of the BA trunk. There is also evidence that cerebral stents within the parent artery across an aneurysm neck may hemodynamically

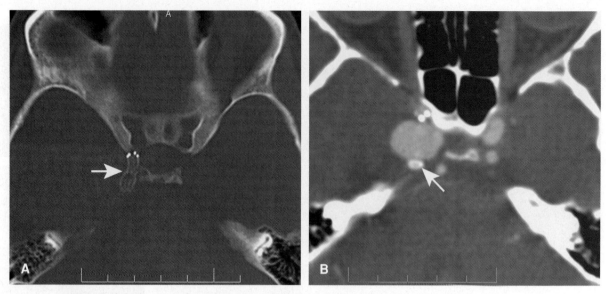

FIGURE 11-41 CTA control after implantation of two overlapping self-expandable nitinol stents for treatment of the large cavernous sinus aneurysm depicted in Figure 11-34B, C. **A:** Using a bone window setting, the stents can be visualized (*arrow*). **B:** After contrast bolus injection, contrast opacification within the stent can be detected (*arrow*). The aneurysm is still present but diminished in size.

uncouple the aneurysm from that parent vessel, leading to thrombosis of the aneurysm (145–147,195).

With the recent availability of flexible self-expandable intravascular nitinol stents (e.g., the Neuroform Stent, Boston Scientific/Target, Fremont, CA), a new therapeutic approach has become possible in the endovascular treatment of intracranial aneurysms (196,197). CTA with thin collimation and appropriate window settings and MRA with ultrashort TE seem to be useful to verify the patency of these stents; however, for a detailed assessment, DSA is required (Fig. 11-41).

Liquid Agents. Embolization with liquid agents has recently been introduced for treatment of aneurysms. This technique seems valuable for treatment of certain fusiform aneurysms or aneurysms with a wide neck. The imaging properties of Onyx (Micro Therapeutics, Inc., Irvine, CA)—a mixture of ethylene vinyl alcohol, dimethyl sulfoxide, and tantalum that is as well used for treatment of arteriovenous malformations—were recently evaluated by Saatci et al. (198).

On CT, the polymer was found to create streak artifacts that impaired the evaluation of the adjacent brain. On MR images, Onyx appeared hypointense, regardless of the sequence used, and no artifacts were observed. As the implant did not interfere with MRA applications, the authors recommended MR imaging with MRA as the first diagnostic workup in patient follow-up.

Vasospasm. Cerebral vasospasm secondary to SAH presents in 40% to 70% of all cases, usually occurs 4 to 9

days after the bleeding, and is reported to double the risk of mortality in SAH (199,200). Detection of vasospasm is important in the prevention of delayed ischemic events. Several studies have shown the feasibility of CTA (201,202) or MRA (203) to detect the arterial narrowing. Multislice CTA, in particular, showed an excellent correlation in the grading of this condition compared with DSA (204). However, at present, transcranial Doppler and DSA dominate for diagnosis: TCD due to its rapidity, noninvasiveness, and amenability to frequent monitoring; DSA, in its excellent visualization of very peripheral arterial segments and its dual utility for therapeutic interventions through intracranial angioplasty (205).

With CTA and MRA, the artifacts from aneurysm clips or endovascular coils can partially or completely impair the assessment of vessels adjacent to the ruptured aneurysm. Thus, visualization of vasospasm by CTA and MRA can be hampered as well (Fig. 11-39). CTA and MRA should be considered for vasospasm detection when Doppler is limited. Since CT and MR can be integrated into a comprehensive workup that provides assessment of brain perfusion and ischemia, a broader utilization is anticipated. These techniques might ultimately yield the best correlation with the degree of symptomatic vasospasm (206–208).

Summing up, multidetector CTA is the recommended noninvasive method of choice for the evaluation of patients with acute SAH. This examination is followed at the author's institution by DSA if (a) no aneurysm is found (e.g., in perimesencephlic hemorrhage), (b) if it is perceived that rotational angiography can provide more details for treatment decision and planning (e.g., information on adjacent small branches), or (c) if the examination provides suboptimal image quality. In patients with vasospasm, Doppler examinations are usually performed first, and DSA examinations are pursued in equivocal cases or in cases requiring subsequent neurovascular interventions. For screening purposes and for the follow-up of patients treated with coiling, we rely on MRA, keeping in mind the somewhat lower detection rate for especially smaller aneurysms.

Intracranial Artery Dissection

Clinical Background

At the cervical portion of the ICA and the extracranial VA, arterial dissection is a well-recognized cause of stroke. Intracranial dissection was not long ago considered as an extremely rare disease but has become increasingly recognized (209). Clinicopathological studies classify dissecting lesions in two categories: (a) dissections between the intima and media, causing luminal narrowing or stenosis (simply termed as *dissection*); and (b) dissections between the media and adventitia, or at the media, causing aneurysmal dilatation (termed *dissecting aneurysms*) (Fig. 11-35) (210).

Headache is a common prodrome and presenting symptom. Neurological deficits are caused either by ischemia or stroke due to stenosis or occlusion, or by SAH due to rupture of the dissected vessel.

The true prevalence of intracranial dissection is unknown. SAH due to rupture of a dissecting aneurysm is believed to be on the order of 1% to 10% (211). In some cases, a (minor) trauma preceding dissection is found. Many predisposing factors including hypertension and fibromuscular dysplasia have been proposed, but often, no history of trauma and no underlying disease can be identified.

According to a nationwide study conducted in Japan in 1996 (210), the vast majority of spontaneous intracranial dissections were found in the posterior circulation—most commonly at the vertebral arteries—however, they might occur as well at the ICA, MCA, or ACA (212–214). In contrast to previous assumptions, intracranial dissection was not mainly confined to young adults: The average age of presentation in this study was 51 years with an age range of 8 to 86 years.

The optimal treatment of intracranial dissection has not yet been determined. The administration of antiplatelet or anticoagulation to patients with ischemic symptoms is controversial. Ruptured dissections have a high incidence of rebleeding. Treatment options include surgical or endovascular parent artery occlusion and, more recently, the use of stents and coils (195,215).

Imaging Strategies

DSA has been the standard of reference for the diagnosis of intracranial dissection. However, the only pathognomonic finding on DSA suggesting a dissection—the double-lumen appearance with an intimal flap—is rarely encountered (216). The presence of the *pearl and string sign*, focal narrowing with a distal site of dilatation, is considered reliable. In contradistinction, the string sign and tapered narrowing are less reliable, as these changes might also be seen in arteriosclerotic disease and in the presence of vasospasm.

The most common location for intracranial dissection is the V4 segment of the VAs. Bilateral involvement is not uncommon as well as the extension of an extracranial dissection to intracranial (178). As it is important to search for an intracranial extension of a dissection starting at the extracranial course of the vessel, it is equally important to analyze the extracranial cervical vessels in patients presenting with ischemia and clinical signs suggestive of ischemia.

In most cases presenting with symptoms of stroke or SAH, or in whom a dissection without these symptoms is clinically suspected, CT or MR is the first imaging modality employed. In addition to the possibility of visualizing the sequela of intracranial dissection, the angiographic aspects of both imaging modalities are capable of raising the suspicion or definitively establishing the diagnosis of intracranial dissection in many cases.

Computed Tomographic and Magnetic Resonance Angiography in Intracranial Artery Dissection

While atherothrombotic lesions are recognized in CTA and MRA by reference to similar criteria as are used in DSA, recognition of dissections of the vessels entails use of additional features: the direct assessment of the vessel wall.

Chen et al. published recently encouraging results on the use of state-of-the-art CTA to detect intracranial dissections. They investigated 17 patients with dissections of the VA—mainly localized in the V4 segment—and 17 control subjects (217). Taking DSA as the standard of reference, they found the technique highly sensitive and accurate (sensitivity, specificity, accuracy—100%, 98%, and 98.5%, respectively) for the diagnosis of these lesions (Fig. 11-42). The principal findings were an increase in the external diameter of the arteries (observed in 100%) and a crescent-shaped mural thickening (observed in 79%). On rare occasions, both signs might be observed in nondissecting arteries. Furthermore, it might not be possible to differentiate an intramural hematoma in an occluded dissection from a mural thrombus in an occluded vessel.

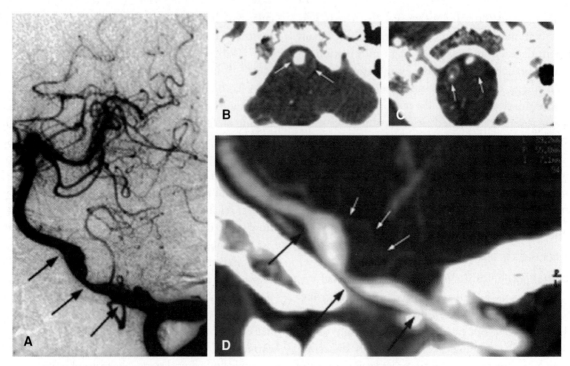

FIGURE 11-42 DSA and CTA images of a 53-year-old woman with a sudden onset of occipital pain and unsteady gait. **A:** DSA of the left VA in an oblique projection shows alternating regions of luminal narrowing and dilatation at the V4 segment (*arrows*). **B, C:** Axial source CT angiograms show a target appearance (narrowed eccentric lumen surrounded by crescent-shaped mural thickening and an enhanced wall) at the bilateral intracranial VAs (*arrows*). An associated increased external diameter of the dissected artery is noted. **D:** MIP CT angiogram demonstrates the same picture of an alternatively narrowed and dilated lumen (*black arrows*) and the intramural hematoma (*white arrows*). Reprinted from Chen CJ, Tseng YC, Lee TH, et al. Multisection CT angiography compared with catheter angiography in diagnosing vertebral artery dissection. *AJNR Am J Neuroradiol.* 2004;25:769–774, with permission.

TOF MRA has the principle advantage over CTA in that the intramural hematoma can more easily be visualized in the subacute stage (Fig. 11-43). Due to the presence of methemoglobin, the hematoma is shown with high signal intensity usually from the second day for up to three months.

In most cases, it poses no problem to distinguish the high signal intensity of the intramural hematoma from the usually slightly higher signal of flowing blood on TOF MRA, especially if the source images are carefully studied. Should there be doubts, the application of an additional caudal presaturation pulse to suppress the high signal intensity from the arterial flow is useful to selectively depict the hematoma (218).

In the very early stage (usually up to two days), the hematoma is isointense to the surrounding tissue, and the thickening of the vessel and narrowing of the patent lumen might be the only signs of dissection. For the recognition of dissections of the larger *extracranial* ICA, this technique is very robust, and DSA is rarely indicated. However, for the visualization of the smaller vertebral arteries that also typically exhibit marked differences in diameter, the technique is less sensitive (219). Problems in diagnosing dissections of the posterior circulation might arise from the venous plexus surrounding the arteries; that might give a flow signal that cannot be suppressed even if a cranial and caudal presaturation pulse is being used (220). Nevertheless, the technique should be applied, as it might disclose complementary information with regard to findings from selective angiography, and if characteristic findings of a dissection are depicted, DSA might be avoided.

The ability of TOF to directly visualize a hematoma represents an advantage compared to the PC technique, where static tissue is entirely suppressed by subtraction. A combination of the PC method with a fat-suppressed, axial T1-weighted spin-echo sequence for depiction of the mural hematoma can be effective.

CE MRA techniques are well suited to visualize residual flow in narrowed vessels. First-pass MRA methods, however, with an inherent high background suppression, have a limited ability to demonstrate a mural hematoma, and the lower spatial resolution compared with TOF MRA is not optimal for a detailed assessment of the intracranial vertebral arteries, particularly the cross-sectional assessment.

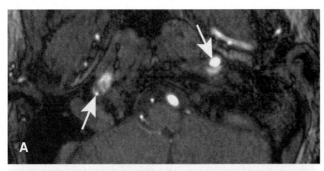

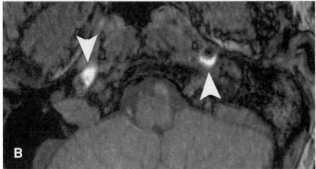

FIGURE 11-43 3D TOF MRA source images in a patient with bilateral dissection of the ICA in the petrous segment. **A:** The patent lumen is depicted with high signal (*arrows*); on the right side, the artery is severely narrowed. **B:** After application of an additional caudal suppression pulse, the flow signal of the arteries is lost, and the hematomas become better apparent. On the left side, a typical crescent-shaped mural hematoma of intermediate signal intensity is depicted (*arrowhead*); on the right side **(B)**, the hematoma is extensive (*arrowhead*).

High-resolution CE MRA in the steady state, on the other hand, has been shown to be effective to depict a double lumen in dissections of the intracranial vertebrobasilar arteries and might be a promising tool (216).

Vascular Malformations

Based on their distinct pathological abnormalities, cerebral vascular malformations traditionally are divided into four types: parenchymal arteriovenous malformations (AVMs), venous angiomas (developmental venous anomaly), cavernous angiomas, and capillary telangiectasias (221). Dural AVMs—acquired vascular lesions—are considered a distinct entity. CTA and MRA are useful tools for the diagnosis and/or the follow-up of AVMs and dural arteriovenous fistulas, which are discussed in the following sections.

Venous angiomas are composed of radially arranged, dilatated veins that drain into a central venous trunk. This collector trunk follows a transcerebral course and drains either to the superficial or deep venous system (Fig. 11-44). Between the veins, normal intervening brain tissue is present, and the venous angiomas provide a physiologically competent venous drainage pathway.

There is strong evidence that venous angiomas, which have an overall incidence of about 2% (222), are not true

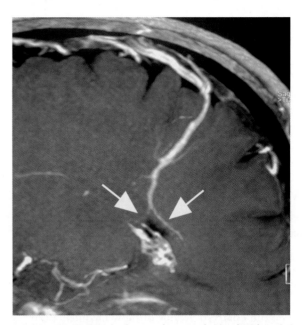

FIGURE 11-44 **CE MRA in the steady state obtained with an interpolated T1-weighted 3D gradient-echo sequence (VIBE).** The MIP slab in the parasagittal plane shows small medullary veins near the lateral ventricle that drain into a transcortical collector vein (*arrows*).

vascular malformations but rather constitute extremes in the variability of venous drainage. Hence, the alternate term *developmental venous anomalies* has been proposed (223). Developmental venous anomalies are most commonly located adjacent to the frontal horn of the lateral ventricle, draining into subependymal veins or the cerebellum, but can be found throughout the cerebrum and cerebellum. CTA or MRA evaluation is usually not necessary, as they can be readily identified on CE conventional CT and MR images in most cases.

Cavernous angiomas and capillary telangiectasias are typically not visible on angiography (DSA) and hence have been termed *occult vascular malformations*. Cavernous angiomas are endothelial-lined sinusoidal vascular spaces containing thrombosed blood and no interposed brain tissue. On CT, these lesions appear as focal high attenuation masses with variable calcification present; no edema or mass effect; and minimal, if any, contrast enhancement. Conventional MR imaging is considered diagnostic, demonstrating centrally heterogeneous lesions, with areas of subacute-to-chronic hemorrhage (methemoglobin) and circumferential rings of hypointense iron storage, but no mass effect or edema.

Capillary telangiectasias, most commonly located in the pons, are nests of pathologically dilated capillaries, containing intervening brain parenchyma. Typical imaging findings include poorly delineated foci of increased signal on CE studies and no abnormality on unenhanced spin-echo images. On gradient-echo sequences, minimal hypointensities, presumably representing residua of subclinical bleeding, might be found.

Apart from the four classically distinct malformations, mixed or unclassified malformations are frequently described as well as associations between the different forms. For example, a high prevalence between occult vascular malformations and venous angiomas has been noted (224).

Arteriovenous Malformations

Clinical Background

AVMs are relatively rare vascular lesions. The prevalence, according to a recent systematic review, is probably less than about 10 per 100,000 people (225). On the other hand, AVMs represent the most common *symptomatic* vascular malformation.

AVMs consist of arterial feeders, coiled and tortuous vascular connections with direct communication, the *nidus*, and enlarged venous outflow channels (226). The vascular structures retain characteristic feeding arterial and venous components, but no interposed capillaries. This results in direct arteriovenous shunting with increased blood flow through the feeding arteries and delivery of increased blood volume under relatively high pressure to the draining veins.

Histologically, cells within the nest show chronic reactive changes and are thought to be nonfunctioning. The arterial and venous elements often show hypertrophy, and the lamina of the arterial intimal layer might show degradation or deficiencies. Regions of thrombosis and recanalization are often present as well as gliosis and hemosiderin staining in the surrounding parenchyma as evidence of prior hemorrhage. Classically, AVMs are located in the supratentorial compartment (over 80%) and extend from the subpial surface of the brain to the deep white matter in the shape of a cone.

Displacement or mass effect on adjacent structures might occur after hemorrhage or by large venous varices that drain the lesion. About 10% of AVMs have associated arterial aneurysms, most of which occur on arteries hemodynamically related to the lesion located at the circle of Willis, the feeding artery, or within the nidus itself (227).

AVMs are most often solitary lesions, but they can be multiple when part of a neurocutaneous syndrome. Rendu-Osler-Weber disease is characterized by multiple capillary telangiectasias of the skin and mucosa, pulmonary arteriovenous fistula, and cerebral AVM. The Wyburn-Mason syndrome is characterized by multiple cutaneous nevi and retinal and brain AVMs.

Although congenital in nature, AVMs, apart from the vein of Galen malformation, are not clinically apparent until the second through the fourth decades of life. The mean age of diagnosis is about 30 years.

Over half of patients with AVMs will present with acute intracranial hemorrhage, and 30% have seizures as the presenting symptom. Another 12% have persistent or progressive neurological deficit, which has been ascribed to a number of potential pathophysiologic mechanisms including "steal" of blood flow from adjacent normal regions of brain into the low-resistance, high-flow vessels feeding the AVM; mass effect from enlarged veins or dilation of arterial supply to the AVM; and venous hypertension (228). Headache as the initial symptom occurs in 1% to 5%.

The yearly risk of hemorrhage after diagnosis of an AVM in patients who present with or without intracranial hemorrhage was thought to be well established at about 1% to 4%, but as high as about 6% to 7% occur within the *first year* after clinical presentation with a hemorrhage, with a 30% risk of death for each hemorrhagic episode and significant long-term morbidity at about 25% (226).

These data were recently challenged by results from a prospective study noting that patients who bled had a risk of rehemorrhage of about 30% in the first year and an overall yearly rehemorrhage rate of about 18%, compared with a yearly hemorrhage rate of 2% in those who had no previous bleeding (229,230). In a second study, performed by the same group, the degree of morbidity after hemorrhage was found to be considerably lower than previously thought, as only 16% of patients were moderately to severely disabled after hemorrhage. Although these rates differed considerably from previous reports, the rate of disability is still greater than the treatment-related morbidity in many modern series and is therefore not necessarily a contraindication to treatment (226).

Apart from previous hemorrhage, hypertension has been found to be positively associated with hemorrhage in patients with AVMs (231,232) as well as numerous angioarchitectural factors: flow-related aneurysm, intranidal aneurysm, deep venous drainage, deep (periventricular) location, small nidus (<3 cm), high feeding artery pressure, slow arterial filling, and venous stenosis.

Various grading systems have been developed in an effort to rank individual AVMs into groups predictive of the difficulty associated with specific treatment and the probable response to that treatment. A widely used and simple AVM grading system is that proposed by Spetzler and Martin (233). In this system, a numerical grade is assigned to the AVM, with higher grades indicating more surgically difficult lesions. Three features are evaluated: the size of the nidus, the location of the nidus, and the venous drainage pattern. The nidus size is rated as small (<3 cm), medium (3 to 6 cm), or large (>6 cm), with 1, 2, or 3 points given, respectively.

The location of the nidus is determined to be within either "eloquent" (score of 1) or "noneloquent" (score of 0) regions of brain. Eloquent areas are those with readily identifiable neurologic function and, by this definition, include the sensorimotor, visual, and language cortex; internal capsule; thalamus; hypothalamus; brain stem; cerebellar peduncles; and deep cerebellar nuclei.

Venous drainage is either superficial, if drainage is entirely into the cortical venous system (score of 0), or deep, if any or all drainage enters the deep system (score of 1). The score from these three features is added to give the overall grade of the AVM. For example, an AVM grade 1 would be small, located in noneloquent cortex, and have only superficial venous drainage.

Because the risk of hemorrhage from the nidus of the AVM persists until the nidus has been completely obliterated (234–236), the goal of management is complete angiographic obliteration of the AVM. A variety of therapeutic options is available to obtain this aim: microsurgery, endovascular embolization, and radiosurgery. Despite advances in all these fields, and the application of multimodality approaches, some AVMs will be judged incurable. In general, the repair of aneurysms associated with AVMs takes priority, and a microsurgical or an endovascular therapy is recommended. The final treatment decision should take into account many factors, such as age, neurological status, clinical risk factors, and angioarchitectural features.

Microsurgical resection is the mainstay for treatment of AVMs. In small (<3 cm) AVMs, there was found to be a high efficacy of obtaining angiographically demonstrated cure (94% to 100%), with little morbidity (1.3% to 10.6%) (237–240). In a prospective validation study of the Spetzler-Martin grading scale, the risk of major neurological morbidity was found to be negligible in patients with grade 1 to 3; however, in patients with grade 4 and 5, the risk of permanent major neurological morbidity was found to be 22% and 17%, respectively (239).

Endovascular treatment, when used in isolation, is the least successful in curing patients with AVMs. In most case series, a complete endovascular obliteration of brain AVMs occurred only in a minority of cases—in AVMs that are small with one or two arterial feeders. Embolization can be extremely beneficial in the context of a multimodality treatment planning, however, usually preceding either microsurgery or radiation (241–243). Prior to surgery, embolization can eliminate deep feeding vessels to the AVM, occlude intranidal fistulas, and reduce the flow through the nidus.

The goal of preradiosurgical embolization is to reduce the size of the radiosurgical target (AVM nidus) to about 3 cm or less in all directions. Radiosurgery, delivered by Gamma Knife, linear accelerator, or heavy charged particles (proton beam or helium ion) uses focused irradiation directed to the AVM. If the nidus has a diameter of less than 3 cm, an angiographic cure can be expected in 65% to 85% of cases. Larger AVMs have a lower obliteration rate (226). Unlike with surgical resection, radiation effect takes months to years until the lesion disappears, during which time the risk of hemorrhage, although reduced, remains present (244).

Imaging Strategies

The information required for optimal therapeutic planning of AVMs requires the delineation of all components of the AVM, specifically the origin and course of feeding arteries and draining veins, and the location, size, and morphology of the nidus. Without question, DSA—with its high spatial and temporal resolution and its ability to selectively evaluate the supplying arteries—at present best serves these requirements and is the most definitive diagnostic tool for the detection and detailed characterization of the angioarchitecture of AVMs.

It should be noted, however, that even DSA examinations may be falsely negative if performed too early after hemorrhage because of compression of the nidus by the hematoma (245). Thus, for the exclusion of an AVM, late DSA, performed three months after the bleeding, is required.

Cross-sectional imaging with CT and MR is mainly used (a) in the initial workup of patients with hemorrhage—the initial detection of AVMs, (b) for localizing AVMs in relation to the surrounding brain parenchyma, (c) for providing volumetric information of AVMs that might include nidus definition for radiation therapy, and (d) for the follow-up of treated patients.

Computed Tomographic and Magnetic Resonance Angiography in Imaging Arteriovenous Malformations

Computed Tomographic Angiography. Most patients with AVMs present with acute neurological symptoms from intracranial hemorrhage and are initially examined with a standard unenhanced CT examination (Fig. 11-45). Findings suggestive of an AVM on this examination include serpiginous isointense or slightly hyperintense vessels and calcifications, which occur in about one third of the cases. These findings may be absent, however, and as the majority of all spontaneous intracranial hemorrhage (ICH) occurs without any demonstrable vascular abnormality, a question arises: Which patients should undergo further diagnostic imaging?

Based on investigations of 206 consecutive patients with spontaneous ICH by CT and DSA, Zhu et al. (246) recommended the consideration of DSA in all patients

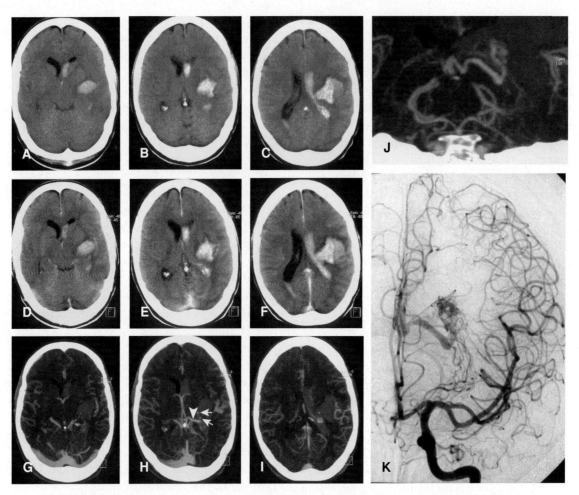

FIGURE 11-45 A–C: Consecutive unenhanced CT slices (10-mm slice thickness) in a young patient with left hemispheric intraparenchymal hemorrhage and intraventricular blood. **D–F:** The CT scan performed five minutes after contrast administration shows no evident underlying pathology. **G–I:** CTA MIP slabs reconstructed with the identical slab thickness and orientation show tubular vascular structures (*arrows*) surrounding the thalamic vein (*arrowhead*). **J:** A coronal MIP slab gives a good overview about the nidus and the draining vein; however, only (**K**) DSA provides the information about the feeding arteries.

except those over 45 years with pre-existing hypertension in thalamic, putaminal, or posterior fossa hemorrhage. Based on the results of this study and our experience, we usually stop the imaging algorithm after the results of the native CT in all patients in whom a "hypertensive hemorrhage" is by far most likely or in whom a further diagnostic evaluation would be without further therapeutic consequences. In the majority of cases, however, we perform CTA as an adjunct, as the examination might establish a first diagnosis of an AVM, facilitating the further workup of the patient in an optimal setting.

For example, DSA might be indicated as an urgent preoperative examination to determine "weak points" such as pseudoaneurysms or if decompressive surgery is indicated because of massive hemorrhage. Alternatively, if the amount of bleeding seen on CT is small, the DSA examination may be delayed and planned in the most appropriate fashion, either as a pure diagnostic examination or as a potentially therapeutic procedure.

The CTA examination should evaluate not only the site of the bleeding, but also the entire circle of Willis as well, to detect flow-related aneurysms and the course of the potential venous drainage path. MPR images and sliding thin-slab MIP images are useful to detect asymmetrically enlarged vessels (the draining veins), the nidus in relation to the hemorrhage, and for the exclusion of larger aneurysms. The arteries feeding the AVM are often not well discriminated within the vessel architecture (247).

For planning of radiosurgery treatment, the optimal determination of the target volume is of importance. For that purpose, the imaging features offered by multimodality MR and MRA techniques are of an advantage and have supplanted CT and CTA in most centers as the primary cross-sectional technique that is applied as an adjunct to DSA.

Magnetic Resonance Angiography. On *conventional* (fast) spin-echo images, an AVM is typically visualized as a cluster of linear or serpentine areas of signal void, reflecting the relatively rapid-flowing blood in dilated vascular channels (Fig. 11-46). However, increased signal intensity associated with flowing blood might be present, especially on gradient-echo sequences. On postcontrast T1 images, enhancement occurs mainly in the enlarged veins with relatively slow flow. Enhancement of the nidus is variable, while the rapidly flowing blood within arterial feeding vessels generally shows no enhancement. Associated parenchymal hemorrhage can be aged on the basis of signal intensity patterns. In clinically asymptomatic AVMs, susceptibility changes in adjacent brain by iron-storage products suggests previous subclinical hemorrhage.

Increased signal intensity indicative of gliosis or secondary demyelination adjacent to the AVM implies chronic vascular ischemia, maybe as result of steal from adjacent brain.

Unenhanced TOF and PC techniques as well as contrast MR techniques have been applied for the evaluation of AVMs. The commonly used 3D TOF MRA is of value in providing 3D representations of AVM architecture in relation to the brain parenchyma. This information is used in many neurosurgical centers in conjunction with DSA to plan stereotactic radiosurgery, as conventional DSA methods provide only projective images that may incompletely define the borders of the nidus. The method is useful to detect associated aneurysms.

The inherent limitations of 3D TOF MRA techniques reduce the diagnostic yield. Due to the limited spatial resolution, small vessels might not be visualized, regions of slow

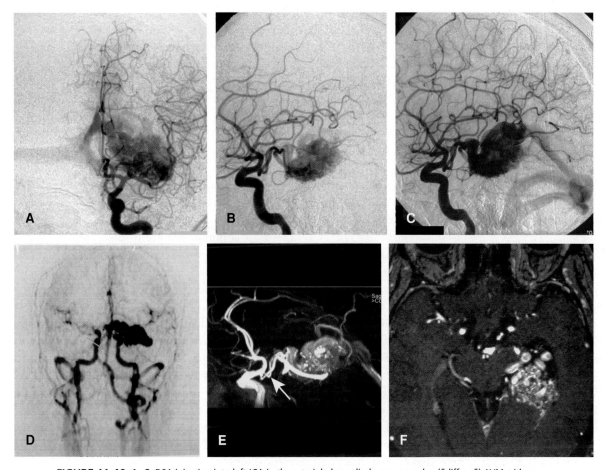

FIGURE 11-46 A–C: DSA injection into left ICA in the arterial phase discloses a complex ("diffuse") AVM with drainage into the deep venous system, as shown in **(A)** anteroposterior and **(B, C)** lateral projection. **D:** On a CE 2D projection MRA image obtained during the arterial phase in coronal orientation, the intense staining of the AVM is depicted as well as the early filling of the straight sinus *(arrow)*—the superior sagittal sinus is not contrast enhanced. **E:** CE 3D MRA MIP projection after contrast administration in the lateral view shows the enlarged feeders nicely but allows no detailed information about the internal architecture of the AVM. **F:** The internal architecture can be better understood by scrolling through MPR images. Larger feeding arteries and draining veins can—to a certain degree—be separated by their course and separated from the diffuse nidus.

blood flow—where saturation from repeated radio frequency pulses occurs—cannot be consistently depicted, and the multidirectional flow of the nidus can cause further signal saturation. Furthermore, within a subacute hematoma, the differentiation of the high signal inherent to blood flow from the high signal inherent to methemoglobin might be impossible.

The negative aspects of 3D PC MRA methods are the dependence of the vessel display on the choice of the VENC and the long measurement times. However, due to the inherent background suppression, the distinction of the malformation from a hematoma might be advantageous (248).

The inconsistent depiction of the nidus and the draining veins can be improved by the use of contrast material with 3D TOF MRA sequences (15,249). Of particular interest, however, are first-pass MRA methods that have been applied for the evaluation of AVMs with diverse features focusing either on high temporal or spatial resolution.

Farb et al. (34), for example, focused on a high spatial resolution technique (voxel size of well below 1 mm³) and used a real time triggered elliptic centric-ordered 3D gadolinium-enhanced MRA sequence that acquires the low-frequency information at the beginning of imaging to improve the vascular contrast. They found the technique superior to 3D TOF MRA for the depiction of the feeding arteries, the nidus, and the veins. Evidently, this high spatial resolution requires long measurement times (here 2 minutes), and information on flow dynamics, which is readily available from DSA, cannot be obtained. On the other side of the spectrum, ultrafast 2D CE MRA techniques with a temporal resolution of up to two images have been applied that can nicely show the hemodynamics of the malformations (250,251).

These 2D CE MRA techniques lack the spatial resolution to identify smaller vascular components of the AVM, however. Superimposition of vascular structures occurs as a slab is excited. Although both approaches have their distinct advantages, a combination of two MRA imaging strategies, an ultrafast sequence with a high-resolution MRA method, might at the present time provide the most complete information that can be obtained with MR to characterize AVMs.

Finally, it is necessary to mention that MR techniques with selective presaturation of individual vessels can be used to indirectly determine the feeding vessels, and that cardiac-gated PC MRA enables measurement of flow velocities in feeding arteries (252,253). These elaborate techniques, however, are mainly used for research purposes.

Dural Arteriovenous Fistulas

Clinical Background

Intracranial dural arteriovenous fistulas (DAVFs) are abnormal arteriovenous shunts consisting of dural branches of the ICA and/or ECA or vertebral arteries, and the dural venous drainage. In contrast to pial AVMs, the site of shunting is confined to the leaflets of the pachymeninges. They account for 10% to 15% of intracranial AVMs and occur mainly in middle-aged patients. The exact pathogenesis for the formation of the fistula is not known. It has been postulated that veno-occlusive disease affecting the dural venous sinus might result in enlargement of normally present microscopic arteriovenous shunts within the sinus wall (254). Conditions associated with the development of DAVFs include pregnancy, sinusitis, trauma, and surgery (255–257).

DAVFs are classified according to their drainage pattern as follows: type I, located in the main sinus, with anterograde flow; type II, located in the main sinus, with reflux into the sinus (type IIa), cortical veins (type IIb), or both (type IIa + b); type III, with direct cortical venous drainage; type IV, with direct cortical venous drainage and venous ectasia; and type V, with spinal venous drainage (258) (Fig. 11-47). In contrast, fistulas with drainage into the cavernous sinus, carotid cavernous fistulas (CCFs), are classified according to the arterial feeding pattern—a classification proposed by Barrow et al. (259). *Direct fistulas* (type A) are often post-traumatic, high-flow shunts between the cavernous portion of the ICA and the cavernous sinus. *Indirect/dural fistulas* (types B–D) have multiple arterial feeders that arise from the ICA (type B), from the ECA (type C), or from both the ICA and ECA (type D).

Depending on the AVF location and the venous drainage, the clinical features are highly variable. Clinical presentations range from asymptomatic to symptomatic (257,260,261). Pulse synchronous bruit and headaches are the most common symptoms of a DAVF involving the transverse or sigmoid sinus, and neurological deficits, venous hypertensive encephalopathy with dementia, and intracranial hemorrhage resulting from venous hypertension might occur.

Proptosis, chemosis, retro-orbital pain, bruit, and opthalmoplegia are usually the leading symptoms observed with cavernous sinus lesions. The venous drainage pattern of a DAVF correlates with progression of neurological deficits. If the venous drainage is unobstructed and drainage occurs directly into a sinus with normal flow direction, the course is benign, whereas parenchymal bleeding or SAH is common in DAVFs with a retrograde cortical venous drainage, especially when there is a venous ectasia (258,262,263).

The decision to treat is based on the severity of presenting symptoms and the venous drainage pattern. The goals of treatment are the prevention of risks and/or the elimination of symptoms. Types of treatment include transvenous or transarterial embolization, surgery, Gamma Knife

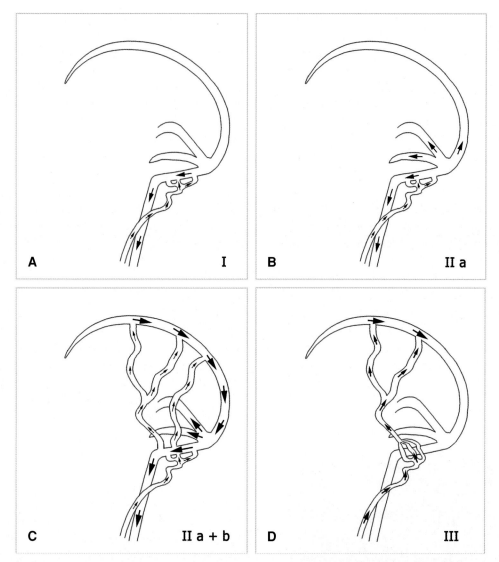

FIGURE 11-47 Schematic drawing of intracranial DAVFs according to the classification proposed by Cognard et al. A: Type I located in the sinus with antegrade flow. **B:** Type IIa located in the sinus with retrograde flow. **C:** Type IIa+b located in the sinus with reflux as well as in cortical veins (type IIb refers to a location in the sinus with retrograde flow in cortical veins only). **D:** Type III with *direct* cortical venous drainage. Not shown are type IV, with direct cortical venous drainage *and* ectasia of the draining veins, and type V, with spinal venous drainage. Adapted from Cognard C, Gobin YP, Pierot L, et al. Cerebral dural arteriovenous fistulas: clinical and angiographic correlation with a revised classification of venous drainage. *Radiology.* 1995;194:671–680.

surgery, or combinations of the three; in selected cases, the lesions can be treated conservatively (264).

Imaging Strategies

DSA is the method of choice for the delineation and grading of fistulas. However, many patients present with symptoms or signs that might be attributable to a fistula, but few have one. Patients are therefore often assigned to the noninvasive imaging modalities of CT or MR.

Conventional CT and MR scans in DAVFs are, however, often normal, and the diagnosis of a DAVF might not be possible. A clue toward the diagnosis can be the presence of dilated or engorged cortical veins in the absence of a parenchymal nidus. DAVFs can be associated with occlusion of a venous sinus and may lead to infarction or hemorrhage.

Computed Tomographic and Magnetic Resonance Angiography in Dural Arteriovenous Fistula.

Both PC MRA and TOF MRA have been reported to be of value for the diagnosis of DAVFs. On TOF MRA source images, curvilinear or nodular structures with high signal intensity adjacent to or within the venous sinus, representing the branches of the feeding arteries or unsaturated flow within the sinus, may indicate the fistula. With PC MR, the flow direction in draining veins and dural sinuses can be demonstrated (265–267).

The presence of flow and the complex flow dynamics of DAVFs can probably best be depicted by the application of ultrafast time-resolved MRA techniques such as 2D CE MR projection angiography (also termed *MR DSA*) (30,31,268) (Fig. 11-48).

Imaging with high temporal resolution allows for visualizing the early filling of a venous sinus, and/or of the cortical veins; an appreciation of the flow direction within the sinus; and a possible determination of larger arterial feeders.

Disadvantages of MR projection angiography compared with conventional DSA include the superimpositions of different cerebral vessels application and the comparably lower resolution. The application of ultrafast 3D CE MRA techniques exploiting the advancement in imaging speed provided by parallel imaging is expected to yield improvements (269) (Fig. 11-49).

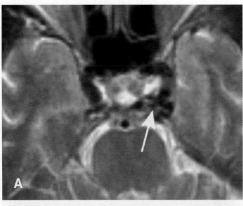
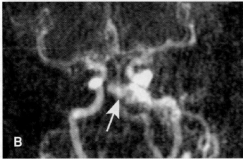

FIGURE 11-48 Patient with headache, tinnitus, and ophthalmoplegia. A: On T2-weighted images, small flow voids adjacent to the left ICA are visualized (*arrow*). **B:** CE MR projection angiography discloses an early filling of the cavernous sinus (*arrow*). DSA confirmed the presence of a carotid cavernous fistula (type C).

DSA is mandatory for treatment planning to document the arterial feeders and, most importantly, to demonstrate the exact relationship of normal cortical veins to the fistula site. On the other hand, the presence or absence of a fistula can be shown with a very high level of confidence using ultrafast 2D or 3D CE MRA techniques and can reduce purely diagnostic DSA examinations for the exclusion of a fistula.

At sites where these MR techniques are available, MR should be considered as the method of choice for the non-invasive detection of DAVFs. CT, with the addition of CTA, can aid in the detection of dural fistulas. The fast image acquisition speed of CTA may show an arterialization of venous structures during arterial phase imaging (Fig. 11-50) (270).

Venous Occlusive Disease

Clinical Background

Cerebral venous thrombosis (CVT) is an elusive and remarkable disease. Its causes include numerous conditions, it can affect all ages from the neonate to the elderly, its clinical presentation and its neuroimaging presentation are diverse, and its potential for recovery is considerable if adequate therapeutic measures are taken early in the course of disease.

The incidence of CVT is not precisely known, but it is likely to be lower than 1 per 1,000 persons per year (271). Recognized etiologies or predisposing factors for the development of cerebral vein and dural sinus thrombosis include pregnancy, puerperium and oral contraceptives, systemic disorders such as dehydration and coagulation disorders, local or general infections, and head injuries or neurosurgical operations. However, about 20% to 30% of patients with CVT do not have any known risk factor (272). If multiple risk factors are present—for example, in a woman who takes oral contraceptives and has a prothrombin-gene mutation—the absolute risk for CVT might substantially increase (271).

CVT can present with any central neurological sign or symptom in isolation or more commonly in combination, and with almost any mode of onset. More typically, the presentation is acute or subacute and can mimic conditions of arterial stroke, tumor, abscess, and benign intracranial hypertension. A focal neurological deficit, such as aphasia, hemiplegia, and/or seizures, often with headache, is the most common clinical onset pattern. Other common patterns are those of isolated intracranial hypertension with headache, papilledema, and sixth nerve palsy, mimicking "benign intracranial hypertension," or a depressed level of consciousness often in combination with seizures. Cavernous sinus thrombosis usually presents with a distinctive

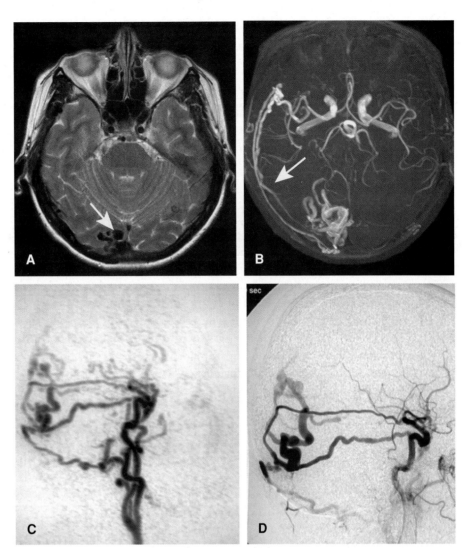

FIGURE 11-49 Dural fistula with drainage via enlarged cortical veins into the superior sagittal sinus. A: On a T2-weighted image, large flow voids but no nidus is observed adjacent to the right superior sagittal sinus. **B:** On 3D TOF MRA data set, arteries that follow the course of the meninges are detected. **C:** Time-resolved 3D CE MRA with high temporal resolution (1.5 seconds per image) in the **(C)** early arterial phase in lateral projection depicts the feeding arteries well as confirmed by **(D)** selective DSA, which allowed characterization of the fistula in detail.

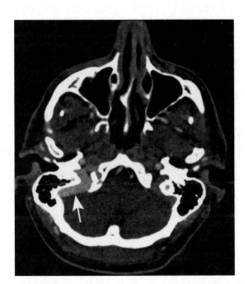

FIGURE 11-50 Patient with right-sided pulsatile bruit. CTA shows an early filling of the right transverse sinus (*arrow*); the left sinus is not contrast enhanced. DSA disclosed a dural fistula.

clinical picture of eyelid edema, chemosis, and proptosis; however, a slowly progressive course with moderately painful third or sixth nerve palsy might occur, often posing diagnostic difficulties.

Heparin administration is considered as first-line treatment of CVT (272–275). Thrombolytic treatment with urokinase or recombinant tissue plasminogen activator (rtPA) directly within the thrombus seems to restore flow more frequently and rapidly than heparin, according to some recent reports (276). However, there is no scientific evidence for the recommendation of that therapy, and the risk of hemorrhage appears to be larger. Thrombolytic therapy is therefore usually reserved for those rare patients who show a rapid deterioration of their symptoms despite proper anticoagulation (274).

The outcome of CVT is largely unpredictable. Even comatose patients might recover without any sequela, while patients presenting only with headache can suddenly develop a severe hemiparesis. Factors that entail poor prognosis have been identified and include clinical features (e.g., extreme age, coma, infectious or malignant courses) and imaging features (e.g., deep venous system involvement or hemorrhagic infarcts).

It is well established that the clinical recovery precedes vessel recanalization and may even occur without visible recanalization. The prognosis of CVT has traditionally been considered poor; but, recent reports have shown mortality rates to be less than 10% (277,278).

Imaging Strategies

Cross-sectional imaging with CT or MR is usually the first examination on an emergency basis in a patient presenting with an unclear neurological symptomatic or clinical suspicion of CVT. Both modalities portray *indirect* signs of CVT—abnormalities of the brain parenchyma—and to a certain extent also offer an assessment of *direct* signs of CVT—the demonstration of the thrombus within a venous sinus or cerebral vein.

Indirect signs that should raise the suspicion of a CVT on a CT scan are hypodense areas in the brain parenchyma that do not correspond to the classic arterial territories and resemble brain edema or brain infarction.

CVT-associated hemorrhage does not localize in the expected distribution of parenchymal hypertensive bleedings. Instead, it typically expands to the cortical surface. Bilateral lesions in a parasagittal location are a common feature of CVT in the SSS; isolated lesions of the temporal lobe are common in CVT of the TS. Bilateral thalamic lesions may be evident in deep venous thrombosis. On enhanced images, the tentorium and the falx might appear thickened and engorged, and will demonstrate a pronounced enhancement that is presumably due to dual venous collaterals.

MR is highly sensitive to brain edema or brain infarction, the parenchymal changes in CVT depicted with signal hyperintensity on T2-weighted images.

Diffusion techniques with assessment of the apparent diffusion coefficient (ADC) can differentiate between cytotoxic and vasogenic edema, offering the potential to distinguish reversible ischemic tissue from irreversible ischemia. Perfusion MR imaging allows for an assessment of the hemodynamic changes—for example, a prolongation of the mean transit time might be seen (279,280).

Direct CT signs for detecting the thrombus are the *cord sign* and *empty delta sign* (Fig. 11-51) (281,282). While the former refers to a hyperdense thrombosed venous sinus on an unenhanced CT scan, the latter refers to a hypoattenuated triangular shape within the posterior part of the SSS on a postcontrast scan. This results from enhancement of the dural leaves surrounding the comparatively less dense

thrombosed components. However, it should be kept in mind that especially in children and young adults, it often appears slightly hyperdense.

On standard MR sequences, the signal characteristics vary with clot age. In the first few days, it is difficult to recognize acute thrombus on conventional MR images. Acute thrombus is isointense to the brain on T1-weighted images and hypointense on T2-weighted images. From 3 days, the thrombus becomes easier to detect, as it is hyperintense on T1-weighted images (up to 3 months), and on T2-weighted images, the absence of the characteristic flow void becomes evident (Fig. 11-52).

While the diagnosis of CVT can be made using CT and MR in many cases, it is recommended that these evaluations be supplemented by CTA and MRA, respectively. Such a comprehensive assessment of the venous cerebral system can now be considered the mainstay for diagnosis.

DSA, once the key diagnostic procedure in CVT, is usually not performed unless endovascular treatment is necessary. A thrombosed sinus appears on DSA as an empty channel surrounded by dilated venous collaterals that are located within the dural wall, and enlarged medullary veins and collaterals via the deep venous system might be present. The diagnosis of a cortical vein thrombosis is easy when the thrombosis affects several veins and adjacent sinus, but it can be difficult in isolated cortical vein thrombosis. A persistence of contrast material into the late venous phase is a well-known sign—these vessels seem to "hang in space" (35).

Computed Tomographic and Magnetic Resonance Angiography in Imaging Venous Occlusive Disease

Although there are no larger studies available analyzing and comparing the performance of CTA and MRA, both modalities seem to be reliable in detecting CVT (283–286). The decision to perform one as opposed to the other depends on the clinical setting, scanner availability, scanner capability, and local expertise.

In most centers, an unenhanced CT scan is the initial imaging modality for patients with an unclear neurological condition frequently supplemented by CTA as the initial angiographic method. The fast acquisition speed of CTA makes the method especially attractive for the examination of severely sick or uncooperative patients. Further advantages include the simple examination protocol and the relative ease to interpret the images for less experienced observers. With CT, the assessment of the venous system is based on the contrast material filling pattern of the vessels and is not affected by the flow effects that can complicate MR assessments.

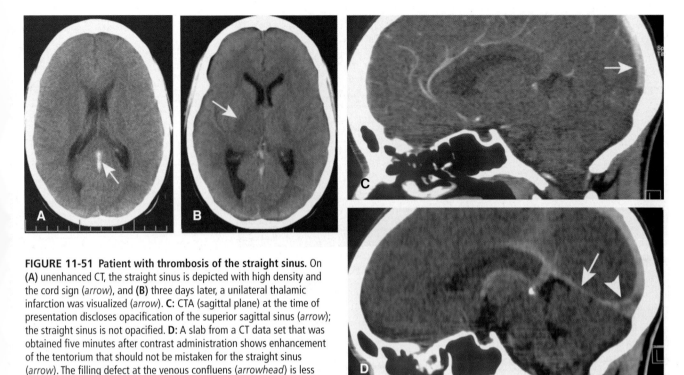

FIGURE 11-51 Patient with thrombosis of the straight sinus. On **(A)** unenhanced CT, the straight sinus is depicted with high density and the cord sign (*arrow*), and **(B)** three days later, a unilateral thalamic infarction was visualized (*arrow*). **C:** CTA (sagittal plane) at the time of presentation discloses opacification of the superior sagittal sinus (*arrow*); the straight sinus is not opacified. **D:** A slab from a CT data set that was obtained five minutes after contrast administration shows enhancement of the tentorium that should not be mistaken for the straight sinus (*arrow*). The filling defect at the venous confluens (*arrowhead*) is less clearly evident but still detectable.

The major findings of a CVT on CTA are a filling defect of the sinus surrounded by an enhancement of the sinus walls and an abnormal pattern of collateral drainage. For correct interpretation, a good knowledge of commonly encountered variants (e.g., a hypoplastic transverse sinus or a high splitting of the superior sagittal sinus) is essential, and filling defects from intrasinus septa (fibrotic bands) and arachnoid (pacchionian granulations) have to be distinguished from filling defects of a venous sinus thrombosis.

Septa are usually thin and have a curvilinear shape along the long axis of the sinus, while arachnoid granulations are sharply circumscribed filling defects that are usually very small (<5 mm). They are encountered in many patients and are predominantly located in the SSS, the TS, and the straight sinus.

The examination of MPR images and MIP slabs allows a detailed and time-efficient analysis, while 3D reconstructions of the entire data set that require segmentation steps can be reserved for documentation purposes in selected cases. The residual enhancement of the arterial structures with superimposition on MIP images cannot be avoided but rarely poses a problem in detecting a CVT. The simultaneous assessment of the arterial vasculature can provide important information in an unclear neurological situation.

While the detection of a thrombosis of a major sinus usually poses no diagnostic problem with CTA, the detection of a thrombosis of the smaller deep cerebral veins or the cortical veins is more demanding. In these cases, it is important to evaluate the unenhanced CT images for the presence of a cord sign and for accompanying parenchymal changes. The cord sign was noted in five out of eight patients with proven thrombosis of the deep cerebral veins in a small study by Lafitte et al. (287).

The clinical hallmarks of a cavernous sinus thrombosis are signs of venous congestion: eyelid edema, chemosis, and proptosis. This relatively rare disease is typically diagnosed on clinical grounds, and CT is mainly performed to evaluate the integrity of the osseous anatomy and to confirm the suspected location of an underlying infectious process. MPR images can reveal signs of a cavernous sinus thrombosis in the form of larger filling defects (>7 mm) of nonfat density, sinus expansion, or dilatation of the tributary veins (288,289).

The flow-dependent TOF and PC techniques have served as a mainstay for evaluating intracranial venous anatomy and pathology (290,291). The slow-flowing venous blood is well demonstrated with TOF using a coronal 2D technique perpendicular to the orientation of most of the intracranial sinuses

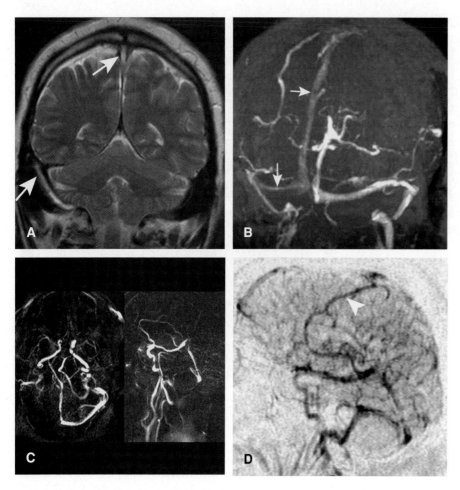

FIGURE 11-52 Patient with headache but no neurological deficits. A: On T2-weighted images, the normal flow void in the SSS and ST is replaced by a high signal intensity thrombus (*arrows*). **B:** 2D TOF MRA shows a high flow signal of the left TS and the deep venous system. The signal of the SSS and of the right TS (*arrows*) is intermediate, representing the extensive subacute thrombus. **C:** On 2D PC MRA (VENC 15 cm/s) in the paraxial and sagittal orientation, no flow signal at all can be observed in the SSS and right TS. **D:** 2D projection MRA during the venous phase depicts flow in the anterior part of the SSS, in the vein of Trolard (*arrowhead*), and in the deep venous system (same patient as in Fig. 11-14).

(292). Nonvisualization of a sinus with TOF MRV indicates a strong likelihood of venous thrombosis.

Knowledge of some pitfalls can help to achieve correct interpretation of the images (Fig. 11-53). Signal loss due to slow flow or in-plane flow might be difficult to distinguish from venous thrombosis. The TS is vulnerable to such a loss since a portion of it runs parallel to a coronal acquisition plane. In this regard, Ayanzen et al. observed flow gaps in the nondominant TS in about one third of patients with otherwise normal MR imaging studies (293).

In cases where the distinction between a flow gap and a thrombosis is problematic, acquisition of 2D TOF images obtained perpendicular to the long axis of the sinus might be helpful (parasagittal). Also, selecting a sequence with a shorter TE or the further workup with CE MRA can be clarifying (Fig. 11-53).

Another pitfall is that the high signal intensity of substances with short T1-relaxation times, such as methemoglobin in a fresh thrombus, might be confused with a flow-related enhancement. However, a thrombus typically does not have the same signal intensity as flowing blood, and images with proper windowing can usually provide distinction.

With PC MRA techniques, signal from stationary tissue is suppressed, a major advantage over the TOF techniques. However, the long acquisition times for the optimal 3D PC technique and the required a priori estimate of blood flow velocity makes this technique less commonly used for the diagnosis of a venous thrombosis. Apart from these shortcomings, with both TOF and PC MRV, only the larger veins and venous sinuses are reliably demonstrated, and the visualization of the cortical veins is usually inadequate.

The visualization of the veins and the detection of CVT can be improved with CE MRA techniques in the steady state (19–21). However, a pitfall with this technique exists—since the measurement time of the sequence employed takes several minutes, a chronic venous thrombus might enhance as a result of vascularization or organization. Thus, it may be difficult to differentiate chronic thrombosis from recanalization of the thrombosis on the CE images.

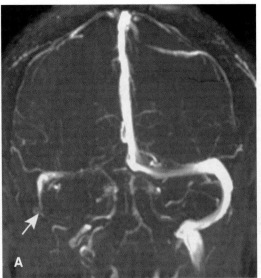 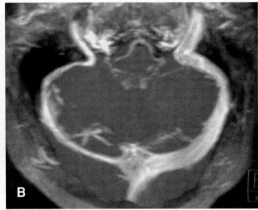

FIGURE 11-53 Patient with headache. A: The distal right TS (*arrow*) is not visualized on 2D TOF MRA. **B:** On a MIP slab of a CE MRA data set in the paraxial orientation, the right sinus is hypoplastic but homogenously enhanced.

Given these points, flow-sensitive and CE MRA techniques with long measurement times can function as complementary methods. Alternatively, in unclear situations, a CE MRA technique in the steady state can be acquired after an ultrafast first-pass CE investigation (Fig. 11-52). Again, the use of MPR images and MIP slabs is an efficient way to analyze the CE data sets, as MIP reconstructions or other 3D visualization techniques showing the entire venous vasculature are time consuming to reconstruct.

Vascular Compression Symptoms

Clinical Background

The most common cranial nerve compression syndromes are hemifacial spasm and trigeminal neuralgia. Hemifacial spasm is clinically characterized by intermittent, painless, involuntary, spasmodic contractions of muscles innervated by the facial nerve in one side of the face only. Patients with trigeminal neuralgia (tic douloureux) suffer from lancinating pains lasting a few seconds that are confined to the distribution of one or more branches of the trigeminal nerve on one side of the phase and are often triggered by sensory stimuli.

While these conditions can be caused by a variety of lesions, including posterior fossa tumors or multiple sclerosis plaques (294,295), the most common cause is the compression of the nerves by vessels. Such compression commonly occurs at the root entry (sensory nerves) or root exit (motor nerves) zone (REZ), the locations where the central myelin of oligodendroglial cells changes to peripheral myelin of Schwann cells.

Microvascular decompression is considered the current procedure of choice for treatment of hemifacial spasm and is one of the therapeutic options in treating trigeminal neuralgia. This procedure has a high success rate, whereby the offending vessel is physically moved off the nerve, and a sponge is interposed as a cushion (296–298). Compared with hemifacial spasm and trigeminal neuralgia, compression syndromes of other cranial nerves by vascular structures are rare but have been described, for example, for the abducens nerve (299).

Although operative indications are greatly influenced by clinical symptoms, MR imaging has become an established method to demonstrate the preoperative neurovascular relationship. "Decompression is relatively straightforward if the surgeon keeps two principles in mind at all times: 1) 'there must be a vessel, and it is my job to find it,' and 2) the . . . REZ can be variable in length, particularly in the case of the trigeminal nerve, and may extend to a more distal portion of the nerve. Therefore the nerve should be inspected from its origin at the brainstem laterally to its exit from the cerebellopontine angle . . ." (300).

Imaging Strategies

The advice from pioneers of microvascular decompression to their fellow neurosurgeons holds true for neuroradiologists as well. To identify an offending vessel or vessels in relation to the nerve, 3D TOF MRA techniques with high resolution are most commonly used (301,302). To define the exact

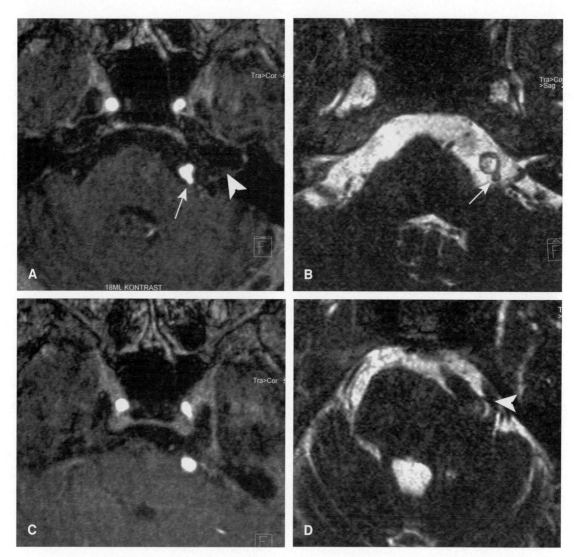

FIGURE 11-54 Patient presenting with trigeminal neuralgia and hemifacial spasm. A: 3D TOF MRA source image shows an enlarged elongated BA with the AICA (*arrow*) compressing the facial nerve (*arrowhead*). The anatomy is depicted in greater detail on the CISS image (**B**), obtained in a nearly identical location. At the level of the trigeminal nerve, the elongation of the basilar artery is well shown on the MRA data set (**C**), while the compression of the nerve (*arrowhead*), however, is more evident on (**D**) the CISS image.

relation and origin of the vessel, it is useful to rely on both the MPR and MIP images obtained from the data set (303).

As a first step, the trigeminal or facial nerve should be identified. Then, using a display that shows MPR images in three planes, the REZ should be carefully evaluated for any contacting vessel as well as for a deviation or bulging of the nerve by the vessel (Fig. 11-54). To identify the origin of the vessel, it can then be useful to place the cursor on the site of contact and change to the MIP display to trace the course of the vessel back to its origin.

The most common arteries that contact the REZ of the trigeminal nerve are a rostroventral SCA loop and the AICA

or PICA for the facial nerve or branches of these vessels. Furthermore, marked elongation and widening of the vertebral or BA with resulting compression of the REZ or compression by two or more vessels might present a situation that makes an operation more difficult (304).

Contact of an artery to the REZ does not always cause symptoms. For example, in a study by Fukuda et al. (305), neurovascular contact was visualized in 15% of asymptomatic nerves, contralateral to the site of compression. However, in only one of their 60 cases was a deformity of the nerve observed. Moreover, on the symptomatic site, a contact was visualized in 71% (trigeminal

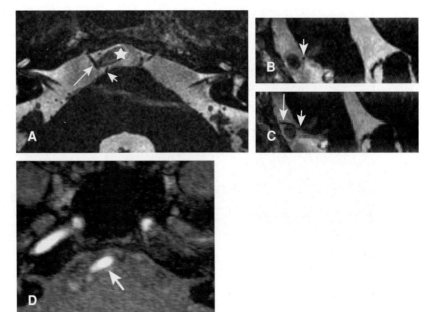

FIGURE 11-55 Patient with compression of the abducens nerve on the right side. On **(A)** the axial CISS image, the abducens nerve (*arrow*) is identified by its course in close relation to the BA (★). A small vascular structure (*small arrow*) that took its origin from the BA—resembling the AICA—was visualized. On CISS images in the parasagittal plane (**B, C**), the vessel (*small arrow*) was found to course superior to the nerve (*arrow*). The nerve was thus stretched by the BA from below, with the root exit zone being compressed by the AICA. **D:** 3D TOF MRA showed the elongated BA (*arrow*) with high signal intensity but failed to show the nerve compression.

nerve) and 90% (facial nerve), respectively, with deformities of the nerves being present in about half of the cases. Vessels identified preoperatively on MRA were present and regarded as causative at surgery in almost all cases.

While 3D TOF MRA is certainly of value if a vessel is identified, what are the possibilities if no artery is visualized? First, there may be no vessel, and the symptoms may be caused by thickened arachnoids around the nerves. Second, the artery or its branches might be too small or have an insufficient flow velocity to be visualized. Third, a petrosal vein might be causative.

To minimize false negative findings, two strategies can be helpful. First, the TOF MRA can be obtained after contrast administration, which might help to visualize distal arterial branches. In this case, the high signal of the venous system may make it difficult to follow the course of the artery (303,306). An MRA acquisition dedicated to first visualizing the arteries can facilitate arterial-venous segmentation on the delayed images.

Second, a 3D MR imaging with constructive interference in steady-state (CISS) sequence with high spatial resolution can be used (Figs. 11-54, 11-55). This sequence provides excellent contrast resolution between the bright CSF and the vascular structures, including arteries *and* veins. In this case, the arteries and veins are distinguished on their anatomical course. In most instances, CISS can supplement a nonenhanced TOF technique, with the two techniques complementing one another (307,308).

Vascular Imaging in Neoplastic Disease

The detection and characterization of brain tumors is a major task in the neuroradiological practice. CT still plays an important role for detection of these lesions in clinical routine. However, there is no doubt that MR imaging is more informative in the detection, localization, and characterization of primary brain tumors and metastases. Moreover, advanced MR techniques such as functional MR imaging using task-activation studies, diffusion MR imaging, and MR spectroscopy offer pathophysiological information about the tumor and its neighboring structures.

Recently, attention has been focused on the evaluation of the tumoral *microcirculation* using perfusion MR imaging techniques, as neovascularity can be important for tumor grading (309).

In the preoperative workup of patients with brain tumors, the course of the large macrovessels in relation to the tumor is often of interest for the neurosurgeon. In particular, knowledge of the venous anatomy is important for minimizing the risk of vascular injury in planning biopsy or resection. Both flow-sensitive MRA and CE MRA techniques are useful for that purpose.

With the unenhanced technique, the patency and displacement of larger arteries and veins by a tumor are usually readily assessable (310). CE techniques offer an improved delineation of smaller vessels—for example, the course of the cortical veins, which are important to plan for access to the lesion. To obtain information about tumor neovascularity as well as about the adjacent vascular anatomy, an MR protocol

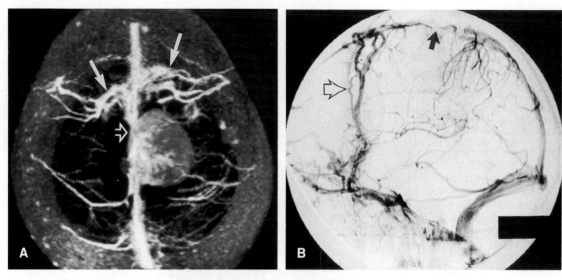

FIGURE 11-56 Patient with a left parasagittal meningioma. A: Para-axial MIP image of a CE MRA data set (*VIBE*) suggests occlusion (*open arrow*) of the SSS by a tumor, which has lower signal intensity compared with that of the sinus. Note the extensive collateral cortical veins (*solid arrows*) draining the frontal part of the sinus. The enhancing tumor blends in with the SSS. **B:** Venous-phase DSA obtained with an injection in the left CCA shows occlusion of the sinus (*solid arrow*) and prominent frontal collateral cortical veins (*open arrow*). Reprinted from Wetzel SG, Cha S, Law M, et al. Preoperative assessment of intracranial tumors with perfusion MR and a volumetric interpolated examination: a comparative study with DSA. *AJNR Am J Neuroradiol.* 2002;23:1767–1774, with permission.

consisting of a T2*-weighted perfusion MR imaging followed by a T1-weighted 3D contrast-enhanced acquisition was found useful to provide most of the information of importance for treatment planning (311) (Fig. 11-56).

The vessels may be difficult to distinguish from contrast-enhancing portions of a tumor. When in close proximity, the ability to follow the course of the vessel may be impaired, which is a limitation of CE MRA. In such cases, flow-sensitive MRA may be more efficient to recognize flow adjacent to a tumor. Ultrafast time-resolved CE MRA sequences emulate features of DSA and thus can demonstrate the temporal passage of the contrast bolus through the cerebral vasculature and reveal the "staining" of a tumor. This approach seems promising, especially if 3D sequences with sufficient spatial and temporal resolution MR DSA are applied, which became possible with parallel imaging techniques (312).

ACKNOWLEDGMENTS

Thanks to Vreni Koch (Basel) for technical assistance and Sean Pierce (New York) for help with the editing process.

REFERENCES

1. Rao VM, Parker L, Levin DC, et al. Use trends and geographic variation in neuroimaging: nationwide Medicare data for 1993 and 1998. *AJNR Am J Neuroradiol.* 2001;22:1643–1649.
2. Cloft HJ, Joseph GJ, Dion JE. Risk of cerebral angiography in patients with subarachnoid hemorrhage, cerebral aneurysm, and arteriovenous malformation: a meta-analysis. *Stroke.* 1999;30:317–320.
3. Aaslid R, Markwalder TM, Nornes H. Noninvasive transcranial Doppler ultrasound recording of flow velocity in basal cerebral arteries. *J Neurosurg.* 1982;57:769–774.
4. Padayachee TS, Gosling RG, Bishop CC, et al. Monitoring middle cerebral artery blood velocity during carotid endarterectomy. *Br J Surg.* 1986;73:98–100.
5. Villablanca JP, Jahan R, Hooshi P, et al. Detection and characterization of very small cerebral aneurysms by using 2D and 3D helical CT angiography. *AJNR Am J Neuroradiol.* 2002;23:1187–1198.
6. Takahashi M, Ashtari M, Papp Z, et al. CT angiography of carotid bifurcation: artifacts and pitfalls in shaded-surface display. *AJR Am J Roentgenol.* 1997;168:813–817.
7. Calhoun PS, Kuszyk BS, Heath DG, et al. Three-dimensional volume rendering of spiral CT data: theory and method. *RadioGraphics.* 1999;19:745–764.
8. Bernstein MA, Huston J 3rd, Lin C, et al. High-resolution intracranial and cervical MRA at 3.0T: technical considerations and initial experience. *Magn Reson Med.* 2001;46:955–962.
9. Willinek WA, Born M, Simon B, et al. Time-of-flight MR angiography: comparison of 3.0-T imaging and 1.5-T imaging—initial experience. *Radiology.* 2003;229:913–920.
10. Pruessmann KP, Weiger M, Scheidegger MB, et al. SENSE: sensitivity encoding for fast MRI. *Magn Reson Med.* 1999;42:952–962.
11. Willinek WA, Gieseke J, von Falkenhausen M, et al. Sensitivity encoding (SENSE) for high spatial resolution time-of-flight MR angiography of the intracranial arteries at 3.0 T. *Rofo Fortschr Geb Rontgenstr Neuen Bildgeb Verfahr.* 2004;176:21–26.
12. Enzmann DR, Ross MR, Marks MP, et al. Blood flow in major cerebral arteries measured by phase-contrast cine MR. *AJNR Am J Neuroradiol.* 1994;15:123–129.
13. Vanninen RL, Manninen HI, Partanen PL, et al. Carotid artery stenosis: clinical efficacy of MR phase-contrast flow

quantification as an adjunct to MR angiography. *Radiology.* 1995;194:459–467.

14. Wetzel SG, Lee VS, Tan AG, et al. Real-time interactive duplex MR measurements: application in neurovascular imaging. *AJR Am J Roentgenol.* 2001;177:703–707.

15. Parker DL, Tsuruda JS, Goodrich KC, et al. Contrast-enhanced magnetic resonance angiography of cerebral arteries. A review. *Invest Radiol.* 1998;33:560–572.

16. Jager HR, Ellamushi H, Moore EA, et al. Contrast-enhanced MR angiography of intracranial giant aneurysms. *AJNR Am J Neuroradiol.* 2000;21:1900–1907.

17. Yang JJ, Hill MD, Morrish WF, et al. Comparison of pre- and postcontrast 3D time-of-flight MR angiography for the evaluation of distal intracranial branch occlusions in acute ischemic stroke. *AJNR Am J Neuroradiol.* 2002;23:557–567.

18. Jung HW, Chang KH, Choi DS, et al. Contrast-enhanced MR angiography for the diagnosis of intracranial vascular disease: optimal dose of gadopentetate dimeglumine. *AJR Am J Roentgenol.* 1995;165:1251–1255.

19. Stevenson J, Knopp EA, Litt AW. MP-RAGE subtraction venography: a new technique. *J Magn Reson Imaging.* 1995;5:239–241.

20. Liang L, Korogi Y, Sugahara T, et al. Evaluation of the intracranial dural sinuses with a 3D contrast-enhanced MP-RAGE sequence: prospective comparison with 2D-TOF MR venography and digital subtraction angiography. *AJNR Am J Neuroradiol.* 2001;22:481–492.

21. Wetzel SJ, Law M, Lee VJ, et al. Imaging of the intracranial venous system with a contrast-enhanced volumetric interpolated examination. *Eur Radiol.* 2003;13:1010–1018.

22. Prince MR. Gadolinium-enhanced MR aortography. *Radiology.* 1994;191:155–164.

23. Remonda L, Heid O, Schroth G. Carotid artery stenosis, occlusion, and pseudo-occlusion: first-pass, gadolinium-enhanced, three-dimensional MR angiography—preliminary study. *Radiology.* 1998;209:95–102.

24. Isoda H, Takehara Y, Isogai S, et al. Technique for arterial-phase contrast-enhanced three-dimensional MR angiography of the carotid and vertebral arteries. *AJNR Am J Neuroradiol.* 1998;19:1241–1244.

25. Wetzel S, Boos M, Bongartz G, et al. Selection of patients for carotid thromboendarterectomy: the role of magnetic resonance angiography. *J Comput Assist Tomogr.* 1999;23[Suppl 1]:S91–S94.

26. Levy RA, Maki JH. Three-dimensional contrast-enhanced MR angiography of the extracranial carotid arteries: two techniques. *AJNR Am J Neuroradiol.* 1998;19:688–690.

27. Lovblad KO, Schneider J, Bassetti C, et al. Fast contrast-enhanced MR whole-brain venography. *Neuroradiology.* 2002;44:681–688.

28. Wang Y, Johnston DL, Breen JF, et al. Dynamic MR digital subtraction angiography using contrast enhancement, fast data acquisition, and complex subtraction. *Magn Reson Med.* 1996;36:551–556.

29. Hennig J, Scheffler K, Laubenberger J, et al. Time-resolved projection angiography after bolus injection of contrast agent. *Magn Reson Med.* 1997;37:341–345.

30. Wetzel SG, Bilecen D, Lyrer P, et al. Cerebral dural arteriovenous fistulas: detection by dynamic MR projection angiography. *AJR Am J Roentgenol.* 2000;174:1293–1295.

31. Klisch J, Strecker R, Hennig J, et al. Time-resolved projection MRA: clinical application in intracranial vascular malformations. *Neuroradiology.* 2000;42:104–107.

32. Metens T, Rio F, Baleriaux D, et al. Intracranial aneurysms: detection with gadolinium-enhanced dynamic three-dimensional MR angiography—initial results. *Radiology.* 2000;216:39–46.

33. Isoda H, Takehara Y, Isogai S, et al. Software-triggered contrast-enhanced three-dimensional MR angiography of the intracranial arteries. *AJR Am J Roentgenol.* 2000;174:371–375.

34. Farb RI, McGregor C, Kim JK, et al. Intracranial arteriovenous malformations: real-time auto-triggered elliptic centric-ordered 3D gadolinium-enhanced MR angiography—initial assessment. *Radiology.* 2001;220:244–251.

35. Osborne A. *Diagnostic Neuroradiology.* St. Louis: Mosby; 1994.

36. Lasjaunias P, Berenstein A, ter Brugge KG. *Surgical Neuroangiography. Clinical Vascular Anatomy and Variations.* 2nd ed. New York: Springer Verlag; 2001.

37. Kretschmann H, Weinrich W. *Cranial Neuroimaging and Clinical Neuroanatomy. Atlas of MR Imaging and Computed Tomography.* 3rd ed., revised and expanded ed. New York: Georg Thieme Verlag; 2003.

38. van der Zwan A, Hillen B, Tulleken CA, et al. Variability of the territories of the major cerebral arteries. *J Neurosurg.* 1992;77:927–940.

39. Bouthillier A, van Loveren HR, Keller JT. Segments of the internal carotid artery: a new classification. *Neurosurgery.* 1996;38:425–432; discussion 432–433.

40. Fischer E. Lageabweichungen der vorderen Hirnarterien im Gefäßbild. *Zbl Neurochir.* 1938;3:300–313.

41. Stock K, Wetzel S, Kirsch E, et al. Anatomic evaluation of the circle of Willis: MR angiography versus intraarterial digital subtraction angiography. *AJNR Am J Neuroradiol.* 1996;17:1495–1499.

42. Schomer DF, Marks MP, Steinberg GK, et al. The anatomy of the posterior communicating artery as a risk factor for ischemic cerebral infarction. *N Engl J Med.* 1994;330:1565–1570.

43. Punt JS. Some observations on aneurysms of the proximal internal carotid artery. *J Neurosurg.* 1979;51:151–154.

44. Gonzalez LF, Walker MT, Zabramski JM, et al. Distinction between paraclinoid and cavernous sinus aneurysms with computed tomographic angiography. *Neurosurgery.* 2003;52:1131–1137; discussion 1138–1139.

45. Uchino A, Sawada A, Takase Y, et al. MR angiography of anomalous branches of the internal carotid artery. *AJR Am J Roentgenol.* 2003;181:1409–1414.

46. Warlow C, Sudlow C, Dennis M, et al. Stroke. *Lancet.* 2003;362:1211–1224.

47. Adams HP Jr., Bendixen BH, Kappelle LJ, et al. Classification of subtype of acute ischemic stroke. Definitions for use in a multicenter clinical trial. TOAST. Trial of Org 10172 in Acute Stroke Treatment. *Stroke.* 1993;24:35–41.

48. Sacco RL, Ellenberg JH, Mohr JP, et al. Infarcts of undetermined cause: the NINCDS Stroke Data Bank. *Ann Neurol.* 1989;25:382–390.

49. Sacco R. Classification of stroke. In: Fisher M, ed. *Clinical Atlas of Cerebrovascular Disorders.* London: Wolfe; 1994.

50. Design, progress and challenges of a double-blind trial of warfarin versus aspirin for symptomatic intracranial arterial stenosis. *Neuroepidemiology.* 2003;22:106–117.

51. Barnett HJ, Gunton RW, Eliasziw M, et al. Causes and severity of ischemic stroke in patients with internal carotid artery stenosis. *JAMA.* 2000;283:1429–1436.

52. Schneider M. Durchblutung und Sauerstoffversorgung des Gehirns. *Verh Dtsch Tes Kreislaufforsch.* 1953:3–12.

53. Zulch K. *The Cerebral Infarct: Pathology, Pathogenesis, and Computed Tomography.* Berlin, Germany: Springer-Verlag; 1985:123–145.

54. van der Zwan A, Hillen B, Tulleken CA, et al. A quantitative investigation of the variability of the major cerebral arterial territories. *Stroke.* 1993;24:1951–1959.

55. Hennerici M, Daffertshofer M, Jakobs L. Failure to identify cerebral infarct mechanisms from topography of vascular territory lesions. *AJNR Am J Neuroradiol.* 1998;19:1067–1074.

56. Derdeyn CP, Khosla A, Videen TO, et al. Severe hemodynamic impairment and border zone–region infarction. *Radiology.* 2001;220:195–201.

57. Bogousslavsky J, Regli F. Borderzone infarctions distal to internal carotid artery occlusion: prognostic implications. *Ann Neurol.* 1986;20:346–350.

58. Pollanen MS, Deck JH. Directed embolization is an alternate cause of cerebral watershed infarction. *Arch Pathol Lab Med.* 1989;113:1139–1141.

59. Waterston JA, Brown MM, Butler P, et al. Small deep cerebral infarcts associated with occlusive internal carotid artery disease. A hemodynamic phenomenon? *Arch Neurol.* 1990;47:953–957.

60. Adams HP Jr., Brott TG, Furlan AJ, et al. Guidelines for thrombolytic therapy for acute stroke: a supplement to the guidelines for the management of patients with acute ischemic stroke: a statement for healthcare professionals from a special writing group of the Stroke Council, American Heart Association. *Stroke.* 1996;27:1711–1718.

61. Tissue plasminogen activator for acute ischemic stroke. The National Institute of Neurological Disorders and Stroke rt-PA Stroke Study Group. *N Engl J Med.* 1995;333:1581–1587.

62. Hacke W, Kaste M, Fieschi C, et al. Intravenous thrombolysis with recombinant tissue plasminogen activator for acute hemispheric stroke. The European Cooperative Acute Stroke Study (ECASS). *JAMA.* 1995;274:1017–1025.

63. Hacke W, Kaste M, Fieschi C, et al. Randomised double-blind placebo-controlled trial of thrombolytic therapy with intravenous alteplase in acute ischaemic stroke (ECASS II). Second European-Australasian Acute Stroke Study Investigators. *Lancet.* 1998;352:1245–1251.

64. Clark WM, Wissman S, Albers GW, et al. Recombinant tissue-type plasminogen activator (Alteplase) for ischemic stroke 3 to 5 hours after symptom onset. The ATLANTIS Study: a randomized controlled trial. Alteplase Thrombolysis for Acute Noninterventional Therapy in Ischemic Stroke. *JAMA.* 1999;282:2019–2026.

65. Libman RB, Wirkowski E, Alvir J, et al. Conditions that mimic stroke in the emergency department. Implications for acute stroke trials. *Arch Neurol.* 1995;52:1119–1122.

66. Fisher M, Bogousslavsky J. Further evolution toward effective therapy for acute ischemic stroke. *JAMA.* 1998;279:1298–1303.

67. Zeumer H, Ringelstein EB, Hassel M, et al. [Local fibrinolysis therapy in subtotal stenosis of the median cerebral artery]. *Dtsch Med Wochenschr.* 1983;108:1103–1105.

68. Provenzale JM, Jahan R, Naidich TP, et al. Assessment of the patient with hyperacute stroke: imaging and therapy. *Radiology.* 2003;229:347–359.

69. Furlan A, Higashida R, Wechsler L, et al. Intra-arterial prourokinase for acute ischemic stroke. The PROACT II study: a randomized controlled trial. Prolyse in Acute Cerebral Thromboembolism. *JAMA.* 1999;282:2003–2011.

70. Lewandowski CA, Frankel M, Tomsick TA, et al. Combined intravenous and intra-arterial r-TPA versus intra-arterial therapy of acute ischemic stroke: Emergency Management of Stroke (EMS) Bridging Trial. *Stroke.* 1999;30:2598–2605.

71. Randomised trial of endarterectomy for recently symptomatic carotid stenosis: final results of the MRC European Carotid Surgery Trial (ECST). *Lancet.* 1998;351:1379–1387.

72. Beneficial effect of carotid endarterectomy in symptomatic patients with high-grade carotid stenosis. North American Symptomatic Carotid Endarterectomy Trial Collaborators. *N Engl J Med.* 1991;325:445–453.

73. Ricci S, Celani MG, Righetti E. Clinical methods for diagnostic confirmation of stroke subtypes. *Neuroepidemiology.* 1994;13:290–295.

74. Barber PA, Demchuk AM, Hudon ME, et al. Hyperdense sylvian fissure MCA "dot" sign: a CT marker of acute ischemia. *Stroke.* 2001;32:84–88.

75. Lovblad KO, Laubach HJ, Baird AE, et al. Clinical experience with diffusion-weighted MR in patients with acute stroke. *AJNR Am J Neuroradiol.* 1998;19:1061–1066.

76. Schellinger PD, Jansen O, Fiebach JB, et al. A standardized MRI stroke protocol: comparison with CT in hyperacute intracerebral hemorrhage. *Stroke.* 1999;30:765–768.

77. Linfante I, Llinas RH, Caplan LR, et al. MRI features of intracerebral hemorrhage within 2 hours from symptom onset. *Stroke.* 1999;30:2263–2267.

78. Kidwell CS, Saver JL, Villablanca JP, et al. Magnetic resonance imaging detection of microbleeds before thrombolysis: an emerging application. *Stroke.* 2002;33:95–98.

79. Tomandl BF, Klotz E, Handschu R, et al. Comprehensive imaging of ischemic stroke with multisection CT. *RadioGraphics.* 2003;23:565–592.

80. Wintermark M, Reichhart M, Cuisenaire O, et al. Comparison of admission perfusion computed tomography and qualitative diffusion- and perfusion-weighted magnetic resonance imaging in acute stroke patients. *Stroke.* 2002;33:2025–2031.

81. Barber PA, Darby DG, Desmond PM, et al. Prediction of stroke outcome with echoplanar perfusion- and diffusion-weighted MRI. *Neurology.* 1998;51:418–426.

82. Ueda T, Yuh WT, Taoka T. Clinical application of perfusion and diffusion MR imaging in acute ischemic stroke. *J Magn Reson Imaging.* 1999;10:305–309.

83. Keir SL, Wardlaw JM. Systematic review of diffusion and perfusion imaging in acute ischemic stroke. *Stroke.* 2000;31:2723–2731.

84. Sunshine JL, Tarr RW, Lanzieri CF, et al. Hyperacute stroke: ultrafast MR imaging to triage patients prior to therapy. *Radiology.* 1999;212:325–332.

85. Schellinger PD, Jansen O, Fiebach JB, et al. Feasibility and practicality of MR imaging of stroke in the management of hyperacute cerebral ischemia. *AJNR Am J Neuroradiol.* 2000;21:1184–1189.

86. Kilpatrick MM, Yonas H, Goldstein S, et al. CT-based assessment of acute stroke: CT, CT angiography, and xenon-enhanced CT cerebral blood flow. *Stroke.* 2001;32:2543–2549.

87. Schellinger PD, Fiebach JB, Hacke W. Imaging-based decision making in thrombolytic therapy for ischemic stroke: present status. *Stroke.* 2003;34:575–583.

88. Ringleb PA, Schellinger PD, Schranz C, et al. Thrombolytic therapy within 3 to 6 hours after onset of ischemic stroke: useful or harmful? *Stroke.* 2002;33:1437–1441.

89. Knauth M, von Kummer R, Jansen O, et al. Potential of CT angiography in acute ischemic stroke. *AJNR Am J Neuroradiol.* 1997;18:1001–1010.

90. Lev MH, Farkas J, Rodriguez VR, et al. CT angiography in the rapid triage of patients with hyperacute stroke to intraarterial thrombolysis: accuracy in the detection of large vessel thrombus. *J Comput Assist Tomogr.* 2001;25:520–528.

91. Shrier D, Tanaka H, Numaguchi Y, et al. CT angiography in the evaluation of acute stroke. *AJNR Am J Neuroradiol.* 1997;18:1011–1020.

92. Skutta B, Furst G, Eilers J, et al. Intracranial stenoocclusive disease: double-detector helical CT angiography versus digital subtraction angiography. *AJNR Am J Neuroradiol.* 1999;20:791–799.

93. Wildermuth S, Knauth M, Brandt T, et al. Role of CT angiography in patient selection for thrombolytic therapy in acute hemispheric stroke. *Stroke.* 1998;29:935–938.

94. Schramm P, Schellinger PD, Fiebach JB, et al. Comparison of CT and CT angiography source images with diffusion-weighted imaging in patients with acute stroke within 6 hours after onset. *Stroke.* 2002;33:2426–2432.

95. Stock KW, Radue EW, Jacob AL, et al. Intracranial arteries: prospective blinded comparative study of MR angiography and DSA in 50 patients. *Radiology.* 1995;195:451–456.

96. Uehara T, Tabuchi M, Mori E. Frequency and clinical correlates of occlusive lesions of cerebral arteries in Japanese patients without stroke. Evaluation by MR angiography. *Cerebrovasc Dis.* 1998;8:267–272.

97. Heiserman JE, Drayer BP, Keller PJ, et al. Intracranial vascular stenosis and occlusion: evaluation with three-dimensional time-of-flight MR angiography. *Radiology.* 1992;185:667–673.

98. Furst G, Hofer M, Steinmetz H, et al. Intracranial stenooc-clusive disease: MR angiography with magnetization trans-fer and variable flip angle. *AJNR Am J Neuroradiol.* 1996;17:1749–1757.

99. Korogi Y, Takahashi M, Mabuchi N, et al. Intracranial vas-cular stenosis and occlusion: diagnostic accuracy of three-dimensional, Fourier transform, time-of-flight MR angiog-raphy. *Radiology.* 1994;193:187–193.

100. Wentz KU, Rother J, Schwartz A, et al. Intracranial verte-brobasilar system: MR angiography. *Radiology.* 1994;190:105–110.

101. Hirai T, Korogi Y, Ono K, et al. Prospective evaluation of suspected stenooclusive disease of the intracranial artery: combined MR angiography and CT angiography compared with digital subtraction angiography. *AJNR Am J Neurora-diol.* 2002;23:93–101.

102. Gondim FA, Cruz-Flores S, Moore J, et al. Angioplasty and stenting for symptomatic basilar artery stenosis. *J Neu-roimaging.* 2002;12:55–58.

103. Lylyk P, Cohen JE, Ceratto R, et al. Angioplasty and stent placement in intracranial atherosclerotic stenoses and dis-sections. *AJNR Am J Neuroradiol.* 2002;23:430–436.

104. Stenting of Symptomatic Atherosclerotic Lesions in the Vertebral or Intracranial Arteries (SSYLVIA): study results. *Stroke.* 2004;35:1388–1392.

105. Hahnel S, Trossbach M, Braun C, et al. Small-vessel stents for intracranial angioplasty: in vitro comparison of differ-ent stent designs and sizes by using CT angiography. *AJNR Am J Neuroradiol.* 2003;24:1512–1516.

106. Furst G, Steinmetz H, Fischer H, et al. Selective MR angiog-raphy and intracranial collateral blood flow. *J Comput Assist Tomogr.* 1993;17:178–183.

107. Hartkamp MJ, van der Grond J, van Everdingen KJ, et al. Circle of Willis collateral flow investigated by magnetic resonance angiography. *Stroke.* 1999;30:2671–2678.

108. Wentz KU, Rother J, Schwartz A, et al. [MR angiography of the vertebrobasilar circulatory area: the potential uses of the saturation technic to determine the direction of the flow]. *Rofo Fortschr Geb Rontgenstr Neuen Bildgeb Ver-fahr.* 1992;156:120–124.

109. Anzola GP, Gasparotti R, Magoni M, et al. Transcranial Doppler sonography and magnetic resonance angiography in the assessment of collateral hemispheric flow in patients with carotid artery disease. *Stroke.* 1995;26:214–217.

110. Jongen JC, Franke CL, Ramos LM, et al. Direction of flow in posterior communicating artery on magnetic resonance angiography in patients with occipital lobe infarcts. *Stroke.* 2004;35:104–108.

111. Siva A. Vasculitis of the nervous system. *J Neurol.* 2001;248:451–468.

112. Moore PM. The vasculitides. *Curr Opin Neurol.* 1999;12:383–388.

113. Ferro JM. Vasculitis of the central nervous system. *J Neurol.* 1998;245:766–776.

114. Moore PM, Richardson B. Neurology of the vasculitides and connective tissue diseases. *J Neurol Neurosurg Psychia-try.* 1998;65:10–22.

115. Wasserman BA, Stone JH, Hellmann DB, et al. Reliability of normal findings on MR imaging for excluding the diagno-sis of vasculitis of the central nervous system. *AJR Am J Roentgenol.* 2001;177:455–459.

116. Pomper MG, Miller TJ, Stone JH, et al. CNS vasculitis in autoimmune disease: MR imaging findings and correla-tion with angiography. *AJNR Am J Neuroradiol.* 1999;20:75–85.

117. Kadkhodayan Y, Alreshaid A, Moran CJ, et al. Primary angiitis of the central nervous system at conventional angiography. *Radiology.* 2004;233:878–882.

118. Nastri MV, Baptista LP, Baroni RH, et al. Gadolinium-enhanced three-dimensional MR angiography of Takayasu arteritis. *RadioGraphics.* 2004;24:773–786.

119. Bley TA, Wieben O, Vaith P, et al. Magnetic resonance imaging depicts mural inflammation of the temporal artery in giant cell arteritis. *Arthritis Rheum.* 2004;51:1062–1063; author reply 1064.

120. Demaerel P, De Ruyter N, Maes F, et al. Magnetic reso-nance angiography in suspected cerebral vasculitis. *Eur Radiol.* 2004;14:1005–1012.

121. Suzuki J, Takaku A. Cerebrovascular "moyamoya" disease. Disease showing abnormal net-like vessels in base of brain. *Arch Neurol.* 1969;20:288–299.

122. Yamada H, Deguchi K, Tanigawara T, et al. The relation-ship between moyamoya disease and bacterial infection. *Clin Neurol Neurosurg.* 1997;99 [Suppl 2]:S221–S224.

123. Ikeda H, Sasaki T, Yoshimoto T, et al. Mapping of a familial moyamoya disease gene to chromosome 3p24.2-p26. *Am J Hum Genet.* 1999;64:533–537.

124. Goto Y, Yonekawa Y. Worldwide distribution of moy-amoya disease. *Neurol Med Chir (Tokyo).* 1992;32:883–886.

125. Natori Y, Ikezaki K, Matsushima T, et al. "Angiographic moyamoya" its definition, classification, and therapy. *Clin Neurol Neurosurg.* 1997;99[Suppl 2]: S168–S172.

126. Gosalakkal JA. Moyamoya disease: a review. *Neurol India.* 2002;50:6–10.

127. Fukui M. Guidelines for the diagnosis and treatment of spontaneous occlusion of the circle of Willis ('moyamoya' disease). Research Committee on Spontaneous Occlusion of the Circle of Willis (Moyamoya Disease) of the Ministry of Health and Welfare, Japan. *Clin Neurol Neurosurg.* 1997;99[Suppl 2]:S238–S240.

128. Calamante F, Ganesan V, Kirkham FJ, et al. MR perfusion imaging in Moyamoya Syndrome: potential implications for clinical evaluation of occlusive cerebrovascular disease. *Stroke.* 2001;32:2810–2816.

129. Wityk RJ, Hillis A, Beauchamp N, et al. Perfusion-weighted magnetic resonance imaging in adult moyamoya syn-drome: characteristic patterns and change after surgical intervention: case report. *Neurosurgery.* 2002;51:1499–1505; discussion 1506.

130. Hasuo K, Mihara F, Matsushima T. MRI and MR angiogra-phy in moyamoya disease. *J Magn Reson Imaging.* 1998;8:762–766.

131. Yamada I, Matsushima Y, Suzuki S. Moyamoya disease: diag-nosis with three-dimensional time-of-flight MR angiogra-phy. *Radiology.* 1992;184:773–778.

132. Houkin K, Aoki T, Takahashi A, et al. Diagnosis of moy-amoya disease with magnetic resonance angiography. *Stroke.* 1994;25:2159–2164.

133. Yamada I, Nakagawa T, Matsushima Y, et al. High-resolu-tion turbo magnetic resonance angiography for diagnosis of moyamoya disease. *Stroke.* 2001;32:1825–1831.

134. Houkin K, Nakayama N, Kuroda S, et al. How does angio-genesis develop in pediatric moyamoya disease after surgery? A prospective study with MR angiography. *Childs Nerv Syst.* 2004;20:734–741.

135. Tsuchiya K, Aoki C, Katase S, et al. Visualization of extracranial-intracranial bypass using multidetector-row helical computed tomography angiography. *J Comput Assist Tomogr.* 2003;27:231–234.

136. Tsuchiya K, Makita K, Furui S. Moyamoya disease: diagno-sis with three-dimensional CT angiography. *Neuroradiol-ogy.* 1994;36:432–434.

137. Murai Y, Takagi R, Ikeda Y, et al. Three-dimensional comput-erized tomography angiography in patients with hypera-cute intracerebral hemorrhage. *J Neurosurg.* 1999;91:424–431.

138. Fogelholm R, Hernesniemi J, Vapalahti MS. Impact of early surgery on outcome after aneurysmal subarachnoid hem-orrhage. A population-based study. *Stroke.* 1993;24:1649–1654.

139. Hop JW, Rinkel GJ, Algra A, et al. Case-fatality rates and functional outcome after subarachnoid hemorrhage: a sys-tematic review. *Stroke.* 1997;28:660–664.

140. Hijdra A, Braakman R, van Gijn J, et al. Aneurysmal sub-arachnoid hemorrhage. Complications and outcome in a hospital population. *Stroke.* 1987;18:1061–1067.

141. Stehbens WES. Etiology of intracranial berry aneurysms. *J Neurosurg.* 1989;70:823–831.

142. Rossitti S, Lofgren JS. Optimality principles and flow order-liness at the branching points of cerebral arteries. *Stroke.* 1993;24:1029–1032.

143. Burleson AC, Strother CM, Turitto VT. Computer modeling of intracranial saccular and lateral aneurysms for the study of their hemodynamics. *Neurosurgery.* 1995;37:774–782; discussion 782–774.

144. Graves VB, Strother CM, Partington CR, et al. Flow dynam-ics of lateral carotid artery aneurysms and their effects on coils and balloons: an experimental study in dogs. *AJNR Am J Neuroradiol.* 1992;13:189–196.

145. Lanzino G, Wakhloo AK, Fessler RD, et al. Efficacy and cur-rent limitations of intravascular stents for intracranial internal carotid, vertebral, and basilar artery aneurysms. *J Neurosurg.* 1999;91:538–546.

146. Geremia G, Haklin M, Brennecke LS. Embolization of experimentally created aneurysms with intravascular stent devices. *AJNR Am J Neuroradiol.* 1994;15:1223–1231.

147. Wakhloo AK, Tio FO, Lieber BB, et al. Self-expanding niti-nol stents in canine vertebral arteries: hemodynamics and tissue response. *AJNR Am J Neuroradiol.* 1995;16: 1043–1051.

148. Perata HJ, Tomsick TA, Tew JM Jr. Feeding artery pedicle aneurysms: association with parenchymal hemorrhage and arteriovenous malformation in the brain. *J Neurosurg.* 1994;80:631–634.

149. Wardlaw JM, White PM. The detection and management of unruptured intracranial aneurysms. *Brain.* 2000;123(Pt 2):205–221.

150. Fox J. *Intracranial Aneurysms.* New York: Springer-Verlag; 1983.

151. Pia HW, Zierski JS. Giant cerebral aneurysms. *Neurosurg Rev.* 1982;5:117–148.

152. Lanzino G, Kaptain G, Kallmes DF, et al. Intracranial dis-secting aneurysm causing subarachnoid hemorrhage: the role of computerized tomographic angiography and mag-netic resonance angiography. *Surg Neurol.* 1997;48: 477–481.

153. Yonas H, Agamanolis D, Takaoka Y, et al. Dissecting intracranial aneurysms. *Surg Neurol.* 1977;8:407–415.

154. Brust JC, Dickinson PC, Hughes JE, et al. The diagnosis and treatment of cerebral mycotic aneurysms. *Ann Neurol.* 1990;27:238–246.

155. Cloud GC, Rich PM, Markus HS. Serial MRI of a mycotic aneurysm of the cavernous carotid artery. *Neuroradiology.* 2003;45:546–549.

156. White PM, Wardlaw J. Unruptured intracranial aneurysms: prospective data have arrived. *Lancet.* 2003;362:90–91.

157. Wiebers DO, Whisnant JP, Huston J 3rd, et al. Unruptured intracranial aneurysms: natural history, clinical outcome, and risks of surgical and endovascular treatment. *Lancet.* 2003;362:103–110.

158. Unruptured intracranial aneurysms—risk of rupture and risks of surgical intervention. International Study of Unruptured Intracranial Aneurysms Investigators. *N Engl J Med.* 1998;339:1725–1733.

159. Chappell ET, Moure FC, Good MC. Comparison of com-puted tomographic angiography with digital subtraction angiography in the diagnosis of cerebral aneurysms: a meta-analysis. *Neurosurgery.* 2003;52:624–631; discussion 630–621.

160. Anxionnat R, Bracard S, Ducrocq X, et al. Intracranial aneurysms: clinical value of 3D digital subtraction angiog-raphy in the therapeutic decision and endovascular treat-ment. *Radiology.* 2001;218:799–808.

161. Yamamoto Y, Asari S, Sunami N, et al. Computed angioto-mography of unruptured cerebral aneurysms. *J Comput Assist Tomogr.* 1986;10:21–27.

162. Mitchell P, Wilkinson ID, Hoggard N, et al. Detection of subarachnoid haemorrhage with magnetic resonance imaging. *J Neurol Neurosurg Psychiatry.* 2001;70:205–211.

163. White PM, Wardlaw JM, Easton V. Can noninvasive imag-ing accurately depict intracranial aneurysms? A systematic review. *Radiology.* 2000;217:361–370.

164. White PM, Teasdale EM, Wardlaw JM, et al. Intracranial aneurysms: CT angiography and MR angiography for detection—prospective blinded comparison in a large patient cohort. *Radiology.* 2001;219:739–749.

165. Yasargil M. *Microneurosurgery.* New York: Georg Thieme Verlag; 1984:299.

166. Ochi T, Shimizu K, Yasuhara Y, et al. Curved planar refor-matted CT angiography: usefulness for the evaluation of aneurysms at the carotid siphon. *AJNR Am J Neuroradiol.* 1999;20:1025–1030.

167. Korogi Y, Takahashi M, Katada K, et al. Intracranial aneurysms: detection with three-dimensional CT angiogra-phy with volume rendering-comparison with conventional angiographic and surgical findings. *Radiology.* 1999;211: 497–506.

168. Villablanca JP, Martin N, Jahan R, et al. Volume-rendered helical computerized tomography angiography in the detection and characterization of intracranial aneurysms. *J Neurosurg.* 2000;93:254–264.

169. Villablanca JP, Hooshi P, Martin N, et al. Three-dimensional helical computerized tomography angiography in the diagnosis, characterization, and management of middle cerebral artery aneurysms: comparison with conventional angiography and intraoperative findings. *J Neurosurg.* 2002;97:1322–1332.

170. Dehdashti AR, Rufenacht DA, Delavelle J, et al. Therapeu-tic decision and management of aneurysmal subarachnoid haemorrhage based on computed tomographic angiogra-phy. *Br J Neurosurg.* 2003;17:46–53.

171. Matsumoto M, Endo Y, Sato M, et al. Acute aneurysm surgery using three-dimensional CT angiography without conventional catheter angiography. *Fukushima J Med Sci.* 2002;48:63–73.

172. Huston J 3rd, Nichols DA, Luetmer PH, et al. Blinded prospective evaluation of sensitivity of MR angiography to known intracranial aneurysms: importance of aneurysm size. *AJNR Am J Neuroradiol.* 1994;15: 1607–1614.

173. Brugieres P, Blustajn J, Le Guerinel C, et al. Magnetic reso-nance angiography of giant intracranial aneurysms. *Neu-roradiology.* 1998;40:96–102.

174. De Jesus O, Rifkinson N. Magnetic resonance angiography of giant aneurysms. Pitfalls and surgical implications. *P R Health Sci J.* 1997;16:131–135.

175. Adams WM, Laitt RD, Jackson A. The role of MR angiogra-phy in the pretreatment assessment of intracranial aneurysms: a comparative study. *AJNR Am J Neuroradiol.* 2000;21:1618–1628.

176. Watanabe Z, Kikuchi Y, Izaki K, et al. The usefulness of 3D MR angiography in surgery for ruptured cerebral aneurysms. *Surg Neurol.* 2001;55:359–364.

177. Okahara M, Kiyosue H, Yamashita M, et al. Diagnostic accuracy of magnetic resonance angiography for cerebral aneurysms in correlation with 3D-digital subtraction angiographic images: a study of 133 aneurysms. *Stroke.* 2002;33:1803–1808.

178. Garnier P, Demasles S, Januel AC, et al. [Intracranial exten-sion of extracranial vertebral artery dissections. A review of 16 cases]. *Rev Neurol (Paris).* 2004;160:679–684.

179. Le Roux PD, Elliott JP, Eskridge JM, et al. Risks and benefits of diagnostic angiography after aneurysm surgery: a retrospective analysis of 597 studies. *Neurosurgery.* 1998;42:1248–1254; discussion 1254–1255.

180. Tsutsumi K, Ueki K, Morita A, et al. Risk of aneurysm recur-rence in patients with clipped cerebral aneurysms: results of long-term follow-up angiography. *Stroke.* 2001;32:1191–1194.

181. Brown J, Lustrin E, Lev M, et al. CT angiography of the circle of Willis: is spiral technology always necessary? *AJNR Am J Neuroradiol.* 1997;18:1794–1797.

182. Vieco P, Morin E 3rd, Gross C. CT angiography in the examination of patients with aneurysm clips. *AJNR Am J Neuroradiol.* 1996;17:455–457.

183. van Loon JJ, Yousry TA, Fink U, et al. Postoperative spiral computed tomography and magnetic resonance angiography after aneurysm clipping with titanium clips. *Neurosurgery.* 1997;41:851–856; discussion 856–857.

184. Molyneux A, Kerr R, Stratton I, et al. International Subarachnoid Aneurysm Trial (ISAT) of neurosurgical clipping versus endovascular coiling in 2143 patients with ruptured intracranial aneurysms: a randomised trial. *Lancet.* 2002;360:1267–1274.

185. Cognard C, Weill A, Spelle L, et al. Long-term angiographic follow-up of 169 intracranial berry aneurysms occluded with detachable coils. *Radiology.* 1999;212:348–356.

186. Hope JKA, Byrne JV, Molyneux AJ. Factors influencing successful angiographic occlusion of aneurysms treated by coil embolization. *AJNR Am J Neuroradiol.* 1999;20:391–399.

187. Hartman J, Nguyen T, Larsen D, et al. MR artifacts, heat production, and ferromagnetism of Guglielmi detachable coils. *AJNR Am J Neuroradiol.* 1997;18:497–501.

188. Derdeyn C, Graves V, Turski P, et al. MR angiography of saccular aneurysms after treatment with Guglielmi detachable coils: preliminary experience. *AJNR Am J Neuroradiol.* 1997;18:279–286.

189. Anzalone N, Righi C, Simionato F, et al. Three-dimensional time-of-flight MR angiography in the evaluation of intracranial aneurysms treated with Guglielmi detachable coils. *AJNR Am J Neuroradiol.* 2000;21:746–752.

190. Boulin A, Pierot L. Follow-up of intracranial aneurysms treated with detachable coils: comparison of gadolinium-enhanced 3D time-of-flight MR angiography and digital subtraction angiography. *Radiology.* 2001;219:108–113.

191. Cottier J-P, Bleuzen-Couthon A, Gallas S, et al. Intracranial aneurysms treated with Guglielmi detachable coils: is contrast material necessary in the follow-up with 3D time-of-flight MR angiography? *AJNR Am J Neuroradiol.* 2003;24:1797–1803.

192. Kahara VJ, Seppanen SK, Ryymin PS, et al. MR angiography with three-dimensional time-of-flight and targeted maximum-intensity-projection reconstructions in the follow-up of intracranial aneurysms embolized with Guglielmi detachable coils. *AJNR Am J Neuroradiol.* 1999;20:1470–1475.

193. Gonner F, Heid O, Remonda L, et al. MR angiography with ultrashort echo time in cerebral aneurysms treated with Guglielmi detachable coils. *AJNR Am J Neuroradiol.* 1998;19:1324–1328.

194. Leclerc X, Navez J-F, Gauvrit J-Y, et al. Aneurysms of the anterior communicating artery treated with Guglielmi detachable coils: follow-up with contrast-enhanced MR angiography. *AJNR Am J Neuroradiol.* 2002;23:1121–1127.

195. Lylyk P, Cohen JE, Ceratto R, et al. Combined endovascular treatment of dissecting vertebral artery aneurysms by using stents and coils. *J Neurosurg.* 2001;94:427–432.

196. Fiorella D, Albuquerque FC, Han P, et al. Preliminary experience using the Neuroform stent for the treatment of cerebral aneurysms. *Neurosurgery.* 2004;54:6–16; discussion 16–17.

197. Howington JU, Hanel RA, Harrigan MR, et al. The Neuroform stent, the first microcatheter-delivered stent for use in the intracranial circulation. *Neurosurgery.* 2004;54:2–5.

198. Saatci I, Cekirge HS, Ciceri EFM, et al. CT and MR imaging findings and their implications in the follow-up of patients with intracranial aneurysms treated with endosaccular occlusion with Onyx. *AJNR Am J Neuroradiol.* 2003;24:567–578.

199. Turjman F, Mimon S, Yilmaz H. [Epidemiology, clinical study and pathology of vasospasm]. *J Neuroradiol.* 1999;26:S10–S16.

200. Schuknecht B, Fandino J, Yuksel C, et al. Endovascular treatment of cerebral vasospasm: assessment of treatment effect by cerebral angiography and transcranial colour Doppler sonography. *Neuroradiology.* 1999;41:453–462.

201. Ochi R, Vieco P, Gross C. CT angiography of cerebral vasospasm with conventional angiographic comparison. *AJNR Am J Neuroradiol.* 1997;18:265–269.

202. Anderson GB, Ashforth R, Steinke DE, et al. CT angiography for the detection of cerebral vasospasm in patients with acute subarachnoid hemorrhage. *AJNR Am J Neuroradiol.* 2000;21:1011–1015.

203. Grandin CB, Cosnard G, Hammer F, et al. Vasospasm after subarachnoid hemorrhage: diagnosis with MR angiography. *AJNR Am J Neuroradiol.* 2000;21:1611–1617.

204. Otawara Y, Ogasawara K, Ogawa A, et al. Evaluation of vasospasm after subarachnoid hemorrhage by use of multislice computed tomographic angiography. *Neurosurgery.* 2002;51:939–942; discussion 942–933.

205. Rosenwasser RH, Armonda RA, Thomas JE, et al. Therapeutic modalities for the management of cerebral vasospasm: timing of endovascular options. *Neurosurgery.* 1999;44:975–979; discussion 979–980.

206. Heiserman JE. MR angiography for the diagnosis of vasospasm after subarachnoid hemorrhage. Is it accurate? Is it safe? *AJNR Am J Neuroradiol.* 2000;21:1571–1572.

207. Condette-Auliac S, Bracard S, Anxionnat R, et al. Vasospasm after subarachnoid hemorrhage: interest in diffusion-weighted MR imaging. *Stroke.* 2001;32:1818–1824.

208. Rordorf G, Koroshetz WJ, Copen WA, et al. Diffusion- and perfusion-weighted imaging in vasospasm after subarachnoid hemorrhage. *Stroke.* 1999;30:599–605.

209. Pelkonen O, Tikkakoski T, Leinonen S, et al. Intracranial arterial dissection. *Neuroradiology.* 1998;40:442–447.

210. Yamaura A, Ono J, Hirai S. Clinical picture of intracranial non-traumatic dissecting aneurysm. *Neuropathology.* 2000;20:85–90.

211. Anxionnat R, de Melo Neto JF, Bracard S, et al. Treatment of hemorrhagic intracranial dissections. *Neurosurgery.* 2003;53:289–300; discussion 300–281.

212. Chaves C, Estol C, Esnaola MM, et al. Spontaneous intracranial internal carotid artery dissection: report of 10 patients. *Arch Neurol.* 2002;59:977–981.

213. Ohkuma H, Suzuki S, Shimamura N, et al. Dissecting aneurysms of the middle cerebral artery: neuroradiological and clinical features. *Neuroradiology.* 2003;45:143–148.

214. Ohkuma H, Suzuki S, Kikkawa T, et al. Neuroradiologic and clinical features of arterial dissection of the anterior cerebral artery. *AJNR Am J Neuroradiol.* 2003;24:691–699.

215. Naito I, Iwai T, Sasaki T. Management of intracranial vertebral artery dissections initially presenting without subarachnoid hemorrhage. *Neurosurgery.* 2002;51:930–937; discussion 937–938.

216. Hosoya T, Adachi M, Yamaguchi K, et al. Clinical and neuroradiological features of intracranial vertebrobasilar artery dissection. *Stroke.* 1999;30:1083–1090.

217. Chen CJ, Tseng YC, Lee TH, et al. Multisection CT angiography compared with catheter angiography in diagnosing vertebral artery dissection. *AJNR Am J Neuroradiol.* 2004;25:769–774.

218. Kirsch E, Kaim A, Engelter S, et al. MR angiography in internal carotid artery dissection: improvement of diagnosis by selective demonstration of the intramural haematoma. *Neuroradiology.* 1998;40:704–709.

219. Levy C, Laissy JP, Raveau V, et al. Carotid and vertebral artery dissections: three-dimensional time-of-flight MR angiography and MR imaging versus conventional angiography. *Radiology.* 1994;190:97–103.

220. Bloem BR, Van Buchem GJ. Magnetic resonance imaging and vertebral artery dissection. *J Neurol Neurosurg Psychiatry.* 1999;67:691–692.

221. McCormick WF. The pathology of vascular ("arteriovenous") malformations. *J Neurosurg.* 1966;24:807–816.

222. Sarwar M, McCormick WF. Intracerebral venous angioma. Case report and review. *Arch Neurol.* 1978;35:323–325.

223. Lasjaunias P, Burrows P, Planet C. Developmental venous anomalies (DVA): the so-called venous angioma. *Neurosurg Rev.* 1986;9:233–242.

224. Abe T, Singer RJ, Marks MP, et al. Coexistence of occult vascular malformations and developmental venous anomalies in the central nervous system: MR evaluation. *AJNR Am J Neuroradiol.* 1998;19:51–57.

225. Berman MF, Sciacca RR, Pile-Spellman J, et al. The epidemiology of brain arteriovenous malformations. *Neurosurgery.* 2000;47:389–396; discussion 397.

226. Fleetwood IG, Steinberg GK. Arteriovenous malformations. *Lancet.* 2002;359:863–873.

227. Cunha e Sa MJ, Stein BM, Solomon RA, et al. The treatment of associated intracranial aneurysms and arteriovenous malformations. *J Neurosurg.* 1992;77:853–859.

228. Hofmeister C, Stapf C, Hartmann A, et al. Demographic, morphological, and clinical characteristics of 1289 patients with brain arteriovenous malformation. *Stroke.* 2000;31:1307–1310.

229. Mast H, Young WL, Koennecke HC, et al. Risk of spontaneous haemorrhage after diagnosis of cerebral arteriovenous malformation. *Lancet.* 1997;350:1065–1068.

230. Hartmann A, Mast H, Mohr JP, et al. Morbidity of intracranial hemorrhage in patients with cerebral arteriovenous malformation. *Stroke.* 1998;29:931–934.

231. Langer DJ, Lasner TM, Hurst RW, et al. Hypertension, small size, and deep venous drainage are associated with risk of hemorrhagic presentation of cerebral arteriovenous malformations. *Neurosurgery.* 1998;42:481–486; discussion 487–489.

232. Pollock BE, Flickinger JC, Lunsford LD, et al. Factors that predict the bleeding risk of cerebral arteriovenous malformations. *Stroke.* 1996;27:1–6.

233. Spetzler RF, Martin NA. A proposed grading system for arteriovenous malformations. *J Neurosurg.* 1986;65:476–483.

234. Steinberg GK, Fabrikant JI, Marks MP, et al. Stereotactic heavy-charged-particle Bragg-peak radiation for intracranial arteriovenous malformations. *N Engl J Med.* 1990;323:96–101.

235. Guo WY, Karlsson B, Ericson K, et al. Even the smallest remnant of an AVM constitutes a risk of further bleeding. Case report. *Acta Neurochir (Wien).* 1993;121:212–215.

236. Miyamoto S, Hashimoto N, Nagata I, et al. Posttreatment sequelae of palliatively treated cerebral arteriovenous malformations. *Neurosurgery.* 2000;46:589–594; discussion 594–595.

237. Heros RC, Korosue K, Diebold PM. Surgical excision of cerebral arteriovenous malformations: late results. *Neurosurgery.* 1990;26:570–577; discussion 577–578.

238. Sisti MB, Kader A, Stein BM. Microsurgery for 67 intracranial arteriovenous malformations less than 3 cm in diameter. *J Neurosurg.* 1993;79:653–660.

239. Hamilton MG, Spetzler RF. The prospective application of a grading system for arteriovenous malformations. *Neurosurgery.* 1994;34:2–6; discussion 6–7.

240. Schaller C, Schramm J, Haun D. Significance of factors contributing to surgical complications and to late outcome after elective surgery of cerebral arteriovenous malformations. *J Neurol Neurosurg Psychiatry.* 1998;65:547–554.

241. Paulsen RD, Steinberg GK, Norbash AM, et al. Embolization of basal ganglia and thalamic arteriovenous malformations. *Neurosurgery.* 1999;44:991–996; discussion 996–997.

242. Paulsen RD, Steinberg GK, Norbash AM, et al. Embolization of rolandic cortex arteriovenous malformations. *Neurosurgery.* 1999;44:479–484; discussion 484–486.

243. Gobin YP, Laurent A, Merienne L, et al. Treatment of brain arteriovenous malformations by embolization and radiosurgery. *J Neurosurg.* 1996;85:19–28.

244. Maruyama K, Kawahara N, Shin M, et al. The risk of hemorrhage after radiosurgery for cerebral arteriovenous malformations. *N Engl J Med.* 2005;352:146–153.

245. Hino A, Fujimoto M, Yamaki T, et al. Value of repeat angiography in patients with spontaneous subcortical hemorrhage. *Stroke.* 1998;29:2517–2521.

246. Zhu XL, Chan MS, Poon WS. Spontaneous intracranial hemorrhage: which patients need diagnostic cerebral angiography? A prospective study of 206 cases and review of the literature. *Stroke.* 1997;28:1406–1409.

247. Aoki S, Sasaki Y, Machida T, et al. 3D-CT angiography of cerebral arteriovenous malformations. *Radiat Med.* 1998;16:263–271.

248. Pant B, Sumida M, Arita K, et al. Usefulness of three-dimensional phase contrast MR angiography on arteriovenous malformations. *Neurosurg Rev.* 1997;20:171–176.

249. Bednarz G, Downes B, Werner-Wasik M, et al. Combining stereotactic angiography and 3D time-of-flight magnetic resonance angiography in treatment planning for arteriovenous malformation radiosurgery. *Int J Radiat Oncol Biol Phys.* 2000;46:1149–1154.

250. Tsuchiya K, Katase S, Yoshino A, et al. MR digital subtraction angiography of cerebral arteriovenous malformations. *AJNR Am J Neuroradiol.* 2000;21:707–711.

251. Griffiths PD, Hoggard N, Warren DJ, et al. Brain arteriovenous malformations: assessment with dynamic MR digital subtraction angiography. *AJNR Am J Neuroradiol.* 2000;21:1892–1899.

252. Wasserman BA, Lin W, Tarr RW, et al. Cerebral arteriovenous malformations: flow quantitation by means of two-dimensional cardiac-gated phase-contrast MR imaging. *Radiology.* 1995;194:681–686.

253. Edelman RR, Wentz KU, Mattle HP, et al. Intracerebral arteriovenous malformations: evaluation with selective MR angiography and venography. *Radiology.* 1989;173:831–837.

254. Halbach VV, Higashida RT, Hieshima GB, et al. Transvenous embolization of dural fistulas involving the transverse and sigmoid sinuses. *AJNR Am J Neuroradiol.* 1989;10:385–392.

255. Newton TH, Cronqvist S. Involvement of dural arteries in intracranial arteriovenous malformations. *Radiology.* 1969;93:1071–1078.

256. Houser OW, Baker HL Jr., Rhoton AL Jr., et al. Intracranial dural arteriovenous malformations. *Radiology.* 1972;105:55–64.

257. Awad IA, Little JR, Akarawi WP, et al. Intracranial dural arteriovenous malformations: factors predisposing to an aggressive neurological course. *J Neurosurg.* 1990;72:839–850.

258. Cognard C, Gobin YP, Pierot L, et al. Cerebral dural arteriovenous fistulas: clinical and angiographic correlation with a revised classification of venous drainage. *Radiology.* 1995;194:671–680.

259. Barrow DL, Spector RH, Braun IF, et al. Classification and treatment of spontaneous carotid-cavernous sinus fistulas. *J Neurosurg.* 1985;62:248–256.

260. Hurst RW, Bagley LJ, Galetta S, et al. Dementia resulting from dural arteriovenous fistulas: the pathologic findings of venous hypertensive encephalopathy. *AJNR Am J Neuroradiol.* 1998;19:1267–1273.

261. Lasjaunias P, Chiu M, ter Brugge K, et al. Neurological manifestations of intracranial dural arteriovenous malformations. *J Neurosurg.* 1986;64:724–730.

262. Davies MA, TerBrugge K, Willinsky R, et al. The validity of classification for the clinical presentation of intracranial dural arteriovenous fistulas. *J Neurosurg.* 1996;85:830–837.

263. Duffau H, Lopes M, Janosevic V, et al. Early rebleeding from intracranial dural arteriovenous fistulas: report of 20 cases and review of the literature. *J Neurosurg.* 1999;90: 78–84.

264. Klisch J, Huppertz HJ, Spetzger U, et al. Transvenous treatment of carotid cavernous and dural arteriovenous fistulae: results for 31 patients and review of the literature. *Neurosurgery.* 2003;53:836–856; discussion 856–857.

265. Cellerini M, Mascalchi M, Mangiafico S, et al. Phase-contrast MR angiography of intracranial dural arteriovenous fistulae. *Neuroradiology.* 1999;41:487–492.

266. Chen JC, Tsuruda JS, Halbach VV. Suspected dural arteriovenous fistula: results with screening MR angiography in seven patients. *Radiology.* 1992;183:265–271.

267. Noguchi K, Melhem ER, Kanazawa T, et al. Intracranial dural arteriovenous fistulas: evaluation with combined 3D time-of-flight MR angiography and MR digital subtraction angiography. *AJR Am J Roentgenol.* 2004;182:183–190.

268. Coley SC, Romanowski CAJ, Hodgson TJ, et al. Dural arteriovenous fistulae: noninvasive diagnosis with dynamic MR digital subtraction angiography. *AJNR Am J Neuroradiol.* 2002;23:404–407.

269. Wetzel SG, Mekle R, Taschner C, et al. Whole-brain MR-DSA using time-resolved 3D contrast-enhanced MRA and parallel imaging. In: *International Society of Magnetic Resonance in Medicine, 12th Scientific meeting.* Kyoto; 2004: Book of abstracts.

270. Meckel S, Lovblad KO, Abdo G, et al. Arterialization of cerebral veins on dynamic multiarray helical CT angiography: a possible sign for a dural arteriovenous fistula. *Am J Roentgenol.* 2005;184:1313–1316.

271. Martinelli I, Sacchi E, Landi G, et al. High risk of cerebral-vein thrombosis in carriers of a prothrombin-gene mutation and in users of oral contraceptives. *N Engl J Med.* 1998;338:1793–1797.

272. Bousser MG. Cerebral venous thrombosis: diagnosis and management. *J Neurol.* 2000;247:252–258.

273. Einhaupl KM, Villringer A, Meister W, et al. Heparin treatment in sinus venous thrombosis. *Lancet.* 1991;338: 597–600.

274. Bousser MG. Cerebral venous thrombosis: nothing, heparin, or local thrombolysis? *Stroke.* 1999;30:481–483.

275. de Bruijn SF, Stam J. Randomized, placebo-controlled trial of anticoagulant treatment with low-molecular-weight heparin for cerebral sinus thrombosis. *Stroke.* 1999;30: 484–488.

276. Frey JL, Muro GJ, McDougall CG, et al. Cerebral venous thrombosis: combined intrathrombus rtPA and intravenous heparin. *Stroke.* 1999;30:489–494.

277. Ameri A, Bousser MG. Cerebral venous thrombosis. *Neurol Clin.* 1992;10:87–111.

278. Brucker AB, Vollert-Rogenhofer H, Wagner M, et al. Heparin treatment in acute cerebral sinus venous thrombosis: a retrospective clinical and MR analysis of 42 cases. *Cerebrovasc Dis.* 1998;8:331–337.

279. Manzione J, Newman GC, Shapiro A, et al. Diffusion- and perfusion-weighted MR imaging of dural sinus thrombosis. *AJNR Am J Neuroradiol.* 2000;21:68–73.

280. Yoshikawa T, Abe O, Tsuchiya K, et al. Diffusion-weighted magnetic resonance imaging of dural sinus thrombosis. *Neuroradiology.* 2002;44:481–488.

281. Grosman H, St Louis EL, Gray RR. The role of CT and DSA in cranial sino-venous occlusion. *Can Assoc Radiol J.* 1987;38:183–189.

282. Virapongse C, Cazenave C, Quisling R, et al. The empty delta sign: frequency and significance in 76 cases of dural sinus thrombosis. *Radiology.* 1987;162:779–785.

283. Ozsvath RR, Casey SO, Lustrin ES, et al. Cerebral venography: comparison of CT and MR projection venography. *AJR Am J Roentgenol.* 1997;169:1699–1707.

284. Wetzel SG, Kirsch E, Stock KW, et al. Cerebral veins: comparative study of CT venography with intraarterial digital subtraction angiography. *AJNR Am J Neuroradiol.* 1999;20:249–255.

285. Casey SO, Alberico RA, Patel M, et al. Cerebral CT venography. *Radiology.* 1996;198:163–170.

286. Hagen T, Bartylla K, Waziri A, et al. [Value of CT-angiography in diagnosis of cerebral sinus and venous thromboses]. *Radiologe.* 1996;36:859–866.

287. Lafitte F, Boukobza M, Guichard JP, et al. Deep cerebral venous thrombosis: imaging in eight cases. 1999;41:410–418.

288. Lee JH, Lee HK, Park JK, et al. Cavernous sinus syndrome: clinical features and differential diagnosis with MR imaging. *AJR Am J Roentgenol.* 2003;181:583–590.

289. Schuknecht B, Simmen D, Yuksel C, et al. Tributary venosinus occlusion and septic cavernous sinus thrombosis: CT and MR findings. *AJNR Am J Neuroradiol.* 1998;19: 617–626.

290. Mattle HP, Wentz KU, Edelman RR, et al. Cerebral venography with MR. *Radiology.* 1991;178:453–458.

291. Tsuruda JS, Shimakawa A, Pelc NJ, et al. Dural sinus occlusion: evaluation with phase-sensitive gradient-echo MR imaging. *AJNR Am J Neuroradiol.* 1991;12:481–488.

292. Liauw L, van Buchem MA, Spilt A, et al. MR angiography of the intracranial venous system. *Radiology.* 2000;214: 678–682.

293. Ayanzen RH, Bird CR, Keller PJ, et al. Cerebral MR venography: normal anatomy and potential diagnostic pitfalls. *AJNR Am J Neuroradiol.* 2000;21:74–78.

294. Gass A, Kitchen N, MacManus DG, et al. Trigeminal neuralgia in patients with multiple sclerosis: lesion localization with magnetic resonance imaging. *Neurology.* 1997;49:1142–1144.

295. Nagata S, Matsushima T, Fujii K, et al. Hemifacial spasm due to tumor, aneurysm, or arteriovenous malformation. *Surg Neurol.* 1992;38:204–209.

296. Jannetta PJ. Neurovascular compression in cranial nerve and systemic disease. *Ann Surg.* 1980;192:518–525.

297. Barker FG 2nd, Jannetta PJ, Bissonette DJ, et al. The long-term outcome of microvascular decompression for trigeminal neuralgia. *N Engl J Med.* 1996;334: 1077–1083.

298. Barker FG 2nd, Jannetta PJ, Bissonette DJ, et al. Microvascular decompression for hemifacial spasm. *J Neurosurg.* 1995;82:201–210.

299. Narai H, Manabe Y, Deguchi K, et al. Isolated abducens nerve palsy caused by vascular compression. *Neurology.* 2000;55:453–454.

300. McLaughlin MR, Jannetta PJ, Clyde BL, et al. Microvascular decompression of cranial nerves: lessons learned after 4400 operations. *J Neurosurg.* 1999;90:1–8.

301. Adler CH, Zimmerman RA, Savino PJ, et al. Hemifacial spasm: evaluation by magnetic resonance imaging and magnetic resonance tomographic angiography. *Ann Neurol.* 1992;32:502–506.

302. Du C, Korogi Y, Nagahiro S, et al. Hemifacial spasm: three-dimensional MR images in the evaluation of neurovascular compression. *Radiology.* 1995;197:227–231.

303. Arbab AS, Nishiyama Y, Aoki S, et al. Simultaneous display of MRA and MPR in detecting vascular compression for trigeminal neuralgia or hemifacial spasm: comparison with oblique sagittal views of MRI. *Eur Radiol.* 2000;10: 1056–1060.

304. Kirsch E, Hausmann O, Kaim A, et al. Magnetic resonance imaging of vertebrobasilar ectasia in trigeminal neuralgia. *Acta Neurochir (Wien).* 1996;138:1295–1298; discussion 1299.

305. Fukuda H, Ishikawa M, Okumura R. Demonstration of neurovascular compression in trigeminal neuralgia and hemifacial spasm with magnetic resonance imaging: comparison with surgical findings in 60 consecutive cases. *Surg Neurol.* 2003;59:93–99; discussion 99–100.

306. Korogi Y, Nagahiro S, Du C, et al. Evaluation of vascular compression in trigeminal neuralgia by 3D time-of-flight MRA. *J Comput Assist Tomogr.* 1995;19:879–884.

307. Akimoto H, Nagaoka T, Nariai T, et al. Preoperative evaluation of neurovascular compression in patients with trigeminal neuralgia by use of three-dimensional reconstruction from two types of high-resolution magnetic resonance imaging. *Neurosurgery.* 2002;51:956–961; discussion 961–962.

308. Yoshino N, Akimoto H, Yamada I, et al. Trigeminal neuralgia: evaluation of neuralgic manifestation and site of neurovascular compression with 3D CISS MR imaging and MR angiography. *Radiology.* 2003;228:539–545.

309. Cha S, Knopp EA, Johnson G, et al. Intracranial mass lesions: dynamic contrast-enhanced susceptibility-weighted echo-planar perfusion MR imaging. *Radiology.* 2002;223:11–29.

310. Wilms G, Bosmans H, Marchal G, et al. Magnetic resonance angiography of supratentorial tumours: comparison with selective digital subtraction angiography. *Neuroradiology.* 1995;37:42–47.

311. Wetzel SG, Cha S, Law M, et al. Preoperative assessment of intracranial tumors with perfusion MR and a volumetric interpolated examination: a comparative study with DSA. *AJNR Am J Neuroradiol.* 2002;23: 1767–1774.

312. Tsuchiya K, Aoki C, Katase S, et al. MR digital subtraction angiography with three-dimensional data acquisition in the diagnosis of brain tumors: preliminary experience. *Magn Reson Imaging.* 2004;22:149–153.

Cervical Vasculature

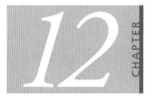

A. Daniel Sasson
Bruce A. Wasserman

Cervical vascular disease is both widespread and highly morbid (1–3). Atherosclerosis of the carotid arteries accounts for the majority of cervical vascular pathology, but the spectrum of disease is broad. It includes vasculitis, trauma, dissection, and congenital vascular pathology such as fibromuscular dysplasia. The most common indications for imaging include a history of transient ischemic attack (TIA), ischemic stroke, or carotid bruit. A history of atherosclerotic disease elsewhere in the body represents an emerging indication for screening the carotid arteries (4).

Several different imaging modalities are commonly used in the evaluation of cervical vascular pathology (5). These include catheter-based digital subtraction angiography (DSA), ultrasonography (US), computed tomographic angiography (CTA), and magnetic resonance angiography (MRA). Each modality has its own particular strengths and limitations (6), though DSA remains the standard against which all other modalities are compared (Fig. 12-1).

In this chapter, we will examine the differences between these modalities, with particular emphasis on CTA and MRA, and their application to different vascular pathologies. By the end of this chapter, the reader should understand the basic principles of CT and MR angiography of the neck, be able to optimize each of these imaging modalities for the assessment of cervical vascular disease, understand their roles in different forms of cervical vascular pathology, and be able to correctly interpret findings on MRA and CTA and compare them with DSA.

IMAGING STRATEGIES

Digital Subtraction Angiography

DSA refers to catheter-based contrast angiography. Routinely performed via common femoral arteriotomy, DSA has many advantages. Of all the available imaging techniques, DSA provides the highest spatial resolution and temporal resolution (TR). It is multiplanar within the limits of rotation of the fluoroscope and can create three-dimensional (3D) images with the use of rotational angiography. Further, DSA provides functional information, including qualitative flow velocity, the presence of arteriovenous shunting, collateral vessel formation, and parenchymal perfusion (7,8).

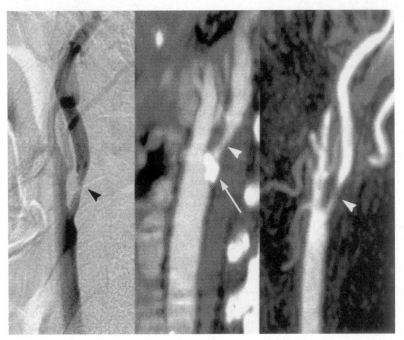

FIGURE 12-1 DSA, CTA, and MRA in the same patient. Oblique digital subtraction (**left**), CT (**middle**), and gadolinium-enhanced MR (**right**) angiograms depict a severe and regular stenosis (*arrowheads*) of the ICA. Note the calcified plaque (*arrow*) on the CT angiogram. (DSA parameters included FOV, 33 cm; matrix, 1,024 × 1,024; spatial resolution, 0.32 × 0.32 mm. CT parameters included FOV, 15 × 15 cm; section thickness, 1 mm; imaging time, 60 seconds. MR parameters included 6/2; signal acquired, 0.5; flip angle, 35 degrees; number of sections, 52; section thickness, 1.6 mm; FOV, 28 × 22 cm; matrix, 256 × 192; imaging time, 32 seconds.) (Adapted from Randoux B, Marro B, Koskas F, et al. Carotid artery stenosis: prospective comparison of CT, three-dimensional gadolinium-enhanced MR, and conventional angiography. *Radiology.* 2001;220:179–185, with permission.)

On the other hand, DSA is also the most expensive and time consuming of the commonly used cervical vascular imaging techniques and has the highest associated procedural risks (9,10). For diagnostic angiography, the risk of stroke ranges from less than 1% to 4%, with a mortality rate of approximately 0.1% (11–14).

Asymptomatic diffusion-weighted imaging (DWI) MRI abnormalities after angiography have been noted and have been seen in up to 26% of cases (15,16). Even higher rates of asymptomatic DWI abnormalities are seen in patients with a pre-existing vasculopathy at the time of DSA (15,16). Further, the neurological complication rates in patients with symptomatic carotid stenosis, a common indication for angiography, have been reported as high as 10% (17).

Though DSA is the standard for carotid endarterectomy (CEA) trials (18–20), it is still an interpreted and qualitative imaging modality. Besides the differences in technique for the measurement of carotid stenosis, the inherent planar nature of DSA can affect interpretation. For example, with the advent of rotational angiography (21), it has been shown that the choice of projection of planar images can over- or underestimate carotid stenosis (22,23) (Figs. 12-2, 12-3).

Ultrasonography

US has developed rapidly as a screening test for carotid stenosis due in part to the superficial location of the cervical carotid arteries as well as the ability to provide functional information with the use of color Doppler and pulsed-wave Doppler imaging (24–26). As a relatively inexpensive (27), rapid, and safe study, US is innocuous to perform. On the other hand, US assessment is operator and equipment dependent.

For the evaluation of carotid stenosis, the diagnosis can be based on grayscale measurements of vessel diameter, which has modest correlation with DSA measurements (28), or on Doppler measurements of carotid artery flow velocity, which is even more prone to technical artifacts than grayscale imaging methods (29–31).

As a stenosis increases in severity to the point where it limits flow, the elevated blood flow velocity will drop. At some point before the vessel occludes, the velocity will fall within the designated normal range and may be interpreted as a false negative (32). Further, in patulous or postendarterectomy carotids, evaluation based solely on velocity measurements can miss the presence of significant atherosclerotic but nonstenotic plaque (33).

While providing a sensitive modality for the detection of carotid stenosis, US remains relatively nonspecific (34,35). Evaluation of the very proximal and distal portions of the carotid arteries, as well as segments of the vertebral arteries, is limited. This can result in a false negative study due to distal stenosis, or ostial stenosis, or failure to detect the presence of a tandem lesion, though the clinical significance of distal tandem carotid lesions is unclear (32,36).

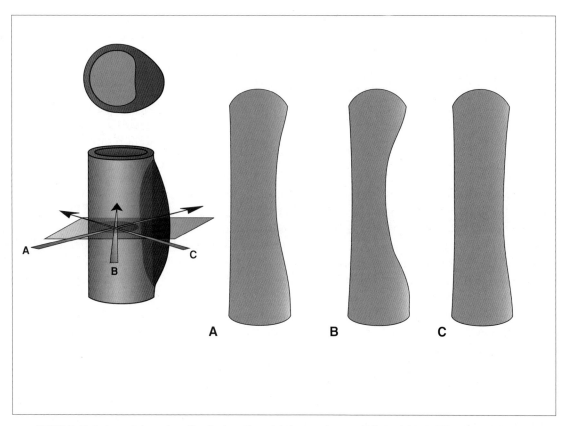

FIGURE 12-2 Stenosis is rarely uniformly circumferential. The complex morphology of the vessel lumen in most areas of stenosis results in different projections **(A–C)** depending on the angle of imaging. In an ovoid stenosis, one projection **(A)** may appear highly stenotic, while another **(C)** may appear almost normal.

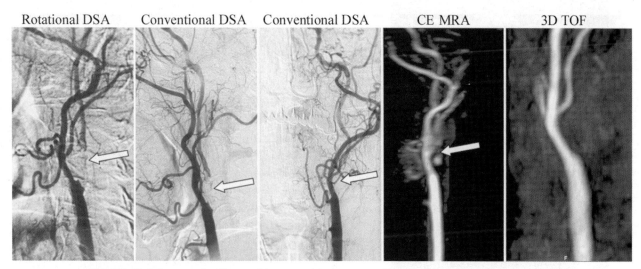

FIGURE 12-3 Images of a 64-year-old woman showing near occlusion of the left internal carotid artery. Minimal slow residual flow (*arrow*), together with normal poststenotic distal ICA, is seen on rotational and conventional DSA projections. CE MRA reveals normal flow in distal ICA and focal intensity (*arrow*) at site of stenosis, which results from delayed contrast material stagnation within possible ulceration. This defect is only partially evident on conventional DSA projection (*arrow*) because of earlier time of acquisition. Later acquisitions demonstrate defect more clearly (*not shown*). On 3D TOF MR angiogram (3D SLINKY MRA), left ICA appears fully occluded. (Reprinted from Anzalone N, Scomazzoni F, Castellano R, et al. Carotid artery stenosis: intraindividual correlations of 3D time-of-flight MR angiography, contrast-enhanced MR angiography, conventional DSA, and rotational angiography for detection and grading. *Radiology.* 2005;236:204–213, with permission.)

Additionally, the presence of large, calcified carotid plaques can cause acoustic shadowing and prevent the adequate evaluation of stenosis (37). The reproducibility of measurements by US is also quite variable (25,35,38).

Due in part to these limitations, US is used more as a screening modality to triage patients for further workup, although some surgeons do operate on the basis of US findings alone (7,25,27).

Computed Tomographic Angiography

CTA of the carotid and vertebral arteries has rapidly evolved over the past decade, especially with the advent of helical multidetector row CT scanners (MDCT). CTA offers several advantages when compared with DSA and other imaging modalities (39). CT technology is widely deployed and readily accessible. MDCT scanners are less widespread but are growing in number. MDCT angiography can be performed at high spatial resolution and is better at detecting calcification than DSA or the MRA techniques used in clinical practice. CTA also provides information about nonvascular structures (Fig. 12-4)

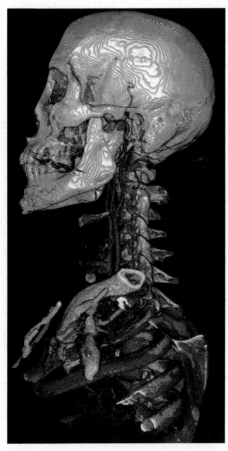

FIGURE 12-4 A volumetric reconstruction of a CTA of the neck demonstrates the detail and coverage of vasculature.

(6,40). In the setting of carotid steno-occlusive disease, CTA is both highly sensitive and specific, with high interobserver reliability and good concordance to both MRA and DSA (7,25). Further, CTA does not suffer from the flow-related artifacts that can affect MRA interpretation.

From a patient safety profile, CTA has a lower complication rate than DSA. Unlike MRA, CTA is not limited by the presence of implanted devices such as cardiac pacemakers. Most patients can tolerate the short scan times of CTA, whereas claustrophobia is a serious limitation of MRA. Patients generally prefer CTA to MRA or DSA from the standpoint of comfort (41). Finally, CTA is less costly than either DSA or MRA (42), though the cost effectiveness for carotid steno-occlusive disease has yet to be established.

There are several disadvantages to the use of CTA in cervical vascular disease. CTA is a contrast-based technique, and thus patients suffer the risk of anaphylactoid contrast reaction or contrast-induced nephrotoxicity (43). CTA using gadolinium as a contrast agent has been described in the carotids (44) and may offer an alternative to iodinated contrast in select patients.

For gadolinium-enhanced CTA, Henson et al. (44) used a 16-detector multisection helical scanner with a 25-second delay after administration of approximately 0.4 mmoL/kg of gadopentetate dimeglumine at 4 mL per second and an 18-gauge cannula followed by a 20-mL normal saline chase. Other parameters for scanning in that study were as follows: 140 kVp, 250 mA, 1.0-second rotation time, 2.5-mm section thickness reconstructed at 1.25-mm intervals, 3.75 mm/rotation table speed, and pitch 0.75:1. A set of images was obtained from the C6 vertebral body level through the circle of Willis followed immediately by a second set of images from the aortic arch through the C6 level.

CTA uses ionizing radiation, and the dose increases with thinner collimation and overlapping slice profiles. The dose of CTA of the carotids is approximately 2 to 3 mSv (200 mrem) (40,45,46). In CTA, the sensitive organs of the neck are the esophagus, thyroid, and skin. The dose to the thyroid, the most radiosensitive of the three, can range from approximately 25 mGy with single detector helical scanners to approximately 75 mGy with MDCT (47,48). When compared with MRA, the postprocessing time required for the generation of 3D images is greater.

The term *computed tomographic angiography* actually encompasses a variety of techniques. Early CT angiograms were performed on single slice "step-and-shoot" scanners. Helical CT scanners, including MDCT, allow for much faster acquisition times and higher spatial resolution (49). This has several advantages: The scan area can be much larger, with less breathing motion artifact; the arterial phase of contrast opacification can be better isolated, with less venous contamination; the dose of contrast required for arterial opacification is reduced; and truly volumetric data sets can be obtained, allowing for 3D image manipulation and postprocessing (49).

Computed Tomographic Angiography Technique

The factors important to achieve acceptable image quality in CT angiography of the cervical vasculature are adequate contrast opacification, minimization of artifacts, and adequate longitudinal or *z*-plane resolution.

Contrast

Although higher intraluminal enhancement may be advantageous (50), the minimum adequate goal for contrast opacification of the arterial system is 150 to 200 Hounsfield Units (HU), with decreased measurement variability above 200 HU (51,52). With this goal in mind, one can adjust the dose, timing, and rate and length of administration of contrast material (CM) to achieve adequate opacification with the minimum dose. To reduce or eliminate venous contamination, the duration of the scan should be short and timed to coincide with the arterial phase of contrast opacification. Approximately 7 seconds are required for recirculation of the intravenous (IV) contrast to reach the arterial compartment in a patient with a normal cardiac output. After that, the arterial attenuation begins to increase. With a uniphasic injector, the attenuation quickly peaks and then fades, resulting in a humplike time-attenuation curve. The ideal time-attenuation curve would be a flat line, with uniform contrast enhancement within a vessel for the duration of the scan. With the use of multiphasic contrast injectors, the time-attenuation curve approaches the ideal plateau, and the issue of timing a scan to coincide with the contrast bolus peak becomes less of an issue (53).

It is important to time the scan precisely in order to minimize the volume of contrast injected and to scan before extensive venous contamination occurs. The three widely used methods are fixed-delay scanning, timing-bolus technique, and bolus tracking (49). *Fixed-delay scanning* simply refers to starting the scan after a standard interval from the beginning of the contrast injection. *Timing bolus*, on the other hand, refers to the use of a separate timing run using a small bolus of contrast and measuring the time of injection to peak enhancement in the region of interest. Bolus tracking combines the timing run and the acquisition in a single scan and is performed by monitoring the time-attenuation curve within a particular vessel after the injection of the CM, with the scan initiated after reaching a particular threshold attenuation.

The enhancement dynamics of contrast administration have been reviewed elsewhere (53), but in short, bolus tracking offers several advantages in the setting of carotid steno-occlusive disease. First, in atherosclerosis, the cardiac output of the patient may not be normal, altering the enhancement dynamics in any individual. Bolus tracking individualizes the contrast timing for each patient. Second, because of individual variability in contrast enhancement, most fixed-delay protocols use longer contrast injection times, increasing the total dose of contrast. This is particularly undesirable, as patients with atherosclerotic disease of the carotids often have impaired renal function. During a scan, the delay between the point at which the attenuation reaches the set threshold and the acquisition of images can range from 4 to 10 seconds, increasing the dose of contrast used and the risk of venous contamination. As a practical step, when the minimization of contrast dose is critical, one can initiate scanning before the time-attenuation curve reaches this threshold by monitoring the curve and initiating the scan when the slope of the attenuation curve abruptly increases, thus decreasing the delay between the start of the scan and the acquisition of the initial images.

For CTA of the carotid arteries, MDCT scanning can cover a field of view from the aortic arch to the skull base in as little as 9 seconds. Because the goal of CTA is not parenchymal enhancement but adequate opacification of the vessel lumen, the dose of contrast can be much less than the often-used 30 to 45 gm of iodine. For a 10-second acquisition performed with a contrast concentration of 350 mg iodine/mL CM, one can use 90 cc injected at 5.0 mL per second, for a total injection time of 18 seconds (53).

The dose can be further reduced by the use of a saline chaser, taking advantage in the recirculation delay to 'push' the contrast through to the arterial system using saline, rather than the tail end of the contrast bolus, which would not reach the arterial system during the scan acquisition. Others (54) have increased the length of the contrast plateau 8 seconds on average with a saline chaser. In this scenario, the total contrast volume would be reduced to 50 cc, for a total iodine dose of 17.7 g, yet it would still maintain the iodine flux of 1.8 g per second for the duration of the scan. Faster scanners can potentially reduce the dose further, though timing becomes more critical, and the potential contrast dose reduction can be offset by the risk of acquiring a nondiagnostic scan. Rather, faster scanners can be used to achieve greater longitudinal resolution for a given scan time or to include the intracranial circulation within the same scan time.

From a practical standpoint, injection rates of 5 to 6 cc per second mandate the placement of a large bore (at least 20 gauge) IV catheter. Ideally, a lower extremity vein should be used, as upper extremity IV injection will result in streak artifact at the level of the brachiocephalic veins; however, this is impractical. The antecubital fossa is the preferred site of IV access.

Artifacts

Several basic steps reduce the amount of artifact in CTA of the cervical vessels. While motion artifact is diminished with the use of rapid scanning technologies, breath holding will reduce motion, especially at the level of the aortic arch. Similarly, instructions to the patient to refrain from swallowing during the scan will reduce artifact. Cardiac pulsation is not a significant source of motion artifact in the cervical vasculature.

Streak artifact in CTA of the neck comes from several sources. While it should go without saying, the arms should be placed at the patient's side for the scan. For combined scans of the body and neck, we advocate split-bolus scanning with repositioning of the arms rather than scanning the entire neck and body in one setting. Streak artifact from the shoulders can be minimized with patient positioning or the use of a shoulder girdle, if necessary.

Artifacts from dental amalgam can be reduced with either neck extension or angling of the gantry to throw off the artifact from the vessels (52,55). With thin-collimation volumetric scanning, reformatted true axial images can be created despite oblique scan planes. This technique can also be used in cases of suboptimal patient positioning.

Streak artifact from dense IV contrast at the level of the subclavian and brachiocephalic veins can be managed by using a lower extremity vein when possible, the use of a saline chaser, and injection of the arm contralateral to suspected pathology (56,57).

Generally, the neck should be scanned in the cranial to caudal direction, which can minimize streak artifact at the brachiocephalic vein, at the risk of venous contamination or breathing motion near the arch. Scanning in the caudal to cranial direction can be performed if a multiphasic contrast injector is not available in order to follow the contrast bolus and avoid excessive variability in the degree of luminal enhancement. Further, with caudocranial scanning, any difficulty with maintaining breath hold should not affect imaging.

Another source of artifact in CTA is the variability in the appearance of a contrast-enhanced vessel with different window and level settings (57–59). This variability is not solely limited to CTA; however, practically it is less of a factor with MRA and DSA. Liu et al. (59) made over 25,000 measurements of vessel caliber in phantoms, using both transverse and maximum-intensity projection (MIP) images. The optimal window and level settings for mea-surement of vessels caliber were found to vary with the degree of luminal opacification and whether transverse or MIP images were examined. It is important to be consistent with whichever display settings are used.

Longitudinal Resolution

Longitudinal resolution, or CT section thickness, is determined by the collimation of the scanner. Helical CT scanners can acquire angiographic images of the neck at 1- to 2-mm slice thickness in 15 to 25 seconds. MDCT scanners can obtain much thinner and essentially isotropic data with much shorter scan times. Higher resolution imaging can provide information for plaque characterization and more accurate assessment of stenosis of the carotid and the origin of the vertebral arteries (Fig. 12-5). With high-resolution imaging, one can potentially visualize dissection flaps, or mural irregularities in the setting of vasculitis. For most purposes, 1- to 2-mm axial reconstructed images provide sufficient diagnostic detail. For the creation of source images for 3D postprocessing, one should use the thinnest possible reconstruction that the collimator settings allow, with 50% overlapping reconstruction, to reduce noise and stair-step artifact (49,57).

CT protocols should be designed based on different clinical priorities. For a given scanner, the section thickness will be inversely proportional to the scan length for a given pitch and longitudinal field of view. Routinely, one may use the thinnest available collimation for the scanner and adjust the pitch (generally between 1 and 2), scan time, mA, and contrast volume appropriately (54). The extracranial circulation, from the aortic arch to the skull base, can be scanned at very thin collimation in a reasonable amount of time, without an excessive contrast dose. If the intracranial circulation is to be included, one can increase the section

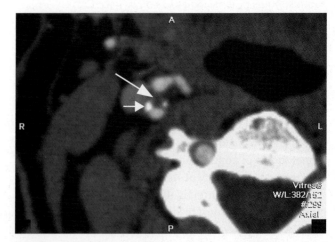

FIGURE 12-5 Axial source image from a CTA shows fatty (*long arrow*) and calcified (*short arrow*) portions of a carotid artery plaque.

thickness for the cervical scan to include the head within the larger scanned area without lengthening the scan time. Some representative scan protocols for different CT scanners can be found online at *www.ctisus.com*. For the patient in whom contrast dose is an issue, the scan time can be adjusted to minimize total contrast dose, with the collimation adjusted proportionately.

Magnetic Resonance Angiography

Sequence Strategies

While an in-depth discussion of the principles underlying the major MRA techniques can be found in Chapter 2, a brief review of the most salient principles and implications is provided herein.

Time-of-flight Imaging

Time-of-flight (TOF) imaging, which is based on differences in the excitation history between flowing protons in blood and the stationary protons in background tissues, can be performed as a two-dimensional (2D) technique, or as a 3D volumetric acquisition. Two-dimensional imaging is rapid but subject to stair-step artifacts due to motion between repeated acquisitions of adjacent slices to cover the area of interest (Fig. 12-6).

TOF imaging with 3D technique offers the ability to achieve a smaller voxel size, resulting in higher resolution, as compared with 2D TOF. However, the smaller voxels result in lower signal-to-noise ratio (SNR), and the use of a larger imaging volume predisposes the technique to signal loss from saturation effects. In addition, 3D imaging offers a shorter allowable echo time (TE), which can minimize signal losses from phase dispersion.

Phase Contrast Imaging

Phase contrast (PC) imaging uses two gradients of equal strength but opposite polarity (a bipolar gradient) to induce a phase change in excited protons. In stationary tissue, the bipolar gradient has no net effect, but in moving blood, the protons acquire a net phase change proportional to the velocity of the blood. PC can thus measure flow velocity as well as directionality. Technical limitations and issues related to scan time limit the clinical application of this technique for cervical arterial disease. In this capacity, PC techniques are largely focused on providing scout information for planning other MRA acquisitions and for showing flow direction, as when subclavian steal physiology is suspected.

Contrast-enhanced Imaging

Contrast-enhanced magnetic resonance angiography (CE MRA) refers to the injection of an intravascular

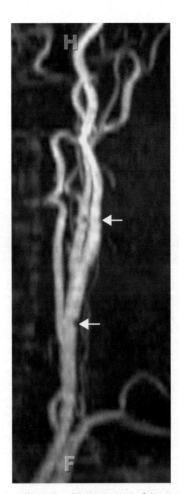

FIGURE 12-6 Two-dimensional TOF MRA MIP of the carotid artery demonstrate stair-step artifact (*arrows*).

contrast agent, typically a chelate of gadolinium, to shorten the T1 of blood and thus provide contrast against surrounding tissue. As with CTA, several techniques can be used to time the administration of contrast and to achieve arterial selectively: A fixed delay time, a timing run, an acquisition triggered off detecting the arrival of contrast, and temporally resolved strategies can all be employed.

Fixed delays are limited by the wide range of circulation times among patients, causing marked differences in the time to peak enhancement and the most vulnerability to venous contamination. Time-resolved imaging (e.g., time-resolved imaging of contrast kinetics [TRICKS]) increases the likelihood of obtaining an arterial phase image but may still benefit from a timing run. Generally, for all these techniques, a noncontrast image is obtained to use as a mask for subtraction.

Black Blood Imaging

Black blood imaging can provide complementary information to TOF and CE MRA. This technique is particularly useful for assessing atherosclerotic plaque (Fig. 12-7). A

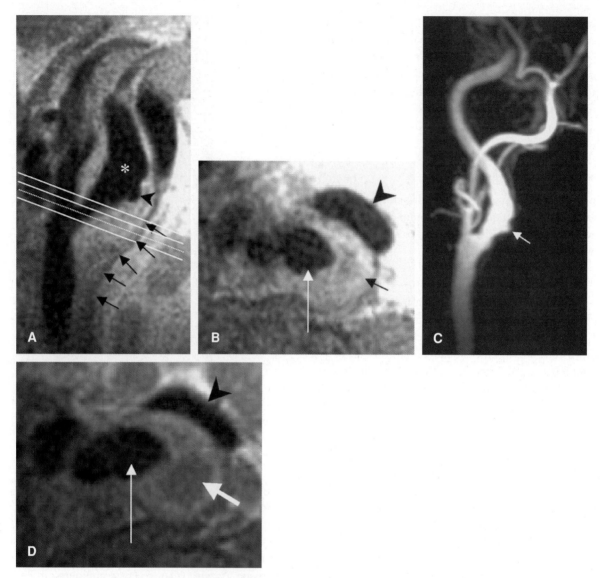

FIGURE 12-7 High-resolution MRI examination from December 2001 of the left carotid artery of a 67-year-old man with hyperlipidemia and left cerebral ischemic events beginning in August 2001. A: Long-axis black blood MRI image through the carotid bifurcation reveals a large plaque along the outer wall of the bulb (*long arrows*) narrowing the ICA lumen (*) with a small ulceration along its distal margin (*arrowhead*). **B:** Double-oblique black blood MRI image oriented through the plaque as shown in (**A**) (*dotted line,* **A**) demonstrates outward expansion of the plaque (*black arrow*) with compression of the adjacent jugular vein (*arrowhead*) and relative preservation of the ICA lumen (*white arrow*) corroborated by the insignificant narrowing seen on the CE MRA MIP. **C:** The small ulceration is again seen on the CE MRA MIP (*arrow*). **D:** Follow-up black blood MRI from July 2002 in the same orientation as the slice shown in (**B**) demonstrates slight expansion of the plaque (*thick arrow*) with continued preservation of the ICA lumen (*thin arrow*) and increasing compression of the adjacent jugular vein (*arrowhead*). (Adapted from Wasserman BA, Wityk RJ, Trout HH 3rd, Virmani R. Low-grade carotid stenosis: looking beyond the lumen with MRI. *Stroke.* 2005;36:2504–2513, with permission.)

common approach to black blood imaging is to use a double-inversion pulse to null signal from flowing blood (33). As such, it is less susceptible to dephasing effects and can help to confirm lumen patency when this effect is present.

Artifact and Signal Loss

Two major sources of artifact and signal loss in MRA are saturation effects and phase dispersion. The different MRA techniques have their own particular strengths and weakness is as well as differing susceptibility to the saturation and dephasing effects.

Saturation Effects

Slower blood protons may become saturated and lead to a signal loss that is caused by the acquisition and not necessarily the vessel morphology. This effect is important for clinical assessment in that it can cause near-occlusive stenosis to appear as complete occlusion.

A similar phenomenon is noted in areas where blood recirculates, crossing the excitation slice repeatedly, as in the carotid bulb. This effect also can be seen from recirculation of blood flow within an ulcer crater. As well, this is the basis for signal dropout from in-plane blood flow: When blood is flowing parallel to the imaging plane rather than perpendicular to it, the blood will be within the imaging slice for a longer period of time, resulting in loss of signal.

Such saturation effects can be minimized by making the imaging slice thinner (decreasing the z) or to increase the TR to prolong the time between excitation pulses, minimizing the number of pulses experienced by the protons when traversing the slice. The ability to obtain a thin z (and increase the sensitivity to demonstrating slow flow) relative to 3D techniques represents an important advantage of 2D imaging. However, a z reduction will require more slices to cover a similar anatomic area of interest and has the potential to increase sensitivity to motion and, thus, stair-step artifacts. Prolonging the TR is problematic, as this will decrease the degree to which the signal from background stationary tissue is suppressed.

MOTSA (multiple overlapping thin-slab acquisition) is a 3D technique that uses a relatively thin-slab thickness to minimize signal loss from saturation while maintaining the advantages of 3D imaging. The saturation effect is less pronounced than with standard 3D imaging, though more pronounced than with the thinner slices used for 2D imaging. TONE (titled optimized nonsaturating excitation), also referred to as *ramped excitation*, is another technique used to reduce signal loss from saturation, which uses a variable flip angle to reduce the saturating effect of the excitation pulse as protons enter the image volume.

The use of gadolinium contrast in CE MRA offers a very effective means of reducing proton magnetization saturation by shortening the T1 of the blood pool. This allows for the use of thick-slab acquisitions without the consequence of saturation. Therefore, a very large field of view (FOV) can be acquired parallel to the vessels of interest, such as a coronal acquisition to cover the aortic arch to the intracranial extent of the cervical arteries without signal loss from in-plane flow (Fig. 12-8). An important advantage of this expanded coverage is that it enables assessment of tandem lesions. It also nullifies the consequent drop in signal when acquiring smaller voxels with 3D imaging.

Phase Dispersion

Phase dispersion, also referred to as *dephasing artifact*, is another source of signal loss in MRA. One solution to phase dispersion artifact is to decrease the size of the voxel

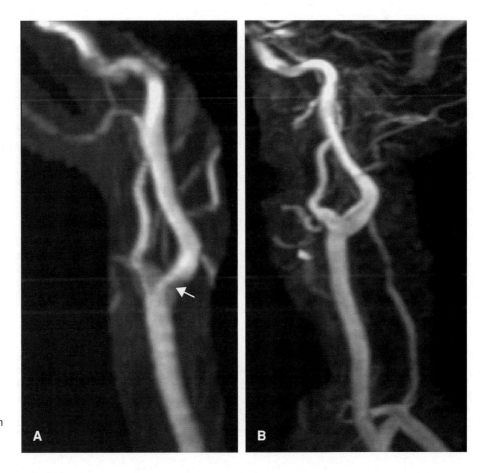

FIGURE 12-8 MRA MIPs of the carotid artery using 2D TOF **(A)** and 3D CE **(B)** techniques. Both techniques minimize saturation effects and allow for increased superior-inferior coverage, though some signal loss is seen in an area of recirculation (*arrow*) that fills in following contrast administration.

so that each voxel contains a smaller range of velocities of flowing blood protons. The smaller distribution of velocities will result in less intravoxel signal loss from dephasing. Furthermore, the phase change is also dependent on the TE, so another approach to decreasing the dephasing artifact is to decrease this parameter. TOF imaging using a 3D technique offers smaller voxels than are generally achievable with 2D techniques. That reduces signal loss from dephasing effects with further benefits from the shorter TE values also achievable relative to 2D imaging. Administering gadolinium compensates for the signal loss in 3D imaging from the saturation effects described earlier while compensating for signal losses from dephasing.

Flow compensation gradients, also known as *gradient moment nulling* (GMN), are refocusing gradients that can be applied to correct for spin dephasing in flowing blood. Phase dispersion from protons flowing at higher orders of velocity can be effectively refocused to recover lost signal by application of more complex gradients, though this is at the expense of longer echo times, which begins to counteract the reduction of dephasing.

It is clear that CE MRA can minimize signal loss from saturation by reducing the T1 relaxation of the entire blood pool, and it can be acquired using a 3D

sequence so that dephasing effects are reduced but the accompanying reduction in signal due to the smaller voxel size and thicker z of 3D imaging is no longer problematic. One might suspect that a TOF MRA sequence is not necessary if a CE MRA is acquired; however, a TOF sequence can complement a contrast study with several added benefits.

The CE MRA is generally acquired as a coronal slab so that a large area can be imaged in order to evaluate for tandem lesions, but the large FOV in the z-direction minimizes the resolution in this plane (Fig. 12-9). A TOF MRA that focuses on the carotid bifurcation allows for a more detailed depiction of stenosis if present because of the smaller FOV in this direction. Furthermore, CE MRA has been shown to overestimate stenosis relative to TOF techniques (60) (Fig. 12-10). Finally, an inadequate CE MRA study is difficult to repeat because of venous contamination and gadolinium dose limitations, so acquiring a TOF MRA prior to contrast administration can serve as a fail-safe measure.

Three-dimensional Postprocessing

Three-dimensional postprocessed images are an essential part of interpretation of MRA and CTA of the

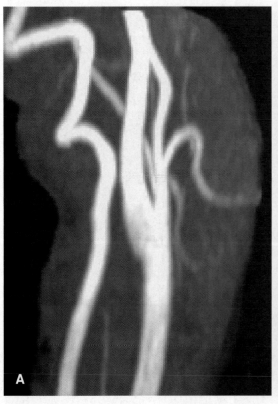
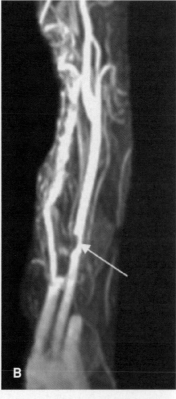

FIGURE 12-9 MRA MIPs of the carotid artery using 3D TOF (**A**) and 3D CE (**B**) techniques. While the TOF technique is more accurate for measuring stenosis, the longer scanning time limits the FOV. In this example, the 3D TOF MRA appears normal, but a proximal stenosis, likely from a focal dissection (*arrow*), is evident on the CE image.

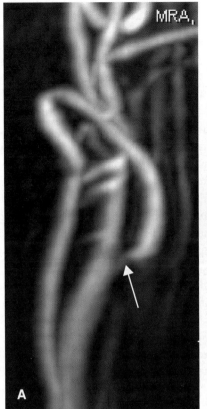
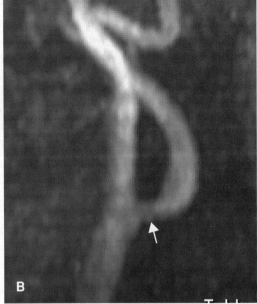

FIGURE 12-10 MRA MIPs of the carotid artery using 3D CE **(A)** and 3D TOF **(B)** techniques. Stenosis is overestimated on the 3D CE-MRA compared with a 3D TOF technique (*arrows*).

cervical vasculature. The essential tools for analysis are multiplanar reformations (MPR), curved planar reformations (CPR), MIP images, and volume-rendered (VR) images (49).

MPR images allow a global overview of the cervical vasculature by examining the coronal and sagittal reformations. MPR axial images can be used to account for obliquity in the scan plane or for tortuous vessels. If it is important to obtain accurate luminal diameters, one must use MPR images to create "double-orthogonal" axial images. Double-orthogonal axial images are created from an axial MPR that is perpendicular to both coronal and sagittal MPR.

CPR images allow one to lay out a tortuous or curving vessel that cannot be imaged in a single plane, however oblique (56). These images can help to visualize a point of narrowing in a vessel. On the other hand, if the center line of the CPR is not in the center of the vessel, one can create an artifactual stenosis. Automated techniques for vessel tracking are now available, with good performance (50,61–65). Again, it is important to examine source images to avoid misinterpretation due to closely adjacent vessels, which can be minimized by reduction of venous opacification (57).

Both MPR and CPR typically refer to planar reformations of an axial data set. MIP refers to the method of displaying data from multiple contiguous planar sections, in this case referring specifically to the highest signal voxel or highest attenuation pixel in a projection of multiple contiguous sections. MIP images are best utilized in combination with either MPR or CPR and have particular utility in carotid imaging.

MIP images are usually easier to create with MRA images, as the signal from the vessel is usually much higher than the background soft tissue. Because MIP images will display the highest attenuation pixel within the selected volume, it is important in CTA to specify a slab that does not include skeletal structures. This can be difficult, especially in evaluation of the vertebral arteries. When this is not possible, one can utilize postprocessing techniques to subtract bone from the image.

For CTA, the attenuation between the enhanced vessel lumen and bone should be distinct enough to allow for segmentation based on attenuation alone (66). Many commercially available 3D postprocessing workstations allow one to select bone, and the software will then subtract out contiguous pixels within the attenuation range specified, leaving discontinuous structures, such as carotid plaque, intact. Alternatively, some advocate the use of a precontrast scan as a mask image for subtraction (66–68).

ASSESSMENT OF STENOSIS

Carotid stenosis is one of the main indications for noninvasive imaging of the neck, either for initial diagnosis or for preoperative assessment, and its assessment is critical for management decisions. Carotid stenosis is quantified on DSA by taking the narrowest luminal measurement of at least two orthogonal projections as a fraction of either the estimated normal luminal diameter at the same level (European Carotid Surgery Trial [ECST]) (19) or by the measured luminal diameter at the next distal diseasefree segment (North American Symptomatic Carotid Endarterectomy Trial [NASCET]; Asymptomatic Carotid Atherosclerosis Study [ACAS]) (18,20) (Fig. 12-11).

For both MRA and CTA, the degree of carotid stenosis should be reported in a way that replicates the measurements used during the NASCET, ECST, and ACAS trials. That is, one should recreate a pseudo-DSA projection using both oblique sagittal and oblique coronal MPR projections that include an MIP of the entire carotid diameter in the projected volume (Fig. 12-12).

Postprocessing methods may be required prior to the creation of the MPR images in those cases where calcification or skeletal structures obscure the lumen on MIP images.

Despite the use of 2D measurements as standards for guiding therapy, the residual lumen of atherosclerotic stenosis is a complex 3D structure (69,70). While the degree of carotid stenosis is reported as a fraction of normal vessel diameter, flow reduction is more a function of absolute vessel caliber (4,70). As the residual lumen drops below 1 mm, the carotid distal to the stenosis will constrict, resulting in diffuse narrowing and asymmetry of the distal carotids on axial images. This finding can be used as an indirect sign of severe stenosis proximal to the point of imaging (4). On flow-dependent MRA techniques, signal dropout has been used as a marker of significant (>70%) stenosis, though in some series, close to 14% of flow voids on TOF imaging were noted in stenosis less than 70% (71) and can vary with imaging parameters (4).

Both CTA and MRA have been variously reported to under- (41,72–79) or overestimate (6,41,60,71,72,74–77, 79–85) the degree of carotid stenosis.

However, meta-analyses (7) have not found any systematic tendency to over- or underestimate carotid stenosis in CTA. The accuracy of MRA is more dependent on the particular technique used (60,71,86,87).

Specifically, TOF imaging has been reported to overestimate stenosis compared with DSA, and CE MRA has been reported to overestimate stenosis with respect to TOF imaging, while black blood imaging may be more

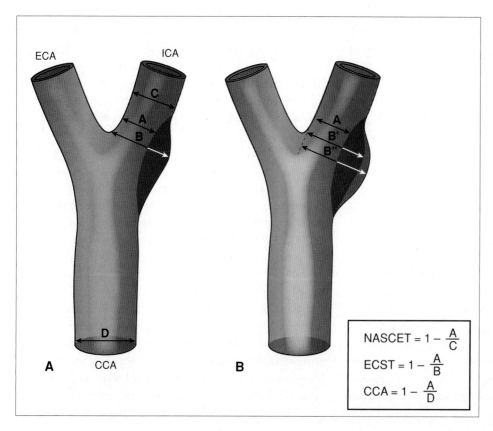

$$NASCET = 1 - \frac{A}{C}$$

$$ECST = 1 - \frac{A}{B}$$

$$CCA = 1 - \frac{A}{D}$$

FIGURE 12-11 Demonstration of the different methodologies for measuring carotid stenosis. **A:** NACSET, ECST, and CCA measurements. The ECST measurement relies on estimation of the outer wall diameter (*B*) at the point of greatest narrowing. **B:** Underestimation of plaque burden can occur using the ECST method since the outer wall remodels (*B'*) during plaque formation. (ECA, external carotid artery; ICA, internal carotid artery; CCA, common carotid artery.)

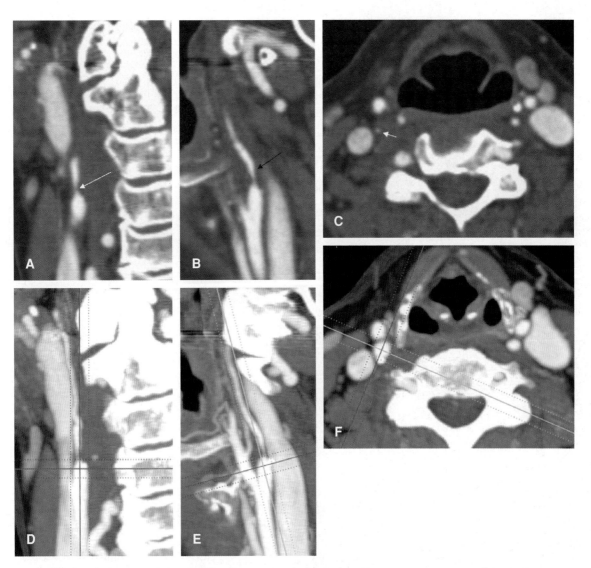

FIGURE 12-12 CTA can be presented as thin-section multiplanar reformations or as MIPs. To recreate the projections obtained on DSA, one must create an MIP that includes the entire vessel within the slab. In cases of eccentric stenosis, a thin-section reformation may appear normal if the slice does not include the area of stenosis. Oblique coronal **(A)**, oblique sagittal **(B)**, and axial **(C)** thin-section MPR images of a stenosis (*arrows*). Cross hairs demonstrating the width of the MIP slabs are shown for these orientations in **(D)**, **(E)**, and **(F)**. The axial image **(F)** is slightly proximal to the area of stenosis **(C)** to demonstrate the vessel diameter at the site of reconstruction. (*Figure 12-12 continues*)

accurate in representing stenosis on axial images (60,88,89). Others (71) have argued that MRA does not overestimate stenosis compared with DSA if appropriate projections are chosen.

One other consideration is the imaging of vessels that have undergone stenting. Both MRA and CTA will suffer from artifacts from stents. MRI-incompatible stents may demonstrate complete dropout of signal along the stented segment of vessel. Thin-section CTA can visualize the contents of a stented vessel, though the stent will cause streak artifact (Figs. 12-13, 12-14). Both Trossbach et al. (90) and Hahnel et al. (91) have examined small stents with CTA and have found that CTA will overestimate the degree of in-stent

stenosis, and that CTA cannot reliably determine patency of a stent smaller than 4 mm in diameter.

There has been extensive debate in the literature concerning the appropriate use of noninvasive imaging methods in the evaluation of carotid stenosis (74,92–95). The debate centers on the accuracy of noninvasive imaging techniques, including CTA and MRA, in the determination of stenosis severity for potential CEA. Some (94,96) have noted that an inappropriate classification of a patient's carotid disease as surgical would result in a 20 times greater risk of disabling stroke. This calculation was based on the assumption of a 2% risk of disabling stroke from carotid endarterectomy in the NASCET trial and 0.1% risk of

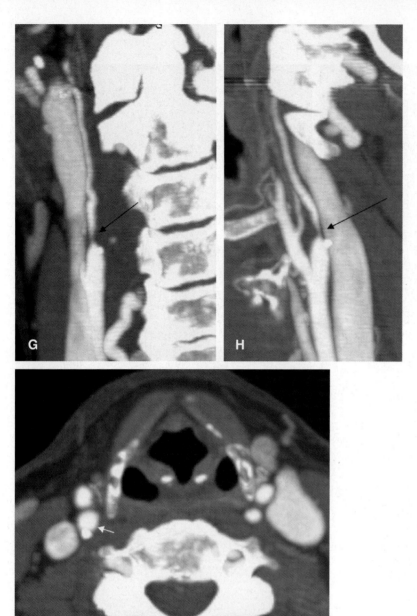

FIGURE 12-12 Continued Oblique coronal (G), oblique sagittal (H), and axial (I) thick-slab MIPs of the stenosis (arrows) with the MIP volumes, including the entire vessel.

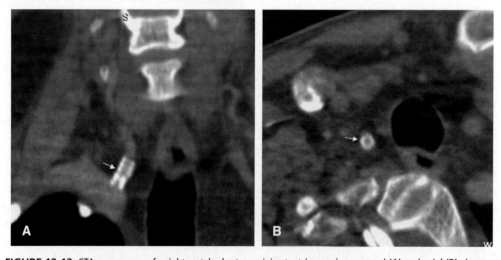

FIGURE 12-13 CTA appearance of a right vertebral artery origin stent (arrows) on coronal (A) and axial (B) views. Despite artifact from the stent, the vessel can be seen to be patent.

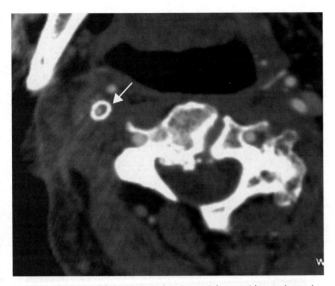

FIGURE 12-14 Axial CTA image showing a right carotid stent (*arrow*). Despite the artifact, the vessel appears to be patent, though there is a suggestion of in-stent restenosis.

disabling stroke from DSA performed during the NASCET trial. The converse, misclassification of an individual's carotid disease as nonsurgical, could result in an increased risk of disabling stroke on best medical therapy alone (36).

The debate revolves around several assumptions that should be examined carefully. The first is the definition of the terms *computed tomographic angiography* (CTA) and *magnetic resonance angiography* (MRA). Unfortunately, the techniques described in the literature for both modalities vary widely, with equally variable clinical accuracies, as described earlier. Certainly, there should be standard minimum acceptable technical criteria for the performance of any noninvasive angiographic method, regardless of location.

Some (10,74,75,97) have argued that the literature results for noninvasive imaging of carotid disease reflect best possible clinical practice and cannot be replicated in the community. In most cases, the methods described here do not require special technology, just attention to technique, and as such are easily achievable by practitioners outside of academic settings.

For example, one study (74) comparing community MRA technique with DSA utilized CE MRA, but with a much higher section thickness and thus lower resolution. These results cannot be taken as the highest practically achievable quality of MRA, even in the community setting. One can speculate that the techniques in the community may be tailored for speed and throughput rather than resolution; however, one must remember that the scan time, postprocessing time, and interpretation time are much less than the time required for cerebral angiography. This is especially true of faster techniques, such as CTA, or dedicated vascular imaging MRI protocols.

Similarly, the operative risks for CEA are the ideal (98). The NASCET contributors, for example, excluded approximately one third of the applicants for participation based on their "track record" (20,36). Regarding risk of disabling stroke, the complication rates of CEA are likely higher than those reported. Specifically, surgery in asymptomatic carotid stenosis is only justified if the operative stroke risk is less than 3% (98). Further, best medical therapy now includes medications not available during the studies, including statins, which may lower risk of stroke even further.

A full discussion of the risks of stroke in CEA versus medical therapy is beyond the scope of this chapter. The point to remember is that, assuming a higher surgical complication rate and a potentially more effective medical therapy, misclassification of a nonsurgical lesion as a surgical one may also have severe consequences.

On the other hand, should the goal for noninvasive evaluation of carotid stenosis be the reproduction of DSA measurements exactly? The CEA trials (NASCET, ECST, and ACAS) all used DSA as a standard. Again, DSA is an interpreted imaging modality. As such, it also suffers from interobserver variability (99–105), variability related to technique (e.g., multiple oblique projections vs. single projection vs. rotational angiography) (23), and variable validity compared with pathology specimens (106,107).

For example, interobserver variability is quite low for severe (70% or greater) carotid stenosis but increases as the severity of stenosis decreases. The variability between observer measurements can approach 9%, certainly enough to change one's classification of a surgical lesion to a nonsurgical lesion, or vice versa. Thus, the same arguments about the risk of misclassification can be made about the "gold standard" test.

Further, the risk of misclassification, multiplied by the lifetime risk of stroke for underclassification of stenosis, or by the surgical risk for overclassification, has to be compared with the procedural risk of DSA in the setting of carotid atherosclerotic disease.

As with many debates in medicine, the devil is in the details. One can come to quite different conclusions regarding CTA or MRA versus DSA depending on the different techniques used, differing rates of complication from DSA and CEA, interobserver reliability, and many other criteria.

We feel that the literature supports the contention that CTA and MRA both are sensitive, specific, and highly accurate in the detection of carotid stenosis. Comparison between invasive and noninvasive methods in carotid stenosis will remain a discussion of apples and oranges, and unless one advocates DSA on all potential CEA patients, there will be a measurable false-positive and false-negative detection rate compared with the CEA trial standards, however small.

It is not unreasonable to suggest the use of multiple imaging modalities when results of a single test are at the edge of significance, as others (4,25,74,78,85,108,109) have noted lower misclassification rates with the use of multiple, concordant imaging modalities. Ultimately, a study is needed examining medical versus surgical or endovascular intervention using CTA or MRA as imaging standards.

NORMAL ANATOMY

The anatomy of the cervical vasculature can be quite variable. Knowledge of some of the more common variations is important for accurate diagnosis and communication to surgeons and interventionalists.

The carotid and vertebral arteries develop from the fusion of several different embryologic arteries. The cervical portion of the carotid arteries originates from multiple branchial arches (110), while the vertebral artery is the remnant of longitudinal collaterals running between the seven cervical intersegmental arteries that have since regressed (110–113).

As a consequence of the embryogenesis of the cephalic great vessels, one should remain aware of the variable origin of the carotid and vertebral arteries (110,114–116). There especially are many potential variants in the origin of the vertebral arteries (111,117–122). The most commonly encountered is an aortic arch origin of the left vertebral artery.

The genesis of the vertebral artery from the fusion of multiple intersegmental arteries allows for the development of fenestrations (113) and duplications (123). The size of the vertebral artery is variable, as it may be hypoplastic and supply only the PICA, or it may be completely absent (112).

Communication can occur between the cervical and vertebral arteries at several levels in the neck via normal variant anastamoses. A persistent proatlantal artery can communicate between the internal or external carotid artery and the vertebral artery. Persistent hypoglossal arteries can communicate between the internal carotid artery (ICA) and the vertebral artery, traveling through the hypoglossal canal (110,124,125). The relative rarity of macroscopic arterial communication is mirrored by the innumerable microscopic anastamoses that are present between the carotid and vertebral artery (126). These microscopic connections can grow and provide significant flow to offset slowly progressive steno-occlusive disease (127,128).

The variability of the level of the carotid bifurcation is one of the better-known anatomic variants. The carotid bifurcation usually occurs at the level of the superior border

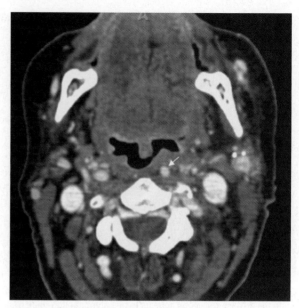

FIGURE 12-15 CE CT demonstrating medial deviation of the left ICA (*arrow*) behind the pharyngeal mucosa at the level of the oropharynx. This anatomic variant should be reported as a guide to avoid iatrogenic injury during certain oropharyngeal surgeries.

of the thyroid cartilage, though it occurs at a higher level in up to 25% of cases (129). Variability in the branching pattern of the carotid bifurcation also can be seen, with external carotid branches such as the ascending pharyngeal, superior thyroid, or the occipital originating from the ICA or from the common carotid artery (CCA) directly (115,128,130). The ICAs also can deviate medially behind the pharyngeal mucosa and should be reported to avoid potential complications during surgery (Fig. 12-15).

Due to the embryology of the carotid artery, fenestrations are quite rare, though they have been described (131). Much more common are pseudofenestrations that actually represent dissection (132,133). Other rare variants include congenital hypoplasia or aplasia of the cervical carotid (131) and separate origins of the internal and external carotid from the aortic arch (114).

Tortuosity and kinking of the cervical carotid artery can be the result of persistent redundancy from embryologic development, particularly when seen in infants and children. However, carotid coils and kinks can be seen as an acquired degenerative disorder associated with atherosclerosis and hypertension and will be discussed in more depth later in this chapter.

CERVICAL VASCULAR DISEASE

Atherosclerosis

Atherosclerosis is a major cause of cervical vascular disease and is a significant cause of stroke morbidity and mortality in the United States. Atherosclerotic cerebrovascular disease accounts for 20% of strokes nationwide (1,134–137). The risk factors for atherosclerosis in the extracranial carotid artery are similar to those for atherosclerosis elsewhere in the body and include hypertension, hyperlipidemia, smoking, and diabetes mellitus (136,138,139).

The prevalence of large vessel atherosclerosis can differ with respect to age, race, or sex. Wityk et al. (139) found a twofold higher rate of extracranial atherosclerosis in white individuals compared with black individuals. White patients also were more likely to have a tandem intracranial lesion. No significant sex differences were found in that study. In contrast, others (2,3,140) found higher rates of carotid atherosclerosis in men than women, with differences disappearing after menopause. In a study of Asian patients, Suwanwela and Chutinetr (138) found that 98% of individuals with cervical atherosclerosis had intracranial atherosclerotic disease.

Kiechl and Willeit (2) noted two distinct patterns of atherosclerotic progression in the carotid artery. The first is described as "diffuse dilative," without a predilection for particular regions of the carotid and characterized by a slowly progressive, nonstenotic course. The second, a "focal stenotic" pattern, was more likely to result in carotid stenosis, particularly at the carotid bulb. This pattern had a more punctuated course, with episodes of rapid progression intermixed with periods of stability. The focal stenotic pattern was more often associated with hypercoagulable states versus the diffuse dilative pattern, which was associated with typical atherosclerotic risk factors. Atherosclerotic disease of the cervical vertebral arteries usually manifests as ostial stenosis (141).

While it can occur anywhere, atherosclerotic plaque has a predilection for certain sites within the cervical vasculature. In the cervical carotid artery, plaque formation tends to occur along the outer wall of the carotid bulb opposite the flow divider (Figs. 12-16, 12-17). Intimal-medial thickening, a precursor to atherosclerotic plaque formation, occurs as a compensatory response to decreased shear stress at these sites due to the alterations in flow dynamics from division of flowing blood at the bifurcation and recirculation of blood at the bulb (142,143).

Vascular remodeling may be a source of discrepancy between CTA or MRA and DSA in the setting of atherosclerosis. Again, as a "luminogram," DSA does not provide direct information about vessel-wall thickness. With early atherosclerosis, vessel-wall thickening may be offset by vascular dilation (140,143,144), resulting in an essentially normal conventional angiogram. Stenosis only becomes evident as the atherosclerotic plaque buildup exceeds the ability of the vessel to compensate (140,145) (Fig. 12-18).

Plaque ulceration is a complex process that requires chronic increase in shear stress at sites of stenosis and sud-

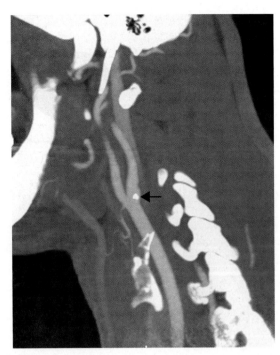

FIGURE 12-16 Multiplanar reconstruction of a CTA through the long axis of the left carotid artery showing a minimally calcified plaque of the carotid bulb (*arrow*).

den changes in intra-arterial pressure; it is invariably associated with activated macrophages and T lymphocytes (146–149). Ulceration represents an important substrate from which thrombus and symptoms may later arise (150). Thrombus, superimposed on ulceration, appears to be important for production of brain ischemia and serves as a key source of cerebral microemboli (151).

Indeed, carotid plaque ulceration is more prevalent in plaques taken from the surgical specimens of symptomatic patients (149). Plaque ulceration and lumen thrombus are

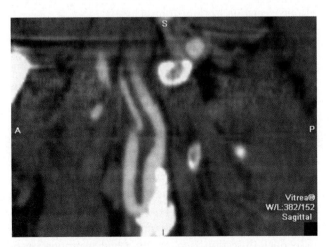

FIGURE 12-17 Multiplanar reconstruction of a CTA through the long axis of the carotid artery showing a highly calcified plaque of the carotid bulb.

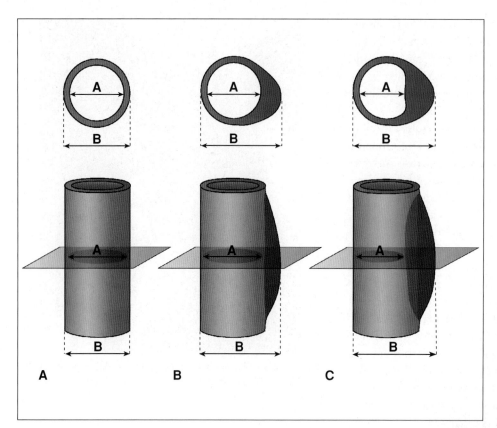

FIGURE 12-18 On luminal studies, such as DSA, compensatory remodeling of the artery may mask early stenosis. As stenosis begins to occur, the vessel will dilate to maintain the lumen (**A**), while the overall vessel diameter (**B**) will increase. Stenosis will be evident angiographically only when the plaque or wall thickening has exceeded the compensatory ability of the vessel.

the main sources of cerebral microemboli in high-grade ICA stenosis (151).

The ability to angiographically depict plaque ulceration thus would seem to carry with it important implications (Fig. 12-19). While ulceration of a symptomatic carotid stenosis as demonstrated with intra-arterial contrast angiography has been shown to be a strong independent predictor of stroke (152,153), the correlation between angiography and surgical observation in detecting carotid plaque ulceration has limitations (154).

CTA and MRA provide unique perspectives that might show ulcerations not seen with conventional angiography and can offer additional information regarding plaque composition. However, further research is required to determine how such CTA and MRA potential will impact therapeutic decisions.

Dissection

Dissection of the cervical arteries is a major cause of cerebrovascular disease, accounting for up to 20% of strokes in patients below the age of 45 (134,155–158). While the risk of dissection is relatively constant throughout the life of an individual, dissection accounts for a higher proportion of strokes in the young (155,156). The etiology of dissection is variable (156,159,160). It can occur as a result of trauma,

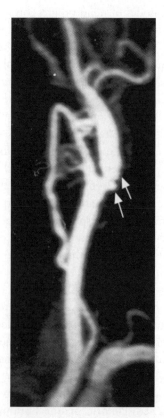

FIGURE 12-19 Gadolinium-enhanced MRA shows ulcerations at the level of the carotid bulb (*arrows*) without a high-grade stenosis. Though not critically narrowed, the ulcerations need to be considered as an at-risk feature for stroke.

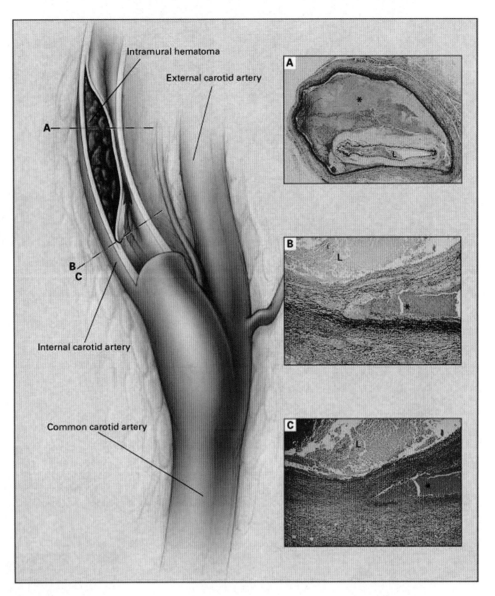

FIGURE 12-20 Pathological findings in a 37-year-old woman with a dissection of the internal carotid artery. Photomicrographs of the right extracranial ICA **(Panels A–C)** show a dissection within the outer layers of the tunica media, resulting in stenosis of the arterial lumen *(L)*. The rectangles outlined in blue **(left)** indicate the sites of the photomicrographs. The intramural hemorrhage *(asterisk)* extends almost entirely around the artery **(Panel A)** (van Gieson's stain, 4×). Higher-power views of the ICA at the point of dissection show fragmentation of elastic tissue **(Panel B)** (van Gieson's stain, 25×), with the accumulation of pale ground-glass substance in the tunica media, indicated by the blue-staining mucopolysaccharides **(Panel C)** (Alcian blue, 25×). These changes are consistent with a diagnosis of cystic medial necrosis. (Reprinted from Schievink WI. Spontaneous dissection of the carotid and vertebral arteries. *N Engl J Med.* 2001;344:898–906, with permission. Copyright © 2001 Massachusetts Medical Society. All rights reserved.)

including minor trauma; as a complication of underlying vasculitis or other vasculopathy; or as a complication of a systemic condition (Fig. 12-20).

The classical angiographic description of an intimal flap is not the most common presenting finding (161). Dissection can present as a focal stenosis, a long-segment stenosis, as a "flame-shaped" occlusion, as a pseudoaneurysm, or even mimicking a fenestration (132,133,156,161–163) (Figs. 12-21, 12-22). Dissections tend to occur in a characteristic location, often in one where a vessel transitions from flexible to fixed, such as at the skull base for the ICAs or at the entry into the foramen transversarium for the vertebral arteries (110,132,159).

In addition to demonstrating the luminal abnormalities seen with DSA in the setting of dissection, CTA and MRA can show mural findings. Furthermore, MRI and MRA can detect intramural hematoma with high conspicuity, evident as bright signal material on unenhanced images, particularly with dark blood techniques (Fig. 12-23). The detection of blood products on axial flow-suppressed MRI images when used with MRA increases the specificity for dissection (156,164–167).

Fibromuscular Dysplasia

Fibromuscular dysplasia (FMD) is a disorder of uncertain etiology that affects medium- to large-sized arteries (131,168–171). The prevalent form of the disease is often seen in young women (170,171). Commonly, the renal arteries are involved, followed by the cervical (carotid and vertebral) arteries (169,170). The disease is

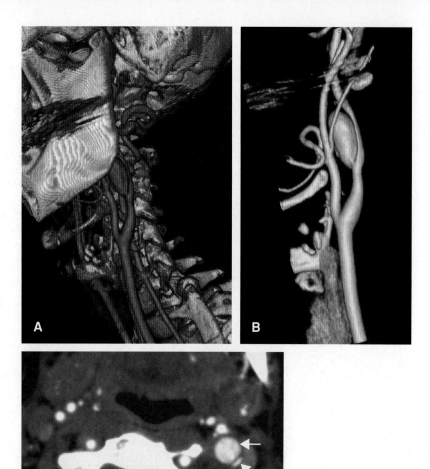

FIGURE 12-21 CTA of a carotid artery dissection with resulting pseudoaneurysm formation. Surface rendered image with **(A)** and without **(B)** bone visualization and axial source image **(C)** show the pseudoaneurysm (*short arrow*) and adjacent narrowed lumen (*long arrow*).

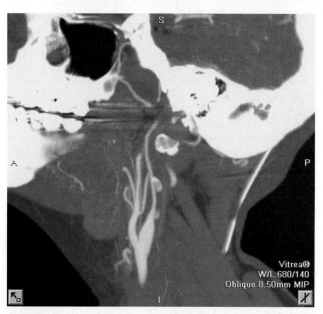

FIGURE 12-22 Carotid dissection. Multiplanar reconstruction of a CTA through the long axis of the carotid artery showing a long-segment stenosis (*arrows*) of the ICA above the bulb (*long arrow*) most consistent with dissection.

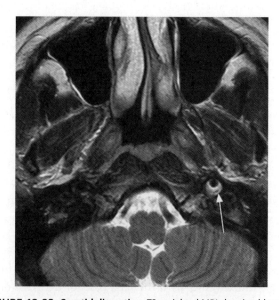

FIGURE 12-23 Carotid dissection. T2-weighted MRI showing blood in the arterial wall (*arrow*) and narrowing of the dark signal lumen of the left ICA. This is also known as the *crescent sign*, a hallmark of ICA dissection. (Adapted from Nautiyal A, Singh S, DiSalle M, et al. Painful Horner syndrome as a harbinger of silent carotid dissection. *PLoS Med.* 2005;2(1):e19)

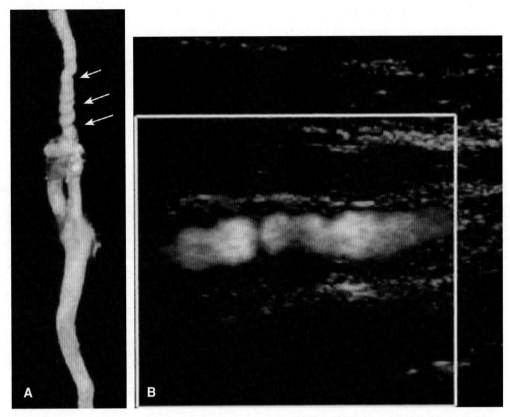

FIGURE 12-24 Fibromuscular dysplasia. A: A 3D reconstructed image from a 16-row-multidetector computed tomographic angiogram of the ICA reveals beading (*arrows*) typical of that seen in medial fibroplasias. (Case courtesy of Corey Goldman, M.D., Ph.D., Ochsner Clinic, New Orleans, LA.) **B:** These findings were also noted on a power Doppler sonogram. (Adapted from Slovut DP, Olin JW. Fibromuscular dysplasia. *N Engl J Med.* 2004;350:1862–1871, with permission. Copyright © 2004 Massachusetts Medical Society. All rights reserved.)

often asymptomatic and is found incidentally. Cervical vascular involvement can present as stroke or TIA, or may mimic inflammatory arteritides (170,171).

FMD of the cervical vasculature typically involves the middle and distal third of the ICA, often beyond the standard area of interrogation on carotid ultrasound examination (131,168,170). Several subtypes exist, classified by the underlying histopathology. The most common type is medial fibroplasia, typified by alternating segments of narrowing and dilation, classically described as a "string of beads" (169,170) (Fig. 12-24). The areas of dilation are wider than the normal vessel luminal diameter. The other subtypes may present as focal, short-segment concentric narrowing; redundant loops of artery; webs; or smooth, tapered narrowing of vessels (131,168,169).

The pathologic changes in the vessel wall are not easily visible on axial imaging. FMD is easier to recognize based on the angiographic appearance and patient demographics. The angiographic appearance of the less common subtypes can overlap with the inflammatory conditions of the carotid but are not associated with systemic signs of inflammation (169,170). FMD is often bilateral and can be associated with intracranial aneurysms (168,170).

Aneurysm

Extracranial carotid artery aneurysm (CAA) is an uncommon clinical disease that can occur as the result of atherosclerotic degeneration, fibromuscular dysplasia, or traumatic injury, or as an uncommon complication following a carotid endarterectomy. It is encountered in 0.2% to 5% of all carotid artery surgeries (172–174).

Atherosclerosis is currently the most common pathology associated with aneurysms, whereas prior to the widespread availability of antibiotics, infectious etiologies were the dominant cause. Atherosclerotic aneurysms are often termed as *degenerative aneurysms* and are true aneurysms. This is to be distinguished from traumatic aneurysms that result from a disruption of the wall and lead to the formation of pseudoaneurysms.

The natural history of CAA is conical growth with the potential for rupture, distal embolization, and local compression. Pulsatile neck swelling is the most common presentation of a carotid artery aneurysm (175–177). Other symptoms include pain, TIA, stroke, hoarseness, and dysphagia (178,179).

Differential diagnoses include carotid body tumor, cervical lymphadenopathy, tortuous (kinked) carotid artery, and cervical abscess. The diagnosis of carotid artery aneurysm often can be confirmed by a noninvasive carotid duplex scan. Arteriography has traditionally been considered the gold standard in preoperative surgical planning (177). CTA and MRA are challenging this notion as both of these modalities, in addition to demonstrating the luminal details, provide important information about the intramural findings and the adjacent soft tissues (Fig. 12-25).

Traditionally, treatment has been surgical, with ligation, external wrapping, and resection being commonly employed techniques. A recent migration to treating these lesions with endovascular intervention has been noted (180,181) (Fig. 12-26). Preliminary data suggest that endovascular treatments offer reduced morbidity and procedural complications along with a reduced length of stay in the hospital (180).

Coiling and Kinking

Tortuosity or redundancy of the extracranial carotid artery appears as coiling or kinking along the course of the vessel and can arise from both developmental and degenerative changes. It commonly affects the ICA but may affect the CCA.

Coiling of the ICA is an elongation in a restricted space, causing tortuosity; it results in a C- or S-shape curvature, or a circular configuration. *Kinking* is a variant of coiling that includes angulation of one or more segments of the ICA often associated with a significant degree of stenosis (182,183). A kinked carotid artery may be seen as a complication of carotid stent procedures (184,185); however, such a history provides a distinction from the redundant form.

Interestingly, a recent study showed that in 78 (56%) of 139 surgical specimens of resected redundant, elongated carotid arteries, both typical and atypical patterns of fibro-

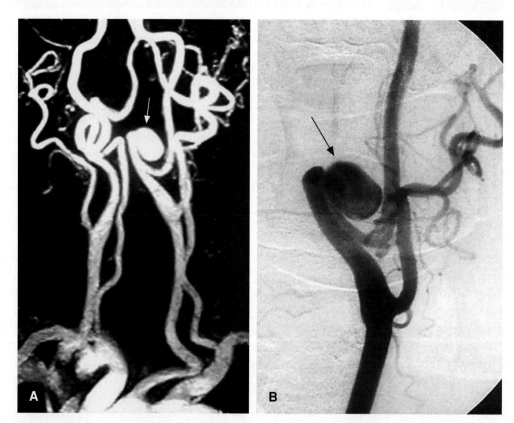

FIGURE 12-25 Carotid artery aneurysm. MRA and DSA images of a patient presenting with crescendo TIAs and no history of neck trauma. **A:** CE 3D MRA shows an extracranial ICA aneurysm (*white arrow*) measuring 3 cm × 3 cm × 2.5 cm. **B:** There is excellent correlation with a catheter carotid angiogram revealing the left ICA aneurysm (*black arrow*). (Adapted Karaman K, Onat L, Sirvanci M, et al. Extracranial carotid artery aneurysm. http://www.eurorad.org/eurorad/case.php?id=1848. Accessed 6/11/06.)

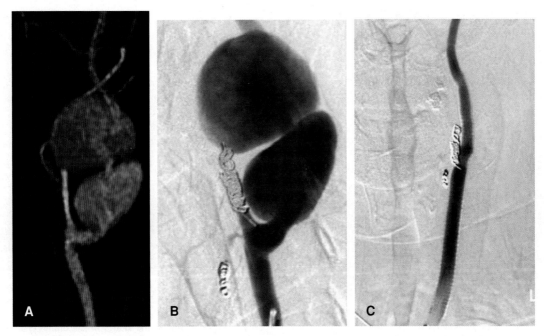

FIGURE 12-26 Aneurysm. A 39-year-old nonsmoking woman presented with a pulsatile swelling in her left neck immediately below the angle of the mandible. There was no prior history of atherosclerotic disease, fibromuscular dysplasia, neck trauma, hypertension, or hyperlipidemia. **A:** A double fusiform aneurysm of the extracranial ICA is well demonstrated with this VR gadolinium-enhanced MRA. **B:** A catheter carotid angiogram of the left CCA following elective embolization of the ECA shows the double fusiform aneurysm of the ICA. The proximity of the aneurysm to the carotid bifurcation prompted ECA embolization to minimize the risk of a type II endoleak. **C:** Post-treatment CCA catheter angiogram demonstrates the success of endovascular treatment with covered stents. (Case courtesy of Dr. Ruben Sebben and Dr. Jones and Partners Medical Imaging, Adelaide, Australia.)

muscular dysplasia were seen at pathologic examination (186). Thus, association suggests a histologic predisposition for the entity.

Angiographic reviews have demonstrated that redundant carotid arteries occur in 10% to 43% of patients studied; kinking is seen in 4% to 16% (187,188). However, the number of patients with hemispheric ischemic symptoms or nonspecific neurologic complaints accounts for a relatively small percentage of cases (4% to 20%) (189,190).

The definitive diagnosis of carotid coils and kinks is made by angiography. CTA and MRA can readily demonstrate these features (186,191) (Figs. 12-27, 12-28, 12-29). With DSA, multiple runs may be required in order to find the adequate projection enabling the diagnosis. It is important to assess for concurrent atherosclerotic features that can coexist and may explain the patient's symptoms.

Surgical correction has been advocated for symptomatic patients (186) and seeks to eliminate the redundancy by partial resection of the CCA or ICA (186,192). Surgery has been shown to be better at preventing stroke when compared with medical treatment and can provide complete symptomatic relief in those patients with nonhemispheric complaints (186).

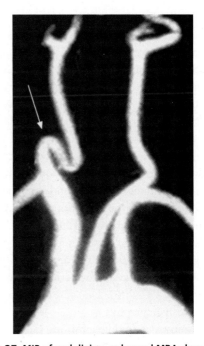

FIGURE 12-27 MIP of gadolinium-enhanced MRA showing a tortuous carotid artery. An ultrasound (*not shown*) initially obtained for a pulsatile neck mass and clinical finding of a bruit was interpreted as showing an aneurysm. The MIP from a gadolinium-enhanced MRA shows a tortuous proximal CCA (*arrow*) to be the cause of the patient's pulsatile neck mass and bruit.

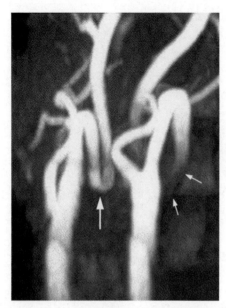

FIGURE 12-28 TOF MRA of bilateral carotid elongation and kinking in a patient with right hemispheric symptoms. An extreme redundancy of the right ICA is noted (*large arrow*). Note the loss of signal in the tortuous portion of the left ICA (*small arrows*) as it courses in a retrograde fashion with an in-plane component posterior to the bifurcation. (Adapted from Ballotta E, Thiene G, Baracchini C, et al. Surgical vs. medical treatment for isolated internal carotid artery elongation with coiling or kinking in symptomatic patients: a prospective randomized clinical study. *J Vasc Surg.* 2005;42:838–846; discussion 846, with permission.)

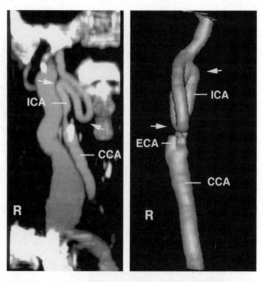

FIGURE 12-29 Kinking of the right internal carotid artery by spiral CT in maximum-intensity projection and shaded-surface display techniques. Shown is severe kinking of the right ICA describing a loop of 360 degrees by MIP **(left)** and shaded-surface display (SSD) reconstruction techniques with 90-degree clockwise rotation on its long axis **(right)**. MIP reconstruction also shows a severe calcified stenosis (70%) at the ICA origin. *Arrows* indicate knee of kinking loop. (Reprinted from Corti R, Ferrari C, Roberti M, et al. Spiral computed tomography: a novel diagnostic approach for investigation of the extracranial cerebral arteries and its complementary role in duplex ultrasonography. *Circulation.* 1998;98:984–989, with permission.)

Vasculitis

The term *vasculitis* encompasses a broad spectrum of inflammatory conditions affecting the vasculature (193). Vasculitides are classified according to their location, underlying pathophysiology and histology, the size of the vessels that are most commonly affected, and by the pattern of clinical features (194,195). In the setting of cervical vascular pathology, we refer to vasculitis as a set of arteritides that affect the large arteries of the neck. These include giant cell (temporal) arteritis, Takayasu arteritis, and Wegener's granulomatosis. Other causes of vasculitis in this location include systemic inflammatory conditions such as systemic lupus erythematosus (SLE), infectious and postinfectious inflammation, and radiation-induced vasculopathy (131,196).

Vasculitis in the large vessels, such as the carotid and vertebral, typically manifests as mural irregularity and multifocal stenosis or aneurysm formation on conventional angiography (131,197–206). The same findings can be seen on noninvasive angiography.

With noninvasive angiography, one can detect inflammatory changes in the vessel wall. These changes will present as wall thickening, wall edema, wall enhancement, and luminal changes such as stenosis, occlusion, or aneurysm formation (131,197–206). MRI has the added capability to detect wall edema in the form of increased signal in the ves-

sel wall on short-T1 inversion-recovery (STIR) images. CT can detect the luminal changes, wall enhancement, and thickening. Vessel-wall enhancement and edema are thought to best reflect the presence of active inflammation, as late fibrosis also can present as vessel-wall thickening, and the luminal changes can persist beyond periods of active inflammation (205,207,208). The use of IV contrast agents, therefore, is essential in the evaluation of suspected vasculitis. Black blood imaging can also be used to image the vessel wall for signs of thickening and inflammation (145).

The classification of the systemic vasculitides is complex (194,195). They are commonly stratified according to the size of the vessels involved; however, there can be considerable overlap, and even the so-called small vessel vasculitides can affect the carotid and vertebral arteries (195). Of note, the features of vasculitis of the smaller branch vessels are often at the limit of CTA and MRA resolution.

Giant Cell (Temporal) Arteritis

Giant cell, or temporal, arteritis is the most common systemic vasculitis in North America (209). It typically occurs after the sixth decade of life, more commonly among women. It is associated with fever, weight loss, carotidynia, jaw claudication, and headache (209). Classically, the disease affects the temporal artery, but involvement can be seen in the aorta and its large branches, including the CCA (198,199,210). Giant cell arteritis can be complicated by dissection, aneurysm formation, and rupture (209,210). The angiographic findings are typically less pronounced than in Takayasu arteritis. On axial images, vessel-wall edema, enhancement, and thickening usually can be seen (198,199,210). The inflammatory changes are important to detect in the aorta, as approximately 20% of cases are associated with clinically silent aortitis (209,210).

Takayasu Arteritis

Takayasu arteritis is a chronic inflammatory condition of unknown etiology that affects the aorta and its branches (211). It is seen most often between the second and fourth decades of life and is more common in women, East Asia, and South Asia (211,212). It is associated with fever, myalagia, weight loss, and arthropathy. Angiographically, the disease is characterized by involvement of the aorta and its branches (200–202,211). Aneurysm formation is noted early in the disease, followed later by long-segment stenosis and occlusion, so-called *pulseless disease* (201,211,213) (Fig. 12-30). The thoracic aorta and cephalic vessels are more commonly involved in the Japanese form, while abdominal aortic involvement is more common in Indian patients (212). On cross-sectional imaging, wall thickening, enhancement, and edema can be detected (200–202,211).

Wegener's Granulomatosis

Wegener's granulomatosis is an inflammatory condition of unknown etiology. Characterized by necrotic granulomatosis and often seen in the head, neck, lungs, and kidneys, it also manifests as a systemic vasculitis of the small to medium vessels (214–216). The peak incidence is in the fourth to fifth decades of life, with a slightly increased prevalence in women. The disease is associated with the circulating antineutrophil cytoplasmic antibody (c-ANCA) serum marker in 95% of cases (214). The disease is often angiographically occult but can be associated with accelerated atherosclerosis of the carotid bulb (216,217). Rarely, wall thickening and stenosis can be seen, similar to that seen in Takayasu arteritis (216).

Postirridation Vasculopathy

Radiation-induced vasculopathy of the cervical arteries can be divided into three categories: acute injury, late fibrosis, and accelerated atherosclerosis (218). Initial injury to the arteries affects the intima and, in the weeks to months following initial exposure, can result in dissection, pseudoaneurysm formation, and fistula formation (131,197,218). Later injury probably reflects disease of the vasa vasorum and results in medial fibrosis and thickening of the endothelium (197,218). This usually occurs 5 to 10 years following irradiation and is characterized angiographically as stenosis and occlusion (218). On axial images, wall thickening and contrast enhancement can be seen (197).

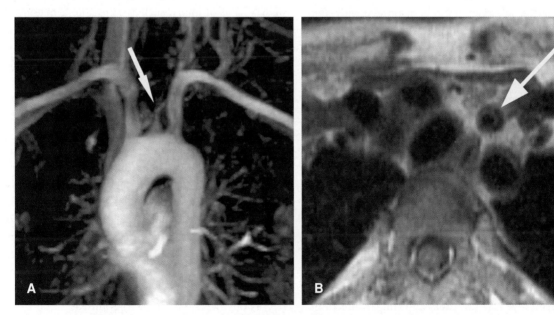

FIGURE 12-30 Takayasu arteritis. A: Coronal MIP 3D MR angiogram of a 35-year-old woman shows high-grade stenosis of the left CCA (*arrow*). **B:** Axial T1-weighted MR image (obtained before administration of gadolinium contrast material) of the same patient shows wall thickening of the left CCA (*arrow*). (Reprinted from Nastri MV, Baptista LP, Baroni RH, et al. Gadolinium-enhanced three-dimensional MR angiography of Takayasu arteritis. *Radiographics.* 2004;24:773–786, with permission.)

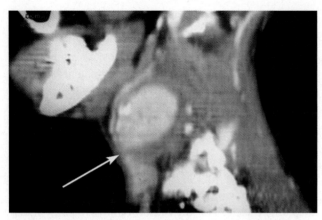

FIGURE 12-31 A 13-year-old male with history of Behçet disease. The patient presented with complaints of severe headaches and a large mass on the right side of his neck. Head and neck CT scan demonstrates a large carotid artery aneurysm (*arrow*) measuring 4 cm in diameter. (Reprinted from Antar KA, Keiser HD, Peeva E. Relapsing arterial aneurysms in juvenile Behçet's disease. *Clin Rheumatol*. 2005;24: 72–75, with permission.)

Fifteen to 20 years following exposure, a pattern quite similar to atherosclerosis will develop, except the findings are typically limited to the irradiated field (218,219).

Behçet Disease

Behçet disease is an inflammatory condition of unknown etiology that is characterized by oral and genital mucosal ulcers and uveitis (220). It is most commonly seen in people of Mediterranean and Near Eastern descent between the third and fifth decades of life. It can be associated with large saccular aneuryms, dissections, and pseudoaneurysms (221–223). Large arterial occlusive disease also can occur. As well, Behçet can be associated with intra-cranial aneurysm formation (220,222,223). The most common site of arterial aneurysms is the aorta, followed by the femoral and pulmonary arteries. Very few cases of Behçet-related extracranial carotid artery aneurysms have been reported (224) (Fig. 12-31).

Infectious and Postinfectious Vasculitis

While infectious and postinfectious vasculitides are usually viral in origin and affect small intracranial vessels, large vessel disease can be seen in the neck (193). While rare, this is usually secondary to spirochetal illness, including syphilis (193). Syphilis is classically associated with aneurysm formation due to medial necrosis from occlusion of the vasa vasorum. Actinomycosis, nocardia, and fungal infections also may directly involve the cephalic great vessels and result in inflammatory changes in the vessel wall and occlusion through direct invasion or pseudoaneurysm formation from damage to the vessel wall (131,225).

TRAUMA

Trauma to the cervical great vessels has traditionally been classified as either blunt or penetrating (7,196,226–228). The distinction is somewhat artificial, as the sequelae of both overlap. Each can result in dissection, pseudoaneurysm formation, vessel occlusion, vessel rupture, or formation of a fistula (196,219,226,228). Blunt trauma is usually the result of motor vehicle accidents or any mechanism that results in sudden neck flexion or extension. As blunt injury to the vessels is often asymptomatic, it may not be diagnosed until well after the initial injury (227–230). Penetrating trauma is usually the result of gunshot or stab wounds to the neck and is usually immediately evident on presentation.

DSA remains the standard for diagnosis of the complications of injury to the cervical vessels; however, DSA is often not immediately available and is rarely the initial imaging test in the setting of trauma. Similarly, MRA is often not available on a 24-hour basis, and the time required for scanning can preclude the use of MRI in an unstable patient. Further, the presence of metallic debris, such as that from a gunshot wound, may also prevent the use of MRI. CT, on the other hand, is widely available, is quick, and is often used in the initial workup of trauma to other parts of the body. With the increasing availability of MDCT, CTA of the neck is becoming the initial method of evaluation for suspected acute injury to the cervical vessels (228,229).

As well, CTA can be used to detect the presence of secondary signs of injury, such as soft-tissue hematoma, laceration, or bullet or knife tract. This is most useful in penetrating injury, as the vessel injury is usually proximate to the wound. Blunt injury, on the other hand, can occur at any point along the length of the vessel. As mentioned in the section on dissection, blunt injury has a predilection for certain segments of the vessels, specifically where the vessel crosses over bone or transitions from a fixed to mobile segment.

Thus far, the performance of CTA in the acute setting has been variable (7,229). Results for penetrating injury have been better than for blunt injury (7,231). Further, the reliability of CTA also varies with the type of injury to the vessel. Small pseudoaneurysms may not be seen easily (7,196,228,229). Arteriovenous fistulas (AVF) can be missed, as they are often small initially. As well, CTA does not have the temporal resolution of DSA, so early venous shunting—the hallmark of AVFs—is not easily noted on CTA.

Though CTA shows great promise (226,227,231,232), the reliability of CTA in the acute setting is still unclear. For these reasons, as the role of CTA develops, DSA should still be performed for suspected injury to the cervical vessels, especially in the setting of blunt injury to the neck.

CAROTID BODY TUMORS

The carotid body is a sensory organ (glomus caroticum) that lines the medial wall of the bifurcation of the CCA and is part of the extra-adrenal neuroendocrine system. Carotid body cells sense changes in arterial partial pressures and are sensitive to changes in oxygen, carbon dioxide, and pH, imparting a role in the autonomic control of the respiratory and cardiovascular systems.

The normal carotid body measures 3 to 5 mm in diameter but is often larger in people living at higher altitudes. Carotid body tumors, also called *glomus tumors, paragangliomas,* and *chemodectomas,* are highly vascular neoplasms that originate from the normal paraganglionic tissue of the carotid body.

The vast majority of carotid body paragangliomas present as slowly enlarging (~5 mm per year), nontender neck masses located just anterior to the sternocleidomastoid muscle at the level of the hyoid. The classic finding is a mass in this location that is mobile in the lateral plane but is limited in the cephalocaudal direction. Occasionally, the mass may transmit the carotid pulse or demonstrate a bruit or thrill. As these tumors enlarge, progressive symptoms of

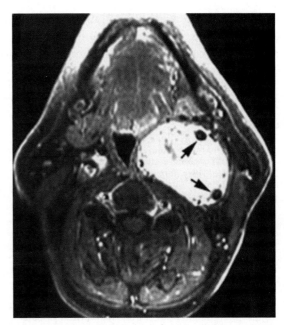

FIGURE 12-33 Carotid body tumor (Glomus tumor). Post contrast T1-weighted axial image shows a large markedly enhancing mass of the upper neck splaying the internal and external (*arrows*) carotids above the common carotid artery bifurcation. Reprinted from Grey ML, Alinani JM. *CT & MRI Pathology: A Pocket Atlas.* New York: McGraw Hill, 2003, with permission from The McGraw-Hill Companies.

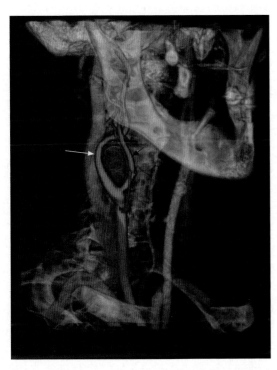

FIGURE 12-32 A 24- × 16-mm ovoid enhancing lesion is demonstrated just above the right carotid bifurcation, splaying the internal (*white arrow*) and external (*black arrow*) carotid branches. The lesion shows dense peripheral rim of enhancement with a relative lack of central enhancement. The location and enhancement characteristics are typical of a carotid body tumor, proven at surgery. (Case courtesy of Dr. Ruben Sebben and Dr. Jones and Partners Medical Imaging, Adelaide, Australia.)

dysphagia, odynophagia, hoarseness, and other cranial nerve (IX–XII) deficits appear.

Fewer than 10% are considered malignant, a designation made by virtue of the presence of metastatic lesions, as malignant behavior cannot be predicted by histologic studies (233,234).

Imaging is indicated for patients suspected of harboring a carotid body paraganglioma, based on the aforementioned clinical presentations, to monitor the size and extension of paragangliomas in patients with known tumors electing a watchful waiting strategy and to screen the asymptomatic kindred of patients with hereditary paragangliomas who are at risk for developing paragangliomas.

Imaging Findings

On angiographic images, the ECA and the ICA are characteristically splayed (Figs. 12-32, 12-33). Multiple small vessels are visible within the region of the mass and appear to arise from a branch of the ECA (usually the ascending pharyngeal artery). Prompt and intense contrast enhancement of a carotid space mass as well as the multiple tiny flow voids on MRI images favor the diagnosis of paraganglioma (235) (Fig. 12-33). Intense enhancement on CT is also characteristic. This enhancement relates to the characteristic vascular blush that typically is seen with conventional angiography (234).

The treatment of choice for most carotid body paragangliomas is surgical excision. However, because of their location in close approximation to important vessels and nerves, there is a recognizable risk of morbidity (mainly cranial nerve X–XII deficits and vascular injuries) and mortality which is estimated at 3% to 9% (236,237).

REFERENCES

1. Self-reported heart disease and stroke among adults with and without diabetes—United States, 1999–2001. *MMWR Morb Mortal Wkly Rep*. 2003;52:1065–1070.
2. Kiechl S, Willeit J. The natural course of atherosclerosis. Part I: incidence and progression. *Arterioscler Thromb Vasc Biol*. 1999;19:1484–1490.
3. Willeit J, Kiechl S. Prevalence and risk factors of asymptomatic extracranial carotid artery atherosclerosis. A population-based study. *Arterioscler Thromb*. 1993;13:661–668.
4. Romero JM, Ackerman RH, Dault NA, et al. Noninvasive evaluation of carotid artery stenosis: indications, strategies, and accuracy. *Neuroimaging Clin N Am*. 2005;15:351–365, xi.
5. Phillips CD, Bubash LA. CT angiography and MR angiography in the evaluation of extracranial carotid vascular disease. *Radiol Clin North Am*. 2002;40:783–798.
6. Randoux B, Marro B, Koskas F, et al. Carotid artery stenosis: prospective comparison of CT, three-dimensional gadolinium-enhanced MR, and conventional angiography. *Radiology*. 2001;220:179–185.
7. Hollingworth W, Nathens AB, Kanne JP, et al. The diagnostic accuracy of computed tomography angiography for traumatic or atherosclerotic lesions of the carotid and vertebral arteries: a systematic review. *Eur J Radiol*. 2003;48:88–102.
8. Derdeyn CP. Conventional angiography remains an important tool for measurement of carotid arterial stenosis. *Radiology*. 2005;235:711–712; author reply 712–713.
9. Berry E, Kelly S, Westwood ME, et al. The cost-effectiveness of magnetic resonance angiography for carotid artery stenosis and peripheral vascular disease: a systematic review. *Health Technol Assess*. 2002;6:1–155.
10. U-King-Im JM, Hollingworth W, Trivedi RA, et al. Contrast-enhanced MR angiography vs intra-arterial digital subtraction angiography for carotid imaging: activity-based cost analysis. *Eur Radiol*. 2004;14:730–735.
11. Berteloot D, Leclerc X, Leys D, et al. [Cerebral angiography: a study of complications in 450 consecutive procedures]. *J Radiol*. 1999;80:843–848.
12. Hankey GJ, Warlow CP, Molyneux AJ. Complications of cerebral angiography for patients with mild carotid territory ischaemia being considered for carotid endarterectomy. *J Neurol Neurosurg Psychiatry*. 1990;53:542–548.
13. Hankey GJ, Warlow CP, Sellar RJ. Cerebral angiographic risk in mild cerebrovascular disease. *Stroke*. 1990;21:209–222.
14. Willinsky RA, Taylor SM, TerBrugge K, et al. Neurologic complications of cerebral angiography: prospective analysis of 2,899 procedures and review of the literature. *Radiology*. 2003;227:522–528.
15. Bendszus M, Koltzenburg M, Burger R, et al. Silent embolism in diagnostic cerebral angiography and neurointerventional procedures: a prospective study. *Lancet*. 1999;354:1594–1597.
16. Heiserman JE. Silent embolism after cerebral angiography—what harm? *Lancet*. 1999;354:1577–1578.
17. Davies KN, Humphrey PR. Complications of cerebral angiography in patients with symptomatic carotid territory ischaemia screened by carotid ultrasound. *J Neurol Neurosurg Psychiatry*. 1993;56:967–972.
18. Endarterectomy for asymptomatic carotid artery stenosis. Executive Committee for the Asymptomatic Carotid Atherosclerosis Study. *JAMA*. 1995;273:1421–1428.
19. Randomised trial of endarterectomy for recently symptomatic carotid stenosis: final results of the MRC European Carotid Surgery Trial (ECST). *Lancet*. 1998;351:1379–1387.
20. Beneficial effect of carotid endarterectomy in symptomatic patients with high-grade carotid stenosis. North American Symptomatic Carotid Endarterectomy Trial Collaborators. *N Engl J Med*. 1991;325:445–453.
21. Tu RK, Cohen WA, Maravilla KR, et al. Digital subtraction rotational angiography for aneurysms of the intracranial anterior circulation: injection method and optimization. *AJNR Am J Neuroradiol*. 1996;17:1127–1136.
22. Anzalone N, Scomazzoni F, Castellano R, et al. Carotid artery stenosis: intraindividual correlations of 3D time-of-flight MR angiography, contrast-enhanced MR angiography, conventional DSA, and rotational angiography for detection and grading. *Radiology*. 2005;236:204–213.
23. Elgersma OE, Buijs PC, Wust AF, et al. Maximum internal carotid arterial stenosis: assessment with rotational angiography versus conventional intraarterial digital subtraction angiography. *Radiology*. 1999;213:777–783.
24. Ho SS, Chan YL, Yeung DK, et al. Blood flow volume quantification of cerebral ischemia: comparison of three noninvasive imaging techniques of carotid and vertebral arteries. *AJR Am J Roentgenol*. 2002;178:551–556.
25. Long A, Lepoutre A, Corbillon E, et al. Critical review of non- or minimally invasive methods (duplex ultrasonography, MR- and CT-angiography) for evaluating stenosis of the proximal internal carotid artery. *Eur J Vasc Endovasc Surg*. 2002;24:43–52.
26. Simonetti G, Bozzao A, Floris R, et al. Non-invasive assessment of neck-vessel pathology. *Eur Radiol*. 1998;8:691–697.
27. Buskens E, Nederkoorn PJ, Buijs-Van Der Woude T, et al. Imaging of carotid arteries in symptomatic patients: cost-effectiveness of diagnostic strategies. *Radiology*. 2004;233:101–112.
28. Wardlaw JM, Lewis S. Carotid stenosis measurement on colour Doppler ultrasound: agreement of ECST, NASCET and CCA methods applied to ultrasound with intra-arterial angiographic stenosis measurement. *Eur J Radiol*. 2005;56:205–211.
29. Arning C, Eckert B. The diagnostic relevance of colour Doppler artefacts in carotid artery examinations. *Eur J Radiol*. 2004;51:246–251.
30. Winkler P, Helmke K. Major pitfalls in Doppler investigations with particular reference to the cerebral vascular system. Part I. Sources of error, resulting pitfalls and measures to prevent errors. *Pediatr Radiol*. 1990;20:219–228.
31. Winkler P, Helmke K, Mahl M. Major pitfalls in Doppler investigations. Part II. Low flow velocities and colour Doppler applications. *Pediatr Radiol*. 1990;20:304–310.
32. Romero JM, Lev MH, Chan ST, et al. US of neurovascular occlusive disease: interpretive pearls and pitfalls. *Radiographics*. 2002;22:1165–1176.
33. Wasserman BA, Wityk RJ, Trout HH 3rd, et al. Low-grade carotid stenosis: looking beyond the lumen with MRI. *Stroke*. 2005;36:2504–2513.
34. Anderson GB, Ashforth R, Steinke DE, et al. CT angiography for the detection and characterization of carotid artery bifurcation disease. *Stroke*. 2000;31:2168–2174.
35. Jahromi AS, Cina CS, Liu Y, et al. Sensitivity and specificity of color duplex ultrasound measurement in the estimation of internal carotid artery stenosis: a systematic review and meta-analysis. *J Vasc Surg*. 2005;41:962–972.
36. Naylor AR, Rothwell PM, Bell PR. Overview of the principal results and secondary analyses from the European and North American randomised trials of endarterectomy for symptomatic carotid stenosis. *Eur J Vasc Endovasc Surg*. 2003;26:115–129.
37. Back MR, Rogers GA, Wilson JS, et al. Magnetic resonance angiography minimizes need for arteriography after inadequate carotid duplex ultrasound scanning. *J Vasc Surg*. 2003;38:422–430; discussion 431.
38. Kuntz KM, Polak JF, Whittemore AD, et al. Duplex ultrasound criteria for the identification of carotid stenosis should be laboratory specific. *Stroke*. 1997;28:597–602.

39. Duddalwar VA. Multislice CT angiography: a practical guide to CT angiography in vascular imaging and intervention. *Br J Radiol*. 2004; 77:S27–S38.
40. Goddard AJ, Mendelow AD, Birchall D. Computed tomography angiography in the investigation of carotid stenosis. *Clin Radiol*. 2001;56:523–534.
41. Patel SG, Collie DA, Wardlaw JM, et al. Outcome, observer reliability, and patient preferences if CTA, MRA, or Doppler ultrasound were used, individually or together, instead of digital subtraction angiography before carotid endarterectomy. *J Neurol Neurosurg Psychiatry*. 2002;73:21–28.
42. van Helvoort-Postulart D, Dirksen CD, Kroon AA, et al. Cost analysis of procedures related to the management of renal artery stenosis from various perspectives. *Eur Radiol*. 2006;16:154–160.
43. Bettmann MA. Frequently asked questions: iodinated contrast agents. *Radiographics*. 2004;24[Suppl 1]:S3–S10.
44. Henson JW, Nogueira RG, Covarrubias DJ, et al. Gadolinium-enhanced CT angiography of the circle of Willis and neck. *AJNR Am J Neuroradiol*. 2004;25:969–972.
45. Ertl-Wagner B, Hoffmann RT, Bruning R, et al. [Diagnostic evaluation of the craniocervical vascular system with a 16-slice multi-detector row spiral CT. Protocols and first experiences.] *Radiologe*. 2002;42:728–732.
46. Cohnen M, Poll LJ, Puettmann C, et al. Effective doses in standard protocols for multi-slice CT scanning. *Eur Radiol*. 2003;13:1148–1153.
47. Chan PN, Antonio GE, Griffith JF, et al. Computed tomography for cervical spine trauma. The impact of MDCT on fracture detection and dose deposition. *Emerg Radiol*. 2005;11:286–290.
48. Rybicki F, Nawfel RD, Judy PF, et al. Skin and thyroid dosimetry in cervical spine screening: two methods for evaluation and a comparison between a helical CT and radiographic trauma series. *AJR Am J Roentgenol*. 2002;179:933–937.
49. Chow LC, Rubin GD. CT angiography of the arterial system. *Radiol Clin North Am*. 2002;40:729–749.
50. Suzuki S, Furui S, Kaminaga T, et al. Measurement of vascular diameter in vitro by automated software for CT angiography: effects of inner diameter, density of contrast medium, and convolution kernel. *AJR Am J Roentgenol*. 2004;182:1313–1317.
51. Claves JL, Wise SW, Hopper KD, et al. Evaluation of contrast densities in the diagnosis of carotid stenosis by CT angiography. *AJR Am J Roentgenol*. 1997;169:569–573.
52. Groell R, Willfurth P, Schaffler GJ, et al. Contrast-enhanced spiral CT of the head and neck: comparison of contrast material injection rates. *AJNR Am J Neuroradiol*. 1999;20:1732–1736.
53. Napoli A, Fleischmann D, Chan FP, et al. Computed tomography angiography: state-of-the-art imaging using multidetector-row technology. *J Comput Assist Tomogr*. 2004;28[Suppl 1]:S32–S45.
54. Prokop M. Multislice CT angiography. *Eur J Radiol*. 2000;36:86–96.
55. Ginsberg LE. Contrast-enhanced spiral CT of the head and neck. *AJNR Am J Neuroradiol*. 2000;21:1365.
56. Prokesch RW, Coulam CH, Chow LC, et al. CT angiography of the subclavian artery: utility of curved planar reformations. *J Comput Assist Tomogr*. 2002;26:199–201.
57. Takhtani D. CT neuroangiography: a glance at the common pitfalls and their prevention. *AJR Am J Roentgenol*. 2005;185:772–783.
58. Dix JE, Evans AJ, Kallmes DF, et al. Accuracy and precision of CT angiography in a model of carotid artery bifurcation stenosis. *AJNR Am J Neuroradiol*. 1997;18:409–415.
59. Liu Y, Hopper KD, Mauger DT, et al. CT angiographic measurement of the carotid artery: optimizing visualization by manipulating window and level settings and contrast material attenuation. *Radiology*. 2000;217:494–500.
60. Townsend TC, Saloner D, Pan XM, et al. Contrast material-enhanced MRA overestimates severity of carotid stenosis, compared with 3D time-of-flight MRA. *J Vasc Surg*. 2003;38:36–40.
61. Okumura A, Araki Y, Nishimura Y, et al. The clinical utility of contrast-enhanced 3D MR angiography for cerebrovascular disease. *Neurol Res*. 2001;23:767–771.
62. Suzuki S, Furui S, Kaminaga T. Accuracy of automated CT angiography measurement of vascular diameter in phantoms: effect of size of display field of view, density of contrast medium, and wall thickness. *AJR Am J Roentgenol*. 2005;184:1940–1944.
63. van Bemmel CM, Elgersma OE, Vonken EJ, et al. Evaluation of semiautomated internal carotid artery stenosis quantification from 3-dimensional contrast-enhanced magnetic resonance angiograms. *Invest Radiol*. 2004;39:418–426.
64. van Bemmel CM, Viergever MA, Niessen WJ. Semiautomatic segmentation and stenosis quantification of 3D contrast-enhanced MR angiograms of the internal carotid artery. *Magn Reson Med*. 2004;51:753–760.
65. Zhang Z, Berg MH, Ikonen AE, et al. Carotid artery stenosis: reproducibility of automated 3D CT angiography analysis method. *Eur Radiol*. 2004;14:665–672.
66. McKinney AM, Casey SO, Teksam M, et al. Carotid bifurcation calcium and correlation with percent stenosis of the internal carotid artery on CT angiography. *Neuroradiology*. 2005;47:1–9.
67. Jayakrishnan VK, White PM, Aitken D, et al. Subtraction helical CT angiography of intra- and extracranial vessels: technical considerations and preliminary experience. *AJNR Am J Neuroradiol*. 2003;24:451–455.
68. Kwon SM, Kim YS, Kim TS, et al. Digital subtraction CT angiography based on efficient 3D registration and refinement. *Comput Med Imaging Graph*. 2004;28:391–400.
69. Hirai T, Korogi Y, Ono K, et al. Maximum stenosis of extracranial internal carotid artery: effect of luminal morphology on stenosis measurement by using CT angiography and conventional DSA. *Radiology*. 2001;221:802–809.
70. Zhang Z, Berg M, Ikonen A, et al. Carotid stenosis degree in CT angiography: assessment based on luminal area versus luminal diameter measurements. *Eur Radiol*. 2005;15:2359–2365.
71. Nederkoorn PJ, Elgersma OE, Mali WP, et al. Overestimation of carotid artery stenosis with magnetic resonance angiography compared with digital subtraction angiography. *J Vasc Surg*. 2002;36:806–813.
72. Alvarez-Linera J, Benito-Leon J, Escribano J, et al. Prospective evaluation of carotid artery stenosis: elliptic centric contrast-enhanced MR angiography and spiral CT angiography compared with digital subtraction angiography. *AJNR Am J Neuroradiol*. 2003;24:1012–1019.
73. Berg M, Zhang Z, Ikonen A, et al. Multi-detector row CT angiography in the assessment of carotid artery disease in symptomatic patients: comparison with rotational angiography and digital subtraction angiography. *AJNR Am J Neuroradiol*. 2005;26:1022–1034.
74. Johnston DC, Eastwood JD, Nguyen T, et al. Contrast-enhanced magnetic resonance angiography of carotid arteries: utility in routine clinical practice. *Stroke*. 2002;33:2834–2838.
75. Johnston DC, Goldstein LB. Clinical carotid endarterectomy decision making: noninvasive vascular imaging versus angiography. *Neurology*. 2001; 56:1009–1015.
76. Link J, Brossmann J, Grabener M, et al. Spiral CT angiography and selective digital subtraction angiography of internal carotid artery stenosis. *AJNR Am J Neuroradiol*. 1996;17:89–94.
77. Magarelli N, Scarabino T, Simeone AL, et al. Carotid stenosis: a comparison between MR and spiral CT angiography. *Neuroradiology*. 1998;40:367–373.
78. Moll R, Dinkel HP. Value of the CT angiography in the diagnosis of common carotid artery bifurcation disease: CT angiography versus digital subtraction angiography and color flow Doppler. *Eur J Radiol*. 2001;39:155–162.

79. Scarabino T, Carriero A, Magarelli N, et al. MR angiography in carotid stenosis: a comparison of three techniques. Eur J Radiol. 1998;28:117–125.

80. Carriero A, Scarabino T, Magarelli N, et al. High-resolution magnetic resonance angiography of the internal carotid artery: 2D vs 3D TOF in stenotic disease. *Eur Radiol.* 1998;8:1370–1372.

81. Cinat M, Lane CT, Pham H, et al. Helical CT angiography in the preoperative evaluation of carotid artery stenosis. *J Vasc Surg.* 1998;28:290–300.

82. Cosottini M, Pingitore A, Puglioli M, et al. Contrast-enhanced three-dimensional magnetic resonance angiography of atherosclerotic internal carotid stenosis as the noninvasive imaging modality in revascularization decision making. *Stroke.* 2003;34:660–664.

83. Cumming MJ, Morrow IM. Carotid artery stenosis: a prospective comparison of CT angiography and conventional angiography. *AJR Am J Roentgenol.* 1994;163:517–523.

84. Herzig R, Burval S, Krupka B, et al. Comparison of ultra-sonography, CT angiography, and digital subtraction angiography in severe carotid stenoses. *Eur J Neurol.* 2004;11:774–781.

85. Serfaty JM, Chirossel P, Chevallier JM, et al. Accuracy of three-dimensional gadolinium-enhanced MR angiography in the assessment of extracranial carotid artery disease. *AJR Am J Roentgenol.* 2000;175:455–463.

86. Heiserman JE. Magnetic resonance angiography and evaluation of cervical arteries. *Top Magn Reson Imaging.* 2001;12:149–161.

87. Nederkoorn PJ, van der Graaf Y, Hunink MG. Duplex ultrasound and magnetic resonance angiography compared with digital subtraction angiography in carotid artery stenosis: a systematic review. *Stroke.* 2003;34:1324–1332.

88. Fellner C, Lang W, Janka R, et al. Magnetic resonance angiography of the carotid arteries using three different techniques: accuracy compared with intraarterial x-ray angiography and endarterectomy specimens. *J Magn Reson Imaging.* 2005;21:424–431.

89. U-King-Im JM, Trivedi RA, Sala E, et al. Evaluation of carotid stenosis with axial high-resolution black-blood MR imaging. *Eur Radiol.* 2004;14:1154–1161.

90. Trossbach M, Hartmann M, Braun C, et al. Small vessel stents for intracranial angioplasty: in vitro evaluation of in-stent stenoses using CT angiography. *Neuroradiology.* 2004;46:459–463.

91. Hahnel S, Trossbach M, Braun C, et al. Small-vessel stents for intracranial angioplasty: in vitro comparison of different stent designs and sizes by using CT angiography. *AJNR Am J Neuroradiol.* 2003;24:1512–1516.

92. Forsting M, Wanke I. Funeral for a friend. *Stroke.* 2003;34: 1324–1332.

93. Hoggard N. Importance of the imaging modality in decision making about carotid endarterectomy. *Neurology.* 2004;63:1340–1341; author reply 1340–1341.

94. Murphy K. Simplicity, voxels, and finding the signal in the noise. *Ann Neurol.* 2005;58:493–494.

95. Powers WJ. Carotid arteriography: still golden after all these years? *Neurology.* 2004;62:1246–1247.

96. Barnett HJ, Meldrum HE, Eliasziw M. The appropriate use of carotid endarterectomy. *CMAJ.* 2002;166:1169–1179.

97. Norris JW, Rothwell PM. Noninvasive carotid imaging to select patients for endarterectomy: is it really safer than conventional angiography? *Neurology.* 2001;56:990–991.

98. Dodick DW, Meissner I, Meyer FB, et al. Evaluation and management of asymptomatic carotid artery stenosis. *Mayo Clin Proc.* 2004;79:937–944.

99. Chow V, Burbridge B, Friedland R, et al. Interobserver variability in the measurement of internal carotid stenosis. *Can Assoc Radiol J.* 1999;50:37–40.

100. Dippel DW, van Kooten F, Bakker SL, et al. Interobserver agreement for 10% categories of angiographic carotid stenosis. *Stroke.* 1997;28:2483–2485.

101. Eliasziw M, Fox AJ, Sharpe BL, et al. Carotid artery stenosis: external validity of the North American Symptomatic

Carotid Endarterectomy Trial measurement method. *Radiology.* 1997;204:229–233.

102. Rothwell PM, Pendlebury ST, Wardlaw J, et al. Critical appraisal of the design and reporting of studies of imaging and measurement of carotid stenosis. *Stroke.* 2000;31:1444–1450.

103. Vanninen R, Manninen H, Koivisto K, et al. The best method to quantitate angiographic carotid artery stenosis? *Stroke.* 1994;25:708–709; author reply 710–702.

104. Vanninen R, Manninen H, Koivisto K, et al. Carotid stenosis by digital subtraction angiography: reproducibility of the European Carotid Surgery Trial and the North American Symptomatic Carotid Endarterectomy Trial measurement methods and visual interpretation. *AJNR Am J Neuroradiol.* 1994;15:1635–1641.

105. Young GR, Sandercock PA, Slattery J, et al. Observer variation in the interpretation of intra-arterial angiograms and the risk of inappropriate decisions about carotid endarterectomy. *J Neurol Neurosurg Psychiatry.* 1996;60: 152–157.

106. Benes V, Netuka D, Mandys V, et al. Comparison between degree of carotid stenosis observed at angiography and in histological examination. *Acta Neurochir (Wien).* 2004; 146:671–677.

107. Schulte-Altedorneburg G, Droste DW, Kollar J, et al. Measuring carotid artery stenosis—comparison of postmortem arteriograms with the planimetric gold standard. *J Neurol.* 2005;252:575–582.

108. Borisch I, Horn M, Butz B, et al. Preoperative evaluation of carotid artery stenosis: comparison of contrast-enhanced MR angiography and duplex sonography with digital subtraction angiography. *AJNR Am J Neuroradiol.* 2003;24:1117–1122.

109. U-King-Im JM, Hollingworth W, Trivedi RA, et al. Cost-effectiveness of diagnostic strategies prior to carotid endarterectomy. *Ann Neurol.* 2005;58:506–515.

110. Morris P. *Practical Neuroangiography.* Baltimore, MD: Williams & Wilkins; 1997.

111. Albayram S, Gailloud P, Wasserman BA. Bilateral arch origin of the vertebral arteries. *AJNR Am J Neuroradiol.* 2002;23:455–458.

112. Sanelli PC, Tong S, Gonzalez RG, et al. Normal variation of vertebral artery on CT angiography and its implications for diagnosis of acquired pathology. *J Comput Assist Tomogr.* 2002;26:462–470.

113. Sim E, Vaccaro AR, Berzlanovich A, et al. Fenestration of the extracranial vertebral artery: review of the literature. *Spine.* 2001;26:E139–E142.

114. Cakirer S, Karaarslan E, Kayabali M, et al. Separate origins of the left internal and external carotid arteries from the aortic arch: MR angiographic findings. *AJNR Am J Neuroradiol.* 2002;23:1600–1602.

115. Gurbuz J, Cavdar S, Ozdogmus O. Trifurcation of the left common carotid artery: a case report. *Clin Anat.* 2001;14: 58–61.

116. Rossitti S, Raininko R. Absence of the common carotid artery in a patient with a persistent trigeminal artery variant. *Clin Radiol.* 2001;56:79–81.

117. Goray VB, Joshi AR, Garg A, et al. Aortic arch variation: a unique case with anomalous origin of both vertebral arteries as additional branches of the aortic arch distal to left subclavian artery. *AJNR Am J Neuroradiol.* 2005;26:93–95.

118. Karcaaltincaba M, Strottman J, Washington L. Multidetector-row CT angiographic findings in the bilateral aortic arch origin of the vertebral arteries. *AJNR Am J Neuroradiol.* 2003;24:157.

119. Lemke AJ, Benndorf G, Liebig T, et al. Anomalous origin of the right vertebral artery: review of the literature and case report of right vertebral artery origin distal to the left subclavian artery. *AJNR Am J Neuroradiol.* 1999;20: 1318–1321.

120. Poultsides GA, Lolis ED, Vasquez J, et al. Common origins of carotid and subclavian arterial systems: report of a rare aortic arch variant. *Ann Vasc Surg.* 2004;18:597–600.

121. Tasar M, Yetiser S, Tasar A, et al. Congenital absence or hypoplasia of the carotid artery: radioclinical issues. *Am J Otolaryngol*. 2004;25:339–349.
122. Yagi K, Satoh K, Satomi J, et al. Primitive vertebrobasilar system associated with a ruptured aneurysm. *AJNR Am J Neuroradiol*. 2004;25:781–783.
123. Nogueira TE, Chambers AA, Brueggemeyer MT, et al. Dual origin of the vertebral artery mimicking dissection. AJNR *Am J Neuroradiol*. 1997;18:382–384.
124. Andoh K, Tanohata K, Moriya N, et al. The posterior inferior cerebellar artery arising from the extracranial segment of the internal carotid artery via the hypoglossal canal without an interposed segment of the basilar artery: a persistent primitive hypoglossal artery variant. *Clin Imaging*. 2001;25:86–89.
125. Nakamura M, Kobayashi S, Yoshida T, et al. Persistent external carotid-vertebrobasilar anastomosis via the hypoglossal canal. *Neuroradiology*. 2000;42:821–823.
126. Ayad M, Vinuela F, Rubinstein EH. The suboccipital carrefour: cervical and vertebral arterial anastomosis. *AJNR Am J Neuroradiol*. 1998;19:925–931.
127. Oguzkurt L, Kizilkilic O, Tercan F, et al. Vertebrocarotid collateral in extracranial carotid artery occlusions: digital subtraction angiography findings. *Eur J Radiol*. 2005;53:168–174.
128. Yamamoto S, Watanabe M. Novel collateral connecting the external and internal carotid arteries. *Clin Anat*. 2004;17:70–72.
129. Lucev N, Bobinac D, Maric I, et al. Variations of the great arteries in the carotid triangle. *Otolaryngol Head Neck Surg*. 2000;122:590–591.
130. Hayashi N, Hori E, Ohtani Y, et al. Surgical anatomy of the cervical carotid artery for carotid endarterectomy. *Neurol Med Chir (Tokyo)*. 2005;45:25–29; discussion 30.
131. Russo CP, Smoker WR. Nonatheromatous carotid artery disease. *Neuroimaging Clin N Am*. 1996;6:811–830.
132. Gailloud P, Carpenter J, Heck DV, et al. Pseudofenestration of the cervical internal carotid artery: a pathologic process that simulates an anatomic variant. *AJNR Am J Neuroradiol*. 2004;25:421–424.
133. Marden FA, Malisch TW. Carotid pseudofenestration: the double-barrel peril. *AJNR Am J Neuroradiol*. 2004;25:1862–1863.
134. Cerrato P, Grasso M, Imperiale D, et al. Stroke in young patients: etiopathogenesis and risk factors in different age classes. *Cerebrovasc Dis*. 2004;18:154–159.
135. De Fabritiis A, Conti E, Coccheri S. Management of patients with carotid stenosis. *Pathophysiol Haemost Thromb*. 2002;32:381–385.
136. Gorelick PB, Sacco RL, Smith DB, et al. Prevention of a first stroke: a review of guidelines and a multidisciplinary consensus statement from the National Stroke Association. *JAMA*. 1999;281:1112–1120.
137. Hankey GJ. Stroke: how large a public health problem, and how can the neurologist help? *Arch Neurol*. 1999;56:748–754.
138. Suwanwela NC, Chutinetr A. Risk factors for atherosclerosis of cervicocerebral arteries: intracranial versus extracranial. *Neuroepidemiology*. 2003;22:37–40.
139. Wityk RJ, Lehman D, Klag M, et al. Race and sex differences in the distribution of cerebral atherosclerosis. *Stroke*. 1996;27:1974–1980.
140. Kiechl S, Willeit J. The natural course of atherosclerosis. Part II: vascular remodeling. Bruneck Study Group. *Arterioscler Thromb Vasc Biol*. 1999;19:1491–1498.
141. Savitz SI, Caplan LR. Vertebrobasilar disease. *N Engl J Med*. 2005;352:2618–2626.
142. Masawa N, Glagov S, Zarins CK. Quantitative morphologic study of intimal thickening at the human carotid bifurcation: I. Axial and circumferential distribution of maximum intimal thickening in asymptomatic, uncomplicated plaques. *Atherosclerosis*. 1994;107:137–146.
143. Montorzi G, Silacci P, Zulliger M, et al. Functional, mechanical and geometrical adaptation of the arterial wall of a

144. Masawa N, Glagov S, Zarins CK. Quantitative morphologic study of intimal thickening at the human carotid bifurcation: II. The compensatory enlargement response and the role of the intima in tensile support. *Atherosclerosis*. 1994;107:147–155.
145. Wasserman BA, Smith WI, Trout HH 3rd, et al. Carotid artery atherosclerosis: in vivo morphologic characterization with gadolinium-enhanced double-oblique MR imaging initial results. *Radiology*. 2002;223:566–573.
146. Dirksen MT, van der Wal AC, van den Berg FM, et al. Distribution of inflammatory cells in atherosclerotic plaques relates to the direction of flow. *Circulation*. 1998;98:2000–2003.
147. Fuster V, Badimon L, Badimon JJ, et al. The pathogenesis of coronary artery disease and the acute coronary syndromes (1). *N Engl J Med*. 1992;326:242–250.
148. van der Wal AC, Becker AE, van der Loos CM, et al. Site of intimal rupture or erosion of thrombosed coronary atherosclerotic plaques is characterized by an inflammatory process irrespective of the dominant plaque morphology. *Circulation*. 1994;89:36–44.
149. Fisher M, Paganini-Hill A, Martin A, et al. Carotid plaque pathology: thrombosis, ulceration, and stroke pathogenesis. *Stroke*. 2005;36:253–257.
150. Rothwell PM, Villagra R, Gibson R, et al. Evidence of a chronic systemic cause of instability of atherosclerotic plaques. *Lancet*. 2000;355:19–24.
151. Sitzer M, Muller W, Siebler M, et al. Plaque ulceration and lumen thrombus are the main sources of cerebral microemboli in high-grade internal carotid artery stenosis. *Stroke*. 1995;26:1231–1233.
152. Rothwell PM, Gibson R, Warlow CP. Interrelation between plaque surface morphology and degree of stenosis on carotid angiograms and the risk of ischemic stroke in patients with symptomatic carotid stenosis. On behalf of the European Carotid Surgery Trialists' Collaborative Group. *Stroke*. 2000;31:615–621.
153. Eliasziw M, Streifler JY, Fox AJ, et al. Significance of plaque ulceration in symptomatic patients with high-grade carotid stenosis. North American Symptomatic Carotid Endarterectomy Trial. *Stroke*. 1994;25:304–308.
154. Streifler JY, Eliasziw M, Fox AJ, et al. Angiographic detection of carotid plaque ulceration. Comparison with surgical observations in a multicenter study. North American Symptomatic Carotid Endarterectomy Trial. *Stroke*. 1994;25:1130–1132.
155. Ahl B, Bokemeyer M, Ennen JC, et al. Dissection of the brain supplying arteries over the life span. *J Neurol Neurosurg Psychiatry*. 2004;75:1194–1196.
156. Guillon B, Levy C, Bousser MG. Internal carotid artery dissection: an update. *J Neurol Sci*. 1998;153:146–158.
157. Leys D, Lucas C, Gobert M, et al. Cervical artery dissections. *Eur Neurol*. 1997;37:3–12.
158. Lucas C, Moulin T, Deplanque D, et al. Stroke patterns of internal carotid artery dissection in 40 patients. *Stroke*. 1998;29:2646–2648.
159. Thanvi B, Munshi SK, Dawson SL, et al. Carotid and vertebral artery dissection syndromes. *Postgrad Med J*. 2005;81:383–388.
160. Schievink WI. Spontaneous dissection of the carotid and vertebral arteries. *N Engl J Med*. 2001;344:898–906.
161. Mokri B, Piepgras DG, Houser OW. Traumatic dissections of the extracranial internal carotid artery. *J Neurosurg*. 1988;68:189–197.
162. Mokri B, Sundt TM Jr., Houser OW, et al. Spontaneous dissection of the cervical internal carotid artery. *Ann Neurol*. 1986;19:126–138.
163. Touze E, Randoux B, Meary E, et al. Aneurysmal forms of cervical artery dissection: associated factors and outcome. *Stroke*. 2001;32:418–423.
164. Auer A, Felber S, Schmidauer C, et al. Magnetic resonance angiographic and clinical features of extracranial vertebral

non-axisymmetric artery in vitro. *J Hypertens*. 2004;22:339–347.

artery dissection. *J Neurol Neurosurg Psychiatry*. 1998;64: 474–481.

165. Felber S, Auer A, Schmidauer C, et al. [Magnetic resonance angiography and magnetic resonance tomography in dissection of the vertebral artery.] *Radiologe*. 1996; 36:872–883.

166. Keller E, Flacke S, Gieseke J, et al. [Craniocervical dissections: study strategies in MR imaging and MR angiography.] *ROFO*. 1997;167:565–571.

167. Oelerich M, Stogbauer F, Kurlemann G, et al. Craniocervical artery dissection: MR imaging and MR angiographic findings. *Eur Radiol*. 1999;9:1385–1391.

168. Furie DM, Tien RD. Fibromuscular dysplasia of arteries of the head and neck: imaging findings. *AJR Am J Roentgenol*. 1994;162:1205–1209.

169. Slovut DP, Olin JW. Fibromuscular dysplasia. *N Engl J Med*. 2004;350:1862–1871.

170. Begelman SM, Olin JW. Fibromuscular dysplasia. *Curr Opin Rheumatol*. 2000;12:41–47.

171. Dayes LA, Gardiner N. The neurological implications of fibromuscular dysplasia. *Mt Sinai J Med*. 2005;72:418–420.

172. Painter TA, Hertzer NR, Beven EG, et al. Extracranial carotid aneurysms: report of six cases and review of the literature. *J Vasc Surg*. 1985;2:312–318.

173. Pulli R, Gatti M, Credi G, et al. Extracranial carotid artery aneurysms. *J Cardiovasc Surg (Torino)*. 1997;38:339–346.

174. Liapis CD, Gugulakis A, Misiakos E, et al. Surgical treatment of extracranial carotid aneurysms. *Int Angiol*. 1994;13:290–295.

175. Welling RE, Taha A, Goel T, et al. Extracranial carotid artery aneurysms. *Surgery*. 1983;93:319–323.

176. McCollum CH, Wheeler WG, Noon GP, et al. Aneurysms of the extracranial carotid artery. Twenty-one years' experience. *Am J Surg*. 1979;137:196–200.

177. Krupski WC, Effeney DJ, Ehrenfeld WK, et al. Aneurysms of the carotid arteries. *Aust N Z J Surg*. 1983;53:521–525.

178. El-Sabrout R, Cooley DA. Extracranial carotid artery aneurysms: Texas Heart Institute experience. *J Vasc Surg*. 2000;31:702–712.

179. Mokri B, Piepgras DG, Sundt TM Jr., et al. Extracranial internal carotid artery aneurysms. *Mayo Clin Proc*. 1982;57:310–321.

180. Zhou W, Lin PH, Bush RL, et al. Carotid artery aneurysm: evolution of management over two decades. *J Vasc Surg*. 2006;43:493–496; discussion 497.

181. Coldwell DM, Novak Z, Ryu RK, et al. Treatment of post-traumatic internal carotid arterial pseudoaneurysms with endovascular stents. *J Trauma*. 2000;48:470–472.

182. Metz H, Murray-Leslie RM, Bannister RG, et al. Kinking of the internal carotid artery. *Lancet*. 1961;1:424–426.

183. Weibel J, Fields WS. Tortuosity, coiling, and kinking of the internal carotid artery. II. Relationship of morphological variation to cerebrovascular insufficiency. *Neurology*. 1965;15:462–468.

184. Willfort-Ehringer A, Ahmadi R, Gschwandtner ME, et al. Single-center experience with carotid stent restenosis. *J Endovasc Ther*. 2002;9:299–307.

185. Lesley WS, Weigele JB, Chaloupka JC. Outcomes for overlapping stents in the extracranial carotid artery. *Catheter Cardiovasc Interv*. 2004;62:375–379.

186. Ballotta E, Thiene G, Baracchini C, et al. Surgical vs medical treatment for isolated internal carotid artery elongation with coiling or kinking in symptomatic patients: a prospective randomized clinical study. *J Vasc Surg*. 2005;42:838–846; discussion 846.

187. Bauer R, Sheehan S, Meyer JS. Arteriographic study of cerebrovascular disease. II. Cerebral symptoms due to kinking, tortuosity, and compression of carotid and vertebral arteries in the neck. *Arch Neurol*. 1961;4:119–131.

188. Vannix RS, Joergenson EJ, Carter R. Kinking of the internal carotid artery. Clinical significance and surgical management. *Am J Surg*. 1977;134:82–89.

189. Koskas F, Bahnini A, Walden R, et al. Stenotic coiling and kinking of the internal carotid artery. *Ann Vasc Surg*. 1993;7:530–540.

190. Vollmar J, Nadjafi AS, Stalker CG. Surgical treatment of kinked internal carotid arteries. *Br J Surg*. 1976;63: 847–850.

191. Corti R, Ferrari C, Roberti M, et al. Spiral computed tomography: a novel diagnostic approach for investigation of the extracranial cerebral arteries and its complementary role in duplex ultrasonography. *Circulation*. 1998;98:984–989.

192. Leipzig TJ, Dohrmann GJ. The tortuous or kinked carotid artery: pathogenesis and clinical considerations. A historical review. *Surg Neurol*. 1986;25:478–486.

193. Siva A. Vasculitis of the nervous system. *J Neurol*. 2001; 248:451–468.

194. Bruce IN, Bell AL. A comparison of two nomenclature systems for primary systemic vasculitis. *Br J Rheumatol*. 1997;36:453–458.

195. Saleh A, Stone JH. Classification and diagnostic criteria in systemic vasculitis. *Best Pract Res Clin Rheumatol*. 2005; 19:209–221.

196. Gandhi D. Computed tomography and magnetic resonance angiography in cervicocranial vascular disease. *J Neuroophthalmol*. 2004;24:306–314.

197. Aoki S, Hayashi N, Abe O, et al. Radiation-induced arteritis: thickened wall with prominent enhancement on cranial MR images report of five cases and comparison with 18 cases of Moyamoya disease. *Radiology*. 2002;223: 683–688.

198. Bley TA, Wieben O, Uhl M, et al. Integrated head-thoracic vascular MRI at 3 T: assessment of cranial, cervical and thoracic involvement of giant cell arteritis. *MAGMA*. 2005;18:193–200.

199. Bley TA, Wieben O, Uhl M, et al. High-resolution MRI in giant cell arteritis: imaging of the wall of the superficial temporal artery. *AJR Am J Roentgenol*. 2005;184:283–287.

200. Choe YH, Kim DK, Koh EM, et al. Takayasu arteritis: diagnosis with MR imaging and MR angiography in acute and chronic active stages. *J Magn Reson Imaging*. 1999;10: 751–757.

201. Gotway MB, Araoz PA, Macedo TA, et al. Imaging findings in Takayasu's arteritis. *AJR Am J Roentgenol*. 2005;184: 1945–1950.

202. Kissin EY, Merkel PA. Diagnostic imaging in Takayasu arteritis. *Curr Opin Rheumatol*. 2004;16:31–37.

203. Ozawa T, Minakawa T, Saito A, et al. MRA demonstration of "periarteritis" in Tolosa-Hunt syndrome. *Acta Neurochir (Wien)*. 2001;143:309–312.

204. Provenzale JM, Barboriak DP, Allen NB, et al. Antiphospholipid antibodies: findings at arteriography. *AJNR Am J Neuroradiol*. 1998;19:611–616.

205. Stanson AW, Friese JL, Johnson CM, et al. Polyarteritis nodosa: spectrum of angiographic findings. *Radiographics*. 2001;21:151–159.

206. Yamazaki K, Suga T, Hirata K. Large vessel arteritis in relapsing polychondritis. *J Laryngol Otol*. 2001;115:836–838.

207. Park JH, Chung JW, Im JG, et al. Takayasu arteritis: evaluation of mural changes in the aorta and pulmonary artery with CT angiography. *Radiology*. 1995;196:89–93.

208. Park JH, Chung JW, Lee KW, et al. CT angiography of Takayasu arteritis: comparison with conventional angiography. *J Vasc Interv Radiol*. 1997;8: 393–400.

209. Calvo-Romero JM. Giant cell arteritis. *Postgrad Med J*. 2003;79:511–515.

210. Narvaez J, Narvaez JA, Nolla JM, et al. Giant cell arteritis and polymyalgia rheumatica: usefulness of vascular magnetic resonance imaging studies in the diagnosis of aortitis. *Rheumatology (Oxford)*. 2005;44:479–483.

211. Cantu C, Pineda C, Barinagarrementeria F, et al. Noninvasive cerebrovascular assessment of Takayasu arteritis. *Stroke*. 2000;31:2197–2202.

212. Ringleb PA, Strittmatter EI, Loewer M, et al. Cerebrovascular manifestations of Takayasu arteritis in Europe. *Rheumatology (Oxford)*. 2005;44: 1012–1015.

213. Tabata M, Kitagawa T, Saito T, et al. Extracranial carotid aneurysm in Takayasu's arteritis. *J Vasc Surg*. 2001;34:739–742.

214. Lamprecht P, Gross WL. Wegener's granulomatosis. *Herz.* 2004;29:47–56.
215. Mentzel HJ, Neumann T, Fitzek C, et al. MR imaging in Wegener granulomatosis of the spinal cord. *AJNR Am J Neuroradiol.* 2003;24:18–21.
216. Schmidt WA, Seipelt E, Molsen HP, et al. Vasculitis of the internal carotid artery in Wegener's granulomatosis: comparison of ultrasonography, angiography, and MRI. *Scand J Rheumatol.* 2001;30:48–50.
217. de Leeuw K, Sanders JS, Stegeman C, et al. Accelerated atherosclerosis in patients with Wegener's granulomatosis. *Ann Rheum Dis.* 2005;64: 753–759.
218. Modrall JG, Sadjadi J. Early and late presentations of radiation arteritis. *Semin Vasc Surg.* 2003;16:209–214.
219. Tsai CF, Jeng JS, Lu CJ, et al. Clinical and ultrasonographic manifestations in major causes of common carotid artery occlusion. *J Neuroimaging.* 2005;15:50–56.
220. Sagduyu A, Sirin H, Oksel F, et al. An unusual case of Behcet's disease presenting with bilateral internal carotid artery occlusion. *J Neurol Neurosurg Psychiatry.* 2002; 73:343.
221. Pannone A, Lucchetti G, Stazi G, et al. Internal carotid artery dissection in a patient with Behcet's syndrome. *Ann Vasc Surg.* 1998;12:463–467.
222. Posacioglu H, Apaydin AZ, Parildar M, et al. Large pseudoaneurysm of the carotid artery in Behcet's disease. *Tex Heart Inst J.* 2005;32:95–98.
223. Gurer O, Yapici F, Enc Y, et al. Spontaneous pseudoaneurysm of the vertebral artery in Behcet's disease. *Ann Vasc Surg.* 2005;19:280–283.
224. Antar KA, Keiser HD, Peeva E. Relapsing arterial aneurysms in juvenile Behcet's disease. *Clin Rheumatol.* 2005;24: 72–75.
225. Aguirre-Sanchez JJ, Portilla-Cuenca JC, Velicia Mata MR, et al. [Internal carotid artery vasculitis originated by cervico-facial actinomycosis as a predisponing factor to stroke.] *Neurologia.* 2005;20:267–270.
226. Munera F, Soto JA, Nunez D. Penetrating injuries of the neck and the increasing role of CTA. *Emerg Radiol.* 2004;10:303–309.
227. Nunez DB Jr., Torres-Leon M, Munera F. Vascular injuries of the neck and thoracic inlet: helical CT-angiographic correlation. *Radiographics.* 2004;24:1087–1098; discussion 1099–1100.
228. Larsen DW. Traumatic vascular injuries and their management. *Neuroimaging Clin N Am.* 2002;12:249–269.
229. Berne JD, Norwood SH, McAuley CE, et al. Helical computed tomographic angiography: an excellent screening test for blunt cerebrovascular injury. *J Trauma.* 2004;57: 11–17; discussion 17–19.
230. Kral T, Schaller C, Urbach H, et al. Vertebral artery injury after cervical spine trauma: a prospective study. *Zentralbl Neurochir.* 2002;63:153–158.
231. Ofer A, Nitecki SS, Braun J, et al. CT angiography of the carotid arteries in trauma to the neck. *Eur J Vasc Endovasc Surg.* 2001;21:401–407.
232. Mutze S, Rademacher G, Matthes G, et al. Blunt cerebrovascular injury in patients with blunt multiple trauma: diagnostic accuracy of duplex Doppler US and early CT angiography. *Radiology.* 2005;237:884–892.
233. Martin CE, Rosenfeld L, McSwain B. Carotid body tumors: a 16-year follow-up of seven malignant cases. *South Med J.* 1973;66:1236–1243.
234. Patetsios P, Gable DR, Garrett WV, et al. Management of carotid body paragangliomas and review of a 30-year experience. *Ann Vasc Surg.* 2002;16:331–338.
235. van den Berg R, Verbist BM, Mertens BJ, et al. Head and neck paragangliomas: improved tumor detection using contrast-enhanced 3D time-of-flight MR angiography as compared with fat-suppressed MR imaging techniques. *AJNR Am J Neuroradiol.* 2004;25:863–870.
236. Kyriakos M. *Pathology of Selected Soft Tissue Tumors of the Head and Neck.* Philadelphia, PA: WB Saunders; 1987.
237. Maves MD. *Vascular Tumors of the Head and Neck.* Philadelphia, PA: JB Lippincott Co.; 1993.

Quantifying Coronary Artery Calcium

CHAPTER 13

Michael A. Brooks
J. Jeffrey Carr

Coronary artery calcified plaque (CACP), a component of coronary atheroma that can be measured with cardiac-gated computed tomography (CT), indicates the presence of advanced atherosclerotic lesions in the coronary arteries and identifies individuals at elevated risk for myocardial infarction and cardiovascular death independent of traditional cardiovascular risk factors. In this chapter, we will explain how calcified plaque is a metabolically active process and has a significant genetic component. We will detail the technical aspects of performing cardiac-gated CT without contrast and for measuring CACP after image acquisition. Finally, we will review the current status of CACP as a clinical tool and indicate how it could be integrated into a cardiovascular disease prevention program.

Atherosclerosis is derived from the Greek words "athera," translated as "gruel" or "porridge," and "sklerosis," meaning "hardening." Thus, from its first description, atherosclerosis was seen as a disease incorporating calcification. Atherogenesis begins in late childhood with the development of fatty streaks, and microcalcifications can be identified in fatty streaks in young individuals in their teens and twenties (1–3). The calcified plaques are located in the intimal layer of the coronary arteries (4) (Fig. 13-1). As atheromata become larger and more complex, the amount of calcified plaque increases. Once the calcified plaque reaches a certain size, it can be imaged by various in vivo modalities, ranging from chest radiographs to cardiac CT, with the threshold for detection dependent on the capability of the imaging devices. Over the years, various imaging modalities, including conventional chest radiography, fluoroscopy, cine fluoroscopy, electron beam computed tomography (EBCT), and more recently, multidetector computed tomography (MDCT) have been used to identify and quantify the amount of CACP.

CACPs are not simply dystrophic calcifications. The existence and maintenance of CACP is a regulated and metabolically active process, which shares a number of similarities with bone formation. Calcified atherosclerotic plaques can recapitulate trabecular bone and marrow elements—osteocytes, chondrocytes, osteoclasts, lymphocytes, mast cells, monocytes, and capillaries have all been identified within calcified coronary plaques (5–8). It is known that proteins found in developing bone are expressed within areas of atherosclerotic plaque undergoing calcification (9–12). There are several proposed models that relate the regulation and homeostasis of atherosclerotic calcification to similar processes involved in bone formation (13).

As further evidence of a connection between atherosclerotic calcification and bone metabolism, it has been known for some time that there is a relationship between atherosclerotic calcification and osteoporosis in humans.

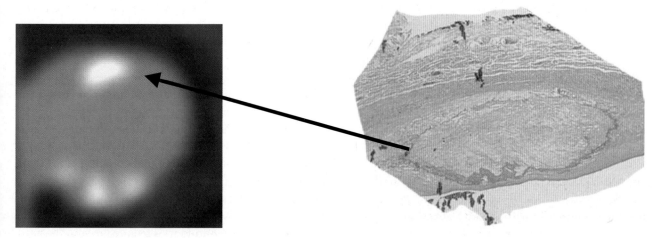

FIGURE 13-1 Ex-vivo specimen CT and histology (H & E section) demonstrating a calcified plaque within the intima of an artery.

Calcified plaque burden in the aorta has been shown to be a predictor both of bone mineral loss and of osteoporotic fracture (14–16). Bone mineral density has also been shown to be inversely correlated with arterial stiffness in dialysis patients (17) and inversely correlated with the presence of echogenic carotid plaque (18). New developments and better understanding of the relationship between atherosclerotic calcification, bone formation and resorption, and inflammation may lead to new therapeutic targets for the prevention and treatment of atherosclerosis.

The presence and extent of atherosclerotic calcification has a significant genetic component that appears to be at least as strong as the known combined environmental risk factors such as smoking and elevated serum cholesterol (19,20). Important ethnic differences in the prevalence and extent of coronary artery calcification exist (21). While the presence of coronary arterial calcification and the presence of atherosclerotic disease are closely correlated (22–24), there are genetic determinants of calcification independent of the genetic determinants of atherosclerotic disease (25,26), indicating that the genetics of CACP are complex and remain to be fully elucidated. At least ten genes are currently implicated in the development of CACP (27).

The American Heart Association and American College of Cardiology have issued several consensus statements which address CACP (28–31). These consensus statements and extensive reviews of the previously published literature are clear in indicating that the presence of coronary artery calcium indicates the presence of coronary artery atherosclerosis, and that increasing amounts of CACP indicate increasing burden of both calcified and noncalcified coronary atherosclerosis. More recently, the data has emerged that CACP predicts cardiovascular events and adds significantly to risk models using traditional cardiovascular risk factors such as the Framingham Risk Score. Autopsy studies have demonstrated a high correlation between the amount of CACP as quantitated by EBCT and the total area of coronary atherosclerotic plaque as determined histologically (32,33). Several studies also demonstrate that CACP predicts and localizes coronary atherosclerotic plaque as depicted by intravascular ultrasound (34,35).

CACP is an indicator of plaque composition and functions as a measure of the total burden of atherosclerotic coronary artery disease. The presence of calcium is seen in atherosclerotic plaques histologically classified as type Vb, according to the American Heart Association (36). Most cases of acute myocardial infarction are precipitated by plaque rupture, and the plaques that rupture and are rupture-prone (the "vulnerable plaque") tend to be lesions that do not contain large amounts of calcium (23,37). However, patterns of calcified plaque may provide insight into segments of the coronary arteries at risk for future events. In a study of patients with acute myocardial infarction, unstable angina pectoris, and stable angina pectoris using intracoronary ultrasound, a "spotty pattern" of calcification was the most highly associated feature with the culprit lesion of acute myocardial infarction (38). CACP has a number of attractive features that make it an excellent marker for use in primary prevention of coronary artery disease. CACP identifies subclinical coronary atherosclerosis, provides a good measure of the total coronary atherosclerosis, can be detected years prior to clinical events, can be measured quantitatively with a standardized protocol, and most importantly predicts future cardiovascular disease (CVD) events, as will be discussed later in this chapter.

MEASUREMENT OF CORONARY ARTERY CALCIFIED PLAQUE BY CT

Cardiac CT allows the standardized measurement of CACP in less than 10 minutes, with little preparation on the part of the patient and no significant risk of complications. It is defined as a CT system that provides for subsecond temporal resolution as well as provides a method for compensation for cardiac motion, most commonly electrocardiogram (ECG) gating. Cardiac CT was initially developed with EBCT in the 1980s. This device could image the heart with 100 ms temporal resolution when performing calcium scoring. More recently, spiral CT and multidetector CT have been utilized. The rapid evolution of MDCT to gantry rotation speeds of 0.3 seconds provides direct temporal resolution of 200 ms. The production of EBCT systems was stopped in 2005, although systems remain operational across the country. The vast majority of cardiac CT, now and in the future, will be performed on MDCT systems designed for cardiac imaging.

Performing CT Scans for Measuring Coronary Artery Calcified Plaque

The basic protocol for measuring coronary calcified plaque was developed in clinical practice and then evolved and has been implemented in several large population-based studies funded by the National Heart, Lung, and Blood Institute (NHLBI) and others. This standardized protocol is being utilized in the Multi-Ethnic Study of Atherosclerosis (MESA) and Coronary Artery Risk Development in Young Adults (CARDIA), two large cohort studies following over 10,000 individuals for cardiovascular outcomes. This protocol is based on using an *axial*, also termed a *sequential* or *cine*, CT acquisition, coupled with prospective ECG gating. With current MDCT systems, the breath-hold time for the patient is less than 15 seconds, during which time the x-ray tube is activated for less than 2 seconds. This allows an extremely low radiation exposure exam to be performed, typically with an effective dose of between 1 to 1.8 mSv, depending on the technique and specific characteristics of the MDCT system. In essence, the ECG tracing triggers the CT scanner to acquire a block of images at a preset window within the cardiac cycle based on the location of the QRS complex. This window has been typically set to late diastole, 70% to 80% of the temporal distance between two R waves. Several alternative approaches to cardiac triggering using an earlier diastolic phase, such as 50% of the R-R interval, have also been successfully used. In setting the R to R offset, it is important to remember that various vendors may define this offset at either the beginning of image acquisition or the temporal center of acquisition, and it is necessary to know the strategy employed by your equipment manufacturer.

To provide a more concrete explanation, we will detail the protocol as implemented on a General Electric Healthcare Lightspeed 16 Pro. On this CT system, there is a 20-mm

wide detector array. For measuring calcified plaque, the standard slice collimation employed is between 2.5 and 3 mm. The GE system uses detector elements of 2.5 mm, and thus an axial scan in which eight 2.5 mm slices are reconstructed utilizes the entire 20 mm detector width (i.e., 8×2.5 mm $= 20$ mm), resulting in the greatest dose efficiency. So, for each heartbeat, the x-ray tube is activated at the appropriate trigger point, and a block of eight slices of 2.5-mm thickness is obtained. Once this acquisition is completed, the CT couch moves to the next level during the subsequent heartbeat. The second scan acquisition is then obtained, and this sequence is repeated until the entire scan volume is covered. For the typical heart, 100 to 120 mm along the z-axis (head-to-foot) is required to scan the heart, resulting in five to six acquisitions. For an individual with a heart rate of 60 beats per minute, each R to R interval occupies one second. Therefore, six cardiac cycles for imaging and five for table movement are needed. This results in a total breath-hold time of 11 seconds.

The LightSpeed Pro 16 has a maximum gantry rotation speed of 0.4 seconds. The cardiac scan mode as previously discussed is in the axial or cine mode. In addition, as detailed in the technical chapter related to CT, a partial or segmental image reconstruction is utilized to maximize temporal resolution. This results in the effective temporal resolution of each image being approximately one half to two thirds the gantry rotation speed, depending on how close one is to the center of the image. In this example, the temporal resolution ranges from .2 to .25 seconds. The exposure useful for calculating mAs is the larger of these. The actual tube-on time for the entire scan acquisition can be estimated by the longer of these values. If six blocks of slices are obtained and the exposure time is approximately 0.25 seconds per exposure, the total tube-on time is equal to 1.5 seconds. Thus, for a breath-hold time of 11 seconds, the participant is only receiving radiation during 1.5 seconds. Gantry speeds slower than 0.5 seconds per rotation are suboptimal for imaging the heart and are not recommended for performing cardiac CT. Ideally, systems capable of gantry speeds between 0.35 and 0.4 seconds (or faster) should be used for cardiac applications.

Preparing and scanning individuals for measuring CACP is straightforward. Prior to the cardiac CT exam, we recommend that subjects avoid caffeine and other stimulants for 12 hours preceding the exam to decrease the incidence of tachycardia. The coronary calcium measurement is relatively tolerant to motion, and therefore administration of oral or IV beta blockade to lower the heart rate is not employed or recommended. The individual is placed on the CT couch; this could be either head or feet first depending on local practice and the manufacturer's recommendations. ECG

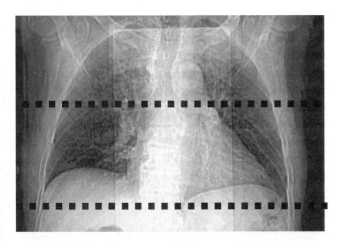

FIGURE 13-2 Scout topogram or scanogram demonstrating the start and end locations for prescribing a noncontrast cardiac CT. The dashed lines indicate superior and inferior extent of the scanning range. The start location should be just below the carina, and the end location should be inferior to the diaphragmatic aspect of the heart. It is important that the individual understand and execute the breathing instructions. Cardiac position varies with respiration, and it is important to the same level of inspiration for both the scout and subsequent cardiac CT acquisition.

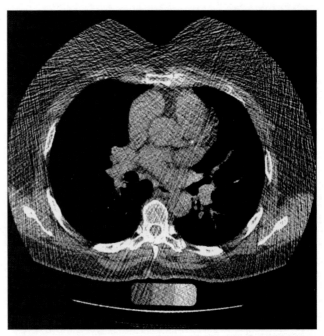

FIGURE 13-3 Patient size and image noise. As the size of the individual within the scan gantry increases, fewer x-ray photons make it through the individual to the detectors. This increased beam attenuation results in an increased signal-to-noise (SNR) ratio. This is manifest in the image as increased "black and white pixels" (image noise) and makes it more difficult to distinguish calcified plaque (or other structures) from noise. In this case, a small calcified plaque in the left anterior descending coronary artery is present and can be distinguished from the surrounding image noise in this large individual.

electrodes are applied to the thorax to provide the necessary gating. A scout tomogram is obtained. The technologist then prescribes the start and stop location based on the frontal scout. The start location is just below the carina, which is generally evident on the scout image. This will place the initial slice generally at the level of the left pulmonary artery and cephalad to the left anterior descending coronary artery. The stop location should be below the diaphragmatic aspect of the heart (Fig. 13-2).

The specific technical factors needed for coronary calcium scanning are CT system specific. There has, however, been work on developing a consensus across vendors toward a standardized protocol. Specific technical factors are kV of 120, slice thickness of between 2.5 and 3 mm, mAs of between 50 and 120 (based on body size considerations to maintain adequate signal-to-noise ratio), reconstruction into a 26-cm field of view centered on the heart, reconstruction using the partial or segmental algorithm, and a medium or standard reconstruction kernel that is vendor specific. Given the low radiation exposure of the prospectively triggered ECG-gated scan, and the improved spatial resolution of current MDCT systems, an adequate mAs should be used to maintain image quality. Various groups have differed on the appropriate mAs value, with suggested values ranging from 50 to 150. It is clear that the size of the individual being scanned is a critical factor in determining the appropriate mAs (Fig. 13-3). In addition, design features of the various CT scanners directly impact the level of noise at a given mAs. Currently, automated exposure tech-

niques are not available for use when cardiac gating is employed on most CT systems. On CT scanners without an automated exposure control, a tiered system of mAs based on an individual's weight is recommended. A weight threshold of 100 kg (220 lb) was selected for use in the MESA and CARDIA studies. Individuals weighing 100 kg or less received the standard mAs value, and those weighing greater than 100 kg received a 25% increase in mAs. To determine the standard mAs value, the specific imaging characteristics of your cardiac CT system need to be understood. Image noise is dependent on several parameters related to the design of the CT scanner and the kernel used for reconstructing the images. One should implement a technique that provides a level of image noise of approximately 18 to 20 CT units. The noise in a given image can be approximated by measuring the standard deviation of a region of interest in the ascending aorta. Once you have determined your base mAs settings, this value can be increased by 25% for individuals greater than 100 kg in weight. If the base mAs for an individual weighing less than 220 lb/100 kg is 100 mAs, the mAs for individuals greater than 100 kg (220 lb) would be 125 mAs.

The nominal slice thickness implemented on the EBCT systems is 3 mm. MDCT systems provide either 2.5 or 3 mm. On the 16-channel and greater MDCT systems, reconstruction of thinner slices at either millimeter or submillimeter slice thickness is possible. Currently, there is little data to support an advantage in measuring calcified plaque with thinner slice thicknesses, although it is clear that the improved spatial resolution in the *z*-axis reduces partial volume averaging of small plaques. In the prospective studies demonstrating the risk assessment benefits of CACP scoring, 2.5- to 3-mm slice thicknesses have been used. Whether thinner slice collimation has a significant role in risk prediction remains to be determined.

Quantifying Coronary Artery Calcified Plaque on a Computer Workstation

Coronary artery calcified plaque, once imaged with cardiac CT, needs to be measured using a software program. CACP is measured in the major (epicardial) coronary arteries, typically the left main, left anterior descending (and diagonal branches), left circumflex (and obtuse marginal branches), and right coronary arteries. These programs are available from several vendors, and all have a similar approach in which the computer and human reader work together in a semiautomated fashion to measure plaque and calculate the "calcium score." Two basic strategies are used. The most common is for the program to highlight potential plaques based on a size criteria and brightness threshold. The human reader then deposits a point or otherwise selects those lesions that are related to the specific coronary artery. The program then grows a region from this seed point in the plaque to its full size based on the connectivity of the adjacent pixels that meet lesion criteria (Fig. 13-4). In most implementations, this is performed on a slice-by-slice ("2-D connectivity") basis; however, newer implementations will connect or grow plaques between slices ("3-D connectivity"). In the second approach, the "reader" identifies the coronary vessels by depositing points along the vessels. These "way points" are used to determine the center of the coronary artery or centroid. The program then automatically selects calcified pixels meeting the threshold and minimum size criteria within a given radius of the center of the vessel. In both cases, the software can then total the amount of calcified plaque by vascular segment. In clinical practice, the total calcium score (TCS) or Agatston score remains the measure of calcified coronary plaque most commonly reported and applied in clinical practice (39). This is a scoring system that combines a threshold of 130 HU with a filter for the minimum lesion size. By lowering the threshold or using a smaller minimum lesion size, sensitivity for smaller, less densely calcified lesions is increased at the cost of decreased specificity. The specificity is decreased because as the threshold is set to a lower HU, say a CT

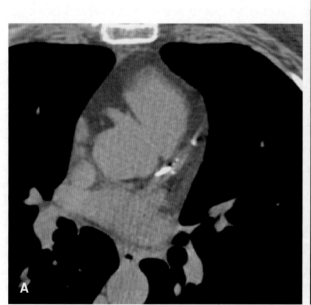
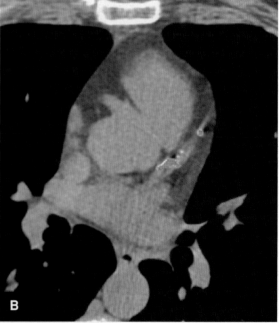

FIGURE 13-4 Calcified plaque identification. Calcified plaques are present in the left anterior descending coronary artery **(A)**. The threshold of 130 CT HU and the minimum lesion size determine which lesions "count" toward the calcium score. After the reader selects the lesions, typically by using the mouse to click or draw a box around the plaque, the "scoreable" lesions are highlighted in pink based on the scoring parameters **(B)**. In this example, the minimum lesion size was set so that the two small plaques do not meet the minimum lesion size criteria and are not color coded or included in the score total.

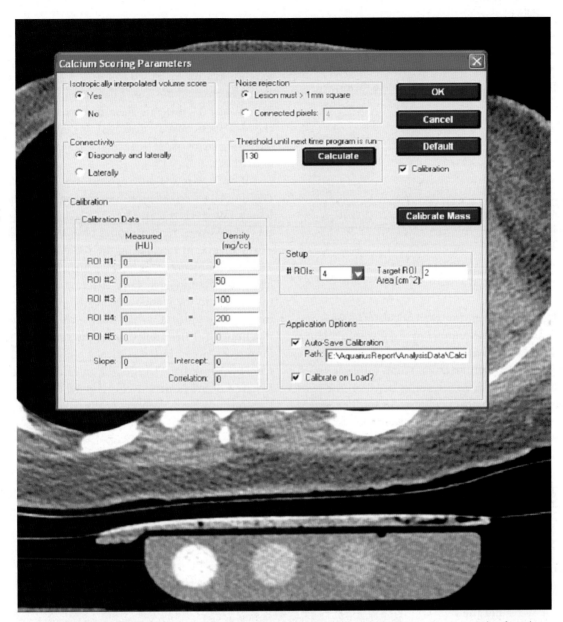

FIGURE 13-5 Options related to calcium scoring parameters. The calcium scoring parameters window from the TeraRecon Aquarius Workstation "Calcium" application is displayed at the top of the figure. Parameters related to minimum lesion size are in essence a filter designed to reduce image noise. In the example shown, the calcified lesions must be greater than 1 mm² to be counted toward the score. The criteria for defining lesion size also must be specified based on whether pixels touch on a full side (i.e., North, South, East, and West) or only on a corner. Additional options allow the volume score to be isotropically interpolated along the slice direction and for using a calibration standard scanned with the patient to create a calibrated mass score.

number of 90 instead of 130, more "noise pixels" will also be identified as possible calcified lesions that the human observer will need to either exclude or accept resulting in more potential false positive lesions. Noise is function of the number of x-ray photons that reach the detector, so lowering the tube current or increasing the size of the patient between the tube and detector will result in increased noise. Therefore, large or obese individuals will have greater image noise if the technique is held constant. As of 2008, clinical practice almost

exclusively uses the standard threshold of 130 HU. The minimum lesion size is more variable, with some implementations based on number of adjacent pixels or absolute lesion size. A minimum lesion size of 1 mm² works well with modern MDCT and EBCT systems. When using the number of adjacent pixels criteria (i.e., 2, 3, or 4 adjacent pixels), images must be reconstructed with a consistent display field of view (dfov), since this will determine pixel size (Fig. 13-5), which in turn will determine minimum lesion size.

TABLE 13-1

Total Calcium Score (TCS) or Agatston Score Weighting Factors for Calcified Plaques

Highest CT # in a Lesion	Weighting Factor
<130	0
130–199	1
200–299	2
300–399	3
≥400	4

Note: When originally proposed, the Agatston or Total Calcium Score did not account for the thickness of CT slice. All current implementation are correct for slice thickness and allow for fractional Agatston Units. Thus, the ranges are more precisely specified as 130 to <200; 200 to <300; 300 to <400, and ≥400.

The TCS or Agatston score then calculates lesion scores based on multiplying the number of pixels within a lesion by a weighting factor based on the brightest pixel in the lesion and then sums all the lesion scores for each vessel. The weighting factor for each lesion is based on the pixel with the highest CT number within the lesion. The weight factors are 0, 1, 2, 3, and 4 and are determined by a step function based on the highest attenuation pixel in the lesion (Table 13-1). This weighting factor is then multiplied by the number of pixels within the lesion (Fig. 13-6). So, as demonstrated in Figure 13-6, there are two calcified plaques located in the proximal left anterior descending coronary

artery. "Plaque 1" consists of five pixels that have CT numbers greater than 130. The highest attenuation pixel in "plaque 1" is 249, and from Table 13-1, the appropriate weighting factor for this lesion is "2." There are five pixels in the lesions, and the score calculation is then $5 \times 2 = 10$. For "plaque 2," there are again five pixels, but in this case, the highest attenuation pixel has a CT number of 346 for a weighting factor of "3." The lesion score would then be calculated as $5 \times 3 = 15$.

If these were the only two plaques in the left anterior descending artery, then the "vessel score" is the sum of the lesions ($10 + 15 = 25$). The TCS is simply the sum of all the "vessel scores," and it utilizes both attenuation and size of the plaque in calculating the score. From this simple example, it becomes clear how the highest attenuation pixel has a disproportionately large effect on the lesion score. A minor shift in the highest attenuation pixel—for example, from 199 to 200 HU—will double the lesion score. The weighting of the entire lesion on the single brightest pixel introduces "noise" into the calculation of the total calcium score by permitting what may be an extreme outlying pixel to have a disproportionate effect on the total score.

Calcified plaque volume or the volume score measures the area of calcified plaque (mm^2) on each slice and then calculates the volume (mm^3) of plaque from the slice thickness. This method ignores the CT density of the plaque above the threshold, and thus plaques with the same number of pixels will have the same volume score. Going back to our example plaques in Figure 13-6, the calculation of a

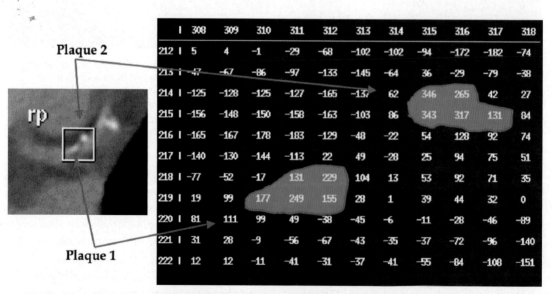

FIGURE 13-6 The calcified plaques visualized on the images are really CT numbers that are used to create the image. Calcium scoring software calculates the calcium scores based on the underlying CT numbers that form the image. In this example, two plaques are demonstrated and outlined based on the 130 CT number threshold.

volume score requires determining the size of each pixel. This is determined from the display field of view of the image and the image matrix size, which is typically 512 rows by 512 columns. Thus, if the image is reconstructed into a 350 mm (35 cm) dfov, each pixel side is 0.68 mm by 0.68 mm (350 mm/512 = 0.68 mm). If the scan data is reconstructed into an image with a 260 mm dfov, the corresponding pixel dimensions are 0.51 mm by 0.51 mm (260 mm/ 512 = 0.51 mm). The area of an individual pixel is 0.46 mm^2 and 0.26 mm^2, respectively. To determine the volume element or voxel size, one simply needs to add the third dimension, which is the slice thickness. If the slice thickness is 3 mm, then the voxel size for the 260 mm dfov image is 0.51 mm $\times$ 0.51 mm $\times$ 3.0 mm = 0.78 mm^3. "Plaque 1" and "plaque 2" are both five pixels or five voxels in size (5 $\times$ 0.78 mm^3 = 3.9 mm^3). The sum of all the individual plaque volumes is the total volume of plaque. From the example, it is clear that spatial resolution is significantly better within the slice than along the slice direction or z-axis. The voxel is anisotropic, meaning that the lengths of the x, y, and z dimensions are different. A variant of the volume score was developed in which the axial slices prior to being analyzed were interpolated to create isotropic voxels. In essence, multiple thin intermediate slices are estimated from the thicker slices, and the resulting data set is used to determine the calcium volumetric score (CVS). Using this methodology, Callister et al. demonstrated improved reproducibility and a reduced rate of calcified plaque progression in individuals receiving statin therapy, although the study was retrospective in design (40,41). Software vendors have implemented the volume score using a variety of algorithms, and the application of the volume score has been largely in the area of clinical research. Several important points about volume scores should be remembered. First, volume scores ignore the CT attenuation values, so whether a plaque is extremely dense or only slightly denser than the 130 threshold has no impact on the "volume" of the lesion or the resulting score. The volume measurements can be reported in SI units of mm^3, which can be compared to histologic morphometry or standardized phantoms to determine measurement error. The volume scores and the TCS (Agatston score) are typically dependent on the threshold value of 130 HU. Error in CT scanner measurement of the 130 HU threshold—which can be related to the technique used, CT system calibration, or to patient characteristics—will introduce an additional source of error into the score calculations.

The *calcium mass* (or *mineral mass*) improves the volume score by weighting of each lesion by its measured attenuation value. This CT attenuation value is mapped to the density of established calcium standard with the resulting calcified plaque reported in milligrams of calcium hydroxyapatite. The first step in determining the calcium mass is performing a linear regression between CT numbers and known samples of calcium. This calibration can be performed on a CT scanner with a standardized phantom. In Figure 13-5, a quantitative CT phantom (Image Analysis, Columbia, KY), used for bone density measurement, is shown in the image posterior to the individual in the CT gantry. This phantom contains four cylinders corresponding to water and 50, 100, and 20 mg/mL of calcium hydroxyapatite. By measuring the CT attenuation values (HU) of these cylinders, a linear regression is then performed, providing the slope and intercept that can be used to convert CT units (HU) to milligrams of calcium. In addition, the phantom calibration can be used to set a standard threshold for measuring calcified plaque based on milligrams of calcium rather than the CT numbers. The calcium mass score, like the volume score, currently is a clinical research tool, and researchers and vendors have implemented various algorithms to calculate a calcium mass. Advantages of this method are that it, like the volume score, uses SI units. The calcium score is calibrated to an external standard, typically a standardized phantom, which should provide greater generalizability. Although the calcium mass score has not been widely implemented, the quality control procedures, developed largely for quantitative CT (QCT) of the spine in which phantoms are used to calibrate the CT images, have been implemented in many research studies, including the NHLBI's MESA. To date there is no evidence that the alternative methods of measuring calcified plaque (volume score, mass score and their variants) improve the ability to predict future risk of cardiovascular events. The development of these methods has been driven by clinical research objectives of improving our understanding of calcified plaque biology or change in calcified plaque over time. Currently, serial studies for measuring change in calcified plaque burden are not recommended for clinical practice secondary to the lack of information about both the biologic and clinical implications of changes in calcified plaque (31).

Measuring coronary artery calcified plaque can be accomplished with a variety of approaches. In clinical practice and in most clinical research applications, the total calcium score, also known as the Agatston score, is used and modified as necessary to correct for slice thickness and the display field of view. As discussed earlier, because of the nonlinear step weighting function employed in its calculation, the TCS has an increased variability relative to the other scoring methods, which is particularly problematic if one intends to measure change in calcified plaque over time. The TCS, though theoretically inferior, is currently the most widely used measure for historical reasons because of the extensive literature documenting its application. The volume scores and calibrated mass score both have properties that make them more robust, as mentioned previously; however, a standardized implementation of these methods has not made its way into clinical practice. Although the scoring methods and parameters such as the threshold and minimum lesion size will alter the absolute score, for the most part, these differences are not clinically important. Previously, we compared six different scoring methodologies (thresholds of 90 and 130 and three different scoring algorithms) to EBCT using the TCS (42). The correlations, both linear and nonparametric, to EBCT-derived TCS as well as between the methods were all >0.96, indicating near perfect correlation. So, in many ways, these scoring methods are like the differences between the Fahrenheit, Kelvin, and Celsius temperature scales. Each will give you different absolute values for a given temperature, and each may be optimally used in specific situations, but all three reflect the same physical state. Likewise, the various measures of calcified plaque, calcium score, volume, mass, and the variants of each quantify the same physical entity with largely the same information content.

REPORTING RESULTS

The amount of coronary artery calcified plaque is typically reported using the Agatston or total calcium score, modified to account for the thickness of the slice. The amount of calcified plaque is highly correlated with total coronary plaque and thus provides a good estimate of total coronary plaque. Guidelines for management that incorporate the calcium score have been proposed but not established in the larger medical community; however, such guidelines are in active development at the time of this writing. A calcium score greater than 100 indicates a moderate burden of plaque, and a score greater than 300 had significant increased risk of events for all levels of Framingham Risk in the South Bay Heart Study (43). In the absence of consensus guidelines, these are reasonable cut points based on the available evidence. For individuals with a calcium score >300, a reasonable recommendation is for further testing for possible obstructive coronary artery disease (CAD) with a functional evaluation including stress. In addition, it is now possible to provide the percentile ranges for individuals asymptomatic for cardiovascular disease specific for age, gender, and ethnicity based on the data from the NHLBI's MESA. These percentiles are available for four ethnic groups: Chinese, Hispanic, White, and African American (http://www.mesa-nhlbi.org/CACReference.aspx (Fig. 13-7). Currently, there is no consensus or guideline for the broad clinical application of percentiles of coronary artery calcified plaque in CVD prevention. However, the National

Cholesterol Education Program Adult Treatment Panel III (NCEP ATP III) update concluded that "measurement of coronary calcium is an option for advanced risk assessment in appropriately selected persons. In persons with multiple risk factors, high coronary calcium scores (e.g., >75th percentile for age and sex) denote advanced coronary atherosclerosis and provide a rationale for intensified LDL-lowering therapy. Moreover, measurement of coronary calcium is promising for older persons in whom the traditional risk factors lose some of their predictive power" (44). As CVD event data becomes available from NHLBI's MESA and other studies, more specific recommendations for age, gender, and ethnicity will likely be developed. The combination of absolute levels of plaque and percentile values specific for age, gender, and ethnicity provide significant information regarding an individual's coronary atherosclerotic burden and CVD risk. Currently, physicians and their patients who choose to use cardiac CT for CVD risk assessment must integrate this information into prevention plans by taking advantage of the extensive albeit incomplete data on coronary artery calcified plaque and CVD events.

APPLICATION FOR CARDIOVASCULAR DISEASE RISK ASSESSMENT

In a joint statement published in 2000, the American College of Cardiology (ACC) and the American Heart Association (AHA) felt that there was insufficient evidence to recommend the use of the calcium score for screening asymptomatic individuals (29). It was recommended that in order for CACP screening to be justified as an aid for risk assessment and primary prevention, it should provide an additive and independent predictive value above the well-established risk factors described in such models as the Framingham score, a position supported by the American Heart Association's Prevention V Conference (45). In addition, there was felt to be insufficient data to justify the use of EBCT to assess for the progression or regression of CAD following preventive intervention.

Since the publication of this statement, there have been several major additions to the scientific literature related to the use of CACP quantification as applied to CAD risk assessment. First, EBCT calcium scoring has been largely supplanted by cardiac-gated MDCT calcium scoring, which utilizes much more widely available equipment. In a number of studies, the calcium score obtained by MDCT has been shown to be equivalent to the EBCT score for range of scores used for clinical decision making (42,46–49), and the reproducibility or measurement errors of these scores are comparable (49). Second, it has been documented that the cardiac CT exam can be introduced into busy clinical practices, and that

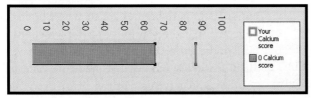

MESA — The Multi-Ethnic Study of Atherosclerosis

Back to MESA CAC

Input your age, select your gender and race/ethnicity, input (optionally) your observed calcium score and click "Calculate".

Age (45-84): 55

Gender: male

Race/Ethnicity: black

Observed Agatston Calcium Score (optional): 50

Calculate

The estimated probability of a non-zero calcium score for a black male of age 55 is 37 %.

Percentiles and Calcium Scores for: black male of age 55

25th	50th	75th	90th
0	0	15	94

The observed calcium score of 50 **is at the** 84th **percentile for subjects of the same age, gender, and race/ethnicity who are free of clinical cardiovascular disease and treated diabetes.**

Chart 1: Percentiles

Your Calcium score
0 Calcium score

FIGURE 13-7 The NHLBI's MESA makes available over the Internet a calculator that determines percentiles for individuals based on an individual's age, gender, and ethnicity. This Web site can be accessed at http://www.mesa-nhlbi.org/CACReference.aspx.

by using a standardized protocol, high quality and comparable results can be obtained across multiple centers using a variety of cardiac CT systems both EBCT and MDCT (50). And lastly, a number of major prospective studies have since provided the evidence for CACP related to cardiovascular events that was lacking in the 2000 ACC/AHA statement. As with many new technologies, the early studies of EBCT calcium scoring were performed at a limited number of pioneering sites. Recruitment strategies often were based on sampling clinical or convenient populations. CVD risk factors were not measured or were obtained by self-report. These early studies, despite their limitations and biases, provided the scientific rationale for funding the subsequent studies with more robust designs.

Currently, there are five published studies that measured CACP with EBCT and other CVD risk factors and prospectively followed individuals for events. Although an initial analysis of EBCT calcium scoring in the prospective South Bay Heart Watch Study showed no benefit of calcium scoring over conventional risk factor analysis (51), further follow-up of subjects in this trial has demonstrated that the CACP score provides additional predictive power above that provided by standard clinical cardiovascular risk factors and serum C reactive protein (43,52). More recently, prospective trials utilizing CACP scoring—the St. Francis Heart Study (53), the Prospective Army Coronary Calcium Project (54), the Cooper Clinic Study (55), and the Rotterdam Heart Study (56)—have all demonstrated independent value for CACP scoring in predicting hard cardiovascular events. The Rotterdam Heart Study demonstrated that the CACP score in the elderly predicts hard and soft coronary events, all cardiovascular events and all cause mortality, and significantly improves prediction above standard cardiovascular risk factors. In the Rotterdam Heart Study, participants and the health care team were blinded to the calcium score, eliminating the calcium score as a source of bias related to participant management and subsequent events. These studies that associate CACP score with clinical events were all performed with EBCT technology, but it is anticipated that CACP scoring performed with cardiac-gated MDCT will demonstrate similar benefits, given the technical equivalence of the two methods of measurement. The initial reports from MESA indicate that coronary artery calcified plaque is a strong predictor of near-term coronary heart disease events in all major American ethnic groups (31). The 6,726 individuals in the study had been followed for an average 3.5 years since the cardiac CT exam. Individuals with calcified plaque burdens of over 100 Agatston units had a 10–20 fold increase in the occurrence of non-fatal myocardial infarction and coronary heart disease death. Calcified plaque added significantly to traditional risk factors, was predictive of cardiovascular events in both men and women as well as four major ethnic groups (Chinese, Hispanic, African American and Caucasian).

CORONARY ARTERY CALCIFIED PLAQUE IN SYMPTOMATIC INDIVIDUALS

In individuals with symptoms, use of cardiac CT to measure CACP has been shown to have diagnostic accuracy comparable to stress treadmill, exercise single photon emission computed tomography (SPECT), and stress echocardiography. As mentioned previously, presence of calcified plaque documents the presence of coronary atherosclerosis and takes an individual from having risk factors to documented coronary artery disease. The diagnostic performance of noncontrast cardiac CT for obstructive coronary disease using the presence of calcified plaque with a cut point of 100 Agatston units in the setting of symptoms has approximately 85% sensitivity and 75% specificity, which is roughly comparable to the performance of the more established tests (stress treadmill, exercise SPECT, and stress echocardiography) used in this population (57–59). Perhaps more important is the potential for noncontrast cardiac CT to improve the diagnostic performance of functional tests such as exercise treadmill, single photon emission tomography, echocardiography, and cardiac magnetic resonance imaging (MRI) by identifying those individuals with CAD and thus dramatically increasing the pretest probability of disease (60). This remains an area of active research and controversy. A calcium score of 0 has also been shown in a large number of studies to have a negative predictive value ranging between 96% to 100% for excluding the presence of obstructive coronary artery disease by coronary angiography (31). However, exercise testing provides a very important assessment of cardiac performance with prognostic implication which extend beyond determining plaque burden and remains a primary tool for evaluating the symptomatic patient. Coronary calcium measurement with cardiac CT can play an important role where functional testing is suboptimal or limited secondary to the inability to exercise, medications, baseline wall motion abnormalities or electrocardiogram abnormalities. Differentiating ischemic cardiomyopathy from primary dilated cardiomyopathy is another role in which the presence of CACP by cardiac CT may play a role. There is significant overlap in the clinical presentations, and the identification of calcified plaque has been shown to be highly sensitive for identifying individuals with ischemic cardiomyopathy (61,62). The presence or absence of CACP has been evaluated as a triage tool in the setting of acute chest pain (63–65). The targeted population is composed of individuals presenting to the Emergency Department with chest discomfort and nondiagnostic ECG and serum markers of myocardial damage. In the studies to date, unstable patients using varying definitions related to blood pressure, congestive heart failure, arrhythmias, and prior CVD have been excluded. These limited studies have documented the feasibility of implementation of cardiac CT in the setting of acute chest pain and have shown a very high sensitivity and negative predictive value for subsequent cardiovascular events. Positive predictive values are significantly lower at approximately 50%. For those individuals found to have calcium scores of zero, a very low rate of subsequent events was observed, although the sample size studied was limited. Given the complex problem of managing acute chest pain, the time urgency, and the alternative diagnostic tests available, further work is needed to determine the potential role, if any, of noncontrast cardiac CT in the setting of acute chest pain.

CONCLUSION

Cardiac CT can be used to measure coronary artery calcified plaque (CACP). The presence of CACP advances an individual from having risk factors to documented subclinical coronary atherosclerosis. The amount of calcified plaque can be measured reproducibly and with sufficient precision with both EBCT and MDCT systems designed for cardiac imaging. CACP can be helpful in guiding the management of individuals with symptoms, but more evidence is required before changes in clinical practice are warranted. However, the continued improvement in temporal resolution of non-cardiac CT means that the presence of CACP should be noted on standard chest CT exams and may play an important role in differential diagnosis. Currently, CACP measured by cardiac CT has strong evidence supporting its use as an assessment tool in determining individuals at risk for cardiovascular disease who could potentially benefit from enhanced prevention strategies. Data from several prospective cohorts demonstrate that the calcium score adds significantly to our ability to prospectively identify individuals at significantly higher risk of CVD events and death. Furthermore, the calcium score adds considerably to the risk prediction of both traditional estimates of CVD risk such as the Framingham Risk Score and novel predictors such as serum C-reactive protein levels. In the National Institutes of Health, Multi-Ethnic Study of Atherosclerosis (MESA) a population-based study of 6,726 individuals across the U.S., it has been documented that the cardiac CT exam can be introduced into busy clinical practices, and that by using a standardized protocol, high quality and comparable results can be obtained across multiple centers using a variety of cardiac CT systems. Importantly, there are established interventions, namely lifestyle changes and lipid lowering with statins, that significantly reduce the risk of myocardial infarction and death in individuals once identified and then treated. The application of cardiac CT to measure calcified plaque as a tool for CVD risk assessment has the potential to significantly improve the prevention of CHD. By identifying those at highest risk for CVD, prevention efforts can be intensified, and the morbidity and mortality from CVD may be reduced.

REFERENCES

1. Bobryshev YV, Lord RSA, Warren BA. Calcified deposit formation in intimal thickenings of the human aorta. *Atherosclerosis.* 1995;118:9–21.
2. Guyton JR, Klemp KF. Transitional features in human atherosclerosis—intimal thickening, cholesterol clefts, and cell loss in human aortic fatty streaks. *Am J Pathol.* 1993;143:1444–1457.
3. Stary HC. The development of calcium deposits in atherosclerotic lesions and their persistence after lipid regression. *Am J Cardiol.* 2001;88(2A): 16E–19E.
4. Stary HC. Natural history of calcium deposits in atherosclerosis progression and regression. *Z Kardiol.* 2000;89[Suppl 2]: 28–35.
5. Abedin M, Tintut Y, Demer LL. Mesenchymal stem cells and the artery wall. *Circ Res.* 2001;95:671–676.
6. Buerger L, Oppenheimer A. Bone formation in sclerotic arteries. *J Exp Med.* 1908;10:354–367.
7. Bunting CH. The formation of true bone with cellular (red) marrow in a sclerotic aorta. *J Exp Med.* 1906;8:365–376.
8. Virchow R. *Die Cellularpathologie in ihrer Begründung auf physiologische und pathologische Gewebelehre.* Berlin: A. Hirschwald.
9. Bini A, Mann KG, Kudryk BJ, et al. Noncollagenous bone matrix proteins, calcification, and thrombosis in carotid artery atherosclerosis. *Arterioscler Throm Vasc Biol.* 1999;19:1852–1861.
10. Fitzpatrick LA, Severson A, Edwards WD, et al. Diffuse calcification in human coronary arteries. Association of osteopontin with atherosclerosis. *J Clin Invest.* 1994;94:1597–1604.
11. Rattazzi M, Bennett BJ, Bea F, et al. Calcification of advanced atherosclerotic lesions in the innominate arteries of apoe-deficient mice. Potential role of chondrocyte-like cells. *Arterioscler Throm Vasc Biol.* 2005;25:1420–1425.
12. Tyson KL, Reynolds JL, Mcnair R, et al. Osteo/chondrocytic transcription factors and their target genes exhibit distinct patterns of expression in human arterial calcification. *Arterioscler Throm Vasc Biol.* 2003;23:489–494.
13. Doherty TM, Asotra K, Fitzpatrick LA, et al. Calcification in atherosclerosis: bone biology and chronic inflammation at the arterial crossroads. *Proc Natl Acad Sci USA.* 2003;100: 11201–11206.
14. Frye MA, Melton LJ, Bryant SC, et al. Osteoporosis and calcification of the aorta. *Bone Miner.* 1992;19:185–194.
15. Kiel DP, Kauppila LI, Cupples LA, et al. Bone loss and the progression of abdominal aortic calcification over a 25-year period: the Framingham Heart Study. *Calcif Tiss Int.* 2001; 68:271–276.
16. Schulz EK, Arfai XD, Liu J, et al. Aortic calcification and the risk of osteoporosis and fractures. *J Clin Endocrinol Metab.* 2004;89:4246–4253.
17. Joki N, Hase H, Shiratake M, et al. Calcaneal osteopenia is a new marker for arterial stiffness in chronic hemodialysis patients. *Am J Nephrol.* 2005;25:196–202.
18. Jorgensen L, Joakimsen O, Berntsen GKR, et al. Low bone mineral density is related to echogenic carotid artery plaques: a population-based study. *Am J Epidemiol.* 2004;160:549–556.
19. O'Donnell CJ, Chazaro I, Wilson PWF, et al. Evidence for heritability of abdominal aortic calcific deposits in the Framingham Heart Study. *Circulation.* 2002;106:337–341.
20. Peyser PA, Bielak LF, Chu JS, et al. Heritability of coronary artery calcium quantity measured by electron beam computed tomography in asymptomatic adults. *Circulation.* 2002;106:304–308.
21. Bild DE, Detrano R, Peterson D, et al. Ethnic differences in coronary calcification. The Multi-Ethnic Study of Atherosclerosis (MESA). *Circulation.* 2005;111:1313–1320.
22. Mautner GC, Mautner SL, Froehlich J, et al. Coronary artery calcification. Assessment with electron-beam CT and histomorphometric correlation. *Radiology.* 1994;192:619–623.
23. Mintz GS, Pichard AD, Popma JJ, et al. Determinants and correlates of target lesion calcium in coronary artery disease: a clinical, angiographic and intravascular ultrasound study. *J Am Coll Cardiol.* 1997;29:268–274.
24. Sangiorgi G, Rumberger JA, Severson A, et al. Arterial calcification and not lumen stenosis is highly correlated with atherosclerotic plaque burden in humans: a histologic study of 723 coronary artery segments using nondecalcifying methodology. *J Am Coll Cardiol.* 1998;31:126–133.
25. Doherty TM., Fitzpatrick LA, Shaheen A, et al. Genetic determinants of arterial calcification associated with atherosclerosis. *Mayo Clin Proc.* 2004;79:197–210.
26. Fischer M, Broeckel U, Holmer S, et al. Distinct heritable patterns of angiographic coronary artery disease in families with myocardial infarction. *Circulation.* 2005;111:855–862.
27. Doherty TM, Fitzpatrick LA, Inoue D, et al. Molecular, endocrine, and genetic mechanisms of arterial calcification. *Endocr Rev.* 2004;25:629–672.
28. Wexler L, Brundage B, Crouse J, et al. Coronary artery calcification: pathophysiology, epidemiology, imaging methods, and clinical implications. A statement for health professionals from the American Heart Association. *Circulation.* 1996;94:1175–1192.

29. O'Rourke RA, Brundage BH, Froelicher VF, et al. American College of Cardiology/American Heart Association expert consensus document on electron-beam computed tomography for the diagnosis and prognosis of coronary artery disease. *J Am Coll Cardiol*. 2000;36:326–340.

30. Carr JJ, et al. Calcified coronary artery plaque measurement with cardiac CT in population-based studies: standardized protocol of Multi-Ethnic Study of Atherosclerosis (MESA) and Coronary Artery Risk Development in Young Adults (CARDIA) study. *Radiology*. 2005;234(1):35–43.

31. Detrano R, et al. Coronary calcium predicts near-term coronary heart disease events in major American ethnic groups: the multi-ethnic study of atherosclerosis. *J Am Coll Cardiol*. 2007;99–183.

32. Rumberger JA, Schwartz RS, Simons B, et al. Relation of coronary calcium determined by electron beam computed tomography and lumen narrowing determined by autopsy. *Am J Cardiol*. 1994;73:1169–1173.

33. Rumberger JA, Simons DB, Fitzpatrick LA, et al. Coronary artery calcium area by electron-beam computed tomography and coronary atherosclerotic plaque area. A histopathologic correlative study. *Circulation*. 1995;92:2157–2162.

34. Baumgart D, Schmermund A, Goerge G, et al. Comparison of electron beam computed tomography with intracoronary ultrasound and coronary angiography for detection of coronary atherosclerosis. *J Am Coll Cardiol*. 1997;30:57–64.

35. Schmermund A, Baumgart D, Gorge G, et al. Coronary artery calcium in acute coronary syndromes: A comparative study of electron-beam computed tomography, coronary angiography, and intracoronary ultrasound in survivors of acute myocardial infarction and unstable angina. *Circulation*. 1997;96:1461–1469.

36. Stary HC, Chandler AB, Dinsmore RE, et al. A definition of advanced types of atherosclerotic lesions and a histological classification of atherosclerosis. A report from the Committee on Vascular Lesions of the Council on Arteriosclerosis, American Heart Association. *Circulation*. 1995;92:1355–1374.

37. Beckman JA, Ganz J, Creager MA, et al.. Relationship of clinical presentation and calcification of culprit coronary artery stenoses. *Arterioscler Thromb Vasc Biol*. 2001;21:1618–1622.

38. Ehara S, Kobayashi Y, Yoshiyama M, et al. Spotty calcification typifies the culprit plaque in patients with acute myocardial infarction: An intravascular ultrasound study. *Circulation*. 2004;110:3424–3429.

39. Agatston AS, Janowitz WR, Hildner FJ, et al. Quantification of coronary artery calcium using ultrafast computed tomography. *J Am Coll Cardiol*. 1990;15:827–832.

40. Callister TQ, Raggi P, Cooil B, et al. Effect of HMG-CoA reductase inhibitors on coronary artery disease as assessed by electron-beam computed tomography. *N Engl J Med*. 1998;339:1972–1978.

41. Callister TQ, Cooil B, Raya SP, et al. Coronary artery disease: improved reproducibility of calcium scoring with an electron-beam CT volumetric method. *Radiology*. 1998;208:807–814.

42. Carr JJ, Crouse JR, Goff DC, et al. Evaluation of subsecond gated helical CT for quantification of coronary artery calcium and comparison with electron beam CT. *Am J Roentgenol*. 2000;174:915–921.

43. Greenland P. Coronary artery calcium score combined with Framingham score for risk prediction in asymptomatic individuals (Vol. 291, p. 210). *JAMA*. 2004;291:563.

44. Third Report of the National Cholesterol Education Program (NCEP) Expert Panel on Detection, Evaluation, and Treatment of High Blood Cholesterol in Adults (Adult Treatment Panel III). Final Report. NIH Publication No. 02-5215. September 2002.

45. Greenland P, Abrams J, Aurigemma GP, et al. Prevention Conference V: Beyond secondary prevention: identifying the high-risk patient for primary prevention: noninvasive tests of atherosclerotic burden: Writing Group III. *Circulation*. 101(1):E16–22.

46. Horiguchi J, Yamamoto H, Akiyama Y, et al. Coronary artery calcium scoring using 16-MDCT and a retrospective ECG-gating reconstruction algorithm. *Am J Roentgenol*. 2004;183:103–108.

47. Knez A, Becker C, Becker A, et al. Determination of coronary calcium with multi-slice spiral computed tomography: a comparative study with electron-beam CT. *Int J Cardiovasc Imaging*. 2002;18:295–303.

48. Stanford W, Thompson BH, Burns TL, et al. Coronary artery calcium quantification at multi-detector row helical CT versus electron-beam CT. *Radiology*. 2004;230:397–402.

49. Detrano RC, Anderson M, Nelson J, et al. Coronary calcium measurements: Effect of CT scanner type and calcium measure on rescan reproducibility—MESA study. *Radiology*. 2005;236:477–484.

50. Carr JJ, Nelson JC, Wong ND, et al. Calcified coronary artery plaque measurement with cardiac CT in population-based studies: standardized protocol of Multi-Ethnic Study of Atherosclerosis (MESA) and Coronary Artery Risk Development in Young Adults (CARDIA) study. *Radiology*. 2005;234:35–43.

51. Detrano RC, Wong ND, Doherty TM, et al. Coronary calcium does not accurately predict near-term future coronary events in high-risk adults. *Circulation*. 1999;99:2633–2638.

52. Park R, Detrano R, Xiang M, et al. Combined use of computed tomography coronary calcium scores and C-reactive protein levels in predicting cardiovascular events in nondiabetic individuals. *Circulation*. 2002;106: 2073–2077.

53. Arad Y, Goodman KJ, Roth M, et al. Coronary calcification, coronary disease risk factors, C-reactive protein, and atherosclerotic cardiovascular disease events—the St. Francis Heart Study. *J Am Coll Cardiol*. 2005;46:158–165.

54. Taylor AJ, Bindeman J, Feuerstein I, et al. Coronary calcium independently predicts incident premature coronary heart disease over measured cardiovascular risk factors: mean three-year outcomes in the Prospective Army Coronary Calcium (PACC) project. *J Am Coll Cardiol*. 2005;46:807–814.

55. Lamonte MJ, Fitzgerald SJ, Church TS, et al. Coronary artery calcium score and coronary heart disease events in a large cohort of asymptomatic men and women. *Am J Epidemiol*. 2005;162:421–429.

56. Vliegenthart R, Oudkerk M, Hofman A, et al. Coronary calcification improves cardiovascular risk prediction in the elderly. *Circulation*. 2005;112: 572–577.

57. Budoff MJ, Georgiou D, Brody A, et al. Ultrafast computed tomography as a diagnostic modality in the detection of coronary artery disease: A multicenter study. *Circulation*. 1996;93:898–904.

58. Budoff MJ, Diamond GA, Raggi P, et al. Continuous probabilistic prediction of angiographically significant coronary artery disease using electron beam tomography. *Circulation*. 2002;105:1791–1796.

59. Haberl R, Becker A, Leber A, et al. Correlation of coronary calcification and angiographically documented stenoses in patients with suspected coronary artery disease: Results of 1,764 patients. *J Am Coll Cardiol*. 2001;37:451–457.

60. Berman DS, Wong ND, Gransar H, et al. Relationship between stress-induced myocardial ischemia and atherosclerosis measured by coronary calcium tomography. *J Am Coll Cardiol*. 2004;44:923–930.

61. Budoff MJ, Shavelle DM, Lamont DH, et al. Usefulness of electron beam computed tomography scanning for distinguishing ischemic from nonischemic cardiomyopathy. *J Am Coll Cardiol*. 1998;32:1173–1178.

62. Shemesh J, Tenenbaum A, Fisman EZ, et al. Coronary calcium as a reliable tool for differentiating ischemic from nonischemic cardiomyopathy. *Am J Cardiol*. 1996;77:191–194.

63. Laudon DA, Vukov LF, Breen JF, et al. Use of electron beam computed tomography in the evaluation of chest pain patients in the emergency department. *Ann Emerg Med*. 1999;33:15–21.

64. Georgiou D, Budoff MJ, Kaufer E, et al. Screening patients with chest pain in the emergency department using electron beam tomography: A follow-up study. *J Am Coll Cardiol*. 2001;38:105–110.

65. McLaughlin VV, Balogh T, Rich S. Utility of electron beam computed tomography to stratify patients presenting to the emergency room with chest pain. *Am J Cardiol*. 1999; 84:327–328.

Coronary Arteries

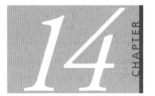

Warren J. Manning
Christoph R. Becker
Neil M. Rofsky

INTRODUCTION

Spectrum and Prevalence of Disease

Despite decades of progress in identification of clinical risk factors, prevention, and early diagnosis, coronary artery disease (CAD) (1) remains the leading cause of mortality for men and women in the United States (2) and throughout the Western world. Overall, CAD results in 700,000 infarctions annually and is responsible for one of every five deaths in the United States (2).

Global View of Unique Aspects and Considerations of Imaging of Coronary Arteries

The small caliber, tortuosity, and rapid motion of the coronary arteries during both the respiratory and cardiac cycle make imaging of the coronary lumen particularly challenging for invasive and noninvasive modalities. Moreover, it is increasingly recognized that conventional x-ray "luminographic" imaging significantly underestimates the true burden of atherosclerotic CAD. The atherosclerotic process is initiated by endothelial injury with local inflammation leading to a focal plaque. In the mid-1980s, Glagov et al. (3) demonstrated that initially, as the plaque expands, the coronary lumen is relatively maintained, but after some period, further plaque enlargement leads to lumen encroachment and development of clinical disease. The definition of *coronary artery disease* is classically taken to include a 50% or greater diameter narrowing of a major coronary artery or branch. This narrowing may correspond to a 75% lumen cross-sectional area loss. A "significant" stenosis that may warrant a mechanical intervention/revascularization is present if the diameter stenosis exceeds 70% (~90% cross-sectional area loss). Improved longevity is generally recognized for patients with left main (LM) or multivessel CAD undergoing coronary artery bypass graft (CABG) surgery.

What Does Computed Tomography and Magnetic Resonance Imaging Bring over Other Imaging and Nonimaging Diagnostic Testing?

For over 40 years, invasive x-ray coronary angiography has been the clinical "gold standard" for the diagnosis of CAD, with almost 1.5 million diagnostic x-ray coronary angiograms performed annually in the United States (2) and nearly a million percutaneous interventions and CABG surgeries. Even higher volumes of diagnostic catheterizations and interventions are performed in Europe and Japan. However, x-ray angiography is a projection technique in which the coronary lumen is viewed from multiple imaging planes.

While numerous noninvasive tests are available to help discriminate among those with and without significant luminographic disease, clinical studies continue to demonstrate that 25% to 40% of patients referred for elective x-ray coronary angiography are found to have no significant stenoses (4,5). Despite the absence of disease, these patients remain subjected to the cost, inconvenience, and potential morbidity of invasive x-ray angiography (6,7). In addition, data suggest that in selected high-risk populations such as patients with aortic valve stenosis, the incidence of subclinical stroke associated with diagnostic cardiac catheterization may exceed 20% (8).

Since surgical revascularization of LM and multivessel proximal coronary disease has the greatest impact on patient mortality and >90% of coronary segments undergoing intervention fall within the proximal/middle segments (9,10), it would be desirable to have a noninvasive method to directly visualize the proximal/midnative coronary vessels for the accurate identification/exclusion of LM/multivessel CAD. In addition, technologies that would permit assessment of subclinical disease of the great vessels and coronary arteries would be desirable so that more intensive therapies could be considered to possibly prevent or delay progression to clinical disease.

The electrocardiogram (ECG) is helpful in diagnosing acute myocardial infarction among patients presenting with chest pain and of inducible ischemia during stress testing, but its findings are less specific to a coronary artery territory. More commonly, the ECG is combined with physiologic stress (treadmill or bicycle ergometry) to identify patients with inducible ischemia, but with only modest

accuracy for identifying patients with CAD. Transthoracic echocardiography is helpful for visualizing the ostia of the native coronary arteries in children and adolescents (11), but identification of focal disease has been limited to transesophageal echocardiography—and then only for the LM coronary artery (12).

Over the last decade, coronary magnetic resonance imaging (MRI) and, more recently, multidector computed tomography (MDCT) and coronary computed tomographic angiography (CTA) have evolved as potential replacements for diagnostic x-ray angiography among patients with suspected anomalous CAD and coronary artery aneurysms, and have now reached sufficient maturity such that they may obviate the need for invasive x-ray angiography when performed at experienced centers.

The rapid advancements in MDCT are yielding relatively uncomplicated and robust assessments of all forms of coronary vascular disease. At the time of this writing, MDCT is undergoing larger scale evaluations for atherosclerotic disease; the results of such studies should more clearly define its role.

IMAGING STRATEGIES

Computed Tomography

Electron Beam

Electron beam CT (EBCT), developed in the late 1980s, was the first CT scanner with exposure times short enough to image the coronary arteries without motion artifacts. In EBCT, electrons are accelerated by an electron gun in a vacuum funnel and are focused on tungsten target rings mounted underneath the patient table. By deceleration of these electrons in the target rings, x-rays are produced that penetrate through the patient. A stationary detector ring above the patient then detects these x-rays (13).

Because of the lack of any moving items, scan time in EBCT for imaging the coronary arteries can be as short as 100 ms. To avoid cardiac motion artifacts, scan acquisition is triggered by the ECG signal at the prospected mid-diastolic phase of the cardiac cycle, typically in between 40% and 80% of the R-R interval (14). The EBCT technique for imaging the coronary arteries is therefore called *prospective ECG triggering*.

As described elsewhere, coronary artery imaging was initially and is still performed by this modality without contrast media to assess coronary calcifications as a surrogate marker of atherosclerosis. Later, contrast-enhanced coronary EBCT showed promising results for also detecting coronary artery stenoses. Because the electron gun always operates at fixed parameters (130 kVp, 63 mAs, and 100 ms), EBCT images may suffer frequently from high image noise and low-contrast resolution, particularly in obese patients. In addition, image acquisition with thinner than 3-mm slices does not allow coverage of the entire coronary artery tree within a single breath hold. Therefore, the spatial resolution is limited, and reliable assessment of the coronary arteries with EBCT is restricted to the proximal part of the coronary artery tree only.

Multidetector Row

In the past, conventional rotating gantry CT did not offer the required temporal resolution to allow for imaging of the coronary arteries. First, single-slice CT scanners with subsecond gantry rotation and prospectively ECG-triggered image acquisition were able to acquire images of the coronary arteries with no or minimal motion artifacts. With the introduction of MDCT, a new acquisition technique was introduced called *retrospective ECG gating*. This technique requires a fast gantry rotation, slow table movement, and multiple detector rows for acquiring a high number of x-ray–projection data from many different angulations and positions of the beating heart in a very short period of time. During the scan acquisition, the ECG signal is recorded simultaneously, and afterward, images are reconstructed retrospectively from the slow-motion diastole phase of the heart.

Retrospective ECG gating with MDCT has several advantages over prospective ECG triggering: (a) the scan time is shorter, (b) the entire volume is acquired continuously and gapless, (c) the image may be reconstructed with overlap, and (d) the optimal individual time point may be selected even after scanning has been completed.

The disadvantage of retrospective ECG gating is that patients are exposed during the systole and diastole, resulting in significantly higher radiation exposure compared with prospective ECG gating. The redundant radiation occurring during the radiation exposure in the systole can substantially be reduced by a technique called *prospective ECG tube current modulation*. On the basis of the ECG signal, the x-ray tube current is switched to its nominal value during the diastole phase and is reduced by 80% during the systole phase of the heart, respectively. This technique reduces the dose by 30% to 50%, depending on heart rate, but is most effective in patients with a low heart rate. For instance, in a patient with a heart rate of around 60 beats per minute (bpm), the radiation exposure will be reduced by approximately 50% (15). For comparison, patients are exposed to approximately 4 mSv by a typical diagnostic coronary catheter procedure (16).

During gantry rotation, x-ray projections of at least 180 degrees are necessary to create an image. The temporal resolution of the image in MDCT therefore depends on the gantry rotation speed. The fastest currently available gantry rotation in MDCT is 330 ms, resulting in a temporal resolution of 165 ms. Attempts have been made to further improve temporal resolution by the so-called multisector-reconstruction algorithm.

For this technique, it may be necessary to reduce the table speed to allow acquisition of x-ray projections from more than one heartbeat to reconstruct an image. The temporal resolution may be improved by up to two to four times compared with 180-degree scan reconstruction but varies with the heart rate. Successful image reconstruction requires absolute consistent data from two or more consecutive heartbeats for successful image reconstruction. However, the rhythm of the human heart may change rapidly, particularly under special conditions such as breath holding and Valsalva maneuver, and reducing the table feed may mean loss of spatial resolution and higher radiation exposure. For these reasons, this technique does not guarantee for consistently good image quality under general clinical conditions.

CT imaging protocols are dependent on the type of scanner. Suggested protocols across a wide variety of platforms can be found in Table 14-1, which includes recommendations for contrast administration and estimations of radiation dose.

Patient Preparation

Optimal scan results with MDCT as well as with EBCT may require some preparation of the patient. Since an image with EBCT is acquired with every heartbeat, acceleration of the heart rate with atropine may help to reduce the scan time and the amount of contrast media. In contrast, in MDCT, deceleration of the heart rate may help to reduce cardiac motion artifacts and to find the optimal image reconstruction interval (17). Prior to a cardiac MDCT examination, patients should avoid the uptake of caffeine or nitroglycerin. Instead, the use of beta-blocker may become necessary for patient preparation, aiming at a heart rate of 65 bpm or less.

To consider a beta-blocker for patient preparation, contraindications (bronchial asthma, atrioventricular [AV] block, severe congestive heart failure, aortic stenosis, etc.) have to be ruled out (18), and informed consent must be obtained from the patient. In a case where the heart rate of a patient is significantly above 60 bpm, 50 to 200 mg of metoprolol tartrate may be administered orally 30 to 90 minutes prior to the investigation. Alternatively, 5 to 20 mg of metoprolol tartrate divided in four doses may be administered intravenously (18) immediately prior to scanning. Monitoring of vital functions, including heart rate and blood pressure, is essential during this approach. Indeed, the positive effect of beta-blocker on cardiac MDCT scanning is fourfold: (a) the sedating effect of

TABLE 14-1

Coronary CTA Technical Factors

Parameter	EBCT Coronary CTA	4-DCT Coronary CTA	16-DCT Coronary CTA	64-DCT Coronary CTA	EBCT Bypass CTA	4-DCT Bypass CTA	16-DCT Bypass CTA	64-DCT Bypass CTA
Slice thickness	3 mm	1.3 mm (4 × 1 mm collimation)	1 mm (16 × 0.75 mm collimation)	0.7 mm (64 × 0.6 mm collimation)	3 mm	3 mm (4 × 2.5 mm collimation)	1 mm (16 × 0.75 mm collimation)	0.7 mm (64 × 0.6 mm collimation)
Scan time	40 s (2 mm/heartbeat and 60 bpm)	40 s (1.5 mm/gantry rotation)	20 s (2 mm/gantry rotation)	10 s (4 mm/gantry rotation)	40 s (3 mm/heartbeat and 60 bpm)	25 s (3 mm/gantry rotation)	25 s (2 mm/gantry rotation)	1.5 s (5 mm/gantry rotation)
Temporal resolution	100 ms	250 ms (500 ms gantry rotation)	185 ms (370 ms gantry rotation)	165 ms (330 ms gantry rotation)	100 ms	250 ms (500 ms gantry rotation)	185 ms (370 ms gantry rotation)	165 ms (330 ms gantry rotation)
ECG-dependent acquisition	Prospective triggering	Retrospective gating	Retrospective gating	Retrospective gating	Prospective triggering	Retrospective gating	Retrospective gating	Retrospective gating
Tube current	63 mAs	400 mAs	500 mAs	700 mAs	63 mAs	400 mAs	500 mAs	700 mAs
Contrast media	120 mL @ 3 mL/s (400 mg iodine/mL)	120 mL @ 3 mL/s (400 mg iodine/mL)	100 mL @ 4 mL/s (300 mg iodine/mL)	80 mL @ 5 mL/s (300 mg iodine/mL)	120 mL @ 3 mL/s (400 mg iodine/mL)	100 mL @ 4 mL/s (300 mg iodine/mL)	100 mL @ 4 mL/s (300 mg iodine/mL)	100 mL @ 5 mL/s (300 mg iodine/mL)
Radiation exposure	2 mSv	4 mSv	5 mSv	7 mSv	2 mSv	5 mSv	6 mSv	8 mSv

EBCT, electron beam computed tomography; DCT, detector-row computed tomography; CTA, computed tomographic angiography; ECG, electrocardiogram; bpm, beats per minute; mAs, milli-Amperes/second; mL, milliliters; mSv, milli Sievert.

beta-blocker results in a better patient compliance and less movement during scanning; (b) the patient is exposed to less radiation, because with lower heart rate, the ECG tube current modulation is working more effectively; (c) cardiac motion artifacts are substantially reduced; and (d) because of the lower cardiac output with a beta-blocker, the contrast enhancement will increase.

Imaging of the coronary arteries and veins with CT requires the highest spatial resolution available. Planning the investigation of the heart from the scout view, the range to be scanned should include the tracheal bifurcation and the inner recess of the diaphragm corresponding to approximately 120 mm. With 4-detector-row CT and 1-mm slice collimation as well as with the EBCT at low heart rates, scanning the entire heart may last up to 40 seconds.

With EBCT prior to scanning the heart, the arrival time of a small contrast media test bolus in the ascending aorta needs to be determined by a series of test scans. With MDCT, the scan acquisition may be triggered automatically by the arrival of the main contrast bolus in the ascending aorta. When contrast injection starts, repeated scanning at the level of the ascending aorta is performed every second. If the enhancement in the ascending aorta reaches 100 Hounsfield units (HU), the MDCT scan acquisition starts with a short delay of 4 to 6 seconds.

Shortly prior to the CT scan acquisition, the patient is instructed to hold their breath. The patients should be instructed not to press down while taking a deep breath in to avoid the Valsalva maneuver, which increases the intra-abdominal pressure leading to an influx of nonenhanced blood from the inferior vena cava into the right atrium. This prevents the influx of blood mixed with contrast media from entering the right atrium. Dense contrast media persisting in the superior vena cava may lead to beam-hardening artifacts, and only inhomogeneous enhancement of the entire cardiac volume may occur.

Bypass Graft Imaging: Technical Considerations

Imaging arterial and venous bypass graft requires also the inclusion of the subclavian artery and the ascending aorta into the scan range. With a 4-detector-row CT scanner, this scan range may only be acquired with a 4 × 2.5-mm collimation in a reasonable breath hold time. Scanning with EBCT requires abandoning overlapping slice acquisition to keep the breath-hold time below 40 seconds.

With EBCT, the time point for image acquisition is the end-systole interval corresponding to approximately 40% of the RR interval in the ECG (14). In retrospect, ECG with MDCT image reconstruction always begins with careful analysis of the ECG trace recorded with the helical scan. The reconstruction interval is best placed in between the T- and P-wave of the ECG corresponding to the mid-diastole interval. The point of time for the least coronary motion may be different for each coronary artery. Reduced motion artifacts may result when reconstructing the right coronary artery (RCA), left anterior descending (LAD) artery, and left circumflex (LCX) coronary artery at 50%, 55%, and 60% of the RR-interval, respectively (17). Individual adaptation of the point of time for reconstruction seems to further improve image quality. However, the lower the heart rate, the easier it is to find the single best interval for all three major branches of the coronary artery tree (19).

Contrast Methods

A timely, accurate, and homogenous vascular lumen enhancement is essential for full diagnostic capability of coronary MDCT angiography studies. Higher contrast enhancement is superior to identify small vessels in MDCT. However, dense contrast material in the right atrium cavity may cause streak artifacts arising from the right atrium that may interfere with the right coronary artery. In addition, high enhancement of the coronary arteries may interfere with coronary calcifications and may therefore hinder the delineation of the residual lumen.

A peripheral venous iodine flow rate of 1 gram per second will result in an enhancement of approximately 250 to 300 HU in the majority of patients (20) and still allows for delineation of coronary calcification. The final vessel enhancement will not only depend on the iodine flow rate but also on the cardiac output and body weight of the patient. In patients with low cardiac output, such as those under beta-blocker medication, the contrast media will accumulate in the cardiac chambers and lead to a higher enhancement than in patients with high cardiac output where the contrast agent will be diluted faster by nonenhanced blood (21). Because patients with higher body weight may have a larger blood volume, there is also an inverse relation between body weight and peak enhancement (22).

The use of dual-head injectors with sequential injection of contrast media and saline may be helpful to keep the contrast bolus compact (21), to reduce the total amount of contrast media (23,24), and to achieve a central venous enhancement profile by the peripheral venous injection (25). Reducing the amount and use of iso-osmolar contrast media may reduce the risk of contrast-induced nephropathy (26). In addition, changes in heart rate have less frequently been observed in cardiac catheterization during the injection of iso-osmolar contrast agent and may therefore be of advantage in CT as well (27). With scan times as short as 20 seconds, the sequential injection of contrast media and saline allows for selective enhancement of the left ventricular cavity (CT levocardio-gram), with wash out of dense contrast media in the right atrium helping to avoid artifacts.

Postprocessing

The primary axial slices are well suited to detect coronary atherosclerosis. However, the detection of coronary artery stenoses in axial CT images may be problematic because every slice displays only a small part of the entire coronary artery, and the course cannot be well followed. The selection of the appropriate postprocessing tool depends on the purpose.

Two-dimensional (2D) postprocessing tools, such as multiplanar reformatting and maximum-intensity projection (MIP), and 3D postprocessing tools, such as volume rendering (VR), virtual coronary endoscopy, and shaded-surface display, have been tested for improving the detection of coronary artery stenosis in CTA images (28). Two-dimensional tools may be of advantage to assess coronary artery stenoses, but 3D tools have their strength in displaying the anatomy and anomalous course of the coronary arteries.

For the assessment of the LM, 3D tools require the segmentation and removal of the left atrium auricle (29) (Fig. 14-1). The newest postprocessing workstations allow for autosegmentation on the base of standard reference models and for angiography, like presentation of the coronary artery tree.

A number of artifacts, such as misalignment of slabs caused by trigger artifacts, may result in artificial coronary stenoses when 2D or 3D postprocessing is performed. New software capabilities allow for a resorting of the data to improve image quality in such circumstances (Fig. 14-2).

A lumen-narrowing scoring system according to Schmermund et al. (30) may be used to describe different grades of coronary artery stenosis in the proximal and middle coronary artery segment: A, angiographically normal segment (0% stenosis); B, nonobstructive disease (1% to 49% lumen diameter stenosis); C, significant (50% to 74% stenosis); D, high-grade (75% to 99% stenosis); E, total occlusion (100% stenosis). The patency of the distal coronary artery segments should also be reported. It is important to emphasize that any finding from postprocessed images has to be confirmed in the original axial CT slices in order to prepare an accurate report.

Magnetic Resonance

Equipment Considerations and Patient Preparation

The small diameter of the coronary arteries and their location within the thorax makes the use of a 1.5T MR system

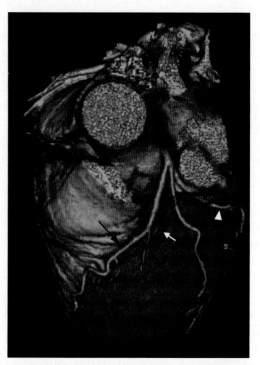

FIGURE 14-1 MDCT 3D volume rendering. This 3D VR image shows normal variant trifurcation anatomy of the LM artery. The left atrial appendage and pulmonary outflow tract have been removed to reveal the LCX artery origin (*white arrowhead*). The LAD is well seen (*black arrow*). The median ramus artery is the middle artery at the point of trifurcation. This artery is also known as the *intermedius*. Note also the great cardiac vein (*colored in red*) passing over the proximal branches (*white arrow*). (Adapted from Manghat NE, Morgan-Hughes GJ, Marshall AJ, et al. Multidetector row computed tomography: imaging congenital coronary artery anomalies in adults. *Heart.* 2005;91(12): 1515–1522, with permission.)

(or potentially greater field strength) and a dedicated thoracic or cardiac phased array receiver coil (with anterior and posterior elements) a requirement for coronary artery imaging. To suppress coronary artery motion during the cardiac cycle, ECG synchronization and QRS detection are absolute necessities (peripheral pulse gating is *not* an adequate alternative). Prominent T waves resulting from the magnetohydrodynamic effect of pulsatile blood (31) and gradient switching noise may lead to ECG signal degradation (Fig. 14-3). Vector ECG approaches appear to be particularly robust for R-wave detection (32). Monitoring of respiration with a thoracic bellows is also desirable.

A critical requirement for successful coronary MRI and magnetic resonance angiography (MRA) is the ability to achieve satisfactory ECG gating via an adequate ECG tracing. The first step toward a satisfactory tracing depends on the placement of the ECG leads. When placing MR compatible leads on the patient's chest, it is recommended to follow the manufacturer's guidelines. In general, leads should first be placed fairly close to one another in order to achieve a strong amplitude. Good contact between the

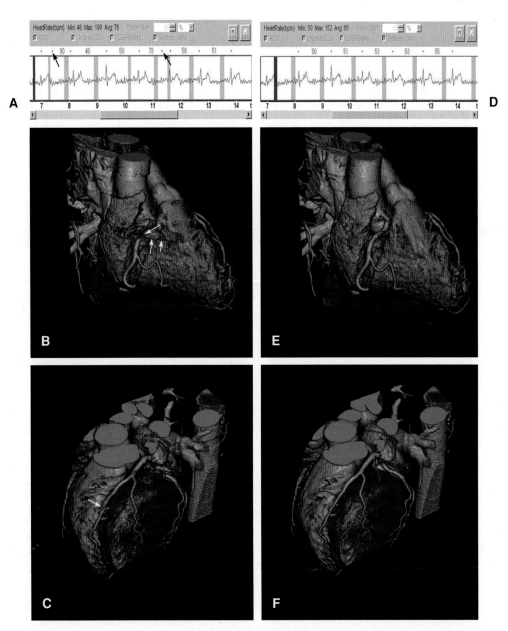

FIGURE 14-2 Influence of ECG tracing on image quality. A: The original ECG tracing, acquired simultaneously with the CT scan, demonstrates a noisy baseline. Ideally, the *red boxes* should be positioned on the R waves, but in this case, not always (*black arrows*). The numbers on top represent the calculated heart rate, which is inaccurate because the R-wave isolation is poor. The *vertical gray bars* correspond to 65% of the calculated R-R interval. **B:** The VR image of the RCA that was reconstructed based on the original ECG data yielded an edge artifact that obscures part of the RCA (*white arrows*). **C:** The VR image of the LAD that was reconstructed based on the original ECG data yielded an image with discontinuity in the LAD that could be misinterpreted as disease (*arrow*). **D:** A feature on contemporary machines enables the user to reposition the *red boxes* to coincide with the R wave. This capability allows for a re-registration and consequent reconstruction of the data at the same point in the cardiac cycle; the result is data uniformity and improved image quality for both the RCA **(E)** and LAD **(F)**. (Courtesy of Stanford University Cardiovascular Imaging).

electrodes and the skin can be accomplished by shaving the skin, when necessary, and by ensuring that there is conductive gel to maximize the contact between the electrode pad and the skin. Twisting or braiding the ECG wires can improve the tracing, but loops of wire must be avoided, as the latter can result in superficial burns.

The R wave is typically the most prominent feature of the ECG tracing and is used to prospectively trigger acquisitions. In addition to poor skin contact, erroneous or poor triggering may occur with excessive respiratory motion, suboptimal lead polarity, heightened T waves (Fig. 14-3), or arrhythmias. To correct gating problems from excessive

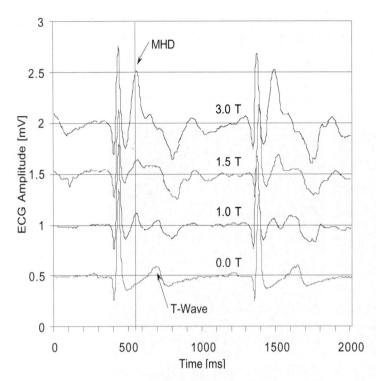

FIGURE 14-3 Effect of field strength on ECG tracing. ECG rhythm strip recorded in the same subject outside of the magnet (0.0T) and at 1.0T, 1.5T, and 3.0T field strengths, demonstrating the associated ST segments and T-wave alterations. These ECG changes are attributed to the magnetohydrodynamic (MHD) effect. (To facilitate the visualization, the DC offsets at the different field strengths were adjusted manually.) (Courtesy of Stefan E. Fischer, PhD.)

respiratory motion, the leads can be placed on the patient's back. Lead polarity can be varied at the machine console to search for the most desirable tracing. Heightened T waves can be minimized with (a) changes in polarity, (b) the use of vectorcardiogram triggering systems, and (c) commercially supplied compensation software, the latter being important at 3T. Patients with arrhythmias present a substantial challenge—when the arrhythmias are severe and lacking periods of regularity, the exam may be nondiagnostic.

As currently implemented, coronary MRI is among the most demanding of patient cooperation, and comprehensive cardiac MR sessions (function, perfusion, viability, flow, coronary imaging) are often relatively lengthy. Thus, to avoid confounders due to patient fatigue, coronary MRI should be performed relatively early in the imaging session. If imaging for coronary artery integrity is desired, administration of sublingual isosorbide dinitrate (2.5 to 5 mg) is suggested both to maximally dilate normal segments and to increase resting blood flow.

Technical Challenges and Solutions

Clinical MRA for the evaluation of similarly sized (e.g., renal, peripheral) vascular beds is now routine, but coronary MRI remains difficult due to several unique technical challenges. These challenges include the small caliber (3- to 6-mm diameter) of the coronary arteries, their near constant motion during both respiratory and cardiac cycles, their high level of tortuosity, and the surrounding signal from adjacent epicardial fat and myocardium.

Cardiac Motion

Bulk epicardial motion can be separated into that related to cardiac contraction/relaxation during the cardiac cycle and that due to a superimposed diaphragmatic and chest wall movement. In-plane coronary motion is maximal at early to midsystole (period of ventricular ejection) with prominent motion again during early diastole (rapid ventricular filling phase). The third component of rapid coronary motion follows atrial systole. During isovolumic relaxation, approximately 350 to 400 msec after the R wave, and again at mid-diastole (immediately prior to atrial systole), coronary motion is minimal and identifies an optimal period for data acquisition as it also corresponds to a period of high coronary blood flow.

While gantry speed limits data acquisition for coronary CTA, MRI techniques offer more flexibility, with acquisitions that may be tailored to an individual patient's heart rate and diastasis period without the need for beta blockade. For a resting heart rate of 70 to 80 bpm, acquisition durations of approximately 80 to 100 ms during each cardiac cycle are utilized (33). With higher heart rates, the duration should be more abbreviated (e.g., <50 msec). With bradycardias, the acquisition interval can be expanded to 150 ms or longer.

Respiratory Motion

The second major motion challenge is suppression of respiratory-related artifacts. With inspiration, the diaphragm descends and the chest wall expands, resulting in an inferior displacement and anterior rotation of the heart (34).

During free breathing in the supine position, diaphragmatic excursion may approach 30 mm, with the predominant dwell time during end expiration (35). Minimizing respiratory motion artifacts can be achieved with several approaches, including sustained end-expiratory breath holding and the use of MR navigators. While repeated, sustained breath holding appears to have a role in healthy volunteers and highly motivated patients, free (uncoached) breathing with right hemidiaphragmatic MR navigators is generally preferred for most subjects, particularly for those with coexistent pulmonary disease (35).

Spatial Resolution

Spatial resolution requirements for coronary MRI depend on whether the goal is to simply identify the origin and proximal course of the coronary artery (e.g., suspected anomalous coronary disease) or whether the goal is to identify focal stenosis. For anomalous disease assessment, in-plane spatial resolution of 1.5 to 2 mm is likely sufficient, while submillimeter spatial resolution is needed for native coronary integrity assessment. Reverse saphenous vein grafts (SVG) are much larger in diameter than the native coronary arteries, with an intermediate spatial resolution likely to be sufficient.

Suppression of Signal from Surrounding Tissue

The coronary arteries are imbedded in epicardial fat. Fat has a relatively short T1 and resultant MR signal intensity similar to that of flowing blood. Frequency selective prepulses can be applied to saturate signal from fat tissue, thereby creating intrinsic contrast and allowing visualization of the underlying coronary arteries (36,37). The coronary arteries also run in close proximity to the myocardium. The myocardium and the coronary blood have relatively similar T1 relaxation values (850 ms and 1200 ms, respectively), making delineation of the coronary arteries difficult. To suppress myocardial signal, both T2 preparation prepulses (33,38,39) and magnetization transfer contrast (MTC) approaches may be used. An added benefit of the T2 prepulse is that it also suppresses deoxygenated blood signal from within the cardiac veins. This suppression is particularly useful if there is minimal epicardial fat and/or the great cardiac vein runs in close proximity to the LAD and LCX coronary arteries. The incremental impact of ECG gating, respiratory gating, and T2 preparation prepulses is displayed in Figure 14-4.

CORONARY MAGNETIC RESONANCE IMAGING ACQUISITION SEQUENCES

Coronary MRI sequences can be conceptualized as being composed of the following building-block components: (a) cardiac (ECG) triggering to suppress bulk cardiac motion,

(b) respiratory motion suppression (breath hold, navigators), (c) prepulses to enhance contrast-to-noise ratio (CNR) of the coronary arterial blood (fat saturation, T2 preparation, MTC), and (d) image acquisition that optimizes coronary arterial signal. The imaging sequences may include bright blood time-of-flight (TOF) (segmented k-space gradient echo), and steady state free precession (SSFP), all implemented as 2D (typically breath hold) and 3D (breath hold or free-breathing navigator) acquisitions. While segmented k-space gradient echo acquisitions have received the most clinical scrutiny, more advanced and less flow-sensitive SSFP methods and intravascular MR contrast agents are receiving increasing attention (40). Similarly, 3T MR systems offer the potential benefits of increased SNR.

Two-dimensional Segmented K-space Gradient Echo

Two-dimensional ECG triggered segmented k-space gradient echo coronary MRI has been available for over a decade and remains useful for older MR systems with slower gradients or those lacking sophisticated navigator technology.

After a coronal or sagittal scout to define the level of the coronary ostia, a series of 10 to 15 axial or oblique overlapping transverse slices (each slice during a single breath hold) are acquired at the level of the origin of the RCA and left coronary artery (LCA). Due to variability in the diaphragmatic position among breath holds, the acquisition of repetitive images with the same spatial coordinates may display adjacent regions of the coronary artery. For imaging of the RCA and more distal LCX, a single- or double-oblique image is acquired along the major axis of the AV groove, as defined in the transverse plane. Both breath-hold variability and coronary vessel tortuosity contribute to the need for 30 to 40 breath holds for a complete 2D coronary MRI examination. The number of breath holds may be reduced by the combination of breath holds with navigator correction (41–43). Spatial resolution, however, remains limited by the breath-hold duration and the need to maintain the acquisition duration during each R-R interval to <100 ms.

Similar breath hold 2D segmented k-space gradient echo acquisitions may also be used to image the larger diameter CABGs. Reverse SVGs are larger in diameter, and both SVGs and internal mammary bypass grafts are less mobile than the native coronary arteries, with predominant flow during ventricular systole. This facilitates data acquisition during a longer period (150 to 200 msec) within each R-R interval and with less rigorous requirements for strict respiratory motion suppression (wider navigator gating window or respiratory bellows gating). In addition, since SV bypass flow is predominantly systolic (44), and TOF

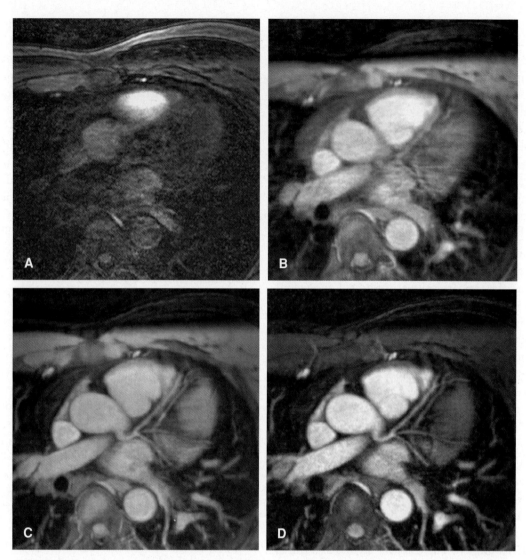

FIGURE 14-4 The importance of motion compensation strategies in MRI. Transverse image at the level of the LM and LAD in the same subject in the absence of cardiac and respiratory gating **(A)**. The incremental value of ECG triggering with mid-diastolic data acquisition **(B)**, navigator gating with real time motion correction **(C)**, and T2 prepulse **(D)** are readily apparent. (Courtesy of Matthias Stuber, PhD.)

methods are dependent on inflow of unsaturated protons, data acquisition during late ventricular systole is often preferred. Susceptibility artifacts from stainless steel bypass graft markers and vascular clips continue to hinder bypass graft coronary MRI (Fig. 14-5).

Targeted Three-dimensional Segmented K-space Gradient Echo

The superior SNR and postprocessing capabilities of 3D coronary MRI make it particularly attractive, though unlike coronary CTA, the voxels are usually anisotropic. The development of free breathing/navigator methods has led to the widespread acceptance of free breathing 3D coronary MRI as the standard at many centers.

As data from an entire volume of tissue surrounding the coronary arteries are acquired, the set-up of free-breathing navigator 3D coronary MRI requires both less operator intervention and less patient cooperation than repetitive 2D breath-hold acquisitions. However, we have found it imperative that the timing and respiratory suppression method for gating of scout images be coherent with the coronary imaging sequences (Fig. 14-6).

For our first scout, we use an ECG-triggered, free-breathing, multislice 2D segmented gradient echo thoracic acquisition with nine transverse, nine coronal, and nine sagittal interleaved acquisitions. From this data set, the navigator is positioned at the dome of the right hemidiaphragm, and the base of the heart is readily identified (Fig. 14-7).

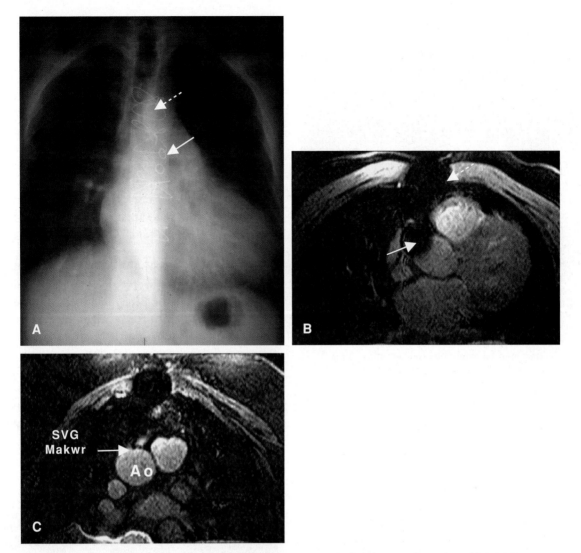

FIGURE 14-5 Magnetic susceptibility artifacts. A: Posterior-anterior (PA) chest x-ray in a patient with CABG. Note the sternal wires (*dashed arrow*) as well as the CABG markers (*solid arrow*). **B:** Transverse coronary MRI in the same patient. Note the large local artifacts (signal voids) related to the sternal wires (*dashed arrow*) and bypass graft markers (*solid arrow*). The size of the artifacts are related to the type of graft marker used. **C:** Barium and tantalum markers (*arrow*) result in the smallest artifacts. The size of the artifacts are also somewhat less with spin echo/black blood MRI as compared with gradient echo imaging. (Ao, ascending aorta.) (Adapted from Applebaum E, Hauser TH, Yeon SB, et al. Coronary artery imaging—clinical applications. In: Higgins CB, de Roos A, eds. *MRI and CT of the Cardiovascular System*. 2nd ed. Philadelphia: Lippincott Williams & Wilkins; 2006:311, with permission.)

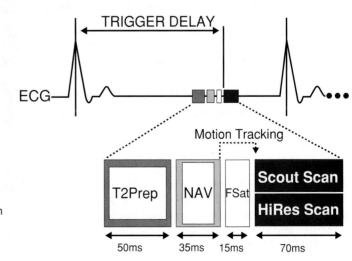

FIGURE 14-6 Schematic for key elements in the scout and high-resolution MR scans. Schematic of the coronary MRI pulse sequence for scout scanning (Scout Scan) and subsequent high-resolution coronary MRI (HiRes Scan). The elements of the sequence (T2-prepulse, anterior chest saturation prepulse [REST], navigator, fat saturation prepulse [FAT SAT], and 3D imaging sequence) are shown in temporal relationshp to the ECG and trigger delay. Note that the ECG timing and respiratory suppression for the Scout Scan and high-resolution coronary MRI are consistent.

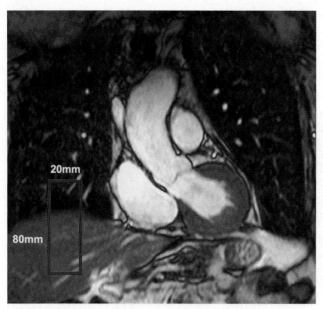

FIGURE 14-7 Navigator for respiratory compensation. Coronal thoracic image with identification of the navigator (*red rectangle*) at the dome of the right hemidiaphragm.

A second scout, consisting of an ECG-triggered 3D fast gradient echo EPI scout, is then acquired with diaphragmatic navigator gating of a volume that includes the coronary arteries, beginning at the cardiac base and extending inferiorly. A free-breathing or breath-hold cine (consistent with the subsequent coronary MRI sequence) is then acquired perpendicular to the proximal/mid-RCA to define the optimal delay and acquisition period (timing and duration of patient specific minimal in-plane motion). Subsequently, a 3D volume is interactively prescribed in the transverse plane centered about the LM coronary artery (identified in the second scout) using the same ECG delay and navigator parameters as the scout. Typically, a 30-mm slab with 20 overlapping slices is acquired using a segmented k-space gradient echo acquisition (TR 7 ms, 8 to 12 phase-encoding lines/R-R interval) with submillimeter in-plane spatial resolution (0.7 $\times$ 1.0 mm) and a temporal acquisition of 56 to 100 ms per heartbeat (33,45). For imaging of the RCA, transverse images from the second scout depicting the proximal, mid, and distal right coronary artery are identified using either a three-point "planscan" software tool (preferred) or in a plane parallel passing through the right and left AV groove. The LCX is often seen in the transverse (left) data set or lies in a plane parallel with the RCA and is therefore seen on the double-oblique RCA data set. Each submillimeter 3D segmented gradient echo acquisition is typically 10 to 12 minutes in duration (assuming a navigator efficiency of 40% to 55%). A similar approach has also been applied for CABGs (46).

Steady-State Free Precession

TOF coronary MRI methods are heavily dependent on inflow of unsaturated protons and blood into the imaging plane. If coronary flow is slow or stagnant, saturation effects will cause a local loss of signal. In contrast, SSFP is relatively insensitive to flow artifacts and, in addition, has superior SNR (47). Three-dimensional SSFP coronary MRI can be implemented with free-breathing/navigator methods (48,49) or with lower resolution prolonged breath holds (50) combined with fat saturation and T2 prepulses for surrounding tissue suppression.

Whole Heart

Both targeted 3D volumes (40,48,50,51) and "whole heart" approaches (49) have been described with segmented k-space methods and SSFP approaches. Right hemidiaphragmatic navigator is used with free breathing and an axial volume extending from approximately 1 cm above the take-off of the LM coronary artery to the diaphragm. Though more lengthy in total acquisition, setup is less complex than the targeted 3D scans, it provides for more distal vessel visualization (49), and is more conducive to advanced postprocessing methods (Fig. 14-8).

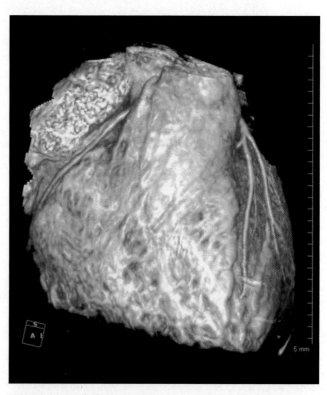

FIGURE 14-8 Whole heart SSFP coronary MRI. Three-dimensional reconstruction of a whole-heart SSFP coronary MRI following computer-assisted image segmentation enables major coronary vessels to be visualized. (Courtesy of Oliver Weber, PhD.)

Contrast Enhanced

Contrast-enhanced MRI has gained widespread acceptance for abdominal, aortic, renal, and peripheral MRI, but the previously described unique constraints for coronary MRI have limited coronary applications of clinically available extracellular agents. Several novel intravascular (blood pool) MR contrast agents are under development and are being evaluated for coronary MRI, including gadolinium-based (52–54) contrast agents with inversion recovery methods. These intravascular agents afford longer scan times with free-breathing or repeated breath-hold methods.

Postprocessing

Postprocessing tools for coronary MRI are relatively rudimentary compared with those available for coronary CTA. As such, they are often used to convey summary results, with primary interpretation of the data set (anomalous coronary artery, focal stenosis) determined from scrolling through the source 3D data set.

Anatomy

Normal Anatomy

The normal coronary vascular anatomy has many variations and can be readily appreciated through the use of diagrams (Figs. 14-9, 14-10), schematics (Fig. 14-11), specimen injected MDCT (Fig. 14-12), and with MDCT from patients (Figs. 14-13–14-16).

The RCA courses in the right AV groove and provides nutrient branches to the right ventricular free wall, extending to the acute margin of the heart. The first branch arising from the RCA is the conal or infundibular branch (55), which courses anteriorly to supply the muscular right ventricular outflow tract or infundibulum. The distal extent of the RCA varies and may extend posteriorly as far as the obtuse margin of the heart. In 90% of patients, the RCA supplies the posterior descending coronary artery branch at the crux of the heart, which supplies the AV node and the posterior aspect of the interventricular septum.

The RCA supplies blood to the atria with a highly variable pattern of small branches. The sinus node artery arises from the proximal RCA in approximately 50% of patients.

The left coronary ostium is usually single, giving rise to a short, common LM artery that promptly branches

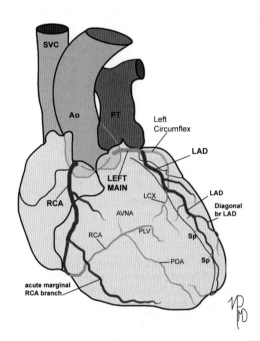

FIGURE 14-9 Diagram of the heart and coronary arteries from an anterior view. The RCA arises from the right aortic sinus, passes first between the right ventricular outflow tract and the right atrial appendage, and then runs in the right AV sulcus. The distal RCA begins just beyond the AM branch and passes horizontally along the diaphragmatic surface of the heart, forming the PDA (which arises from a dominant RCA in 85% of individuals), and the PLV. The AVNA is also commonly seen arising from the diaphragmatic portion of the RCA. Note that the apex of the left ventricle is supplied by the LAD and the anterior left ventricular wall by diagonals from the LAD. The inferior left ventricular wall receives its supply of blood flow by the PDA arising from the RCA; individuals with this coronary artery configuration are known as *right dominant*. Note also that the AV node is supplied by a short vessel at the bend of the RCA before the take-off of the PDA at a position known as the *crux* of the heart. (SVC, superior vena cava; Ao, aorta; AVNA, atrioventricular nodal artery; LAD, left anterior descending artery; LCX, left circumflex coronary artery; PDA, posterior descending coronary artery; PLV, posterior left ventricular artery.)

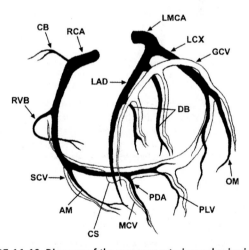

FIGURE 14-10 Diagram of the coronary arteries and veins in left anterior oblique view. The left coronary system consists of the left main coronary artery *(LMCA)*, left circumflex artery *(LCX)*, left anterior descending artery *(LAD)*, diagonal branches *(DB)*, and obtuse marginal branch *(OM)*. The right coronary system consists of the right coronary artery *(RCA)*, conus branch *(CB)*, right ventricular branch *(RVB)*, acute marginal branch *(AM)*, posterior descending artery *(PDA)*, and posterior left ventricular branch *(PLV)*. The coronary venous system is composed of the coronary sinus *(CS)*, great cardiac vein *(GCV)*, middle cardiac vein *(MCV)*, and small cardiac vein *(SCV)*. (Reprinted from Sevrukov A, Jelnin V, Kondos GT. Electron beam CT of the coronary arteries: cross-sectional anatomy for calcium scoring. *AJR Am J Roentgenol.* 2001;177(6):1437–1445, with permission.)

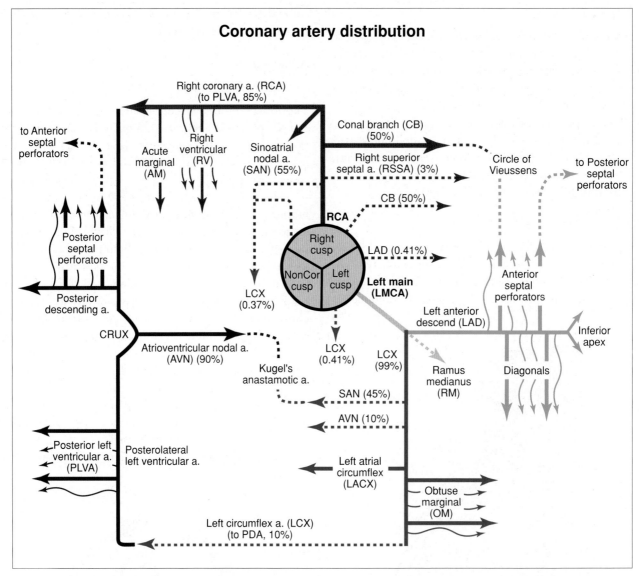

FIGURE 14-11 Schematic of coronary artery anatomy and common variants. The LM coronary artery is shown (*yellow line*). The three main systems, the RCA coronary system (*red lines*), the LAD coronary system (*green lines*), and the LCX coronary system (*blue line*) and associated branches are depicted. The *purple lines* indicate the variable contributions influenced by coronary artery dominance, where roughly 70% of the time the supply is from the RCA, 20% from the LCX, and 10% as a balanced contribution from both. (Adapted from Frandics Chan, MD.)

into the LAD and LCX coronary arteries. The LAD courses in the anterior interventricular groove, giving rise to diagonal branches that course at downward angles to supply the anterolateral free wall of the left ventricle. More distally, the LAD gives rise to the anterior septal perforating branches as it extends toward the cardiac apex. Small branches may arise from the LAD and supply the anterior wall of the right ventricle.

The LCX coronary artery courses along the left AV groove, around the obtuse margin, and posteriorly toward the crux of the heart. When the LCX coronary artery reaches the crux of the heart and supplies the posterior descending

coronary artery, the left coronary system is termed *dominant*, occurring in approximately 10% of patients. Atrial branches may arise from the LCX coronary artery and supply the sinus node in 40% of patients. Obtuse marginal branches arise from the LCX system to supply the posterolateral aspect of the left ventricle. In approximately 70% of patients, a coronary branch arises early off the left coronary system (referred to as the *ramus medianus, intermedius,* or *intermediate branch*) to supply an area between diagonal branches from the LAD and obtuse branches from the LCX.

The normal coronary arteries situated subepicardially can be subdivided into coronary segments that are numbered

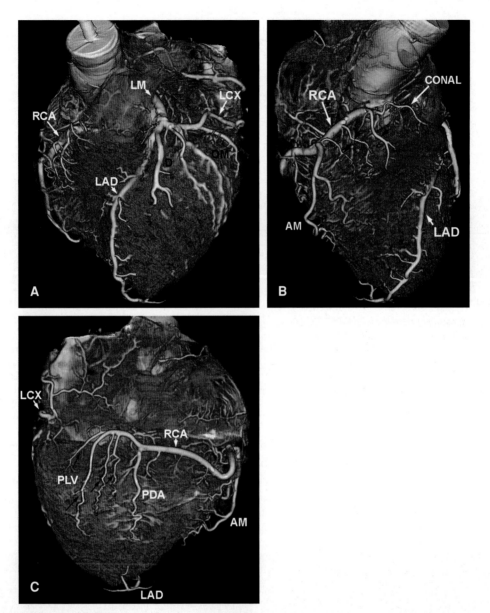

**FIGURE 14-12 Coronary artery anatomy as demonstrated by MDCT of a human heart specimen injected
with dilute iodinated solution into the aortic root. A:** VR frontal reconstruction emphasizing the LCA. The LM
appears from under the pulmonary outflow track and gives rise to the LAD and LCX. Left ventricular branches that arise
from the LCX artery are designated as marginal branches, whereas those arising from the LAD are designated as diagonal (D) branches. In this case, the large D artery originates close to the LAD/LCX bifurcation and can be referred to as
an *intermediate branch.* **B:** VR frontal oblique reconstruction emphasizing the LAD and RCA. The first branch is the
conus, which extends anteriorly from the RCA. Of the many branches supplying the right ventricular wall (*arrowheads*),
the largest vessel can typically be identified—the acute marginal branch. The LAD is well seen in this projection, including numerous septal perforators (*arrows*). **C:** VR reconstruction emphasizes the coronary anatomy on the posterior surface of the heart. The RCA, after having given off the AM branch, is seen tracking posteriorly along the right AV sulcus.
The PDA extends toward the apex along the interventricular septum, and multiple PLV branches (*black arrows*) are seen
in the terminus of the RCA. The posterior extension of the LCX is seen giving off posterior atrial branches toward the base.
The distal aspect of the LAD is seen as it curves around the apex of the heart. (RCA, right coronary artery; LAD, left anterior descending artery; LCX, left circumflex coronary artery; LM, left main artery; AM, acute marginal branch; PDA, posterior descending coronary artery; PLV, posterior left ventricular artery.) (Courtesy of Stanford Cardiovascular Imaging.)

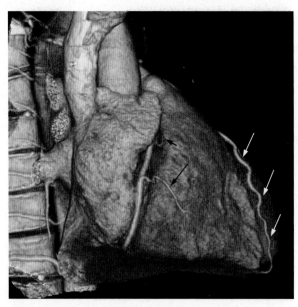

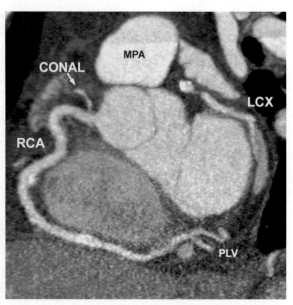

FIGURE 14-13 Normal coronary anatomy with MDCT. This ECG-triggered MDCT VR image shows segments the RCA with a conus branch (*short black arrow*) and an acute marginal branch (*long black arrow*). The acute marginal branch is the point of reference for division of the RCA into segments 1 and 2. The proximal RCA is obscured by the right atrium. Also note that the distal LAD can be seen as well (*white arrows*). (Courtesy of Stanford Cardiovascular Imaging.)

FIGURE 14-14 Normal coronary anatomy with MDCT. This thin-slab restricted MIP image from a MDCT study shows a tortuous RCA with its conal branch. The right conus artery (conal branch) is the first ventricular branch of the RCA, which courses anteriorly to supply the muscular right ventricular outflow tract or infundibulum. The RCA is well visualized in this projection to the base of the heart, where the PLV origin is seen. (RCA, right coronary artery; MPA, main pulmonary artery; LCX, left circumflex artery; PLV, posterior left ventricular branch.) (Courtesy of Stanford Cardiovascular Imaging.)

according to a model suggested by the American Heart Association (56). The right coronary artery is situated at the right AV sulcus and is divided into four segments. The proximal segment (segment 1) begins at the ostium of the right coronary sinus and ends at the acute marginal branch, the middle segment (segment 2) continues to the bottom of the heart, followed by the distal segment (segment 3) that ends at the crux cordis. At the crux cordis, the right coronary artery turns by 90 degrees and runs into the posterior interventricular sulcus and is then called the *posterior descending coronary artery*

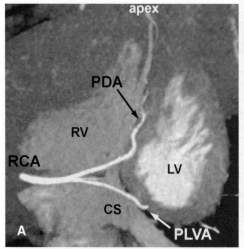

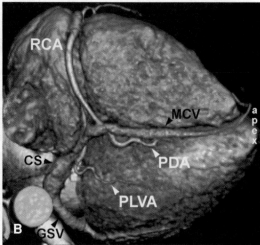

FIGURE 14-15 Normal coronary anatomy with MDCT. A: Thin-slab restricted MDCT MIP showing that the inferior surface of the heart nicely demonstrates the RCA and its distal branching into the PLVA branch and the anteriorly coursing PDA, the latter running in the posterior interventricular sulcus. Note the relationships to the right ventricle and the coronary sinus (CS). **B:** A VR image from the inferior surface of the heart shows the RCA and its distal branches, the PLVA, and the PDA partially obscured by the CS and the middle cardiac vein, respectively. The PDA courses toward the cardiac apex. (LV, left ventricle; PLVA, posterior left ventricular artery; RCA, right coronary artery; PDA, posterior descending artery.) (Courtesy of Stanford Cardiovascular Imaging.)

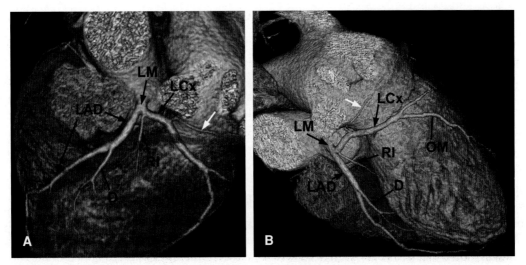

FIGURE 14-16 Normal left coronary anatomy with MDCT. VR left ventricular view in the frontal/cranial projection **(A)** and a steeper oblique projection **(B)** from an MDCT acquisition. The LM bifurcates into the LAD and the LCX. Note the ramus intermedius, an early branch off the left coronary system supplying the area between diagonal branches from the LAD and obtuse marginal branches from the LCX. Given its small size and origin just beyond the bifurcation at the proxima LCX, this vessel could also be considered as a very proximal obtuse marginal. The *white arrow* depicts an atrial branch off the LCX. (Courtesy of Stanford Cardiovascular Imaging.)

(segment 4). It is often necessary to generate several renderings to display all features of the RCA (Fig. 14-15).

Numbering continues with the LM coronary artery (segment 5) originating from the left coronary sinus. This LM may vary in size and branches early into the LAD (segment 6) and LCX (segment 11). The LAD coronary artery is situated in the anterior interventricular sulcus and is divided into the proximal (segment 6), middle (segment 7), and distal (segment 8) segment. This vessel also provides the first (segment 9) and second (segment 10) diagonal branch as well as penetrating septal branches. The proximal (segment 11) and distal (segment 13) part of the circumflex coronary artery is situated in the left AV sulcus and provides the obtuse marginal branch (segment 12). The most distal branches of the circumflex coronary artery are the posterolateral and posterior descending branch (segments 14 and 15).

Commonly, the coronary vein can be identified in the anterior interventricular sulcus accompanying the LAD coronary artery. At the level of the proximal segment of the LAD coronary artery, the coronary vein turns 90 degrees to dorsal, crossing over the circumflex coronary artery. Here, it runs parallel to the circumflex coronary artery in the left AV sulcus to the bottom of the heart opening up to the coronary sinus and draining into the right atrium.

Dominant Coronary Artery

The vessel and branches of the coronary artery tree—in particular, the most distal branches—may vary widely from patient to patient. Commonly, one of the three major coronary arteries is larger, has more side branches, and provides a larger portion of the myocardium with blood than the others. This coronary artery is called the *dominant coronary artery*, and stenoses in this vessel may be of higher clinical relevance than in other vessels.

The lateral wall of the myocardium is furthest away from the coronary artery ostium and most of the coronary variances are seen here. As described previously, the right as well as the circumflex coronary artery may both provide a posterior descending coronary branch (segments 4 and 15). In this indeterminate type, the lateral wall of the myocardium is supplied by both the right and left coronary artery. In fact, this type accounts for only 8% of all coronary supplying types. The right-supplying type with segments 4 and 14 coming from the right coronary artery accounts for approximately 89%. The left-supplying type with both branches coming from the circumflex coronary artery is only rarely found in approximately 3% of patients (57).

Asymptomatic Anatomy Variant

The incidence of coronary anomalies is variable and has been reported for up to 5.6% of all patients undergoing coronary angiography (57). Most of the coronary anomalies are asymptomatic and only found incidentally. In normal coronary anatomy, the left and the right coronary artery originate from the left and right coronary sinus, respectively. However, in coronary anomalies, the left and right coronary artery may originate from any other: right, left, or noncoronary sinus. When the aberrant coronary artery is situated posterior the aortic root, it is currently considered as a benign course with usually no therapeutic implication.

Symptomatic Anatomy Variant

Coronary anomalies may be a significant cause of chest pain, myocardial ischemia, and sudden cardiac death. For instance, in young athletes, coronary anomalies may account for up to 20% of unheralded deaths (58). In these instances, the aberrant left or right coronary artery is situated in between the aortic root and pulmonary outflow tract. Currently, the hypothesis exists that the aberrant coronary artery may be squeezed within the two major vessels—in particular, under high pressure or stress leading to myocardial ischemia. Depending on the anatomical situation, these kinds of coronary anomalies may require reinsertion or protection against ischemia by bypass grafting.

Bland-White-Garland Syndrome

With an incidence of 1 in 3,000 newborns, Bland-White-Garland syndrome describes a coronary in which the left coronary artery (LCA) starts from the pulmonary artery (PA) instead of the ascending aorta, leading to left ventricular failure, either congenitally or shortly after birth. Symptoms include failure to thrive, dyspnea, tachypnea, precordial pain, sweating, pallor, and crying after feeding and exertion. If untreated, death is likely in childhood or adolescence. Treatment may require surgical correction by reinsertion or bypass grafting. It is only rarely described that the right coronary may originate from the PA (reverse Bland-White-Garland syndrome), leading to atypical symptoms in the adolescent.

CLINICAL STUDIES

At the time of this writing, the largest body of published clinical experience has been with the ECG-triggered 2D or targeted 3D segmented k-space gradient-echo coronary MRI approaches, with increasing preliminary reports on whole heart SSFP, intravascular contrast, and 3T methods. MDCT studies are rapidly proliferating, with data available using 4 through 64 detectors and steady improvements being realized with higher detector systems.

Evaluation of Normal Coronary Arteries

Contrast-enhanced MDCT with submillimeter collimation and retrospective ECG-gated image reconstruction permits successful noninvasive visualization of the coronary arteries (Fig. 14-17). For MRI, a relatively low spatial resolution (1.5 × 2.0 mm) breath-hold 2D segmented k-space gradient echo approach (36) was the first robust approach for imaging the native coronary arteries. As implemented across numerous vendor platforms, the LM, LAD, and RCA are visualized in nearly all subjects (59–64), with proximal coronary artery diameter similar to that reported by x-ray angiography and pathology.

Currently, both targeted 3D segmented k-space gradient echo and whole-heart SSFP coronary MRI methods have reported successful visualization of all the major vessels in nearly every subject and predominate in current practice. A distinct advantage of the 3D approaches is increased contiguous visualization of length/distal segments (33,49).

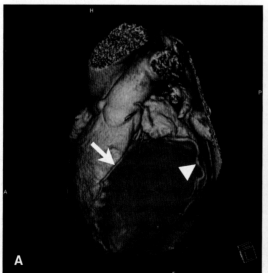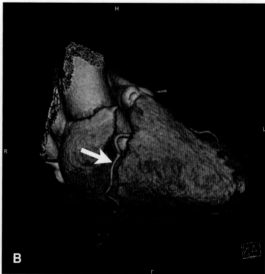

FIGURE 14-17 Normal anatomy in a 64-year-old female, depicted with MDCT. A: VR nicely displays the course of the LCX coronary artery (*arrow*) and the circumflex coronary artery (*arrowhead*). **B:** The RCA courses in the right AV groove.

Anomalous Coronary Disease

The detection and exact anatomic definition of coronary artery anomalies is necessary for establishing a prognosis and initiating upcoming therapeutic procedures. The potential association with myocardial ischemia and sudden cardiac death highlights the need to identify those individuals with at-risk aberrant vasculature, often referred to as the *malignant variety*. Moreover, the capacity to distinguish benign anomalies from those associated with serious complications represents an important contribution from both CT and MRI, and these modalities can be clarifying when other imaging studies, including conventional angiography, are suggestive.

While the majority of coronary artery anomalies are not thought to be hemodynamically significant, the origin of a coronary artery from the contralateral side with subsequent passage between the aorta and PA has the potential to impair myocardial perfusion (65,66) (Figs. 14-18, 14-19).

Invasive coronary angiography is limited to a projectional 2D view of the coronary arteries and can lead to misinterpretations (67). Contrast-enhanced electron beam tomography has a lower spatial but higher temporal resolution than MDCT and has considerably lower radiation

exposure. MRI offers a noninvasive, nonionizing radiation method that does not require contrast media. It does, however, require expertise for consistent results.

Computed Tomography

The reliability of MDCT coronary CTA for the evaluation of anomalous coronary arteries has been shown (68–70). In a recent study, all patients with coronary artery anomalies and all controls with normal coronary anatomy were identified by MDCT (70). In that study, the origins and course concerning their anatomical relationship to adjacent cardiac structures were visualized in all patients (Figs. 14-20, 14-21). Interestingly, one study showed that selective cannulation and final diagnosis was possible in only 11 of the 20 catheter angiograms performed, suggesting that MDCT may outperform conventional catheter angiography for this application (68).

Coronary Magnetic Resonance Imaging for Anomalous Coronary Disease

Coronary MRI has several advantages in the diagnosis of coronary anomalies. In addition to not employing ionizing

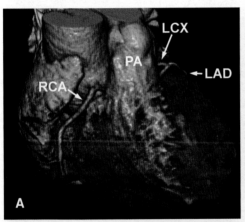
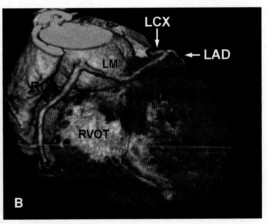
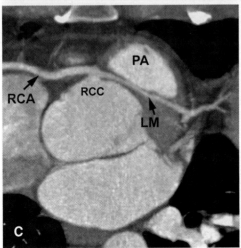

FIGURE 14-18 Aberrant left main coronary artery (malignant variety). VR and curved reformatted images from gated multislice CTA (64-slice scanner); 0.6-mm detector width with 0.75-mm reconstruction. **A:** The LM coronary artery arises from the anterior or right coronary cusp of the aorta and courses between the aorta and pulmonary outflow tract. The PA obscures the proximal LM. **B:** With an anterior cut plane, the PA has been removed from the image, revealing the right ventricular outflow tract (RVOT) and allowing for a better demonstration of the aberrant LM coronary artery. In both images, the LM can be seen to bifurcate into the LCX and LAD. **C:** This curved reformatted image nicely shows the malignant course of the LM in a format that is readily appreciated. (RCA, right coronary artery; LCX, left circumflex coronary artery; LAD, left anterior descending artery; RCC, right coronary cusp; PA, pulmonary artery.) (Courtesy of Stanford Cardiovascular Imaging.)

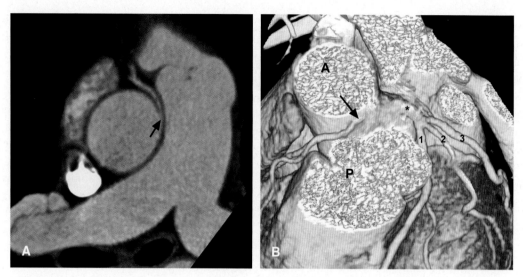

FIGURE 14-19 Aberrant RCA (malignant variety) and left main trifurcation shown with CTA. A: This source image offers a straightforward demonstration of an anomalous RCA (*arrow*), insinuating between the aorta and PA. **B:** This VR view shows the aberrant origin of the RCA (*arrow*) coming off between the aorta (*A*) and pulmonary artery (*P*). The LM coronary artery (*∗*) is seen as well, trifurcating into the LAD (*1*), intermediate branch (*2*), and LCX (*3*). (Courtesy of Stanford Cardiovascular Imaging.)

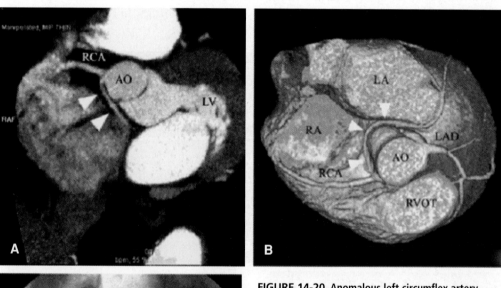

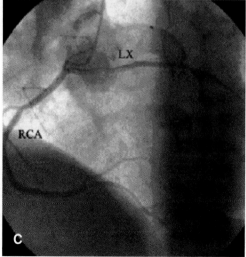

FIGURE 14-20 Anomalous left circumflex artery depicted by MDCT. A 42-year-old male patient with a right-sided LCX following a retroaortic course. **A:** MDCT reconstruction (MIP, slice thickness 5 mm) demonstrates the origin of the LCX (*arrowheads*) from the proximal RCA and the initial retroaortic path. This retroaortic course creates a risk for LCX damage by sutures placed in the mitral valve surgery. **B:** The origin and subsequent course with the anatomical relationship of the anomalous LCX (*arrowheads*) to adjacent cardiac structures is clearly visualized by 3D MDCT reconstruction with VR technique. **C:** Corresponding invasive angiogram in left anterior oblique straight projection. (AO, ascending aorta; LAD, left anterior descending coronary artery; LX, left circumflex coronary artery; LA, left atrium; LV, left ventricle; RA, right atrium; RVOT, right ventricular outflow tract.) (Adapted from Schmid M, Achenbach S, Ludwig J, et al. Visualization of coronary artery anomalies by contrast-enhanced multidetector row spiral computed tomography. *Int J Cardiol.* 2006;111(3):430–435.)

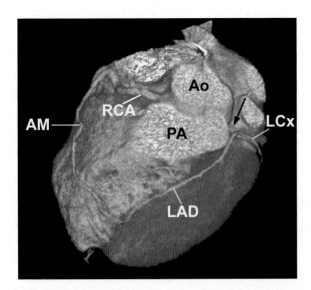

FIGURE 14-21 Congenitally absent left main coronary artery. VR images from gated multislice CTA (16-slice scanner); 0.625-mm detector width with 1-mm reconstructions. A large RCA originates from the aorta, giving rise to an acute marginal branch. The AM fills both the LAD and LCX in a retrograde manner. Note that the LM is congenitally absent (*black arrow* points to the empty fossa where the LM is normally seen). (AM, acute marginal branch; RCA, right coronary artery; Ao, aorta; PA, pulmonary artery; LAD, left anterior descending artery; LCX, left circumflex artery.) (Courtesy of Stanford Cardiovascular Imaging.)

radiation (an important consideration among children, adolescents, and younger adults), coronary MRI also does not require placement of an intravenous catheter or administration of contrast (Fig. 14-22).

There have been at least five published series (71–75) of patients who underwent a blinded comparison of coronary MRI data with x-ray angiography (Table 14-2). Early studies used a 2D breath-hold ECG-triggered segmented k-space gradient echo approach with uniformly excellent accuracy, including several studies in which coronary MRI was determined to be superior to x-ray angiography (74,75). Most centers now utilize 3D coronary MRI because of superior reconstruction capabilities with similar excellent results (73). As a result, clinical coronary MRI is now the preferred test for young patients in whom anomalous disease is suspected or known anomalous disease needs to be further clarified, or if the patient has another cardiac anomaly associated with coronary anomalies (e.g., tetralogy of Fallot).

MYOCARDIAL BRIDGING

Myocardial bridging is a nonatherosclerotic anatomic abnormality of the coronary arteries and is generally considered a

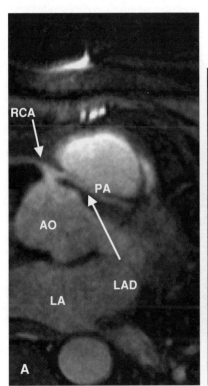
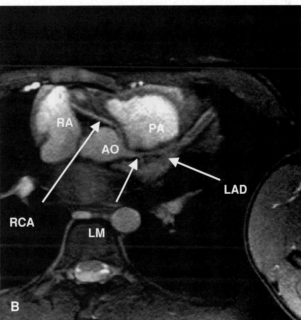

FIGURE 14-22 Anomalous coronary arteries demonstrated with MR. Free-breathing 3D coronary MRI using T2 prepulse navigator gating with real time motion correction. **A:** Transverse orientation depicting a malignant-type anomalous LAD originating from the RCA and traversing between the aortic root and the PA. **B:** Transverse image in another patient with a malignant-type anomalous origin of the RCA from the left coronary cusp. (PA, pulmonary artery; LA, left atrium; RA, right atrium.) (From Applebaum E, Hauser TH, Yeon SB, et al. Coronary artery imaging—clinical applications. In: Higgins CB, de Roos A, eds. *MRI and CT of the Cardiovascular System.* 2nd ed. Philadelphia: Lippincott Williams & Wilkins; 2006.)

TABLE 14-2

Anomalous Coronary Magnetic Resonance Imaging

Study	Points (number)	Correctly Classified Vessels (%)
McConnell et al. (71)	15	14 (93)
Post et al. (74)	19	19 (100)[a]
Vliegen et al. (75)	12	11 (92)[b]
Taylor et al. (72)	25	24 (96)
Bunce et al. (73)	26	26 (100)[c]

[a]Including three patients originally misclassified by x-ray angiography.
[b]Including five patients unable to be classified by x-ray angiography.
[c]Including 11 patients unable to be classified by x-ray angiography.

benign condition that is a common angiographic and autopsy finding (76). Muscle overlying a segment of a coronary artery causes this type of bridging, and the artery coursing within the myocardium is referred to as a *tunneled artery* (77). The tunneled artery runs intramurally through the myocardium (Figs. 14-23, 14-24).

There are two morphologic variants, *superficial* and *deep*, as described by Ferreira et al. (78). The superficial variant exists when the LAD is in the interventricular groove and is crossed by the muscle bundle perpendicularly or at an acute angle before it deviates to the apex of the heart. The deep variant exists when the LAD is situated deeply on the interventricular septum, where it is crossed transversely, obliquely, or helically by a longitudinal muscle bundle arising from the apex of the right ventricle and inserting into the interventricular septum. Typically, the LAD is deviated toward the right ventricle.

The diagnosis of clinically important myocardial bridging must be considered in patients at low risk for coronary atherosclerosis who have angina or established myocardial ischemia.

Myocardial bridging has been associated with a variety of clinical manifestations, including angina, arrhythmia, depressed left ventricular function, myocardial stunning, early death after cardiac transplantation, and sudden death (76). However, there is a discrepancy between the limited frequency of myocardial bridging observed angiographically, reported as 0.5% to 16% (79) and that seen at autopsy, the latter reported as 40% to 80% (80,81).

This discrepancy contributes to the controversy surrounding the clinical significance of myocardial bridging. The bridging often occurs without overt symptoms, so patients are rarely referred for coronary angiography. As an example, Kramer et al. reviewed 658 normal coronary

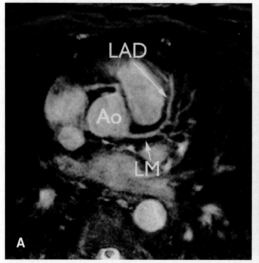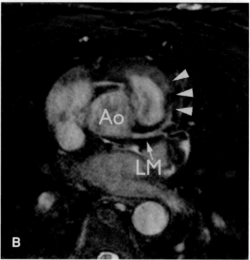

FIGURE 14-23 Myocardial bridging demonstrated with MRA in a 52-year-old man. Proximal and midsegment of the LAD in diastole (**A**), disappearing during systole (**B**; *arrowheads*). (Ao, aorta; LAD, left anterior descending artery; LM, left main artery.) (From Bekkers SC, Leiner T. Images in cardiovascular medicine. Myocardial bridging. *Circulation*. 2006;113(9):e390–e391, with permission.)

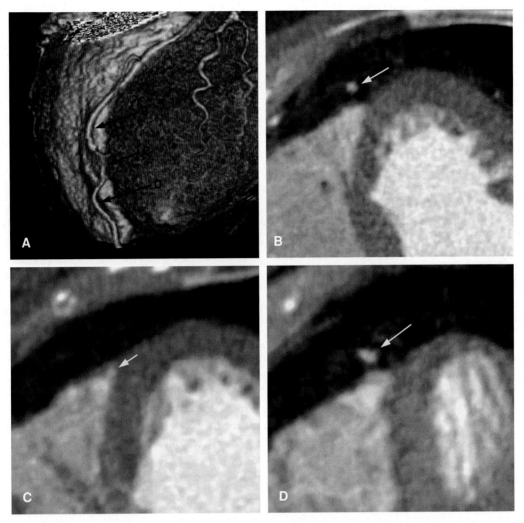

FIGURE 14-24 Myocardial bridging as demonstrated with MDCT. A: VR image of the LAD shows the levels at which axial source images are taken. **B:** This axial image is just above the myocardial bridge and shows the LAD (*arrow*) in the epicardial fat. **C:** The intramural portion of the LAD (*arrow*) is seen at the level where the vessel is narrowed and slightly deviated to the left on the VR image. **D:** Immediately below the bridge, the vessel returns to normal caliber (*arrow*) and is again seen in the epicardial fat. (Courtesy of Stanford University Cardiovascular Imaging).

angiograms of patients with normal left ventricular function and found that 81 (12%) had a myocardial bridge of the LAD (82). Of these 81 patients, only 11 had a systolic reduction in luminal diameter >50%, and 15 presented with typical angina.

Imaging

The typical angiographic finding in myocardial bridging is systolic narrowing of an epicardial artery (83). More recently, the capacity to detect myocardial bridging with MDCT and MRA has been reported (77,84–86).

In one study with MDCT coronary angiography, 22 cases (3.5%) of myocardial bridging were detected among 626 patients (86). Fifteen myocardial bridging cases (2.4%) were located at the middle third, five (0.8%) at the distal third, and two (0.3%) at the proximal third of the LAD.

The length of tunneled artery was between 6 and 22 mm (mean, 17 mm). The depth of tunneled artery was between 1.2 and 3.3 mm (mean, 2.5 mm).

Treatment

In symptomatic patients, treatment is usually medical and rarely surgical. In the past few years, angioplasty and stenting have been used more frequently in cases resistant to medical therapy, and they appear to be an effective alternative to surgery (87–90).

Nitrates generally should be avoided, because they increase the angiographic degree of systolic narrowing and can lead to worsening of the symptoms (91). Beta-blockers should be beneficial, as these agents decrease tachycardia and increase diastolic time, with a decrease in contractility and compression of the coronary arteries.

However, to date, there have been no randomized controlled trials to validate this. Additional research is needed to define patients in whom myocardial bridging is potentially pathologic, and randomized multicenter long-term follow-up studies are needed to assess the natural history, patient selection, and therapeutic approaches.

CORONARY ARTERY ANEURYSMS/KAWASAKI DISEASE

The vast majority of acquired coronary aneurysms in children and younger adults are due to mucocutaneous lymph node syndrome (Kawasaki disease), a generalized vasculitis of unknown etiology usually occurring in children under 5 years of age, with nearly 20% developing coronary artery aneurysms. Approximately 50% of children with coronary aneurysms during the acute phase of the disease will have angiographically normal-appearing vessels 1 or 2 years later (92,93). For afflicted young children, transthoracic echocardiography is usually adequate for diagnosing and following these aneurysms, but transthoracic echocardiography is often inadequate after adolescence and in obese children. These patients are therefore often referred for serial x-ray coronary angiography.

Computed Tomography

A recent study using MDCT in 16 adolescents and young adults with Kawasaki disease assessed coronary artery abnormalities (94). In the Kanamaru study, adequate images were obtained for 96% of major coronary segments. MDCT showed a sensitivity of 100% for the ability to detect coronary artery aneurysms, and for significant stenoses and occlusions, sensitivity was 87.5% (94) (Figs. 14-25, 14-26). False-positive results due to severe calcification was present in five arteries, and those due to cardiac motion artifact were present in two, resulting in a specificity of 92.5%.

Magnetic Resonance Imaging

Data from a series of adolescents and young adults with coronary artery aneurysms defined on x-ray angiography have confirmed the high accuracy of coronary MRI for both the identification and the characterization (diameter, length) of these aneurysms (95,96) (Figs. 14-27, 14-28). Good correlation between coronary MRI and x-ray coronary angiography has also been reported for ectatic coronary arteries (distinct from Kawaski disease) among adults (97).

CORONARY ARTERY FISTULAS

A coronary artery fistula (CAF) is a sizable communication between a coronary artery and either a chamber of the heart (coronary-cameral fistula) or any segment of the systemic or pulmonary circulation (coronary AV fistula). These fistulas are congenital or acquired coronary artery abnormalities in which blood is shunted into a cardiac

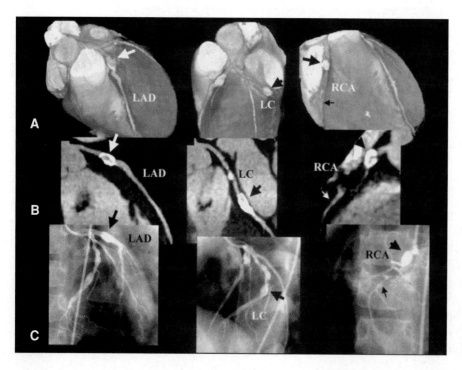

FIGURE 14-25 Kawasaki disease as shown by MDCT. VR **(A)**, curved multiplanar reformatted **(B)**, and angiographic **(C)** images from a 20-year-old man. Multiple coronary artery aneurysms involving the LAD, LCX, and RCA are well visualized (*large arrows*). Multislice spiral computed tomographic and angiographic images of the RCA show complete occlusion distal to the aneurysm and distal enhancement (*small arrows*). Well-developed collateral vessels are demonstrated on the angiogram. (LAD, left anterior descending artery; LC, left circumflex artery; RCA, right coronary artery.) (Reprinted from Kanamaru H, Sato Y, Takayama T, et al. Assessment of coronary artery abnormalities by multislice spiral computed tomography in adolescents and young adults with Kawasaki disease. *Am J Cardiol.* 2005;95(4):522–525, with permission.)

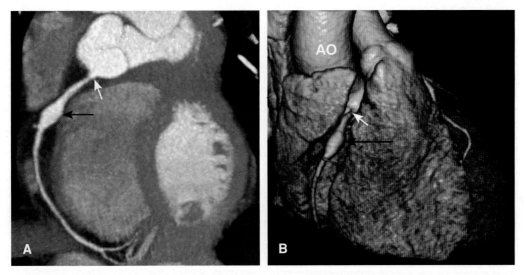

FIGURE 14-26 Kawasaki disease—MDCT. Curved multiplanar reformatted **(A)** and VR **(B)** images of a focal RCA aneurysm (*black arrow*). The origin of the RCA (*white arrow*) is more easily seen on the multiplanar reformatted image. (AO, aorta.) (Courtesy of Stanford Cardiovascular Imaging.)

chamber, great vessel, or other structure, bypassing the myocardial capillary network (98). They often are collectively termed *coronary arteriovenous fistulas* (CAVF).

The pathophysiologic implication of CAF is a reduction in myocardial blood flow distal to the site of the CAF connection. The mechanism is related to the diastolic pressure gradient and run-off from the coronary vascula-

ture to a low-pressure–receiving cavity. With large fistulas, the intracoronary diastolic perfusion pressure may be diminished.

CAFs can occur from any of the three major coronary arteries, including the LM trunk (99). The majority of these fistulas arise from the RCA and the LAD coronary artery; the LCX is rarely involved. The RCA, or its branches, is the

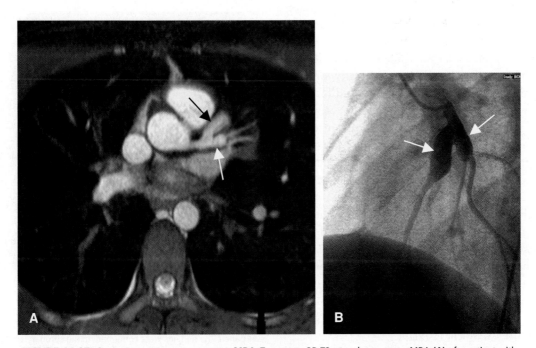

FIGURE 14-27 Coronary artery aneurysm on MRA. Transverse 3D T2 prepulse coronary MRA **(A)** of a patient with an LCA aneurysm and corresponding x-ray angiogram **(B)**, demonstrating good correlation of coronary MRI findings. (*Black arrow*, LAD aneurysm; *white arrow*, LCX aneurysm.) (From Applebaum E, Hauser TH, Yeon SB, et al. Coronary artery imaging—clinical applications. In: Higgins CB, de Roos A, eds. *MRI and CT of the Cardiovascular System.* 2nd ed. Philadelphia: Lippincott Williams & Wilkins; 2006, p. 303.)

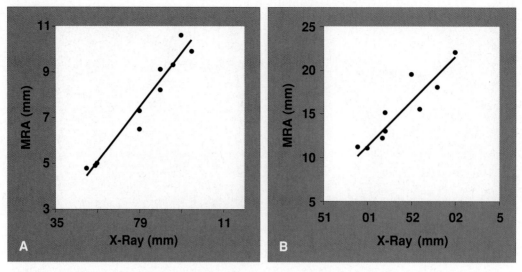

FIGURE 14-28 X-ray angiogram and coronary MRI aneurysm correlations. Correlation of coronary artery aneurysm length **(A)** and diameter **(B)** as determined by coronary x-ray angiography and coronary MRI. (Adapted from Greil GF, Stuber M, Botnar RM, et al. Coronary magnetic resonance angiography in adolescents and young adults with Kawasaki disease. *Circulation.* 2002;105(8):908–911, with permission.)

site of the fistula in about 55% of cases, the LCA in about 35%, and both coronary arteries in 5% (100,101).

Clinical manifestations vary considerably, dominated by the severity of the left-to-right shunt, and the long-term outcome is not fully known (102). Patients may present with dyspnea, congestive heart failure, angina, endocarditis, arrhythmias, or myocardial infarction, although the majority of patients are asymptomatic. A highly suggestive clinical clue is the presence of a continuous murmur.

Treatment, or closure of the fistulous connections, is advocated for symptomatic patients, particularly for those with heart failure and myocardial ischemia, and for those asymptomatic patients who are at risk for future complications. Therapeutic options include surgical correction (102–104) and transcatheter embolization (105–108). The management is controversial, and recommendations are based on anecdotal cases or small retrospective series (101).

Although noninvasive imaging may facilitate the diagnosis and identification of the origin and insertion of CAFs, cardiac catheterization and coronary angiography is often considered necessary to precisely delineate the coronary anatomy, for assessment of hemodynamics, and to detail concomitant atherosclerosis and other structural anomalies. The capacity for MR to accurately determine Qp/Qs data adds value to the assessment (109).

To date, contrast-enhanced MDCT (110–112), EBCT (69,113) or MR have been used primarily as an adjunct to coronary angiography (114–118). A larger dependence on CT and MR is predicted following improvements in spatial and temporal resolution (Figs. 14-29–14-31). The demonstration of the course of blood vessels and the sites of influx and outflow of abnormal blood vessels is facilitated with multiplanar reconstructions, targeted thin-slab MIPs, and VR techniques (111).

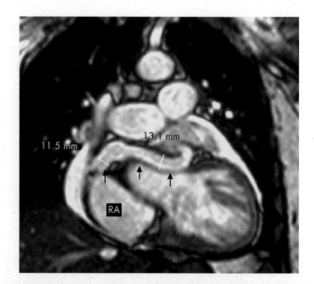

FIGURE 14-29 Left coronary to right atrium fistula demonstrated by MR. A 68-year-old woman presented with dyspnea and chest tightness. A fistula (*arrows*) from the left coronal ostium to the right atrium (*RA*) is seen (length 77.4 mm, proximal width 13.1 mm, distal width 11.5 mm—see panel). The findings were confirmed during coronary and aorta arteriography (not shown) and revealed that there was no significant stenosis in the coronary arteries. The Qp/Qs ratio was 2.1. (Adapted from Yoda M, Minami K, Koerfer R. Images in cardiology. Left coronal ostium to right atrium fistula causing right ventricular failure and pulmonary hypertension. *Heart.* 2006;92(3):330, with permission.)

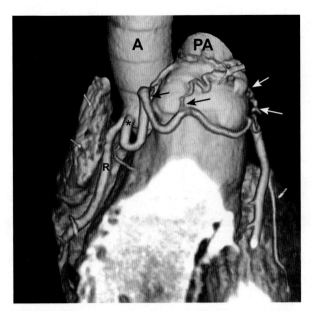

FIGURE 14-30 Right coronary artery system—pulmonary outflow tract fistulas. This VR MDCT image was modified with an anterior cut plane and shows the RCA (*R*) arising from the aorta (*A*). A markedly enlarged conal branch (*) is the site of origin for three feeding vessels (*arrows*), each connecting with the pulmonary outflow tract (*PA*). Coronary artery fistulas most commonly arise from the right system (~55%). (Courtesy of Stanford Cardiovascular Imaging.)

The prognosis following successful closure of CAFs is excellent. Long-term follow-up is necessary to assess for the postoperative recanalization, persistent dilation of the coronary artery and ostium, thrombus formation, calcification, and myocardial ischemia (119). Patients treated conservatively should be followed-up closely for the appearance of

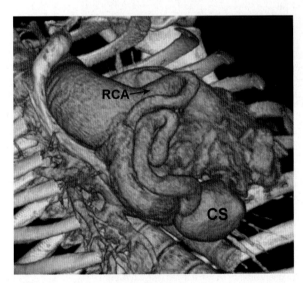

FIGURE 14-31 Right coronary artery to coronary sinus fistula. This obliquely oriented VR MDCT viewed from below shows a markedly enlarged RCA (*arrow*) with a tortuous and redundant course, extending to the inferior surface of the heart and forming a fistulous communication with the aneurysmal coronary sinus. (Courtesy of Stanford Cardiovascular Imaging.)

symptoms. Most asymptomatic adult patients remain free of symptoms for long periods (120,121).

IDENTIFICATION OF NATIVE VESSEL CORONARY STENOSIS

Computed Tomography

A major strength of CTA is the ability to display wall changes of the coronary arteries. Coronary calcifications can easily be assessed even without contrast media and represent an advanced stage of atherosclerosis. However, as different stages of coronary atherosclerosis may be present simultaneously, calcifications may also be associated with more early stages of coronary atherosclerosis. Therefore, the entire extent of coronary atherosclerosis will be underestimated by assessing coronary calcifications alone (122). With contrast enhancement, coronary atherosclerosis identified by calcified as well as noncalcified lesions can more completely be assessed by MDCT.

The current gold standard to assess coronary atherosclerosis in vivo is coronary intravascular ultrasound (IVUS). In a segmental analysis, Achenbach et al. reported that segments containing noncalcified plaque, alone or in combination with calcified plaque, were detected with a sensitivity of 78% and specificity of 87%. However, the sensitivity to exclusively detect noncalcified plaques showed MDCT to have a sensitivity of 53% only (123). Schroeder et al. (124) reported that coronary lesions classified as soft, intermediate, and dense in IVUS correspond to coronary artery wall plaques in MDCT with a density of 14 ± 26, 91 ± 21, and 419 ± 194 HU, respectively.

In heart specimen studies, it was demonstrated that noncalcified plaques with a low (40 to 60 HU) and intermediate (80 to 90 HU) density may correspond to lipid- and fibrous-rich plaques, respectively (1). In patients with an acute coronary syndrome, a noncalcified plaque with low density (40 HU) may also correspond to an intracoronary thrombus (125). In patients after acute myocardial infarction, noncalcified plaques are more common than in patients with stable angina. On the other hand, the number of calcified plaques is significantly higher in patients with stable angina.

Commonly, spotty calcified lesions may be present in MDCT angiography studies that may correlate to minor wall changes in conventional coronary angiography only (126). However, it is known from pathologic studies that such calcified nodules may also be the source of unheralded plaque rupture and consecutive thrombosis, which may lead to sudden coronary death in very rare cases (127).

Achenbach et al. reported a sensitivity and specificity of 92% and 94%, respectively, for evaluating coronary artery stenoses with CTA using EBCT as compared with cardiac catheterization (128). For coronary EBCT, Schmermund

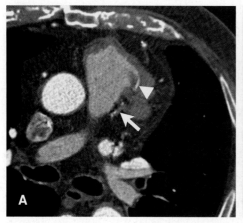
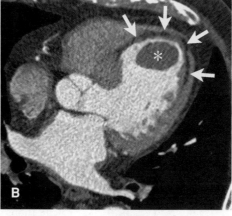

FIGURE 14-32 LAD disease and myocardial infarct with MDCT. A: Male patient with an occluded mid-segment of the LAD (*arrow*) and an intramural course of the distal LAD (*arrowhead*). **B:** A large infarction with scar is seen in the anterior wall of the myocardium (*arrows*) along with thrombus in the apex (∗).

et al. (30) reported that small vessel diameter may lead to false-positive findings for coronary artery stenoses. Furthermore, extensive calcifications might interfere with the detection of coronary artery stenoses, resulting in false-negative results compared with selective coronary angiography. The reported results for detecting stenoses with the 16 MDCT (129,130) are comparable to EBCT.

The assessment of the coronary artery tree is no longer limited to the most proximal part of the coronary artery tree. Furthermore, adjunctive information including the depiction of myocardial scar can be visualized (131–133) (Figs. 14-32, 14-33).

In selected patient populations, MDCT has performed well in demonstrating stenotic disease with an ability to show strong comparisons with conventional angiography (Figs. 14-34, 14-35).

Using a 64-detector system in a study of 52 patients (34 men; mean age 59.6 ± 12.1 years) with atypical chest

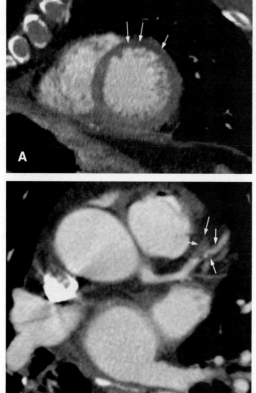
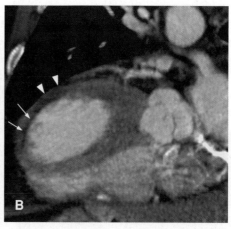

FIGURE 14-33 Acute coronary syndrome. This patient presented to the emergency department with chest pain, and a CT was ordered to assess for aortic dissection. While dissection was ruled out, the radiologist noted anterior wall perfusion deficits on short axis **(A)** and vertical long axis **(B)** reconstructions are seen, including subendocardial components (*thin arrows*). **C:** A reconstructed image to detail the coronary arteries shows a filling defect (*yellow arrows*) occluding the LAD and smaller nonocclusive plaques (*white arrows*) in a large diagonal branch. Note the cardiac vein (*blue arrowhead*) immediately posterior to the diagonal branch. (Courtesy of Stanford Cardiovascular Imaging.)

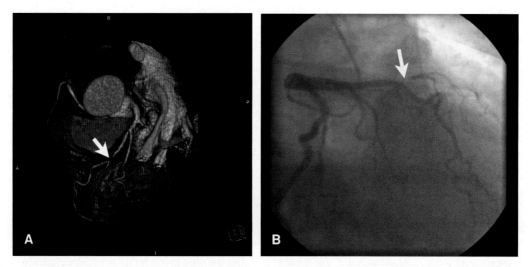

FIGURE 14-34 Stenosis of LAD demonstrated with MDCTA. A: 55-year-old male patient with a single-vessel disease in the LAD (*arrow*). **B:** Finding of CTA confirmed by cardiac catheter with a high-grade stenosis in the midsegment of the LAD.

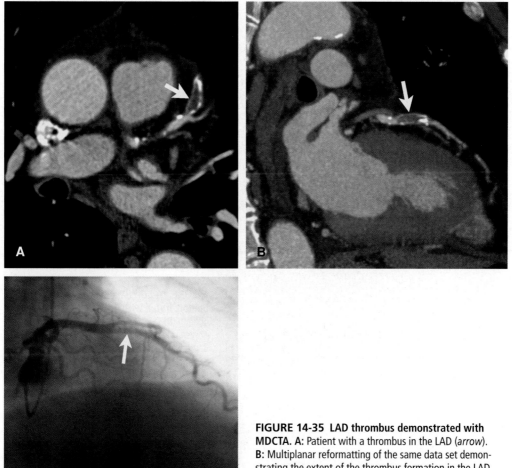

FIGURE 14-35 LAD thrombus demonstrated with MDCTA. A: Patient with a thrombus in the LAD (*arrow*). **B:** Multiplanar reformatting of the same data set demonstrating the extent of the thrombus formation in the LAD. **C:** In the coronary angiogram, only slightly diminished enhancement is visible at the corresponding location (*arrow*).

pain, stable or unstable angina pectoris, or non–ST-segment elevation myocardial infarction, the sensitivity, specificity, and positive and negative predictive values for detecting significant stenoses on a segment-by-segment analysis were 99% (93 of 94; 95% CI [confidence interval], 94 to 99), 95% (601 of 631; 95% CI, 93 to 96), 76% (93 of 123; 95% CI, 67 to 89), and 99% (601 of 602; 95% CI, 99 to 100), respectively (134).

Coronary MDCT, like EBCT, still suffers from limitations in respect to dense calcifications and precise accuracy in determining the degree of localization of coronary artery stenoses. Therefore, coronary MDCT is currently not suited to determine the progression in patients with known CAD or typical angina, or in those with obvious myocardial ischemia on exercise testing. These patients are better approached by cardiac catheter examination with the option to perform percutaneous coronary interventions in the same session (135).

A drawback of all the current studies is that MDCT has, to date, been tested in a heterogeneous group of patients with suspicion of CAD or with established CAD with recurrent symptoms (high CAD pretest probability). Because of the high negative predictive value reported for coronary CTA (97% to 99%), this modality seems to be ideally suited to rule out CAD. However, further studies are required to determine the accuracy in a patient cohort with an unknown history of CAD and ambiguous coronary symptoms or stress tests (low CAD pretest probability).

Magnetic Resonance Imaging

While data support a broad clinical role for coronary MRI in the assessment of suspected anomalous CAD (and CABG patency, discussed later), data are currently in evolution regarding clinical coronary MRI for routine identification of coronary artery stenoses among patients

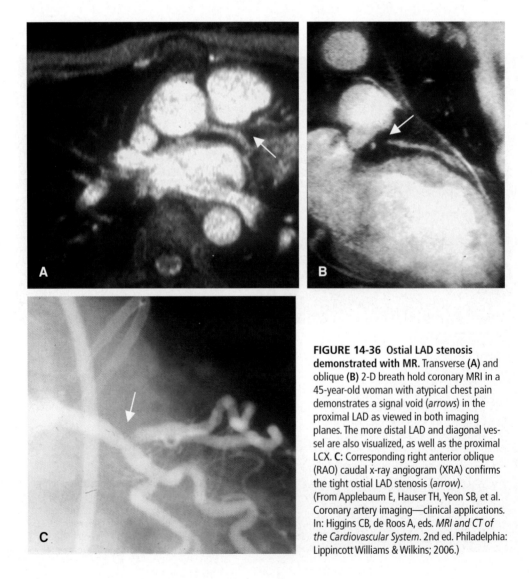

FIGURE 14-36 Ostial LAD stenosis demonstrated with MR. Transverse **(A)** and oblique **(B)** 2-D breath hold coronary MRI in a 45-year-old woman with atypical chest pain demonstrates a signal void (*arrows*) in the proximal LAD as viewed in both imaging planes. The more distal LAD and diagonal vessel are also visualized, as well as the proximal LCX. **C:** Corresponding right anterior oblique (RAO) caudal x-ray angiogram (XRA) confirms the tight ostial LAD stenosis (*arrow*). (From Applebaum E, Hauser TH, Yeon SB, et al. Coronary artery imaging—clinical applications. In: Higgins CB, de Roos A, eds. *MRI and CT of the Cardiovascular System.* 2nd ed. Philadelphia: Lippincott Williams & Wilkins; 2006.)

presenting with chest pain who are under consideration for x-ray angiography, and no efficacy data have been reported regarding "screening" coronary MRI in low- or high-risk populations. However, current data support a clinical role for patients in whom the concern is LM or multivessel CAD. Though coronary MRI methods may not depict the more distal vessels, data suggest that only a small minority (<5%) of patients undergoing intervention have an isolated lesion in the distal or minor side branches (9).

As previously discussed, gradient echo sequences depict flow in the coronary lumen, with rapidly moving laminar blood flow appearing "bright," while areas of stagnant flow and/or focal turbulence appear "dark" due to local saturation (stagnant flow) or dephasing (turbulence) (Fig. 14-36).

Areas of focal stenoses produce varying severity of "signal void" in the coronary MRI, with the severity of the signal loss related to the angiographic stenosis (136) (Fig. 14-37).

However, gradient echo coronary MRI may sometimes be misleading. If there is slow blood flow distal to a stenosis, there may be complete loss of signal in the segment distal to the lesion, despite the absence of a total occlusion. Similarly, as lumen signal is insensitive to the direction of blood flow, a total occlusion with adequate retrograde (or antegrade collateral blood flow) to the distal segment may result in signal in the lumen distal to the occlusion. SSFP sequences are less dependent on blood flow for signal intensity, but the overall depiction of stenoses is similar.

Due to time constraints of a breath hold, 2D breath-hold coronary MRI has relatively limited in-plane spatial resolution, but the technique has successfully demonstrated proximal coronary stenoses (61,136–139) with good correlation between the distance from the vessel origin to the focal stenosis (136) (Table 14-3) (Fig. 14-38).

However, there has been wide variation in reported sensitivity and specificity of this approach. These differences are likely due to technical issues or methodology, including the wide variation in patient selection, presence of arrhythmias, prevalence of disease and technical issues (MR vendor, echo time, receiver coils, timing of the acquisition, acquisition duration, breath-hold maneuvers), and the need for somewhat exhausting 20- to 40-second breath holds to complete a study.

With the increasing availability of MR navigators, many cardiac magnetic resonance (CMR) imaging centers have migrated to a free-breathing targeted 3D gradient echo or whole heart SSFP coronary MRI for ease in patient acceptance (free breathing) and for improved SNR with facilitated multiplanar reconstructions. Early studies using *retrospective* diaphragmatic navigators incorporated relatively prolonged acquisition times (260 msec/R-R interval) (140–142), while more recent reports have

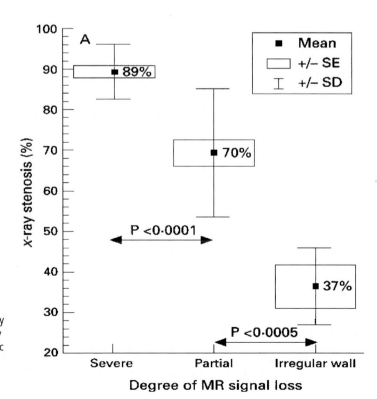

FIGURE 14-37 MR signal loss and x-ray angiography correlation. Breath-hold 2D segmented k-space gradient echo coronary MRI comparison of focal MR signal loss versus x-ray coronary artery diameter stenosis. Note the strong correlation between the severity of signal loss by coronary MRI and the degree of x-ray angiographic stenosis. (From Pennell DJ, Bogren HG, Keegan J, et al. Assessment of coronary artery stenosis by magnetic resonance imaging. *Heart.* 1996;75(2): 127–133, with permission.)

TABLE 14-3

Two-Dimensional Breath-hold Coronary Magnetic Resonance Imaging for Identification of ≥50%-Diameter Focal Coronary Stenoses

Study	Number of Subjects	Number of CAD Vessels (%)	Sensitivity	Specificity
Manning et al. (137)	39	52 (35)	90% (71–100)	92% (78–100)
Duerinckx & Urman (61)	20	27 (34)	63% (0–73)	— (37–82)
Pennell et al. (136)	39	55 (35)	85% (75–100)	
Post et al. (138)	35	35 (28)	63% (0–100)	89% (73–96)
Nitatori et al. (139)	57[a]		87%	94%
	13[b]		43%	90%

[a]With ≥90%–diameter stenosis.
[b]With 50% to 75%–diameter stenosis.

utilized acquisition intervals of <120 msec (143–145). These single-center reports were encouraging with overall sensitivity and specificity of up to 90% for proximal coronary disease (145) (Table 14-4). Subsequently, single-center targeted 3D k-space segmented gradient echo studies using more sophisticated prospective diaphragmatic navigators with real-time motion correction have shown

improved results, especially for the proximal coronary segments and in subjects with high image-quality scans (146) (Fig. 14-39).

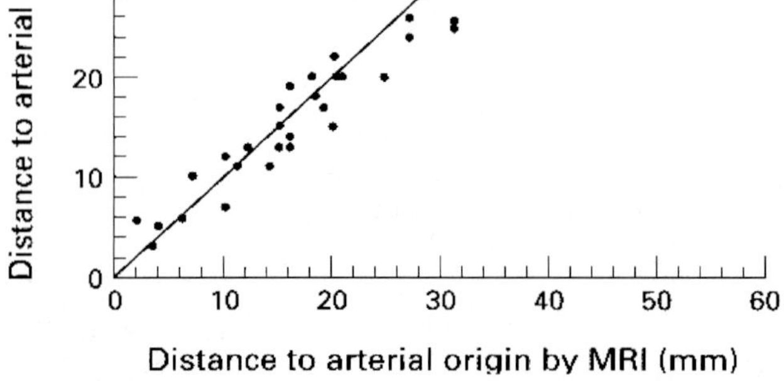

An international multicenter, free-breathing 3D volume-targeted coronary MRI study of 109 patients without prior x-ray angiography using common hardware and software demonstrated high sensitivity (though only modest specificity) and high negative predictive value of coronary MRI for the identification of coronary disease (as defined as ≥50%-diameter stenosis by quantitative coronary angiography) (5) (Table 14-5). The sensitivity and negative predictive value were particularly high for the identification of LM or multivessel disease, demonstrating a clinical role for coronary MRI for this subset. Accordingly, we have found coronary MRI to be especially valuable for patients who present with a dilated cardiomyopathy/congestive heart failure in the absence of clinical infarction to determine the etiology (ischemic vs. nonischemic) (150). For this group, more conventional noninvasive tests often have suboptimal diagnostic accuracy, with coronary MRI also being superior to delayed enhancement CMR methods.

Despite inferior in-plane spatial resolution, single-center data using free-breathing, navigator-gated, and corrected whole heart SSFP among patient series are particularly impressive for reconstruction and suggest superior accuracy for this approach (151–153), with sensitivities of 80% to 90% and specificity exceeding 90% (Fig. 14-8). An approach that uses the affine prospective navigator algorithm (compensates for motion in both the inferior-superior and the anterior-posterior orientations) offers theoretical

FIGURE 14-38 MR and x-ray angiography correlation: distance to stenosis. Scatterplot comparing the distance from the coronary origin to the stenosis as measured by x-ray and magnetic resonance coronary angiography. (From Danias PG, McConnell MV, Khasgiwala VC, et al. Prospective navigator correction of image position for coronary MR angiography. *Radiology*. 1997;203(3):733–736, with permission.)

TABLE 14-4

Free-breathing Three-dimensional K-space Segmented Gradient Echo Coronary Magnetic Resonance Imaging Using *Retrospective* and *Prospective* Navigators for Identification of Focal ≥50%-Diameter Coronary Stenoses

Study	Number of Subjects	Number of CAD Vessels (%)	For $50%-diameter Stenosis Specificity	For $50%-diameter Stenosis Sensitivity
Retrospective Navigator Gating				
Post et al. (140)	20	21 (27)	38% (0–57)	95% (85–100)
Muller et al. (142)	35	—	83%[a]	94%[a]
Woodard et al. (141)	10	10 (100)	70%	—
Sandstede et al. (198)	30	30 (100)	81%[b]	89%[b]
van Geuns et al. (143)	32	—	50% (50–55)[c]	91% (73–95)[c]
Huber et al. (144)	40	20 (50)	73% (25–100)	50% (25–82)
Sardanelli et al. (145)	42	40% of segments	82% (57–100) 90% proximal	89% (72–100) 90% proximal
Prospective Navigators with Real Time Motion Correction				
Bunce et al. (146)	34	—	88%	72%
Moustapha et al. (147)	25	—	92% 90% (proximal)	55% 92% (proximal)
Sommer (173)	112	—	74% 88% (good quality)	63% 91% (good quality)
Bogaert et al. (148)	19	—	85%–92%	50%–83%
Plein et al. (149)	10	—	75%	85%
Osgun et al. (199)	14	TFE SSFP	91% 76%	57% 85%

CAD, coronary artery disease.
[a]Excluding five patients for "lack of cooperation" and 15 segments for being uninterpretable.
[b]Based on 23 (77%) with high-quality scans.
[c]Based on 74% of coronary artery segments analyzable by MRI.

advantages (152), but no direct comparison with a single diaphragmatic navigator is available. A comparative study of segmented k-space gradient echo versus SSFP did confirm the expected improvement of SNR and CNR but no benefit with regard to accuracy for identification of CAD (40).

Comparative data for noncontrast and inversion recovery contrast-enhanced coronary MRA in patients are currently few. In small series, overall sensitivity and specificity of free-breathing navigator-corrected Gadomer-17 [Schering, Berlin, Germany] (154) coronary MRI was 80% and 93%, respectively, and similar to that of noncontrast single-center studies.

High (3T)-field coronary MRI offers the theoretical benefit of a doubling of SNR. In practice, the SNR gain is more modest, owing to lack of optimization of surface coils, shimming, and the like. Only preliminary comparative data regarding the clinical utility of 3T coronary MRI have been reported. These suggest superior SNR but demonstrate similar sensitivity and specificities of 82% and 89%, respectively, for detection of significant CAD (155) (Fig. 14-40).

An alternative method for increasing SNR that also provides a long imaging window is the use of blood pool MR contrast agents (156). These agents reside in the vascular system for much longer time periods than traditional

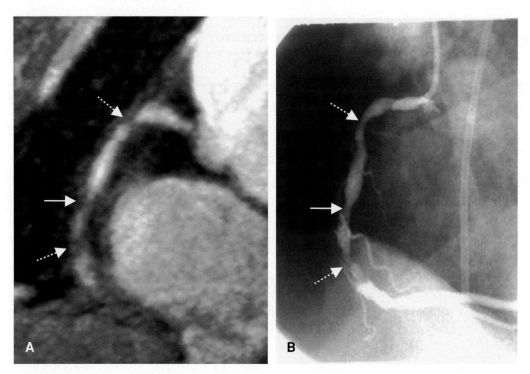

FIGURE 14-39 MR and x-ray angiography correlation. Free-breathing 3D T2 prepulse coronary MRI with navigator gating and real time motion correction **(A)** and corresponding x-ray angiography (XRA) **(B)** in a patient with proximal (*dashed arrow*) and mid-RCA stenoses (*solid and dashed arrows*). (From Stuber M, Botnar RM, Danias PG, et al. Double-oblique free-breathing high resolution three-dimensional coronary magnetic resonance angiography. *J Am Coll Cardiol.* 1999;34(2):524–531, with permission.)

extracellular MR contrast agents, and early data suggest benefits for visualizing smaller and more distal vessels (Fig. 14-41).

POSTOPERATIVE AND POSTINTERVENTIONAL EVALUATION

Until the advent of intracoronary stents a decade ago, CABG surgery was among the most common procedures performed in the United States. Unfortunately, early (<1 month) vein graft occlusion occurs in up to 10% of patients

due to mechanical issues, and an accelerated atherosclerotic process often leads to late (5- to 10-year) stenoses/occlusion in the majority of grafts (157,158). Improvements in long-term patency rates for percutaneous coronary interventions using conventional and drug-eluting intracoronary stents has resulted in their widespread use in over 80% of the growing number of percutaneous coronary artery revascularizations.

In general, the evaluation of patients following coronary intervention can be difficult with cardiac CT and MR. Because of their present coronary artery disease, many of

TABLE 14-5

Identification of Coronary Artery Disease in Multicenter Coronary Magnetic Resonance Imaging Trial

	Patient (%)	Left Main/3VD (%)
Sensitivity	93	100
Specificity	58	85
Prevalence	42	15
Positive predictive value	70	54
Negative predictive value	81	100

Adapted from Kim WY, Danias PG, Stuber M, et al. Coronary magnetic resonance angiography for the detection of coronary stenoses. *N Engl J Med.* 2001;345(26):1863–1869.

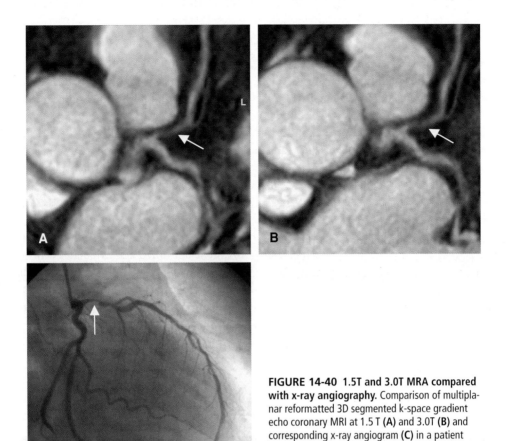

FIGURE 14-40 1.5T and 3.0T MRA compared with x-ray angiography. Comparison of multiplanar reformatted 3D segmented k-space gradient echo coronary MRI at 1.5 T **(A)** and 3.0T **(B)** and corresponding x-ray angiogram **(C)** in a patient with a proximal stenosis (*arrow*) of the LAD. At both field strengths, there is good correlation between coronary MRI and the x-ray angiogram. (Images courtesy of Thorsten Sommer, MD, PhD.)

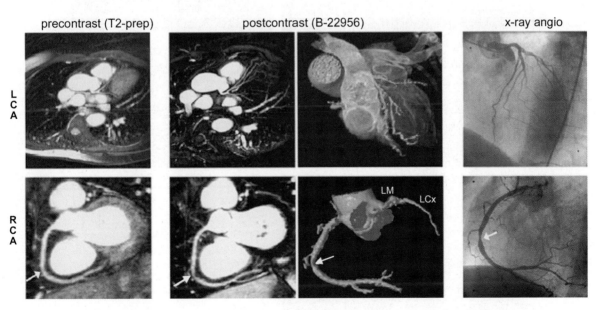

FIGURE 14-41 Coronary artery imaging with a blood pool contrast agent. Imaging of the right (*RCA*) and left (*LCA*) coronary artery system of a patient. The multiplanar reformatted precontrast T2 prep scan, the postcontrast B-22956 (0.075 mmol/kg) enhanced scan (**left:** multiplanar reformatted image; **right:** surface-rendered image), and corresponding x-ray angiography are shown. **Upper row:** The precontrast scan does not visualize the distal LAD and side branches. The postcontrast scan shows a normal LCA system. **Bottom row:** On the precontrast scan, the lumen of the mid-RCA appears normal, while the postcontrast scan gives clear evidence of obstructive coronary disease in this segment. (Adapted from Paetsch I, Jahnke C, Barkhausen J, et al. Detection of coronary stenoses with contrast enhanced, three-dimensional free breathing coronary MR angiography using the gadolinium-based intravascular contrast agent gadocoletic acid (B-22956). *J Cardiovasc Magn Reson.* 2006;8(3):509–516, with permission.)

these patients have severe calcification, and coronary stents are commonly implanted after angioplasty. Any of this dense material can hinder the detection of stenoses or in-stent stenoses with CT. Metallic artifacts from hemostatic clips, ostial stainless steel graft markers, sternal wires, coexistent prosthetic valves and supporting struts or rings, and graft stents can pose limitations to MR evaluations.

Evaluation after Stent Placement

Computed Tomography

MDCT provides limited direct visualization of coronary in-stent restenosis but shows a capacity to differentiate between stent patency and stent occlusion (159). MDCT can be limited primarily by partial volume effects and beam hardening, the latter induced by the stent material (159,160). One report has described value in measuring the CT contrast-density curve behind stents to demonstrate the success of a reintervention (161).

More encouraging results have been reported with the use of ≥16-slice MDCT. While stent material impacts the ability to demonstrate the stent lumen, 16-slice MDCT can detect in-stent restenoses of assessable stents with high accuracy in comparison to conventional coronary angiography (162).

The introduction of 64-slice CT has demonstrated superior visualization of the stent lumen and in-stent stenosis compared with 16-slice CT, especially when the stent is orientated parallel to the x-ray beam (163). Furthermore, artificial lumen narrowing (ALN) was significantly reduced with 64-slice CT compared with 16-slice CT (163). Even with the improved spatial resolution of 64-slice CT, the use of a stent-optimized kernel remains beneficial for stent visualization when compared with the standard medium-soft CTA protocol (164). Regardless, the use of multiplanar reformation (MPR) can facilitate the assessment by offering a cross-sectional evaluation (Fig. 14-42).

Magnetic Resonance

Typically made from high-grade stainless steel, preliminary data demonstrate no short or long-term adverse events for

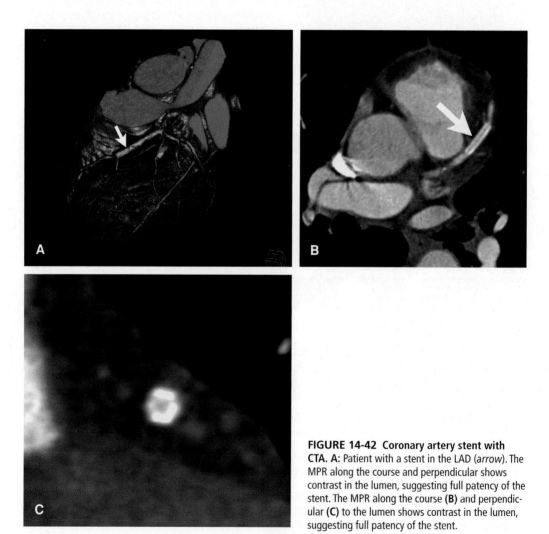

FIGURE 14-42 Coronary artery stent with CTA. A: Patient with a stent in the LAD (*arrow*). The MPR along the course and perpendicular shows contrast in the lumen, suggesting full patency of the stent. The MPR along the course (**B**) and perpendicular (**C**) to the lumen shows contrast in the lumen, suggesting full patency of the stent.

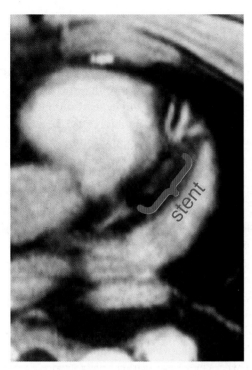

FIGURE 14-43 Coronary artery stent with MRA: susceptibility.
Transverse, 2D breath-hold gradient echo coronary MRI at the level of the LAD in a patient with a patent stent. Note the signal void corresponding to the site of the stent. (Courtesy of Christopher Kramer, MD.)

patients who undergo "early" MR scanning after stent implantation (165,166), but the stents do pose local imaging problems. Though the attractive force and local heating are negligible at 1.5T (167–172) and 3T (173), the local susceptibility effects lead to substantial signal voids/artifacts at the site of the stent (Fig. 14-43).

The size of the artifact is dependent on the stent material (increased with stainless steel and less with titanium stents) (174,175) as well as the MR sequence (increased with gradient echo sequences). A novel MR-lucent stent has also been reported (176) but remains to be clinically tested for durability and restenosis (Fig. 14-44).

Though signal void/artifact precludes direct evaluation of intrastent and peristent coronary integrity, assessment of blood flow/direction proximal and distal to the stent using MR flow methods or spin-labeling methods may provide indirect evidence of a patency by documentation of antegrade flow.

Evaluation after Coronary Artery Bypass Graft Assessment

The conduits used for CABG surgery may be divided into arterial and venous grafts (177). SV conduits are harvested

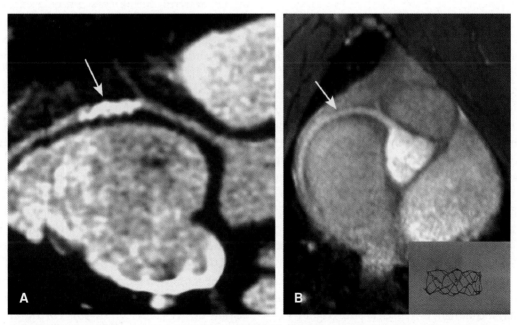

FIGURE 14-44 MR-lucent stent. A: Multidetector CT (MDCT) with Aachen Resonance prototype MR stent in the RCA. **B:** 3D coronary MRI in the same animal. Note the absence of local susceptibility effects on the MR image. The hand-woven stent is shown as inlay. (Reprinted from Buecker A, Spuentrup E, Ruebben A, et al. New metallic MR stents for artifact-free coronary MR angiography: feasibility study in a swine model. *Invest Radiol.* 2004;39(5):250–253, with permission.)

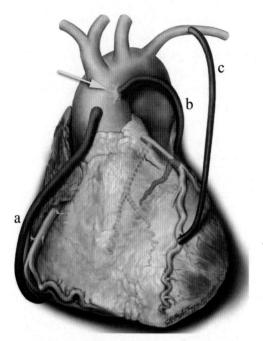

FIGURE 14-45 Diagrammatic examples of CABGs. Drawing shows examples of CABGs. A right SVG **(a)** is attached to the anterior aorta proximally and to the posterior descending artery distally. A left SVG **(b)** has an altered appearance because it is attached to the aorta with an aortic connector device (*arrow*); the origin of this SVG is moved laterally to prevent kinking. A typical left IMA graft **(c)** is left intact at its origin and is grafted to the LAD artery distally. (From Frazier AA, Qureshi F, Read KM, et al. Coronary artery bypass grafts: assessment with multidetector CT in the early and late postoperative settings. *Radiographics.* 2005;25(4): 881–896, with permission.)

from the legs and are grafted from the ascending aorta to the distal coronary artery beyond the point of stenosis or obstruction (Fig. 14-45).

The vein graft usually originates the anterior aspect of the aorta. Left-sided grafts are typically anastomosed distally to the LAD artery, diagonal artery, circumflex artery, or the obtuse marginal branches of the circumflex artery.

Right coronary artery grafts are typically attached to the anterior aorta, or lower on the anterior aorta, so that the graft lies in the right AV groove. Grafts for the LCA are brought from the left side of the aorta so as to be supported by their course over the PA.

Internal mammary artery (IMA) grafts offer decreased postoperative mortality and improved cardiac eventfree survival rates as compared with SV grafts; thus, the IMA has become the preferred bypass graft. Typically, the left IMA is used as the graft, and the right IMA is left in place (Fig. 14-45). The left IMA is typically separated from the chest wall, and its relative proximity to the LAD artery favors the LAD for a revascularization target. The origin of the left IMA from the subclavian artery remains intact.

The right IMA may be used as direct graft to the RCA, LAD artery, or LCX artery. It may also be removed from the subclavian artery and used as a free or composite graft. One configuration of composite graft attaches the right IMA proximally to a left IMA graft so that the left IMA inflow supplies both grafted vessels. In this configuration, total arterial myocardial revascularization can be accomplished (instead of using a left IMA and an additional SVG) when two-vessel bypass is necessary.

The assessment of graft patency is the most common clinical request for CT and MR following CABG surgery. However, aneurysms and pseudoaneurysms of grafts are complications that are well demonstrated with noninvasive vascular imaging.

Graft Aneurysms and Pseudoaneurysms

Aneurysms and pseudoaneurysms of SVGs to the coronary arteries are rare (178) and are more commonly seen as a delayed complication (179). True aneurysms are more likely to be asymptomatic, whereas pseudoaneurysms more often present with chest pain. Either entity carries a significant morbidity or mortality rate and should be considered in the differential diagnosis of a patient with a hilar mass on chest x-ray, presenting after CABG.

In one review of 50 cases, the mean length of time that postcoronary artery bypass aneurysms were diagnosed was 10 years after surgery (range, 7 days to 21 years) (179). Typically, SVG aneurysms present as asymptomatic chest masses detected during chest imaging or with ischemic symptoms secondary to graft occlusion or distal embolization from intraluminal thrombus. Mycotic or infected CABG aneurysms are only a small fraction of the reported cases (178).

True aneurysms typically are fusiform and involve the body of the graft and also commonly result from graft arteriosclerosis. Pseudoaneurysms, in contrast, are saccular, usually present at the anastomotic site, and often related to technical issues (179).

Once an SVG aneurysm is suspected or detected, CT or MRI of the chest should be performed to determine patency of the graft lumen as well as the precise location of the graft within the mediastinum to guide the surgical approach (Figs. 14-46, 14-47).

Computed Tomography. The use of CT in the assessment of bypass grafts continues to grow with advances in CT technology and has accelerated with the rapid dissemination of MDCT (Fig. 14-48). For the morphological assessment of bypass graft patency with MDCT compared with cardiac catheterization, Ropers et al. reported a sensitivity and specificity of 97% and 98%, respectively (180). For the detection of bypass graft stenosis, the sensitivity and

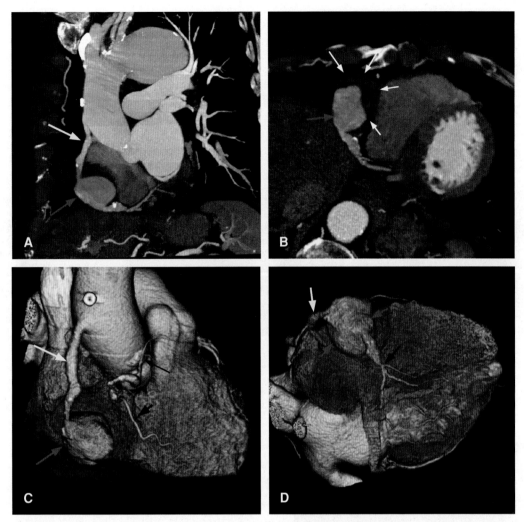

FIGURE 14-46 CTA of a right coronary artery saphenous vein graft pseudoaneurysm. A: Oblique thin-slab MIP image shows the origin of the SVG (*yellow arrow*) with the pseudoaneurysm (PsA) seen more distally (*red arrow*). **B:** An alternate projection of a thin-slab MIP shows the PsA (*red arrow*) bounded by clot (*white arrows*). **C:** A VR image displays the SVG (*yellow arrow*) and PsA (*red arrow*) and includes a demonstration of a conal branch (*thin black arrow*) off the RCA and a ventricular branch (*short black arrow*). **D:** VR image of the inferior surface of the heart shows the distal SVG (*yellow arrow*) as it expands into the PsA (*red arrow*). The distal portion of the native RCA beyond the PsA (*black arrow*) is seen as it bifurcates into the posterior descending and posterior left ventricular arteries. (Courtesy of Stanford Cardiovascular Imaging.)

specificity was significantly lower with 75% and 92%, respectively.

The diameter of an occluded bypass graft may give a hint for a subacute or chronic occlusion. Enzweiler et al. (181) reported that the mean diameter of patent, subacute, and chronic occluded bypass grafts was 3.9, 5.4, and 0.3 mm, respectively. This finding may be explained by the fact that venous bypass grafts may widen by the clot, and later fibrous organization will lead to a shrinkage of the graft.

Sequential scanning and administration of a small contrast bolus has already been shown to allow determination of a spiral CT flow index with a single-detector CT. This index agreed with angiographically determined coronary

bypass flow in 85% of the grafts investigated (182) but is difficult to routinely obtain.

More recently, improved imaging of all bypass types was demonstrated using 16- to 64-row MDCT as compared with 4-row MDCT, but the assessment of the distal anastomosis yielded no difference between 4- and 16-row technology (183). Still, beam hardening from vascular metal clips and partial volume effects can limit the proper assessment of arterial bypass grafts, particularly when located along the course of vessels with smaller diameters (184). An excellent review of the use of MDCT for assessing CABG patients is recommended to the interested reader (177).

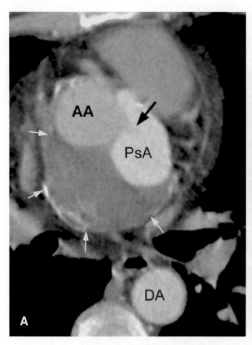

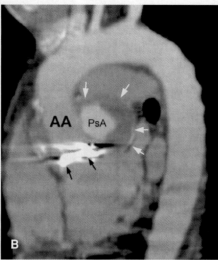

FIGURE 14-47 Pseudoaneurysm from dehisced coronary artery button. A: Axial CT scan demonstrates the pseudoaneurysm *(PsA)* emanating *(black arrow)* from the ascending aorta *(AA)*. The PsA attenuation, higher than the AA and similar to the descending aorta *(DA)*, is consistent with relative stasis of the opacified blood into the PsA. Note the thrombus bounding the PsA *(yellow arrows)*. **B:** This sagittal reformation shows the PsA near the aortic root, just above an aortic valve prosthesis *(thin black arrows)*. (Courtesy of Stanford Cardiovascular Imaging.)

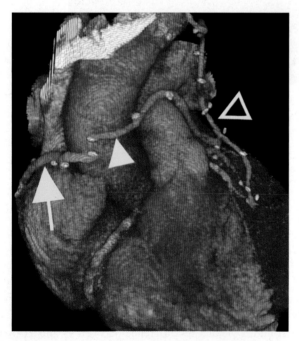

FIGURE 14-48 CTA of saphenous vein grafts. Three-dimensional VR image shows the typical appearances of right *(arrow)* and left *(solid arrowhead)* SVGs sutured to the anterior aorta. The left SVG is attached to the diagonal artery distally; the distal anastomosis of the right SVG to the posterior descending artery is not seen. There is also a left IMA graft *(open arrowhead)*, which is connected to the LAD artery. (From Frazier AA, Qureshi F, Read KM, et al. Coronary artery bypass grafts: assessment with multidetector CT in the early and late postoperative settings. *Radiographics*. 2005;25(4):881–896, with permission.)

Magnetic Resonance. In comparison with the native coronary arteries, reverse SV and IMA grafts are easier to image (in the absence of adjacent vascular clips) due to their relatively stationary position during the cardiac and respiratory cycle as well as their larger lumen.

With schematic knowledge of the origin and touchdown site of each graft, conventional free-breathing ECG-gated 2D spin echo (157,158,186–189) and 2D gradient echo (190–192) MR in the transverse plane have both been utilized to reliably assess bypass graft patency (Table 14-6) (Fig. 14-49).

Patency is determined by visualizing a patent graft lumen in at least two contiguous transverse levels along its expected course. If a patent lumen is only seen at one level, the graft is considered indeterminate. If a patent graft lumen is not seen at any level, the graft is considered occluded. Combining spin echo and gradient echo imaging in the same patient does not appear to improve accuracy (189). Both 3D noncontrast (193–194) and contrast-enhanced coronary MRI have been described for the assessment of graft patency (195,196), with slightly improved results. The accuracy of ECG-gated SSFP sequences appears to be similar to that of spin echo and gradient echo approaches (194) (Figs. 14-50, 14-51). Data suggest that the use of phase velocity mapping for assessment of CABG flow may be superior to graft imaging (197,198).

TABLE 14-6

Sensitivity, Specificity, and Accuracy of Coronary Magnetic Resonance Imaging for Assessment of Coronary Artery Bypass Graft Patency

Study	Technique	Grafts	Patency (%)	Sensitivity (%)	Specificity (%)	Accuracy
White et al. (186)	2D SE	72	69	86	59	78
Rubenstein et al. (187)	2D SE	47	62	90	72	83
Jenkins et al. (188)	2D SE	41	63	89	73	83
Galjee et al. (189)	2D SE	98	74	98	85	89
White et al. (190)	2D GRE	28	50	93	86	89
Aurigemma et al. (191)	2D GRE	45	73	88	100	91
Galjee et al. (189)	2D GRE	98	74	98	88	96
Engelmann et al. (192)	2D GRE	55	100 (IMA)	100		100
			66 (SVG)	92	85	89
Molinari et al. (193)	3D GRE	51	76.5	91	97	96
Bunce et al. (194)	3D SSFP	56 SVG	82	84	45	78
		23 IMA	96			
Wintersperger et al. (195)	CE-3D GRE	39	87	97	100	97
Vrachliotis et al. (196)	CE-3D GRE	45	67	93	97	95

SE, spin echo; GRE, gradient-recalled echo; IMA, internal mammary artery; SVG, saphenous vein graft; CE, contrast enhanced; SSFP, steady state free precession.

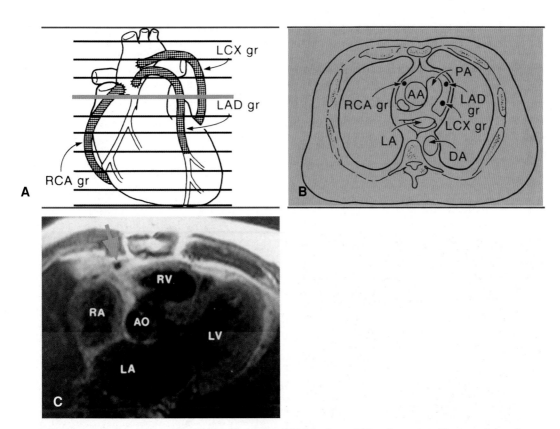

FIGURE 14-49 Schematics and axial black blood MR of CABGs. Coronal **(A)** and transverse **(B)** schematic (at colored slice level) of the anatomic location of CABGs (*RCA gr, LAD gr, LCX gr*) originating from the aortic root and anastomosing with the distal native coronary arteries with location of contiguous transverse slices. **C:** Transverse ECG-gated conventional spin echo coronary MRI image demonstrating flow (*arrow*) in an anatomic area corresponding to the RCA vein graft, indicating graft patency at that level. (RCA gr, right coronary artery graft; AA, aortic root; PA, pulmonary artery; LAD gr, left anterior descending artery graft; LCX gr, left circumflex artery graft; DA, descending artery; LA, left anterior; RA, right anterior; AO, aorta; RV, right ventricle; LV, left ventricle.) (Adapted from Rubinstein RI, Askenase AD, Thickman D, et al. Magnetic resonance imaging to evaluate patency of aortocoronary bypass grafts. *Circulation*. 1987;76(4): 786–791, with permission.)

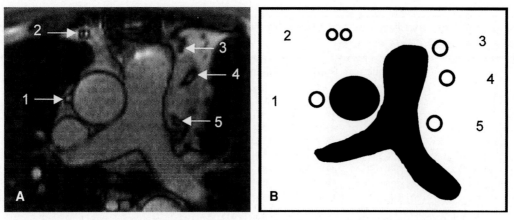

FIGURE 14-50 CABG grafts with SSFP MR. A: Transverse steady state free precession (SSFP) MR angiographic image. **B:** Graphic representation of image. Patent grafts can be seen in their typical anatomic positions. (1, venous graft to RCA or posterior descending artery; 2, right IMA without a graft; 3, arterial graft from left IMA to LAD; 4, venous graft to LAD or diagonal vessels; 5, venous graft to the circumflex artery or obtuse marginal vessels.) (From Bunce NH, Lorenz CH, John AS, et al. Coronary artery bypass graft patency: assessment with true ast imaging with steady-state precession versus gadolinium-enhanced MR angiography. *Radiology*. 2003;227(2):440–446, with permission.)

A practical limitation of coronary MRI bypass graft assessment is related to local signal loss/artifacts due to nearby metallic objects (hemostatic clips, ostial stainless steel graft markers, sternal wires, coexistent prosthetic valves and supporting struts or rings, and graft stents) (Figs. 14-5, 14-43). The inability to identify severely diseased yet patent grafts is also a hindrance to clinical utility and acceptance.

Langerak et al. (46) reported on the use of free-breathing T2 prep submillimeter 3D coronary MRI for assessment of SVG stenoses (Fig. 14-52). There was very good agreement between quantitative x-ray angiography for assessment of both graft occlusion and graft stenoses (Table 14-7). This group also advocated assessment of rest and adenosine stress coronary artery flow assessment using phase velocity MR techniques (199, 200).

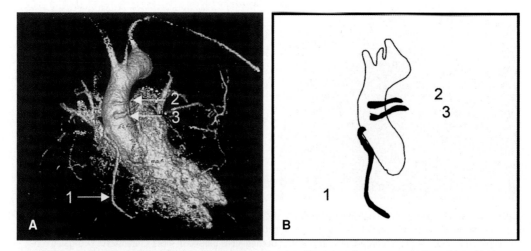

FIGURE 14-51 CABG grafts with SSFP MR. A: Three-dimensional VR image from a coronal MR angiographic data set. **B:** Graphic representation of image. Patent grafts are seen in their typical anatomic positions. IMAs are located more anteriorly and are not depicted. (1, venous graft to RCA or posterior descending artery; 2, venous graft to LAD or diagonal vessels; 3, venous graft to the circumflex or obtuse marginal vessels.) (From Bunce NH, Lorenz CH, John AS, et al. Coronary artery bypass graft patency: assessment with true ast imaging with steady-state precession versus gadolinium-enhanced MR angiography. *Radiology*. 2003;227(2):440–446, with permission.)

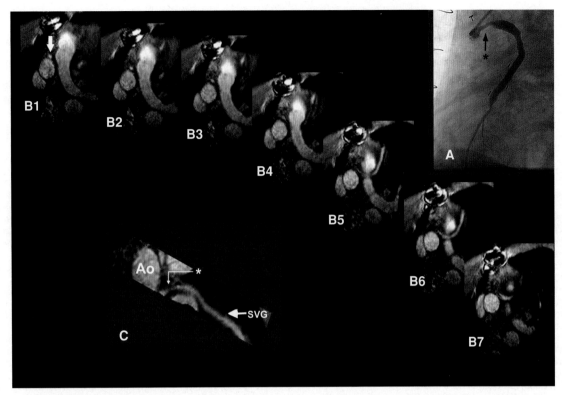

FIGURE 14-52 Saphenous vein graft—MR correlation to x-ray angiography. X-ray angiogram (XRA) of SVG to the LAD *(A)* with a 56% proximal stenosis (*). Individual slices of the MRI obtained in the oblique plane *(B1–7)*. MPR of the 3D scan demonstrating the loss of graft lumen (tapering graft contour) *(C)* corresponding to the x-ray angiographic stenosis (*). (Adapted from Langerak SE, Vliegen HW, de Roos A, et al. Detection of vein graft disease using high-resolution magnetic resonance angiography. *Circulation*. 2002;105(3):328–333, with permission.)

TABLE 14-7

Diagnostic Accuracy of Coronary Magnetic Resonance Imaging for Saphenous Vein Graft Disease

	Sensitivity (%)	Specificity (%)
Graft occlusion	83 (36%–100%)	100 (92%–100%)
Graft stenosis ≥50%	82 (57%–96%)	88 (72%–97%)
Graft stenosis ≥70%	73 (39%–94%)	80 (64%–91%)

Percentages following Sensitivity and Specificity are confidence intervals.
Adapted from Langerak SE, Vliegen HW, de Roos A, et al. Detection of vein graft disease using high-resolution magnetic resonance angiography. *Circulation*. 2002;105(3):328–333.

REFERENCES

1. Becker CR, Nikolaou K, Muders M, et al. Ex vivo coronary atherosclerotic plaque characterization with multi-detector-row CT. *Eur Radiol*. 2003;13(9): 2094–2098.
2. Rosamond W, Flegal K, Friday G, et al. Heart disease and stroke statistics—2007 update: a report from the American Heart Association Statistics Committee and Stroke Statistics Subcommittee. *Circulation*. 2007;115:e69–171.
3. Glagov S, Weisenberg E, Zarins CK, et al. Compensatory enlargement of human atherosclerotic coronary arteries. *N Engl J Med*. 1987;316(22):1371–1375.
4. Budoff MJ, Georgiou D, Brody A, et al. Ultrafast computed tomography as a diagnostic modality in the detection of coronary artery disease: a multicenter study. *Circulation*. 1996;93(5):898–904.
5. Kim WY, Danias PG, Stuber M, et al. Coronary magnetic resonance angiography for the detection of coronary stenoses. *N Engl J Med*. 2001;345(26):1863–1869.
6. Johnson LW, Lozner EC, Johnson S, et al. Coronary arteriography 1984–1987: a report of the Registry of the Society for Cardiac Angiography and Interventions. I. Results and complications. *Cathet Cardiovasc Diagn*. 1989;17(1):5–10.
7. Davidson CJ, Mark DB, Pieper KS, et al. Thrombotic and cardiovascular complications related to nonionic contrast media during cardiac catheterization: analysis of 8,517 patients. *Am J Cardiol*. 1990;65(22):1481–1484.
8. Omran H, Schmidt H, Hackenbroch M, et al. Silent and apparent cerebral embolism after retrograde catheterisation of the aortic valve in valvular stenosis: a prospective, randomised study. *Lancet*. 2003;361(9365):1241–1246.
9. Kelle S, Hug J, Kohler U, Fleck E, Nagel E. Potential intrinsic error of noninvasive coronary angiography. *J Cardiovasc Magn Reson* 2005;7:401–407.
10. Rizzo MJ, Ryan K, McLean C, et al. Distance from the ostium to the culprit coronary lesion: implications for new non-invasive coronary imaging technologies. *Circulation*. 1997;96:I-306.
11. Douglas PS, Fiolkoski J, Berko B, et al. Echocardiographic visualization of coronary artery anatomy in the adult. *J Am Coll Cardiol*. 1988;11(3):565–571.
12. Yamagishi M, Yasu T, Ohara K, et al. Detection of coronary blood flow associated with left main coronary artery stenosis by transesophageal Doppler color flow echocardiography. *J Am Coll Cardiol*. 1991;17(1):87–93.

13. Boyd DP. New horizons in cardiac imaging. Screening for coronary artery disease using ultrafast computed tomography. *Invest Radiol*. 1993;28[Suppl 3]:S148.
14. Lu B, Mao SS, Zhuang N, et al. Coronary artery motion during the cardiac cycle and optimal ECG triggering for coronary artery imaging. *Invest Radiol*. 2001;36(5):250–256.
15. Jakobs TF, Becker CR, Ohnesorge B, et al. Multislice helical CT of the heart with retrospective ECG gating: reduction of radiation exposure by ECG-controlled tube current modulation. *Eur Radiol*. 2002;12(5):1081–1086.
16. Leung KC, Martin CJ. Effective doses for coronary angiography. *Br J Radiol*. 1996;69(821):426–431.
17. Hong C, Becker CR, Huber A, et al. ECG-gated reconstructed multi-detector row CT coronary angiography: effect of varying trigger delay on image quality. *Radiology*. 2001;220(3):712–717.
18. Ryan TJ, Anderson JL, Antman EM, et al. ACC/AHA guidelines for the management of patients with acute myocardial infarction. A report of the American College of Cardiology/American Heart Association Task Force on Practice Guidelines (Committee on Management of Acute Myocardial Infarction). *J Am Coll Cardiol*. 1996;28(5):1328–1428.
19. Herzog C, Abolmaali N, Balzer JO, et al. Heart-rate-adapted image reconstruction in multidetector-row cardiac CT: influence of physiological and technical prerequisite on image quality. *Eur Radiol*. 2002;12(11):2670–2678.
20. Becker CR, Hong C, Knez A, et al. Optimal contrast application for cardiac 4-detector-row computed tomography. *Invest Radiol*. 2003;38(11):690–694.
21. Fleischmann D. Use of high-concentration contrast media in multiple-detector-row CT: principles and rationale. *Eur Radiol*. 2003;13[Suppl 5]:M14–M20.
22. Awai K, Hiraishi K, Hori S. Effect of contrast material injection duration and rate on aortic peak time and peak enhancement at dynamic CT involving injection protocol with dose tailored to patient weight. *Radiology*. 2004;230(1):142–150.
23. Hopper KD, Mosher TJ, Kasales CJ, et al. Thoracic spiral CT: delivery of contrast material pushed with injectable saline solution in a power injector. *Radiology*. 1997;205(1):269–271.
24. Haage P, Schmitz-Rode T, Hubner D, et al. Reduction of contrast material dose and artifacts by a saline flush using a double power injector in helical CT of the thorax. *AJR Am J Roentgenol*. 2000;174(4):1049–1053.
25. Hittmair K, Fleischmann D. Accuracy of predicting and controlling time-dependent aortic enhancement from a test bolus injection. *J Comput Assist Tomogr*. 2001;25(2):287–294.
26. Aspelin P, Aubry P, Fransson SG, et al. Nephrotoxic effects in high-risk patients undergoing angiography. *N Engl J Med*. 2003;348(6):491–499.
27. Bergstra A, van Dijk RB, Brekke O, et al. Hemodynamic effects of iodixanol and iohexol during ventriculography in patients with compromised left ventricular function. *Catheter Cardiovasc Interv*. 2000;50(3):314–321.
28. Vogl TJ, Abolmaali ND, Diebold T, et al. Techniques for the detection of coronary atherosclerosis: multi-detector row CT coronary angiography. *Radiology*. 2002;223(1):212–220.
29. Manghat NE, Morgan-Hughes GJ, Marshall AJ, et al. Multi-detector row computed tomography: imaging congenital coronary artery anomalies in adults. *Heart*. 2005;91(12):1515–1522.
30. Schmermund A, Rensing BJ, Sheedy PF, et al. Intravenous electron-beam computed tomographic coronary angiography for segmental analysis of coronary artery stenosis. *Am J Cardiol*. 1998;31:1547–1554.
31. Polson MJ, Barker AT, Gardiner S. The effect of rapid rise-time magnetic fields on the ECG of the rat. *Clin Phys Physiol Meas*. 1982;3(3):231–234.
32. Fischer SE, Wickline SA, Lorenz CH. Novel real-time R-wave detection algorithm based on the vectorcardiogram for accurate gated magnetic resonance acquisitions. *Magn Reson Med*. 1999;42(2):361–370.
33. Botnar RM, Stuber M, Danias PG, et al. Improved coronary artery definition with T2-weighted, free-breathing, three-dimensional coronary MRA. *Circulation*. 1999;99(24):3139–3148.
34. Wang Y, Riederer SJ, Ehman RL. Respiratory motion of the heart: kinematics and the implications for the spatial resolution in coronary imaging. *Magn Reson Med*. 1995;33(5):713–719.
35. Taylor AM, Jhooti P, Wiesmann F, et al. MR navigator-echo monitoring of temporal changes in diaphragm position: implications for MR coronary angiography. *J Magn Reson Imaging*. 1997;7(4):629–636.
36. Edelman RR, Manning WJ, Burstein D, et al. Coronary arteries: breath-hold MR angiography. *Radiology*. 1991;181(3):641–643.
37. Li D, Paschal CB, Haacke EM, et al. Coronary arteries: three-dimensional MR imaging with fat saturation and magnetization transfer contrast. *Radiology*. 1993;187(2):401–406.
38. Brittain JH, Hu BS, Wright GA, et al. Coronary angiography with magnetization-prepared T2 contrast. *Magn Reson Med*. 1995;33(5):689–696.
39. Shea SM, Deshpande VS, Chung YC, et al. Three-dimensional true-FISP imaging of the coronary arteries: improved contrast with T2-preparation. *J Magn Reson Imaging*. 2002;15(5):597–602.
40. Maintz D, Aepfelbacher FC, Kissinger KV, et al. Coronary MR angiography: comparison of quantitative and qualitative data from four techniques. *AJR Am J Roentgenol*. 2004;182(2):515–521.
41. McConnell MV, Khasgiwala VC, Savord BJ, et al. Comparison of respiratory suppression methods and navigator locations for MR coronary angiography. *AJR Am J Roentgenol*. 1997;168(5):1369–1375.
42. McConnell MV, Khasgiwala VC, Savord BJ, et al. Prospective adaptive navigator correction for breath-hold MR coronary angiography. *Magn Reson Med*. 1997;37(1):148–152.
43. Danias PG, McConnell MV, Khasgiwala VC, et al. Prospective navigator correction of image position for coronary MR angiography. *Radiology*. 1997;203(3):733–736.
44. Langerak SE, Kunz P, Vliegen HW, et al. Improved MR flow mapping in coronary artery bypass grafts during adenosine-induced stress. *Radiology*. 2001;218(2):540–547.
45. Stuber M, Botnar RM, Danias PG, et al. Double-oblique free-breathing high resolution three-dimensional coronary magnetic resonance angiography. *J Am Coll Cardiol*. 1999;34(2):524–531.
46. Langerak SE, Vliegen HW, de Roos A, et al. Detection of vein graft disease using high-resolution magnetic resonance angiography. *Circulation*. 2002;105(3):328–333.
47. Balaban RS, Ceckler TL. Magnetization transfer contrast in magnetic resonance imaging. *Magn Reson Q*. 1992;8(2):116–137.
48. Spuentrup E, Bornert P, Botnar RM, et al. Navigator-gated free-breathing three-dimensional balanced fast field echo (TrueFISP) coronary magnetic resonance angiography. *Invest Radiol*. 2002;37(11):637–642.
49. Weber OM, Martin AJ, Higgins CB. Whole-heart steady-state free precession coronary artery magnetic resonance angiography. *Magn Reson Med*. 2003;50(6):1223–1228.
50. Deshpande VS, Shea SM, Laub G, et al. 3D magnetization-prepared true-FISP: a new technique for imaging coronary arteries. *Magn Reson Med*. 2001;46(3):494–502.
51. Niendorf T, Saranathan M, Lingamneni A, et al. Short breath-hold, volumetric coronary MR angiography employing steady-state free precession in conjunction with parallel imaging. *Magn Reson Med*. 2005;53(4):885–894.
52. Stuber M, Botnar RM, Danias PG, et al. Contrast agent-enhanced, free-breathing, three-dimensional coronary magnetic resonance angiography. *J Magn Reson Imaging*. 1999;10(5):790–799.
53. Huber ME, Paetsch I, Schnackenburg B, et al. Performance of a new gadolinium-based intravascular contrast agent in free-breathing inversion-recovery 3D coronary MRA. *Magn Reson Med*. 2003;49(1):115–121.

54. Herborn CU, Barkhausen J, Paetsch I, et al. Coronary arteries: contrast-enhanced MR imaging with SH L 643A—experience in 12 volunteers. *Radiology*. 2003; 229(1):217–223.

55. Sevrukov A, Jelnin V, Kondos GT. Electron beam CT of the coronary arteries: cross-sectional anatomy for calcium scoring. *AJR Am J Roentgenol*. 2001;177(6):1437–1445.

56. Austen WG, Edwards JE, Frye RL, et al. A reporting system on patients evaluated for coronary artery disease. Report of the Ad Hoc Committee for Grading of Coronary Artery Disease, Council on Cardiovascular Surgery, American Heart Association. *Circulation*. 1975;51[Suppl 4]: 5–40.

57. Angelini P. Coronary artery anomalies—current clinical issues: definitions, classification, incidence, clinical relevance, and treatment guidelines. *Tex Heart Inst J*. 2002; 29(4):271–278.

58. Angelini P, Velasco JA, Flamm S. Coronary anomalies: incidence, pathophysiology, and clinical relevance. *Circulation*. 2002;105(20):2449–2454.

59. Pennell DJ, Keegan J, Firmin DN, et al. Magnetic resonance imaging of coronary arteries: technique and preliminary results. *Br Heart J*. 1993;70(4):315–326.

60. Manning WJ, Li W, Boyle NG, et al. Fat-suppressed breath-hold magnetic resonance coronary angiography. *Circulation*. 1993;87(1):94–104.

61. Duerinckx AJ, Urman MK. Two-dimensional coronary MR angiography: analysis of initial clinical results. *Radiology*. 1994;193(3):731–738.

62. Sakuma H, Caputo GR, Steffens JC, et al. Breath-hold MR cine angiography of coronary arteries in healthy volunteers: value of multiangle oblique imaging planes. *AJR Am J Roentgenol*. 1994;163(3):533–537.

63. Masui T, Isoda H, Mochizuki T, et al. MR angiography of the coronary arteries. *Radiat Med*. 1995;13(1):47–50.

64. Davis SF, Kannam JP, Wielopolski P, et al. Magnetic resonance coronary angiography in heart transplant recipients. *J Heart Lung Transplant*. 1996;15(6):580–586.

65. Levin DC, Fellows KE, Abrams HL. Hemodynamically significant primary anomalies of the coronary arteries. Angiographic aspects. *Circulation*. 1978;58(1):25–34.

66. Chaitman BR, Lesperance J, Saltiel J, et al. Clinical, angiographic, and hemodynamic findings in patients with anomalous origin of the coronary arteries. *Circulation*. 1976;53(1):122–131.

67. Ishikawa T, Brandt PW. Anomalous origin of the left main coronary artery from the right anterior aortic sinus: angiographic definition of anomalous course. *Am J Cardiol*. 1985; 55(6):770–776.

68. Schmitt R, Froehner S, Brunn J, et al. Congenital anomalies of the coronary arteries: imaging with contrast-enhanced, multidetector computed tomography. *Eur Radiol*. 2005; 15(6):1110–1121.

69. Ropers D, Moshage W, Daniel WG, et al. Visualization of coronary artery anomalies and their anatomic course by contrast-enhanced electron beam tomography and three-dimensional reconstruction. *Am J Cardiol*. 2001;87(2): 193–197.

70. Schmid M, Achenbach S, Ludwig J, et al. Visualization of coronary artery anomalies by contrast-enhanced multi-detector row spiral computed tomography. *Int J Cardiol*. 2006;111(3):430–435.

71. McConnell MV, Ganz P, Selwyn AP, et al. Identification of anomalous coronary arteries and their anatomic course by magnetic resonance coronary angiography. *Circulation*. 1995;92(11):3158–3162.

72. Taylor AM, Thorne SA, Rubens MB, et al. Coronary artery imaging in grown up congenital heart disease: complementary role of magnetic resonance and x-ray coronary angiography. *Circulation*. 2000;101(14):1670–1678.

73. Bunce NH, Lorenz CH, Keegan J, et al. Coronary artery anomalies: assessment with free-breathing three-dimensional coronary MR angiography. *Radiology*. 2003;227(1):201–208.

74. Post JC, van Rossum AC, Bronzwaer JG, et al. Magnetic resonance angiography of anomalous coronary arteries. A new gold standard for delineating the proximal course? *Circulation*. 1995;92(11):3163–3171.

75. Vliegen HW, Doornbos J, de Roos A, et al. Value of fast gradient echo magnetic resonance angiography as an adjunct to coronary arteriography in detecting and confirming the course of clinically significant coronary artery anomalies. *Am J Cardiol*. 1997;79(6):773–776.

76. Alegria JR, Herrmann J, Holmes DR Jr, et al. Myocardial bridging. *Eur Heart J*. 2005;26(12):1159–1168.

77. Bekkers SC, Leiner T. Images in cardiovascular medicine. Myocardial bridging. *Circulation*. 2006;113(9):e390–e391.

78. Ferreira AG Jr, Trotter SE, Konig B Jr, et al. Myocardial bridges: morphological and functional aspects. *Br Heart J*. 1991;66(5):364–367.

79. Soran O, Pamir G, Erol C, et al. The incidence and significance of myocardial bridge in a prospectively defined population of patients undergoing coronary angiography for chest pain. *Tokai J Exp Clin Med*. 2000;25(2):57–60.

80. Kosinski A, Grzybiak M. Myocardial bridges in the human heart: morphological aspects. *Folia Morphol (Warsz)*. 2001;60(1):65–68.

81. Venkateshu KV, Mysorekar VR, Sanikop MB. Myocardial bridges. *J Indian Med Assoc*. 2000;98(11):691–693.

82. Kramer JR, Kitazume H, Proudfit WL, et al. Clinical significance of isolated coronary bridges: benign and frequent condition involving the left anterior descending artery. *Am Heart J*. 1982;103(2):283–288.

83. Amplatz K, Anderson R. Angiographic appearance of myocardial bridging of the coronary artery. *Invest Radiol*. 1968;3(3):213–215.

84. Goitein O, Lacomis JM. Myocardial bridging: noninvasive diagnosis with multidetector CT. *J Comput Assist Tomogr*. 2005;29(2):238–240.

85. Rychter K, Salanitri J, Edelman RR. Multifocal coronary artery myocardial bridging involving the right coronary and left anterior descending arteries detected by ECG-gated 64 slice multidetector CT coronary angiography. *Int J Cardiovasc Imaging*. 2006;22:713–717.

86. Kantarci M, Duran C, Durur I, et al. Detection of myocardial bridging with ECG-gated MDCT and multiplanar reconstruction. *AJR Am J Roentgenol*. 2006;186[6 Suppl 2]: S391–S394.

87. Walters DL, Aroney CN, Radford DJ. Coronary stenting for a muscular bridge in a patient with hypertrophic obstructive cardiomyopathy. *Cardiol Young*. 2003;13(4): 377–379.

88. Antonellis IP, Patsilinakos SP, Pamboukas CA, et al. Intracoronary stent placement proximal to a myocardial bridge: immediate and long-term results. *Catheter Cardiovasc Interv*. 1999;46(3):363–367.

89. Stables RH, Knight CJ, McNeill JG, et al. Coronary stenting in the management of myocardial ischaemia caused by muscle bridging. *Br Heart J*. 1995;74(1):90–92.

90. Hurst RT, Askew JW, Lee R. Resolution of myocardial bridge-related wall motion abnormality and associated myocardial perfusion defect with beta-blocker therapy. *J Invasive Cardiol*. 2005;17(12):E40–E42.

91. Hongo Y, Tada H, Ito K, et al. Augmentation of vessel squeezing at coronary-myocardial bridge by nitroglycerin: study by quantitative coronary angiography and intravascular ultrasound. *Am Heart J*. 1999;138[2 Pt 1]:345–350.

92. Akagi T, Rose V, Benson LN, et al. Outcome of coronary artery aneurysms after Kawasaki disease. *J Pediatr*. 1992;121[5 Pt 1]:689–694.

93. Kato H, Ichinose E, Yoshioka F, et al. Fate of coronary aneurysms in Kawasaki disease: serial coronary angiography and long-term follow-up study. *Am J Cardiol*. 1982;49(7):1758–1766.

94. Kanamaru H, Sato Y, Takayama T, et al. Assessment of coronary artery abnormalities by multislice spiral computed tomography in adolescents and young adults with Kawasaki disease. *Am J Cardiol*. 2005;95(4):522–525.

95. Greil GF, Stuber M, Botnar RM, et al. Coronary magnetic resonance angiography in adolescents and young adults with Kawasaki disease. *Circulation.* 2002;105(8):908–911.

96. Mavrogeni S, Papadopoulos G, Douskou M, et al. Magnetic resonance angiography is equivalent to X-ray coronary angiography for the evaluation of coronary arteries in Kawasaki disease. *J Am Coll Cardiol.* 2004;43(4):649–652.

97. Mavrogeni SI, Manginas A, Papadakis E, et al. Correlation between magnetic resonance angiography (MRA) and quantitative coronary angiography (QCA) in ectatic coronary vessels. *J Cardiovasc Magn Reson.* 2004(6):17–23.

98. Gowda RM, Vasavada BC, Khan IA. Coronary artery fistulas: clinical and therapeutic considerations. *Int J Cardiol.* 2006;107(1):7–10.

99. Iadanza A, del Pasqua A, Fineschi M, et al. Three-vessel left-ventricular microfistulization syndrome: a rare case of angina. *Int J Cardiol.* 2004;96(1):109–111.

100. Garcia-Rinaldi R, Von Koch L, Howell JF. Successful repair of a right coronary artery-coronary sinus fistula with associated left coronary arteriosclerosis. *Bol Asoc Med P R.* 1977;69(5):156–159.

101. Umana E, Massey CV, Painter JA. Myocardial ischemia secondary to a large coronary-pulmonary fistula—a case report. *Angiology.* 2002;53(3):353–357.

102. Balanescu S, Sangiorgi G, Castelvecchio S, et al. Coronary artery fistulas: clinical consequences and methods of closure. A literature review. *Ital Heart J.* 2001;2(9):669–676.

103. Kamiya H, Yasuda T, Nagamine H, et al. Surgical treatment of congenital coronary artery fistulas: 27 years' experience and a review of the literature. *J Card Surg.* 2002;17(2):173–177.

104. Wang S, Wu Q, Hu S, et al. Surgical treatment of 52 patients with congenital coronary artery fistulas. *Chin Med J (Engl).* 2001;114(7):752–755.

105. Hartnell GG, Jordan SC. Balloon embolisation of a coronary arterial fistula. *Int J Cardiol.* 1990;29(3):381–383.

106. Qureshi SA, Tynan M. Catheter closure of coronary artery fistulas. *J Interv Cardiol.* 2001;14(3):299–307.

107. Alekyan BG, Podzolkov VP, Cardenas CE. Transcatheter coil embolization of coronary artery fistula. *Asian Cardiovasc Thorac Ann.* 2002;10(1):47–52.

108. Armsby LR, Keane JF, Sherwood MC, et al. Management of coronary artery fistulae. Patient selection and results of transcatheter closure. *J Am Coll Cardiol.* 2002;39(6):1026–1032.

109. Arheden H, Holmqvist C, Thilen U, et al. Left-to-right cardiac shunts: comparison of measurements obtained with MR velocity mapping and with radionuclide angiography. *Radiology.* 1999;211(2):453–458.

110. Schmid M, Achenbach S, Ludwig J, et al. Visualization of coronary artery anomalies by contrast-enhanced multidetector row spiral computed tomography. *Int J Cardiol.* 2006;111(3):430–435.

111. Datta J, White CS, Gilkeson RC, et al. Anomalous coronary arteries in adults: depiction at multi-detector row CT angiography. *Radiology.* 2005;235(3):812–818.

112. Katayama T, Yasu T, Saito M. Aneurysm of coronary-pulmonary artery fistula diagnosed non-invasively by contrast echocardiography and multi-detector computed tomography. *Heart.* 2005;91(3):e20.

113. Yoshimura N, Hamada S, Takamiya M, et al. Coronary artery anomalies with a shunt: evaluation with electron-beam CT. *J Comput Assist Tomogr.* 1998;22(5):682–686.

114. Aydogan U, Onursal E, Cantez T, et al. Giant congenital coronary artery fistula to left superior vena cava and right atrium with compression of left pulmonary vein simulating cor triatriatum—diagnostic value of magnetic resonance imaging. *Eur J Cardiothorac Surg.* 1994;8(2):97–99.

115. Sato Y, Ishikawa K, Sakurai I, et al. Magnetic resonance imaging in diagnosis of right coronary arteriovenous fistula—a case report. *Jpn Circ J.* 1997;61(12):1043–1046.

116. Sparrow P, Reid S, Sivananthan M. Magnetic resonance imaging of a coronary fistula manifesting as a pericardial effusion. *J Comput Assist Tomogr.* 2006;30(2):250–253.

117. Rathi VK, Mikolich B, Patel M, et al. Coronary artery fistula; non-invasive diagnosis by cardiovascular magnetic resonance imaging. *J Cardiovasc Magn Reson.* 2005;7(4):723–725.

118. Yoda M, Minami K, Koerfer R. Images in cardiology. Left coronal ostium to right atrium fistula causing right ventricular failure and pulmonary hypertension. *Heart.* 2006;92(3):330.

119. Pettersen MD, Ammash NM, Hagler DJ, et al. Endovascular stent implantation in a coronary artery to pulmonary artery fistula in a patient with pulmonary atresia with ventricular septal defect and severe cyanosis. *Catheter Cardiovasc Interv.* 2001;54(3):358–362.

120. Said SA, Landman GH. Coronary-pulmonary fistula: long-term follow-up in operated and non-operated patients. *Int J Cardiol.* 1990;27(2):203–210.

121. Sunder KR, Balakrishnan KG, Tharakan JA, et al. Coronary artery fistula in children and adults: a review of 25 cases with long-term observations. *Int J Cardiol.* 1997;58(1):47–53.

122. Wexler L, Brundage B, Crouse J, et al. Coronary artery calcification: pathophysiology, epidemiology, imaging methods, and clinical implications. A statement for health professionals from the American Heart Association. *Circulation.* 1996;94(5):1175–1192.

123. Achenbach S, Moselewski F, Ropers D, et al. Detection of calcified and noncalcified coronary atherosclerotic plaque by contrast-enhanced, submillimeter multidetector spiral computed tomography: a segment-based comparison with intravascular ultrasound. *Circulation.* 2004;109(1):14–17.

124. Schroeder S, Kopp A, Baumbach A, et al. Noninvasive detection and evalutation of atherosclerotic coronary plaque with multislice computed tomography. *J Am Coll Cardiol.* 2001;37:1430–1435.

125. Becker CR, Knez A, Ohnesorge B, et al. Imaging of noncalcified coronary plaques using helical CT with retrospective ECG gating. *AJR Am J Roentgenol.* 2000;175(2):423–424.

126. Kajinami K, Seki H, Takekoshi N, et al. Coronary calcification and coronary atherosclerosis: site by site comparative morphologic study of electron beam computed tomography and coronary angiography. *J Am Coll Cardiol.* 1997;29(7):1549–1556.

127. Virmani R, Kolodgie FD, Burke AP, et al. Lessons from sudden coronary death. A comprehensive morphological classification scheme for atherosclerotic lesions. *Arterioscler Thromb Vasc Biol.* 2000;20:1262–1275.

128. Achenbach S, Moshaqe W, Ropers D, et al. Value of electron-beam computed tomography for the noninvasive detection of high-grade coronary-artery stenoses and occlusions. *N Engl J Med.* 1998;339(27):1964–1971.

129. Nieman K, Cademartiri F, Lemos PA, et al. Reliable noninvasive coronary angiography with fast submillimeter multislice spiral computed tomography. *Circulation.* 2002;106(16):2051–2054.

130. Ropers D, Baum U, Pohle K, et al. Detection of coronary artery stenoses with thin-slice multi-detector row spiral computed tomography and multiplanar reconstruction. *Circulation.* 2003;107(5):664–666.

131. Nikolaou K, Sanz J, Poon M, et al. Assessment of myocardial perfusion and viability from routine contrast-enhanced 16-detector-row computed tomography of the heart: preliminary results. *Eur Radiol.* 2005;15(5):864–871.

132. Lardo AC, Cordeiro MA, Silva C, et al. Contrast-enhanced multidetector computed tomography viability imaging after myocardial infarction: characterization of myocyte death, microvascular obstruction, and chronic scar. *Circulation.* 2006;113(3):394–404.

133. Mahnken AH, Koos R, Katoh M, et al. Assessment of myocardial viability in reperfused acute myocardial infarction using 16-slice computed tomography in comparison to magnetic resonance imaging. *J Am Coll Cardiol.* 2005;45(12):2042–2047.

134. Mollet NR, Cademartiri F, van Mieghem CA, et al. High-resolution spiral computed tomography coronary

angiography in patients referred for diagnostic conventional coronary angiography. *Circulation*. 2005;112(15): 2318–2323.

135. Nakanishi T, Ito K, Imazu M, et al. Evaluation of coronary artery stenoses using electron-beam CT and multiplanar reformation. *J Comput Assist Tomogr*. 1997;21(1):121–127.

136. Pennell DJ, Bogren HG, Keegan J, et al. Assessment of coronary artery stenosis by magnetic resonance imaging. *Heart*. 1996;75(2):127–133.

137. Manning WJ, Li W, Edelman RR. A preliminary report comparing magnetic resonance coronary angiography with conventional angiography. *N Engl J Med*. 1993;328(12):828–832.

138. Post JC, van Rossum AC, Hofman MB, et al. Clinical utility of two-dimensional magnetic resonance angiography in detecting coronary artery disease. *Eur Heart J*. 1997;18(3): 426–433.

139. Nitatori T, Yokoyama K, Hachiya J, et al. Comparison of 2D coronary MR angiography with conventional angiography—difference in imaging accuracy according to the severity of stenosis. *Asian Oceanian J Radiol*. 1998;3:15–19.

140. Post JC, van Rossum AC, Hofman MB, et al. Three-dimensional respiratory-gated MR angiography of coronary arteries: comparison with conventional coronary angiography. *AJR Am J Roentgenol*. 1996;166(6):1399–1404.

141. Woodard PK, Li D, Haacke EM, et al. Detection of coronary stenoses on source and projection images using three-dimensional MR angiography with retrospective respiratory gating: preliminary experience. *AJR Am J Roentgenol*. 1998;170(4):883–888.

142. Muller MF, Fleisch M, Kroeker R, et al. Proximal coronary artery stenosis: three-dimensional MRI with fat saturation and navigator echo. *J Magn Reson Imaging*. 1997;7(4): 644–651.

143. van Geuns RJ, de Bruin HG, Rensing BJ, et al. Magnetic resonance imaging of the coronary arteries: clinical results from three dimensional evaluation of a respiratory gated technique. *Heart*. 1999;82(4):515–519.

144. Huber A, Nikolaou K, Gonschior P, et al. Navigator echo-based respiratory gating for three-dimensional MR coronary angiography: results from healthy volunteers and patients with proximal coronary artery stenoses. *AJR Am J Roentgenol*. 1999;173(1):95–101.

145. Sardanelli F, Molinari G, Zandrino F, et al. Three-dimensional, navigator-echo MR coronary angiography in detecting stenoses of the major epicardial vessels, with conventional coronary angiography as the standard of reference. *Radiology*. 2000;214(3):808–814.

146. Bunce N, Rahman S, Jhooti P, et al. The assessment of coronary artery disease by combined magnetic resonance coronary arteriography and perfusion [abstract]. *J Cardiovasc Magn Reson*. 2001;3:118(abst).

147. Moustapha AI, Pereyra M, Muthupillai R, et al. Coronary magnetic resonance angiography using a free breathing, T2 weighted, three-dimensional gradient echo sequence with navigator respiratory and ECG gating can be used to detect coronary artery disease [abstract]. *J Am Coll Cardiol*. 2001;37:380(abst).

148. Bogaert J, Kuzo R, Dymarkowski S, et al. Coronary artery imaging with real-time navigator three-dimensional turbo-field-echo MR coronary angiography: initial experience. *Radiology*. 2003;226(3):707–716.

149. Plein S, Ridgway JP, Jones TR, et al. Coronary artery disease: assessment with a comprehensive MR imaging protocol—initial results. *Radiology*. 2002;225(1):300–307.

150. Hauser TH, Yeon SB, Appelbaum E, et al. Multimodality cardiovascular magnetic resonance discrimination of ischemic vs. non-ischemic cardiomyopathy among patients with heart failure (abstr). *J Cardiovasc Magn Reson*. 2005;7:94.

151. Sakuma H, Ichikawa Y, Chino S, et al. Detection of coronary artery stenosis with whole-heart coronary magnetic resonance angiography. *J Am Coll Cardiol*. 2006;48:1946–1950.

152. Jahnke C, Paetsch I, Nehrke K, et al. Rapid and complete coronary arterial tree visualization with magnetic reso-

nance imaging: feasibility and diagnostic performance. *Eur Heart J*. 2005;26:2313–2319.

153. Cheng L, Gao Y, Guaricci AI, et al. Breath-hold 3D steady-state free precession coronary MRA compared with conventional X-ray coronary angiography. *J Magn Reson Imaging*. 2006;23(5):669–673.

154. Herborn CU, Schmidt M, Bruder O, et al. MR coronary angiography with SH L 643 A: initial experience in patients with coronary artery disease. *Radiology*. 2004;233(2): 567–573.

155. Hackenbroch M, Meyer C, Schmiedel A, et al. Coronary MRA at 3.0 Tesla compared to 1.5 Tesla: initial results in patients with suspected coronary artery disease. *J Cardiovasc Magn Reson*. 2005;7(1):6–7.

156. Paetsch I, Jahnke C, Barkhausen J, et al. Detection of coronary stenoses with contrast enhanced, three-dimensional free breathing coronary MR angiography using the gadolinium-based intravascular contrast agent gadocoletic acid (B-22956). *J Cardiovasc Magn Reson*. 2006;8(3): 509–516.

157. Goldman S, Copeland J, Moritz T, et al. Saphenous vein graft patency 1 year after coronary artery bypass surgery and effects of antiplatelet therapy. Results of a Veterans Administration Cooperative Study. *Circulation*. 1989; 80(5):1190–1197.

158. Fitzgibbon GM, Kafka HP, Leach AJ, et al. Coronary bypass graft fate and patient outcome: angiographic follow-up of 5,065 grafts related to survival and reoperation in 1,388 patients during 25 years. *J Am Coll Cardiol*. 1996;28(3): 616–626.

159. Kruger S, Mahnken AH, Sinha AM, et al. Multislice spiral computed tomography for the detection of coronary stent restenosis and patency. *Int J Cardiol*. 2003;89(2–3):167–172.

160. Mahnken AH, Buecker A, Wildberger JE, et al. Coronary artery stents in multislice computed tomography: in vitro artifact evaluation. *Invest Radiol*. 2004;39(1):27–33.

161. Storto ML, Marano R, Maddestra N, et al. Images in cardiovascular medicine. Multislice spiral computed tomography for in-stent restenosis. *Circulation*. 2002;105(16):2005.

162. Kitagawa T, Fujii T, Tomohiro Y, et al. Noninvasive assessment of coronary stents in patients by 16-slice computed tomography. *Int J Cardiol*. 2006;109(2):188–194.

163. Seifarth H, Ozgun M, Raupach R, et al. 64- versus 16-slice CT angiography for coronary artery stent assessment: in vitro experience. *Invest Radiol*. 2006;41(1):22–27.

164. Maintz D, Seifarth H, Raupach R, et al. 64-slice multidetector coronary CT angiography: in vitro evaluation of 68 different stents. *Eur Radiol*. 2006;16(4):818–826.

165. Syed MA, Carlson K, Murphy M, et al. Long-term safety of cardiac magnetic resonance imaging performed in the first few days after bare-metal stent implantation. *J Magn Reson Imaging*. 2006;24(5):1056–1061.

166. Patel MR, Albert TS, Kandzari DE, et al. Acute myocardial infarction: safety of cardiac MR imaging after percutaneous revascularization with stents. *Radiology*. 2006;240(3): 674–680.

167. Strohm O, Kivelitz D, Gross W, et al. Safety of implantable coronary stents during 1H-magnetic resonance imaging at 1.0 and 1.5 T. *J Cardiovasc Magn Reson*. 1999;1(3):239–245.

168. Kramer CM, Rogers WJ Jr, Pakstis DL. Absence of adverse outcomes after magnetic resonance imaging early after stent placement for acute myocardial infarction: a preliminary study. *J Cardiovasc Magn Reson*. 2000;2(4):257–261.

169. Gerber TC, Fasseas P, Lennon RJ, et al. Clinical safety of magnetic resonance imaging early after coronary artery stent placement. *J Am Coll Cardiol*. 2003;42(7):1295–1298.

170. Hug J, Nagel E, Bornstedt A, et al. Coronary arterial stents: safety and artifacts during MR imaging. *Radiology*. 2000;216(3):781–787.

171. Scott NA, Pettigrew RI. Absence of movement of coronary stents after placement in a magnetic resonance imaging field. *Am J Cardiol*. 1994;73(12):900–901.

172. Shellock FG, Shellock VJ. Metallic stents: evaluation of MR imaging safety. *AJR Am J Roentgenol*. 1999;173(3):543–547.

173. Sommer T, Maintz D, Schmiedel A, et al. [High field MR imaging: magnetic field interactions of aneurysm clips, coronary artery stents and iliac artery stents with a 3.0 Tesla MR system]. *Rofo*. 2004;176(5):731–738.

174. Spuentrup E, Ruebben A, Schaeffter T, et al. Magnetic resonance–guided coronary artery stent placement in a swine model. *Circulation*. 2002;105(7):874–879.

175. Maintz D, Botnar RM, Fischbach R, et al. Coronary magnetic resonance angiography for assessment of the stent lumen: a phantom study. *J Cardiovasc Magn Reson*. 2002;4(3):359–367.

176. Spuentrup E, Ruebben A, Mahnken A, et al. Artifact-free coronary MR angiography and coronary vessel wall imaging in the presence of a new metallic coronary MRI stent. *Circulation*. 2005;111(8):1019–1026.

177. Frazier AA, Qureshi F, Read KM, et al. Coronary artery bypass grafts: assessment with multidetector CT in the early and late postoperative settings. *Radiographics*. 2005;25(4):881–896.

178. Hirsch GA, Johnston PV, Conte JV Jr, et al. Mycotic aorto-coronary saphenous vein graft aneurysm presenting with unstable angina pectoris. *Ann Thorac Surg*. 2004;78(4): 1456–1458.

179. Kalimi R, Palazzo RS, Graver LM. Giant aneurysm of saphenous vein graft to coronary artery compressing the right atrium. *Ann Thorac Surg*. 1999;68(4):1433–1437.

180. Ropers D, Ulzheimer S, Wenkel E, et al. Investigation of aortocoronary artery bypass grafts by multislice spiral computed tomography with electrocardiographic-gated image reconstruction. *Am J Cardiol*. 2001;88(7):792–795.

181. Enzweiler CN, Wiese TH, Petersein J, et al. Diameter changes of occluded venous coronary artery bypass grafts in electron beam tomography: preliminary findings. *Eur J Cardiothorac Surg*. 2003;23(3):347–353.

182. Tello R, Hartnell GG, Costello P, et al. Coronary artery bypass graft flow: qualitative evaluation with cine single-detector row CT and comparison with findings at angiography. *Radiology*. 2002;224(3):913–918.

183. Khan MF, Herzog C, Landenberger K, et al. Visualisation of non-invasive coronary bypass imaging: 4-row vs. 16-row multidetector computed tomography. *Eur Radiol*. 2005;15(1):118–126.

184. Nieman K, Pattynama PM, Rensing BJ, et al. Evaluation of patients after coronary artery bypass surgery: CT angiographic assessment of grafts and coronary arteries. *Radiology*. 2003;229(3):749–756.

185. van Geuns RJ, Wielopolski PA, de Bruin HG, et al. MR coronary angiography with breath-hold targeted volumes: preliminary clinical results. *Radiology*. 2000;217(1):270–277.

186. White RD, Caputo GR, Mark AS, et al. Coronary artery bypass graft patency: noninvasive evaluation with MR imaging. *Radiology*. 1987;164(3):681–686.

187. Rubinstein RI, Askenase AD, Thickman D, et al. Magnetic resonance imaging to evaluate patency of aortocoronary bypass grafts. *Circulation*. 1987;76(4):786–791.

188. Jenkins JP, Love HG, Foster CJ, et al. Detection of coronary artery bypass graft patency as assessed by magnetic resonance imaging. *Br J Radiol*. 1988;61(721):2–4.

189. Galjee MA, van Rossum AC, Doesburg T, et al. Value of magnetic resonance imaging in assessing patency and function of coronary artery bypass grafts. An angiographically controlled study. *Circulation*. 1996;93(4):660–666.

190. White RD, Pflugfelder PW, Lipton MJ, et al. Coronary artery bypass grafts: evaluation of patency with cine MR imaging. *AJR Am J Roentgenol*. 1988;150(6):1271–1274.

191. Aurigemma GP, Reichek N, Axel L, et al. Noninvasive determination of coronary artery bypass graft patency by cine magnetic resonance imaging. *Circulation*. 1989;80(6): 1595–1602.

192. Engelmann MG, Knez A, von Smekal A, et al. Non-invasive coronary bypass imaging after multivessel revascularisation. *Int J Cardiol*. 2000;76(1):65–74.

193. Molinari G, Sardanelli F, Zandrino F, et al. Value of navigator echo magnetic resonance angiography in detecting occlusion/patency of arterial and venous, single and sequential coronary bypass grafts. *Int J Card Imaging*. 2000;16(3):149–160.

194. Bunce NH, Lorenz CH, John AS, et al. Coronary artery bypass graft patency: assessment with true ast imaging with steady-state precession versus gadolinium-enhanced MR angiography. *Radiology*. 2003;227(2):440–446.

195. Wintersperger BJ, Engelmann MG, von Smekal A, et al. Patency of coronary bypass grafts: assessment with breath-hold contrast-enhanced MR angiography—value of a non-electrocardiographically triggered technique. *Radiology*. 1998;208(2):345–351.

196. Vrachliotis TG, Bis KG, Aliabadi D, et al. Contrast-enhanced breath-hold MR angiography for evaluating patency of coronary artery bypass grafts. *AJR Am J Roentgenol*. 1997;168(4):1073–1080.

197. Langerak SE, Kunz P, Vliegen HW, et al. MR flow mapping in coronary artery bypass grafts: a validation study with Doppler flow measurements. *Radiology*. 2002;222(1): 127–135.

198. Langerak SE, Vliegen HW, Jukema JW, et al. Value of magnetic resonance imaging for the noninvasive detection of stenosis in coronary artery bypass grafts and recipient coronary arteries. *Circulation*. 2003;107(11):1502–1508.

199. Sandstede JJ, Pabst T, Beer M, et al. Three-dimensional MR coronary angiography using the navigator technique compared with conventional coronary angiography. *AJR Am J Roentgenol*. 1999;172(1):135–139.

200. Osgun M, Quante M, Kouwenhoven M, et al. Comparison of spoiled TFE and balanced TFE coronary MR angiography [abstract]. *J Cardiovasc Magn Reson*. 2004;6:268–269(abst).

Thoracic Vascular Anomalies

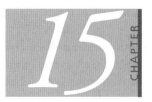

Marilyn J. Siegel
James P. Earls

Since their introduction, computed tomography (CT) and magnetic resonance imaging (MRI) have been widely used for evaluating both congenital and acquired abnormalities of the thoracic great vessels. Both imaging methods can clearly demonstrate the morphology of the aorta, systemic veins, and pulmonary vascular supply, and in many clinical scenarios, they have reduced the need for angiography. Each method has its strengths and limitations. Regardless of the imaging method used, however, the technique of performing the examination is crucial to its diagnostic performance.

This chapter highlights the use of CT and MRI for evaluating congenital anomalies of the thoracic great vessels. Various CT and MRI techniques are addressed, with an emphasis on angiography, and the rationale for choosing between CT and MRI as well as other imaging studies in different clinical situations is explained. The clinically relevant embryology and anatomy of the systemic and pulmonary vasculature and the CT and MRI appearances of important congenital anomalies involving these vessels are detailed.

METHODS FOR IMAGING THE THORACIC GREAT VESSELS

There are a number of imaging methods available for investigating a suspected mediastinal vascular anomaly, all of which have advantages and disadvantages. Recognition of the strengths and limitations of these studies is crucial in order to decide which examination is appropriate for a specific patient and clinical scenario.

For many years, chest radiography, echocardiography, and catheter angiography were the only proven diagnostic methods for evaluating disorders of the thoracic vessels. In the last two to three decades, however, CT and MRI also have been shown to be essential tools in the radiologic evaluation of the systemic and pulmonary vessels. Both cross-sectional techniques are particularly useful in establishing the diagnosis of a vascular abnormality, evaluating its full extent, and detecting the presence of associated abnormalities (1–3).

In many instances, plain chest radiography still remains the method of choice for the initial detection of a thoracic vascular anomaly, as it is simple, readily available, and inexpensive and can serve to confirm the presence and position of an arch abnormality, an anomalous vessel coursing through the pulmonary parenchyma, and abnormal pulmonary vasculature. Although such information may be helpful in planning other investigative procedures, the plain radiograph often is not diagnostic and cannot precisely characterize vascular anomalies or determine their extent.

With improvements in techniques, echocardiography is still useful for evaluating thoracic anomalies in neonates

and infants, but its use in adults is largely limited because of its small field of view and lack of an adequate acoustic window. Transesophageal echocardiography has overcome some of these deficiencies. The close proximity of the esophageal probe to cardiac and aortic structures has resulted in improved image quality in the evaluation of the aortic arch and descending aorta. However, this technique is somewhat invasive, has potential morbidity, and still has limitations in examining the distal ascending aorta and its branch vessels and the pulmonary vessels. Therefore, it has not gained widespread use as a primary diagnostic imaging tool.

Catheter angiography still remains a first-line tool for providing accurate anatomic definition of many intra- and extracardiac abnormalities, but it is not without significant risk. The results of multi-institutional studies have shown the frequency of complications associated with cardiac catheterization to be as high as 10%, with vascular access complications being the most common. The usual major complication is arrhythmia, with death occurring at a rate of 0.1% to 0.5% (4). Virtually all patients undergoing catheter angiography require sedation, and some patients require active airway support. Conventional angiography also results in exposure to both relatively high radiation doses, which is particularly problematic in young children, and relatively high volumes of contrast material. With technical improvements in noninvasive diagnostic studies such as echocardiography, CT, and MRI, the performance of conventional catheter angiography is now largely restricted to those situations where the results of noninvasive studies are equivocal or when hemodynamic assessment is needed.

The cross-sectional depiction of vascular anatomy achieved with CT and MRI has transformed the diagnostic investigation of suspected vascular pathology. These techniques are superior to echocardiography for evaluating thoracic vessels because they can provide images unobscured by overlying structures such as gas-filled lung or bone. Compared with conventional angiography, abnormalities are shown to better advantage on both CT and MRI because of the ability of these techniques to separate structures that may be superimposed on angiography. The volumetric acquisition of CT and MRI allows clear delineation of the aorta, superior vena cava, and pulmonary arteries and veins and their branches. Other advantages over conventional angiography include shorter acquisition times, superior three-dimensional (3D) renderings, and greater range of coverage, which increases the conspicuity of vascular lesions. In addition, compared with the radiation dose for angiography, the radiation dose for CT angiography is at least two to three times less.

The introduction of multidetector-row CT has been largely responsible for the increasing utilization of this technique in imaging the thoracic vessels in adults and children (1,2). The advantages of multidetector-row CT, compared with single detector CT, include improved temporal and spatial resolution, greater anatomic coverage, more consistent contrast enhancement, and higher quality reconstructions. These benefits have dramatically expanded the applications of CT in the evaluation of vascular diseases of the thorax.

CT is gaining increasing acceptance as an alternative method to MRI in the diagnosis of vascular anomalies. An important advantage of CT angiography over MR angiography relates to the shorter scan time, which means reduction in the need for sedation in the pediatric population and the ability to scan extremely ill patients who cannot tolerate the long imaging times for MR examinations. However, CT is not without certain drawbacks. One significant limitation, especially compared with MRI, is the exposure to ionizing radiation, but in the critically ill patient, the risk of a prolonged MR examination may be greater than that of radiation. Other limitations of CT are the use of intravenous contrast material, which needs to be avoided in patients with known allergies and in other patients with renal compromise, and the inability to provide functional data. In such settings, MRI is recommended.

MRI, like CT, can provide a wealth of morphologic and functional information in an accurate and noninvasive fashion without the use of ionizing radiation (3). The great vessels and pulmonary circulation can be easily evaluated, and detailed assessment of anatomy, size, and function are accurately obtained. Like elsewhere in the body, MR offers superior parenchymal imaging characteristics and is by and large able to portray more subtle differences in tissues than CT, ultrasound (US), or other noninvasive imaging tech-

niques. Images can also be acquired in any axis, optimizing the in-plane resolution for structures that may have complex orientation and geometry.

Unlike CT, there are no known permanent adverse biological effects from MRI. Transient effects of tissue heating and peripheral nerve stimulation can be easily monitored and controlled by limiting the system's radio frequency (RF) power deposition. The most commonly used MR contrast media, the gadolinium chelates, have very safe adverse event profiles and can be employed safely in patients with renal insufficiency (5).

There are many techniques available for imaging the thoracic vessels. Most studies use a combination of 2D "dark blood," cine "bright blood," and 3D contrast-enhanced MR angiography. Additional sequences are also performed as needed for functional analysis; most commonly a velocity-encoded cine PC technique is employed.

MR systems have evolved fairly rapidly in the last several years. Advances in hardware and software have increased the rate of data acquisition, reducing scan times considerably. Higher gradient strength and faster slew rates continue to push the envelope of MR techniques well beyond what was achievable just a few years ago. Many sequences have imaging times of less than 1 second per slice, and several new techniques for dynamic studies have acquisition times approaching 0.02 to 0.05 seconds (20 to 50 msec) per slice. Complete sequences covering the entire chest can now be acquired in the time allowed for a routine breath hold. Some high performance systems are now fast enough for time-resolved "4D MRA" techniques that acquire multiple dynamic 3D MR angiographic images of the thorax in a single breath hold (Fig. 15-1).

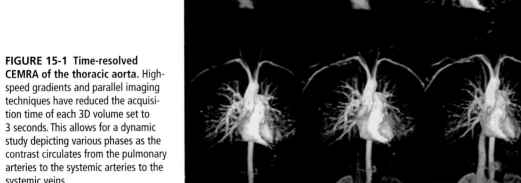

FIGURE 15-1 Time-resolved CEMRA of the thoracic aorta. High-speed gradients and parallel imaging techniques have reduced the acquisition time of each 3D volume set to 3 seconds. This allows for a dynamic study depicting various phases as the contrast circulates from the pulmonary arteries to the systemic arteries to the systemic veins.

New eight-channel and higher systems continue to increase the spatial and temporal resolution of the studies. Many older techniques such as spin echo and cine fast gradient echo (cine GRE) have been replaced by faster and more robust techniques such as dual inversion recovery T2 (DIR) and steady state free precession (SSFP). These new sequences have fewer artifacts and better imaging characteristics, and they are acquired much more rapidly than the techniques they replaced.

While very rapid comprehensive assessments of the thoracic aorta, requiring less than 4 minutes, have been reported, most thoracic MR angiographic studies currently take 20 to 30 minutes (6). These examination times, however, are short enough to decrease patient motion, which improves study quality and reduces the rate of repeat examinations, and increase patient throughput.

TECHNICAL ASPECTS OF COMPUTED TOMOGRAPHIC ANGIOGRAPHY

An understanding of the technical factors for performing CT angiography, including anatomic coverage, contrast administration, acquisition parameters, and reconstruction techniques, is essential in order to achieve consistently high-quality results. This section describes a practical approach for optimizing each of these factors.

Anatomic Coverage

One of the initial steps in performing thoracic CT angiography is to select the anatomic coverage needed to address the clinical question. At a minimum, the anatomic coverage should extend from just above the thoracic inlet so that the proximal portions of the vascular structures in the neck are included in the CT scan. Caudally, the scan should extend at least 1 to 2 cm below the diaphragm. A greater degree of coverage may be needed in some clinical settings. For instance, in the evaluation of sequestration, imaging through the upper abdomen is often necessary because the anomalous artery may rise from the upper abdominal aorta. Similarly, a greater degree of abdominal coverage is needed when assessing hemiazygous continuation of the inferior vena cava.

To ensure that all important anatomic structures are included in the CT angiogram, the study begins with a frontal topogram of the chest and upper abdomen. Nonenhanced axial scans are not routinely acquired. However, in some clinical scenarios, nonenhanced scans should be acquired. Specifically, when a bicuspid aortic valve is a diagnostic consideration, nonenhanced views can be valuable for identifying valvular calcification.

Nonenhanced scans are also useful in the evaluation of surgical shunts to assess for contrast leakage and calcification.

Contrast Medium

The goal in optimizing contrast delivery is to achieve the highest contrast enhancement with the least amount of contrast material. However, no single approach to contrast administration is effective in all patients, as there are several factors that influence the degree of contrast enhancement. These factors can be divided into three major groups: the patient, the contrast injection, and the scan factors.

Patient factors that influence contrast enhancement are the patient's body size, cardiac output, renal function, and route of vascular access. Factors related to the contrast injection include the volume and concentration of the contrast material, the type of injection technique (power injector or manual injection), and the flow rate. Factors related to scanning are the delay between the start of the contrast injection and the initiation of scanning, the method of triggering the examination (empiric, bolus tracking, or a test injection), and whether scanning should be performed during multiple phases of contrast enhancement.

Optimal vascular enhancement for thoracic CT angiography requires a fast injection of contrast medium via a power injector at a high flow rate of 3 to 4 mL per second. A contrast volume of 100 to 150 mL with concentrations of 280 to 320 mg I/mL usually results in an excellent degree of vascular opacification.

The contrast material is given through a 20- or 22-gauge antecubital vein. Because CT angiography requires high flow rates and large volumes of contrast, the iodinated contrast medium should be nonionic. The use of nonionic agents minimizes gastrointestinal side effects (nausea and vomiting), discomfort at the site of injection, patient motion during intravenous contrast administration, and complications arising from contrast extravasation (7,8).

The delay time between the start of the contrast injection and the initiation of data acquisition is one of the most important factors in optimizing contrast delivery in CT. To time image acquisition, we use real time bolus tracking (Fig. 15-2). This method monitors the attenuation value of a target vessel during the contrast injection and displays the attenuation graphically in a real time fashion. Once the desired attenuation value, usually 120 HU, is reached, the scan sequence is automatically triggered. An alternative method of initiating the CT angiogram is the use of an

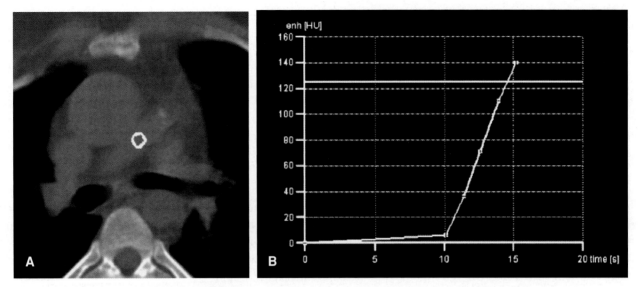

FIGURE 15-2 Automated computer technique for contrast administration. A: After an initial scout topogram is obtained, a cursor is placed within the region of interest, in this case, on the pulmonary artery. **B:** Graphic display of time (*x*-axis) and enhancement in HU (*y*-axis) after the initiation of the low-dose sampling scans. Scan initiation begins when the threshold level of 120 HU is reached.

empiric delay of 25 to 30 seconds after the start of the injection. Empiric timing is used mainly as a default method if the bolus tracking fails to trigger. A third method to time image acquisition is the use of a 15- to 20-mL test bolus of contrast material administered at a rate of 3 to 4 mL per second. After an 8- to 10-second delay, images are acquired every 2 seconds for a total of 30 seconds. A time-attenuation curve is generated, and the image with the greatest contrast density is used to select the time delay. Although a test bolus is effective, it is more time consuming than the alternative methods and has the added disadvantage of an increased radiation exposure and a slight increase in background attenuation value because of the test-bolus injection. In our experience, bolus tracking has proved most reliable for timing scan initiation.

Computed Tomographic Angiographic Acquisition Parameters

Thoracic CT angiography should be performed with a 0.5 to 1.5 collimation thickness and a fast table speed (24 to 36 mm) per rotation. The gantry rotation time should be the lowest possible to minimize the duration of the CT acquisition. CT angiography should be performed with a single breath hold.

Image Reconstruction

Reconstruction thicknesses for axial viewing are 1 to 5 mm, depending on the clinical scenario. For example, if arch positioning is of clinical interest, then images at 5-mm thickness usually suffice for diagnosis. If thrombus within a

surgical systemic-to-arterial shunt or the presence of a small anomalous vessel is of clinical concern, then 1-mm reconstructions may be more appropriate.

The reconstruction field of view should be minimized to include only the relevant anatomic structures. A standard reconstruction algorithm is used to reconstruct the enhanced data set. This algorithm minimizes noise in the data set and therefore can optimize the creation of 3D images. Images should also be viewed with a high-resolution algorithm if associated abnormalities of the airways are suspected.

Two- and Three-dimensional Rendering Techniques

Axial images are usually sufficient for diagnosis, but multiplanar or 3D reconstructions, particularly when viewed in a cine mode, provide better anatomic detail about anatomic relationships between the great vessels and adjacent soft tissue structures and the tracheobronchial tree. There are a number of 3D reconstruction techniques available to reconstruct the volume data (9–13). A detailed description of the various rendering techniques is beyond the scope of this chapter and has been described elsewhere in this book. However, a brief review of the various reconstruction techniques is presented below.

Multiplanar Reformatting

Multiplanar reformatting—the simplest reformation technique—is used to assess the extent of disease processes in the craniocaudal direction. Its advantages are that it is fast; it can be easily performed at the CT scanner; and it uses all of the attenuations in the data set, presenting them in off-axis views. The major disadvantage of this technique is that it provides only a 2D display of data; thus, it lacks depth cues. However, it does provide a quick road map of an abnormality and can be used to provide information about the nature of a disorder almost immediately after examination.

Shaded-surface Display

The shaded-surface representation displays data in a 3D format based on an assigned threshold. All structures within the threshold range are displayed, while other tissues are deleted. The principle application of the shaded-surface display is the evaluation of osseous structures of the thorax.

Variable Thickness Maximum and Minimum Intensity Projections

Small peripheral vessels and airways are often better seen as an assimilation of sections in a volume slab rather than in individual sections of equivalent thickness (12). The variable thickness technique uses thin collimation (1 mm) and low milliamperage and then combines the volumetric data in multiples or "slabs" to create a thicker image. The volume slab technique can be used with either maximum-intensity projections (MIP), which display data based on the maximum attenuation value, or minimum-intensity projections (MINIP), which display data based on the minimum attenuation value. The former has been applied to the examination of pulmonary vessels, while the latter technique can be used to enhance evaluation of the airways. The variable thickness technique does not replace volume rendering, but it can be useful in demonstrating vascular anatomy at the subsegmental level. In particular, it can be useful to demonstrate small arteriovenous malformations in the lung.

Volume Rendering

Volume rendering (VR) has largely replaced other 3D reformatting techniques in evaluating vascular pathology. Whereas the shaded-surface display and the MIP and MINIP reconstructions use only a portion of the attenuation values and their spatial relationships, VR uses the entire attenuation composition and spatial relationships in the data set. The user can interactively alter the window width and level in order to customize the display and rapidly achieve a variety of attenuation ranges. Opacity and brightness also can be altered. Both can be varied from 0% to 100%. *Opacity* refers to the degree in which struc-

tures close to the user obscure structures that are farther away. Higher opacity values produce an appearance similar to surface rendering. Lower opacity values allow a transparency view that is useful to evaluate the lumen of the airway. Brightness settings affect the appearance of the image and are largely based on the preference of the individual user. A setting of 100% usually is adequate for all applications.

Special Considerations for Pediatric Patients

Pediatric patients have several inherent problems that are not present in adults, in particular, patient motion, small body size, lack of perivisceral fat, and increased sensitivity to radiation exposure. These problems can be minimized or eliminated by the appropriate use of sedation and intravenous contrast medium, and by the selection of optimal technical factors for performing the CT examination (14–17).

Sedation

As the speed of CT increases, the need for sedation in the pediatric age group decreases (18). Although the frequency has diminished, sedation has not been eliminated. Sedation will likely still be required for some infants and children 5 years of age and younger to prevent motion artifacts during scanning. Children older than 5 years of age generally will cooperate after verbal reassurance and explanation of the procedure and will not need immobilization or sedation.

Standards of care for sedation are based on recommendations from the Committee on Drugs, the American Academy of Pediatrics (AAP), and the American Society of Anesthesiologists (ASA) Task Force (19,20). Sedation for imaging examinations is nearly always conscious sedation. Conscious sedation is defined as a minimally depressed level of consciousness that retains the patient's abilities to maintain a patent airway, independently and continuously, and respond appropriately to physical stimulation and/or verbal command.

The sedatives used most widely for CT are oral chloral hydrate and intravenous pentobarbital sodium. Oral chloral hydrate (Pharmaceutical Associates, Inc., Greenville, S.C.) is the drug of choice for children younger than 18 months. It is given in a dose of 50 to 100 mg/kg, with a maximum dosage of 2,000 mg. Onset of action is usually within 20 to 30 minutes. Intravenous pentobarbital (Nembutal, Abbot Laboratories, North Chicago, IL) is preferred in children 18 months of age and older. Intravenous pentobarbital, up to 6 mg/kg, with a maximum dose of 200 mg, is injected slowly in aliquots, starting at 2 to 3 mg/kg, and is titrated against the patient's response. Onset of action is usually within 5 to 10 minutes.

Patients who are to receive parenteral sedation should have no liquids by mouth for 3 hours and no solid foods for 6 hours prior to their examination. Patients who are not sedated but are to receive intravenous contrast medium should be NPO (nothing per mouth) for 3 hours to minimize the likelihood of nausea or vomiting with possible aspiration during a bolus injection of intravenous contrast medium.

Regardless of the choice of drug, the use of parenteral sedation requires personnel experienced in maintaining adequate cardiorespiratory support during and after the examination. Intravenous access must be continuously maintained, and continuous monitoring of vital signs must be performed and recorded.

Intravenous Contrast Medium

The performance of CT angiography administration in children requires that an intravenous line be placed. The largest-gauge cannula that can be placed is recommended. An antecubital catheter is preferred, but this is usually not possible in neonates and small infants. Ideally, intravenous access should be in place before the child arrives in the CT suite. This reduces patient agitation that otherwise would be associated with a venipuncture performed immediately prior to administration of contrast material and thus increases patient cooperation.

The contrast volume is 2 mL/kg (not to exceed 4 mL/kg) with concentrations of 280 to 300 mg I/mL (21). The use of nonionic contrast medium is now standard accepted practice. The advantages of nonionic agents over ionic agents in children are similar to those in adults and include less discomfort at the injection site, fewer side effects such as nausea and vomiting, and decreased patient motion during contrast administration.

Intravenous contrast medium can be administered with a power injector or manual (hand) injection. The benefits of power injection over manual injection are the uniformity of enhancement and the ability to determine precisely the timing of contrast delivery. A power injector is used when a 22-gauge or larger cannula can be placed in an antecubital vein. The contrast injection rate is determined by the caliber of the intravenous catheter. Suggested flow rates are 1.5 to 2.0 mL per second for a 22-gauge catheter and 3.0 mL per second for a 20-gauge catheter. The site of injection is closely monitored during the initial injection of contrast in order to minimize the risk of contrast extravasation. A power injection also can be used to administer contrast media via a central venous catheter if the rate of injection is slow (1 mL per second).

Although a power injector is preferred for the intravenous delivery of contrast material, a manual injection is used when intravenous access is via a catheter placed in the dorsum of the hand or wrist. The contrast is injected as quickly as possible. The ability to inject quickly is affected by the viscosity of the contrast material, which increases directly with high iodine concentrations. This is probably the main reason for the use of contrast with lower iodine concentrations in children. The complication rates from manual and power injections are similar (<0.4%), provided that the catheter is properly positioned and functions well (22).

Scan Delay Time

As in adults, the determination of the scan initiation time can be made by an empiric method, bolus-tracking method, or test bolus of contrast material (14–17,21). In pediatric patients weighing less than 10 kg, we use an empiric scan delay of 12 to 15 seconds after the start of the intravenous contrast injection. A bolus-tracking method can be used in very small patients, but it may not always trigger scan initiation because of the intrinsically small volumes of contrast material that can be administered.

Precontrast scans and multiphasic imaging are not routine for CT angiography in children in order to minimize the radiation dose. The exceptions are the evaluation of endoluminal stents for repair of coarctation and systemic-to-pulmonary surgical shunts. In these scenarios, calcification around the graft, which can mimic an endoleak on the contrast-enhanced scans, will be seen best on nonenhanced scans. High-attenuation thrombus also can be seen on the nonenhanced CT scans.

Breath-hold Techniques

CT examinations are performed with breath holding at suspended inspiration in cooperative patients, usually children over 5 to 6 years of age. Scans are obtained during quiet respiration in children who are unable to cooperate with breath-holding instructions and in patients who are sedated.

Radiation Dose

For CT of the thorax in children, it is critical to tailor the selection of CT parameters, including milliamperage and kilovoltage, to patient size (23–27). Additionally, multiphasic studies should be performed only when necessary, rather than being used as a routine protocol.

The tube currents recommended for thoracic CT examinations in children are shown in Table 15-1. In neonates and infants weighing less than 15 kg, the maximal suggested dose is 25 mA. This limit gradually increases until the patient reaches approximately 50 kg, when it becomes possible to use adult radiographic standards.

TABLE 15-1

Milliamperage and Kilovoltage Settings versus Patient Weight

Weight (Kg)	mA	kVP
<15	25	80
15–24	30	80
25–34	45	80
35–44	75	80
45–54	100	80–120
>54	120–140	100–120

Another factor to consider is kVp. In patients weighing less than 50 kg, 80 kVp can be successfully used. In patients who weigh 50 kg or more, the kVp should be increased to 100 or 120. The use of 80 kVp in smaller patients (compared with the standard 120 kVp protocols) decreases the radiation dose by approximately 30% with better contrast visualization (27).

TECHNICAL ASPECTS OF MAGNETIC RESONANCE ANGIOGRAPHY

MR is a flexible and accurate method for depicting cardiovascular morphology and for quantitating vascular function. Numerous techniques have been developed to depict the structure and blood flow within the heart, pulmonary arteries, and the great vessels. Both unenhanced and gadolinium-enhanced methods are available, and many examinations use a combination of approaches to obtain a comprehensive evaluation of the vasculature. Three-dimensional contrast-enhanced MR angiography (CEMRA) is a fast sequence that generates a 3D data set with high signal to images of the intravascular space following a rapid bolus of gadolinium chelate. Noncontrast-enhanced methods are generally referred to as "black blood" and "bright blood" techniques, depending on the signal intensity of the blood within the vessels.

Special Considerations for Pediatric Patients

There are several considerations that need to be addressed for pediatric patients prior to start of an MR scan. Choice of imaging coils can have significant impact on image quality. Because small children and infants require very small field-of-view to obtain adequate spatial resolution, local or phased array coils are required for the study. Infants can often be scanned within the head coil. This provides sufficient space for the child while guaranteeing satisfactory signal-to-noise ratios (SNR) for the examination. Larger children are usually imaged within the torso or cardiac coils. Use of the body coil, especially in children, should be avoided because of lower SNRs.

Sedation is still required for the majority of MR studies of infants and children 5 years of age and younger to prevent motion artifacts during scanning. Older children can usually be scanned successfully as long as there is continued verbal reassurance and explanation of the procedure. Some developmentally delayed older children may still require sedation for MR studies, and they need to be evaluated on an individual basis. Children undergoing conscious sedation should have no liquids by mouth for 3 to 6 hours and no solid foods for 6 hours prior to their study. Conscious sedation requires the presence of health care providers trained in maintaining adequate cardiorespiratory support during and after the examination. Patients' vital signs are continuously monitored and recorded throughout the procedure and through the recovery period.

Contrast-enhanced Magnetic Resonance Angiography

CEMRA is a fast, accurate, and flexible method for noninvasive imaging of the arterial and venous system. In the 10 years since its development, the method has been continually refined (28,29). Because of its great clinical utility, it migrated from academic centers into the community within a short period of time and is now the workhorse of non-neurological vascular MR imaging. In patients with complex anomalies involving the thoracic vessels, CEMRA can be useful for simultaneous evaluation of both arterial and venous anomalies as well as complications of surgical intervention (Fig. 15-3).

CEMRA is performed by acquiring a 3D gradient echo sequence following a rapid bolus of gadolinium. It is both reliable and relatively easy to perform given the automation and speed of current MR systems. Unlike iodinated contrast agents, gadolinium chelates can be used safely, even at high doses, in patients with renal failure (5). CEMRA depicts the relevant arteries and, when desired, venous structures in a 10- to 30-second acquisition, depending on the strength and other technical factors of the MR system used for the study. This can be performed during a breath hold if the patient is nonsedated and able to comply with breath-holding instructions.

For most thoracic cardiovascular applications, a 3D spoiled gradient echo (SPGR) volume that includes the heart, pulmonary arteries, thoracic aorta, and proximal great vessels is used. The parameters for the 3D SPGR sequence are optimized to attain the highest-quality images. In general, faster is better for data acquisition with 3D CEMRA, and low temporal resolution (TR) and echo time (TE) values are usually selected. Too much spin dephasing can cause signal loss at stenoses, although this can be reduced or eliminated by selection of a TE less than 3 msec. Faster data acquisitions

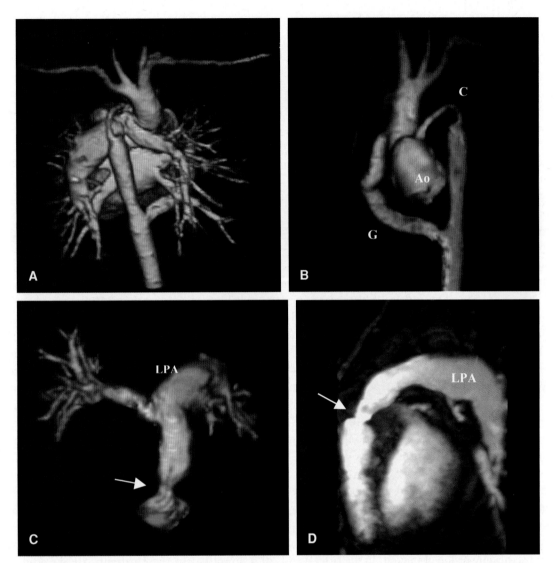

FIGURE 15-3 Complex thoracic vascular disease depicted with CEMRA in a patient with a truncus arteriosus, interrupted aortic arch, and multiple prior surgeries. A: Volume rendering of entire 3D data set depicts numerous overlapping structures. **B:** Postprocessed volume rendering of the arterial system depicts enlargement of the ascending aorta (*Ao*), a small transverse arch conduit (*C*), and a large ascending aorta to descending aorta bypass graft (*G*). **C:** Volume rendering of the pulmonary arteries depicts stenosis at the level of the pulmonary valve (*arrow*) and enlargement of the left PA (*LPA*). **D:** Sagittal MIP of the pulmonary artery confirms the proximal stenosis (*arrow*) and the dilatation of the left PA (*LPA*).

allow the gadolinium contrast material to be injected with a higher injection rate, producing a higher arterial gadolinium concentration and optimized enhancement of the relevant anatomy. The high arterial signal to noise (S/N) may then compensate for reduced T1 relaxation and signal averaging.

Fast data acquisition minimizes motion artifacts and makes it easier for patients to successfully suspend breathing for the entire data acquisition window. In addition to minimizing TR and TE, one needs to select the smallest number of sections sufficient to cover the arterial anatomy and to keep the acquisition time to a minimum. Widening

the bandwidth also makes the acquisition faster, but it may also reduce S/N, especially if a very small field-of-view is used, as required for small children and infants. The signal of background tissue is also reduced or eliminated by obtaining a 3D data set "mask" before gadolinium administration to use for digital subtraction (30).

Contrast-enhanced Magnetic Resonance Angiography in Pediatric Patients

In young children who are either sedated or are unable to perform a successful breath hold, we have altered our

CEMRA technique to help minimize artifacts associated with respiration. Rather than reduce acquisition time by using a partial Fourier technique, as done with older children and adults, we have effectively lengthened the acquisition time by sampling all of the k-space. This allows for effective signal averaging, reduces motion related artifacts, and increases the SNR. Because children have rapid circulation times, it is difficult or impossible to obtain a pure arterial phase acquisition with this approach. The veins are often enhanced to the same degree as the arteries. To generate only arterial-phase images, the veins can be removed by postprocessing techniques. Often, especially in cases of complex congenital heart disease, it is very useful to have the veins and arteries enhanced simultaneously because it helps depict the anatomical relationship between the structures.

The flip angle of the 3D sequence is optimized for T1 contrast on the basis of the repetition time and expected blood gadolinium concentration. In practice, a flip angle of 30 to 45 degrees works well in nearly all cases. The flip angle may need to be larger for higher doses of contrast material and longer repetition time or smaller for lower doses of contrast material and shorter repetition time. Zero filling in the section direction is useful because it doubles the number of sections, which is useful for image reconstruction, without increasing imaging time.

The imaging volume is prescribed to depict all of the relevant anatomy while minimizing the actual acquisition time. In almost all cases, a coronal imaging volume is used, the exception being larger children or adults in whom the thoracic aorta is the only region of interest. In the latter scenario, a sagittal imaging volume is used.

Timing of Contrast Infusion

In larger patients, correct timing coordination of the bolus injection with peak vascular enhancement during acquisition of central k-space data is essential for good quality studies. There are several ways to time contrast delivery. Each has its own advantages—the best guess method is simplest, the automated detection method is the most operator independent (31), and the timing run method is the most reliable (32). Fluoroscopic triggering, although not yet widely available, is reliable and fast for achieving optimal enhancement in every case (33–35). As MR systems become faster, 4D MRA will likely become the dominant method. This will acquire multiple complete 3D acquisitions, and the optimally enhanced acquisition will be chosen retrospectively. Although some current scanners have this capability, the resolution is limited compared with other methods.

In infants and small children, it is difficult to achieve a well-timed examination that results in a pure arterial- or venous-phase acquisition. Because the circulation time is so rapid, both the arteries and veins enhance within a short period of time following contrast infusion. Reducing the acquisition time to a point where a timed acquisition can be effective may sacrifice image resolution and reduce SNR. We have found that simultaneous initiation of contrast infusion and data acquisition result in diagnostic CEMRA studies that have adequate resolution and SNRs, although both venous and arterial structures are enhanced.

Contrast Dosage and Administration

The dose of gadolinium is an important determinant of image quality, and widely ranging doses have been advocated. Three-dimensional CEMRA studies have used doses of gadolinium ranging from 0.5 mmol/kg ("half dose") to 0.3 mmol/kg ("triple dose"). For adult patients, we routinely use 30 mL of gadolinium per patient. For most adults in the United States, this dose is equivalent to approximately 0.15 to 0.25 mmol/kg. High-dose bolus injection of gadolinium for MR angiography is still not approved by the U.S. Food and Drug Administration. However, given the preponderance of studies supporting the safety and efficacy of these doses in the literature, we feel that this dose is medically justifiable. We do not exceed a total weight-based dose of 0.3 mmol/kg for any study.

In children and infants, careful attention must be given to the volume of infused gadolinium chelate in order to not exceed the clinically accepted upper limit of 0.3 mmol/kg. In these patients, unlike adults, we use a weight-based dosing of 0.2 mmol/kg for CEMRA studies. In some small infants, only 1 or 2 mL of gadolinium may be needed. This volume is so small that it can often be preloaded into the intravenous line tubing prior to infusion, simplifying the injection process. After the gadolinium has been injected, a saline flush of approximately twice the gadolinium volume is infused to clear the line and to ensure that the patient receives the entire gadolinium dose.

Contrast may be administered either by hand or by a MR compatible power injector. For larger children or adults, a 20- or 22-gauge angiocatheter is routinely inserted in an antecubital vein prior to the start of the study. In smaller children or infants, a smaller angiocatheter can be used if needed, and this can be positioned elsewhere as long as it can handle a rapid bolus of 1 to 2 mL per second. A long extension tube is used to connect to hand-held syringes or a power injector located outside of the MR scanning room. Since CEMRA is a first-pass technique, the contrast must be infused while the patient is in the magnet, thus the need for the long extension tubing. The power injector ensures a reliable rate of contrast delivery and eliminates the need for a second technologist during the study. Contrast is usually infused as a bolus at a rate of 1 to 2 mL per second and is followed immediately by a saline flush.

Image Processing

As discussed in the CT section above, accurate interpretation of CEMRA requires interactive manipulation of the 3D data sets. It is not possible to rely solely on the source images because they are subject to partial volume effects. The reconstructed images greatly enhance diagnostic confidence. In the past, the most widely used postprocessing technique for CEMRA was maximum-intensity projection. The diagnostic accuracy of contrast-enhanced MR angiography using the MIP technique is well described and accepted clinically (36–40). In the thorax, subvolume MIPs, made from only a selected portion of the original data set, are useful to exclude nonrelevant anatomy.

Multiplanar reconstructions are useful in the evaluation of thoracic vascular anomalies. Because both MIPs and volume-rendered images are projectional images, adjacent structures may overlap and may obscure the relevant anatomy. MPRs are generated using any angle through the original data set. Orientations that depict the blood vessel(s) of interest in an optimal manner are selected interactively. This is a very practical method to accurately determine the size of a vessel or its angulation and relationship to other structures.

Volume rendering is another useful method for depicting thoracic vessels. Recent studies have shown that the VR technique has significant advantages for CEMRA (39–40). Mallouhi et al. (39) found that VR performed slightly better than MIP for quantification of renal stenoses greater than 50% and significantly better for severe stenoses. VR also had a substantial improvement in positive predictive value, and renal vascular delineation on VR images was significantly better. In another series, MIPs were statistically less reliable for determining renal artery stenoses compared with digital subtraction angiography (40).

The MIP algorithm selects only the voxel with the highest attenuation along a ray projected through the data set; volume-averaged voxels may be erroneously excluded from the final image, resulting in overestimation of stenosis. VR is based on the percentage classification technique, which is used to estimate the probability of a material being homogeneously present in a voxel (39). This provides an accurate determination of the amounts of materials when the voxel consists of two or more materials, which are volume averaged. With VR, the volume-averaged voxels are included in the final image because VR calculates a weighted sum of data from all voxels along a ray projected through the data set.

Black Blood Techniques

Spin echo (SE) was the first sequence used for evaluating cardiac and thoracic vascular morphology. The development of ECG-gating made SE technique especially useful by substantially reducing motion artifacts (41–43). Spin echo sequences generally provide good contrast between the vessel wall and blood. These are called *black blood* images because of the signal void created by flowing blood. Blood signal may appear brighter in slowly flowing areas, such as areas immediately adjacent to the vessel wall. Presaturation with radio frequency and reduction of the echo time minimizes blood signal and increases contrast on gated SE images (43). Although widely available, SE imaging has limited temporal resolution and is degraded by respiratory and other motion-related artifacts.

Shorter acquisition times are achieved with fast (or turbo) spin echo (FSE) pulse sequences, also known as rapid-acquisition relaxation enhancement (RARE) (42). Although faster, soft tissue contrast can be less than that with SE techniques because of the wide range of acquired TEs inherent in FSE technique (43). Numerous modifications to the basic FSE sequence have been made, including the use of one or more inversion pulses, increased echo train length, half-Fourier reconstruction, and echo planar techniques.

Single-shot FSE (SSFSE) sequences use a very long echo train in tandem with half-Fourier reconstruction (44). The center of k-space is acquired in a short time, minimizing motion blurring. The rapid acquisition of multiple phase lines for a single TR allows for coverage of the entire heart and thorax in the time frame of one or two breath holds. SSFSE technique has the advantage of being faster than the FSE technique in the evaluation of thoracic aortic disease (45,46). The SSFSE sequence can be modified for better cardiac results by reducing the echo train length, lowering the effective TE, and using a blood-suppressed preparation method (47,48).

T2-weighted inversion recovery imaging is now used as the front-line sequence for depiction of cardiac and thoracic vascular morphology. This technique uses a selective and a nonselective 180-degree inversion pulse followed by a long inversion time to null blood magnetization (49,50). A second selective 180-degree inversion pulse can also be applied to null fat. This is referred to as double (or triple) inversion recovery (DIR and TIR, respectively). The sequence is acquired either with breath hold or a non-breath-hold technique and provides for excellent delineation of vessel wall or myocardial blood interfaces. It effectively nulls blood and depicts blood vessel interfaces so well that the sequence has even been useful for performing coronary angiography (50).

Bright Blood Techniques

Bright blood imaging yields both morphologic and functional data. In this sequence, blood has a bright signal intensity. Multiple consecutive images are acquired and can be viewed dynamically to depict cardiac motion. Sequences include gradient echo (GRE), fast GRE, segmented k-space fast GRE, and steady state free precession (SSFP) (true FISP, FIESTA) techniques.

Gradient echo imaging is well suited for cardiac and vascular imaging because of its short echo and repetition times. Blood appears bright compared with adjacent myocardium due to time-of-flight effects as well as the relatively long T2. Markedly turbulent blood loses signal due to intravoxal dephasing, a helpful artifact for assessing areas of stenosis or valvular regurgitation (51).

A segmented k-space approach provides high-resolution dynamic images and can be performed much more rapidly than other techniques (52–54). Using short echo times (2 msec) and short TRs (<10 msec), multiple lines (segments) of k-space are acquired during each cardiac cycle. In contradistinction, in the GRE techniques, only a single line of k-space is acquired per cycle. Segmented k-space fast GRE imaging remains a mainstay for dynamic cardiac and vascular imaging and has been improved and adapted for even faster acquisition times (55–57). However, the technique is limited by the need to maintain adequate enhancement of inflowing blood. At lower TRs, now available with high-performance gradient systems, inflow enhancement of the cardiac blood pool diminishes and saturation occurs, reducing vessel wall–blood contrast. The inability to further reduce TR effectively limits achievable spatial and temporal resolution.

Steady state free precession is a state-of-the-art approach to the improvement of cine imaging (Fig. 15-4). Image contrast in SSFP depends on the T1/T2 ratio of tissue and, unlike GRE techniques, is less dependent on flow. SSFP uses the available blood signal very efficiently and accurately depicts blood, myocardium, and epicardial fat (58). First described in 1986, it was not used for cardiac or vascular applications for some years (59,60). SSFP is susceptible to magnetic field inhomogeneities and requires very short TRs, limiting its use until recently. With techni-

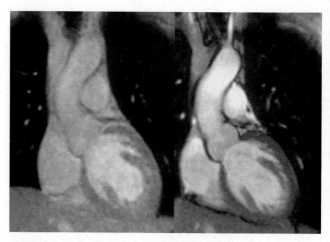

FIGURE 15-4 Steady state free precession imaging compared with fast cine GRE. The SSFP sequences result in improved contrast between the blood pool and vascular wall and myocardium (**right**). The signal-to-noise and contrast-to-noise ratios of SSFP are substantially higher than that of the conventional techniques (**left**).

cal improvements in magnetic field homogeneity and the development of higher performance gradient systems, diagnostic SSFP images can now be obtained with limited artifacts (61–64). This technique is also known as BFFE (balanced fast field echo), FIESTA (fast imaging employing steady state acquisition), FISP (fast imaging with steady precession), and trueFISP.

In the heart, SSFP sequences result in improved contrast between myocardium and ventricular cavities with clearer delineation of trabeculation and papillary muscles as compared with segmented k-space fast GRE techniques. The signal-to-noise and contrast-to-noise (C/N) ratios of SSFP are substantially higher than conventional techniques (65–67). Barkhausen et al. found that the mean C/N ratio improved by an average of 46% and 100% in short- and long-axis images, respectively, compared with the standard cine gradient echo sequences (67). The reported C/N ratios are also higher than those obtained with contrast-enhanced gradient echo techniques (68). Pereles et al. found that SSFP depicts morphologic and functional abnormalities with greater precision and provides greater diagnostic confidence than conventional techniques (66). The other advantage of SSFP is improved temporal resolution (67,69). Reduction in acquisition time by a factor of two to three at similar spatial resolutions is possible. Shorter acquisition times also can be exploited to improve spatial resolution.

Phase Contrast

Phase contrast (PC) techniques allow for depiction of blood flow and quantitative analysis of the velocity and volume of flow through a vessel (Fig. 15-5). Image data regarding the

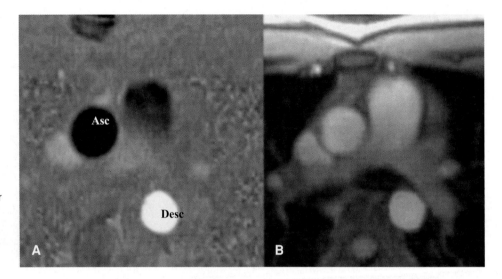

FIGURE 15-5 Phase contrast depiction of aortic flow. A: Phase image depicts blood flow in the ascending aorta away from the viewer as black (*Asc*) and blood flow toward the viewer in the descending aorta (*Desc*) as white. **B:** Magnitude image depicts aortic and pulmonary arterial morphology.

phase and magnitude of spin vectors are routinely acquired in MR imaging, but the phase data are usually discarded. PC MRI allows phase information to be saved and displayed. Pixels corresponding to spins moving across a magnetic gradient, as occurs with active blood flow, are assigned bright or dark signal intensity, while stationary spins are assigned an intermediate (grey) value.

This can be used to determine patency of vessels and can be quantitatively evaluated to determine a profile of spin velocities across a vessel lumen. Spins moving across a magnetic gradient accumulate a phase shift proportional to their velocity. Most recent MR systems can now accurately calculate the velocity profile by analyzing the phase shift in a pixel using an equation that uses the gyromagnetic ration, time interval between gradient lobes, and the area of the bipolar gradient pulse (70).

Velocity-encoded (VEC) PC techniques are used to determine flow, peak flow rates, and the volume of flow per unit time. Once the velocity profile is acquired, the area of the vessel lumen of interest is measured, and the volume of blood moving through a vessel is quantitatively determined. ECG-gated velocity-encoded PC is used to calculate cardiac output. A region of interest placed on the ascending aorta can be used to accurately calculate the volume of blood flow per minute. A similar region of interest placed on the pulmonary artery can be used to calculate pulmonary blood flow, which generally is equal to that determined in the aorta. If there is an intra- or extracardiac shunt present, the ratio of pulmonary to systemic flow can be calculated. Peak flow rates across an area of stenosis can also be used to determine the pressure gradient. Using a modified Bernoulli equation, the pressure gradient, in millimeters of mercury (mmHg) across

a stenosis is calculated as the product of the cube of the peak velocity as measured in meters per second.

VEC PC imaging is a valuable technique for quantitative assessment of flow dynamics in congenital heart disease. Clinical applications include the measurement of collateral flow and pressure gradients in coarctation of the aorta (Fig. 15-6), differentiation of blood flow in the left and right pulmonary arteries, quantification of shunts, and evaluation of valvular regurgitation and stenosis. After surgical conduit placement, VEC PC is used to monitor blood flow, restenosis, and flow dynamics. With VEC PC imaging, there are some potential pitfalls such as potential underestimation of velocity and flow, aliasing, inadequate depiction of very small vessels, and possible errors in pressure gradient measurements (71). Nevertheless, VEC MR imaging is a valuable tool for preoperative planning and postoperative monitoring in patients with coronary heart disease (CHD).

Parallel Imaging Techniques

A new method of spatial encoding referred to as *parallel imaging* is helpful for MR of the thoracic vessels (72,73). This type of imaging uses arrays of radio frequency detector coils to acquire multiple data points simultaneously rather than sequentially, as has been traditionally performed. This results in faster imaging speeds that can be used to increase either temporal or spatial resolution.

An R factor (parallel factor) is used to describe the order of factor used. For a given R factor, data acquisition time is reduced to approximately 1/R if the imaging matrix is unchanged. A factor of two is currently the most widely available factor, although higher factors are now being utilized by some centers. At a factor of two, a typical acquisition time

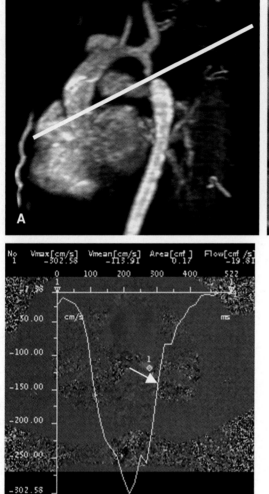

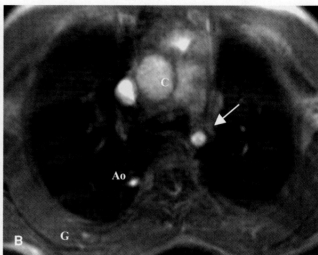

FIGURE 15-6 Velocity-encoded phase contrast determination of pressure gradient in a child with coarctation. A: Oblique 2D PC image is positioned orthogonal to the region of maximal narrowing as depicted on the CEMRA study. **B:** Magnitude image from the PC data depicts a small descending aorta (*arrow*). **C:** Graphic depiction of aortic velocities superimposed on the phase image captures peak systolic velocity of 306 cm per second, equal to a gradient of 36 mmHg.

will be reduced by 50%. Alternatively, image resolution could be doubled, by acquiring more phase lines or thinner partitions, without changing the study acquisition time.

In the thorax, the scan times of many sequences can be reduced by a factor of two or four given the current technology, and larger reductions in scan time will likely be possible in the future. The increased speed associated with parallel imaging does not come without a price. The SNR of parallel imaging is always reduced compared with the SNR ratio of other sequences obtained using the same coil array. The SNR of accelerated studies is lower by approximately 20% at a parallel factor of two and is further reduced by the square root of the parallel factor at greater levels.

EMBRYOLOGIC DEVELOPMENT OF THE THORACIC GREAT VESSELS

Knowledge of the embryology of the thoracic great vessels is helpful in understanding the variations in the number, size,

and position of the thoracic great vessels. Therefore, the embryology of the mediastinal great vessels is reviewed briefly. For more detail, the reader is referred to general texts of embryology (74,75).

Arterial System

The normal left aortic arch and its branches develop from paired pharyngeal arches, which are bilateral bars of mesoderm, separated by ectodermal clefts. The pharyngeal arches form during the fourth and fifth weeks of development and undergo a process of orderly regression. Each arch has its own cranial nerve as well as its own artery. These arteries are known as aortic arches and arise from the aortic sac, which is the most distal part of the truncus arteriosus. There are five aortic arches in the human embryo, numbered craniocaudally as I, II, III, IV, and VI. Arch V either never forms or forms incompletely and then regresses. The aortic arches course dorsally from the aortic sac to terminate in the right and left dorsal aortas. The ventral portion of the

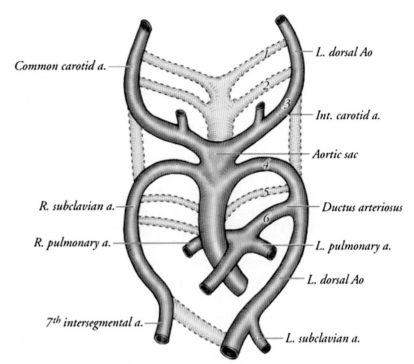

FIGURE 15-7 Diagram of primitive arch. At 6 weeks of intrauterine life, the first and second pairs of arches have virtually disappeared (*dotted lines*). The third arch forms the common carotid arteries. The fourth pair of arches forms different structures. The right fourth arch becomes the proximal part of the right subclavian artery, and the left arch becomes part of the normal aortic arch. The distal part of the right subclavian develops from the seventh intersegmental artery. The left subclavian forms from the left seventh intersegmental artery. The fifth arch never forms or involutes early. The sixth pair of arches forms the pulmonary arteries bilaterally. The left sixth arch also gives rise to the ductus arteriosus.

aortic sac develops into the truncus arteriosus, which is divided by the aorticopulmonary septum into the proximal aortic root and the main pulmonary artery.

By the sixth week of intrauterine life, most of the first and second aortic arches have atrophied, except for small portions that persist to form the maxillary artery and stapedial arteries, respectively. The third, fourth, and sixth arches remain and develop into the great arteries (Figs. 15-7, 15-8).

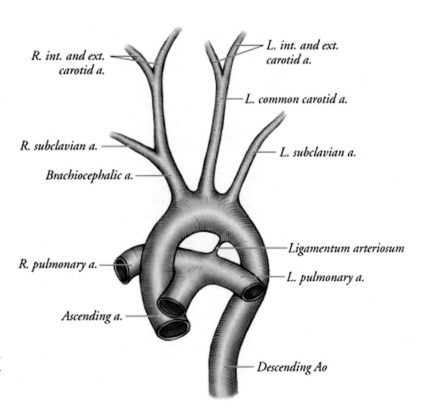

FIGURE 15-8 Normal adult aortic arch. The right subclavian and carotid arteries join to form the right brachiocephalic artery. The left subclavian and carotid arteries arise separately from the aorta.

The third aortic arch forms the common carotid arteries and the first part of the internal carotid arteries. The fourth aortic arches form asymmetric structures. The right fourth arch forms the most proximal segment of the right subclavian artery. The distal part of the subclavian artery forms from a portion of the right dorsal aorta and the seventh intersegmental artery. The left fourth arch forms the portion of the aortic arch between the left common carotid and the left subclavian arteries. The sixth aortic arches also develop asymmetrically. The right arch forms the right pulmonary artery, and the left arch forms the left pulmonary artery and the ductus arteriosus.

In the fifth week of intrauterine life, the right dorsal aorta disappears between the origin of the seventh intersegmental artery and the junction with the left dorsal aorta. The two aortas fuse caudally below T4 to form a single aorta in the distal thorax and abdomen.

Regression of a segment of arch that should have persisted or persistence of a segment of arch that should have regressed explains the development of most arch anomalies (74–76). These anomalies include left aortic arch with aberrant left subclavian artery, double aortic arch, right aortic arch with mirror image branching, right aortic arch with aberrant left subclavian artery, and cervical aortic arch. Aortic arch anomalies are of clinical importance when they produce symptoms.

Venous System

The three major venous systems of the thorax—cardinal, subcardinal, and supracardinal veins—develop during the early embryonic period (Figs. 15-9, 15-10). The cardinal veins form the main venous drainage system of the embryo. This system consists of the anterior cardinal veins, which drain the cephalic part of the embryo, and the posterior cardinal veins, which drain the remaining part of the fetal body. The intersegmental veins drain into the anterior and posterior cardinal veins. Through anastomoses, the cardinal venous system becomes the superior vena cava and brachiocephalic, subclavian, internal jugular, and superior intercostal veins.

The subcardinal system is a paired longitudinal venous plexus located in the developing fetal abdomen. This network mainly drains the kidneys and gonads in the urogenital ridge. Numerous ventrodorsal anastomoses unite the subcardinal with the supracardinal venous system.

The supracardinal veins lie lateral to the dorsal aorta and drain the body wall via the intercostal veins. By the sixth intrauterine week, they take over the functions of the posterior cardinal veins. The supracardinal veins are the origin of the adult azygos venous system. The fourth to 11th right intercostal veins empty into the right supracardinal vein, which, together with a portion of the posterior cardinal vein, forms the azygos vein. On the left side, the fourth to seventh intercostal veins enter into the left supracardinal vein, and

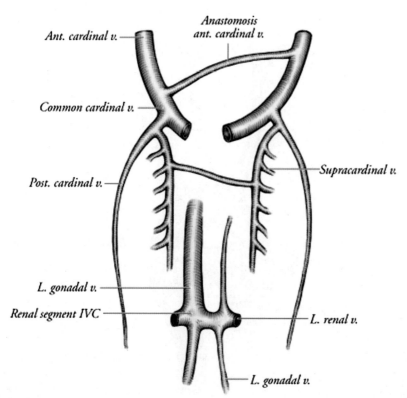

FIGURE 15-9 Development of the venous system. The cardinal and supracardinal veins form the main venous drainage system for the thorax.

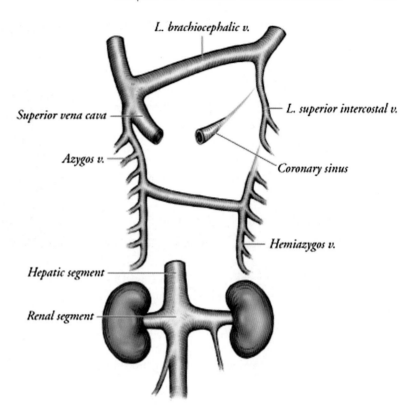

FIGURE 15-10 Normal adult venous drainage. The cardinal system has become the superior vena cava, its main tributaries, and the superior intercostal veins. The supracardinal veins form the azygous and hemiazygous systems.

the left supracardinal vein empties into the azygos vein and is then known as the hemiazygous vein.

Variations in venous anatomy are the result of regression of a channel that should have persisted or persistence of a channel that should have regressed. The common deviations from the normal developmental pattern are the left superior vena cava, which is caused by persistence of the left anterior cardinal vein and obliteration of the common cardinal and proximal part of the right anterior cardinal vein, and the absence of the inferior vena cava, which occurs when the right subcardinal vein fails to establish a connection with the liver and shunts its blood directly into the right supracardinal vein (75).

Fetal and Postnatal Circulation

In utero, blood from the placenta, which is 80% to 85% saturated with oxygen, returns to the fetus via the umbilical vein. Most of this blood flows into the ductus venosus and then into the inferior vena cava. In the inferior vena cava, the saturated placental blood mixes with deoxygenated blood (30% saturated) returning from the lower limbs. The mixed blood (70% saturated) from the inferior vena cava enters the right atrium, where it passes through the oval foramen into the left atrium. In the left atrium, it mixes with the pulmonary venous flow.

From the left atrium, the blood enters the left ventricle. Blood from the left ventricle (65% saturated) enters the aortic arch and supplies the head and neck. The desaturated venous blood from the head is drained by the superior vena cava. From the superior vena cava, it flows by way of the right ventricle into the pulmonary trunk. Since pulmonary vascular resistance is high during fetal life, the main portion of this blood passes directly through the ductus arteriosus into the descending aorta, where it mixes with blood from the proximal aorta, before being distributed to the trunk, lower extremities, and placenta.

At birth, there is the cessation of placental blood flow and the beginning of respiration, which results in closure of the ductus arteriosus by contraction of its muscular wall. As a result, blood in the ductus arteriosus no longer flows into the aortic arch. However, a small left-to-right shunt is not unusual during the first few days after birth. Complete anatomical closure by intimal proliferation occurs after 1 to 3 months, resulting in the ligamentum arteriosum (74,75). The return of oxygenated blood from the lungs also increases pressure in the left atrium, which, combined with a decrease in pressure in the right atrium, closes the foramen ovale. Fibrous union occurs in several months, although in approximately 30% of individuals anatomical closure may never be obtained, resulting in a patent foramen ovale.

NORMAL MEDIASTINAL VASCULAR ANATOMY

Knowledge of the CT and MR appearances of the thoracic great vessels allows discovery of previously unsuspected vascular anomalies on studies performed for other reasons. Familiarity with the position and shape of the normal systemic and pulmonary vessels and their many anatomic variations also is important so as not to mistake them for masses or other abnormalities (77). Therefore, a discussion of normal vascular anatomy, including anatomic variations, is offered below.

Systemic Mediastinal Arteries and Veins

At the level of the sternal notch, there are usually six vascular structures, the left and right carotid and subclavian arteries and the bilateral brachiocephalic veins (Fig. 15-11). At a more caudal level, the right subclavian and right common carotid arteries join, such that there are usually five vessels at the level of the sternoclavicular joint: the right brachiocephalic artery, the left common carotid and left subclavian arteries, and the right and left brachiocephalic (innominate) veins (Fig. 15-12).

The right brachiocephalic artery, which is the largest of the arch vessels, lies anterior or just to the right of the trachea. The left common carotid and the subclavian arteries course just to the left of the trachea. The left subclavian artery may also contact the mediastinal pleural reflection of the left upper lobe and may indent it in a convex fashion.

The right and left brachiocephalic veins are located anterior to the arch vessels (Figure 15-13). The right bra-

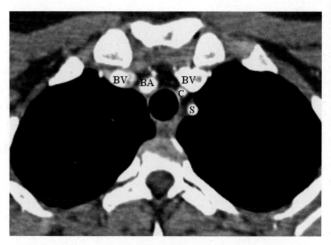

FIGURE 15-12 Normal anatomy; level of sternoclavicular joint. Five major vessels are noted around the trachea: the brachiocephalic artery (*BA*), left carotid artery (*C*), left subclavian artery (*S*), and right and left brachiocephalic veins (*BV*).

chiocephalic vein has a nearly vertical course throughout its length and thus is seen in cross section on axial images. It usually lies anterior and to the right of the trachea. The left brachiocephalic vein usually has a horizontal course. It crosses the anterior mediastinum from left to right to join the right brachiocephalic vein.

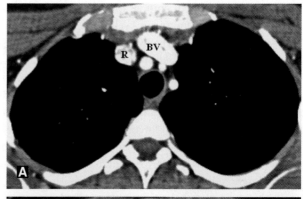

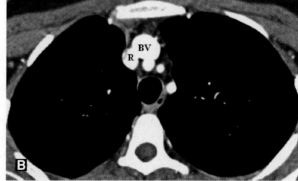

FIGURE 15-13 Brachiocephalic veins. A, B: Two transverse CT scans show the left brachiocephalic vein (*BV*) crossing the anterior mediastinum from left to right to join the right brachiocephalic vein (*R*).

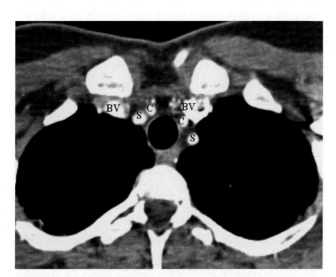

FIGURE 15-11 Normal anatomy, sternal notch. Six vessels are noted at this level. The left jugular and carotid arteries are noted along with both brachiocephalic veins. (*C*, carotid arteries; *S*, subclavian arteries; *BV*, brachiocephalic veins.)

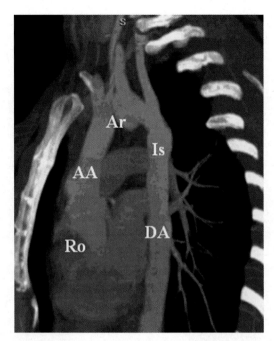

FIGURE 15-14 Thoracic aorta. Sagittal MIP shows the five aortic segments: the aortic root (*Ro*), ascending aorta (*AA*), aortic arch (*Ar*), aortic isthmus (*Is*), and descending aorta (*DA*).

None of the major systemic vessels is normally located posterior to the trachea. Except for the esophagus, any other extra soft-tissue structure in the superior mediastinum behind the trachea likely represents an aberrant vessel, lymph node, or mass.

Thoracic Aorta

The thoracic aorta can be divided into five segments: the aortic root, ascending aorta, proximal aortic arch, posterior aortic arch, and descending thoracic aorta (Fig. 15-14).

The aortic root is the short segment that arises from the base of the heart and contains the aortic valve and annulus. The ascending aorta begins at the aortic root and extends to the origin of the right brachiocephalic artery. The aortic arch extends from the origin of the right brachiocephalic artery to the attachment of the ligamentum arteriosum. This is divided into two segments: the proximal arch extending between the right brachiocephalic artery and the origin of the left subclavian artery, and the posterior arch or isthmus extending from the left subclavian artery to the ligamentum arteriosum. The descending thoracic aorta begins below the ligamentum and extends to the aortic hiatus in the diaphragm.

Anatomic Variations

Common anatomic variants that are of no clinical significance include the aortic spindle, ductus diverticulum, and pseudocoarctation (78,79). All three variations are found in

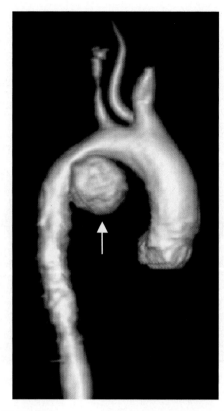

FIGURE 15-15 Ductus aneurysm depicted by CEMRA in a 67-year-old. Large focal aneurysm (*arrow*) arises from the underside of the distal arch and proximal descending aorta.

the posterior arch. The aortic spindle is a small, circumferential outpouching, whereas the ductus diverticulum appears as a focal convex bulge with smooth, obtuse margins along the ventral surface of the posterior aortic arch (Fig. 15-15).

Pseudocoarctation appears as a buckle in the arch at the insertion of the site of the ligamentum arteriosum (Fig. 15-16). This anomaly is usually found in elderly patients with an elongated, redundant aortic arch. Luminal obstruction is absent. The blood pressures in the upper and lower extremities are nearly always similar, although minor differences have been reported. There is no collateral circulation.

Superior Vena Cava

The superior vena cava lies anterior and to the right of the trachea, separated from it by the pretracheal space. On transaxial images, the superior vena cava has an oval, round, or elliptical configuration. Its diameter is usually one third to two thirds the diameter of the ascending aorta (77).

Azygous and Hemiazygous Veins

The azygous and hemiazygous veins represent continuations of the right and left ascending lumbar veins, respectively.

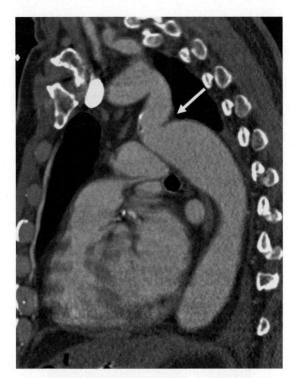

FIGURE 15-16 Aortic pseudocoarctation. The proximal descending aorta just distal to the arch is elongated and kinked (*arrow*).

The azygous vein courses through the aortic hiatus into the thorax, where it then ascends in the right prevertebral area. It lies to the right of the descending aorta and just posterolateral to the esophagus. At the level of the T5 or T6 vertebra, the azygous vein passes over the mainstem bronchus to drain into the posterior aspect of the superior vena cava (Fig. 15-17). Just before the formation of the azygous arch, the azygous vein is joined by the right superior intercostal vein. The right superior intercostal vein receives drainage from the right second through fourth intercostal veins, descending along the right anterolateral edge of the vertebra before draining into the azygous vein posteriorly.

The hemiazygous and accessory hemiazygous veins, which are left-sided structures, also course along the vertebral bodies. After penetrating the diaphragm, they course in a more posterior plane, usually just behind the descending aorta. The hemiazygous vein usually crosses the midline anterior to the vertebra, passing posterior to the aorta to join the azygous vein at about the T8 level. The accessory hemiazygous vein crosses the midline to join the azygous vein one or two vertebral body levels higher. The accessory hemiazygous vein, which collects flow from the left fourth through eighth posterior intercostal veins, may or may not communicate with the hemiazygous vein.

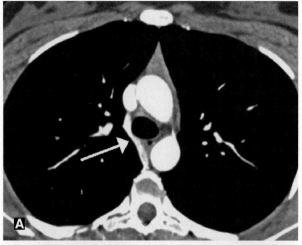

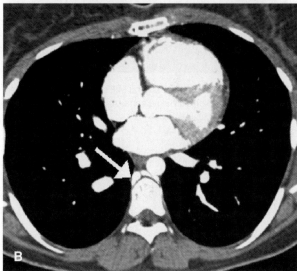

FIGURE 15-17 Azygous vein. A: The azygous vein (*arrow*) is seen emptying into the superior vena cava. **B:** At a lower level, the vein (*arrow*) lies lateral to the aorta. It joins with the hemiazygous vein.

At or just above the level of the aortic arch, the accessory hemiazygous vein may communicate with the left superior intercostal vein. The left superior intercostal vein, which drains the left second to fourth intercostal veins, then forms a horizontal arch (also referred to as the *arch of the hemiazygous vein*) that courses anteriorly along the superolateral border of the aortic arch to join the posterior aspect of the left brachiocephalic vein (Fig. 15-18). This produces the "aortic nipple" on frontal chest radiographs.

Pulmonary Arteries

The main pulmonary artery lies entirely within the pericardium. It divides into the right and left pulmonary arteries behind and to the left of the ascending aorta (Fig. 15-19). The normal diameter of the main pulmonary artery usually is about two thirds that of the ascending aorta and should not exceed 28 mm (77). The

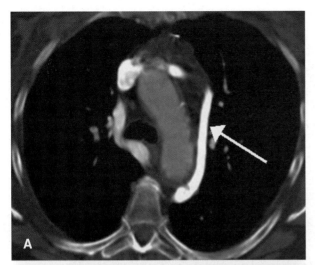

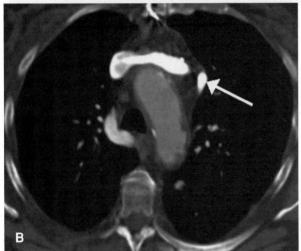

FIGURE 15-18 Left superior intercostal vein. A: The superior intercostal vein (*arrow*) is seen coursing lateral to the aorta. **B:** At a higher level, the vein (*arrow*) drains into the brachiocephalic vein.

right pulmonary artery extends posteriorly and to the right from the main pulmonary artery, coursing posterior to the superior vena cava and anterior to the right main and intermediate bronchus. The intrapericardial portion of the right pulmonary artery normally measures 12 to 15 mm in diameter. The left pulmonary artery extends posteriorly from the main pulmonary artery and courses in a transverse plane. It lies 1 to 2 cm above the right pulmonary artery at about the level of the carina. The left pulmonary artery normally measures 18 to 24 mm in diameter and has a shorter intrapericardial course than the right pulmonary artery (77).

Pulmonary Veins

Four pulmonary veins (two superior and two inferior) with four independent ostia are found in about 70% of the general population (80,81) (Fig. 15-20). The superior pul-

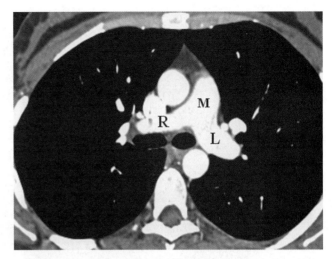

FIGURE 15-19 Normal pulmonary arteries. After arising from the main pulmonary artery (*M*), the right pulmonary artery (*R*) extends posteriorly and to the right, coursing behind the superior vena cava. The left pulmonary artery (*L*) extends posteriorly and to the left of the main pulmonary artery.

monary veins course inferiorly and lie anterior to their accompanying pulmonary arteries. The inferior pulmonary veins course superiorly and are located below their accompanying bronchi. Each vein receives three to five major venous tributaries from the lungs.

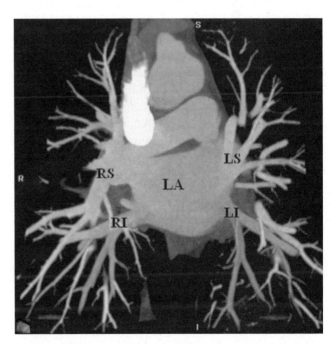

FIGURE 15-20 Normal pulmonary veins. 3D display of the left atrium and pulmonary veins in the posterior projection from an electrocardiogram-gated multidetector CT study shows the four pulmonary veins draining into the left atrium. (LA, left atrium; RS, right superior pulmonary vein; RI, right inferior pulmonary vein; LS, left superior pulmonary artery; LI, left inferior pulmonary artery.)

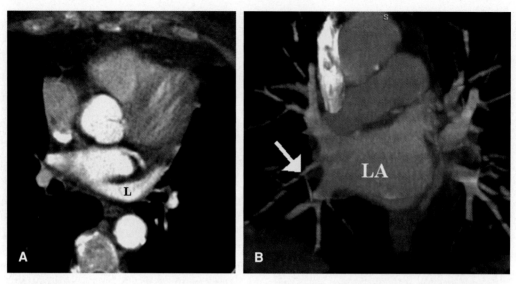

FIGURE 15-21 Pulmonary veins, normal anatomic variations. A: Left common pulmonary vein (*L*) formed by the confluence of the two inferior pulmonary veins. **B:** Accessory right middle lobe pulmonary vein draining independently into the left atrium (*LA*).

Anatomic Variations

There are two common types of anatomic variations: conjoined veins and accessory veins (Fig. 15-21). A conjoined or common vein occurs when two veins form a common trunk before draining into the left atrium. The confluence may involve both superior veins, both inferior veins, or the superior and inferior pulmonary veins on one side. The latter variant is the most common, occurring in 12% to 15% of the general population (80). Conjoined veins occur more commonly on the left side (81). They are usually widened at their site of insertion into the atrium.

Accessory or supernumerary veins are extra veins with atrial insertions that are separate from the superior and inferior pulmonary veins. Accessory drainage is more often right-sided than left-sided, with separate drainage of the right middle lobe into the left atrium being most common. However, accessory lingular veins have been described. Accessory veins usually narrow at their site of insertion into the left atrium (81). The right middle lobe and lingular veins also may have anomalous drainage into the superior or inferior pulmonary veins.

THORACIC AORTIC ANOMALIES

Persistence of a segment of arch that should have regressed or regression of a segment that should have normally persisted explains the development of most arch anomalies. Congenital anomalies of the aorta and its branch vessels are found in 0.5% to 3% of the population (82). The common anomalies are the left arch with aberrant right subclavian artery,

right aortic arch with aberrant left subclavian artery, right aortic arch with mirror image branching, double aortic arch, cervical aortic arch, coarctation, and interrupted aortic arch (82,83).

CT and MR have been shown to be reliable in the detection of aortic arch anomalies. Axial images can usually establish the diagnosis of a vascular anomaly, but 3D reconstructions are of value in demonstrating the precise anatomy of the malformation and the associated tracheobronchial anomalies, which is critical information for treatment planning (84,85).

Left Arch With Aberrant Right Subclavian Artery

The left aortic arch with an aberrant right subclavian artery is the most common congenital abnormality of the aortic arch vessels and occurs in about 0.5% to 2% of the general population (83). The right subclavian artery is the last of the major arteries to arise from the aortic arch, and so the order of arterial branching is the following: right common carotid, left common carotid, left subclavian, and aberrant right subclavian (Figs. 15-22, 15-23). The anomalous subclavian artery courses cephalad from left to right crossing the mediastinum obliquely behind the trachea and esophagus to reach the right arm. Often, there is dilatation of the origin of the aberrant vessel, termed a *diverticulum of Kommerell*. Atherosclerotic changes and intramural thrombus formation can occur within this diverticulum (83).

This type of anomaly is usually asymptomatic and is found incidentally on imaging examinations. However,

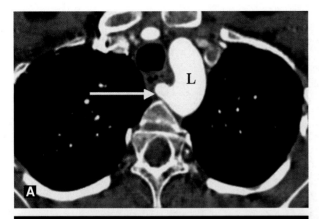

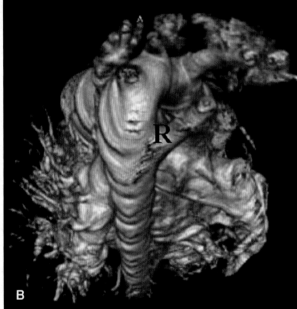

FIGURE 15-22 Left aortic arch with an aberrant right subclavian artery. A: Axial CT image shows left aortic arch (*L*) and an aberrant right subclavian artery (*white arrow*) coursing posterior to the esophagus and trachea. **B:** Posterior view of a 3D volume rendered image depicts the origin of the aberrant right subclavian artery (R) arising from the posterior arch.

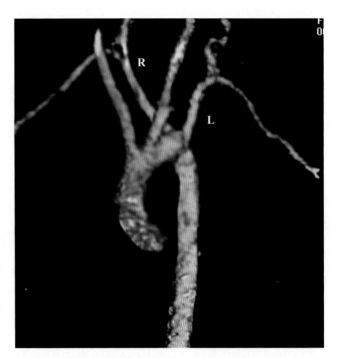

FIGURE 15-23 Left arch with aberrant left (L) and right (R) subclavian arteries. CEMRA in a 3-month-old infant depicts both the left and right subclavian arteries originating from the posterior arch.

when the aberrant subclavian artery becomes tortuous or ectatic, usually in the elderly population, it can compress the esophagus, resulting in dysphagia (dysphagia lusoria) (83). Symptoms of dysphagia and dyspnea also may develop if there is a right rather than a left ligamentum arteriosum, resulting in a vascular ring encircling the esophagus and trachea. In the latter instance, the vascular ring is formed by the anomalous subclavian artery, right ligamentum arteriosum, left aortic arch, and main pulmonary arteries.

Right Aortic Arch Anomalies

A right aortic arch occurs in approximately 0.05% to 0.2% of the population (83,86,87). There are two main types of right arch: the right arch with aberrant left subclavian artery

and the right arch with mirror image branching. The former is more commonly seen in adults; the latter is more often seen in children.

Right Arch With Aberrant Subclavian Artery

In a right aortic arch anomaly with an aberrant left subclavian artery, the great arteries originate from the arch in the following order: left common carotid artery, right common carotid artery, right subclavian artery, and left subclavian artery (Figs. 15-24, 15-25). The aberrant subclavian artery often arises from an associated diverticulum of Kommerell, representing the distal remnant of the left arch. The descending aorta is more commonly right-sided (82).

Patients are symptomatic when there is a left ligamentum arteriosum (Fig. 15-26). If the ligamentum arteriosum is on the left, a vascular ring is formed by the right arch, left subclavian artery, and ligamentum arteriosum, which attaches to the left pulmonary artery. If the ligamentum arteriosum is on the right, there is no vascular ring. Approximately 10% of patients have associated heart disease (82).

Right Arch With Mirror Imaging

In the right arch with mirror image branching, the great arteries originate from the right arch in the following order: left innominate artery, right carotid artery, and right subclavian

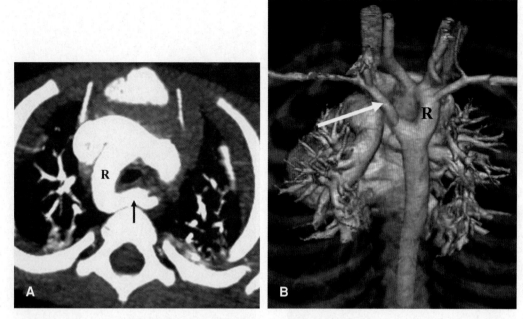

FIGURE 15-24 Right aortic arch with aberrant left subclavian artery. A: Axial CT image demonstrates right aortic arch (*R*) with aberrant left subclavian artery (*arrow*) crossing the mediastinum posterior to the trachea. **B:** 3D coronal reconstruction showing the right arch (*R*) and an aberrant left subclavian vessel (*arrow*), which is the last vessel arising from the arch.

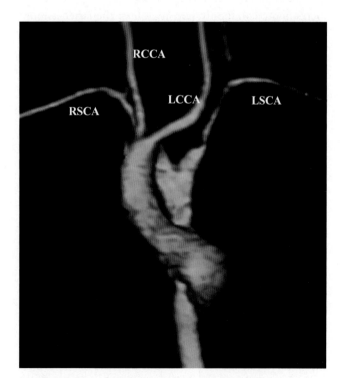

FIGURE 15-25 Right aortic arch with aberrant left subclavian artery depicted on CEMRA. The great arteries originate from the arch in the following order: left common carotid artery (*LCCA*), right common carotid artery (*RCCA*), right subclavian artery (*RSCA*), and left subclavian (*LSCA*). The latter artery arises from a diverticulum of Kommerell.

artery (Fig. 15-27). The descending aorta usually descends on the right. This is not a true vascular ring because there is no structure posterior to the trachea.

Most patients with this anomaly come to clinical attention because of associated heart disease, which is usually cyanotic. The common heart anomalies associated with a mirror image right arch are tetralogy of Fallot, truncus arteriosus, pulmonary artery atresia with ventricular septal defect, tricuspid atresia, double outlet right ventricle, and transposition of the great arteries (82). Because of the concomitant heart disease, the right arch with mirror image branching usually is discovered in infancy. The diagnosis of right arch with mirror image branching is unusual in adulthood, and this population either has no heart disease or disease that is not hemodynamically significant. In this subgroup, the diagnosis is an incidental finding on chest radiographs or CT obtained for other clinical indications.

Double Aortic Arch

A double arch occurs in 0.05% to 3% of the population (82,87). The double aortic arch is characterized by the presence of two aortic arches arising from a single ascending aorta (Fig. 15-28). Each arch gives rise to its own subclavian and carotid arteries before uniting to form a single descending aorta, which is usually left-sided. Both limbs of the double arch are usually patent and functioning. The right limb

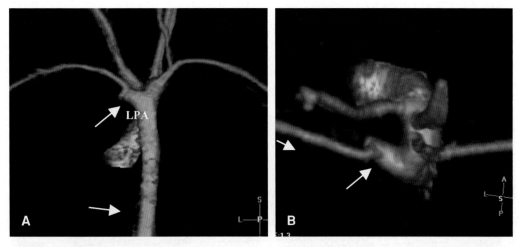

FIGURE 15-26 Right arch with aberrant left subclavian and persistent ligamentum arteriosum. A: Posterior view of a CEMRA in a 2-year-old child with dysphagia depicts a large diverticulum of Kommerell (*arrow*), an aberrant left subclavian artery, and a right aortic arch. **B:** Superior view depicts the large diverticulum (*arrow*) compressing the esophagus posteriorly. A ligamentum arteriosum was found and ligated at surgery.

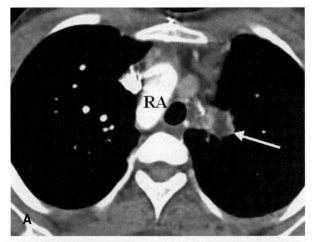

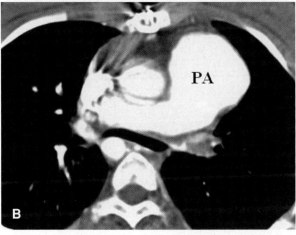

FIGURE 15-27 Right aortic arch with mirror image branching. A: Axial image shows a right aortic arch (*RA*). A thrombosed Blalock-Taussig shunt (*arrow*) is noted in this patient with a repaired tetralogy of Fallot. **B:** At a lower level, the arch descends on the right. There is no anomalous vessel crossing the mediastinum. Also noted is a dilated main pulmonary artery (*PA*) following a patch graft for treatment of pulmonic stenosis.

is typically larger and more cephalad than the left arch (Fig. 15-29). Occasionally, the left arch can be equal in size or larger than the right arch.

In rare instances, a portion of the left limb is atretic with a fibrous band completing the ring. In this circumstance, it can be difficult to separate a double arch with an atretic segment from the right arch with an aberrant left subclavian artery (87,88) (Fig. 15-30). With 3D imaging techniques, the effect of the atretic arch can sometimes be appreciated on a superior view of the arch, where the vessels can appear to be pulled toward each other by the fibrous band (Fig. 15-31).

Patients with double arch are often symptomatic and show symptoms of esophageal or tracheal compression. Double arch is usually diagnosed in childhood, although it can be discovered incidentally if the ring formed by the double arch is loose (87). This is generally an isolated anomaly, and associated heart disease is rare.

Cervical Aortic Arch

A cervical aortic arch is a rare anomaly characterized by a high-riding elongated aortic arch, which extends cephalad in the mediastinum before turning downward to descend in the thorax. The arch often projects above the level of the clavicles and extends into the cervical soft tissues. Associated anomalies are common and include absence of the innominate artery, origin of the contralateral subclavian artery from the descending proximal aorta, and a retroesophageal course of the descending aorta with the aorta descending on the right side contralateral to the arch. When the ligamentum arterious is on the side opposite the arch, a vascular ring is formed. A right-sided

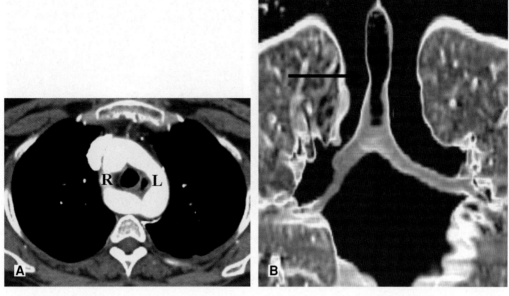

FIGURE 15-28 Double aortic arch. **A:** Axial CT image demonstrating right (*R*) and left (*L*) arches encircling the trachea and esophagus. **B:** 3D volume-rendered image shows mild compression of the right lateral tracheal wall (*arrow*).

cervical arch is more common than a left-sided cervical arch (82).

Most patients are asymptomatic, and the diagnosis is an incidental finding on imaging examinations. Clinical symptoms include dysphagia from the retroesophageal course of the aorta or from a vascular ring and a pulsatile neck mass.

Aortic Coarctation

Coarctation of the aorta occurs in 3.2 of 10,000 births, with an overall incidence of approximately 5% to 8% of all

congenital cardiac disease (75,89). Two major types of coarctation are recognized: preductal and postductal. These are also known as the infantile and adult forms of coarctation, respectively. Both forms are easily shown on CT and MR angiography (18–20,85,90).

In the preductal form of coarctation, the narrowing of the aorta occurs immediately below the origin of the left subclavian artery at the insertion of the ductus arteriosus or ligamentum arteriosum (Fig. 15-32). This form of coarctation is associated with hypoplasia of the transverse aortic

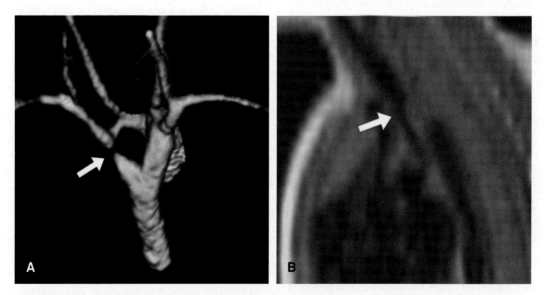

FIGURE 15-29 Double arch with mirror image branching. **A:** Posterior view of a CEMRA depicts a large right arch and a smaller left arch with focal stenosis (*arrow*) distal to the left subclavian origin. **B:** Sagittal reformat of DIR images depicts tracheal narrowing (*arrow*) secondary to extrinsic compression by the vascular ring.

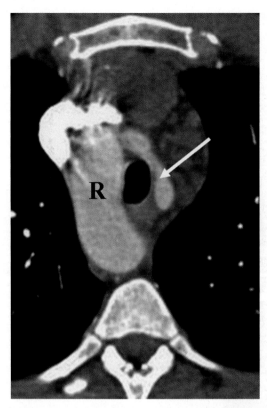

FIGURE 15-30 Double aortic arch and atretic left aortic arch. Axial CT scan at the level of the superior vena cava shows a smaller left aortic arch (*arrow*) and a larger right aortic arch (*R*).

arch and left subclavian artery and congenital heart lesions, including ventricular septal defects, patent ductus arteriosus, and hypoplastic left heart (Figs. 15-33–15-35). Affected patients usually present in the first 6 months of life with heart failure.

In the postductal form, which is more common after the neonatal period, the coarctation is almost always located at the junction of the distal aortic arch and the descending aorta, immediately below the obliterated ductus arteriosus (89) (Fig. 15-36). The coarctation is usually localized and caused by a shelflike folding of the posterior aortic wall into the aortic lumen opposite the ductus (Fig. 15-37). The ascending aorta is usually dilated, and the descending aorta just below the coarctation shows poststenotic dilatation (Fig. 15-38). In the latter case, collateral circulation between the proximal and distal parts of the aorta is established via large intercostal and internal thoracic arteries. In this manner, the lower part of the body is supplied with blood. Rib notching due to erosion of the undersurface of the ribs by the dilated intercostal vessels is common. The third to sixth ribs are most often affected.

Patients with postductal coarctations are usually asymptomatic, and the condition is recognized during evaluation of hypertension or a coexistent cardiac anomaly, usually a bicuspid aortic valve, which is found in up to 85% of patients. The blood pressure in the upper extremities is typically higher than that in the lower extremities. If there also is an aberrant right subclavian artery, the pressure in the right upper arm may be lower than that in the left upper arm.

MR can provide a quantitative analysis of blood flow across the area of vessel narrowing. VEC MR imaging is used to estimate peak flow velocity through the most severely narrowed segment. The pressure gradient across this site can be calculated with the modified Bernoulli equation (Fig. 15-5) (91). The pressure gradient is used to determine the need for repair of the coarctation. Typically, a pressure gradient greater than 15 mmHg is considered an indication for intervention. However, this threshold is arbitrary. Other clinical and laboratory considerations are also included when determining the need for surgical intervention. The depiction of collateral vessel formation is one such important consideration.

The identification of collateral flow is important for two reasons. First, it can help to plan operative repair. If there are insufficient numbers of collateral vessels, cross clamping of the aorta may be contraindicated because it can result in spinal cord ischemia. Second, the extent of collateral vessel formation can indicate the severity of the narrowing. A large number of collateral vessels suggests that the coarctation is more likely to be clinically significant (Fig. 15-39). Direct visualization of collateral vessels by MRA is a more reliable indicator of hemodynamic significance than the commonly performed arm-leg blood pressure gradient (92).

Treatment for coarctation is either open surgical repair or catheter interventions, including angioplasty and stent implantation (89). The choice of procedure depends on the site and extent of the coarctation and the patient's age. After surgical repair or postballoon angioplasty, CT or MR can be used to demonstrate complications, such as residual stenosis or restenosis, aneurysm formation, and dissection (Fig. 15-40). The prevalence of recoarctation is between 3% and 41% and is associated with smaller patient size or younger age at operation and the presence of associated transverse arch hypoplasia (89) (Fig. 15-41). The frequency of aneurysms is reported to be 5% to 9% after end-to-end anastomosis, 33% to 51% after Dacron patch aortoplasty, and 4% to 12% after angioplasty (89).

Coarctation is commonly associated with complex congenital and acquired cardiac pathology, such as aortic valve disease, that may require surgical intervention (93,94). In addition, 5% to 30% of patients who have previously undergone a coarctation repair will present with

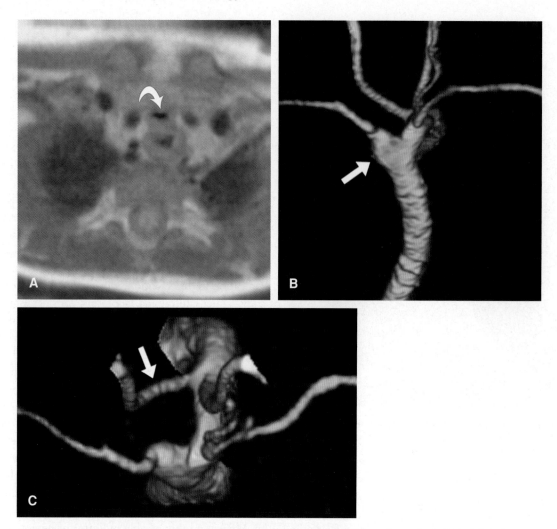

FIGURE 15-31 Double arch with an atretic left arch, values of superior view of vessels on 3D imaging. A: Seven-month-old male presented with airway compromise, depicted as a narrowed trachea (*arrow*) on axial DIR image. **B:** Posterior view of CEMRA exam depicts an aberrant right subclavian artery and a diverticulum of Kommerell (*arrow*), but a double arch is not appreciated. **C:** Superior view of the arch reveals that the right common carotid artery (*arrow*) is pulled posteriorly toward the right subclavian artery. At surgery, a double arch with an atretic left arch completed by a fibrous band was found. When the band was ligated, the trachea distended normally.

recoarctation requiring intervention (95–97). There is no consensus on the optimal approach for these patients (98). Several extra-anatomic bypass grafting techniques have been described, including an anastomosis between the proximal aorta and descending thoracic aorta, supraceliac abdominal aorta, or infrarenal abdominal aorta (98). MR has been useful in the postoperative evaluation of these patients. It can evaluate graft patency and associated surgical complications, and it also can assess the native aorta and other vessels (Fig. 15-42) (99).

Interruption of the Aortic Arch

Interruption of the aortic arch is a rare anomaly, accounting for about 1.5% of cases of congenital heart disease (82). Embryologically, this is related to regression of portions of the arch on two sides. There are three basic types of

interrupted arch, depending on the site of interruption. In descending order of frequency, these are Type A, interruption distal to the left subclavian artery; Type B, interruption between the left common carotid artery and the left subclavian artery; and Type C, interruption between the brachiocephalic trunk and the left carotid artery (100). A dilated patent ductus arteriosus supplies the descending aorta beyond the interruption (Fig. 15-43). Recognizing the dilated ductus is important so that it is not mistaken for the aortic arch.

Almost all patients with interrupted aortic arch present in the early neonatal period with respiratory distress, cyanosis, and congestive heart failure. Congenital heart disease is usually present and includes ventricular septal defect, bicuspid aortic valve, aortopulmonary window, truncus arteriosus, transposition of the great arteries,

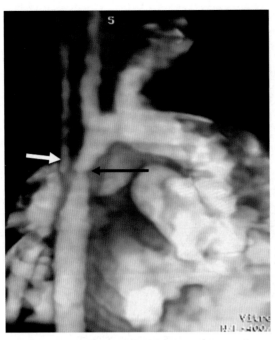

FIGURE 15-32 Preductal aortic coarctation. Sagittal 3D volume-rendered CT demonstrates focal constriction (*black arrow*) of the aortic lumen just proximal to the left subclavian artery, which is also narrowed (*white arrow*). Subclavian artery narrowing was not appreciated on the axial views.

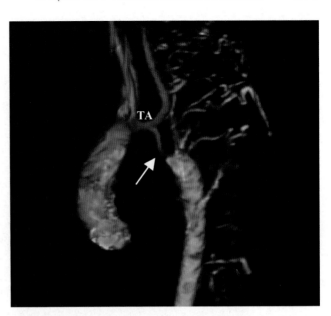

FIGURE 15-34 Preductal aortic coarctation associated with a hypoplastic aortic arch. CEMRA depicts narrowing of the transverse arch (*TA*) and a high-grade long segment coarctation beginning at the left subclavian artery (*arrow*). Note extensive collaterals.

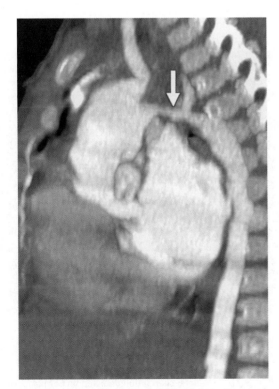

FIGURE 15-33 Preductal aortic coarctation. Sagittal image demonstrates constriction and hypoplasia (*arrow*) of the aortic lumen just proximal to the left subclavian artery.

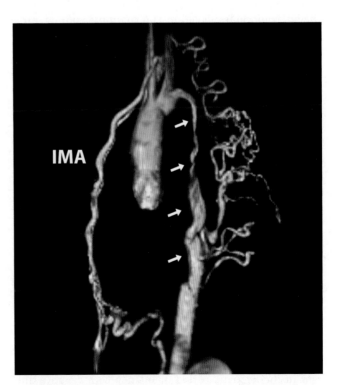

FIGURE 15-35 Long segment aortic coarctation. CEMRA depicts extensive narrowing of the distal aortic arch to the mid to distal descending thoracic aorta (*arrows*). Note extensive collateral development, including the internal mammary arteries (*IMA*).

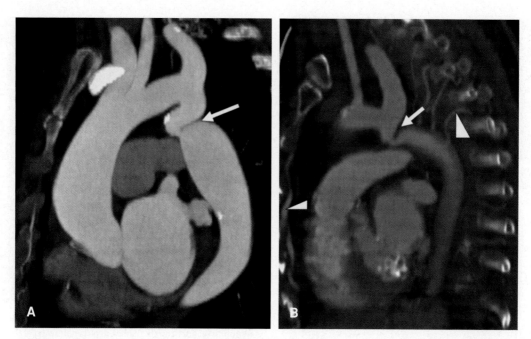

FIGURE 15-36 Postductal aortic coarctation. A: Thin-slab MIP of a CTA shows a dilated ascending aorta and a high-grade coarctation (*arrow*) of the proximal descending aorta. **B:** Lateral slab VR in another patient also demonstrates the characteristic narrowing (*arrow*) of the aortic lumen below the origin of the left subclavian artery. Also noted are dilated internal mammary and posterior intercostal arteries (*arrowheads*).

double-outlet right ventricle, and single ventricle (89). Type B interruption has also been associated with the DiGeorge syndrome (82). Treatment is surgical repair of the interruption by an end-to-end anastomosis or by interposition of a conduit.

Aortic Valvular Stenosis

Aortic valvular stenosis can be isolated or associated with bicuspid aortic valve. The bicuspid aortic valve can become stenotic as a result of thickening and calcification. Hemodynamically significant aortic stenosis can result in dilatation of the ascending aorta (Fig. 15-44) and cardiac failure.

AORTOPULMONARY ANOMALIES

Common Arterial Trunk

Common arterial trunk, also known as truncus arteriosus, persistent truncus arteriosus, and truncus arteriosus communis, is an uncommon vascular lesion, accounting for 1% to 4% of all congenital heart disease (101). In this lesion, a single artery (truncus) arises from the base of the heart because of failure of proximal division into the aorta and the pulmonary artery. Thus, both pulmonary and systemic arteries arise from the common trunk. Most patients present in the neonatal period or infancy with cyanosis and congestive heart failure.

Early classifications of this anomaly were based primarily on its morphologic features. The Society of Thoracic

Surgeons classification is the most recent classification scheme and is an attempt to provide a system that reflects both the anatomy and features that affect surgical outcome (102). In this classification, there are three types of

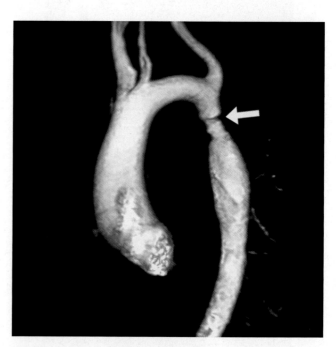

FIGURE 15-37 Postductal coarctation depicted on CEMRA. Focal shelflike narrowing, most prominent posteriorly, at the junction of the distal aortic arch and the descending aorta (*arrow*). There is mild poststenotic dilatation of the descending aorta, but no significant collaterals are present.

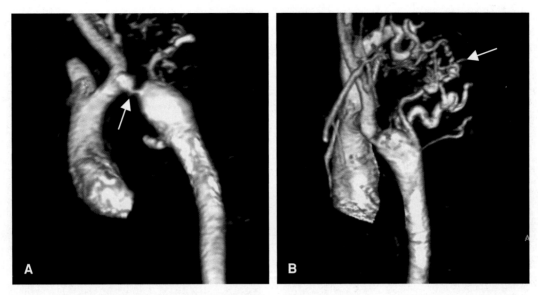

FIGURE 15-38 High-grade coarctation with extensive collateral development. A: CEMRA depicts a very small lumen at the site of coarctation (*arrow*) and poststenotic dilatation of the descending aorta. **B:** Large collateral vessels are also depicted (*arrow*).

common arterial trunks based on the origin of the pulmonary arteries: Type I, a common arterial trunk with confluent pulmonary arteries; Type II, a common arterial trunk with absence of one pulmonary artery; and Type III, a common arterial trunk with interrupted aortic arch or severe coarctation. The common trunk is larger than the normal aorta and is the only vessel exiting the heart. It

gives rise to the pulmonary and systemic arteries as well as the coronary arteries. There is a single semilunar valve (101). A ventricular septal defect is invariably present. Treatment is surgical repair using an aortic homograft with an aortic valve and a pulmonary conduit with a porcine valve or a homograft.

Hemitruncus Arteriosus

In hemitruncus arteriosus, one of the pulmonary arteries originates from the ascending aorta, while the other arises from the right ventricle. Affected patients usually present in the neonatal period or infancy with congestive heart failure secondary to a large left-to-right shunt (103).

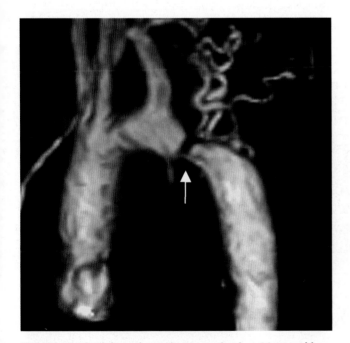

FIGURE 15-39 High-grade aortic coarctation in a 14-year-old patient without prior treatment. Large collaterals have developed secondary to the restrictive coarctation that has a lumen of approximately 2 mm (*arrow*).

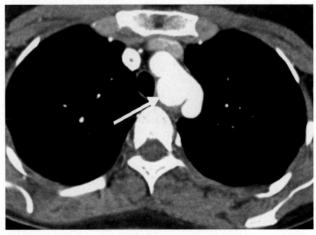

FIGURE 15-40 Aortic coarctation repair. Axial image shows pseudoaneurysm (*arrow*) at the site of prior anastomosis.

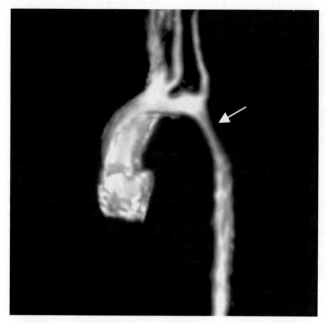

FIGURE 15-41 Restenosis of the aorta following surgical repair for coarctation. CEMRA depicts a long segment narrowing of the descending aorta 12 years following surgical repair performed at 18 months of age.

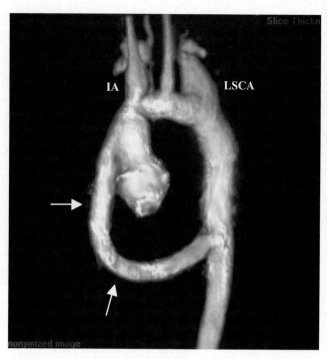

FIGURE 15-42 Ascending to descending aorta shunt depicted by CEMRA. The shunt (*arrows*) was placed following coarctation repair in a child with aneurysms of the innominate (*IA*) and left subclavian arteries (*LSCA*).

The anomalous pulmonary artery, most commonly the right, usually arises from the posterior wall of the ascending aorta and enters the pulmonary hilus to supply the ipsilateral lung (Fig. 15-45). The left pulmonary artery arises from the right ventricle to supply its ipsilateral lung. Associated anomalies include patent ductus arterious and ventricular septal defect.

Patent Ductus Arteriosus

The ductus arteriosus represents persistence of the distal part of the sixth aortic arch. In most instances, the ductus functionally closes shortly after birth through contraction of the muscular wall. Patent ductus arteriosus is a common

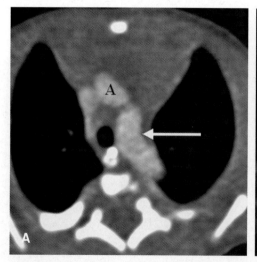
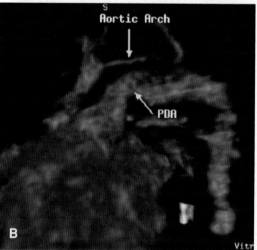

FIGURE 15-43 Interrupted aortic arch and severe congestive heart failure in a 2 kg neonate. A: Axial CT section demonstrates a normal caliber aortic arch (*A*). The vessel lateral and posterior to the aorta is a dilated patent ductus arteriosus (*arrow*). **B:** 3D volume-rendered reconstruction shows a markedly hypoplastic transverse arch (*Aortic Arch*) and a large patent ductus arteriosus (*PDA*) that supplies the distal aorta.

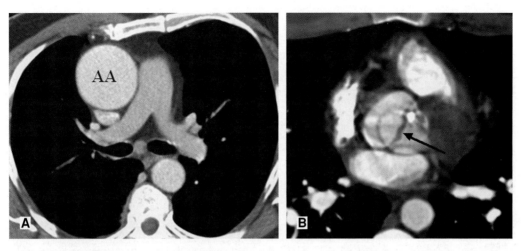

FIGURE 15-44 Poststenotic aortic dilatation. A: Axial image shows a dilated ascending aorta (*AA*). The descending aorta is normal. **B:** Axial image at a lower level shows a calcified bicuspid valve (*arrow*).

lesion in pediatric patients, especially in those with hyaline membrane disease and severe congenital heart disease, particularly pulmonary atresia and hypoplastic left heart syndrome. Except for neonates, most patients with patent ductus arteriosus are asymptomatic, and the lesion is usually diagnosed by the discovery of a murmur (104).

The diagnostic CT and MR finding is that of a small tubular structure connecting the descending proximal aorta with the distal main or proximal left pulmonary artery (105) (Fig. 15-46). The ductus may massively dilate in severe congenital heart disease, particularly when there are

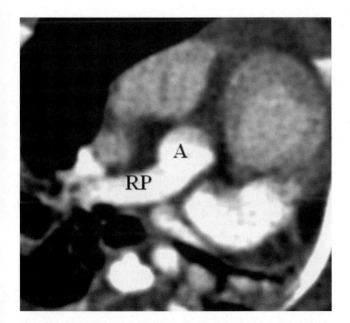

FIGURE 15-45 Right hemitruncus. Axial CT image shows right pulmonary artery (*RP*) arising from the ascending aorta (*A*).

defects that cause large differences between aortic and pulmonary pressure, thus substantially increasing blood flow through the ductus. Treatment is either device closure or operative repair.

Aortopulmonary Window

Aortopulmonary window is a direct communication between the proximal ascending aorta and the main pulmonary artery. This lesion is rare and results from incomplete division of the common arterial trunk. This defect is usually large, so most patients are diagnosed in infancy, presenting with congestive heart failure. Occasionally, the lesion is relatively small (about 10%), and the diagnosis is made later in life based on the detection of a murmur or findings of pulmonary hypertension (104). CT and MRI can easily demonstrate the aortopulmonary connection (Fig. 15-47). Treatment is surgical, either with direct suture or the use of a patch.

Transposition of the Great Arteries

Complete transposition of the great vessels, also known as *D-transposition*, is characterized by a discordant connection of the great arteries and ventricles, such that the pulmonary artery arises from the left ventricle, and the aorta arises from the right ventricle. There usually is an associated ventricular septal defect. This lesion causes cyanosis from birth and is virtually always diagnosed in the first few days of life. Survival until adolescence or adulthood is highly unlikely without surgical palliation or correction. Diagnosis is based on clinical and conventional angiographic findings, but CT or MRI have a role in defining the anatomy after surgical repair and in evaluating

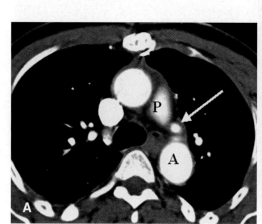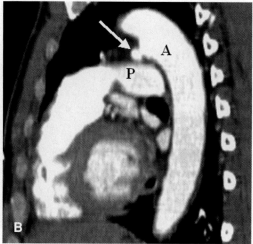

FIGURE 15-46 Patent ductus arteriosus. A: Axial CT shows an enhancing vessel (*arrow*) between the pulmonary artery (*P*) and descending aorta (*A*). **B:** Coronal multiplanar image also demonstrates the patent ductus (*arrow*) between the main pulmonary artery (*P*) and proximal descending aorta (*A*).

postoperative complications (Fig. 15-48). Therefore, recognition of the characteristic morphology can be of importance.

Corrected transposition, also known as *L-transposition*, is characterized by double discordance, both ventriculoarterial and atrioventricular, resulting in normal physiologic flow of blood. In such cases, the pulmonary artery arises from the anatomic left ventricle and the aorta from the anatomic right ventricle. In addition, the left atrium connects to the right ventricle, and the right atrium connects to the left ventricle. Thus, blood from the right atrium goes through a (right-sided) left ventricle and into the pulmonary arteries. Blood flowing through a (left-sided) right ventricle goes out the aorta. Although these patients have minimal hemodynamic alterations, they have a high frequency of arrhythmias.

On CT and MRI, the aorta usually lies anterior and to the right of the pulmonary artery (Figs. 15-49, 15-50). On rare occasion, it is positioned anterior but to the left of the pulmonary artery.

PULMONARY ARTERY

Idiopathic Dilatation of the Pulmonary Artery Trunk

Idiopathic dilatation of the pulmonary artery refers to enlargement of the pulmonary outflow tract without pulmonary valvular stenosis. This is a rare condition and usually is detected incidentally on imaging studies (106) (Figs. 15-51, 15-52).

Absence or Proximal Interruption

Absence or proximal interruption of a main pulmonary artery affects the right or left pulmonary artery. In this disorder, there is interruption of the right or left pulmonary artery, usually within 1 cm of its origin from the main pulmonary artery (106–109). The vessels distally are usually diminutive and are supplied by systemic collateral vessels. Pulmonary venous drainage is normal. In most instances, interruption of the left pulmonary artery is associated with

FIGURE 15-47 Aorticopulmonary window in a neonate in congestive failure. Axial multiplanar reformatted image (MPR) from a CEMRA depicts direct communication (*arrow*) between the main pulmonary artery (*MPA*) and the posterior wall of the ascending aorta (*Ao*).

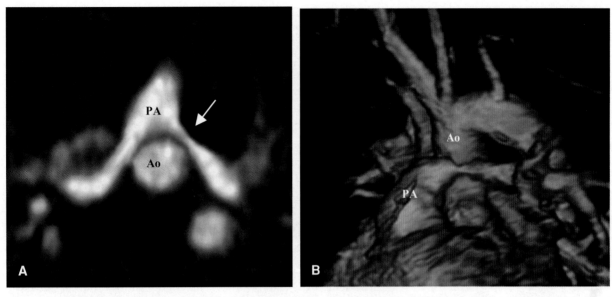

FIGURE 15-48 Transposition of the great vessels following surgical arterial switch procedure. A: Axial MPR from a CEMRA depicts the switched aorta (*Ao*) posterior to the pulmonary artery (*PA*). The pulmonary arteries branch around the aorta, and there is narrowing of the left pulmonary artery (*arrow*). **B:** Volume-rendered image confirms the narrowing of the left pulmonary artery.

other congenital cardiovascular anomalies, including right aortic arch, septal defects, patent ductus arteriosus, and tetralogy of Fallot. Right pulmonary artery interruption is usually an isolated finding.

Most affected patients come to clinical attention in the first year of life and present with dyspnea or recurrent pulmonary infections. However, patients can be asympto-

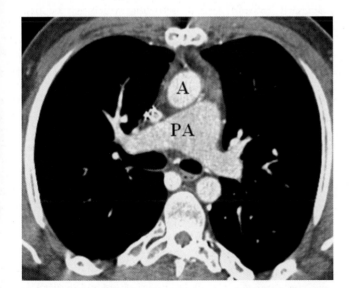

FIGURE 15-49 D-transposition of the great vessels. Contrast-enhanced CT scan at the level of the carina shows the aorta (*A*) lying anterior to the main pulmonary artery (*PA*).

matic, and the diagnosis is made in adolescence or adulthood as an incidental detection on chest radiographs or CT obtained for other clinical indications. Occasionally, adults with this disorder present with hemoptysis due to systemic-to-pulmonary arterial shunting.

The abnormal termination of the proximal pulmonary artery and the collateral arteries supplying the normal lung are usually easy to identify on CT and MR. Collateral pathways include aortopulmonary anastomoses from the thoracic aorta, direct origin of a pulmonary artery from the aorta, and coronary to left pulmonary artery anastomoses. Other findings include decreased size of the affected lung, diminished ipsilateral pulmonary vascularity, and scoliosis (Fig. 15-53).

Pulmonary Arterial Stenosis

Pulmonary artery stenosis can occur anywhere from the pulmonary valve to the peripheral arteries (106,110,111). These stenoses can be single or multiple and unilateral or bilateral. They can involve the trunk, main pulmonary artery branches (Figs. 15-2, 15-54, 15-55), segmental pulmonary branches, or a combination of these areas. Central and peripheral stenoses also can occur in combination. In children, these lesions are frequently associated with congenital syndromes including Williams, Noonan, Alagille, and Ehlers-Danlos, and in utero exposure to rubella virus. In adults, the lesions are usually isolated. Patients are often asymptomatic unless they have elevated

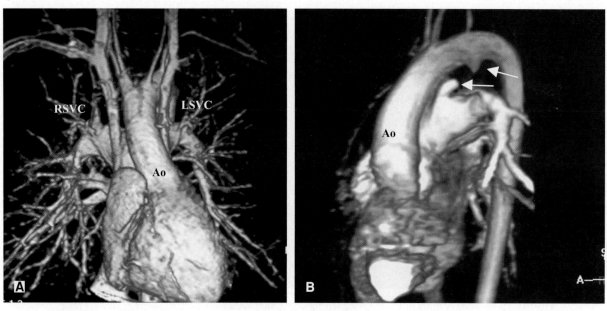

FIGURE 15-50 Corrected (L-)Transposition in a 34-year-old. A: Volume-rendered CEMRA study depicts that the aorta (*Ao*) arises anteriorly. Note left and right superior vena cava (*LSVC, RSVC*). **B:** Lateral view confirms the anterior aorta (*Ao*) and depicts small ductus aneurysms arising from both the aorta and the pulmonary trunk (*arrows*).

right ventricular pressures, usually manifesting as dyspnea or associated heart disease (111).

Pulmonary Sling

In pulmonary sling, the left pulmonary artery originates from the right pulmonary artery and crosses the medi-

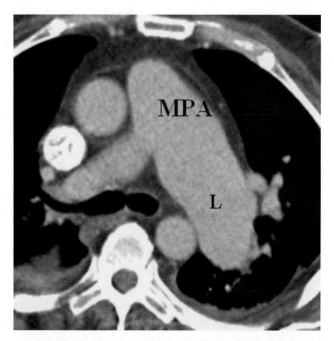

FIGURE 15-51 Idiopathic dilatation of the pulmonary artery trunk. Axial contrast-enhanced CT scan shows a dilated main (*MPA*) and left (*L*) pulmonary artery.

astinum, extending between the trachea and esophagus to reach the left hilum (106,109). This anomaly usually comes to clinical attention in neonates and young infants because of the compressive effect of the artery on the airway and/or the associated tracheal or bronchial stenosis due to cartilaginous rings. On occasion, it is an incidental finding in asymptomatic adults (106,109,112).

Multidetector CT and MRI can easily show the abnormal origin and course of the left pulmonary artery and the associated tracheobronchial narrowing, which may be focal or diffuse (106,109,113) (Fig. 15-56). In addition, dynamic CT during forced inspiration and expiration can show air trapping, further confirming the presence of bronchial obstruction.

PULMONARY ARTERIOVENOUS MALFORMATION

Pulmonary arteriovenous malformation (AVM) is characterized by a direct communication between a pulmonary artery and vein without an intervening capillary bed. This anomaly is most often congenital and associated with Rendu-Osler-Weber disease (hereditary hemorrhagic telangiectasia). Acquired pulmonary AVMs are less common, but they have been associated with chronic liver disease and surgically repaired congenital heart disease. Pulmonary AVMs are a cause of right-to-left shunting. As the size and number of lesions increase, patients are at risk for hypoxemia, stroke, and cerebral or abdominal abscess

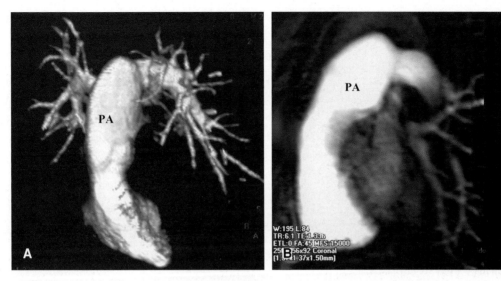

FIGURE 15-52 Idiopathic pulmonary artery (PA) enlargement in a young adult. A: Volume-rendered CEMRA depicts a large main PA segment with normal branch pulmonary arteries. **B:** Sagittal MIP depicts the 5.4-cm dilatation of the distal main PA.

related to the right-to-left shunt (106,114,115). Small lesions may be asymptomatic. Approximately 80% of pulmonary AVMs have a single feeding arterial branch (simple angioarchitecture) (116–118). The remaining 20% have two or more feeding arteries.

At CT, AVMs appear as rounded or lobular masses with rapid enhancement and wash out after intravenous contrast medium administration (Fig. 15-57). Enhancement typically occurs immediately after enhancement of the right ventricle. At least one feeding artery and one draining vein must be seen to establish the diagnosis. Slid-ing thin-slab maximum intensity projection images and 3D reconstructions are useful to optimize the precise anatomy of the feeding arteries and draining veins, which may course perpendicular or obliquely to the axial sections (12,116–118). In one study, it was shown that approximately 98% of AVMs were detected on transaxial contrast-enhanced CT examinations, and 38.5% of the lesions were seen only on CT, compared with unilateral pulmonary angiography. The majority of the lesions seen only on CT were less than 5 mm in diameter (117). Another study has shown that the combination of axial sections and 3D

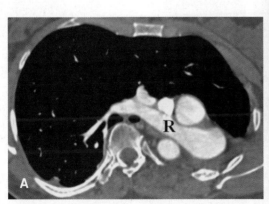

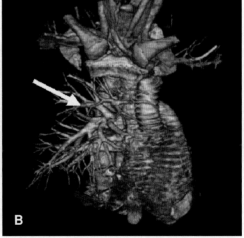

FIGURE 15-53 Agenesis of the left pulmonary artery. A: Axial CT image shows the right pulmonary artery (*R*) crossing over to the left hemithorax and herniation of the right lung across the midline anteriorly. The left lung and left pulmonary artery are absent. **B:** Coronal 3D volume-rendered image demonstrates the main branches (*arrow*) of the right pulmonary artery and absence of the left pulmonary artery.

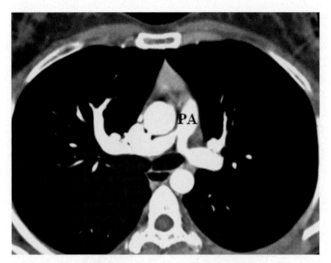

FIGURE 15-54 Pulmonary artery stenosis. Transverse CT section shows narrowing of the proximal left and right pulmonary arteries after their take-off from the main pulmonary artery (*PA*).

shaded-surface display reconstructions results in an accurate diagnosis of pulmonary AVM in 95% of cases (116).

MR also can be used to depict and diagnose pulmonary AVMs (119–123). Artifacts caused by respiratory motion represent the most significant limitation of pulmonary MR angiography (124). CEMRA has permitted assessment of the pulmonary arteries to a subsegmental level (125,126). Although this has required rather lengthy breath holds, excellent results have been reported in detection of pulmonary

emboli (127). Recently, a time-resolved contrast-enhanced 3D CEMRA technique for depicting pulmonary AVM has been described (128). The technique requires less than 4 seconds for each single 3D MRA data set displaying the entire pulmonary arterial tree. Multiple successive time-resolved data sets can therefore be acquired during a single breath hold lasting less than 20 seconds. This time-resolved approach is fast enough to document early enhancement of the draining veins that are characteristic of pulmonary AVMs.

PULMONARY VEINS

Total Anomalous Pulmonary Venous Connection

In total anomalous pulmonary venous connection, the veins from both lungs do not connect to the left atrium but instead connect to a systemic venous structure that returns to the right heart. An atrial septal defect is present and allows blood to reach the left heart. Total anomalous pulmonary venous connection is classified as supracardiac, cardiac, infracardiac, or mixed, depending on the site or sites of connect (Fig. 15-58). Pulmonary venous obstruction is usually present in the infracardiac form. Virtually all patients present in the neonatal period with cyanosis and congestive heart failure. Treatment is surgical anastomosis of the confluence of pulmonary veins to the left

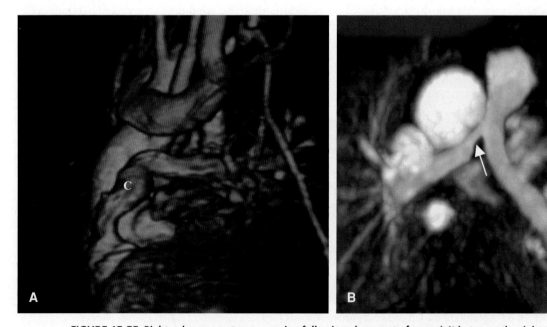

FIGURE 15-55 Right pulmonary artery narrowing following placement of a conduit between the right ventricle and the main pulmonary artery in a patient with pulmonary atresia. A: CEMRA depicts the patent conduit (*C*). **B:** Axial MPR depicts narrowing of the native right pulmonary artery near its origin (*arrow*).

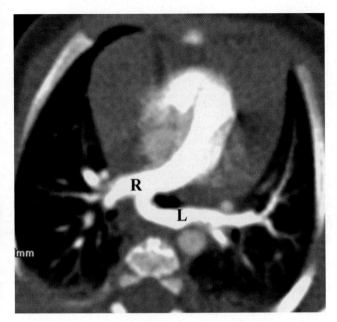

FIGURE 15-56 Pulmonary artery sling. Contrast-enhanced axial CT scan demonstrates the left pulmonary artery (*L*) arising posterior from the right pulmonary artery (*R*) before crossing behind the trachea to reach the left lung.

atrium. In adults, CT and MRI are useful to show the postoperative anatomy and to evaluate associated complications.

Partial Anomalous Venous Connection

Partial anomalous venous connection of one or more lobes produces a left-to-right shunt because the abnormal vein enters either the right heart or the systemic circulation. This anomaly may occur in isolation or with other cardiovascular

defects. Right-sided anomalous venous return is twice as common as left-sided anomalous return. As an isolated anomaly in an otherwise healthy individual, partial anomalous drainage is usually asymptomatic (106).

There are three common patterns of anomalous drainage: anomalous right superior pulmonary venous drainage to the superior vena cava, anomalous left superior pulmonary venous return into the left brachiocephalic vein or innominate vein, and anomalous right lower lobe drainage into the inferior vena cava or portal vein. Anomalous return is diagnosed based on recognition of the abnormal course of the intraparenchymal pulmonary vein. This is especially well seen on 3D reconstructions (129).

Partial Anomalous Drainage of the Left Upper Lung

In this anomaly, the left upper lobe pulmonary vein usually empties into the left brachiocephalic or innominate vein. CT and MRI show a vertical vein coursing lateral to the aortic arch and aortopulmonary window (Fig. 15-59). A normal left superior pulmonary vein is not identified in the left hilum, but instead, a small lingular vein will be seen anterior to the left main bronchus. Blood flow is caudocranial. Partial anomalous venous return needs to be distinguished from a persistent left superior vena cava (see below). Two vessels will be seen in the left hilar region in the latter anomaly (the left cava and the left pulmonary vein), whereas only one vessel will be found in this location in anomalous venous return. In addition, the persistent left superior vena cava usually drains into a dilated coronary sinus (130).

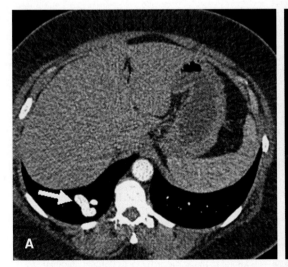
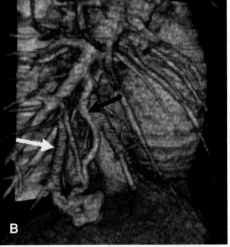

FIGURE 15.57 Pulmonary arteriovenous malformation. A: Axial CT image shows a contrast-enhanced nodular opacity in the right lower lobe (*arrow*). **B:** Oblique coronal 3D volume-rendered image. The feeding artery (*white arrow*) originates from the right lower lobe artery. The draining vein (*black arrow*) drains into the right inferior pulmonary vein.

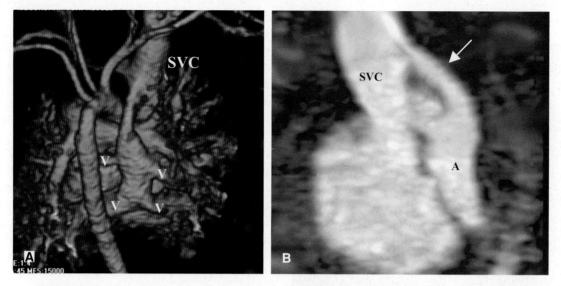

FIGURE 15-58 Supracardiac total anomalous pulmonary venous return (TAPVR). A: Posterior view of a CEMRA depicts the four pulmonary veins (*V*) forming a chamber that then drains into the superior vena cava (*SVC*). **B:** Sagittal MPR depicts the communication (*arrow*) between the atrium (*A*) and the superior vena cava (*SVC*).

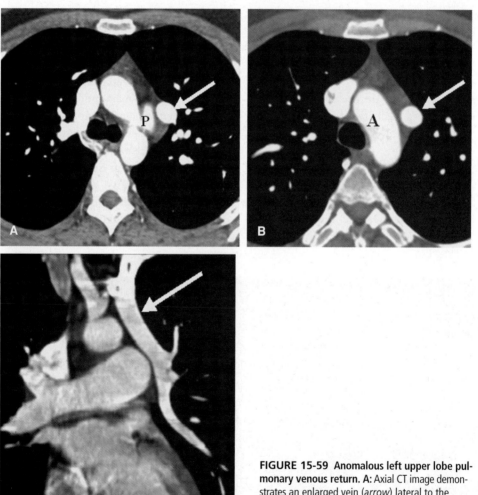

FIGURE 15-59 Anomalous left upper lobe pulmonary venous return. A: Axial CT image demonstrates an enlarged vein (*arrow*) lateral to the main pulmonary artery (*P*). **B:** A more cranial axial CT image shows the enlarged vein (*arrow*) lying lateral to the aortic arch (*A*). **C:** Coronal multiplanar reformation shows the full course of the anomalous left upper lobe vein (*arrow*), which empties into the brachiocephalic vein.

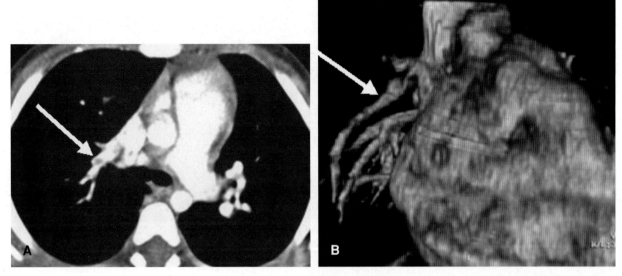

FIGURE 15-60 Anomalous right upper lobe venous return. A: Axial CT image shows an anomalous vein (*arrow*) in the right upper lobe. **B:** Coronal 3D image shows the vein emptying into the superior vena cava (*arrow*).

Partial Anomalous Drainage of the Right Upper Lobe

In this form of anomaly, the right upper lobe drains into the superior vena cava, usually near the caval-right atrial junction. A communication located posterosuperior to the oval fossa, termed a *sinus venosus defect*, is a common associated finding, occurring in up to 90% of patients with anomalous right upper lobe drainage (129,131) (Figs. 15-60, 15-61).

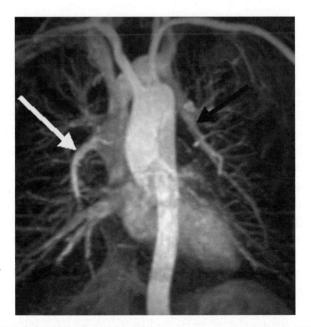

FIGURE 15-61 Bilateral upper lobe anomalous venous drainage. MIP MR image shows anomalous right (*white arrow*) and left (*black arrow*) upper lobe veins.

Less often, anomalous drainage from the right lung is into the right atrium or azygous vein or to the azygous arch.

Abnormal Drainage of the Right Lower Lobe

In this anomaly, an anomalous pulmonary vein from the right lung drains to the inferior vena cava, hepatic vein, or portal vein (Fig. 15-62). The scimitar or hypogenetic lung syndrome is a special form of anomalous pulmonary venous return that is associated with a hypoplastic right lung and pulmonary artery, mediastinal shift, systemic arterial supply to the small lung, and partial anomalous pulmonary venous return from the right lung (132–134). Anomalous return is usually to the inferior vena cava, although it may join with the suprahepatic part of the inferior vena cava, hepatic vein, portal vein, azygous vein, coronary sinus, or right atrium (109). Other associated anomalies include systemic arterial blood supply from the thoracic or abdominal aorta to the hypogenetic lung and horseshoe lung. Horseshoe lung is a rare anomaly in which the posterobasal segments of both lungs are fused behind the pericardial sac.

Pulmonary Varix

A varicosity of the pulmonary vein can be congenital or the result of chronic pulmonary hypertension. Patients may be asymptomatic or present with hemoptysis. Contrast-enhanced helical CT shows filling of the varix concurrently with the normal pulmonary veins and continuity between the varix and the adjacent pulmonary veins or the left atrium (Fig. 15-63).

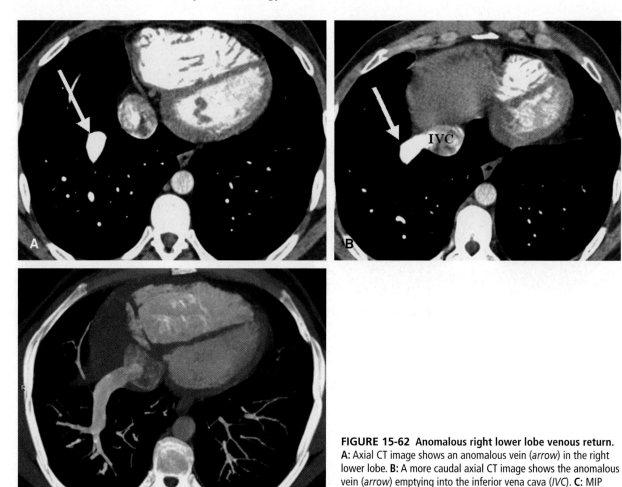

FIGURE 15-62 Anomalous right lower lobe venous return.
A: Axial CT image shows an anomalous vein (*arrow*) in the right lower lobe. **B:** A more caudal axial CT image shows the anomalous vein (*arrow*) emptying into the inferior vena cava (*IVC*). **C:** MIP demonstrates the entire course of the anomalous vein as it courses through the lung to enter the inferior vena cava.

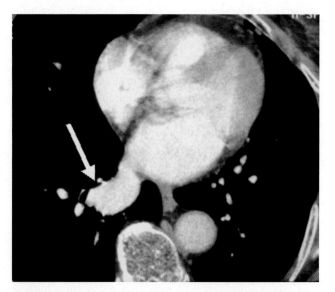

FIGURE 15-63 Pulmonary varix. Axial contrast-enhanced CT shows a dilated right inferior pulmonary vein (*arrow*).

SYSTEMIC THORACIC VEINS

Left-sided Superior Vena Cava

The common anomalies of the systemic thoracic veins are the left-sided superior vena cava and azygous/hemiazygous continuation of the inferior vena cava (135). The persistent left superior vena cava represents persistence of the embryologic common cardinal and left anterior cardinal veins. It has been reported to occur in 1% to 3% of the general population. In most cases, it is an isolated finding, but it can be associated with congenital heart disease, usually atrial septal defects. A left-sided SVC usually is not hemodynamically significant unless it is associated with congenital heart anomalies.

The persistent left superior vena cava lies anterior to the left subclavian artery and lateral to the left common carotid artery. As it descends, it passes lateral to the aortic arch, lateral to the main pulmonary artery, and anterior to

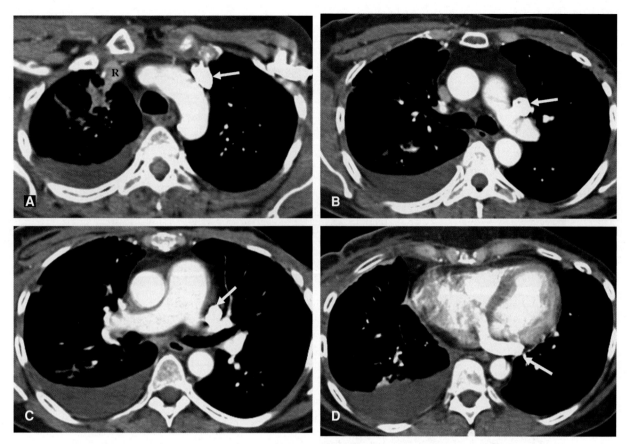

FIGURE 15-64 Persistent left superior vena cava. A: Contrast-enhanced CT scan shows the left superior vena cava (*arrow*) lateral to the aortic arch. Also noted is a right superior vena cava (*R*). **B, C:** At lower levels, the left superior vena cava (*arrow*) courses lateral to the left hilum. **D:** At the level of the left atrium, the cava drains into the coronary sinus (*arrow*). The patient also has a right pleural effusion and right upper lobe atelectasis.

the left hilum. Most commonly, it drains into the coronary sinus posterior to the left ventricle (Fig. 15-64). On rare occasions, it drains into the left atrium, which results in a right-to-left shunt. In many cases, there is an associated right-sided superior vena cava, which is usually smaller than the left. In this scenario, this anomaly is more appropriately termed the *double superior vena cava.*

A left-sided superior vena cava can mimic partial anomalous pulmonary venous drainage from the left upper lobe at the level of the aortic arch. In both disorders, a vessel is seen lateral to the aortic arch. These two conditions can be differentiated by noting the course of the anomalous vessel on serial images. In left-sided superior vena cava, a normal size left upper lobe pulmonary vein can be seen at the level of the left main stem bronchus. In partial anomalous return, the only vessel anterior to the bronchus is a small lingular vein. Most often, the left-sided superior vena cava empties into the coronary sinus, whereas the anomalous left upper lobe pulmonary vein empties into the brachiocephalic vein (Fig. 15-59).

Azygous Continuation of the Inferior Vena Cava

Azygous continuation of the inferior vena cava results when the suprarenal segment of the inferior vena cava fails to develop. Thus, blood from the lower half of the body is returned to the heart via the retrocrural azygous and hemiazygous veins, which are derived from the right supracardinal vein. The prevalence of this anomaly is about 0.6% (136). Previously, it was thought that this condition was virtually always associated with congenital heart disease and asplenia or polysplenia, but with the increasing utilization of cross-sectional imaging, it is now recognized that azygous continuation is often an incidental finding in an otherwise asymptomatic individual.

CT and MRI findings are dilatation of the azygous arch, the azygous vein, and the superior vena cava caudal to the azygous junction; enlargement of the azygous and hemiazygous veins in the paraspinal and retrocrural areas; and absence of the suprarenal and intrahepatic portions of the inferior vena cava (Fig. 15-65). CT and MRI also can provide useful information about abdominal situs, particularly splenic status.

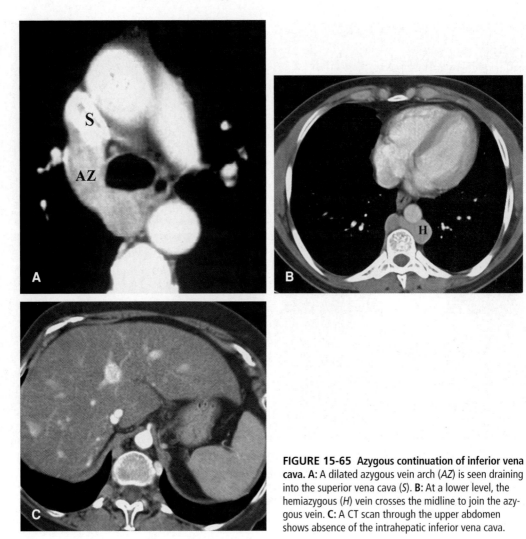

FIGURE 15-65 Azygous continuation of inferior vena cava. A: A dilated azygous vein arch (*AZ*) is seen draining into the superior vena cava (*S*). **B:** At a lower level, the hemiazygous (*H*) vein crosses the midline to join the azygous vein. **C:** A CT scan through the upper abdomen shows absence of the intrahepatic inferior vena cava.

BRONCHOPULMONARY SEQUESTRATION

Bronchopulmonary sequestration is a congenital mass of pulmonary tissue that has no normal connection with the tracheobronchial tree and is supplied by an anomalous artery, usually arising from the aorta (133,134,137). Sequestration is classically divided into intralobar (acquired) and extralobar (congenital) types. In both the intra- and extralobar forms, the arterial supply is usually from the descending aorta, but in approximately 20% of cases, it comes from the infradiaphragmatic aorta, other systemic arteries such as the celiac and splenic arteries, and even from the coronary arteries (137,138). The venous drainage of the two types of sequestration differs. In the intralobar type, venous drainage is typically via an inferior pulmonary vein (Fig. 15-66). In extralobar sequestration, venous drainage is usually via the azygous vein, hemiazygous vein, and inferior vena cava, although unusual drainage routes such as drainage into the portal vein have been reported (139) (Fig. 15-67).

Intralobar sequestration accounts for approximately 75% of all pulmonary sequestrations (133,140). It is contained within the visceral pleura of the normal lobe and is surrounded by normal lung. Most affected patients present with recurrent pneumonias and are diagnosed in adolescence or adulthood. Associated anomalies, usually diaphragmatic hernias, occur in approximately up to 15% of cases (133,140).

Extralobar sequestration is contained within a separate pleural investment, and most cases are diagnosed within the first 6 months of life (141). This anomaly is often asymptomatic and is discovered during the evaluation of associated anomalies, which occur in approximately 65% of cases (133). The most common anomalies are congenital diaphragmatic hernia or eventration and a fistula between the sequestrated lung and the esophagus or stomach.

Both intra- and extralobar sequestrations are more common on the left side. Nearly all intralobar sequestrations

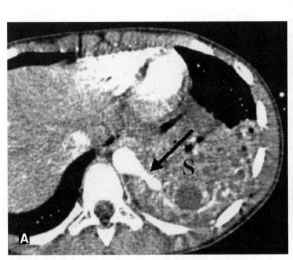
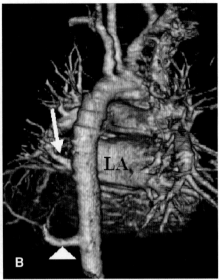

FIGURE 15-66 Intralobar sequestration. A: Axial CT image shows a feeding artery (*arrow*) originating from the descending thoracic aorta and extending into left lower lobe sequestration (*S*). **B:** Coronal 3D volume-rendered image from a posterior orientation shows the feeding artery (*arrowhead*) originating from the descending thoracic aorta. Also noted is a draining vein (*arrow*) going to the left atrium (*LA*).

arise in the lower lobe. The typical location of an extralobar sequestration is within the pleural space in the posterior costodiaphragmatic sulcus between the diaphragm and the lower lobe.

CT and MR, particularly with 3D reconstructions, are helpful to establish the diagnosis and show the morphology

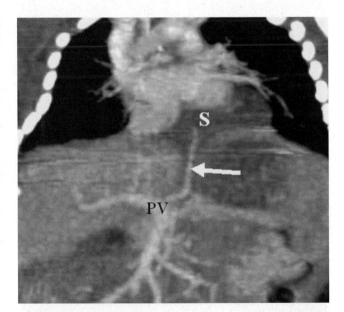

FIGURE 15-67 Extralobar sequestration in a 6-day-old neonate girl with a mass in the left lower hemithorax on prenatal sonography. Coronal MIP demonstrates a small vein (*arrow*) from the sequestered lung (*S*) draining into the portal vein (*PV*).

of the sequestration and its feeding artery and draining vein (142–145). The CT appearance of the pulmonary parenchyma depends on whether or not the sequestered lung is aerated. When the sequestration communicates with the remainder of the lung, usually after being infected, it appears cystic; a sequestration that does not communicate appears as a homogeneous density, usually in the posterior portion of the lower lobe. Hyperinflated or emphysematous lung often surrounds the sequestered lung.

Vascular Sequestration

In a purely vascular sequestration, the only anomaly is the systemic arterial supply to the lung (146,147). The aberrant artery supplies normal lung tissue that communicates with the tracheobronchial tree. There are no associated parenchymal or tracheobronchial anomalies. This anomaly usually occurs in the basal segments of the lung and is more common on the left than the right. Affected patients may be asymptomatic and the lesion detected incidentally, or they may present with hemoptysis due to focal pulmonary hypertension in the involved lung or to intrabronchial rupture of the abnormal systemic artery.

The anomalous artery usually replaces the normal pulmonary arterial supply to the lower lobe. Less often, it is an accessory artery and accompanies the normal pulmonary artery supply. The anomalous artery usually arises from the descending aorta and enters the lung through the pulmonary ligament (142,146,147). Typically, it has a sigmoid-shaped configuration before it ramifies into its peripheral branches (146). The proximal portion of the abnormal artery is often narrowed, while the distal portion often appears dilated. Mural calcifications and intramural thrombus also have been noted (106). The intralobar branches of the anomalous artery follow the course of the normal bronchi in the basal segments of the lower lobes. Early filling of the corresponding inferior pulmonary vein has been noted on CT, reflecting the left-to-right shunting that characterizes this malformation (106).

SYSTEMIC ARTERIAL SUPPLY TO THE LUNGS

Anomalous systemic arterial supply to the lungs has been described in congenital heart diseases, usually the cyanotic heart diseases, and in congenital lung diseases, most commonly the hypogenetic lung syndrome and bronchopulmonary sequestration (148). It also has been described in association with normal lung (the avascular sequestration). In patients with cyanotic heart disease, normal branches of the thoracic aorta, usually the bronchial arteries, hypertrophy and anastomose with pulmonary arteries within the lung parenchyma to allow blood flow to the lungs (149). In bronchopulmonary sequestration and the hypogenetic lung syndrome, a systemic artery with an anomalous origin supplies the involved lung.

The normal bronchial arteries supply the airways of the lungs, the esophagus, and hilar lymph nodes and are usually less than 2 mm in diameter (149,150). There are usually three bronchial arteries, two for the left lung and one for the right lung. The left bronchial artery usually arises directly from the aorta, whereas the right bronchial artery originates either from the first intercostal artery (43% of cases) or directly from the aorta. In the majority of individuals, right and left bronchial arteries originate around the level of the fifth and sixth thoracic vertebra. Occasionally, subclavian, innominate, internal mammary, and coronary arteries are sources of bronchial vessels (149). The bronchial arteries course for a variable distance in the mediastinum before reaching their respective hilum.

Hypertrophied bronchial arteries are larger than 2 mm in diameter and in some instances may dilate to 1 cm or more in diameter (150). They appear as nodular or linear structures within the mediastinum, usually in the retrotracheal area, retroesophageal area, posterior wall of the main bronchi, and the aortopulmonary window (150,151) (Fig. 15-68). Curved reformation techniques have been shown useful in demonstrating the origin and course of bronchial arteries (151).

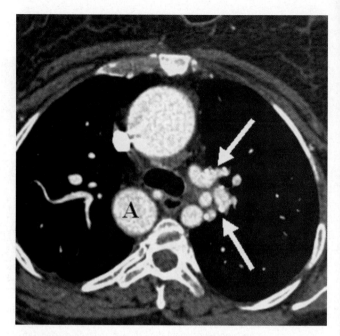

FIGURE 15-68 Bronchial collaterals associated with left pulmonary artery atresia. Axial CT image demonstrates multiple bronchial collateral vessels (*arrows*) in the region of the left hilum. Also noted is a right descending aorta (*A*).

SURGICAL SHUNTS

Most surgical shunts are palliative procedures that are done to augment pulmonary blood flow and thus decrease cyanosis.

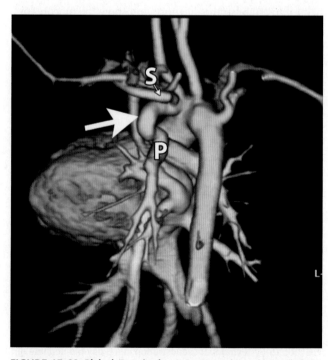

FIGURE 15-69 Blalock Taussig shunt. Contrast-enhanced coronal 3D CT reconstruction viewed posteriorly shows a patent Blalock-Taussig shunt (*arrow*) between the left subclavian artery (*S*) and left pulmonary artery (*P*).

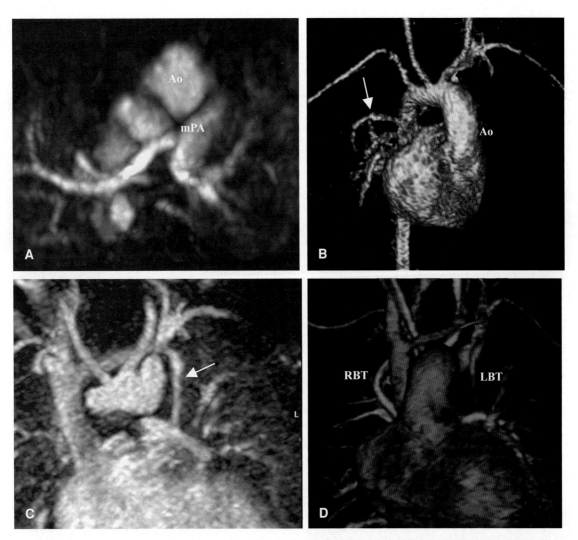

FIGURE 15-70 Blalock-Taussig shunts used with staged repair in pulmonary atresia. A: Axial MPR from a CEMRA depicts a large aortic root (*Ao*) and a short main pulmonary artery (*mPA*) without communication with the right ventricle. **B:** CEMRA reveals a large ascending aorta (*Ao*) and systemic collaterals arising from the descending aorta (*arrow*). **C:** Patent left Blalock-Taussig shunt (*arrow*), placed to increase blood supply to the lungs, can be noted. **D:** A subsequent MR examination shows interval placement of a right Blalock-Taussig shunt (*RBT*) and stenosis of the older left Blalock-Taussig shunt (*LBT*).

These include both systemic artery to pulmonary artery shunts and systemic vein to pulmonary artery shunts (152,153).

Systemic Artery to Pulmonary Artery Shunts

The Blalock-Taussig shunt is an anastomosis between a subclavian artery and the ipsilateral pulmonary artery, either with an end-to-side anastomosis or using an interposed graft. Pulmonary hypertension is an occasional complication. CT or MR is useful to evaluate the shunts postoperatively (Figs. 15-69, 15-70).

The Waterston shunt is a direct side-to-side anastomosis between the ascending aorta and right pulmonary artery. This is often complicated by both pulmonary arterial hypertension, usually because the shunt is too large, and distortion of the right pulmonary artery, resulting in an acquired stenosis.

The Potts shunt is a direct side-to-side anastomosis between the pulmonary artery and the descending aorta (Fig. 15-71). Complications include pulmonary vascular hypertension and distortion of the left pulmonary artery, the latter leading to acquired stenosis.

Systemic Vein to Pulmonary Artery Shunts

The Glenn shunt is a direct anastomosis between the superior vena cava and a pulmonary artery. This procedure does not cause ventricular volume overload. The classic Glenn

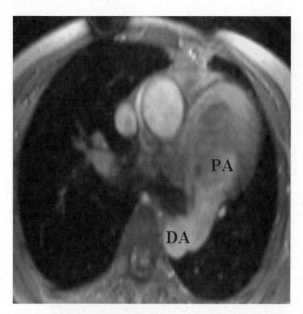

FIGURE 15-71 Potts shunt. MR angiogram scans show a patent connection between the descending aorta (*DA*) and main pulmonary artery (*PA*).

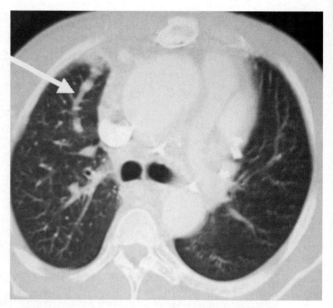

FIGURE 15-73 Arteriovenous malformation following a Glenn procedure. CT image shows an AVM in the right lower lobe.

anastomosis was between the superior vena cava and the distal end of the divided right pulmonary artery with ligation of the superior vena cava below the anastomosis (Fig. 15-72). Pulmonary AVMs were a common complication of this procedure due to the chronic systemic arterial desaturation (Fig. 15-73).

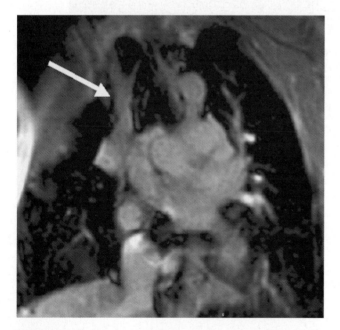

FIGURE 15-72 Glenn procedure. MR angiogram shows the Glenn shunt (*arrow*) extending from the superior vena cava to the right pulmonary artery.

The classic Glenn shunt was subsequently replaced by the bidirectional Glenn shunt, which is an end-to-side anastomosis of the divided superior vena cava to the undivided pulmonary artery. This allows both lungs to be perfused by the superior vena caval blood, which is hemodynamically more physiologic. Pulmonary AVMs are still a complication of this procedure.

The Fontan procedure involves diversion of all venous return to the pulmonary artery without the interposition of the right ventricle. The classic Fontan operation consisted of a valved conduit between the right atrium or right atrial appendage and left pulmonary artery. Subsequently, this was replaced by a direct anastomosis between the right atrium or right atrial appendage and the main pulmonary artery (Fig. 15-74). Following the original Fontan procedure, there has been the evolution of at least seven other variants of this procedure (152). More recent modifications include inferior vena cava to pulmonary artery anastomosis with a tube graft (extracardiac Fontan) and anastomosis of the inferior vena cava and superior vena cava to each other and then to the pulmonary artery (lateral tunnel or total cavopulmonary Fontan). Complications intrinsic to all Fontan procedures include narrowing or leaks in the Fontan graft (Fig. 15-75), ventricular outflow obstruction, and right atrial enlargement (153).

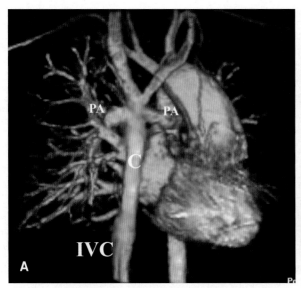

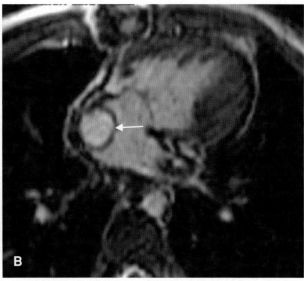

FIGURE 15-74 **Extra-cardiac Fontan procedure in a 10 year-old with pulmonary atresia and a single ventricle.** **A:** CEMRA depicts a conduit (C) connecting the inferior vena cava (IVC) and the pulmonary arteries (PA). **B:** Steady state free precession (SSFP) image shows the conduit passing through the right artium (*arrow*).

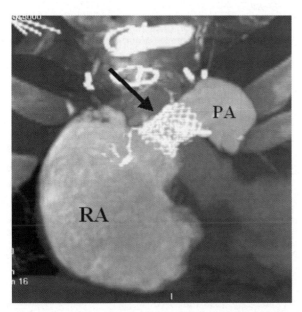

FIGURE 15-75 **Fontan procedure with postoperative graft stenosis treated with a stent.** CT performed to evaluate graft position shows a stent (*arrow*) between the right atrium (*RA*) and main pulmonary artery (*PA*). Note the marked right atrial enlargement characteristic of tricuspid atresia.

CONCLUSION

Advances in technology have led to a changing role for CT and MR imaging in the evaluation of the thoracic vasculature. Axial images often can make the diagnosis of aortic anomalies, but 3D reconstructions can provide additional information about the character and extent of a lesion. They also can help in surgical planning and can obviate more invasive conventional angiography.

REFERENCES

1. Gilkeson RC, Ciancibello L, Zahka K. Multidetector CT evaluation of congenital heart disease in pediatric and adult patients. *AJR Am J Roentgenol.* 2003;180:973–980.
2. Gup HW, Park I-S, Ko JK, et al. CT of congenital heart disease: normal anatomy and typical pathologic conditions. *Radiographics.* 2003;23:S147–S165.
3. Steiner RM, Reddy GP, Flicker S. Congenital cardiovascular disease in the adult patient. *J Thorac Imaging.* 2002;17:1–17.
4. King KM, Ghali WA, Faris PD, et al. Sex differences in outcomes after cardiac catheterization. *JAMA.* 2004;291: 1220–1225.
5. Prince MR, Arnoldus C, Frisoli JK. Nephrotoxicity of high-dose gadolinium compared with iodinated contrast. *J Magn Reson Imaging.* 1996;6:162–166.
6. Pereles FS. Thoracic aortic dissection and aneurysm: evaluation with nonenhanced true FISP MR angiography in less than 4 minutes. *Radiology.* 2002;223(1)(April):270–274.
7. Cohan RH, Ellis JH, Garner WL. Extravasation of radiographic contrast material: recognition, prevention and treatment. *Radiology.* 1996;200:593–604.
8. Stockberger SM, Hickling JA, Liang Y, et al. Spiral CT with ionic and nonionic contrast material: evaluation of patient motion and scan quality. *Radiology.* 1998;206:631–636.
9. Calhoun PS, Kuszyk B, Heath DG, et al. Three-dimensional volume rendering of spiral CT data: theory and method. *RadioGraphics.* 1999;19:745–764.
10. Cody DD. Image processing in CT. *RadioGraphics.* 2002;22: 1255–1268.
11. Lawler LP, Fishman EK. Multi-detector row CT of thoracic disease with emphasis on 3D volume rendering and CT angiography. *RadioGraphics.* 2001;21:1257–1273.
12. Napel S, Rubin GD, Jeffrey RB. STS-MIP: a new reconstruction technique for CT of the chest. *J Comput Assist Tomogr.* 1993;17:832–838.
13. Rubin GD. Data explosion: the challenge of multidetector CT. *Eur J Radiol.* 2000;36:74–81.
14. Bhalla S, Siegel MJ. Multislice computed tomography in pediatrics. In: Silverman PM, ed. *Multislice Computed Tomography: A Practical Approach to Clinical Protocols.* Philadelphia: Lippincott Williams & Wilkins; 2002:231–282.

15. Siegel MJ. Multiplanar and three-dimensional row CT of thoracic vessels and airways in the pediatric population. *Radiology.* 2003;229:641–650.

16. Siegel MJ. Pediatric chest applications. In: Fishman E, Jeffrey RB, eds. *Multislice Helical CT.* 3rd ed. Philadelphia: lippincott Williams & Wilkins; 2003:159–182.

17. Siegel MJ. Pediatric multislice CT of the chest. In: Schoeph UJ, ed. *Multidetector-Row CT of the Chest.* Heidelberg: Springer Verlag; 2003;371–390.

18. Pappas JN, Donnelly LF, Frush DP. Reduced frequency of sedation of young children using new multi-slice helical CT. *Radiology.* 2000;215:897–899.

19. Committee on Drugs, American Academy of Pediatrics. Guidelines for monitoring and management of pediatric patients during and after sedation for diagnostic and therapeutic procedures. *Pediatrics.* 1992;89:1110–1115.

20. American Society of Anesthesiologists Task Force. Practice guidelines for sedation and analgesia by non-anesthesiologists: a report by the American Society of Anesthesiologists Task Force on sedation and analgesia by non-anesthesiologists. *Anesthesiology.* 1996;84:459–471.

21. Siegel MJ. CT angiography: optimizing contrast use in pediatric patients. *Appl Radiol.* 2003;32(12):S43–S49.

22. Kaste SC, Young CW. Safe use of power injectors with central and peripheral venous access devices for pediatric CT. *Pediatr Radiol.* 1995;26:499–501.

23. Donnelly LF, Emery KH, Brody AS, et al. Minimizing radiation dose for pediatric body applications for single-detector helical CT: strategies at a large children's hospital. *AJR Am J Roentgenol.* 2001;176:303–306.

24. Pages J, Buls N, Osteaux M. CT doses in children: a multi-centre study. *Br J Radiol.* 2003;76:803–811.

25. Patterson A, Frush DP, Donnelly L. Helical CT of the body: are settings adjusted for pediatric patients? *AJR Am J Roentgenol.* 2001;176:297–301.

26. Slovis TL. The ALARA concept in pediatric CT: myth or reality. *Radiology.* 2002;223:5–6.

27. Siegel MJ, Suess C, Schmidt B, et al. Radiation dose and image quality in pediatric CT: effect of technical factors and phantom size and shape. *Radiology.* 2004;233: 515–522.

28. Prince MR, Yucel EK, Kaufman JA, et al. Dynamic gadolinium-enhanced three-dimensional abdominal MR arteriography. *J Magn Reson Imaging.* 1993;3:877–881.

29. Prince MR. Gadolinium-enhanced MR aortography. *Radiology.* 1994;191:155–164.

30. Lee VS, Flyer MA, Weinreb JC, et al. Image subtraction in gadolinium-enhanced MR imaging. *AJR Am J Roentgenol.* 1996;167:1427–1432.

31. Foo TK, Saranathan M, Prince MR, et al. Automated detection of bolus arrival and initiation of data acquisition in fast, three-dimensional, gadolinium-enhanced MR angiography. *Radiology.* 1997;203:275–280.

32. Earls JP, Rofsky NM, DeCorato DR, et al. Breath-hold single-dose gadolinium-enhanced three-dimensional MR aortography: usefulness of a timing examination and MR power injector. *Radiology.* 1996;201:705–710.

33. Fain SB, King BF, Breen JF, et al. High-spatial-resolution contrast-enhanced MR angiography of the renal arteries: A prospective comparison with digital subtraction angiography. *Radiology.* 2001;218:481–490.

34. Riederer SJ, Fain SB, Kruger DG, et al. Real-time imaging and triggering of 3D contrast-enhanced MR angiograms using MR fluoroscopy. *MAGMA.* 1999;8:196–206.

35. Riederer SJ, Fain SB, Kruger DG, et al. 3D contrast-enhanced MR angiography using fluoroscopic triggering and an elliptical centric view order. *Int J Card Imaging.* 1999;15:117–129.

36. De Cobelli F, Vanzulli A, Sironi S, et al. Renal artery stenosis: evaluation with breath-hold, three-dimensional, dynamic, gadolinium-enhanced versus three-dimensional, phase-contrast MR angiography. *Radiology.* 1997;205: 689–695.

37. De Cobelli F, Venturini M, Vanzulli A, et al. Renal arterial stenosis: prospective comparison of color Doppler US and breath-hold, three-dimensional, dynamic, gadolinium-enhanced MR angiography. *Radiology.* 2000;214:373–380.

38. Grist T. MR angiography of the renal arteries during a breath-hold using gadolinium-enhanced 3D TOF with k-space zero-filling and a contrast timing scan. *Proceedings of the Fourth Meeting of the International Society for Magnetic Resonance in Medicine.* Berkeley, CA; 1996: 163.

39. Mallouhi A, Schocke M, Judmaier W, et al. 3D MR angiography of renal arteries: Comparison of volume rendering and maximum intensity projection algorithms. *Radiology.* 2002;23:509–516.

40. Baskaran V, Pereles FS, Nemcek AA, Jr., et al. Gadolinium-enhanced 3D MR angiography of renal artery stenosis: a pilot comparison of maximum intensity projection, multiplanar reformatting, and 3D volume-rendering postprocessing algorithms. *Acad Radiol.* 2002;9:50–59.

41. Pettigrew RI. Dynamic cardiac MR imaging. Techniques and applications. *Radiol Clin North Am.* 1989;27: 1183–1203.

42. Haddad JL, Rofsky NM, Ambrosino MM, et al. T2-weighted MR imaging of the chest: comparison of electrocardiograph-triggered conventional and turbo spin-echo and nontriggered turbo spin-echo sequences. *J Magn Reson Imaging.* 1995;5:325–329.

43. Pettigrew RI, Oshinski JN, Chatzimavroudis G, et al. MRI techniques for cardiovascular imaging. *J Magn Reson Imaging.* 1999;10:590–601.

44. Semelka RC, Kelekis NL, Thomasson D, et al. HASTE MR imaging: description of technique and preliminary results in the abdomen. *J Magn Reson Imaging.* 1996;6: 698–699.

45. Stemerman DH, Krinsky GA, Lee VS, et al. Thoracic aorta: rapid black-blood MR imaging with half-Fourier rapid acquisition with relaxation enhancement with or without electrocardiographic triggering. *Radiology.* 1999;213:185–191.

46. Stehling MK, Holzknecht NG, Laub G, et al. Single-shot T1- and T2-weighted magnetic resonance imaging of the heart with black blood: preliminary experience. *MAGMA.* 1996;4(3–4):231–240.

47. Vignaux OB, Augui J, Coste J, et al. Comparison of single-shot fast spin-echo and conventional spin-echo sequences for MR imaging of the heart: initial experience. *Radiology.* 2001;219:545–550.

48. Le Roux P, Gilles RJ, McKinnon CG, et al. Optimized outer volume suppression for single-shot fast spin echo cardiac imaging. *J Magn Reson Imaging.* 1998;8:1022–1032.

49. Edelman RR, Chien D, Kim D. Fast selective black-blood MR imaging. *Radiology.* 1991;181:655–660.

50. Simonetti OP, Finn JP, Withe RD, et al. "Black blood" T2-weighted inversion recovery MR imaging of the heart. *Radiology.* 1996;199:49–57.

51. Stuber M, Botnar RM, Kissinger KV, et al. Free-breathing black-blood coronary MR angiography: initial results. *Radiology.* 2001;219:278–283.

52. Utz JA, Herfkens RJ, Heinsimer JA, et al. Valvular regurgitation: dynamic MR imaging. *Radiology.* 1988;168:91–94.

53. Atkinson DJ, Edelman RR. Cineangiography of the heart in a single breath hold with a segmented turboFLASH sequence. *Radiology.* 1991;178:357–360.

54. Edelman RR, Wallner B, Singer A, et al. Segmented turbo FLASH: method for breath-hold MR imaging of the liver with flexible contrast. *Radiology.* 1990;177:515–521.

55. Chien D, Atkinson D, Edelman RR. Strategies to improve contrast in turboFLASH imaging: reordered phase encoding and k-space segmentation. *J Magn Reson Imaging.* 1991;1:63–70.

56. Leung DA, Debatin JF, Wildermuth S, et al. Cardiac imaging: comparison of two-shot echo-planar imaging with fast segmented K-space and conventional gradient-echo cine acquisitions. *J Magn Reson Imaging.* 1995;5:684–688.

57. Reeder SB, Atalar E, Faranesh AZ, et al. Multi-echo segmented k-space imaging: an optimized hybrid sequence for ultrafast cardiac imaging. *Magn Reson Med.* 1999;41:375–385.

58. Epstein FH, Wolff SD, Arai AE. Segmented k-space fast cardiac imaging using an echo-train readout. *Magn Reson Med.* 1999;41:609–613.

59. Zur Y, Wood ML, Neuringer LJ. Motion-insensitive, steady-state free precession imaging. *Magn Reson Med.* 1990;16:444–459.

60. Oppelt A, Graumann R, Barfu H, et al. FISP—A new fast MRI sequence. *Electromedica.* 1986;54:15–18.

61. Haacke EM, Wielopolski PA, Tkack JA, et al. Steady-state free precession imaging in the presence of motion: application for improved visualization of the cerebrospinal fluid. *Radiology.* 1990;175:545–552.

62. Haacke EM, Tkach JA. Fast MR imaging: techniques and clinical applications. *Am J Radiol.* 1990;5:951–964.

63. Deimling M, Heid O. Magnetization prepared True FISP imaging [Abstract]. *Proceedings of the 2nd Annual Meeting of ISMRM.* San Francisco; 1994:495.

64. Bundy J, Simonetti O, Laub G, et al. Segmented TrueFISP cine imaging of the heart [Abstract]. *Proceedings of the 7th Annual Meeting of the ISMRM.* Philadelphia;1999: 1282.

65. Fang W, Pereles FS, Bundy J, et al. Evaluating LV function using real-time True FISP: A comparison with conventional MR techniques [Abstract]. *Proceedings of the 8th Annual Meeting of ISMRM.* Denver; 2000: 308.

66. Pereles FS, Kapoor V, Carr JC, et al. Usefulness of segmented trueFISP cardiac pulse sequence in evaluation of congenital and acquired adult cardiac abnormalities. *AJR Am J Roentgenol.* 2001;177:1155–1160.

67. Barkhausen J, Ruehm SG, Goyen M, et al. MR evaluation of ventricular function: true fast imaging with steady-state precession versus fast low-angle shot cine MR imaging: Feasibility study. *Radiology.* 2001;219:264–269.

68. Stillman AE, Wilke N, Jerosch-Herold M. Use of an intravascular T1 contrast agent to improve MR cine myocardial-blood pool definition in man. *J Magn Reson Imaging.* 1997;7:765–767.

69. Plein S, Bloomer TN, Ridgway JP, et al. Steady-state free precession magnetic resonance imaging of the heart: comparison with segmented k-space gradient-echo imaging. *J Magn Reson Imaging.* 2001;14:230–236.

70. Rebergen SA, van der Wall EE, Doornbos J, et al. Magnetic resonance measurement of velocity and flow: technique, validation, and cardiovascular applications. *Am Heart J.* 1993;126(6)(December):1439–1456.

71. Varaprasathan GA, Araoz PA, Higgins CB, et al. Quantification of flow dynamics in congenital heart disease: applications of velocity-encoded cine MR imaging. *Radiographics.* 2002;22(4)(July/August):895–905.

72. Sodickson DK, Manning WJ. Simultaneous acquisition of spatial harmonics (SMASH): fast imaging with radiofrequency coil arrays. *Magn Reson Med.* 1997;38(4):591–603.

73. Pruessmann KP, Weiger M, Scheidegger MB, et al. SENSE: sensitivity encoding for fast MRI. *Magn Reson Med.* 1999;42(5):952–962.

74. Brooks M, Zietman A. *Clinical Embryology. A Color Atlas and Text.* Boca Raton: CRC Press; 1998.

75. Sadler TW. *Langman's Medical Embryology.* 7th ed. Baltimore: Williams & Wilkins;1995.

76. Bisset GS. Anomalies of the great vessels. In: Siegel BA, Proto AV, eds. *Pediatric Disease (Fourth Series) Test and Syllabus.* Reston, VA: American College of Radiology; 1993:199–219.

77. Molina PL. Mediastinum: CT. In: Shirkhoda A, ed. *Variants and Pitfalls in Body Imaging.* Philadelphia: Lippincott Williams & Wilkins;2000:3–35.

78. Fisher RG, Sanchez-Torres M, Whigham CT, et al. Lumps and bumps that mimic acute aortic and brachiocephalic vessel injury. *Radiographics.* 1997;17:825–834.

79. Gotway MB, Dawn SK. Thoracic aorta imaging with multislice CT. *Radiol Clinics North Am.* 2003;41:521–543.

80. Ghaye B, Szapiro D, Dacher J-N, et al. Percutaneous ablation for atrial fibrillation: The role of cross-sectional imaging. *Radiographics.* 2003;23:S19–S33.

81. Lacomis JM, Wigginton W, Fuhrman C, et al. Multi-detector row CT of the left atrium and pulmonary veins before radio-frequency catheter ablation for atrial fibrillation. *Radiographics.* 2003;23:S35–S50.

82. VanDyke CW, White RD. Congenital abnormalities of the thoracic aorta presenting in the adult. *J Thorac Imaging.* 1994;9:230–245.

83. Remy-Jardin M, Remy J, Mayo JR, et al. Thoracic aorta. In: *CT Angiography of the Chest.* Philadelphia: Lippincott Williams & Wilkins;2001;29–50.

84. Katz M, Konen E, Rozenman, et al. Spiral CT and 3D image reconstruction of vascular rings and associated tracheo-bronchial anomalies. *J Comput Assist Tomogr.* 1995;19:564–568.

85. Lee EY, Siegel MJ, Hildebolt CF, et al. (in press). Multidetector CT evaluation of pediatric thoracic aortic anomalies: comparison of axial, multiplanar, and three-dimensional images. *AJR Am J Roentgenol.*

86. Raymond GS, Miller RM, Muller NL, et al. Congenital thoracic lesions that mimic neoplastic disease on chest radiographs of adults. *AJR Am J Roentgenol.* 1997;168:763–769.

87. Predey TS, McDonald V, Demos TC, et al. CT of congenital anomalies of the aortic arch. *Semin Roentgenol.* 1989;14:96–111.

88. Hopkins KL, Patrick LE, Simoneaux SF, et al. Pediatric great vessel anomalies: Initial clinical experience with spiral CT angiography. *Radiology.* 1996;200:811–815.

89. Kaemmerer H. Aortic coarctation and interrupted aortic arch. In: Gatzoulis MA, Wevbb GD, Daubeney PEF, eds. *Adult Congenital Heart Disease.* Edinburgh: Churchill Livingstone; 2003:253–264.

90. Becker C, Soppa C, Fink U, et al. Spiral CT angiography and 3D reconstruction in patients with aortic coarctation. *Eur Radiol.* 1997;7:1473–1477.

91. Mohiaddin RH, Kilner PT, Rees S, et al. Magnetic resonance volume flow and jet velocity mapping in aortic coarctation. *J Am Coll Cardiol.* 1993;22:1515–1521.

92. Araoz PA, Reddy GP, Tarnoff H, et al. MR findings of collateral circulation are more accurate measures of hemodynamic significance than arm-leg blood pressure gradient after repair of coarctation of the aorta. *J Magn Reson Imaging.* 2003;17(2)(February):177–183.

93. Maron B, Humphries J, Rowe R, et al. Prognosis of surgically corrected coarctation of the aorta: A 20-year postoperative appraisal. *Circulation.* 1973;47:119–126.

94. Swan L, Wilson N, Houston A, et al. The long-term management of the patient with an aortic coarctation repair. *Eur Heart J.* 1998;19:382–386.

95. Foster E. Reoperation for aortic coarctation. *Ann Thorac Surg.* 1984;38:81–89.

96. Sweeney M, Walker W, Duncan J, et al. Reoperation for aortic coarctation: Techniques, results, and indications for various approaches. *Ann Thorac Surg.* 1985;40:46–49.

97. Cohen M, Fuster V, Steele P, et al. Coarctation of the aorta: long-term follow-up and prediction of outcome after surgical correction. *Circulation.* 1989;80:840–845.

98. Connolly HM, Schaff HV, Izhar U, et al. Posterior pericardial ascending-to-descending aortic bypass: an alternative surgical approach for complex coarctation of the aorta. *Circulation.* 2001;104:I133–I137.

99. Almeida de Oliveira S, Lisboa LA, Dallan LA, et al. Extraanatomic aortic bypass for repair of aortic arch coarctation via sternotomy: midterm clinical and magnetic resonance imaging results. *Ann Thorac Surg.* 2003;76(6): 1962–1966.

100. Celoria CG, Patton RB. Congenital absence of the aortic arch. *Am Heart J.* 1959;58:407–413.

101. Connelly M. Common arterial trunk. In: Gatzoulis MA, Wevbb GD, Daubeney PEF, eds. *Adult Congenital Heart Disease*. Edinburgh: Churchill Livingstone; 2003:265–271.
102. Jacobs ML. Congenital heart surgery nomenclature and database project: truncus arteriosus. *Ann Thorac Surg*. 2000;69:S50–S55.
103. Amplatz K, Moller JH. *Radiology of Congenital Heart Disease*. St. Louis: Mosby–Year Book; 1993:315–320.
104. Stella VB, Toutouzas P. Patent arterial duct and aortopulmonary window. In: Gatzoulis MA, Wevbb GD, Daubeney PEF, eds. *Adult Congenital Heart Disease*. Edinburgh: Churchill Livingstone; 2003:247–252.
105. Morgan-Hughes GJ, Marshall AJ, Roobottom C. Morphologic assessment of patent ductus arteriosus in adults using retrospectively ECG-gated multidetector CT. *AJR Am J Roentgenol*. 2003;181:749–754.
106. Remy-Jardin M, Remy J, Mayo JR, et al. Vascular anomalies of the lung. In: *CT Angiography of the Chest*. Philadelphia: Lippincott Williams & Wilkins; 2001:97–114.
107. Bouros D, Pare P, Panagou P, et al. The varied manifestation of pulmonary artery agenesis in adulthood. *Chest*. 1995;18:244–247.
108. Mahnken AH, Wildberger JE, Spuntrup E, et al. Unilateral absence of the left pulmonary artery associated with coronary-to-bronchial artery anastomosis. *J Thorac Imaging*. 2000;17:187–190.
109. Zylak CJ, Eyler WR, Spizarny DL, et al. Developmental lung anomalies in the adult: radiologic-pathologic correlation. *Radiographics*. 2002;22:S25–S43.
110. Gupta H, Mayo-Smith WW, Mainiero MB, et al. Helical CT of pulmonary vascular abnormalities. *AJR Am J Roentgenol*. 2002;178:487–492.
111. Kreutzer J, Landzberg MJ, Preminger TJ, et al. Isolated peripheral pulmonary artery stenoses in the adult. *Circulation*. 1996;93:1417–1423.
112. Procacci C, Residori E, Bertocco M, et al. Left pulmonary artery sling in the adult: case report and review of literature. *Cardiovasc Intervent Radiol*. 1993;16:388–391.
113. Park HS, Im JG, Jung JW, et al. Anomalous left pulmonary artery with complete cartilaginous ring. *J Comput Assist Tomogr*. 1997;21:478–480.
114. Gossage JR, Kanj G. Pulmonary arteriovenous malformations. *Am J Respir Crit Care Med*. 1998;158:643–661.
115. Shovlin C, Letarte M. Hereditary haemorrhagic telangiectasis and pulmonary arteriovenous malformations: issues in clinical management and review of pathogenic mechanisms. *Thorax*. 1999;54:714–729.
116. Remy J, Remy-Jardin M, Giraud F, et al. Angioarchitecture of pulmonary arteriovenous malformations: clinical utility of three-dimensional helical CT. *Radiology*. 1994;191:657–664.
117. Remy J, Remy-Jardin M, Wattinee L, et al. Pulmonary arteriovenous malformations: evaluation with CT of the chest before and after treatment. *Radiology*. 1992;182:809–816.
118. Hoffman LV, Kuszyk BS, Mitchell SE, et al. Angioarchitecture of pulmonary arteriovenous malformation: characterization using volume-rendered 3D CT angiography. *Cardiovasc Intervent Radiol*. 2000;23:165–170.
119. Silverman JM, Julien PJ, Herfkens RJ, et al. Magnetic resonance imaging evaluation of pulmonary vascular malformations. *Chest*. 1994;106:1333–1338.
120. Gossage JR, Kanj G. Pulmonary arteriovenous malformations. A state of the art review. *Am J Respir Crit Care Med*. 1998;158:643–661.
121. Dinsmore BJ, Gefter WB, Hatabu H, et al. Pulmonary arteriovenous malformation: diagnosis by gradient-echo MR imaging. *J Comput Assist Tomogr*. 1990;14:918–923.
122. Rotondo A, Scialpi M, Scapati C. Pulmonary arteriovenous malformation: evaluation by MR angiography. *AJR Am J Roentgenol*. 1997;168:847–849.
123. Vrachliotis TG, Kostaki GB, Kirsch MJ, et al. Contrast-enhanced MRA in pre-embolization assessment of a pulmonary arteriovenous malformation. *J Magn Reson Imaging*. 1997;7:434–436.
124. Meaney JF, Johansson LO, Ahlstrom H, et al. Pulmonary magnetic resonance angiography. *J Magn Reson Imaging*. 1999;10:326–338.
125. Prince MR, Yucel EK, Kaufman JA, et al. Dynamic gadolinium-enhanced three-dimensional abdominal MR arteriography. *J Magn Reson Imaging*. 1993;3:877–881.
126. Steiner P, McKinnon GC, Romanowski B, et al. Contrast-enhanced, ultrafast 3D pulmonary MR angiography in a single breath-hold: initial assessment of imaging performance. *J Magn Reson Imaging*. 1997;7:177–182.
127. Meaney JF, Weg JG, Chenevert TL, et al. Diagnosis of pulmonary embolism with magnetic resonance angiography. *N Engl J Med*. 1997;336:1422–1427.
128. Goyen M, Ruehm SG, Jagenburg A, et al. Pulmonary arteriovenous malformation: characterization with time-resolved ultrafast 3D MR angiography. *J Magn Reson Imaging*. 2001;13(3)(March):458–460.
129. Zwetsch B, Wicky S, Meuli R, et al. Three-dimensional image reconstruction of partial anomalous pulmonary venous return to the superior vena cava. *Chest*. 1995;108:1743–1735.
130. Dillon EH, Camputaro C. Partial anomalous pulmonary venous drainage of the left upper lobe vs duplication of the superior vena cava: distinction based on CT findings. *AJR Am J Roentgenol*. 1993;160:375–379.
131. Van Praagh S, Carrera ME, Sanders S, et al. Partial or total direct pulmonary venous drainage to the right atrium due to malposition of septum primum. *Chest*. 1995;107:1488–1498.
132. Ko K-H, Goo JM, Im J-G, et al. Systemic arterial supply to the lungs in adults: spiral CT findings. *Radiographics*. 2001;21:387–402.
133. Konen E, Raviv-Zilka L, Cohen RA, et al. Congenital pulmonary venolobar syndrome: Spectrum of helical CT findings with emphasis on computerized reformatting. *RadioGraphics*. 2003;23:1175–1184.
134. Woodring JH, Howard TS, Kanga JF. Congenital pulmonary venolobar syndrome revisited. *Radiographics*. 1994;14:349–369.
135. Remy-Jardin M, Remy J, Mayo JR, et al. Superior vena cava syndromes. In: *CT Angiography of the Chest*. Philadelphia: Lippincott Williams & Wilkins; 2001:130–139.
136. Bass JE, Redqine MD, Kramer LA, et al. Spectrum of congenital anomalies of the inferior vena cava: cross-sectional imaging findings. *Radiographics*. 2000;20:639–652.
137. Felker RE, Tonkin IL. Imaging of pulmonary sequestration. *AJR Am J Roentgenol*. 190;154:241–249.
138. Bertsch G, Markert T, Hahn D, et al. Intralobar lung sequestration with systemic coronary arterial supply. *Eur Radiol*. 1999;9:1324–1326.
139. Kamata S, Sawai T, Nose K, et al. Extralobar pulmonary sequestration with venous drainage to the portal vein: a case report. *Pediatr Radiol*. 2000; 30:492–494.
140. Frazier AA, Rosado de Christenson ML, Stocker JT, et al. Intralobar sequestration: radiologic-pathologic correlation. *RadioGraphics*. 1997;17:725–745.
141. Rosado-de-Christenson ML, Frazier AA, Stocker JT, et al. Extralobar sequestration: radiologic-pathologic correlation. *RadioGraphics*. 1993; 13:425–441.
142. Franco J, Aliaga R, Domingo ML, et al. Diagnosis of pulmonary sequestration by spiral CT angiography. *Thorax*. 1998;53:1089–1092.
143. Frush DP, Donnelly LF. Pulmonary sequestration spectrum: a new spin with helical CT. *AJR Am J Roentgenol*. 1997;169:679–682.
144. Ko SF, Ng SH, Lee TY, et al. Noninvasive imaging of bronchopulmonary sequestration. *AJR Am J Roentgenol*. 2000;175:1005–1012.
145. Lee E, Siegel MJ, Sierra LM, et al. (in press). Original report: evaluation of angioarchitecture of pulmonary sequestration in pediatric patients using multidetector CT angiography. *AJR Am J Roentgenol*.

146. Ko SF, Ng SH, Lee TY, et al. Anomalous systemic arterialization to normal basal segments of the left lower lobe: helical CT and CTA findings. *J Comput Assist Tomogr*. 2000;24:971–976.

147. Miyake H, Hori Y, Takeoka H, et al. Systemic arterial supply to normal basal segments of the left lung: characteristic features on chest radiography and CT. *AJR Am J Roentgenol*. 1998;171:387–392.

148. Do J-H, Goo JM, Im J-G, et al. Systemic arterial supply to the lungs in adults: spiral CT findings. *Radiographics*. 2001;21:387–402.

149. Deffebach ME, Charan NB, Lakshminarayan S, et al. The bronchial circulation: small, but a vital attribute of the lung. *Am Rev Respir Dis*. 1987;135:463–481.

150. Furose M, Saito K, Kunieda E, et al. Bronchial arteries: CT demonstration with arteriographic correlation. *Radiology*. 1987;162:393–398.

151. Murayama S, Hashiguchi N, Murakami J, et al. Helical CT imaging of bronchial arteries with curved reformation technique in comparison with selective bronchial arteriography: preliminary report. *J Comput Assist Tomogr*. 1996;20:749–755.

152. Mavroudis C, Backer CL, Deal BJ. Venous shunts and the Fontan circulation in adult congenital heart disease. In: Gatzoulis MA, Wevbb GD, Daubeney PEF, eds. *Adult Congenital Heart Disease*. Edinburgh: Churchill Livingstone; 2003:79–83.

153. Freedom RM, Li J, Yoo S-J. The complications following the Fontan operation. In: Gatzoulis MA, Wevbb GD, Daubeney PEF, eds. *Adult Congenital Heart Disease*. Edinburgh: Churchill Livingstone; 2003:85–91.

Pulmonary Vasculature

U. Joseph Schoepf
James F. M. Meaney

SPECTRUM AND PREVALENCE OF DISEASES

Pulmonary vascular conditions span the gamut from common, everyday disorders to rare but important medical problems. By far and away, the clinical suspicion of pulmonary embolism (PE) drives the most diagnostic concern for imaging the pulmonary vasculature. Indeed, the mortality rate associated with PE exceeds 15% in the first 3 months after diagnosis and brings one of the most common medical problems in the Western world (1,2).

However, other pulmonary vascular disorders are increasingly recognized, such as pulmonary hypertension (PH) with a wide array of etiologies, ranging from idiopathic to chronic thromboembolic PH (3), various types of arteritis (4), large vessel arteritis such as Takayasu disease (4), and pulmonary arteriovenous malformations (5) (often in the context of systemic disorders such as polyarteritis nodosa, Churg-Strauss syndrome, and Wegener's disease) and a host of other less common vascular pathologies. Furthermore, some vascular assessment may be required prior to novel interventional therapy, such as radio frequency ablation for heart rhythm disorders or its complications. (6,7)

GLOBAL VIEW OF UNIQUE ASPECTS AND CONSIDERATIONS OF IMAGING OF THIS ORGAN SYSTEM

The pulmonary vasculature has a wide range of vessel caliber; a complex, multiplanar course; and is impacted by respiratory and cardiac motion. In contradiction to most vascular beds in which atherosclerotic disease predominates, the pulmonary vessels are dominated by embolic disease.

WHAT DO COMPUTED TOMOGRAPHY AND MAGNETIC RESONANCE BRING OVER OTHER IMAGING AND NONIMAGING DIAGNOSTIC TESTING?

The maturation of computed tomography (CT) and magnetic resonance (MR) technology has dramatically modified the evaluation of pulmonary arteries in routine clinical practice. Prior to imaging of the pulmonary vasculature with these approaches being the routine, an assessment of pulmonary vascular disorders was based either on a noninvasive, indirect method: ventilation-perfusion scintigraphy; or on an invasive and sparingly used study, that is, pulmonary angiography.

The cross-sectional information available from CT and MR provides direct visualization of the vasculature and parenchyma, improving greatly on the informational content from nuclear medicine with newer CT and MR tech-

niques capturing pulmonary perfusion (8–13). Furthermore, CT and MR present a minimal risk to patients when compared with that associated with conventional pulmonary angiography.

IMAGING STRATEGIES

Advantages of Computed Tomography for Pulmonary Vasculature Imaging

There are several inherent advantages that made CT the preferred modality for imaging the pulmonary vasculature. First and foremost, the ability to directly visualize thrombus with cross-sectional technique in a rapid manner is the attribute that has propelled its widespread use in patients who are suspected of having PE. In addition to the direct visualization of thrombus (Fig. 16-1), both mediastinal and parenchymal structures are well evaluated. Furthermore, other manifestations of PE can readily be visualized with spiral CT, including parenchymal infarction (Fig. 16-2), pleural effusion, vascular remodeling (dilation, pouches, thrombotic wall thickening), and oligemia.

Alternative diagnoses, some potentially life-threatening, such as aortic dissection, pneumonia, lung cancer, and pneumothorax, are readily established with CT (14–16).

Multidetector-row spiral CT offers fast and high-resolution imaging and, at the time of this writing, close to 4,000 units are installed in the United States. With current generation of 4-slice, 16-slice, and 64-slice multidetector-row

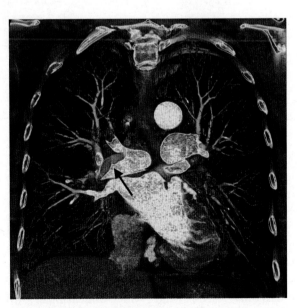

FIGURE 16-1 Contrast-enhanced (CE) multidetector-row CT scan in a 54-year-old woman presenting to the emergency department with acute chest pain. Volume rendering seen from an anterior coronal perspective shows extensive acute PE (*arrow*) in the right main pulmonary artery.

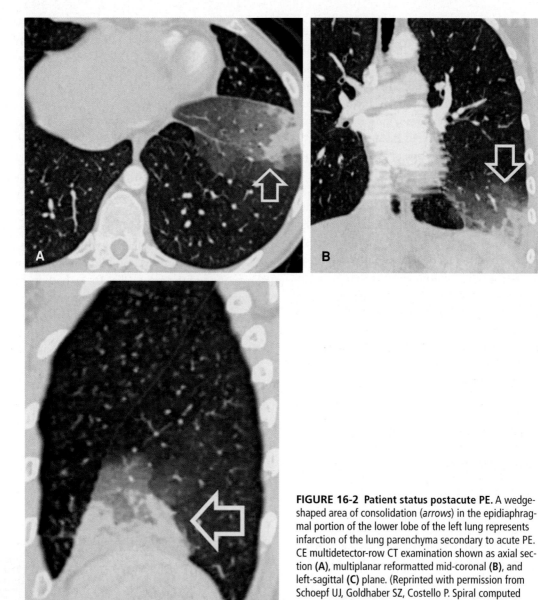

FIGURE 16-2 Patient status postacute PE. A wedge-shaped area of consolidation (*arrows*) in the epidiaphragmal portion of the lower lobe of the left lung represents infarction of the lung parenchyma secondary to acute PE. CE multidetector-row CT examination shown as axial section (**A**), multiplanar reformatted mid-coronal (**B**), and left-sagittal (**C**) plane. (Reprinted with permission from Schoepf UJ, Goldhaber SZ, Costello P. Spiral computed tomography for acute pulmonary embolism. *Circulation.* 2004;109:2160–2167.)

spiral CT scanners, the entire chest can be imaged with 1-mm or submillimeter resolution within a short single breath-hold; in the case of 64-slice CT, that breath-hold can be less than 5 seconds (Table 16-1).

Shorter breath-hold times benefit patients with underlying lung disease and reduce the percentage of non-diagnostic CT scans (17). High-resolution multidetector-row spiral CT data can be transformed easily for two-dimensional (2D) and three-dimensional (3D) visualization. This may, in some instances, improve diagnosis but is generally of greater importance for conveying information on localization and extent of disease in a more intuitive display format.

Technical Considerations, Problems, and Limitations of Computed Tomography

Contrast Media Injection and Artifacts

Despite advances in CT technology, there are still several factors that can render CT pulmonary angiography inconclusive. The most common reasons for nondiagnostic CT studies are poor contrast opacification of pulmonary vessels, patient motion, and increased image noise due to excessive patient obesity.

The advent of multidetector-row CT necessitates an extensive revision of contrast material injection protocols. Faster acquisition times allow scanning during maximal

TABLE 16-1

Comparison of Acquisition Parameters for Computed Tomographic Pulmonary Angiography Using Different Scanners

Parameter	Single-slice CTPA	EBCT CTPA	4-DCT CTPA	16-DCT CTPA	64-DCT CTPA
Collimation	2 to 3 mm, depending on patient breath-hold capability	3 mm	4 × 1 to 2 mm, depending on gantry rotation speed	16 × 0.75 mm	64 × 0.6 mm
Reconstructed section thickness	1 to 2 mm	1.5 mm	1 mm	1 mm	0.75 mm
Scan time	≈30 seconds	≈30 seconds	≈25 seconds	≈15 seconds	≈8 seconds
Tube current	200 mA	640 mA	120 mA	300 mA	250 mA
Contrast media	120 mL @ 4 mL/ second (300 to 400 mg iodine/mL)	120 mL @ 4 mL/ second (300 to 400 mg iodine/mL)	120 mL @ 4 mL/ second (300 to 400 mg iodine/mL)	100 mL @ 5 mL/ second (300 to 400 mg iodine/mL)	80 mL @ 5 mL/second (300 to 400 mg iodine/mL)
Radiation exposure	≈3 mSv	≈2 mSv	≈5 mSv	≈5 mSv, lower with automatic tube current modulation	≈5 mSv, lower with automatic tube current modulation

CTPA, computed tomographic pulmonary angiography; EBCT, electron-beam computed tomography; DCT, detector computed tomography.

contrast opacification of the pulmonary vessels but pose an increased challenge for precise timing of the contrast bolus.

Strategies that have the potential to improve the delivery of contrast media for high and consistent vascular enhancement during CT pulmonary angiography currently include use of a test bolus or automated bolus triggering techniques (18,19). Saline flushing has been used for effective utilization of contrast media and for reduction of streak artifacts arising from dense contrast material in the superior vena cava. Multiphasic injection protocols have proved beneficial for general CT angiography (CTA) (19) but have not been scientifically evaluated for the pulmonary circulation.

Motion artifacts due to patient respiration or transmitted cardiac pulsation can adversely impact diagnostic outcome. The shorter breath-holds feasible with multidetector-row CT reduce respiratory motion artifacts and facilitate investigation of dyspneic patients (20). Similarly, artifacts arising from transmitted cardiac pulsation appear amenable to improved temporal resolution with fast CT acquisition techniques (19).

Electrocardiogram (ECG) synchronization of CT scan acquisition effectively reduces cardiac pulsation artifacts. Thus, the evaluation of cardiac structures, the thoracic aorta, and pulmonary structures is improved. With retrospective ECG-gating and the previous generation of 4-slice multidetector-row CT scanners, the relatively long scan duration inherent to data oversampling limited the achiev-

able spatial resolution. Thus, high-resolution acquisition could only be achieved for relatively small volumes (e.g., the coronary arterial tree) but not for extended coverage of the entire chest.

However, with 16-slice multidetector-row CT, the entire thorax can be covered with submillimeter resolution in a single breath-hold while using retrospective ECG-gating. In this manner, potential diagnostic pitfalls arising from cardiac motion can be avoided. It still remains to be seen whether this technology increases the accuracy of CT for detecting small emboli in the vicinity of the heart, as would be predicted.

Radiation Dose

When high-quality multidetector computed tomography (MDCT) establishes an unequivocal diagnosis, the overall radiation burden to patients can be reduced by eliminating the need for further workup with other ionizing radiation tests. However, it is important to consider the impact of MDCT on radiation exposure.

As an example, if a 4-slice multidetector-row CT protocol with 4×1-mm collimation is chosen to replace a single-detector CT protocol based on a 1×5-mm collimation, the increase in radiation dose ranges between 30% and 100%. Similar increases in radiation dose, however, are not to be expected with 16-slice multidetector-CT technology and submillimeter resolution capabilities. The addition of detector elements should improve tube output utilization compared with current 4-slice CT scanners and reduce the ratio of excess radiation dose that does not contribute to actual image generation.

Technologies that modulate and adapt tube output relative to the geometry and x-ray attenuation of the scanned object, that is, the patient, can substantially reduce the dose without compromising diagnostic quality. However, the effect of such devices on the diagnostic performance has not been scientifically evaluated in some specific scenarios (21).

A critical factor for ensuring responsible utilization of MDCT is the increased awareness of the protocols that can be used by technologists and radiologists. For example, it has been shown that diagnostic quality of chest CT is not compromised if tube output is adjusted to the body type of the individual patient. Furthermore, when the concept of volume imaging is applied to MDCT, an effective trade-off between increased spatial resolution and image noise can result.

Given the great flexibility and diagnostic benefit that a high-resolution, near-isotropic multidetector-row CT data set provides, radiologists are increasingly willing to compromise on the degree of image noise in an individual axial thin-section image in order to keep radiation dose within reasonable limits.

Data Management

Although multidetector-row CT increases diagnostic capabilities, the massive amount of data generated by this technique creates significant strain on image analysis and archiving systems. A high-resolution 16-slice multidetector-row CT study in a patient with suspected PE, for instance, routinely results in 500 to 600 individual axial images from which the diagnosis is most commonly established.

Interpretation of such large volume studies is only feasible by use of digital workstations that allow viewing in "scroll-through" or "cine" mode. Large and accessible storage capacities are an essential requirement for successful routine performance of multidetector-row CT in a busy clinical environment. In the future, development of dedicated computer-aided detection algorithms may be helpful for the identification of PE in large volume multidetector-row CT data sets (Fig. 16-3).

However, extensive or isolated abnormal findings as well as normal pulmonary vasculature can be visualized in an alluring, comprehensive manner by means of 3D reconstructions generated from high-resolution multidetector-row CT.

3D visualization of multidetector-row CT data may aid diagnosis in some instances and help to avoid diagnostic pitfalls (e.g., for the correct interpretation of hilar lym-

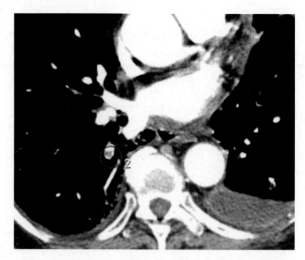

FIGURE 16-3 Prototype software platform for the automated detection of embolic filling defects at CT pulmonary angiography. An isolated peripheral filling defect in the right lower lobe of a patient with acute PE is automatically detected by the computer software (marked by a *red circle*).

phatic tissue adjacent to central pulmonary arteries in patients suspected of having PE). Furthermore, focal lung disease can be accurately diagnosed by use of MIP reconstructions that beneficially "condense" large volume multidetector-row CT data sets.

Magnetic Resonance Imaging and Magnetic Resonance Angiography

At the time when the early experience with CT was showing great promise for vascular assessment, there was widespread pessimism regarding the use of noncontrast magnetic resonance imaging (MRI) and magnetic resonance angiography (MRA) (22–27). Diaphragmatic and cardiac motion artifacts, long scan times, susceptibility artifacts at air-tissue interfaces, and poor contrast between flowing blood and emboli limited these early approaches.

The introduction of contrast-enhanced (CE) MR techniques circumvented many of those limitations, enabling high-quality diagnostic images of the pulmonary arteries to be generated during one breath-hold (28–30) (Fig. 16-4).

Initial studies reported good success for detection of PE compared with catheter angiography to the segmental level, but in common with early CTA, spatial resolution was suboptimal and detection of PE in smaller subsegmental arteries was limited (28–30).

Recent improvements in gradient technology, introduction of parallel imaging techniques, and use of optimized imaging protocols have generated a technique that now matches the spatial and temporal resolution of MDCT (Fig. 16-5) but that still lags behind that of digital subtraction angiography (DSA) (30).

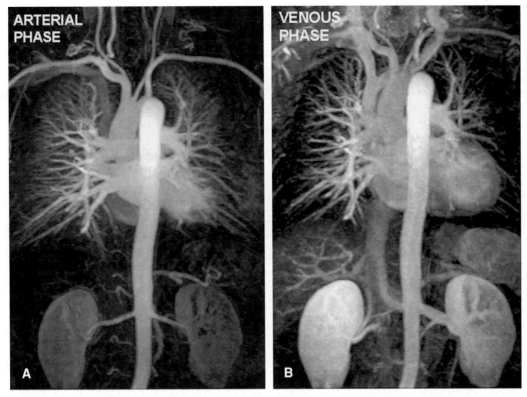

FIGURE 16-4 CE MRA/venography. A,B: Because of the short transit time from pulmonary artery to pulmonary vein, both arteries and veins are typically depicted on 3D data sets unless a time-resolved approach is employed. Therefore, even on CE MRA examinations "timed" to the pulmonary arteries **(A)**, the pulmonary veins are also well depicted as demonstrated, as they are also on the "venous" phase **(B)**.

Acquisition parameters for pulmonary MRA and MR perfusion imaging are different among institutions and depend on the clinical scenario and scanner capabilities. Nevertheless, some sequences constitute the basis of the most widely accepted protocols. A flow rate of 2 mL/second is generally used to ensure a longer imaging time and more homogeneous contrast enhancement. First, a test-bolus sequence takes place to determine the exact circulation time of the contrast material bolus from the injection site to the region of interest. Then, breath-hold pre- and post-contrast 3D fast MR imaging is performed in the preferred orientation (in most cases, in the coronal or oblique sagittal plane) by using parallel imaging techniques whenever possible.

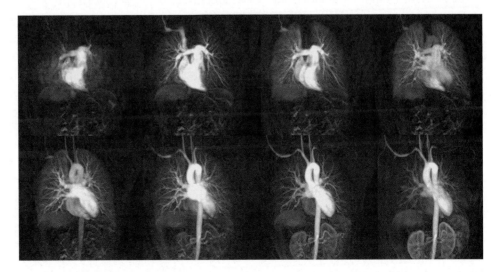

FIGURE 16-5 Coronal MIP images from 3D time-resolved MRA at 3T (2/0.84; flip angle, 17°), with a sample interval of 1.5 seconds show sequential filling of pulmonary arteries, pulmonary parenchyma, and systemic arteries. (Reprinted with permission from Nael K, Michaely HJ, Kramer U, et al. Pulmonary circulation: Contrast-enhanced 3.0T MR angiography-initial results. *Radiology* 2006;240:858–868.)

TABLE 16-2

Example of Acquisition Parameters for Pulmonary Magnetic Resonance Angiography and Magnetic Resonance Perfusion Imaging

Modality (MRA)	TR/TE (msec)	Spatial Resolution (mm)	Section Thickness (mm)	Number of Sections	Slab Thickness (mm)	Number of Phases	Acquisition Time per Phase (sec)	Total Acquisition Time (sec)
Without parallel acquisition	3.3/1.2	1.4 × 0.7 × 2.0	2.0	64	128	1	21	21
With parallel acquisition	2.9/1.2	1.0 × 0.7 × 1.6	1.6	88	144	1	22	22

MRA, magnetic resonance angiography; TR, repetition time; TE, echo time.
Reprinted with permission from Hatabu H, Tadamura E, Levin DL, et al. Quantitative assessment of pulmonary perfusion with dynamic contrast-enhanced MRI. *Magn Reson Med.* 1999;42:1033–1038.

Fast imaging is essentially accomplished with short repetition time (TR) (typically 5 msec) and short echo time (TE) (typically 2 msec) 3D sequences. With strong gradients, extremely short TR/TE combinations can be achieved (e.g., 2.9/1.2 msec, respectively). Generally speaking, a flip angle of 15 to 25 degrees will be satisfactory for these sequences. Table 16-2 presents further details of acquisition parameters proposed by Nikolaou et al. (31) for patients suspected of having pulmonary arterial hypertension.

Acquisition time for one 3D data set is usually in the range of 15 to 30 seconds. The data set is acquired during breath-hold (inspiration), and the k-space readout scheme is usually centrically reordered. Because of the asymmetric sequential k-space readout scheme, image acquisition should begin a few seconds before the estimated arrival of the contrast material bolus. Precontrast MR angiograms, acquired before the administration of the larger amount of contrast material, are then subtracted from the postcontrast images, and for image analysis, multiplanar reformation (MPR) and maximum-intensity projection (MIP) reconstructions of the complete data are obtained.

Other Magnetic Resonance Imaging Techniques for Pulmonary Vasculature Assessment

Initial attempts with MR imaging to evaluate the pulmonary arteries solely focused on "first-pass" data with an injection of an extra-cellular contrast agent. More recently, investigators have reported several other techniques as follows:

1. Perfusion imaging
2. Time-resolved MRA
3. Blood-pool contrast agents
4. True fast imaging with steady-state precession (FISP) MRA
5. Direct thrombus imaging

Perfusion Imaging and Ventilation

Phase-contrast techniques (8) have given way to CE acquisitions (9,10,32,33) and potentially to new techniques such as arterial spin labeling (11). Despite the fact that perfusion imaging with isotope scintigraphy is limited for the diagnosis of PE, perfusion imaging with MRI offers substantial benefit in terms of spatial and temporal resolution (Fig. 16-6). Several studies compare scintigraphic and MR pulmonary perfusion in a variety of disorders. Although results with both techniques are similar, reproducibility is significantly greater with MR. Differential lung perfusion, which may be of value in assessing patients with chronic obstructive pulmonary disease prior to and after lung volume reduction surgery, is also well demonstrated with MR lung perfusion (12,34–37).

Time-resolved Magnetic Resonance Angiography

Because of the short transit time from pulmonary artery to pulmonary vein, some researchers have implemented extremely rapid imaging of the pulmonary vasculature, in an effort to capture an arterial phase (38,39) (Fig. 16-7). In order to achieve this goal, however, images must be acquired in 4 seconds or less per scan, thus requiring lower resolution than might otherwise have been employed. With this approach, a "clean" arterial phase is acquired in favor of a higher resolution scan that can depict subsegmental arteries. Often, in-plane resolution is sacrificed to achieve a sufficient combination of in-plane spatial resolution and rapid temporal resolution. That will limit the number of useful projections that can be generated.

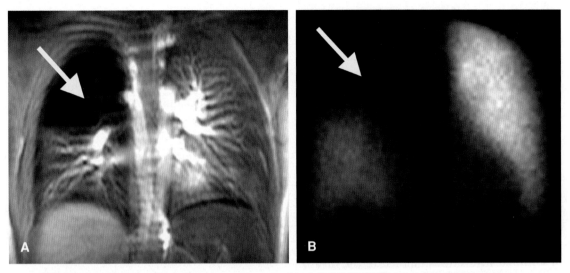

FIGURE 16-6 A 65-year-old male patient with upper right lobe PE. A: Gadolinium-enhanced MR imaging shows perfusion defect (*arrow*) involving the upper lobe of the right lung. **B:** The same perfusion defect (*arrow*) is confirmed by Tc 99m-macroaggregated albumin scan. (Courtesy of Qun Chen, PhD, New York University Medical Center.)

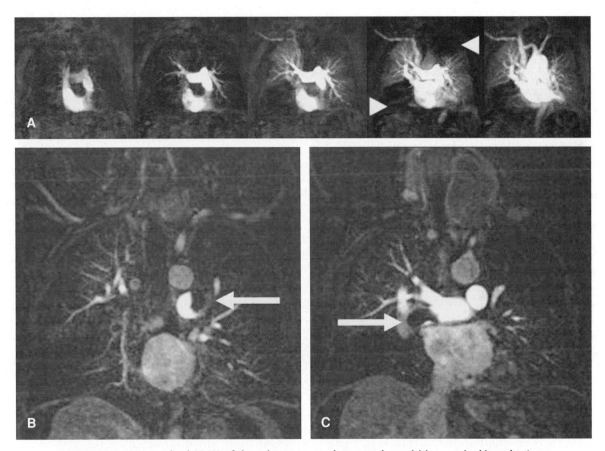

FIGURE 16-7 Time-resolved CE MR of the pulmonary vasculature, each acquisition acquired in under 4 seconds. Note sequential enhancement of the pulmonary arteries and veins during a single breath-hold or several shorter breath-holds. There is a perfusional deficit in the lower right and upper left pulmonary lobes (*arrowheads* in **A**) secondary to PE (*arrows* in **B** and **C**). (Courtesy of S. Schoenberg, MD, Munich, Germany.)

Blood-pool Imaging

Currently, no blood-pool contrast agent has been released commercially within the United States, but in 2006, MS-325 received a license for vascular use in Europe (40–42). Blood-pool agents offer a promising role in pulmonary vascular diagnosis, especially in situations where higher resolution is required. To date, no prospective comparative study of blood-pool agent compared with DSA has been performed. Because of their long vascular persistence time, repeated breath-hold studies targeted to a suspected abnormal area can be performed at higher resolution after an initial screening examination performed at lower resolution (40–42). Alternatively, high-resolution breath-hold images of the entire pulmonary vasculature can be performed in multiple acquisitions tailored to the breath-hold capability of the patient. Another possibility that is attractive for patients with severe respiratory compromise is the use of navigator-echo techniques to eliminate the need for breath-holding. The long vascular persistence of blood-pool agents offers the potential to detect clots within the lower extremities (43) in patients with suspected PE.

True-FISP Imaging

True-FISP imaging is a "balanced" technique that depicts vessels as bright structures and shows promise for diagnosis of both deep venous thrombosis (DVT) and PE. Kluge et al. recently reported promise for detection of PE with True-FISP MRA (44). Images can be acquired in any plane, and although breath-holding is essential, small imaging volumes tailored to the breath-hold capability can be acquired. However, a recent article suggests that some clots may go undetected with True-FISP imaging (45).

Direct Thrombus Imaging

Direct thrombus imaging, based on the principle that changes in MR signal intensity occur due to reproducible changes in blood clots over time, offers a whole new vista for noninvasive diagnosis of PE (46–51). One of the intermediate products of this process is methemoglobin, which has a characteristic appearance on MRI due to a significant reduction in T1 values that can be highlighted with a heavily T1-weighted sequence (48,50). This truly noninvasive technique (does not require injection of contrast material) holds promise for the detection of both DVT and PE. Also, as time-dependent changes in MR appearance reflect evolution of the clot, high signal is seen in new clots only (46–49). Further advantages include the ability to scan in the coronal plane, thus allowing time-efficient coverage of the lower extremity

veins with two coronally overlapping acquisitions in a relatively short scan time.

Normal Anatomy: Pulmonary Arteries

The pulmonary arteries, one on each side, arise from the bifurcation of the pulmonary trunk (1–3). The left main pulmonary artery is a direct posterior continuation of the pulmonary trunk and describes a course from anteroinferior to posterosuperior as it arches over the left main bronchus before diving into upper and lower trunks. The right main pulmonary artery, longer than the left, forms a graceful sweep toward the right lung from its point of origin from the pulmonary trunk and follows a horizontal or slightly inferior course passing under the concavity of the aortic arch before dividing into a smaller upper and a larger lower trunk (Figs. 16-8, 16-9).

The subsequent branching pattern of the pulmonary arteries then mirrors that of the segmental bronchi. The right gives rise to the apicoposterior, anterior, and posterior segmental arteries that feed the right upper lobe, a middle lobe artery that immediately divides into medial and lateral segmental arteries, and five segmental arteries to the right lower lobe (apical, anterior, posterior, medial, and lateral).

On the left side, the arrangement is analogous with the following variations—the lingular artery, a branch of the left upper lobe pulmonary artery, divides into superior and inferior branches. The apical and posterior arteries are shared on the left (the apicoposterior segmental artery) as are the medial and posterior segmental arteries on the left (the mesiobasal segmental artery), thus giving a total of 10 segmental arteries on the right but only 8 on the left.

The segmental arrangement of the pulmonary arteries is important and impacts the original research evaluating the role of CTA and MRA for PE—only the segmental arteries and larger were evaluated while ignoring the subsegmental arteries. This was appropriate for the time, considering first the (now largely irrelevant) spatial resolution limitations of both CT and MR and second the fact that the importance of isolated subsegmental embolism remains unknown.

A nomenclature of the pulmonary arteries respecting the distance from the right ventricle is widely used as follows: first order branch, the pulmonary trunk; second order, the left and right main pulmonary arteries; third order, the upper and lower trunks and "lobar" arteries; fourth order, all 10 segmental arteries; fifth order, subsegmental arteries arising directly from a segmental artery; sixth order, arteries arising directly from the first division of a subsegmental artery; and so on.

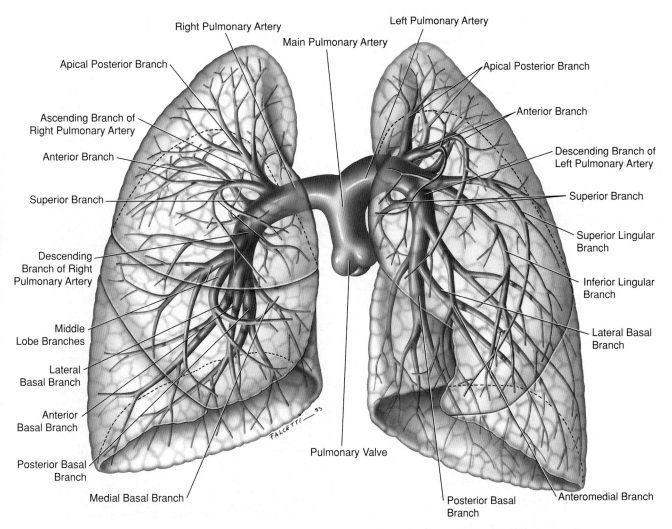

FIGURE 16-8 Diagram of the distribution of the pulmonary arteries in both lungs. (Reprinted with permission from Uflacker R. Pulmonary arterial circulation. In: Uflacker R, ed. *Atlas of Vascular Anatomy: An Angiographic Approach.* 2nd ed. Philadephia: Lippincott Williams & Wilkins; 2007:234.)

Bronchial Artery Anatomy

Although bronchial artery anatomy is extremely variable, most (>70%) originate from the descending thoracic aorta close but usually slightly below the carina (T5-T6 level). Anomalous bronchial arteries are defined as bronchial arteries that originate outside the T5-T6 range. Bronchial arteries typically run parallel to the bronchovascular axes (Fig. 16-10).

The largest published anatomic series, based on the assessment of cadaveric specimens, described four classical branching patterns, as follows (52) (Fig. 16-11):

I. (40.6%) Two arteries on the left and one on the right that arises as an intercostobronchial trunk (ICBT)
II. (21.3%) One artery on the left and one ICBT on the right
III. (20.6%) Two on the left and two on the right, one of which is an ICBT

IV. (9.7%) One on the left and two on the right, one of which is an ICBT

Variant Anatomy: Arteries

Transposition of the great arteries is a condition where the pulmonary trunk arises from the left ventricle and the aorta from the right ventricle. Despite the abnormal arrangement, the arteries otherwise appear normal (3,4).

Anomalous origin of the left pulmonary artery ("pulmonary sling") is usually diagnosed in infancy because of the effect of the aberrant artery on the airway and because of the frequent association of tracheal or bronchial stenosis due to complete cartilage rings (5). This can result in obstruction, feeding problems, and respiratory tract infections. Occasionally, the abnormality may be detected as an incidental finding in an asymptomatic adult or in the adult with respiratory complaints.

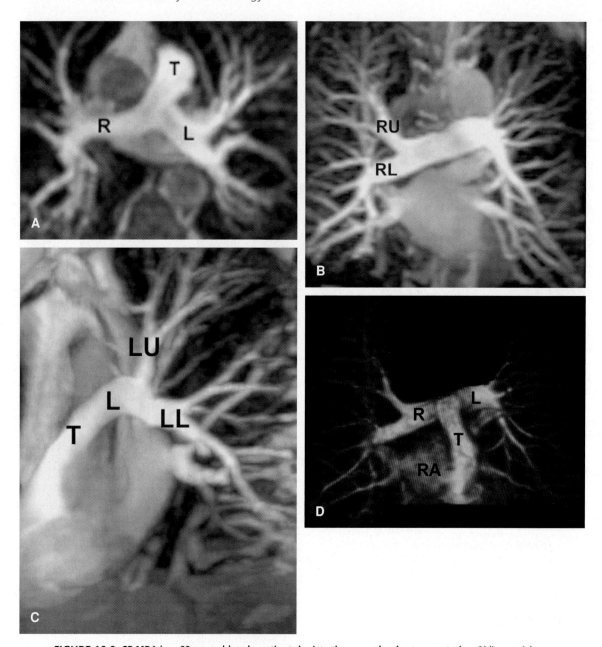

FIGURE 16-9 CE MRA in a 69-year-old male patient depicts the normal pulmonary arteries. Oblique axial **(A)**, coronal **(B)**, and sagittal **(C)** subvolume MIPs demonstrate the pulmonary branches and their branches. Volume rendering reformat **(D)** also allows a good demonstration of these structures and their interrelation. (T, pulmonary trunk; R, right pulmonary artery; L, left pulmonary artery; RU, right upper trunk; RL, right lower trunk; LU, left upper trunk; LL, left lower trunk; RA, right atrium.) (Courtesy of Neil M. Rofsky, MD, Beth Israel Deaconess Medical Center, Boston.)

The aberrant left pulmonary artery originates from the right pulmonary artery and travels across the midline posterior to the distal trachea or right main bronchus, where it turns abruptly to the left, passing between the esophagus and trachea to its destination in the left hilum (Fig. 16-12). CT and MRA with 3D visualization of complicated vascular anatomy are vital prerequisites for appropriate surgical planning of this and similar congenital disorders (5) (Fig. 16-13).

Systemic Arterial Supply to the Lung

A pulmonary sequestration consists of nonfunctioning lung tissue that is not in normal continuity with the tracheobronchial tree; it derives its blood supply from systemic vessels (Figs. 16-14, 16-15). Depending on the pleural coverage, the condition is described as "intralobar" or "extralobar." Intralobar sequestrations account for 75% of all pulmonary sequestrations. An intralobar sequestration consists of an abnormal segment of lung tissue that shares

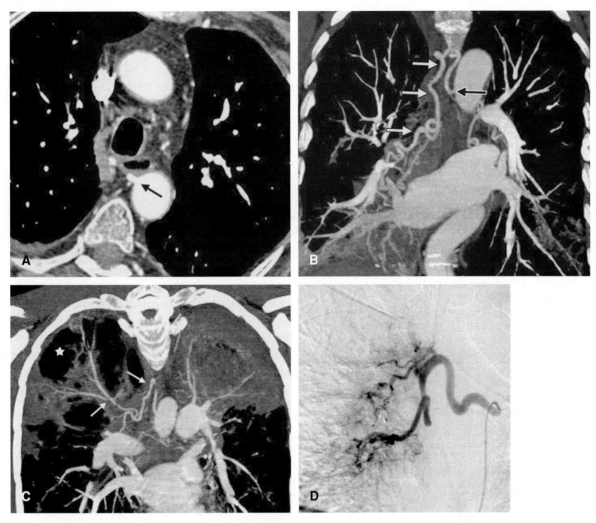

FIGURE 16-10 Images from a thoracic CT angiographic study performed with a 16-detector-row scanner.
A: Axial 1-mm-thick CT scan obtained just below the aortic arch (window center, 50 HU; window width, 350 HU) shows enlarged bronchial arteries (*arrow*) manifesting as avidly enhancing nodules in the paratracheal and retrobronchial regions of the mediastinum. These findings represent the typical appearance of enlarged bronchial arteries on axial images. Although the origins of the bronchial arteries are well depicted on axial images, their further course is very tortuous, and the intrapulmonary direction of the artery can be difficult to ascertain. **B:** Coronal thin-section MIP image clearly demonstrates an enlarged intercostobronchial artery (*arrows*) coursing into the pulmonary parenchyma parallel to the bronchial airways. **C:** Coronal thin-section MIP image obtained in a different patient provides a detailed analysis of the entire intrapulmonary course of an intercostobronchial artery (*arrows*). (★, intracavitary mycetoma.) **D:** Reformatted image demonstrates how CTA can provide anatomic information that is useful for planning subsequent bronchial artery embolization. (Reprinted with permission from Bruzzi JF, Remy-Jardin M, Delhaye D, et al. Multidetector row CT of hemoptysis. *Radiographics.* 2006;26:3–22.)

the visceral pleural covering of an otherwise normal pulmonary lobe and that lacks a normal communication to the tracheobronchial tree.

Extralobar sequestrations are a completely distinct entity and constitute 25% of all pulmonary sequestrations (Fig. 16-16). The malformation is typically found during the patients' first days to weeks of life and less frequently in late infancy or early childhood. An extralobar sequestration consists of a discrete, accessory lobe of nonaerated lung tissue that is invested in its own pleural envelope (53–55).

Disorders of the systemic arterial supply to the lung are an infrequent cause of massive hemoptysis that can lead to death, mainly by asphyxiation. Systemic arterialization of the lung parenchyma is most often congenital, in which case an aberrant systemic artery supplies the parenchyma involved in congenital pulmonary venolobar syndrome or bronchopulmonary sequestration (56). Often, these congenital conditions go unnoticed until hemoptysis occurs, leading to diagnostic workup and detection of the disorder.

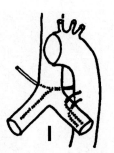 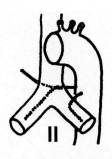 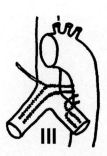 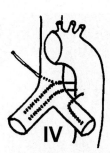

FIGURE 16-11 Diagrams illustrating the types of bronchial arterial supply. Type I, two bronchial arteries on the left and one on the right that manifests as an ICBT (40.6% of cases); Type II, one on the left and one ICBT on the right (21.3%); Type III, two on the left and two on the right (one ICBT and one bronchial artery) (20.6%); and Type IV, one on the left and two on the right (one ICBT and one bronchial artery) (9.7%). (Adapted with permission from Yoon W, Kim JK, Kim YH, et al. Bronchial and nonbronchial systemic artery embolization for life-threatening hemoptysis: a comprehensive review. *Radiographics*. 2002;22:1395–1409.)

Pulmonary Veins: Normal Anatomy

Pulmonary venous anatomy does not mirror pulmonary artery anatomy. Four pulmonary veins drain typically into the left atrium (Figs. 16-17, 16-18). Normally, the right and left upper lobe pulmonary veins drain the right upper and middle lobe, and the left upper lobe and lingula, respectively (Fig. 16-19). The lower lobe pulmonary veins drain their corresponding lower lobe (57–59).

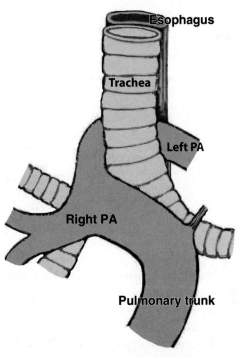

FIGURE 16-12 Diagram shows an anterior view of the anomalous origin of a left pulmonary artery (*PA*) that arises from the posterior aspect of the right pulmonary artery and reaches the left hilum by passing between the trachea and the esophagus. (Reprinted with permission from Castaner E, Gallardo X, Rimola J, et al. Congenital and acquired pulmonary artery anomalies in the adult: radiologic overview. *Radiographics*. 2006;26:349–371.)

The course of the pulmonary veins is quite different from that of the pulmonary arteries. The upper lobe (superior) pulmonary veins course downward, posteriorly and medially, the left superior pulmonary vein lies in the angle between the left main pulmonary artery and the left upper lobe pulmonary artery. On the right side, the upper pulmonary vein lies adjacent and lateral to the superior vena cava, and medial to the right upper lobe pulmonary artery (Fig. 16-18).

The middle lobe pulmonary vein, which is considerably smaller that the other main pulmonary veins, normally empties into the right superior pulmonary vein just before it empties into the left atrium (Figs. 16-17, 16-19). The lingular pulmonary vein almost always empties into the left superior pulmonary vein and only rarely empties directly into the left atrium.

Unlike the superior pulmonary veins, the inferior pulmonary veins describe a horizontal course for several centimeters prior to emptying into the left atrium. Also, the plane of the inferior pulmonary veins is substantially more posterior to that of the superior pulmonary veins. The pulmonary vein trunk, defined as the distance from the ostium to the first tributary, is usually longer for the upper lobe than the lower lobe pulmonary veins.

Pulmonary Vein Mapping Prior to Radio Frequency Ablation for Atrial Fibrillation

An increased interest in the assessment of the anatomic configuration and size of the pulmonary veins is the result of new therapies for treatment of atrial fibrillation with radio frequency ablation. Arrythmogenic foci are commonly located at the ostium of the pulmonary veins, and they are an important source of ectopic atrial electrical activity (60–62). Selective radio frequency ablation of arrythmogenic foci in the pulmonary veins is increasingly being performed to treat patients with

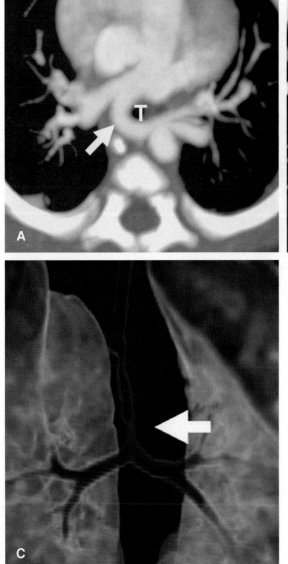
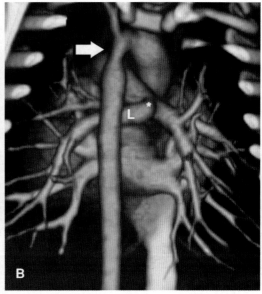
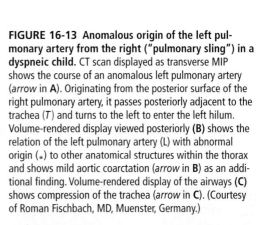

FIGURE 16-13 Anomalous origin of the left pulmonary artery from the right ("pulmonary sling") in a dyspneic child. CT scan displayed as transverse MIP shows the course of an anomalous left pulmonary artery (*arrow* in **A**). Originating from the posterior surface of the right pulmonary artery, it passes posteriorly adjacent to the trachea (*T*) and turns to the left to enter the left hilum. Volume-rendered display viewed posteriorly (**B**) shows the relation of the left pulmonary artery (L) with abnormal origin (*) to other anatomical structures within the thorax and shows mild aortic coarctation (*arrow* in **B**) as an additional finding. Volume-rendered display of the airways (**C**) shows compression of the trachea (*arrow* in **C**). (Courtesy of Roman Fischbach, MD, Muenster, Germany.)

refractory atrial fibrillation (63). The size and shape of the pulmonary venous ostium is an important consideration in selection of the optimal diameter of the radio frequency catheter.

CE CT (64) and gadolinium-enhanced MR imaging (65) provide accurate demonstration of pulmonary vein location, number, ostial size, branching pattern, and length of the pulmonary vein trunk prior to ablation being performed and additionally offer an ideal method for detection of procedure-related complications such as pulmonary vein stenosis (61,62) (Fig. 16-20) and occlusion (Fig. 16-21). In addition, atrial or atrial appendage thrombus, an absolute contraindication to the procedure, can be excluded. A reduction in pulmonary vein diameter, circumference, and

cross-sectional area can occur as a result of radio frequency ablation therapy for atrial fibrillation (66), and it is more pronounced with increasing number of therapeutic radio frequency ablations (67). The left inferior pulmonary vein normally narrows as it enters the left atrium, and therefore, diagnosis of stenosis in this vessel should be made with caution (64).

Gadolinium-enhanced MRI provides a detailed examination of the pulmonary vasculature and possible collateral pathways in the chest in a single breath-hold, without using ionizing radiation or iodinated contrast. There is excellent correlation between the MR findings and those at cardiac catheterization, echocardiogram, and intraoperative findings. MR provides additional information regarding the

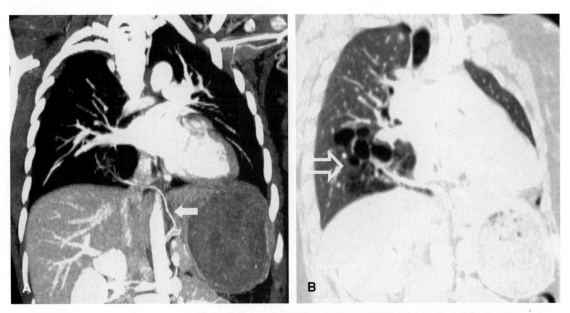

FIGURE 16-14 High-resolution CE multidetector-row CT. A: A coronal MIP, which allows for visualization of an aberrant vessel (*arrow*) of the abdominal aorta supplying a bronchopulmonary sequestration. **B:** Lung window settings enable evaluation of the sequestration (*arrow*) with cystic components from the same scan. (Courtesy of James Ravenel, MD, Charleston, SC.)

anatomy of the pulmonary veins (number and size), presence of stenosis, or aneurysmal dilatation as well as presence of additional vascular anomalies (68).

2D cine steady-state free precession pulse sequences demonstrate significant changes in the location and size of the pulmonary vein ostium that occur during the cardiac cycle (69,70). A comparison between 2D cine sequences and a 3D gadolinium-enhanced MR approach showed an increased sharpness of the pulmonary vein borders with cine sequences. In addition, cine images can resolve differences in diameter across the cardiac cycle.

3D gadolinium-enhanced MR images tend to overestimate the size of the ostium and suffer from blurriness at the edges of the pulmonary veins due to pulsatile motion. Nevertheless, 3D gadolinium-enhanced MRI provides a comprehensive display of the pulmonary vein anatomy that simplifies understanding of the anatomy, particularly in patients with complex anatomic variants. Furthermore, 3D acquisitions are significantly faster than 2D cine acquisitions for the same anatomic coverage (71).

Since many of these patients have an implanted pacemaker or defibrillator, CT plays an important role. CT of the pulmonary veins can be performed without gating. Retrospectively gated images can compensate for cardiac motion and do produce sharper images. Whether or not the uncertain clinical benefit of these sharper images offsets the increased radiation dose and contrast load remains to be determined. A bolus tracking cursor is placed in the left atrium. A craniocaudal field from the aortic arch to the diaphragm is prescribed. The amount of contrast needed is determined by the product of the injection rate (usually 4 to 5 mL/second) and the scan duration; 10 mL can be added to offset the small pause between the detection of the bolus and the initiation of scanning. A saline flush is used. It is recommended for scanning to occur from inferior to superior to minimize artifacts from the superior vena cava.

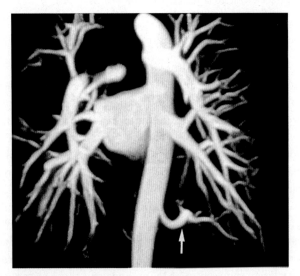

FIGURE 16-15 Pulmonary sequestration. Subvolume MIP from 3D CE MRA shows a feeding vessel (*arrow*) from the aorta to a pulmonary sequestration.

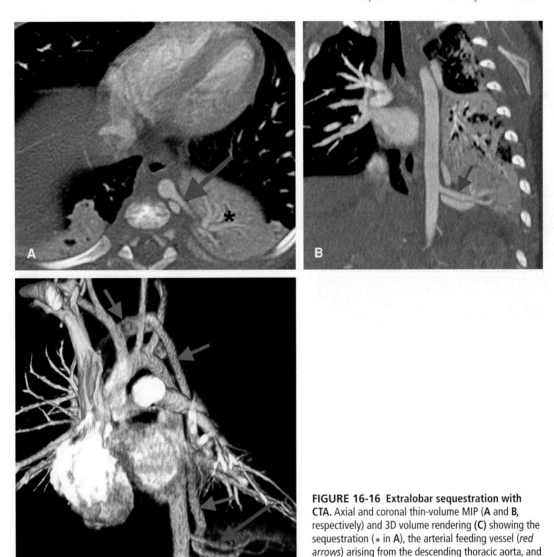

FIGURE 16-16 Extralobar sequestration with CTA. Axial and coronal thin-volume MIP (**A** and **B**, respectively) and 3D volume rendering (**C**) showing the sequestration (∗ in **A**), the arterial feeding vessel (*red arrows*) arising from the descending thoracic aorta, and an aberrant vein connecting with the brachiocephalic vein (*blue arrows*). (Courtesy of Stanford Cardiovascular Imaging.)

Variant Anatomy: Veins

Developmental anomalies of the pulmonary veins are common (60–62) (Fig. 16-22). A common pulmonary vein on one side (representing conjoined upper and lower pulmonary veins) occurs in up to 25% of individuals; however, in clinical practice, a single common vein on the left is quite common whereas a common right pulmonary vein is extremely uncommon. As expected, a common pulmonary vein trunk has a significantly larger diameter (Fig. 16-23B) than individual upper or lower lobe pulmonary veins. The middle lobe pulmonary vein usually drains into the upper lobe pulmonary vein proximal to the left atrium but drains separately into the left atrium in 19% of patients (Fig. 16-23A), shares a common ostium to

the proximal part of the right superior pulmonary vein in 69% of patients, and joins with the right inferior pulmonary vein in 8% of cases (61).

Anomalous Pulmonary Venous Drainage

The term *anomalous pulmonary venous drainage* describes the condition where part or all of the venous drainage of one or both lungs drains into the right atrium or its tributaries (72,73). Several anomalous pulmonary and systemic connections exist. These anomalous drainages can be partial or total.

Abnormalities can be classified into four categories: supracardiac, cardiac, infracardiac, and mixed. The

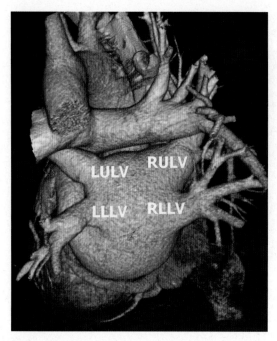

FIGURE 16-17 CE ECG-gated cardiac CT displayed as volume rendering seen from posterior shows normal configuration of the pulmonary venous return to the left atrium with the left upper lobe vein (*LULV*) and the left lower lobe vein (*LLLV*) draining the left lung and the right upper lobe vein (*RULV*) and the right lower lobe vein (*RLLV*) draining the right lung.

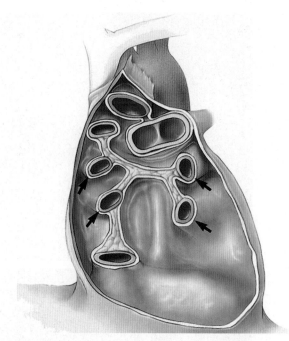

FIGURE 16-18 Drawing of the pulmonary veins as they reach the left atrium. The heart has been removed, and the relationship of the four pulmonary veins can be appreciated (*arrows*). (Reprinted with permission from Lawler LP, Corl FM, Fishman EK. Multi-detector row and volume-rendered CT of the normal and accessory flow pathways of the thoracic systemic and pulmonary veins. *Radiographics.* 2002;22:S45–S60.)

supracardiac drains to the superior vena cava or azygous vein; the cardiac type drains to the coronary sinus or right atrium; the infracardiac type drains to the portal vein, ductus venosus, or the inferior vena cava; and mixed type (~5%) represents some combination of two or more of the above anomalies.

Totally Anomalous Pulmonary Venous Drainage

In totally anomalous pulmonary venous drainage (TAPVD), there is complete failure of the pulmonary veins to reach the left atrium. Instead, the pulmonary veins coalesce into a common pulmonary vein behind the heart.

Onward drainage is then via one of three routes—(a) a vertical vein that ultimately empties into the right atrium via the left brachiocephalic vein and SVC (supracardiac type, Fig. 16-24), (b) direct drainage into the right atrium or coronary sinus (intracardiac type), or (c) via a vertically draining inferior vein that passes through the diaphragm and enters into the portal vein or ductus venosus (infracardiac type).

In all such cases, survival depends on an obligatory right-to-left shunt. Associated anomalies such as atrial septal defect (ASD), ventricular septal defect (VSD), aortic coarctation, or interrupted arch are present in up to 30% of

cases. Patients with asplenia syndrome always have associated TAPVD (60).

Partially Anomalous Pulmonary Venous Drainage

In most instances, the anomalous veins follow a normal course within the lung; it is only the "termination" of the vein that is anomalous (74). Physiologically, an extracardiac physiologic left-to-right shunt ensues but is commonly asymptomatic. Clinical presentation is similar to individuals with an ASD.

Examples include partially anomalous pulmonary venous drainage (PAPVD), where an upper lobe pulmonary vein drains into the superior vena cava, azygous vein, right atrium, left-sided SVC, left brachiocephalic vein (Fig. 16-25), or coronary sinus. This anomaly is frequently associated with an atrial septal defect (74).

Scimitar Syndrome

The hypogenetic lung (or Scimitar) syndrome is an example of PAPVD in which the right lung, usually in its entirety (although occasionally only the right middle or lower lobe) drains via a large vein (the so-called "scimitar" vein because of its shape) that parallels the right cardiac

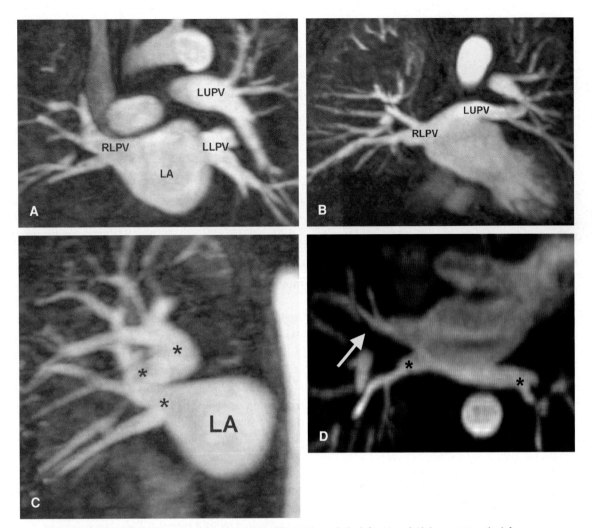

FIGURE 16-19 CE MRA/venography. A: Coronal reformat through the left atrium *(LA)* demonstrates the left upper and left and right lower pulmonary veins *(LUPV, LLPV,* and *RLPV,* respectively). **B:** At a slightly different level the left upper *(LUPV)* and right lower pulmonary veins *(RLPV)* are optimally demonstrated. **C:** Sagittal oblique image demonstrates the right upper pulmonary vein (∗) as it enters the left atrium *(LA).* **D:** Axial reformat demonstrates the typical orientation of the lower pulmonary veins (∗) as they course anteriorly and medially to the left atrium. Also, note the two tributaries from the middle lobe *(arrow)* that join together to form a common trunk, which usually joins with the right upper pulmonary vein just before emptying into the left atrium.

border to the inferior cava, just above the diaphragm (72,73) (Fig. 16-26).

This condition is usually discovered incidentally on imaging studies of the thorax. With the Scimitar syndrome, a proportion of oxygenated blood passes around in an "endless" loop from pulmonary vasculature to right atrium to pulmonary vasculature, an extracardiac left-to-right shunt. This condition may assume clinical relevance in patients with abnormal lung function or in patients in whom resection of another lobe or lobes might result in cardiorespiratory compromise.

In most instances, the finding is part of a more global syndrome involving pulmonary and systemic vascular anomalies. Frequently associated anomalies include small right pulmonary artery, right lung hypoplasia, bilobed right lung, and intrapulmonary sequestration (73,74).

CLINICAL APPLICATIONS

Acute Pulmonary Embolism

Background

PE has a suspected incidence of three cases in 1,000 persons per year in Western society and an estimated 600,000 cases per year in the United States (75–79). Unsuspected PE is the cause of death in 5% of unselected autopsies, and PE contributes to the cause of death in another 10% (79–81).

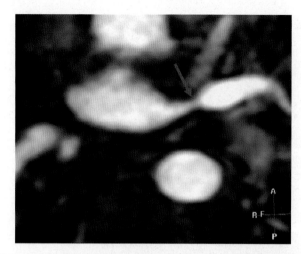

FIGURE 16-20 Postablation pulmonary vein stenosis. This oblique reformatted image from a CE MRA exam reveals a stenosed left inferior pulmonary vein (*arrow*) following ablation therapy for atrial fibrillation. (Courtesy of Thomas Hauser, MD, and Warren Manning, MD, Beth Israel Deaconess Medical Center, Boston, MA.)

PE is said to be the cause of death in 15% of inpatients (79), although this figure is disputed (80). Additionally, in those patients shown at autopsy to have died of unsuspected massive PE, it has been estimated that 21% would have had a favorable prognosis had the diagnosis been established, while the remainder were split evenly between those in whom establishing a diagnosis would not have made a difference due to severe associated comorbid conditions and those who would have a favorable prognosis in any case (80–84).

The importance of establishing a diagnosis of PE is paramount, owing to a 10-fold difference in mortality between untreated PE (30%) and treated PE (3%) (75,78,82–84). However, the imperative to treat PE must be tempered by the fact that PE is infrequently present even in patients with a high clinical suspicion (most studies report a prevalence of 20% to 40%) (79), and treatment must be withheld in patients without PE due to a high prevalence of (potentially fatal) hemorrhagic complications in patients undergoing anticoagulation (85,86).

Because the definitive diagnostic test, catheter angiography, is invasive and has an attendant but rare fatal complication risk (87–90), diagnostic strategies for PE are often complex and focus initially on determining whether a PE might be present without recourse to imaging the pulmonary arteries (15,91–98).

Strategies aimed at eliminating the need for catheter angiography include ventilation-perfusion lung scanning (94,98), estimation of blood D-dimer levels (15,91,95–97), and/or a search for lower extremity DVT by noninvasive evaluation of the lower limb veins with sonography (15,91–93,95,96). However, in the many cases where indirect, noninvasive testing fails to give the definitive information necessary to allow a therapeutic decision to be made, evaluation of the pulmonary arteries becomes essential (20,99).

The advent of spiral CT heralded a new horizon for direct visualization of PE (14,18,100–116) (Fig. 16-27). The interobserver agreement for spiral CT is better than for nuclear scintigraphy (16,100). Spiral CT also appears to be the most

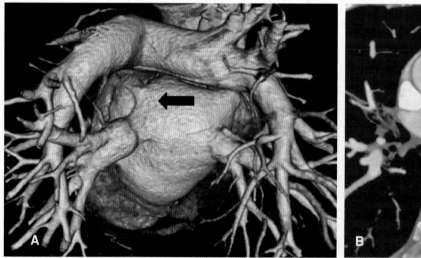
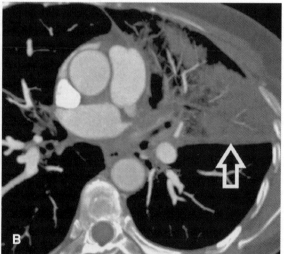

FIGURE 16-21 *A* 64-year-old woman's status following pulmonary vein ablation therapy for cardiac arrhythmia. CE ECG-gated multidetector-row CT scan displayed as volume rendering **(A)** seen from posterior demonstrates occlusion of the left upper lobe pulmonary vein (*arrow* in **A**) as a complication of the procedure. Display as axial MIP **(B)** shows consolidation of the left upper lobe (*arrow* in **B**) due to pulmonary venous infarction.

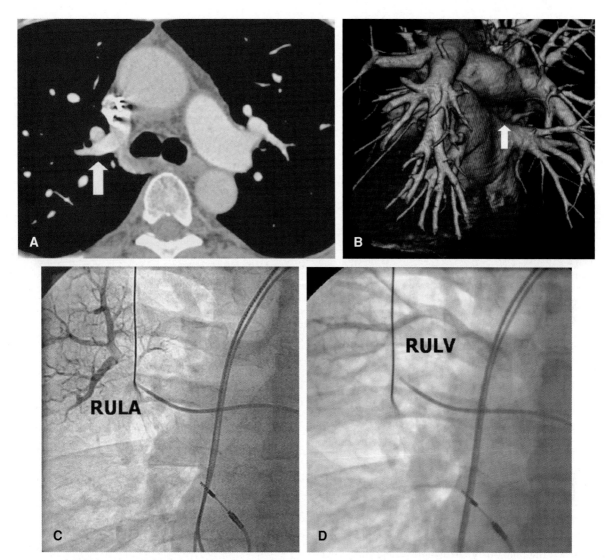

FIGURE 16-22 CE ECG-gated multidetector-row CT scan prior to ablation therapy for cardiac arrhythmia. Transverse section (**A**) and volume-rendered display (**B**) show anomalous pulmonary venous return (*arrows*) with drainage of the right upper lobe pulmonary vein into the superior vena cava. These findings are confirmed at conventional DSA (**C** and **D**), which demonstrates the drainage of contrast via the anomalous right upper lobe vein (*RULV*) after selective injection of the right upper lobe artery (*RULA*).

cost-effective modality in the diagnostic algorithm of PE compared with algorithms that do not include spiral CT (117).

While CT avoids the more invasive component of catheter angiography (catheterization), it retains some of its drawbacks, including use of iodinated contrast material and exposure to ionizing radiation. However, as CT is clinically proven, widely available, and generally accepted by clinicians, a steady increase in its usage has been paralleled by a decline in referrals for pulmonary angiography, to a point where conventional pulmonary angiography is rarely performed in clinical practice.

Despite the fact that single-slice spiral CT has excellent accuracy for detection of main, lobar, and segmental PE, variable accuracy for subsegmental PE has been reported

(99,103,112,114) with a risk that subsegmental PEs may be overlooked (103,114). The accuracy for the detection of emboli in subsegmental pulmonary arteries with single-slice, dual-slice, and electron-beam CT scanners ranges between 61% and 79% (18,103,106,110). Multi-detector technologies offer further enhancements with the potential to demonstrate smaller arteries and possibly improve diagnosis of subsegmental emboli (18,19,102).

The lack of unequivocal acceptance of noninvasive angiography for PE diagnosis largely stems from concerns surrounding the perceived limitations in detecting small peripheral emboli. In the absence of central emboli, the clinical significance of such isolated peripheral emboli is uncertain, as will be discussed in the next section.

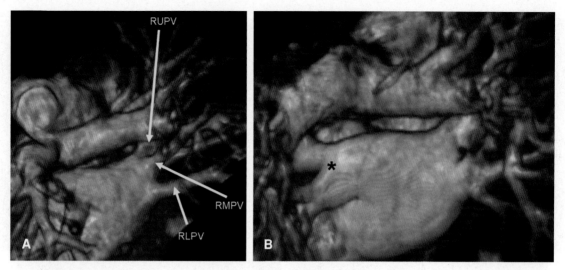

FIGURE 16-23 Variant anatomy of the pulmonary veins with MRA. These are normal variants of the pulmonary veins depicted by Gd-enhanced MRA volume-rendering reformats obtained prior to radio frequency ablation. **A:** Note the presence of three pulmonary veins draining the right lung on this posterior view. **B:** The veins draining the left lung form a common trunk (∗) before reaching the left atrium. (RUPV, right upper pulmonary vein; RMPV, right middle pulmonary vein; RLPV, right lower pulmonary vein.)(Courtesy of Eli Gelfand, MD, and Warren Manning, MD, Beth Israel Deaconess Medical Center, Boston.)

Controversies Regarding the Significance of Subsegmental Emboli

As a background to this issue, it is appropriate to look to the mechanism by which emboli reach the lung. It appears that when a clot breaks away from a site of attachment (usually within the lower extremity), it becomes macerated by the churning motion of the heart as it passes through the right-sided heart chambers and tricuspid value. The fragments thus produced reach the pulmonary circulation, where they lodge in an artery. In the majority of patients, the embolic fragments vary in size, but in some cases, multiple small fragments shower into the pulmonary circulation. In this case, the importance of subsegmental artery evaluation is paramount.

Evidence cited in favor of subsegmental PE being unimportant can be summarized accordingly:

1. There is a substantial interobserver difference on DSA for demonstrating subsegmental PE. This implies the existence of false-negative and false-positive results in clinical practice (118,119). Moreover, very few patients with negative DSA have a proven episode of PE or sudden death related to PE on follow-up. Thus, it is assumed that a missed diagnosis of subsegmental PE may be unimportant, at least in some patients (118,119). This is supported by the fact that there was only one death in 20 patients with isolated subsegmental PE missed on initial evaluation of angiograms in the Prospective Investigation of Pulmonary Embolism Diagnosis (PIOPED) Study but was picked up at subsequent review (120).

2. Autopsy studies in patients who have had no clinical episodes suggestive of PE and who have died from causes unrelated to PE frequently demonstrate multiple old, small subsegmental PE. This observation underlines one of the functions of the lung, namely to remove small embolic particles from the circulation and prevent them reaching the brain (79–81).

3. Single-slice spiral CT, which is limited for detection of subsegmental PE, has been used as the "de facto" standard for diagnosis of PE for many years. Its very acceptance as an arbiter in clinical practice attests to a clinical reality that chooses to ignore small emboli (15,92,95).

4. There is an impressive body of literature that assesses patient outcome following the withholding of treatment with negative test results (14,100,101,104,105,107,108, 113,115,116). A pooled assessment of the outcome in 3,500 patients who did not receive anticoagulation based on a negative spiral CT showed that the negative predictive value of CT approaches 100% and in fact exceeds that of pulmonary angiography (111). More practically, the results of these trials clearly show that patient outcome is not adversely affected when anticoagulation is withheld because of a negative spiral CT test.

Evidence cited in favor of subsegmental PE being just as important as embolism to larger arteries includes:

1. Logic—This dictates that an embolus broken up into multiple tiny fragments that lodge within subsegmental arteries only because of their small size probably has the

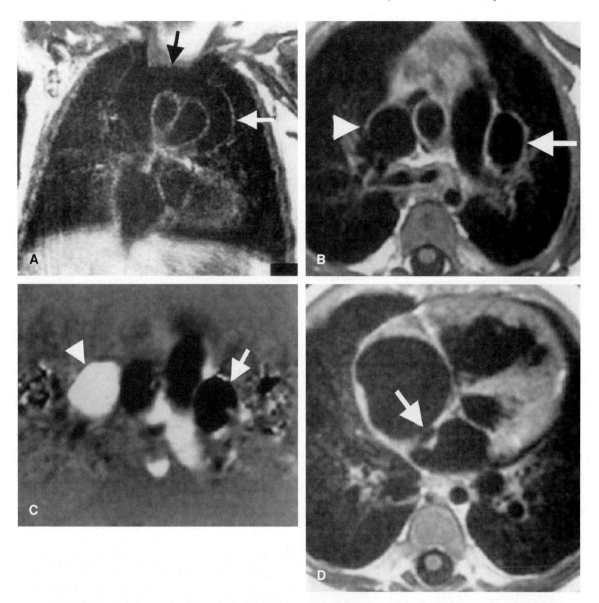

FIGURE 16-24 Supracardiac form of total APVD in a 7-month-old boy. Although the vertical vein was well visualized at echocardiography, the individual pulmonary veins could not be delineated adequately. **A:** Coronal T1-weighted (512/13) SE MR image demonstrates a large vertical vein (*white arrow*) draining into the left brachiocephalic vein (*black arrow*). The enlarged vertical vein, brachiocephalic vein, and SVC form the top part of the "snowman" that occurs in supracardiac total APVC. **B:** Axial T1-weighted (504/16) SE MR image shows the markedly enlarged vertical vein (*arrow*) and SVC (*arrowhead*) in cross section at the level of the left main pulmonary artery. **C:** Axial cine phase-contrast (30/8, 30° flip angle, velocity encoding = 180) MR image obtained at the same level as (**B**) reveals cephalic flow (low signal intensity) in the vertical vein (*arrow*) that is opposite in direction (high signal intensity) from that in the SVC (*arrowhead*). **D:** Axial T1-weighted (512/13) SE MR image obtained through the left atrium demonstrates absent pulmonary veins and a patent foramen ovale (*arrow*). Findings were confirmed surgically. (Reprinted with permission from White CS, Baffa JM, Haney PJ, et al. MR imaging of congenital anomalies of the thoracic veins. *Radiographics.* 1997;17:595–608.)

same clinical significance as the "same" embolus broken into fewer but larger fragments that lodge within segmental and larger arteries.

2. Autopsy studies in patients dying from PE often reveal smaller recent PEs, raising the possibility that a small PE may "herald" a larger, potentially fatal one (118–121).

Technical Advances Impacting Subsegmental Pulmonary Embolism Assessment

The limited ability for demonstrating subsegmental pulmonary arteries and for detecting emboli within is based on data using single-slice, dual-slice, and electron-beam CT (18,103,106,110). The advent of MDCT improves

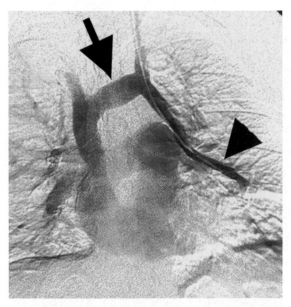

FIGURE 16-25 A 50-year-old woman after intraoperative placement of central venous line. Contrast material injection through a left-sided central venous catheter shows opacification of left upper lobe vessel (vertical vein) that drains left upper lobe (*arrowhead*) into left innominate vein (*arrow*). (Reprinted with permission from Klecker RJ, Christoforidis AJ, Sinclair DS. Case 2. Vertical vein (partial anomalous pulmonary venous drainage). *AJR Am J Roentgenol.* 2000;175:867, 869–870.)

visualization of the pulmonary arteries and the diagnoses of small peripheral emboli.

The high spatial resolution (i.e., 0.6 × 0.6 × 0.6 mm in x-, y- and z-direction) of multidetector-row spiral CT data sets now allows evaluation of pulmonary vessels down

to sixth-order branches and significantly increases the detection rate of segmental and subsegmental PEs (18,102). Interestingly, the interobserver correlation for confident diagnosis of subsegmental emboli with high-resolution multidetector-row spiral CT exceeds the reproducibility of selective pulmonary angiography (18,120,122).

Thus, with high-resolution imaging capabilities, small peripheral clots that may have gone unnoticed in the past are now frequently seen, often in patients with minor symptoms. The impact of this "improved" capacity is unknown and returns us to the previous discussion regarding whether patients with such minimal thromboembolic disease should be exposed to the inherent risks of anticoagulation therapy. Research directed toward outcomes analyses will be important in the coming years.

Challenges in Determining the Accuracy of Noninvasive Angiography

Comparison studies to catheter pulmonary angiography are impacted by the inability to exceed the performance of the gold standard, unless endpoints other than imaging are used. Based on imaging comparisons alone, the unique ability to visualize clots on cross-sections may be misrepresented with false-positives.

Furthermore, the dramatic curtailment in the use of catheter pulmonary angiography, even as single-slice CTA was being accepted in clinical practice (103,106,112), has challenged further comparisons with the traditional reference standard. Thus, there is no level

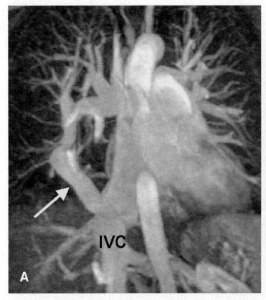
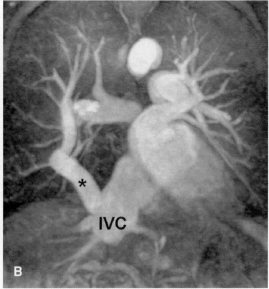

FIGURE 16-26 CF MRA in a patient with Scimitar syndrome with venous drainage of the right lung to the inferior vena cava (IVC). The pulmonary arteries are normal. A: Whole volume MIP demonstrated an abnormal vessel (*arrow*) descending inferiorly toward the right diaphragm and inferior vena cava (*IVC*). **B:** Subvolume coronal reformat demonstrates that the entire venous drainage of the right lung is to the IVC through the abnormal vessel (*∗*).

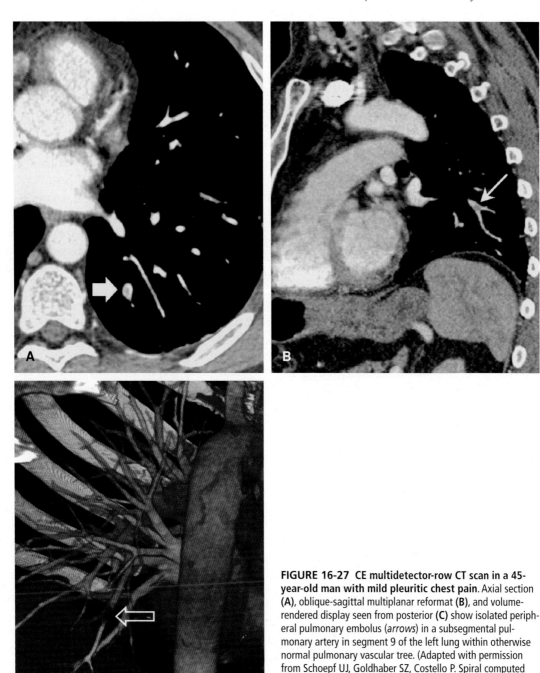

FIGURE 16-27 CE multidetector-row CT scan in a 45-year-old man with mild pleuritic chest pain. Axial section **(A)**, oblique-sagittal multiplanar reformat **(B)**, and volume-rendered display seen from posterior **(C)** show isolated peripheral pulmonary embolus (*arrows*) in a subsegmental pulmonary artery in segment 9 of the left lung within otherwise normal pulmonary vascular tree. (Adapted with permission from Schoepf UJ, Goldhaber SZ, Costello P. Spiral computed tomography for acute pulmonary embolism. *Circulation*. 2004;109:2160–2167.)

playing field for assessing diagnostic accuracy as the technologies evolve.

Hence, there are only a handful of prospective studies comparing MRA with DSA, and the assessment of the latest technological innovations for MDCT and MRA cannot be subjected to the same scientific scrutiny as was single-slice CTA (18,19,102,109).

It is widely acknowledged that there are several limitations of pulmonary angiography that may adversely impact the imaging endpoint itself. These limitations include:

1. Catheter-directed pulmonary angiography is inherently a projectional technique. As such, it has no through-plane resolution and can only offer a limited number of perspectives for interpretation.
2. DSA is not feasible in up to 20% of patients due to renal impairment and iodine hypersensitivity (20,89).
3. The use of selective injections of each pulmonary artery is clearly preferred by experts, and yet, this approach is not the routine across clinical practices (87–89,121).

4. It is claimed that balloon occlusion with injection into the isolated arterial segment is the angiographic method that gives the greatest likelihood of demonstrating subsegmental emboli, but in contemporary practice, this approach is almost never used (121).

5. Substantial interobserver variability has been reported when interpreting catheter pulmonary angiography images. This phenomenon is observed even when a cohort of experienced operators performs the interpretation. For example, in the PIOPED study, the observed variability for main, lobar, and segmental arteries was low; however, there was agreement between all three reviewer pairs on the presence of subsegmental embolism in only 13% of cases (88,120).

Computed Tomography–based Algorithm for Evaluation of Patients with Suspected Pulmonary Embolism

What follows is a proposal for a simple CT-based algorithm to evaluate patients with clinically suspected PE. At the Medical University of South Carolina, D-dimer testing is the most important first line clinical tool for PE diagnosis; a negative result is usually accepted for ruling out the presence of PE, especially if during further workup other causes for the patient's signs and symptoms can be established.

A diagnosis of DVT is pursued, and if this can be established (e.g., by a positive lower extremity ultrasound) in a patient with clinically suspected PE, usually no further diagnostic workup of the pulmonary circulation is pursued. The reason is that in clinically stable patients, the same regimen of anticoagulation is usually chosen for treatment of both PE and DVT.

If a diagnosis of DVT cannot be established in a patient with suspected PE, a CT pulmonary angiogram (CTPA) of the pulmonary circulation is then performed, and if positive for PE, the patient is treated accordingly. If a good-quality CTPA study does not reveal PE, the workup for PE typically stops at this point, and other diagnostic routes for elucidating the source of the patient's signs and symptoms should be pursued.

In the unlikely case of a persisting high clinical suspicion of PE in the face of a good-quality, negative CT pulmonary angiogram, there is the theoretical option of pursuing a definitive diagnosis by means of catheter pulmonary angiography as the last resort to exhaust all diagnostic means available. However, to date, this has not occurred in our practice.

In those few cases where a poor-quality CTPA study does not allow confidently establishing or ruling out a diagnosis of PE as the source of the patient's symptoms, a repeat CTPA is usually attempted, if at all feasible, in view of the patient's clinical presentation. In many instances, analyzing and remedying factors responsible for failed CTPA (e.g., improved intravenous access, higher contrast media injection rates, use of automated bolus-triggering techniques, adaptation of tube output to patient's body type, use of ECG-synchronized scan acquisition, etc.) yields a repeat CTPA as being diagnostic.

Computed Tomography Assessment of Cardiac Function

The main cause of death within 30 days from acute PE is right ventricular (RV) failure. Rapid risk stratification is paramount for identifying high-risk patients and helps to select the appropriate management strategy. Thrombolysis, catheter intervention, or surgical embolectomy as adjuncts to anticoagulation may rapidly reverse RV failure and reduce the risk of recurrence and death. Reperfusion therapy is indicated in patients with cardiogenic shock and may be considered in selected patients with preserved systemic pressure and RV dysfunction.

Echocardiography has emerged as an important risk stratification tool, because RV dysfunction is a powerful and independent predictor of mortality. However, echocardiography has limited availability at many institutions, and occasionally, the RV may be difficult to image with the transthoracic approach.

With newer generation CT scanners, standardized cardiac views are easily obtained in almost all patients who undergo routine, nongated CE chest CT. It has been shown that the presence of RV enlargement on the initial chest CT scan helps to predict 30-day mortality (123).

A ratio of RV diameter over LV diameter of greater than 0.9 proved sensitive to predict major complications (cardiopulmonary resuscitation, mechanical ventilation, vasopressors, thrombolysis, catheter intervention, surgical embolectomy) or death within 30 days. Conversely, in the absence of RV enlargement on CT, most patients survived. Thus, from the same scan used to diagnose PE, important prognostic information can be obtained, obviating the time and cost associated with additional tests, such as echocardiography.

Magnetic Resonance Imaging and Angiography for Acute Pulmonary Embolism

MRA offers an alternative to CTA while avoiding ionizing radiation and iodinated contrast material. MRA's safety advantages can capture some patients who might otherwise be relegated to indirect diagnostic methods. A key consideration is in validating the accuracy of MRA for detection of PE, as is demonstrated by the results in Table 16-3 (28–30).

TABLE 16-3

Magnetic Resonance Angiography versus Digital Subtraction Angiography for Pulmonary Embolism: Results of Clinical Studies

Author	Year	Number of Patients	Scan Time (sec)	Sensitivity (%)	Specificity (%)
Meaney (28)	1997	23	27	87	95
Gupta (29)	1999	46	23	85	96
Oudkerk (30)	2002	141	15 to 17	77	98

The initial studies (28,29) used coronal plane acquisition to image both lungs simultaneously. Because of breath-holding considerations, in-plane resolution, through-plane resolution, and spatial coverage were compromised in order to achieve breath-hold scan times. Accurate imaging of the subsegmental small arteries in these studies was hampered by inadvertent exclusion of distal arteries within the anterior and posterior reaches of the lung from the coronal imaging volume. In addition, resolution constraints meant that even those subsegmental arteries enclosed within the imaging volume were poorly visualized.

In order to improve spatial resolution and coverage, Oudkerk et al. devised a sagittal plane two-injection protocol (30). The tailored sagittal imaging volume enclosed all of the pulmonary arteries within each lung in a 3D volume that gave higher resolution than was possible with a coronal study. The residual contrast from a first injection is not problematic for pulmonary MRA.

The most comprehensive evaluation of MRA versus DSA for diagnosis of PE available at the time of this writing date compared 115 of 141 patients recruited (30). There was a prevalence of PE of 30%, and MRA correctly diagnosed 27 of 35 patients with PE for a sensitivity of 77% but missed PE in 3 of 5 patients with subsegmental PE only. Also of note, MRA detected PE in 2 patients with normal DSA, for a specificity of 98%.

Technological advances in MRA are closing the gap between the competing demands of achieving adequate spatial resolution (both in-plane and through-plane), adequate anatomic coverage, and a scan time within a comfortable breath-hold. Advances such as improvements in gradient technology in combination with more efficient k-space filling methods (124), parallel imaging techniques (125,126), and optimized injection protocols (127) are continuously improving diagnostic possibilities.

Parallel MRI allows for a substantial reduction in scan time with the possibility of achieving acceleration improvements by an order of magnitude (128). The marked reduction in acquisition can be translated into either improved spatial resolution, improved temporal resolution, or a combination of both such that an accurate evaluation of subsegmental arteries is becoming feasible.

Comparison of Magnetic Resonance Angiography and Computed Tomographic Angiography for Diagnosis of Pulmonary Embolism

At the time of this writing, there has been only a single prospective study of MRA compared with CTA for diagnosis of PE. Ohno et al. compared MDCT (4-slice), CE MRA (4-second time-resolved technique), and ventilation-perfusion (VQ) scanning in patients with suspected PE by using what was, at that time, state-of-the-art technology for both CT and MR and compared the results to catheter pulmonary angiography (129). The superiority of MRA over CTA demonstrated in that study and as summarized in Table 16-4 is, of course, based on but a moment in the continuum of technological evolution.

Relevance of Animal Studies in Determining Validity of New Approaches

Data from animal studies offer some insights into the performance of improved cross-sectional imaging modalities for PE diagnosis and allow for comparisons with catheter angiography. However, it should be noted that such comparisons are carried out under "ideal" conditions of suspended respiration during general anesthesia. As such, the applicability of these results to in vivo human studies can certainly be questioned.

Three published studies have compared CTA and MRA in animal models (Table 16-5). The first study (130), which compared single-slice CT with CE MRA reported superiority of CTA over MRA. Two more recent studies using an improved MR technique (higher spatial resolution and shorter scan times) reported superiority of MRA over CTA (131,132). One study (132) reported detection rates of 97.7% for real time MR for both readers (Table 16-5) (130–132).

TABLE 16-4

Magnetic Resonance Angiography and Four-slice Multidetector Computed Tomographic Angiography versus Angiography: Diagnostic Capability of Data Sets per Vascular Zone

Vascular Zone	Sensitivity (%)	Specificity (%)	PPV (%)	NPV (%)	Accuracy (%)
Overall					
MRA	83	97	64	99	96
CTA	75	97	64	98	96
Central					
MRA	100	99	92	100	99
CTA	100	99	97	100	99
Peripheral					
MRA	68	96	47	98	95
CTA	54	96	42	98	94

PPV, positive predictive value; NPV, negative predictive value; MRA, magnetic resonance angiography; CTA, computed tomographic angiography.

Other Magnetic Resonance Imaging Techniques for Pulmonary Embolism Diagnosis

Perfusion Imaging and Ventilation

Several studies compare scintigraphic and MR pulmonary perfusion in a variety of disorders. Although results between the two techniques are similar, reproducibility is significantly greater with MR. Differential lung perfusion, which may be of value in assessing patients with chronic obstructive pulmonary disease prior to and after lung volume reduction surgery, is also well demonstrated with MR lung perfusion (12,34–37).

Time-resolved Magnetic Resonance Angiography

In a unique study using catheter pulmonary angiography as the gold standard in 48 consecutive studies, time-resolved MRA, a 4-detector-row spiral CT (4-MDCT), combined CE MRA plus 4-MDCT, VQ scanning alone, and VQ scanning plus 4-MDCT were compared (129). In that study, Ohno et al. reported that time-resolved CE MRA with a 4-second acquisition had significantly higher sensitivity for PE in the overall and peripheral vascular zones than the other noninvasive modalities including 4-MDCT, but not significantly different in the central vascular zone (Table 16-6A). Per patient results from that study are shown in Table 16-6B.

Of note, in the Ohno study, the use of 4-MDCT likely underestimates the capability of higher detector MDCT systems. However, Ohno expressed skepticism, suggesting that the resolution capability of both time-resolved CE MRA (optimized by parallel imaging) and CT (optimized by multidetector technology) are not sufficient for detection of embolism in the small, peripheral arteries (129).

TABLE 16-5

Animal Studies of Computed Tomographic Angiography versus Magnetic Resonance Angiography for Diagnosis of Pulmonary Embolism

Author	Year	Number/ Species	CTA Sensitivity (%)	CTA Specificity (%)	MRA Sensitivity (%)	MRA Specificity (%)	Size of Emboli	Gold Standard
Hurst (130)	1999	7/Dog	64 to 76	98 to 99	48 to 52	98 to 99	3.7 mm	DSA + autopsy
Haage (132)	2003	9/Pig	69 to 72	—	79 to 81	—	3.0 mm	DSA
Seo (131)	2003	5/Pig	57 to 66	95 to 98	88 to 92	85 to 90	3.0 mm	Autopsy

CTA, computed tomographic angiography; MRA, magnetic resonance angiography; DSA, digital subtraction angiography.

TABLE 16-6A

Accuracy of Contrast-enhanced Magnetic Resonance Angiography, Multidetector Computed Tomography, and Combined Contrast-enhanced Magnetic Resonance Angiography and Multidetector Computed Tomography on a Per Vascular Zone Basis in Forty-eight Patients Using Catheter Pulmonary Angiography as the Gold Standard

Modality	Sensitivity (%)	Specificity (%)	PPV (%)	NPV (%)	Accuracy (%)
Overall					
CE MRA	83	97	64	99	96
MDCT	75*	97	64	98	96
CE MRA + MDCT	83	97	65	99	96
Central					
CE MRA	100	99	92	100	99
MDCT	100	99	97	100	99
CE MRA + MDCT	100	99	95	100	99
Peripheral					
CE MRA	68	96	47	98	95
MDCT	54*	96	42	98	94
CE MRA + MDCT	68	96	47	98	95

PPV, positive predictive value; NPV, negative predictive value; CE MRA, contrast-enhanced magnetic resonance angiography; MDCT, multidetector computed tomography.

*Significant difference with CE MRA.

Overall results (all vascular segments) and results for central and peripheral segments are presented from Ohno Y, Higashino T, Takenaka D, et al. MRA with sensitivity encoding (SENSE) for suspected pulmonary embolism: comparison with MDCT and ventilation-perfusion scintigraphy. *AJR AM J Roentgenol.* 2004;183:91–98.

Direct Thrombus Imaging

Moody et al. have evaluated both the lower extremity veins and pulmonary vasculature for clots bright on T1-weighted images, indicating recent thrombosis (48–51). Using a water-excitation only magnetization prepared gradient-echo sequence (inversion time chosen to suppress flowing blood), they reported sensitivity of 94% to 96% and specificity of 90% to 92% in a large study of patients with DVT.

The same authors recently reported a study assessing the role of direct thrombus imaging in patients with PE. Because of problems related to use of the gold standard in all patients, they randomized patients into several arms by

TABLE 16-6B

Accuracy of Contrast-enhanced Magnetic Resonance Angiography, Multidetector Computed Tomography, Combined Contrast-enhanced Magnetic Resonance Angiography and Multidetector Computed Tomography, Ventilation-perfusion Scanning, and Combined Ventilation-perfusion and Multidetector Computed Tomography on a Per Patient Basis

Modality	Sensitivity (%)	Specificity (%)	PPV (%)	NPV (%)	Accuracy (%)
CE MRA	92	94	85	97	94
MDCT	83	94	83	94	92
CE MRA + MDCT	92	94	85	97	94
VQ scanning	67	78*	50	88	75*
MDCT + VQ	92	94	85	97	94

PPV, positive predictive value; NPV, negative predictive value; CE MRA, contrast-enhanced magnetic resonance angiography; MDCT, multidetector computed tomography; VQ, ventilation-perfusion.

*Significant difference compared with CE MRA.

using a multiplicity of tests (VQ scanning, spiral CTA, pulmonary angiography, direct thrombus imaging) and used outcome measures instead of comparison with the gold standard. The outcome of MR direct thrombus imaging (157 patients were included in the MRI arm) was similar to that of other investigative strategies (51). The use of such surrogate parameters conveys a clinical relevance to the investigation.

Blood-pool and True-FISP Imaging

To date, no prospective comparisons with DSA for diagnosis of PE have been reported.

Magnetic Resonance Imaging for Pulmonary Embolism in Current Practice

MR continues to evolve at a dramatic pace, and with the widespread availability of isotropic or near submillimeter data sets, the depiction of subsegmental arteries will be routine (Fig. 16-28). Until such a time, MRA will probably remain a second-line investigation in patients in whom CTA is contraindicated. However, if proxy arbiters of MRA accuracy for subsegmental embolism are accepted and if MRA and CTA are deemed equivalent or identical in terms of ability to image small arteries successfully, MR will offer benefit over CTA from a safety perspective.

The many options for imaging strategies with MRA demand that the trade-off between complexity and opportunity be tipped in favor of practical clinical implementation.

Scanner availability is a prime consideration in considering the role for MRI/MRA when evaluating patients suspected of having PE. The impact of newer techniques incorporating ventilation imaging, in association with MR perfusion and MRA, will need to be assessed as they continue to emerge into clinical practice (8–12,32–44,46–51).

PULMONARY ARTERIAL HYPERTENSION

Pulmonary arterial hypertension comprises a group of clinical and physiopathological entities with similar features but a variety of underlying causes. Because the range of medical conditions and environmental exposures associated with pulmonary arterial hypertension is wide, it is difficult to identify a unifying pathogenic mechanism (133). Clinically apparent pulmonary arterial hypertension is likely a final common manifestation of multiple preclinical conditions.

Pulmonary arterial hypertension is defined as a sustained elevation of pulmonary arterial pressure to more than 25 mmHg at rest or to more than 30 mmHg with exercise, with a mean pulmonary-capillary wedge pressure and left ventricular end-diastolic pressure of less than 15 mmHg (134).

It is usually classified as primary (idiopathic) or secondary (135). Since it has been recognized that there are conditions within the category of secondary PH that resemble primary PH in their histopathological features and their response to treatment, the World Health Organization

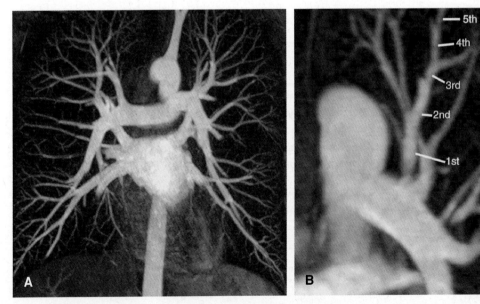

FIGURE 16-28 A: Coronal thin (20-mm-thick) MIP from high-spatial-resolution CE MRA (3/1.1; flip angle, 22°) in a volunteer reveal up to the fifth-order pulmonary branches with good definition. **B:** Image shows the order (1st to 5th) of the pulmonary arterial branches in left upper lobe. (Reprinted with permission from Nael K, Michaely HJ, Kramer U, et al. Pulmonary circulation: contrast-enhanced 3.0T MR angiography-initial results. *Radiology* 2006; 240: 858–868.)

TABLE 16-7

The Revised World Health Organization Classification of Pulmonary Hypertension

Group I. Pulmonary Arterial Hypertension
- Idiopathic (primary)
- Familial
- Related conditions: collagen vascular disease, congenital systemic-to-pulmonary shunts, portal hypertension, HIV infection, drugs, and toxins (e.g., anorexigens, rapeseed oil, L-tryptophan, methamphetamine, and cocaine). Other conditions: thyroid disorders, glycogen storage diseases, Gaucher disease, hereditary hemorrhagic telangiectasia, hemoglobinopathies, myeloproliferative disorders, splenectomy.
- Associated with significant venous or capillary involvement:
  Pulmonary veno-occlusive disease
  Pulmonary-capillary hemangiomatosis
- Persistent pulmonary hypertension of the newborn

Group II. Pulmonary Venous Hypertension
- Left-sided atrial or ventricular heart disease
- Left-sided valvular heart disease

Group III. Pulmonary Hypertension Associated with Hypoxemia
- Chronic obstructive pulmonary disease
- Interstitial lung disease
- Sleep-disordered breathing
- Alveolar hypoventilation disorders
- Chronic exposure to high altitude
- Developmental abnormalities

Group IV. Pulmonary Hypertension Due to Chronic Thrombotic Disease, Embolic Disease, or Both
- Thromboembolic obstruction or proximal pulmonary arteries
- Thromboembolic obstruction of distal pulmonary arteries
- Pulmonary embolism (tumor, parasites, foreign material)

Group V. Miscellaneous
- Sarcoidosis, pulmonary Langerhans cell histiocytosis, lymphangiomatosis, compression of pulmonary vessels (adenopathy, tumor, fibrosing mediastinitis)

Adapted from Simonneau G, Galie N, Rubin LJ, et al. Clinical classification of pulmonary hypertension. *J Am Coll Cardiol*. 2004;43:5S–12S. Copyright 2004, reprinted with permission from American College of Cardiology Foundation.

(WHO) has classified PH into five groups on a mechanistic basis rather than on the basis of associated conditions (Table 16-7).

PH of the precapillary pulmonary circulation is a diagnostic challenge (136–138). The host of potential underlying disorders includes idiopathic disease, recurrent embolism, and structural lung changes among other more readily identifiable causes. In 0.1% to 0.5% of survivors of acute PE, emboli do not resolve completely but are replaced by weblike constrictions and stenoses within arteries (136–138).

Chronic Thromboembolic Pulmonary Hypertension

In patients predisposed to recurrent PE, chronic thromboembolic pulmonary hypertension (CTEPH) occurs when approximately 60% of the pulmonary vascular bed is affected. Once mean pulmonary arterial pressures reach 30 mmHg, patients are usually severely dyspneic with right-sided heart failure and anticipated 5-year survival is 30%. Surgical thromboendarterectomy offers the only hope of

cure in these patients but can only be performed if organized thrombi are located proximal to the origins of the segmental arteries.

Catheter pulmonary angiography is still being used for preoperative evaluation of the severity of disease and determining the technical feasibility of surgery in patients being considered for endarterectomy, but it gives at best limited functional information. Today, most information required for therapeutic planning can be obtained noninvasively by cross-sectional imaging with MRA or CTA, which provides excellent information regarding the location of the relevant (proximal) clots.

Cross-sectional Imaging of Patients with Pulmonary Hypertension

Regardless of etiology, the cardinal sign of PH on cross-sectional imaging by both CT and MR is dilatation of the pulmonary trunk and the proximal (main and lobar) pulmonary arteries on both sides (Figs. 16-29, 16-30). A distal pulmonary trunk diameter greater than the diameter

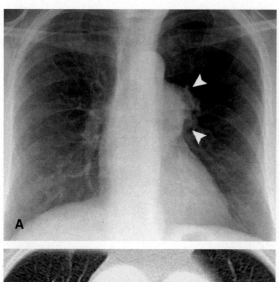
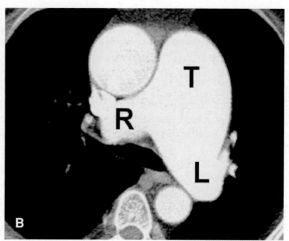
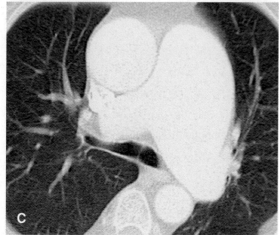

FIGURE 16-29 Idiopathic dilatation of the pulmonary trunk in a 55-year-old asymptomatic woman. A: Posteroanterior chest radiograph shows an abnormal bulge in the left mediastinal border (*arrowheads*), a feature suggestive of a mediastinal mass identical to that observed on radiographs obtained 6 years earlier (not shown). **B:** CE CT scan shows abnormal enlargement of the main pulmonary trunk (T), with mild dilatation of the right (R) and left (L) pulmonary arteries. **C:** CT scan obtained with a lung window setting at the same level as **(B)** shows normal vessels and parenchyma. (Reprinted with permission from Castaner E, Gallardo X, Rimola J, et al. Congenital and acquired pulmonary artery anomalies in the adult: radiologic overview. *Radiographics*. 2006;26:349–371.)

of the ascending aorta or a main pulmonary artery diameter of 29 mm on either side is diagnostic of PH. Additional signs include distal pulmonary artery tapering and enlargement of right-sided cardiac structures (Figs. 16-30, 16-31). Although the diagnosis of PH can be easily established by both CTA and MRA, both offer additional but very different benefit to patients with PH—in the case of CT, many nonvascular causes can be inferred by evaluating the lung parenchyma on appropriate windows; in the case of MRA, valuable information on lung perfusion and cardiac function can be noninvasively obtained.

Computed Tomography Evaluation of Patients with Pulmonary Hypertension

CT plays a much wider role than MRA in the evaluation of patients with PH, as it can demonstrate nonvascular causes in many cases. For example, evaluation of the nonvascular structures gives a number of clues about the etiology of PH as follows:

1. Widespread interstitial lines with distortion of the normal lung architecture and traction bronchiectasis in patients with established pulmonary fibrosis. The location and pattern in some instances may suggest a specific cause.
2. Interlobular septal thickening is also seen in patients with sarcoidosis and veno-occlusive disease.
3. Diffuse or focal decreased lung capacity points toward emphysema.
4. Parenchymal nodules (e.g., centrilobular opacities) are present in patients with long-standing sarcoidosis and extrinsic allergic alveolitis.
5. Enlarged mediastinal lymph nodes in patients with sarcoidosis.
6. Smooth masses with two associated vessels in patients with arteriovenous malformations.
7. Altered contrast dynamics are present in patients with mitral stenosis or left heart failure.
8. Segmental mosaic perfusion (oligaemia) pattern, which in association with pulmonary artery abnormality to that segment (usually a small artery) is virtually pathognomonic of chronic PE.

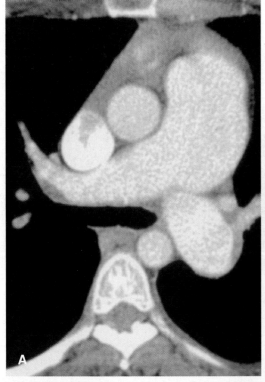

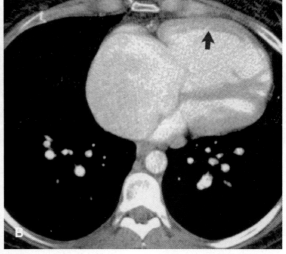

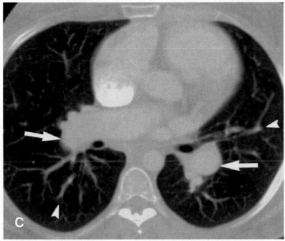

FIGURE 16-30 Primary PH in a young adult woman.
A: CE chest CT scan (mediastinal window) demonstrates a widened pulmonary trunk. **B:** CE chest CT scan (mediastinal window) obtained at a lower level shows right ventricular dilatation and thickening of the free right ventricular wall (*arrow*). **C:** Chest CT scan (lung window) shows large-caliber central pulmonary arteries (*arrows*) with abrupt tapering of the peripheral vessels (*arrowheads*). (Reprinted with permission from Frazier AA, Galvin JR, Franks TJ, et al. From the archives of the AFIP: pulmonary vasculature: hypertension and infarction. *Radiographics.* 2000;20:491–524; quiz 530–531, 532.)

Computed Tomography for Chronic Thromboembolic Pulmonary Hypertension

CT has traditionally been an important tool in the diagnostic algorithm of CTEPH, allowing for an accurate assessment of both pathogenesis and extent of the disease (137,139–142). High-resolution CT (HRCT) is the gold standard to evaluate a patient with suspected PH for structural lung changes that may cause increased pre- or postcapillary pressure within the lung vessels in the absence of recurrent thromboembolism as the etiology for increased pulmonary pressure. Mosaic attenuation on HRCT, combined with distal pruning of pulmonary arteries, is a sign of impaired pulmonary perfusion due to recurrent peripheral embolism as the underlying cause.

CE CT allows for direct visualization of chronic thromboembolic changes (Fig. 16-32). If neither structural lung changes nor signs of thromboembolism are found in the absence of other identifiable etiologies for PH, such as congenital heart disease or tumor embolism, a diagnosis of primary PH is usually considered. Since the differential diagnosis of PH includes diseases with both focal and diffuse character, the entire pathology frequently cannot be appreciated with a single CT technique. Thick collimation single-slice CT may not suffice to assess interstitial changes.

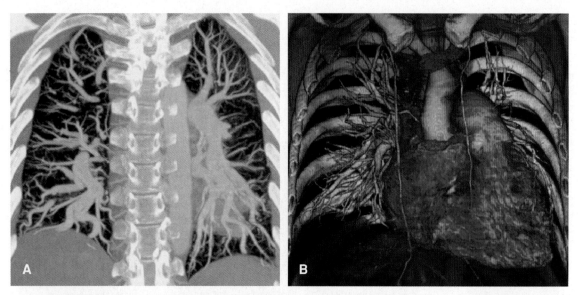

FIGURE 16-31 Patient with long-standing idiopathic PH. MIP **(A)** and volume rendering **(B)** of a CE multidetector-row CT study show tortuous, corkscrewlike appearance of the pulmonary arteries and massive dilatation of the
right heart in response to the increased pulmonary arterial pressure.

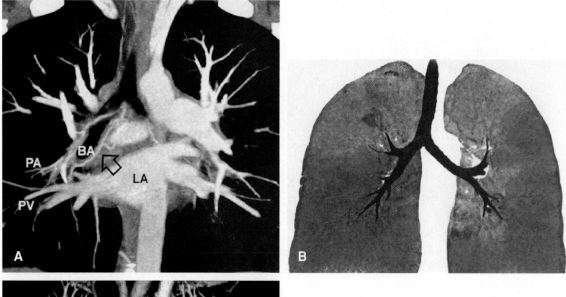

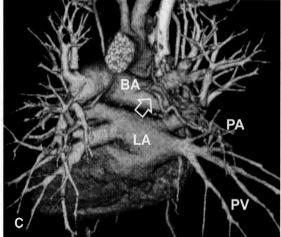

FIGURE 16-32 CE multidetector-row CTA in a patient with
recurrent thromboembolic disease displayed as coronal MIP **(A)**,
coronal minimum-intensity projection **(B)**, and using volume-
rendered technique **(C)** seen from posterior. The pulmonary arteries (*PA*) in the right lower lobe appear obliterated by recurrent
PE, with normal-sized pulmonary veins (*PV*) returning to the left
atrium (*LA*) **(A)**. Lung perfusion in the affected lower lobes of the
lung is diminished but maintained in the upper lobes **(B)**. Blood
flow to the right lower lobe is maintained via the bronchial arteries (*BA*) , which are hypertrophied (*arrow* in **A** and **C**) and have
formed collaterals bypassing occluded and obliterated pulmonary
arteries. (Reprinted with permission from Schoepf UJ, Goldhaber
SZ, Costello P. Spiral computed tomography for acute pulmonary
embolism. *Circulation*. 2004;109:2160–2167.)

If only HRCT is performed, focal pathology, such as thromboembolism, is easily missed due to the high-frequency reconstruction algorithms and because scans are acquired at only every 10 to 20 mm.

If single-slice CT is used for evaluation of patients with suspected PH, it is therefore often necessary to perform both a CE spiral acquisition and HRCT for a comprehensive assessment of the underlying pathology. Now, a thin-collimation multidetector-row CT acquisition during a single breath-hold generates a set of raw data that provides all options for image reconstruction, addressing multiple diagnostic problems by performing a single CE scan.

In patients with suspected PH, we routinely perform a thin-slice reconstruction of the entire chest, which can detect PEs with high accuracy. In addition, from the same set of raw data, 5-mm contiguous lung sections and HRCT sections at every 1 cm are routinely performed. Thus, from a single set of raw data, a comprehensive analysis of gross and diffuse lung changes and of thromboembolic disease becomes feasible.

Magnetic Resonance for Chronic Thromboembolic Pulmonary Hypertension

In addition to structural information (Figs. 16-33–16-35), MRA has the potential to also provide information on functional parameters, such as pulmonary perfusion and myocardial dysfunction (Fig. 16-36). Kreitner et al. recently reported combined morphological assessment of the pulmonary arteries with CE MRA and functional assessment by MR with short-axis cine gradient refocused echo (GRE)

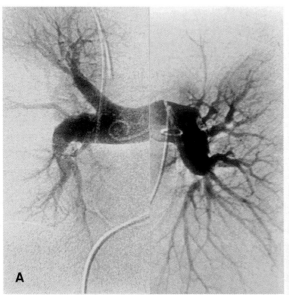
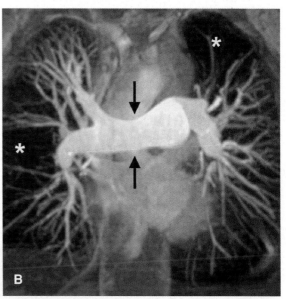
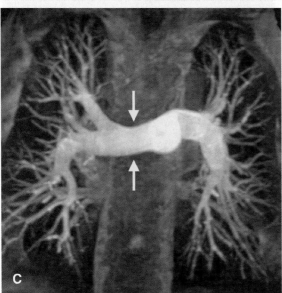

FIGURE 16-33 Selective DSA images versus MIPs of CE MR angiographic data obtained in 63-year-old man.
A: Selective DSA image of right and left pulmonary arteries in anteroposterior projections; images from two separate injections in right and left pulmonary arteries have been juxtaposed. MIPs of preoperative **(B)** and postpulmonary thromboendarterectomy **(C)** MR angiographic data (4.6/1.8; flip angle, 30°) have excellent overall image quality. Nearly complete normalization of pulmonary arterial vasculature is seen postoperatively (especially comparing the areas marked with an * in **B**). Note postoperative decrease in diameters of right (*arrows*) and left pulmonary arteries. (Adapted with permission from Kreitner KF, Ley S, Kauczor HU, et al. Chronic thromboembolic pulmonary hypertension: pre- and postoperative assessment with breath-hold MR imaging techniques. *Radiology.* 2004;232:535–543.)

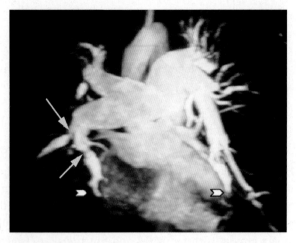

FIGURE 16-34 3D CE MRA in a CTEPH patient with webs and stenoses (*arrows*). Notice the enlarged main pulmonary artery and acute caliber changes at lobar and segmental levels with cut-off vessels (*arrowheads*). (Reprinted with permission from Pedersen MR, Fisher MT, van Beek EJ. MR imaging of the pulmonary vasculature—an update. *Eur Radiol.* 2006;16:1374–1386.)

images and ECG-gated phase-contrast velocity-encoded segmented k-space acquisitions in 34 patients with CTEPH (136).

They reported that CE MRA revealed all 533 arteries to segmental level depicted by DSA and 681 of 733 (93%) patent subsegmental arteries shown by DSA. Functional assessment confirmed typical findings of CTEPH, such as

reduced right ventricular ejection fraction, paradoxical septal motion, normal left ventricular ejection fraction, and differences in flow rates through the pulmonary arteries and ascending aorta (attributed to recruitment from the bronchial circulation in CTEPH) (136–138). Follow-up MRI/MRA also allowed a comprehensive assessment of morphology and functional characteristics in patients who had undergone surgery.

PRETREATMENT EVALUATION FOR HEMOPTYSIS

The planning and successful performance of bronchial arterial embolization, as a treatment for massive and recurrent hemoptysis, depends on exact knowledge of the pulmonary vascular anatomy and the location of the hemorrhage (143). CT is readily available at most institutions, allowing for a fast diagnosis, even in patients with acute hemoptysis (144,145).

Thin-section multidetector-row CT of the thorax is capable of providing high-resolution images and CT angiograms in a single session. Two recent studies (144,145) reported successful visualization of the bronchial arteries with 16-slice MDCT in almost all patients.

This enables evaluation of structural changes of the lung parenchyma as well as of pulmonary vessels, which makes this technology quite suitable for comprehensive imaging of disorders of the systemic arterial supply of the lung (Fig. 16-37).

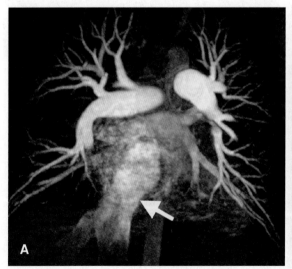
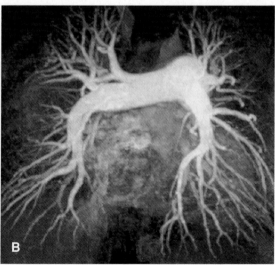

FIGURE 16-35 Chronic thromboembolism with Gd-enhanced MRA. Coronal thin (**A**) and full-thickness (**B**) MIPs from high-spatial-resolution pulmonary CE MRA (3/1.1; flip angle, 22°) show proximal dilatation of the central pulmonary arteries in a patient with PAH. Because the pulmonary transit time was prolonged, pulmonary venous enhancement was delayed. Note hepatic venous reflux (*arrow* in **A**) secondary to the high pressures in the right heart. (Reprinted with permission from Nael K, Michaely HJ, Kramer U, et al. Pulmonary Circulation Contrast-enhanced 3.0T MR Angiography-Initial Results. *Radiology* 2006;240:858–868.)

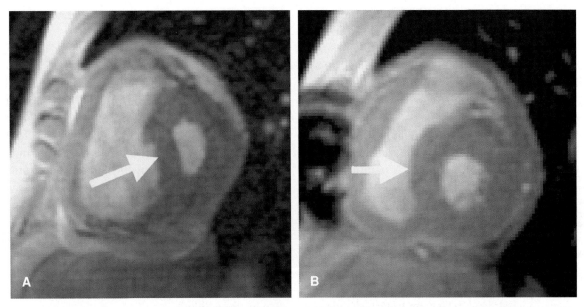

FIGURE 16-36 Short-axis cine MR images (echo time, 4.8 milliseconds; temporal resolution, 50 milliseconds) in 48-year-old man show interventricular septum (*arrow*) during systole. **A:** Preoperative image shows paradoxical movement of interventricular septum, with bulging into the left ventricle. **B:** Image obtained 10 days after surgery shows normal movement of interventricular septum. (Reprinted with permission from Kreitner KF, Ley S, Kauczor HU, et al. Chronic thromboembolic pulmonary hypertension: pre- and postoperative assessment with breath-hold MR imaging techniques. *Radiology.* 2004;232:535–543.)

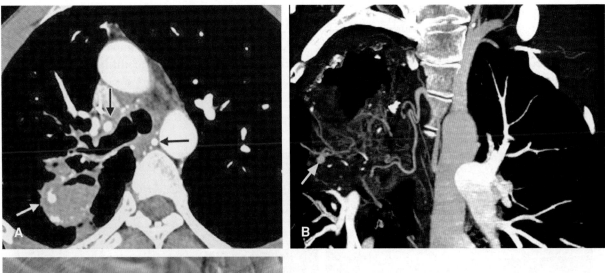

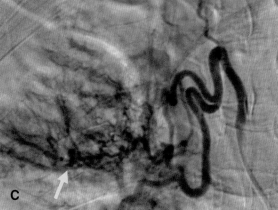

FIGURE 16-37 Bronchial artery aneurysm in a 37-year-old man with acute hemoptysis of 300 mL in 24 hours. **A:** Axial CT scan (1-mm-thick section) obtained with mediastinal soft-tissue window settings (window center, 50 HU; window width, 350 HU) depicts a dense nodular lesion (*white arrow*) within a necrotic mass in the right upper lobe. Enlarged bronchial arteries (*black arrows*) can be identified in the mediastinum. **B:** Thoracic CTA study performed with a 16-detector-row scanner. In the coronal MIP image, the dense nodule (*arrow*) can be clearly identified as a bronchial artery aneurysm. **C:** Arteriogram shows the aneurysm (*arrow*) arising from a branch of the intercostobronchial artery, which was later successfully embolized. (Reprinted with permission from Bruzzi JF, Remy-Jardin M, Delhaye D, et al. Multi-detector row CT of hemoptysis. *Radiographics.* 2006;26:3–22.)

Although no study has evaluated the role of MRA in patients with hemoptysis who might require bronchial artery embolization, O'Keefe et al. reported visualization of the right and left bronchial arteries in 82.5% and 12.5%, respectively, in subjects undergoing pulmonary MRA for evaluation of pulmonary vein architecture prior to radio frequency ablation (146).

Since that study was not optimized for bronchial artery technique (observations were made while studying the pulmonary veins), the true ability for MRA to visualize the right and left bronchial arteries is unknown.

SYSTEMIC ARTERIALIZATION OF THE LUNGS

Chronic inflammatory disease can result in acquired systemic arterialization of the lungs by causing anastomoses between pulmonary and systemic arteries (147). Most often, the anastomoses develop between bronchial and pulmonary arteries within the lung parenchyma. Transpleural anastomoses between pulmonary and systemic nonbronchial arteries may occur in response to an inflammatory pleural adhesion, resulting in neovascularization from regional systemic arteries (147,148).

Chronic vascular obstruction by inflammatory disorders (e.g., Takayasu arteritis) or chronic thromboembolic changes of the pulmonary arteries can also cause anastomoses between the bronchial and pulmonary arterial systems, resulting in collateralization of the stenosed or obstructed pulmonary arterial bed by the systemic bronchial component of the dual pulmonary blood supply with subsequent hypertrophy of the bronchial arteries (149–152).

VASCULAR INVOLVEMENT IN PULMONARY MALIGNANCY

Primary Neoplasms of the Pulmonary Arteries

Pulmonary artery sarcomas are rare malignancies of the pulmonary vasculature (153–155). The etiology of these tumors is obscure. Histopathologically, most pulmonary artery sarcomas are leiomyosarcomas or "undifferentiated spindle cell sarcomas." Histopathologic classification, however, does not seem to be useful clinically or prognostically.

Most pulmonary artery sarcomas arise from the dorsal area of the pulmonary trunk, although the tumors also may arise from the right and left pulmonary arteries, the pulmonary valve, and the right ventricular outflow tract. Because of its rarity and insidious growth characteristics, pulmonary artery sarcoma is often mistaken for PE, resulting in inappropriate therapy such as prolonged anticoagulation or thrombolysis.

Symptoms and signs such as weight loss, fever, anemia, and digital clubbing may be subtle clues to diagnosis. Other characteristics, such as the absence of risk factors for DVT, high sedimentation rate, nodular parenchymal infiltrates, and lack of response to anticoagulation should raise the suspicion of a process other than PE.

Cross-sectional imaging for a precise preoperative assessment is crucial for the appropriate exploration of the pulmonary artery to ensure complete resection and reconstruction. Subtle features of infiltration as opposed to thromboembolic occlusion and contrast enhancement on delayed CT (Fig. 16-38) or MR imaging (Fig. 16-39) may provide clues as to the malignant character of these lesions;

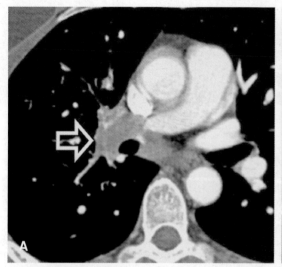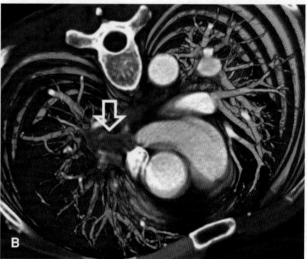

FIGURE 16-38 A 52-year-old woman with dyspnea. Multidetector-row CTA images shown as axial section **(A)** and volume rendering **(B)** depict an endoluminal filling defect in the right pulmonary artery (*arrow*) that was initially felt to be consistent with chronic thromboembolism. Surgical exploration after failure of specific treatment established a diagnosis of pulmonary artery sarcoma. Volume rendering **(B)** may be better suited for appreciating the masslike and slightly infiltrative nature of the right pulmonary artery lesion.

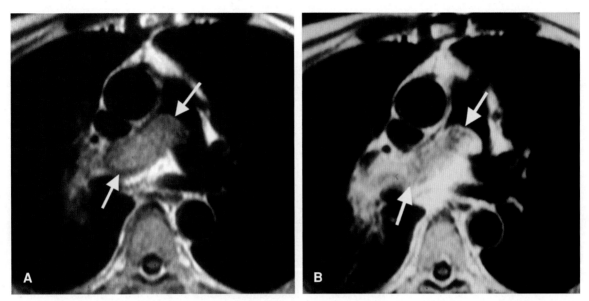

FIGURE 16-39 Pulmonary artery sarcoma with MRI. A: Axial ECG-triggered T1-weighted spin echo image shows an intermediate signal intensity mass filling the right main pulmonary artery (*arrows*). **B:** Identical image after intravenous Gd-DTPA demonstrates marked enhancement of the mass (*arrows*). Following surgical removal, this mass was shown to be a pulmonary artery sarcoma. (Images courtesy of Neil M. Rofsky, MD, Beth Israel Deaconess Medical Center, Boston.)

however, in many cases, a straightforward differentiation from pulmonary thromboembolism will remain elusive.

Primary Neoplasms of the Pulmonary Veins

Primary neoplasms of the pulmonary veins are rare. Most primary tumors are sarcomas, although those originating in the pulmonary arteries are much more common than those with origin in the pulmonary veins (156). Pulmonary vein leiomyosarcoma is the most common primary neoplasm originating in the pulmonary vein. Pulmonary vein leiomyosarcomas are more common in women, and they can express hormone receptors. Extension into the left atrium is common at the time of diagnosis. Prognosis is poor, although complete surgical excision can provide long-term survival (157).

Secondary Tumor Involvement

Cross-sectional imaging of the pulmonary circulation has a premier role in pre- and post-therapeutic evaluation of the vascular status of thoracic malignancies (153,158,159). The correct staging of tumors of the lung and of the mediastinum, foremost of bronchogenic carcinoma, is a cardinal prerequisite for appropriate tumor management (158).

CE CT and MR pulmonary angiography of the pulmonary circulation enable a determination of the exact location and extent of tumor mass with respect to pulmonary vessels and tumor vascularity (Figs. 16-40, 16-41).

Over the course of treating bronchogenic carcinoma, therapeutic effects can be accurately monitored by follow-up imaging. Furthermore, when the tumor mass is located in the immediate proximity of vessels or when invasion of vessels has already occurred, crucial information about the risk of hemorrhage can be provided (153).

Visualization of the pulmonary vessels also guides surgical planning. When tumor invasion of central structures such as the main bronchi and the central pulmonary vessels is diagnosed, a more radical surgical approach becomes necessary. Centrally located tumors that do not invade or surround adjacent vessels are usually resected by a sleeve lobectomy and an end-to-end anastomosis of the main stem bronchus. If, however, tumor invasion of more centrally located pulmonary arteries is determined, angioplastic pulmonary artery reconstruction or pneumonectomy is indicated.

Any postsurgical complications, such as arterial strictures and bronchoarterial fistulas following pulmonary artery reconstruction, or clot in the pulmonary artery stump after lobectomy are usually readily identified on cross-sectional imaging follow-up (160,161).

Pulmonary Venous Thrombosis with Intrathoracic Malignancy

Pulmonary venous thrombosis can occur in patients with intrathoracic malignancies, particularly lung cancer, and can affect surgical approach. Thrombus in the pulmonary veins can be the source for systemic embolism, including patients with stroke or distal extremity arterial occlusion (162). Preoperative recognition of this condi-

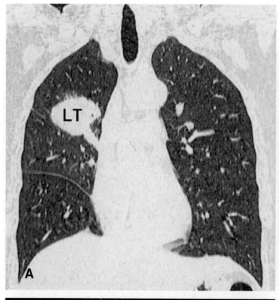

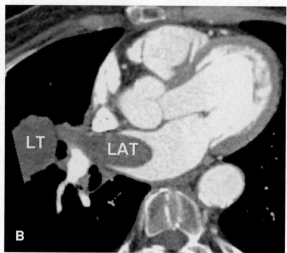

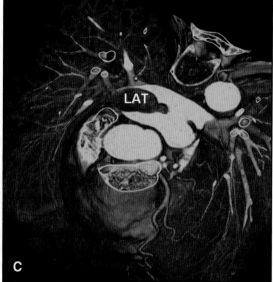

FIGURE 16-40 CE ECG-gated multidetector-row CT scan in a 62-year-old woman with a lung tumor (*LT*). Display as coronal MPR in lung window settings (**A**) shows the tumor in the right upper lobe invading the right upper lobe pulmonary vein. Transverse-oblique MPR (**B**) and volume rendered display (**C**) show the left atrial extension of the tumor mass (*LAT*) via the right upper lobe pulmonary vein.

tion is important, as systemic tumor emboli can occur during the resection of the intravenous component of the tumor, which can lead to a life-threatening complication (163).

Extension of the tumor thrombus into the left atrium may require a different surgical approach. Pulmonary venous thrombus can be recognized with CT (164) (Fig. 16-40), transesophageal echo (165), and positron emission tomography (PET). PET imaging can demonstrate direct extension of the tumor into the left atrium and confirm the tumoral nature of the thrombus (166). 3D gadolinium-enhanced MR imaging provides excellent evaluation of the pulmonary veins in patients with lung cancer (167). Thrombus in the pulmonary vein remnant

after lobectomy can also be seen on cross-sectional imaging (Fig. 16-42).

PULMONARY ARTERIOVENOUS MALFORMATION

Arteriovenous malformations are abnormal communications between arteries and veins (168–170). Between 70% and 90% of patients with pulmonary arteriovenous malformations (PAVMs) have hereditary hemorrhagic telangiectasia (HHT, also known as Osler-Rendu-Weber syndrome), which has an autosomal dominant pattern of transmission; the remainder are sporadic. Conversely, only 35% of patients with HHT have PAVMs. Although the PAVMs in

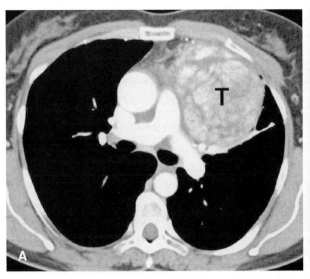
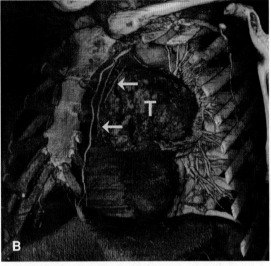

FIGURE 16-41 Invasive thymoma (T). CE transverse CT image **(A)** shows an intensely enhancing nodular mediastinal mass with adjacent atelectasis. Display as volume rendering **(B)** shows feeding neovasculature (*arrows*) arising from the left internal mammary artery and other thoracic collaterals in this hypervascular tumor.

HHT are inherited and should be present at birth, they seldom manifest clinically until adult life (90%). There is a steady increase through the fifth and sixth decades, a female predominance (2:1) apart from cases presenting in infancy, where males predominate.

Between 50% and 75% of PAVMs are found in the lower lobes, 75% are unilateral disease, and 36% have multiple lesions. Individual PAVMs are typically from 1 to 5 cm in size, although they are occasionally greater than 10 cm.

Seven to 11% of patients have diffuse microvascular PAVMs (telangiectasia—almost always present in childhood), which are often in combination with larger, radiographically visible PAVMs (168).

In the pulmonary circulation, arteriovenous malformations short circuit the capillary bed with three main clinical consequences, as follows: (a) The blood passing through these right-to-left shunts remains deoxygenated, resulting in hypoxemia that cannot be reversed even with

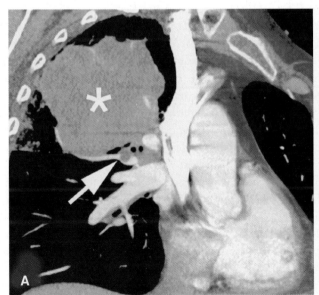
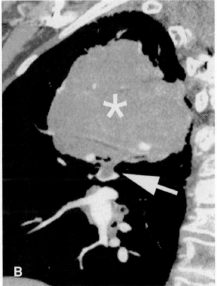

FIGURE 16-42 CE multidetector-row CT scan in a patient with a primary lung tumor (∗). Coronal **(A)** and sagittal **(B)** MPR in soft tissue window shows the tumor in the right upper lobe invading the right upper lobe pulmonary vein (*arrows*).

100% oxygen; (b) the normal filtering capacity of the pulmonary capillary bed is bypassed, thus allowing matter (air bubbles and blood clots) to reach the systemic circulation directly, causing paradoxical embolism (transient ischemic attack, stroke, cerebral or systemic abscess); (c) rupture into a bronchus (hemoptysis) or pleural cavity (hemothorax) occasionally occurs, most commonly in pregnant women.

Arteriovenous malformations are categorized as "simple" (where one or multiple feeding arteries originate from a single segmental artery) or "complex" (where feeding arteries always originate from two or more segmental arteries). In some patients, diffuse pattern of a lobe may occur (168,169). By CT criteria, the majority (approximately 90%) are simple (169).

The incidence of symptoms is said to be greater in patients with multiple rather than single PAVM. It is unusual for a single PAVM <2 cm in diameter to cause symptoms. Patients with diffuse microvascular PAVM are uniformly symptomatic.

The most common complaint in symptomatic patients with PAVM is epistaxis, related to bleeding from mucosal telangiectases and reflecting the high incidence of HHT in patients with PAVM.

Dyspnea, the second most common complaint in patients with PAVM, is more common in patients with large or multiple PAVMs. Platypnea, symptomatic improvement in breathing on reclining (secondary to a decrease in blood flow through PAVM in the dependent portions of the lungs upon assuming the supine position), should raise the possibility of an underlying AVM. Hemoptysis, the third most common symptom, is usually mild but occasionally massive and can be fatal.

Cross-sectional imaging has proved useful and highly sensitive for the detection of PAVM and is accepted as the method of choice for routine detection of this vascular abnormality. Morphologically, PAVMs are similar to AVMs elsewhere in the body and present one of three typical appearances: a large, single sac; a plexiform mass of dilated vascular channels; or a dilated and often tortuous direct artery-vein communication (Fig. 16-43). Mural thrombi or calcification within the sac is uncommon.

Apart from detection, CT and MRA are also crucial for pretherapeutic evaluation of the angioarchitecture of PAVMs, especially for assessing the number and configuration of feeding and draining vessels connected to the aneurysmal sac (Fig. 16-44). The therapy of choice consists in embolization of the vascular nidus and the number, course, and orientation of the feeding

arteries are the most important factors that determine the technical difficulty and success rate of this procedure (170).

PULMONARY ARTERY STENOSES, OCCLUSIONS, ANEURYSMS, AND PSEUDOANEURYSMS

Pulmonary Artery Stenosis

Pulmonary artery stenosis is usually due to pulmonary vasculitis, associated with a cardiac anomaly, or secondary to direct invasion by a lung tumor (171,172). Treatment is that of the underlying condition, and intravascular stent deployment has become the treatment of choice for a flow-limiting pulmonary stenosis accompanying a cardiac anomaly (170,171).

Pulmonary Vasculitis

Although pulmonary vasculitis is associated with a variety of disorders such as Takayasu arteritis, Behçet disease, polyarteritis nodosa, Wegener disease, Churg-Strauss syndrome, systemic lupus erythematous, and microscopic angiitis, only the first two of these produce abnormalities within the pulmonary arteries that can be demonstrated with imaging. The remaining disorders are usually manifested only as pulmonary parenchymal abnormalities on imaging (149,150,173–176).

Takayasu Arteritis

This inflammatory disease of larger- and medium-sized arteries characterized by arterial stenoses and occlusions (and occasionally aneurysms) shows a strong female preponderance (10:1) and strong predilection for the thoracic aorta, its branches, and the pulmonary arteries (149,150,173). Although more common in Asia, it is not geographically restricted. The highest incidence is in adolescent and young adult women. Histologically, there is a pan-arteritis with inflammatory mononuclear infiltrates with occasional giant cells. Although immunopathogenic mechanisms are implicated due to the demonstration of circulating immune complexes, their precise mechanism in the etiology of this disorder remains unclear.

Takayasu arteritis is a systemic disease of insidious onset with malaise, fever, night sweats, arthralgias, anorexia, and weight loss. In the early stages, there are no specific indicators of vascular involvement; however, tenderness of superficial arteries such as the common femoral artery may point to the diagnosis.

Cardiac enlargement and cardiac failure, secondary to aortic or PH, are common; however, the coronary arteries are uncommonly involved.

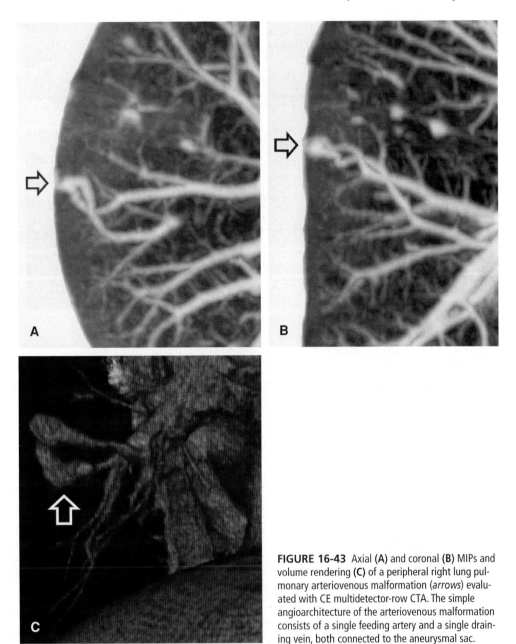

FIGURE 16-43 Axial **(A)** and coronal **(B)** MIPs and volume rendering **(C)** of a peripheral right lung pulmonary arteriovenous malformation (*arrows*) evaluated with CE multidetector-row CTA. The simple angioarchitecture of the arteriovenous malformation consists of a single feeding artery and a single draining vein, both connected to the aneurysmal sac.

Chest radiographic findings are usually noncontributory, although occasionally, irregularity of the outline of the descending thoracic aorta is noted. In the early stages, the lumen may be entirely normal on catheter angiography of thoracic aorta or pulmonary arteries; however, increased distance between the normal-appearing descending aortic lumen and the lung may indicate mural inflammation. In the late stages, characteristic angiographic findings include stenoses and occlusions.

Pulmonary artery involvement, once thought rare, is present in 50% of severe cases. Coinvolvement of the pulmonary arteries in a patient with aortitis is unique to Takayasu disease. However, symptomatic pulmonary involvement is uncommon, and typically, respiratory function remains normal even in patients with extensive pulmonary involvement.

Cross-sectional imaging with both CTA and MRA is as effective as catheter angiography in demonstrating

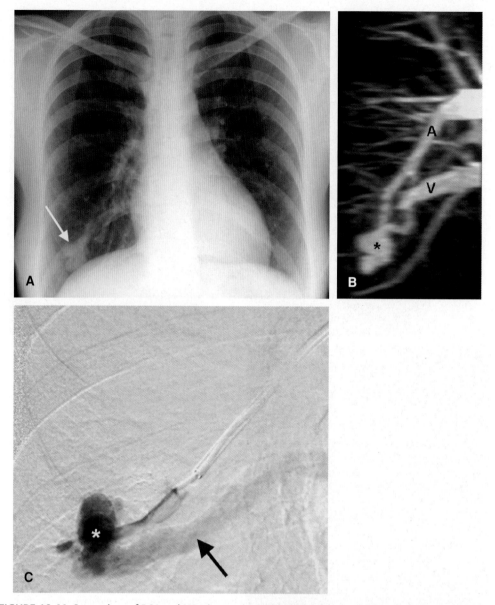

FIGURE 16-44 Comparison of DSA and MRA in a patient with HHT. A: Chest x-ray demonstrates a "mass" at the right base (*arrow*) along with an elongated structure typical of a draining vein. **B:** Oblique reformat clearly demonstrates the feeding artery (*A*), the nidus (*∗*) and enlarged vein (*V*). **C:** Selective DSA with injection into the feeding artery demonstrates enhancement of the nidus (*∗*) and also early filling of an enlarged inferior pulmonary vein (*arrow*).

stenoses, occlusions, aneurysms, and mural thrombi but have the distinct advantage of being able to demonstrate mural thickening (149,150) (Fig. 16-45). The diagnosis is frequently established nowadays by demonstration of vascular abnormalities in a patient with nonspecific symptoms undergoing CT to exclude an inflammatory process or underlying malignancy (149).

Behçet Disease and Hughes-Stovin Syndrome

Behçet disease is a chronic, multisystem inflammatory disorder of unknown cause. In addition to the classic triad of oral

ulceration, genital ulceration, and ocular abnormalities, skin, joint, gastrointestinal, genitourinary, neurological, cardiovascular, and lung involvement may be present (173–175).

Vascular involvement occurs in 20% to 40%, and there may be pulmonary involvement in 1% to 10% of cases. The disease typically presents at between 20 and 30 years of age, is much more common in males, and has a predilection for Mediterranean regions with a highest recorded prevalence in Turkey (173).

Behçet disease is the most common cause of pulmonary artery aneurysms (Fig. 16-46). The underlying

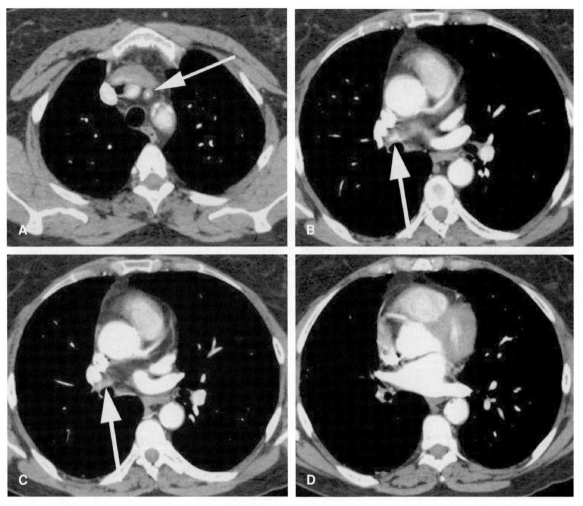

FIGURE 16-45 Type IIb Takayasu arteritis with pulmonary artery involvement in a 30-year-old woman.
A: Axial contrast material-enhanced multidetector-row CT scan shows stenosis and wall thickening of the left common carotid artery at its origin (*arrow*). **B,C:** Axial CE multidetector-row CT scans (**B** obtained at a higher level than **C**) show occlusion of the right descending interlobar artery (*arrow*). **D:** Axial CE multidetector-row CT scan from the same examination shows absence of enhanced vessels in the right lower lobe. There is also mild wall thickening of the descending thoracic aorta. (Reprinted with permission from Nastri MV, Baptista LP, Baroni RH, et al. Gadolinium-enhanced three-dimensional MRA of Takayasu arteritis. *Radiographics.* 2004;24:773–786.)

pathology is destruction of the elastic media secondary to vasculitis affecting the vasa vasorum, the arteries providing the blood supply to the pulmonary artery wall.

Although DVT is common in Behçet disease, PE is rare, as clots are tightly adherent to the vessel wall, and the frequent observation of clots within pulmonary arteries is believed to represent in-situ thrombosis.

Unlike Takayasu arteritis where pulmonary involvement, although common, rarely leads to symptoms, in Behçet disease, pulmonary involvement is almost always associated with severe symptoms such as life-threatening hemoptysis—possible causes include rupture into a bronchus or thrombosis of an artery with distal infarc-tion. Pulmonary aneurysm formation carries a very poor prognosis, with a death rate of 30% of patients within 2 years (173).

Associated parenchymal abnormalities in Behçet disease, including infarcts, atelectasis, hemorrhage, organizing pneumonia, eosinophilic pneumonia, and nonspecific fibrosis, are common and easily detectable by CT.

Hughes-Stovin syndrome is likely a form fruste of Behçet disease, manifesting as pulmonary artery aneurysms, DVT, and cerebral venous sinus thrombosis but without oral or genital ulceration. Imaging findings within the pulmonary arteries are identical to those described for Behçet syndrome (176,177).

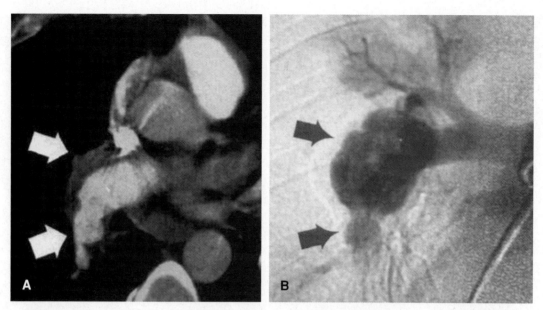

FIGURE 16-46 A 28-year-old man with Behçet disease, hemoptysis, and dyspnea. A: CT scan shows partially thrombosed main and lobar pulmonary artery aneurysms (*arrows*). **B:** DSA shows multiple right pulmonary artery aneurysms (*arrows*). (Reprinted with permission from Tunaci M, Ozkorkmaz B, Tunaci A, et al. CT findings of pulmonary artery aneurysms during treatment for Behçet's disease. *AJR Am J Roentgenol.* 1999;172:729–733.)

Pulmonary Artery Aneurysms

Although the cause of true pulmonary artery aneurysms is not well known, they may be congenital or acquired (178). Most cases reported in the literature are found incidentally at autopsy. PH is present in the majority of cases, and pulmonary aneurysms outside this setting are extremely rare. The major complication is rupture (Fig. 16-47), presenting as severe hemoptysis, which is frequently fatal. Evidence-based guidelines for treatment do not exist, but serial increase in size merits treatment. Transcatheter embolization is a safe and effective method for preventing rupture (170,178).

Other Nontraumatic Causes of Pulmonary Artery Aneurysms and Occlusions

Other causes of pulmonary artery pseudoaneurysms are few but include pneumonia, tuberculosis, aspergillosis, mucormycosis, endocarditis, pulmonary sequestration, and malignancy (170,179–181). The term *Rasmussen aneurysm* describes a pseudoaneurysm and results from disruption of the media of segmental pulmonary arteries by granulation tissue in patients with active tuberculosis (170,181). A Rasmussen pseudoaneurysm typically forms months to years after the initial exposure to tuberculosis or reactivation of the disease and the development of cavitation. The majority of patients with active tuberculosis who develop hemoptysis bleed from the bronchial and not from the pulmonary circulation. However, the pulmonary circulation should be evaluated in cases with a normal bronchial angiogram or if the pseudoaneurysm is sufficiently large to have been diagnosed at CT.

Massive hemoptysis in patients with carcinoma of the lung is usually secondary to a pulmonary artery pseudoaneurysm within a necrotic tumour cavity lesion (158,159).

Traumatic Causes of Pulmonary Artery Aneurysms

Rupture of the pulmonary artery or one of its branches occurs in 0.001% to 0.5% of cases of Swan-Ganz catheter placement (Fig. 16-48) and carries with it a mortality rate as high as 50% (182–185). Factors identified as important in patients with pulmonary artery rupture include penetration of the pulmonary artery by the catheter tip, distal migration of the catheter during balloon deflation, retraction while the balloon remains inflated, and high-pressure inflation of the balloon in excess of the tensile strength of the vessel wall. Risk factors include PH, systemic anticoagulation, long-term steroid use, surgically induced hypothermia, age older than 60 years, female sex, and cardiac manipulation during surgery (170,182,183). Acute presentation with brisk hemoptysis or hemothorax requires immediate catheter-directed delivery of *n*-butyl-cyanoacrylate and/or metal coils (184,185). Delayed presentation

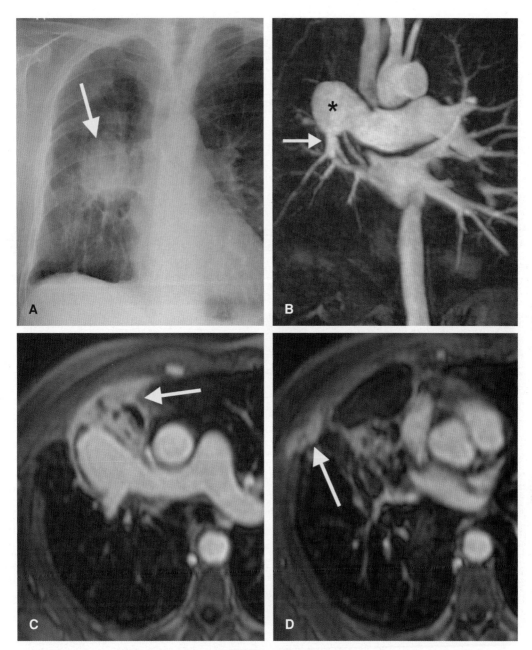

FIGURE 16-47 CE MRA demonstrating a large pseudoaneurysm of the distal right main pulmonary artery in a patient who previously underwent right upper lobectomy. Patient complained of intermittent bloody discharge from the right lateral chest wall. **A:** Chest x-ray demonstrates a large right-sided mass, presumed to represent a new lung tumor (*arrow*). **B:** Coronal subvolume MIP reformat from a CE MRA demonstrates that the "mass" represents a pseudoaneurysm of the distal right main pulmonary artery (∗). Note the relationship of the aneurysm to the lower lobe pulmonary artery (*arrow*). **C:** Postcontrast axial images demonstrate extensive consolidation (*arrow*) surrounding the pseudoaneurysm. **D:** At a more inferior level, note enhancement within the lateral chest wall (*arrow*) consistent with extension of the inflammatory process into the chest wall.

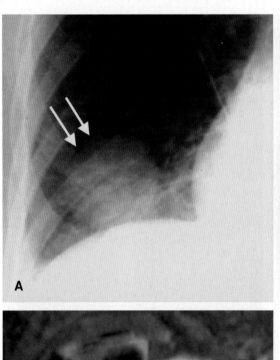

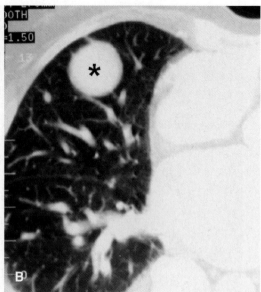

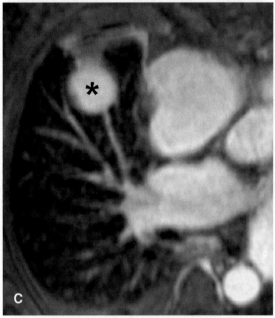

FIGURE 16-48 Patient who experienced massive hemoptysis in intensive care; several months earlier, a Swan-Ganz catheter had been inserted. **A:** Chest x-ray demonstrates a well-circumscribed "mass" in the middle lobe (*arrows*) that was not present on earlier chest x-rays. **B:** Lung windows from a CT thorax demonstrate a well-circumscribed middle lobe mass (∗). **C:** Axial reformat from a CE MRA demonstrates a well-circumscribed uniform enhancing mass (∗). Catheter angiography confirmed a pseudoaneurysm of the pulmonary artery, presumably secondary to Swan-Ganz catheter–induced pulmonary artery rupture.

with hemoptysis secondary to pseudoaneurysm formation may also occur.

CONCLUSION

Cross-sectional angiography of the chest with CT and MR today offers the possibility for evaluation of almost all pulmonary vascular disorders in a noninvasive fashion. The inexorable progress in technology will strengthen existing techniques and offer novel methods to add to the already enormous scope of noninvasive angiographic imaging.

REFERENCES

1. Jackson CL, Huber JF. Correlated applied anatomy of the bronchial tree and lungs with a system of nomenclature. *Dis Chest.* 1943;9:319–326.
2. Boyden EA. *Segmental Anatomy of the Lungs.* New York, NY: McGraw-Hill; 1955.
3. Remy-Jardin M, Remy J, Mayo JR, et al. Anatomy and normal variants. In: *CT Angiography of the Chest.* Philadelphia, PA: Lippincott Williams & Wilkins; 2001:15–17.
4. Castaner E, Gallardo X, Rimola J, et al. Congenital and acquired pulmonary artery anomalies in the adult: radiologic overview. *Radiographics.* 2006;26:349–371.
5. Siripornpitak S, Reddy GP, Schwitter J, et al. Pulmonary artery sling: anatomical and functional evaluation by MRI. *J Comput Assist Tomogr.* 1997;21:766–768.

6. Do KH, Goo JM, Im JG, et al. Systemic arterial supply to the lungs in adults: spiral CT findings. *Radiographics*. 2001;21:387–402.

7. Livingston DR, Mehta AC, O'Donovan PB, et al. An angiographic dilemma: bronchopulmonary sequestration versus pseudosequestration: case reports. *Angiology*. 1986;37:896–904.

8. Mai VM, Chen Q, Bankier AA, et al. Imaging pulmonary blood flow and perfusion using phase-sensitive selective inversion recovery. *Magn Reson Med*. 2000;43:793–795.

9. Amundsen T, Torheim G, Kvistad KA, et al. Perfusion abnormalities in pulmonary embolism studied with perfusion MRI and ventilation-perfusion scintigraphy: an intramodality and inter-modality agreement study. *J Magn Reson Imaging*. 2002;15:386–394.

10. Halliburton SS, Paschal CB, Rothpletz JD, et al. Estimation and visualization of regional and global pulmonary perfusion with 3D magnetic resonance angiography. *J Magn Reson Imaging*. 2001;14:734–740.

11. Lin YR, Wu MT, Huang TY, et al. Comparison of arterial spin labeling and first-pass dynamic contrast-enhanced MR imaging in the assessment of pulmonary perfusion in humans: the inflow spin-tracer saturation effect. *Magn Reson Med*. 2004;52:1291–1301.

12. Nakagawa T, Sakuma H, Murashima S, et al. Pulmonary ventilation-perfusion MR imaging in clinical patients. *J Magn Reson Imaging*. 2001;14:419–424.

13. Nael K, Michaely HJ, Lee M, et al. Dynamic pulmonary perfusion and flow quantification with MR imaging, 3.0T vs. 1.5T: initial results. *J Magn Reson Imaging*. 2006;24:333–339.

14. Garg K, Welsh CH, Feyerabend AJ, et al. Pulmonary embolism: diagnosis with spiral CT and ventilation-perfusion scanning—correlation with pulmonary angiographic results or clinical outcome. *Radiology*. 1998;208:201–208.

15. Hull RD, Raskob GE, Ginsberg JS, et al. A noninvasive strategy for the treatment of patients with suspected pulmonary embolism. *Arch Intern Med*. 1994;154:289–297.

16. van Rossum AB, Pattynama PM, Mallens WM, et al. Can helical CT replace scintigraphy in the diagnostic process in suspected pulmonary embolism? A retrolective-prolective cohort study focusing on total diagnostic yield. *Eur Radiol*. 1998;8:90–96.

17. Remy-Jardin M, Tillie-Leblond I, Szapiro D, et al. CT angiography of pulmonary embolism in patients with underlying respiratory disease: impact of multislice CT on image quality and negative predictive value. *Eur Radiol*. 2002;12:1971–1978.

18. Schoepf UJ, Holzknecht N, Helmberger TK, et al. Subsegmental pulmonary emboli: improved detection with thin-collimation multi-detector row spiral CT. *Radiology*. 2002;222:483–490.

19. Schoepf UJ, Costello P. CT angiography for diagnosis of pulmonary embolism: state of the art. *Radiology*. 2004;230:329–337.

20. van Beek EJ, Reekers JA, Batchelor DA, et al. Feasibility, safety and clinical utility of angiography in patients with suspected pulmonary embolism. *Eur Radiol*. 1996;6:415–419.

21. Klingenbeck-Regn K, Schaller S, Flohr T, et al. Subsecond multi-slice computed tomography: basics and applications. *Eur J Radiol*. 1999;31:110–124.

22. MacFall JR, Sostman HD, Foo TK. Thick-section, single breath-hold magnetic resonance pulmonary angiography. *Invest Radiol*. 1992;27:318–322.

23. Wielopolski PA, Haacke EM, Adler LP. Three-dimensional MR imaging of the pulmonary vasculature: preliminary experience. *Radiology*. 1992;183:465–472.

24. Grist TM, Sostman HD, MacFall JR, et al. Pulmonary angiography with MR imaging: preliminary clinical experience. *Radiology*. 1993;189:523–530.

25. Wielopolski P, Haacke E, Adler L. Evaluation of the pulmonary vasculature with three-dimensional magnetic resonance imaging techniques. *MAGMA*. 1993;1:21–34.

26. Schiebler ML, Holland GA, Hatabu H, et al. Suspected pulmonary embolism: prospective evaluation with pulmonary MRA. *Radiology*. 1993;189:125–131.

27. Erdman WA, Peshock RM, Redman HC, et al. Pulmonary embolism: comparison of MR images with radionuclide and angiographic studies. *Radiology*. 1994;190:499–508.

28. Meaney JF, Weg JG, Chenevert TL, et al. Diagnosis of pulmonary embolism with magnetic resonance angiography. *N Engl J Med*. 1997;33:6:1422–1427.

29. Gupta A, Frazer CK, Ferguson JM, et al. Acute pulmonary embolism: diagnosis with MRA. *Radiology*. 1999;210:353–359.

30. Oudkerk M, van Beek EJ, Wielopolski P, et al. Comparison of contrast-enhanced magnetic resonance angiography and conventional pulmonary angiography for the diagnosis of pulmonary embolism: a prospective study. *Lancet*. 2002;359:1643–1647.

31. Nikolaou K, Schoenberg SO, Attenberger U, et al. Pulmonary arterial hypertension: diagnosis with fast perfusion MR imaging and high-spatial-resolution MRA—preliminary experience. *Radiology*. 2005;236:694–703.

32. Hatabu H, Tadamura E, Levin DL, et al. Quantitative assessment of pulmonary perfusion with dynamic contrast-enhanced MRI. *Magn Reson Med*. 1999;42:1033–1038.

33. Fink C, Bock M, Puderbach M, et al. Partially parallel three-dimensional magnetic resonance imaging for the assessment of lung perfusion—initial results. *Invest Radiol*. 2003;38:482–488.

34. Kauczor HU, Chen XJ, van Beek EJ, et al. Pulmonary ventilation imaged by magnetic resonance: at the doorstep of clinical application. *Eur Respir J*. 2001;17:1008–1023.

35. Suga K, Ogasawara N, Okada M, et al. Regional lung functional impairment in acute airway obstruction and pulmonary embolic dog models assessed with gadolinium-based aerosol ventilation and perfusion magnetic resonance imaging. *Invest Radiol*. 2002;37:281–291.

36. Moller HE, Chen XJ, Saam B, et al. MRI of the lungs using hyperpolarized noble gases. *Magn Reson Med*. 2002;47:1029–1051.

37. Jalali A, Ishii M, Edvinsson JM, et al. Detection of simulated pulmonary embolism in a porcine model using hyperpolarized 3He MRI. *Magn Reson Med*. 2004;51:291–298.

38. Goyen M, Laub G, Ladd ME, et al. Dynamic 3D MRA of the pulmonary arteries in under four seconds. *J Magn Reson Imaging*. 2001;13:372–377.

39. Korosec FR, Frayne R, Grist TM, et al. Time-resolved contrast-enhanced 3D MRA. *Magn Reson Med*. 1996;36:345–351.

40. Ahlstrom KH, Johansson LO, Rodenburg JB, et al. Pulmonary MRA with ultrasmall superparamagnetic iron oxide particles as a blood pool agent and a navigator echo for respiratory gating: pilot study. *Radiology*. 1999;211:865–869.

41. Bremerich J, Roberts TP, Wendland MF, et al. Three-dimensional MR imaging of pulmonary vessels and parenchyma with NC100150 injection (Clariscan). *J Magn Reson Imaging*. 2000;11:622–628.

42. Grist TM, Korosec FR, Peters DC, et al. Steady-state and dynamic MRA with MS-325: initial experience in humans. *Radiology*. 1998;207:539–544.

43. Hoffmann U, Loewe C, Bernhard C, et al. MRA of the lower extremities in patients with pulmonary embolism using a blood pool contrast agent: initial experience. *J Magn Reson Imaging*. 2002;15:429–437.

44. Kluge A, Muller C, Hansel J, et al. Real-time MR with True-FISP for the detection of acute pulmonary embolism: initial clinical experience. *Eur Radiol*. 2004;14:709–718.

45. Pedrosa I, Morrin M, Oleaga L, et al. Is true FISP imaging reliable in the evaluation of venous thrombosis? *AJR Am J Roentgenol*. 2005;185:1632–1640.

46. Cohen MD, McGuire W, Cory DA, et al. Society for Pediatric Radiology John Caffey Award. MR appearance of

blood and blood products: an in vitro study. *AJR Am J Roentgenol.* 1986;146:1293–1297.

47. Sostman D, Pope CF, Smith GJ, et al. Proton relaxation in experimental clots varies with method of preparation. *Invest Radiol.* 1987;22:509–512.

48. Moody AR, Pollock JG, O'Connor AR, et al. Lower-limb deep venous thrombosis: direct MR imaging of the thrombus. *Radiology.* 1998;209:349–355.

49. Moody AR, Liddicoat A, Krarup K. Magnetic resonance pulmonary angiography and direct imaging of embolus for the detection of pulmonary emboli. *Invest Radiol.* 1997;32:431–440.

50. Fraser DG, Moody AR, Morgan PS, et al. Diagnosis of lower-limb deep venous thrombosis: a prospective blinded study of magnetic resonance direct thrombus imaging. *Ann Intern Med.* 2002;136:89–98.

51. Moody AR, Crossley I, Moorby S, et al. Magnetic resonance direct thrombus imaging (MRDTI) as a first line investigation for pulmonary embolism—the PDQ trial. In: 11th Annual Meeting of ISMRM. Toronto, Canada, 2003.

52. Cauldwell EW, Siekert RG, Lininger RE. The bronchial arteries: an anatomic study of 150 human cadavers. *Surg Gynecol Obstet.* 1948;86:395–412.

53. DeParedes CG, Pierce WS, Johnson DG, et al. Pulmonary sequestration in infants and children: a 20-year experience and review of the literature. *J Pediatr Surg.* 1970;5:136–147.

54. Rosado-de-Christenson ML, Frazier AA, Stocker JT, et al. From the archives of the AFIP. Extralobar sequestration: radiologic-pathologic correlation. *Radiographics.* 1993;13:425–441.

55. Savic B, Birtel FJ, Tholen W, et al. Lung sequestration: report of seven cases and review of 540 published cases. *Thorax.* 1979;34:96–101.

56. Ellis K. Fleischner lecture. Developmental abnormalities in the systemic blood supply to the lungs. *AJR Am J Roentgenol.* 1991;156:669–679.

57. Marom EM, Herndon JE, Kim YH, et al. Variations in pulmonary venous drainage to the left atrium: implications for radiofrequency ablation. *Radiology.* 2004;230:824–829.

58. Bharati S, Lev M. Congenital anomalies of the pulmonary veins. *Cardiovasc Clin.* 1973;5:23–41.

59. Budorick NE, McDonald V, Flisak ME, et al. The pulmonary veins. *Semin Roentgenol.* 1989;24:127–140.

60. Lawler LP, Corl FM, Fishman EK. Multi-detector row and volume-rendered CT of the normal and accessory flow pathways of the thoracic systemic and pulmonary veins. *Radiographics.* 2002;22[Spec No]:S45–S60.

61. Cronin P, Sneider MB, Kazerooni EA, et al. MDCT of the left atrium and pulmonary veins in planning radiofrequency ablation for atrial fibrillation: a how-to guide. *AJR Am J Roentgenol.* 2004;183:767–778.

62. Mansour M, Holmvang G, Sosnovik D, et al. Assessment of pulmonary vein anatomic variability by magnetic resonance imaging: implications for catheter ablation techniques for atrial fibrillation. *J Cardiovasc Electrophysiol.* 2004;15:387–393.

63. Haissaguerre M, Jais P, Shah DC, et al. Spontaneous initiation of atrial fibrillation by ectopic beats originating in the pulmonary veins. *N Engl J Med.* 1998;339:659–666.

64. Kim YH, Marom EM, Herndon JE II, et al. Pulmonary vein diameter, cross-sectional area, and shape: CT analysis. *Radiology.* 2005;235:43–49; discussion 49–50.

65. Hauser TH, Yeon SB, McClennen S, et al. A method for the determination of proximal pulmonary vein size using contrast-enhanced magnetic resonance angiography. *J Cardiovasc Magn Reson.* 2004;6:927–936.

66. Robbins IM, Colvin EV, Doyle TP, et al. Pulmonary vein stenosis after catheter ablation of atrial fibrillation. *Circulation.* 1998;98:1769–1775.

67. Hauser TH, Yeon SB, McClennen S, et al. Subclinical pulmonary vein narrowing after ablation for atrial fibrillation. *Heart.* 2005;91:672–673.

68. Prasad SK, Soukias N, Hornung T, et al. Role of magnetic resonance angiography in the diagnosis of major aortopulmonary collateral arteries and partial anomalous pulmonary venous drainage. *Circulation.* 2004;109:207–214.

69. Hauser TH, Yeon SB, Kissinger KV, et al. Variation in pulmonary vein size during the cardiac cycle: implications for non-electrocardiogram-gated imaging. *Am Heart J.* 2006;152:974.e1–6.

70. Lickfett L, Dickfeld T, Kato R, et al. Changes of pulmonary vein orifice size and location throughout the cardiac cycle: dynamic analysis using magnetic resonance cine imaging. *J Cardiovasc Electrophysiol.* 2005;16:582–588.

71. Syed MA, Peters DC, Rashid H, et al. Pulmonary vein imaging: comparison of 3D magnetic resonance angiography with 2D cine MRI for characterizing anatomy and size. *J Cardiovasc Magn Reson.* 2005;7:355–360.

72. Brody H. Drainage of the pulmonary veins into the right side of the heart. *Arch Pathol Lab Med.* 1942;33:221–240.

73. Woodring JH, Howard TA, Kanga JF. Congenital pulmonary venolobar syndrome revisited. *Radiographics.* 1994;14:349–369.

74. White CS, Baffa JM, Haney PJ, et al. MR imaging of congenital anomalies of the thoracic veins. *Radiographics.* 1997;17:595–608.

75. Dalen JE, Alpert JS. Natural history of pulmonary embolism. *Prog Cardiovasc Dis.* 1975;17:259–270.

76. Bell WR, Simon TL. Current status of pulmonary thromboembolic disease: pathophysiology, diagnosis, prevention, and treatment. *Am Heart J.* 1982;103:239–262.

77. Silverstein MD, Heit JA, Mohr DN, et al. Trends in the incidence of deep vein thrombosis and pulmonary embolism: a 25-year population-based study. *Arch Intern Med.* 1998;158:585–593.

78. Coon WW, Willis PW. Deep venous thrombosis and pulmonary embolism: prediction, prevention and treatment. *Am J Cardiol.* 1959;4:611–621.

79. Stein PD, Henry JW. Prevalence of acute pulmonary embolism among patients in a general hospital and at autopsy. *Chest.* 1995;108:978–981.

80. Saeger W, Genzkow M. Venous thromboses and pulmonary embolisms in post-mortem series: probable causes by correlations of clinical data and basic diseases. *Pathol Res Pract.* 1994;190:394–399.

81. Morpurgo M, Schmid C. Clinico-pathological correlations in pulmonary embolism: a posteriori evaluation. *Prog Respir Dis.* 1980;13:8–15.

82. Prevention of venous thrombosis and pulmonary embolism. NIH Consensus Development. *JAMA.* 1986;256:744–749.

83. Ginsberg JS. Management of venous thromboembolism. *N Engl J Med.* 1996;335:1816–1828.

84. Stein PD, Henry JW, Relyea B. Untreated patients with pulmonary embolism. Outcome, clinical, and laboratory assessment. *Chest.* 1995;107:931–935.

85. van der Meer FJ, Rosendaal FR, Vandenbroucke JP, et al. Bleeding complications in oral anticoagulant therapy. An analysis of risk factors. *Arch Intern Med.* 1993;153:1557–1562.

86. Zidane M, Schram MT, Planken EW, et al. Frequency of major hemorrhage in patients treated with unfractionated intravenous heparin for deep venous thrombosis or pulmonary embolism: a study in routine clinical practice. *Arch Intern Med.* 2000;160:2369–2373.

87. Mills SR, Jackson DC, Older RA, et al. The incidence, etiologies, and avoidance of complications of pulmonary angiography in a large series. *Radiology.* 1980;136:295–299.

88. Stein PD, Athanasoulis C, Alavi A, et al. Complications and validity of pulmonary angiography in acute pulmonary embolism. *Circulation.* 1992;85:462–468.

89. Hudson ER, Smith TP, McDermott VG, et al. Pulmonary angiography performed with iopamidol: complications in 1,434 patients. *Radiology.* 1996;198:61–65.

90. Zuckerman DA, Sterling KM, Oser RF. Safety of pulmonary angiography in the 1990s. *J Vasc Interv Radiol*. 1996;7: 199–205.

91. Wells PS, Ginsberg JS, Anderson DR, et al. Use of a clinical model for safe management of patients with suspected pulmonary embolism. *Ann Intern Med*. 1998;129: 997–1005.

92. Weg JG. Current diagnostic techniques for pulmonary embolism. *Semin Vasc Surg*. 2000;13:182–188.

93. Turkstra F, Kuijer PM, van Beek EJ, et al. Diagnostic utility of ultrasonography of leg veins in patients suspected of having pulmonary embolism. *Ann Intern Med*. 1997;126: 775–781.

94. Tetalman MR, Hoffer PB, Heck LL, et al. Perfusion lung scan in normal volunteers. *Radiology*. 1973;106:593–594.

95. Perrier A, Desmarais S, Miron MJ, et al. Non-invasive diagnosis of venous thromboembolism in outpatients. *Lancet*. 1999;353:190–195.

96. Perrier A, Bounameaux H, Morabia A, et al. Diagnosis of pulmonary embolism by a decision analysis-based strategy including clinical probability, D-dimer levels, and ultrasonography: a management study. *Arch Intern Med*. 1996;156:531–536.

97. Becker DM, Philbrick JT, Bachhuber TL, et al. D-dimer testing and acute venous thromboembolism. A shortcut to accurate diagnosis? *Arch Intern Med*. 1996;156:939–946.

98. Value of the ventilation/perfusion scan in acute pulmonary embolism. Results of the prospective investigation of pulmonary embolism diagnosis (PIOPED). The PIOPED Investigators. *JAMA*. 1990;263:2753–2759.

99. Smith TP. Pulmonary embolism: what's wrong with this diagnosis? *AJR Am J Roentgenol*. 2000;174:1489–1497.

100. Blachere H, Latrabe V, Montaudon M, et al. Pulmonary embolism revealed on helical CT angiography: comparison with ventilation-perfusion radionuclide lung scanning. *AJR Am J Roentgenol*. 2000;174:1041–1047.

101. Donato AA, Scheirer JJ, Atwell MS, et al. Clinical outcomes in patients with suspected acute pulmonary embolism and negative helical computed tomographic results in whom anticoagulation was withheld. *Arch Intern Med*. 2003;163:2033–2038.

102. Ghaye B, Szapiro D, Mastora I, et al. Peripheral pulmonary arteries: how far in the lung does multi-detector row spiral CT allow analysis? *Radiology*. 2001;219:629–636.

103. Goodman LR, Curtin JJ, Mewissen MW, et al. Detection of pulmonary embolism in patients with unresolved clinical and scintigraphic diagnosis: helical CT versus angiography. *AJR Am J Roentgenol*. 1995;164:1369–1374.

104. Goodman LR, Lipchik RJ, Kuzo RS, et al. Subsequent pulmonary embolism: risk after a negative helical CT pulmonary angiogram—prospective comparison with scintigraphy. *Radiology*. 2000;215:535–542.

105. Gottsater A, Berg A, Centergard J, et al. Clinically suspected pulmonary embolism: is it safe to withhold anticoagulation after a negative spiral CT? *Eur Radiol*. 2001;11:65–72.

106. Mayo JR, Remy-Jardin M, Muller NL, et al. Pulmonary embolism: prospective comparison of spiral CT with ventilation-perfusion scintigraphy. *Radiology*. 1997;205:447–452.

107. Ost D, Rozenshtein A, Saffran L, et al. The negative predictive value of spiral computed tomography for the diagnosis of pulmonary embolism in patients with nondiagnostic ventilation-perfusion scans. *Am J Med*. 2001;110:16–21.

108. Perrier A, Roy PM, Sanchez O, et al. Multidetector-row computed tomography in suspected pulmonary embolism. *N Engl J Med*. 2005;352:1760–1768.

109. Prokop M. Multislice CT angiography. *Eur J Radiol*. 2000; 36:86–96.

110. Qanadli SD, Hajjam ME, Mesurolle B, et al. Pulmonary embolism detection: prospective evaluation of dual-section helical CT versus selective pulmonary arteriography in 157 patients. *Radiology*. 2000;217:447–455.

111. Quiroz R, Kucher N, Zou KH, et al. Clinical validity of a negative computed tomography scan in patients with suspected pulmonary embolism: a systematic review. *JAMA*. 2005;293:2012–2017.

112. Remy-Jardin M, Remy J, Wattinne L, et al. Central pulmonary thromboembolism: diagnosis with spiral volumetric CT with the single-breath-hold technique—comparison with pulmonary angiography. *Radiology*. 1992;185:381–387.

113. Swensen SJ, Sheedy PF II, Ryu JH, et al. Outcomes after withholding anticoagulation from patients with suspected acute pulmonary embolism and negative computed tomographic findings: a cohort study. *Mayo Clin Proc*. 2002;77: 130–138.

114. Teigen CL, Maus TP, Sheedy PF II, et al. Pulmonary embolism: diagnosis with electron-beam CT. *Radiology*. 1993;188:839–845.

115. Tillie-Leblond I, Mastora I, Radenne F, et al. Risk of pulmonary embolism after a negative spiral CT angiogram in patients with pulmonary disease: 1-year clinical follow-up study. *Radiology*. 2002;223:461–467.

116. van Strijen MJ, de Monye W, Kieft GJ, et al. Diagnosis of pulmonary embolism with spiral CT as a second procedure following scintigraphy. *Eur Radiol*. 2003;13:1501–1507.

117. van Erkel AR, van Rossum AB, Bloem JL, et al. Spiral CT angiography for suspected pulmonary embolism: a cost-effectiveness analysis. *Radiology*. 1996;201:29–36.

118. Henry JW, Relyea B, Stein PD. Continuing risk of thromboemboli among patients with normal pulmonary angiograms. *Chest*. 1995;107:1375–1378.

119. Forauer AR, McLean GK, Wallace LP. Clinical follow-up of patients after a negative digital subtraction pulmonary arteriogram in the evaluation of pulmonary embolism. *J Vasc Interv Radiol*. 1998;9:903–908.

120. Stein PD, Henry JW, Gottschalk A. Reassessment of pulmonary angiography for the diagnosis of pulmonary embolism: relation of interpreter agreement to the order of the involved pulmonary arterial branch. *Radiology*. 1999;210:689–691.

121. Quinn MF, Lundell CJ, Klotz TA, et al. Reliability of selective pulmonary arteriography in the diagnosis of pulmonary embolism. *AJR Am J Roentgenol*. 1987;149:469–471.

122. Diffin DC, Leyendecker JR, Johnson SP, et al. Effect of anatomic distribution of pulmonary emboli on interobserver agreement in the interpretation of pulmonary angiography. *AJR Am J Roentgenol*. 1998;171:1085–1089.

123. Ghaye B, Ghuysen A, Bruyere PJ, et al. Can CT pulmonary angiography allow assessment of severity and prognosis in patients presenting with pulmonary embolism? What the radiologist needs to know. *Radiographics*. 2006;26:23–39; discussion 39–40.

124. Peters DC, Korosec FR, Grist TM, et al. Undersampled projection reconstruction applied to MRA. *Magn Reson Med*. 2000;43:91–101.

125. Sodickson DK, Manning WJ. Simultaneous acquisition of spatial harmonics (SMASH): fast imaging with radiofrequency coil arrays. *Magn Reson Med*. 1997;38:591–603.

126. Pruessmann KP, Weiger M, Scheidegger MB, et al. SENSE: sensitivity encoding for fast MRI. *Magn Reson Med*. 1999;42:952–962.

127. Sonnet S, Buitrago-Tellez CH, Schulte AC, et al. Dose optimization for dynamic time-resolved contrast-enhanced 3D MRA of pulmonary circulation. *AJR Am J Roentgenol*. 2003;181:1499–1503.

128. Sodickson DK, Hardy CJ, Zhu Y, et al. Rapid volumetric MRI using parallel imaging with order-of-magnitude accelerations and a 32-element RF coil array: feasibility and implications. *Acad Radiol*. 2005;12:626–635.

129. Ohno Y, Higashino T, Takenaka D, et al. MRA with sensitivity encoding (SENSE) for suspected pulmonary embolism: comparison with MDCT and ventilation-perfusion scintigraphy. *AJR Am J Roentgenol*. 2004;183:91–98.

130. Hurst DR, Kazerooni EA, Stafford-Johnson D, et al. Diagnosis of pulmonary embolism: comparison of CT angiography and MRA in canines. *J Vasc Interv Radiol.* 1999;10:309–318.
131. Seo JB, Im JG, Goo JM, et al. Comparison of contrast-enhanced CT angiography and gadolinium-enhanced MRA in the detection of subsegmental-sized pulmonary embolism. An experimental study in a pig model. *Acta Radiol.* 2003;44:403–410.
132. Haage P, Piroth W, Krombach G, et al. Pulmonary embolism: comparison of angiography with spiral computed tomography, magnetic resonance angiography, and real-time magnetic resonance imaging. *Am J Respir Crit Care Med.* 2003;167:729–734.
133. Farber HW, Loscalzo J. Pulmonary arterial hypertension. *N Engl J Med.* 2004;351:1655–1665.
134. Gaine SP, Rubin LJ. Primary pulmonary hypertension. *Lancet.* 1998;352:719–725.
135. Barst RJ. Medical therapy of pulmonary hypertension. An overview of treatment and goals. *Clin Chest Med.* 2001;22:509–515, ix.
136. Kreitner KF, Ley S, Kauczor HU, et al. Chronic thromboembolic pulmonary hypertension: pre- and postoperative assessment with breath-hold MR imaging techniques. *Radiology.* 2004;232:535–543.
137. Ley S, Kreitner KF, Fink C, et al. Assessment of pulmonary hypertension by CT and MR imaging. *Eur Radiol.* 2004;14:359–368.
138. Prince MR, Alderson PO, Sostman HD. Chronic pulmonary embolism: combining MRA with functional assessment. *Radiology.* 2004;232:325–326.
139. Heinrich M, Uder M, Tscholl D, et al. CT scan findings in chronic thromboembolic pulmonary hypertension: predictors of hemodynamic improvement after pulmonary thromboendarterectomy. *Chest.* 2005;127:1606–1613.
140. King MA, Ysrael M, Bergin CJ. Chronic thromboembolic pulmonary hypertension: CT findings. *AJR Am J Roentgenol.* 1998;170:955–960.
141. Bergin CJ, Sirlin CB, Hauschildt JP, et al. Chronic thromboembolism: diagnosis with helical CT and MR imaging with angiographic and surgical correlation. *Radiology.* 1997;2004:695–702.
142. Schwickert HC, Schweden F, Schild HH, et al. Pulmonary arteries and lung parenchyma in chronic pulmonary embolism: preoperative and postoperative CT findings. *Radiology.* 1994;191:351–357.
143. Remy J, Voisin C, Ribet M, et al. [Treatment, by embolization, of severe or repeated hemoptysis associated with systemic hypervascularization.] *Nouv Presse Med.* 1973;2:2060.
144. Remy-Jardin M, Bouaziz N, Dumont P, et al. Bronchial and nonbronchial systemic arteries at multi-detector row CT angiography: comparison with conventional angiography. *Radiology.* 2004;233:741–749.
145. Yoon YC, Lee KS, Jeong YJ, et al. Hemoptysis: bronchial and nonbronchial systemic arteries at 16-detector row CT. *Radiology.* 2005;234:292–298.
146. O'Keeffe SA, McGrath A, Farrelly CT, et al. Bronchial artery visualization on contrast-enhanced MRA of the pulmonary vasculature. In: 91st Scientific Meeting and Annual Assembly RSNA. Chicago, 2005.
147. Webb WR, Jacobs RP. Transpleural abdominal systemic artery-pulmonary artery anastomosis in patients with chronic pulmonary infection. *AJR Am J Roentgenol.* 1977;129:233–236.
148. North LB, Boushy SF, Houk VN. Bronchial and intercostal arteriography in non-neoplastic pulmonary disease. *Am J Roentgenol Radium Ther Nucl Med.* 1969;107:328–342.
149. Yamato M, Lecky JW, Hiramatsu K, et al. Takayasu arteritis: radiographic and angiographic findings in 59 patients. *Radiology.* 1986;161:329–334.
150. Yamada I, Numano F, Suzuki S. Takayasu arteritis: evaluation with MR imaging. *Radiology.* 1993;188:89–94.
151. Boushy SF, North LB, Trice JA. The bronchial arteries in chronic obstructive pulmonary disease. *Am J Med.* 1969;46:506–515.
152. Kauczor HU, Schwickert HC, Mayer E, et al. Spiral CT of bronchial arteries in chronic thromboembolism. *J Comput Assist Tomogr.* 1994;18:855–861.
153. Engelke C, Riedel M, Rummeny EJ, et al. Pulmonary haemangiosarcoma with main pulmonary artery thrombosis imitating subacute pulmonary embolism with infarction. *Br J Radiol.* 2004;77:623–625.
154. Parish JM, Rosenow EC III, Swensen SJ, et al. Pulmonary artery sarcoma. Clinical features. *Chest.* 1996;110:1480–1488.
155. Baker PB, Goodwin RA. Pulmonary artery sarcomas. A review and report of a case. *Arch Pathol Lab Med.* 1985;109:35–39.
156. Yi ES. Tumors of the pulmonary vasculature. *Cardiol Clin.* 2004;22:431–440, vi–vii.
157. Oliai BR, Tazelaar HD, Lloyd RV, et al. Leiomyosarcoma of the pulmonary veins. *Am J Surg Pathol.* 1999;23:1082–1088.
158. DiPerna CA, Wood DE. Surgical management of T3 and T4 lung cancer. *Clin Cancer Res.* 2005;11:5038s–5044s.
159. Khanavkar B, Stern P, Alberti W, et al. Complications associated with brachytherapy alone or with laser in lung cancer. *Chest.* 1991;99:1062–1065.
160. Chae EJ, Seo JB, Kim SY, et al. Radiographic and CT findings of thoracic complications after pneumonectomy. *Radiographics.* 2006;26:1449–1468.
161. Kim EA, Lee KS, Shim YM, et al. Radiographic and CT findings in complications following pulmonary resection. *Radiographics.* 2002;22:67–86.
162. Gandhi AK, Pearson AC, Orsinelli DA. Tumor invasion of the pulmonary veins: a unique source of systemic embolism detected by transesophageal echocardiography. *J Am Soc Echocardiogr.* 1995;8:97–99.
163. Mansour KA, Malone CE, Craver JM. Left atrial tumor embolization during pulmonary resection: review of literature and report of two cases. *Ann Thorac Surg.* 1988;46:455–456.
164. Dore R, Alerci M, D'Andrea F, et al. Intracardiac extension of lung cancer via pulmonary veins: CT diagnosis. *J Comput Assist Tomogr.* 1988;12:565–568.
165. Tassan S, Chabert JP, Tassigny C, et al. [Peripheral embolic arterial accident due to pulmonary vein thrombosis revealing bronchial carcinoma.] *Ann Cardiol Angeiol (Paris).* 1998;47:11–13.
166. Pitman AG, Solomon B, Padmanabhan R, et al. Intravenous extension of lung carcinoma to the left atrium: demonstration by positron emission tomography with CT correlation. *Br J Radiol.* 2000;73:206–208.
167. Takahashi K, Furuse M, Hanaoka H, et al. Pulmonary vein and left atrial invasion by lung cancer: assessment by breath-hold gadolinium-enhanced three-dimensional MRA. *J Comput Assist Tomogr.* 2000;24:557–561.
168. Gossage JR, Kanj G. Pulmonary arteriovenous malformations. A state of the art review. *Am J Respir Crit Care Med.* 1998;158:643–661.
169. Remy J, Remy-Jardin M, Giraud F, et al. Angioarchitecture of pulmonary arteriovenous malformations: clinical utility of three-dimensional helical CT. *Radiology.* 1994;191:657–664.
170. Pelage JP, El Hajjam M, Lagrange C, et al. Pulmonary artery interventions: an overview. *Radiographics.* 2005;25:1653–1667.
171. Fogelman R, Nykanen D, Smallhorn JF, et al. Endovascular stents in the pulmonary circulation. Clinical impact on management and medium-term follow-up. *Circulation.* 1995;92:881–885.
172. Takahashi M, Shimoyama K, Murata K, et al. Hilar and mediastinal invasion of bronchogenic carcinoma: evaluation by thin-section electron-beam computed tomography. *J Thorac Imaging.* 1997;12:195–199.

173. Hamzaoui A, Hamzaoui K. [Pulmonary complications of Behcet's disease and Takayasu's arteritis.] *Rev Mal Respir.* 2005;22:999–1019.

174. Uzun O, Akpolat T, Erkan L. Pulmonary vasculitis in Behçet disease: a cumulative analysis. *Chest.* 2005;127:2243–2253.

175. Hiller N, Lieberman S, Chajek-Shaul T, et al. Thoracic manifestations of Behcet disease at CT. *Radiographics.* 2004;24:801–808.

176. Ketchum ES, Zamanian RT, Fleischmann D. CT angiography of pulmonary artery aneurysms in Hughes-Stovin syndrome. *AJR Am J Roentgenol.* 2005;185:330–332.

177. Balci NC, Semelka RC, Noone TC, et al. Multiple pulmonary aneurysms secondary to Hughes-Stovin syndrome: demonstration by MRA. *J Magn Reson Imaging.* 1998;8: 1323–1325.

178. Tsui EY, Cheung YK, Chow L, et al. Idiopathic pulmonary artery aneurysm: digital subtraction pulmonary angiography grossly underestimates the size of the aneurysm. *Clin Imaging.* 2001;25:178–180.

179. Mody GN, Lau CL, Bhalla S, et al. Mycotic pulmonary artery pseudoaneurysm. *J Thorac Imaging.* 2005;20: 310–312.

180. Choong CK, Meyers BF. Lung mass after pulmonary artery catheterization: beware of the pulmonary artery false aneurysm. *J Thorac Cardiovasc Surg.* 2005;130:899–900.

181. Kim HY, Song KS, Goo JM, et al. Thoracic sequelae and complications of tuberculosis. *Radiographics.* 2001;21: 839–858; discussion 859–860.

182. Poplausky MR, Rozenblit G, Rundback JH, et al. Swan-Ganz catheter-induced pulmonary artery pseudoaneurysm formation: three case reports and a review of the literature. *Chest.* 2001;120:2105–2111.

183. Abreu AR, Campos MA, Krieger BP. Pulmonary artery rupture induced by a pulmonary artery catheter: a case report and review of the literature. *J Intensive Care Med.* 2004;19:291–296.

184. Dimarakis I, Thorpe JA, Papagiannopoulos K. Successful treatment of a posttraumatic pulmonary artery pseudoaneurysm with coil embolization. *Ann Thorac Surg.* 2005;79:2134–2136.

185. Block M, Lefkowitz T, Ravenel J, et al. Endovascular coil embolization for acute management of traumatic pulmonary artery pseudoaneurysm. *J Thorac Cardiovasc Surg.* 2004;128:784–785.

Thoracic Aorta

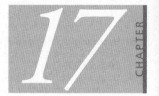

Daniel Nóbrega Costa
Geoffrey D. Rubin
Neil M. Rofsky
Richard L. Hallett

SPECTRUM AND PREVALENCE OF DISEASES

Thoracic aortic diseases are often life-threatening conditions that require immediate diagnosis and treatment. Despite continuous progress in identification of clinical risk factors, prevention, and early diagnosis of these conditions, they remain major causes of morbidity and mortality throughout the world (1–3). These include aneurysms, acute aortic syndromes (which comprise aortic dissection, intramural hematoma [IMH], and penetrating ulcer), occlusive diseases, vasculitides, trauma, and congenital abnormalities.

GLOBAL VIEW OF UNIQUE ASPECTS AND CONSIDERATIONS OF IMAGING

Although assessment of the aorta has traditionally relied on conventional angiography, the cross-sectional information available with computed tomography (CT) and magnetic resonance (MR) extends its diagnostic possibilities and has been shown to provide benefits beyond angiography (4–11). Isotropic acquisitions in multidetector computed tomography (MDCT), as well as volumetric and multiplanar capabilities of magnetic resonance imaging (MRI), have overcome the challenging issue of vessel tortuosity, enable a truly transverse aortic plane (useful especially in aneurysms and dissections), facilitate understanding of the relation between the aorta and its branches, and provide supplementary assessment of intramural and perivascular abnormalities.

CT scanning provides a rapid assessment in emergent conditions and has been an important tool for evaluating patients presenting with chest pain. Transesophageal echocardiography (TEE), while readily available in many centers, is less commonly applied, as it is invasive and more operator-dependent than CT or MR. MR as an emergent tool is less attractive due to concerns of compatibility with the MR environment; however, recent technologic developments have allowed fast acquisition of high-quality data sets and the potential to view them in MPR and real-time fashion.

Advantages of CT and MR

Despite the fact that transverse images are adequate for diagnosis in most cases, volume-rendered three-dimensional (3D) and multiplanar reformatted images can provide more information about the nature of the disease and better communication with clinicians (12,13).

Evaluation of the aortic wall is a critical part of the vascular assessment and is best appreciated with cross-sectional imaging (14–18). The same holds true to the evaluation of aortic wall distensibility and quantitative flow measurements that are achievable by using MRI (14,19–21).

Important additional information unique to CT imaging includes the detection of bony and other nonvascular abnormalities associated to trauma. MRI, on the other hand, provides assessment of flow dynamics in coarctation and real-time analyses of dynamic processes that can be used to extract functional data (e.g., intimal flap, aortic valve flow, and wall stress).

Imaging Strategies

A comprehensive assessment of the aorta requires that one examine its course, caliber, and contour along with visualization of the intraluminal and intramural details. The first step in performing CT and MR angiography is to define the imaging volume of interest, which depends on the anatomic territory to be studied and the clinical questions to be answered (22).

Computed Tomography

Although the thoracic aorta is the largest artery in the body, assuming that simple thick-section acquisition and borderline luminal enhancement will suffice for obtaining diagnostic studies would be a critical error. The diseases of the thoracic aorta and its branches necessitate high-resolution volumetric examinations that allow clear delineation of both the lumen as well as the wall of the vessel and offer the possibility in specific circumstances to compensate for pulsatile motion.

Computed Tomography Acquisition

Virtually all thoracic aortic examinations are performed with the patient lying in a supine position and centered so that the isocenter of the gantry corresponds to the center of the mediastinum. The patient's arm should be placed above his or her head, but care should be taken to avoid extreme shoulder abduction, which can pinch the subclavian vein and hinder delivery of contrast medium. Exceptions to this positioning protocol include imaging of the thoracic aorta in association with an upper extremity in the setting of suspected cardiac source for upper extremity thromboembolism, in which case the symptomatic arm is abducted but the arm to be injected is held at the patient's side. Another exception is when the primary focus of the examination are the carotid and intracranial arteries and only the upper portions of the thoracic aorta are to be imaged. In these circumstances, it may be desirable to image the patient with both arms at his or her sides.

A scout view is always obtained first and is sufficient for defining the scan range for thoracic aortic computed tomographic angiography (CTA). The scan range for thoracic CTA should begin in the lower neck to allow imaging of the proximal common carotid and vertebral arteries as well as the subclavian arteries. Inferiorly, the scan should not end above the celiac origin. Establishment of these proximal and distal landmarks is important in accurately locating aortic lesions as well as in detecting coexistent disease in the supra-aortic branches.

Prior to acquiring the CT angiogram, an unenhanced, thin-section (1 to 1.5 mm) acquisition should be performed whenever hemorrhage is suspected, particularly in the setting of an acute aortic syndrome. One notable exception to this acquisition strategy is in the setting of blunt or penetrating trauma, where an unenhanced scan is usually not required. Unenhanced scans are particularly sensitive for detecting intramural and periaortic blood. Another important reason for acquiring a preliminary unenhanced acquisition is when assessing the aorta following stent-graft placement, particularly for treating thoracic aortic aneurysms. Because calcifications within the aortic wall or within thrombus lining the aortic wall can mimic the appearance of small endoleaks, an unenhanced scan allows definitive characterization of potentially ambiguous opacities, as their presence on the unenhanced scan is diagnostic of calcification.

While 64-row and greater CT scanners are capable of acquiring images through the thorax with submillimeter section thickness, accurate characterization of aortic diseases rarely necessitates submillimeter section thickness unless a detailed assessment of the coronary arteries is desired simultaneously. As a result, most thoracic aortic CTA can be performed with 1- to 1.5-mm section thickness. Thicker sections are never advised. As with all CTA, overlapping reconstruction is recommended to improve the quality of multiplanar reformation (MPR) and 3D visualization. Section intervals equal to half of the effective section thickness are a good compromise between optimized longitudinal spatial resolution and overall image number. The CT angiogram should be acquired during breath holding whenever possible; however, due to its relatively fixed position within the thorax, high-quality images of the thoracic aorta can be obtained while the patient is breathing. Quiet ventilation is preferred to hyperventilation.

Pulsatile motion and its effect on ascending aortic visualization, in particular, has been a reality of thoracic aortic CTA since its beginnings. The recognition of typical motion artifacts is critical to an accurate diagnosis of thoracic aortic CTA, lest incorrect diagnoses including aortic dissection are made. If the appearance of the aorta is ambiguous despite consideration of pulsatile artifacts, reconstruction of the helical acquisition by using a half scan interpolation algorithm rather than standard helical interpolation algorithms can substantially diminish the artifact and clarify the presence of motion versus intrinsic disease (Fig. 17-1).

With the introduction of 16-row MDCT, it is now practical to routinely image the thoracic aorta by using electrocardiogram (ECG)-gating. Because patients are often critically ill and because myocardial and cardiac valve function are frequently valuable adjunctive data to thoracic aortic imaging, retrospective gating of the thoracic aorta is preferred to prospective gating; however, a formal comparison of prospectively gated thoracic aortic CT angiograms relative to retrospectively gated acquisitions has not been performed to date. Because of the substantially greater radiation exposure associated with a retrospectively gated CTA even when implementing tube current modulation, a gated acquisition is not advised for all thoracic aortic CTA.

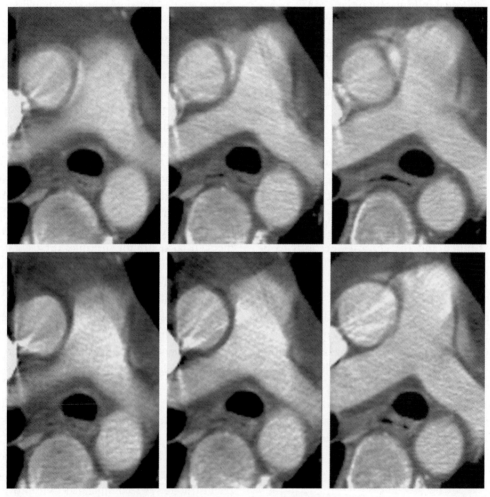

FIGURE 17-1 Contiguous transverse MDCT sections obtained through the ascending aorta in a patient who had been run over by a tractor. Acquisition parameters are 4 × 3.75 mm, pitch 1.5, table speed of 22.5 mm per rotation, and 0.8 seconds per rotation. **Top Row:** An apparent linear filling defect is present within the ascending aorta on all three sections. This filling defect persisted even with the reconstruction of overlapping sections (not shown). **Bottom Row:** Identical image locations from the same CT acquisition reconstructed with a half scan or segmented reconstruction algorithm. The segmented reconstruction requires approximately 220 degrees of data, resulting in an effective temporal resolution of 0.5 seconds. By reconstructing the sections using this algorithm, the apparent linear filling defects are revealed to be motion-related artifacts, and thus there is no suspicion for ascending aortic injury. (Reprinted with permission from Rubin GD. CT angiography of the thoracic aorta. *Semin Roentgenol.* 2003;38:115–134.)

At Stanford University, we gate all CT angiograms where there is suspected or known ascending aortic pathology or any presentation of an acute aortic syndrome. We have found gated acquisitions to be critical in completely characterizing ascending aortic dissection and demonstrating the relationship of intimal flaps to the structures of the aortic root, assessing the aortic valve, and assessing for intracoronary extension of aortic dissection. Gated acquisitions are also very valuable postoperatively, when subtle dehiscence of graft anastomoses near the aortic root can be blurred due to motion artifacts. Gated acquisitions are also helpful in pinpointing the specific location of anastomotic dehiscence even in the setting of broad-based pseudo-

aneurysms that on static images do not allow clear delineation of the point of communication between the lumen and the pseudoaneurysm. In unusual circumstances, cardiac gating, by eliminating motion-related artifacts, may unmask lesions otherwise hidden within the motion-related artifacts (Figs. 17-2 and 17-3).

When assessing the thoracic aorta both for aneurysms and acute aortic syndromes, imaging of the abdominal aorta and iliac arteries is highly advisable. In the setting of thoracic aortic aneurysms, there is a high prevalence of coexistent abdominal aortic aneurysm, and in the setting of acute aortic syndromes, aortic dissection—particularly type B—can extend into the abdominal aorta and iliac

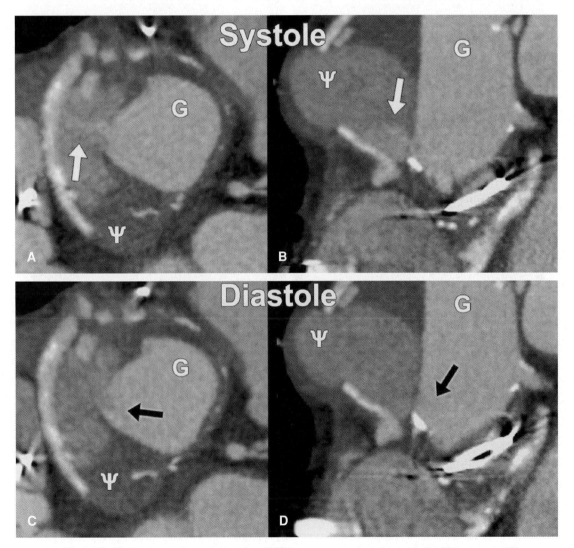

FIGURE 17-2 Cardiac-gated CTA acquired 6 days following aortic root aneurysm repair with an interposition graft above a preexisting St. Jude aortic valve prosthesis. The left and right coronary arteries were transplanted onto the graft. Transverse and coronal sections at the proximal graft anastomosis were acquired in mid-systole (**A** and **B**, respectively) and mid-diastole (**C** and **D**, respectively). There is a pseudoaneurysm (ψ) that contains thrombus and an enhancing lumen. The pseudoaneurysm has a broad region of contiguity with the graft (G). The specific point of anastomotic dehiscence is identified by a jet of high concentration contrast entering the pseudoaneurysm in systole (*white arrows*) and reversal of flow with filling of the graft by less enhanced blood from the pseudoaneurysm in diastole (*black arrows*).

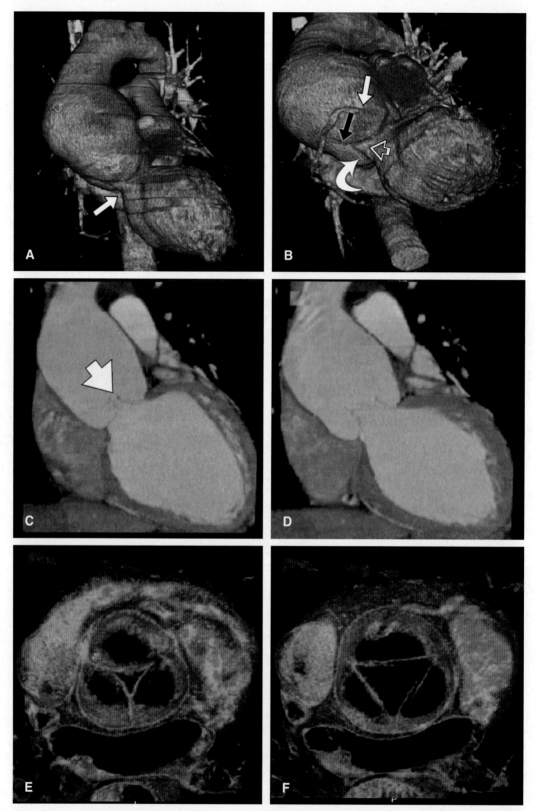

FIGURE 17-3 Gated CTA of patient with Marfan syndrome and anuloaortic ectasia. Frontal volume rendering with an opacity transfer function that renders the myocardium transparent and the contrast-enhanced arterial blood opaque (**A**). There is a 6.5-cm ascending aortic aneurysm with effacement of the sinotubular junction and dilation of the aortic root. The narrowest portion of the left ventricular outflow is in the subvalvular region below the annulus (*arrow*). The anatomy of the root is clearly visualized for surgical planning (**B**) (*white arrow*, right coronary artery origin; *black arrow*, commissure between right and noncoronary cusps; *curved arrow*, aortic annulus, illustrating that the annulus is not a simple ring but a complex three-crowned "coronet" shape; *open arrow*, subanular "interleaflet triangle"). Coronal MPR in diastole (**C**) and systole (**D**) demonstrate the movement of the aortic valve leaflets and the incomplete coaptation of the leaflets in diastole (*arrow*) due to the dilated annulus, resulting in aortic insufficiency. Three-centimeter thick-slab volume-rendered images in diastole (**E**) and systole (**F**) were created with an opacity transfer function that renders the aortic lumen transparent and allows delineation of the interior of the aortic root and the 3D relationships of the valve leaflets.

arteries where malperfusion of abdominal and pelvic viscera and the lower extremities can be a critical cause of morbidity and must be considered in treatment planning. Moreover, because an important treatment option is endoluminal therapy with stent-graft placement, imaging of the abdominal aorta and iliac arteries provides visualization of the access route for these large thoracic aortic devices. The identification of iliac arterial stenoses and aneurysms within the abdominal aorta and iliac arteries are important to planning the delivery of the endovascular device both from the standpoint of determining the feasibility of device passage and the selection of the side for device insertion.

Contrast Medium

When performing thoracic aortic CTA, it is always preferable to inject into the right arm instead of the left arm. This assures that the left brachiocephalic vein is not filled with undiluted, high-attenuation contrast medium. When the left arm is used, a high degree of opacification of the left brachiocephalic vein and associated streak artifacts can obscure the origins of the supra-aortic branches and limit the assessment of occlusive disease and extension of intimal flaps into these branches as well as the possibility for streak artifacts mimicking lesions that are not present. Although a saline flush should always be employed when performing thoracic aortic CTA to clear the inflowing veins of high-

attenuation contrast medium, because the CT angiogram is acquired from a cranial to caudal direction, the supra-aortic branches and aortic arch are acquired during the earlier phase of the acquisition prior to the clearing of the veins with the saline flush.

Another important consideration when delivering contrast medium for thoracic aortic CTA concerns the position of a region of interest for automated bolus triggering. Although it is tempting to place a region of interest within the largest vessel cross section (the aortic arch), this strategy has an important pitfall in the setting of aortic dissection and aneurysmal disease of the aortic arch. Because of the frequent coexistence of mural thrombus in the setting of both aortic dissection and arch aneurysm, the positioning of a region of interest on unenhanced views can result in its placement within an area of thrombus. If the images acquired during the course of the bolus monitoring are not carefully examined directly, the scan may not trigger at the appropriate time. A more reliable method for bolus monitoring and automated scan triggering relies on placement of the region of interest within the descending thoracic aorta approximately 2 cm distal to the aortic arch (Fig. 17-4). Because a near-orthogonal cross section of the vessel is acquired at this point, the inclusion of the true vessel lumen in at least a portion of the region of interest is much more likely than in the aortic arch, where the true lumen may pass above or below the plane selected for region-of-interest

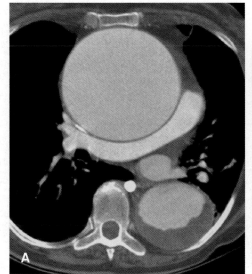
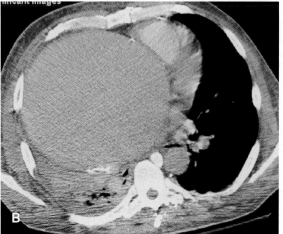

FIGURE 17-4 Transverse MDCT sections from a patient with an 11-cm ascending aortic aneurysm **(A)** and a 16-cm ascending aortic aneurysm **(B)**. In both cases, the superior vena cava has been compressed into a slitlike configuration with contrast reaching the heart via the hemiazygous vein. Case **(A)** was acquired after bolus monitoring and scan triggering in the descending thoracic aorta. Case **(B)** was performed with an empiric 20-second delay. The capacious aneurysm and obstructed inflow combine to hinder aortic opacification. Bolus monitoring should be employed always to assure adequate contrast enhancement. ([A] Reprinted with permission from Rubin GD. CT angiography of the thoracic aorta. *Semin Roentgenol.* 2003;38:115–134.)

placement. Once opacification achieves a threshold above 100 Hounsfield units (HU), the scan is triggered after the table is repositioned to allow initiation of the acquisition in the lower neck.

Postprocessing

Because the bony thorax completely surrounds the thoracic aorta, it is not possible to visualize the thoracic aorta with 3D rendering methods without some form of segmentation. However, region-of-interest editing and more recently automated chest wall removal tools can be used to facilitate thoracic aortic visualization. The limitation of these tools is that they may remove portions of the supra-aortic branches and internal mammary arteries. Perhaps the most expedient means for volume rendering the thoracic aorta is the use of a 2- to 5-cm thick slab. By dynamically translating and rotating the slab, all branches can be visualized and the visualization is not subjected to the idiosyncrasies of automated algorithms. It is also an easy means to eliminate the overlying pulmonary vessels, which automated chest wall removal tools may not remove effectively.

Because of the complex spatial relationships of the thoracic aorta and the overall thickness of the vessel, maximum intensity projections (MIPs) are rarely valuable and volume rendering is preferred. MPRs, particularly curved planar reformation (CPR), can be very useful for assessing the thoracic aorta and its branches, especially in the setting of multiple lumina or mural hematoma in the acute aortic syndromes.

Magnetic Resonance

Nuances of Acquisition Strategies

A comprehensive assessment of the aorta with MR requires that one assesses accurately the course, caliber, and contour of the aorta and visualizes the intraluminal and intramural details. Since ECG-triggering is commonly utilized in many approaches, a brief digression to address lead placement will be pursued.

A practical consideration of time constraints, patient compliance, and efficacy mandate the prescription of diagnostic and time-efficient strategies for MR aortography. The combination of dark blood techniques, cine MRI, and 3D gadolinium-enhanced MRA (or some other bright blood strategy) constitutes a comprehensive evaluation of the thoracic aorta that can be performed in a reasonable time frame. In certain circumstances, a subset of these techniques can be applied.

It is useful to divide MR aortic techniques in two broad groups: dark blood and bright blood strategies. Both groups can benefit from synchronizing the acquisition to the cardiac cycle in order to compensate for cardiovascular motion.

ECG-triggered sequences are used when quantifying aortic valve insufficiency and stenosis, for a clear and uniform assessment with dark blood sequences, for distinguishing flow from thrombus, and for minimizing pulsation artifacts.

Dark blood strategies consist of cardiac-triggered spin-echo (SE) imaging, cardiac-triggered echo-train imaging, half-Fourier single-shot turbo SE, with or without cardiac-triggering and magnetization prepared gradient echo (GRE) imaging. These techniques provide an excellent depiction of the anatomy and simultaneous evaluation of the lumen, vessel wall, and periaortic structures. With techniques that render the blood pool as low signal, excellent contrast also facilitates visualization of IMH and dissection (Fig. 17-5). This approach has had a long history beginning with nonbreath-hold SE imaging of the chest.

Traditional SE imaging has a demonstrated high accuracy for diagnosis of aortic dissection but offers limited assessment of the branch vessels and entails lengthy acquisition times. Breath-hold imaging is not possible with SE techniques, and therefore, effective resolution is compromised. In SE imaging, ECG-triggering is essential for obtaining images of diagnostic quality. The R-wave is used to trigger the acquisition and thus achieve a uniform synchronization for gathering data with respect to the cardiac cycle.

The weighting of the image is not essential, but trade-offs in the echo time (TE) selection should be highlighted. The selection of shorter TE values provides a greater

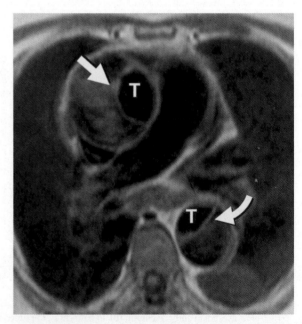

FIGURE 17-5 Dissection of the ascending, arch, and descending aorta in a 63-year-old patient. On this ECG-triggered SE T1-weighted MR image, the intimal flap is readily identified (*arrows*). Note the heterogeneous signal secondary to slow flow in the false lumen, making it easy to identify the true lumen (*T*).

number of slices for a given repetition time (TR). The selection of a longer TE allows for more spin dephasing and therefore often yields a better dark blood image. Saturation bands applied above and below the slices can improve the uniformity of the dark blood (23). All SE sequences tend toward a dark blood appearance by virtue of an exit phenomenon. That is, excitation of the slice includes a plug of blood with substantial components exiting the slice prior to the ability to encode it.

In cardiac-triggered black blood imaging, an R-wave spike is used to trigger image acquisition at a specific point during the cardiac cycle in order to minimize motion artifacts of the heart and the other mediastinal structures. The early success of ECG-triggered SE sequences for aortography was achieved with dark blood imaging (24–28). In such older versions of black blood imaging, the outflow phenomenon was exploited—excited spins in blood left the slice of interest before it was possible to apply the refocusing pulse, thus leaving a signal void; saturation bands placed above and below the extreme sections were often used to minimize flow-related enhancement (23).

Faster acquisitions are achievable by using echo train imaging techniques, with less sensitivity to cardiac and respiratory motion. During a TR interval, a series of echoes with unique phase-encoding information is acquired, with contrast determined by those echoes featured in the center of the k-space data matrix. With this family of sequences, referred to as fast spin echo (FSE) or turbo spin echo (TSE), one can reduce acquisition times to a breath-hold. For aortic protocols, this is most often employed as an ECG-triggered strategy that benefits from saturation bands.

Inversion pulses can be used to facilitate black blood imaging. Inversion pulses can be applied to echo train SE imaging or to GRE imaging. In each case, the inversion pulse is a preparation pulse that sets up the condition for black blood imaging. For TSE imaging, a double inversion pulse is used. This is really a misnomer, as the pulse sequence is actually an inversion–reversion strategy. A nonselective inversion pulse inverts the magnetization over a broad range of the body. This is followed by a slice-selective reversion that restores the magnetization in the slice only while leaving the magnetization outside the slice inverted. During systole, blood in the imaging slice flows out while blood outside the imaging slice, with inverted magnetization, flows in. This sequence can be properly timed so that data acquisition is initiated as the T1 recovery of blood crosses the null point. Thus, blood will lack the longitudinal magnetization necessary for signal generation. This allows for uniform dark blood. When combined with a half-Fourier reconstruction readout, robust and rapid black blood imaging is obtainable (Fig. 17-6). Alternatively, single-shot without half-Fourier reconstruction can obtain one to two slices per breath hold, which trades off improved resolution for less efficient anatomic coverage per unit of time as compared with the half-Fourier approach.

An inversion pulse preparation can be applied to GRE imaging. This is often known as magnetization preparation GRE and has also been referred to as Turbo FLASH. This rapid acquisition can be a useful strategy when ECG-triggering is not practical and strong T1 contrast is desired (29). Since each slice can be obtained in less than 1 second, ECG-triggering is not a strict constraint.

Bright blood strategies include gadolinium-enhanced angiography, GRE flow-sensitive imaging, steady-state free precession imaging, and phase-contrast MRI.

Gadolinium-enhanced MRA is especially useful for studying the branch vessels of the thoracic aorta, with

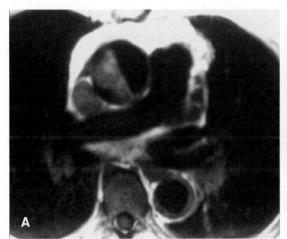
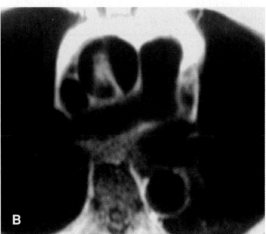

FIGURE 17-6 Dissection of the ascending aorta in a 67-year-old male. Compare the diagnostic quality of images obtained with turbo SE T1-weighted (**A**, imaging time: 3 minutes) and dark blood HASTE (**B**, imaging time: 31-second breath hold) ECG-triggered images, despite the difference in the acquisition times. (HASTE, half-Fourier turbo spin-echo.)

improved resolution, signal-to-noise ratio, speed, and overall quality of vascular images. The entire thoracic aorta can be covered in <20 seconds with minimal flow artifacts and with sufficiently thin sections for versatile data displays. These displays include an infinite number of projections and MPR images of the aorta.

A sagittal or oblique sagittal acquisition with a large field of view can cover the entire aorta, offering its maximal resolution in a familiar projection. It can be done by using non-breath-hold technique with slower sequences or with a breath-hold technique that exploits the benefits of high-performance gradient systems. Despite the respiratory motion that degrades the quality of images, the non-breath-hold technique provides diagnostic images in almost all cases (30). The breath-hold technique uses a spoiled 3D GRE with very short TRs and TEs to encompass the entire aorta in a single breath-hold, typically within 15 to 25 seconds.

The application of ECG-triggering to ensure diagnostic quality images for GRE strategies requires further discussion (see section below). The effective TR is calculated first based on the R-R interval. Conventional GRE images without the use of saturation bands can be acquired at different phases of the cardiac cycle and displayed in dynamic fashion. Flow is visualized as changes in signal intensity through the cardiac cycle on the cine display, which is useful for demonstrating altered flow at the aortic valve. The TR depends on the heart rate of the patient, the SE is the minimum achievable with flow compensation (in the range of 4 to 10 ms), the flip angle is 30 to 40 degrees, and matrix is typically 128×256 (phase $\times$ frequency encoding). The data are acquired in peak systole immediately following the R-wave to maximize inflow into the imaging section. The number of heartbeats and breath-hold duration required is determined by the number of phase-encoding steps per section, the number of lines of k-space sampled per R-R interval, and the heart rate of the patient (30).

ECG-Triggering and Gating

The heart contracts in a rhythmic manner, and cardiac contraction motion artifacts may be eliminated by application of an electrocardiographic gate to cardiac image acquisition. In this approach, each phase-encoding step in an acquisition is obtained at the same phase of the cardiac cycle. Then, when the image is processed, it will be coherent and free from cardiac motion–related artifacts. By convention, the R-wave is chosen as the gating signal because it has the greatest amplitude and is therefore more easily identified in the ECG. In addition, because the R-wave immediately precedes ventricular contraction, it represents the end of ventricular diastole and thus the images are obtained when the ventricular chambers are most dilated (31). Certain calculations must be made in order to set up the MR sequence correctly.

It is important to define the terms applied to the use of ECG leads in MRI/MRA: ECG-triggering and ECG-gating. These terms are often used interchangeably. The term *ECG-triggering* can be used to describe prospective acquisitions during which data accumulation is initiated based on synchronization with the ECG-tracing. This differs from *ECG-gating*, a term that refers to the continuous acquisition of image data during an independent recording of the ECG. With retrospective gating, the sequence is initiated by using the minimum TR without being synchronized to the ECG. The points in the cardiac cycle at which the data are acquired are monitored and later referenced to the ECG for reconstruction.

Lead placement can be time consuming when trying to achieve a trace that will provide reliable information for triggering the acquisition. However, the time investment is important and can be facilitated by some helpful tips.

The objective is to achieve a tracing in which the R-wave is substantially taller than the T-wave of the tracing. The T-wave elevation that is characteristically seen in the MR environment results from the magnetoelectrodynamic effect that scales with field strength (32). This can lead to data acquisition triggered off the T-wave. Thus, data will not be adequately synchronized to the mechanical-temporal features needed for optimized flow and quantitative evaluations.

Depending on the system, typically three or four electrodes are used. Optimized electrode contact is important. Thorough cleansing of the contact area with alcohol and/or acetone is recommended. Body hair should be removed in the area where the electrode is placed.

Lead placement typically represents a compromise between optimizing signal (wider spacing of the electrodes) and minimizing gradient artifacts (narrower spacing of the electrodes). The latter typically dominates, and therefore it is common to begin the procedure with the leads relatively close together on the anterior chest wall. In cases when a poor tracing dominates, it can be helpful to position the electrodes on the patient's back.

The recent implementation of vectorcardiography improves the efficiency which adequately identifies the QRS complex correctly (32). This approach examines the 3D orientation of the ECG signal and uses the calculated vector of the QRS complex as a filter mechanism to ignore electrical signals that are of a similar timing in the cardiac cycle or of a similar magnitude but different vector.

When setting up the parameters for imaging, it is important to understand the relationship of heart rate with the TR. In triggered echoes, the TR is equal to the R-R interval. The R-R interval is calculated by multiplying (1/patient's heart rate) by 60,000 (msec/minute).

$$\underset{\text{(or effective TR)}}{\text{R-R interval}} = 60{,}000/\text{Heart rate (in beats per min [BPM])}$$

For example, considering determining the effective TR for a patient with a heart rate of 80 BPM. If the patient's heart rate is 80 BPM, there are 80 beats occurring for every 60 × 1,000 msec (1 second); stated inversely, during 60,000 msec, there will be 80 heart beats. We wish to solve for msec/beat (each beat yields one R-R interval), and in this example, the R-R interval is 60,000/80 = 750 msec. To obtain images with T2-weighting, longer TR values are needed—usually >2,000 msec at 1.5T. Thus, for T2-weighted images, triggering occurs every two to three R-R intervals.

When triggering, the slices are sampled once during the effective TR in the same way as in conventional imaging. However, multiple slices can be sampled in a given R-R interval, and the number of slices is influenced by the patient's heart rate. That is, with slower heart rates, there is a longer TR allowing for more slices to be sampled. The important limitation to be recognized is that each slice of a multislice acquisition will be imaged during a different portion of the cardiac cycle.

To reduce pulsatile flow artifacts when quantification of aortic valve disease is not needed, the application of pulse-triggering can be effective and is much simpler to set up as compared with ECG-triggering.

Functional Assessment

The ability to provide accurate assessments of flow velocities along with a comprehensive anatomic evaluation extends the role of MRI in aortography when an aortic valve assessment is being considered. As previously commented, however, echocardiography is the modality of choice for aortic valve evaluation in most instances, as it provides sufficient temporal and spatial resolution for structural and functional information in a noninvasive and readily obtainable format.

For aortic flow measurement with MR, a plane transecting the aortic root immediately distal to the aortic valve cusps has been recommended. Through-plane, flow measurements are obtained with velocity encoded along the slice select gradient. Such phase velocity mapping, also referred to as phase-contrast MR, is acquired at multiple points throughout the cardiac cycle, emphasizing the cross-sectional through-plane mean directed velocity. This provides measurements of systolic forward flow and diastolic reversed flow, the latter after valve closure (Fig. 17-7).

Nuances of Contrast Methods

Although detailed discussion can be found in Chapter 5, following is a summary of the key points regarding the use of intravenous contrast in thoracic aorta MRA.

Because the right brachiocephalic vein courses more directly into the right atrium, facilitating more rapid and coherent delivery of contrast to the heart, the right arm should be used for the injection of the contrast media whenever possible. Besides, the left brachiocephalic vein has been known to obscure visualization of the arch vessels due to its proximity to these vessels as it crosses left to right (33).

In order to deliver all of the contrast from the venous circulation into the heart in one efficient, tight, and coherent bolus, use of *saline bolus* (or *flush*) is recommended (34). There is no consensus about the volume to be used, but most protocols suggest around 20 mL at the same rate as the contrast injection (35). It is important to remember that a variety of injection approaches are available, and further details can be found in Chapter 5.

Different *timing strategies* are also available, including timing bolus, automated bolus detection (such as SmartPrep, developed by GE Healthcare), operator-dependent bolus detection (also known as FluoroTrigger, BolusTrak, and CareBolus, respectively developed by GE Healthcare, Philips Medical Systems, and Siemens Solutions), and time-resolved sequences (e.g., TRICKS and TREAT, developed by GE Healthcare and Siemens Solutions, respectively) (36–39).

Although general guidelines can be found in the literature, choices usually depend on available equipment, previous experience and success, level of expertise, individual preferences, and careful coordination in the data sampling (k-space filling strategy).

Nuances of Postprocessing

Because of the complexity of thoracic aortic disease and the importance of aortic branch assessment, 3D visualization is often mandatory to fully interpret MR data (Fig. 17-8). For further details on this topic, please refer to Chapter 6.

Magnetic Resonance Imaging and Angiography Pitfalls

Pseudostenosis can result from susceptibility artifacts secondary to metallic stents, surgical clips, and prostheses. These can cause signal loss within a vessel, mimicking stenosis or occlusion. Clinical information is crucial, and sometimes source images reveal a blooming or susceptibility artifact near the suspicious vascular segment (33).

Another cause of signal loss on contrast-enhanced MRA reported more recently is the suppression of intravascular

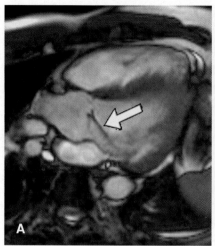
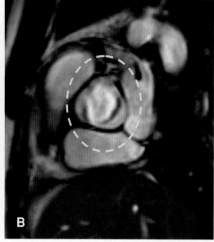
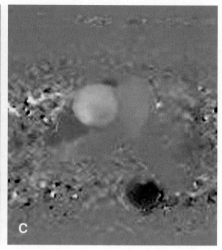

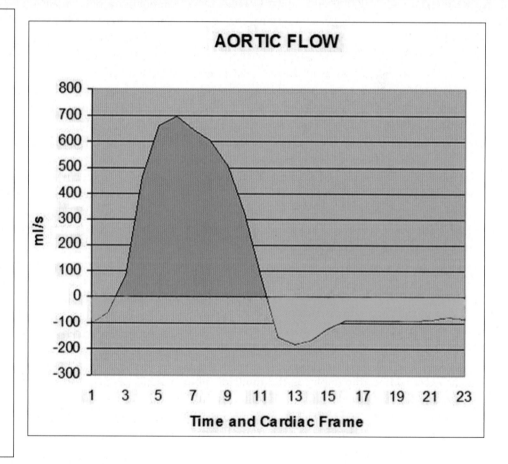

Time	ml/s
0	-97,9
34	-60,7
69	79,4
103	465,2
137	662,2
172	696,4
206	642,2
240	602,9
274	501,3
309	323,3
343	80,1
377	-154,4
412	-180,9
446	-164,4
480	-122,3
515	-91,4
549	-89,5
583	-91,5
618	-88,7
652	-89,3
686	-84,2
720	-76,6
755	-81,6

FIGURE 17-7 Aortic regurgitation. MRI for quantification of left ventricular systolic function and aortic valve assessment in a 39-year-old man with known aortic regurgitation. **A:** This cine image shows a signal void (*arrow*) during diastole in the left ventricular outflow tract directed toward the anterior mitral leaflet, consistent with aortic regurgitation. **B:** In this cine image in a plane transverse to the aortic valve, note that this is bicuspid valve (*dashed circle*). **C:** Phase-contrast cine image was obtained transverse to the ascending aorta. In this image, flow in the caudocranial direction (as in the ascending aorta, in this case) appears bright whereas flow in the opposite direction (as in the descending aorta) appears dark. The measured aortic regurgitant fraction (the *green areas* over the sum of the *green* and *blue areas*) was consistent with moderate to severe aortic regurgitation.

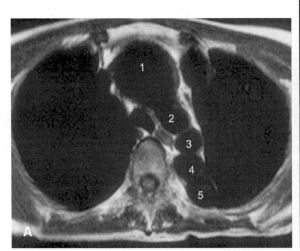
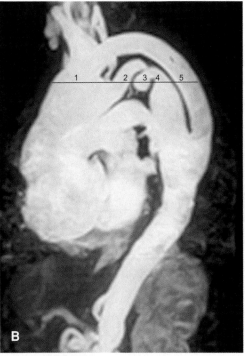

FIGURE 17-8 Postoperative findings in a patient with aortic coarctation surgically corrected by using an extra-anatomic bypass. In the axial dark blood HASTE image **(A)**, a curious image results of the contiguous multiple lumina (*numbers*). It is not easy to appreciate their meaning in this single image. On the other hand, the sagittal MIP **(B)** allows the understanding of these different structures as the oblique section of a single redundant and tortuous aortic arch and the circumjacent bypass. (1, prearch ascending aorta; 2, proximal branch of coarctation; 3, pseudo-aneurysm of coarctation; 4, distal portion of coarctation; 5, lumen of extra-anatomic bypass graft.)

signal on fat-saturated sequences (Fig. 17-9). Magnetic susceptibility effects from aerated lung result in frequency shifts in adjacent fat- and water-containing tissues. Thus, when a spectrally selective fat-saturation technique is used, regions of water, and not adjacent fat, may be saturated. In order to identify this as an artifact, it is important to recognize the lack of luminal narrowing and the absence of collateral vessels. Because of this artifact, one should avoid the routine use of fat saturation with contrast-enhanced MR angiographic studies of the chest (40).

ANATOMY

Normal Anatomy

The thoracic aorta is divided into four regions: the aortic root, the ascending aorta, the transverse aorta or aortic arch, and the descending aorta (Fig. 17-10).

The *aortic root* is the region of the aorta from the aortic annulus to the sinotubular junction (STJ). The normally trileaflet aortic valve is attached to the aorta at the annulus, which is a complex 3D coronet or crown-shaped structure

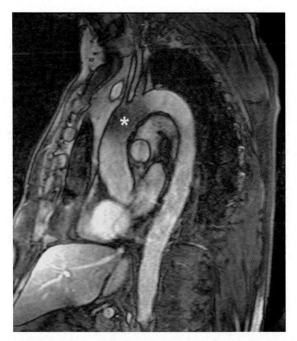

FIGURE 17-9 Fat-suppression artifact. Sagittal thin-slab MIP from a fat-saturated 3D MR angiographic examination demonstrates moderate loss of signal intensity within the proximal aortic arch (∗).

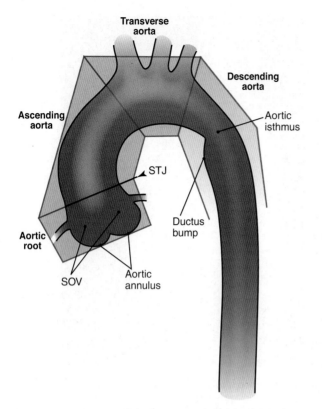

Transverse aorta

Descending aorta

Ascending aorta

Aortic isthmus

STJ

Aortic root

Ductus bump

SOV

Aortic annulus

FIGURE 17-10 Diagram of the segments of thoracic aorta, their anatomical references, and adjacent structures. (*SOV*, sinuses of Valsalva; *STJ*, sinotubular junction.)

rather than a simple two-dimensional (2D) ring. The three sinuses of Valsalva are outpouchings above the annulus that terminate distally at the sinotubular junction or STJ. The left main and right coronary arteries typically originate at the apex of the left and right sinuses of Valsalva, respectively. The third sinus is referred to as the posterior or noncoronary sinus.

The *ascending aorta* comprises the tubular segment of the aorta, extending from the aortic root to the brachiocephalic or innominate artery. The ascending aorta is anterior to the left atrium, right pulmonary artery, and right main bronchus. The superior vena cava and right atrial appendage are located to the right of the ascending aorta, and the pulmonary trunk is on its left. Most of the ascending aorta lies within the pericardial sac.

The *transverse aorta* or *aortic arch* extends from the proximal aspect of the brachiocephalic arterial origin to the distal aspect of the left subclavian arterial origin and thus contains the three supra-aortic branches—the brachiocephalic, left common carotid, and left subclavian arteries, which provide oxygenated blood to the neck, head, and upper extremities (further details can be found in Chapter 15). In 5% of subjects, the left vertebral artery can be seen originating separately from the aorta between the left common carotid and the left subclavian arteries. The bifurca-

tion of the pulmonary trunk, the left main bronchus, and the left recurrent laryngeal nerve lie within the concavity of the arch. To the right are the trachea and the esophagus.

The *descending aorta* extends from the left subclavian artery to the aortic hiatus of the diaphragm. The *aortic isthmus* is that segment of the aorta between the origin of the left subclavian artery and the ligamentum arteriosum. Just distal to the isthmus, a bulge on the lesser curve of the aorta is a ductus bump, which is a normal finding and should not be confused for an aneurysm (Fig. 17-11). The esophagus is on the right of the proximal two thirds of the descending aorta. The esophagus crosses the aorta anteriorly and, distal to this, is on the left side of the descending aorta (41).

In adults, the ascending aorta is typically 5 cm in length, the arch 4.5 cm, and the descending aorta 20 cm. The diameter of the thoracic aorta is largest at the aortic root and gradually decreases distally: 3.6 cm is the average diameter of the aortic root, 3.5 cm in the ascending aorta, and 2.4 cm in the distal descending aorta (42). The diameter increases progressively with age. The aorta is smaller in females and also varies with body habitus (41).

The branches of the descending aorta are divided into visceral (pericardial, bronchial, esophageal, and mediastinal arteries) and parietal (intercostal, subcostal, and superior

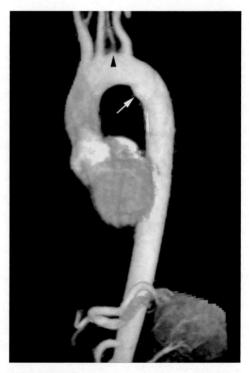

FIGURE 17-11 Image of a 39-year-old woman allergic to iodinated contrast and complaining of severe chest pain. Thick-slab sagittal oblique MIP demonstrates a normal ductus bump (*arrow*) in an otherwise unremarkable aorta. Incidentally seen is a separate origin of the left vertebral artery off the arch (*arrowhead*).

phrenic arteries) branches. The *pericardial branches* consist of a few small vessels that are distributed to the posterior aspect of the pericardium. The *bronchial arteries* vary in number, size, and origin and are further discussed elsewhere in this text. The *esophageal arteries* are four or five in number, arise from the anterior wall of the aorta, and travel obliquely downward to the esophagus, creating a net of anastomoses along the esophagus. The *mediastinal branches* are multiple small vessels that supply the lymphatic tissue in the posterior mediastinum.

The *intercostal arteries* are usually nine pairs that arise from the posterior wall of the aorta and course along the lower nine intercostal spaces. The first two spaces are supplied by the highest intercostal artery, a branch of the costocervical trunk of the subclavian artery. The aortic intercostal branches are longer on the right side because of the position of the aorta on the left side of the spine. They pass across the vertebral bodies, posterior to the esophagus, thoracic duct, and vena azygos, and are covered by the right lung and pleura.

The *subcostal arteries* lie below the last ribs and are the lowest pair of branches arising from the thoracic aorta. Each passes along the lower border of the twelfth rib, posterior to the kidney. After passing forward between the transversus abdominis muscle and the obliquus internus muscle, it anastomoses with the superior epigastric, lower intercostal, and lumbar arteries. The *superior phrenic branches* are small vessels that arise from the lower part of the thoracic aorta. They are distributed to the posterior part of the upper surface of the diaphragm, and anastomose with the musculophrenic and pericardiacophrenic arteries (43).

It is also important to recognize the contribution of the descending thoracic aorta to the circulation of the spinal cord (Fig. 17-12). The major arterial circulation to the

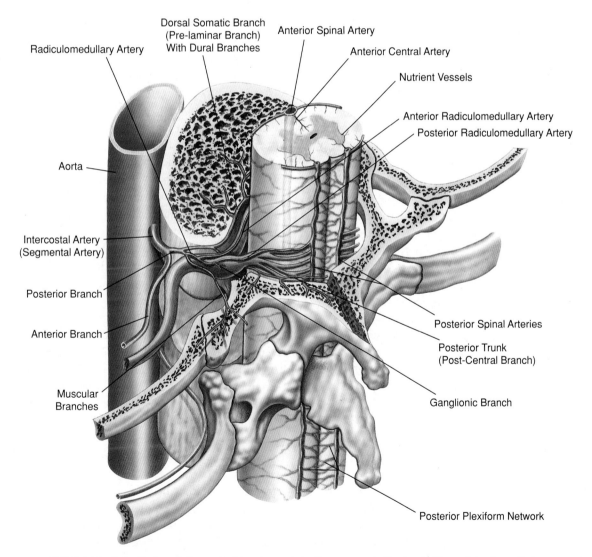

FIGURE 17-12 Radiculomedullary, spinal arteries, and plexiform network. (Reprinted with permission from Uflacker R. *Atlas of Vascular Anatomy: An Angiographic Approach*. 2nd ed. Philadelphia: Lippincott Williams & Wilkins; 2007.)

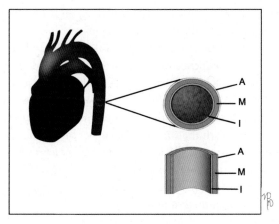

FIGURE 17-13 Schematic illustration of the layers constituent of the aortic wall. (*I*, intima; *M*, media; *A*, adventitia.)

spinal cord is the anterior longitudinal spinal artery and the paired posterior longitudinal spinal arteries with the great anterior medullary artery (the *artery of Adamkiewicz*, arteria radicularis magna or ARM) serving as the dominant feeder of the spinal cord (44). In anatomical studies, the ARM most often originated from the left side in 72% to 78% of patients (45,46), between T8 and L1 levels in 91% of patients (45), and between T7 and L1 levels in 94% of patients (46). Koshino and colleagues (45) reported that there was no significant correlation between the diameter of the ARM and the diameters of the intercostal artery and lumbar artery from which the ARM originated.

The aortic wall is composed of three layers: the inner layer of intima, the middle layer of media, and the outer layer of adventitia (Fig. 17-13). Studies evaluating the aortic wall thickness *in vivo* are far less common than those of the carotid arteries. Li and associates (47) used MRI to measure aortic wall thickness in 196 individuals without clinical evidence of cardiovascular disease. According to their results, wall thickness increases with age and is greater in men. There is no statistically significant difference between whites and blacks. The average thickness was 2.32 mm and 2.11 mm, respectively, in men and women (47).

ANEURYSMAL DISEASE

Definition and Epidemiology

An *aneurysm* is defined as a permanent localized enlargement of an artery to more than 1.5 times its expected diameter. Aneurysms can be seen in any location of the arterial tree but are more common in the aorta, especially in the infrarenal aorta (48). In general, the ascending and transverse aorta are considered aneurysmal when their diameter exceeds 4 cm, and the descending aorta is considered aneurysmal when its diameter exceeds 3.5 cm.

Thoracic aortic aneurysms (TAAs) are less common than abdominal aortic aneurysms but are becoming increasingly prevalent as the population ages, with an incidence of 6 per 100,000 persons per year. It is the most common condition of the thoracic aorta requiring surgical treatment. TAAs are more equally distributed between the genders than abdominal aneurysms, with a male-to-female ratio of 2:1. The afflicted population is usually elderly, and familial incidence is also present (3,49,50).

Classification and Pathogenesis

Aneurysms can be described further according to their location, morphology, and etiology.

Location is used commonly to classify aortic aneurysms for clinical significance and surgical approach. Typically, the aneurysm can be localized to the aortic root, an individual sinus of Valsalva, ascending, arch, descending, and abdominal portions of the aorta.

The *morphology* of an aneurysm is either fusiform or saccular. Fusiform aneurysms are sausage-like in shape; they are dilated symmetrically throughout the full circumference of the aorta. Saccular aneurysms are asymmetric and involve an outpouching of a portion of the circumference of the aortic wall.

Aneurysms also may be classified morphologically as either true or false (pseudoaneurysm). True aneurysms involve all layers of the aortic wall. A pseudoaneurysm is a contained rupture that extends through all layers of the aortic wall. The integrity of the vasculature is maintained by surrounding tissues and the chronic inflammatory reaction to extravasated blood. Pseudoaneurysms are the second most common form of TAA and the most common type in younger patients. They are contained arterial disruptions usually caused by blunt nonpenetrating trauma, most often due to rapid deceleration in motor vehicle collisions (41).

Aneurysms can be classified according to their *etiology* as congenital or acquired, although the pathogenesis of aortic aneurysms is complex and not completely understood. A number of hypotheses have been proposed, but no single theory has been universally accepted. Acquired aneurysms may be due to atherosclerosis, cystic medial degeneration, infection, trauma, iatrogenic, or inflammatory processes. Atherosclerosis is the most common cause of aortic aneurysms (Fig. 17-14).

The pathologic basis of atherosclerotic aneurysm is a diseased intima with secondary degeneration and fibrous replacement of the media beneath it. Following aortic dilatation, the wall is exposed to increasing tension due to the increasing lateral hydrostatic pressure as the velocity of blood flow diminishes. These factors compromise mural vascular nutrition. Increased mechanical stress and poor nutrition lead to further degeneration and progressive

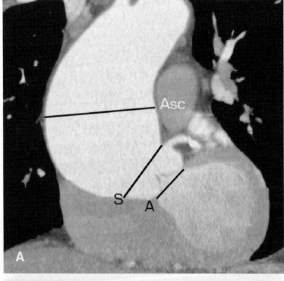

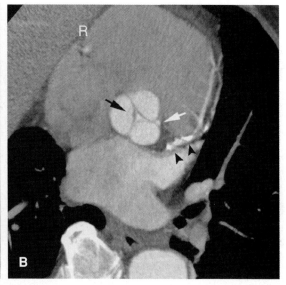

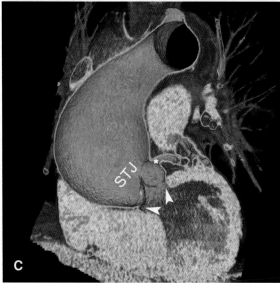

FIGURE 17-14 Ascending aortic aneurysm with sparing of the annulus and sinuses. A 77-year-old male with aortic stenosis and regurgitation. **A:** Orthogonal MPR image from a cardiac-gated MDCT angiogram shows marked dilatation of the ascending thoracic aorta, from the sinotubular junction through the arch. Annulus (*A*) measurement was 24 mm, sinuses (*S*) measured 40 mm, and ascending aorta (*Asc*) measured 88 mm maximally. **B:** Orthogonal short-axis image of the aortic valve in maximal closed position shows incomplete coaptation of the right and left leaflets (*white arrow*) as well as lack of central coaptation (*black arrow*). Note severe left coronary artery calcification (*black arrowheads*). The patient was found to have a significant right coronary artery stenosis, which was treated by saphenous vein bypass grafting at the time of aortic valve replacement. The right coronary artery (*R*) is seen in cross section in the right atrioventricular groove. **C:** Volume-rendered image shows sparing of the annulus (*white arrowheads*) and preferential dilatation from the sinotubular junction (*STJ*) cephalad. The left main coronary artery is also noted in normal position (*).

dilatation. Ultimately, the aneurysm wall consists of acellular and avascular connective tissue (51–53).

Medial degeneration resulting from repetitive aortic injury and repair encountered in aging, sometimes accelerated by connective disorders (such as Marfan and Ehlers-Danlos syndromes), is the most common cause of degenerative aneurysms. These are the most common aneurysms in the ascending aorta (52,54).

Connective disorders (such as Marfan and Ehlers-Danlos syndromes) are genetic conditions that affect the connective tissues throughout the body. In Marfan syndrome, a major elastic fiber protein found in the wall of the aorta is defective, and most patients with this disease develop aneurysms of the ascending aorta with subsequent malfunctioning of the aortic valve (Figs. 17-15–17-17). In contrast to ascending aortic aneurysms in patients without underlying connective tissue disease, which tend not to involve the aortic root, patients with Marfan disease often manifest annuloaortic ectasia and aortic root aneurysms (Fig. 17-15). The annular dilation results in incomplete coaptation of the aortic valve leaflets and aortic valvular insufficiency (Fig. 17-16).

Another important and independent risk factor for the development of ascending aortic and aortic root aneurysms is bicuspid aortic valve disease. The disease has a prevalence of approximately 1:1,000 with a 4:1 male predominance and familial aggregation. The disease is associated with aortic coarctation, coronary artery anomalies, and patent ductus arteriosus. Aortic root dilation is present in approximately 50% of individuals and is a precursor to aneurysm and dissection. Aortic dissection occurs in 5% of affected individuals. Routine surveillance of subjects with bicuspid aortic valve by using echocardiography is advised (55).

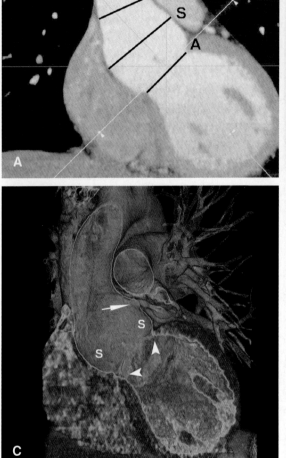

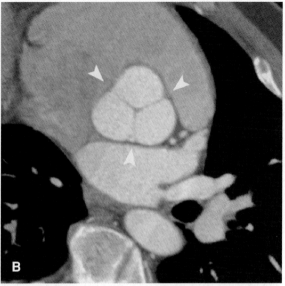

FIGURE 17-15 Utility of cardiac-gated MDCT angiography for evaluation of aortic root pathology in a 43-year-old male with Marfan syndrome. A: Orthogonal MPR image from retrospectively gated MDCT angiogram shows dilatation of the aortic annulus, reaching 34 mm in size (normal range 23 to 27 mm). There is dilatation of the sinuses of Valsalva (*S*), reaching 48-mm orthogonal dimension. At the sinotubular junction (*STJ*), there is less dilatation, measuring 33 mm. Annuloaortic ectasia may be seen in Marfan syndrome, forme-fruste Marfan, Ehlers-Danlos syndrome, osteogenesis imperfecta, and other connective tissue disorders; it may also be idiopathic. **B:** Orthogonal short-axis image of the aortic valve shows trileaflet configuration (*arrowheads*). The ability to create a "cine" loop of the retrospectively reconstructed gated MDCT series allows excellent detail of valvular motion and coaptation. **C:** Volume-rendered image shows dilatation of the aortic annulus (*arrowheads*) and sinuses (*S*). The left main coronary artery (*arrow*) arises high from the left sinus of Valsalva, which is important for planning of valve-sparing surgery. Aortic dilatation in Marfan syndrome may be complicated by dissection and aortic regurgitation.

Although primary aortic infection may result in aortic aneurysmal disease (commonly seen in patients with syphilis in the preantibiotic era), secondary infection is more common. An aneurysm caused by nonsyphilitic infection of the arterial wall is known as mycotic aneurysm, a misnomer generally adopted and originally applied based on the gross pathologic appearance (mushroom-like morphology) (56). The most common pathogens for blood-borne infection are *Staphylococcus* and *Salmonella*, and contiguous spread is rare but most commonly due to tuberculosis extending from the spine (57,58). Mycotic aneurysms are often insidious and may lead to sepsis and aortic rupture if untreated. The normal arterial intima is extremely resistant to infection, and the development of a mycotic aneurysm requires prior damage to the aortic wall. Its prevalence is increased in immunocompromised patients, and predisposing factors include contiguous bacterial endocarditis, atherosclerosis, drug abuse, and aortic trauma (caused by accidents, surgery, or catheterization) (59).

Other noninfective generalized inflammatory processes are associated with TAAs, including Takayasu arteritis, giant cell arteritis, ankylosing spondylitis, psoriatic arthritis, rheumatic fever, rheumatoid arthritis, relapsing polychondritis, Reiter syndrome, systemic lupus erythematosus, scleroderma, ulcerative colitis and Behçet disease. (41).

Clinical Presentation and Natural History

Because no large-scale screening programs for aortic aneurysm are in place and TAAs seldom produce symptoms, most of them are discovered on imaging during investigation of an unrelated problem. Although uncommon,

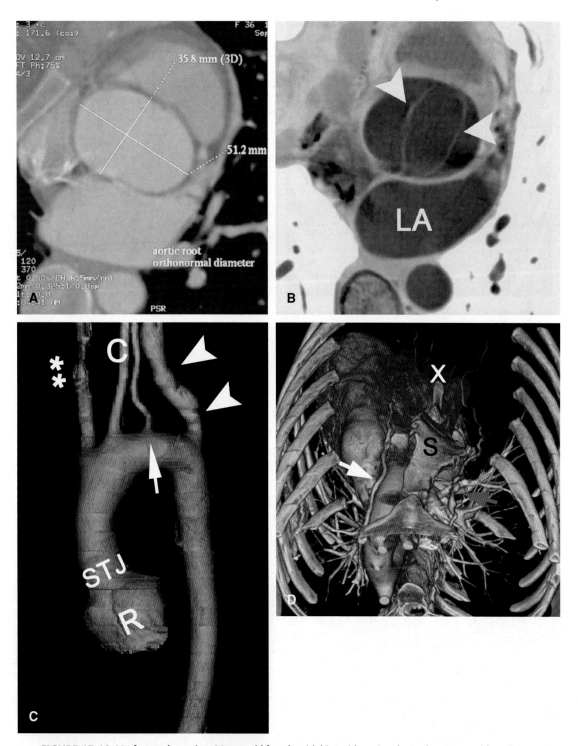

FIGURE 17-16 Marfan syndrome in a 36-year-old female with bicuspid aortic valve and aneurysms of aortic root and left subclavian artery. Images from ECG-gated CTA of the chest. **A:** Orthonormal (obtained orthogonal to vessel center-line) measurement at sinuses of Valsalva demonstrates aneurysmal dilatation of the aortic root, reaching 51 mm in dimension. **B:** MPR with inverted grayscale, obtained orthogonal to aortic valve in systole. The two aortic valve leaflets are well demonstrated (*arrowheads*), assuming a "fish-mouth" appearance typical of bicuspid aortic valve. (*LA*, left atrium.) **C:** Volume-rendered image of thoracic aorta with bone segmentation shows the typical "onion-bulb" appearance of the aortic root (*R*). There is dilation of the aortic annulus and sinuses of Valsalva, with preservation of the sinotubular junction (*STJ*). There is a fusiform aneurysm of the left subclavian artery (*arrowheads*). There is separate origin of the left vertebral artery directly from the aortic arch (*arrow*), which represents variant anatomy. An artifact from the bone segmentation process is created in the innominate artery (∗∗), secondary to streak artifact from dense contrast in the venous system on the source images. (*C*, left common carotid artery.) **D:** Volume-rendered image viewed from the head shows a severe pectus excavatum deformity with depression and angulation of the sternum (*S*). There are focal aneurysms of the right internal mammary artery (*purple arrow*). There is ectasia of the left internal mammary artery (*white arrow*) but no focal aneurysm. (*X*, xyphoid process.) (*Figure 17-16 continues*)

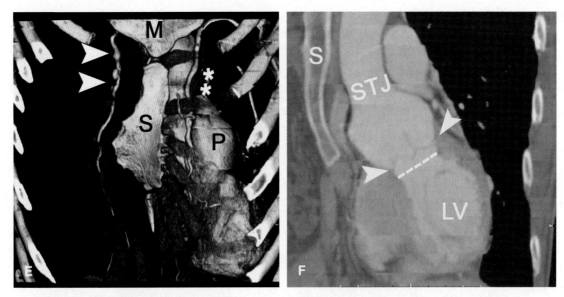

FIGURE 17-16 Continued E: Volume-rendered image viewed anteriorly shows the right internal mammary aneurysm (*arrowheads*). The sternal deformities are again seen (*S*). (∗∗, left internal mammary artery; *M*, manubrium; *P*, pulmonary outflow tract.) **F:** Oblique coronal thin-slab MIP image demonstrates widening of the aortic annulus (-----), measuring 31 mm. There is good coaptation of the aortic valve on this image in diastole (*arrowheads*). There is preservation of the sinotubular junction (*STJ*). (*LV*, left ventricle; *S*, sternum.)

symptoms usually are the result of a large aneurysm compressing (Fig. 17-18) or eroding adjacent structures, including superior vena cava syndrome, stridor or dyspnea due to tracheobronchial compression, dysphagia due to esophageal compression, and hoarseness secondary to recurrent compression of the laryngeal nerve. Acutely expanding aneurysms produce severe deep back pain. This presentation often precedes rupture, and urgent treatment is required. Rarely, the first clinical manifestation is embolization to the lower extremity. This complication is not related to the size of the aneurysm and constitutes itself an independent indication for repair (41,60,61).

The natural history of aortic aneurysms is to enlarge and rupture (Fig. 17-19), and treatment strategies are designed to prevent this complication since an overall mortality rate of 94% is found following rupture (50). Unlike

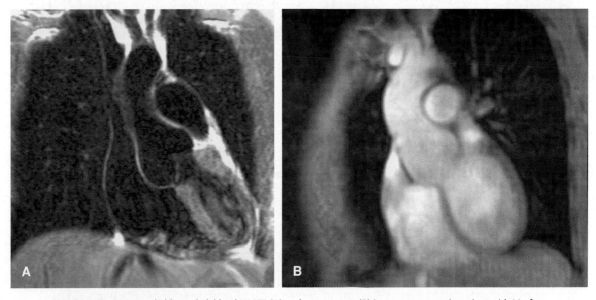

FIGURE 17-17 Coronal oblique dark blood HASTE **(A)** and postcontrast **(B)** in an asymptomatic patient with Marfan syndrome show a dilated tulip-bulb appearance of the aortic root.

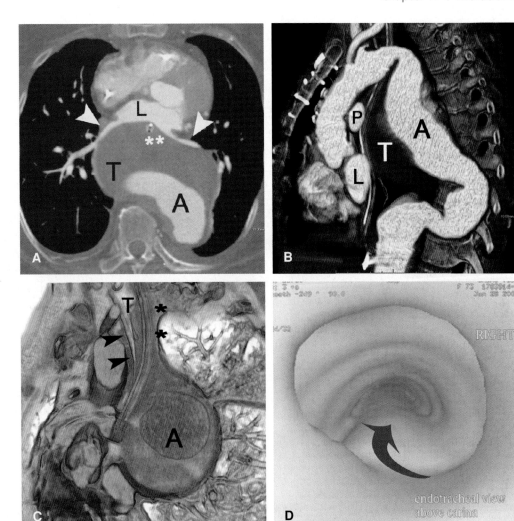

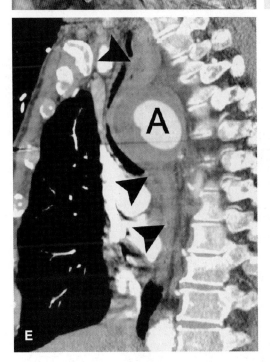

FIGURE 17-18 A 73-year-old female with thoracic aortic aneurysm causing compression of mediastinal structures. A: Axial image at level of the left atrium (*L*) depicts an aneurysm of the descending thoracic aorta (*A*), which contains a large amount of thrombus (*T*). There is marked compression of the pulmonary veins (*arrowheads*) and left atrium. A nasogastric tube in the esophagus is displaced anteriorly (**). **B:** Oblique sagittal volume-rendered image demonstrates the large aneurysm (*A*) and anterior thrombus (*T*). There is marked elongation and tortuosity of the descending thoracic aorta. Mass effect on the left atrium (*L*), pulmonary artery (*P*), and nasogastric tube is noted again. **C:** Oblique volume-rendered image is rendered with airway opacity, viewed from left posterior oblique. There is marked mass effect on the nasogastric tube (**) by the aneurysm (*A*). The trachea (*T*) is also narrowed along its inferior portion (*arrowheads*). **D:** Virtual bronchoscopic view of the trachea reconstructed from the CTA data set shows the degree of compression of the distal trachea (*arrow*), near the carina. **E:** Sagittal thin-slab MIP image demonstrates high-density esophageal contents (*arrowheads*) draped around the aneurysm (*A*). At surgery, an aortoesophageal fistula was found.

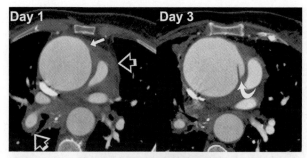

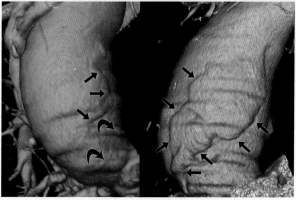

FIGURE 17-19 A 73-year-old man with chest pain referred to CT to assess for pulmonary embolism. The transverse section and volume rendering on the left were obtained at the time of initial presentation, and the transverse section and volume rendering on the right were obtained 2 days later. Initially, the transverse section demonstrated a 6-cm ascending aortic aneurysm with thrombus in the mediastinum extending around the left interlobar pulmonary artery (*open arrows*). A subtle contour irregularity is present on the anteromedial surface of the ascending aorta (*small arrow*), corresponding to the only direct manifestation of mural instability at this time. The volume rendering below reveals an obvious longitudinal "crack" (*small black arrows*) at the site of the contour abnormality on the transverse section. It is distinguished from transverse ridges (*curved arrows*) that are caused by aortic pulsation in this ungated acquisition. Two days later, the rupture has progressed with aneurysm expansion and undermining of the intimomedial complex (*curved white arrow*) and early pseudoaneurysm formation (*black arrows*). The patient underwent ascending aortic replacement where a ruptured aneurysm was identified with only the aortic adventitia preventing exsanguinations.

rupture of abdominal aortic aneurysms, which can be contained in the retroperitoneal compartment, rupture of TAAs is usually unrestrained and rapidly fatal. The single most important factor associated with rupture is maximal cross-sectional aneurysm diameter. Equal in significance but less commonly used is maximal cross-sectional area (48,62–65).

Imaging Findings

The criteria for diagnosing aortic aneurysm with CT are well established. Information regarding the focal or diffuse nature of aortic dilatation and deformity, as well as the length of the aneurysm, is readily available on unenhanced scans. Unenhanced CT scans are also important for identifying calcification and acute hematomas. Peripheral calcifications have been reported in about 75% of aortic aneurysms. It is important to remember that peripheral calcification on the surface of the false lumen in a chronic dissection can mimic an aneurysm (41,66).

Mural thrombus is frequently present with aneurysmal disease. There is a direct relationship between the size of the aneurysm and the amount of thrombus. Thrombus may be circumferential or crescentic. Since the thrombus is usually removed in the open surgical approach, and inadequate manipulation of the thrombus may result in embolization to distal vessels, knowledge of the position and amount of mural thrombus may be important in surgical planning. The injection of intravenous contrast material is usually required to differentiate between the patent lumen and mural thrombus (41,66,67) (Fig. 17-20).

The aorta can be dilated or normal in caliber following dissection. Aortic dissection can be accurately differentiated from aneurysms when an intimal flap and two aortic lumens are demonstrated. Intravenous contrast material is usually required for visualization of an intimal flap on CT,

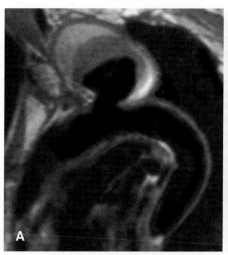

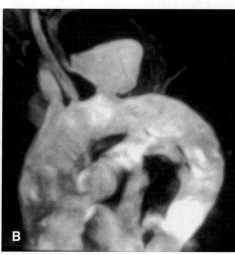

FIGURE 17-20 Arch aneurysm. Note the distinct layers with high and intermediate signal within the mural thrombus that represent blood in different stages of decomposition in the black blood image (**A**) and the remaining patent region of the aneurysm in the postcontrast MIP image (**B**). (Courtesy of Mark Flyer, MD.)

but it is sometimes visible on unenhanced images. It may be challenging to distinguish an aneurysm with thrombus from an aortic dissection with a thrombosed false lumen. In this setting, the most reliable sign of dissection is the presence of a recent thrombus within the aortic wall (41,68).

CT and MRI are superior to angiography in evaluating the true size of an aneurysm because of the ability to demonstrate mural thrombus with cross-sectional techniques (for further details, refer to Chapter 6). Furthermore, CT and MRI have the advantage of being minimally invasive. CT and angiography can better depict the coronary arteries. MRI and angiography can better demonstrate aortic insufficiency. In comparison to conventional angiography, CT and MRI are usually capable of better depicting the relationship of an aortic aneurysm to adjacent structures and the attendant complications that may be present. Subtle erosion of bone, compression of the tracheobronchial tree, pulmonary vessels or the superior vena cava, and esophageal displacement or obstruction may be appreciated (41,60) (Fig. 17-21).

As discussed previously, atherosclerosis is the leading cause of TAAs. *Atherosclerotic aneurysms* usually begin distal to the left subclavian artery and are relatively uncommon in the ascending aorta. Saccular aneurysms of the ascending thoracic aorta should prompt consideration of an infectious etiology. Whereas syphilis was formerly the major cause of eccentric ascending aortic aneurysms, currently, the most common cause of a saccular ascending thoracic aortic aneurysm is atherosclerosis. TAAs may extend into the abdomen, or a second aneurysm in the abdominal aorta can

be present. Most of them are fusiform, but up to 20% are saccular (41).

Degenerative aneurysms are the most common in the ascending aorta. Involvement of the aortic sinuses and concurrent cardiovascular diseases are frequent. The aneurysmal dilatation generally decreases at higher levels in the ascending aorta, and the aortic arch is usually normal. Aortic calcifications are rare. Aortic valve regurgitation is common, occurring in all patients with a diameter over 6 cm. Annuloaortic ectasia is the combination of an aneurysm of the aortic root and aortic valve regurgitation due to dilatation of the aortic annulus (41).

Most *traumatic pseudoaneurysms* of the thoracic aorta occur near the aortic isthmus. Acute aortic transection can be diagnosed as subtle changes in aortic contour with CT and MRI, but CT is the preferred method in the emergency setting. Nevertheless a mediastinal hematoma, even in a periaortic location, does not mean that the aorta is traumatized (69). Angiography is the definitive method of making or excluding the diagnosis of aortic injury. If secondary rupture of the aorta does not occur, a chronic pseudoaneurysm will develop. These usually calcify and may contain thrombus (41).

In its classical appearance, *mycotic aneurysms* are saccular, with an irregular lumen, perianeurysmal fluid, gas and/or hematoma, osteomyelitis in adjacent vertebral bodies, and disruption of intimal calcification (70).

Thoracic aortic aneurysms may rupture into the mediastinum (Fig. 17-22), pericardium, pleural sac, or the extrapleural space. Aortobronchopulmonary fistula is rare

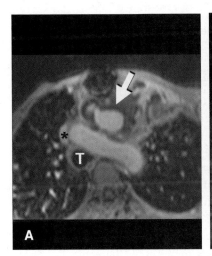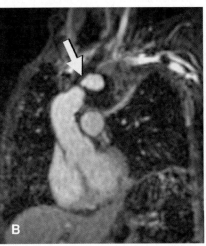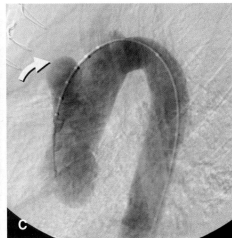

FIGURE 17-21 Post-traumatic pseudoaneurysm in a 50-year-old male patient, a victim of a motor vehicle accident 30 years before, now complaining of a pulsatile left neck mass. The axial (**A**) and oblique MPR (**B**) contrast-enhanced MRA of the chest reveal a pseudoaneurysm (*arrows*) arising from the arch, also seen in the conventional aortography (**C**). The pseudoaneurysm is anterior to the aortic arch and exerts mass effect, pushing the trachea (*T* in **A**) and superior vena cava (⋆) toward the right. (**C** is courtesy of Melvin Clouse, MD.)

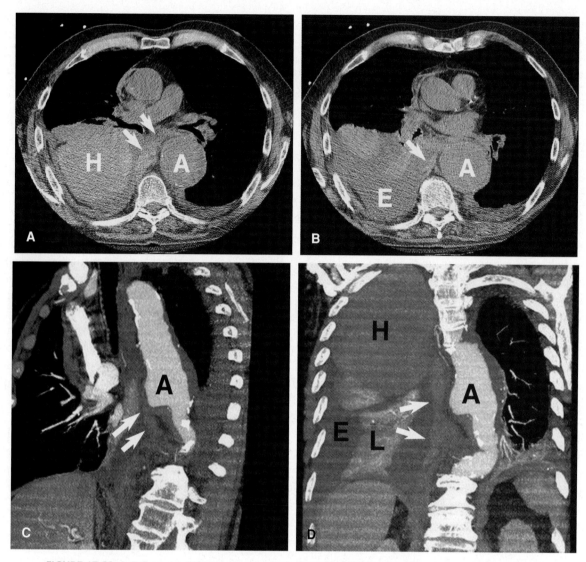

FIGURE 17-22 A, B: Transverse MDCT sections obtained prior to the administration of intravenous contrast material demonstrate a descending aortic aneurysm (*A*) with high-attenuation blood present anteriorly and medially (*arrows*). Both pleural effusion (*E*) and a large pleural hematoma (*H*) are present. **C:** Curved planar reformation during the arterial phase of an intravenous iodinated contrast material injection demonstrates the mid descending aortic aneurysm (*A*) with high-attenuation blood in the middle mediastinum anteromedial to the aneurysm (*arrows*). **D:** A coronal oblique slab MIP positioned posteriorly in the thorax demonstrates the periaortic blood (*arrows*) as well as the large pleural effusion (*E*), a large pleural hematoma (*H*), and enhancing atelectatic lung (*L*).

and is demonstrated as a consolidation of the lung adjacent to the aneurysm (71,72).

Basics of Treatment

Therapeutic options for aortic disorders fall into three major categories: (a) surgical, (b) endovascular, and (c) medical/expectant. The approach is greatly influenced by the surgical risk assessment of the patient, the segment of aorta that is involved, its possible association with aortic valve disease, and whether or not branch vessel repair is required. The latter includes the coronary arteries as well as the arch vessels. A combination of procedures may be

required in one surgery. Recently, hybrid approaches using both traditional surgical methods and endovascular techniques have emerged as important treatment options.

Since the risk of rupture increases rapidly, elective aneurysm repair should be warranted when an aneurysm reaches a diameter equal to or greater than 2.5 times the diameter of adjacent normal aorta or when the aneurysm becomes more than 6 to 7 cm in diameter. Peripheral embolization originating from the aneurysm is an indication for repair, regardless of aneurysm size. Patients with evidence of rapid expansion, tenderness in the region of the aneurysm, and/or symptoms that can be related to the aneurysm should also undergo repair (49). Aneurysms in patients with connective disorders are prone to rupture at smaller sizes when compared with aneurysms of other etiologies, so a threshold of 5.5 cm was advocated and has now come down to 5 cm in some units (73).

Despite advances in surgical technique, the risk of serious complications and mortality remains substantial (5% to 20% in elective cases and up to 50% in emergency situations) (49). This risk is higher in comparison to that associated with the repair of abdominal aortic aneurysms. Knowledge of the surgical technique performed and its anatomic consequences is critical to an adequate postoperative imaging evaluation. This may permit to distinguish between normal postoperative findings and those indicative of a postoperative complication.

Surgery involving the *ascending aorta* and/or *arch* typically requires an anterior approach, whereas repair of the descending aorta is generally accomplished via a lateral thoracotomy. A comprehensive treatment of the myriad surgical techniques and nuances is beyond the scope of this book. Nonetheless, an appreciation of the common surgical procedures can facilitate communication and consultation and an effective understanding of postsurgical anatomy.

Aneurysms affecting the ascending aorta are treated with one of two general methods: an interposition graft or an inclusion graft (or CSGIT, continuous-suture graft inclusion technique).

The *interposition* graft technique consists of resection of the pathologic aortic segment and reconstruction of the vessel with graft material, usually made of Dacron (Figs. 17-23–17-25). When the sinuses of Valsalva need to be replaced, the coronary arteries must be transplanted onto the graft. Composite grafts that contain an integrated mechanical aortic valve may be used when aortic valve replacement is necessary.

When aneurysms of the ascending, transverse, and descending aorta coexist, repair of both regions in a single operation is rarely attempted, as ascending aortic repair is approached through a median sternotomy and descending aortic repair is approached through a thoracotomy or endovascularly. The prolonged anesthesia time and complex access makes a staged approach to the lesions preferred. Neurologic injury is another important cause of morbidity and a factor in many perioperative deaths associated with total aortic arch replacement. Such insults can be either global or focal in nature. Global insults typically

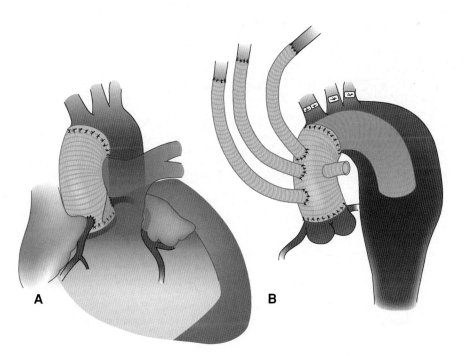

FIGURE 17-23 **Diagram illustrating examples of surgical procedures performed by using synthetic interposition grafts. A:** Root replacement with the distal anastomosis at the level of the brachiocephalic (innominate) artery. **B:** Complete root and arch replacement with the elephant trunk technique used as a staged procedure for complete replacement of the aorta. In this example, three separate graft conduits revascularize the brachiocephalic branches, and the native branches are tied off. A short segment of graft material projecting off the lateral aspect of the graft is used to vent the aorta when transitioning from circulatory arrest on the cardiopulmonary bypass pump. Because the heart and aorta are filled with air during the open procedure, the air is removed through an anterolateral vent, which is then sutured closed. Recognition of this feature is important to avoid suggesting the presence of a pseudoaneurysm on postoperative imaging, seen in Figure 17-24.

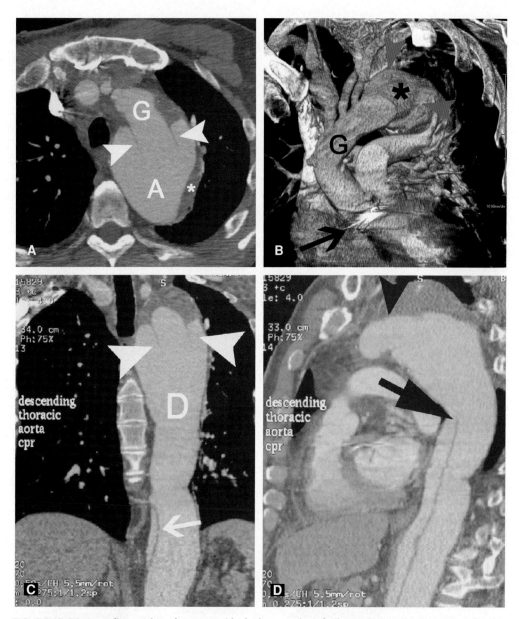

FIGURE 17-24 Ascending aortic replacement with elephant trunk graft placement into the descending thoracic aorta in a 54-year-old male with history of type A dissection. A: Axial image at the level of the surgically reconstructed arch shows the elephant trunk (*arrowheads*) "dangling" into the aneurysmal proximal descending thoracic aorta (*A*). The distal portion of the graft reconstruction is also seen (*G*). A small amount of thrombus in the residual false lumen is also seen (***). **B:** Oblique coronal volume-rendered image shows the surgical replacement of the ascending aorta and arch by graft (*G*), with reimplantation of the great vessels and placement of a prosthetic aortic valve (*arrow*). The elephant trunk can be seen (***) entering the native, aneurysmal descending thoracic aorta (*arrowheads*). **C:** CPR reconstruction viewed in coronal orientation shows the elephant trunk (*arrowheads*) ending in the descending thoracic aorta (*D*). A small dissection flap can be visualized in the distal descending thoracic aorta (*arrow*). **D:** Sagittal CPR shows the origin of the residual type B dissection in the descending thoracic aorta (*arrow*). The surgical anastamosis is noted (*arrowhead*).

reflect diffuse hypoperfusion, whereas focal insults are often embolic in nature.

A recent innovation in arch replacement consists of transecting the cerebral vessels cephalad to their origins and anastomosing them separately to a trifurcated graft (74). This technique employs antegrade selective cerebral perfusion (SCP) as an adjunct to hypothermic circulatory arrest (HCA) during arch reconstruction, an approach that reduces many of the cerebral sequelae of global cerebral injury and avoids manipulation of the often-diseased vessel ostia, which may help prevent embolic stroke.

Arch replacement can be performed as a staged procedure when in addition to an arch aneurysm there is also an aneurysm in the descending aorta, the distal extent of

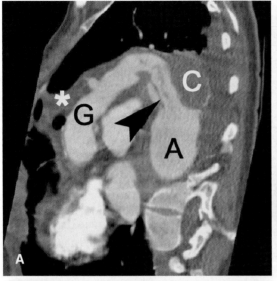

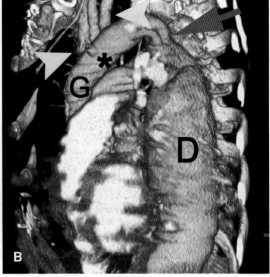

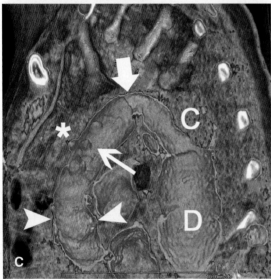

FIGURE 17-25 Elephant trunk repair with infolding of the trunk in a 38-year-old female with Marfan syndrome and previous repair of type A aortic dissection with aneurysm. A: Oblique sagittal MPR image from CTA shows a narrowed, folded appearance of the elephant trunk graft (*arrowhead*). The elephant trunk dangles into the descending thoracic aortic aneurysm (*A*). A focal outpouching in the ascending aortic graft (*G*) reflects a cannulation port (⋆) used to vent air from the aorta after discontinuation of circulatory arrest. There is clot (*C*) noted in the widely fenestrated false lumen of the residual type B dissection. **B:** Volume-rendered thick-slab sagittal image demonstrates the elephant trunk (*arrow*), reimplanted great vessels (*arrowheads*), and surgical graft replacement of ascending aorta (*G*). The cannulation port is again seen (⋆). (*D*, descending thoracic aorta.) **C:** Volume-rendered thin-slab sagittal image with opacity-transfer functions set for virtual endoluminal view shows the surgical anastomosis (*thick arrow*) and reimplanted great vessels (*thin arrow*). Felt around the ascending aorta is noted (*arrowheads*). (*D*, descending thoracic aorta; ⋆, cannulation port of graft.)

which cannot be easily reached. Thus, in anticipation of subsequent descending thoracic aortic repair, a surplus intravascular graft length is used during the first stage arch repair, a procedure known as the elephant trunk technique (Fig. 17-23, part B) (75).

The elephant trunk technique has several variants, with the common feature being the presence of a length of graft material within the descending aorta extending beyond a suture line in the distal aortic arch or proximal descending aorta. The supra-aortic branches are revascularized either with one or more graft conduits off the ascending aortic limb of the graft or by direct implantation onto the apex of the graft along with a single unifying patch of native aortic tissue. The specific approach is dictated by the patient's anatomy and access considerations. Patients with elephant trunk grafts may undergo secondary completion of the graft with open or endovascular extension of the

intradescending aortic graft segment to the distal descending aorta after recovery from the primary procedure. However, oftentimes, patients do not undergo immediate descending aortic repair in favor of regular monitoring of the descending aortic dimensions. In circumstances where the progression of the descending aortic dilation is modest, the completion of the descending aortic graft may be postponed for many years or may never occur at all. It is thus important to be familiar with the imaging features of elephant trunk grafts, as the free graft within the descending aorta can be confused for an intimal flap associated with an aortic dissection. In order to avoid this pitfall, unenhanced scans will show high-attenuation graft material whereas an intimal flap will be isoattenuative with the aortic lumen. Another key feature of the graft is that it is tubular and terminates abruptly within the middle of an aneurysmal segment of the descending aorta.

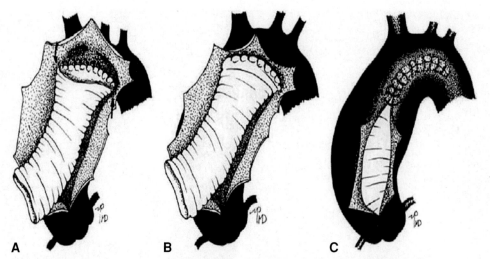

FIGURE 17-26 A–C: Diagrams illustrate the continuous suture graft-inclusion technique. After aortotomy, graft material is placed within the native aorta. The distal anastomosis is created first (**A** and **B**), followed by the proximal anastomosis. The native aortic sac is wrapped around the prosthesis (**C**), and its cut edges are sutured together. (Adapted with permission from Rofsky NM, Weinreb JC, Grossi EA, et al. Aortic aneurysm and dissection: normal MR imaging and CT findings after surgical repair with the continuous-suture graft-inclusion technique. *Radiology.* 1993;186:195–201, Figures 1a–c.)

Occasionally, high-attenuation felt rings are employed to reinforce the anastomosis of interposition grafts; these rings indicate the site of anastomosis. If such rings are not used, the site of the anastomosis may be deducted by an abrupt change in diameter of the aorta or an abrupt change in an atherosclerotic native aorta versus a disease-free graft. Felt pledgets are also sometimes employed with interposition grafts to reinforce the sites of cannula placement. These felt pledgets, like felt rings, are high in attenuation and can resemble a pseudoaneurysm. The coronary artery anastomosis is another pitfall of composite interposition grafts that may simulate pathology. Often, the coronary arteries are reimplanted into the aortic graft with a portion of native aortic root known as coronary buttons. These buttons may occasionally appear somewhat prominent and may simulate a pseudoaneurysm if the true nature of the finding is not understood (76,77).

The use of *inclusion* graft technique entails insertion of graft material within the native, diseased aorta (Fig. 17-26). First described by Bentall and De Bono, this technique or one of its modifications has become the procedure of choice in patients with annuloaortic ectasia or aortic dissection involving the aortic sinuses. It consists of direct suture of coronary arteries to the conduit and wrapping of the native aortic wall around the prosthetic conduit (Fig. 17-27). Other commonly proposed approaches are the button technique (reimplantation of coronary arteries with a small button of surrounding tissue to the conduit, without wrapping) and Cabrol technique (interposition of Dacron T tube between coronary arteries and the main conduit) (78–80) (Figs. 17-28, 17-29). This form of reconstruction

creates a potential space between the graft material and aorta. These potential spaces may thrombose or contain flowing blood. Blood flow within the perigraft space does not mandate surgery unless the situation is associated with hemodynamic instability.

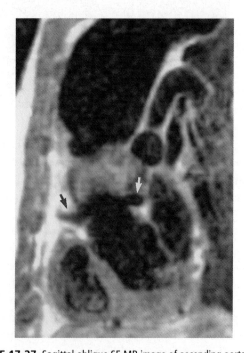

FIGURE 17-27 Sagittal oblique SE MR image of ascending aorta replaced with the Bentall technique (direct suture of coronary arteries [*arrows*] to the conduit). (Adapted with permission from Fattori R, Descovich B, Bertaccini P, et al. Composite graft replacement of the ascending aorta: leakage detection with gadolinium-enhanced MR imaging. *Radiology.* 1999;212:573–577, Figure 1.)

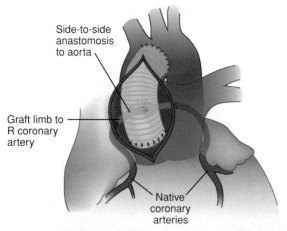

FIGURE 17-28 Diagrammatic representation of Cabrol procedure.
A small Dacron tube graft that connects the right and left coronary arteries is attached to the aortic graft by a side-to-side anastomosis. The native aortic wall surrounds both grafts. (Adapted with permission from Posniak HV, Demos TC, Olson MC. Coronary artery interposition graft simulating pseudoaneurysm of the ascending aorta on CT. *AJR Am J Roentgenol.* 1994;163:1368–1370, Figure 2.)

Serious postoperative complications include dehiscence of the surgical suture line, more commonly at the proximal site. Dehiscence may result in pseudoaneurysm formation. Pseudoaneurysm at the site of coronary artery reimplantation may result in myocardial ischemia and infarction. Aneurysm formation and dissection may also occur, particularly in patients with cystic medial necrosis. CT or MR surveillance of aortic grafts is therefore routinely recommended.

Suture line dehiscence and subsequent refilling of the aneurysm sac may be silent following CSGIT until the expanding aortic mass compresses adjacent structures, such as the superior vena cava, causing symptoms (Fig. 17-30).

Innocuous findings commonly encountered following aortic repair include left lower lobe atelectasis, pleural and pericardial effusions, and mediastinal adenopathy. These findings usually resolve over time. With interposition grafts, low-attenuation material within the mediastinum surrounding the graft is often encountered, even in late follow-up examinations. This material may represent hematoma

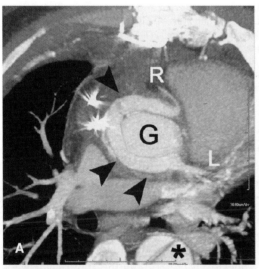

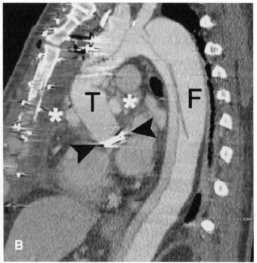

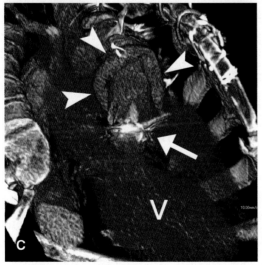

FIGURE 17-29 Repair of type A dissection utilizing composite valve-graft with Cabrol coronary reimplantation. A: Axial 5-mm MIP image at level of neoaortic root shows placement of a composite graft (*G*) with reimplantation of the coronary arteries wrapping around the graft (*arrowheads*). A single coronary graft tube then is anastomosed to the right (*R*) and left (*L*) coronary arteries. Residual type B dissection is noted in the descending thoracic aorta (*). **B:** Oblique sagittal 5-mm MIP image demonstrates the coronary graft (*) wrapped around the tube (*T*) graft portion of the composite valve graft. The prosthetic aortic valve is seen (*arrowheads*), as is residual dissection in the descending thoracic aorta with larger false lumen (*F*). **C:** Volume-rendered image viewed from below and obliquely shows the characteristic "pair of pants" appearance of the Cabrol reconstruction (*arrowheads*). The valve is also seen (*arrow*). (*V,* left ventricle.)

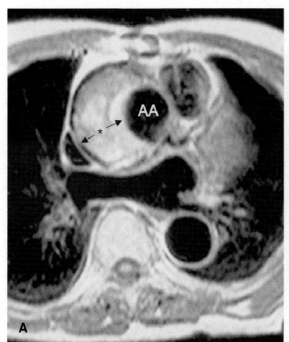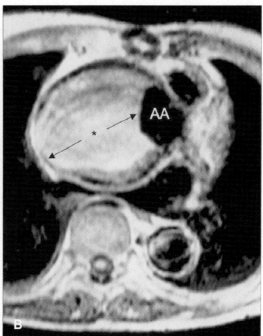

FIGURE 17-30 **81-year-old man, 3 years following correction of aortic root aneurysm by using the CSGIT, presenting with progressive swelling and redness of face, neck, and arms. A:** Axial ECG-triggered T1-weighted image at the level of the left atrium demonstrates perigraft thrombus (∗) surrounding the ascending aorta *(AA)*. Although there is mild displacement of the superior vena cava, the flow void suggests patency. One year later **(B)**, there is marked increase in the overall diameter of the ascending aorta with mass effect on the right atrium and distal superior vena cava, consistent with the symptomatology. (Reprinted with permission from Haddad JL, Rofsky NM, Weinreb JC, et al. SVC syndrome as a late complication of ascending aortic aneurysm repair: MR diagnosis. *J Comput Assist Tomogr.* 1993;17:982–985, Figures 1a, 2a.)

organizing into fibrous tissue, and it may never completely resolve in some patients.

Complications of these techniques of replacement of the ascending aorta include perivalvular leakage and false aneurysm formation as well as leakage or chronic partial dehiscence due to tension at the anastomosis of the coronary arteries. Postoperative assessment has been performed with angiography, echocardiography, and CT, but MRI has been shown to be the most effective procedure, providing MPR evaluation of the entire aorta and its surrounding structures (81).

Aneurysms of the *descending aorta* benefit from endovascular stent-graft placement as a less invasive alternative. The treatment of aortic arch aneurysm is more complex, and surgical replacement and endovascular procedure can be combined (49).

Endovascular grafts have the distinct advantage of being a less invasive technique as compared with conventional arterial reconstructions, owing to the unique ability to insert these grafts through a small incision from remote arterial access sites. This minimally invasive approach results in several advantages to the patient as compared with

conventional aortic repair. Avoiding thoracotomy eliminates the need for extensive perioperative aortic dissection. This technique obviates the need for extensive and prolonged aortic occlusion, decreases blood loss, and avoids the significant fluid shifts that occur with manipulation, thus lowering the risk of significant hemodynamic changes perioperatively (82,83). But this approach depends on morphologic criteria for patient selection, and only aneurysms with suitable necks and adequate vascular access can be treated with this technique. The dimensions of the stent graft used are determined on the basis of preoperative imaging evaluation, and aortic diameter and length of the aneurysm are considered (49).

ACUTE AORTIC SYNDROMES

Definition and Epidemiology

Patients presenting with chest and/or back pain in the setting of hypertension prompt the consideration of three conditions of the aorta: penetrating atherosclerotic aortic ulcer, intramural aortic hematoma, and the classic aortic dissection. The pathophysiological mechanism that precipitates each of these entities is different. Occasionally, however, some patients exhibit several or all of these lesions, demonstrating a link among them. In such cases, it is difficult to know which one is the initiating event. Given the overlap in clinical presentation, it has been recommended that the term *acute aortic syndrome* (AAS) be used to embrace this heterogeneous group (84).

Aortic dissection is a disruption of the tunica media of the aorta. Flowing blood enters this space, or false channel, via one or more disruptions of the intima (85) (Fig. 17-31). The proximal tear in the intima has been termed the *entry* tear, and more distal tears are designated as *exit* or *re-entry* tears. Most notably in patients with connective tissue diseases, *redissection* may occur, and multiple false lumina can be found (Fig. 17-32). The media can also be dissected by thrombosed blood without evidence of disruption of the intima. This abnormal condition has been termed an *intramural hematoma*. The false channel is most easily seen when it contains flowing blood, because its motion within the lumen produces a high contrast between the blood and surrounding stationary tissue on SE images (86). However, extremely slow or sluggish flow and complete thrombosis

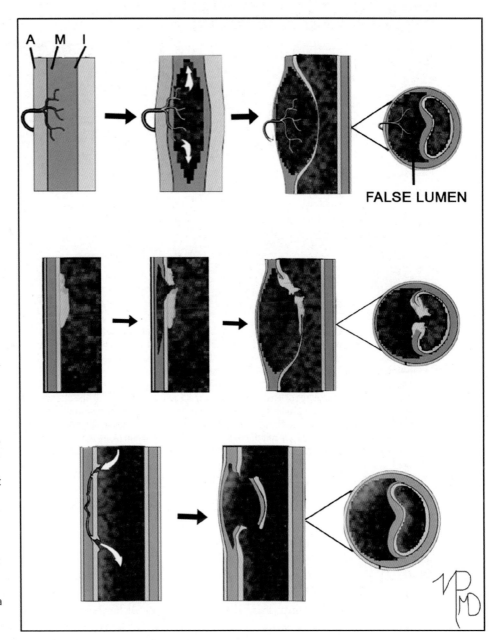

FIGURE 17-31 Mechanism underlying development of intramural hemotoma and dissection. In the first example, spontaneous rupture of aortic vasa vasorum is responsible for hematoma formation within the aortic wall. In this case, IMH is not secondary to intimal disruption. Illustrated below, the other type of IMH is related to an atherosclerotic ulcer that penetrates into the internal elastic lamina and allows hematoma formation within the media of the aortic wall. Lastly, the third diagram illustrates the origin of dissection, where there is disruption of the tunica media of the vessel. Blood flows into this space, creating a false lumen.

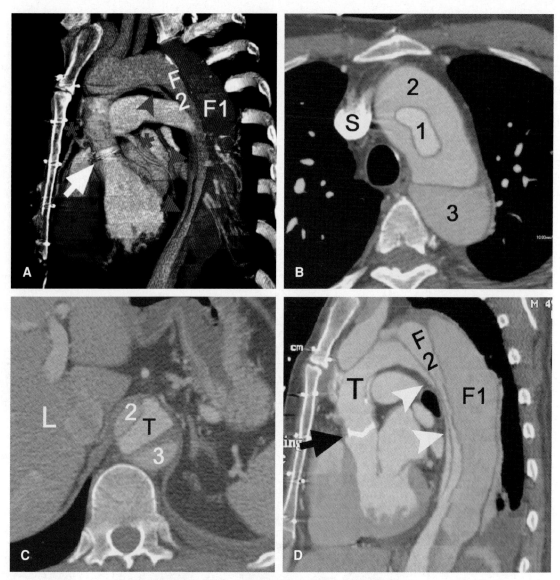

FIGURE 17-32 Complex residual type B dissection with multiple false lumina due to redissection, status post repair of type A dissection with composite valve graft in a 49-year-old male with Marfan syndrome.
A: Oblique sagittal volume-rendered image demonstrates prior composite valve-graft repair of the ascending aorta. The prosthetic valve is noted (*arrow*), as are patent reimplanted coronary arteries (*∗*). There is a type B dissection, with appearance suggesting three different lumens—a compressed true lumen (*arrowheads*) and two false channels (F1, F2). **B:** Axial image at aortic arch demonstrates three different densities within different sections (1, 2, 3). The true lumen is labeled number 1. (*S,* superior vena cava.) **C:** Axial image at level of upper abdominal aorta demonstrates the true lumen (*T*), again surrounded by two false lumina (2, 3) with differing contrast densities. A small amount of thrombus is seen in one of the channels (3). (*L,* liver.) **D:** Oblique sagittal curved planar reconstruction along the true lumen shows severe compression of the descending aortic true lumen (*arrowheads*) by the false channels (F1, F2). A portion of the prosthetic valve is noted (*arrow*).

will exhibit an increased intraluminal signal (87) and should be considered during interpretation.

Intramural aortic hematoma and *penetrating atherosclerotic ulcer* lack a mobile intimomedial flap and a double aortic lumen (88) (Fig. 17-33). Two different pathophysiological processes can lead to IMH formation. One is IMH without intimal disruption; in this entity, it is believed that spontaneous rupture of aortic vasa vasorum is responsible for hematoma formation within the aortic wall (89). The other type of IMH is associated and sometimes hidden within an atherosclerotic ulcer that penetrates into the internal elastic lamina and allows hematoma formation within the media of the aortic wall (15,90,91) (Figs. 17-34, 17-35).

It has been shown that IMH with penetrating atherosclerotic ulceration (PAU) is associated significantly with a

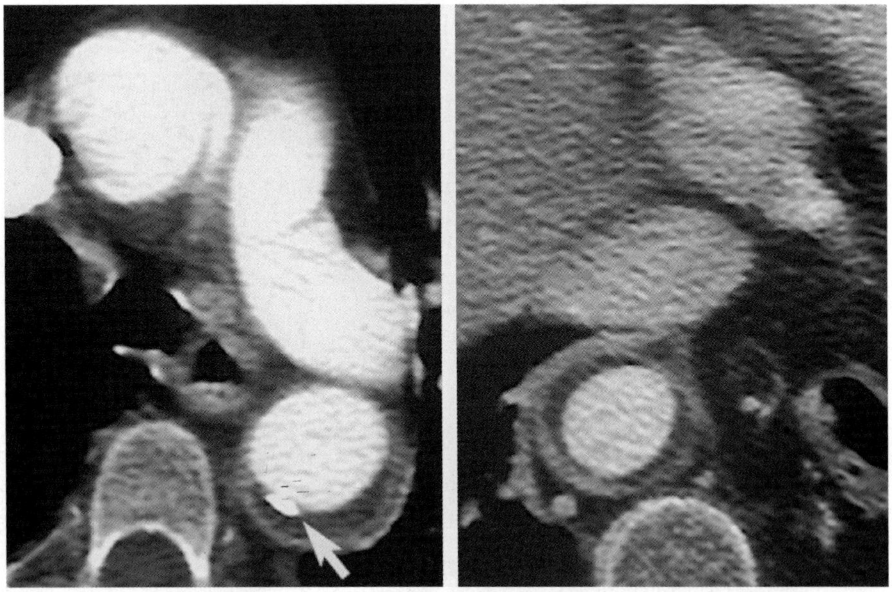

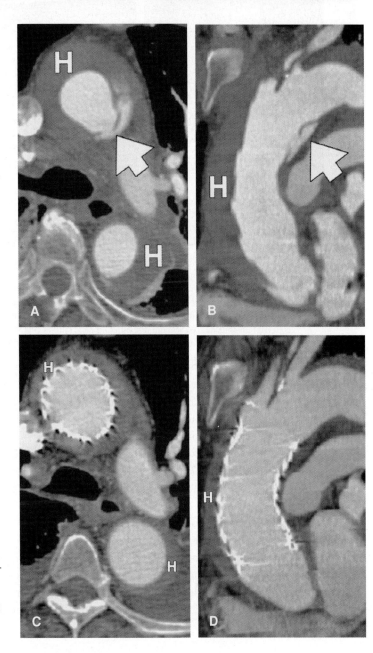

FIGURE 17-33 Transverse CTA sections demonstrate a descending thoracic aortic IMH associated with marked aortic wall enhancement and thickening. The subintimal location of the hematoma is confirmed by the presence of intimal calcium on its internal surface (*arrow*). Ulceration was not identified.

FIGURE 17-34 Ascending aortic penetrating ulcer with IMH. Transverse (**A**) and sagittal (**B**) CTA sections illustrate a penetrating ulcer (*arrows*) in the ascending aorta. There is a large IMH (*H*) surrounding the ulcer in the ascending aorta and extending into the descending aorta. One day following placement of a stent graft over the ulcer, the ulcer no longer fills and the IMH (*H*) has diminished (**C**). Two weeks later, it resolved completely (**D**).

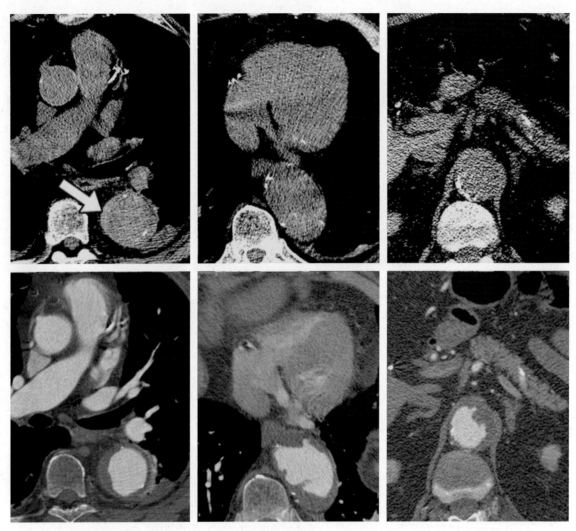

FIGURE 17-35 Acute chest pain in a patient with descending aortic ectasia. The top row of transverse CT images are unenhanced and photographed with narrow "thrombus" windows (w = 100 HU). A smoothly marginated crescent of high attenuation is present in the medial aspect of the descending aortic wall on the first image, corresponding to an acute IMH (*arrow*). The second row contains the corresponding sections following intravenous contrast enhancement. There is extensive mural atheroma and thrombus at all levels, presenting an irregular contour with the lumen. When correlated with the unenhanced sections, the atheroma and chronic mural thrombus is isoattenuative with the unenhanced lumen in distinction to the acute IMH. The IMH is very difficult to distinguish on the contrast-enhanced sections.

progressive disease course, whereas IMH without PAU typically has a stable course, especially when limited to the descending thoracic aorta (92). Sustained or recurrent pain, increasing pleural effusion, and both the maximum diameter and maximum depth of the PAU are reliable predictors of disease progression (92). Data suggest that cases of PAU confined to the descending thoracic aorta may be managed expectantly (93,94).

AAS is characterized clinically by a severely intense, acute, searing or tearing, throbbing, and migratory chest pain. Anterior chest, neck, throat, and even jaw pain suggest involvement of the ascending aorta, whereas back and abdominal pain more often indicate that the descending aorta is involved (95).

Moderate to severe hypertension is a universal risk factor for the development of AAS. Inheritable disorders of elastic tissues also predispose to the development of classic aortic dissection, but hypertension is the most frequently associated condition. Hypertension is also the most common comorbid disease associated with penetrating aortic ulcers and intramural aortic hematomas (50).

Classification and Pathogenesis

The clinical progress of these patients is unpredictable and, in many cases, unfavorable. Therefore, an early diagnosis is essential. Patients presenting with suspected AAS should be evaluated by using noninvasive diagnostic modalities, and echocardiography is often performed initially (96).

Classic *aortic dissection* is characterized by the presence of an intimal flap, a double lumen, an entry tear, and one or more reentry sites. It is thought to begin with a laceration of the aortic intima and inner layer of the aortic media that allows entering blood to split the aortic media. The most common location of an intimal tear is a few centimeters above the aortic valve at the right anterolateral aspect, likely related to the substantial hydrodynamic and stress forces (97). The next most frequent entry site is in the descending aorta, just beyond the ligamentum arteriosum, the latter an anchor point just beyond the relatively mobile arch. Although an intimal tear is the characteristic feature of aortic dissection, intimal atherosclerotic disease is not universally present. Rather, disease of the media with degeneration of the elastic fibers and smooth muscles is the rule (98–102).

In most instances, aortic dissection is related to degeneration of an aging aorta and may be accelerated by hypertension. In younger patients, there is often an underlying process such as bicuspid or unicuspid aortic valve, coarctation, pregnancy, connective tissue disorders such as Marfan syndrome, relapsing polychondritis, thoracic cage deformities, and rarely, systemic lupus erythematosus or giant cell arteritis. Dissection may also occur at sites of iatrogenic trauma such as at the location of a prior aortic incision, cross clamping, or traumatic catheterization (103,104). The two most common sites for the initiation of aortic dissection are the proximal ascending aorta and the descending aorta just distal to the left subclavian artery. These sites reflect areas of maximal mechanical strain on the aorta caused by flexion. The dissection channel generally is seen spiraling, as the false lumen in the ascending aorta is usually anterior and to the right, and then in the arch, the false lumen takes a superior and slightly posterior direction and continues posterior and to the left in the descending aorta. The false channel may compress the true lumen. Branch arteries may be perfused by the false lumen, the true lumen, or both.

The breach and splitting of the media forms the double-channel aorta, with an aortic dissection flap dividing the aortic lumen into true and false lumens (Fig. 17-36). The "intimal flap" is really an intimomedial flap, formed by the intima and the inner part of the aortic wall, and is mainly composed of delaminated aortic media (84). This forms the inner boundary between the true and false lumens. The outer portion of the aortic media and adventitia form the outer wall of the false channel. Typically, the true lumen is relatively small with high-velocity flow, whereas the false lumen is larger with slower velocity and turbulent blood flow (Fig. 17-37).

Exit tears typically occur at the site of aortic branches. A circumferential tear at the ostium of the branch results in a local communication and source of pressure equalization between the true and false aortic lumina (Fig. 17-38).

The dissecting column of blood propagates most often in an anterograde direction under the influence of systolic forces, although retrograde extension can and does occur with the possibility of a retrograde conversion of type B into type A dissection (Fig. 17-39).

Alternatively, the dissecting column of blood can rupture through the adventitia, which, depending on its location, can result in any one of several well-recognized clinical complications: hemopericardium with cardiac tamponade

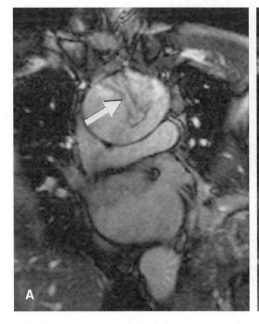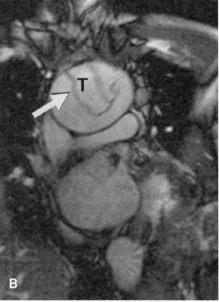

FIGURE 17-36 Changes in morphology of the complex intimal flap (*arrows*) during different phases of the cardiac cycle. These images obtained from a cine MRI sequence demonstrate the reduced size of the true lumen (*T*) during diastole (**A**), in comparison to systole (**B**).

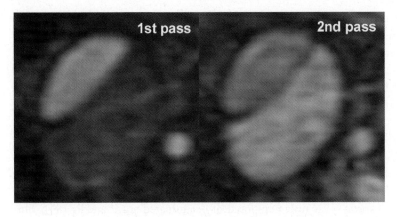

FIGURE 17-37 Images at the level of the descending aorta during first and second postcontrast dynamic MRI phases show distinct signal of the true and false lumina. During the earlier phase, true lumen appears with higher signal. Afterward, the contrast media in this rapid flowing portion is washed out resulting in the reverse appearance (false lumen becomes brighter).

(type A involvement) or hemothorax with circulatory collapse (type A or B involvement). Distortion or disruption of the aortic valve may lead to varying degrees of aortic regurgitation. It has a mortality rate of 1% per hour during the first 24 hours after onset and a mortality rate of 75% at 2 weeks in untreated cases (87,97,105,106).

In a review of the Stanford experience in 725 symptomatic patients with a working diagnosis of aortic dissection between January 1990 and June 2000, 663 (91%) had a classic "double-barreled" dissection and 66 (9%) had an aortic IMH (93).

The Stanford and older DeBakey classification schemes are commonly ascribed to aortic dissection. The Stanford

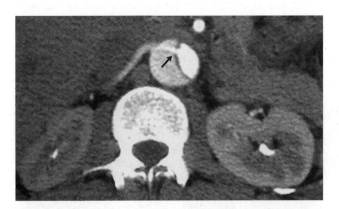

FIGURE 17-38 Aortic dissection exit tear and intimal flap fenestration. Transverse CTA section illustrates an exit tear at the origin of a right accessory renal artery. A fenestration (*arrow*) in the intimal flap corresponds to the site of the accessory renal artery ostium. This exit tear and resulting fenestration enables communication between the true and false lumina, equalizing the pressure across the flap and protecting against true luminal collapse. Higher attenuation contrast medium is present in the true lumen and is flowing across the fenestration into the false lumen. Note the differential renal parenchymal enhancement. The greater enhancement in the left kidney is a reflection of greater iodine delivery from faster blood flow within the true lumen when compared with the right kidney, which is supplied by the false lumen. It is important not to confuse this phenomenon of differential opacification in the renal parenchyma due to differential iodine delivery rates in the true and false lumina from differential opacification due to renal ischemia.

classification divides dissections into two types, type A and type B (107). Type A includes all cases in which the ascending aorta is involved by the dissection, with or without involvement of the arch or the descending aorta. Type B includes cases in which the ascending thoracic aorta is not involved and thus begins distal to the brachiocephalic artery origin. This system also helps to delineate treatment. Type A dissections are almost always considered to require surgery, while type B dissections may be managed medically under most circumstances.

The DeBakey classification includes three types (108,109). In type I, the intimal tear usually originates in the ascending aorta, and the dissection involves the ascending aorta, the arch, and variable lengths of the descending and abdominal aorta. In type II, the dissection is confined to the ascending aorta. Type III dissection is confined to the descending aorta distal to the left subclavian artery. In type III, the dissection may be limited to the descending thoracic aorta (type IIIA) or extend into the abdominal aorta and iliac arteries (type IIIB). A widespread misconception is that Stanford type B and DeBakey type III are the same. It should be evident from the above that they are not, as dissection of the aortic arch is included in the Stanford type B but not as a DeBakey type III.

In addition to describing the extent of the dissection, localization of the primary intimal tear can have an important bearing on the management of the patient (110), particularly when considering stent-graft repair to occlude the entry tear.

IMH of the aorta results either from spontaneous rupture of the vasa vasorum of the aortic wall or from a *penetrating atherosclerotic ulcer*. In a prospective study by Evangelista and associates (111), the most frequent long-term evolution of IMH is to aortic aneurysm or pseudoaneurysm (54% of cases). Complete regression without changes in aorta size was observed in 34% of cases, and progression to classical dissection was less common, seen in 12% of cases. A normal aortic diameter in the acute phase was the best

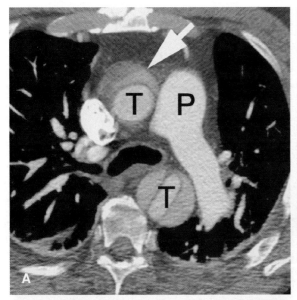

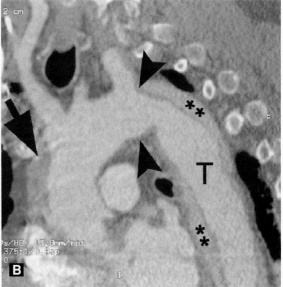

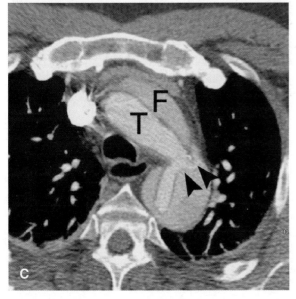

FIGURE 17-39 Retrograde conversion of type B dissection into type A dissection. A: Axial image from CTA shows a Stanford type A dissection. The true lumen (*T*) is moderately effaced by the false lumen in both the ascending and descending aorta. The false lumen in the ascending aorta shows low-density thrombus or slow flow (*arrow*). P, pulmonary trunk. **B:** Sagittal CPR image from CTA shows flap extending distal to the left subclavian artery (*arrowheads*) into the descending thoracic aorta. The true (*T*) and false (**) lumina can be seen. The great vessels arise from the true lumen. **C:** Axial image at the level of the ligamentum arteriosum shows the site of the intimal tear (*arrowheads*). The true (*T*) and false (*F*) lumina are noted. The tear site at this location is consistent with retrograde extension of a type B dissection to form a type A dissection. The patient was treated with replacement of the ascending aorta with elephant trunk, subsequent stent grafting of the elephant trunk and descending aorta, and a jump graft to the left subclavian artery.

predictor of IMH regression without complications, and in the experience of these investigators, it was an echocardiographic finding—the absence of echolucent areas and atherosclerotic ulcerated plaque—that was highly associated with evolution to aortic aneurysm. A life-threatening complication of IMH is aortic rupture (Fig. 17-40).

Clinical Presentation and Natural History

Suzuki and colleagues (112) found that an assay of smooth-muscle myosin heavy-chain protein had a high sensitivity (90.9%) and acceptable specificity (98% compared with healthy controls, 83% compared with patients who had acute myocardial infarction) in patients with aortic dissection who presented within the first 3 hours after symptom onset. The assay performed best in patients with proximal lesions and

was less sensitive in patients who presented at a later point in the disease and had decreased levels of smooth-muscle myosin heavy-chain protein. Important issues surround the practicality of this assay in clinical settings. At present, it appears that this biochemical test would be most useful at the initial decision-making stage (triaging) in the emergency department or clinic. When examining patients presenting with acute chest pain, physicians can use the assay to help determine whether aortic dissection is a possibility. The assay may be most effective in its negative predictive role, given the low prevalence of aortic dissection in patients with chest pain (1% to 2%). It is important to note that the assay is best at detecting proximal lesions, which are more often associated with an unfavorable outcome and are therefore more likely to have devastating consequences if overlooked.

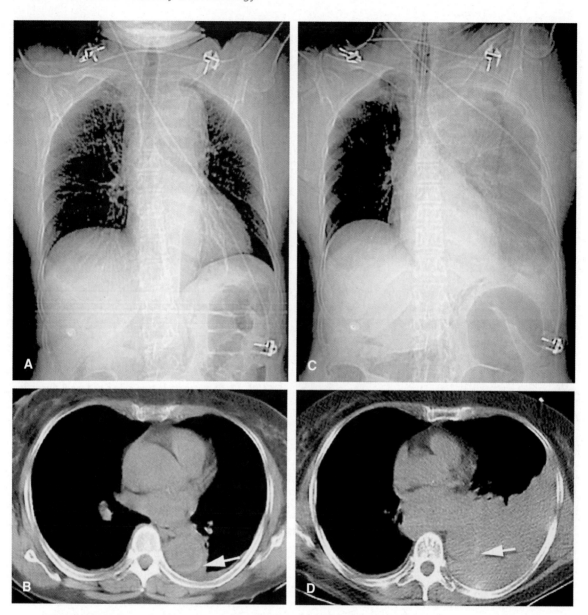

FIGURE 17-40 A: Frontal projectional radiograph of the chest demonstrates a widened aortic arch in a patient with acute chest pain. **B:** Unenhanced transverse CT section obtained in anticipation of performing a CT angiogram demonstrates a high-attenuation crescent within the posterior wall of the descending aorta (*arrow*). A small left pleural effusion is present. This high-attenuation crescent is pathognomonic for an IMH. Prior to performing the ensuing CT angiogram, the patient became acutely hemodynamically unstable on the CT table, necessitating cardiopulmonary resuscitation. **C:** Forty-five minutes after the initial acquisition (**A, B**), the patient was stabilized hemodynamically. A repeat frontal projectional radiograph demonstrates that the left hemothorax is now filled with fluid. **D:** Transverse CT section at this time demonstrates a large left pleural effusion, which was subsequently demonstrated to represent blood due to acute rupture of the aorta at the site of the IMH. The high-attenuation crescent within the aorta wall, which is now displaced anteriorly compared with the earlier cross section, is still visible (*arrow*). (Reprinted with permission from Rubin GD. CT angiography of the thoracic aorta. *Semin Roentgenol.* 2003;38:115–134.)

For patients with type A aortic dissection who do not receive immediate treatment, mortality is estimated to be approximately 25% during the first 24 hours after the initial presentation, 70% during the first week, and 80% at 2 weeks (113). Therefore, rapid diagnosis and timely management play an essential role in patient survival (Fig. 17-41). The most life-threatening complications are mediastinal hematoma, hemopericardium, and acute aortic valve insufficiency. Ischemic signs and symptoms may appear when a flap extends into the ostia of branch vessels, when there is intermittent or persistent coverage of an ostium by the intimal flap, or when increased pressure in the false lumen leads to narrowing or collapse of the true lumen (Fig. 17-42).

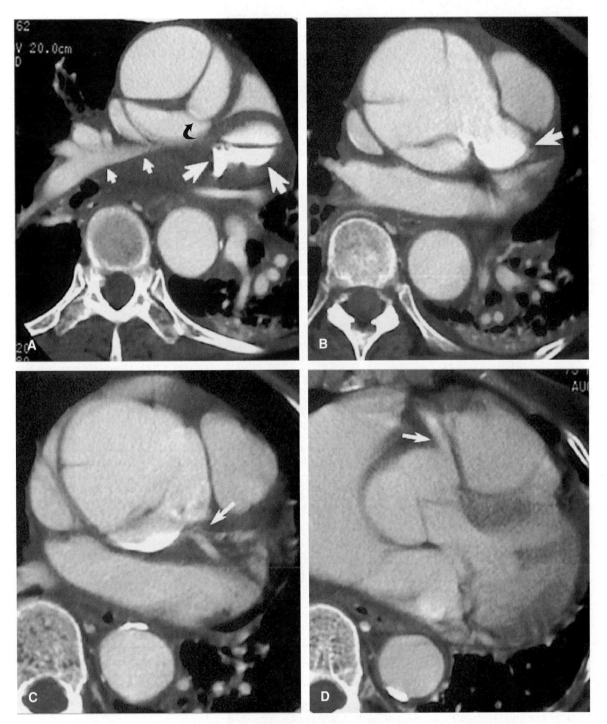

FIGURE 17-41 A, B: Transverse CT sections in a patient with acute chest pain demonstrates a type A aortic dissection with posteromedial rupture of the proximal ascending aorta and active extravasation of arterial contrast medium into the mediastinum through a pseudoaneurysm (*larger arrows*). A mediastinal hematoma is resulting in substantial right pulmonary arterial compression (*small arrows*). An aortic cobweb (*curved arrow*) tethers the intimal flap and gives the appearance of a tripartite aorta. **C:** The origin of the left main coronary artery could be visualized one section below this image, which demonstrates the proximal left and circumflex coronary arteries (*arrow*) originated immediately below the pseudoaneurysm from the left sinus of Valsalva. **D:** The right coronary artery origin (*arrow*) is clearly uninvolved, as is the aortic valve. (Reprinted with permission from Rubin GD. CT angiography of the thoracic aorta. *Semin Roentgenol.* 2003;38:115–134.)

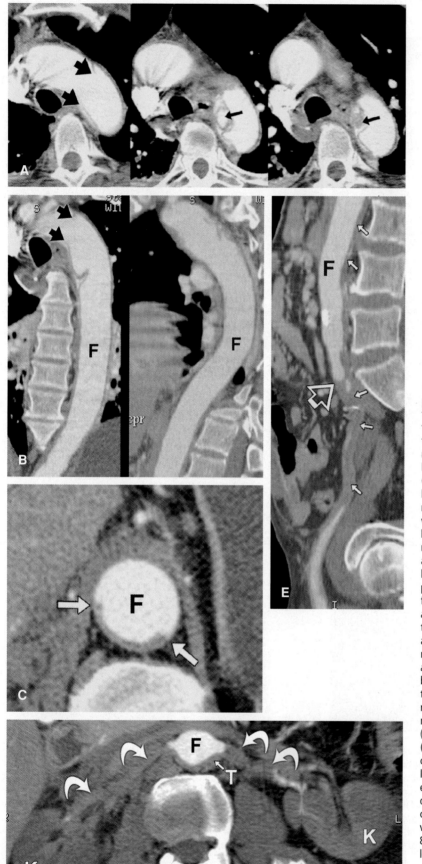

FIGURE 17-42 37-year-old man with acute chest pain, cold left leg, and anuria. A: Transverse CT sections through the aortic arch demonstrate a type B aortic dissection with a large entry tear (space between the *wide arrows*). The intimal flap is highly redundant, resulting in a large portion prolapsing into the true lumen and producing an intimo-intimal intussusception (*small arrows*) and obstructing flow into the true lumen. **B:** Coronal and sagittal MPRs illustrate the normal caliber of the descending thoracic aorta, free of a visible intimal flap distal to the entry tear (space between the *black arrows*). This apparent normality is misleading, as the true lumen is completely collapsed and only the false lumen is visible (*F*). **C:** At the aortic hiatus of the diaphragm, the true lumen remains completely collapsed. The two opposing layers of intima form a region of wall thickening between the *white arrows*. Only the false lumen (*F*) has flowing blood and thus enhances. **D:** There are no exit tears at the renal arteries to allow false luminal blood (*F*) to reach the renal arteries. Therefore, the renal arteries (*curved arrows*) and the renal parenchyma (*K*) do not enhance, because no blood or contrast material is reaching them through the collapsed true lumen (*T*). **E:** Curved sagittal reformation through the abdominal aorta and left common and external iliac arteries shows the false lumen (*F*) terminating in the proximal common iliac artery (*open arrow*). The true lumen (*small arrows*), which is collapsed posteriorly, cannot deliver blood to the left leg, and therefore the distal common and proximal external iliac arteries are not enhanced. Opacification of the distal external iliac artery is due to filling from collaterals supplied by the left internal mammary artery via the left inferior epigastric artery. The patient died 8 hours after presentation with high serum myoglobin levels and multiorgan system failure despite aggressive attempts to revascularize the kidneys and fenestrate the dissection to create true luminal flow. The preferred therapy of placing a stent graft over the large entry tear was not available.

An important uncommon consequence of type B dissection is the *malperfusion syndrome*, which occurs when the true lumen collapses, preventing blood flow into abdominal aortic branches that originate from the true lumen. The specific pathophysiologic mechanism of this is that a large entry tear combined with a paucity of exit tears creates a diastolic pressure gradient across the intimal flap, because the false lumen will have a higher pressure than the true lumen after the aortic valve has closed due to the absence of pressure-relieving exit tears from the false lumen. The higher false luminal pressure causes the false lumen to expand, collapsing the true lumen and occluding blood flow (Fig. 17-43 and 17-44). Malperfusion syndrome has a high mortality, as it is often accompanied by intestinal ischemia, renal ischemia, and lower extremity ischemia. Within the ascending aorta, true luminal collapse can occur under similar circumstances; however, the collapse typically persists through diastole only with the true lumen opening in systole to allow perfusion of the brachiocephalic branches.

In type B aortic dissection, the affected aortas have shown a high incidence of enlargement during the follow-up period. This was greatest for those cases with flowing blood in the false channel, and in one study, the mean growth rate of aortic dissections in thoracic aorta was 4.1 mm/year (114).

Imaging Findings

The diagnostic strategy for aortic dissection often involves chest radiography, echocardiography (preferably transesophageal), and an imaging procedure such as computed tomography (preferably helical), MRI, or angiography.

Aortography was considered the reference standard for diagnosis of aortic dissection but has been supplanted by CT and MRI. The sensitivity of aortography has been found to be 88% and the specificity 94%, with positive and negative predictive values of 96% and 84%, respectively. The diagnostic accuracy of angiography approaches 98% in some series. Angiography allows evaluation of the aortic valve and aortic branch vessel involvement. The high frame rates of arterial digital subtraction angiography facilitate identification of the intimal tear and the degree of aortic insufficiency. Cineangiography has been used, but the field of view is usually limited. False-negative arteriograms may occur when the false lumen is not opacified, when there is simultaneous opacification of the true and false lumen, and when the intimal flap is not seen. Disadvantages of angiography are that it is invasive, iodinated contrast material is required, and there is typically a delay in implementing the procedure. Nonetheless, of all the imaging techniques used

in the diagnosis of aortic dissection, conventional angiography provides an excellent means of characterizing complex patterns of aortic branch supply, particularly when guided by a CT or MR angiogram, and is a key element in directing endoluminal therapy.

CTA is less invasive, faster, safer, cheaper, and less resource intensive than conventional aortography. CTA affords high-quality thin sections that demonstrate mural changes, detailed assessment of aortic branch involvement (Chapters 10, 19, and 20), the perfusion status of adjacent organs, extraluminal complications including hemorrhage, and demonstration of extrinsic causes of vascular compromise. The use of cardiac-gated MDCT allows a detailed assessment of the aortic root and coronary arterial involvement (Fig. 17-43). CT allows exclusion of other causes of mediastinal widening, detection of intraluminal and periaortic thrombus (Fig. 17-45), and diagnosis of pericardial and pleural effusions, and allows diagnosis of other causes of chest pain, such as pulmonary embolism and acute coronary syndrome when the MDCT scan is ECG-gated. Factors reducing the diagnostic accuracy of CTA are poor opacification of the aorta due to inadequate contrast injection or improper bolus timing and misinterpretation of streak artifacts or motion artifacts as an intimal flap (Fig. 17-1). When the false lumen is not opacified, differentiation from an IMH may be difficult. These limitations are almost always eliminated with proper CTA technique using thin-section acquisition and timing of the scan to the contrast injection. One notable limitation of CT is the inability to directly detect aortic insufficiency; however, as seen previously in this chapter, CT offers the greatest morphological detail of the aortic root among currently available imaging techniques. There are no studies rigorously comparing MDCT with other imaging modalities, so specific diagnostic performance data are unavailable. Published literature reporting sensitivities of 90% to 100% and specificity of 87% are attributable to prehelical conventional CT, which is now 15 years out of date. However, the superior volumetric spatial resolution, intersubject consistency, ready availability to the emergency patient, and exquisite detail of complex moving structures afforded by ECG-gating have made MDCT the diagnostic test of choice for aortic dissection in many institutions.

MRI provides for noninvasive visualization of the thoracic and abdominal aorta in multiple projections without the use of contrast agents or ionizing radiation. A variety of pulse sequences are available, as previously discussed and illustrated. ECG-triggered SE images provide anatomic detail of the heart and aorta. Cine MRI and other GRE techniques allow visualization of flowing

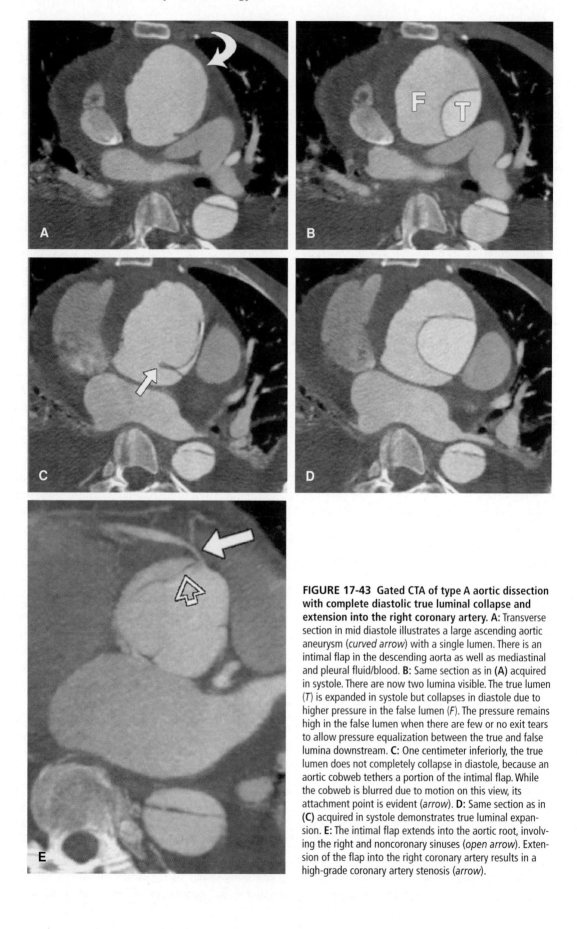

FIGURE 17-43 Gated CTA of type A aortic dissection with complete diastolic true luminal collapse and extension into the right coronary artery. A: Transverse section in mid diastole illustrates a large ascending aortic aneurysm (*curved arrow*) with a single lumen. There is an intimal flap in the descending aorta as well as mediastinal and pleural fluid/blood. **B:** Same section as in **(A)** acquired in systole. There are now two lumina visible. The true lumen (*T*) is expanded in systole but collapses in diastole due to higher pressure in the false lumen (*F*). The pressure remains high in the false lumen when there are few or no exit tears to allow pressure equalization between the true and false lumina downstream. **C:** One centimeter inferiorly, the true lumen does not completely collapse in diastole, because an aortic cobweb tethers a portion of the intimal flap. While the cobweb is blurred due to motion on this view, its attachment point is evident (*arrow*). **D:** Same section as in **(C)** acquired in systole demonstrates true luminal expansion. **E:** The intimal flap extends into the aortic root, involving the right and noncoronary sinuses (*open arrow*). Extension of the flap into the right coronary artery results in a high-grade coronary artery stenosis (*arrow*).

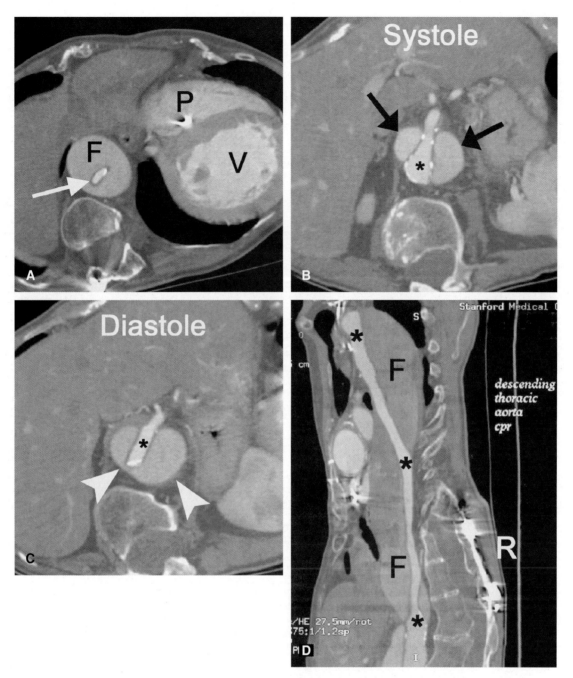

FIGURE 17-44 The "floating true lumen" and imaging of dynamic lumen compression in a 51-year-old male with type B aortic dissection, evaluated by ECG-gated CTA of the chest and abdomen for clinical question of true lumen compromise. A: Axial image through the lower chest demonstrates dissection of the distal descending thoracic aorta with marked compression of the true lumen (*arrow*). The true lumen is surrounded circumferentially by the false lumen (*F*), giving the appearance that the true lumen is freely floating in the false lumen. (*V*, left ventricle; *P*, pacer lead traversing right ventricle.) **B, C:** Axial images at the level of the celiac axis origin in systole (**B**) and diastole (**C**). The celiac axis arises from the true lumen (*). Note the increased compression in diastole (*arrowheads* in **C**), when true lumen pressure decreases and pressure in the false lumen (*arrows* in **B**) remains high. This finding indicates the presence of a mobile flap and dynamic luminal compression. **D:** CPR of the descending thoracic and abdominal aorta demonstrates long-segment compression of the true lumen (*) by the dilated false lumen (*F*). Differential opacity of the false lumen allows identification of the site of communication between the true and false lumen in the abdomen. The opacity gradient in the thoracic aortic false lumen from inferior to superior indicates slow retrograde flow. Dural ectasia is noted. (*R*, spine fixation rod.)

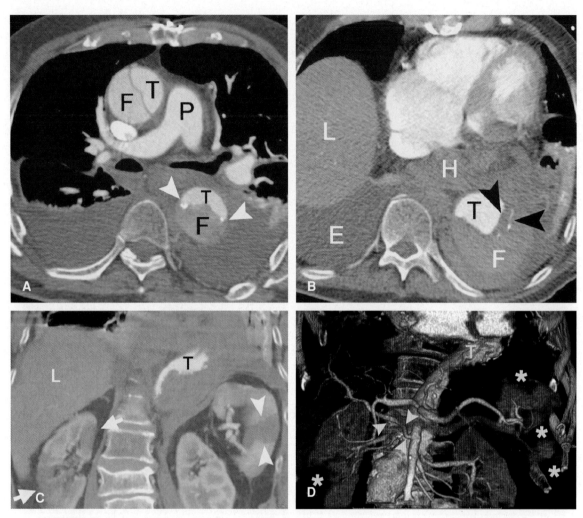

FIGURE 17-45 Thrombus in true and false lumina of type A dissection. A: Axial image at the level of the pulmonary trunk *(P)* shows a Stanford type A dissection with differential opacification of the true *(T)* and false *(F)* lumina. Lower opacity in the false lumen of the descending aorta represents thrombus. Displaced intimal calcium is present *(arrowheads)*. **B:** Axial image at a level inferior to **(A)** demonstrates thrombus in the true lumen *(T)*, anterior to displaced intimal calcium *(arrowheads)*. The false lumen *(F)* also shows thrombus. There is a mediastinal hematoma *(H)* from retrograde extension. *(L,* liver; *E,* pleural effusion.) **C:** Coronal image through the upper abdomen demonstrates evidence of splenic *(arrowheads)* and renal *(arrows)* infarctions secondary to embolic phenomena from thrombus in the true lumen *(T)*. *(L,* liver.) **D:** Coronal volume-rendered image shows that the major mesenteric and renal arteries arise from the true lumen *(T)*. There is a replaced right hepatic artery arising from the superior mesenteric artery *(arrowheads)*. Multiple infarcts are again noted (*).

blood, facilitating the differentiation of slow-flowing blood and clot, and determination of the presence of aortic insufficiency. The sensitivity and specificity of MRI for the diagnosis of aortic dissection has recently been reported to be 100%. For identifying the site of entry, sensitivity was 85% and specificity 100%; for identifying thrombus and the presence of a pericardial effusion, sensitivity and specificity were both 100% (115). Gadolinium-enhanced 3D MRA techniques permit rapid acquisition of MR angiograms of the thoracic and abdominal aorta and their branch vessels. 3D MRA permits identification of both the true and false lumen, enables identification of the type of dissection, and assessment of patency of the false lumen (Fig. 17-46). Although MR has the potential to provide information about the coronary arteries, currently it cannot rapidly and routinely do so. Limitations of MRI/MRA include longer examination times compared with CT and less access to the patient. Further, patients with cardiac pacemakers, ferromagnetic aneurysm clips, and ocular or otologic implants cannot undergo MRI. Studies may be suboptimal in patients with cardiac arrhythmias and limited in unstable patients, and motion artifact in uncooperative patients can result in nondiagnostic images. Currently, MRI is more expensive than

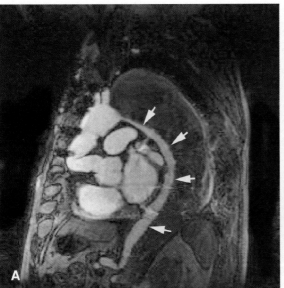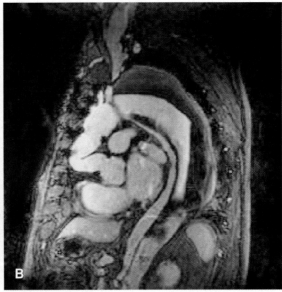

FIGURE 17-46 Complex aortic dissection. Complex residual dissection following repair of type A dissection. **A:** An oblique sagittal section from the first-pass gadolinium-enhanced MRA study shows a kinked portion of the ascending aortic graft and enhancement in the compressed true lumen (*arrows*). **B:** Same orientation during the second pass after gadolinium administration shows the nonuniform filling of the false lumen with thrombus posteriorly. The intimal flap separates the true and false lumina.

other imaging techniques and may not be routinely available in emergencies. However, MRI is extremely well suited for the study of patients with stable or chronic dissection, and there is growing consensus that it will become the gold standard in defining the anatomy in such patients. Faster scanning times may extend its use in unstable patients.

In the diagnosis of aortic dissection, *echocardiography* has the advantage of being readily available and easily performed at the bedside. Transthoracic echocardiography has been found to have a sensitivity of 59% to 85% and a specificity of 93% to 96%. It is useful in the diagnosis of dissection involving the ascending aorta, but due to limitations in echocardiographic windows, it is of limited value in the diagnosis of distal dissections. Transesophageal echocardiography overcomes many of these limitations and can image almost the entire thoracic aorta. It is also useful for detecting coronary artery involvement with the dissection and has sensitivity similar to MRI and CT for detecting dissection. With single-plane units, the sensitivity of transthoracic echocardiography and transesophageal echocardiography is lower than CT and MR, mainly as a result of false-positive findings in the ascending aorta. Biplane units allow improved visualization of the ascending aorta. Multiplane transesophageal echocardiography permits a 3D understanding of the condition of the aorta, and these units are becoming more widely available. The additional views pro-

vided by MPR transesophageal echocardiography considerably reduce the blind spot of monoplanar transesophageal echocardiography, leaving only a small portion between the ascending aorta and proximal aortic arch that is suboptimally shown. A limitation of transesophageal echocardiography is the lack of visualization of the abdominal aorta and the strong dependence on the investigator's experience. Nonetheless, in most cases of acute dissection, transesophageal echocardiography provides immediate, sufficient information for the decision to perform surgery. In descending aortic dissection, angiography, CT, and MRI/MRA have a larger role because they allow evaluation of branch vessel involvement and assessment of the distal extension of the aneurysm—parameters not well evaluated by transesophageal echocardiography (115).

Because patients with acute dissection are critically ill and potentially in need of an emergency operation, the selection of a given modality will depend on clinical circumstances and availability. In centers where experienced cardiologists are available to perform state-of-the-art transesophageal echocardiography in the emergency room, this type of imaging may be the preferred first-line imaging because it can provide sufficient information to determine whether emergency surgery is needed. However, CTA is likely to be more readily available on a 24-hour basis and can provide information on branch vessel involvement. Although it does not provide information regarding aortic insufficiency, this can be obtained with transthoracic echocardiography or transesophageal echocardiography while the operating room is being prepared.

The differentiation of the true and false lumen is crucial to treatment planning (116–121). In classic aortic dissection, the true lumen tends to be smaller than the false lumen. Spontaneous contrast and some degree of thrombosis can be seen in the false lumen. In the true lumen, early laminar systolic flow is usually detected, whereas in the false lumen, diastolic, late systolic, or slow-swirling flow can be documented with transesophageal 2D and color-coded Doppler echocardiography (90). Finally, aortic cobwebs, when detected, represent a pathognomonic sign of the false lumen (122–124).

The classic appearance of aortic dissection is that of a double-barrel aorta with two channels separated by a thin flap of intimomedial tissue. Often seen as straight or lenticular in appearance, on occasion the dissected tissue appears quite complex, with redundancy and herniation (Fig. 17-42). Recently recognized variants of classical dissection such as limited intimal tears (80) have been notoriously difficult to diagnose on imaging studies, but improvements in imaging capabilities are allowing them to be diagnosed more noninvasively (Fig. 17-47).

The presence of an IMH within the aortic wall is most often recognizable as a crescentic or circular local aortic wall thickening and the absence of a visible intimal flap or tear (Fig. 17-48). Characteristic features for CT include displacement of intimal calcifications, higher attenuation of the thickened wall as compared with the blood pool as seen on unenhanced imaging (Fig. 17-49), and no contrast enhancement of the thickened aortic wall with enhanced imaging (Figs. 17-50, 17-51) (125). With MRI, no flow within the locally thickened aortic wall and increased signal intensity of thickened aortic wall for T1-weighted MRI characterize an IMH (Figs. 17-49, 17-52). A 5- to 10-mm communication between the aortic lumen and the IMH within the ascending aorta or aortic arch typically represents the residua of a penetrating atherosclerotic ulcer, causing the IMH (Fig. 17-53).

A final cause of AAS is a PAU with pseudoaneurysm formation. In the absence of frank arterial extravasation or perianeurysmal hemorrhage, the stability of a PAU is difficult to ascertain based on imaging characteristics alone. Its association with acute chest pain with or without hypertension should raise concern for an acutely expanding pseudoaneurysm, and frequent monitoring is advised (Fig. 17-54).

OCCLUSIVE DISEASES

With the exception of congenital aortic coarctation, (Chapter 15), hemodynamically significant occlusive disease of the thoracic aorta is rare. Nevertheless, atherosclerosis is highly prevalent within the thoracic aorta and is frequently admixed with thrombus. When particularly exuberant and irregular, small pieces of atheroma and thrombus may embolize distally into the arterial system, a process known as *atheroembolism* and the cause of occlusion of primary aortic branches as well as smaller vessels, resulting in segmental end-organ infarctions (Fig. 17-55) and clinical syndromes such as the blue toe syndrome. Another important cause of occlusive disease of the thoracic aorta and in particular its

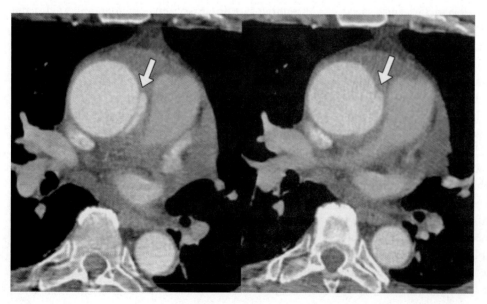

FIGURE 17-47 Serial ECG-gated CT sections in a patient with acute chest pain. A limited intimal tear presents as a focal transverse filling defect with bulging of the aortic wall (*arrows*). There is mediastinal hemorrhage associated with this dissection variant that is easily overlooked on suboptimal CT and MR examinations. The lesion is highly unstable, and surgical repair should be performed urgently.

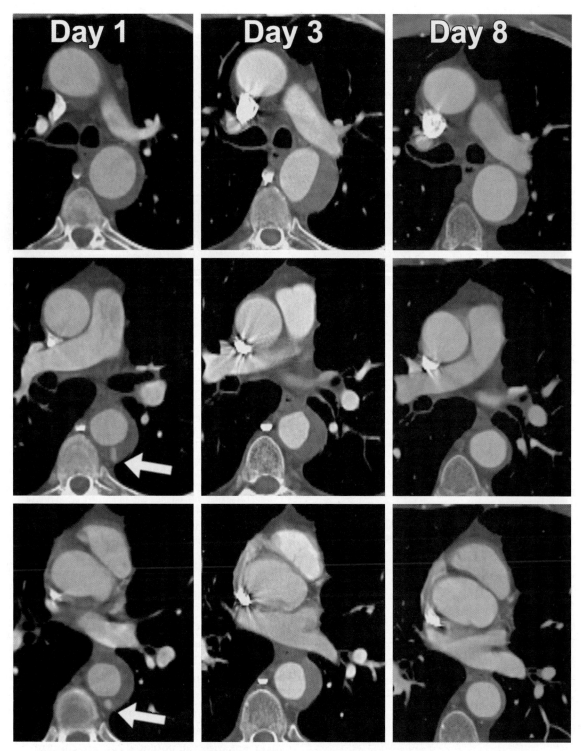

FIGURE 17-48 Evolution of a descending aortic IMH over a 7-day period. Transverse CT sections are presented at three levels on the day of presentation with acute chest pain (Day 1), 2 days later (Day 3), and 1 week after presentation (Day 8). Throughout this time frame, the patient was closely monitored in the hospital with a mean arterial pressure of 70 mmHg. On initial presentation, the proximal descending aorta is mildly dilated. There is a crescentic mural thickening corresponding to the IMH at each of the three levels. Intramural contrast collections (*arrows*) do not correspond to ulcers, as is commonly and wrongly suggested, but instead correspond to regions of flow through sheared-off intercostal artery origins, either prograde through tears in the aortic intima or retrograde from the intercostal arteries. On Day 3, the intramural contrast collections have spontaneously resolved, but the IMH is larger at its proximal extent. On Day 8, the IMH has almost completely resolved, but dilation of the proximal descending aorta persists.

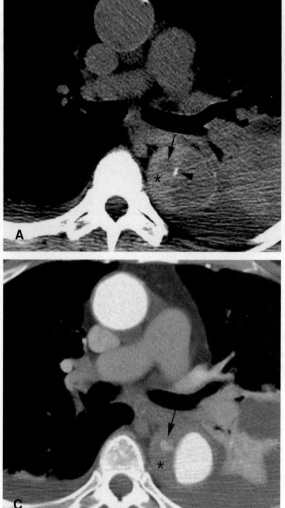

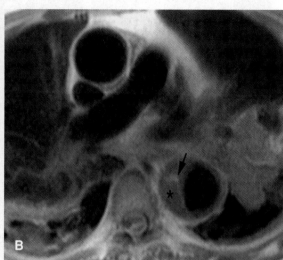

FIGURE 17-49 74-year-old man with bilateral pleural effusion and chest pain, with CTA ordered to rule out pulmonary embolism. The precontrast CT image **(A)** shows a hyperattenuating lenticular area suggestive of an IMH in the right aspect of the descending aorta (*). There is also a centrally located calcification (*arrowhead*) indicating displaced intima and a small communication with the blood-filled lumen (*arrow*). Note a similar appearance on the noncontrast dark blood HASTE image **(B)** and the contrast-enhanced CT **(C)**. In this case, the distinction between segmental dissection and IMH is difficult. Regardless, this type B anatomic configuration confers conservative management.

proximal branches is radiation-induced arteriopathy and fibrosis, which should be considered in patients with a history of thoracic neoplasia treated with radiation therapy (Fig. 17-56). Abnormalities will conform to the radiation portal.

VASCULITIDES

The manifestations and imaging of vasculitides involving the thoracic aorta are presented in Chapter 10.

TRAUMA

Traumatic injury of the thoracic aorta is a major clinical concern in patients with penetrating trauma (Fig. 17-57) or in those who sustained deceleration or crush injuries, as in motor vehicle collisions or falls from great heights. When

these injuries are full-thickness tears, rapid exsanguination follows, resulting in death before medical intervention is available (126,127).

It is estimated that among patients with incomplete or contained lesions, about 20% may survive and reach the trauma center. If left untreated, these lesions may progress to complete rupture or may lead to pseudoaneurysm with the potential for late rupture. The good news is that of the patients with thoracic aortic injury who reach the hospital alive, 60% to 70% will survive once they receive the proper treatment (126,127). Nevertheless, clinical awareness is critical, given the fact that there are usually no clinical signs or symptoms that cause suspicion for aortic injury (128).

Classically, the initial screening for acute traumatic aortic rupture relied on chest radiography. Some critics to this

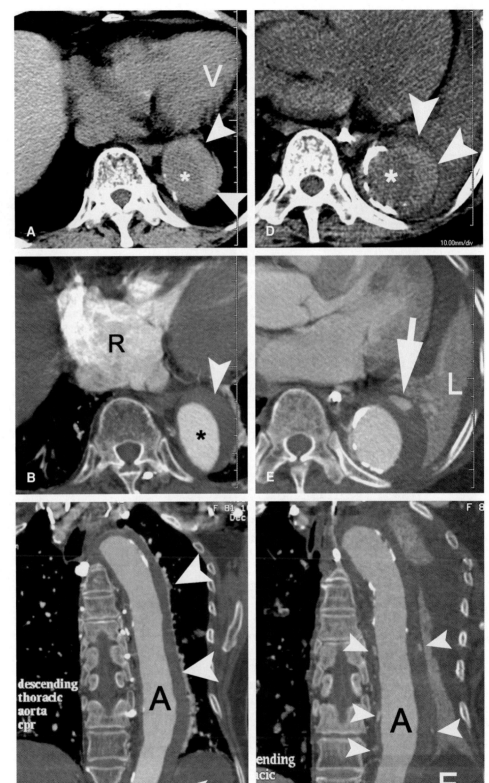

FIGURE 17-50 Temporal evolution of IMH in an 81-year-old female with malignant hypertension and back pain. A: Axial unenhanced image at the level of the diaphragm demonstrates an eccentric hyperdense IMH along the left lateral aspect of the aortic wall (*arrowheads*). The aortic lumen is not compressed (*). (*V*, ventricle.) **B:** Axial image from CTA at a similar level shows the eccentric hematoma (*arrowhead*) adjacent to the aortic lumen (*). Note the potential difficulty in differentiation of IMH versus thrombus in false lumen if noncontrast images are not acquired. (*R*, dilated right atrium.) **C:** Curved planar reconstruction of the descending thoracic aorta (*A*) demonstrates the extent of the IMH (*arrowheads*) extending along the entire descending aorta. Note the lack of arterial enhancement or vascular puddling. **D:** Axial noncontrast image obtained 1 week later. The amount of hyperdense IMH has increased (*arrowheads*). The aortic lumen (*) remains noncompressed at this level. **E:** Corresponding axial image from CTA demonstrates a new focal area of arterial phase puddling in the intramural abnormality (*arrow*). (*L*, atelectatic lung.) **F:** CPR image of descending thoracic aorta (*A*) demonstrates puddling at multiple levels (*arrowheads*), with some expansion of IMH thickness throughout. These findings often herald the conversion of IMH toward a more classical type B aortic dissection. (*E*, subpulmonic pleural effusion.)

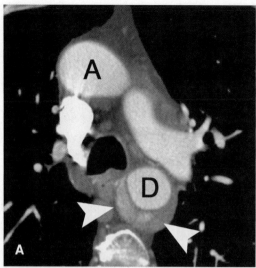

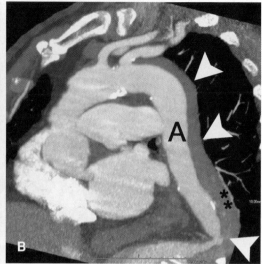

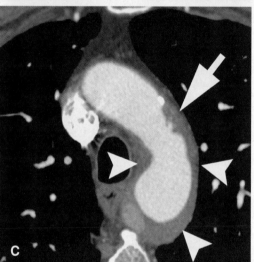

FIGURE 17-51 IMH versus type B dissection in a 79-year-old male presenting with chest pain. A CTA to exclude pulmonary embolus was performed. No pulmonary emboli were found. **A:** Axial image at level of proximal descending thoracic aorta demonstrates a focal, eccentric mixed attenuation intimal separation (*arrowheads*) associated with the posterior aspect of the descending thoracic aorta (*D*). The ascending aorta (*A*) is not involved. **B:** Oblique sagittal thin-slab MIP reconstruction demonstrates that the intramural abnormality (*arrowheads*) extends for the length of the descending thoracic aorta (*A*), but only a very small focus of enhancement is seen (******). Differential diagnosis for this appearance includes both extensive IMH and type B dissection with near-complete thrombosis of false lumen. **C:** Axial image at level of aortic arch shows localized irregularity laterally, near the origin of left subclavian artery (*arrow*), with abnormal soft-tissue thickening involving the more distal arch (*arrowheads*), similar to that seen in (**B**).

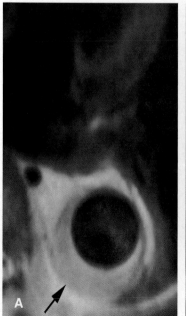

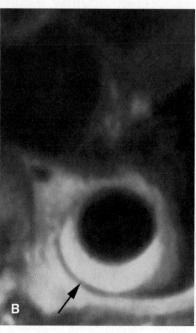

FIGURE 17-52 This patient presented with hypertension and chest pain radiating to the back. The initial dark blood HASTE image (**A**) obtained at presentation shows a lenticular-shaped signal collection (*arrow*) within the posterior wall of the descending aorta, which is classic for IMH. A follow-up image obtained 10 days later (**B**) shows transition to a higher signal intensity within the mural collection (*arrow*).

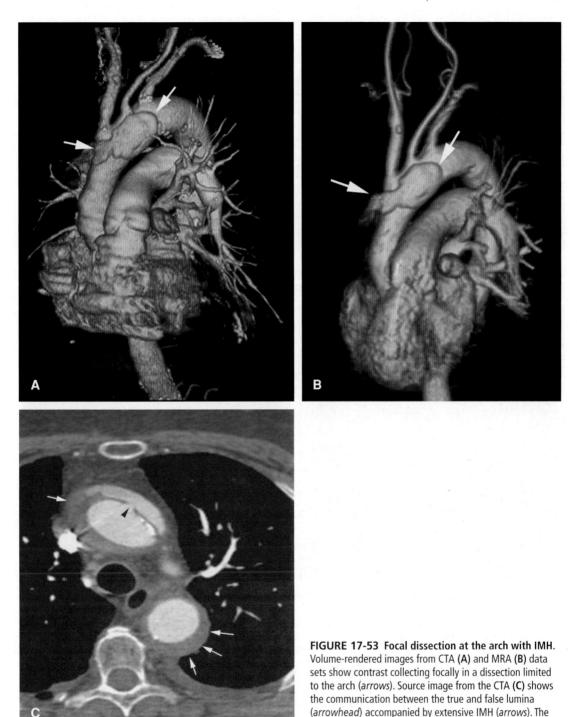

FIGURE 17-53 Focal dissection at the arch with IMH.
Volume-rendered images from CTA **(A)** and MRA **(B)** data
sets show contrast collecting focally in a dissection limited
to the arch (*arrows*). Source image from the CTA **(C)** shows
the communication between the true and false lumina
(*arrowhead*) accompanied by extensive IMH (*arrows*). The
latter is only appreciated on the source images.

approach, however, claim that there is no consensus about
the criteria for calling the mediastinum normal or
"widened," as well as on further imaging strategies for
patients with abnormal findings (128). Besides, chest x-ray
findings are interpreted as normal at the time of initial evaluation in 9% to 40% of patients with aortic rupture in
major trauma centers (129). In this scenario, CT aortography is becoming popular as the one-stop strategy in patients
with positive mechanism of injury (130). Although most
attention is devoted to the aorta, CT may show unsuspected lesions involving the chest wall (Fig. 17-58) and aortic branches (Fig. 17-59). Careful scrutiny of all vascular
(and nonvascular) structures is important in the setting of
thoracic trauma.

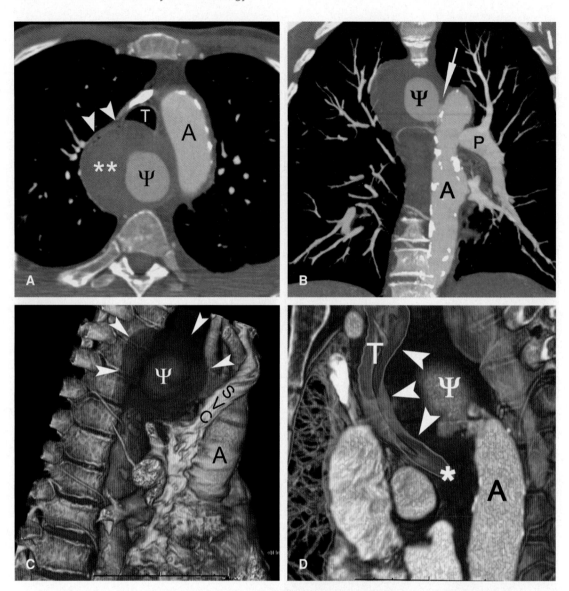

FIGURE 17-54 Pseudoaneurysm of the descending thoracic aorta arising from a penetrating atherosclerotic ulcer. A: Axial image at level of aortic arch shows a large pseudoaneurysm (ψ) arising from the medial border of the descending thoracic aorta (A). There is a large amount of thrombus (∗∗) as well as flowing blood within the lesion. Bubbles of gas are seen in the esophagus (*arrowheads*), which is displaced anteriorly. There is mass effect on the trachea (T) as well. **B:** Coronal 10-mm MIP image shows communication (*arrow*) between the descending thoracic aorta (A) and the pseudoaneurysm (ψ), which was created by erosion of a penetrating ulcer. (P, left pulmonary artery.) **C:** Thick-slab volume-rendered image viewed from the patient's right shows the flow lumen of the pseudoaneurysm (ψ) arising from the aorta (A). Careful selection of opacity transfer functions allows visualization of the thrombus with the lesion as well (*arrowheads*). (SVC, superior vena cava.) **D:** Oblique sagittal volume-rendered image viewed from the patient's left shows extensive mass effect (*arrowheads*) on the trachea (T) by the pseudoaneurysm (ψ). (A, aorta; ∗, left main stem bronchus.)

The terminology used to describe aortic injuries is inconsistent and includes *tear* (the result of pulling apart or into pieces by force), *laceration* (the consequence of tearing or a torn, ragged, or mangled wound), *transection* (a section made across a long axis or a division by cutting transversely) (Fig. 17-60), and *rupture* (forcible tearing or disruption) (127).

Ninety percent of thoracic aortic injuries in patients presenting to the hospital alive occur at the aortic isthmus—the portion of the proximal descending thoracic aorta located between the origin of the left subclavian artery and the site of attachment of the ligamentum arteriosum (Fig. 17-61). Although uncommon in clinical practice, the

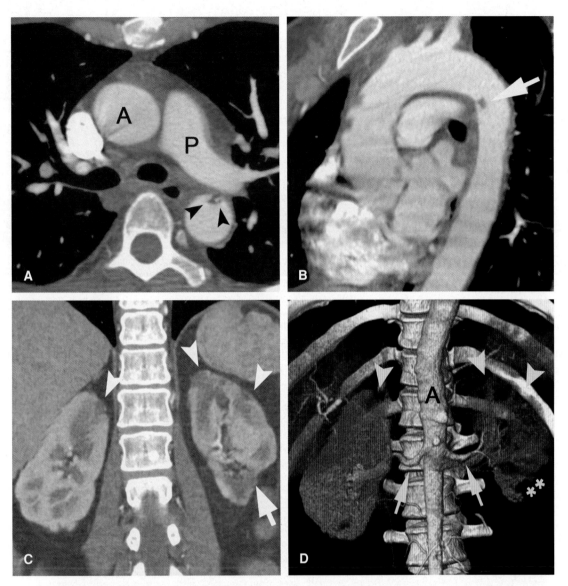

FIGURE 17-55 Emboligenic plaque causing end-organ infarcts. A: Axial image from CTA exam shows focal area of eccentric atheroma within the descending thoracic aorta (*arrowheads*) with a configuration irregular contour, morphology suggesting a high risk of embolization. (*A*, ascending aorta; *P*, left pulmonary artery.) **B:** Sagittal 5-mm MIP image shows the focal plaque appearing to float in the aortic lumen (*arrow*). Note the lack of other plaque in the thoracic aorta and proximal great vessels. **C:** Coronal MPR image at the level of the kidneys shows focal acute renal infarcts bilaterally (*arrowheads*), with cortical edema and swelling. There is also evidence of an old vascular insult showing cortical atrophy in the lower pole of the left kidney (*arrow*). The patient did not suffer from arrhythmia. **D:** Coronal thick-slab volume-rendered image shows widely patent single bilateral renal arteries (*arrows*) arising from the aorta (*A*). The abdominal aorta also shows a lack of other significant plaque or ulceration. The renal infarcts are again seen (*arrowheads*), as is the chronic infarct in the lower pole of the left kidney (**).

descending aorta at its diaphragmatic hiatus or the ascending aorta at the aortic root are also preferential sites for primary injury (127) (it should be noted that up to 25% of aortic injuries found in autopsy studies are in the ascending aorta, emphasizing the higher mortality rate of these injuries) (131).

A number of forces may be involved in blunt thoracic trauma and result in aortic injury. Primary mechanisms include shearing stress, bending stress, and the osseous pinch mechanism for the isthmic injuries (Fig. 17-62). Given the fact that the aortic arch is mobile, in contrast to the descending aorta (relatively fixed to the spine), shearing

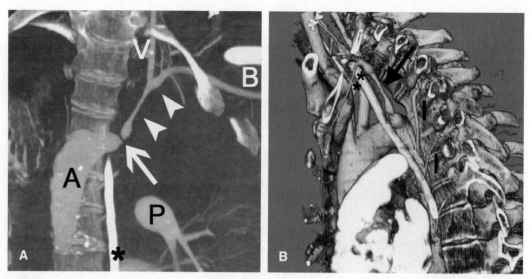

FIGURE 17-56 Aberrant left subclavian artery arising from right aortic arch, with radiation-induced vascular stenosis in a 37-year-old patient with shortness of breath and blood pressure changes in the left arm. A CTA was performed to exclude pulmonary embolus and venous thrombosis (none was found). Patient has a remote history of radiation therapy to the left chest for Hodgkin lymphoma. **A:** Oblique coronal 10-mm MIP image demonstrates marked narrowing at the origin of the left subclavian artery (*arrow*), which arises aberrantly from a right-sided aortic arch. The aorta descends on the right (*A*). The remainder of the left subclavian artery shows tubular narrowing (*arrowheads*). This region corresponded to a previous radiation portal site. The CTA findings are consistent with radiation-induced vasculitis/fibrosis. The left vertebral artery (*V*) and left brachial artery (*B*) have normal caliber. (*P,* left lower lobe pulmonary artery; *,* nasogastric tube.) **B:** Thin-slab oblique sagittal volume-rendered image shows the tubular narrowing of the aberrant left subclavian artery (*arrow*). The origin of the left internal mammary artery is spared (**). Note the presence of dilated intercostal collateral vessels (*I*).

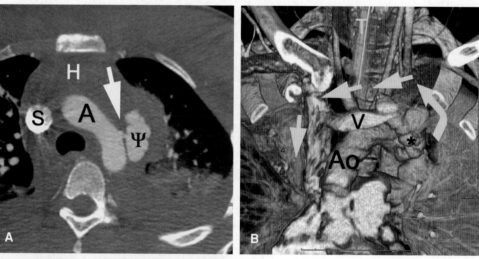

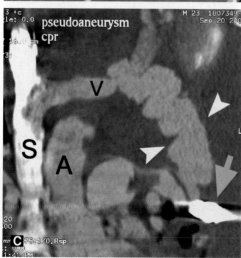

FIGURE 17-57 Gunshot wound in a 23-year-old male, resulting in pseudoaneurysm and arteriovenous fistula. **A:** Axial CTA image at the level of the aortic arch (*A*). There is a narrow-necked communication (*arrow*) between the aortic arch and a pseudoaneurysm (ψ). Adjacent mediastinal hematoma is also seen (*H*). (*S,* superior vena cava.) **B:** Volume-rendered image shows course of blood in arteriovenous fistula. Blood flows through the aorta (*Ao*), into the pseudoaneurysm at the level of injury (*), into the left subclavian and innominate veins (*V*), returning to the right heart via the superior vena cava (*arrows*). (*T,* endotracheal tube.) **C:** Curved planar reconstruction of arteriovenous fistula shows filling of the pseudoaneurysm (*arrowheads*) and draining venous system (*V*). Streak artifact from the offending bullet is noted (*arrow*). (*S,* superior vena cava; *A,* ascending aorta.)

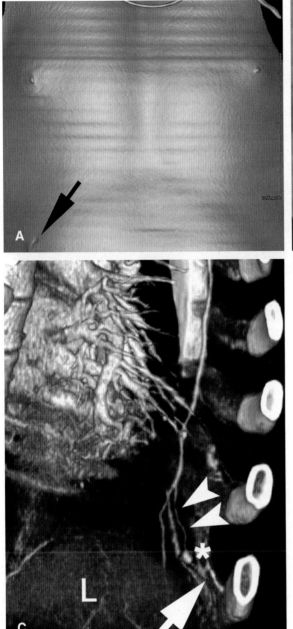

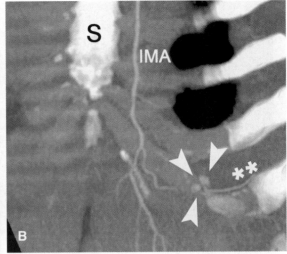

FIGURE 17-58 Penetrating trauma with pseudoaneurysm of intercostal artery in a 28-year-old male with knife wound. A: Volume-rendered CTA image with opacity transfer function set for skin evaluation shows a laceration from a penetrating knife wound in the right lower chest (*arrow*). **B:** Coronal 20-mm MIP image viewed posteriorly shows a bilobed pseudoaneurysm (*arrowheads*) arising from the anterior aspect of an intercostal artery (**). The internal mammary artery (*IMA*) is noted. (*S,* sternum.) **C:** Oblique sagittal volume-rendered slab shows the pseudoaneurysm (*) with supply from the intercostal (*arrow*) as well as a small supply arising from a branch of the right internal mammary (*arrowheads*). (*L,* liver.)

stress occurs when the rates of deceleration of these two aortic segments are different. Bending stress results in the flexion of the aorta over the left pulmonary artery and left main bronchus (132,133). In the osseous pinch mechanism, following compression of the chest, the aorta is squeezed between the anterior osseous structures and the spine (134).

Torsion and water-hammer effect are used to explain injuries to the ascending aorta. Torsion is created by displacement of the heart during impact. The water-hammer effect occurs by an abrupt increase in intra-aortic pressure (127).

Since chest radiography alone is not sufficient to rule out aortic injury and its positive predictive value is also low (only 10% to 20% of confirmatory thoracic aortograms are positive for aortic injury in patients with abnormal chest x-ray), CT has become the method of choice in the initial evaluation of suspected aortic trauma in hemodynamically stable patients. The findings include mediastinal hematoma, tear of the intima and media, rupture with extravasation of contrast material, posttraumatic dissection, pseudoaneurysm, and coarctation (127,130).

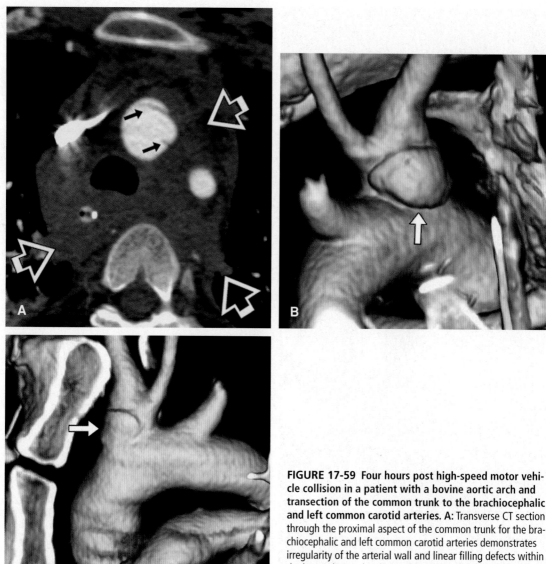

FIGURE 17-59 Four hours post high-speed motor vehicle collision in a patient with a bovine aortic arch and transection of the common trunk to the brachiocephalic and left common carotid arteries. A: Transverse CT section through the proximal aspect of the common trunk for the brachiocephalic and left common carotid arteries demonstrates irregularity of the arterial wall and linear filling defects within the lumen (*arrows*). Adjacent hematoma is present in the mediastinum (*open arrows*). **B, C:** Volume-renderings provide better delineation of the pseudoaneurysm (*arrows*). The aorta was normal.

Mediastinal hematoma (Fig. 17-63) is an indirect sign of aortic injury and is characterized by a soft-tissue attenuation material surrounding the aorta and/or other mediastinal structures. It should raise higher suspicion when located immediately adjacent to the aorta. It is important to recognize pitfalls that can mimic mediastinal hematomas, especially motion artifacts and atelectasis of segments of the left lung in close contact to the aorta (127,130).

On the other hand, to avoid false-positives, radiologists should be able to recognize the normal appearance of the ductus bump or diverticulum, or a penetrating atherosclerotic ulcer (Fig. 17-10). The typical ductus diverticulum has smooth and regular contour, obtuse angles with the wall of the aorta, and lack of an intimal flap (127,130).

PRIMARY AORTIC TUMORS

Primary aortic neoplasms are rare but typically are angiosarcomas when they occur (135,136). They are five times more common in veins than in arteries (136), with about 145 cases of aortic sarcomas published in the literature (137). Although they usually carry an unfavorable prognosis, successful surgical resection is becoming more common, and clinical awareness and MRI can aid in the early diagnosis (136). In a report of 11 cases, Akiyama and colleagues found a mean age at the time of presentation of 59.5 years, with a male-to-female ratio of 9:5 (137).

Aortic neoplasms can be divided into two groups, according to the site of occurrence in the aortic wall (138).

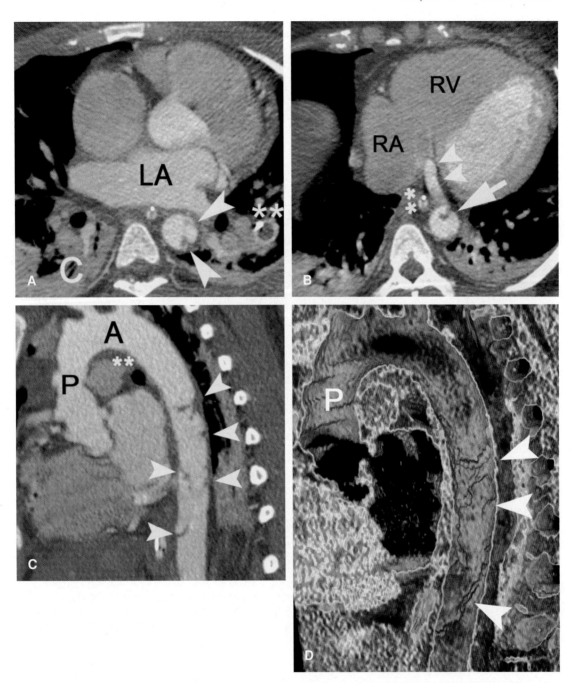

FIGURE 17-60 Transection of the descending thoracic aorta in a patient with history of deceleration injury.
A: Axial CT image at level of left atrium (*LA*) shows a focal transection of the descending thoracic aorta (*arrowheads*).
There is extensive pulmonary contusion (*C*) bilaterally. A left-sided chest tube is noted (∗∗). **B:** Axial image inferior to
(A) shows extension of the full-thickness tear in **(A)** as a flap consisting of a portion of intima and media (*arrow*). The
coronary sinus (*arrowheads*) is noted entering the right atrium (*RA*). (RV, right ventricle; ∗∗, nasogastric tube.) **C:** Sagittal MPR image shows the craniocaudal extent of the transection (*arrowheads*), which extends to the level of the
diaphragmatic hiatus. There is no evidence of injury or hematoma at the ligamentum arteriosum (∗∗). (*A*, aortic arch; *P*,
pulsation artifact in the ascending aorta.) **D:** Sagittal 20-mm slab volume-rendered image with "hollow lumen" opacity
transfer settings demonstrates a wrinkled appearance of the transection.

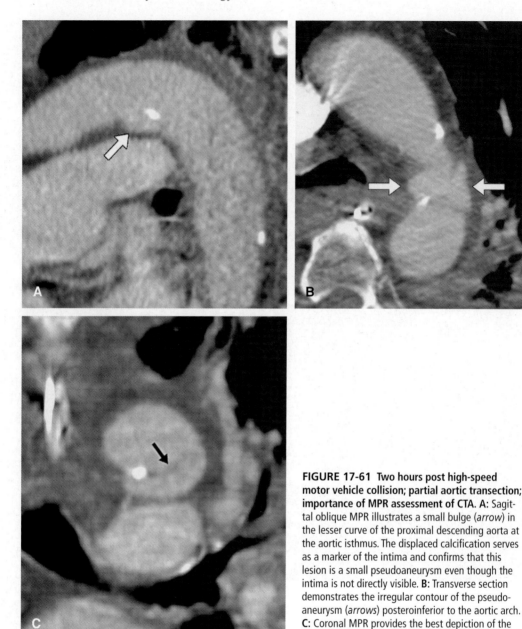

FIGURE 17-61 Two hours post high-speed motor vehicle collision; partial aortic transection; importance of MPR assessment of CTA. **A:** Sagittal oblique MPR illustrates a small bulge (*arrow*) in the lesser curve of the proximal descending aorta at the aortic isthmus. The displaced calcification serves as a marker of the intima and confirms that this lesion is a small pseudoaneurysm even though the intima is not directly visible. **B:** Transverse section demonstrates the irregular contour of the pseudo-aneurysm (*arrows*) posteroinferior to the aortic arch. **C:** Coronal MPR provides the best depiction of the intimal flap (*arrow*) and associated calcification.

The first is the luminal type, which involves the intima and grows in the direction of the aortic lumen (Fig. 17-64), causing symptoms due to luminal obstruction and embolic events. It may be difficult to distinguish them from atherosclerosis. In this case, hematogenous metasta-sis is quite frequent, especially to the spine, liver, adrenal glands, pancreas, lung, and soft tissues (138–141). The second group is the mural type, whose growth pattern is extravascular, arising in the media and adventitia. Clinical signs are nonspecific and more indolent, sometimes simi-lar to those of aortic dissection or ruptured or dissecting aneurysm (142).

The value of MRI and transesophageal echography in the diagnosis of aortic leiomyosarcoma has been reported (139,140). MRI is superior to CT in detecting the tumoral origin of the symptoms, better depicting wall nodules and periaortic and vertebral extensions. These lesions show con-trast enhancement, which is also useful to achieve the correct diagnosis (Fig. 17-64). TEE may aid in the diagnosis and depiction of wall thickness and nodules, but it is less helpful than MRI on the assessment of periaortic extension (136).

Because aortic tumors are uncommon, it is not easy to establish the optimal treatment—even when proper diagno-sis is established before surgery (136,139,141). Therapeutic

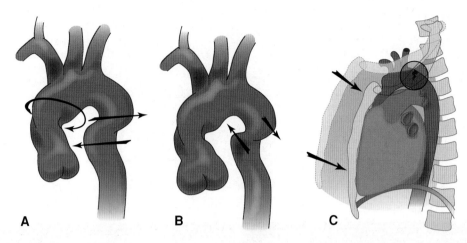

FIGURE 17-62 Diagrams illustrate the mechanisms of injury at the ascending aorta and at the aortic isthmus. A: Torsion stress and the water-hammer effect are proposed mechanisms of injury affecting the ascending aorta. **B:** Shearing stress and bending stress are forces that involve the aortic isthmus. **C:** Diagram of the osseous pinch mechanism, in which the aorta is pinched between the anterior bony structures and the thoracic spine, shows resultant tear of the aorta within the highlighted area. (Adapted with permission from Creasy JD, Chiles C, Routh WD, et al. Overview of traumatic injury of the thoracic aorta. *Radiographics*. 1997;17:27–45, Figures 3, 4.)

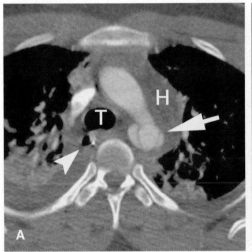

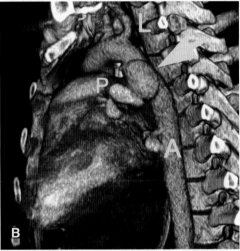

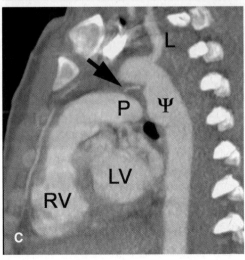

Figure 17-63 Traumatic aortic injury in a 32-year-old patient involved in a high-speed motor vehicle accident. A: Axial CT image at the level of the aortic arch demonstrates a focal flaplike tear in the aorta at the ligamentum arteriosum (*arrow*), with adjacent mediastinal hematoma (*H*). There is rightward displacement of the trachea (*T*) and nasogastric tube (*arrowhead*). **B:** Oblique sagittal thick-slab volume-rendered image shows a typical location and appearance of a pseudoaneurysm (*arrow*) in traumatic aortic injury. The lesion begins immediately distal to the left subclavian artery (*L*). The main pulmonary artery (*P*) and descending thoracic aorta (*A*) are also indicated. **C:** Oblique sagittal 10-mm MIP image shows a mildly calcified ligamentum arteriosum (*arrow*) extending between the pulmonary trunk (*P*) and the aortic pseudoaneurysm (ψ). (*L*, left subclavian artery; *RV*, right ventricle; *LV*, left ventricle.)

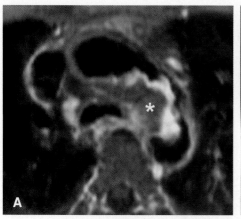

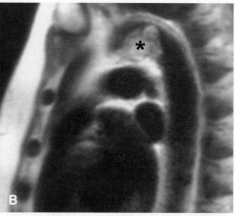

Figure 17-64 48-year-old woman with intimal aortic sarcoma. A: Axial gadolinium-enhanced fat-saturated T1-weighted SE MR image shows peripheral enhancement of lobulated aortic tumor mass (*). B: Half-Fourier acquisition single-shot turbo SE MR image shows high signal on T2-weighted image within mass. (Reprinted with permission from Mohsen NA, Haber M, Urrutia VC, et al. Intimal sarcoma of the aorta. *AJR Am J Roentgenol*. 2000;175: 1289–1290, Figures 1a, 1b.)

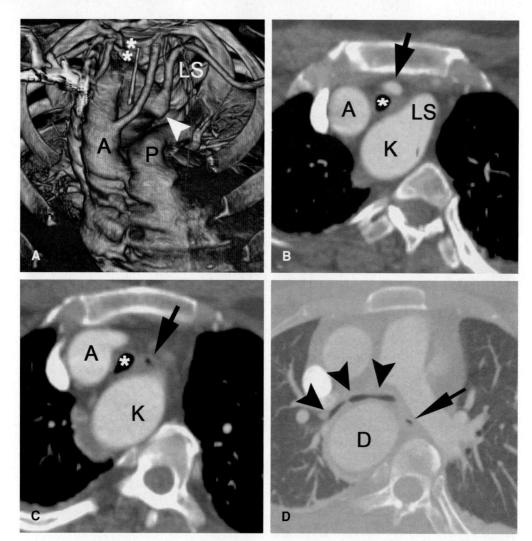

Figure 17-65 Right aortic arch and aberrant left subclavian artery and diverticulum of Kommerell in a 44-year-old female with respiratory failure and dysphagia. A: Volume-rendered image viewed obliquely from the front shows a right-sided aortic arch (*A*) with aberrant left subclavian artery (*LS*). There is an outpouching at the origin of the aberrant vessel consistent with a diverticulum of Kommerell (*arrowhead*). An endotracheal tube is noted (**). (*P*, main pulmonary artery.) B: Axial image near the thoracic inlet shows the trachea (*) surrounded by the large diverticulum of Kommerell (*K*), aberrant left subclavian artery (*LS*), right arch (*A*), and right common carotid artery (*arrow*). C: Axial image slightly lower than (B) shows the esophagus (*arrow*) and trachea (*) narrowed by the vascular ring. (*A*, right arch; *K*, diverticulum of Kommerell.) D: Axial image at the carina shows marked compression of the carina and proximal main stem bronchi (*arrowheads*) from the enlarged descending thoracic aorta (*D*). The esophagus is displaced leftward and posteriorly (*arrow*). A midline descending aorta has been shown in approximately 75% of patients with right arch and aberrant left subclavian artery and may contribute to airway narrowing. (*Figure 17-65 continues*)

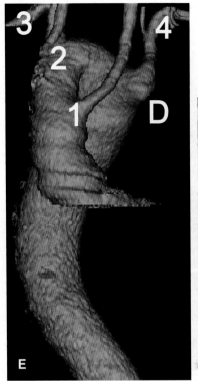
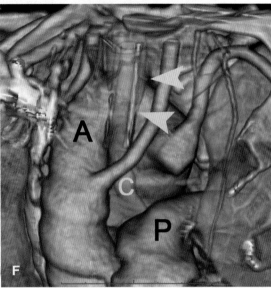

FIGURE 17-65 Continued E: Volume-rendered image with bone segmentation shows typical branching pattern. The left common carotid artery (*1*) originates first, followed by the right subclavian (*2*) and common carotid (*3*) arteries. The aberrant left subclavian then arises (*4*) with a diverticulum of Kommerell (*D*). Descending aorta is midline. **F:** Oblique coronal volume-rendered image shows the relationship of the endotracheal tube (*arrowheads*) and carina (*C*) to the aorta (*A*) and arch vessels. (*P,* main pulmonary artery.)

options may be surgical, combining primary resection with reconstruction. Other reported options are association of radiotherapy and chemotherapy, with or without surgical resection. Life expectancy usually lies between 8 and 14 months (143,144).

CONGENITAL ANOMALIES

Knowledge of the most common congenital anomalies plays a crucial role in the interpretation of vascular studies (Fig. 17-65). This topic is discussed in detail in Chapter 23.

POSTOPERATIVE FINDINGS AND COMPLICATIONS

CT and MRI play an important role when following up patients after surgical repair of aortic disease. Follow-up protocol varies, but it seems reasonable to include imaging before discharge, at 6 and 12 months postoperatively, and annually thereafter or whenever complications are suspected (49).

Postoperative *paraplegia* or paraparesis is a serious complication of reconstructive surgery of the thoracoabdominal or descending aorta and is thought to result from spinal cord ischemia related to the procedure. Advances in anesthetic and surgical techniques have lessened the inci-

dence of intractable neurologic complications, but the rate of paraplegia or paraparesis is still substantial, reported to be between 5% and 15% (146–147). The most important reasons for spinal neurologic deficits are related to reduced blood flow to the spinal cord during aortic cross clamping and permanent disruption of delicate and variable arteries to the spinal cord. The duration of cross clamping influences the magnitude of spinal cord ischemia and reperfusion (148–150). Although not universally accepted (151,152), some investigators emphasize the importance of identifying the artery of Adamkiewicz preoperatively in patients with thoracoabdominal aortic aneurysm to aid in surgical planning and to prevent postoperative paraplegia or paraparesis. Regardless, there are benefits to surgical planning that can be achieved by knowing the origin of this vessel. The segment bearing the identified spinal vessel may be spared from resection if the aorta is not severely aneurysmal; residual mild dilatation is preferable to paraplegia. Alternatively, a bevel in the resection may preserve the crucial vessel yet still extirpate the neighboring aneurysmal tissue. Knowledge of the location of the spinal vessel may aid in intelligent placement of the lower cross clamp so that the vital vessel is not excluded from distal perfusion by the left atrial–femoral artery bypass setup. And, for most surgeons who believe strongly in

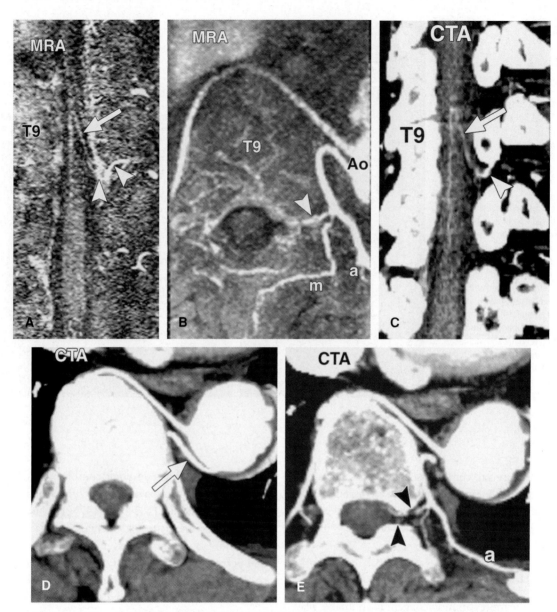

Figure 17-66 True thoracoabdominal aortic aneurysm in a 63-year-old woman. A: Oblique coronal MPR image from MRA shows the artery of Adamkiewicz (*arrow*), which branches from the left ninth radiculomedullary artery (*arrowheads*). The anterior spinal artery is continuous with the artery of Adamkiewicz, creating a hairpin turn. **B:** Axial partial MPR image from MRA demonstrates continuity between the aorta (*Ao*) and the radiculomedullary artery (*arrowhead*). The anterior (*a*) and muscular (*m*) branches are also visualized. **C:** Oblique coronal MPR image from CTA shows the artery of Adamkiewicz (*arrow*) and the radiculomedullary artery (*arrowhead*). **D:** Oblique axial MPR image from CTA shows the proximal portion of the left ninth intercostal artery (*arrow*). **E:** Oblique axial MPR image from CTA shows the radiculomedullary artery (*arrowheads*). The anterior branch (*a*) is also visualized. (Reprinted with permission from Yoshioka K, Niinuma H, Ohira A, et al. MR angiography and CT angiography of the artery of Adamkiewicz: noninvasive preoperative assessment of thoracoabdominal aortic aneurysm. *Radiographics.* 2003;23:1215–1225, Figure 3.)

reimplantation, intelligent selection of implanted vessel(s) can be made—in contradistinction to the "roulette wheel."

However, the artery of Adamkiewicz is difficult to visualize and may be impossible or dangerous to evaluate with selective intercostal or lumbar angiography. It can be identified on the basis of continuity from the aorta to the anterior spinal artery with a fairly characteristic hairpin turn. Some investigators have reported on the usefulness of preoperative evaluation of the artery of Adamkiewicz with selective conventional angiography, which will be very helpful in planning surgical repair of thoracoabdominal

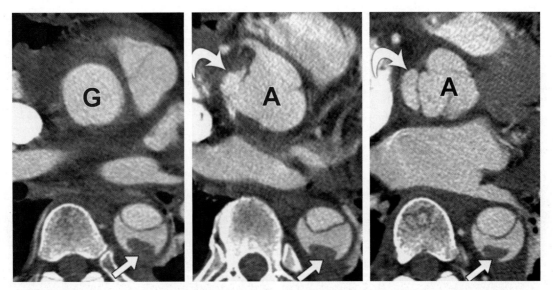

FIGURE 17-67 Proximal anastomotic dehiscence of ascending aortic interposition graft in a patient with repaired type A dissection. Transverse CTA sections from cranial to caudal **(left to right)** demonstrate the inferior aspect of the aortic graft (G). The lateral aspect of the anastomosis between the graft and the sinotubular junction has broken down, resulting in a pseudoaneurysm (*curved arrow*). The three sinuses of Valsalva are identifiable on the rightmost image and distinct from the inferior extent of the pseudoaneurysm (*curved arrow*). An intimal flap is present in the descending aorta with a thrombus on the posterior wall of the false lumen (*straight arrows*), serving as a potential source of distal embolization to any aortic branch originating from the false lumen. (*A*, aorta.)

aortic aneurysms and improving the surgical outcome with respect to paralysis (151,153–155). In these studies, no paraplegia occurred during examination, and the detection rate for the artery of Adamkiewicz was 65%. Recent data from a report comparing both MRA and CTA detected the artery of Adamkiewicz at a similar rate (156). While successful demonstration of the ARM is possible with both CT and MRA (Fig. 17-66), the demands of spatial resolution must be carefully considered. This is particularly germane to the use of MRA in the context of a comprehensive examination. The resolution used with MDCT is sufficient to study the aorta and the ARM; however, with MRA, separate acquisitions are needed. The latter places a burden on patient throughput, as the ARM study and aortic study are best performed at separate times. It is possible to perform both evaluations in one sitting, focusing first on the ARM evaluation by using a spine coil and focusing second on the aortic evaluation by using a body phased-array coil.

Imaging Findings after Aortic Repair

Knowledge of the types of aortic repair and their expected postoperative findings is essential in the postoperative assessment. After repair of aortic disease, the anastomoses between the graft and native aorta are often reinforced with Teflon felt, which appears on CT scans as a thick curvilinear

area of high attenuation. After the graft is secured, the aortic wall is often wrapped around it and the incision is sutured. This technique creates a potential space between the graft and the native aorta. A small amount of blood and gas may normally accumulate in this space in the immediate postoperative period (41).

The presence of gas between the graft and the native aorta later than 2 to 3 weeks after surgery is highly suggestive of *infection*. Any fluid detected between the graft and native aorta 6 weeks after surgery is virtually pathognomonic of graft infection.

Suture dehiscence (Fig. 17-67), either proximally or distally, can lead to the development of a *pseudoaneurysm* by allowing blood to enter the space between the graft and native aorta (Fig. 17-68). Although rare, pseudoaneurysms can also arise from infected endovascular repair. The pseudoaneurysm is identified on scans as the presence of contrast material within the perigraft space (157–159).

Graft material is readily recognized on unenhanced CT images, as it is slightly hyperattenuative compared with the native aortic wall. *Folds* or *kinks* in graft material are common (Fig. 17-69). Mild folding or kinking of the graft may simulate dissection depending on the plane observed (Fig. 17-70). Care must be taken to avoid this pitfall.

Endovascular aneurysm repair is associated with a unique set of complications. Incomplete exclusion of the

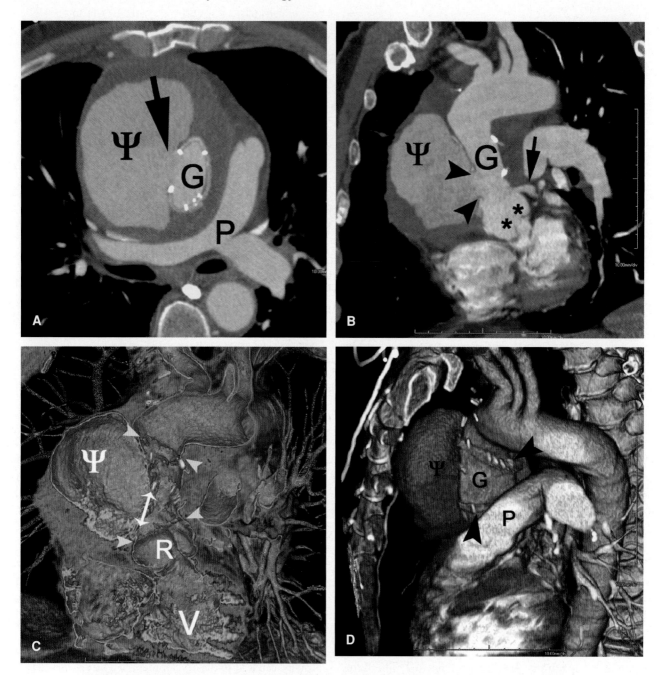

FIGURE 17-68 Postoperative pseudoaneurysm after ascending aortic replacement with tube graft. A: Axial CTA image in mid-ascending aortic region shows a large pseudoaneurysm (*ψ*) arising from a wide dehiscence (*arrow*) of the proximal anastomosis between the aortic tube graft *(G)*. There is mass effect on the pulmonary arteries *(P)*. **B:** Oblique coronal thin-slab MIP image demonstrates the craniocaudal length of the dehiscence (*arrowheads*), with free communication from the graft anastomosis *(G)* to the large pseudoaneurysm (*ψ*). The native aortic valve leaflets are seen (*⋆*), as is the origin of the left coronary artery (*arrow*). **C:** Thin-slab volume-rendered image with opacity-transfer functions set for virtual endoluminal view shows the wide communication (*double-sided arrow*) from the graft anastomosis to the pseudoaneurysm (*ψ*). The proximal and distal anastomosis sites are marked by surgical clips (*arrowheads*). The native aortic root *(R)* is well visualized. *(V*, left ventricle.) **D:** Right posterior oblique view of a volume-rendered image demonstrates the tube graft *(G)* with intact posterior surgical anastomosis (*arrowheads*) and posterior portion of pseudoaneurysm (*ψ*). The arch and great vessels are unaffected. (*P*, pulmonary trunk.)

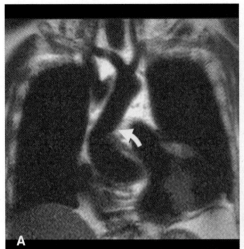
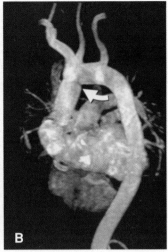
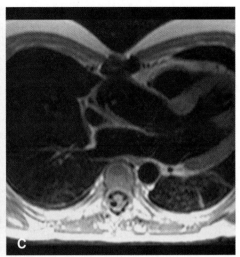

FIGURE 17-69 Bentall procedure for correction of dissection of the ascending aorta in a 45-year-old male patient with Marfan syndrome. Note the presence of the graft just beyond the aortic valve and before the origin of the innominate artery. There is some degree of kinking in both anastomoses (*curved arrows*), as demonstrated in the coronal single-shot FSE **(A)** and thick-slab sagittal oblique MIP **(B)**. The patient also had some residual pectus excavatum **(C)** despite surgical correction.

aneurysm sac with continued perfusion is referred to as *endoleak* (Fig. 17-71) and is the most common complication after stent-graft implantation. Endoleak classification is summarized in Table 17-1. Type I and II are the most concerning, as they indicate instability of fixation or breakdown of the stent graft (157,160). Other key observations include assessment of the stability of the stent-graft position to exclude *migration*; assessment of the metallic component for *fracture*, which can lead to instability and migration (Fig. 17-71); and most important, aneurysm enlargement.

The presence of thrombus within the stent graft is reported to occur at rates of 3% to 19%. On contrast-enhanced scans, *graft thrombus* is recognized as an intraluminal, parietal, circular, or semicircular filling defect within the stent graft. The prognosis varies from spontaneous shrinkage to development of complete thrombosis; therefore, follow-up studies at short intervals are necessary (157).

Some complications of vascular interventions in the thoracic aorta may be seen in the abdominal aortoiliac arteries, including sequelae of stent-graft delivery-induced

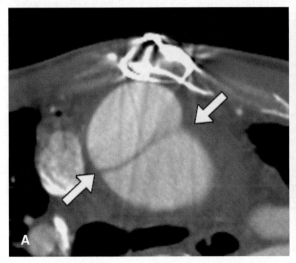
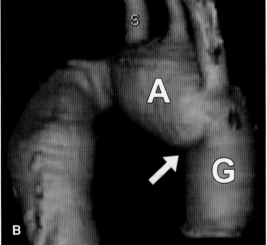

FIGURE 17-70 Graft fold simulating an intimal flap. A: Transverse CT section with a linear filling in the ascending aorta (*arrows*). Note that the outer contour of the aorta is deviated inward at the medial intersection with the linear filling defect. This contour abnormality is a clue that the filling defect is a graft fold and not an intimal flap. **B:** Volume rendering of the same CTA demonstrates a fold (*arrow*) at the distal anastomosis of the ascending aortic graft (*G*) with an aneurysmal aortic arch (*A*) (*arrow*). This corresponds to the contour abnormality seen in **(A)**.

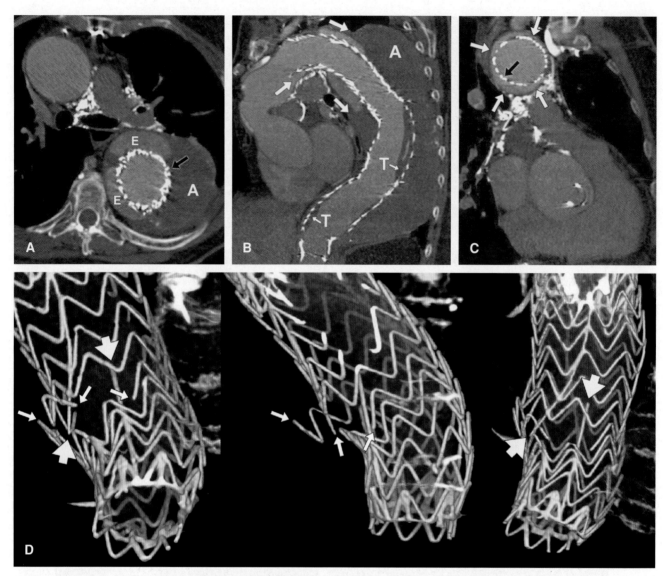

FIGURE 17-71 CTA 1 year following deployment of a stent-graft to treat a descending thoracic aortic aneurysm. A: Transverse section demonstrates a 9-cm descending aortic aneurysm (the aneurysm had measured 7 cm at the time of stent-graft deployment). Although the majority of the aneurysm (*A*) is thrombosed, there is an endoleak (*E*). The stent-graft is indicated by a *black arrow*. **B:** Sagittal oblique MPR enables characterization of the endoleak as type Ia, a proximal attachment site leak. The proximal aspect of the stent-graft is displaced from the lesser curve of the distal aortic arch, allowing contrast-enhanced luminal blood to flow around the stent-graft initially, inferiorly, and then in a spiraling direction distally (*arrows*). Small amounts of thrombus (*T*) within the stent-graft are commonly observed in the thoracic aorta and are of no known clinical consequence. **C:** Coronal oblique MPR through the proximal stent-graft (*black arrow*) demonstrates the poor fixation of the stent-graft at this level with the endoleak channel filling over the majority of the aortic circumference (*white arrows*). **D:** Three volume-renderings of the distal stent-graft by using an opacity transfer function to accentuate detail in the metallic skeleton of the stent-graft illustrates multiple fractures of the transverse stent rings (*small arrows*) and the distal longitudinal strut (*wide arrows*). The ends of the fractured strut and rings are highly distracted, suggesting substantial motion and loss of structural integrity on the distal device, possibly leading to migration of the proximal device and the subsequent type Ia endoleak and aneurysm expansion.

TABLE 17-1

Classification of Endoleaks Following Endovascular Repair

Type	Description
Ia	Perigraft leak from poor proximal attachment or seal
Ib	Perigraft leak from poor distal attachment or seal
II	Collateral backflow or retrograde endoleak
III	Midgraft fabric tear, or modular disconnection or poor seal
IV	Porosity—graft-wall porosity or suture holes

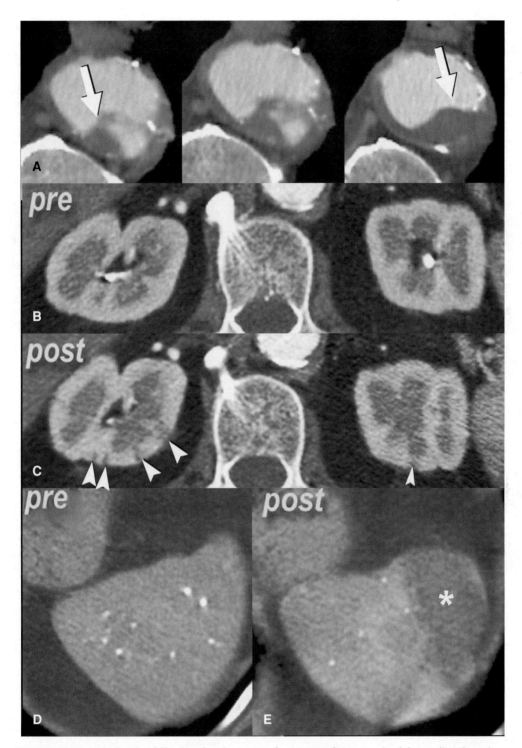

FIGURE 17-72 Embolization following the placement of a stent-graft in a proximal descending thoracic aortic aneurysm. In the preprocedure transverse CT sections **(A)**, irregular plaques are present in the posterior aspect of the distal descending thoracic aorta along the delivery route for the stent-graft (*arrows*). Predeployment, the enhancement pattern of the renal parenchyma is normal **(B)**. Following stent-graft deployment, there are multiple discrete peripheral renal infarcts (*arrowheads* in **C**) secondary to embolization. In addition (**D** and **E**, respectively, pre- and postprocedure transverse CT images of the upper left abdomen), the initially normal spleen **(D)** shows a well-demarcated lateral infarct (∗ in **E**). This case illustrates the importance of scanning the abdomen and pelvis following thoracic interventional vascular procedures.

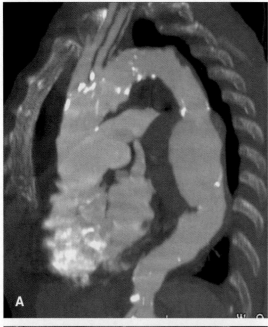

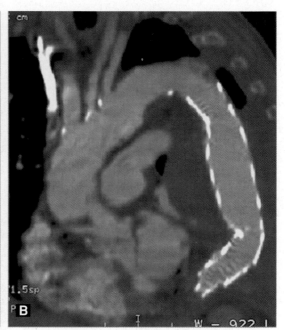

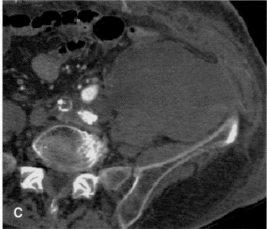

FIGURE 17-73 A: Curved thin-slab parasagittal MIP demonstrates a large descending thoracic aortic aneurysm with mural thrombus. **B:** Curved planar reformation following deployment of a descending aortic stent-graft demonstrates successful isolation of the aneurysm. **C:** Transverse sections through the pelvis demonstrate a large retroperitoneal hematoma as well as a complete thrombosis of the right common iliac artery that occurred following deployment of the stent-graft. An oval enhancing structure anterior to the common iliac arteries represents a small graft conduit sutured to the distal aorta into which the stent-graft was introduced for primary deployment. (Reprinted with permission from Rubin GD. CT angiography of the thoracic aorta. *Semin Roentgenol.* 2003;38:115–134.)

atheroembolism (Figs. 17-72, 17-73), iliac arterial injury, and retroperitoneal hematoma. Thus, the abdomen and pelvis should always be included in any perioperative scanning following thoracic aortic stent-graft deployment.

REFERENCES

1. Olsson C, Thelin S, Stahle E, et al. Thoracic aortic aneurysm and dissection: increasing prevalence and improved outcomes reported in a nationwide population-based study of more than 14,000 cases from 1987 to 2002. *Circulation.* 2006;114:2611–2618.
2. Lederle FA, Johnson GR, Wilson SE, et al. Prevalence and associations of abdominal aortic aneurysm detected through screening. Aneurysm Detection and Management (ADAM) Veterans Affairs Cooperative Study Group. *Ann Intern Med.* 1997;126:441–449.
3. Kouchoukos NT, Dougenis D. Surgery of the thoracic aorta. *N Engl J Med.* 1997;336:1876–1888.
4. Rubin GD. Helical CT angiography of the thoracic aorta. *J Thorac Imaging.* 1997;12:128–149.
5. Thurnher SA, Dorffner R, Thurnher MM, et al. Evaluation of abdominal aortic aneurysm for stent-graft placement: comparison of gadolinium-enhanced MR angiography versus helical CT angiography and digital subtraction angiography. *Radiology.* 1997;205:341–352.
6. Pavone P, Di Cesare E, Di Renzi P, et al. Abdominal aortic aneurysm evaluation: comparison of US, CT, MRI, and angiography. *Magn Reson Imaging.* 1990;8:199–204.
7. Hertz SM, Baum RA, Owen RS, et al. Comparison of magnetic resonance angiography and contrast arteriography in peripheral arterial stenosis. *Am J Surg.* 1993;166:112–116.
8. Hany TF, Debatin JF, Leung DA, et al. Evaluation of the aortoiliac and renal arteries: comparison of breath-hold, contrast-enhanced, three-dimensional MR angiography with conventional catheter angiography. *Radiology.* 1997;204:357–362.
9. Fox AD, Whiteley MS, Murphy P, et al. Comparison of magnetic resonance imaging measurements of abdominal aortic aneurysms with measurements obtained by other imaging techniques and intraoperative measurements: possible

implications for endovascular grafting. *J Vasc Surg*. 1996; 24:632–638.

10. Fain SB, King BF, Breen JF, et al. High-spatial-resolution contrast-enhanced MR angiography of the renal arteries: a prospective comparison with digital subtraction angiography. *Radiology*. 2001;218:481–490.

11. Rubin GD. CT angiography of the thoracic aorta. *Semin Roentgenol*. 2003;38:115–134.

12. Lawler LP, Fishman EK. Multi-detector row CT of thoracic disease with emphasis on 3D volume rendering and CT angiography. *Radiographics*. 2001;21:1257–1273.

13. Calhoun PS, Kuszyk BS, Heath DG, et al. Three-dimensional volume rendering of spiral CT data: theory and method. *Radiographics*. 1999;19:745–764.

14. Berry CL, Sosa-Melgarejo JA, Greenwald SE. The relationship between wall tension, lamellar thickness, and intercellular junctions in the fetal and adult aorta: its relevance to the pathology of dissecting aneurysm. *J Pathol*. 1993;169:15–20.

15. Harris JA, Bis KG, Glover JL, et al. Penetrating atherosclerotic ulcers of the aorta. *J Vasc Surg*. 1994;19:90–98; discussion 98–99.

16. Hayashi H, Matsuoka Y, Sakamoto I, et al. Penetrating atherosclerotic ulcer of the aorta: imaging features and disease concept. *Radiographics*. 2000;20:995–1005.

17. Merickel MB, Berr S, Spetz K, et al. Noninvasive quantitative evaluation of atherosclerosis using MRI and image analysis. *Arterioscler Thromb*. 1993;13:1180–1186.

18. Yamada I, Numano F, Suzuki S. Takayasu arteritis: evaluation with MR imaging. *Radiology*. 1993;188:89–94.

19. Rebergen SA, van der Wall EE, Doornbos J, et al. Magnetic resonance measurement of velocity and flow: technique, validation, and cardiovascular applications. *Am Heart J*. 1993;126:1439–1456.

20. Shipkowitz T, Rodgers VG, Frazin LJ, et al. Numerical study on the effect of secondary flow in the human aorta on local shear stresses in abdominal aortic branches. *J Biomech*. 2000;33:717–728.

21. Lotz J, Meier C, Leppert A, et al. Cardiovascular flow measurement with phase-contrast MR imaging: basic facts and implementation. *Radiographics*. 2002;22:651–671.

22. Rubin GD. Three-dimensional helical CT angiography. *Radiographics*. 1994;14:905–912.

23. Felmlee JP, Ehman RL. Spatial presaturation: a method for suppressing flow artifacts and improving depiction of vascular anatomy in MR imaging. *Radiology*. 1987;164: 559–564.

24. Nienaber CA, von Kodolitsch Y, Nicolas V, et al. The diagnosis of thoracic aortic dissection by noninvasive imaging procedures. *N Engl J Med*. 1993;328:1–9.

25. Mohiaddin RH, Schoser K, Amanuma M, et al. MR imaging of age-related dimensional changes of thoracic aorta. *J Comput Assist Tomogr*. 1990;14:748–752.

26. Link KM, Lesko NM. The role of MR imaging in the evaluation of acquired diseases of the thoracic aorta. *AJR Am J Roentgenol*. 1992;158:1115–1125.

27. Gaubert JY, Moulin G, Mesana T, et al. Type A dissection of the thoracic aorta: use of MR imaging for long- term follow-up. *Radiology*. 1995;196:363–369.

28. Rofsky NM, Weinreb JC, Grossi EA, et al. Aortic aneurysm and dissection: normal MR imaging and CT findings after surgical repair with the continuous-suture graft-inclusion technique. *Radiology*. 1993;186:195–201.

29. Lee YJ, Chung TS, Joo JY, et al. Suboptimal contrast-enhanced carotid MR angiography from the left brachiocephalic venous stasis. *J Magn Reson Imaging*. 1999;10:503–509.

30. Krinsky GA, Rofsky NM, DeCorato DR, et al. Thoracic aorta: comparison of gadolinium-enhanced three-dimensional MR angiography with conventional MR imaging. *Radiology*. 1997;202:183–193.

31. Boxt LM. How to perform cardiac MR imaging. *Magn Reson Imaging Clin N Am*. 1996;4:191–216.

32. Fischer SE, Wickline SA, Lorenz CH. Novel real-time R-wave detection algorithm based on the vectorcardiogram for accurate gated magnetic resonance acquisitions. *Magn Reson Med*. 1999;42:361–370.

33. Lee VS, Martin DJ, Krinsky GA, et al. Gadolinium-enhanced MR angiography: artifacts and pitfalls. *AJR Am J Roentgenol*. 2000;175:197–205.

34. Maki JH, Prince MR, Chenevert TC. Optimizing three-dimensional gadolinium-enhanced magnetic resonance angiography. Original investigation. *Invest Radiol*. 1998; 33:528–537.

35. Maki JH, Chenevert TL, Prince MR. Contrast-enhanced MR angiography. *Abdom Imaging*. 1998;23:469–484.

36. Earls JP, Rofsky NM, DeCorato DR, et al. Breath-hold single-dose gadolinium-enhanced three-dimensional MR aortography: usefulness of a timing examination and MR power injector. *Radiology*. 1996;201:705–710.

37. Prince MR, Chenevert TL, Foo TK, et al. Contrast-enhanced abdominal MR angiography: optimization of imaging delay time by automating the detection of contrast material arrival in an artery. *Radiology*. 1997;203:109–114.

38. Riederer SJ, Tasciyan T, Farzaneh F, et al. MR fluoroscopy: technical feasibility. *Magn Reson Med*. 1988;8:1–15.

39. Korosec FR, Frayne R, Grist TM, et al. Time-resolved contrast-enhanced 3D MR angiography. *Magn Reson Med*. 1996;36:345–351.

40. Siegelman ES, Charafeddine R, Stolpen AH, et al. Suppression of intravascular signal on fat-saturated contrast-enhanced thoracic MR arteriograms. *Radiology*. 2000;217:115–118.

41. Posniak HV, Olson MC, Demos TC, et al. CT of thoracic aortic aneurysms. *Radiographics*. 1990;10:839–855.

42. Aronberg DJ, Glazer HS, Madsen K, et al. Normal thoracic aortic diameters by computed tomography. *J Comput Assist Tomogr*. 1984;8:247–250.

43. Gray H, Lewis WH. *Anatomy of the Human Body*. 20th ed. Philadelphia: Lea & Febiger; 1918.

44. Brockstein B, Johns L, Gewertz BL. Blood supply to the spinal cord: anatomic and physiologic correlations. *Ann Vasc Surg*. 1994;8:394–399.

45. Koshino T, Murakami G, Morishita K, et al. Does the Adamkiewicz artery originate from the larger segmental arteries? *J Thorac Cardiovasc Surg*. 1999;117:898–905.

46. Morishita K, Murakami G, Fujisawa Y, et al. Anatomical study of blood supply to the spinal cord. *Ann Thorac Surg*. 2003;76:1967–1971.

47. Li AE, Kamel I, Rando F, et al. Using MRI to assess aortic wall thickness in the multiethnic study of atherosclerosis: distribution by race, sex, and age. *AJR Am J Roentgenol*. 2004;182:593–597.

48. Johnston KW, Rutherford RB, Tilson MD, et al. Suggested standards for reporting on arterial aneurysms. Subcommittee on Reporting Standards for Arterial Aneurysms, Ad Hoc Committee on Reporting Standards, Society for Vascular Surgery and North American Chapter, International Society for Cardiovascular Surgery. *J Vasc Surg*. 1991;13:452–458.

49. Garzon G, Fernandez-Velilla M, Marti M, et al. Endovascular stent-graft treatment of thoracic aortic disease. *Radiographics* 2005;25[Suppl 1]:S229–S244.

50. Coady MA, Rizzo JA, Goldstein LJ, et al. Natural history, pathogenesis, and etiology of thoracic aortic aneurysms and dissections. *Cardiol Clin*. 1999;17:vii, 615–635.

51. Bickerstaff LK, Pairolero PC, Hollier LH, et al. Thoracic aortic aneurysms: a population-based study. *Surgery*. 1982;92:1103–1108.

52. Frist WH, Miller DC. Repair of ascending aortic aneurysms and dissections. *J Card Surg*. 1986;1:33–52.

53. Joyce JW, Fairbairn JF 2nd, Kincaid OW, et al. Aneurysms of the thoracic aorta. A clinical study with special reference to prognosis. *Circulation*. 1964;29:176–181.

54. Moreno-Cabral CE, Miller DC, Mitchell RS, et al. Degenerative and atherosclerotic aneurysms of the thoracic aorta. Determinants of early and late surgical outcome. *J Thorac Cardiovasc Surg*. 1984;88:1020–1032.

55. Fedak PW, Verma S, David TE, et al. Clinical and pathophysiological implications of a bicuspid aortic valve. *Circulation*. 2002;106:900–904.

56. Osler W. The Gulstonian lectures on malignant endocarditis. *Br Med J*. 1885;1:467–472.
57. Long R, Guzman R, Greenberg H, et al. Tuberculous mycotic aneurysm of the aorta: review of published medical and surgical experience. *Chest*. 1999;115:522–531.
58. Silbergleit A, Arbulu A. Tuberculous mycotic aneurysms. *Chest*. 1999;116:1142.
59. Gomes MN, Choyke PL, Wallace RB. Infected aortic aneurysms. A changing entity. *Ann Surg*. 1992;215:435–442.
60. Duke RA, Barrett MR 2nd, Payne SD, et al. Compression of left main bronchus and left pulmonary artery by thoracic aortic aneurysm. *AJR Am J Roentgenol*. 1987;149:261–263.
61. Penner C, Maycher B, Light RB. Compression of the left main bronchus between a descending thoracic aortic aneurysm and an enlarged right pulmonary artery. *Chest*. 1994;106:959–961.
62. Englund R, Hudson P, Hanel K, et al. Expansion rates of small abdominal aortic aneurysms. *Aust N Z J Surg*. 1998; 68:21–24.
63. Rasmussen TE, Hallett JW Jr. Inflammatory aortic aneurysms. A clinical review with new perspectives in pathogenesis. *Ann Surg*. 1997;225:155–164.
64. Brown LC, Powell JT. Risk factors for aneurysm rupture in patients kept under ultrasound surveillance. UK Small Aneurysm Trial Participants. *Ann Surg*. 1999;230:289–296.
65. Lederle FA, Johnson GR, Wilson SE, et al. The aneurysm detection and management study screening program: validation cohort and final results. Aneurysm Detection and Management Veterans Affairs Cooperative Study Investigators. *Arch Intern Med*. 2000;160:1425–1430.
66. Machida K, Tasaka A. CT patterns of mural thrombus in aortic aneurysms. *J Comput Assist Tomogr*. 1980;4: 840–842.
67. Heiberg E, Wolverson MK, Sundaram M, et al. CT characteristics of aortic atherosclerotic aneurysm versus aortic dissection. *J Comput Assist Tomogr*. 1985;9:78–83.
68. Demos TC, Posniak HV, Churchill RJ. Detection of the intimal flap of aortic dissection on unenhanced CT images. *AJR Am J Roentgenol*. 1986;146:601–603.
69. Godwin JD. Examination of the thoracic aorta by computed tomography. *Chest*. 1984;85:564–567.
70. Vogelzang RL, Sohaey R. Infected aortic aneurysms: CT appearance. *J Comput Assist Tomogr*. 1988;12:109–112.
71. Kucich VA, Vogelzang RL, Hartz RS, et al. Ruptured thoracic aneurysm: unusual manifestation and early diagnosis using CT. *Radiology*. 1986;160:87–89.
72. Coblentz CL, Sallee DS, Chiles C. Aortobronchopulmonary fistula complicating aortic aneurysm: diagnosis in four cases. *AJR Am J Roentgenol*. 1988;150:535–538.
73. Treasure T. Cardiovascular surgery for Marfan syndrome. *Heart*. 2000;84:674–678.
74. Spielvogel D, Halstead JC, Meier M, et al. Aortic arch replacement using a trifurcated graft: simple, versatile, and safe. *Ann Thorac Surg*. 2005;80:90–95.
75. Borst HG, Walterbusch G, Schaps D. Extensive aortic replacement using "elephant trunk" prosthesis. *Thorac Cardiovasc Surg*. 1983;31:37–40.
76. Posniak HV, Demos TC, Olson MC. Coronary artery interposition graft simulating pseudoaneurysm of the ascending aorta on CT. *AJR Am J Roentgenol*. 1994;163: 1368–1370.
77. Quint LE, Francis IR, Williams DM, et al. Synthetic interposition grafts of the thoracic aorta: postoperative appearance on serial CT studies. *Radiology*. 1999;211:317–324.
78. Bentall H, De Bono A. A technique for complete replacement of the ascending aorta. *Thorax*. 1968;23:338–339.
79. Cabrol C, Pavie A, Gandjbakhch I, et al. Complete replacement of the ascending aorta with reimplantation of the coronary arteries: new surgical approach. *J Thorac Cardiovasc Surg*. 1981;81:309–315.
80. Svensson LG, Crawford ES, Hess KR, et al. Composite valve graft replacement of the proximal aorta: comparison of techniques in 348 patients. *Ann Thorac Surg*. 1992;54: 427–437.
81. Fattori R, Descovich B, Bertaccini P, et al. Composite graft replacement of the ascending aorta: leakage detection with gadolinium-enhanced MR imaging. *Radiology*. 1999;212:573–577.
82. Mitchell RS. Endovascular stent graft repair of thoracic aortic aneurysms. *Semin Thorac Cardiovasc Surg*. 1997;9:257–268.
83. Greenberg R, Risher W. Clinical decision making and operative approaches to thoracic aortic aneurysms. *Surg Clin North Am*. 1998;78:805–826.
84. Vilacosta I, Roman JAS. Acute aortic syndrome. *Heart*. 2001;85:365–368.
85. Reddy GP, Higgins CB. MR imaging of the thoracic aorta. *Magn Reson Imaging Clin N Am*. 2000;8:vii, 1–15.
86. Nienaber CA, Eagle KA. Aortic dissection: new frontiers in diagnosis and management. Part I: From etiology to diagnostic strategies. *Circulation*. 2003;108:628–635.
87. Solomon SL, Brown JJ, Glazer HS, et al. Thoracic aortic dissection: pitfalls and artifacts in MR imaging. *Radiology*. 1990;177:223–228.
88. Vilacosta I. Acute aortic syndrome. *Rev Esp Cardiol*. 2003; 56:29–39.
89. Murray JG, Manisali M, Flamm SD, et al. Intramural hematoma of the thoracic aorta: MR image findings and their prognostic implications. *Radiology*. 1997;204: 349–355.
90. Kreitner KF, Kunz RP, Kalden P, et al. Contrast-enhanced three-dimensional MR angiography of the thoracic aorta: experiences after 118 examinations with a standard dose contrast administration and different injection protocols. *Eur Radiol*. 2001;11:1355–1363.
91. Stanson AW, Kazmier FJ, Hollier LH, et al. Penetrating atherosclerotic ulcers of the thoracic aorta: natural history and clinicopathologic correlations. *Ann Vasc Surg*. 1986;1: 15–23.
92. Ganaha F, Miller DC, Sugimoto K, et al. Prognosis of aortic intramural hematoma with and without penetrating atherosclerotic ulcer: a clinical and radiological analysis. *Circulation*. 2002;106:342–348.
93. Absi TS, Sundt TM 3rd, Camillo C, et al. Penetrating atherosclerotic ulcers of the descending thoracic aorta may be managed expectantly. *Vascular*. 2004;12:307–311.
94. Cho KR, Stanson AW, Potter DD, et al. Penetrating atherosclerotic ulcer of the descending thoracic aorta and arch. *J Thorac Cardiovasc Surg*. 2004;127:1393–1399; discussion 1399–1401.
95. Wooley CF, Sparks EH, Boudoulas H. Aortic pain. *Prog Cardiovasc Dis*. 1998;40:563–589.
96. Miller JS, Lemaire SA, Coselli JS. Evaluating aortic dissection: when is coronary angiography indicated? *Heart*. 2000;83:615–616.
97. Roberts WC. Aortic dissection: anatomy, consequences, and causes. *Am Heart J*. 1981;101:195–214.
98. Tiessen IM, Roach MR. Factors in the initiation and propagation of aortic dissections in human autopsy aortas. *J Biomech Eng*. 1993;115:123–125.
99. Takagi H, Umemoto T. Homocysteinemia is a risk factor for aortic dissection. *Med Hypotheses*. 2005;64:1007–1010.
100. Muller BT, Modlich O, Prisack HB, et al. Gene expression profiles in the acutely dissected human aorta. *Eur J Vasc Endovasc Surg*. 2002;24:356–364.
101. Ishii T, Asuwa N. Collagen and elastin degradation by matrix metalloproteinases and tissue inhibitors of matrix metalloproteinase in aortic dissection. *Hum Pathol*. 2000;31:640–646.
102. Gutierrez PS, de Almeida IC, Nader HB, et al. Decrease in sulphated glycosaminoglycans in aortic dissection—possible role in the pathogenesis. *Cardiovasc Res*. 1991;25: 742–748.
103. Flamm SD, VanDyke CW, White RD. MR imaging of the thoracic aorta. *Magn Reson Imaging Clin N Am*. 1996;4: 217–235.
104. Sakamoto I, Hayashi K, Matsunaga N, et al. Aortic dissection caused by angiographic procedures. *Radiology*. 1994;191:467–471.

105. Meszaros I, Morocz J, Szlavi J, et al. Epidemiology and clinicopathology of aortic dissection. *Chest.* 2000;117:1271–1278.
106. Nienaber CA, Eagle KA. Aortic dissection: new frontiers in diagnosis and management. Part II: Therapeutic management and follow-up. *Circulation.* 2003;108:772–778.
107. Kouchoukos NT, Daily BB, Rokkas CK, et al. Hypothermic bypass and circulatory arrest for operations on the descending thoracic and thoracoabdominal aorta. *Ann Thorac Surg.* 1995;60:67–76.
108. DeBakey ME, McCollum CH, Crawford ES, et al. Dissection and dissecting aneurysms of the aorta: twenty-year follow-up of five hundred twenty-seven patients treated surgically. *Surgery.* 1982;92:1118–1134.
109. DeBakey ME, Henly WS, Cooley DA, et al. Surgical management of dissecting aneurysms of the aorta. *J Thorac Cardiovasc Surg.* 1965;49:130–148.
110. Ergin MA, O'Connor J, Guinto R, et al. Experience with profound hypothermia and circulatory arrest in the treatment of aneurysms of the aortic arch. Aortic arch replacement for acute arch dissections. *J Thorac Cardiovasc Surg.* 1982;84:649–655.
111. Evangelista A, Dominguez R, Sebastia C, et al. Long-term follow-up of aortic intramural hematoma: predictors of outcome. *Circulation.* 2003;108:583–589.
112. Suzuki T, Katoh H, Tsuchio Y, et al. Diagnostic implications of elevated levels of smooth-muscle myosin heavy-chain protein in acute aortic dissection. The smooth muscle myosin heavy chain study. *Ann Intern Med.* 2000;133:537–541.
113. Khan IA, Nair CK. Clinical, diagnostic, and management perspectives of aortic dissection. *Chest.* 2002;122:311–328.
114. Sueyoshi E, Sakamoto I, Hayashi K, et al. Growth rate of aortic diameter in patients with type B aortic dissection during the chronic phase. *Circulation.* 2004;110:II256–II261.
115. Gomes AS, Bettmann MA, Casciani T, et al. Expert Panel on Cardiovascular Imaging. *Acute Chest Pain—Suspected Aortic Dissection.* Reston, VA: American College of Radiology (ACR), 2005.
116. Nienaber CA, Fattori R, Lund G, et al. Nonsurgical reconstruction of thoracic aortic dissection by stent-graft placement. *N Engl J Med.* 1999;340:1539–1545.
117. Hernandez-Gonzalez M, Solorio S, Conde-Carmona I, et al. Intraluminal aortoplasty vs. surgical aortic resection in congenital aortic coarctation. A clinical random study in pediatric patients. *Arch Med Res.* 2003;34:305–310.
118. von Kodolitsch Y, Csosz SK, Koschyk DH, et al. Intramural hematoma of the aorta: predictors of progression to dissection and rupture. *Circulation.* 2003;107:1158–1163.
119. Eggebrecht H, Naber CK, Bruch C, et al. Value of plasma fibrin D-dimers for detection of acute aortic dissection. *J Am Coll Cardiol.* 2004;44:804–809.
120. Dake MD, Kato N, Mitchell RS, et al. Endovascular stent-graft placement for the treatment of acute aortic dissection. *N Engl J Med.* 1999;340:1546–1552.
121. Fattori R, Napoli G, Lovato L, et al. Descending thoracic aortic diseases: stent-graft repair. *Radiology.* 2003;229:176–183.
122. Lee DY, Williams DM, Abrams GD. The dissected aorta: part II. Differentiation of the true from the false lumen with intravascular US. *Radiology.* 1997;203:32–36.
123. Hayashi H, Onda M, Takagi R, et al. [CT analysis of aortic cobwebs in aortic dissection.] *Nippon Igaku Hoshasen Gakkai Zasshi.* 1995;55:402–408.
124. Williams DM, Joshi A, Dake MD, et al. Aortic cobwebs: an anatomic marker identifying the false lumen in aortic dissection—imaging and pathologic correlation. *Radiology.* 1994;190:167–174.
125. Sueyoshi E, Matsuoka Y, Sakamoto I, et al. Fate of intramural hematoma of the aorta: CT evaluation. *J Comput Assist Tomogr.* 1997;21:931–938.
126. Blackmore CC, Zweibel A, Mann FA. Determining risk of traumatic aortic injury: how to optimize imaging strategy. *AJR Am J Roentgenol.* 2000;174:343–347.
127. Creasy JD, Chiles C, Routh WD, et al. Overview of traumatic injury of the thoracic aorta. *Radiographics.* 1997;17:27–45.
128. Parmley LF, Mattingly TW, Manion WC, et al. Nonpenetrating traumatic injury of the aorta. *Circulation.* 1958;17:1086–1101.
129. Gleason TG, Bavaria JE. Trauma to the great vessels. In: Cohn LH, Edmunds LH, eds. *Cardiac Surgery in the Adult.* New York: McGraw-Hill; 2003:1229–1250.
130. Alkadhi H, Wildermuth S, Desbiolles L, et al. Vascular emergencies of the thorax after blunt and iatrogenic trauma: multi-detector row CT and three-dimensional imaging. *Radiographics.* 2004;24:1239–1255.
131. Groskin SA. Selected topics in chest trauma. *Radiology.* 1992;183:605–617.
132. Beel T, Harwood AL. Traumatic rupture of the thoracic aorta. *Ann Emerg Med.* 1980;9:483–486.
133. Sevitt S. The mechanisms of traumatic rupture of the thoracic aorta. *Br J Surg.* 1977;64:166–173.
134. Crass JR, Cohen AM, Motta AO, et al. A proposed new mechanism of traumatic aortic rupture: the osseous pinch. *Radiology.* 1990;176:645–649.
135. Burke AP, Virmani R. Sarcomas of the great vessels. A clinicopathologic study. *Cancer.* 1993;71:1761–1773.
136. Golli M, Said M, Gamra H, et al. Primary leiomyosarcoma of the thoracic aorta mimicking aortic dissection. *Ann Saudi Med.* 2000;20:265–266.
137. Akiyama K, Nakata K, Negishi N, et al. Intimal sarcoma of the thoracic aorta; clinical-course and autopsy finding. *Ann Thorac Cardiovasc Surg.* 2005;11:135–138.
138. Schipper J, van Oostayen JA, den Hollander JC, et al. Aortic tumours: report of a case and review of the literature. *Br J Radiol.* 1989;62:35–40.
139. Glock Y, Laghzaoui A, Wang J, et al. [Fissured leiomyosarcoma of the descending thoracic aorta. Apropos of a case and review of the literature.] *Arch Mal Coeur Vaiss.* 1997;90:1317–1320.
140. Iorgulescu DG, White AL. Leiomyosarcoma of the thoracic aorta. *Aust N Z J Surg.* 1999;69:537–540.
141. Navarra G, Occhionorelli S, Mascoli F, et al. Primary leiomyosarcoma of the aorta: report of a case and review of the literature. *J Cardiovasc Surg (Torino).* 1994;35:333–336.
142. Kevorkian J, Cento DP. Leiomyosarcoma of large arteries and veins. *Surgery.* 1973;73:390–400.
143. Pompilio G, Tartara P, Varesi C, et al. Intimal-type primary sarcoma of the thoracic aorta: an unusual case presenting with left arm embolization. *Eur J Cardiothorac Surg.* 2002;21:574–576.
144. Seelig MH, Klingler PJ, Oldenburg WA, et al. Angiosarcoma of the aorta: report of a case and review of the literature. *J Vasc Surg.* 1998;28:732–737.
145. Cambria RP, Clouse WD, Davison JK, et al. Thoracoabdominal aneurysm repair: results with 337 operations performed over a 15-year interval. *Ann Surg.* 2002;236:471–479.
146. Safi HJ, Campbell MP, Ferreira ML, et al. Spinal cord protection in descending thoracic and thoracoabdominal aortic aneurysm repair. *Semin Thorac Cardiovasc Surg.* 1998;10:41–44.
147. Hollier LH, Money SR, Naslund TC, et al. Risk of spinal cord dysfunction in patients undergoing thoracoabdominal aortic replacement. *Am J Surg.* 1992;164:210–213.
148. von Oppell UO, Dunne TT, De Groot KM, et al. Spinal cord protection in the absence of collateral circulation: meta-analysis of mortality and paraplegia. *J Card Surg.* 1994;9:685–691.
149. Berendes JN, Bredee JJ, Schipperheyn JJ, et al. Mechanisms of spinal cord injury after cross-clamping of the descending thoracic aorta. *Circulation.* 1982;66:I112–I116.
150. Safi HJ, Winnerkvist A, Miller CC 3rd, et al. Effect of extended cross-clamp time during thoracoabdominal aortic aneurysm repair. *Ann Thorac Surg.* 1998;66:1204–1209.
151. Griepp RB, Ergin MA, Galla JD, et al. Looking for the artery of Adamkiewicz: a quest to minimize paraplegia after operations for aneurysms of the descending thoracic and thoracoabdominal aorta. *J Thorac Cardiovasc Surg.* 1996;112:1202–1213.

152. Biglioli P, Roberto M, Cannata A, et al. Upper and lower spinal cord blood supply: the continuity of the anterior spinal artery and the relevance of the lumbar arteries. *J Thorac Cardiovasc Surg*. 2004;127:1188–1192.

153. Heinemann MK, Brassel F, Herzog T, et al. The role of spinal angiography in operations on the thoracic aorta: myth or reality? *Ann Thorac Surg*. 1998;65:346–351.

154. Williams GM, Perler BA, Burdick JF, et al. Angiographic localization of spinal cord blood supply and its relationship to postoperative paraplegia. *J Vasc Surg*. 1991;13:23–33.

155. Kieffer E, Richard T, Chiras J, et al. Preoperative spinal cord arteriography in aneurysmal disease of the descending thoracic and thoracoabdominal aorta: preliminary results in 45 patients. *Ann Vasc Surg*. 1989;3:34–46.

156. Yoshioka K, Niinuma H, Ohira A, et al. MR angiography and CT angiography of the artery of Adamkiewicz: noninvasive preoperative assessment of thoracoabdominal aortic aneurysm. *Radiographics*. 2003;23:1215–1225.

157. Mita T, Arita T, Matsunaga N, et al. Complications of endovascular repair for thoracic and abdominal aortic aneurysm: an imaging spectrum. *Radiographics*. 2000;20:1263–1278.

158. Jacobs NM, Godwin JD, Wolfe WG, et al. Evaluation of the grafted ascending aorta with computed tomography. *Radiology*. 1982;145:749–753.

159. Mark AS, McCarthy SM, Moss AA, et al. Detection of abdominal aortic graft infection: comparison of CT and in-labeled white blood cell scans. *AJR Am J Roentgenol*. 1985;144:315–318.

160. Wain RA, Marin ML, Ohki T, et al. Endoleaks after endovascular graft treatment of aortic aneurysms: classification, risk factors, and outcome. *J Vasc Surg*. 1998;27:69–78.

Abdominal Aorta

CHAPTER
18

W. Dennis Foley
F. Scott Pereles

COMPUTED TOMOGRAPHIC ANGIOGRAPHY

Computed tomographic angiography (CTA) has become a standard technique for preoperative evaluation of patients with abdominal aortic abnormalities. In the presence of abdominal aortic aneurysm (AAA), information provided by CTA includes aneurysm dimension (both longitudinal and transverse) and lumen size; length and diameter of superior and inferior neck; patency of aortic branch vessels, particularly mesenteric and renal; and degree and extent of atherosclerotic disease involving the iliac arteries. CTA has been used to study infrarenal, juxtarenal, and suprarenal AAAs as well as thoracoabdominal aneurysms. CTA implemented with a multidetector row CT system has now replaced conventional catheter arteriography for preoperative and preintervention evaluation.

Exam Technique

Based on the principles discussed in Chapters 1 and 4, abdominal aortic CTA should result in an intraluminal attenuation of the abdominal aorta and iliac arteries of at least 250 Hounsfield units (HU) and preferably 300 to 400 HU throughout the duration of acquisition.

Aortoiliac studies for juxtarenal and infrarenal AAAs are designed to cover the region from the supraceliac aorta to the femoral artery bifurcation and proximal superficial and profunda femoral arteries (Fig. 18-1). In patients with suprarenal aneurysms that may incorporate the celiac and superior mesenteric arteries, the imaging test should include the full extent of the thoracoabdominal aorta and iliac vessels in order to determine the presence of a coexistent ectatic or aneurysmal thoracic aorta, particularly one that is in continuity with a suprarenal aneurysm at the level of the aortic hiatus (Fig. 18-2).

There are three general principles in designing an aortoiliac CTA protocol. These relate to arterial enhancement, coverage speed and breath-hold interval, and z-axis resolution.

Arterial Enhancement

As stated above, uniform aortoiliac enhancement of 250 to 300 HU throughout the full longitudinal extent of the vasculature

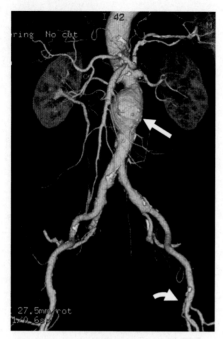

FIGURE 18-1 Typical area coverage for aortoiliac CT angiographic study of patient with suspected abdominal aortic aneurysm. VR in a frontal projection demonstrates anatomic coverage from the supraceliac aorta to proximal thigh (up to the level of the common femoral arteries bifurcation, *curved arrow*). All abdominal visceral branch vessels (including the IMA, which is patent and emerges from the aneurysm, *arrow*) and the bilateral common iliac, internal iliac, external iliac, common femoral and proximal superficial and profunda femoral arteries are displayed.

is an important goal. This provides adequate contrast between vessel lumen, lining thrombus, and mural calcification and is necessary for adequate segmentation of the aortoiliac vasculature for three-dimensional (3D) rendering (Fig. 18-3). In addition, delineation of abdominal visceral branch vessels, including celiac, mesenteric, and renal, is likewise improved with a 250 to 300 HU intraluminal arterial enhancement.

Arterial enhancement in conjunction with z-axis resolution are important factors in delineating arterial stenoses, particularly in branch vessels that are parallel to the primary transverse section, such as the renal arteries.

Empiric observation has demonstrated that an injection rate of 5 cc/second of 300 to 370 mg iodine/mL contrast concentration and a minimum 50-cc contrast volume will result in elevation of abdominal aortic attenuation to 250 to 300 HU in the majority of patients. Physiological variables that affect enhancement include heart rate and stroke volume (the two factors that determine cardiac output) and total blood volume. Relative contrast dilution will occur in patients with increased cardiac output and blood volume, whereas relative contrast enhancement will occur in patients with decreased cardiac output and blood volume. Elderly patients with relatively poor cardiac output may have surprisingly good aortoiliac contrast enhancement, although the bolus arrival is relatively delayed, the bolus is more compact related to relatively low stroke volume and cardiac output. However, flow deceleration and poor admixture in the relatively static blood pool of an AAA is not unusual and may result in suboptimal opacification (Fig. 18-4).

Patient arm positioning is an important consideration in that elevating the arm by placing the palm of the hand against the face of the gantry allows for a relatively smooth flow of the injected contrast bolus from the upper extremity venous circulation into the superior vena cava. If the arm is placed behind the patient's head in the same axis as the body, venous constriction at the thoracic inlet between the clavicle and the first costoclavicular junction may result in significant delay in delivery of the contrast bolus to the superior vena cava and right heart. In conjunction with proper arm position, a saline flush system that follows the administered

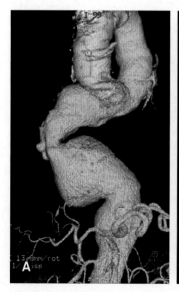
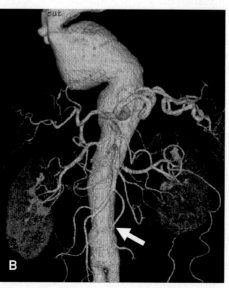

FIGURE 18-2 Thoracoabdominal aortic aneurysm. A: VR display in frontal projection of tortuous aneurysmal descending thoracic and suprarenal abdominal aortic aneurysm. There is marked tortuosity and multifocal aneurysmal disease of the descending thoracic aorta in contiguity with a suprarenal aneurysm incorporating the celiac and superior mesenteric arteries. **B:** VR display in frontal projection of the distal thoracic aorta and abdominal aorta demonstrates the ectatic juxta and infrarenal aorta caudal to the aneurysmal thoracic and suprarenal aorta. Proximal margin of an aortobiiliac graft is seen in the distal aorta (*arrow*).

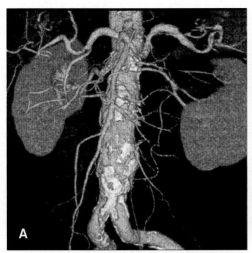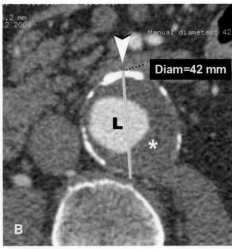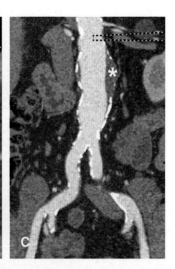

FIGURE 18-3 Intraluminal contrast attenuation as compared with lining mural thrombus and mural calcification. A: VR in a mild left anterior oblique projection of fusiform infrarenal aortic aneurysm demonstrates mural calcification as white plaque and vessel contrast in light yellow. **B:** Axial scans through the midsection of the aneurysm demonstrating aortic lumen (*L*), lining thrombus (*∗*), and circumferential mural calcification (*arrowhead*). External AP diameter of the aneurysm is 42 mm. **C:** Curved planar reformation in a frontal projection of the abdominal aorta and right common and external iliac arteries demonstrates lining mural thrombus (*∗*) and mural calcification in this infrarenal aneurysm. Linear measurements with *dotted lines* represent the measurement of the superior neck length—in this patient less than 10 mm and unsuitable for stent grafting.

bolus with a 20 to 30 mL saline flush injected at the same rate as the contrast bolus will effectively clear the administered contrast medium from the upper extremity venous circulation, allowing the full injected contrast bolus to be delivered to the aortoiliac system during acquisition. When saline flush is not used, some of the injected bolus will remain as a relatively static contrast column in the upper extremity veins following the end of the power injection.

The length of the contrast bolus injection approximates the length of the acquisition interval plus an additional 4 to

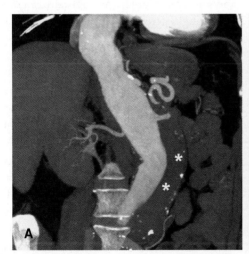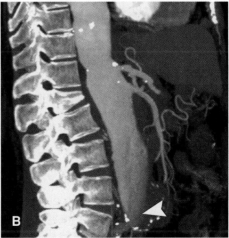

FIGURE 18-4 Contrast layering in an AAA of an elderly patient with thoracoabdominal aneurysm, marginal renal function, and a prior episode of contrast-induced nephropathy. The study was performed with limited contrast volume—60 mL of IsoVue 370 (Bracco Diagnostics, Princeton, NJ)—on a 64-channel scanner (LightSpeed VCT—General Electric Medical Systems, Waukesha, WI) at a table speed of 11 cm/second. **A:** Thin-section planar MIP in frontal projection demonstrates extensive fusiform aneurysm of the inferior thoracic and the abdominal aorta extending to the aortic bifurcation. There is prominent lining mural thrombus (*∗*) and mural calcification. Contrast opacity in the infrarenal aorta is suboptimal. **B:** Thin-section planar MIP in lateral projection. Note the contrast layering and poor admixture in the infrarenal aorta (*arrowhead*). This appearance is probably due to "poor mixing" of the contrast bolus and relatively slow arterial flow within the aneurysm sac. There are normally patent celiac and superior mesenteric arteries. Note the wedge compression of T12 vertebral body. Despite the contrast layering in the abdominal aortic component of the aneurysm, the study was adequate for preoperative planning.

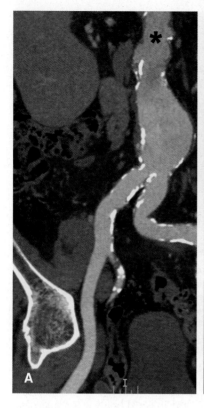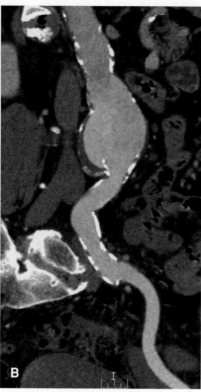

FIGURE 18-5 Progressively increasing enhancement in the cephalocaudal dimension of the aorta and iliac arteries. If a 4-channel MDCT system is used and acquisition interval is greater than 10 seconds, increasing arterial attenuation can be secondary to recirculation of the contrast bolus. In this patient studied with the 64-channel scanner and a short injection duration interval of 8 seconds, the table speed is lower than the arterial flow velocity. The low attenuation contrast medium in the proximal aorta represents the front end of the contrast bolus. **A:** Curved planar reformation of the aorta and the right common and external iliac arteries in an oblique projection. There is a fusiform infrarenal aortic aneurysm. Note the relatively decreased attenuation in the cephalad aspect of the abdominal aorta (*) and the progressive increase in arterial attenuation from the supraceliac aorta to the distal external iliac artery. **B:** Curved planar reformation of the aorta and left common and external iliac arteries in an oblique projection. Similar findings of a progressive increase in arterial attenuation from the supraceliac aorta to the distal external iliac artery.

6 seconds that accounts for the up slope of enhancement after contrast arrival in the aorta and is due to spreading of the contrast bolus in the arterial tree. This approach to injection/acquisition aims to image the aortoiliac arterial tree during a relative plateau of sustained enhancement. The acquisition interval will depend on the cephalocaudad distance of the imaging field and the coverage speed, which in turn is dependent on beam width, pitch, and scan rotation speed. For injection durations and acquisition intervals greater than 10 seconds, contrast recirculation through the cerebral and renal circuits can result in incremental increases in aortic and iliac attenuation in the more caudal aspect of the imaging field (1) (Fig. 18-5).

Coverage Speed and Breath-hold Interval

Volume coverage speed should be related to the cephalocaudad dimension of the imaging field, which for an aortoiliac acquisition extending from the supraceliac aorta to the proximal thigh can approximate 40 to 50 cm, depending on individual patient body habitus. A practical factor in determining coverage speed is a suitable breath-hold interval. If an upper limit of suitable breath-hold interval of 20 seconds is accepted, this will then determine the acquisition parameters for a 4-, 8- or 16-channel multidetector computed tomography (MDCT) systems. Patient breath holding is necessary for a satisfactory abdominal CT angiographic study,

though acceptable CT rendering of the iliac and proximal thigh circulation can be obtained with the patient in quiet breathing. This switch to quiet breathing midway through the scan was utilized when aortoiliac studies were obtained with single-detector helical CT systems but is generally unnecessary with MDCT.

Circulation Timing

Individual patient circulation time may be obtained for a preliminary mini bolus, usually 5 cc/second for 15 cc total. Single-level low-dose imaging of the aorta at the level of the celiac artery is performed beginning 10 seconds after the beginning of injection with one image every 2–3 seconds. This will provide an aortic time-attenuation curve, consisting of arrival time, up slope, time to peak, and washout. Computer modeling with verification in a porcine model has demonstrated that the delay time between aortic peak on a 3-second mini bolus and aortic peak on an 8- to 12-second injection bolus approximates 4 to 6 seconds (2). If time from beginning of injection to 4 seconds after aortic peak on the mini bolus is chosen as the injection to scan delay for the subsequent CT angiogram, it is appropriate to make the injection interval equal to the acquisition interval plus 4 seconds and to achieve adequate and relatively uniform aortoiliac enhancement throughout the cephalocaudad extent of acquisition.

An alternative approach is to utilize online bolus tracking software to determine aortic arrival by establishing a preset threshold of enhancement. If 150 HU is the threshold, then acquisition may be initiated within a relatively short time after aortic arrival of the contrast bolus. This delay time will vary with individual vendors and will depend on image reconstruction interval and time to initiate helical scanning. If reconstruction and display takes 2 seconds and time for helical scan initiation an additional 3 seconds, there will be a 5-second delay between aortic arrival and initiation of scanning. This can be compensated by increasing the total injection duration by 5 seconds. A slower initial rate of injection can be utilized with this approach.

Two additional pharmacokinetic factors influence aortic attenuation throughout the duration of injection. These are (a) relative lengthening of the contrast bolus in the pulmonary and systemic circulation prior to aortic arrival and (b) as previously stated, the recirculation of the contrast bolus in the cerebral and renal circuits that can incrementally increase aortic attenuation in the more caudal aspect of the imaging field (1).

Protocol Development (4-, 8-, and 16-Channel Computed Tomography Scanners)

For a cephalocaudad coverage of 30 cm (supraceliac aorta to femoral artery bifurcation) and a 4-channel MDCT system with a detector collimation of 1.25 mm, beam width 5 mm, gantry rotation speed of 0.5 seconds, and pitch value of 1.5, the table speed is 15 mm/second and acquisition duration is 20 seconds. Acquisition duration is increased with an increase in the gantry rotation time or cephalocaudad coverage or with

a decrease in pitch. If the contrast injection duration is made equal to the acquisition duration (20 seconds) plus a delay time between aortic arrival and the beginning of scanning (4 seconds) and a contrast injection rate of 5 mL/second into an antecubital vein is used, then the total contrast volume is 120 mL (Table 18-1). Acquisition duration will increase with increasing gantry rotation time and increased cephalocaudad coverage, and contrast load will be increased proportionately. Contrast concentration may vary from 300 to 370 mg iodine/mL. Increased contrast concentration will result in increased aortic attenuation, all other acquisition and physiological factors being equal.

In the progression from a 4- to 8-channel MDCT system (e.g., General Electric LightSpeed Plus to General LightSpeed Ultra, General Electric Healthcare, Milwaukee, Wisconsin), beam width is doubled for the same detector collimation (1.25-mm). For the same scan rotation speed and pitch value, acquisition duration is halved. In actual practice, the pitch value for the 8-channel system can be set at 1.35 as compared to 1.5 for the 4-channel system. For 0.5-second scan rotation speed, 30-cm cephalocaudad coverage is accomplished in 12-seconds as compared to 20-seconds for the 4-channel system. Using the paradigm of mini bolus timing and making injection interval equal to acquisition interval plus 4-seconds, total contrast load is reduced to 80-ml (5-ml/second for 16-seconds) (Table 18-1).

For a 16-channel MDCT system (e.g., General Electric LightSpeed 16), detector collimation can be reduced to 0.625 mm for the same 10-mm beam width as utilized for the 8-channel systems. This results in identical acquisition interval for a 16-channel CT system as the 8-channel

TABLE 18-1

Generalized Parameters Commonly Recommended for Abdominal Aorta Coverage (Cephalocaudad Coverage 300 mm)[a]

	Number of Channels				
	4	**8**	**16**	**16**	**64**
Acquisition parameters					
Detector collimation (mm)	1.25	1.25	0.625	1.250	0.625
Beam width (mm)	5.0	10.0	10.0	20.0	40.0
Pitch	1.5	1.35	1.375	1.375	1.375
Scan rotation speed (second)	0.5	0.5	0.5	0.5	0.5
Table speed (mm/second)	15.0	27.0	27.5	55.0	110.0
Injection parameters					
Rate (mL/sec)	5	5	5	5	6
Volume (mL)	120	80	80	50 to 60	60

[a]Cephalocaudad coverage may vary between 300 and 400 mm, depending on the body habitus of the patient. Increasing cephalocaudad coverage and using slower scan rotation speeds (e.g., 0.6 to 0.8 seconds) will result in longer acquisition intervals and proportionately increased contrast load requirements. The numbers in this table relate to coverage of 300 mm and a gantry rotation speed of 0.5 seconds. Example parameters specifically given for General Electric (Milwaukee, Wisconsin) CT scanners are generalizable to similar scanners from other manufacturers.

system but an improvement in z-axis resolution and provides a nearly isotropic volume data set (Table 18-1). For a 30-cm field of view with a 512 × 512 matrix, voxel dimensions are 0.6 × 0.6 in the *xy*-plane and 0.625 mm in the longitudinal axis. Actual measured longitudinal resolution approximates 0.8 mm.

With 4- and 8-channel MDCT systems, improved longitudinal resolution can be obtained by overlapping reconstructions utilizing 50% overlap. However, the longitudinal resolution of overlapped 1.25-mm axial sections is still inferior to contiguous 0.625-mm sections.

Although an 80-mL contrast injection (supplemented by 15-mL preliminary mini bolus) is an acceptable contrast load for patients with marginal renal function, further reduction in contrast load can be achieved when the 16-channel scanner is operated with 1.25-mm detector collimation and a 20-mm beam width. This will double the coverage speed for the 16-channel system if the same pitch value and scan rotation speed are used. Acquisition interval can approximate 6 seconds. Satisfactory patient studies may be obtained with a minimum of 50 cc of contrast material injected at 5 cc/second. For these very short acquisition times, precise determination of circulation time is an absolute prerequisite (Table 18-1).

For patients with suprarenal aneurysms involving the aortic hiatus or patients with suspected or known thoracoabdominal aneurysms, a total thoracoabdominal aortic and iliac study are required. In this circumstance, the cephalocaudad coverage is approximately 60 cm. For a 4-channel MDCT system utilizing 2.5-mm detector collimation, pitch value 1.5, and gantry rotation speed 0.5-seconds, z-axis coverage is 3 cm/second and the total study can be obtained in a 20-second time interval, corresponding to a comfortable breath-hold interval for most patients (Table 18-2).

If the paradigm of preliminary mini bolus timing is used, the aortic time-attenuation curve is obtained from the level of the mid ascending aorta, again using a 5-cc bolus injection over 3 seconds.

For the 8-channel MDCT system, the same beam width of 10 mm as a 4-channel system (with detector collimation 2.5 mm) can be utilized and the detector collimation reduced from 2.5 to 1.25 mm. With pitch value set at 1.35 (8-channel) in comparison to 1.5 (4-channel), acquisition duration approximates 22 seconds and contrast load 130 mL (Table 18-2).

For a 16-channel MDCT system, two options are possible. If the same detector collimation (1.25 mm) as the 8-channel approach is used, beam width is increased from 10 to 20 mm, and if approximately the same pitch value (1.375) and gantry rotation speed (0.5 seconds) are used, acquisition duration approximates 12 seconds with contrast load of 80 mL (Table 18-2). Alternatively, detector collimation can be reduced to 0.625 mm, and with otherwise identical acquisition parameters, acquisition duration will be equivalent to an 8-channel system with the same beam width (i.e., 22 seconds). In patients with aneurysmal disease, the thinner detector collimation approach (0.625 mm) will have the advantage of improved display of abdominal visceral branch vessels, particularly the renal arteries, which are parallel to the slice plane (Table 18-2).

Further technical progression in CT scanner performance has resulted in the production of 32, 40, and 64-channel systems. Dependent on the choice of technical factors already stressed (i.e., detector collimation, pitch value, and scan rotation speed), such systems can significantly decrease scan acquisition duration for both thoracoabdominal and aortoiliac CTA. In thoracic studies, retrospective electrocardiogram (ECG) gating can be implemented in patients in

TABLE 18-2

Thoracoabdominal Aorta (Cephalocaudad Coverage 600 mm)[a]

Number of Channels	4	8	16	16	64
Acquisition parameters					
Detector collimation (mm)	2.5	1.25	1.250	0.625	0.625
Beam width (mm)	10.0	10.0	20.0	10.0	40.0
Pitch	1.5	1.35	1.375	1.375	1.375
Scan rotation speed (sec)	0.5	0.5	0.5	0.5	0.5
Table speed (mm/sec)	30.0	27.0	55.0	27.5	110.0
Injection parameters					
Rate (mL/sec)	5	5	5	5	6
Volume (mL)	120	130	65	130	70 to 80

[a]Cephalocaudad coverage is not usually greater than 600 mm. If the scan rotation speed is slower than 0.5 seconds (e.g., 0.6 to 0.8 seconds), the acquisition interval will be longer and the contrast load requirements will be increased proportionately. The numbers in this table relate to coverage of 600 mm and a gantry rotation speed of 0.5 seconds. Example parameters specifically given for General Electric (Milwaukee, Wisconsin) CT scanners are generalizable to similar scanners from other manufacturers.

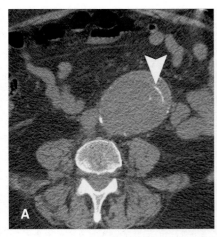 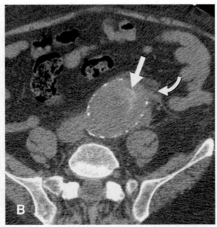 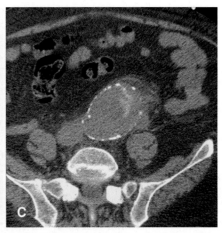

FIGURE 18-6 CT crescent sign. A: Precontrast axial scan in the more cephalad aspect of an infrarenal aortic aneurysm demonstrates laminated calcification in lining mural thrombus (*arrowhead*). **B:** Axial scan at a more caudal level demonstrates a focal curvilinear high-attenuation material consistent with coagulum in a dissecting channel of the lining thrombus (*arrow*). Anterolateral periaortic stranding is consistent with an aortic leak (*curved arrow*). **C:** Scan at a more caudal level demonstrates both the intra thrombotic "crescent" and periaortic blood to greater effect.

whom a combined study of the coronary and aortic vasculature is desired. ECG-gated cardiac studies are acquired with a lower pitch value (approximately 0.18 to 0.25) increasing acquisition duration in order to obtain appropriate sampling of the heart during a chosen diastolic interval. Thus, if ECG gating is implemented with a 64-channel MDCT system employing a low pitch value of 0.25, total acquisition time for a thoracoabdominal aortic study would approximate that of a 16-channel system with a

pitch value of 1.0. Patient radiation dose can be kept within diagnostically acceptable limits with simultaneous tube current modulation in the x-, y- and z-axes.

For aortic aneurysm CTA studies, a precontrast imaging sequence is obtained. This delineates arterial calcification and can demonstrate higher attenuation thrombus in a mural dissection (Fig. 18-6). Precontrast imaging is critical in patients who present with suspected aortic rupture, as in a hemodynamically compromised patient. An immediate diagnosis can be obtained and the patient transferred without delay to the operating room (Fig. 18-7) or a rapid dynamic contrast-enhanced study obtained to delineate the site of rupture and obtain a vascular road map for emergency surgery. In patients with periaortic hematoma whose clinical history suggests a "slow leak" and who are hemodynamically stable, a contrast-enhanced study is of value in providing a multiplanar and 3D display for the patient who would be transferred to the operating room in a semiemergent fashion (Fig. 18-8).

CTA of patients who have an endovascular stent graft in general conforms to the same imaging guidelines just described with the exception that an additional "early delayed" aortoiliac acquisition is acquired immediately following the dynamic angiographic sequence in order to increase sensitivity to endoleak (3) (Fig. 18-9). This issue is discussed later in this chapter under the section on postintervention findings.

Image Postprocessing

Postprocessing of abdominal aortic CTA follows the principles outlined in Chapter 6. For volume rendering (VR) and maximum-intensity projection (MIP), the liver, spleen,

FIGURE 18-7 Ruptured infrarenal AAA. Axial precontrast image demonstrates the aneurysm sac (*A*) and a large right retroperitoneal hematoma predominantly in the anterior pararenal space (*H*). The right psoas outline is obscured (∗). Oval-shaped fibrofatty tissue in the right retroperitoneum (*F*) represents the inferior extent of the right perinephric space.

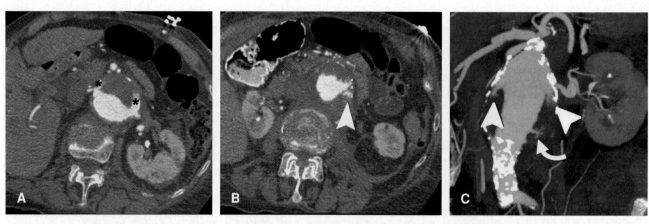

FIGURE 18-8 Large juxta renal/infrarenal abdominal aortic aneurysm with contrast opacification of a "neochannel" in lining mural thrombus. This may be a prelude to aortic rupture. **A:** Axial image at level of renal artery origins demonstrates flow channels between the lining mural thrombus and aortic wall (∗), larger on the left. **B:** Axial scan at a more caudal level demonstrates an additional irregular flow channel in the left side lining mural thrombus (*arrowhead*). **C:** Thin section planar MIP in a frontal projection demonstrates the juxtarenal/infrarenal fusiform aneurysm with two prominent flow channels (*arrowheads*) in the lining mural thrombus caudal to the renal vascular pedicle. There is an additional horizontally directed flow channel (*curved arrow*). The morphology of these flow channels suggests an increased risk for aortic rupture.

pancreas, and intestines are generally removed. It is also useful to eliminate all but the origins of the celiac axis and superior mesenteric artery (SMA). Prior to removal of the spine and bony pelvis, projection of aneurysmal disease over the background spine and pelvis may provide useful anatomic reference landmarks for subsequent correlation with fluoroscopic images during intervention (Fig. 18-10).

AAAs are frequently tortuous. Conventional 3D displays as outlined previously do not provide an accurate representation of longitudinal dimensions of a tortuous aorta. Point-to-point measurements on coronal plane reformatted images are thus inherently inaccurate, and discrepancies are to be expected between these planar measurements on a CTA display and a measurement obtained at catheter arteriography by using a calibrated catheter. Software techniques that use centerline tracking and automatic edge detection have been implemented to evaluate the aortoiliac arterial system in potential stent-

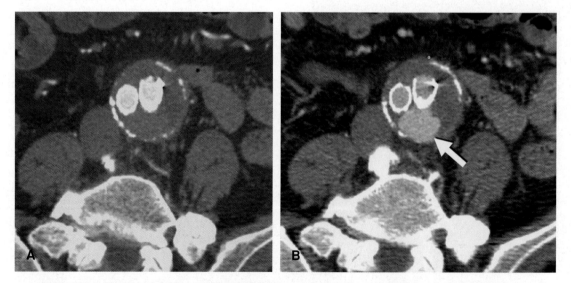

FIGURE 18-9 Type 2 endoleak in a patient with a bifurcated aortoiliac endovascular stent graft. In this patient, the endoleak is only evident on the early delayed scan and not on the initial dynamic scan. **A:** First-pass dynamic scan obtained during the first circulation of the injected contrast bolus does not demonstrate an endoleak. **B:** "Early delayed" second-pass study obtained immediately following the completion of the first circulation study demonstrates a prominent posterior endoleak in the aneurysm sac secondary to lumbar artery inflow (*arrow*).

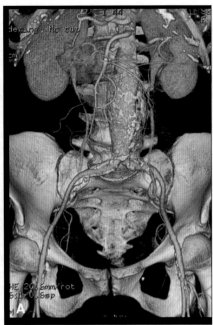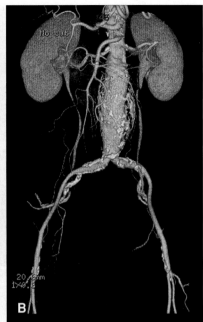

FIGURE 18-10 Aortoiliac CTA in patient with fusiform infrarenal AAA; pre- and postbone segmentation. A: Prebone segmentation. VR of the abdominal aorta and iliac arteries superimposed on background skeletal anatomy. Note the upper margin of the aneurysm at mid L2 level and the lower margin of the aneurysm at the aortic bifurcation at L5 level. **B:** VR with the same projection and area coverage as in **(A)** following bone segmentation. This illustrates the value of 3D volume display with the option of selective bone removal.

graft candidates. The software provides a true longitudinal dimension of tortuous aortoiliac vessels as well as diameter and area measurements that are orthogonal to the artery. One such software technique available commercially ("Advanced Vessel Analysis," General Electric Healthcare, Milwaukee, Wisconsin) requires placement of a cursor in the supraceliac aorta and both common femoral arteries as well as additional aortic branch vessels as desired. The software then automatically displays a 3D image indicating the location of the centerline and true orthogonal images of the aorta at any selected point (Fig. 18-11). After the operator selects designated anatomic levels from a rotatable stretched longitudinal image, the software is programmed to provide length and transverse dimensions of the superior neck (at upper, mid, and lower neck) (Fig. 18-12), length, transverse dimension and endoluminal volume of aneurysm (Fig. 18-13), and the length and transverse dimensions of the common iliac arteries, the usual distal placement zone for an endovascular stent graft (Fig. 18-14). Additional measurements of the suprarenal aorta and the external iliac arteries can be obtained, depending on individual patient anatomy and type of stent-graft option. Finally, the angle between the superior neck and the long axis of the aneurysm is calculated (Fig. 18-15). An angle of less than 60 degrees is desirable for most endovascular stent grafts.

In addition to the above measurements, the images that are generated by this program include curved planar reformations through the vessel centerline of the aortoiliac vasculature. This allows a determination of iliac artery

stenosis and an assessment of iliac artery tortuosity, both important factors in stent-graft planning (Fig. 18-16). In conventional MIP and subvolume MIP, circumferential mural calcification does not allow an accurate assessment of the iliac arterial lumen. This issue is addressed with the curved planar reformations.

An assessment of change in aneurysm sac size following endovascular stent grafting may be obtained by using either diameter or volume measurements. Although the automated centerline tracking technique provides a true longitudinal dimension of the aortoiliac arterial system, the centerline measurement may be misleading in relation to the choice of an appropriate stent graft. Following proximal and distal fixation, stent grafts do not usually lie within the center of the aortic lumen but are relatively posterior and do not conform to the curvature of the aorta. However, after placement, assume the shortest longitudinal dimension between the proximal and distal placement zones that accommodates underlying tortuosity. Researchers at Stanford University have determined that moving the longitudinal centerline away from center of the aorta so that it is closer to the inner curve of the vessel is a good practical accommodation (4).

The automated centerline tracking technique has most value in measurement of the length of the superior neck. The superior neck may be angulated anteriorly with reference to the juxtarenal and suprarenal aorta and relatively foreshortened in a series of axial images (Fig. 18-17). In addition to the perception of foreshortening in axial images, the superior neck may be angulated obliquely with reference to both

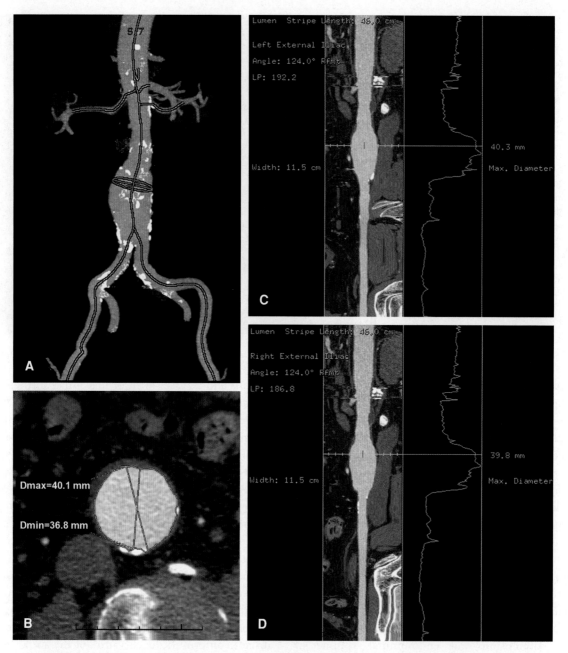

FIGURE 18-11 Automated centerline tracking and edge detection algorithm applied to a mildly tortuous aortoiliac arterial system in a patient with a fusiform infrarenal aneurysm. A: Centerline tracking of the abdominal aorta and right and left common and external iliac arteries together with celiac, superior mesenteric, and both renal arteries. Measurements of aortic diameter and area (*green circle*) are obtained by using a true cross section of the aorta rather than utilizing a transverse abdominal section. **B:** Measurements of maximum diameter (40.1 mm) and minimum diameter (36.8 mm) obtained from a true orthogonal projection of the abdominal aorta. Note that the automated edge detection algorithm has separated mural calcification and lining mural thrombus from contrast-enhanced blood in the vessel lumen. **C:** A stretched lumen view of the abdominal aorta and right common and external iliac arteries. This image is rotatable on the long axis of the vessel to allow imaging of side branches. The *green line* to the right of the image represents the mean diameter at any selected cephalocaudal level. A numerical value is provided depending on the level of the "slider." **D:** A stretched lumen view of the abdominal aorta and the left common and external iliac arteries. As in **(C)**, graphical representation of lumen diameter at any selected level is provided.

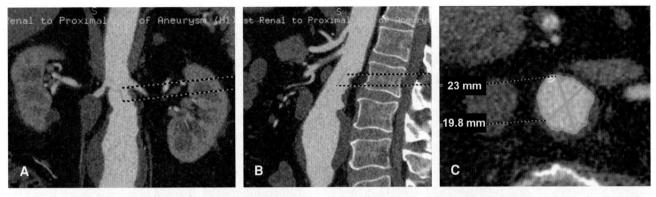

FIGURE 18-12 Semiautomated measurements of the superior neck of an infrarenal AAA. Measurements of the neck (12 mm) in the frontal **(A)** and lateral **(B)** projections of the aorta (not of the body) and automated measurements of the maximum and minimum diameter (23 mm and 19.8 mm, respectively) in a cross section of the aorta in that segment **(C)**, with an average diameter of 21.1 mm.

the juxtarenal and suprarenal aorta and the long axis of the aneurysm. Proper placement in the superior neck is critical to maintaining stability of a stent graft, and knowledge of the true dimensions and orientation of the superior neck are vital.

In addition to measurement of the superior neck, the shape and wall characteristics of the superior neck are also important. Stent-graft devices usually fixate well in superior necks that are relatively straight. However, fixation and stability over time are questionable if the shape of the superior neck is relatively conical or flared. Stent grafts that are fixated by friction may migrate proximally or distally over time if fixation is to a conical or flared superior neck. In addition, fixation either with friction devices or barb devices into a superior neck with significant atherosclerotic plaque and/or ulceration may lead to distal embolization during procedure, poor fixation, and/or possible endoleak.

MAGNETIC RESONANCE ANGIOGRAPHY

Equipment Considerations

Not all magnetic resonance (MR) machines are created equal, but a large percentage of MR equipment is capable of diagnostic-quality examination of the abdominal aorta. High field ($\geq$1T) strength magnets are certainly preferable to low field examination of the abdominal aorta, and therefore discussion that follows will mostly relate to examination

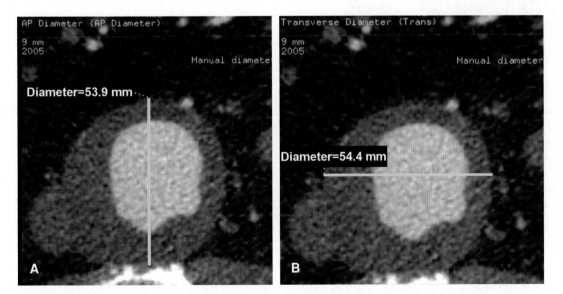

FIGURE 18-13 Anteroposterior and transverse dimensions of an infrarenal AAA. A: Manual measurement of external AP diameter obtained from a true cross-sectional view of the aorta. Measurement is 53.9 mm. **B:** Manual measurement of transverse diameter of an aortic aneurysm (including aortic lumen and lining mural thrombus). Measurement was obtained from a true cross-sectional image of the aorta. Measurements of true aneurysm volume, including lumen and lining thrombus, may provide more clinically meaningful estimates of aneurysm dimensions.

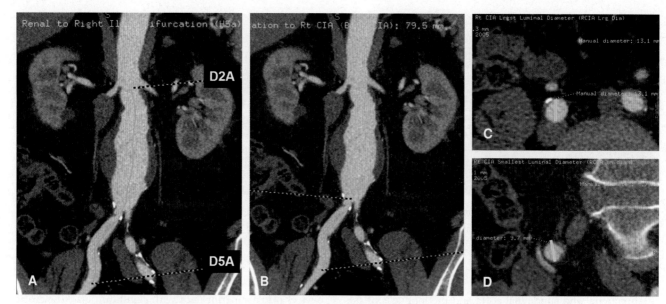

FIGURE 18-14 Linear measurement of the infrarenal abdominal aorta and common iliac artery and length and transverse dimensions of the common iliac artery. A: Automated centerline measurement obtained from the inferior margin of a renal vascular pedicle (D2A) to level of the right common iliac artery bifurcation (D5A). This measurement is a true linear longitudinal distance that accounts for vessel tortuosity. Measured length is 191.2 mm. **B:** Automated centerline measurement of length of the right common iliac artery. Measurement accounts for vessel tortuosity. Measured length is 79.5 mm. **C:** Anteroposterior diameter measurement of largest lumen diameter of the right common iliac artery from a true orthogonal display. Measured dimension is 13.1 mm. **D:** Anteroposterior diameter measurement of the smallest dimension of the right common iliac artery obtained from a true orthogonal projection of the vessel. Diameter measurement is 9.7 mm.

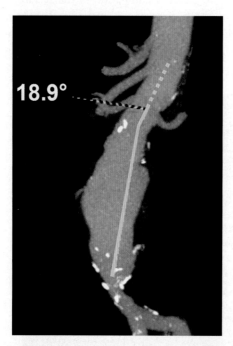

FIGURE 18-15 Angulation of the superior neck in relation to the long axis of the infrarenal AAA. The intersection of the long axis of the superior neck and the infrarenal aneurysm results in an angle of 18.9 degrees. The long axis of both the superior neck and the infrarenal aneurysm were determined from the 3D image data. For endovascular stent grafts, angulation of the superior neck in relation to the long axis of the aneurysm should ideally be less than 60 degrees.

at 1.5 and 3T. This is not to say that low field examinations of the abdominal aorta are not possible or are always nondiagnostic.

Techniques

Early MR techniques focused on comprehensive evaluation of the aorta by employing both bright blood and dark blood pulse sequences. However, these examinations had been hampered by severe motion artifact from respiration, bowel peristalsis, and vascular pulsations. Newer breath-hold acquisitions and snapshot techniques, which are to large measure breathing independent, can reliably evaluate acute pathology within the aorta. These techniques include incoherent gradient echo imaging with ultrashort TR (TR <4 milliseconds) with and without gadolinium contrast (often referred to as contrast-enhanced 3D magnetic resonance angiography [MRA]), and steady state gradient echo (e.g., True fast imaging with steady state free procession [FISP], balanced fast field echo [FFE], and fast imaging employing steady state acquisition [FIESTA]). More comprehensive interrogation can include dark blood preparation strategies and high spatial resolution imaging if plaque morphology and quantitation are to be assessed.

Rapid aortic imaging is no longer the sole domain of CT. Although MDCT is truly stunning in its speed, interrogation

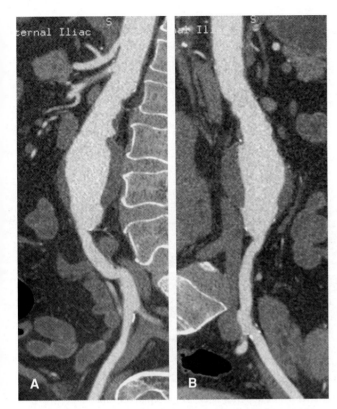

FIGURE 18-16 Automated curved planar reformation of the abdominal aorta and both common iliac and external iliac arteries. A: Curved planar reformation of the abdominal aorta and right common and external iliac arteries. There is mild tortuosity of the common iliac artery and minimal atheromatous plaque disease. **B:** Curved planar reformation of the abdominal aorta and left common and external iliac arteries. Minimal tortuosity and atheromatous wall thickening of the left common iliac artery. A fusiform infrarenal aneurysm with lining mural thrombus is present. Posterior wall atheroma is noted in the superior neck. The mildly tortuous iliac vessels in this patient are suitable for percutaneous access for aortic endovascular stent grafting.

of the entire abdominal aorta in a single breath hold is also possible by magnetic resonance imaging (MRI). Using a combination of noncontrast-enhanced single-slice and cine-balanced gradient echo images, the abdominal aorta can be screened in a matter of minutes for critical pathology. More detailed evaluation, including contrast-enhanced MRA and evaluation for complications surrounding the aorta, can be completed in a matter of a few additional minutes.

Nuances of Acquisition Strategies

Noncontrast Techniques

Historically, spin echo techniques dominated noncontrast MR aortic imaging; however, the advent of high-performance gradients (slew rates >100 mT/m/milliseconds) coupled with development of balanced gradient echo techniques shifted aortic imaging strategies from spin echo to gradient echo. Occasionally, black blood turbo spin-echo (TSE,

FSE) or its single shot analogs (HASTE, SSFSE) imaging is still performed for an overall anatomical appreciation of the abdominal aorta course and caliber. These single-shot techniques can also provide strong anatomic definition of the periaortic tissues as well as a more overall view of the regional organs including the bowel. In general, however, flow heterogeneity can present a problem for most dark blood preparations, making them somewhat less reliable than bright blood gradient echo techniques and contrast-enhanced MRA for luminal evaluation, including detection of dissection.

Noncontrast bright blood aortic imaging with time of flight is still performed on occasion on older units but has mostly been abandoned in favor of faster and more robust balanced gradient echo techniques and contrast-enhanced MRA. Some people espouse using phase contrast imaging at sites of stenosis to determine if the stenosis is hemodynamically significant. A significant stenosis will create a flow void at and just distal to the stenosis due to intravoxel spin dephasing. This is certainly true and may be of value in smaller vessels (i.e., renal arteries) but is relatively time-consuming and of dubious necessity in an artery the caliber of the aorta.

Balanced gradient echo techniques can be used without dark blood preparations and have a robust contrast-to-noise ratio, making them ideal for evaluation of the blood pool (5). TrueFISP was specifically shown to be extremely well suited for evaluation of the thoracic aorta and can also be applied to abdominal aortic evaluation (see rapid aortic protocol below) (6). The aorta is typically imaged in at least two planes (i.e., the axial and coronal planes). Sagittal imaging can be obtained in place of coronal images, if desired. In the interest of time conservation in the protocols, three-plane evaluation is usually not critical. An axial stack of single-shot images is obtained from the diaphragm to the bifurcation. A coronal stack of images is obtained to cover the aorta alone (usually, thin slices of 3 to 4 mm) or the entire abdomen, if desired. Axial images take approximately 350 to 600 milliseconds to acquire, while coronal images take approximately 500 to 900 milliseconds to acquire. This extremely fast acquisition speed means that breath holding is helpful for slice registration but is not crucial for maintenance of relatively high image quality. Thus, critically ill patients unable to breath hold still produce reliable images.

Because of their extremely rapid gradient reversals, balanced gradient echo images are prone to certain predictable artifacts. The two most common artifacts are phase cancellation and dark band artifacts. Phase cancellation artifacts are the result of rapid gradient reversals, typically performed at a recovery time (TR) of approximately 2 milliseconds. As a result of the phase cancellation created between fat and

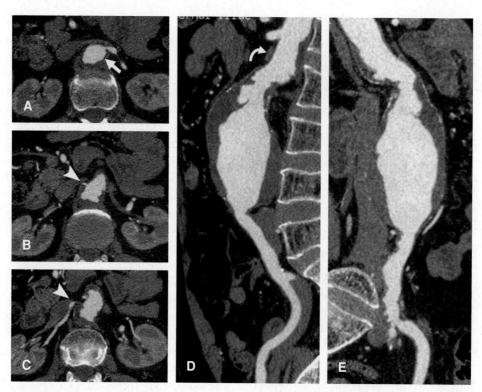

FIGURE 18-17 Measurement, shape, and wall characteristics of the superior neck, as determinants in stent-graft planning. A: Axial scan of the aorta at the level of the origin and proximal segment of the left renal artery. Note the prominent circumferential mural thrombus, predominantly posterior, in the aorta at this level (*arrow*). **B:** Anterior and leftward angulation of the superior neck, as demonstrated in a more caudal axial scan. The origin and proximal segment of one of two right renal arteries is seen (*arrowhead*). Prominent atherothrombotic wall thickening is noted. **C:** More caudal axial CT scan demonstrates anterior and leftward projection of the aorta and the takeoff of a more inferior right renal artery (*arrowhead*). **D:** Curved planar reformation of the abdominal aorta and left common iliac artery in a lateral projection. Caudal to the left renal vein (*curved arrow*), there is anterior angulation, flaring, and atherothrombosis of the aorta as it becomes progressively aneurysmal. **E:** Curved planar reformation of the abdominal aorta and left common and external iliac arteries in an oblique projection. Angulation, flaring, and tortuosity of the supra-aneurysmal aorta with prominent atherothrombosis is demonstrated. This sequence of axial images and curved planar reformations demonstrates relatively caudal origin of the right renal arteries and extensive irregular circumferential atherothrombosis of the superior neck, factors that could preclude use of endovascular stent grafting.

water when a TR of approximately 2.1 milliseconds is used, any interface between fat and water (muscle, blood, etc.) produces black lines like India ink etching. An example where this property is used to the imager's advantage is in adrenal imaging, where gradient echo imaging with roughly the same TR is used to delineate voxels that contain both fat and water such as the micromolecular composition of adrenal adenomas.

The second artifact of dark bands occurs as a result of off resonance effects from minor field inhomogeneity. These dark bands are usually harmless when they occur outside the area of interest, but to the untrained observer, they can be mistaken for true pathology. One example is if a dark band fell within the area of interest, such as through the aortic lumen, where it could be mistaken for a dissection

flap. However, one should note that a dark band artifact will usually continue beyond the lumen. Additionally, shifting the tuning frequency of the magnet will change the position of dark band artifacts within the image but will not change the position of a true dissection flap. Although the same phase cancellation and dark band artifacts exist in both single-shot and cine gradient echo techniques, it is often useful to perform a few cine-balanced gradient echo slices in addition to the single-shot images. These dynamic imaging sequences usually give the observer a sense for whether the abnormality seen on the single-shot images is artifact or true pathology.

After balanced gradient echo images are obtained, a single breath-hold set of fat-saturated low flip angle incoherent gradient echo images (two-dimensional [2D]

FMPSPGR/FLASH) can be obtained. This sequence will demonstrate subacute blood products such as extracellular methemoglobin, which will manifest bright signal intensity. It will also serve as a precontrast baseline for comparison to postcontrast imaging, if this is to be performed. Lastly, it is a sensitive evaluator of pancreatitis, whose clinical presenting symptoms of abdominal and/or back pain can often mimic aortic symptomatology.

In the setting of examination for acute or immediate life-threatening aortic abnormalities, the above noncontrast sequences are accurate for making a determination of the presence and extent of aortic pathology (6).

At this point, if a patient's exam is negative for aortic pathology, he or she can be safely returned to the emergency room for further evaluation. If an aortic abnormality is present, a decision can be made as to whether further imaging is warranted or whether immediate surgical attention is most prudent. For the more stable patients that present with positive aortic pathology, completion of a comprehensive abdominal exam can be performed, including fast-spin echo HASTE/SSFSE images, postcontrast time-resolved MRA and/or 3D MRA and 2D postcontrast fat-saturated FLASH/FMPSPGR.

Flow Quantification

Although flow quantification is frequently used in cardiac MR regarding shunts and valvular function and its use has been described to measure renal artery stenosis and mesenteric blood flow, flow quantification is rarely performed on the abdominal aorta itself. In cases of severe aortic stenosis, the same principles of flow quantification can be applied that apply elsewhere. Namely, a gradient echo quantified phase contrast sequence can be implemented to determine flow parameters, including peak velocity, across a stenosis (perpendicular to the direction of flow). The modified Bernoulli equation "$4V^2$" can be applied where "V" equals the velocity, as measured in meters per second, is squared and then multiplied by 4 to yield the approximate gradient across a stenosis. Normal velocity in the aorta is less than 1.25 meters per second (m/s).

Contrast-enhanced Magnetic Resonance Angiography

Postcontrast imaging of the aorta can be performed in several different ways. Time-resolved imaging can be performed with a modicum of contrast on many newer machines (hardware/software packages after the year 2000). One example is projectional MRA, often referred to as "freeze-frame" or "subsecond angiography" after its subsec-

ond temporal resolution capabilities. In subsecond MRA, 4 to 6 cc of gadolinium contrast is injected at 5 to 6 cc per second followed by a 15- to 20-cc saline flush. Although technically a 3D MRA acquisition, the images are acquired with the shortest TR (preferably <2 milliseconds), a wide bandwidth (>1,000 hz/pixel), and a small number (<12) of thick partitions (>8 mm) so that images are really only viewable in one axis and thus become projectional 2D angiograms in reality. The ultrashort TR gadolinium-enhanced imaging with a sacrifice of through-plane resolution coupled with in-line subtraction of mask images from the postcontrast frames is what enables this technique's high-contrast, high temporal resolution performance. Subsecond MRA (Fig. 18-18) has been shown to demonstrate luminal course and caliber as well as differential flow patterns within aneurysms and dissections of the aorta (7).

More commonly, high spatial resolution contrast-enhanced 3D MRA is employed for accurate evaluation of the abdominal aorta. The standard 3D MRA sequence is a spoiled gradient-recalled echo sequence run with the minimum possible echo time (TE) and TR achievable (typically TR <4 milliseconds). The 3D volume (sometimes referred to as a slab) is placed in the coronal orientation and is typically 60 to 120 mm thick. This volume allows anterior–posterior coverage to include the entire abdominal aorta and its major branches, including the celiac trunk, splenic, hepatic, gastric, superior mesenteric, renal, and inferior mesenteric arteries. This volume also usually includes much of the descending thoracic aorta as well as the common iliac arteries. The slab can easily be tailored and placed slightly more anteriorly or posteriorly to focus on branch vessels such as the superior mesenteric artery (SMA) or renals, respectively (Fig. 18-19). The slab is composed of multiple partitions of thickness generally ranging from 0.8 mm to 4 mm, depending on individual MR unit capabilities. Some type of slice interpolation scheme is always used in the through-plane direction to help palliate partial volume averaging effects. Generally, somewhere between 30 and 45 actual partitions are acquired, and this is interpolated to 60 to 90 partitions of the aforementioned thickness.

Three breath-hold 3D MRA acquisitions are generally obtained—mask, arterial phase, and venous phase. The first 3D acquisition is prior to contrast administration and has a dual function to insure proper position and coverage as well as to serve as the mask acquisition. The mask will be the background image subtracted from subsequent postcontrast acquisitions to produce a higher contrast ratio

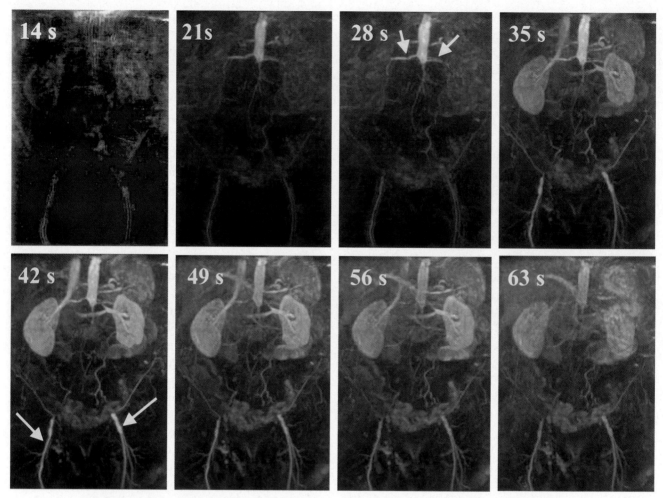

FIGURE 18-18 TRICKS imaging demonstrated in a 69-year-old man with aortic occlusion. 3D TRICKS time frames (TR = 7.8/TE = 1.7), demonstrating the peak arterial filling of the aortorenal arteries just above the occlusion at 28 seconds (*short arrows*) and the maximum signal intensity of the common femoral arteries at 42 seconds (*long arrows*). (Reprinted with permission from Swan JS, Carroll TJ, Kennell TW, et al. Time-resolved three-dimensional contrast-enhanced MR angiography of the peripheral vessels. *Radiology.* 2002; 225:43–52.)

image, which truly mimics conventional digital subtraction angiograms. The angiographic 3D MRA is acquired at the time of maximal enhancement of the abdominal aorta and its branches. The start of this acquisition is predetermined by either a timing run preceding the 3D MRA or some type of fluoroscopic triggering. After a small period of breathing (generally, 10 to 20 seconds), the third breath-held 3D MRA is obtained coinciding with the venous phase of circulation. This acquisition typically displays the splenic, mesenteric, and renal veins to good advantage. The shortest possible delay between arterial and venous phase imaging is suggested to demonstrate splenic and renal veins

to the greatest advantage. A 20-second delay after the arterial phase is suggested if mesenteric and portal veins are of greatest interest.

Contrast Enhancement Schemes

Dozens of contrast enhancement schemes have been proposed to leverage the intricacies of MRA. What follows is a general approach that can be tailored depending on exact equipment specifications. Double-dose gadolinium (0.2 mmol/kg) is useful for aortic imaging, although diagnostic images can often be created with far less contrast (as low as 0.05 mmol/kg). The aortic MRA itself only requires single

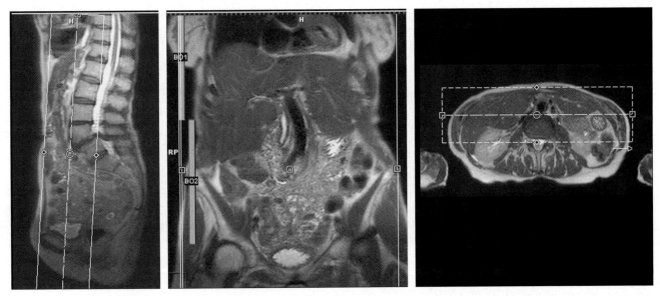

FIGURE 18-19 MRI screen capture showing positioning of the 3D MRA slabs on the sagittal and axial scout images for an abdominal aorta MRA. The lateral limits of the field are demonstrated in the coronal plane image. In this example, the mesenteric circulation as well as the main renal arteries to the renal hilar are included.

dose (0.1 mmol/kg); however, there are numerous reasons to use double dose instead of single dose if contrast cost is not the overriding issue in your practice. First, a typical aortic injection scheme is to inject contrast at 2 to 3 cc per second. If one injects 20 cc of contrast (single dose for a 100-kg person) at 2 cc per second, then the bolus duration is only about 12 to 15 seconds (10 seconds of infusion plus a few seconds of leeway due to the fact that the injected bolus dilutes or spreads out to a larger volume and time as it is injected and carried in the blood). Most MR machines require a greater length of time to make an adequate 3D image than 12 seconds. If one injects double-dose contrast, then the imaging window lengthens to roughly 25 to 30 seconds, depending on cardiac output and various other factors influencing circulation time. This longer bolus makes it easier for the technologist to obtain images during an appropriately contrasted window. Furthermore, although the arterial phase images may have adequate contrast in the aorta at 0.1 mmol/kg injections, venous images of the mesenteric, renal, and portal veins benefit from the higher initial concentration of gadolinium (0.2 mmol/kg), as it is diluted to a vastly larger volume by the venous phase of imaging.

Subtraction Imaging

Subtraction imaging is typically performed where a non-contrast (mask) 3D MRA data set is subtracted from subsequent contrast-enhanced 3D MRA data sets. The importance of this step is related to how robust the contrast enhancement is and the availability and capability of post-processing tools. The strength of MRI is that the contrast differential between gadolinium-enhanced arterial signal and background is much greater than the differential seen between iodinated CT contrast attenuation values of arteries versus background.

Multiple vendors sell hardware and software systems that are designed to import raw data (DICOM) and process these data into realistic 3D images. The most common modes of display include MIP, multiplanar reformatting (MPR), and VR (see Chapter 6 for further details). If a contrast-enhanced MRA has a particularly high contrast signal within arteries and a relatively low background tissue signal, then actual subtraction imaging is often not necessary. Some 3D workstations are capable of auto segmentation and through a series of complex algorithms perform their own scaling to remove background tissue signals and only display the vascular tree. If arterial signal is not greatly higher than background, then subtraction techniques help to raise the contrast level between the artery in question and the background. This is more critical with imaging smaller branch vessels and is less important when imaging the aorta itself due to its relatively large size.

Caution must be exercised when performing evaluation of aortic MRA just as with any MRA. Source images and MPR interrogation of the data set must be performed, otherwise intraluminal abnormalities such as dissection and shelflike plaque will be missed during viewing of projectional images (MIP) only (Fig. 18-20).

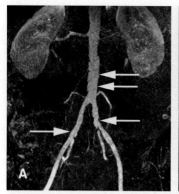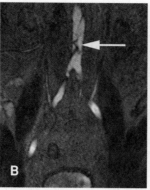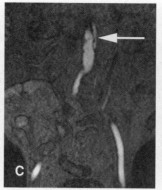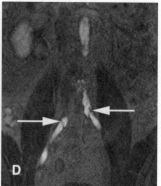

FIGURE 18-20 A: MIP of aortoiliac MRA showing mild atherosclerotic irregularity (*arrows*) but does not demonstrate underlying dissection. **B, C:** Source MRA images demonstrating aortic dissection (*arrows*). **D:** Source MRA image better demonstrating bilateral common iliac dissections (*arrows*) not well seen on MIP.

Postcontrast Two-dimensional Imaging

Although not mandatory, it is often extremely beneficial to obtain at least a limited number of 2D images after a 3D MRA is performed. For the abdominal aorta, these are typically obtained in axial and coronal planes although sagittal is acceptable as well. These delayed 2D images are obtained with a fat-saturated spoiled gradient-recalled echo sequence like FLASH or FMPSPGR and can reasonably be obtained any time within 20 minutes after contrast administration.

They are most beneficial to show mural abnormalities of the aorta, periaortic pathology, and more diffuse abdominal abnormalities in neighboring organs. One must bear in mind that the 3D MRA is really a lumenogram, only demonstrating the aortic lumen in any detail. Critical pathology such as mural thrombus, aneurysm, wall thickening, and plaquing is only demonstrated through additional standard 2D sequences. Furthermore, a small but important percentage of incidental disease (e.g., renal, hepatic, pancreatic, adrenal, and bowel tumors) is detected in the solid and hollow organs as a result of these additional sequences.

Multiphase Exams

Clinical Protocols

Rapid Aorta Protocol for Emergent Evaluation

1. Axial stack of single-slice steady state gradient echo images
2. Coronal stack of single-slice steady state gradient echo images
3. Axial cine steady state gradient echo at the level of the renal arteries
4. Coronal cine steady state gradient echo

Comprehensive Aorta Protocol (add to the above Rapid Aorta Protocol)

1. Axial or coronal precontrast HASTE/SSFSE images for evaluation of surrounding abdominal structures, including bowel
2. Axial and coronal precontrast-enhanced fat-saturated, fast incoherent gradient echo images
3. (Optional for cases with stenosis) Phased contrast flow quantification sequence at site of stenosis if spin dephasing is noted on cine sequences
4. (Optional) Contrast-enhanced coronal subsecond MRA
5. Contrast-enhanced 3D gradient echo MR angiogram acquired in coronal plane (3D-efgre, 3D-FLASH, can use time-resolved sequences like TRICKS or TREAT, if available). The anterior margin of the scan volume is typically positioned based on whether the hepatic and superior mesenteric arteries are to be included. If hepatic arteries and SMA are in question, then the anterior margin of the scan volume is placed 4 to 6 cm anterior to the aorta. The posterior margin of the 3D volume is generally positioned based on whether the renal arteries are of significant interest. If renal arteries are of main interest, then the posterior border of the scan volume is usually extended to the posterior margin of the kidneys. In addition, the coronal plane can be obliqued slightly to follow the course of the aorta, if desired.
6. Axial and coronal postcontrast-enhanced fat-saturated, fast incoherent gradient echo images (FMPSPGR, FLASH) for evaluation of the aortic wall and surrounding abdominal structures, including bowel.

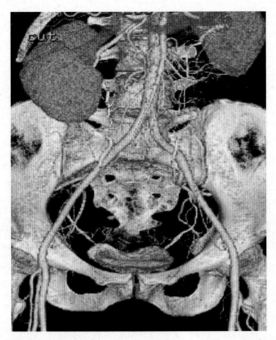

FIGURE 18-21 VR display in frontal projection of the aortoiliac arterial system without bone segmentation. The bifurcation of the abdominal aorta is at the level of the L4-L5 intervertebral space.

ABDOMINAL AORTIC ANATOMY

Normal Anatomy

The normal abdominal aorta is defined at its superior extent by the aortic hiatus of the diaphragm (at approximately the T12 level) and at its inferior extent by bifurcation into the common iliac arteries (at approximately the L4 level). Major branches consist of the celiac axis (left gastric, hepatic, splenic arteries), superior and inferior mesenteric arteries, renal, phrenic, suprarenal, spermatic or testicular in male and ovarian in female, lumbar, and medial sacral artery. These branches are classified as visceral (celiac, superior and inferior mesenteric, renal, suprarenal, and gonadal) and parietal (phrenic, lumbar, and middle sacral arteries).

The aortic bifurcation is usually at L4 level, though the bifurcation tends to "migrate" inferiorly with increase in tortuosity and lengthening of the aorta accompanying the aging process (Fig. 18-21).

The common and external iliac arteries are a direct conduit from the abdominal aorta to the common femoral artery. The iliac artery bifurcation with origin of the hypogastric arteries is at the level of the pelvic brim. At this point, the iliac arteries are crossed by the ureters.

The hypogastric arteries divide into anterior and posterior divisions, the posterior division forming the lateral sacral, iliolumbar, and superior gluteal arteries and the anterior division forming the inferior gluteal, obturator, vesicle, middle hemorrhoidal, internal pudendal, uterine (female), and deferential

(male). Multiple variations of the branching pattern of both the posterior and anterior division vessels are common. The pelvic arteries form an important potential collateral network in patients with aortoiliac occlusive disease. Major potential connections include lumbar to iliolumbar, medial to lateral sacral, and superior to middle hemorrhoidal, the superior hemorrhoidal being a branch of the inferior mesenteric artery (IMA).

Three important arterial branches arise from the distal external iliac artery immediately proximal to the common femoral artery. These are the circumflex iliac, inferior epigastric, and external pudendal. The circumflex iliac and inferior epigastric arteries also make important contributions to arterial collateral networks, the circumflex artery communicating with parietal branches of the lumbar arteries and the inferior epigastric with the superior epigastric branches in turn deriving inflow from the internal mammary arteries (Fig. 18-22).

Variant Anatomy

Variant anatomy of the abdominal aorta is uncommon, mainly reflecting abnormal situs and branch variants. Patients with *situs inversus* may have associated anomalies, including azygous continuation of the inferior vena cava (Fig. 18-23). Some patients with normal abdominal situs will have a left inferior vena cava, usually incomplete and continuing as a right-sided inferior vena cava at the level of the renal vascular pedicle with the left inferior vena cava ending in the left renal vein. Double inferior vena cavas are even more uncommon (Fig. 18-24).

An important but very rare congenital anomaly is absence of the common and external iliac and femoral arteries with replacement by a persistent sciatic artery. The sciatic artery usually regresses during development with the residual vessel forming the superior gluteal artery. A persistent sciatic artery runs adjacent to the nerve, exiting the pelvis via the sciatic notch and continuing superficial to the adductor magnus muscle (Fig. 18-25). A sciatic artery is associated with the clinical conundrum of absent femoral pulse and normal pulse pressure in the distal extremity arteries. Importance relates to recognition of a congenital variation and avoidance of attempted femoral catheterization.

Congenital variation in origin and branching pattern of abdominal aortic visceral arterial branches is not uncommon. Thirty percent of patients have more than one renal artery, the accessory artery most commonly supplying the lower pole. Lower pole accessory arteries usually arise from the mid-abdominal aorta but may arise from the distal aorta or common iliac artery. Accessory renal arteries may arise from an abdominal aorta or iliac aneurysm, posing issues in terms of vessel sacrifice or reimplantation for endovascular stent grafting or open aneurysmectomy, respectively (Fig. 18-26). The number of accessory renal arteries is variable and usually not more than four. Multiple renal arteries are

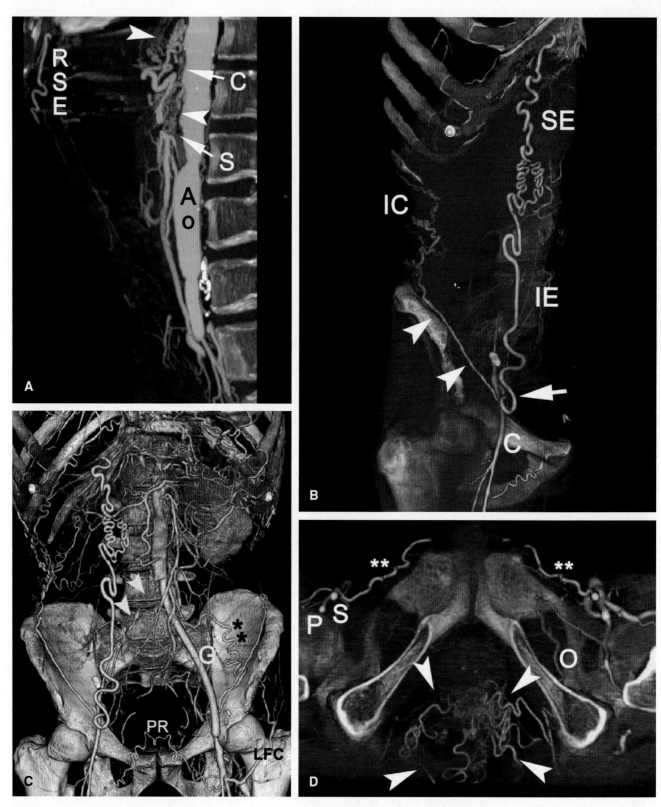

FIGURE 18-22 Collateral pathways in a patient with multiple vascular occlusions, including occlusion of the celiac and superior mesenteric arteries, right iliac system, and right renal artery. A: Sagittal 10-mm MIP along long axis of aorta shows occlusion of the celiac axis (*C*) and superior mesenteric artery (*S*) at their respective origins (*arrows*). There are multiple tiny, serpentine collateral vessels (*arrowheads*). There is an enlarged, tortuous right superior epigastric artery (*RSE*). **B:** Thick-slab VR image, showing the enlarged tortuous course of the right superior epigastric (*SE*) to inferior epigastric (*IE*) pathway, providing collateral flow to the external iliac artery (*arrow*). There are also corkscrew intercostal collaterals (*IC*), which provide collateral flow to the deep iliac circumflex artery (*arrowheads*). (*C,* common femoral artery.) **C:** Full-slab VR image shows additional collateral pathways, including left iliolumbar collateral (∗∗), left lateral femoral circumflex (*LFC*), and perirectal collateral (*PR*). Long-segment right common/external iliac occlusion is seen (*arrowheads*), as is a vascular graft (*G*) in the left pelvis. Collateral pathways described in **(B)** can also be appreciated. **D:** Axial thick-slab VR image shows in exquisite detail the perirectal collaterals (*arrowheads*), which arise from superior hemorrhoidal and inferior gluteal collaterals. Note the enlarged external pudendal arteries bilaterally (∗∗), receiving pelvic collateral flow and dumping into the proximal superficial femoral artery (*S*). An enlarged obturator artery (*O*) is noted on the left. (*P,* profunda femoris artery.) (Figure courtesy of Richard L. Hallett, MD.)

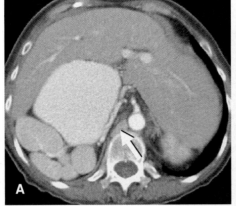
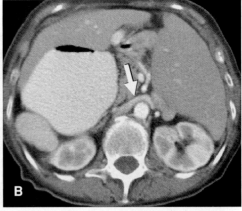

FIGURE 18-23 Situs inversus with polysplenia and azygous continuation of the inferior vena cava.
A: There is a large right azygous vein in the right retrocrural space adjacent to the aorta (*arrow*). There are prominent gastric vessels adjacent to the lesser curvature of the stomach. **B:** Axial scan at a more caudal level demonstrates the left renal vein anterior to the aorta and communicating with the upper extent of the abdominal inferior vena cava (*arrow*).

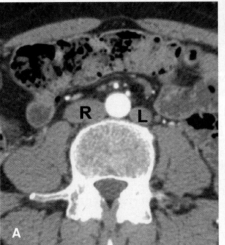
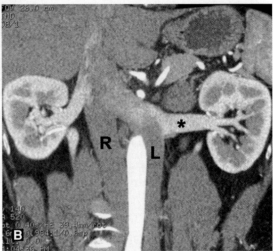

FIGURE 18-24 Potential renal donor with a double inferior vena cava. A: Axial CT scan of the abdomen at the level of the takeoff of the inferior mesenteric artery demonstrates a right (*R*) and left (*L*) inferior vena cava. **B:** Planar reformation of the abdomen demonstrates the two unopacified inferior vena cavas on either side of the aorta, with the left inferior vena cava emptying into the proximal left renal vein (*).

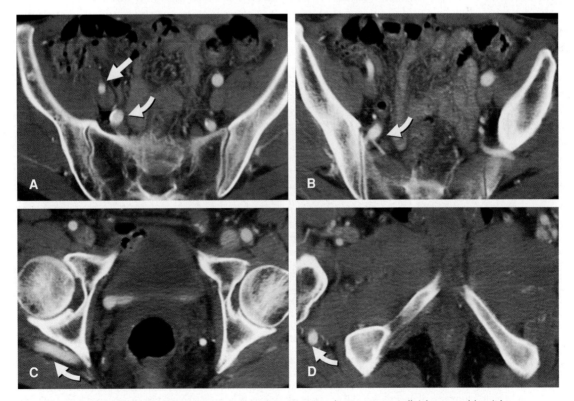

FIGURE 18-25 Persistent sciatic artery. A: Transverse CT section demonstrates small right external (*straight arrow*) and large right internal (*curved arrow*) iliac arteries. **B–D:** The course of the right internal iliac artery can be followed inferiorly as it exits the pelvis to become the right sciatic artery (*curved arrow* in **C** and **D**). Note the tiny right superficial femoral artery in (**D**). (Images courtesy of Geoffrey D. Rubin, MD.)

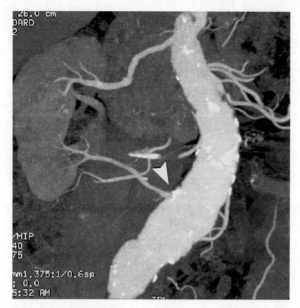

FIGURE 18-26 Thin-section planar MIP image of the abdominal aorta and right renal arteries in a patient with a fusiform aneurysm. The inferior right renal artery arises from the aneurysm (*arrowhead*) and supplies the inferior third of the kidney. This precluded intentional devascularization of the inferior third of the right kidney as would occur with the placement of an endovascular stent graft. This patient had surgical repair of the aneurysm and right renal artery reimplantation.

usual in patients with horseshoe kidney. In patients with both horseshoe kidney and AAA, a major renal arterial branch may arise from the aortic midline to supply both lower pole moieties and poses a technical challenge in an open aneurysmectomy procedure (Fig. 18-27).

The celiac axis is usually a single trunk, but separate aortic origins of the hepatic, left gastric, and splenic arteries do occur (Fig. 18-28). Combined origin of the celiac and superior mesenteric artery is unusual (Fig. 18-29). Multiple congenital variations in hepatic arterial branching have been classified by Michel and are outlined in Chapter 19.

Arterial communication between the middle colic branch of the superior mesenteric artery and the superior left colic branch of the IMA is important in maintaining left colon perfusion in patients with an occluded IMA (Fig. 18-30). Arterial communication between the two colic arterial branches at the splenic flexure has been labeled as "Griffith's Point." Integrity of this communication maintains left colon perfusion when the IMA is either deliberately occluded (as when an AAA is excluded by an endovascular stent graft) or when the IMA is ligated (at open aneurysmectomy). Collateral communication between the middle hemorrhoidal branch of the hypogastric artery and superior hemorrhoidal branch of the IMA also contributes to left colon perfusion.

ABDOMINAL AORTIC ANEURYSM

An *aneurysm* is defined as a more than 50% increase in diameter compared with the expected normal diameter vessel (8). A less than 50% increase is termed *ectasia*. The accepted upper limit of normal values for the juxtarenal aorta is 28 mm and for the infrarenal aorta is 20 mm. Thus, an infrarenal aorta may be considered to be aneurysmal if it is 3 cm in diameter or greater. Some authors consider 3.5 cm in diameter to be a better "cut off point."

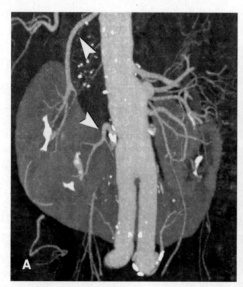 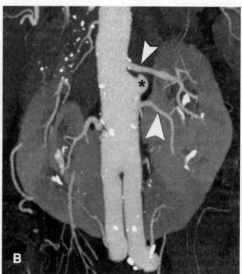

FIGURE 18-27 Patient with horseshoe kidney and aortobifemoral surgical tube graft. A: Thin-section MIP in a slight right anterior oblique (RAO) projection demonstrates both a superior and inferior artery to the right moiety of the horseshoe kidney (*arrowheads*). The inferior right renal artery arises from the aorta immediately proximal to the aortic graft anastomosis. **B:** Thin-section MIP in a slight left anterior oblique (LAO) projection. Superior and inferior left renal arteries arise from the aorta proximal to the surgical anastomosis and supply the left moiety of the horseshoe kidney (*arrowheads*). The focal irregular projection of the aorta between the two left renal arteries (*) could represent focal atheromatous ulceration.

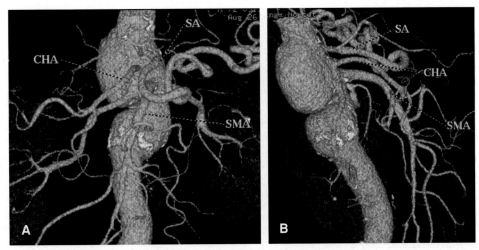

FIGURE 18-28 **Anomalous direct aortic origin of celiac branch vessels from a suprarenal AAA. A:** VR in frontal projection demonstrates separate aortic origins of the hepatic and splenic arteries. The left gastric artery arises from the splenic artery. (*CHA*, common hepatic artery; *SA*, splenic artery; *SMA*, superior mesenteric artery.)
B: VR in a lateral projection demonstrating the splenic, common hepatic, and superior mesenteric arteries arising in stepwise progression from the anterior border of the aneurysmal aorta. (*SA*, splenic artery; *CHA*, common hepatic artery; *SMA*, superior mesenteric artery.)

Aortic wall degeneration secondary to atherosclerotic disease is probably not the primary mechanism responsible for formation of AAAs. Fragmentation and degeneration of elastin, which has been observed histologically in aneurysm walls, may be the primary pathogenic mechanism (9). Elastin is the principal load-bearing element in the aortic wall. An increase in proteolytic enzymes in the distal aorta, specifically matrix metalloproteinase (MMP) has also been observed and may contribute to the observed degeneration and fragmentation of elastic fibers (10,11). Other less common causes of aortic aneurysms include penetrating aortic ulcer (Fig. 18-31), inflammatory aortoarteritis such as Takayasu disease (12) (Fig. 18-32), and the rare inflammatory aneurysm (Figs. 18-33, 18-34) characterized by medial inflammatory infiltrate associated with aortic wall thickening, perianeurysmal fibrosis, and adhesion to adjacent abdominal organs. Aortic pseudoaneurysms may develop at tube graft anastomotic sites. Finally, aneurysms may develop with aortic dissection, either focal in the aortoiliac system or secondary to distal extension of a classic thoracoabdominal aortic dissection.

In patients over the age of 50 years, the prevalence of aneurysm (greater than 3 cm in diameter) is 3% to 10% (13). The vast majority of aneurysms occur in the male population. Aneurysms are more common in whites and in patients with a history of smoking and hypertension, a positive family history, hypercholesterolemia, peripheral vascular disease, coronary artery disease, and diabetes.

Twelve percent of patients with AAAs have thoracic aneurysms, whereas 60% of patients with thoracic aneurysms have other aneurysms, including AAAs (14). One third of patients with femoral popliteal aneurysms have AAAs (15). These are important considerations in patients who have a clinical finding of a femoral popliteal aneurysm or who have a thoracic aneurysm discovered incidentally on chest radiography or CT scanning.

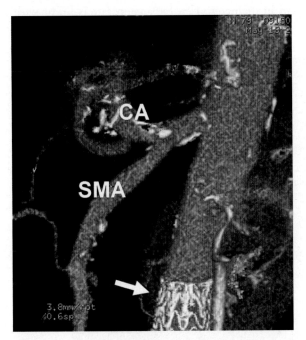

FIGURE 18-29 **Conjoint origin of the celiac and superior mesenteric arteries.** VR in lateral projection demonstrates a single trunk dividing into a separate celiac (*CA*) and superior mesenteric (*SMA*) arteries. The upper segment of an aortoiliac endovascular stent graft is seen in the more caudal aorta (*arrow*).

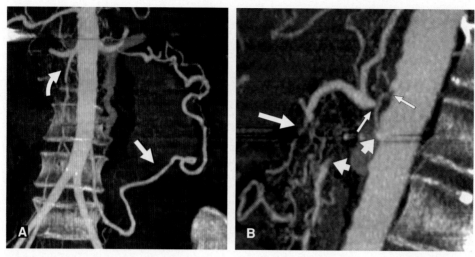

FIGURE 18-30 Communication of the inferior and superior mesenteric arterial systems via the superior left colic to middle colic arterial anastomosis. A: A hypertrophied superior left colic branch of the IMA (*thin arrows*) extends to the splenic flexure with a direct connection to the left branch of the middle colic artery. The superior mesenteric artery is a small caliber vessel (*curved arrow*). The central left renal vein and an opacified left gonadal vein at the left border of the aorta are seen. **B:** Thin-section planar MIP in lateral projection demonstrates proximal occlusion of the celiac artery (*thin arrows*) and a longer segment occlusion of the proximal superior mesenteric artery (*wide arrows*). There are extensive transpancreatic arterial collateral connections between the superior mesenteric and celiac arteries.

The clinical presentation of AAAs may be catastrophic related to aneurysm rupture. The classic clinical presentation is back pain, hypotension, and a palpable pulsatile abdominal mass. Immediate mortality rate approximates 80% with cumulative mortality rate over the next 30 days approximating 50% of survivors (16). Rupture risk relates to aneurysm dimension, being 0% per year for aneurysms less than 4 cm in diameters, 0.5% to 3% per year for aneurysms 4 to 5 cm in diameter, 3% to 15% per year for aneurysms 5 to 6 cm in diameter, 10% to 20% per year for aneurysms 6 to 7 cm in diameter, 20% to 40% per year for aneurysms 7 to 8 cm in diameter, and 30% to 50% per year for aneurysms greater than 8 cm in diameter (17). Expansion rate is linear with an

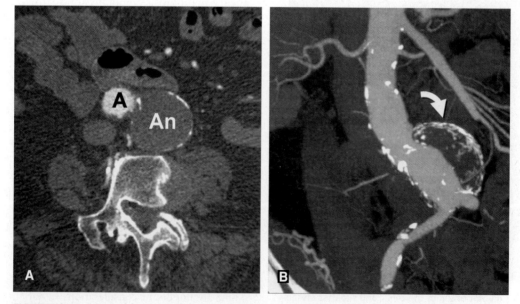

FIGURE 18-31 Eccentric focal saccular aneurysm of the distal infrarenal aorta, presumed secondary to a penetrating aortic ulcer. A: Axial CT scan at the level of the inferior aorta *(A)* demonstrates a thrombus-filled saccular aneurysm *(An)* arising from the left aortic margin. **B:** Thin-section MIP in a slight RAO projection demonstrates the peripherally calcified thrombus-filled aneurysm (*curved arrow*).

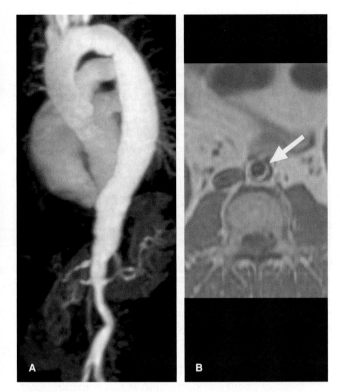

FIGURE 18-32 Type 3 Takayasu arteritis. A: Oblique MIP 3D MR angiogram of a 34-year-old woman shows irregular dilatation of the descending thoracic aorta and proximal abdominal aorta and narrowing of the infrarenal aorta. **B:** Axial T1-weighted MR image of the same patient as in **(A)** shows the narrowed infrarenal aorta (*arrow*). There is mural thickening of the narrowed infrarenal aorta with relatively high signal intensity. (Reprinted with permission from Nastri MV, Baptista LP, Baroni RH, et al. Gadolinium-enhanced three-dimensional MR angiography of Takayasu arteritis. *Radiographics.* 2004;24:773–786.)

average increase of 10% per year (18). Hypertension, obstructive pulmonary disease, and smoking are independent risk factors for aneurysm rupture (19). The mortality

rate after elective AAA repair is 5% or less and after ruptured AAA repair is 50% (20). Based on the preceding figures of rupture risk and the morbidity and mortality of intervention, 5.5-cm external anteroposterior (AP) diameter of an AAA is now considered the threshold above which aneurysmectomy or endovascular stent grafting should be considered.

The 5-year survival rate after successful AAA repair approximates 70%, and 10-year survival rate is 40% (21). The survival rate reflects comorbidity, most commonly cardiovascular and pulmonary disease. Survival rates after successful repair in patients with ruptured AAA are comparable to elective surgery if the patient survives the initial 30 days. In general, survival after AAA repair is reduced in comparison to an age-matched and sex-matched population because of greater associated comorbidity in patients with aneurysms (22).

The minority of aneurysms present with distal thromboembolism or with aortoiliac thrombosis (23). In a population at risk that is selected for screening, presymptomatic aortic aneurysms may be diagnosed by sonography (24). On occasion, AAAs may be detected as incidental findings in patients having abdominal radiography or abdominal CT or MRI for other clinical indications.

Imaging Findings

Both CT and MR are definitive noninvasive diagnostic angiographic tests that provide a template for therapy, either operative or endovascular. Neither CT nor MR is a screening examination, that role being played by a clinical examination and ultrasound imaging. Clinical examination is unreliable in the detection of AAA, being limited by patient body habitus and the unreliable quantitative estimations that derive from a physical examination (25). Ultrasound is a reliable screening strategy, and there is an increasing consensus that application

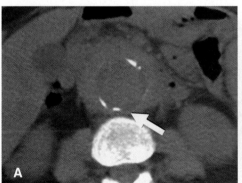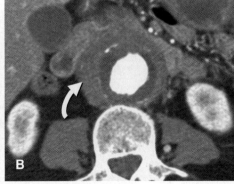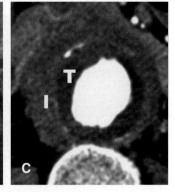

FIGURE 18-33 Inflammatory aneurysm. A: Transverse CT section without intravenous contrast medium illustrates an AAA with a mantle of soft tissue peripheral to the aneurysm but sparing the posterior aspect adjacent to the lumbar spine (*arrow*). **B:** Following administration of intravenous contrast medium, the soft tissue around the aneurysm enhances (*curved arrow*), which identifies it as inflammatory tissue rather than thrombus from a leaking aneurysm. **C:** The enhancement is best appreciated by noting the increased attenuation difference between the unenhancing mural thrombus (*T*) lining the aneurysm and the inflammatory tissue (*I*) following administration of iodinated contrast medium. This difference is easiest to identify when using a narrow window width. (Courtesy of Geoffrey D. Rubin, MD.)

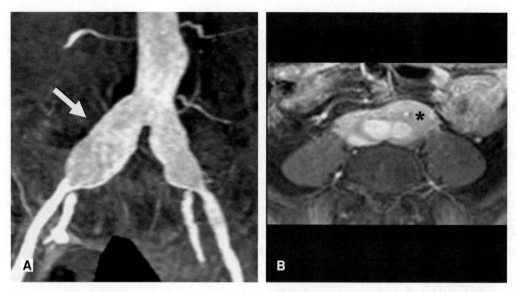

FIGURE 18-34 Inflammatory aneurysm. A: MIP of a gadolinium-enhanced 3D MRA demonstrates bilateral common iliac artery aneurysms (*arrow*). **B:** Transverse MPR demonstrates hyperintense soft tissue around the proximal common iliac arteries due to avidly enhancing inflammatory tissue (∗). (Courtesy of Thomas M. Grist, MD.)

of ultrasound in a population at risk will lead to detection and management of the presymptomatic AAA (26) (Fig. 18-35). An undiagnosed AAA that ruptures has an 80% immediate mortality rate and a cumulative additional 30-day mortality rate of approximately 50% in survivors (27). Ultrasound is useful for detection of infrarenal AAAs. However, the technique is unreliable in determining whether an aneurysm may be juxtarenal or suprarenal and whether an aneurysm involves the common iliac artery or extends to the iliac artery bifurcation. Furthermore, additional aneurysmal disease or stenotic disease of abdominal visceral vessels generally is not evaluated.

Although ultrasound is useful in the detection of AAAs, interobserver variability in estimation of anteroposterior aortic dimension is on the order of ±5 mm (28).

This interobserver variability requires a more precise measurement of aneurysm dimension if a therapeutic intervention is considered. Both precise measurement and display of regional vascular anatomy are provided by either CT or MR.

Both CT and MR are noninvasive, meaning that vascular access is via the peripheral vein, and intra-arterial puncture is avoided. In addition, both techniques are inherently 3D and quantitative, allowing for a full range of imaging projections and measurements from a single acquisition. These two factors, noninvasiveness and inherent 3D quantitation, are the principal reasons why CTA and MRA are preferred over conventional diagnostic arteriography for preoperative planning for patients with AAA.

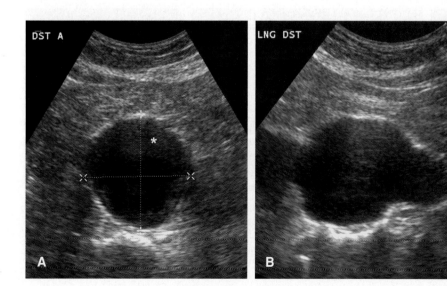

FIGURE 18-35 Transverse (**A**) and longitudinal (**B**) sonographic images of an infrarenal AAA.

Quantitative measurements from conventional arteriography can be obtained by using a calibrated catheter to provide length measurements between designated anatomic levels (Fig. 18-36)—for example, between the renal vascular pedicle and each iliac artery bifurcation (29). This information can be supplemented by intravascular ultrasound to provide diameter and area measurements at selected anatomic levels—for example, at the proximal mid and distal extent of the superior neck (30). Although this information may be accurate, the relatively inexpensive and noninvasive angiography provided by CTA and MRA has rapidly gained acceptance for preintervention assessment and planning (Fig. 18-37). In essence, both CTA and MRA provide information comparable to that provided by diagnostic arteriography with a calibrated catheter and supplemental intravascular ultrasound but in a manner that provides a vascular 3D model. The potential morbidity of conventional arteriography associated with catheter-related complications at the puncture site (femoral artery), vessel access site (iliac arteries), and definitive injection site (abdominal aorta) are avoided. These complications are well known and include pseudoaneurysm, dissection, and thromboembolism related to the puncture site; arterial dissection and thrombosis related to the access site; and dissection and microembolism related to the injection site.

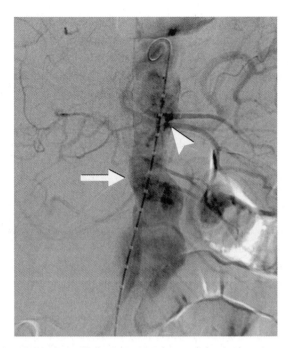

FIGURE 18-36 **Preliminary transcatheter abdominal aortogram in frontal projection prior to placement of endovascular stent graft.** Pigtail catheter tip placed in the suprarenal aorta. The 1-cm marker scale on the catheter demarcates the distance between the lower margin of the renal vascular pedicle (*arrowhead*) and the upper margin of the aneurysm (*arrow*).

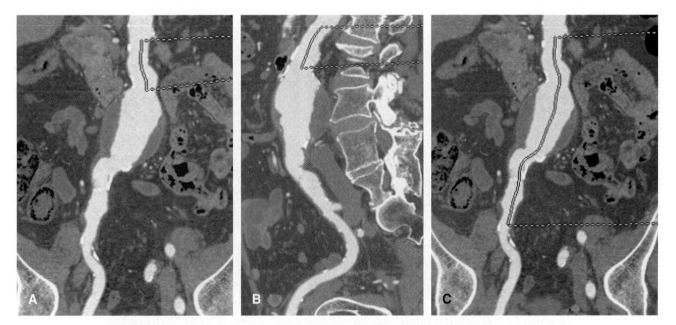

FIGURE 18-37 **Quantitative measurement of length of superior neck provided by CTA (same patient as illustrated in Figure 18-36). A:** Curved coronal reformation of the abdominal aorta and right common iliac artery. The aneurysm involves the infrarenal aorta extending to bifurcation and the proximal common iliac arteries. Measured length of superior neck (using automated centerline tracking) is 47.3 mm, in good agreement with the estimation provided by the calibrated catheter, as illustrated in Figure 18-36. Curved sagittal **(B)** and coronal **(C)** reformations of the abdominal aorta and right iliac arteries. The automated extraction of the aortic centerline provides a more accurate measurement than estimations obtained from serial axial scans of the lordotically curved aorta.

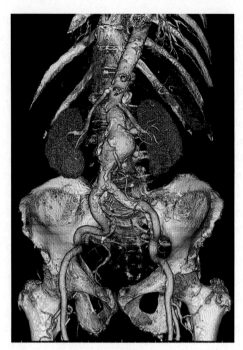

FIGURE 18-38 Typical appearance of infrarenal AAA using volume rendering. (Courtesy of Geoffrey D. Rubin, MD.)

Patients selected for noninvasive abdominal aortic CTA or MRA usually have the diagnosis of significant aneurysm established by preliminary sonography. However, not all patients will proceed to an endovascular or operative interven-

tion. This may be due to a combination of factors, including anatomy that prevents effective endovascular stent grafting (31) or systemic factors, in particular cardiovascular and renal disease that make the patient a relatively high operative risk for an open procedure. For these patients, the reproducibility of noninvasive angiography is a significant advantage.

The typical AAA is an infrarenal fusiform aneurysm, in which the upper margin is at least one centimeter distal to the renal vascular pedicle and the aneurysm terminates above or extends to the aortic bifurcation with ectatic or normal diameter common iliac arteries (Fig. 18-38). The aneurysm may be relatively straight but it is frequently torturous, and the presence of lining mural thrombus, particularly at the posterior aspect, is common. Mural calcification is frequent. Some degree of angulation to the superior neck in relation to both the juxtarenal aorta and the long axis of the aneurysm is common.

Distal extension of the aneurysm into the common iliac arteries is not unusual. Such aneurysms usually involve the proximal common iliac arteries with normal diameter distal common iliac arteries and hypogastric arteries. As with aortic aneurysms, lining mural thrombus and mural calcification are relatively common. Although most aneurysms are fusiform in shape, saccular aneurysms also occur and may be eccentric in relation to the long axis of the aorta (Fig. 18-39). Saccular aneurysms are more likely

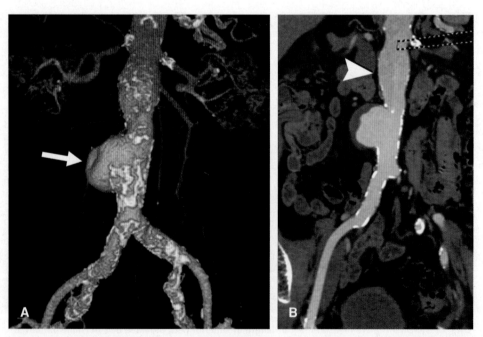

FIGURE 18-39 Eccentric sacular infrarenal aortic aneurysm. A: VR in frontal projection demonstrating mild fusiform dilatation of the immediate infrarenal aorta and an eccentric saccular aneurysm of the more caudal abdominal aorta projecting to the right (*arrow*). There is extensive atherosclerotic calcification involving the abdominal aorta, the ostia and proximal segments of both main renal arteries, and the common iliac and proximal internal iliac arteries. **B:** Curved planar reformation of the abdominal aorta and right common and external iliac arteries. The eccentric saccular aneurysm with lining mural thrombus is at the caudal aspect of a more proximal fusiform aneurysm (*arrowhead*). The linear intraluminal measurement in the supra-aneurysmal aorta is the length of the superior neck obtained by the vessel analysis program.

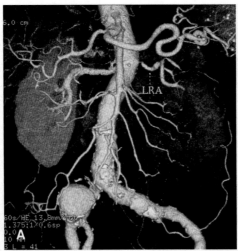
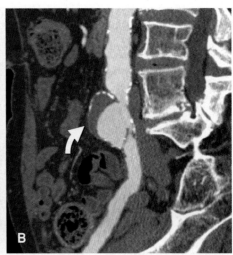

FIGURE 18-40 Common iliac artery saccular aneurysm. A: VR in frontal projection of the aortoiliac arterial system demonstrates a prominent saccular right common iliac artery aneurysm involving the common iliac artery bifurcation. There is a proximal stenosis of the left renal artery (*LRA*). The left internal iliac artery is occluded. **B:** Curved sagittal reformation of the abdominal aorta and right common and external iliac arteries. Prominent lining thrombus and mural calcification are noted in the saccular right common iliac artery aneurysm (*curved arrow*). The external iliac artery distal to the aneurysm shows a high-grade stenosis.

in instances of isolated common iliac artery aneurysms or hypogastric artery aneurysms (Fig. 18-40).

The superior neck of an infrarenal aortic aneurysm is usually relatively straight and smooth in contour, though superior necks may be ectatic and have significant atherosclerotic disease and ulceration, a possible source of peripheral microembolization during angiography and stent-graft placement. Besides being angulated in relation to both the proximal aorta and the more caudal aneurysm, a superior neck may be either flared or conical in shape and present relative risk in terms of stability of an implanted stent graft, particularly one with a friction seal.

Approximately 5% of AAAs are juxtarenal (within one centimeter below the renal arteries) or suprarenal (extending

above the renal arteries) (32). Both juxtarenal and suprarenal aneurysms are unsuitable for conventional endovascular stent grafting.

Important issues in relation to operative or endovascular repair are the presence of accessory renal arteries arising from the aneurysm, patency of the IMA arising from the aneurysm, and stenosis or occlusion of the superior mesenteric and/or hypogastric arteries. An accessory renal artery arising from the aneurysm may be sacrificed by an endoluminal stent-graft procedure if the artery supplies a relatively small portion of the kidney, the patient has normal renal function, and the main renal arteries are not stenotic (33).

A patent IMA arising from an aneurysm (Fig. 18-41) may be implanted into an aortic graft during surgery or may

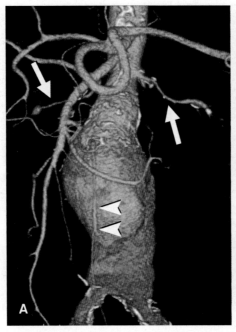
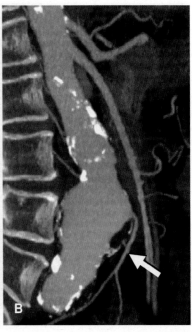

FIGURE 18-41 IMA arising from an AAA. A: VR in slight LAO projection demonstrates the IMA arising from a large fusiform infrarenal AAA (*arrowheads*). The small-caliber renal arteries (*arrows*) reflect chronic renal disease. **B:** Thin-section planar MIP in lateral projection of another patient with the IMA (*arrow*) arising from the anterior surface of a fusiform infrarenal aortic aneurysm.

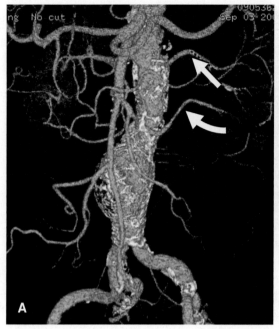
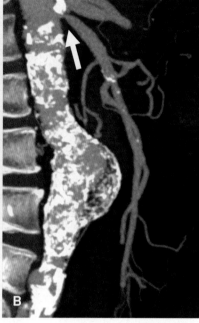

FIGURE 18-42 AAA, occluded IMA, and stenosis of the superior mesenteric artery. A: Extensively calcified infrarenal abdominal aorta with a fusiform aneurysm of the distal aorta. The IMA is occluded. Patient has two left renal arteries (*straight* and *curved arrows*), the most inferior of which arises from the upper margin of the fusiform aneurysm. **B:** Thin-section planar MIP in lateral projection demonstrates the fusiform aneurysm with anterior lining mural thrombus and a high-grade orifice stenosis of the superior mesenteric artery (*arrow*) immediately caudal to a prominent anterior wall calcified plaque.

be ligated if there is adequate collateral circulation from the middle colic to the left colic artery via the marginal colonic circulation (34). Such assessments can be made intraoperatively by evaluating pulse pressure in the stump of an IMA after separation from the aorta. In patients treated with endovascular stent grafting, in whom the IMA is patent off the aneurysm, a preintervention display of the middle colic and superior left colic arteries is important in determining the likelihood of adequate left colon perfusion after aneurysm exclusion. In addition to evaluating colic artery patency, stenosis of the superior mesen-

teric artery and/or hypogastric artery is also important. A stenosed superior mesenteric artery may not provide adequate pulse pressure through the meandering mesenteric arterial circulation to provide sufficient left colon perfusion following aneurysm exclusion (Fig. 18-42). The hypogastric artery through its middle hemorrhoidal to superior hemorrhoidal anastomoses also contributes to sigmoid and left colonic arterial perfusion, and stenosis of the hypogastric arteries in the presence of a patent IMA arising from the aneurysm introduces a relative risk of postendograft colonic ischemia.

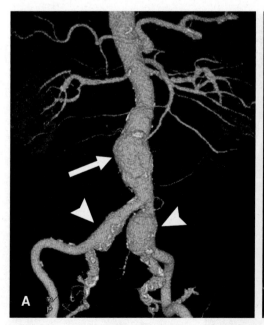
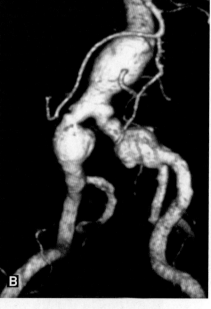

FIGURE 18-43 Aortic and iliac aneurysms proximal to and incorporating the iliac artery bifurcations. A: Frontal perspective of a VR CT image shows a fusiform infrarenal aortic aneurysm (*arrow*) and bilateral fusiform common iliac artery aneurysms (*arrowheads*). **B:** In another patient, very similar findings are depicted by using MRI. (Courtesy of Neil M. Rofsky, MD.)

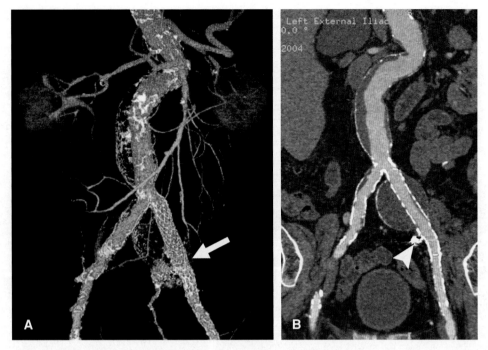

FIGURE 18-44 Endovascular therapy of a discrete common iliac artery aneurysm. A: VR in frontal projection of the aortoiliac vessels demonstrates a fusiform infrarenal aortic aneurysm caudal to an angulated superior neck and an endovascular stent graft in an isolated left common iliac artery aneurysm. The endovascular graft is extended into the proximal external iliac artery (*arrow*). **B:** Curved planar reformation in the frontal projection of the abdominal aorta and left common iliac and external iliac arteries. Endovascular stent-graft exclusion of the left common iliac artery aneurysm with extension into the left external iliac artery. There is a coil occluder (*arrowhead*) in the proximal left internal iliac artery placed before endovascular stenting to prevent reflow endoleak.

Aortoiliac aneurysms, in which the common iliac aneurysms extend to the iliac artery bifurcation, require the use of a bifurcated endovascular stent graft with extenders into the external iliac artery on the involved side. Concomitantly, occlusion of the ipsilateral hypogastric artery has to be performed to prevent reflow endoleak into the distal graft (35). In this circumstance, arterial inflow into the pelvis should be maintained by a patent opposite hypogastric artery, thus requiring any contralateral common iliac artery aneurysm to have a distal margin proximal to the iliac artery bifurcation (Fig. 18-43).

Isolated common iliac artery aneurysm that is not in continuity with an aortic aneurysm can be treated by a separate iliac endovascular stent graft (36) (Fig. 18-44).

An isolated hypogastric artery aneurysm with a normal-diameter patent hypogastric artery of the opposite side can be treated with coil embolization (37) (Fig. 18-45).

In general, juxtarenal AAAs are not treated with conventional stent grafts. Clinical experimentation relates to incorporating fenestrations in a suprarenally fixated stent graft to allow perfusion of the renal arteries (38). At present, suprarenal aneurysms are treated by surgical tube-graft replacement with implantation of the abdominal visceral branches.

A suprarenal AAA may be combined with a thoracoabdominal aneurysm. A classification scheme for such aneurysms was proposed by Crawford, who developed four categories (Fig. 18-46) of descending thoracic/abdominal aortic aneurysm (39). These are:

I. Complete descending and suprarenal aortic aneurysm with nonaneurysmal juxta and infrarenal aorta

II. Complete descending thoracic aortic aneurysm and AAA to aortic bifurcation

III. Distal descending thoracic aortic aneurysm and complete AAA to bifurcation

IV. Suprarenal, juxtarenal, and infrarenal AAA with proximal margin at aortic hiatus

At present, there are no endograft solutions for these complex thoracoabdominal aneurysms. Surgical therapy involves tube-graft replacement of the aneurysmal aorta with implantation of intercostal and abdominal visceral branches, the latter as appropriate (39). This surgical procedure carries the risk of spinal cord ischemia and paraplegia, as the artery of Adamkiewicz may arise from an intercostal or upper lumbar vessel most commonly at the levels of T9-L2.

Aortic aneurysmal disease may develop after surgical or endovascular therapy. Following surgical aortobiiliac or

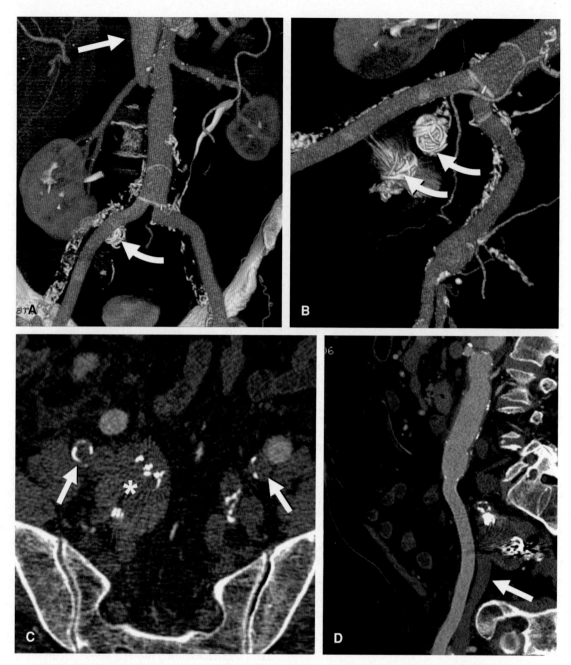

FIGURE 18-45 Hypogastric artery aneurysm with coil embolization. A: Patient with an aortobiiliac surgical tube graft (proximal anastomosis end to side) and extensively calcified infrarenal aorta and iliac vessels. There is a thoracoabdominal aortic dissecting aneurysm extending to the upper margin of the graft (*arrow*). The right renal artery arises from the false lumen and the left renal artery from the true lumen. Embolic coils are seen in the right hypogastric artery (*curved arrow*). **B:** A "tilt rotate" image demonstrating the extensive packing of embolic coils in the hypogastric artery aneurysm (*curved arrows*). **C:** Axial CT scan at the level of the mid pelvis demonstrates the large thrombosed hypogastric artery aneurysm containing embolic coils (∗). Both native external iliac arteries and the left hypogastric artery are occluded (*arrows*). The patent iliac artery graft limbs are immediately anterior to the native iliac vessels. **D:** Curved planar reformation of the aortic and right iliac component of the surgical tube graft in a lateral projection. The native thrombosed hypogastric artery aneurysm and occluded right external iliac artery (*arrow*) are posterior to the surgical tube graft.

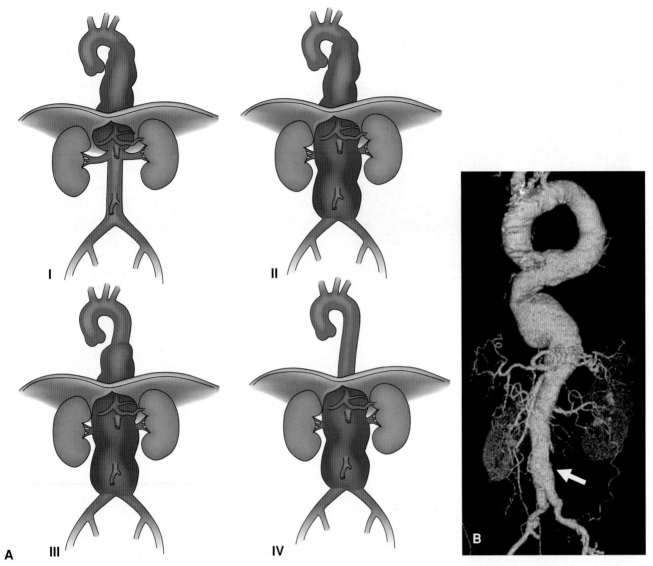

FIGURE 18-46 Crawford classification of thoracoabdominal aortic aneurysm. A: (I) Complete descending thoracic aortic aneurysm and suprarenal aortic aneurysm with nonaneurysmal juxta and infrarenal aorta. (II) Complete descending thoracic aortic aneurysm and AAA to aortic bifurcation. (III) Distal descending thoracic aortic aneurysm and complete AAA to bifurcation. (IV) Suprarenal juxtarenal and infrarenal AAA with proximal margin at aortic hiatus. **B:** VR in left anterior oblique projection demonstrates diffuse aortic ectasia with aneurysmal dilatation beginning at mid descending thoracic aorta and extending inferiorly to renal vascular pedicle. There is a short-segment aortoiliac tube graft (*arrow*). This patient's aneurysm would have been categorized as type III by the Crawford classification. The patient's infrarenal aortic aneurysm had been treated surgically.

aorto bifemoral tube grafting, a pseudoaneurysm may develop at the proximal anastomotic site, or an atherosclerotic aneurysm may develop either in the infrarenal, juxtarenal, or suprarenal aorta (Figs. 18-47, 18-48) (40). Both anastomotic and atherosclerotic postsurgical aneurysms may be treated by endovascular techniques (41). Anastomotic aneurysms tend to be saccular, whereas atherosclerotic aneurysms are usually fusiform. Anastomotic aneurysms may be infected, particularly if associated with an aortoenteric fistula, either aortoduodenal or more distal aortoenteric (42).

Infected anastomotic aneurysms frequently contain intraaneurysmal thrombus and may be associated with perianeurysmal gas bubbles and fluid (Fig. 18-49). An infected anastomotic aneurysm requires antibiotic therapy and surgical correction—in the latter, most frequently, removal and extra anatomic surgical bypass using an axillofemoral and femorofemoral crossover graft in combination with an infrarenal aortic occlusion (43) (Fig. 18-50). In some patients in whom a stump aneurysm involves the level of the renal vascular pedicle, the renal arteries are implanted separately

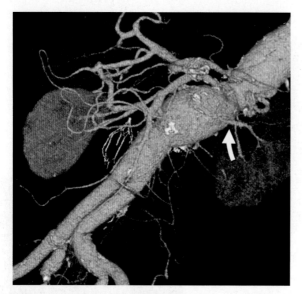

FIGURE 18-47 Supra anastomotic juxtarenal aortic aneurysm in a patient with prior aortobiiliac tube graft. VR demonstrates fusiform dilatation of the upper abdominal aorta incorporating the left renal artery (*curved arrow*) with the inferior margin of the aneurysm at the proximal anastomotic site of the aortobiiliac tube graft.

into the hepatic, splenic, or superior mesenteric arteries, and the aortic stump is closed below the level of the superior mesenteric artery (Fig. 18-51).

Patients with proximal anastomotic aneurysms should also be evaluated for distal anastomotic aneurysms, either iliac or femoral (Fig. 18-52). Noninfected proximal and distal aneurysms may be treated by endovascular stenting of the proximal anastomoses and surgical aneurysmorrhaphy for a distal iliac aneurysm (44).

A focal saccular AAA may be secondary to a penetrating aortic ulcer. A penetrating atherosclerotic ulcer and focal aneurysm may be treated with an endovascular graft if the anatomy at the level of the aneurysm is suitable. Such locations include the supraceliac abdominal aorta and the infrarenal abdominal aorta (45). If a penetrating aortic ulcer results in an infected saccular aneurysm, antibiotic therapy and subsequent surgical treatment are usually deemed advisable.

Aortocaval fistula may develop after penetrating trauma, including iatrogenic trauma related to diskectomy, or be secondary to an infected penetrating aortic ulcer with focal aneurysm formation (46). Patients with aneurysm and aortocaval fistula have a high-flow arteriovenous communication with an associated hyperdynamic state which, in the presence of coronary artery disease, may be associated with left and right heart failure. Aortocaval fistula may be diagnosed with ultrasound and Doppler imaging, CTA, MRA, or conventional arteriography.

Focal saccular aneurysms of the infrarenal aorta may result in localized vertebral body compression. A thrombus-filled saccular aortic aneurysm compressing a vertebral body may be mistaken for a periaortic malignant mass such as multiple myeloma or plasmocytoma (47). Awareness of this entity and appropriate noninvasive imaging is essential for diagnosis.

Important concomitant abdominal visceral pathology may be present in patients who have aortoiliac arterial vascular disease. Although CTA/MRA is designed as a vascular imaging study, all abdominal organs and compartments should be evaluated. Occult malignancies, when detected, may require additional CT study during parenchymal phase enhancement to best delineate tumor for local and regional staging (48) (Fig. 18-53). Either a CT or, if appropriate, ultrasound can be used for guided percutaneous biopsy.

Most patients with renal cell carcinoma are now detected serendipitously during imaging studies performed

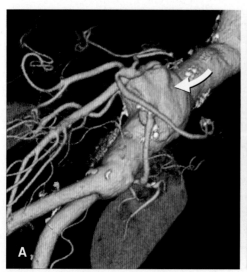
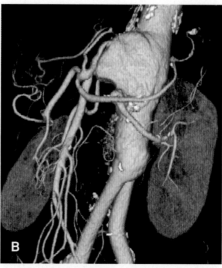

FIGURE 18-48 A: VR of a patient with focal saccular aneurysm of the juxtarenal/suprarenal aorta (*curved arrow*) following replacement of the descending thoracic aorta with a surgical graft and an abdominal aortobiiliac tube graft previously placed for aneurysmal disease. The celiac, superior mesenteric, and left and right renal arteries are all patent from the isolated aneurysmal segment of the aorta. **B:** VR in LAO projection demonstrates the isolated aneurysmal juxtarenal/suprarenal aortic segment situated between the thoracic aortic graft and the aortoiliac tube graft.

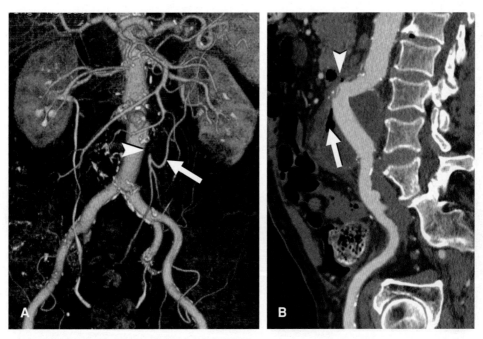

FIGURE 18-49 Infected aortic tube graft with perigraft abscess in the aneurysm sac. A: VR in frontal projection demonstrates normal patency of the aorta, aortic tube graft, and iliac arterial vessels. The IMA is occluded (*arrowhead*), and the sigmoid and superior hemorrhoidal branches are reconstituted by inflow from the superior left colic artery (*arrow*). **B:** Curved sagittal reformation of the abdominal aorta and right common and external iliac arteries. There is a prominent gas bubble in the infected aortic aneurysm sac (*arrow*). A small focus of gas in the cephalad aspect of the sac is contiguous to the transverse duodenum (*arrowhead*). Aortoduodenal fistulas are not an infrequent cause of a perigraft aortic abscess.

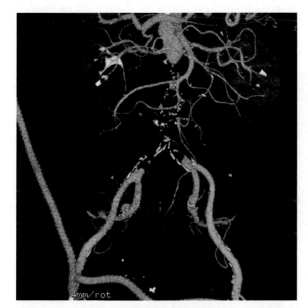

FIGURE 18-50 Same patient illustrated in Figure 18-49 following removal of the infected aortoiliac graft, surgical infrarenal aortic occlusion, and axillofemoral and femorofemoral bypass graft.

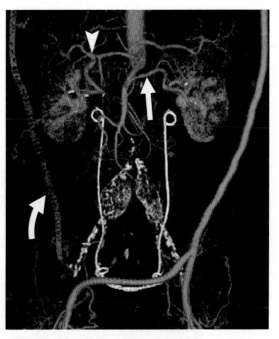

FIGURE 18-51 Patent left axillofemoral and femorofemoral bypass graft in a patient with bilateral renal artery reimplantation following aortic aneurysmectomy. VR demonstrates the patent left axillofemoral and femorofemoral bypass grafts, the right renal artery attached to the proper hepatic artery (*arrowhead*), and the left renal artery to the proximal superior mesenteric artery (*arrow*). There are calcified thrombosed common iliac artery aneurysms in situ and bilateral internal ureteral stents. A previously placed and occluded right axillofemoral graft is noted (*curved arrow*).

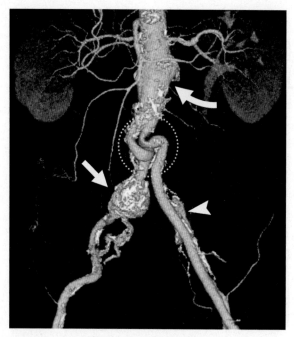

FIGURE 18-52 Supra-anastomotic and infra-anastomotic aneurysms in patient with aorto right iliac and aorto left femoral arterial bypass grafts. VR demonstrates redundant tortuous right iliac and left femoral distal limbs of the bypass graft (*dashed circle*). There is a fusiform aneurysm of the distal right common iliac artery (*arrow*) extending to the iliac artery bifurcation. A fusiform infrarenal aortic aneurysm above the proximal anastomotic site is seen (*curved arrow*). There are two renal arteries to the right kidney and a single renal artery to the left kidney. The native left iliac artery (*arrowhead*) was opacified by retrograde flow from the distal left graft anastomosis to the common femoral artery.

for other reasons, including vascular CT examinations. When detected and confirmed, the approach to patient management requires careful consideration of survival benefit with appropriate triaging of therapy for both aortoiliac vascular disease as well as the occult neoplasm.

Alternatively, a parenchymal phase CT may demonstrate disease of solid or hollow abdominal organs and in addition have incidentally discovered vascular disease, including AAA or aortoiliac atheromatous stenosis/occlusion with or without ulceration or focal dissection. Additional dedicated intravenous CT or MR arteriography may be necessary in these patients before deciding on a treatment approach.

Endovascular Aneurysm Repair

Endovascular aortic stent grafting was introduced in the mid 1990s. The major value of the endovascular technique is avoidance of (i) laparotomy, (ii) cross clamping of the aorta, and (iii) the obligatory blood loss associated with opening of the aneurysm sac (49). In addition, the endovascular technique avoids the problem of cross clamping of the infrarenal aorta in the presence of a retroaortic renal vein, which has a well-documented history of surgical catastrophe when surgeons are unaware of this anatomic anomaly in their patient (50). Both CTA and MRA clearly define both retroaortic (less than 5%) and circumaortic (5% to 10%) renal veins as well as the uncommon anomaly of a left-sided inferior vena cava, thus allowing the surgeon to make appropriate preoperative planning.

A randomized, controlled clinical trial of surgical tube grafting versus endovascular stenting for treatment of AAAs has not been performed. Endovascular stent grafting can be offered to good risk patients who are considered fit for conventional open repair. Patient suitability for endovascular stent grafting, then, depends on anatomical and technical considerations. At present, approximately 50% of the

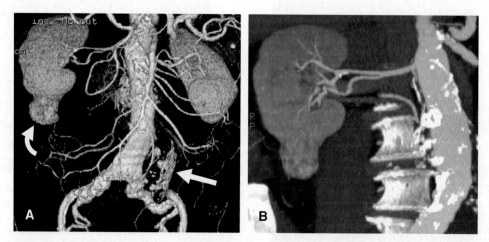

FIGURE 18-53 Image from an 82-year-old patient with a large fusiform infrarenal AAA extending to bifurcation and an incidental right lower pole exophytic renal cell carcinoma. A: VR in frontal projection demonstrates peripheral calcification at the left margin of the large aneurysm (*arrow*). There is an exophytic right lower pole renal cell carcinoma (*curved arrow*). **B:** Thin-section subvolume MIP demonstrates prominent aortic atheromatous calcification, the single right renal artery and its segmental intrarenal branches, and the exophytic lower pole.

patient population with AAA are suitable for endovascular grafting. All patients with a high surgical risk for treatment of an AAA that is 5.5 cm in diameter or greater can, if technically feasible, be offered endovascular therapy.

An endovascular graft is anchored in place by a balloon expandable or self-expanding metal frame that supports all or part of the graft and provides a watertight seal proximal and distal to the dilated segment of the artery. In addition to avoiding surgery and potential complications of laparotomy and aortic cross clamping, the stent-graft procedure decreases the hospital length of stay and has a lower perioperative morbidity and mortality rate (51). However, the technique requires repeat imaging at relatively close intervals in the first 2 years and probably a yearly evaluation after that time. During this interval, patients may require repeat procedures for closure of endoleak. Occasionally, patients may require conversion to open repair in instances of persistent endoleak, particularly type 1, infected endograft, or outflow obstruction. At this time, the long-term durability of the endograft prosthesis produced by the various manufacturers is unknown.

Major problems recognized during endovascular stent-graft placement are microembolization of the renal and peripheral circulation and type 1 endoleak. Microembolization is likely secondary to catheter manipulation abrading the surface of an ulcerated atherosclerotic aorta or secondary to the manipulation of the stent-graft device during deployment.

Anatomic Suitability and Sizing

The essential anatomic features of an angiography study that determines suitability for endovascular stent grafting of AAAs are adequate iliac access, dimensions of potential proximal and distal placement zones, and angulation of the superior neck in relation to long axis of the aneurysm.

For the Aneuryx (Medtronic, Sunnyvale, CA) (Fig. 18-54), a nickel titanium stent graft with friction seal, and the Excluder (WL Gore, Flagstaff, AZ), a nickel titanium device with friction seal and staggered barbs that is introduced by a lower profile delivery system, the following dimensions are acceptable:

- Proximal neck 28 mm in maximum external AP and transverse diameter, 15 mm in length with a 60 degrees or less angulation in relation to the long axis of the aneurysm. The aneurysm neck should not be excessively conical or flared and should be free of excessive atherothrombosis (<25% of neck circumference and <2-mm thrombus thickness).
- Distal placement zone in the iliac arteries should be 13 to 15 mm in maximal external AP diameter, 20 mm in length, and proximal to iliac artery bifurcation.

- Both external and common iliac arteries should allow access; have no focally significant stenosis, particularly a calcific stenosis; and have a maximum allowable angle of tortuosity of less than 120°.

Talent (Medtronic/World Medical, Sunrise, FL), a nickel titanium, modular, self-expanding prosthesis with a woven Dacron fabric, is designed for transrenal fixation and a wider aneurysm neck.

Zenith (Cook, Bloomington, IN), a stainless steel, self-expanding (Fig. 18-54) fully supported, modular endograft with friction seal and staggered barbs, is designed for transrenal fixation and accommodates wider aneurysm neck (up to 32 mm) and wider iliac diameter (up to 20 to 24 mm). These specific tolerances are applicable at the time of writing this chapter. Manufacturers web sites should be consulted for updated values.

Either automated software measurement or manual technique by using curved planar reformation and subsequent length measurement should be used to determine true linear distance from the level of the renal vascular pedicle to the aortic bifurcation and the length of each common iliac artery to the iliac artery bifurcation.

As in all potential stent grafting, careful assessment of patency of the mesenteric, renal, and hypogastric arteries should be performed for reasons as detailed previously.

Post Stent-graft Imaging

Computed Tomographic Angiography

Follow-up imaging after endovascular repair may be performed after the procedure, at 3, 6, 12, and 18 months. Annual follow-up is advised. In CTA, a post–stent-graft imaging examination employs precontrast, dynamic first circulation helical imaging and "immediate delayed" postcontrast imaging. Both the precontrast and "immediate delayed" postcontrast imaging can be performed with relatively thick sections of 2 to 3 mm, although thinner sections may be of value for resolving mural calcium. The dynamic first circulation helical study is performed with maximum z-axis resolution, which depending on MDCT system employed can vary from 0.5- to 1.25-mm detector collimation. As with preoperative imaging, a first circulation study requires accurate circulation timing, equivalence of injection and acquisition intervals, and sufficiently rapidly injected contrast bolus to elevate aortic CT attenuation by 250 to 300 HU throughout acquisition. Images are evaluated in stacked axial cine mode, full-volume and subvolume MIP, VR, multiplanar reformations, and curved planar reformations (Fig. 18-55). In addition to measuring the maximum external AP and

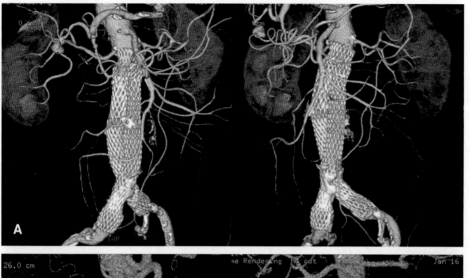

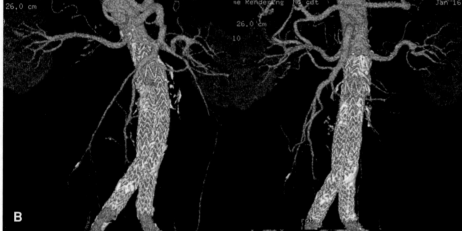

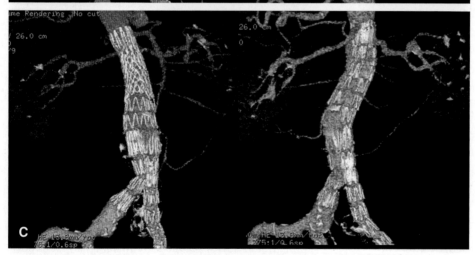

FIGURE 18-54 Aortic endovascular stent grafts. A: AneuRx aortoiliac endovascular stent graft in a RAO (*1*) and LAO (*2*) projection. The upper margin of the device is immediately caudal to the renal arteries and the lower margin immediately cephalad to each iliac artery bifurcation. Arterial wall calcification is superimposed on the metallic endoskeleton. **B:** VR in RAO (*1*) and LAO (*2*) projections of a Gore aortoiliac endovascular stent graft. There is immediate infrarenal fixation of the proximal margin with the lower margins in the common iliac arteries. **C:** Cook Zenith aortoiliac endovascular stent graft with suprarenal fixation. VR in RAO (*1*) and LAO (*2*) projection demonstrates single patent renal arteries bilaterally overlain by the uncovered proximal segment of the stent graft. The superior mesenteric artery likewise is overlain by the uncovered proximal segment of the stent graft. Distal margin of the right iliac limb is in an ectatic common iliac artery. The left iliac limb is extended into the external iliac artery, as the left iliac aneurysm had involved the iliac artery bifurcation.

transverse dimensions of the aneurysm sac and the endoluminal measurements of the aortic stent graft and its two limbs, the distance between the proximal margin of the stent graft and the inferior margin of the most inferior renal artery, and the lower margin of the stent graft and the iliac artery bifurcation of each side are measured (Fig. 18-56).

In endovascular aortic stent-graft imaging, attention should be directed to the following important issues.

* *Aneurysm Dimension.* Aneurysm dimension, particularly comparison of external AP and transverse dimension on sequential imaging studies. Aneurysm volume may be a useful measure in some cases.

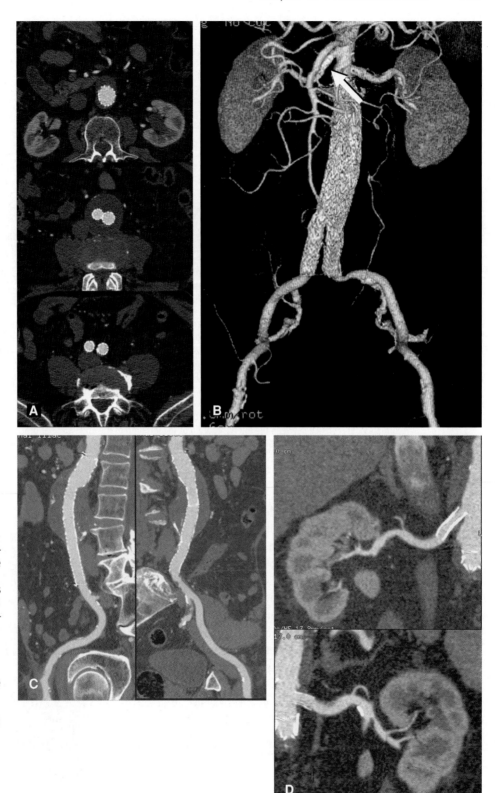

FIGURE 18-55 Patient with aorto-biiliac endovascular stent graft (Gore Excluder). A: Selected axial images demonstrating (*1*) the aortic component of the endovascular graft in the more cephalad segment of the aneurysm, (*2*) the proximal aspect of the bifurcated distal limbs in the more caudal aspect of the aortic aneurysm, and (*3*) the bifurcated distal limbs in each common iliac artery. **B:** VR in frontal projection of the aortoiliac system demonstrating placement of the bifurcated stent graft, upper margin in the superior neck and both lower margins in the common iliac arteries proximal to the iliac artery bifurcation. Note the right renal artery stent (*arrow*). **C:** Selected curved planar reformations of the aortoiliac vessels. (*1*) Abdominal aorta and right iliac artery. (*2*) Abdominal aorta and left iliac artery. **D:** Selective curved planar reformations of both renal arteries. (*1*) Right renal artery visualized from the ostium to the renal hilum. Normal patency at the endovascular stent site. At the renal hilum, the curved plane continues in a segmental branch vessel. (*2*) Left renal artery visualized from the aortic ostium to the left renal hilum. Eccentric calcific plaque is in the distal left main renal artery. At the renal hilum, the centerline tracking continues in a segmental renal artery.

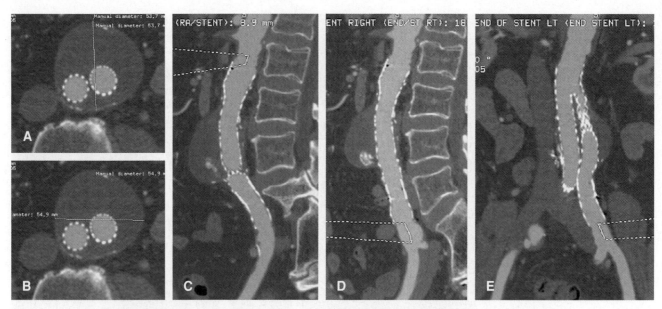

FIGURE 18-56 Measurements of the aneurysm sac and the endovascular graft; images obtained from curved planar reformation. Transverse images portrayed in **(A)** and **(B)** are perpendicular to the long axis of the aneurysm, not perpendicular to the patient's long axis. **A:** AP diameter of the aneurysm sac is 53.7 mm. **B:** Transverse dimension of the aneurysm sac is 54.9 mm. **C:** Distance between the inferior margin of the lowest renal artery and the upper margin of the endovascular graft is 8.9 mm. Renal artery origins were localized in a frontal projection with the same spatial location recorded on the sagittal view. The sagittal view best portrays the true linear distance in the slightly anteriorly angulated aorta. **D:** Distance between the inferior margin of the right limb of the endovascular graft and the right iliac bifurcation is 18.4 mm. Only the origin of the right hypogastric artery is seen on this curved sagittal reformation. **E:** Distance between the inferior margin of the left limb of the endovascular graft and the left iliac bifurcation is 14.7 mm. Only the proximal segment of the left hypogastric artery is seen on the curved coronal reformation.

- *Endoleak.* There are five types of endoleak (Fig. 18-57), which can be summarized as follows:

A type 1 endoleak is an attachment site endoleak, either proximal or distal. This is usually recognized following stent-graft placement (Fig. 18-58A). Type 1 endoleaks maintain arterial pressure inside the sac and if untreated can eventually lead to aortic enlargement and rupture (52). Type 1 endoleaks require treatment either by placement of aortic extender cuffs at the proximal or distal attachment site or by open surgical suture closure.

A type 2 endoleak is a re-entry endoleak via an aortic branch, typically the lumbar or IMA (Figs. 18-58B, 18-59). Lumbar arteries are not embolized or ligated in an endovascular repair, and although small, they may continue to communicate with the aneurysm sac. A type 2 endoleak usually requires both an inflow and outflow vessel, and both lumbar and inferior mesenteric arteries may function as either inflow or outflow vessels (53).

A type 3 endoleak is due to mechanical disruption involving either the fabric of an endograft or mechanical separation of an iliac module or exten-

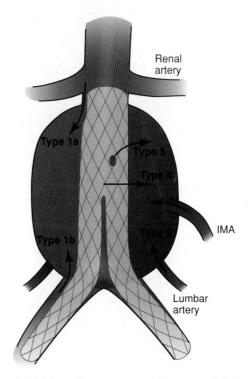

FIGURE 18-57 Schematic representation of common endoleak types (1–3).

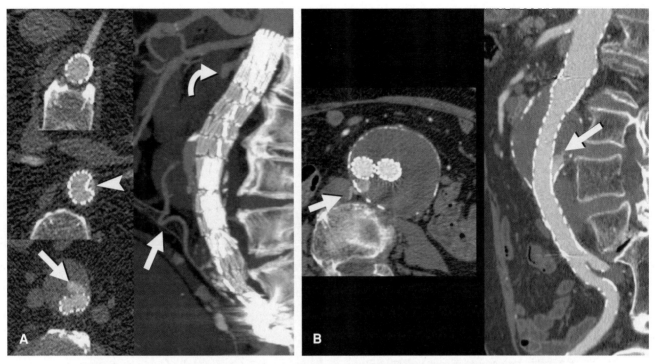

FIGURE 18-58 Examples of different types of endoleak. A: Type I endoleak following suprarenal fixation with a Cook Zenith endograft. (*1*) Axial CT scan at the level of the superior mesenteric artery takeoff. Uniform opacification of aortic lumen inside the uncovered first segment of the stent graft. (*2*) Crenated appearance of the second segment of the stent graft with contrast opacification between the covered stent graft and the aortic wall (*arrowhead*). (*3*) Contrast opacification of the aneurysm sac anterior to the two adjacent distal graft limbs (*arrow*). (*4*) Thin-section planar MIP in lateral projection demonstrates contrast opacification of the aneurysm sac from the inflow site at the upper margin of the second segment of the graft (*curved arrow*). Cephalad to caudad flow in the aneurysm sac opacifies the IMA, the outflow vessel (*arrow*). The crenation of the second segment of the graft was secondary to slight oversizing. This was corrected with use of a Palmaz internal stent, and the endoleak was closed. **B:** (*1*) Type II aortic endoleak with contrast opacification of the aneurysm sac via inflow from a lumbar artery (*arrow*). (*2*) Curved planar reformation of the abdominal aorta and right common and external iliac arteries in a lateral projection. The posterior leak into the inferior aneurysm sac is clearly defined (*arrow*).

der from the main graft (54). Type 3 endoleaks may be treated by placement of an additional endograft to seal the local leak or may require conversion to open procedure.

A type 4 endoleak is secondary to graft porosity, a condition that may occur immediately after placement before the graft material has been sealed by incorporation of fibrin. A type 4 endoleak is by its nature self-healing.

A type 5 endoleak, described as "endotension," occurs when arterial pressure is recorded in the aneurysm sac, but there is no identifiable cause (55). Endotension is a diagnosis of exclusion in that both noninvasive and catheter arteriography (with injection of all potential feeders to supply a possible reflow endoleak) has been performed. Endotension, associated with expansion of the aneurysm sac, usually requires conversion to open repair.

If an endoleak is detected, this should be categorized into types 1, 2, 3, 4 or 5 as determined by the imaging study. It is important to compare precontrast, dynamic bolus postcontrast, and "immediate delayed" postcontrast CTA to identify laminated calcium, to distinguish laminated calcium from endoleak, and to maximize sensitivity to endoleak. Laminated calcium as seen on the dynamic bolus study may be mistaken for endoleak if not compared with the precontrast image at the same level. A type 2 endoleak may only be evident on the "delayed" postcontrast study and not evident on the dynamic bolus study (Figs. 18-60, 18-61). This may relate to slower circulation through the feeding arteries (i.e., lumbar and inferior mesenteric) and continued enhancement of the endoleak cavities secondary to continued slow inflow of contrast-enhanced blood.

Another key strategy for maximizing endoleak detection is the use of a "thrombus window," which has a narrow

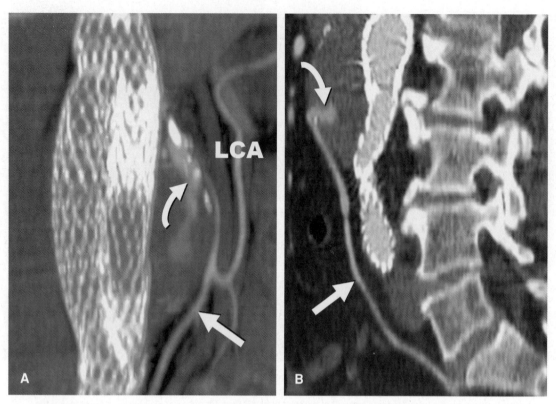

FIGURE 18-59 Type 2 endoleak (*curved arrows*) fed by the IMA (*straight arrows*) in different patients, displayed on subvolume MIP **(A)** and curved planar reformation **(B)**. In **(A)**, also note the role of the left colic artery (*LCA*) in the retrograde filling of the IMA. (Courtesy of Geoffrey D. Rubin, MD.)

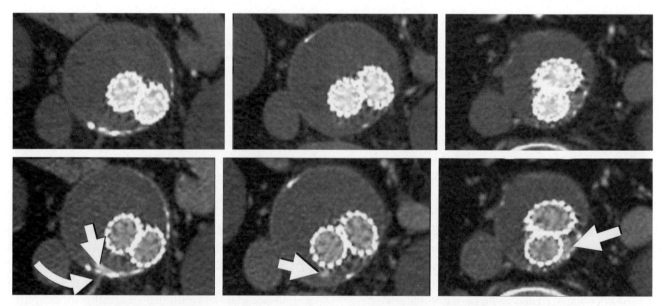

FIGURE 18-60 Comparison of early (top row, 28-second delay) and delayed (bottom row, 70-second delay) postcontrast axial CT images emphasize the relevance of the latter in the detection of subtle endoleaks. Note that this type 2 endoleak (*arrows*) fed by a lumbar artery (*curved arrow*) seen on the delayed phase is not readily identified in the early images. (Courtesy of Geoffrey D. Rubin, MD.)

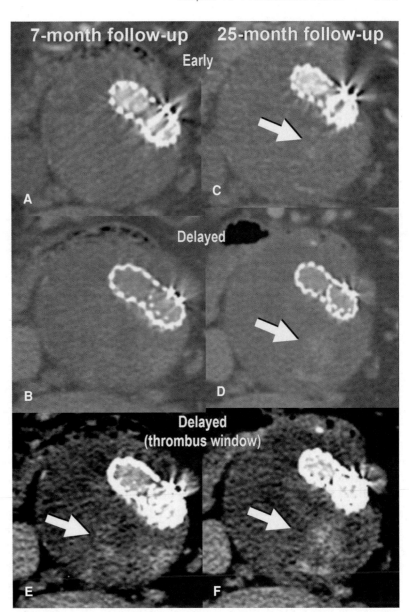

FIGURE 18-61 Transverse postcontrast CT images for follow-up of an aortoiliac stent-graft (**A** and **B**, 7 months; **C** and **D**, 25 months following stent-graft deployment). Seven months after stent-graft deployment, an increase in the aneurysm sac size was observed, but no endoleak was found (**A, B**). When the patient returned for follow-up 25 months following stent-graft deployment, a faint endoleak can be seen (*arrow* in **C**), which can be better depicted by using proper window levels (**F**). Retrospective review of the first exam with adequate window levels (**E**) show that the endoleak was already detectable at that point (*arrow*). This example illustrates the importance of using proper window levels when assessing potential endoleaks. (Courtesy of Geoffrey D. Rubin, MD.)

window width (<100 HU) and is centered on thrombus attenuation (Fig. 18-61).

Graft Limb Thrombosis

Graft limb thrombosis is uncommon and may be secondary to kinking of the aortic component of the stent graft within the aneurysm sac or kinking of the iliac limbs within the iliac arteries (Fig. 18-62). Iliac artery dissection by the catheter or delivery system during initial placement of the endovascular graft may result in ipsilateral iliac artery thrombosis distal to the graft. Iliac graft limb thrombosis may require use of a femorofemoral crossover graft to provide ipsilateral lower limb perfusion. An aortic thrombosis requires urgent conversion to open repair.

Endovascular Stent-graft Migration and Kinking

If an endovascular stent graft is not adequately fixated proximally, it can migrate, leading to the late development of a type 1 endoleak and be associated with prominent kinking in the aortic or iliac limb. Improper proximal fixation may occur if the superior neck is not anatomically suitable as a proximal placement zone, being either too conical or flared in shape. This is a subjective area of evaluation, and absolute parameters for degree of flare or conical shape for each of the different endovascular stent-graft devices has not been developed.

Rarely, aneurysm shrinkage can result in extreme aortic conformational changes. Because the stent-graft is a relatively stiff arterial element, conformational changes are concentrated at the arterial segments proximal and, in particular,

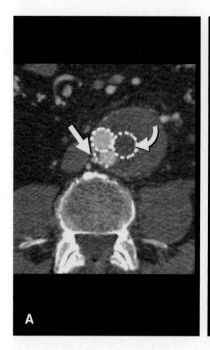
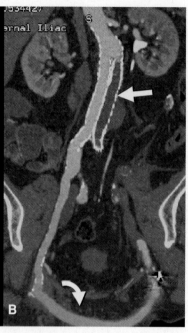

FIGURE 18-62 Graft limb thrombosis. A: Thrombosed left limb of an aortobiiliac endovascular stent graft (*curved arrow*). There is a concomitant type II endoleak in the posterior aneurysm sac filled by a lumbar artery (*arrow*). **B:** Curved planar reformation of the abdominal aorta, right common and external iliac arteries, and femorofemoral crossover graft. There is a full-length thrombotic occlusion of the left limb of the graft (*arrow*). Arterial circulation to the left lower limb was maintained by the femorofemoral crossover graft (*curved arrow*).

distal to the stent-graft, which may cause late appearance of outflow stenosis (Fig. 18-63).

Branch Vessel Occlusion

Branch vessel occlusion (Fig. 18-64) should not occur if there is proper preprocedural patient selection and appropriate placement of a suitable endovascular stent graft. If the proximal margin of a covered stent graft overlays a renal artery, renal artery occlusion and infarction can occur. More commonly, inferior accessory renal arteries are overlain by the covered portion of the stent graft and are occluded if they supply a relatively small proportion of kidney parenchyma in a patient with normal renal function and without main renal artery stenosis.

The success rate of endovascular stent grafting approximates 90%, and the 5-year survival rate of treated patients is 83% (56). This is equivalent to the reported 5-year survival rate of surgical repair of AAA. At most medical institutions, patients who have suitable anatomy for endovascular stent-graft repair are treated endovascularly, and the proportion of patients who will, in the future, be suitable for the endovascular approach will increase as new types of endovascular stent grafts are developed.

Magnetic Resonance Angiography

As this chapter demonstrates, the majority of attention for stent-graft planning and follow-up has focused on MDCT examination; however, several have demonstrated MRA/MRI examination as a viable alternative for planning and surveillance in patients with nonferrous-containing grafts (31,57,58). Essentially, all aortic stent grafts are compatible

with MR examination, meaning the patient will not suffer ill effects if he or she is scanned. However, not all stent grafts themselves can actually be interrogated in the magnet. Many stainless steel–containing grafts produce far too much susceptibility artifact to yield diagnostic examination in the immediate vicinity of the stent graft. In contrast, stents composed of novel alloys such as nickel titanium (sometimes called *nitinol*) have variable but often minimal susceptibility artifact-yielding diagnostic images, including in-stent and immediately adjacent portions of the aorta.

According to a review by Thurnher (31), imaging evaluation of stent grafts should be able to show aneurysm size, change in size, position, change in position, structural integrity, endoleak, and change in endoleak characteristics (52). CTA obviously performs admirably for these tasks; however, CTA is not without its drawbacks. Beam-hardening artifact from stent material and aortic wall calcifications can obscure subtle endoleaks. The CT exam itself uses ionizing radiation, usually of little consequence given the typical age of patients undergoing stent-graft procedures but possibly of greater concern in younger patients who will receive serial exams for a lifetime. The use of iodinated contrast material in patients whose renal function is in any way compromised poses a mild risk of nephrotoxicity. The incidence of iodinated contrast material reactions, although rare, is far greater than the incidence of serious reactions to gadolinium MR contrast agents.

There are now reported cases where MR is more sensitive than CT for the detection of aortic endoleak (59). As mentioned above, the surveillance of stent grafts is aimed at assessment of aneurysm size, detection of endoleaks, and

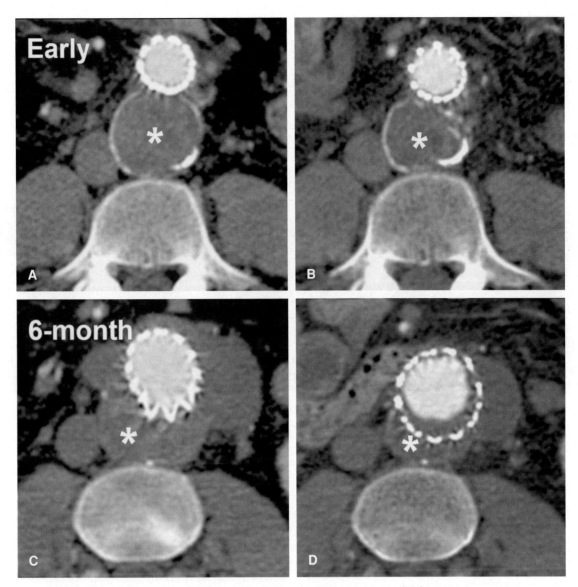

FIGURE 18-63 Kinking of the distal anastomotic site secondary to aneurysm shrinkage. Transverse postcontrast CT images 5 days (**A, B**) and 6 months (**C, D**) following stent-graft deployment to repair a proximal perianastomotic pseudoaneurysm that had developed following aortobifemoral bypass grafting. Aneurysm shrinkage is demonstrated (*). (*Figure 18-63 continues*)

evaluation of positional and structural integrity. A plain film evaluation can reveal important pathology related to stent-graft position and integrity but cannot reliably reveal endoleak information (60). Admittedly, no single modality always answers all of these questions optimally. Practical considerations such as cost, radiation and contrast exposure risks, invasiveness, equipment availability, imaging, and operator experience affect the preferred method of follow-up. For any of the previously listed reasons, CT will continue to be the predominant method of endograft surveillance, but for nonferrous stents, MRI likely answers all of the questions reliably except for structural integrity of the device. MRI alone might miss subtle structural fatigue or device fracture without significant displacement. Theoretically, a combined modality

strategy of MRI at 3 months postprocedure followed by semiannual plain film examination and annual MRI may serve as an adequate surveillance scheme. However, this has not yet been documented by medical trials.

Aortic Graft Aneurysms

Aortic or iliac arterial pseudoaneurysm may develop at the anastomotic site of an aortobiiliac graft (61) (Fig. 18-65). As with atherosclerotic ulcers, these pseudoaneurysms may be associated with distal thromboembolism. Intravenous CTA and/or MRA is the preferred technique to evaluate suspected intra-abdominal or pelvic complications of surgical tube grafts or endovascular grafts. The intravenous technique avoids graft

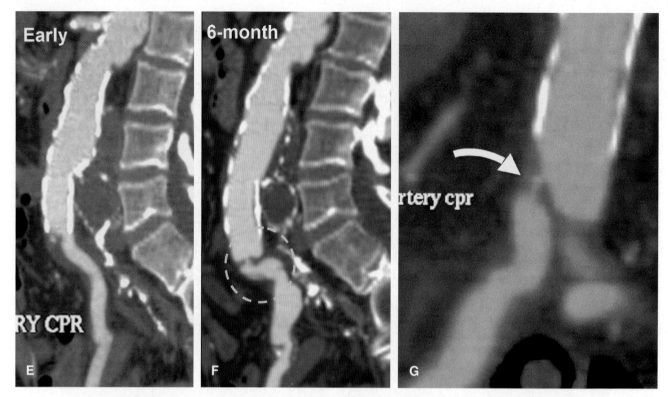

FIGURE 18-63 (Continued) This also can be observed in curved sagittal reformations (**E** and **F**, early and late follow-up images, respectively). When aneurysm growth or shrinkage occurs, movement of the aorta is expected. Because of the relatively high columnar strength of the metallic stent graft, bending forces are translated to the arteries immediately proximal and distal to the stent graft. As a consequence of the pseudoaneurysm shrinkage in this case, the distal end of the stent graft shifted posteriorly, resulting in a kink and high-grade stenosis of the right common iliac artery (*dashed area* in **F**). The coronal MPR (**G**) of this area demonstrates the kinking in the second plane (*curved arrow*). (Courtesy of Geoffrey D. Rubin, MD.)

puncture, an important advantage in patients who may have graft infection or infected pseudoaneurysms at anastomotic sites.

AORTIC STENOSIS/OCCLUSION

Classic aortoiliac atherosclerotic occlusive disease involves the distal abdominal aorta and proximal common iliac arteries with circumferential stenosis (62). The proximal aorta and the distal extremity arteries are usually normal. Predominant collateral circulation is via inferior mesenteric to hemorrhoidal branches, median to lateral sacral arteries, and intercostal and lumbar to iliolumbar and cirumflex iliac vessels. This disease pattern, classified as type 1, is relatively uncommon and more predominant in middle-aged females with a smoking history. Type 2 is more extensive, involving common and external iliac arteries as well as the aorta with predominant collateral circulation from intercostal and lumbar arteries to circumflex iliac and superior epigastric to inferior epigastric arteries as well as utilizing the other pelvic collateral circulations enumerated for type 1 disease. In type 2 disease, the arterial vessels below the inguinal ligament are normal.

Type 3 disease is diffuse aortoiliac disease as in type 2, with additional involvement of the femoropopliteal vessels. This type is most common, accounting for 65% of patients. Pelvic collateral circulation includes the conduits listed for type 1 and type 2, but with more distal disease involving the proximal superficial femoral artery, additional pelvic to thigh collateral circulation utilizing interconnections between the inferior gluteal and profunda system is recruited (63).

The clinical presentation may be the classic Leriche syndrome of claudication; weak femoral pulses; and in male patients, impotence. Ulcerated atherothrombotic disease may lead to concomitant peripheral atheroembolism (64).

Takayasu arteritis is a nonspecific aortoarteritis that may result in a focal "abdominal coarctation," usually in the vicinity of the renal vascular pedicle (Fig. 18-67). Patients may have concomitant renal, iliac, and mesenteric arterial stenoses and present with abdominal angina or hypertension in addition to buttock claudication (65).

CTA and MRA are ideal techniques for the study of patients with predominant aortoiliac stenotic or occlusive disease in that peripheral intravenous injection results in uniform opacification of all potential collateral pathways with

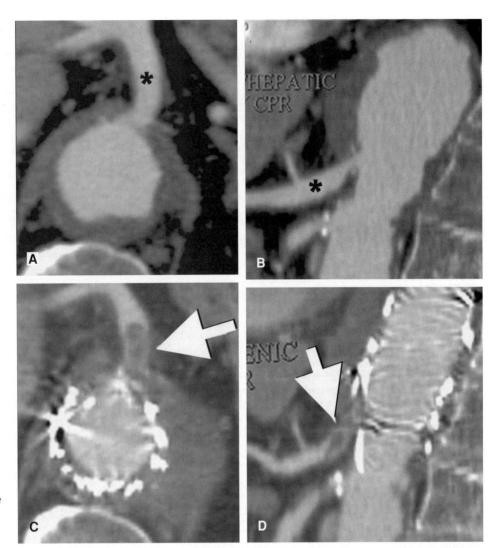

FIGURE 18-64 Supraceliac AAA with juxtaceliac distal extension in transverse (**A**) and sagittal (**B**) post-contrast CT images. Although the aneurysm with associated mural thrombus extends to involve the celiac (∗) origin, it remains patent. One day following stent-graft deployment (**C, D**), the distal end of the stent graft covers the celiac origin, where a thrombus has formed and occludes the vessel proximal to the left gastric artery (*arrows*). (Courtesy of Geoffrey D. Rubin, MD.)

good demonstration of the reconstituted extremity circulation. This occurs in the mid pelvis with retrograde flow in the hypogastric arteries to reconstitute the external iliac arteries or in the distal pelvis via circumflex iliac and inferior epigastric arteries to reconstitute flow in the common femoral arteries and via the "cruciate anastomosis" of inferior gluteal to profunda circulation to reconstitute the proximal profunda femoris artery.

Attempting to perform common femoral angiographic approaches prior to upper extremity arterial approaches can be frustrating and potentially morbid. The occlusion of the distal aorta and bilateral iliacs, therefore, puts catheter digital subtraction angiography at a distinct disadvantage in this diagnosis. Conventional catheter arteriography is limited in that brachial or axillary access may be necessary in patients with bilateral iliac disease and that separate infrarenal and descending thoracic aortic injections may be required to define the focal aortoiliac disease as well as to opacify collateral circulation. Opacification of the distal femoropopliteal

and calf circulation from either of the two separate injection sites is often suboptimal.

CTA and MRA, by virtue of the fact that they are accomplished by venous contrast injection, are ideally suited to make this diagnosis. The advantage of CTA is that a complete display of all the potential collateral arteries in the anteroposterior dimension of the subject can be portrayed. MRA is limited by the thickness of the coronal plane slab that is employed (Fig. 18-66). Both CTA and MRA may be employed as a localized aortoiliac study with inferior extension of imaging to the proximal thigh or be part of an inflow/outflow extremity arterial study extending to the feet.

AORTOILIAC ATHEROMATOUS ULCERATION

The most common locations for ulcerated aortoiliac atherosclerotic plaque are the infrarenal aorta and proximal iliac arteries. Peripheral atheroembolism from these sites usually results in unilateral showering of the distal extremity circulation. The less common suprarenal atherosclerotic ulcer may

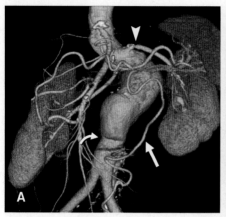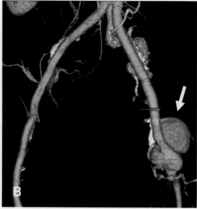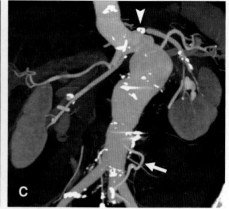

FIGURE 18-65 Patient with aortobifemoral graft (end-to-side proximal anastomosis) and multiple aneurysms. There is a supra-anastomotic infrarenal fusiform AAA **(A)** extending to the proximal margin of the surgical graft, an onlay site aneurysm in the left groin at the junction of the left graft limb and common femoral artery **(B)**, and a native left iliac artery aneurysm. **A:** Frontal projection of VR demonstrates the infrarenal fusiform aneurysm. The upper margin of the aneurysm is immediately caudal to the left renal artery (*arrowhead*). The right renal artery is more caudal but cephalad to the aneurysm and overlain by the superior mesenteric artery. The lower margin of the aneurysm is at the proximal graft anastomosis (*curved arrow*). Note the prominent middle colic to left colic arterial connection (*arrow*) reconstituting the IMA and its superior hemorrhoidal branch. **B:** Frontal projection of VR at a more caudal level demonstrates the femoral artery onlay site and pseudoaneurysm (*arrow*). The native left common iliac artery aneurysm is overlain by the left graft limb. **C:** Thin-slab MIP image of the infrarenal aortic aneurysm and proximal aspect of the aortobifemoral graft. Note the upper margin of the aneurysm caudal to the renal vascular pedicle and a proximal left renal artery stenosis (*arrowhead*). The aneurysm sac contains lining mural thrombus and scattered calcification. The reconstituted IMA is demonstrated crossing the left iliac graft limb (*arrow*).

result in bilateral embolic showering. Atheroembolism results from microembolization of platelet aggregates and cholesterol-laden debris. Emboli may be very small, of the order of 10 to 20 microns in size, with distal ischemic changes secondary to arteriolar obstruction in the presence of normal distal pedal pulses. The condition has been misdiagnosed as vasospasm, cold injury, localized Raynaud phenomenon, or connective tissue disorders including vasculitis and polyarteritis. Although most atheroembolic episodes are spontaneous in onset, precipitating events can include surgical aortic cross clamping or arterial catheterization.

Patients with focal aortoiliac atherosclerotic ulceration, in the absence of coexistent stenosis or aneurysm, may present with abdominal pain or distal thromboembolism, the classic clinical presentation being blue toe syndrome (45,64). In patients presenting with blue toe syndrome, ultrasound is a useful first step to evaluate for occult aortoiliac aneurysm, which in a limited number of patients may be the source of distal thromboembolism. However, a survey arteriogram of the thoracoabdominal aorta and iliac circulation is generally warranted. Intravenous CTA or MRA is ideal for this purpose, providing diagnostic arteriography without the risk of catheter-induced thromboembolism. CTA, in particular, can depict ulceration and associated thrombosis, often in association with focal mural calcification. The wide dynamic range of CTA that enables the depiction of a contrast-enhanced lumen, lining thrombus with superficial ulceration, and

mural calcification is not replicated in a conventional arteriogram. Furthermore, both CTA and MRA provide 3D volume data sets in which the most appropriate projection for demonstrating atherosclerotic ulceration can be chosen from a rotatable model following a single contrast injection. Both stenotic and nonstenotic iliac arterial atherosclerotic ulcers can be treated by covered percutaneously inserted stents. The surgical alternative is thromboendarterectomy or focal arterial resection and grafting.

On occasion, patients with penetrating aortic atherosclerotic ulcers will develop focal aneurysms (66). The aortic or iliac ulcerations may be multifocal. Rotatable 3D renderings are important in profiling penetrating ulcers and saccular aneurysms and assessing relationships to important branch vessels (Fig 18-68). On occasion, such penetrating ulcers may result in arteriovenous fistulas, including aortocaval fistula (67). Pseudoaneurysms resulting from a penetrating aortic ulcer may become thrombosed. A radiologist who is interpreting routine CT/MR studies of the abdomen may interpret such findings as a periaortic solid mass lesion. A high index or suspicion is required, particularly in cases where percutaneous needle aspiration biopsy is being considered.

Aortocaval fistula may be secondary to a penetrating aortic ulcer with focal aneurysm formation or may develop after penetrating trauma, including iatrogenic trauma related to diskectomy. Patients with aneurysm and aortocaval fistula have a high-flow arteriovenous communication

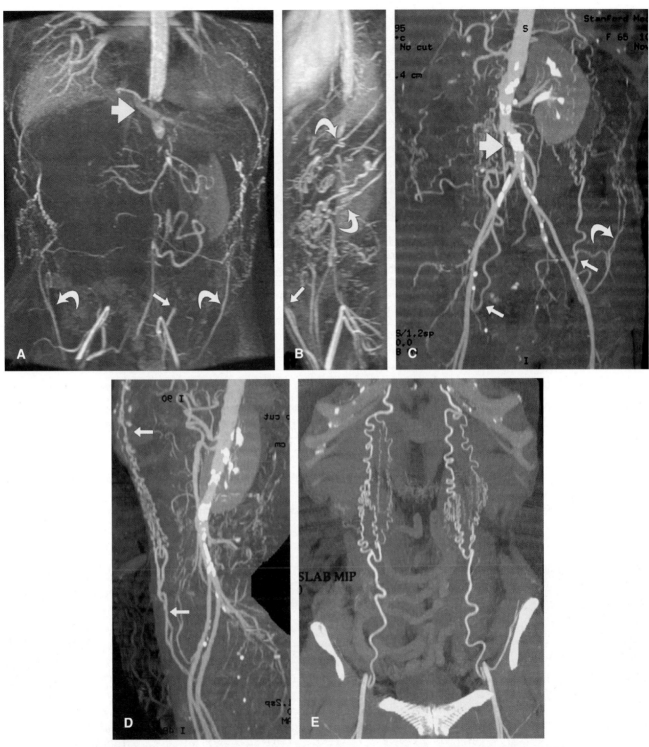

FIGURE 18-66 Two example of Leriche syndrome. (A, B) Frontal and lateral MIPs of an MRA in a patient with complete infrarenal aortic and common iliac arterial occlusion (*wide arrow*). Reconstritution of flow in the external iliac arteries is via circumflex iliac arteries (*curved arrows*) and inferior epigastric arteries (*thin arrows*). To balance between achieving sufficient anteroposterior coverage, while achieving adequate section thickness, an imaging subvolume was selected, which while imaging the entire aorta and iliac arteries, misses the anterior abdominal wall, and the majority of the internal mammary and inferior epigastric arteries. **(C, D)** Frontal and lateral MIPs of a CTA in a different patient with focal, calcified distal aortic occlusion (*wide arrow*). While the lateral circumflex iliac arteries contribute less to collateral flow (*curved arrow*), the internal mammary and inferior epigastric arteries are the dominate collateral network (*thin arrows*). The full field-of-view available with CTA does not compromise spatial resolution and enables visualization of the internal mammary and inferior epigastric arteries in the anterior abdominal wall **(E).**

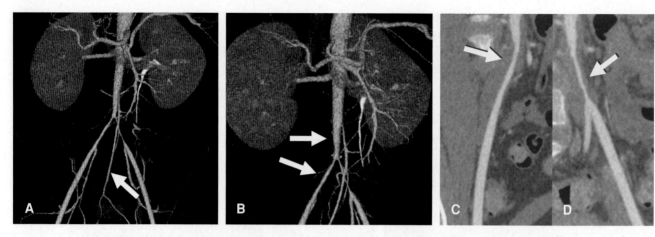

FIGURE 18-67 Takayasu aortoarteritis in an 8-year-old male with systemic symptoms and elevated erythrocyte sedimentation rate but no vascular symptomatology. **A:** VR in frontal projection with circumferential smooth stenoses of the distal aorta and both common iliac arteries, more marked on the left. Note the enlarged IMA (*arrow*) and its superior hemorrhoidal branch acting as visceral collateral circulation. **B:** VR of aortoiliac circulation in a slight RAO projection demonstrating the focal smoothly stenotic disease of the distal abdominal aorta and both common iliac arteries (*arrows*). The disease begins immediately distal to the orifice of the enlarged IMA. **C:** Right common and external iliac arteries demonstrated by curved planar reformation. Prominent mural thickening of the right common iliac artery is evident (*arrow*). **D:** Curved sagittal reformation of the distal aorta left common external iliac and proximal internal iliac arteries. Note the prominent mural thickening of the left common iliac artery (*arrow*).

with an associated hyperdynamic state which, in the presence of coronary artery disease, may be associated with left and right heart failure.

FOCAL AORTOILIAC ARTERIAL DISSECTION

The most common cause of dissection of the abdominal aorta and iliac arteries is a thoracoabdominal dissection, either type A or type B. Localized aortoiliac dissection,

unassociated with the classic aortic dissection beginning in the thoracic aorta, is an uncommon entity.

Atherosclerosis, aortoarteritis, trauma, and connective tissue disorder including Marfan and Ehlers-Danlos syndrome and fibrodysplasia (Fig. 18-69) may all result in a focal aortoiliac dissection. These dissections are usually limited to the aortoiliac vasculature and do not extend into the extremity vessels. Important imaging features are to recognize the

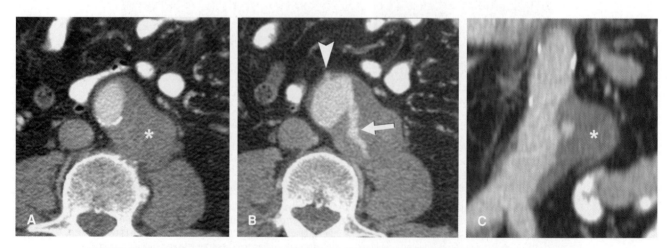

FIGURE 18-68 A 4.5-cm pseudoaneurysm of the distal abdominal aorta, considered to be a contained rupture from an ulcerated plaque. **A:** Transverse image of the infrarenal aorta at the level of the transverse duodenum demonstrates a thrombus-filled saccular aneurysm (***) projecting posteriorly and laterally to the anterior surface of the left psoas muscle. **B:** Transverse scan at a more caudal level demonstrates opacification of the serpiginous lumen in the center of the aneurysm sac (*arrow*). Note the origin of the IMA (*arrowhead*) from the anterior margin of the aorta. **C:** Coronal plane reformation demonstrating a localized saccular aneurysm projecting from the left margin of the infrarenal aorta immediately above the aortic bifurcation (***).

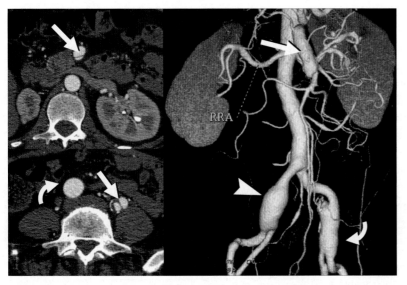

FIGURE 18-69 Fibrodysplasia. (*1*) Axial CT scan of an abdominal CTA examination demonstrates a dilated dissected proximal superior mesenteric artery (*arrow*). (*2*) Axial CT scan at the level of the pelvic brim demonstrates aneurysmal right common iliac artery (*curved arrow*) and dissected partly thrombosed aneurysm of the left common iliac artery (*arrow*). (*3*) VR of the aortoiliac arterial vessels in RAO projection. (*RRA*, right renal artery.) Note the dissection and aneurysm of the proximal superior mesenteric artery (*arrow*) and the isolated aneurysm of the right common iliac artery (*arrowhead*) and dissection with aneurysm of the left common iliac artery (*curved arrow*). This 40-year-old female also had focal dissection with aneurysm of a high cervical internal carotid artery.

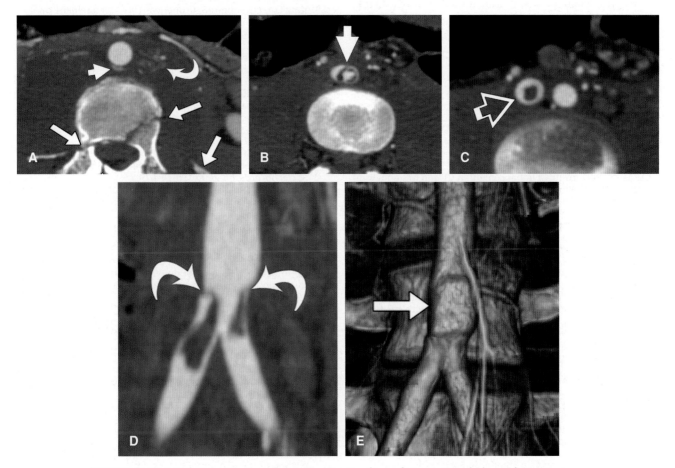

FIGURE 18-70 Aortic dissection secondary to deceleration force after a motor vehicle accident. Transverse CTA of the distal aorta (**A**) demonstrates vertebral fractures (*long arrows*) and irregularity of the aortic posterior contour (*short arrow*) with contrast extravasation (*curved arrow*) forming an extensive perivertebral hematoma. At a lower level (**B**), an intimal flap is noted (*arrow*), which becomes a central rounded filling defect in the right common iliac artery (*arrow* in **C**). The intimal flap and its extension into the aortoiliac bifurcation and the right common iliac artery are observed in a coronal MPR (*curved arrows* in **D**). The VR (**E**) depicts a bulging aortic contour in the region where the intimo-medial complex has transected, and the aortic wall integrity is compromised. (Images courtesy of Geoffrey D. Rubin, MD.)

presence of an intimal flap, flow, or thrombosis in the false lumen and involvement of branch vessels. As with other arterial dissections, focal aneurysm, thrombosis of false lumen, and occlusion of branch vessels are possible sequelae.

Clinical manifestations of aortoiliac dissection relate to stenoses/occlusion of abdominal visceral branch vessels resulting in mesenteric ischemia, hypertension, or iliac dissection and extremity ischemia. On occasion, aortoiliac dissection will result in focal aneurysmal disease.

The advantage of CT and MR arteriography is the combination of cross-sectional and 3D display to outline precisely the site and extent of arterial dissection, flow, or occlusion in the false channel and the status of branch vessels.

TRAUMATIC AORTOILIAC DISRUPTION

Traumatic disruption of the aortoiliac vasculature, either intimal or intimal/medial disruption with focal false aneurysm formation, is very uncommon. Intimal disruption may be secondary to blunt trauma and intimal/medial disruption secondary to either blunt or penetrating trauma. Blunt trauma injuries usually involve the infrarenal aorta or proximal iliac arteries (68) (Fig. 18-70).

REFERENCES

1. Fleischmann D. Use of high concentration contrast media: principles and rationale-vascular district. *Eur J Radiol.* 2003;45[Suppl 1]:S88–S93.
2. Bae KT. Peak contrast enhancement in CT and MR angiography: when does it occur and why? Pharmacokinetic study in a porcine model. *Radiology.* 2003;227:809–816.
3. Rozenblit AM, Patlis M, Rosenbaum ET, et al. Detection of endoleaks after endovascular repair of abdominal aortic aneurysm: value of unenhanced and delayed helical CT acquisitions. *Radiology.* 2003;227(2):426–433.
4. Tillich M, Hill BB, Paik DS, et al. Prediction of aortoiliac stent-graft length: comparison of measurement methods. *Radiology.* 2001;220:475–483.
5. Carr JC, Simonetti O, Bundy J, et al. Cine MR angiography of the heart with segmented true fast imaging with steady-state precession. *Radiology.* 2001;219:828–834.
6. Pereles FS, McCarthy RM, Baskaran V, et al. Thoracic aortic dissection and aneurysm: evaluation with nonenhanced true FISP MR angiography in less than 4 minutes. *Radiology.* 2002;223:270–274.
7. Finn JP, Baskaran V, Carr JC, et al. Thorax: low-dose contrast-enhanced three-dimensional MR angiography with subsecond temporal resolution—initial results. *Radiology.* 2002;224:896–904.
8. Johnston KW, Rutherford RB, Tilson MD, et al. Suggested standards for reporting on arterial aneurysms. Subcommittee on Reporting Standards for Arterial Aneurysms, Ad Hoc Committee on Reporting Standards, Society for Vascular Surgery and North American Chapter, International Society for Cardiovascular Surgery. *J Vasc Surg.* 1991;13:452–458.
9. Grange JJ, Davis V, Baxter BT. Pathogenesis of abdominal aortic aneurysm: an update and look toward the future. *Cardiovasc Surg.* 1997;5:256–265.
10. McMillan WD, Tamarina NA, Cipollone M, et al. Size matters: the relationship between MMP-9 expression and aortic diameter. *Circulation.* 1997;96:2228–2232.
11. Wills A, Thompson MM, Crowther M, et al. Pathogenesis of abdominal aortic aneurysms—cellular and biochemical mechanisms. *Eur J Vasc Endovasc Surg.* 1996;12:391–400.
12. Nastri MV, Baptista LP, Baroni RH, et al. Gadolinium-enhanced three-dimensional MR angiography of Takayasu arteritis. *Radiographics.* 2004;24:773–786.
13. Wilmink TB, Quick CR, Hubbard CS, et al. The influence of screening on the incidence of ruptured abdominal aortic aneurysms. *J Vasc Surg.* 1999;30:203–208.
14. Crawford ES, Cohen ES. Aortic aneurysm: a multifocal disease. Presidential address. *Arch Surg.* 1982;117:1393–1400.
15. Dent TL, Lindenauer SM, Ernst CB, et al. Multiple arteriosclerotic arterial aneurysms. *Arch Surg.* 1972;105:338–344.
16. Stone PA, Hayes JD, AbuRahma AF, et al. Ruptured abdominal aortic aneurysms: 15 years of continued experience in a southern West Virginia community. *Ann Vasc Surg.* 2005;19:851–857.
17. Guirguis EM, Barber GG. The natural history of abdominal aortic aneurysms. *Am J Surg* 1991;162:481–483.
18. Cronenwett JL, Sargent SK, Wall MH, et al. Variables that affect the expansion rate and outcome of small abdominal aortic aneurysms. *J Vasc Surg.* 1990;11:260–268; discussion 268–269.
19. Cronenwett JL, Murphy TF, Zelenock GB, et al. Actuarial analysis of variables associated with rupture of small abdominal aortic aneurysms. *Surgery.* 1985;98:472–483.
20. Katz DA, Littenberg B, Cronenwett JL. Management of small abdominal aortic aneurysms. Early surgery vs watchful waiting. *JAMA.* 1992;268:2678–2686.
21. Rohrer MJ, Cutler BS, Wheeler HB. Long-term survival and quality of life following ruptured abdominal aortic aneurysm. *Arch Surg.* 1988;123:1213–1217.
22. Hollier LH, Plate G, O'Brien PC, et al. Late survival after abdominal aortic aneurysm repair: influence of coronary artery disease. *J Vasc Surg.* 1984;1:290–299.
23. Baxter BT, McGee GS, Flinn WR, et al. Distal embolization as a presenting symptom of aortic aneurysms. *Am J Surg.* 1990;160:197–201.
24. Bruce CJ, Spittell PC, Montgomery SC, et al. Personal ultrasound imager: abdominal aortic aneurysm screening. *J Am Soc Echocardiogr.* 2000;13:674–679.
25. Lederle FA, Simel DL. The rational clinical examination. Does this patient have abdominal aortic aneurysm? *JAMA.* 1999;281:77–82.
26. Lin PH, Bush RL, McCoy SA, et al. A prospective study of a hand-held ultrasound device in abdominal aortic aneurysm evaluation. *Am J Surg.* 2003;186:455–459.
27. Katz DJ, Stanley JC, Zelenock GB. Operative mortality rates for intact and ruptured abdominal aortic aneurysms in Michigan: an eleven-year statewide experience. *J Vasc Surg.* 1994;19:804–815; discussion 816–817.
28. Singh K, Bonaa KH, Solberg S, et al. Intra- and interobserver variability in ultrasound measurements of abdominal aortic diameter. The Tromso Study. *Eur J Vasc Endovasc Surg.* 1998;15:497–504.
29. Coenegrachts K, Rigauts H, De Letter J. Prediction of aortoiliac stent graft length: comparison of a semiautomated computed tomography angiography method and calibrated aortography. *J Comput Assist Tomogr.* 2003;27:284–288.
30. Garret HE Jr, Abdullah AH, Hodgkiss TD, et al. Intravascular ultrasound aids in the performance of endovascular repair of abdominal aortic aneurysm. *J Vasc Surg.* 2003;37:615–618.
31. Thurnher SA, Dorffner R, Thurnher MM, et al. Evaluation of abdominal aortic aneurysm for stent-graft placement: comparison of gadolinium-enhanced MR angiography versus helical CT angiography and digital subtraction angiography. *Radiology.* 1997;205:341–352.
32. Schermerhorn ML, Cronenwett JL. Abdominal aortic and iliac aneurysms. In: Rutherford RB, ed. *Vascular Surgery.* Philadelphia, PA: Elsevier Saunders; 2005:1408–1451.
33. Aquino RV, Rhee RY, Muluk SC, et al. Exclusion of accessory renal arteries during endovascular repair of abdominal aortic aneurysms. *J Vasc Surg.* 2001;34:878–884.

34. Ernst CB. Prevention of intestinal ischemia following abdominal aortic reconstruction. *Surgery.* 1983;93:102–106.
35. Lee WA, O'Dorisio J, Wolf YG, et al. Outcome after unilateral hypogastric artery occlusion during endovascular aneurysm repair. *J Vasc Surg.* 2001;33:921–926.
36. Parsons RE, Marin ML, Veith FJ, et al. Midterm results of endovascular stented grafts for the treatment of isolated iliac artery aneurysms. *J Vasc Surg.* 1999;30:915–921.
37. Wolpert LM, Dittrich KP, Hallisey MJ, et al. Hypogastric artery embolization in endovascular abdominal aortic aneurysm repair. *J Vasc Surg.* 2001;33:1193–1198.
38. Stanley BM, Semmens JB, Lawrence-Brown MM, Goodman MA, et al. Fenestration in endovascular grafts for aortic aneurysm repair: new horizons for preserving blood flow in branch vessels. *J Endovasc Ther.* 2001;8:16–24.
39. Safi HJ, Huynh TT, Estrera AL, et al. Thoracoabdominal aortic aneurysms. In: Rutherford RB, ed. *Vascular Surgery.* Philadelphia, PA: Elsevier Saunders; 2005:1490–1511.
40. Baker DM, Hinchliffe RJ, Yusuf SW, et al. True juxta-anastomotic aneurysms in the residual infra-renal abdominal aorta. *Eur J Vasc Endovasc Surg.* 2003;25:412–415.
41. Tiesenhausen K, Hausegger KA, Tauss J, et al. Endovascular treatment of proximal anastomotic aneurysms after aortic prosthetic reconstruction. *Cardiovasc Intervent Radiol.* 2001;24:49–52.
42. Sessa C, Farah I, Voirin L, et al. Infected aneurysms of the infrarenal abdominal aorta: diagnostic criteria and therapeutic strategy. *Ann Vasc Surg.* 1997;11:453–463.
43. Moneta GL, Taylor LM Jr, Yeager RA, et al. Surgical treatment of infected aortic aneurysm. *Am J Surg.* 1998;175:396–399.
44. van Herwaarden JA, Waasdorp EJ, Bendermacher BL, et al. Endovascular repair of paraanastomotic aneurysms after previous open aortic prosthetic reconstruction. *Ann Vasc Surg.* 2004;18:280–286.
45. Tsuji Y, Tanaka Y, Kitagawa A, et al. Endovascular stent-graft repair for penetrating atherosclerotic ulcer in the infrarenal abdominal aorta. *J Vasc Surg.* 2003;38:383–388.
46. Lau LL, O'Reilly MJ, Johnston LC, et al. Endovascular stent-graft repair of primary aortocaval fistula with an abdominal aortoiliac aneurysm. *J Vasc Surg.* 2001;33:425–428.
47. Kapoor V, Kanal E, Fukui MB. Vertebral mass resulting from a chronic-contained rupture of an abdominal aortic aneurysm repair graft. *AJNR Am J Neuroradiol.* 2001;22:1775–1777.
48. Hafez KS, El Fettouh HA, Novick AC, et al. Management of synchronous renal neoplasm and abdominal aortic aneurysm. *J Vasc Surg.* 2000;32:1102–1110.
49. White GH, May J. Basic techniques of endovascular aneurysm repair. In: Rutherford RB, ed. *Vascular Surgery.* Philadelphia, PA: Elsevier Saunders; 2005:784–797.
50. Karkos CD, Bruce IA, Thomson GJ, et al. Retroaortic left renal vein and its implications in abdominal aortic surgery. *Ann Vasc Surg.* 2001;15:703–708.
51. Bosch JL, Lester JS, McMahon PM, et al. Hospital costs for elective endovascular and surgical repairs of infrarenal abdominal aortic aneurysms. *Radiology.* 2001;220:492–497.
52. Thurnher S, Cejna M. Imaging of aortic stent-grafts and endoleaks. *Radiol Clin North Am.* 2002;40:799–833.
53. Baum RA, Carpenter JP, Golden MA, et al. Treatment of type 2 endoleaks after endovascular repair of abdominal aortic aneurysms: comparison of transarterial and translumbar techniques. *J Vasc Surg.* 2002;35:23–29.
54. Tutein Noltheniius RP, van Herwaarden JA, van den Berg JC, et al. Three year single centre experience with the AneuRx aortic stent graft. *Eur J Vasc Endovasc Surg.* 2001;22:257–264.
55. Lin PH, Bush RL, Katzman JB, et al. Delayed aortic aneurysm enlargement due to endotension after endovascular abdominal aortic aneurysm repair. *J Vasc Surg.* 2003;38:840–842.
56. May J, White GH, Yu W, et al. Concurrent comparison of endoluminal versus open repair in the treatment of abdominal aortic aneurysms: analysis of 303 patients by life table method. *J Vasc Surg.* 1998;27:213–220; discussion 220–211.
57. Insko EK, Kulzer LM, Fairman RM, et al. MR imaging for the detection of endoleaks in recipients of abdominal aortic stent-grafts with low magnetic susceptibility. *Acad Radiol.* 2003;10:509–513.
58. Ludman CN, Yusuf SW, Whitaker SC, et al. Feasibility of using dynamic contrast-enhanced magnetic resonance angiography as the sole imaging modality prior to endovascular repair of abdominal aortic aneurysms. *Eur J Vasc Endovasc Surg.* 2000;19:524–530.
59. Wicky S, Fan CM, Geller SC, et al. MR angiography of endoleak with inconclusive concomitant CT angiography. *AJR Am J Roentgenol.* 2003;181:736–738.
60. May J, White GH, Yu W, et al. Importance of plain x-ray in endoluminal aortic graft surveillance. *Eur J Vasc Endovasc Surg.* 1997;13:202–206.
61. White RA, Donayre CE, Walot I, et al. Endoluminal graft exclusion of a proximal para-anastomotic pseudoaneurysm following aortobifemoral bypass. *J Endovasc Surg.* 1997;4:88–94.
62. Cynamon J, Marin ML, Veith FJ, et al. Stent-graft repair of aorto-iliac occlusive disease coexisting with common femoral artery disease. *J Vasc Interv Radiol.* 1997;8:19–26.
63. Brewster DC. Direct reconstruction for aortoiliac occlusive disease. In: Rutherford RB, ed. *Vascular Surgery.* Philadelphia, PA: Elsevier Saunders; 2005:1106–1107.
64. Farooq MM, Kling K, Yamini D, et al. Penetrating ulceration of the infrarenal aorta: case reports of an embolic and an asymptomatic lesion. *Ann Vasc Surg.* 2001;15:255–259.
65. Hata A, Noda M, Moriwaki R, et al. Angiographic findings of Takayasu arteritis: new classification. *Int J Cardiol.* 1996;54(suppl):S155–S163.
66. Saiki M, Nishimura K, Ikebuchi M, et al. Mycotic abdominal aortic pseudoaneurysm caused by a penetrating atherosclerotic ulcer: report of a case. *Surg Today.* 2003;33:698–701.
67. Vetrhus M, McWilliams R, Tan CK, et al. Endovascular repair of abdominal aortic aneurysms with aortocaval fistula. *Eur J Vasc Endovasc Surg.* 2005;30:640–643.
68. Gupta N, Auer A, Troop B. Seat belt-related injury to the common iliac artery: case report and review of the literature. *J Trauma.* 1998;45:419–421.

Mesenteric Vasculature

CHAPTER 19

Nicole M. Hindman
Christoph U. Herborn
R. Brooke Jeffrey

INTRODUCTION: SPECTRUM AND PREVALENCE OF DISEASE

Mesenteric Arteries

A broad spectrum of disorders may affect the mesenteric arteries, including such diverse conditions as collagen vascular disease, vasculitis, fibromuscular dysplasia, trauma, and neoplastic encasement. However, by far, the most common pathologic process is occlusive disease caused by atherosclerosis. The vast majority of patients with atherosclerotic disease of the mesenteric arteries are elderly and asymptomatic (1,2). The celiac axis (CA), superior mesenteric artery (SMA), and inferior mesenteric artery (IMA) comprise the three major branch vessels arising off the aorta that supply the abdominal gastrointestinal (GI) viscera.

Atherosclerotic occlusive disease of the mesenteric arteries carries the potential risk for life-threatening bowel ischemia and infarction. Yet, despite the widespread prevalence of mesenteric atherosclerosis in the adult population, the actual incidence of clinically significant intestinal ischemia is remarkably low in clinical practice. Surgery for acute mesenteric ischemia (AMI) represents <1% of all laparotomies (3).

The low incidence of clinically significant intestinal ischemia is undoubtedly due to the ability of the mesenteric arterial circulation to form extensive collateral pathways, given the slow progressive nature of the disease. The one exception to this is acute occlusion of the SMA due to embolic disease, usually from a cardiac source. This is an important etiology of acute intestinal ischemia, representing 50% of all cases (4).

The development of chronic mesenteric ischemia typically requires disease progression in two of the three major branch vessels. Chronic mesenteric ischemia (CMI) is an unusual but important cause of abdominal pain. Although this condition accounts for only 5% of all intestinal ischemic events, it can have significant morbidity (5).

All other disease processes involving the mesenteric arteries—including arteritis, collagen vascular disease, fibromuscular dysplasia, and intestinal dissection—are clinically exceedingly rare.

Portal Veins

The hemodynamic effect of cirrhosis and portal hypertension is far and away the most common disease process to affect the portal venous system. Anatomic changes accompany the prolonged raised pressure within the intra- and extrahepatic portal veins, including dilation of the main portal vein and the development of numerous venous collaterals, most notably esophageal varices. In the United States for the year 2003, cirrhosis was the twelfth leading cause of death, representing 1.1% of all fatalities (6,7). Although alcoholism still represents an important cause of cirrhosis worldwide, its incidence in the United States is currently declining (8). The prevalence of portal hypertension now most closely parallels the development of cirrhosis due to the worldwide epidemic of viral hepatitis, particularly in Asia. It is estimated that chronic hepatitis B infection occurs in 0.5% of the population of the United States and Europe but infects approximately 10% of the population of Asia and nearly 350 million people worldwide (9). Hepatitis C is estimated to infect 3% of the global population, or approximately 170 million individuals (9,10). The incidence of hepatitis C in the United States is approximately 3.8 million (10). Even if a very small percentage of individuals go on to develop clinically significant cirrhosis from hepatitis B and C, the dimension of the problem is enormous, given the worldwide prevalence of infection.

The most clinically significant effects of cirrhosis and portal hypertension are the development of esophageal varices and the risk of acute life-threatening variceal hemorrhage. Approximately half of all patients with cirrhosis will develop esophageal varices, and one third of these patients will have a clinically significant GI hemorrhage from these varices within 2 years of the diagnosis (11). Compared with other causes of upper GI bleeding, hemorrhage from esophageal varices carries an unusually high mortality rate of 30% to 60%, thus underscoring the clinical severity of this entity (12–14).

The second most clinically important disease process to involve the portal veins is thrombosis. Thrombus formation within the portal or superior mesenteric veins may be classified as acute or chronic and either partially or totally occlusive. Patients may be entirely asymptomatic if the thrombus is nonobstructive or may have symptoms of intestinal ischemia if there is acute total occlusion of the superior mesenteric vein (SMV). Venous thrombosis accounts for 15% to 20% of all cases of bowel infarction (15). Primary or idiopathic thrombosis of the portal venous system is actually quite rare, and the vast majority of cases are secondary to identifiable risk factors such as hypercoagulable states, pancreatitis, abdominal surgery, trauma, portal hypertension, and bowel obstruction from volvulus or intussusception (15).

GLOBAL VIEW OF UNIQUE ASPECTS AND CONSIDERATIONS OF IMAGING OF THIS ORGAN SYSTEM

The early diagnosis of acute occlusive mesenteric ischemia is essential to minimize the associated high mortality rates. A liberal use of conventional, catheter-based angiography is thus frequently advocated. Depending on resource availability, some patients presenting acutely can be well served with multidetector computed tomography (MDCT) or computed tomographic angiography (CTA).

CMI is a condition that can be clinically elusive and greatly benefits from the physiologic assessments available with duplex sonography and phase contrast (PC) MRA, comparing velocity and flow values prior to and after a prescribed caloric intake (16–19).

For cases that require a rapid evaluation of the vasculature and parenchyma, such as trauma, computed tomography (CT)/CTA is the preferred technique (20–22), whereas in an elective assessment, such as for malignancy or portal hypertension, both CT/CTA and magnetic resonance (MR)/magnetic resonance angiography (MRA) are most effective (20).

Venous imaging is the clear domain of CTA/CTV (CT venography) and MRA/MRV (MR venography), as delineation of the relevant vasculature is most reliable with these techniques (15).

WHAT DO COMPUTED TOMOGRAPHY AND MAGNETIC RESONANCE BRING OVER OTHER IMAGING AND NONIMAGING DIAGNOSTIC TESTING?

Digital Subtraction Angiography

When evaluating patients suspected of having a mesenteric vascular disease, it is the clinical presentation of the patient that guides the choice of a specific diagnostic modality. For patients presenting with AMI, digital subtraction angiography (DSA) is typically the diagnostic modality of choice offering the opportunity for diagnosis and treatment of many conditions. Depending on the particular diagnosis, vasodilators (23), thrombolytics (24), and angioplasty (+/− stent) (25) can be applied to achieve revascularization and restoration of blood flow at the time of diagnosis.

DSA is an invasive and expensive technique that is capable of providing high-quality images of the mesenteric vasculature but is associated with a small but finite morbidity, including arterial dissection and thrombosis (26,27). In addition to abdominal aortography, selective injections into the celiac and SMA are routinely required for comprehensive evaluation. In selected patients, this results in a considerable radiation dose and contrast burden. Arteriography was used in the past to diagnosis both embolic disease to the SMA (cutoff sign) and arterial stenoses in CMI (Fig. 19-1). With DSA, information about blood flow can only be inferred. In addition, global assessment of intra-abdominal processes is relatively poor with angiography, with only limited information about the bowel wall, mesentery, peritoneal cavity, and solid viscera.

Duplex Sonography

Duplex sonography is a noninvasive means to provide quantitative data about the flow velocity in the larger mesenteric vessels of interest. This has been of value in CMI, but its success depends on operator expertise. A combination of increased peak systolic velocity (greater than 275 cm/second in the SMA) and increased end diastolic velocity correlates with a greater than 70% stenosis with sensitivities in the 80% to 90% range (28–30). This may be useful information to screen for CMI, but it does not provide sufficient anatomic information to direct therapy (either stent placement or surgical reconstruction). A combination of color flow imaging with duplex sonography and ultrasound (US) contrast agents may be a rapid and inexpensive screening technique for patients with CMI (31,32).

Pre- and postprandial studies can provide physiologic information regarding the ability to mount a normal postprandial hyperemia (33). Direct imaging of the major branch vessels can be limited by body habitus and bowel gas and may not benefit greatly from the use of US contrast agents (34).

Color Doppler sonography, however, may be highly effective to screen patients for suspected portal vein thrombosis (31,32). Yet, sonography often fails to visualize the entire length of the SMV, and, therefore, in patients with possible SMV thrombosis, CT and MR are the imaging techniques of choice.

Computed Tomographic Angiography

Both contrast-enhanced (CE) CT and magnetic resonance imaging (MRI) may provide exquisite anatomic displays of the mesenteric arteries and portal venous system. The acuity of patient symptoms, therefore, often dictates the choice of imaging modality. In patients with sudden onset of severe abdominal pain, AMI is one of many important diagnostic considerations, including such diverse entities as perforated duodenal ulcer, pancreatitis, bowel obstruction, peritonitis, and cholecystitis. In general, CT is the preferred diagnostic modality in acutely ill patients. CT can visualize not only the mesenteric arterial circulation and portal venous system but can also detect important secondary findings involving the liver, bowel wall, and mesentery—such as pneumotosis, portal venous gas, bowel wall thickening, and other secondary findings of intestinal ischemia—thus providing comprehensive information for diagnosis and treatment planning.

The net iodinated contrast media load administered to the patient and its attendant risks must be considered in the context of possible follow-up with catheter-based interventional techniques.

Magnetic Resonance Angiography

Although not frequently used in the emergent setting (due to instability of patients, remote location of MRI scanners, and relatively long imaging times compared with CT), MRA provides excellent contrast resolution of the mesenteric vasculature, bowel, and mesentery. Acquisition of images utilizing three-dimensional (3D) volumetric sequences allows for reconstruction in multiple planes, facilitating the visualization of subtle vascular abnormalities. Despite advances in limiting motion of the bowel, the resolution of the distal vasculature is still limited, but application of advanced techniques combined with pharmacologic preparation (e.g., glucagon, hyoscyamine sulfate) offers exciting future possibilities in this arena.

In patients with suspected abdominal angina and CMI, CT and MRI often provide complementary diagnostic information. CE MDCT and gadolinium-enhanced MRI in combination with image displays such as volume

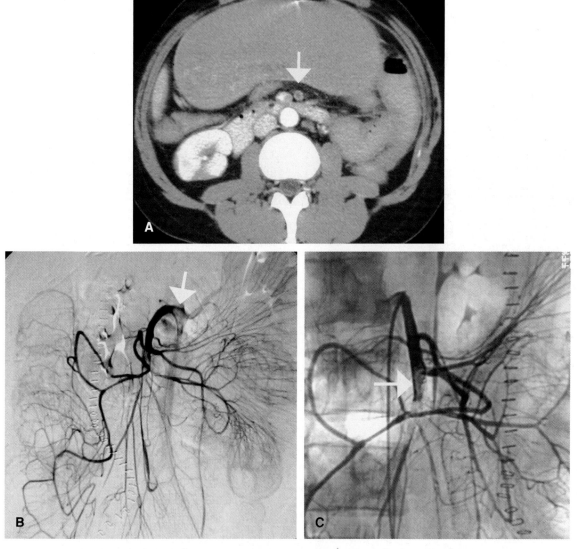

FIGURE 19-1 SMA cut-off sign in a 77-year-old man presenting with acute severe abdominal pain. A: Axial CE CT demonstrates a filling defect within the proximal SMA (*arrow*) as well as a wedge-shaped infarct in the right kidney, compatible with prior embolic disease. **B** and **C:** DSA images demonstrate a filling defect in the proximal SMA (*arrows*), also called the *cut-off sign.*

rendering (VR), maximum-intensity projection (MIP), and curved planar reformations (CPRs) provide excellent anatomic displays of the mesenteric arterial and portal venous systems and resultant collaterals forming in response to chronic occlusion (2,35–44).

In addition to this high-resolution anatomic information, MRI has the additional advantage of providing quantitative functional information about mesenteric arterial and venous blood flow. Using PC angiography, quantitative flow information can be provided that may be useful in documenting CMI (39). In addition, novel MRI techniques have been developed to measure postprandial oxy-

gen extraction in the SMV that may provide physiologic confirmation in conjunction with anatomically demonstrated mesenteric arterial stenoses (36–38,41,43,44).

IMAGING STRATEGIES

Computed Tomography

In order to evaluate both the mesenteric arteries and the portal venous system with CE MDCT, a biphasic scan is required. An initial high-resolution arterial study is performed during peak arterial enhancement following a rapid intravenous (IV) injection (4 to 5 mL/second) from an IV

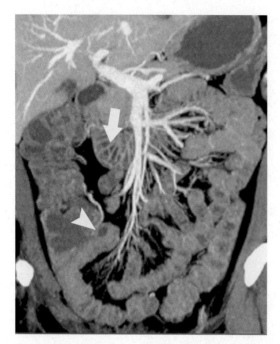

FIGURE 19-2 Bowel with negative intraluminal contrast. Coronal MIP image obtained in a 58-year-old woman displays both mesenteric arterial supply and venous drainage of small bowel. Note the uniform distention of the entire length of the small bowel. Folds in the duodenal sweep (*arrow*) can be seen. Terminal ileal region is displayed (*arrowhead*). (Reprinted with permission from Megibow AJ, Babb JS, Hecht EM, et al. Evaluation of bowel distention and bowel wall appearance by using neutral oral contrast agent for multi-detector row CT. *Radiology.* 2006; 238:87–95.)

breath for at least 25 seconds. Because of the scan acquisition in the craniocaudal direction, shallow breathing can be performed during the latter part of the scan, when images are obtained through the lower abdomen, without significant motion artifact.

Careful attention should be given to the contrast bolus administration and timing of image acquisition for optimal arterial opacification. Although in thinner patients with low body mass index, as little as 80 mL of contrast may provide adequate enhancement, in general, approximately 100 to 120 mL of warm iodinated contrast is administered via a 20- or 18-gauge IV cannula placed in an antecubital vein. This is to accommodate a power injection of 4 to 5 mL/second, which is essential for adequate arterial opacification. A saline flush of 40 to 50 mL is quite valuable to ensure complete delivery of all the iodinated contrast. Bolus tracking to determine peak arterial enhancement is the most efficient method of determining the appropriateness of scan delay. This is generally performed by obtaining a series of low-dose scans at the level of the upper abdominal aorta and placing a region-of-interest cursor within the aorta. Once a triggering threshold reaches 150 Hounsfield units (HU) above the baseline noncontrast scans, the patient is instructed to perform a breath hold. Image acquisition is then obtained for delineation of the mesenteric arteries. The scanning region of interest for the arterial acquisition is from just above the CA to the symphysis pubis. Following a 60- to 70-second delay from the initial injection, another breath-hold acquisition is obtained of the entire upper abdomen and pelvis to delineate the portal veins and solid abdominal viscera. Scanning parameters for both a 4- and 16-detector row MDCT scanner will differ slightly. Typically, collimation is 1 to 1.25 mm for the 4-detector row scanner and 0.75 mm for the 16-detector row scanner. Venous phase scans should be obtained at 2.5- to 5.0-mm collimation.

To obtain the highest quality volumetric imaging with voxels, there should be at least a 30% to 50% overlap in reconstruction interval. This substantially improves z-axis resolution and the quality of multiplanar and 3D reformations. A variety of postprocessing techniques should be performed routinely for optimal mesenteric arterial imaging. This includes obtaining MIP and VR images, as well as CPRs of the celiac, and SMA (Fig. 19-3).

CPRs are particularly useful to delineate individual vessels such as the SMA and celiac and may be invaluable in the presence of metallic stents to determine precise positioning of the stent and intraluminal thrombus formation (Fig. 19-4). In patients with extensive calcification within the abdominal aorta and splanchnic vessels, CPRs may

power injection. This is followed by a delayed scan (60 to 70 seconds from the start of the injection) to acquire images during the portal venous phase to assess the portal venous system and solid abdominal viscera (42).

The use of negative oral contrast agent represents a practical means of marking the bowel, facilitating the visualization of bowel wall enhancement, and the presentation of the vascular structures (45,46) (Fig. 19-2).

The initial patient preparation should involve only water (500 to 700 mL) as a negative oral contrast agent prior to scanning. Positive oral contrast agents will substantially interfere with reconstructions such as MIPs to delineate the mesenteric arteries and should always be avoided. In addition, water distention of the bowel lumen facilitates evaluation of focal or diffuse mural abnormalities and perfusion of the small bowel, stomach, and duodenum. As with all CTA techniques, newer multidetector scanners (either 16- or 64-detector row) offer the distinct advantage of thinner collimation and shorter scan times, and therefore shorter breath-holding requirements for patients. However, adequate imaging can be provided with a 4-detector row CT if the patient is able to hold their

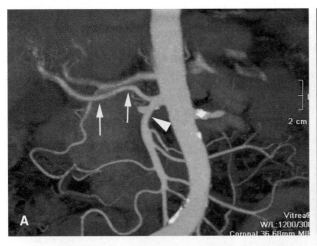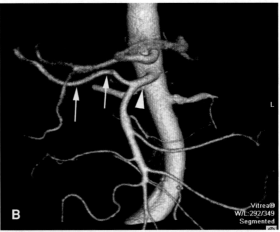

FIGURE 19-3 Replaced right hepatic artery on MIP and VR MDCT images. A: MIP image showing the origin of the SMA (*white arrowhead*) supplying a replaced right hepatic artery (*thin white arrows*). **B:** VR image better differentiating the origin of the SMA (*arrowhead*) from the similarly opacified aorta; again seen is the replaced right hepatic artery.

more accurately delineate the assessment of arterial stenoses. The patient with extensive calcification may provide unique challenges for MIP or VR; therefore, CPR should be done routinely to precisely assess the degree of luminal narrowing. Similarly, in patients with suspected tumor encasement of the mesenteric vessels, CPRs are quite useful to assess perivascular tumor extension (33–35,47–49).

Magnetic Resonance

MRI has been successfully established as an outstanding diagnostic tool for the morphological and functional evaluation of the mesenteric and portal venous system since the early 1990s. Besides offering excellent analysis of the parenchymal and hollow organs in the abdomen with unsurpassed soft tissue contrast, 3D CE MRA also permits accurate assessment of the abdominal aorta and particularly the splanchnic arteries, that is, the celiac trunk and its branches as well as the SMA and the IMA (40,50–55).

Recent improvements in gradient capabilities and new parallel imaging techniques allow for rapid image acquisition with submillimeter spatial resolution acquired in a single short breath hold (56). Therefore, it is anticipated that there will be a shift toward utilizing MRA examinations for evaluation of the visceral arteries and portal vessels for many clinical indications, including vascular diseases, functional disorders, and neoplasms (57).

The gains in gradient power capabilities have laid foundation for a variety of new fast MRI techniques for the abdominal vasculature. In patients suspected of having CMI, patient preparation is not as important for routine MRA as it is for catheter-based arteriography, CT, or US. Patients do not need to fast prior to the MR examination nor does intraluminal gas in the small bowel impair image quality. Application of glucagon (0.5 to 1 mg IV or intramuscularly [IM]) or scopolamine (40 mg IV) prior to the MR examination has been proposed as a means for reducing bowel motion and augmenting splanchnic flow. However, with a fast scanner capable of high-resolution imaging during a mere breath hold, arresting bowel motion is not deemed mandatory. Alternatively, a high-caloric meal prior to the examination can transiently increase splanchnic flow, thereby enhancing visibility of the smaller branch vessels (58). Patients with chronic abdominal symptoms, suspected of AMI, should be considered surgical emergencies. MRA should only be performed in patients presenting with an acute abdomen under unusual circumstances and only if adequate monitoring is available. An abdominal surgeon should be nearby in case the patient decompensates and requires immediate surgical exploration.

Patients suspected of CMI are often very thin and thus well suited to MRI with surface array coils, such as a body array or torso phased array coils. Large patients may be easier to image by using the body coil. The patient is placed in the supine position. The arms may be in a comfortable position by the patient's side during the initial localizer sequence and throughout the 3D CE MRA acquisition in the coronal plane. However, if the patient is able to elevate the arms

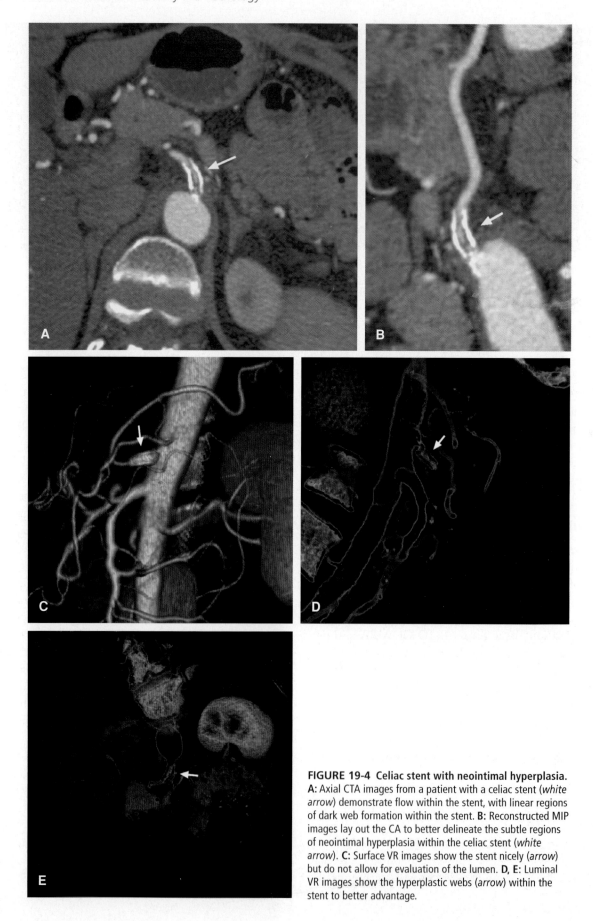

FIGURE 19-4 Celiac stent with neointimal hyperplasia.
A: Axial CTA images from a patient with a celiac stent (*white arrow*) demonstrate flow within the stent, with linear regions of dark web formation within the stent. **B:** Reconstructed MIP images lay out the CA to better delineate the subtle regions of neointimal hyperplasia within the celiac stent (*white arrow*). **C:** Surface VR images show the stent nicely (*arrow*) but do not allow for evaluation of the lumen. **D, E:** Luminal VR images show the hyperplastic webs (*arrow*) within the stent to better advantage.

over the head throughout the examination, this might help to minimize aliasing.

Time-of-flight Magnetic Resonance Angiography

Time-of-flight (TOF) MRA enables high-contrast views of the abdominal arteries with the use of presaturation bands (53,59). However, being one of the oldest techniques used, TOF MRA has not been established in current clinical practice for the evaluation of the mesenteric arteries due to several limitations. Images have to be acquired orthogonal to flow, thereby complicating the depiction of the ostia of both the celiac trunk and the SMA because the flow within the aorta is at right angles to that in the proximal part of both vessels. This often results in artifacts at the vessel origins where most of the pathology in patients with CMI is located. Reflecting the anatomic predisposition of the celiac artery and the SMA, it is impossible to optimize a single TOF-sequence for the depiction of the two arteries. In addition, misregistration artifacts may arise from the need to acquire images during suspended respiration in patients with limited breath-holding capabilities.

Phase Contrast Magnetic Resonance Angiography

PC MRA techniques require relatively long imaging times, as at least two data sets are acquired by using flow-encoding gradients of opposite polarity, and at least three measurements in the orthogonal planes are needed for detection of flow. However, PC MRA can be used to assess the mesenteric vasculature by using either 3D (60) or two-dimensional (2D) approaches (16,36,61,62); the aforementioned technique allows for image acquisition in any desired plane (60).

Wasser and associates (60) reported their experience with a systolically gated PC MRA technique in patients with suspected mesenteric ischemia. Only 66% of stenoses seen on catheter-based arteriography could be visualized by MRA, and false-positive results were encountered. The limitations include problems with phase ghosting, motion artifacts, and uncertainty as to choice of appropriate velocity-encoding (VENC) gradient value.

The long scan times of PC MRA predisposed the study to respiratory motion artifacts. In addition, ghost artifacts caused by diminished and reversed flow during systole can severely hamper image quality. Cardiac triggering can counter the latter limitation, albeit with a further increase in scan time. Thus, respiratory motion artifacts remain a major problem with PC MRA. Combinations of cardiac triggering and respiratory compensation strategies can be quite successful.

Cardiac-gated 2D PC MRA techniques have been implemented for the mesenteric vasculature to provide functional information. This approach segments the phase data acquired at different time points throughout the cardiac cycle and thereby permits quantitative flow measurements, including velocities and volumes. However, accurate contrast is poorly achieved due to flow and saturation effects within visceral vessels that course in different directions, bowel peristalsis, and motion artifacts owing to long acquisition times.

Contrast-enhanced Magnetic Resonance Angiography

3D CE MRA does not depend on flow effects of unsaturated spins and flow phenomena and thus overcomes the saturation problems encountered with the above-mentioned techniques. CE MRA relies on heavily T1-weighted gradient echo sequences with very short repetition times and echo times, which produce high contrast between vessels and the surrounding tissue. Short repetition times result in fast acquisition times and, therefore, fewer motion artifacts and greater coverage of the area of interest. Inherent complexity of CE MRA leads to a trade-off between spatial resolution, volume coverage, and acquisition time for each respective examination. Subtraction of pre- and postcontrast examinations, as is commonly used in MRA imaging of the vasculature of the extremities, does not always improve image quality owing to bowel motion between the data acquisitions. However, the introduction of CE MRA enables the generation of high-quality images of the mesenteric vasculature (54,63,64).

3D imaging in the coronal acquisition plane permits evaluation of the aorta, splanchnic arteries, and portal vein in a single examination. A slice partition thickness between 3 and 5 mm is acceptable if zero padding of the k-space is available for interpolation. In the absence of an interpolation algorithm, the slice thickness should be kept to less than 3 mm in order to depict smaller branches of the mesenteric arteries. To determine stenotic disease of the proximal portions of the SMA and IMA, imaging in the sagittal plane leads to improved image quality. Aliasing is less of a concern when scanning in the sagittal plane, and it is possible to prescribe an aggressive rectangular field-of-view volume with a high-resolution acquisition matrix (Fig. 19-5).

When using magnets with slower gradients, it might be advantageous to acquire data in the sagittal plane with fewer sections required to cover the aorta, celiac SMA, and IMA. A relatively short breath-hold scan performed in the sagittal plane is preferable to a comparably longer coronal acquisition that may be hampered by respiratory artifacts. Imaging parameters should be individually adjusted to

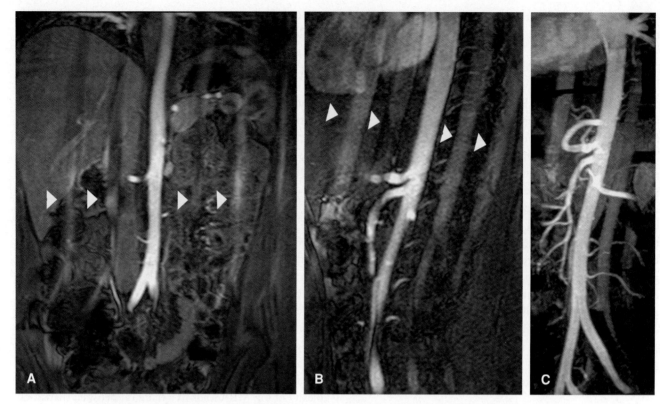

FIGURE 19-5 Aliasing. A: Coronal acquisition of the aorta demonstrating aliasing. **B:** Acquiring the images in the sagittal plane with an aggressive rectangular field of view will switch the direction of aliasing (*arrowheads*) from right to left to anterior to posterior and allow a higher resolution acquisition matrix because of the aggressive rectangular field of view used. **C:** Reformatted images of the coronal acquisition in this patient still reveal excellent depiction of the mesenteric vessels, despite the aliasing seen on the source images in **(A)**.

allow for data acquisition within reasonable breath holds for the patient being studied. Axial imaging may be useful if the primary goal is evaluation of the hepatic arteries, hepatic parenchyma, and portal venous system. One difficulty with the axial orientation is aliasing in the slice direction, which tends to be severe with the extremely short radio frequency (RF) pulses typically used in 3D CE MRA. To minimize aliasing, coils with S-I dimensions only slightly larger than the S-I dimension of the imaging volume tend to provide better image quality. Fat saturation or chemically selective fat inversion pulses might also be applicable. This will help to minimize unwanted signal from pericardial and abdominal fat wrapping onto the bottom and top of the image volume. A 3D CE MRA image data set should be collected before, during, and following completion of the IV contrast administration. Precontrast images should be checked to be sure that the imaging volume is positioned correctly.

The use of 3D sequences structured to achieve excellent delineation of both the vasculature and soft tissues, such as volumetric interpolated breath-hold examination (VIBE; Siemens Medical Systems, Erlangen, Germany) and

liver acquisition with volume acceleration (LAVA; General Electric, Giles, United Kingdom), is recommended (65).

Manual versus automated contrast material injection has been as much debated as the amount of gadolinium, the rate of injection, and the optimal synchronization of contrast material injection and data acquisition. A single dose of contrast material (i.e., 0.1 mmol/kg) is feasible for high-quality contrast enhancement of the mesenteric arteries, but many choose to use double-dose (0.2 mmol/kg) administrations. Above all, proper gadolinium bolus timing is essential for arterial phase acquisitions. This can easily be accomplished with automatic triggering (SmartPrep by General Electric, Waukesea, WI, or CARE Bolus by Siemens Medical Systems, Erlangen, Germany) or fluoroscopic triggering (Bolus Track by Philips Medical Systems, Best, Netherlands) or with a test bolus to the mid abdominal aorta (66–68) (see Chapter 2). After arterial phase imaging, a delayed image data set is useful for showing the portal venous and hepatic venous anatomy.

Arterial phase 3D CE MRA is best analyzed by first performing multiple overlapping thin-slice MIPs in the coronal plane. Subsequently, reformations and subvolume MIPs can be reconstructed in perpendicular planes through each major abdominal aortic branch vessel, including the celiac trunk, SMA, and IMA. It might also be useful to assess the iliac arteries, especially internal iliac arteries, as they may represent an important collateral pathway in patients with CMI.

By means of CE 3D MRA, an accurate morphologic assessment of the proximal mesenteric vessels can be accomplished. Meaney et al. (63) examined 65 patients with suspected mesenteric ischemia by using a 3D CE MRA technique. In all 14 patients with catheter-based angiographic correlation, all significant stenoses of the celiac artery and the SMA were identified. Twenty-eight of 30 arteries with correlation were correctly graded; therefore, despite disagreement between MRA and catheter-based arteriography in two patients, MRA had both sensitivity and specificity of 100% for diagnosis of mesenteric ischemia compared with catheter-based arteriography or surgery, and the specificity was 95%. The authors concluded that CE 3D MRA is accurate for the evaluation of the origins of the mesenteric and celiac arteries, although the image resolution is too low for a reliable assessment of the IMA. In addition, the delineation of the small mesenteric branch vessels is still hampered by the limited spatial resolution of MRA (52). Furthermore, the development of a strong collateral circulation can prevent major abdominal symptoms in patients with severe alterations of the mesenteric arteries (38,69,70).

Complementary Sequences

If the patient is capable of lying still in the magnet for a short while, additional T1- and T2-weighted turbo spin echo images covering the liver and upper abdomen may be acquired before and after contrast material injection to search for other relevant pathology that might account for the patient's abdominal symptoms.

3D CE MRA provides a morphological analysis of the mesenteric arteries. The high incidence of visceral artery stenosis in the asymptomatic population makes it difficult to determine the clinical significance of a morphologic finding. For patients with mesenteric artery stenosis or an equivocal history of mesenteric ischemia, it may be difficult to predict whether correcting the mesenteric artery stenosis will alleviate symptoms. Functional MRI may complement 3D CE MRA in this regard. A cine PC sequence can assess blood flow in the SMV following caloric stimulation. Postprandial blood flow is increased within the SMV out of proportion to SMA blood flow with mesenteric ischemia (16,61). This effect is due to recruitment of collateral flow. By exploiting the known paramagnetic effect of deoxyhemoglobin, correlation can be made between flow-independent

T2 measurement of blood in the SMV and oxygen saturation in an in vivo animal model (71,72). Identifying low oxygen saturation in the SMV compared with that in the inferior vena cava (IVC) suggests ischemia (71,72).

When the celiac and the SMA are patent, the possibility of branch vessel stenosis and regional ischemia can be assessed by looking at bowel wall enhancement before and after IV application of contrast material. Bowel mucosa normally enhances avidly immediately after gadolinium injection. Regional areas of diminished or delayed bowel enhancement are suggestive of regional ischemia. The combination of morphologic 3D contrast MRA of the splanchnic vasculature with functional assessment of mesenteric flow holds considerable promise as the emerging modality of choice for evaluation of patients suspected of mesenteric ischemia.

Portal Venous Magnetic Resonance Angiography

Both 2D and 3D TOF and PC techniques provide accurate evaluation of the portal venous system. However, they have been widely replaced by fast CE MRA due to their inherent limitations (motion artifacts, acquisition time). Nevertheless, PC MRA can still be used to determine the direction of portal venous blood flow by acquisition of an axial or an oblique plane, perpendicular to the portal vein with a VENC between 30 and 50 cm/second. Alternatively, a simple and fast assessment of flow direction can be achieved by using TOF with a saturation band to suppress a given direction of flow (Fig. 19-6).

The imaging plane for CE MRA of the portal venous system can be set to either coronal or axial. The axial plane permits a more thorough evaluation of the hepatic parenchyma and displays the main portal vein and its branches in-plane, which generates higher resolution as compared with reformats. However, the coronal plane has the advantage of including the mesenteric veins as well as the retroperitoneal collaterals in case of portal vein obstruction. As CE MRA of the portal venous system often is accomplished at the end of an MRA examination, the acquisition time should be kept as short as possible (i.e., below 30 seconds) in order for patients to perform satisfactory breath holds. Slice thickness should not be more than 5 mm. This approach provides sufficient coverage of the portal venous anatomy and the liver in the majority of patients.

In patients with suspected concomitant parenchymal pathology of the liver, additional T1- and T2-weighted MRI is beneficial in order to identify and characterize hepatic lesions. In case of biliary obstruction, pancreatitis, or ampullary carcinoma, a turbo spin echo magnetic resonance cholangiopancreatography (MRCP) sequence acquired in oblique coronal planes is useful.

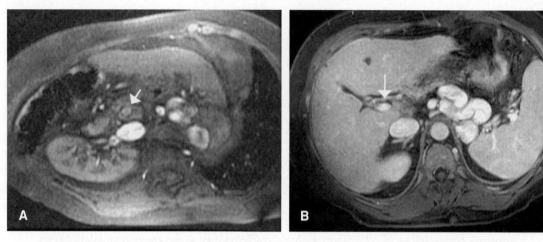

FIGURE 19-6 TOF hepatofugal flow. A: TOF image obtained with a superior saturation band (saturating out aortic flow from above) through the liver in a patient with a history of cirrhosis and hepatitis B. Note the lack of signal in the portal vein, indicating either thrombosis of the portal vein or hepatofugal flow (*arrow*). **B:** Postcontrast portal venous phase images demonstrate flow within the main portal vein (*arrow*), proving patency and hepatofugal flow.

NORMAL ANATOMY AND CONGENITAL ANATOMIC VARIANTS

Mesenteric Arteries

The blood flow to the viscera and the intestinal tract is supplied through the three major anterior branches of the abdominal aorta: the CA, the SMA, and the IMA (Fig. 19-7). A multitude of variants exists with regard to the origin of these vessels from the aorta and their branches. With CE 3D MRA and CTA, the detailed assessment of the normal and abnormal vascular anatomy in the majority of cases can readily be displayed and analyzed.

Celiac Axis

The CA arises from the ventral surface of the aorta at the thoracolumbar level. It supplies the upper abdominal viscera. In as many as two thirds of patients, the CA has a classic branching pattern into three major vessels: the splenic artery, common hepatic artery (CHA), and left gastric artery (LGA) (Fig. 19-8). The branching pattern of the CA in the remaining third of patients is highly variable. In the most common variants, the splenic, the CHA, or the LGA may arise directly from the aorta or from the SMA. The proper hepatic artery is the distal continuation of the CHA, arising after the origin of the gastroduodenal artery (GDA).

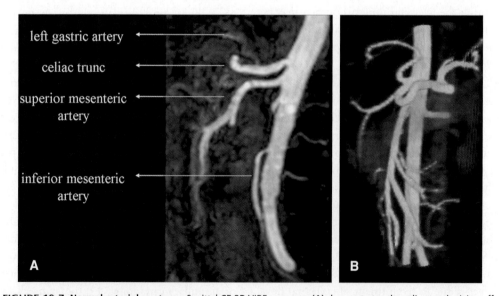

left gastric artery

celiac trunk

superior mesenteric artery

inferior mesenteric artery

FIGURE 19-7 Normal arterial anatomy. Sagittal CE 3D VIBE sequence **(A)** demonstrates the celiac trunk giving off the LGA and the SMA and IMA. Coronal MIP reformatted image **(B)** from the sagittal 3D volume set demonstrates an alternative projection of the branch vessels.

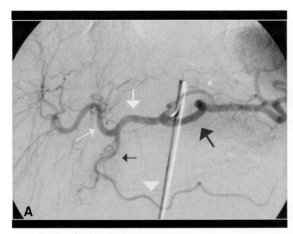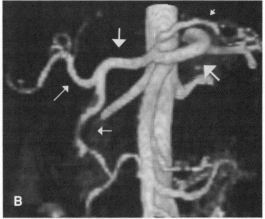

FIGURE 19-8 Celiac axis. Selective celiac arteriography **(A)** demonstrates the normal celiac axis and its branches: the common hepatic artery (*big white arrow*), the splenic artery (*big black arrow*), the left gastric artery (*small short white arrow*), the proper hepatic artery (*small white arrow*), the gastroduodenal artery (*small black arrow*), and the right gastroepiploic artery (*white arrowhead*). Coronal 3D MIP VIBE image **(B)** demonstrates the identical vessels, with their corresponding *arrows*.

The CHA normally divides into the left and right hepatic artery, a branching pattern that is present in approximately 55% of all individuals; the other half have replaced or accessory hepatic arterial branches. The GDA arises from the CHA in roughly 75% of patients and usually presents two main branches: the superior pancreaticoduodenal artery and the right gastroepiploic artery. The superior pancreaticoduodenal artery forms an anastomotic arcade with the inferior pancreaticoduodenal artery that arises from the SMA. The GDA-pancreaticodoudenal arcade serves as an important collateral pathway in the setting of visceral artery occlusion.

In approximately 3% of individuals, there is a large anastomotic connection between the proximal celiac, common hepatic, or splenic artery and the proximal SMA, called the arc of Buhler (73,74). The arc of Buhler represents a persistent embryologic channel and serves as a collateral from the SMA to the proximal celiac (Fig. 19-9). Note is made that the arc of Buhler is frequently confused with the dorsal pancreatic arteries, and differentiation is sometimes difficult (73).

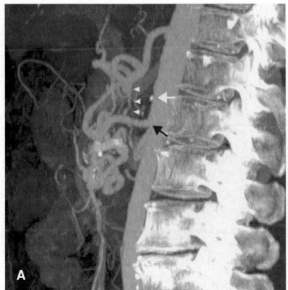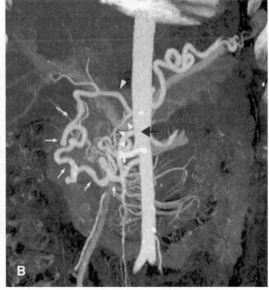

FIGURE 19-9 Arc of Buhler. A: Sagittal MIP image of the aorta demonstrates an absent celiac artery (*white arrow*) with a patent origin of the SMA (*black arrow*) and reconstitution of the proximal celiac trunk by an arc of Buhler (*small white arrowheads*). **B:** Coronal MIP image demonstrates the arc of Buhler (*white arrowheads*) arising from the SMA (*black arrow*), reconstituting the proximal celiac trunk, with a patent CHA seen (*gray arrowhead*). Also noted is an enlarged gastroduodenal-pancreaticoduodenal collateral (*white arrows*).

Splenic Artery

The splenic artery usually stems from the CA, but it may occasionally arise from the aorta or SMA. The course of this vessel varies because of its high degree of tortuousity. According to a classification by Kupic et al. (75), the splenic artery can be divided into four main segments including: (a) the suprapancreatic part, which is the first 1 to 3 cm directly behind the origin; (b) the most tortuous pancreatic part, which lies on the dorsal surface of the pancreas; (c) the prepancreatic section, which runs on the anterior surface of the pancreas; and finally, (d) the prehilar part, which courses between the pancreas and the spleen. Between 2 to 10 short gastric branches arise from the splenic artery and supply the cardia and the fundus of the stomach. The most frequent origin of these vessels is the splenic terminals.

The splenic artery usually gives off the dorsal pancreatic artery (superior pancreatic branch of Testut), which sustains the dorsal and ventral surfaces of the pancreas in the region of the neck. Two right branches arise from the dorsal pancreatic artery, one anastomosing with the superior pancreaticoduodenal artery, the other directly supplying the uncinate process of the pancreas.

Additional pancreatic branches off the splenic artery include the irregularly observed transverse pancreatic artery as well as small splenic branches to the body and the tail of the pancreas. These small branches run in an almost vertical direction and can be the only vessels demonstrated to the left part of the body and the tail of the pancreas. The largest artery of the latter is named the *pancreatic magna artery*. This artery frequently courses obliquely to the left after entering the pancreas. Then, it subdivides into right branches, which anastamose with terminal branches of the transverse pancreatic artery. Another more or less constant branch is the caudal pancreatic artery, which originates either from the distal splenic artery in the hilum of the spleen or from the left gastroepiploic artery. However, these rather small vessels can hardly ever be appreciated with cross-sectional imaging techniques.

The left epiploic branch arises from the distal part of the splenic artery and descends along the left side of the greater curvature of the stomach in an anterior layer of the omentum and anastomoses with the right gastroepiploic arch to form the arcus arteriosus ventriculi inferior of Hyrtl. This vessel may supply a rather large amount of blood to the spleen through inferior polar branches. The left epiploic branch is an important branch of the left gastroepiploic artery, which descends in the posterior layer of the greater omentum inferior to the transverse colon and constitutes the left limb of the arcus epiploicus magnus of Barkow. The right limb is formed by the right epiploic branch arising from the right gastroepiploic branch or the transverse pancreatic artery. The arch of Barkow supplies the transverse colon with multiple ascending branches.

Accessory superior or inferior polar splenic arteries might be encountered arising as a branch from various parts of the splenic artery. Rarely, polar arteries originate from the CA. Polar arteries have a tortuous course and give off multiple small branches to adjacent viscera.

Gastroduodenal Artery

The GDA arises from the CHA in most cases; however, it may also originate from an aberrant right or left hepatic artery. The GDA has a relatively variable course in a caudal direction, largely depending on the degree of filling of the stomach and on the size and position of the liver and the gallbladder (Fig. 19-10).

Pancreaticoduodenal Arcades

The superior and inferior pancreaticoduodenal arteries represent the pancreaticoduodenal arcades, which show wide interconnections through anterior and posterior branches forming single or double arcades on the corresponding sites of the pancreas. While the superior arcades often arise directly from the GDA, the inferior arteries arise as a common branch directly from the posterior aspect of the SMA or, more frequently, from the first branch of the jejunal artery coursing behind the SMA.

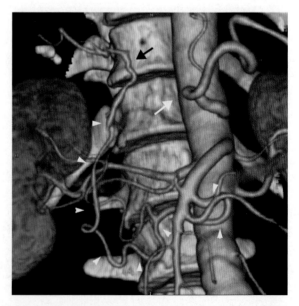

FIGURE 19-10 Occluded CHA. VR CTA images demonstrate occlusion of the origin of the CHA (*white arrow*). There is reconstitution of the proper hepatic artery (*black arrow*) from the gastroduodenal-pancreatico-duodenal collateral system (*white arrowheads*) from the SMA.

TABLE 19-1

Hepatic Arterial Variants According to Michels (N = 200)

Variant Type	Description	Number of Cases (%)
I	Conventional anatomy: proper HA arising from common HA and then giving rise to right and left HAs as the sole supply of arterial blood to liver	110 (55.0)
II	Replaced left HA arising from LGA	20 (10.0)
III	Replaced right HA arising from SMA	22 (11.0)
IV	Both replaced left and right HAs as described for types II and III	2 (1.0)
V	Accessory left HA arising from LGA	16 (8.0)
VI	Accessory right HA arising from SMA	14 (7.0)
VII	Accessory right HA arising from SMA and accessory left HA arising from left gastric artery	2 (1.0)
VIII	Replaced right HA and accessory left HA or replaced left HA and accessory right HA	4 (2.0)
IX	Entire hepatic trunk arising from LGA	9 (4.5)
X	Entire hepatic trunk arising from LGA	1 (0.5)

HA, hepatic artery; LGA, left gastric artery; SMA, superior mesenteric artery.

Common Hepatic Artery

The CHA also shows a highly variable course along the cranial border of the body and the head of the pancreas. The course is variable in direction, but tortuous courses are usually not observed. According to Michels (76–79), anatomic variations most often affect the origin of the hepatic artery. Table 19-1 provides a list of the variations, as noted on the autopsy series by Michels (80).

Most commonly, the CHA arises from the celiac trunk, gives off the GDA and the right gastric and supraduodenal artery, and then becomes the proper hepatic artery, which courses obliquely within the anterior hepatoduodenal ligament. The proper hepatic artery then gives off the cystic artery and bifurcates into the right and left hepatic arteries, with a middle hepatic artery that may arise from either the right or left hepatic arterial branch (79). As described in Table 19-1, this conventional arterial pattern occurs only 55% of the time.

The replaced right hepatic artery is a common variant that traverses the pancreatic head as it passes from the SMA to the liver, providing branches to the pancreas (Fig. 19-11). Another common variant is the replaced left hepatic artery, which arises from the LGA, usually associated with the right and middle hepatic artery arising from the proper hepatic artery (Fig. 19-12). Less frequent variations include an accessory left hepatic artery from the LGA, an accessory right hepatic artery from the SMA, and the entire CHA arising from the SMA without any hepatic artery arising from the CA. Many of the major variations described by Michels in his dissection of the arterial trees of cadavers have also been detected in vivo with CTA and MRA techniques, and some additional variations have been demonstrated as well (81) (Figs. 19-13, 19-14).

Superior Mesenteric Artery

The SMA arises from the ventral aspect of the aorta approximately 1 to 20 mm below the origin of the celiac trunk at the level of the twelfth thoracic to the second lumbar

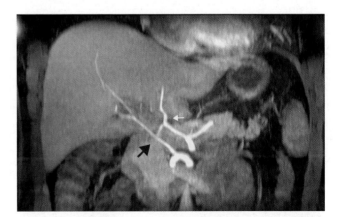

FIGURE 19-11 Replaced right hepatic artery. Coronal reformatted image from the arterial phase of a routine liver MRI examination demonstrates a replaced right hepatic artery arising from the SMA (*black arrow*), supplying the right lobe of the liver. The left hepatic artery (*white arrow*) arises from the proper hepatic artery.

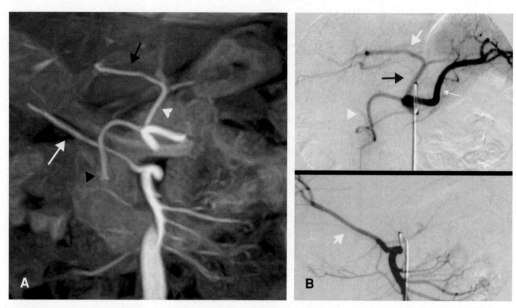

FIGURE 19-12 Replaced right and left hepatic arteries. (A) MIP image from a 3D CE MRA examination demonstrates a prominent left gastric artery (*white arrowhead*), a replaced left hepatic artery (*black arrow*), a replaced right hepatic artery (*white arrow*), and the gastroduodenal artery (*black arrowhead*). Selective celiac angiography (**B**-top image) and selective SMA angiography (**B**-bottom image) redemonstrates the variant anatomy. (**B**-top) an enlarged LGA (*black arrow*) supplies the replaced left hepatic artery (*white arrow*); incidentally seen is the GDA (*white arrowhead*). (**B**-bottom image) the replaced right hepatic artery (*white arrow*) is seen arising from the SMA.

vertebral bodies. It courses ventrally and caudally over the uncinate process of the pancreas and follows the small bowel mesentery into the right lower quadrant. A single celiomesenteric trunk rarely arises directly from the aorta and divides into the respective vessels. The first part of the SMA is immediately behind the body of the pancreas and can also be completely surrounded by this organ when the uncinate process of the pancreas extends medially. The relationship of the SMA to the surrounding tissue can nicely be

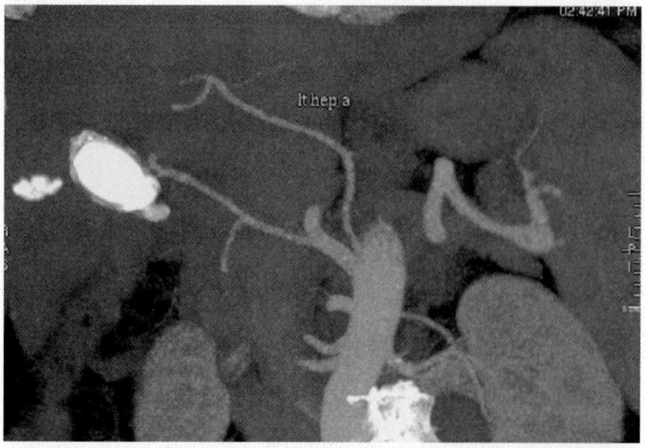

FIGURE 19-13 Replaced left hepatic artery arising from the aorta. MDCT volume reformatted images demonstrate an unusual variant where the left hepatic artery (*lt hep a*) arises directly from the aorta. (Courtesy of Ivan Pedrosa, MD, BIDMC, Boston.)

studied with CE CT and MR. US permits detection of this vessel in as much as 91% of cases (82). The width of the main stem of the SMA varies from 6 to 13 mm in diameter (83). The course of the very proximal SMA varies from a 45- to 90-degree angle to the aorta, depending on the amount of adipose tissue in the abdomen.

The first branch of the SMA normally is the inferior pancreaticoduodenal artery, which passes from the right side directly to the duodenum and the pancreas. This vessel normally arises from the main stem of the SMA or from the first jejunal artery. Less frequently, it may arise as a single artery or as one posterior and one anterior branch, each with separate origins. An intercommunicating arterial arcade between the inferior pancreaticoduodenal artery and the first jejunal artery can be found in roughly 60% of individuals (76). This arcade supplies the fourth part of the duodenum and simultaneously represents an important anastomotic collateral in the case of arterial occlusive disease (77).

The jejunal and ileal branches vary in size and number. These arteries originate from the left side of the SMA. As no strict anatomic border between the jejunum and ileum exists, there is no way to discriminate where jejunal arteries end and ileal arteries begin. Therefore, the simplest rule is to regard those arteries arising proximal to the ileocolic artery as jejunal branches and those distal to this landmark as ileal arteries. There are between 2 and 7 jejunal arteries but up to 17 ileal arteries (excluding those supplying the

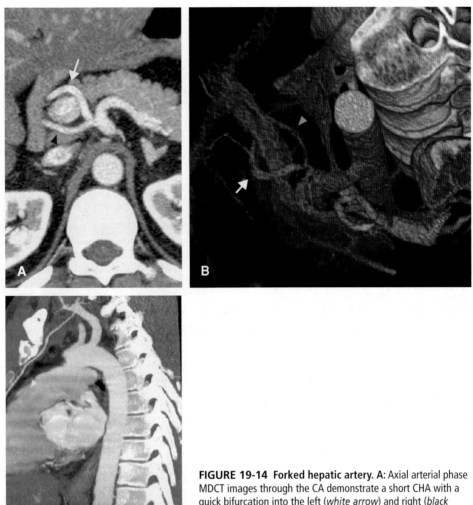

FIGURE 19-14 Forked hepatic artery. A: Axial arterial phase MDCT images through the CA demonstrate a short CHA with a quick bifurcation into the left (*white arrow*) and right (*black arrowhead*) hepatic arteries, surrounding the portal vein. **B:** VR MIP MDCT images show the left (*white arrow*) and right (*blue arrowhead*) from a different vantage point. **C:** Sagittal MIP images from the arterial phase demonstrate the right (*white arrow*) and left (*black arrowhead*) hepatic artery entering directly into the right and left lobes, respectively.

terminal ileum). The size and the width of the ileal arteries decrease distally, and the smallest vessels are observed in the terminal ileum. The latter is supplied by three to fifteen separate branches arising from the ileal branch of the ileocolic artery. This ileal arch anastomoses directly with the most distal part of the SMA to form a distal arcade.

Such intra-arterial arcades are a characteristic feature of the mesenteric circulation. However, the number and extent of such arcades differs between distinct parts of the bowel: While the midportion of the small bowel shows the largest number of arcades, they are rare in the terminal ileum. Those arcades close to the mesenteric border let off the long vasa recta, which penetrate the bowel wall and enter the submucosa layer. The short vasa recta arise from the last arcade or

directly from the long vasa recta and enter the submucosa of the intestinal wall from the mesenteric border. A rather tight interarterial anastomotic network among the vasa recta is present in the small bowel wall, while the number of such connections in the large bowel is comparatively low (Fig. 19-15).

The only constant artery arising from the right side of the SMA is the ileocolic artery, which supplies the terminal ileum, the appendix, the cecum, and the proximal part of the ascending colon. Extension of supply to more distal bowel regions may occur when the right colonic artery is absent, occluded, or directly originates from the ileocolic artery. The ileocolic artery gives off an ileal and a colic artery, which usually communicate through an ileocolic arcade. The ileal artery communicates directly with the SMA. The

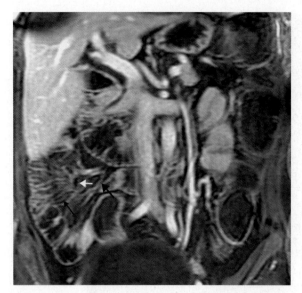

FIGURE 19-15 Normal vasa recta. Coronal CE 3D LAVA acquisition from a 36-year-old female patient with colicky abdominal pain demonstrates the normal vasa recta in the small bowel. The ileal artery (*larger black arrow*) supplies several anastomotic loops (*white arrow*) that then supply the vasa recta (*small black arrow*).

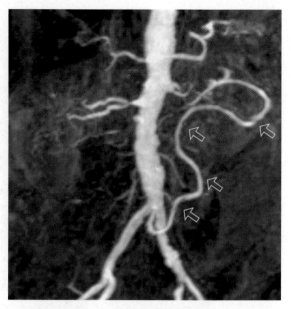

FIGURE 19-16 Left colic collateral in a 67-year-old man with vague abdominal pain. Coronal 3D MIP images acquired during the arterial phase demonstrate diffuse atherosclerotic disease of the abdominal aorta, with moderate stenosis in the origin of the SMA (not shown). Note is made of an enlarged left colic artery (*open arrows*) supplying the middle colic branch of the SMA.

right colic artery has a highly variable origin from the SMA, the middle colic, or ileocolic artery. It supplies the ascending colon and the hepatic colonic flexure. The middle colic artery usually arises from the first part of the SMA at the level of the first jejunal artery and supplies the transverse colon. Rarely, an accessory middle colonic artery is present and is then named the middle mesenteric artery. The left branch of the middle colic artery is in direct communication with the left colic artery, which originates from the IMA and herewith forms the most important collateral pathway for the mesenteric circulation (38,69,70) (Fig. 19-16). The next most functionally important collateral is the arc of Riolan, also called the *central anastomotic artery*, or the meandering mesenteric artery, a short, direct, and retroperitoneal connection from the root of the SMA (or one of its primary branches) to the IMA (or one of its branches). The marginal artery of Drummond is an additional collateral pathway that supplies the arterial arcades along the mesenteric border of the colon.

Pancreatic and pancreaticoduodenal arteries may also serve as collateral pathways in cases of stenosis or occlusion of the main stem of the SMA (Figs. 19-17, 19-18). Further collaterals for bowel supply in case of vascular occlusion include the epiploic arteries, retroperitoneal parietal arteries, renal capsular arteries, inferior phrenic arteries, and arteries for the adipose tissue of the mesentery. Dilatation of such collateral vessels may be extreme and lead to aneurysms as indirect signs of occlusive disease. In addition to these three more common collaterals, more than 50 collateral pathways in the small and

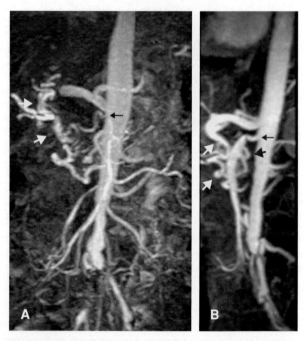

FIGURE 19-17 Moderate stenosis of the SMA with collateral flow from the GDA. Coronal (**A**) and sagittal (**B**) 3D MIP VIBE images in a patient with diffuse atherosclerotic disease demonstrate a moderate stenosis of the origin of the SMA (*small black arrow*). Flow distal to the stenosis is increased, secondary to retrograde supply via the GDA (*large white arrows* in **A** and **B**) and the inferior pancreaticoduodenal artery (*large black arrow* in **B**).

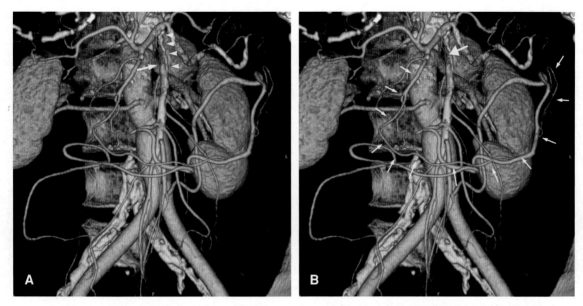

FIGURE 19-18 Occluded SMA origin. VR CT images of the mesenteric vasculature demonstrate occlusion of the origin of the SMA (*white arrow* in **A**, *large white arrow* in **B**), with flow seen distally. The SMA is reconstituted distally by the arc of Buhler (*small white arrowheads* in **A**) and by the GDA, inferior pancreaticoduodenal arcade supplying the left colic (*small white arrows* in **B**).

large bowels have been listed by Michels (77), and a detailed description of these anastomoses can be found in his work.

Superior Mesenteric Vein

The SMV follows the course of the corresponding artery. Anatomy and flow are displayed to best extent on CT, MRI, and MRA or duplex and color Doppler US. The SMV usually can be observed on cross-sectional imaging being to the right and anterior to the SMA.

Inferior Mesenteric Artery

The IMA arises from the left anterior wall of the abdominal aorta approximately at the level of the third lumbar vertebra. After descending parallel to the aorta for 2 to 4 cm, it gives off the left colic artery, which has an ascending course. The left colic artery then gives off sigmoid arterial branches. The remaining IMA gives off additional sigmoid branches not originating from the left colic artery. Below the iliac arteries, the IMA becomes the superior hemorrhoidal artery. Branches of the left colic artery and the sigmoid arteries form the large arterial channel of the mesocolon, the marginal artery of Drummond. This artery represents a complex arcade fed by branches from the ileocolic, right colic, middle colic, left colic, and upper sigmoid arteries and thereby represents an important collateral in case of occlusion in the aforementioned vascular territories. There is great variability in the size of the IMA in adults (1 to 6 mm in diameter). Reflecting the small size of the IMA and its

subtle branches, these vessels are difficult to consistently image with MRA (84).

Clinical Relevance of Splanchnic Arterial Anatomic Variations

Variations in the splanchnic arterial anatomy occur in more than 40% of patients. For this reason, pretherapeutic planning for hepatic resections, liver transplantations, resection of retroperitoneal lymph nodes, chemoinfusion pump placement, surgical shunting, or other abdominal operations may require mapping of the visceral arterial anatomy. In the past, this was done by conventional angiography for the fine detail necessary to identify variations involving tiny arteries. However, for evaluation of the splanchnic artery origins and major branches, 3D contrast MRA in its latest implementation is sufficient. In those patients being considered for a surgical renal revascularization, it is important to know the status of the splanchnic arterial anatomy as the source of inflow to a splenorenal or hepatorenal bypass graft.

Portal Venous System

The liver has a double blood supply: the proper hepatic artery divides into the right and left hepatic artery and carries oxygenated blood to the liver, and the portal vein carries venous blood from the GI tract to the liver (Fig. 19-19). The venous blood from the GI tract drains into the superior and inferior mesenteric veins; these two vessels are then joined by the splenic vein (whose tributaries include the short gastric

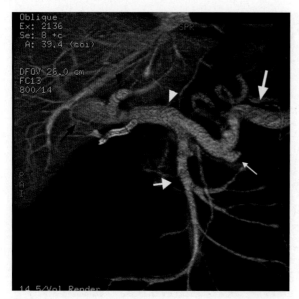

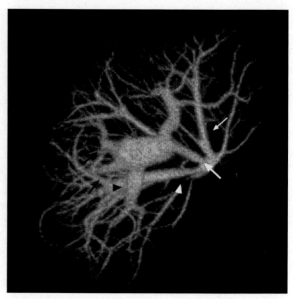

FIGURE 19-19 Normal portal vein. VR images of a 56-year-old man demonstrate the portal venous anatomy well. The splenic vein (*long large white arrow*) receives the IMV (*long small white arrow*) and the SMV (*short white arrow*) to form the main portal vein (*white arrowhead*), which then branches into the left (*black arrowhead*) and right (*black arrow*) portal veins.

FIGURE 19-20 Projection image. VR CT image of the hepatic veins and the portal veins demonstrates the left (*small white arrow*), middle (*large white arrow*), and right (*white arrowhead*) hepatic veins as well as the portal venous anatomy, with the left portal vein (*gray arrowhead*) branching into its medial (*red arrowhead*) and lateral (*red arrow*) components. The right portal vein (*gray arrow*) branches into the right anterior veins (*black arrow* and *red arrow*) and posterior vein (*black arrowhead*).

veins, the gastroepiploic vein and pancreatic veins) just posterior to the neck of the pancreas to form the portal vein, which runs cephalad and obliquely toward the right to the hilum of the liver, where it is the most posterior structure in the hepatoduodenal ligament. The main portal vein receives the coronary vein and then splits to form the right and left branches, each supplying about half of the liver.

In adults, the length of the main portal vein is typically 8 cm, and the diameter of the portal vein after its confluence ranges from 9 to 11 mm in diameter. Variations in the branching pattern of the main portal vein are less common than variations in the hepatic arteries, veins, and bile ducts, with a reported incidence of 0.09% to 24% (85–87). For the majority of cases, the main portal vein divides into a short, oblique right portal vein and a transversely oriented left portal vein (88). The right portal vein quickly branches within the right lobe of the liver to supply the anterior segment (V and VIII, and, variably, IV), and the posterior segment (VI and VII) of the right lobe (Fig. 19-20). The cystic vein drains into the right portal vein before the right portal vein enters into the right lobe of the liver. As a single trunk, the left branch of the portal vein turns transversely to the left between the quadrate and caudate lobe. Portal branches to the caudate lobe arise from the transverse portion of the left portal vein, from the first part of the right portal vein, and/or

directly from the portal trunk. The left portal vein has a long transverse course to the level of the umbilical fissure, where it gives off medial branches to segment IV and lateral branches to segments II and III.

Hepatic Veins

On entering the liver, the blood drains into the hepatic sinusoids. Three major hepatic veins originating from the right and left lobe and from the middle portion of the liver join the IVC just inferior to the diaphragm (76–79).

The right, middle, and left hepatic veins enter the retrohepatic IVC just below the diaphragm, usually 2 cm inferior to the right atrium (89). The right hepatic vein drains separately into the IVC, but the middle hepatic vein and the left hepatic vein may share a common trunk (65% to 85%) (90). In addition to the three main hepatic veins, small accessory (short) hepatic veins from the pericaval liver segments drain directly into the IVC inferior to the drainage of the three major veins (91) (Fig. 19-21). These short hepatic veins usually drain the right lobe or caudate lobe and need to be accounted for when a living donor hepatic transplant candidate is being evaluated (92–94). The major short hepatic veins are the inferior or middle right hepatic veins. All of the venous drainage, major hepatic venous and accessory venous drainage, exits the liver in its bare area.

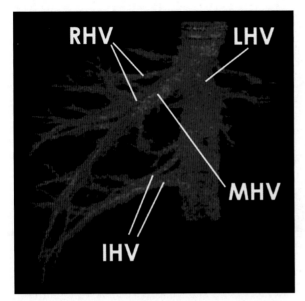

FIGURE 19-21 Short hepatic veins (Nakamura and Tsuzuki's classification).[a] VR reconstructions show hepatic venous drainage pattern at the right liver lobe. Pattern is classified according to dominant development among the right hepatic vein (*RHV*), inferior right hepatic vein (*IHV*), and middle hepatic vein (*MHV*). (*LHV*, left hepatic vein.) In type 3 (*n* = 1, 2%), large middle hepatic vein is present and drains paramedian sector and inferior part of lateral sector. The right hepatic vein is small and drains superior part of lateral sector. Also, the thick inferior hepatic vein is present. (Reprinted with permission from Onodera Y, Omatsu T, Nakayama J, et al. Peripheral anatomic evaluation using 3D CT hepatic venography in donors: significance of peripheral venous visualization in living-donor liver transplantation. *AJR Am J Roentgenol.* 2004;183:1065–1070.)

[a]This classification describes a dominant hepatic vein in the right lobe and venous drainage from the right hepatic vein, inferior hepatic vein, and middle hepatic vein.

Portal Vein Variants

Portal venous variants are primarily important for interventionalists performing transjugular intrahepatic portosystemic shunt (TIPS) procedures and for transplant surgeons evaluating candidacy of patients. Venous anomalies include early branching of the portal vein, a trifurcation of the portal vein (late origin of the left portal vein at the bifurcation of the right portal vein into its anterior and posterior branches), an anomalous origin of the left portal vein from the right anterior portal vein branch, and early origin of the right posterior portal vein. These venous anomalies are important preoperative findings. The more branches, the more anastomoses the surgeon must make, increasing the potential complications (96,97).

The right anterior portal vein (which supplies segments V and VIII, and variably IV), may arise from the left portal vein distal to the bifurcation. This poses a problem for living donor donation of either the right or the left lobe of the liver. If this variant is not appreciated preoperatively, resection of the left portal vein will devascularize segments V,

VIII, and, variably, IV. In these patients, resection of the left portal vein must follow the takeoff of the aberrant right anterior portal vein.

The left portal vein may have a very short extraparenchymal segment. When explanted, the small extrahepatic segment will be insufficient in length for anastomosis to the recipient's portal vein, and an interpositioned venous graft will need to be placed.

Some venous anomalies are absolute contraindications to liver transplantation. Portal vein trifurcation is considered a contraindication to living related liver transplantation of the right lobe of the liver (segments V–VIII). Additionally, absence of the living donor's right portal vein is a contraindication to liver transplantation.

Hepatic Vein Variants

Similar to portal venous variants, hepatic venous variants are most important for delineating aberrant drainage prior to transplantation. In evaluation of hepatic venous variants prior to right lobe living donor transplantation, the caliber of the right main hepatic vein should be determined. If the right main hepatic vein is small, portions of the right lobe may be drained via tributaries leading to the middle hepatic or inferior right hepatic veins (Fig. 19-22). Thus, viability of the donated right lobe will depend on preservation of all the venous drainage.

Common anatomic hepatic venous variants are an accessory inferior right hepatic vein, which drains Couinaud segment VI (18% of the normal population) (Fig. 19-23), and a middle right hepatic vein, which drains Couinaud segment V (5.5%) (90). The accessory inferior right hepatic vein is commonly seen deep to the posterior division of the right portal vein.

CLINICAL APPLICATIONS

With 3D contrast MRA and multidetector spiral CTA, the main visceral vessels are displayed with excellent diagnostic accuracy. However, neither achieves the spatial resolution of selective catheter angiography, limiting visualization of smaller branch vessels.

Mesenteric Ischemia

Reflecting the dramatic increase of life expectation and a growing number of elderly patients, the last decades have seen an increasing frequency in the diagnosis of ischemic disorders of the intestines. Partly, this is due to a real increase in incidence of atherosclerotic changes of the arterial tree in an aging population. However, this is also a result of the increasing awareness (and thus, increasing diagnosis) of clinical syndromes that have secondary changes of the intestinal blood flow.

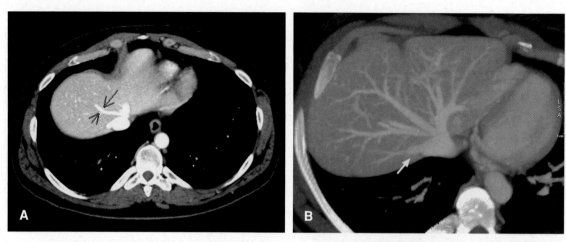

FIGURE 19-22 Accessory hepatic veins. A: Axial CT image through the level of the hepatic veins demonstrates an accessory hepatic vein (*black arrows*), entering the middle hepatic vein. **B:** Axial CT image in a different patient demonstrates an accessory vein from segment VI draining into the IVC directly (*white arrow*). (Images courtesy of Ivan Pedrosa, MD, BIDMC, Boston.)

The demonstration of significant stenoses in two of the three main mesenteric vessels in conjunction with appropriate clinical symptoms underscores the diagnosis of mesenteric ischemia (63). However, many patients with stenoses in the mesenteric vessels are asymptomatic. Autopsy series in unselected patient populations document significant mesenteric atherosclerosis in 35% to 70% of patients (98). This incidence is greater in selected patient populations with risk factors for atherosclerosis, including diabetes, hyperlipidemia, smoking, and hypertension. In performing duplex sonography of the mesenteric arteries in 184 asymptomatic patients, Roobottom and Dubbins (1) found total occlusion or >70% stenosis in 3% of adult patients under age 65 and an 18% incidence in patients over age 65. In 11% of patients, the disease was found in only one vessel; 7% had disease in both the celiac or SMA (1). The most common site of significant atherosclerotic disease is the origin of the celiac artery (86%), followed by the IMA (70%) and SMA (55%) (98).

Heretofore, selective angiography has been considered the gold standard for establishing the diagnosis of this disease (99). However, CTA and CE MRA have the potential to become a definitive noninvasive tool for the diagnosis of CMI. These cross-sectional techniques not only can provide information about anatomy, patency, and stenosis of mesenteric vessels but are also becoming a modality of

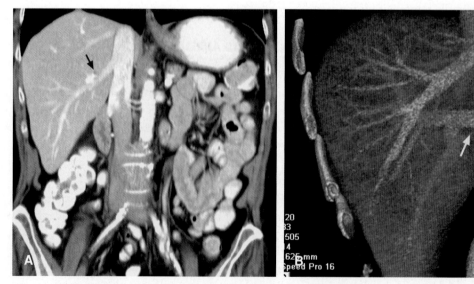

FIGURE 19-23 Accessory inferior right hepatic vein. A: Coronal MDCT images obtained during the portal venous phase demonstrate a prominent accessory inferior right hepatic vein (*black arrow*) draining into the IVC. **B:** Coronal VR MDCT images demonstrate a replaced right hepatic vein (*white arrow*) draining into the IVC.

choice in the selection of patients suspected of having mesenteric ischemia who may benefit from endovascular therapy or surgery.

Pathophysiology

Mesenteric ischemia results from any reduction in blood flow to the intestine, as in shock or heart failure, as well as from either local morphologic or functional changes. Such inadequate circulation may derive from focal atheromatous emboli, luminal narrowing of the mesenteric vessels, vasculitis as part of a systemic disease, mesenteric venous thrombosis, and mesenteric vasoconstriction (nonocclusive mesenteric ischemia). Independent of the cause, intestinal ischemia has the same end results, ranging from completely reversible functional changes to total hemorrhagic necrosis of the bowel. However, numerous collateral pathways exist between the small and large bowel. The major vascular supply of the bowel depends on the CA and the SMA, while the supply source for the lower intestine is the IMA. In case of stenosis or occlusion to one of these vessels, the development of a rich collateral circulation between these arteries can mostly prevent major abdominal symptoms (38,69,70) (Fig. 19-24).

Most patients will not become clinically symptomatic unless blood flow in at least two major vessels is compromised (63,100). Occlusion of two of the three vessels occurs frequently without evidence of ischemia, and total occlusion of all three vessels has also been observed in totally asymptomatic patients. Collateral pathways around occlusions of small arterial branches in the mesentery are provided by the primary, secondary, and tertiary arcades in the small bowel and the arc of Riolan and the marginal artery of Drummond in the colon. Within the bowel wall, a tight network of closely intercommunicating arteries provides a second level of arterial supply to short intestinal segments when extramural supply has been stopped.

At rest, intestinal blood flow is estimated between 50 and 1,200 mL/minute, which equates to approximately 10% to 20% of the cardiac output (101). This volume may modestly increase after eating or may decrease during exercise, but major changes are induced by the level of sympathetic activity. Short-term vascular constriction as modulated by alpha- and beta-adrenergic receptors can be tolerated by the intestine. Similarly, the lumen of the SMA might be reduced by 80% without appreciable diminution in blood flow. Interestingly, intestinal ischemia can be present without intestinal necrosis, and intestinal necrosis may be present with normal blood flow if blood flow is measured after a transient episode of ischemia has been relieved.

Splanchnic ischemia syndromes are classified for simplicity as either acute or chronic. However, the term *chronic*

is somewhat of a misnomer, in that the majority of "chronic" cases are caused by acute mesenteric ischemic events that exhibit immediate or delayed effects of the circulatory insult.

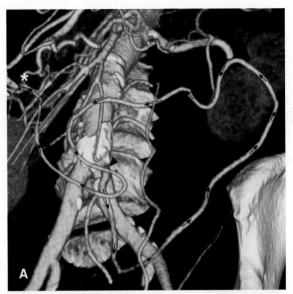
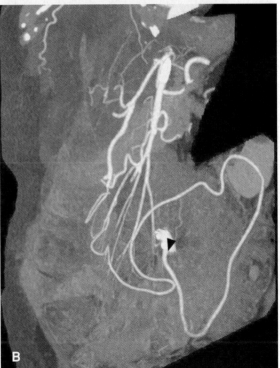

FIGURE 19-24 Meandering artery. VR CTA (**A**) shows the meandering artery (also called the anastomosis of Riolan) arising from the IMA (*arrowhead*) for retrograde perfusion (*arrows*) of the SMA via an enlarged branch of the left colic artery connecting centrally (∗) with the middle colic artery. This collateral pathway expresses itself in the event of occlusion of the origin of the SMA. **B:** MIP images from the same patient demonstrate the origin of the left colic artery at the IMA (*black arrowhead*). (Figure courtesy of Stanford University Cardiovascular Imaging.)

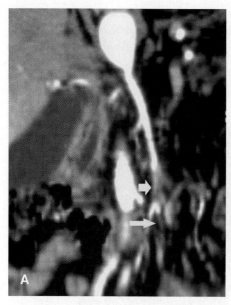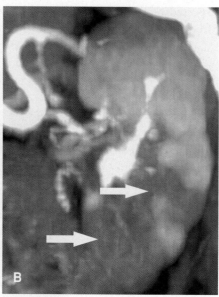

FIGURE 19-25 Endocarditis with emboli to the SMA and left kidney. **A:** Coronal CPR demonstrating embolus within SMA (*short arrow*) and proximal jejunal branch (*long arrow*). **B:** VR image of the left kidney revealing multiple renal infarcts (*arrows*).

Acute Mesenteric Ischemia

Acute obstruction of mesenteric arteries or their branches causes symptoms that are difficult to interpret clinically. Hence, the correct diagnosis is likely to be delayed, potentially with serious consequences. Abdominal pain of sudden onset is the most often clinical presentation of AMI. Occlusive emboli, thromboses, mesenteric vasoconstriction (nonocclusive ischemia), vasculitis, and mesenteric venous thrombosis are known causes for AMI. The clinical symptoms are basically the same for all causes and depend mainly on the duration of the ischemia. Concomitant renal artery or splenic artery occlusion with associated renal or splenic infarction has to be considered in such a clinical scenario. While occlusion of small peripheral arterial arcades or separate colic arteries cannot be visualized with CT or MR, indirect signs of mesenteric vascular occlusion have to be appreciated. Parts of the bowel wall prone to hemorrhagic necrosis are usually swollen, and the lumen is compressed. In addition, one might encounter effusion or hemorrhage in the compromised bowel and mesentery. Numerous lymph nodes with pathologically increased diameters can be appreciated. Mortality is extremely high in this disease. Treatment includes catheter angiography with intra-arterial administration of vasodilators or thrombolytic agents. In the majority of cases, patients with AMI are referred to a surgical procedure.

Emboli

As much as 50% of cases of AMI are caused by SMA emboli, which usually originate from a mural or an atrial thrombus in patients with atrial fibrillation (Fig. 19-25). While rheumatic valvular disease was most commonly associated with such thrombi in the past, atherosclerotic changes have become much more important today. Paradoxical embolism to the SMA from deep venous thrombosis has also been observed. Twenty-five percent of patients with acute onset of abdominal pain and suspected mesenteric emboli have a previous history of peripheral arterial embolism, and many patients will present with concomitant emboli in other arteries (101). Depending on the localization of the embolus, it can be visualized with CT or MR in the proximal part of the SMA. Using catheter angiography, emboli can be delineated as sharp, rounded filling defects. The artery may be completely occluded, but more often, the embolus only partially obstructs the blood flow. In addition, mild vasoconstriction might be detected proximal and distal to the embolus (102,103). Emboli tend to lodge at points of vascular divisions and narrowings—for example, distal to the origin of a major branch, such as the origin of the inferior pancreaticoduodenal artery, the origin of the middle colic artery, or the origin of the ileocolic artery. Lodging distal to the inferior pancreaticoduodenal artery or the middle colic artery is problematic, as it isolates the distal small bowel from collaterals that connect to these arteries.

Thrombosis

An acute thrombosis of the SMA may also lead to acute ischemia of the intestine. SMA thrombosis is less common than embolic disease. Thrombosis is almost always superimposed on severe atherosclerotic narrowing, most commonly in the region where the main artery arises. Since the acute onset of the episode represents the end stage of a chronic process of luminal narrowing, as much as 50% of patients have experienced abdominal pain during the preceding weeks or months. These patients typically suffer from severe atherosclerotic changes throughout the arterial system, and a prior history of coronary, cerebral, or peripheral arterial ischemia is frequently present. Apart from local intestinal pathologies, both MRA and CTA nicely display the extent of atherosclerosis throughout the arterial tree. However, the differentiation between an older thrombus and an embolus may be demanding. The absence of dilated collateral vessels or the presence of inadequate contrast enhancement within the SMA indicates an acute occlusion. Prompt surgical intervention is indicated irrespective of additional findings in these cases.

Nonocclusive Mesenteric Ischemia

Nonocclusive mesenteric ischemia occurs in patients with low-flow syndromes. Thus, when it occurs, it is observed in elderly and/or extremely ill patients who are hospitalized in coronary/intensive care units. These patients develop vasoconstriction in response to a decrease in cardiac output, hypovolemia, dehydration, vasopressor agents, or arterial hypotension. Predisposing conditions include myocardial infarction, congestive heart failure, aortic or mitral insufficiency, renal and hepatic disease, and recent cardiac or major abdominal operations. Additionally, pulmonary edema, cardiac arrhythmia, or shock has been present. Digitalis, a commonly prescribed drug, has a constrictive effect on the mesenteric circulation and may produce bowel necrosis if given in too high a dose. In the majority of cases, the underlying cause of the inadequate blood flow is not amenable to interventional or surgical correction. Diagnosis of the nonocclusive subtype of AMI is demanding. Severe pancreatitis may display features like those of a nonocclusive mesenteric ischemia. On MRA or CTA imaging, findings suggestive of a nonocclusive etiology of mesenteric ischemia include findings of luminal irregularities of the splanchnic vasculature in conjunction with indirect imaging signs of mesenteric ischemia (i.e., ascites, impaired contrast enhancement of circumscribed bowel wall areas). If this diagnosis is suggested early, treatment is the optimization of the patient's hemodynamic and volume status, with treatment of the underlying medical condition. Selective injection of the mesenteric vasculature with IV papaverine or glucagon may also increase blood flow to the bowel. If the patient demonstrates a surgically correctable lesion, an emergent operation should be performed.

Vasculitis and Iatrogenic Causes

In addition to embolus and thrombosis secondary to atherosclerosis, a wide variety of other vascular disorders may cause acute occlusion of small mesenteric arteries. High-resolution CTA and MRA can provide information about abnormalities due to lupus erythematosus, rheumatoid disease, and other types of vasculitis (104,105). Intimal arterial hyperplasia and thrombus formation in small mesenteric arteries may also cause infarction. Bowel ischemia secondary to abdominal surgery, catheterization, and trauma are other important causes of vascular occlusions that can be detected and defined by cross-sectional imaging.

Mesenteric Venous Thrombosis

Mesenteric vascular occlusion is usually subacute in presentation, with a vague clinical prodrome that may last days to weeks prior to disease recognition. The most common causes of venous thrombosis include inflammation, peritonitis, portal hypertension, and hypercoagulable states associated with various malignancies and the use of oral contraceptives. Paraneoplastic syndromes most commonly affect the SMV. Since the diagnosis of an SMV thrombus with angiography is notoriously difficult and the angiographic findings are indistinct, cross-sectional imaging techniques play an important role in diagnosing this form of mesenteric ischemia (Figs. 19-26, 19-27). Surgical therapy consists of thrombectomy, resection of infarcted bowel, and anticoagulation. Correction of the underlying medical condition (such as investigation for Factor V Leiden antibodies, antithrombin III deficiency, protein C and S deficiency, etc.) is essential. An extensive discussion on venous thrombosis can be found within Chapter 24).

Inferior Mesenteric Artery

The incidence of acute embolic occlusion of the IMA is much lower than occlusion of the SMA. The larger diameter of the SMA and its nearly parallel course to the aorta combine to invoke a much higher risk for collecting emboli. Acute occlusion of the IMA is generally well tolerated if limited to the proximal portion of the vessel and collateral flow from the SMA is sustained. If this is not the case, occlusion of the IMA may cause infarction of variable segments of the left colon. In some patients, IMA occlusion relates to preceding surgery; in others, it may be associated with atheromatous plaques, blood dyscrasias, saccular aortic aneurysms, and sepsis. Clinically, patients with an acute occlusion of the IMA present with sudden, severe, lower abdominal pain and often bloody rectal discharge. Iatrogenic ligation of the IMA alone during a surgical procedure (e.g., resection of abdominal aortic aneurysms [AAAs]) might be well tolerated when the marginal artery of Drummond is intact. However, if the hypogastric arteries are also ligated and the channels between IMA and SMA are not well established, the outcome may be disastrous.

With acute obstruction of the SMA, the IMA may maintain arterial supply through the aforementioned

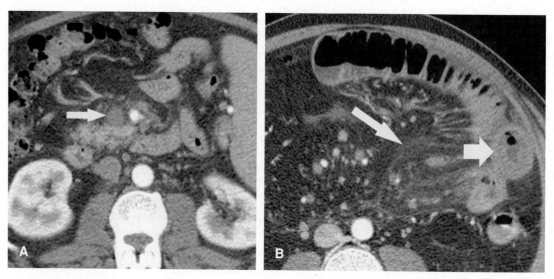

FIGURE 19-26 Acute SMV thrombus. In **(A)**, note thrombus within the proximal SMV (*arrow*). **B:** Scan at a more caudal level reveals thickening of small bowel loops (*short arrow*) and mesenteric edema (*long arrow*) from venous occlusion.

marginal artery of Drummond; however, the supply is unlikely to be adequate in most cases.

Imaging Diagnosis of Acute Mesenteric Ischemia

Helical CT and CTA (especially when performed with multidetector row scanners) and MRI (particularly gadolinium-enhanced MRA) enable volumetric acquisitions in a single breath hold. MDCT should be considered the primary diagnostic modality for patients with a high clinical suspicion of AMI due to its wide availability, rapid acquisition,

and ability to demonstrate air. Conventional angiography is reserved for equivocal cases at noninvasive imaging and is also used in conjunction with transcatheter therapeutic techniques in management of symptomatic portal and mesenteric venous thrombosis (15). With MRA, thrombus in the SMV can easily be delineated on contrast-enhanced T1-weighted transverse images as hypointense luminal filling defect with peripheral contrast uptake. The peripheral contrast enhancement and central hypodense demarcation of the thrombus can also be appreciated on CT images. In

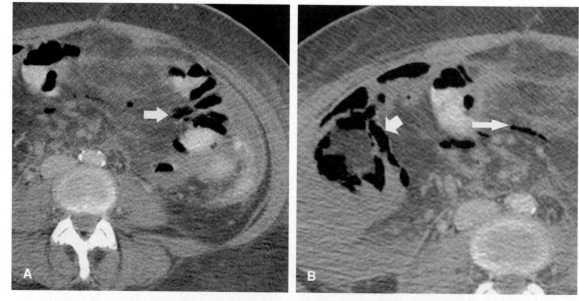

FIGURE 19-27 SMV thrombus with infarction. Mesenteric venous infarction with peritonitis. In **(A)**, extraluminal free air (*arrow*) adjacent to the small bowel (*arrow*) with extensive surrounding inflammatory change in the mesentery. Part **(B)** reveals pneumatosis of the cecum (*short arrow*), with linear gas extending into the mesenteric veins (*long arrow*).

addition to venous thrombosis detection, cross-sectional imaging often detects displacement of the SMV in relation to the SMA. Both CT and MR permit detection of the underlying pathologic condition—for example, external compression from pancreatic tumors or lymph nodes. Vascular compromise—particularly venous but also arterial—is also noted in bowel intussusception, strangulated bowel obstruction, intestinal volvulus, and midgut malrotation.

Chronic Mesenteric Ischemia

The diagnosis of CMI includes a host of various conditions in which there is insufficient blood flow to the intestine to satisfy the demands of increased motility, secretion, and absorption that develop after meals. The clinical syndrome of CMI is rare. Symptoms include abdominal pain, weight loss, and food aversion (53,63,106,107). The pain is somewhat similar to that arising in the myocardium with angina pectoris or that in the calf muscles in patients with intermittent claudication. Atherosclerotic wall changes of the splanchnic arteries are reported to be the main pathophysiologic mechanism for CMI (40). Although partial or complete occlusions of the CA, SMA, and IMA have been identified frequently in autopsy and angiographic studies, there have been relatively few patients with clinically documented chronic intestinal ischemia. There are many patients with occlusion of two or even all three vessels who remain asymptomatic. Therefore, the diagnosis of mesenteric ischemia remains challenging in clinical practice. Reflecting the risks associated with arterial catheterization, the clinical diagnosis of mesenteric ischemia has been mostly one of exclusion. In addition, the clinical significance of the angiographic demonstration of one or more of these vessels being occluded remains controversial. The dearth of objective means of determining the inadequacy of intestinal blood flow before any morphologic changes of mesenteric ischemia is the major obstacle to identifying patients with CMI.

CMI has been reported with aneurysms of the aorta, the CA, the SMA, congenital and traumatic arteriovenous fistulas involving the hepatic arteries, coarctation of the aorta, and congenital anomalies of the splanchnic vessels. Such cases are rare, however, and atherosclerotic disease in the mesenteric vasculature is the usual cause of intestinal ischemia.

Atherosclerosis commonly affects the splanchnic arteries in individuals over 45 years of age. Luminal narrowing of the major mesenteric vessels is mostly due to a plaque at the aortic origin or within the first 1 to 3 cm of the artery, respectively. Severe stenosis is mostly associated with marked aortic atherosclerosis. As may be expected, patients with severe atherosclerotic changes of the mesenteric vessels have a higher incidence of coronary artery disease and diabetes mellitus (98).

Due to the lack of a specific and reliable diagnostic test for abdominal angina, the diagnosis is based on clinical symptoms, noninvasive cross-sectional imaging, and catheter angiography in selected cases and the exclusion of other GI disease. The median time span between clinical presentation and diagnosis of CMI is more than 18 months for patients with new symptoms and approximately 1 month for patients with recurrent symptoms. Symptoms of mesenteric ischemia may overlap with those of more common intestinal disorders such as peptic ulcer or chronic cholecystitis.

Recent advances in MR technology permit a comprehensive assessment of the splanchnic arterial system (50,51,60,63,84). Hence, MRA in combination with flow quantification (16,36,39,61) or oximetry (72) has been proposed for the diagnosis of mesenteric ischemia. Despite the availability of noninvasive MRA, a reliable diagnosis remains difficult in a high percentage of cases: atherosclerotic changes are often based on the level of arterioles and therefore cannot be safely detected by luminographic procedures (108). In addition, the mesenteric circulation very often is supported by arterial collaterals, especially under long-lasting clinical circumstances. Therefore, severe stenotic changes might be present in the main mesenteric vessels in an asymptomatic population (69,70). A way out of this dilemma might be the more subtle evaluation of mesenteric ischemia using perfusion values of the small bowel wall before and after caloric stimulation (51,109) (Fig. 19-28).

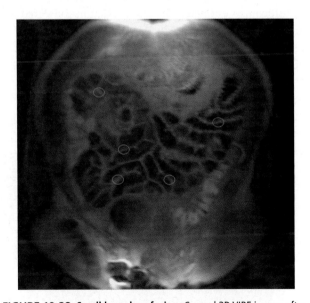

FIGURE 19-28 Small bowel perfusion. Coronal 3D VIBE images after the administration of oral contrast demonstrate dark fluid filling the small bowel. ROIs placed on the small bowel wall can yield information about perfusion as it relates to enhancement. Measurements with physiologic challenges such as before and after caloric stimulation may help in detecting subtle mesenteric ischemia.

Portal Hypertension

Portal hypertension is defined as a portal venous pressure exceeding 10 mmHg and is caused by increased resistance to portal blood flow. Causes for this increased resistance are classified into prehepatic (presinusoidal), hepatic (sinusoidal), and posthepatic (postsinusoidal) etiologies. Mechanical venous obstruction (e.g., portal/splenic vein thrombosis, hepatic venous obstruction) is primarily responsible for the prehepatic and posthepatic etiologies, while cirrhosis is the primary etiology of hepatic portal hypertension (110).

In the normal physiologic state, the liver offers very little resistance to portal venous flow. Intrahepatic resistance with subsequent portal hypertension is most frequently found in cirrhosis of the portal, biliary, or postnecrotic type. The pathologic changes (including collagen deposits in the space of Disse) cause distortion of the hepatic parenchyma with intermingling of necrotic, fibrotic, and regenerating areas of liver tissue. This progressive process eventually results in impaired circulation of blood through the liver and portal hypertension. With cirrhotic livers, the portal intrahepatic ramifications are often involved to such a degree as to cause venous stasis and portal hypertension. When the vascular obstruction is intrahepatic, the collateral vessels will drain the congested vascular area toward the low-pressure systemic veins and not to the liver, which constitutes a hepatofugal collateral circulation.

Collateral vessels form in patients with liver disease and portal hypertension (Fig. 19-29). The extent, number, and size of collateral vessels as well as the velocity of flow are difficult to estimate. The large variations observed are due mainly to differences in the duration and severity of the portal venous hypertension, to individual differences in the duration and severity of an obstruction, and to individ-

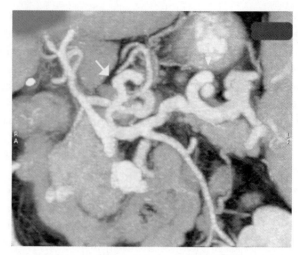

FIGURE 19-29 Portal hypertension. Coronal MIP MRA images from a patient with portal hypertension demonstrate the coronary (*arrow*) and splenic (*arrowhead*) varices.

ual differences in the rapidity with which a collateral circulation can be formed. Even in cases where a collateral circulation is well developed, an inability to drain the congested vascular bed adequately is apparent when low-flow velocities and pathologically high pressures are observed.

The function of collaterals in the portal circulation is to decompress the hepatic circulation and divert splanchnic blood flow from the portal to the systemic circulation. The most common of the connections establish communication with the superior caval system via the coronary vein and short gastric veins on the one hand and the esophageal venous plexus on the other (Fig. 19-30).

Demonstrable communications with the inferior caval system via the inferior mesenteric vein (IMV) and hemor-

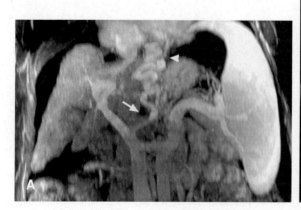 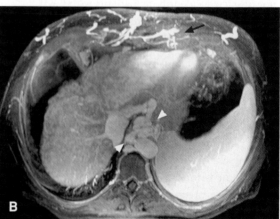

FIGURE 19-30 Coronary varices. A: Coronal reformatted MIP images from a gadolinium-enhanced MR study demonstrate the coronary vein (*arrow*), with extensive variceal formation connecting to the gastroesophageal venous plexus (*arrowhead*). **B:** Axial MIP images of the same patient demonstrate the gastroesophageal varices (*white arrowheads*) as well as anterior abdominal wall varices (*black arrow*) forming the "caput medusa" of portal hypertension.

rhoidal vein plexus or via retroperitoneal connections with the left renal vein are less common (Fig. 19-31). These are formed by vessels that are normally present but that are unused in the absence of elevated portal pressure, rather than from the growth of new vessels. In advanced manifestations of intrahepatic obstruction and portal hypertension, a collateral communication between the left anterior branch of the portal vein and the caval system via recanalized remnants of the umbilical vein and veins in the abdominal wall may be demonstrated, a constellation of findings that can also be seen with the Cruveilhier-Baumgarten syndrome. (The latter is designated when any organic disease causes portal hypertension and splenomegaly with umbilical collateral circulation that is audible to auscultation as a venous hum.) The portosystemic collateral may even be intrahepatic, from the portal vein to a hepatic vein (Fig. 19-32).

The collaterals represent a natural mechanism that attempts to reduce portal pressure by diverting the portal circulation away from the abnormal liver. The development of hematemesis, melena, and ascites reflects a failure of the collateral to fully compensate for the dysregulated physiology. MDCTA and CE MRA can facilitate the presurgical planning in patients who require a portal-systemic shunt. In addition, spontaneous portal-systemic shunts (e.g., splenorenal shunts) can be detected and accurately displayed (Fig. 19-33). As long as metallic clips do not obscure the anatomy, CE MRA can be used to assess patency of both surgical and spontaneous shunts. With MRA PC techniques, flow

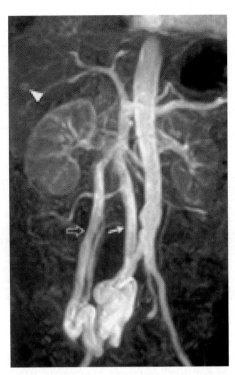

FIGURE 19-31 Mesenteric-gonadal shunt in a 68-year-old man with liver cirrhosis and hepatic encephalopathy. CE 3D MR portogram reveals a portosystemic collateral pathway from the ileocolic vein (*solid arrow*) to the right testicular vein (*open arrow*). CE CT included only the upper abdomen and thus did not reveal this mesenteric-gonadal shunt. Note the small hepatic hemangioma (*arrowhead*). (Reprinted with permission from Okumura A, Watanabe Y, Dohke M, et al. Contrast-enhanced three-dimensional MR portography. *Radiographics.* 1999;19:973–987.)

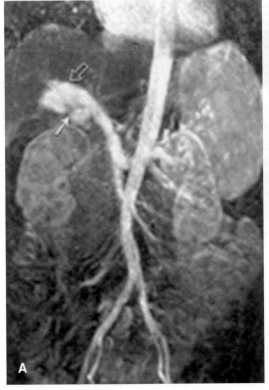

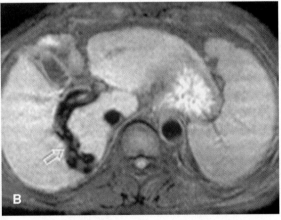

FIGURE 19-32 Intrahepatic portosystemic shunt in a 62-year-old man with alcoholic liver cirrhosis and hepatic encephalopathy. A: CE 3D MR portogram shows a large intrahepatic portosystemic collateral pathway (*solid arrow*) from the right portal vein (*open arrow*) to an accessory hepatic vein. Note that the intrahepatic portal vein branches are small. **B:** Axial fat-suppressed T1-weighted MR image (500/18) clearly demonstrates the collateral pathway (*arrow*). (Reprinted with permission from Okumura A, Watanabe Y, Dohke M, et al. Contrast-enhanced three-dimensional MR portography. *Radiographics.* 1999;19:973–987.)

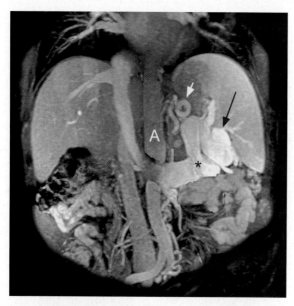

FIGURE 19-33 Spontaneous splenorenal shunt. Coronal thin-slab MIP of a gadolinium MRA study with a portion of the aorta (*A*) removed to demonstrate the enlarged left renal vein connecting with the IVC. Note the enlarged tangle of veins (*black arrow*) emanating from the left upper quadrant that drain (∗) into the left renal vein. Additional varices are seen in the region of the lesser sac (*white arrow*).

volumes and velocities supplement the depiction of the vasculature. For more detailed discussion of venous imaging techniques, please refer to Chapter 24.

Portal Vein Thrombosis

Extrahepatic obstruction of the portal venous system is usually caused by thrombosis, malformations, or both, which are long-standing conditions with well-developed signs of stasis. The underlying pathophysiology includes local infection, appendicitis, pancreatitis, portal hypertension, malignancy, trauma, coagulopathy, and surgery (Figs. 19-34, 19-35), to mention a few.

Malignant tumors and pancreatic cysts can easily be detected with CT and MR, whereas display with US may be hampered by bowel gas, motion artifacts, or obesity. In most patients with complete obstruction of the portal vein, hepatopetal collateral flow toward the liver can be appreciated as cavernous transformation. Portal vein thrombosis and collateral circulation can be accurately demonstrated with both CT and MR. Acute thrombosis generally presents with an expanded portal vein diameter, central thrombus material, and flow void on PC MRA images. Perivascular enhancement, when seen, reflects inflammatory changes of the adjacent interstitial tissue. The liver parenchyma shows a weak and patchy enhancement. In due course, small collaterals bypass portal venous occlusion, also known as cavernous transformation. This network of fine collaterals shows a characteristic enhancement pattern in the hepatic hilum during portal venous and equilibrium phases of CE CTA and CE MRA (Fig. 19-36). Additional discussion of the imaging findings on MRI of portal thrombosis is included in Chapter 24.

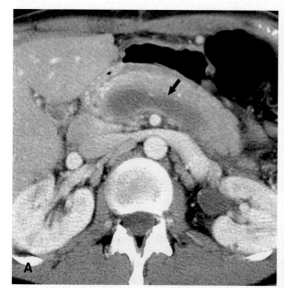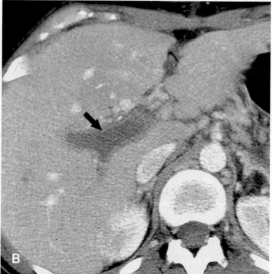

FIGURE 19-34 Splenic and portal vein thrombosis. Acute splenic and portal vein thrombosis after splenectomy. In **(A)**, note low-attenuation thrombus slightly distending splenic and portal veins (*arrow*). In **(B)**, thrombus extends into the right portal vein (*arrow*). The cluster of vessels seen anterior to the portal vein thrombus represents cavernous transformation.

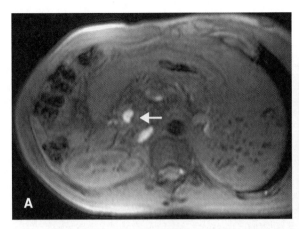
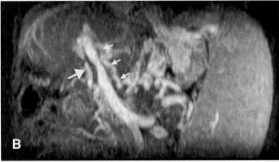

FIGURE 19-35 Partial thrombosis portal vein. A: Axial TOF images through the portal vein demonstrate a crescentic, partial filling defect (*white arrow*) along the posteromedial aspect of the main portal vein. **B:** Coronal MIP images from the portal venous phase of a 3D LAVA acquisition demonstrate eccentric, partially circumferential, non-occlusive thrombus along the walls of the portal vein (*large and small white arrows*).

When intrahepatic obstruction is coupled with extra-hepatic obstruction (e.g., cirrhosis complicated by portal thrombosis), all collaterals run to the caval system. In these cases, a surgically established shunt between the portal vein and the IVC aims at relieving portal hypertension and its complications (i.e., GI bleeding, encephalopathy, and refractory ascites) by reducing the portal pressure through the creation of iatrogenic portosystemic shunts. Surgical shunts can be structured as portocaval, splenorenal, or mesocaval connections. These shunts are directly demonstrable with MRA and CTA when a vascular graft is inserted. In patients with a history of implantation of a TIPS, evaluation of the metallic intrahepatic stent can be impaired by artifacts on both MR and CT (Fig. 19-37). Generally, the artifacts are more severe on MRI, but the severity depends on the material and orientation of the device. MR and color-coded duplex US can also provide flow quantification, an additional assessment of the functional status of such devices.

Splenic Vein Thrombosis and Budd-Chiari Syndrome

These two relatively common causes of prehepatic and posthepatic obstruction are discussed in Chapter 24.

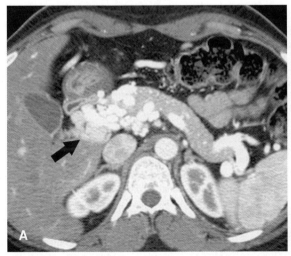
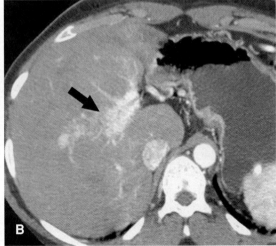

FIGURE 19-36 Chronic portal vein occlusion with cavernous transformation. In **(A)**, note numerous periportal collaterals (*arrow*). In **(B)**, a tangle of collateral veins in seen in the porta hepatis (*arrow*).

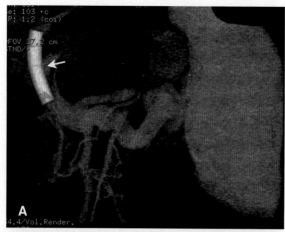

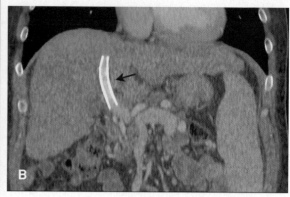

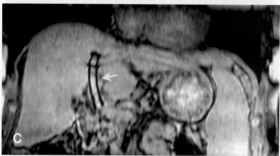

FIGURE 19-37 TIPS. A: Volume reformatted CT image demonstrates TIPS stent (*white arrow*) in place but does not demonstrate internal flow. **B:** Coronal reformatted CT images demonstrate probable flow within the stent (*black arrow*). **C:** Coronal reformatted MR images demonstrate minimal artifact from the stent, with widely patent internal flow within the stent (*white arrow*).

Extrinsic Compression Syndromes

Median Arcuate Ligament Syndrome

The median arcuate ligament is a fibrous band that connects the left and right diaphragmatic crura and forms the anterior aspect of the diaphragmatic aortic hiatus (Fig. 19-38). Usually, the median arcuate ligament arises at the L1 vertebral body, superior to the CA, but 24% of the time, it inserts low and crosses the proximal portion of the celiac artery (112). A characteristic impression on the proximal celiac artery at end-expiration, which simulates stenosis of the celiac artery, may be seen in a variety of individuals, including those who are asymptomatic. With varying degrees of respiration, the stenosis will appear more or less severe. When symptomatic, the condition has been referred to as the median arcuate ligament syndrome or as celiac artery compression syndrome (113) (Figs. 19-39, 19-40).

The characteristic configuration in median arcuate ligament syndrome is that of a "hooked" abrupt turn of the CA as it courses under the low insertion of the median arcuate ligament. This characteristic appearance distinguishes this syndrome from atherosclerotic disease (114). The diagnosis has traditionally been made utilizing conventional angiography but now is being made more frequently on CTA and MRA. Often, these examinations are not targeted for detection of this entity, and without careful atten-

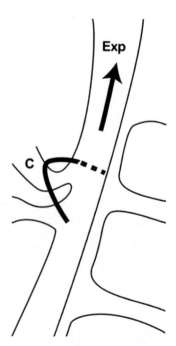

FIGURE 19-38 Cartoon median arcuate ligament. Diagram of a sagittal view of the abdominal aorta shows celiac artery compression by the median arcuate ligament (*solid and dashed line*). At expiration *(Exp)*, the aorta and its major branches, including the celiac artery *(C)*, move cephalad (*arrow*). This typically causes worsening of compression by the median arcuate ligament. (Image courtesy of Martha Helmers, BS, New York University Medical Center, New York, NY. Reprinted with permission from Lee VS, Morgan JN, Tan AG, et al. Celiac artery compression by the median arcuate ligament: a pitfall of end-expiratory MR imaging. *Radiology*. 2003;228:437–442.)

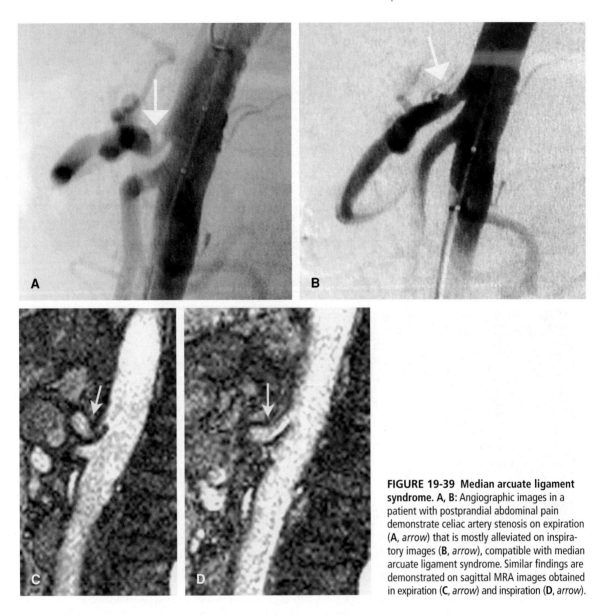

FIGURE 19-39 Median arcuate ligament syndrome. A, B: Angiographic images in a patient with postprandial abdominal pain demonstrate celiac artery stenosis on expiration (**A**, *arrow*) that is mostly alleviated on inspiratory images (**B**, *arrow*), compatible with median arcuate ligament syndrome. Similar findings are demonstrated on sagittal MRA images obtained in expiration (**C**, *arrow*) and inspiration (**D**, *arrow*).

tion to technique and respiratory phase, the diagnosis may be either exaggerated or missed (115). It is important to note that the appearance can be produced in asymptomatic individuals (115).

Historically, there has been controversy in the medical and surgical community as to the existence of this syndrome (116,117). In a review of 51 symptomatic patients who underwent celiac artery decompression operations, surgery was found to have the most benefit for patients that had the following symptoms: postprandial pain pattern (81% cure rate), age between 40 and 60 years (77%), and weight loss of 20 pounds or more (67%) (118). These criteria for operative success have been validated by additional surgical studies (119–121). Symptoms that are not predictive of operative success include atypical pain pattern with

periods of remission, a history of psychiatric disorder or alcohol abuse, age greater than 60 years, and weight loss of less than 20 pounds (118). Surgical therapies most predictive of long-term success are those that establish definitive vascular patency of the CA (e.g., vascular bypass operations or celiac stent placement) and not just celiac decompression through division of the sympathetic fibers and the median arcuate ligament.

Superior Mesenteric Artery Syndrome

SMA syndrome (also called *Wilkie's disease*) is a rare clinical entity characterized by compression of the third portion of the duodenum between the SMA and the aorta, resulting in complete or partial duodenal obstruction (122,123). The SMA syndrome was first described in 1861 by Von

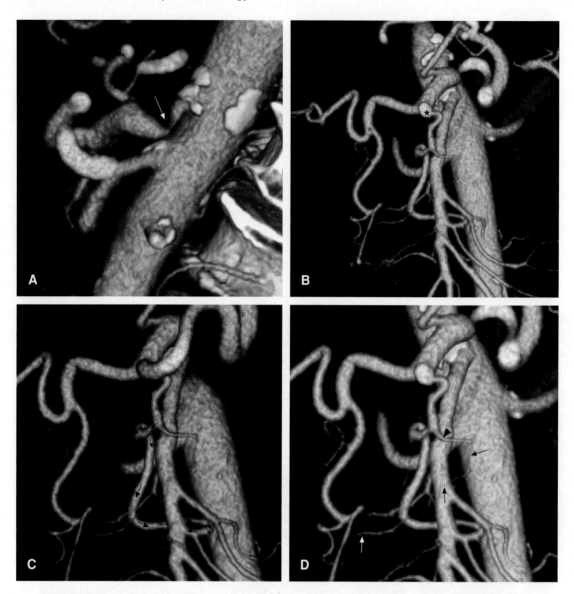

FIGURE 19-40 Median arcuate ligament with collaterals. Volume reformatted CTA images demonstrate severe stenosis of the celiac origin (*white arrow* in **A**) secondary to compression from the median arcuate ligament. Manipulation of the source images allows us to remove the splenic artery (∗) to better visualize the dorsal pancreatic collaterals (*small black arrows* in **C** and **D**) allowing collateral flow between the celiac and SMA. (Courtesy of Stanford University Cardiovascular Imaging.)

Rokitansky and later by Wilkie in 1927, with the pathogenesis thought to be secondary to the rapid loss of mesenteric and retroperitoneal fat (124,125).

Patients are typically young with a thin body habitus. The syndrome is associated with severe rapid weight loss due to hospitalization, cancer, or burns; body casting for scoliosis or vertebral fractures; dietary disorders; and exaggerated lumbar lordosis (126). Patients present with nonspecific symptoms, including epigastric pain, postprandial discomfort, nausea, bilious vomiting, early satiety, duodenal obstruction, and weight loss (127,128). Symptoms are exacerbated by eating and by supine position, with improvement by left lateral decubitus, prone, or knee–chest positioning (129).

Angiographic measurements of the aorta–SMA angle and aorta–SMA distance at the point where the SMA crosses the duodenum have been tabulated and can be measured by utilizing CTA, MRA, or conventional angiographic techniques (123,130). In control subjects, the SMA forms an angle of 25 to 60 degrees with the abdominal aorta and has an aortic–SMA distance of 10 to 28 mm. When this angle is narrowed to less than 22 degrees (most commonly between 6 and 15 degrees) and the aortic–SMA distance decreases to 2 to 8 mm, the third portion of the duodenum can become compressed (127,130,131).

The diagnosis of SMA syndrome has been made by utilizing upper GI series, noting dilatation of the first and second portions of the duodenum (with or without gastric dilatation), retention of barium within the duodenum with emptying after postural changes, antiperistaltic waves of barium in the proximal duodenum, and vertical linear extrinsic pressure on the transverse duodenum (132) (Fig. 19-41).

CTA or MRA can simultaneously evaluate the abdominal findings of duodenal dilatation/loss of retroperitoneal fat with the arterial findings of decreased aortic–SMA angle and/or decreased aorta–SMA distance (127). This demonstration is facilitated by administration of oral contrast prior to the angiographic study. Additionally, CTA and MRA are useful in evaluating other causes of the patient's pain. The imaging findings in SMA syndrome are nonspecific and can be seen with a variety of conditions, including diabetes, pancreatitis, peptic ulcer disease, scleroderma, enlarged

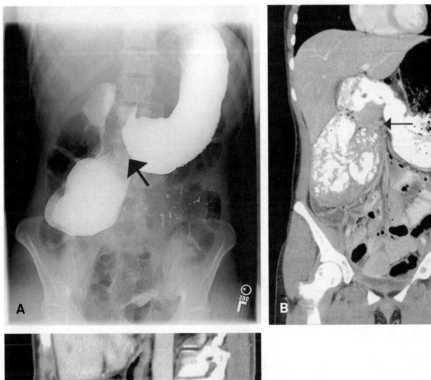

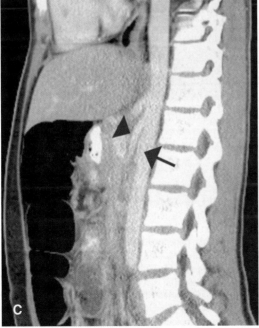

FIGURE 19-41 SMA syndrome. A: Overhead image from an upper GI series demonstrates marked distention of the stomach and first and second portions of the duodenum, with rapid tapering of the lumen size at the level of the crossing of the SMA. **B:** Coronal MDCT reformatted image again demonstrates distention of the stomach and first and second portions of the duodenum, with visualization of the SMA at the level of transition. **C:** Sagittal MDCT reformatted image demonstrates a sharp angle of the SMA with the aorta (*black arrowhead*), along with compression of the third portion of the duodenum (*black arrow*).

lymph nodes, and tumors in the root of the mesentery (132–135). Therefore, the clinical context is an important part of the evaluation.

Treatment for SMA syndrome is usually conservative, with high success rates after nasogastric drainage, IV fluid administration, and peroral or parenteral hyperalimentation (128). Weight gain is associated with improvement in clinical symptoms. When conservative therapy fails, and when other causes of pseudo-obstruction have been eliminated (idiopathic megaduodenum, neurologic conditions, diabetic gastroparesis), surgical therapy is usually considered. These patients usually display a long history of progressive weight loss, often with peptic ulcer disease resulting from chronic duodenal distention. There are several surgical options, including transposition of the third portion of the duodenum anterior to the SMA (130,136,137) or duodenojejunostomy. Alternative therapies include lysis of the ligament of Treitz, with mobilization of the duodenum.

Nutcracker Syndrome (Renal Vein Entrapment Syndrome)

The left renal vein can be compressed as it crosses between the aorta and the SMA (Fig. 19-42). This condition leads to elevated pressure within the left renal vein, collateral vessel formation, and hematuria from left renal vein hypertension. Orthostatic proteinuria has also been documented (138). The hematuria is thought to occur by rupture of thin-walled veins into the calyceal fornix. Collateral venous circulation can occur rarely, with associated enlargement of the left gonadal vein, causing vulvar varices or a varicocele (139). A variant of the nutcracker syndrome can occur with circumaortic or retroaortic left renal veins, when the left renal vein is compressed between the aorta and spine, a condition sometimes referred to as the "posterior nutcracker phenomenon." Usually, the patients are young and previously healthy, who experience new onset hematuria or proteinuria (140).

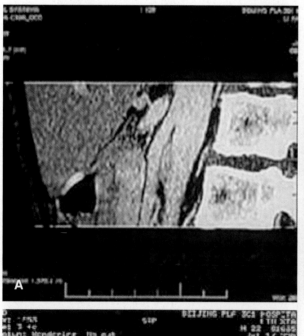

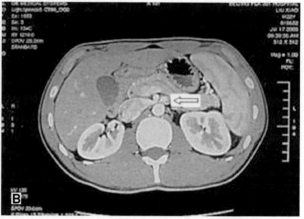

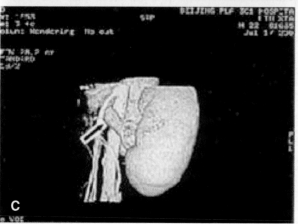

FIGURE 19-42 Nutcracker syndrome I. A: Sagittal CT in a patient with the nutcracker phenomenon showing that the angle between the SMA and the aorta was almost at 35 degrees. **B:** Coronal CT in a patient with the nutcracker phenomenon. The distance between the SMA and the aorta at the level of the renal vein was shorter (*arrow*). **C:** 3D helical CTV in a patient with the nutcracker phenomenon. The LRV was compressed by the aorta and the SMA (*arrow*). (Reprinted with permission from Fu WJ, Hong BF, Gao JP, et al. Nutcracker phenomenon: a new diagnostic method of multislice computed tomography angiography. *Int J Urol.* 2006;13:870–873.)

Classically, this condition has been diagnosed with left renal venography and is considered in patients with greater than 3 mmHg difference in pressure measurements between the left renal vein and the IVC (141). Ultrasonographic technique can also be used to make the diagnosis, via measurement of the diameter ratio between dilated and narrowed portions of the left renal vein, via Doppler measurement of the increase in flow velocity at the aortomesenteric angle or via Doppler detection of flow within collateral veins (138,142,143). These two methods of evaluation are invasive and time-consuming, respectively.

The diagnosis is most commonly suggested by CT or MR, obtained for unexplained hematuria in a previously asymptomatic patient, when searching for other abnormalities. The nutcracker syndrome may be suggested by the imaging findings of a small aortomesenteric angle (less than 22 degrees) and absence of visualization of the left renal vein with retroperitoneal collateral visualization (143). Treatment of the nutcracker syndrome can be achieved surgically by transposition of the left renal vein, nephrectomy, or autotransplantation of the left kidney (144,145).

Aneurysms

Patients with AAAs frequently have aneurysms of the iliac, common femoral, and popliteal arteries. Less frequently, there will be concomitant aneurysmal dilatation of the proximal CA or SMA. Even more infrequently, representing 0.1% to 0.2% of all vascular aneurysms, isolated visceral artery aneurysms occur in the splenic, hepatic, gastroduodenal,

gastric, gastroepiploic, and inferior mesenteric arteries (148) (Fig. 19-43).

Visceral artery aneurysms are a rare form of vascular disease with a predisposition to rupture, resulting in life-threatening hemorrhage. The mortality rate of these splanchnic aneurysms is 8.5% (149). The classic distribution of aneurysms in the visceral arteries is splenic artery (60%); hepatic artery (20%); SMA (5.5%); celiac artery (4%); gastric and gastroepiploic arteries (4%); jejunal, ileal, and colic (3%); pancreaticoduodenal and pancreatic arteries (2%); GDA (1.5%); and IMA (<1%) (149,150).

Splenic Artery Aneurysm

Of visceral artery aneurysms, splenic artery aneurysms are thought to be the most frequent in natural incidence, seen in approximately 0.8% of arteriograms and in up to 10.4% of autopsies (151,152) (Fig. 19-44). These aneurysms are usually smaller than 2.0 cm and are located in the mid to distal splenic artery. Most splenic artery aneurysms are found in women (4:1 female-to-male ratio), with an increased incidence in multiparous women (150). Although most splenic artery aneurysms are asymptomatic, occasionally patients may present with epigastric, left upper quadrant, or back pain or with GI hemorrhage secondary to erosion into an adjacent viscus. The risk of rupture increases with size. Splenic artery aneurysms that are diagnosed during pregnancy are usually discovered because of rupture (95%), with a maternal mortality rate of 70% and a fetal mortality rate of 95% (149).

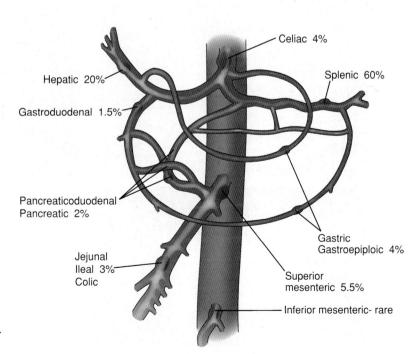

FIGURE 19-43 Incidence of aneurysms affecting the arteries of the splanchnic circulation. (Adapted from Upchurch GR, Zelenock GB, Stanley JC. Splanchnic artery aneurysms. In: Rutherford R (ed). *Vascular Surgery.* 6th ed. Philadelphia: Elsevier Saunders; 2005:1566.

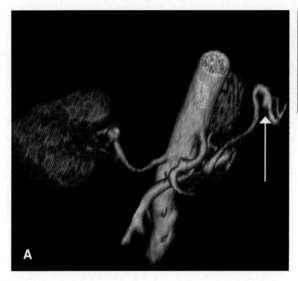

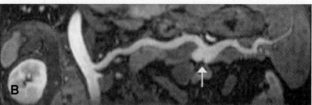

FIGURE 19-44 Splenic artery aneurysms. A: Volume reformatted image of the splenic artery demonstrates a distal aneurysm (*long white arrow*). **B:** MIP MRA image from a different patient with a history of pancreatitis demonstrates a distal splenic aneurysm (*white arrow*).

The etiology of splenic artery aneurysm formation is thought to be due to defects in the media of the artery, with loss of elasticity and smooth muscle. In pregnant women, the etiology is thought to be secondary to increased splenic blood flow and weakening of the vascular wall secondary to increased hormonal circulation. Splenic artery aneurysms are also seen with increased incidence in patients with pancreatitis, medial fibroplasia, portal hypertension, splenomegaly, status post liver transplantation, and atherosclerosis (153–156). Vasculitides (e.g., polyarteritis nodosa [PAN] and necrotizing angiitis) and infection (e.g., bacterial endocarditis) have also been reported as causes of splenic artery aneurysm formation (157–159). Splenic artery aneurysms are most commonly discovered incidentally on imaging examinations performed for other reasons (Fig. 19-45).

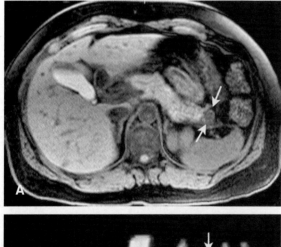

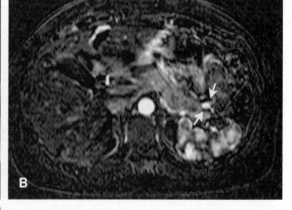

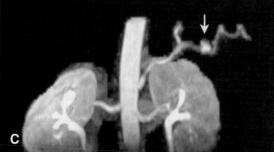

FIGURE 19-45 Splenic artery aneurysm mimicking a pancreatic tail cancer in a 52-year-old male patient with vague abdominal pain, with outside CT stating "mass in pancreatic tai—rule out pancreatic cancer." Axial 3D LAVA precontrast (**A**) images and arterial phase postcontrast subtraction images (**B**) demonstrate a hypointense well-circumscribed mass in the pancreatic tail (**A**, *arrows*) that demonstrates brisk arterial enhancement (**B**, *arrows*) after the administration of contrast, compatible with a small splenic arterial aneurysm. Coronal MIP image (**C**) demonstrates the aneurysm (*white arrow*) communicating with the splenic artery.

Imaging findings that predict the risk of rupture have been proposed, such as peripheral calcification, but this has not been definitively proven (Fig. 19-46). Repair is warranted in patients with a symptomatic aneurysm or contained rupture and has been advocated for certain asymptomatic lesions: splenic artery aneurysms in patients who may become pregnant or who are waiting for a liver transplant, aneurysms greater than 2.0 cm in diameter, and pseudoaneurysms of splenic or hepatic arteries. Interestingly, multiplicity is not a current stated indication for resection (160) (Fig. 19-47). The treatment of choice has been surgical resection, although percutaneous embolization is increasing in utilization, with good outcomes (161).

Hepatic Artery Aneurysms

Hepatic artery aneurysms are thought to be the second most common visceral aneurysm after splenic aneurysms but are the most commonly reported aneurysm. This discrepancy between (presumed) natural incidence and reported frequency is thought to be due to the rising number of interventional diagnostic and therapeutic procedures (photothermoacoustic [PTA] imaging, biopsies, TIPS, intra-arterial chemotherapy, etc.) increasing the rate of pseudoaneurysm formation (162). Additionally, increased imaging of stable blunt trauma patients has increased the incidence of detection of post-traumatic intrahepatic aneurysms. In fact, the incidence of hepatic arterial

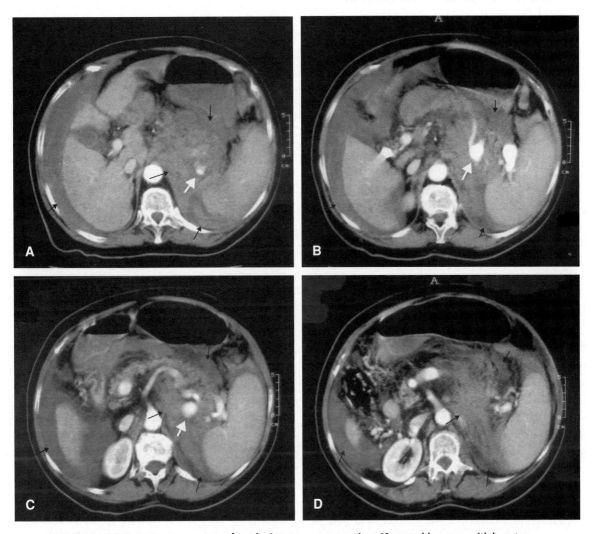

FIGURE 19-46 Spontaneous rupture of a splenic artery aneurysm in a 40-year-old woman with hypotension and abdominal pain. Emergent abdominal CT during the arterial phase demonstrates a large aneurysm in the distal splenic artery (*white arrow* in **A**, **B**, and **C**). A large amount of blood is seen within the abdomen (*black arrows* in **A**, **B**, **C**, and **D**). The patient was emergently taken to surgery for ligation of the splenic artery and splenectomy. (Images courtesy of Ivan Pedrosa, MD, BIDMC, Boston.)

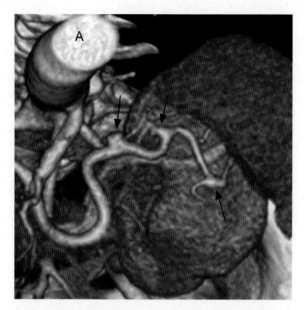

FIGURE 19-47 Multiple splenic artery aneurysms. This VR CTA study shows the abdominal aorta (*A*) seen on end and three splenic artery aneurysms (*arrows*). In general, the indications for removal include the presence of symptoms, pregnancy or plan to become pregnant, increasing size, and a diameter of 2 cm or greater. Interestingly, multiplicity is not an established indication for removal.

aneurysm formation is now equally divided between naturally occurring aneurysms and false aneurysms (152). Atherosclerosis, infection, and inflammation also contribute to the formation of hepatic arterial aneurysms; however, the incidence of hepatic mycotic aneurysms has decreased due to improved therapy of bacterial endocarditis in IV drug users. The pathogenesis of these aneurysms is unknown, partly because these lesions are asymptomatic until they rupture.

Hepatic aneurysms occur more often in men than women and, like all visceral artery aneurysms, are typically asymptomatic. For the rare hepatic aneurysm that is symptomatic, the most frequent clinical presentation is abdominal pain, followed by intestinal hemorrhage (from rupture of an extrahepatic aneurysm into the peritoneal cavity) or hemobilia (from rupture of an intrahepatic aneurysm into the biliary tree). There is a wide variation in the reported incidence of hepatic arterial aneurysm rupture, ranging from 20% to 80% (149,163).

Usually, hepatic aneurysms are detected on CT examinations evaluating a blunt trauma patient or a patient with right upper quadrant pain/hematobilia after an interventional procedure involving the liver. Additional imaging modalities that can detect hepatic arterial anatomy include MRA (with breath-hold techniques), traditional angiography (which offers the therapeutic benefit of

coiling the aneurysm), and ultrasonography (164) (Fig. 19-48).

Hepatic artery aneurysms are treated based on their location, feeding vessels, and importance relative to liver parenchymal supply. Excision or obliteration of most aneurysms can be justified based on the 20% to 44% incidence of rupture that has been reported (150,165). Treatment is clearly recommended for hepatic artery aneurysms greater than 2.0 cm in diameter, for those in patients with PAN or fibromuscular dysplasia, and in all cases of pseudoaneurysms (160).

The goal of treatment is to eliminate the risk of rupture of the aneurysm without overly disrupting the blood supply to the liver, and this is most commonly accomplished with percutaneous embolization. Surgical therapy (ligation, bypass, revascularization, aneurysmectomy, or aneurysmorrhaphy) can also be offered, with technical difficulty increasing as the aneurysms become intrahepatic. Complications of therapy include rupture, abscess formation, and hepatic necrosis.

Most of these aneurysms are inaccessible surgically (intrahepatic location, intrapancreatic location, perianeurysmal inflammation), which has led to the widespread use of transcatheter embolization as the primary treatment. But even transcatheter embolization may be treacherous due to multiple prior interventions, atherosclerotic disease, and anatomic variations, necessitating direct percutaneous embolization (166).

Superior Mesenteric Artery Aneurysms

SMA aneurysms (5.5% of all visceral aneurysms) typically are saccular or fusiform and are nearly always located in the first 5 cm of the SMA (152). In the past, the dominant etiology of SMA aneurysms was infection, usually due to hematogenous or direct spread from the small intestine (Fig. 19-49). However, improved antibiotic therapy and increase in cardiovascular diseases has led to a decrease in the proportion of SMA aneurysms caused by infection, with an increase in the proportion caused by atherosclerosis or connective tissue disease, and pseudoaneurysms caused by trauma, dissection, and pancreatitis (148). CTA and MRA provide innumerable perspectives that can facilitate the demonstration of complex anatomy and overlapping structures (167) (Figs. 19-50, 19-51).

SMA aneurysms are frequently symptomatic, presenting with progressive moderate to severe abdominal pain that mimics mesenteric ischemia or nausea, vomiting, GI hemorrhage, hemobilia, or jaundice. Some patients present with a palpable mass. SMA aneurysms are at risk for both rupture and thrombosis, either leading to exsanguination or mesenteric ischemia.

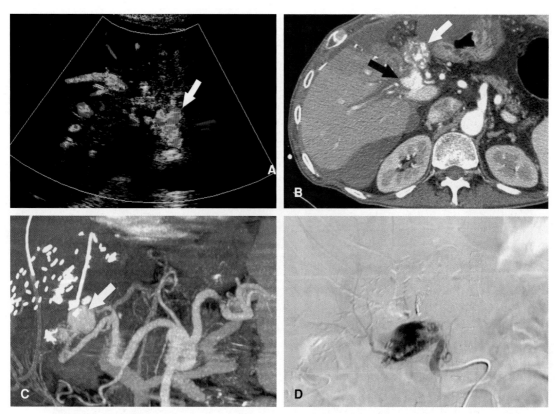

FIGURE 19-48 Hepatic artery pseudoaneurysm rupture in a 63-year-old man with hepatic artery pseudo-aneurysm detected on Doppler sonography. A: Color Doppler sonogram at postoperative day 7 shows periportal round structure with turbulent flow (*white arrow*). **B:** Sudden hypotension developed the next day. Hepatic artery phase CT scan shows pseudoaneurysm (*black arrow*), extravasation of contrast material (*white arrow*), and acute hematoma adjacent to graft. **C:** MIP image shows a pseudoaneurysm (*white arrow*) at hepatic artery anastomosis. **D:** Hepatic arteriogram shows similar appearance as seen on MIP image. (Reprinted with permission from Kim HJ, Kim KW, Kim AY, et al. Hepatic artery pseudoaneurysms in adult living-donor liver transplantation: efficacy of CT and Doppler sonography. *AJ Am J Roentgenol.* 2005;184:1549–1555.)

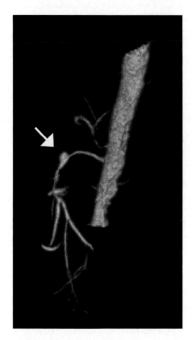

FIGURE 19-49 SMA aneurysm. VR MRA of the SMA in a patient with a history of prior recurrent pancreatitis demonstrates an aneurysm of the proximal SMA.

Treatment is usually surgical ligation. Bypass grafting is often difficult, due to the extensive atherosclerotic disease present within the vessel distal to the aneurysm site. Transcatheter occlusion of saccular aneurysms with discrete necks arising from the side of the SMA has been reported (168). If infection or inflammation is the cause (Fig. 19-52), therapy is very hazardous, and a saphenous vein bypass may be necessary (152,169). In general, preintervention evaluation of adequate collateral supply to the small bowel is necessary.

Celiac Artery Aneurysms

Celiac artery aneurysms (4% of all visceral aneurysms) are usually associated with atherosclerosis (170). Less common causes include trauma, increased pressure secondary to aortic dissection, and mycotic aneurysms (due to *Staphylococcus* and *Streptococcus*) (171). Celiac aneurysms are frequently asymptomatic, but patients may present with vague abdominal pain, nausea, vomiting, or symptoms of mesenteric ischemia. Celiac aneurysms are often found in association with additional visceral or peripheral aneurysms.

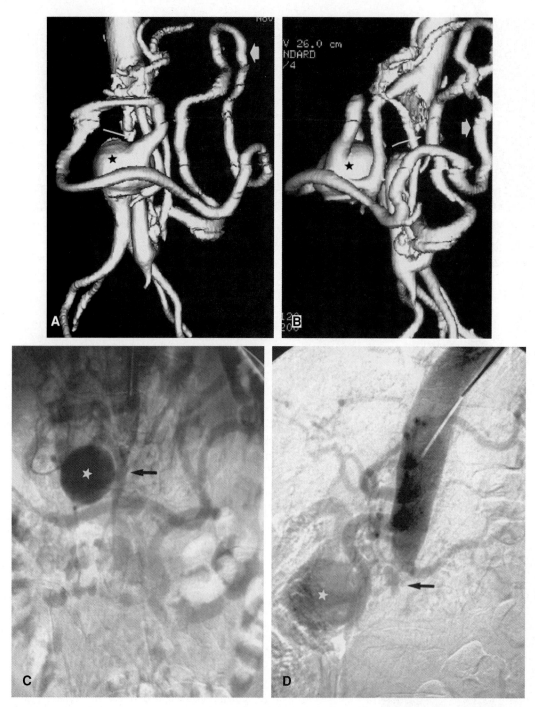

FIGURE 19-50 CTA rendering of an SMA aneurysm in patient with Leriche's syndrome. A: Frontal view and **(B)** oblique view 3D VR images of the abdominal aorta. 3D CT angiogram performed with SmartPrep software (Light Speed Qx/I, General Electric Medical Systems, Milwaukee, WI) after a bolus injection of 120 mL iodinated contrast (Iopamidol, Bracco, Milan, Italy) at 3 mL/second, showing the infrarenal aortic occlusion (*white arrow*), the concomitant SMA aneurysm (*black star*), and the arc of Riolan collateral pathway. Note the tortuous and meandering aspect of the artery (*large white arrow*) coursing in the left hypochondrium. **C, D:** DSA rendering of an SMA aneurysm in anteroposterior view **(C)** and lateral view **(D)**. DSA of the abdominal aorta was performed via a transbrachial approach with a 5-French straight catheter. The SMA aneurysm (*white star*) and infrarenal aortic occlusion (*black arrow*) are shown, but details of the SMA–inferior mesenteric artery collateral pathway could not be shown. (Reprinted with permission from Chan HH, Tai KS, Yip LK. Patient with Leriche's syndrome and concomitant superior mesenteric aneurysm: evaluation with contrast-enhanced three-dimensional magnetic resonance angiography, computed tomography angiography and digital subtraction angiography. *Australas Radiol.* 2005;49:233–237.)

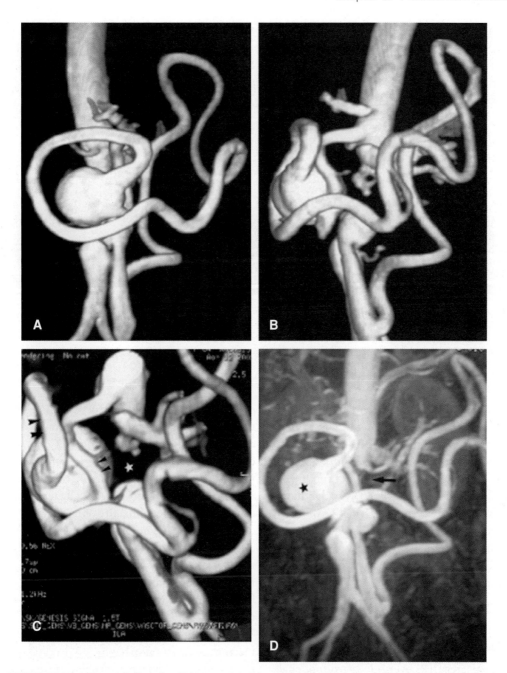

FIGURE 19-51 MRA rendering of an SMA aneurysm in patient with Leriche's syndrome. A: Frontal view and **(B)** oblique view 3D VR images of the abdominal aorta. **C:** Magnified view of the aortic occlusion (*white star*) and the feeding (*small black arrowheads*) and the draining arteries (*large black arrowheads*) of the SMA aneurysm. **D:** MIP image of CE 3D MRA acquisition of the abdomen also shows the infrarenal aortic occlusion (*black arrow*) and SMA aneurysm (*black star*). 3D CE MRA performed on a 1.5-T system with the SmartPrep software (Signa EchoSpeed Lx, General Electric Medical Systems, Milwaukee, WI) with the use of a torso coil. Gadolinium-diethylene triamine penta-acetic acid (DTPA) was injected at a dose of 0.2 mmol/kg body weight and at an injection rate of 2.5 mL/second. 3D contrast-enhanced MRA shows superior image quality when compared with CTA and DSA. (Reprinted with permission from Chan HH, Tai KS, Yip LK. Patient with Leriche's syndrome and concomitant superior mesenteric aneurysm: evaluation with contrast-enhanced three-dimensional magnetic resonance angiography, computed tomography angiography and digital subtraction angiography. *Australas Radiol.* 2005;49:233–237.)

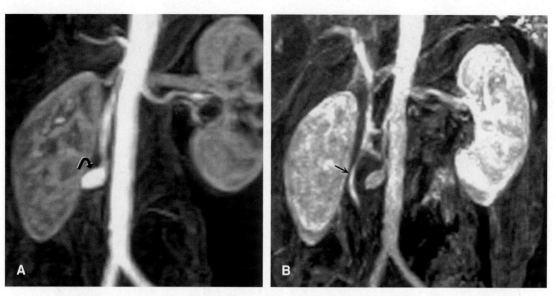

FIGURE 19-52 Mycotic aneurysm of the SMA in a 62-year-old asymptomatic man. Arterial-phase **(A)** and portal-phase **(B)** CE 3D MR portograms clearly show a mycotic aneurysm of the SMA (*arrow* in **A**) displacing the SMV (*arrow* in **B**). (Reprinted with permission from Okumura A, Watanabe Y, Dohke M, et al. Contrast-enhanced three-dimensional MR portography. *Radiographics.* 1999;19:973–987.)

Like other visceral aneurysms, celiac artery aneurysms are often diagnosed as an incidental finding when imaging the abdomen. Further evaluation of the aneurysm can be performed with sonography, MDCTA, MRA, or traditional angiography (172–177) (Fig. 19-53). The risk of rupture of celiac artery aneurysms is approximately 20%, with a mortality rate of 35% to 80% after rupture (170). The primary treatment of celiac artery aneurysms is surgical repair, including aneurysmectomy, aneurymorrhaphy, reimplantation, and ligation, although endovascular repair has been increasingly utilized (178).

Pancreaticoduodenal and Gastroduodenal Artery Aneurysms

Pancreaticoduodenal atery (PDA) and gastroduodenal artery (GDA) aneurysms (3.5% of all visceral artery aneurysms) are most often false aneurysms caused by pancreatitis. Up to 7% of these aneurysms are infected (152). The majority of these patients are symptomatic at the time of diagnosis, typically with abdominal or epigastric pain, and clinically, the symptoms can mimic those from pancreatitis. Additional presentations include GI hemorrhage and jaundice. There is a very high incidence of rupture of these pseudoaneurysms at the time of clinical presentation: 56% of GDA and 38% of PDA aneurysms (152).

Imaging, if the patient is stable, is usually via angiography with the goal of therapeutic embolization at the time of

diagnosis. Ruptured PDA aneurysms suspected on CT scan require emergent visceral angiography and selective embolization as definitive treatment (179). The evaluation of associated pancreatic disease is facilitated with CT and MR. Since the aneurysms are often caused by periarterial inflammation, the artery may be adherent to adjacent structures, increasing the difficulty of repair.

A report that employed a 4-row MDCT demonstrated a sensitivity of CTA for the detection of arterial complications of pancreatitis as 94.7% and a specificity of 90.0% (180). In that study, all of the major arterial extravasations including all the ten pseudoaneurysms were correctly identified on CTA (180) (Fig. 19-54).

Treatment options include surgical ligation, aneurysmectomy, aneurysmorrhaphy, or percutaneous embolization. The choice of repair depends on the location of the aneurysm and the degree of surrounding inflammation. For pancreaticoduodenal aneurysms, percutaneous interventional repair is more frequently attempted than for GDA aneurysms, as the isolation of small aneurysms embedded in the pancreatic tissue is technically difficult for surgical open repair (181). Complications of repair include rupture and bleeding.

Inferior Mesenteric and Colic Artery Aneurysms

Aneurysms of the IMA and distal colic branches are extremely rare (<2%) and are usually isolated and less than 1 cm in size. These aneurysms are most commonly due to atherosclerosis (often secondary to occlusion of the celiac

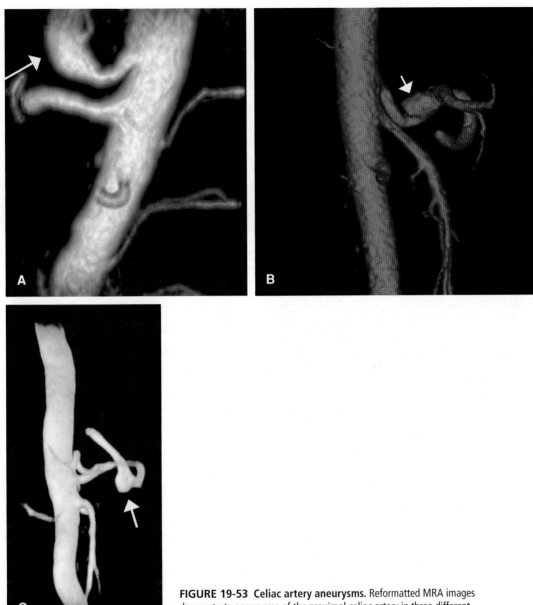

FIGURE 19-53 Celiac artery aneurysms. Reformatted MRA images demonstrate aneurysms of the proximal celiac artery in three different patients (*white arrows* in **A–C**).

and SMA origins, with IMA hypertrophy supplying the bowel), with less common etiologies including inflammation, vasculitis, and infection (182) (Fig. 19-55). The majority of patients with IMA/distal colic aneurysms are symptomatic, presenting with abdominal pain and hypovolemic shock (50%) and GI hemorrhage (15%). The majority of affected patients are men. Surgical treatment is advocated because of the high risk of rupture. IMA aneurysms are treated by revascularization, while colic artery aneurysms are too distal for feasible revascularization and usually are treated by aneurysmectomy or ligation.

Dissection

Dissection of the visceral arteries usually occurs as an extension of aortic dissection, with spontaneous dissection much more rare. Symptomatic malperfusion of the visceral arteries occurs in up to 6% of aortic dissections (183). This complication is secondary to thrombosis of the supplying lumen or from extension of the dissection flap into the visceral artery, with associated stenosis of the true lumen of the visceral artery. Mesenteric ischemia in aortic dissection has a mortality rate of 25% to 50% at 30 days, even with intervention (183). The celiac, SMA, and right renal arteries are

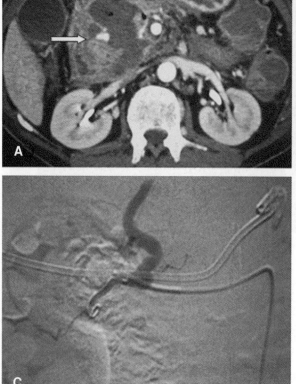
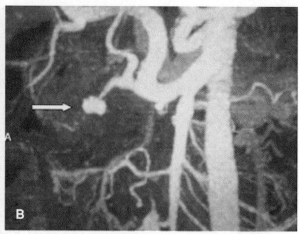

FIGURE 19-54 GDA pseudoaneurysm in a 44-year-old male with acute pancreatic necrosis and pseudocyst in head of pancreas. A: Axial arterial phase, contrast-enhanced CT demonstrates pseudoaneurysm in head of the pancreas (*arrow*). **B:** Coronal oblique MIP demonstrates the site of bleeding as the GDA (*arrow*). **C:** Selective GDA angiogram confirms the site and type of bleed, and a single coil to the pseudoaneurysm causes cessation of flow. (Reprinted with permission from Hyare H, Desigan S, Nicholl H, et al. Multi-section CT angiography compared with digital subtraction angiography in diagnosing major arterial hemorrhage in inflammatory pancreatic disease. *Eur J Radiol.* 2006;59:295–300.)

usually supplied by the true lumen and the left renal artery by the false lumen.

Isolated spontaneous dissection of the visceral arteries is rare, but when it occurs, the SMA is most frequently involved. This can be associated with acute or chronic mesenteric ischemia, with most acute cases presenting with epigastric pain and sudden onset of nausea and vomiting (184). Patients may present with profound shock after rupture of the dissection. The etiology is unknown, with links having been found to trauma, atherosclerosis, fibrodysplasia, and congenital connective tissue disorders (185). Dissection usually occurs approximately 1.5 to 3 cm from the origin of the SMA, sparing the origin (186) (Fig. 19-56).

This segment of the SMA is the fixed retropancreatic portion, and it is thought that shearing forces from the more mobile distal SMA are transmitted here. There is controversy in the surgical community as to the best way to manage this condition, with most recommending urgent operative or interventional repair (with bypass grafting, thrombectomy, percutaneous fenestration, or stent place-

ment) (184,187) and others suggesting watchful waiting (188) (Fig. 19-57).

Vascular Malformations and Fistulas

Congenital arteriovenous malformations of the liver, spleen, pancreas, and bowel are very rare, accounting for only 1% of all such malformations. The most common locations of arteriovenous malformations throughout the body are the head and neck (40%), extremities (40%), and trunk (20%) (189,190). There have been many different classification systems for vascular anomalies, divided either by histopathology, vascular flow dynamics, or therapy (191,192). The International Society for the Study of Vascular Anomalies has developed a widely accepted classification system that divides the anomalies by cellular features, flow characteristics, and clinical behavior (193). In this system, the malformation is divided into arterial, lymphatic, and venous subtypes and is considered either a tumor, a simple malformation, or a combined malformation (Table 19-2). Vascular malformations develop secondary to abnormal embryonic

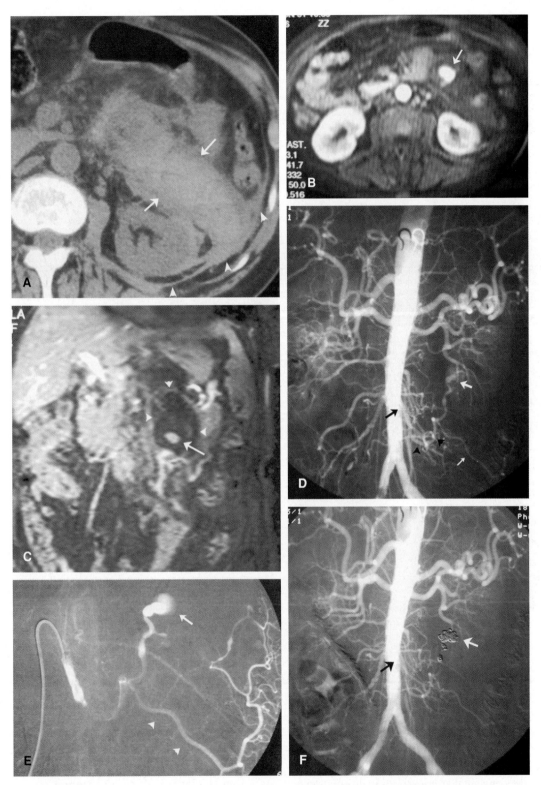

FIGURE 19-55 Pseudoaneurysm of the left colic branch of the IMA in a 60-year-old man with recurrent pancreatitis and abdominal pain. A: Axial noncontrast CT scan demonstrates an enlarged pancreas (*white arrows* in **A**), with high-density fluid tracking along the lateralconal fascia (*arrowheads*). **B:** Axial 3D VIBE images during the arterial phase demonstrates a large pseudoaneurysm (*white arrow*) enhancing to the same degree as the aorta posterior and inferior to the pancreas. **C:** Coronal reconstructed VIBE image demonstrates the vascular component of the pseudoaneurysm (*white arrow*), with surrounding low intensity acute hemorrhage (*arrowheads*). **D:** Angiographic images demonstrate a rapid blush in the IMA (*black arrow*) and its left colic branch (*black arrowheads*) distribution, indicating the pseudoaneurysm (*thick white arrow*). Incidentally noted is the sigmoid branch (*thin white arrow*). **E:** Selective injection of the left colic artery better delineates the pseudoaneurysm (*white arrow*). Again noted is the sigmoid branch off the IMA (*white arrowheads*). **F:** Coils were placed distal and proximal to the left colic pseudoaneurysm (*white arrow*), with no filling seen after injection of contrast. (Images courtesy of Ivan Pedrosa, MD, BIDMC, Boston.)

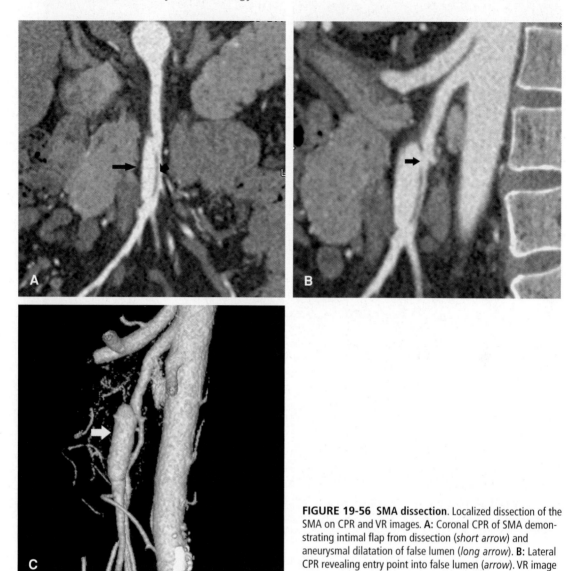

FIGURE 19-56 SMA dissection. Localized dissection of the SMA on CPR and VR images. **A:** Coronal CPR of SMA demonstrating intimal flap from dissection (*short arrow*) and aneurysmal dilatation of false lumen (*long arrow*). **B:** Lateral CPR revealing entry point into false lumen (*arrow*). VR image (**C**) demonstrates dilated false lumen (*arrow*).

differentiation of the vascular system. They are due to a communication between arterial, venous, and lymphatic systems without an intervening capillary bed. They may be localized or diffuse in location. Recurrence rates are high because of the abnormal nature of their embryonic precursors that persist after local removal (190).

Although the congenital arteriovenous malformation is the most common true vascular lesion, congenital syndromes such as hereditary hemorrhagic telangiectasia (HHT) and Osler Weber Rendu account for many of the inherited abnormalities. In HHT, liver lesions predominate (either arterioportal or arteriovenous) and typically have a delayed presentation with portal hypertension, liver dysfunction, biliary obstruction, or high-output congestive heart failure.

A large variety of arterial malformations affect the stomach, small bowel, and colon. These vascular lesions include hemangiomas, angiodysplasia, gastric antral vascular ectasia, vascular ectasia, arteriovenous malformations, and the Dieulafoy lesion. The most common presentation of these lesions is GI bleeding.

Angiodysplasia is the most common vascular malformation of the GI tract. Pathologically, the lesion is an arteriovenous fistula between distal arterial branches and adjacent submucosal veins, venules, or capillaries. The lesion is thought to develop from degenerative changes within the vascular walls from stress through repeated colonic contractions. It occurs most frequently in the cecum and ascending colon (77%), with 15% occurring in the jejunum and ileum and the remainder occurring in equal amounts

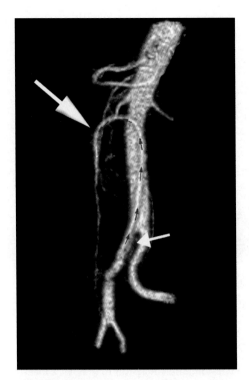

FIGURE 19-57 Iliac–SMA bypass graft. MIP images from a VIBE sequence obtained during the arterial phase demonstrate a graft originating from the right common iliac artery (*small white arrow*) extending to the SMA (*small red arrows*). The proximal SMA is attenuated and small in caliber from its origin to the level of its anastomosis with the bypass graft (*large white arrow*). Distal to the graft, the SMA caliber is minimally increased.

commonly diagnosed at endoscopy. Treatment is through cautery or direct injection.

The Dieulafoy lesion is an isolated large (1 to 3 mm) artery that lies close to the mucosal surface of the bowel. This lesion is most commonly diagnosed in elderly patients. Although initially described in the stomach, this lesion occurs in equal prevalence from the esophagus to the colon.

Arteriovenous fistulas are usually post-traumatic, occurring after either blunt or penetrating trauma, or secondary to iatrogenic procedures or infection. These lesions occur in the liver, spleen, pancreas, and bowel. These may be occult originally or present with portal hypertension, biliary hemorrhage, variceal bleeding, or high output cardiac failure (Fig. 19-58).

Diagnosis of vascular malformations has traditionally been via conventional angiography; however, US, CTA, and MRA are now preferential diagnostic options, as these modalities are less invasive. US is useful in evaluation of lesions in surface organs that have a good acoustic background (liver and spleen) but is not useful for evaluation of the bowel. Color Doppler imaging allows dynamic analysis of the arterial and venous flow as well as determination of flow velocities. US is a useful modality for evaluating treatment response. CTA allows for detection of enhancement, calcification, and thrombosis as well as excellent depiction of multifocality. Its high temporal resolution allows for improved accuracy in detecting small lesions. Bowel lesions may be more easily seen in CT, as there are fewer artifacts than in US and MRA from air within the lumen. Drawbacks of CTA include ionizing radiation and limitations in blood flow characterization. MRA can detect and classify vascular malformations. Slow-flow venous malformations have high

throughout the GI tract. Angiodysplasia is thought to account for 6% of cases of GI bleeding (194). Diagnosis has traditionally been made angiographically, through visualization of a vascular tuft/tangle with an early, dense draining vein (see Fig. 19-60). Currently, angiodysplasia is most

TABLE 19-2

ISSVA Classification of Vascular Anomalies[a]

| | Vascular Malformation | |
Vascular Tumor	Simple	Combined
Hemangioma	Capillary malformation	Arteriovenous fistula, arteriovenous malformation, capillary-venous malformation,capillary-lymphatic-venous malformation
Other	Lymphatic malformation	Lymphatic-venous malformation, capillary-lymphatic-arteriovenous malformation
	Venous malformation	

[a]ISSVA, International Society for the Study of Vascular Anomalies.
Reprinted with permission from Hyodoh H, Hori M, Akiba H, et al. Peripheral vascular malformations: imaging, treatment approaches, and therapeutic issues. *Radiographics*. 2005;25[Suppl 1]:S159–S171.

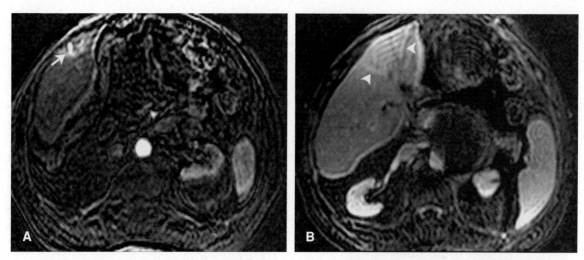

FIGURE 19-58 AVF liver. Subtraction images obtained in the arterial **(A)** and portal **(B)** phases in a patient after liver biopsy demonstrate an arterial-phase enhancing vessel (*arrow* in **A**) that rapidly fades and is followed by diffuse venous enhancement (*arrowheads* in **B**), compatible with an arteriovenous fistula, as was proven on subsequent Doppler evaluation (not shown).

signal intensity on T2-weighted images, and high-flow arteriovenous malformations/arteriovenous fistulas will create a flow void (190) (Fig. 19-59). There is limited detection of calcification and phleboliths, which present as signal voids (190). Dynamic gradient echo sequences are typically utilized for their speed of acquisition and ability to separate the various vascular malformations (190).

Obscure Overt Gastrointestinal Bleeding

Obscure GI bleeding is bleeding that occurs without an obvious source after standard endoscopic evaluation. For clinicians, this is further subdivided into obscure occult and obscure overt bleeding, where obscure occult bleeding is idiopathic, persistently positive fecal occult blood tests, and obscure overt bleeding is clinically evident bleeding for which the source cannot be found on endoscopic evaluation (195). Radiographic analysis is generally directed toward finding the source of the bleed of the latter entity, obscure overt GI bleeding. This can be a challenging endeavor for imaging and for imagers.

Causes of obscure overt GI bleeding include neoplasms, inflammation (ulcers, ulcerative colitis, Crohn disease, radiation proctitis, ischemic colitis), vascular malformations, colonic varices, and Meckel diverticula. Bleeding in the left colon is most commonly associated with diverticulosis and angiodysplasia (Fig. 19-60). In idiopathic bleeding, associated factors include immunosuppression, chemotherapy, and anticoagulation for various disorders. The problem in locating the occult bleed is that the lesion may no longer be bleeding (or may be bleeding very slowly or intermittently), there may be postbleed volume contrac-

tion of the lesion, and the lesion may be in a location that is difficult to evaluate (small bowel) (196).

Small bowel follow through (SBFT) and enteroclysis are not very sensitive unless there is high suspicion of a small bowel mass or Crohn disease (195). CTA and MRA examinations have not proven very sensitive in the detection of obscure overt GI bleeds, and bleeding rates of over 6 mL/minute are believed to be necessary to detect active bleeding (197). Contrast-enhanced CTA and MRA examinations may demonstrate lesions with active bleeding (such as a Meckel diverticulum) when extravasation or accumulation of contrast material in the ectopic gastric mucosa can be observed. CTA has a reported sensitivity of 70%, with a specificity of 100% in detecting colonic vascular lesions, when compared with traditional angiography (198). Ileal varicosities may be seen in patients with portal hypertension as large and dilated veins in the ileal bowel wall.

Scintigraphy is most useful in patients with active bleeding at the time of nuclear analysis and is useful when endoscopy has failed. Scintigraphy can detect bleeding at a rate of 0.1 mL/minute, and the patient can be rescanned for up to 12 to 24 hours after the initial tracer administration. However, the localization of the bleed is frequently nonoptimal, as the blood pool agent may move in any direction in the bowel after it has bled. Angiography is able to diagnose and treat the bleed if there is active bleeding at the time of patient evaluation. Angiography detects extravasation of contrast if the bleeding rate is greater than 0.5 mL/minute. Diagnostic yields of angiography are approximately 40% within the literature, although widely varying success rates have been reported (199,200).

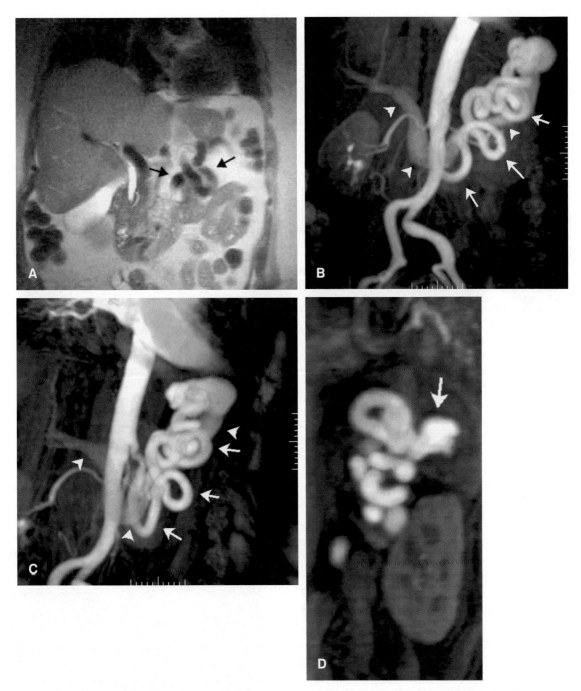

FIGURE 19-59 Splenic high-flow arteriovenous malformation. A: Coronal half-Fourier acquisition single-shot turbo spin-echo (HASTE) image demonstrates a flow void in a tortuous enlarged splenic artery (*black arrows*), with the dark signal on T2-weighted images indicative of fast flow. **B, C:** Coronal MIP images demonstrate an enlarged splenic artery (*white arrows*) with early enhancement of the splenic and portal veins (*arrowheads*). **D:** Sagittal MIP image through the spleen demonstrates a large collection of contrast within the hilum of the spleen (*arrow*).

To date, there is no ideal technique to diagnose the source of bleeding in patients with chronic or recurrent GI hemorrhage in the small bowel. The use of a blood pool contrast agent for MRA might overcome the limitation of GI hemorrhage evaluation of the small bowel. Such blood pool MR contrast agents make it possible to replicate the concept of labeled red cell nuclear medicine examinations by using 3D contrast MRA. Although MR blood pool agents are as of yet experimental, the higher SNR and resolution of MR compared with nuclear medicine makes this a promising future technique for use in patients suspected of GI bleeding. Arterial and venous mesenteric anatomy

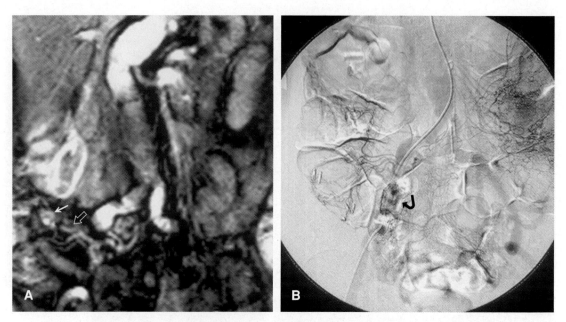

FIGURE 19-60 Ileal angiodysplasia in an 84-year-old woman with massive gastrointestinal hemorrhage.
A: Coronal source image reveals the bleeding point as a hypervascular lesion (*solid arrow*) with dilated ileal veins (*open arrow*) in the right lower quadrant. **B:** Superior mesenteric arteriogram also reveals angiodysplasia of the terminal ileum (*arrow*). (Reprinted with permission from Okumura A, Watanabe Y, Dohke M, et al. Contrast-enhanced three-dimensional MR portography. *Radiographics.* 1999;19:973–987.)

can be evaluated during the arterial and venous phases of blood pool contrast agent injection. By periodically reimaging the patient over time, the accumulation of blood in the GI tract can be imaged to identify the site of GI bleeding. When bleeding is intermittent, the patient can be scanned periodically, every hour or two, until a bleeding episode is detected. The 3D nature of MRI makes it easier to identify the specific loop of bowel that is bleeding (201,202).

Inflammatory diseases of the small bowel are associated with changes in mesenteric blood flow. Active bowel inflammation is associated with increased blood flow, while chronic fibrotic inflammation is associated with normal to decreased blood flow (203). Increased blood flow can manifest by enlargement of the mesenteric vessels supplying diseased loops of small bowel (45) (Fig. 19-61).

Vasculitis

Vasculitis has varied presentations in the GI tract, ranging from submucosal edema and hemorrhage, stricture, mesenteric ischemia, and ileus to bowel perforation. The extent of the involved bowel and the resultant symptoms depend on the size and location of the affected vessel. Vasculitis may affect large vessels (giant cell arteritis, Takayasu arteritis), medium-sized vessels (PAN, Kawasaki disease, primary granulomatous disease), or small vessels (systemic lupus crythematosus [SLE], rheumatoid vasculitis, Behçet syndrome, Wegener granulomatosis, Churg-Strauss, microscopic

polyangiitis, Henoch-Schönlein syndrome, Burger disease). Clinical symptoms (e.g., weight loss, fever, night sweats, arthralgias) and laboratory values (e.g., erythrocyte sedimentation rate, C-reactive protein, anti-neutrophilic cytoplasmic antibodies [ANCA]) are independently nonspecific, but

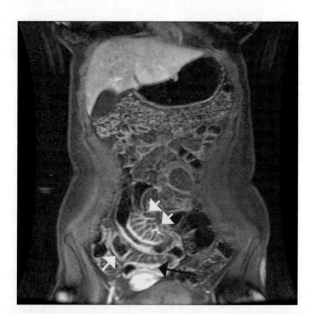

FIGURE 19-61 Crohn exacerbation in a 26-year-old female patient with Crohn disease. Coronal LAVA images obtained through the small bowel demonstrates narrowing and thickening of the terminal ileum with surrounding hyperemia (*white arrows*).

when combined with classic vascular distributions on radiologic studies, the specific type of vasculitis can be diagnosed. In the absence of a suggestive clinical history, vasculitis should be considered when mesenteric ischemic changes occur in young patients, at unusual sites (e.g., stomach, duodenum, rectum), and involve varied vascular territories (both the small and large bowel) or the genitourinary system (204).

CTA and MRA techniques are very useful in the diagnosis of large vessel vasculitides, as they readily depict the luminal irregularities, vascular wall thickening, and physiologic changes (degree of wall thickness and edema) of the aorta and its major branch vessels (205). However, for medium and small vessel vasculitides (e.g., PAN, SLE, Wegener, rheumatoid, Behçet, Churg-Strauss, etc.), imaging studies are mainly used for demonstrating bowel wall thickening, submucosal hemorrhage, and segmental involvement of the bowel (clinically useful for determining disease extent, activity, and localizing for biopsy), but the vasculitic lesions, for the most part, are not directly visualized. This is because the small arterioles and end-arteries affected by these diseases are typically below the resolution of all current radiographic modalities: digital angiography, CTA, and MRA (206).

Rarely is there isolated involvement of the mesenteric vasculature (celiac, SMA, or IMA) by a vasculitis. Frequently, the patient has a known primary vasculitic diagnosis (Takayasu, PAN, rheumatoid, SLE, etc.), and the mesenteric vessels are interrogated because of new abdominal complaints. Of the vasculitides, giant cell arteritis notably spares the mesenteric circulation (207,208). The most common mesenteric artery involved in vasculitis is the SMA. When the SMA is involved, primary diagnostic considerations are Takayasu, PAN, SLE, rheumatoid arthritis, and Henoch-Schönlein purpura and Kawasaki disease (204). Of these, Takayasu arteritis and PAN are the most frequent primary vasculitides encountered when the mesenteric vasculature is involved.

Takayasu Arteritis

Takayasu arteritis is a rare granulomatous vasculitis that affects large- and medium-sized arteries. The disease can affect any portion of the aorta in isolation, may be segmental in its distribution, and can affect branches off the aorta. Detailed characteristics of this disease can be found in Chapter 10. Mesenteric angina from SMA stenosis typically is a symptom associated with late-phase disease.

Because the clinical presentation and laboratory results are nonspecific, accurate diagnosis depends on imaging studies. In the past, angiography was used for diagnosis, but CTA and MRA improve sensitivity for

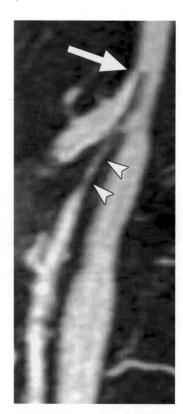

FIGURE 19-62 Takayasu SMA narrowing, type IV Takayasu arteritis. Sagittal 3D MR angiogram of a 30-year-old man shows a long stenotic segment of the SMA (*arrowheads*) and focal stenosis of the celiac trunk (*arrow*). (Reprinted with permission from Nastri MV, Baptista LP, Baroni RH, et al. Gadolinium-enhanced three-dimensional MR angiography of Takayasu arteritis. *Radiographics.* 2004;24:773–786.)

early-stage Takayasu, where there is inflammation and thickening of the vascular wall without luminal narrowing. Later-stage radiographic features (stenosis, post-stenotic dilatation, aneurysm formation, occlusion, and collateral formation) can be diagnosed with multiple imaging modalities, including angiography, US, CTA, and MRA (209) (Fig. 19-62).

Mesenteric involvement occurs with types III, IV, or V of the Numano disease classification system, Chapter 10 (210,211). When the SMA origin becomes occluded, collateral flow via the meandering artery re-establishes flow from the IMA to the distal SMA branches (212) (Fig. 19-63).

When the infrarenal abdominal aorta becomes completely occluded, the meandering artery can be dilated to the same size as the aorta (212). Aortograms in late-stage Takayasu can show dilatation of the vasa vasorum in the wall of the descending thoracic aorta. These structures become a collateral pathway to the pulmonary or systemic circulation. Aneurysms and dissections can be seen as complications.

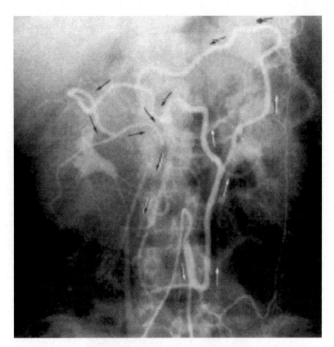

FIGURE 19-63 Takayasu meandering artery collateral. Development of a meandering mesenteric artery in a 19-year-old woman with late-phase Takayasu arteritis. Inferior mesenteric catheter angiogram shows the typical appearance of a meandering mesenteric artery due to severe stenosis or occlusion of the SMA at its origin. *Arrows* indicate the direction of blood flow. (Reprinted with permission from Matsunaga N, Hayashi K, Sakamoto I, et al. Takayasu arteritis: protean radiologic manifestations and diagnosis. *Radiographics.* 1997;17:579–594.)

Medium Vessel Vasculitis

Polyarteritis Nodosa

PAN is a necrotizing vasculitis that affects blood vessels of medium to small caliber, causing multiple microaneurysms (by segmental erosion of the arterial wall) as well as arterial occlusions and ectasia of medium to small arteries. Men are affected twice as commonly as women, and it is most commonly diagnosed in the fifth to seventh decades. The kidneys are most commonly involved (70% to 80%), followed by the GI tract, peripheral nerves, and skin (50%), liver (50%), spleen (45%), and pancreas (25% to 35%) (204,213).

In the GI tract, the small intestine is most commonly affected. Nonspecific symptoms are present, including fatigue, fever, weight loss, weakness, headache, and malaise, with 70% of patients having abdominal pain, nausea, and vomiting (secondary to bowel ischemia and/or infarction). GI hemorrhage, bowel perforation, and bowel infarction are rare complications. Laboratory tests are nonspecific, with reports of patients presenting with hypergammaglobulinemia, hepatitis B surface Ag positivity (30%) and positive ANCA titers. Visualization of aneurysms up to 1 cm in size in the visceral vasculature is suggestive of the diagnosis of PAN; however, definitive diagnosis is made by end-organ

biopsy, as other vasculitides can present similarly (rheumatoid vasculitis, Wegener granulomatosis, SLE, Churg-Strauss, and drug abuse). Radiographic studies with high resolution (digital angiography) are necessary for detecting subtle findings, such as small microaneurysms, or evidence for occlusive manifestations of the disease, such as minimal luminal irregularity or narrowing. However, CT and MR can offer suggestive findings (Fig. 19-64). If untreated, the disease is fatal (5-year survival of 15%). But if treated with steroids, survival approaches 80% (213).

Trauma

Liver

The liver and spleen are the most commonly injured intra-abdominal organs, with roughly equal incidence of 30% to 40%. Hepatic vascular trauma can be secondary to blunt (motor vehicle accidents) or penetrating (stab wounds, bullet wounds) trauma. The incidence of penetrating trauma in trauma admissions has been declining, while the incidence of blunt trauma has been steadily increasing (214). Additionally, there has been an increase in iatrogenic injuries secondary to liver biopsies and interventional radiology procedures. The overall mortality from liver trauma is approximately 10% (215). There has been a trend toward nonoperative management of hemodynamically stable blunt liver injuries (80% of stable blunt trauma patients are currently managed nonoperatively), with successful outcomes in 92% to 97% of patients (216,217). Patients with penetrating injuries are still treated surgically.

Patients with hemodynamic instability (systolic blood pressure <90 mmHg) who do not respond to fluid resuscitation are taken to the operating room emergently without imaging studies, regardless of mechanism of injury. Hemodynamically stable patients are typically evaluated with CT as a first-line diagnostic test. Findings of liver injury are classified by the grading system developed by the American Association for the Surgery of Trauma (AAST) liver injury scale (218,219) (Table 19-3).

The grading scale ranges from grade I to VI, where I represents superficial lacerations and small subcapsular hematomas and grade VI represents avulsion of the vascular pedicle from the liver. Injuries that fall into grades I to III tend to be managed nonoperatively, but injuries that involve more parenchymal damage and the hepatic/juxtahepatic veins are more concerning. Grade VI injuries are lethal.

Vascular trauma to the liver may present as active extravasation, hemoperitoneum, subcapsular hematoma, arteriovenous fistula (from the hepatic artery to either the

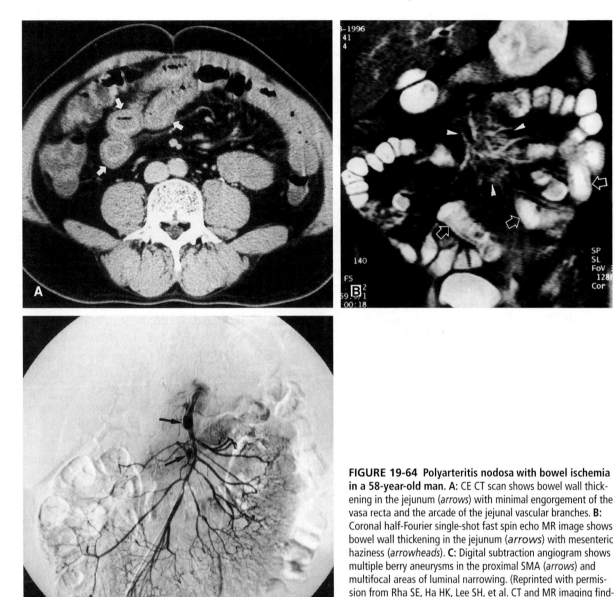

FIGURE 19-64 Polyarteritis nodosa with bowel ischemia in a 58-year-old man. A: CE CT scan shows bowel wall thickening in the jejunum (*arrows*) with minimal engorgement of the vasa recta and the arcade of the jejunal vascular branches. **B:** Coronal half-Fourier single-shot fast spin echo MR image shows bowel wall thickening in the jejunum (*arrows*) with mesenteric haziness (*arrowheads*). **C:** Digital subtraction angiogram shows multiple berry aneurysms in the proximal SMA (*arrows*) and multifocal areas of luminal narrowing. (Reprinted with permission from Rha SE, Ha HK, Lee SH, et al. CT and MR imaging findings of bowel ischemia from various primary causes. *Radiographics*. 2000;20:29–42.)

portal or hepatic veins), pseudoaneurysm, thrombosis, and hemobilia.

Active contrast material extravasation seen at angiography, CTA, or MRA is indicative of an ongoing, severe hemorrhage (Fig. 19-65). This finding on imaging studies is predictive of failure of nonsurgical management and requires emergent intervention (surgical or interventional) (220,221). Emergent angiography is a safe and effective intervention in active arterial hemorrhage (222). There is a current trend in nonoperative surgical management toward angiographic embolization, either as definitive therapy or as conjunctive therapy prior to surgery (223–225).

The use of focused abdominal sonography for trauma (FAST) US to evaluate patients with blunt trauma is based on the assumption that clinically important abdominal injuries are associated with free intraperitoneal fluid or hemoperitoneum (226). However, substantial numbers of high-grade intraperitoneal or extraperitoneal injuries can occur without associated hemoperitoneum (226). Thus, management based on FAST US assessment is limited, and additional imaging modalities should be utilized according to clinical suspicion.

Subcapsular hematomas are uncommon and arise when the liver parenchyma is disrupted by blunt trauma, with preservation of Glisson capsule. Grades I and II subcapsular

TABLE 19-3

Liver Injury Scale (1994 Revision)

Grade[a]	Type of Injury	Description of Injury
I	Hematoma	Subcapsular, <10% surface area
	Laceration	Capsular tear, <1 cm parenchymal depth
II	Hematoma	Subcapsular, 10% to 50% surface area intraparenchymal <10 cm in diameter
	Laceration	Capsular tear 1 to 3 parenchymal depth, <10 cm in length
III	Hematoma	Subcapsular, >50% surface area of ruptured subcapsular or parenchymal hematoma; intraparenchymal hematoma >10 cm or expanding
	Laceration	>3 cm parenchymal depth
IV	Laceration	Parenchymal disruption involving 25% to 75% hepatic lobe or one to three Couinaud's segments
V	Laceration	Parenchymal disruption involving >75% of hepatic lobe or >3 Couinaud's segments within a single lobe
	Vascular	Juxtahepatic venous injuries; that is, retrohepatic vena cava/central major hepatic veins
VI	Vascular	Hepatic avulsion

[a]Advance one grade for multiple injuries up to grade III.

Reprinted with permission from Moore EE, Cogbill TH, Jurkovich GJ, et al. Organ injury scaling: spleen and liver (1994 revision). *J Trauma.* 1995;38:323–324.

hematomas (hematomas involving less than 50% of the surface of the liver) are managed nonoperatively. Grades III and IV hematomas are treated with exploration and selective ligation, frequently with packing of the denuded surface of the liver.

A rare complication (1%) of blunt injury to the liver is the formation of a hepatic artery pseudoaneurysm (227). This complication occurs from disruption of the arterial wall with subsequent fibrous capsule formation. On angiography, CTA, and MRA, this appears a focal region of contrast material that follows the arteries in attenuation/signal characteristics. Frequently, these rare complications are found on delayed, follow-up imaging studies (228). Pseudoaneurysms have a high incidence of complications (intraparenchymal hemorrhage, arteriovenous fistula formation, rupture into a bile duct) associated with enlargement and rupture, and angiographic coiling is the treatment of choice.

Hepatic venous injuries are life threatening and should be managed surgically. Active venous extravasation, if seen, is indicative of severe hepatic injury (Fig. 19-66). Venous injury can be suspected if a liver laceration is seen extending into a hepatic vein or into the IVC. Additionally, the detection of venous injury often indicates associated, nonvisualized arterial injury (229).

The mortality for liver injury is 10%, with exsanguination the most common cause of death, followed by multisystem organ dysfunction and intracranial injury. Risk factors increasing morbidity and mortality in liver trauma include injury grade, mechanism of injury (with blunt trauma having a higher mortality than penetrating trauma), and risk of infection (higher with penetrating trauma, due to enteric contamination) (230).

Spleen

Penetrating and blunt splenic injuries were both historically treated by splenic repair (splenorrhaphy), partial splenectomy, or resection, depending on the grade of injury and condition of the patient. For penetrating trauma, surgical repair is still the standard of care. In children, however, preservation of the spleen has been a priority for many years because of the rare risk of overwhelming postsplenectomy infection. Thus, nonoperative management of blunt splenic injury in children has been the standard of care for many years. However, the application of similar management strategies to adult patients has been heavily debated in the literature. The risk of nonoperative management of splenic injuries is rapid exsanguination, which can lead to death if not quickly recognized. Stratifying patients into those at high risk for hemorrhage and those at low risk has been difficult. Initially, CT grading of splenic injuries was thought to represent a promising way to stratify patients into risk groups (219). Surgical grading is done by the Spleen Injury Scale of the AAST, with multiple CT grading systems devised to correlate to this scale (218,219) (Table 19-4).

However, the 1989 study by Mirvis and associates (231) showed that while CT was able to accurately localize, quantify, and track progression/healing of splenic injury, CT was not able to reliably predict outcome in blunt splenic injury. The foremost predictor of outcome is hemodynamic stability.

To confirm stability, patients must be monitored with frequent assessment of vital signs and hematocrit. Hypotension can develop several days after the initial splenic injury.

A current recommended management strategy for patients with blunt splenic trauma is as follows: (a) if the patient is hemodynamically unstable, surgery is recommended; (b) if the patient is stable but has a contrast blush on CT (either from a pseudoaneurysm or active extravasation), angiographic coiling is necessary (Fig. 19-67); and (c) if neither a blush nor instability is observed, the patient can be managed nonoperatively with close monitoring

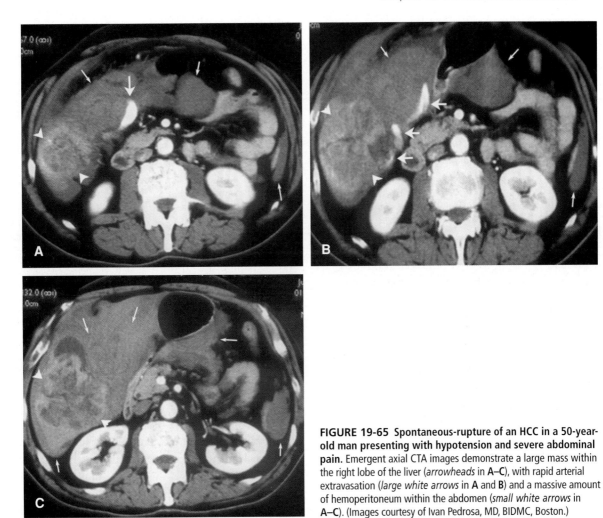

FIGURE 19-65 Spontaneous-rupture of an HCC in a 50-year-old man presenting with hypotension and severe abdominal pain. Emergent axial CTA images demonstrate a large mass within the right lobe of the liver (*arrowheads* in **A–C**), with rapid arterial extravasation (*large white arrows* in **A** and **B**) and a massive amount of hemoperitoneum within the abdomen (*small white arrows* in **A–C**). (Images courtesy of Ivan Pedrosa, MD, BIDMC, Boston.)

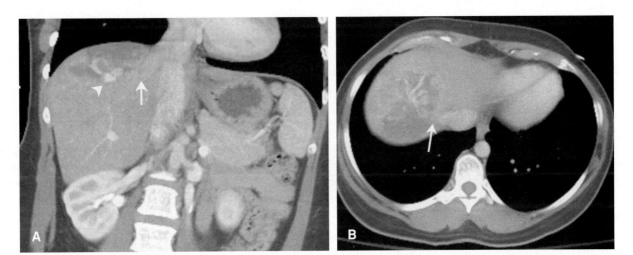

FIGURE 19-66 Hepatic vein avulsion in liver trauma in a young, male patient with blunt trauma to the abdomen. Arterial-phase images from MDCT obtained in the emergency department demonstrate a large hematoma in the right lobe of the liver (occupying <50% of the liver parenchyma) with active extravasation (*white arrowhead* in **A**) from a disrupted hepatic vein that is avulsed from the IVC (*white arrow* in **A** and **B**). The liver injury was classified as grade V liver injury due to the avulsion of the right hepatic vein. (Images courtesy of Ivan Pedrosa, MD, BIDMC, Boston.)

TABLE 19-4

Spleen Injury Scale (1994 Revision)

Grade[a]	Injury Type	Description of Injury
I	Hematoma	Subcapsular, <10% surface area
	Laceration	Capsular tear, <1 cm parenchymal depth
II	Hematoma	Subcapsular, 10% to 50% surface area intraparenchymal, <5 cm in diameter
	Laceration	Capsular tear, 1 to 3 cm parenchymal depth that does not involve a trabecular vessel
III	Hematoma	Subcapsular, >50% surface area or expanding; ruptured subcapsular or parenchymal hematoma; intraparenchymal hematoma ≤5 cm or expanding
	Laceration	>3 cm parenchymal depth or involving trabecular vessels
IV	Laceration	Laceration involving segmental or hilar vessels producing major devascularization (>25% of spleen)
V	Laceration	Completely shattered spleen
	Vascular	Hilar vascular injury with devascularized spleen

[a]Advance one grade for multiple injuries up to grade III.
Reprinted with permission from Moore EE, Cogbill TH, Jurkovich GJ, et al. Organ injury scaling: spleen and liver (1994 revision). *J Trauma.* 1995;38:323–324.

TABLE 19-5

Small Bowel Injury Scale

Grade[a]	Type of Injury	Description of Injury
I	Hematoma	Contusion or hematoma without devascularization
	Laceration	Partial thickness, no perforation
II	Laceration	Laceration <50% of circumference
III	Laceration	Laceration ≤50% of circumference without transection
IV	Laceration	Transection of the small bowel
V	Laceration	Transection of the small bowel with segmental tissue loss
	Vascular	Devascularized segment

[a]Advance one grade for multiple injuries up to grade III.
Reprinted with permission from Moore EE, Cogbill TH, Jurkovich GJ, et al. Organ injury scaling: spleen and liver (1994 revision). *J Trauma.* 1995;38:323–324.

(Fig. 19-68) (232–234). Success was reported with this management strategy in 98% of children and in 83% of adults (233).

Complications of nonoperative management for both blunt hepatic and splenic injuries include missed abdominal injuries, parenchymal infarction, infected hematomas, and (for hepatic injuries) bilomas (233–236).

Bowel

Bowel injury occurs in less than 1% to 4% of cases of blunt trauma to the abdomen. However, enteric injuries are found in a high percentage of patients with aortoiliac artery injuries from blunt or penetrating trauma. CT diagnosis of injuries to the bowel and mesentery relies on the following radiographic findings: bowel wall discontinuity, pneumoperitoneum, bowel wall thickening, mural hematoma, pneumatosis, mesenteric hematoma, triangle-shaped fluid collections in the mesentery, mural enhancement, extravasation of contrast from mesenteric vessels, the sentinel clot sign, and extravasation of oral contrast material (237,238) (Fig. 19-69). Vascular injuries include thrombosis, arteriovenous fistula, avulsion of the mesenteric pedicle, or transection of the mesenteric arteries. Surgical grading is done via the AAST grading system and is different for the duodenum, small bowel, rectum, and colon. The AAST small bowel injury grading system is shown in Table 19-5 (239).

Neoplastic Diseases

Hepatocellular Carcinoma

Hepatocellular carcinoma (HCC) has a variable incidence that is determined by geographic location. It is the most common primary liver malignancy and usually occurs in patients with chronic liver disease (most commonly from cirrhosis secondary to alcohol abuse or from infection with hepatitis B or C) (240,241).

These tumors are vascular, with primary blood supply from the hepatic artery with arterioportal shunting (242,243). There is a propensity to invade the portal vein, with less common invasion of the hepatic veins. There are many different proposed staging systems for HCC (244). A suggested algorithm for management of HCC has been proposed by the Barcelona Cancer of the Liver Clinic, which clearly shows the importance of diagnosing portal venous invasion (or lack thereof), as portal vein involvement eliminates most of the treatment options for patients (245,246) (Fig. 19-70).

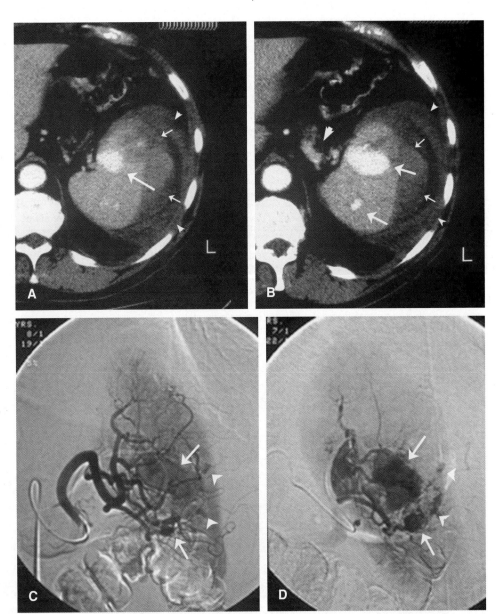

FIGURE 19-67 Grade III splenic laceration with pseudoaneurysm and active extravasation in a young, male patient who was in a motor vehicle accident. Axial arterial phase CT scan images (**A, B**) demonstrate a large pseudoaneurysm in the hilum of the spleen, (*long, white arrow*) with a second pseudoaneurysm in the medial spleen (*medial white arrow*) as well as active extravasation from the splenic hilum (*large white arrowhead*). There is a subcapsular hematoma (*small white arrows*) and hemorrhage tracking along the flank (*small arrowheads*). Angiographic images in the arterial (**C**) and venous (**D**) phases demonstrate early filling of the pseudoaneurysms (*arrows* in **C**), with early foci of arterial hemorrhage (*arrowheads* in **C**), persistent opacification on more delayed images (*arrows* in **D**), and increasing hemorrhage (*arrowheads* in **D**). The patient went to angiography for coiling of the pseudoaneurysms. (Images courtesy of Ivan Pedrosa, MD, BIDMC, Boston.)

CTA and MRA both demonstrate the hepatic arterial supply, arterioportal shunting, and vascular invasion associated with hepatomas (242,247,248). However, MRA may be preferable to CTA in imaging hepatoma, as MR is better at defining the primary tumor's morphology (249,250).

Arterioportal shunting of hepatomas typically appears as early/prolonged flow with a portal venous branch supplying the tumor, with wedge-shaped hyperenhancement peripheral to the tumor (Fig. 19-71).

On CTA and MRA, portal or hepatic vein tumor invasion demonstrates a low-density or low-signal intraluminal filling defect with expansion of the vein. When this filling defect demonstrates contrast enhancement, tumor thrombus is distinguished from bland thrombus, as the latter does not enhance (251,252) (Figs. 19-72, 19-73).

Pancreatic Carcinoma

In pancreatic adenocarcinoma, the infiltrative tumor can spread to involve the larger vessels about the pancreatic head and even the smaller intrapancreatic vessels, such as the dorsal or transverse pancreatic arteries. In the absence of metastases or local extension of tumor, tumor resectability will depend on the extent of vascular involvement.

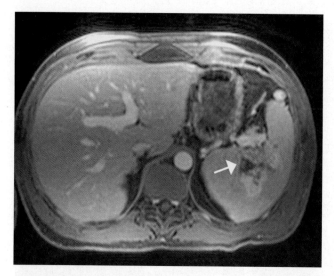

FIGURE 19-68 Grade II splenic injury in a 42-year-old patient with blunt trauma to the abdomen. Portal venous axial images from a VIBE sequence demonstrate a wedge-shaped hypointensity (*arrow*) in the mid-portion of the spleen, compatible with a grade II splenic injury. Patient was managed conservatively.

Involvement of the major arteries (SMA, CHA, proper hepatic artery, neural plexus around the CA) or venous structures (portal vein, splenic vein, SMV) can preclude surgical resection (253). Isolated involvement of smaller arteries (gastroduodenal or pancreaticoduodenal) can be resected (254,255). Most institutions grade vascular involvement by degree of circumferential encasement of the vessels by tumor, with more than 180-degree involvement of the vessel indicating unresectable disease (256,257). Care must be taken to exclude benign fibrous scarring and inflammatory stranding from tumor involvement of the peripancreatic vessels (such as the celiac, hepatic, and superior mesenteric arteries), as studies have shown an increased incidence of benign reactive changes around these vessels in pancreatic cancer (257). Thus, evaluation of vascular involvement with tumor must include not only circumferential soft tissue encasement but also caliber change of the vessel lumen and associated soft tissue mass (254). Additional findings suggestive of vascular involvement include increased attenuation

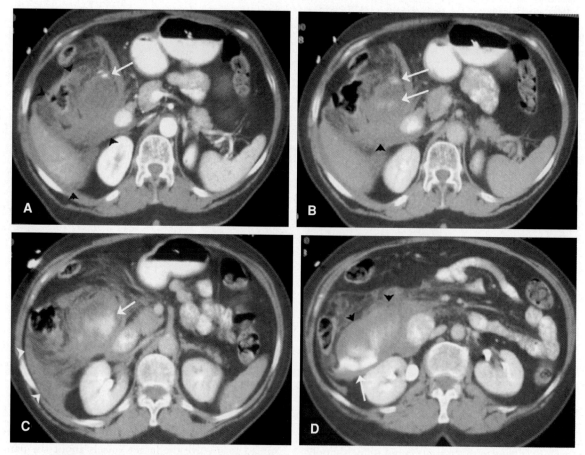

FIGURE 19-69 Traumatic middle colic injury in a young, male patient who had been in a motor vehicle accident. Axial CE images demonstrate active arterial extravasation (*white arrows* in **A–C**) in the right upper quadrant, adjacent to the ascending colon in the middle colic artery distribution. There is a large amount of adjacent hemorrhage (*white arrowheads* in **C**; *black arrowheads* in **D**), with high-density extravasated contrast seen layering dependently (*white arrow* in **D**). The patient was taken to the operating room for ligation of the bleeding middle colic artery. (Images courtesy of Ivan Pedrosa, MD, BIDMC, Boston, MA.)

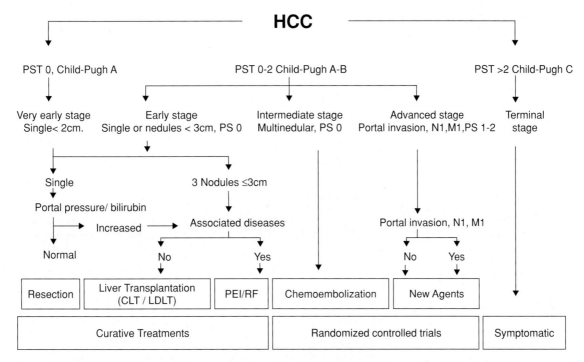

HCC

PST 0, Child-Pugh A   PST 0-2 Child-Pugh A-B   PST >2 Child-Pugh C

Very early stage
Single< 2cm.

Early stage
Single or nedules < 3cm, PS 0

Intermediate stage
Multinedular, PS 0

Advanced stage
Portal invasion, N1,M1,PS 1-2

Terminal
stage

Single   3 Nodules ≤3cm

Portal pressure/ bilirubin

Increased → Associated diseases   Portal invasion, N1, M1

Normal   No   Yes   No   Yes

| Resection | Liver Transplantation (CLT / LDLT) | PEI/RF | Chemoembolization | New Agents |

| Curative Treatments | Randomized controlled trials | Symptomatic |

FIGURE 19-70 The Barcelona staging and treatment classification. (PST, performance status; CLT, cadaveric liver transplant; HCC, hepatocellular carcinoma; LDLT, living donor liver transplant; PEI, percutaneous ethanol injection; PS, prognostic score; RF, radio frequency.) (From Bruix J, Sherman M. Management of hepatocellular carcinoma. *Hepatology.* 2005;42:1218; Marrero JA, Pelletier S. Hepatocellular carcinoma. *Clin Liver Dis.* 2006;10:ix, 339–351.)

of the normal perivascular fat (termed *perivascular cuffing*), which when seen correlates with nonresectable vascular invasion and absence of the fat plane around the superior mesenteric and celiac arteries (253) (Figs. 19-74, 19-75). Additionally, the finding of enlarged nodes surrounding the celiac, SMA, or para-aortic chains suggests lymphatic involvement.

The location of the pancreatic tumor will affect the vessels that are involved. Tumors in the pancreatic head may encase the portal vein, SMV, and medial splenic vein as well as the SMA (Fig. 19-76). Tumors in the pancreatic body and tail are closer in proximity to the celiac artery and its major branch vessels (hepatic artery, splenic artery, GDA) as well as the splenic vein and SMA.

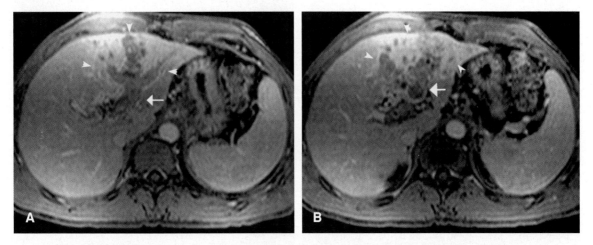

FIGURE 19-71 HCC with portal vein thrombus MRI. Portal venous phase subtraction images from a patient with known HCC demonstrate an ill-defined tumor with wedge-shaped hyperenhancement indicative of arterioportal shunting (*white arrowheads* in **A** and **B**) within the medial left lobe of the liver, infiltrating and expanding the left portal vein (*white arrow*). Enhancement is seen within the thrombus (*white arrows*, **A** and **B**), indicating tumor, not bland, thrombus.

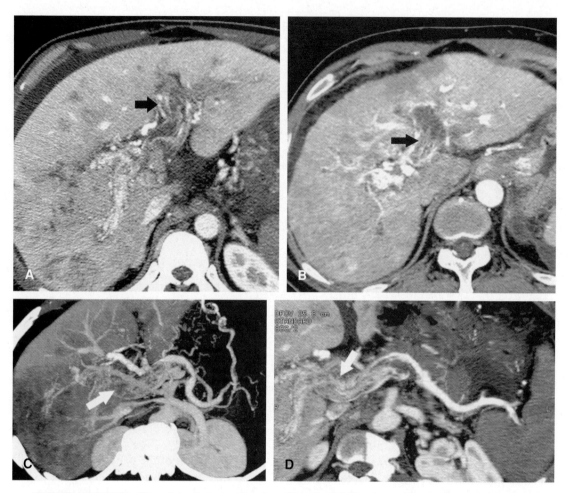

FIGURE 19-72 HCC with portal vein tumor thrombus, CT. A: Arterial-phase image demonstrating neovascularity within left portal vein thrombus (*arrow*). **B:** Venous-phase image demonstrating enhancing thrombus in left portal vein (*arrow*). MIP in **(C)** reveals tumor neovascularity in the main portal vein (*arrow*). CPR in **(D)** demonstrates enhancing tumor thrombus on the main portal vein (*arrow*).

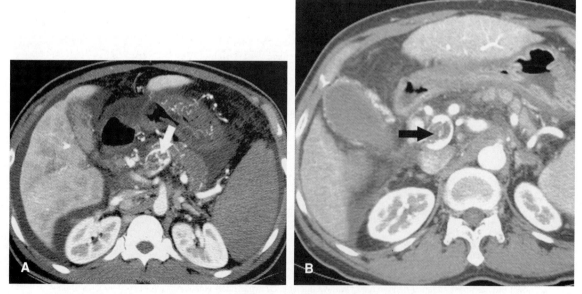

FIGURE 19-73 Extrahepatic tumor thrombus involving portal vein from hepatoma. A: Arterial-phase image with visible neovascularity in the portal vein thrombus (*arrow*). **B:** Later-phase image demonstrating enhancing thrombus in the portal vein (*arrow*).

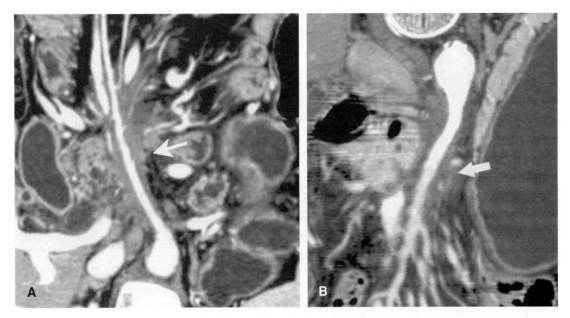

FIGURE 19-74 Pancreatic carcinoma with arterial encasement on CPR. Axial **(A)** and sagittal **(B)** CPR images demonstrate soft tissue infiltration (*white arrow* in **A** and **B**) along mesenteric fat on coronal CPR.

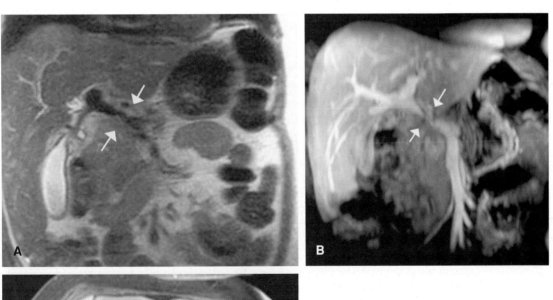

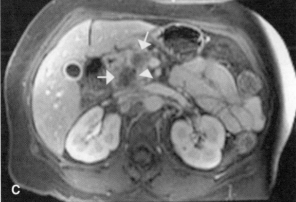

FIGURE 19-75 Pancreatic cancer encasing the portal vein. Coronal HASTE image **(A)** and coronal VIBE MIP image from the portal venous phase **(B)** demonstrate an extensive soft tissue mass from the patient's pancreatic cancer encasing the main portal vein (*arrows* in **A** and **B**). **C:** Axial VIBE image from the same patient demonstrates low signal intensity masses (*arrows*) in the head of the pancreas, as well as soft tissue (*arrowhead*) abutting the SMV. This soft tissue does not contact the SMV for the >180 degrees, which alone would favor resectibility; the concomitant portal vein encasement needs to be considered as the dominant driver for treatment options.

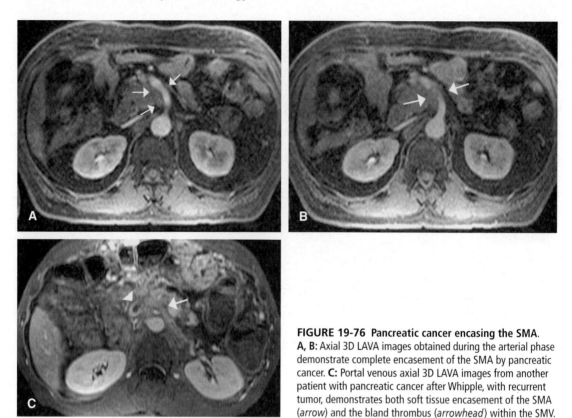

FIGURE 19-76 Pancreatic cancer encasing the SMA.
A, B: Axial 3D LAVA images obtained during the arterial phase demonstrate complete encasement of the SMA by pancreatic cancer. **C:** Portal venous axial 3D LAVA images from another patient with pancreatic cancer after Whipple, with recurrent tumor, demonstrates both soft tissue encasement of the SMA (*arrow*) and the bland thrombus (*arrowhead*) within the SMV.

Splenic vein occlusion due to tumor infiltration from the pancreatic body and tail often causes short gastric varices serving as venous collaterals that can be appreciated as briskly enhancing vessels in equilibrium phase CE MRA. Gaa and colleagues (258) reported promising results by using a comprehensive "all-in-one" approach for assessing patients with pancreatic cancer combining CE MRA with fast MRCP techniques and parenchymal imaging.

For unresectable pancreatic carcinoma, helical CT has a positive predictive value of 100%, a negative predictive value of 56%, and 70% overall accuracy (259). The sensitivity of small vessel involvement improves with the use of thin sections (259,260). MRI is sensitive for the detection of resectable and unresectable pancreatic neoplasms, with the most useful sequences utilizing T1-weighted fat-suppressed and dynamic gadolinium-enhanced spoiled gradient echo images and T2-weighted fat suppressed and T2-weighted breath-hold images. Additionally, MRI is helpful as an adjunct to CT imaging, especially in patients with the following scenarios: (a) history of CT imaging demonstrating a focally enlarged pancreas without a definable mass, (b) patients with a clinical history concerning for malignancy with equivocal findings

on CT, and (c) in patients with chronic pancreatitis and a questionable mass (261).

Liver Transplantation

Liver transplantation is a lifesaving procedure for patients with end-stage liver disease (defined as a damaged liver with minimal function and no potential for recovery) (262) or limited involvement of the liver with hepatoma (limited involvement, according to the Milan criteria, includes either a single hepatocellular carcinoma smaller than 5 cm in diameter or up to three tumor nodules, each 3 cm or less in diameter) (263). The current options for liver transplantation include cadaveric or living related donor transplantation.

In traditional orthotopic liver transplantation, the recipient's liver is excised, with careful transection of the inferior and superior vena cava, portal vein, hepatic artery, and common bile duct. The recipient is placed on venovenous bypass (diverting flow from the portal vein and IVC to the superior vena cava) during the anhepatic phase of liver explantation. The cadaveric donor liver is then anastomosed at the vascular and biliary sites with particular attention to preserve hepatic arterial flow (262,264) (Figs. 19-77, 19-78).

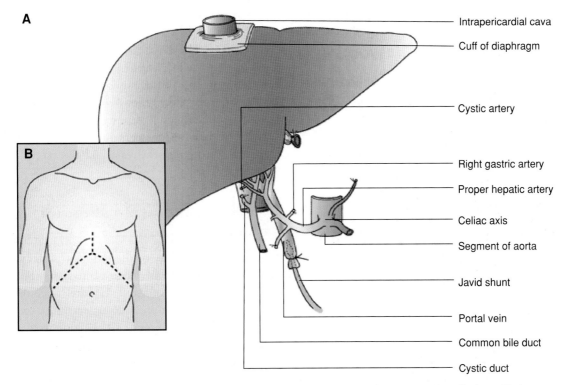

A

Intrapericardial cava

Cuff of diaphragm

Cystic artery

Right gastric artery

Proper hepatic artery

Celiac axis

Segment of aorta

Javid shunt

Portal vein

Common bile duct

Cystic duct

B

FIGURE 19-77 Donor liver. A: The donor liver after excision and before transplantation. **B:** Bilateral subcostal incision with a subxiphoid extension. (Reprinted with permission from Punch J. Hepatic transplantation. In: Mulholland MW, Lillemoe KD, Doherty GM, et al., eds. *Greenfield's Surgery: Scientific Principles and Practice.* Philadelphia: Lippincott Williams & Wilkins; 2006:590–609.)

In living donor liver transplantation, a portion of the donor's liver is removed, with careful attention to preservation of the vascular supply and function of the remaining organ. Resection of either the larger right hepatic lobe or smaller left hepatic lobe is determined by the recipient size. For pediatric recipients, the lateral segment or entire left lobe of the liver is resected; for adult recipients, the right lobe of the liver is resected. For donation of the lateral segment of the left lobe of the liver (segments II and III), the left hepatic vein, left portal vein, left hepatic artery, and left bile duct are resected (Fig. 19-79). The left hepatic vein of the donor liver is anastomosed to the common origin of the recipient's middle and left hepatic vein; the left donor portal vein is anastomosed to the main recipient portal vein, and the bile duct is anastomosed to the jejunum.

For right lobe transplantation, the entire right lobe is resected, including the right hepatic vein, the right portal vein, right hepatic artery, and right bile duct (Fig. 19-80). The right hepatic vein is then anastomosed to the recipient's right hepatic vein; the donor right portal vein is anastomosed to the main recipient portal vein, and the bile duct is anastomosed to the Roux-en-Y loop (86,262).

Preoperative Imaging

Preoperative noninvasive imaging is attractive for both living liver donor and recipient (obviously, preoperative imaging of the cadaveric donor is impossible). Limitations of US and duplex sonography (i.e., operator dependency and physical restraints) and inherent risks of catheter angiography and CT (i.e., arterial puncture, radiation, and nephrotoxic contrast material) have given rise to MRA as the alternative imaging modality of choice for a safe, accurate, and comprehensive assessment of the liver vasculature (265). The goals of preoperative recipient imaging are calculation of the hepatic volume, determination of the size and patency of the portal and superior mesenteric veins, evaluation of surgical or spontaneous portosystemic shunts, location of varices, and detection of fatty infiltration and focal hepatic masses (264,266).

Calculation of Liver Volume

The goal of liver transplantation is to transplant a liver that is the same size as the native organ. This goal is rarely completely reached, and a donor liver up to 20% larger than the

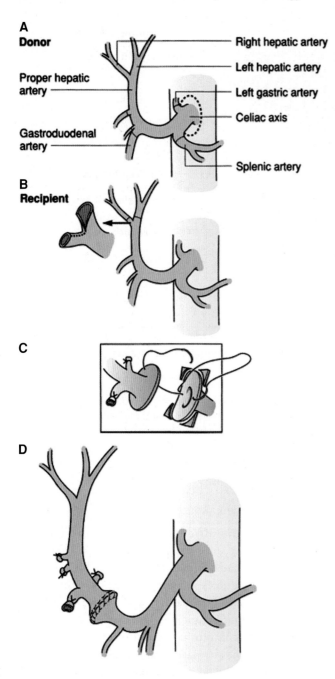

FIGURE 19-78 Donor hepatic artery. A: The donor hepatic artery is procured with a Carrel patch of aorta. **B:** The recipient hepatic artery bifurcation is used to fashion a branch patch for a larger anastomosis. **C:** The anastomosis is carried out by using continuous monofilament suture material. **D:** The completed anastomosis. (Reprinted with permission from Punch J. Hepatic transplantation. In: Mulholland MW, Lillemoe KD, Doherty GM, et al., eds. *Greenfield's Surgery: Scientific Principles and Practice.* Philadelphia: Lippincott Williams & Wilkins; 2006:590–609.)

estimated optimal volume is allowed (266). For recipients of partial livers from living donors, the minimum graft-to-recipient body weight ratio (GRBW) is 0.8% after correction for steatosis and diffuse liver disease. For living donors,

a residual liver volume of 30% to 40% of the total liver volume is adequate for survival (266,267).

MRA and CTA techniques acquire images of the liver parenchyma with clear depiction of the intrahepatic and extrahepatic vascular anatomy, allowing accurate determination of the size of the various Couinaud liver segments. These volumes are classically determined on reconstruction software, by tracing the segment size on consecutive slices through the liver parenchyma, and give excellent estimation of organ size.

Preoperative Vascular Assessment

Portal Vein

The size and patency of the recipient portal vein must be determined prior to liver transplantation, while other variables, such as hepatofugal flow and elevated or slow portal vein velocity, do not preclude patients from candidacy. Previously, portal vein thrombosis was considered a contraindication to liver transplantation. Currently, this is no longer an absolute contraindication, as there are several options for portal revascularization in the recipient as long as the SMV is patent. For example, a venous bypass graft can be used to direct flow from the SMV to the portal vein as long as a 5 cm length of SMV is patent proximal to the graft (262,268).

The donor portal vein size should optimally be within ±3 to 4 mm of the recipient's portal vein diameter. The diameter of the portal vein should be measured at the extrahepatic portion of the portal vein proximal to the portal confluence, as this is the anastomotic site. If the size discrepancy is greater than 3 to 4 mm, a cadaveric donor iliac vein graft can be used to connect the recipient SMV and the donor portal vein.

Anatomical variations in the portal vein bifurcation must be identified in the preoperative living donor (96). Certain anomalies of the donor portal vein anatomy such as absence of the right portal vein and a trifurcation of the portal vein can preclude liver donation. Twenty percent of liver donors are estimated to be excluded from the donor pool because of portal venous anomalies (96). Other anomalies such as early branching or trifurcation of the donor portal vein increase the complexity of living donor liver transplantation, requiring additional anastomoses with the recipient's main portal vein. Origin of the right anterior portal vein from the left portal vein distal to the main portal bifurcation must be recognized preoperatively so that the resection occurs after the origin of the aberrant right anterior portal vein. If this variant is not recognized and the surgeon ligates the left portal vein *proximal* to the takeoff of the aberrant right anterior portal vein, then the territory of

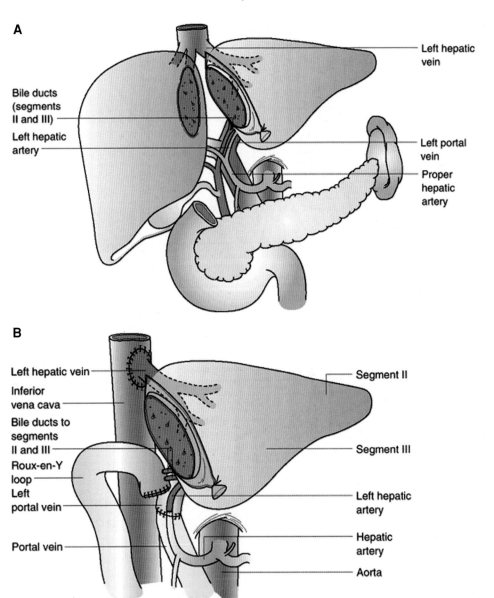

FIGURE 19-79 Left lateral segment (segments II and III) living donor transplantation. A: Donor operation. **B:** Recipient operation completed. (Reprinted with permission from Punch J. Hepatic transplantation. In: Mulholland MW, Lillemoe KD, Doherty GM, et al., eds. *Greenfield's Surgery: Scientific Principles and Practice.* Philadelphia: Lippincott Williams & Wilkins; 2006:590–609.)

this aberrant right anterior portal vein (segments IV, V, and VIII) will be devascularized.

Hepatic Arteries

For living donors, hepatic arterial supply must be evaluated preoperatively. In particular, the origin and location of the artery supplying segment IV of the liver must be determined, as inadvertent ligation will devascularize flow to the donor's medial segment. The traditional origin of this artery is from the CHA (25% of patients [79]). In 11% of the population, segment IV is supplied by a replaced right hepatic artery arising from the SMA (79).

Preoperative evaluation of the hepatic arterial supply of the recipient is not essential but provides useful infor-

mation in predicting postoperative hepatic arterial flow. Particularly in patients with severe atherosclerotic disease, intraoperative grafting of a donor cadaveric iliac artery can be performed, connecting the recipient aorta and the donor hepatic artery.

Hepatic Veins

Preoperative evaluation of the living donor's hepatic veins is important, with attention to the patency, size, and number. In particular, the middle hepatic vein origin (which can arise directly from the IVC or from a common trunk with the left hepatic vein) must be documented so that it is carefully preserved at the time of transplantation. If the middle hepatic vein clots after placement of the graft in the recipient,

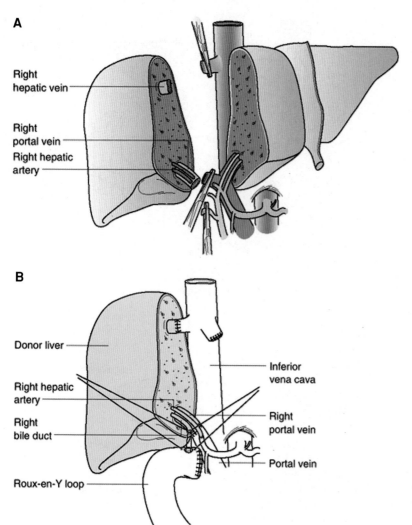

A

Right
hepatic vein

Right
portal vein

Right hepatic
artery

B

Donor liver

Right hepatic
artery

Right
bile duct

Roux-en-Y loop

Inferior
vena cava

Right
portal vein

Portal vein

**FIGURE 19-80 Right lobe (segments V to VIII) living
donor transplantation. A:** Donor operation. **B:** Recipient operation completed. (Reprinted with permission
from Punch J. Hepatic transplantation. In: Mulholland
MW, Lillemoe KD, Doherty GM, et al., eds. *Greenfield's
Surgery: Scientific Principles and Practice.* Philadelphia:
Lippincott Williams & Wilkins; 2006:590–609.)

a Budd-Chiari syndrome will develop in the donor's remaining left lobe, leading to congestion, reversed flow in the portal vein, and eventual atrophy of the donor's remaining liver (Fig. 19-81). The veins that drain segment IV of the liver and supply the middle hepatic vein can have multiple variations, including accessory venous drainage directly into the IVC, and must be identified preoperatively to avoid transection during surgery.

Portosystemic Shunts and Varices

Patients with cirrhosis frequently have surgical or spontaneous portosystemic shunts. Preoperative evaluation of the presence of these shunts and their functionality is important, as these shunts are typically eradicated during the transplant procedure to stop the diversion of portal flow from the newly transplanted liver (86). The exception to this standard of shunt eradication is the presence of a distal splenorenal shunt, which is technically complex to

eradicate and frequently associated with increased postoperative morbidity (excessive blood loss, splenectomy, portal vein thrombosis). Therefore, ligation of shunts is limited to the technically less complex portacaval or mesocaval shunts.

The surgical approach and technique utilized is not significantly swayed by the presence of portosystemic varices. Typically, the surgeon ligates varices as they are encountered, but their obliteration will not affect transplantation outcome. In fact, ligation of very large varices may be unsuccessful and lead to serious hemorrhagic complications. Thus, the decision to ligate or ignore varices is usually made intraoperatively by the surgeon.

There is debate within the radiology community over the best imaging modality for optimizing an "all-in-one" imaging protocol for the assessment of potential living donor liver transplants (92,266,269–276). When CTA was performed with the addition of a biliary contrast agent,

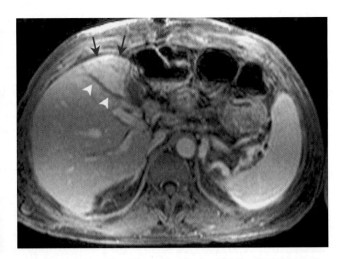

FIGURE 19-81 Accessory hepatic vein thrombosis transplant recipient. Axial delayed phase post-contrast VIBE image demonstrates delayed hapatic outflow and thus prolonged enhancement (*black arrows*) from segment 4B secondary to a thrombosed accessory hepatic vein (*white arrowheads*).

Yeh and colleagues (274) and Schoeder and associates (275) reported improved visualization of second order biliary tract anatomy as compared with conventional MRA and excretory MRA (performed with mangafodipir trisodium). However, these two studies describe the comparable ability of both CTA and MRA to detect accurate vascular anatomy (274,275). Additionally, a potential drawback of biliary-enhanced CTA is the relatively high incidence of moderate adverse reactions to the CT biliary agent (275). Other investigators advocate the superiority of MRA over CTA in detecting liver parenchymal lesions (272). All studies comparing the two modalities demonstrate equivalent depiction of hepatic arterial variations and portal and hepatic venous variations with both CTA and MRA (92,266,272,274,275).

Thus, both MRA and CTA imaging of the preoperative liver donor and recipient allows comprehensive evaluation of the liver parenchyma, biliary tree (when using either a CT or an MRI biliary contrast agent), and vascular variants. 3D MRA has also been shown to be valuable in depicting vascular anomalies with regard to the aortic branch vessels (81).

The main problem in MRI, motion artifacts, can be reduced by fast spin echo, breath-hold GRE, and echo planar imaging.

Using 3D breath-hold CE MRA, the complete liver volume can be obtained in one breath hold during the arterial phase of contrast administration. Previous limitations of MRI in depicting terminal arterial branches like the segment IV artery due to older MRI techniques (such as TOF, which was limited by in-plane saturation, phase dispersion,

and long acquisition times) have been eliminated by the use of thin-section, 3D volumetric postcontrast imaging. Additionally, MRV allows excellent resolution of portal and hepatic venous anomalies, along with assessment of vessel size (277). Vascular complications of liver transplantation are another indication for visceral artery imaging. CE MRA has been reported to be useful for the evaluation of vascular complications following liver transplantation (265,278).

Postoperative Imaging Evaluation of the Transplant Recipient

Vascular complications occur in 8% to 12% of liver transplant recipients (279). Hepatic artery thrombosis occurs in 5% to 10% of liver transplantation recipients and is more common in children (due to the smaller hepatic arteries and increased technical difficulty) (280) and in partial liver transplant recipients (279) (Fig. 19-82). Risk factors for hepatic arterial thrombosis include size discrepancy between the donor and recipient hepatic artery, reconstructive arterioplasty performed intraoperatively, and acute rejection in the first postoperative week as well as history of smoking and other hypercoagulable states. This complication is usually suspected clinically secondary to elevated liver transaminases or biliary abnormalities on laboratory

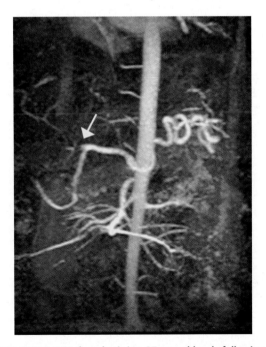

FIGURE 19-82 CHA thrombosis in a 37-year-old male following complicated partial hepatectomy of a hepatoma invading the IVC. This is not a transplant patient, but it demonstrates the appearance of a cut-off in the arterial vasculature nicely, even in a noncooperative, postoperative patient. MIP images from the arterial phase of a 3D LAVA acquisition demonstrate an abrupt cut-off in the proper hepatic artery (*arrow*), compatible with thrombosis. Not shown is extensive clot within the IVC.

testing. The presence of hepatic arterial thrombosis is readily made by radiologic evaluation with Doppler sonography, MRA, or traditional angiography.

If diagnosed within the first week of transplantation, urgent thrombectomy and revision of the anastomosis are warranted, as there is rapid progression to biliary necrosis and graft failure (262). However, if hepatic arterial thrombosis is seen months to years after transplantation, intervention is less emergent, as up to one third of patients will do well without intervention (281).

Thrombosis of the portal veins is less common than hepatic arterial thrombosis, accounting for 1% to 3% of cases (262). Clinically, patients present with liver dysfunction, uncontrollable ascites, and variceal bleeding. If portal vein thrombosis is suspected early, then patients will undergo operative thrombectomy and revision of the anastomosis. However, if the diagnosis is subacute or late, collateral vessels and left-sided (splenic and IMV) portal hypertension has often occurred, limiting the usefulness of intervention (279).

Thrombosis of the IVC is a rare complication after liver transplantation, usually secondary to size discrepancies between the donor and recipient livers. Hepatic vein outflow obstruction occurs more frequently, in up to 2% to 4% of transplant recipients (262). These rare complications are classically described on sonography but are readily diagnosed with MRV techniques. Treatment is via interventional radiology with balloon angioplasty (282).

OUTLOOK: FUTURE PERSPECTIVES OF MESENTERIC AND PORTAL VENOUS MAGNETIC RESONANCE ANGIOGRAPHY

Functional Assessment of Mesenteric Flow/Oximetry

MR flow quantification has been proposed as an indirect parameter for the evaluation of mesenteric ischemia. Using PC MRI, flow characteristics of the celiac trunk, SMA, and IMA can be qualitatively and quantitatively assessed. A reciprocal correlation between the degree of stenosis in the SMA and the flow augmentation after a caloric stimulation can be determined. Likewise, flow in the SMV can be quantified, which is an accurate indicator of flow in the visceral arteries and mirrors changes in each of the three main arterial branches.

Perfusion Magnetic Resonance Imaging of the Small Bowel to Assess Mesenteric Ischemia

As in cardiac imaging where a perfusion reserve can be determined after exposing the patient to a physiologic challenge (283–285), comparable findings can be pursued for

evaluating patients with mesenteric ischemia (286). Instead of a pharmacologic increase of blood flow through IV application of pharmaceutical drugs, as is done for coronary assessments, the mesenteric blood flow can be increased after the oral administration of a high-caloric meal. In fact, in one study the mesenteric reserve capacity of bowel wall perfusion proved to be the most reliable parameter for identifying patients with mesenteric ischemia during the first-pass period of the contrast agent (286).

CONCLUSION

The last decade has seen continuous development of CE MRA techniques for evaluation of the mesenteric and portal venous vasculature. The technique is useful for evaluating a wide spectrum of abdominal pathology. In many centers worldwide, it is the technique of choice for evaluating patients with suspected CMI, assessing operability of patients with pancreatic cancer, and investigating the portal system. Further indications include the assessment of liver transplant patients before and after transplant and of living related liver transplant donors. Functional assessment utilizing perfusion sequences is evolving as an attractive adjunct to the examination.

REFERENCES

1. Roobottom CA, Dubbins PA. Significant disease of the celiac and superior mesenteric arteries in asymptomatic patients: predictive value of Doppler sonography. *AJR Am J Roentgenol.* 1993;161:985–988.
2. Cademartiri F, Raaijmakers RH, Kuiper JW, et al. Multidetector row CT angiography in patients with abdominal angina. *Radiographics.* 2004;24:969–984.
3. Bjorck M, Bergqvist D, Troeng T. Incidence and clinical presentation of bowel ischaemia after aortoiliac surgery—2930 operations from a population-based registry in Sweden. *Eur J Vasc Endovasc Surg.* 1996;12:139–144.
4. Sachs SM, Morton JH, Schwartz SI. Acute mesenteric ischemia. *Surgery.* 1982;92:646–653.
5. Sreenarasimhaiah J. Chronic mesenteric ischemia. *Best Pract Res Clin Gastroenterol.* 2005;19:283–295.
6. Yoon YH, Yi H. *Surveillance Report #75: Liver Cirrhosis Mortality in the United States, 1970–2003.* NIAAA, Division of Epidemiology and Prevention Research, Alcohol Epidemiologic Data System, Rockville, MD: DHHS, PHS, 2006. Available at: http: pubs.niaaa.nih.gov/publications/surveillance75/Cirr03.htm. [Accessed Oct 1, 2007].
7. Yoon YH, Yi H, Grant B. *Surveillance Report #57: Liver Cirrhosis Mortality in the United States, 1970–98.* NIAA, Division of Epidemiology and Prevention Research. Alcohol Epidemiology Data System, Rockville, MD: DHHS, PHS, 2001.
8. Mann RE, Smart RG, Govoni R. The epidemiology of alcoholic liver disease. *Alcohol Res Health.* 2003;27:209–219.
9. Custer B, Sullivan SD, Hazlet TK, et al. Global epidemiology of hepatitis B virus. *J Clin Gastroenterol.* 2004;38:S158–S168.
10. Alter MJ. The epidemiology of acute and chronic hepatitis C. *Clin Liver Dis.* 1997;1:vi–vii, 559–568.

11. El-Serag HB, Everhart JE. Improved survival after variceal hemorrhage over an 11-year period in the Department of Veterans Affairs. *Am J Gastroenterol*. 2000;95: 3566–3573.

12. Fleischer D. Etiology and prevalence of severe persistent upper gastrointestinal bleeding. *Gastroenterology*. 1983;84:538–543.

13. Groszmann RJ, de Franchis R. Portal hypertension. In: Schiff ER, Sorrel MF, Maddrey WX, eds. *Schiff's Diseases of the Liver*. 8th ed. New York: Lippincott-Raven; 1999;387–422.

14. Pinto HC, Abrantes A, Esteves AV, et al. Long-term prognosis of patients with cirrhosis of the liver and upper gastrointestinal bleeding. *Am J Gastroenterol*. 1989;84:1239–1243.

15. Bradbury MS, Kavanagh PV, Chen MY, et al. Noninvasive assessment of portomesenteric venous thrombosis: current concepts and imaging strategies. *J Comput Assist Tomogr*. 2002;26:392–404.

16. Li KC, Whitney WS, McDonnell CH, et al. Chronic mesenteric ischemia: evaluation with phase-contrast cine MR imaging. *Radiology*. 1994;190:175–179.

17. Jager K, Bollinger A, Valli C, et al. Measurement of mesenteric blood flow by duplex scanning. *J Vasc Surg*. 1986;3: 462–469.

18. Giovagnorio F, Picarelli A, Di Giovambattista F, et al. Evaluation with Doppler sonography of mesenteric blood flow in celiac disease. *AJR Am J Roentgenol*. 1998;171:629–632.

19. Cognet F, Ben Salem D, Dranssart M, et al. Chronic mesenteric ischemia: imaging and percutaneous treatment. *Radiographics*. 2002;22:863–879; discussion 879–880.

20. Shih MC, Hagspiel KD. CTA and MRA in mesenteric ischemia: part 1. Role in diagnosis and differential diagnosis. *AJR Am J Roentgenol*. 2007;188:452–461.

21. Chan FP, Rubin GD. MDCT angiography of pediatric vascular diseases of the abdomen, pelvis, and extremities. *Pediatr Radiol*. 2005;35:40–53.

22. Rubin GD. Three-dimensional helical CT angiography. *Radiographics*. 1994;14:905–912.

23. Meilahn JE, Morris JB, Ceppa EP, et al. Effect of prolonged selective intramesenteric arterial vasodilator therapy on intestinal viability after acute segmental mesenteric vascular occlusion. *Ann Surg*. 2001;234:107–115.

24. Savassi-Rocha PR, Veloso LF. Treatment of superior mesenteric artery embolism with a fibrinolytic agent: case report and literature review. *Hepatogastroenterology*. 2002;49: 1307–1310.

25. Matsumoto AH, Angle JF, Spinosa DJ, et al. Percutaneous transluminal angioplasty and stenting in the treatment of chronic mesenteric ischemia: results and longterm followup. *J Am Coll Surg*. 2002;194:S22–S31.

26. Giswold ME, Landry GJ, Taylor LM, et al. Iatrogenic arterial injury is an increasingly important cause of arterial trauma. *Am J Surg*. 2004;187:590–592; discussion 592–593.

27. Lazarides MK, Arvanitis DP, Liatas AC, et al. Iatrogenic and noniatrogenic arterial trauma: a comparative study. *Eur J Surg*. 1991;157:17–20.

28. Moneta GL, Lee RW, Yeager RA, et al. Mesenteric duplex scanning: a blinded prospective study. *J Vasc Surg*. 1993;17:79–84; discussion 85–86.

29. Perko MJ. Duplex ultrasound for assessment of superior mesenteric artery blood flow. *Eur J Vasc Endovasc Surg*. 2001;21:106–117.

30. Zwolak RM. Can duplex ultrasound replace arteriography in screening for mesenteric ischemia? *Semin Vasc Surg*. 1999;12:252–260.

31. Marshall MM, Beese RC, Muiesan P, et al. Assessment of portal venous system patency in the liver transplant candidate: a prospective study comparing ultrasound, microbubble-enhanced colour Doppler ultrasound, with arteriography and surgery. *Clin Radiol*. 2002;57:377–383.

32. Santana P, Jeffrey RB Jr, Bastidas A. Acute thrombosis of a giant portal venous aneurysm: value of color Doppler sonography. *J Ultrasound Med*. 2002;21:701–704.

33. Gentile AT, Moneta GL, Lee RW, et al. Usefulness of fasting and postprandial duplex ultrasound examinations for predicting high-grade superior mesenteric artery stenosis. *Am J Surg*. 1995;169:476–479.

34. Blebea J, Volteas N, Neumyer M, et al. Contrast enhanced duplex ultrasound imaging of the mesenteric arteries. *Ann Vasc Surg*. 2002;16:77–83.

35. Iannaccone R, Laghi A, Passariello R. Multislice CT angiography of mesenteric vessels. *Abdom Imaging*. 2004;29: 146–152.

36. Burkart DJ, Johnson CD, Reading CC, et al. MR measurements of mesenteric venous flow: prospective evaluation in healthy volunteers and patients with suspected chronic mesenteric ischemia. *Radiology*. 1995;194: 801–806.

37. Chan FP, Li KC, Heiss SG, et al. A comprehensive approach using MR imaging to diagnose acute segmental mesenteric ischemia in a porcine model. *AJR Am J Roentgenol*. 1999;173:523–529.

38. Chow LC, Chan FP, Li KC. A comprehensive approach to MR imaging of mesenteric ischemia. *Abdom Imaging*. 2002;27: 507–516.

39. Debatin JF. MR quantification of flow in abdominal vessels. *Abdom Imaging*. 1998;23:485–495.

40. Hagspiel KD, Leung DA, Angle JF, et al. MR angiography of the mesenteric vasculature. *Radiol Clin North Am*. 2002;40: 867–886.

41. Heiss SG, Li KC. Magnetic resonance angiography of mesenteric arteries. A review. *Invest Radiol*. 1998;33:670–681.

42. Kirkpatrick ID, Kroeker MA, Greenberg HM. Biphasic CT with mesenteric CT angiography in the evaluation of acute mesenteric ischemia: initial experience. *Radiology*. 2003;229:91–98.

43. Li KC. MR angiography of abdominal ischemia. *Semin Ultrasound CT MR*. 1996;17:352–359.

44. Li KC. Mesenteric occlusive disease. *Magn Reson Imaging Clin N Am*. 1998;6:331–350.

45. Horton KM, Fishman EK. Volume-rendered 3D CT of the mesenteric vasculature: normal anatomy, anatomic variants, and pathologic conditions. *Radiographics*. 2002;22:161–172.

46. Megibow AJ, Babb JS, Hecht EM, et al. Evaluation of bowel distention and bowel wall appearance by using neutral oral contrast agent for multi-detector row CT. *Radiology*. 2006;238:87–95.

47. Brugel M, Rummeny EJ, Dobritz M. Vascular invasion in pancreatic cancer: value of multislice helical CT. *Abdom Imaging*. 2004;29:239–245.

48. Prokesch RW, Schima W, Chow LC, et al. Multidetector CT of pancreatic adenocarcinoma: diagnostic advances and therapeutic relevance. *Eur Radiol*. 2003;13:2147–2154.

49. Vargas R, Nino-Murcia M, Trueblood W, et al. MDCT in pancreatic adenocarcinoma: prediction of vascular invasion and resectability using a multiphasic technique with curved planar reformations. *AJR Am J Roentgenol*. 2004;182:419–425.

50. Baden JG, Racy DJ, Grist TM. Contrast-enhanced three-dimensional magnetic resonance angiography of the mesenteric vasculature. *J Magn Reson Imaging*. 1999;10:369–375.

51. Hany TF, Schmidt M, Schoenenberger AW, et al. Contrast-enhanced three-dimensional magnetic resonance angiography of the splanchnic vasculature before and after caloric stimulation. Original investigation. *Invest Radiol*. 1998;33:682–686.

52. Laissy JP, Trillaud H, Douek P. MR angiography: noninvasive vascular imaging of the abdomen. *Abdom Imaging*. 2002;27:488–506.

53. Meaney JF. Non-invasive evaluation of the visceral arteries with magnetic resonance angiography. *Eur Radiol*. 1999;9:1267–1276.

54. Prince MR, Yucel EK, Kaufman JA, et al. Dynamic gadolinium-enhanced three-dimensional abdominal MR arteriography. *J Magn Reson Imaging*. 1993;3:877–881.

55. Vosshenrich R, Fischer U. Contrast-enhanced MR angiography of abdominal vessels: is there still a role for angiography? *Eur Radiol.* 2002;12:218–230.

56. Pruessmann KP, Weiger M, Scheidegger MB, et al. SENSE: sensitivity encoding for fast MRI. *Magn Reson Med.* 1999;42:952–962.

57. Weiger M, Pruessmann KP, Kassner A, et al. Contrast-enhanced 3D MRA using SENSE. *J Magn Reson Imaging.* 2000;12:671–677.

58. Matheson PJ, Wilson MA, Garrison RN. Regulation of intestinal blood flow. *J Surg Res.* 2000;93:182–196.

59. Miyazaki T, Yamashita Y, Shinzato J, et al. Two-dimensional time-of-flight magnetic resonance angiography in the coronal plane for abdominal disease: its usefulness and comparison with conventional angiography. *Br J Radiol.* 1995;68:351–357.

60. Wasser MN, Geelkerken RH, Kouwenhoven M, et al. Systolically gated 3D phase contrast MRA of mesenteric arteries in suspected mesenteric ischemia. *J Comput Assist Tomogr.* 1996;20:262–268.

61. Li KC, Hopkins KL, Dalman RL, et al. Simultaneous measurement of flow in the superior mesenteric vein and artery with cine phase-contrast MR imaging: value in diagnosis of chronic mesenteric ischemia. Work in progress. *Radiology.* 1995;194:327–330.

62. Naganawa S, Cooper TG, Jenner G, et al. Flow velocity and volume measurement of superior and inferior mesenteric artery with cine phase contrast magnetic resonance imaging. *Radiat Med.* 1994;12:213–220.

63. Meaney JF, Prince MR, Nostrant TT, et al. Gadolinium-enhanced MR angiography of visceral arteries in patients with suspected chronic mesenteric ischemia. *J Magn Reson Imaging.* 1997;7:171–176.

64. Prince MR, Narasimham DL, Stanley JC, et al. Breath-hold gadolinium-enhanced MR angiography of the abdominal aorta and its major branches. *Radiology.* 1995;197:785–792.

65. Rofsky NM, Lee VS, Laub G, et al. Abdominal MR imaging with a volumetric interpolated breath-hold examination. *Radiology.* 1999;212:876–884.

66. Earls JP, Rofsky NM, DeCorato DR, et al. Breath-hold single-dose gadolinium-enhanced three-dimensional MR aortography: usefulness of a timing examination and MR power injector. *Radiology.* 1996;201:705–710.

67. Foo TK, Saranathan M, Prince MR, et al. Automated detection of bolus arrival and initiation of data acquisition in fast, three-dimensional, gadolinium-enhanced MR angiography. *Radiology.* 1997;203:275–280.

68. Wilman AH, Riederer SJ, King BF, et al. Fluoroscopically triggered contrast-enhanced three-dimensional MR angiography with elliptical centric view order: application to the renal arteries. *Radiology.* 1997;205:137–146.

69. Cunningham CG, Reilly LM, Stoney R. Chronic visceral ischemia. *Surg Clin North Am.* 1992;72:231–244.

70. Kurland B, Brandt LJ, Delany HM. Diagnostic tests for intestinal ischemia. *Surg Clin North Am.* 1992;72:85–105.

71. Li KC, Dalman RL, Wright GA. In vivo flow-independent T2 measurements of superior mesenteric vein blood in diagnosis of chronic mesenteric ischemia: a preliminary evaluation. *Acad Radiol.* 1999;6:530–534.

72. Li KC, Dalman RL, Ch'en IY, et al. Chronic mesenteric ischemia: use of in vivo MR imaging measurements of blood oxygen saturation in the superior mesenteric vein for diagnosis. *Radiology.* 1997;204:71–77.

73. Saad WE, Davies MG, Sahler L, et al. Arc of Buhler: incidence and diameter in asymptomatic individuals. *Vasc Endovascular Surg.* 2005;39:347–349.

74. Buhler A. Uber eine Anastomose zwischen den Stammen der Art. Coeliaca und der Art. Mesenterica superior. *Gegenbaurs Morph JB.* 1904;32:185–188.

75. Kupic EA, Marshall WH, Abrams HL. Splenic arterial patterns angiographic analysis and review. *Invest Radiol.* 1967;2:70–98.

76. Michels NA. Constitutional arterial variations as exemplified in the blood supply of the liver. *J Int Coll Surg.* 1953;20:213–220.

77. Michels NA. Collateral arterial pathways to the liver after ligation of the hepatic artery and removal of the celiac axis. *Cancer.* 1953;6:708–724.

78. Michels NA. Variational anatomy of the hepatic, cystic, and retroduodenal arteries; a statistical analysis of their origin, distribution, and relations to the biliary ducts in two hundred bodies. *AMA Arch Surg.* 1953;66:20–34.

79. Michels NA. Newer anatomy of the liver and its variant blood supply and collateral circulation. *Am J Surg.* 1966;112:337–347.

80. Michels NA. *Blood Supply and Anatomy of the Upper Abdominal Organs.* Philadelphia: JB Lippincott Co.; 1955.

81. Lavelle MT, Lee VS, Rofsky NM, et al. Dynamic contrast-enhanced three-dimensional MR imaging of liver parenchyma: source images and angiographic reconstructions to define hepatic arterial anatomy. *Radiology.* 2001;218:389–394.

82. Kolmannskog F, Schrumpf E, Valnes K. Computed tomography and angiography in pancreatic apudomas and cystadenomas. *Acta Radiol Diagn (Stockh).* 1982;23:365–372.

83. Boijsen E, Redman HC. Effect of bradykinin on celiac and superior mesenteric angiography. *Invest Radiol.* 1966;1:422–430.

84. Ernst O, Asnar V, Sergent G, et al. Comparing contrast-enhanced breath-hold MR angiography and conventional angiography in the evaluation of mesenteric circulation. *AJR Am J Roentgenol.* 2000;174:433–439.

85. Atasoy C, Ozyurek E. Prevalence and types of main and right portal vein branching variations on MDCT. *AJR Am J Roentgenol.* 2006;187:676–681.

86. Erbay N, Raptopoulos V, Pomfret EA, et al. Living donor liver transplantation in adults: vascular variants important in surgical planning for donors and recipients. *AJR Am J Roentgenol.* 2003;181:109–114.

87. Kamel IR, Kruskal JB, Pomfret EA, et al. Impact of multidetector CT on donor selection and surgical planning before living adult right lobe liver transplantation. *AJR Am J Roentgenol.* 2001;176:193–200.

88. Schulick RD. Hepatobiliary anatomy. In: Mulholland MW, Lillemoe KD, Doherty GM, et al., eds. *Greenfield's Surgery: Scientific Principles and Practice.* Philadelphia: Lippincott Williams & Wilkins; 2006:892–909.

89. Desser TS, Sze DY, Jeffrey RB. Imaging and intervention in the hepatic veins. *AJR Am J Roentgenol.* 2003;180:1583–1591.

90. Cheng YF, Huang TL, Chen CL, et al. Variations of the middle and inferior right hepatic vein: application in hepatectomy. *J Clin Ultrasound.* 1997;25:175–182.

91. Sato TJ, Hirai I, Murakami G, et al. An anatomical study of short hepatic veins, with special reference to delineation of the caudate lobe for hanging maneuver of the liver without the usual mobilization. *J Hepatobiliary Pancreat Surg.* 2002;9:55–60.

92. Lee MW, Lee JM, Lee JY, et al. Preoperative evaluation of the hepatic vascular anatomy in living liver donors: comparison of CT angiography and MR angiography. *J Magn Reson Imaging.* 2006;24:1081–1087.

93. Lee SG. Techniques of reconstruction of hepatic veins in living-donor liver transplantation, especially for right hepatic vein and major short hepatic veins of right-lobe graft. *J Hepatobiliary Pancreat Surg.* 2006;13:131–138.

94. Varotti G, Gondolesi GE, Goldman J, et al. Anatomic variations in right liver living donors. *J Am Coll Surg.* 2004;198:577–582.

95. Onodera Y, Omatsu T, Nakayama J, et al. Peripheral anatomic evaluation using 3D CT hepatic venography in donors: significance of peripheral venous visualization in living-donor liver transplantation. *AJR Am J Roentgenol.* 2004;183:1065–1070.

96. Atri M, Bret PM, Fraser-Hill MA. Intrahepatic portal venous variations: prevalence with US. *Radiology*. 1992;184:157–158.
97. Cheng YF, Huang TL, Chen CL, et al. Anatomic dissociation between the intrahepatic bile duct and portal vein: risk factors for left hepatectomy. *World J Surg*. 1997;21:297–300.
98. Reiner L, Jimenez FA, Rodriguez FL. Atherosclerosis in the mesenteric circulation. Observations and correlations with aortic and coronary atherosclerosis. *Am Heart J*. 1963;66:200–209.
99. Char D, Hines G. Chronic mesenteric ischemia: diagnosis and treatment. *Heart Dis*. 2001;3:231–235.
100. Chang JB, Stein TA. Mesenteric ischemia: acute and chronic. *Ann Vasc Surg*. 2003;17:323–328.
101. Zelenock S. Splanchnic vascular occlusive and aneurysmal disease. In: Mulholland MW, Lillemoe KD, Doherty GM, et al., eds. *Greenfield's Surgery: Scientific Principles and Practice*. Philadelphia: Lippincott Williams & Wilkins; 2006;1614–1632.
102. Aakhus T, Brabrand G. Angiography in acute superior mesenteric arterial insufficiency. *Acta Radiol Diagn (Stockh)*. 1967;6:1–12.
103. Aakhus T, Evensen A. Angiography in acute mesenteric arterial insufficiency. *Acta Radiol Diagn (Stockh)*. 1978;19:945–951.
104. Kato T, Fujii K, Ishii E, et al. A case of polyarteritis nodosa with lesions of the superior mesenteric artery illustrating the diagnostic usefulness of three-dimensional computed tomographic angiography. *Clin Rheumatol*. 2005;24:628–631.
105. Rha SE, Ha HK, Lee SH, et al. CT and MR imaging findings of bowel ischemia from various primary causes. *Radiographics*. 2000;20:29–42.
106. Moawad J, Gewertz BL. Chronic mesenteric ischemia. Clinical presentation and diagnosis. *Surg Clin North Am*. 1997;77:357–369.
107. Williams LF Jr. Mesenteric ischemia. *Surg Clin North Am*. 1988;68:331–353.
108. Tassi G, Maggi G, de Nicola P. Microcirculation in the elderly. *Int Angiol*. 1985;4:275–283.
109. Dalman RL, Li KC, Moon WK, et al. Diminished postprandial hyperemia in patients with aortic and mesenteric arterial occlusive disease. Quantification by magnetic resonance flow imaging. *Circulation*. 1996;94:II206–II210.
110. Budd G. *On Diseases of the Liver*. London: John Churchill; 1845.
111. Okumura A, Watanabe Y, Dohke M, et al. Contrast-enhanced three-dimensional MR portography. *Radiographics*. 1999;19:973–987.
112. Lindner HH, Kemprud E. A clinicoanatomical study of the arcuate ligament of the diaphragm. *Arch Surg*. 1971;103:600–605.
113. Harjola PT. A rare obstruction of the coeliac artery. Report of a case. *Ann Chir Gynaecol Fenn*. 1963;52:547–550.
114. Horton KM, Talamini MA, Fishman EK. Median arcuate ligament syndrome: evaluation with CT angiography. *Radiographics*. 2005;25:1177–1182.
115. Lee VS, Morgan JN, Tan AG, et al. Celiac artery compression by the median arcuate ligament: a pitfall of end-expiratory MR imaging. *Radiology*. 2003;228:437–442.
116. Szilagyi DE, Rian RL, Elliott JP, et al. The cardiac artery compression syndrome: does it exist? *Surgery*. 1972;72:849–863.
117. Cornell SH. Severe stenosis of the celiac artery. Analysis of patients with and without symptoms. *Radiology*. 1971;99:311–316.
118. Reilly LM, Ammar AD, Stoney RJ, et al. Late results following operative repair for celiac artery compression syndrome. *J Vasc Surg*. 1985;2:79–91.
119. Daskalakis MK. Celiac axis compression syndrome. *Int Surg*. 1982;67:442–444.
120. Kernohan RM, Barros D'Sa AA, et al. Further evidence supporting the existence of the celiac artery compression syndrome. *Arch Surg*. 1985;120:1072–1076.
121. Moawad J, McKinsey JF, Wyble CW, et al. Current results of surgical therapy for chronic mesenteric ischemia. *Arch Surg*. 1997;132:613–618; discussion 618–619.
122. Jones SA, Carter R, Smith LL, et al. Arteriomesenteric duodenal compression. *Am J Surg*. 1960;100:262–277.
123. Mansberger AR Jr, Hearn JB, Byers RM, et al. Vascular compression of the duodenum. Emphasis on accurate diagnosis. *Am J Surg*. 1968;115:89–96.
124. Rokitansky C. *Handbuch der Pathologischen Anotomie*. Vienna: Branmiller and Siedel; 1842.
125. Wilkie D. Chronic duodenal ileus. *Am J Med Sci*. 1927;173:643–649.
126. Hutchinson DT, Bassett GS. Superior mesenteric artery syndrome in pediatric orthopedic patients. *Clin Orthop Relat Res*. 1990;250:250–257.
127. Konen E, Amitai M, Apter S, et al. CT angiography of superior mesenteric artery syndrome. *AJR Am J Roentgenol*. 1998;171:1279–1281.
128. Lippl F, Hannig C, Weiss W, et al. Superior mesenteric artery syndrome: diagnosis and treatment from the gastroenterologist's view. *J Gastroenterol*. 2002;37:640–643.
129. Akin JT Jr, Gray SW, Skandalakis JE. Vascular compression of the duodenum: presentation of ten cases and review of the literature. *Surgery*. 1976;79:515–522.
130. Gustafsson L, Falk A, Lukes PJ, et al. Diagnosis and treatment of superior mesenteric artery syndrome. *Br J Surg*. 1984;71:499–501.
131. Applegate GR, Cohen AJ. Dynamic CT in superior mesenteric artery syndrome. *J Comput Assist Tomogr*. 1988;12:976–980.
132. Hines JR, Gore RM, Ballantyne GH. Superior mesenteric artery syndrome. Diagnostic criteria and therapeutic approaches. *Am J Surg*. 1984;148:630–632.
133. Wilson-Storey D, MacKinlay GA. The superior mesenteric artery syndrome. *J R Coll Surg (Edinb)*. 1986;31:175–178.
134. Gondos B. Duodenal compression defect and the "superior mesenteric artery syndrome" 1. *Radiology*. 1977;123:575–580.
135. Anderson WC, Vivit R, Kirsh IE, et al. Arteriomesenteric duodenal compression syndrome. Its association with peptic ulcer. *Am J Surg*. 1973;125:681–689.
136. Strong EK. Mechanics of arteriomesenteric duodenal obstruction and direct surgical attack upon etiology. *Ann Surg*. 1958;148:725–730.
137. Duvie SO. Anterior transposition of the third part of the duodenum in the management of chronic duodenal compression by the superior mesenteric artery. *Int Surg*. 1988;73:140–143.
138. Park SJ, Lim JW, Cho BS, et al. Nutcracker syndrome in children with orthostatic proteinuria: diagnosis on the basis of Doppler sonography. *J Ultrasound Med*. 2002;21:39–45; quiz 46.
139. Wendel RG, Crawford ED, Hehman KN. The "nutcracker" phenomenon: an unusual cause for renal varicosities with hematuria. *J Urol*. 1980;123:761–763.
140. Chang CT, Hung CC, Ng KK, et al. Nutcracker syndrome and left unilateral haematuria. *Nephrol Dial Transplant*. 2005;20:460–461.
141. Nishimura Y, Fushiki M, Yoshida M, et al. Left renal vein hypertension in patients with left renal bleeding of unknown origin. *Radiology*. 1986;160:663–667.
142. Takebayashi S, Ueki T, Ikeda N, et al. Diagnosis of the nutcracker syndrome with color Doppler sonography: correlation with flow patterns on retrograde left renal venography. *AJR Am J Roentgenol*. 1999;172:39–43.
143. Kim SH, Cho SW, Kim HD, et al. Nutcracker syndrome: diagnosis with Doppler US. *Radiology*. 1996;198:93–97.
144. Hohenfellner M, Steinbach F, Schultz-Lampel D, et al. The nutcracker syndrome: new aspects of pathophysiology, diagnosis and treatment. *J Urol*. 1991;146:685–688.

145. Shokeir AA, el-Diasty TA, Ghoneim MA. The nutcracker syndrome: new methods of diagnosis and treatment. *Br J Urol.* 1994;74:139–143.

146. Fu WJ, Hong BF, Gao JP, et al. Nutcracker phenomenon: a new diagnostic method of multislice computed tomography angiography. *Int J Urol.* 2006;13:870–873.

147. Beinart C, Sniderman KW, Saddekni S, et al. Left renal vein hypertension: a cause of occult hematuria. *Radiology.* 1982;145:647–650.

148. Drescher R, Koster O, von Rothenburg T. Superior mesenteric artery aneurysm stent graft. *Abdom Imaging.* 2006;31(1):113–116.

149. Stanley JC. Splanchnic artery aneurysms. In: Rutherford R, ed. *Vascular Surgery.* 4th ed. Philadelphia: WB Saunders; 1995:1124.

150. Stanley JC, Thompson NW, Fry WJ. Splanchnic artery aneurysms. *Arch Surg.* 1970;101:689–697.

151. Bedford PD, Lodge B. Aneurysm of the splenic artery. *Gut.* 1960;1:312–320.

152. Messina LM, Shanley CJ. Visceral artery aneurysms. *Surg Clin North Am.* 1997;77:425–442.

153. Kobori L, van der Kolk MJ, de Jong KP, et al. Splenic artery aneurysms in liver transplant patients. Liver Transplant Group. *J Hepatol.* 1997;27:890–893.

154. Feist JH, Gajaraj A. Extra- and intrasplenic artery aneurysms in portal hypertension. *Radiology.* 1977;125:331–334.

155. White AF, Baum S, Buranasiri S. Aneurysms secondary to pancreatitis. *AJR Am J Roentgenol.* 1976;127:393–396.

156. Tandon V, Shanna R, Pande GK. Post-traumatic pancreatitis with associated aneurysm of the splenic artery: report of 2 cases and review of the literature. *Can J Surg.* 1999;42:215–219.

157. Das CJ, Pangtey GS. Images in clinical medicine. Arterial microaneurysms in polyarteritis nodosa. *N Engl J Med.* 2006;355:2574.

158. Imai MA, Kawahara E, Katsuda S, et al. Berry splenic artery aneurysm rupture in association with segmental arterial mediolysis and portal hypertension. *Pathol Int.* 2005;55:290–295.

159. Adajar MA, Painter T, Woloson S, et al. Isolated celiac artery aneurysm with splenic artery stenosis as a rare presentation of polyarteritis nodosum: a case report and review of the literature. *J Vasc Surg.* 2006;44:647–650.

160. Berceli SA. Hepatic and splenic artery aneurysms. *Semin Vasc Surg.* 2005;18:196–201.

161. Carr SC, Pearce WH, Vogelzang RL, et al. Current management of visceral artery aneurysms. *Surgery.* 1996;120:627–633; discussion 633–624.

162. Shanley CJ, Shah NL, Messina LM. Common splanchnic artery aneurysms: splenic, hepatic, and celiac. *Ann Vasc Surg.* 1996;10:315–322.

163. Oddi A, Borgna E, Tomassetti S, et al. [Aneurysm of the hepatic artery. Case report and review of the literature.] *G Chir.* 1997;18:277–282.

164. Kim HJ, Kim KW, Kim AY, et al. Hepatic artery pseudoaneurysms in adult living-donor liver transplantation: efficacy of CT and Doppler sonography. *AJR Am J Roentgenol.* 2005;184:1549–1555.

165. Busuttil RW, Brin BJ. The diagnosis and management of visceral artery aneurysms. *Surgery.* 1980;88:619–624.

166. Araoz PA, Andrews JC. Direct percutaneous embolization of visceral artery aneurysms: techniques and pitfalls. *J Vasc Interv Radiol.* 2000;11:1195–1200.

167. Chan HH, Tai KS, Yip LK. Patient with Leriche's syndrome and concomitant superior mesenteric aneurysm: evaluation with contrast-enhanced three-dimensional magnetic resonance angiography, computed tomography angiography and digital subtraction angiography. *Australas Radiol.* 2005;49:233–237.

168. Baker KS, Tisnado J, Cho SR, et al. Splanchnic artery aneurysms and pseudoaneurysms: transcatheter embolization. *Radiology.* 1987;163:135–139.

169. Sessa C, Tinelli G, Porcu P, et al. Treatment of visceral artery aneurysms: description of a retrospective series of 42 aneurysms in 34 patients. *Ann Vasc Surg.* 2004;18:695–703.

170. Connell JM, Han DC. Celiac artery aneurysms: a case report and review of the literature. *Am Surg.* 2006;72:746–749.

171. Porcu P, Marongiu GM, Bacciu PP. [Aneurysms of the celiac artery: case report and review of the literature.] *J Mal Vasc.* 2002;27:88–92.

172. Pilleul F, Beuf O. Diagnosis of splanchnic artery aneurysms and pseudoaneurysms, with special reference to contrast enhanced 3D magnetic resonance angiography: a review. *Acta Radiol.* 2004;45:702–708.

173. Gilfeather M, Holland GA, Siegelman ES, et al. Gadolinium-enhanced ultrafast three-dimensional spoiled gradient-echo MR imaging of the abdominal aorta and visceral and iliac vessels. *Radiographics.* 1997;17:423–432.

174. Soudack M, Gaitini D, Ofer A. Celiac artery aneurysm: diagnosis by color Doppler sonography and three-dimensional CT angiography. *J Clin Ultrasound.* 1999;27:49–51.

175. Winter TC, Ager JD, Nghiem HV, et al. Upper gastrointestinal tract and abdomen: water as an orally administered contrast agent for helical CT. *Radiology.* 1996;201:365–370.

176. Lubbers PR, Goff WB, Volpe RJ, et al. CT diagnosis of celiac artery aneurysm. *J Comput Assist Tomogr.* 1988;12:352–354.

177. Serafino G, Vroegindeweij D, Boks S, et al. Mycotic aneurysm of the celiac trunk: from early CT sign to rupture. *Cardiovasc Intervent Radiol.* 2005;28:677–680.

178. Atkins BZ, Ryan JM, Gray JL. Treatment of a celiac artery aneurysm with endovascular stent grafting—a case report. *Vasc Endovascular Surg.* 2003;37:367–373.

179. Bageacu S, Cuilleron M, Kaczmarek D, et al. True aneurysms of the pancreaticoduodenal artery: successful non-operative management. *Surgery.* 2006;139:608–616.

180. Hyare H, Desigan S, Nicholl H, et al. Multi-section CT angiography compared with digital subtraction angiography in diagnosing major arterial hemorrhage in inflammatory pancreatic disease. *Eur J Radiol.* 2006;59:295–300.

181. Murata S, Tajima H, Fukunaga T, et al. Management of pancreaticoduodenal artery aneurysms: results of superselective transcatheter embolization. *AJR Am J Roentgenol.* 2006;187:W290–W298.

182. Araji O, Barquero JM, Marcos F, et al. Inferior mesenteric artery aneurysm associated with occlusion of the superior mesenteric and celiac arteries. *Ann Vasc Surg.* 2001;15:399–401.

183. Kaufman JLM. *Vascular and Interventional Radiology: The Requisites.* Philadelphia: Mosby; 2004.

184. Hirai S, Hamanaka Y, Mitsui N, et al. Spontaneous and isolated dissection of the main trunk of the superior mesenteric artery. *Ann Thorac Cardiovasc Surg.* 2002;8:236–240.

185. Guthrie W, Maclean H. Dissecting aneurysms of arteries other than the aorta. *J Pathol.* 1972;108:219–235.

186. Solis MM, Ranval TJ, McFarland DR, et al. Surgical treatment of superior mesenteric artery dissecting aneurysm and simultaneous celiac artery compression. *Ann Vasc Surg.* 1993;7:457–462.

187. Sparks SR, Vasquez JC, Bergan JJ, et al. Failure of nonoperative management of isolated superior mesenteric artery dissection. *Ann Vasc Surg.* 2000;14:105–109.

188. Nakamura K, Nozue M, Sakakibara Y, et al. Natural history of a spontaneous dissecting aneurysm of the proximal superior mesenteric artery: report of a case. *Surg Today.* 1997;27:272–274.

189. Dubois J, Soulez G, Oliva VL, et al. Soft-tissue venous malformations in adult patients: imaging and therapeutic issues. *Radiographics.* 2001;21:1519–1531.

190. Hyodoh H, Hori M, Akiba H, et al. Peripheral vascular malformations: imaging, treatment approaches, and therapeutic issues. *Radiographics.* 2005;25[Suppl 1]:S159–S171.

191. Mulliken JB, Glowacki J. Hemangiomas and vascular malformations in infants and children: a classification based

on endothelial characteristics. *Plast Reconstr Surg.* 1982;69:412–422.

192. Jackson IT, Carreno R, Potparic Z, et al. Hemangiomas, vascular malformations, and lymphovenous malformations: classification and methods of treatment. *Plast Reconstr Surg.* 1993;91:1216–1230.

193. Enjolras O. Classification and management of the various superficial vascular anomalies: hemangiomas and vascular malformations. *J Dermatol.* 1997;24:701–710.

194. Howard OM, Buchanan JD, Hunt RH. Angiodysplasia of the colon. Experience of 26 cases. *Lancet.* 1982;2:16–19.

195. Lin S, Rockey DC. Obscure gastrointestinal bleeding. *Gastroenterol Clin North Am.* 2005;34:679–698.

196. Leighton JA, Goldstein J, Hirota W, et al. Obscure gastrointestinal bleeding. *Gastrointest Endosc.* 2003;58:650–655.

197. Ettorre GC, Francioso G, Garribba AP, et al. Helical CT angiography in gastrointestinal bleeding of obscure origin. *AJR Am J Roentgenol.* 1997;168:727–731.

198. Junquera F, Quiroga S, Saperas E, et al. Accuracy of helical computed tomographic angiography for the diagnosis of colonic angiodysplasia. *Gastroenterology.* 2000;119:293–299.

199. Rollins ES, Picus D, Hicks ME, et al. Angiography is useful in detecting the source of chronic gastrointestinal bleeding of obscure origin. *AJR Am J Roentgenol.* 1991;156:385–388.

200. Cohn SM, Moller BA, Zieg PM, et al. Angiography for preoperative evaluation in patients with lower gastrointestinal bleeding: are the benefits worth the risks? *Arch Surg.* 1998;133:50–55.

201. Hilfiker PR, Zimmermann-Paul GG, Schmidt M, et al. Intestinal and peritoneal bleeding: detection with an intravascular contrast agent and fast three-dimensional MR imaging—preliminary experience from an experimental study. *Radiology.* 1998;209:769–774.

202. Weishaupt D, Hetzer FH, Ruehm SG, et al. Three-dimensional contrast-enhanced MRI using an intravascular contrast agent for detection of traumatic intra-abdominal hemorrhage and abdominal parenchymal injuries: an experimental study. *Eur Radiol.* 2000;10:1958–1964.

203. Ludwig D, Wiener S, Bruning A, et al. Mesenteric blood flow is related to disease activity and risk of relapse in Crohn's disease: a prospective follow-up study. *Am J Gastroenterol.* 1999;94:2942–2950.

204. Ha HK, Lee SH, Rha SE, et al. Radiologic features of vasculitis involving the gastrointestinal tract. *Radiographics.* 2000;20:779–794.

205. Atalay MK, Bluemke DA. Magnetic resonance imaging of large vessel vasculitis. *Curr Opin Rheumatol.* 2001;13: 41–47.

206. Schmidt WA, Both M, Reinhold-Keller E. [Imaging in vasculitis.] *Z Rheumatol.* 2006;65:652–661.

207. Lockhart ME, Robbin ML. Case 58: giant cell arteritis. *Radiology.* 2003;227:512–515.

208. Srigley JR, Gardiner GW. Giant cell arteritis with small bowel infarction. A case report and review of the literature. *Am J Gastroenterol.* 1980;73:157–161.

209. Nastri MV, Baptista LP, Baroni RH, et al. Gadolinium-enhanced three-dimensional MR angiography of Takayasu arteritis. *Radiographics.* 2004;24:773–786.

210. Moriwaki R, Noda M, Yajima M, et al. Clinical manifestations of Takayasu arteritis in India and Japan—new classification of angiographic findings. *Angiology.* 1997;48:369–379.

211. Numano F, Okawara M, Inomata H, et al. Takayasu's arteritis. *Lancet.* 2000;356:1023–1025.

212. Matsunaga N, Hayashi K, Sakamoto I, et al. Takayasu arteritis: protean radiologic manifestations and diagnosis. *Radiographics.* 1997;17:579–594.

213. Stanson AW, Friese JL, Johnson CM, et al. Polyarteritis nodosa: spectrum of angiographic findings. *Radiographics.* 2001;21:151–159.

214. Parikh MS, Pachter HL. Liver injury. In: Asensio, JA and Trunkey AA, eds., *Current Therapy of Trauma and Surgical Critical Care.* St. Louis: Mosby; 2008 (in press).

215. Burch JME. Injuries to the liver, biliary tract, spleen, and diaphragm. In: Souba W, ed. *ACS Surgery: Principles and Practice.* Chicago, IL: American College of Surgeons; 2006.

216. Pachter HL, Spencer FC, Hofstetter SR, et al. The management of juxtahepatic venous injuries without an atriocaval shunt: preliminary clinical observations. *Surgery.* 1986;99: 569–575.

217. David Richardson J, Franklin GA, Lukan JK, et al. Evolution in the management of hepatic trauma: a 25-year perspective. *Ann Surg.* 2000;232:324–330.

218. Moore EE, Shackford SR, Pachter HL, et al. Organ injury scaling: spleen, liver, and kidney. *J Trauma.* 1989;29:1664–1666.

219. Moore EE, Cogbill TH, Jurkovich GJ, et al. Organ injury scaling: spleen and liver (1994 revision). *J Trauma.* 1995;38: 323–324.

220. Fang JF, Chen RJ, Wong YC, et al. Pooling of contrast material on computed tomography mandates aggressive management of blunt hepatic injury. *Am J Surg.* 1998;176: 315–319.

221. Wong YC, Wang LJ, See LC, et al. Contrast material extravasation on contrast-enhanced helical computed tomographic scan of blunt abdominal trauma: its significance on the choice, time, and outcome of treatment. *J Trauma.* 2003;54:164–170.

222. Hagiwara A, Yukioka T, Ohta S, et al. Nonsurgical management of patients with blunt hepatic injury: efficacy of transcatheter arterial embolization. *AJR Am J Roentgenol.* 1997;169:1151–1156.

223. Asensio JA, Roldan G, Petrone P, et al. Operative management and outcomes in 103 AAST-OIS grades IV and V complex hepatic injuries: trauma surgeons still need to operate, but angioembolization helps. *J Trauma.* 2003;54: 647–653; discussion 653–654.

224. Mohr AM, Lavery RF, Barone A, et al. Angiographic embolization for liver injuries: low mortality, high morbidity. *J Trauma.* 2003;55:1077–1081; discussion 1081–1082.

225. Wahl WL, Ahrns KS, Brandt MM, et al. The need for early angiographic embolization in blunt liver injuries. *J Trauma.* 2002;52:1097–1101.

226. Shanmuganathan K, Mirvis SE, Sherbourne CD, et al. Hemoperitoneum as the sole indicator of abdominal visceral injuries: a potential limitation of screening abdominal US for trauma. *Radiology.* 1999;212:423–430.

227. Croce MA, Fabian TC, Spiers JP, et al. Traumatic hepatic artery pseudoaneurysm with hemobilia. *Am J Surg.* 1994;168:235–238.

228. Yoon W, Jeong YY, Kim JK, et al. CT in blunt liver trauma. *Radiographics.* 2005;25:87–104.

229. Poletti PA, Mirvis SE, Shanmuganathan K, et al. CT criteria for management of blunt liver trauma: correlation with angiographic and surgical findings. *Radiology.* 2000;216:418–427.

230. Kozar RA, Moore FA, Cothren CC, et al. Risk factors for hepatic morbidity following nonoperative management: multicenter study. *Arch Surg.* 2006;141:451–458; discussion 458–459.

231. Mirvis SE, Whitley NO, Gens DR. Blunt splenic trauma in adults: CT-based classification and correlation with prognosis and treatment. *Radiology.* 1989;171:33–39.

232. Pachter HL, Guth AA, Hofstetter SR, et al. Changing patterns in the management of splenic trauma: the impact of nonoperative management. *Ann Surg.* 1998;227:708–717; discussion 717–719.

233. Cogbill TH, Moore EE, Jurkovich GJ, et al. Nonoperative management of blunt splenic trauma: a multicenter experience. *J Trauma.* 1989;29:1312–1317.

234. Meredith JW, Young JS, Bowling J, et al. Nonoperative management of blunt hepatic trauma: the exception or the rule? *J Trauma.* 1994;36:529–534; discussion 534–535.

235. Pachter HL, Hofstetter SR. The current status of nonoperative management of adult blunt hepatic injuries. *Am J Surg.* 1995;169:442–454.

236. Kass JB, Fisher RG. The Seurat spleen. *AJR Am J Roentgenol.* 1979;132:683–684.
237. Stuhlfaut JW, Soto JA, Lucey BC, et al. Blunt abdominal trauma: performance of CT without oral contrast material. *Radiology.* 2004;233:689–694.
238. Shuman WP. CT of blunt abdominal trauma in adults. *Radiology.* 1997;205:297–306.
239. Moore EE, Cogbill TH, Malangoni MA, et al. Organ injury scaling. II: Pancreas, duodenum, small bowel, colon, and rectum. *J Trauma.* 1990;30:1427–1429.
240. Stuart KE, Anand AJ, Jenkins RL. Hepatocellular carcinoma in the United States. Prognostic features, treatment outcome, and survival. *Cancer.* 1996;77:2217–2222.
241. Huang MA, Marrero JA. Hepatocellular carcinoma. *Curr Opin Gastroenterol.* 2002;18:345–350.
242. Mathieu D, Grenier P, Larde D, et al. Portal vein involvement in hepatocellular carcinoma: dynamic CT features. *Radiology.* 1984;152:127–132.
243. Murphy BJ, Casillas J, Ros PR, et al. The CT appearance of cystic masses of the liver. *Radiographics.* 1989;9:307–322.
244. Daniele B, Perrone F. Staging for liver cancer. *Clin Liver Dis.* 2005;9:vi, 213–223..
245. Marrero JA, Pelletier S. Hepatocellular carcinoma. *Clin Liver Dis.* 2006;10:ix, 339–351.
246. Bruix J, Sherman M, Llovet JM, et al. Clinical management of hepatocellular carcinoma. Conclusions of the Barcelona–2000 EASL conference. European Association for the Study of the Liver. *J Hepatol.* 2001;35:421–430.
247. Inamoto K, Sugiki K, Yamasaki H, et al. CT of hepatoma: effects of portal vein obstruction. *AJR Am J Roentgenol.* 1981;136:349–353.
248. LaBerge JM, Laing FC, Federle MP, et al. Hepatocellular carcinoma: assessment of resectability by computed tomography and ultrasound. *Radiology.* 1984;152:485–490.
249. Sherman M, Takayama Y. Screening and treatment for hepatocellular carcinoma. *Gastroenterol Clin North Am.* 2004;33:xi, 671–691.
250. Haliloglu M, Hoffer FA, Gronemeyer SA, et al. 3D gadolinium-enhanced MRA: evaluation of hepatic vasculature in children with hepatoblastoma. *J Magn Reson Imaging.* 2000;11:65–68.
251. Kreft B, Strunk H, Flacke S, et al. Detection of thrombosis in the portal venous system: comparison of contrast-enhanced MR angiography with intraarterial digital subtraction angiography. *Radiology.* 2000;216:86–92.
252. Nguyen BD. Pancreatic neuroendocrine tumor with portal vein tumor thrombus: PET demonstration. *Clin Nucl Med.* 2005;30:628–629.
253. Kalra MK, Maher MM, Sahani DV, et al. Current status of imaging in pancreatic diseases. *J Comput Assist Tomogr.* 2002;26:661–675.
254. Horton KM, Fishman EK. Multidetector CT angiography of pancreatic carcinoma: part I, evaluation of arterial involvement. *AJR Am J Roentgenol.* 2002;178:827–831.
255. Raptopoulos V, Steer ML, Sheiman RG, et al. The use of helical CT and CT angiography to predict vascular involvement from pancreatic cancer: correlation with findings at surgery. *AJR Am J Roentgenol.* 1997;168:971–977.
256. Lu DS, Reber HA, Krasny RM, et al. Local staging of pancreatic cancer: criteria for unresectability of major vessels as revealed by pancreatic-phase, thin-section helical CT. *AJR Am J Roentgenol.* 1997;168:1439–1443.
257. Nakayama Y, Yamashita Y, Kadota M, et al. Vascular encasement by pancreatic cancer: correlation of CT findings with surgical and pathologic results. *J Comput Assist Tomogr.* 2001;25:337–342.
258. Gaa J, Wendl K, Tesdal IK, et al. [Combined use of MRI and MR cholangiopancreatography and contrast enhanced dual phase 3-D MR angiography in diagnosis of pancreatic tumors: initial clinical results.] *Rofo.* 1999;170:528–533.
259. McNulty NJ, Francis IR, Platt JF, et al. Multi-detector row helical CT of the pancreas: effect of contrast-enhanced multiphasic imaging on enhancement of the pancreas, peripancreatic vasculature, and pancreatic adenocarcinoma. *Radiology.* 2001;220:97–102.
260. Fishman EK, Horton KM, Urban BA. Multidetector CT angiography in the evaluation of pancreatic carcinoma: preliminary observations. *J Comput Assist Tomogr.* 2000; 24:849–853.
261. Pamuklar E, Semelka RC. MR imaging of the pancreas. *Magn Reson Imaging Clin N Am.* 2005;13:313–330.
262. Punch J. Hepatic transplantation. In: Mulholland MW, Lillemoe KD, Doherty GM, et al., eds. *Greenfield's Surgery: Scientific Principles and Practice.* Philadelphia: Lippincott Williams & Wilkins; 2006;590–609.
263. Mazzaferro V, Regalia E, Doci R, et al. Liver transplantation for the treatment of small hepatocellular carcinomas in patients with cirrhosis. *N Engl J Med.* 1996;334:693–699.
264. Redvanly RD, Nelson RC, Stieber AC, et al. Imaging in the preoperative evaluation of adult liver-transplant candidates: goals, merits of various procedures, and recommendations. *AJR Am J Roentgenol.* 1995;164:611–617.
265. Pandharipande PV, Lee VS, Morgan GR, et al. Vascular and extravascular complications of liver transplantation: comprehensive evaluation with three-dimensional contrast-enhanced volumetric MR imaging and MR cholangiopancreatography. *AJR Am J Roentgenol.* 2001;177:1101–1107.
266. Sahani D, D'Souza R, Kadavigere R, et al. Evaluation of living liver transplant donors: method for precise anatomic definition by using a dedicated contrast-enhanced MR imaging protocol. *Radiographics.* 2004;24:957–967.
267. Urata K, Kawasaki S, Matsunami H, et al. Calculation of child and adult standard liver volume for liver transplantation. *Hepatology.* 1995;21:1317–1321.
268. Tokunaga Y, Tanaka K, Uemoto S, et al. Experience with vascular grafts in living related liver transplantation. *Transplant Proc.* 1994;26:896–897.
269. Dalen K, Day DL, Ascher NL, et al. Imaging of vascular complications after hepatic transplantation. *AJR Am J Roentgenol.* 1988;150:1285–1290.
270. Cheng YF, Chen CL, Huang TL, et al. Single imaging modality evaluation of living donors in liver transplantation: magnetic resonance imaging. *Transplantation.* 2001;72: 1527–1533.
271. Schroeder T, Nadalin S, Stattaus J, et al. Potential living liver donors: evaluation with an all-in-one protocol with multi-detector row CT. *Radiology.* 2002;224:586–591.
272. Eubank WB, Wherry KL, Maki JH, et al. Preoperative evaluation of patients awaiting liver transplantation: comparison of multiphasic contrast-enhanced 3D magnetic resonance to helical computed tomography examinations. *J Magn Reson Imaging.* 2002;16:565–575.
273. Goyen M, Barkhausen J, Debatin JF, et al. Right-lobe living related liver transplantation: evaluation of a comprehensive magnetic resonance imaging protocol for assessing potential donors. *Liver Transpl.* 2002;8:241–250.
274. Yeh BM, Breiman RS, Taouli B, et al. Biliary tract depiction in living potential liver donors: comparison of conventional MR, mangafodipir trisodium-enhanced excretory MR, and multi-detector row CT cholangiography—initial experience. *Radiology.* 2004;230:645–651.
275. Schroeder T, Malago M, Debatin JF, et al. "All-in-one" imaging protocols for the evaluation of potential living liver donors: comparison of magnetic resonance imaging and multidetector computed tomography. *Liver Transpl.* 2005;11:776–787.
276. Schroeder T, Radtke A, Kuehl H, et al. Evaluation of living liver donors with an all-inclusive 3D multi-detector row CT protocol. *Radiology.* 2006;238:900–910.
277. Cheng YF, Huang TL, Lui CC, et al. Magnetic resonance venography in potential pediatric liver transplant recipients. *Clin Transplant.* 1997;11:121–126.
278. Stafford-Johnson DB, Hamilton BH, Dong Q, et al. Vascular complications of liver transplantation: evaluation with gadolinium-enhanced MR angiography. *Radiology.* 1998;207:153–160.

279. Humar A, Dunn DL. Transplantation. In: Brunicardi FC, Anderson DK, Billiar TR, et al., eds. *Schwartz's Principles of Surgery*. 8th ed. New York: McGraw-Hill Companies Inc. 2005:295–331.
280. Oh CK, Pelletier SJ, Sawyer RG, et al. Uni- and multi-variate analysis of risk factors for early and late hepatic artery thrombosis after liver transplantation. *Transplantation*. 2001;71:767–772.
281. Bhattacharjya S, Gunson BK, Mirza DF, et al. Delayed hepatic artery thrombosis in adult orthotopic liver transplantation—a 12-year experience. *Transplantation*. 2001;71:1592–1596.
282. Borsa JJ, Daly CP, Fontaine AB, et al. Treatment of inferior vena cava anastomotic stenoses with the Wallstent endoprosthesis after orthotopic liver transplantation. *J Vasc Interv Radiol*. 1999;10:17–22.
283. Wilke N, Jerosch-Herold M, Wang Y, et al. Myocardial perfusion reserve: assessment with multisection, quantitative, first-pass MR imaging. *Radiology*. 1997;204:373–384.
284. Wilke NM, Jerosch-Herold M, Zenovich A, et al. Magnetic resonance first-pass myocardial perfusion imaging: clinical validation and future applications. *J Magn Reson Imaging*. 1999;10:676–685.
285. Penzkofer H, Wintersperger BJ, Knez A, et al. Assessment of myocardial perfusion using multisection first-pass MRI and color-coded parameter maps: a comparison to 99mTc Sesta MIBI SPECT and systolic myocardial wall thickening analysis. *Magn Reson Imaging*. 1999;17:161–170.
286. Lauenstein TC, Ajaj W, Narin B, et al. MR imaging of apparent small-bowel perfusion for diagnosing mesenteric ischemia: feasibility study. *Radiology*. 2005;234:569–575.

Renal Vasculature

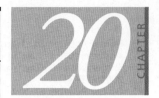

Stefan O. Schoenberg
Henrik J. Michaely
Christoph R. Becker

BACKGROUND

Spectrum and Prevalence of Diseases

The renal arteries can be affected by virtually any type of disease ranging from atherosclerotic occlusive diseases such as renal artery stenosis (RAS), dysplastic changes of the renal artery wall, aneurysmal disease, and vasculitis. The diagnostic evaluation of the renal arteries plays a pivotal role in the comprehensive clinical assessment of various systemic diseases such as hypertension. Also, a multitude of systemic diseases such as essential hypertension, rheumatologic, and infectious diseases as well as various urologic disorders can affect the kidneys with potentially life-threatening consequences such as renal failure with lifelong dialysis (1). In this context, imaging of the renal arteries repre-

sents only one facet of diagnostic requirements for detection and staging of disease. Multiple imaging techniques may need to be applied to integrate the evaluation of the renal arteries into a larger diagnostic concept also addressing the renal parenchyma in terms of malignant disease; inflammatory changes; and functioning in terms of perfusion, filtration, and excretion (2) (Fig. 20-1). In addition, morphologic and functional assessment of the urinary out-flow tract may be required.

Unique Considerations for Imaging of the Renal Vasculature

Cross-sectional imaging of the renal arteries has been challenging over the last decade and remains until today. The reason for this is threefold. First, there have been established

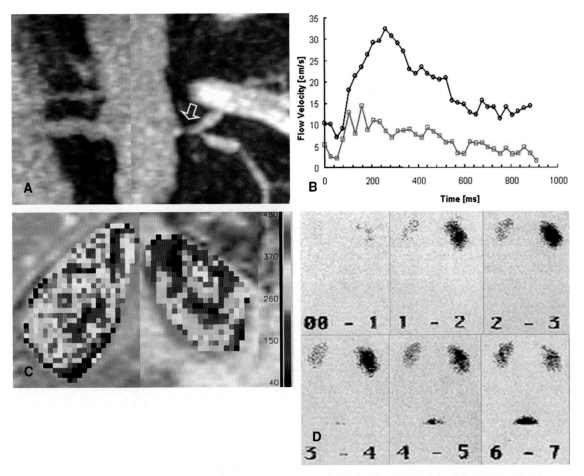

FIGURE 20-1 Comprehensive renal MR examination in a patient with high-grade left RAS (*arrow*) in the MRA **(A)**, which was acquired in the steady state after the administration of an ultrasmall superparamagnetic iron oxide (USPIO) intravascular contrast agent (NC100150). **B:** The phase-contrast flow measurements revealed a normal flow of the right renal artery (*black line*) and a pathologic flow profile on the left side with loss of the early systolic peak and diminished flow volume (*red line*). **C:** The T2*-renal perfusion measurement during the first-pass of NC100150 shows a substantially reduced perfusion of the left kidney, as shown in this color-coded parameter map of the renal blood flow per 100 g of tissue per minute. **D:** This patient also underwent renal scintigraphy, which confirmed the MR findings of a delayed perfusion and decreased function of the left kidney (dorsoposterior projection).

invasive and noninvasive imaging techniques such as intraarterial digital subtraction angiography (DSA), Doppler ultrasound (US), and scintigraphy, which have managed to maintain their role for diagnostic evaluation until today. The advantages of DSA are the high temporal and spatial resolution as well as the possibility to directly intervene in the renal artery pathology such as dilating of a RAS, coiling of a renal artery aneurysm, fenestration and renal artery dissection, or embolization of arterial segment in a trauma setting. Doppler US is a readily available, noninvasive bedside technique. In addition to the hemodynamic evaluation of the renal arteries, it also allows for an assessment of the renal parenchymal morphology and blood flow. Renal scintigraphy was the first technique that allowed semiquantitative assessment of renal function by measurements of the clearance rate including filtration and excre-

tion kinetics. This method has been the established modality for a preinterventional assessment of renal function prior to dilatation of RAS or assessment of the contralateral kidney prior to donor or tumor nephrectomy.

Compared with the diagnostic information available from the combined use of these three modalities, MR angiography initially played almost no role in the evaluation of the renal arteries. The reason for this is the particularly challenging anatomy of the renal arteries and the substantial effects of motion on this vessel territory during the cardiac and respiratory cycles. The initially available time-of-flight (TOF) techniques required scanning times of several minutes leading to substantial motion artifacts, which made a large fraction of all exams virtually uninterpretable. In addition, the tortuous course of the renal arteries resulted in artifacts from in-plane saturation of slow flow. Stenosis or focal dilatations with acceleration or deceleration of flow resulted in severe dephasing artifacts mimicking complete occlusion of the vessel. Overall, only the proximal portions of the renal arteries were usually well seen, while the smaller intrarenal branches were not adequately displayed (4). Although functional MR techniques such as flow measurements were already available in the early days of MR imaging, the long acquisition times did not allow integration of these various techniques into a single comprehensive morphologic and function exam.

The spatial resolution of magnetic resonance imaging (MRI) has been about 10-fold lower than that of DSA over most of the decade, which made the grading of small pathologic changes such as wall irregularities in fibromuscular dysplasia (FMD) virtually impossible, in particular when intrarenal branches are affected. On the other hand, computed tomography angiography (CTA) immediately started off with high spatial resolution within the imaging plane of less than 0.5 mm; however, the slice thickness of the individual cross-sectional images was 3 mm for the initial spiral CT scanners. With the advent of multidetector computed tomography (MDCT) scanners, the acquisition of thinner sections has enabled the rapid acquisition of high-resolution scans (Fig. 20-2). Despite short scan times and high resolution, however, the benefits of a functional assessment of the renal arteries has limited the role of CT in the primary evaluation of some renal arterial disorders. Also, patients undergoing evaluation of the renal arteries may be azotemic, limiting the use of iodinated contrast agents in larger amounts.

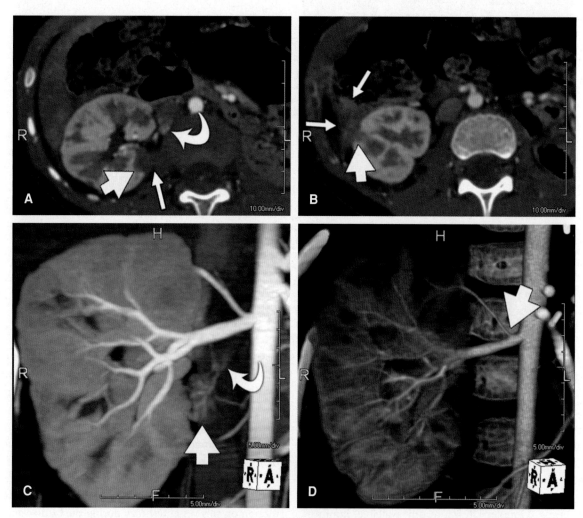

FIGURE 20-2 Intrarenal and intralymph node arterial visualization in a 5-year-old boy with nephroblastomatosis. A: Transverse CT section from a 4-row MDCT scan obtained with 1.25-mm section thickness demonstrates an abnormal infiltrative soft tissue density involving the posterior midzone of the right kidney (*wide arrow*) and abutting the right psoas muscle (*small arrow*). There is a hypervascular lymph node in the renal hilum (*curved arrow*). **B:** A second area of infiltrative soft tissue density involves the lateral aspect of the lower pole (*wide arrow*) involving the lateral conal fascia (*small arrows*). **C:** Slab MIP demonstrates the lymph node and its internal arteries (*wide arrow*) as well as its vascular pedicle (*curved arrow*). **D:** Volume-rendered image demonstrates prehilar branching of the right renal artery (*arrow*). (Figure courtesy of Pietro Sedati and Geoffrey D. Rubin.)

Advantages of CT and MR

Despite the described challenges for cross-sectional imaging of the renal arteries due to the difficulties from the influence of vascular anatomy and physiologic effects, dramatic technical improvements within the last 5 years have led to a key role of CT and MR imaging for the assessment of renal artery disease. With the introduction of three-dimensional gadolinium-enhanced magnetic resonance angiography (3D Gd-MRA), the limitations of spatial resolution and long scan times as well as artifacts due to in-plane saturation and turbulent blood flow have diminished. Within a single breath-hold, high-resolution data sets of the renal arteries can now be acquired with isotropic spatial resolution of less than 1 mm, thereby coming close to the spatial resolution of DSA. Due to the short scan times and relatively easy set-up, 3D Gd-MRA can now be combined with other morphological and functional MR techniques within one patient examination for a comprehensive assessment of renal disease. These additional techniques include high-resolution imaging with morphologic sequences for detection and characterization of benign and malignant renal masses, phase-contrast (PC) flow measurements for detection and grading of RAS, time-resolved measurements of renal perfusion, and excretion and infiltration for detection of underlying parenchymal disease as well as high-resolution MR urography for detection and grading of urinary outflow obstruction, congenital abnormalities, or transitional cell carcinoma of the urinary tract. Due to the high gradient strength of current state-of-the-art MR scanners, as well as the introduction of parallel acquisition, all of these techniques can now be limited to exam times of a few minutes, allowing for a comprehensive assessment within less than 1 hour (5).

For CT, similar revolutionary achievements have been made within the last 10 years. These include the transition from single row to MDCT, which now allows to not only assess the territory of the renal arteries with isotropic spatial resolution of approximately 0.5 mm in all directions but also to cover a large scan volume of the human body within a short period of time (6). Thus, MDCT plays a pivotal role in the emergency evaluation of acute vascular injury, such as blunt trauma or dissection, since not only the renal arteries, but also the entire aorta can be scanned within less than 20 seconds (Fig. 20-3). CT also plays a key role when high-resolution imaging of the arterial wall or lumen is required to correctly characterize complex renal arterial abnormalities (Fig. 20-4).

CT IMAGING STRATEGIES

Within the last decade, CTA of the renal arteries improved significantly by the introduction of MDCT.

With more detector rows and faster gantry rotation, these new CT scanners allow for both at the same time, faster acquisition of a certain scan volume, and higher spatial resolution. Short scan times also allow for condensed contrast bolus administration in order to improve the enhancement of the vascular structures. Both high spatial resolution and high-contrast enhancement lead to an improved visualization of even the smallest vessels in the periphery of pole arteries of the kidney. Because of the short scan time and fast contrast injection, administration of contrast media in CTA of the renal arteries with MDCT is of special concern. High-pressure contrast injectors are mandatory for MDCT and are commonly combined with a dual-syringe system for sequential injection of contrast media and a saline flush.

Reconstruction with a soft tissue kernel can lead to "blooming" of renal arterial calcium, which may hinder the detection of stenoses or tent to overestimate the degree of stenoses in particular at the origin of the renal arteries. Higher spatial resolution in MDCT and the use of sharper reconstruction kernels may help to reduce the "blooming artifact"; however, image noise increases with sharper kernels.

CTA provides detailed morphologic information of the renal arteries such as aneurysm, dissection, or thrombosis; yet, it provides little functional information beyond qualitative regional perfusion.

CT Acquisition

Nuances of Acquisition Strategies

The optimal scan range of the renal arteries begins at the level of the diaphragm and extends down to include the internal iliac arteries. This ensures that all accessory renal arteries are included in the scan volume. A precontrast low-dose scan may help to differentiate a renal hematoma or calcification of the renal arteries.

The optimal acquisition parameters for a renal CTA depend on the MDCT scanner used. The slice thickness should be in the range of 0.5 and 1.25 mm, pitch 1 and 1.5, rotation time 0.33 and 0.8 seconds. X-ray exposure parameters, kVp, and mAs, may then be adapted to patients' habitus, body weight, and size to result in images with low image noise. Automatic attenuation adapted x-ray tube current modulation allows for constant image quality throughout different patients. To avoid the necessity to segment and cut out bowel loops for postprocessing and visualization of the renal arteries, positive oral contrast should not be given.

A delayed scan may help to assess the renal parenchyma for any infarction, tumor, or cystic lesion and also to determine the course and filling of the renal veins, renal pelvis, and ureters. Delayed scans may also help to detect contrast

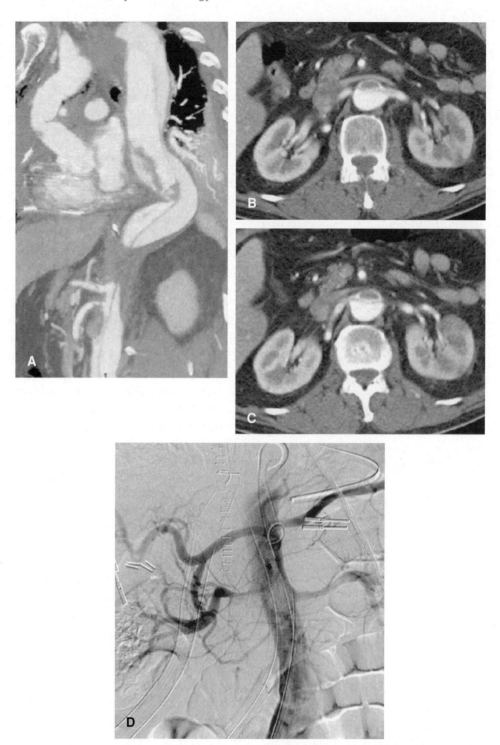

FIGURE 20-3 A 64-year-old man who presented with an acute dissection of the abdominal aorta extending to the superior mesenteric artery as well as to the left and right renal artery. Three-millimeter-thick sagittal **(A)** and transverse **(B, C)** views from a 64-row multidetector CTA with a collimation of 0.6 mm and the DSA in coronal view **(D)** during the intervention are shown. There is a large thrombus in the true lumen (seen en face in the DSA as an oval filling defect). MDCT clearly demonstrates the thrombus partially occluding the ostium of both renal arteries and leading to a tapering appearance of the right renal artery on DSA. Pigtail catheters have been placed into the true and the false lumen of the aorta prior to fenestration.

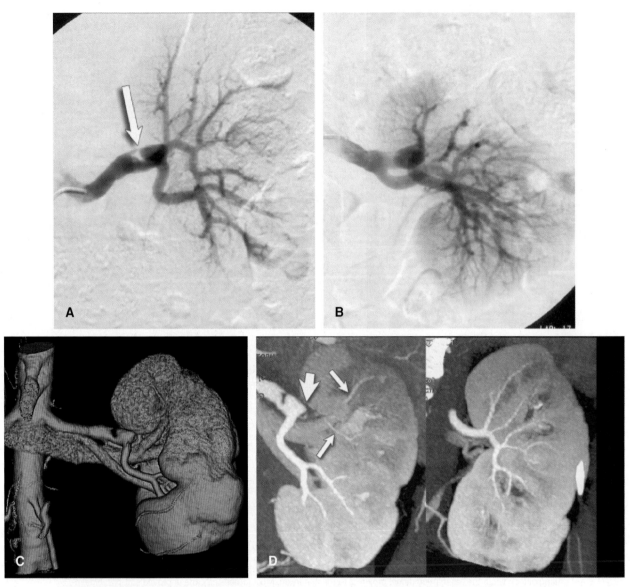

FIGURE 20-4 A 33-year-old male with 6-month history of refractory hypertension. An initial MRA examination (not shown) performed at 1.5T with gadolinium enhancement failed to allow prospective recognition of any renal vascular abnormality; however, irregularities in the renal parenchyma suggested a diagnosis of chronic pyelonephritis. Inconsistencies between this imaging diagnosis and the clinical presentation led to a catheter arteriogram. **A:** Selective left renal arterial injection demonstrates an abnormality of the distal right main renal artery (*arrow*). It was difficult to ascertain at the time of the examination whether this represented multiple branching structures that were overlapping or whether this represented an aneurysm with a filling defect. **B:** Image obtained in the early nephrographic phase of the arteriogram demonstrates poor parenchymal opacification in the lateral aspect of the upper pole extending to the midzone. Although five different projections of the renal artery were obtained during the course of the examination, greater clarity of the anatomic relationship of the renal artery abnormality could not be ascertained. The specific nature of the abnormality, which was felt to most likely represent aneurysm and the mechanism of regional renal arterial hypoperfusion, were not clear. The appearance of a web-like filling defect proximal to the aneurysmal abnormality was considered as a possible intrinsic renal lesion due to vasculitis or fibromuscular dysplasia but was only visualized on the single view **(B)**. Finally, the relationship of the abnormality to the renal parenchyma was important to determine, as it was likely that an operation would be required to treat this lesion, and its relationship to the renal parenchyma was critical to determining whether the operation could be performed in situ or ex vivo. **C:** Volume rendering from a CT angiogram provides a 3D representation of the abnormality and most notably establishes its presence within the renal hilum, though external to the renal parenchyma. The color scale with purplish tones representing lower attenuation and pinker tones representing higher attenuation indicates the zone of poor renal perfusion to a much greater extent than is evident from the arteriogram. **D:** Three-centimeter thick-slab MIPs of the anterior and posterior halves of the kidney illustrate the complex anatomy that was difficult to separate on the projection arteriogram **(A, B)**. The posterior half of the kidney **(right)** is perfused by a single branch with segmental branches reaching all posterior renal lobes. On the anterior image **(left)**, two thin arrows indicate sequestered intrarenal branches, which are separated from the apparent apex of the aneurysm (*wide arrow*) by 1 to 2 cm distance. The parenchyma distal to the small intrarenal branches is hypoperfused. Note that a branch from the aneurysm to the lower pole provides adequate supply to the anterior lower pole. (*Figure 20-4 continues*)

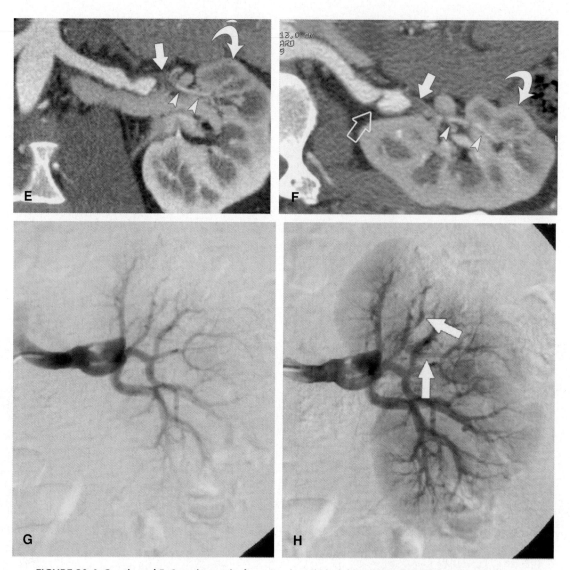

FIGURE 20-4 Continued E: Curved coronal reformation through the left renal artery establishes that there is no filling defect within the renal artery defect proximal to the aneurysm. Most importantly, the improved soft tissue delineation available from the single voxel thick reformation illustrates thrombus at the apex of the aneurysm (*wide arrow*) extending to one of the small intrarenal branches (*arrowheads*), which in turns supplies a zone of the anterior upper pole, which is both hypoattenuative and demonstrates cortical thinning (*curved arrow*). These abnormalities are similarly displayed on a curved transverse reformation **(F)** with the additional visualization of a weblike filling defect within the aneurysm (*open arrow*), likely representing partial recanalization of thrombus within the aneurysm. The mechanism of hypertension is now evident, as two anterior upper polar segmental renal branches that once were in direct contiguity with the main renal artery are being supplied through intrarenal collaterals because thrombus at the apex of the aneurysm has blocked prograde flow to these branches. The resulted ischemia to the anterior upper pole is presumably the cause of hypertension. **G, H:** In retrospect, the two intrarenal branches can be observed (*white arrows*) to fill on delayed images only from the arteriogram. The patient underwent an ex vivo repair with resection of the aneurysmal segment and transplantation of the intrarenal branches with subsequent resolution of hypertension. (Images courtesy of Geoffrey D. Rubin.)

media extravasation, laceration, rupture, and contusion after traumatic renal injury.

For CTA scanning of the renal arteries in transplanted kidneys, the scan field needs to be adapted to the pelvis.

Contrast Medium

The amount of contrast media mainly depends on the scan time and contrast media flow rate. Contrast media flow rates may range between 3 and 5 mL/second depending on location and diameter of the intravenous access. The higher flow rates improve the visualization of smaller vessels by higher opacification. Highly concentrated contrast media (370 or 400 mg/mL iodine) may also improve the visualization but requires administration at body temperature because of the high viscosity of these contrast media. A saline flush may help to reduce the amount of contrast media necessary for a CTA and improves the opacification of the renal arteries by keeping the contrast bolus compact.

Postprocessing

The exclusive use of transverse reconstructions for interpreting renal arterial CTA is challenging and fraught with peril (Fig. 20-5). The high-resolution data set by MDCT is ideally suited for postprocessing to improve visualization of the findings. Curved multiplanar reformation (MPR) allows one to visualize the entire course of both arteries within the same image. A disadvantage of curved MPR is the manual pathfinding process that is time consuming. In the worst case, MPR may create "pseudo-stenoses" by off-center reconstruction. Automatic pathfinding is superior in this respect and creates a stretched view of the arteries from a centerline position. The reconstruction angle can be changed to any direction to enable visualization from any perspective. This kind of reconstruction also allows for curved measurements of the degree and length of the renal artery stenoses in order to provide important information prior to an intervention. It is also important to assess the composition of the underlying atherosclerosis prior to the invasive therapy. Perpendicular MPR at the location of the stenosis may help to differentiate between eccentric and concentric manifestation of plaques in the renal artery wall, giving a hint for the differential diagnosis between atherosclerosis and vasculitis (Fig. 20-6).

Maximum intensity projections (MIP) should be generated along the course and separated for both renal arteries, in left and right anterior oblique projection. MIP reconstruction will fail to visualize RAS in case of severe calcifications.

Volume rendering (VR) is primarily suited to display the anatomy of the vessels, such as in the case of complex multivessel supply and drainage of the kidney (Fig. 20-7). In particular, in renal transplants, VR is helpful and allows for easy assessment of renal artery anatomy and pathology such as kinking and stenoses. Calcifications may cause false-negative results in VR, and renal artery stenoses are commonly overestimated. Manual segmentation of the bones may become necessary to display the renal arteries from any perspective.

VR should not be used to grade stenoses, as it will not display the interface between calcium and the arterial lumen accurately and can both under- or overestimate non-calcified stenoses (Fig. 20-8). In many other pathologies (e.g. renal artery dissection and thrombosed aneurysms), however, it is essential to review the planar reformations.

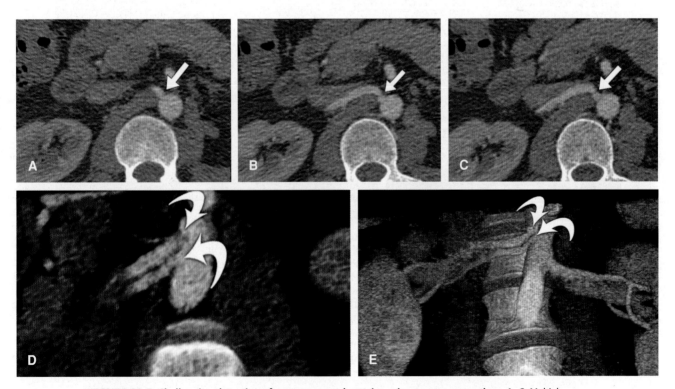

FIGURE 20-5 Challenging detection of accessory renal arteries using transverse sections. A–C: Multiple transverse CTA sections suggest the presence of two right renal arteries, but they are difficult to distinguish from one another in the transverse plane (*small arrows*). **D, E:** Two coronal oblique volume-rendered images with a 5-mm slab **(D)** and a 40-mm slab **(E)** clearly demonstrate two distinct right renal arteries (*curved arrows*). (Figure courtesy of Pietro Sedati and Geoffrey D. Rubin.)

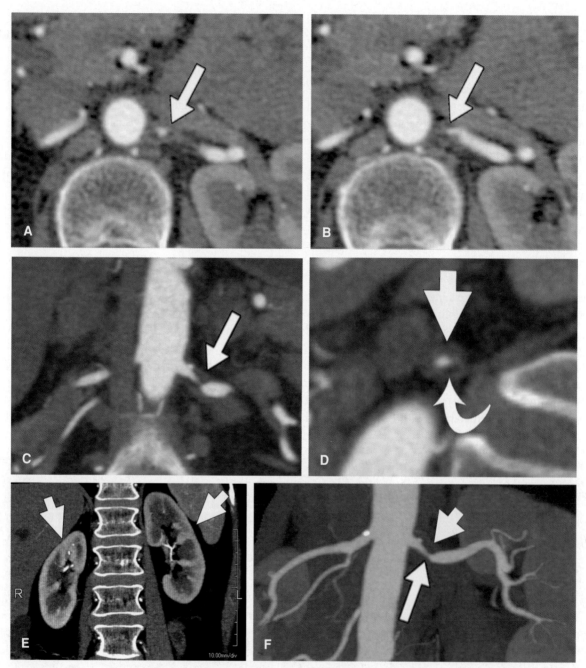

FIGURE 20-6 Renal artery CTA: comparison of visualization techniques. A, B: Contiguous transverse images demonstrate proximal left RAS (*arrows*). **C:** Oblique MPR parallel to the long axis of the left renal artery provides an orientation that demonstrates a greater portion of the artery in the region of the stenosis (*arrow*), but neither displays the entire artery nor does it document the full degree of luminal narrowing. **D:** Oblique MPR perpendicular to the right RAS documents the absolute luminal restriction but does not provide context for the narrowing relative to a normal segment of the artery. Both fatty and soft tissue attenuation components of the mural atheroma are visible (*curved arrow*). Expansion of the outer wall of the artery is a manifestation of positive remodeling (*big arrow*). When stenosis measurements are made relative to the outer wall, percent luminal narrowing may be overestimated relative to normal luminal dimensions. **E:** Coronal MPR image demonstrates less enhancement of the left renal parenchyma compared with the right (*arrows*). **F:** Coronal MIP demonstrates a portion of the atheroma (*short arrow*) without the possibility to evaluate the inferior margin of the plaque due to the superimposed left renal vein (*long arrow*). (*Figure 20-6 continues*)

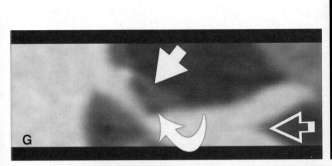

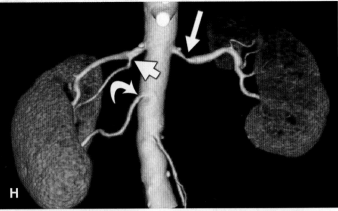

FIGURE 20-6 Continued G: Curved planar reformat (CPR) demonstrates the fatty elements within the atheroma (*curved arrow*) and the extent of positive remodeling (*big arrow*). Open arrow indicates a loop artifact. **H:** Coronal 3D volume-rendered image demonstrates proximal left RAS (*long arrow*) within the context of adjacent arterial anatomy, including prehilar branching of the main right renal artery (*wide arrow*), and an accessory right renal artery (*curved arrow*). The atheroma is not visualized on the volume rendering. Note the decreased enhancement of the left kidney compared with the right. (Figure courtesy of Pietro Sedati and Geoffrey D. Rubin.)

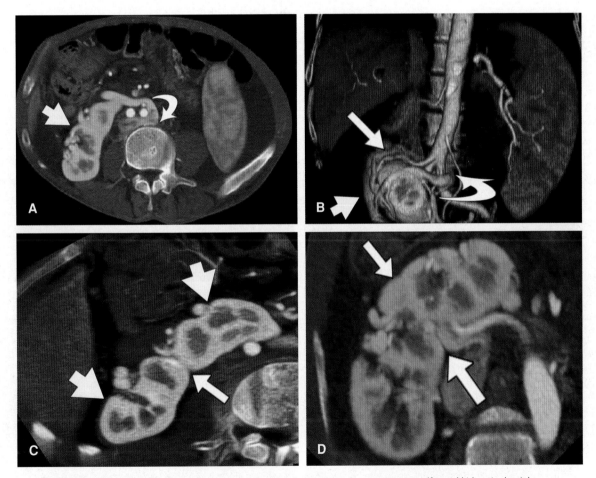

FIGURE 20-7 Cross-fused renal ectopia. A: Transverse CT section demonstrates a malformed kidney in the right renal fossa (*big arrow*) and large circumiliac draining vein entering the inferior vena cava (*curved arrow*). **B:** Volume rendering documents absence of the left kidney and presence of the abnormal kidney in the right renal fossa (*short arrow*). There are multiple large venous channels (*long arrow*) draining into the inferior vena cava and one of the renal veins via the circumiliac course (*curved arrow*). **C:** Transverse volume rendering through the inferior aspect of the kidney (*wide arrows*) demonstrates an indentation at the level of the fusion between right and left kidneys (*thin arrow*). **D:** Coronal oblique MPR image shows the plane between the fused kidneys (*arrows*). (*Figure 20-7 continues*)

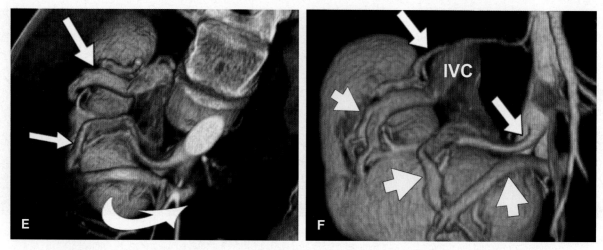

FIGURE 20-7 Continued E: Oblique volume rendering illustrates the complex relationships of both the arterial supply and the venous drainage (*straight arrows*). The curved arrow indicates the circumiliac course of the renal vein. **F:** There are two renal arteries (*long arrows*) and three renal veins (*wide arrows*). (Figure courtesy of Pietro Sedati and Geoffrey D. Rubin.)

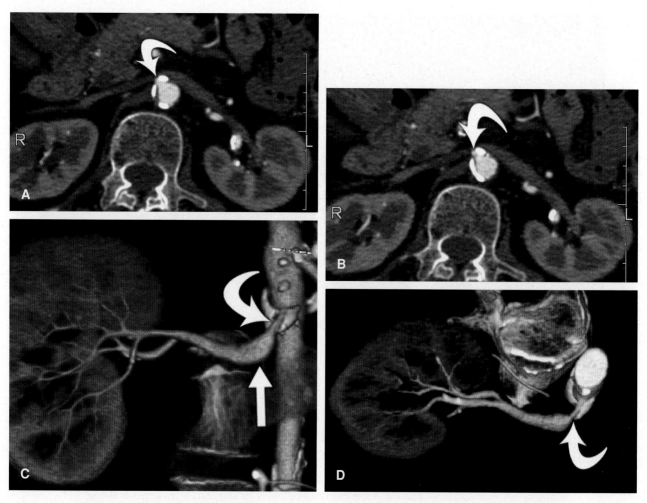

FIGURE 20-8 Right RAS and calcification. A, B: Contiguous transverse sections from a CTA illustrate the challenge of detecting and characterizing RAS (*curved arrow*) when the artery has an oblique course. **C, D:** Volume renderings allow identification of the renal artery along its entire course and provide a clearer display of the stenosis (*curved arrow*) and associated poststenotic dilation (*straight arrow*). Appropriate selection of view angles allows the stenosis to be visualized free of overlying calcifications. (*Figure 20-8 continues*)

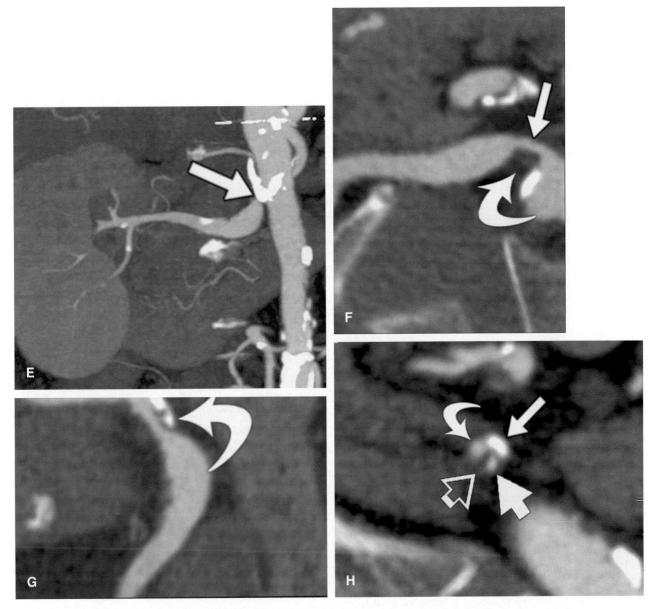

FIGURE 20-8 Continued E: MIP does not allow visualization of the stenosis through the calcification (*arrow*). **F, G:** Curved planar reformations generated 90° apart provide the best depiction of the stenosis (*straight arrow*) relative to the calcified and noncalcified plaques (*curved arrows*), while also showing the aorta and the distal renal artery. **H:** Oblique MPR generated perpendicular to the center line of the renal artery at the point of maximal stenosis illustrates the cross-sectional area of the residual stenosis (*curved arrow*), varying degrees of calcification in plaque (*thin and wide arrows*), and noncalcified plaque (*open arrow*). (Figure courtesy of Pietro Sedati and Geoffrey D. Rubin.)

Transverse sections and MPRs of the abdominal aorta allow determination of the renal arterial supply from the false or true lumen. Eccentric thrombus formation and calcifications in an aneurysm sac may be best seen in the axial slices.

MR IMAGING STRATEGIES

MR Acquisition

Generally, it has to be stated that an optimized protocol of 3D Gd-MRA balances three factors—anatomic cover-age, spatial resolution, and scan time. Current results on the accuracy for stenosis grading require a spatial resolution of less than 1 mm isotropic in all anatomic directions and breath-hold times of less than 20 seconds. For this reason, MR scanners with a high gradient strength of a minimum of 30 mT/m and a rise time of 200 μsec or less should be used in conjunction with techniques for faster k-space acquisition, such as parallel acquisition techniques, asymmetric k-space sampling, or spiral echo-planar imaging.

To fulfill the requirements of anatomic coverage and spatial resolution, 3D contrast-enhanced MRA with fast 3D gradient-echo (GRE) sequences and bolus administration of gadolinium chelates is the only technique that is reliable and accurate in clinical routine. Standard TOF techniques have virtually disappeared from clinical use due to the multitude of artifacts and long scan times. However, currently evolving free-breathing navigator-corrected steady-state free precession (SSFP) techniques might play a role in the near future for high-resolution imaging of the renal arteries without contrast agents (8). Likewise, 3D Gd-MRA can be applied in a free-breathing high-resolution mode when intravascular blood-pool contrast agents have been applied; however, none of these agents is currently approved for clinical use (9), although the strong albumin-binding Gd-chelate MS-325 is on the doorstep of clinical availability.

Breath-hold 3D Gd-MRA is usually performed with a field of view of approximately 40 cm and a thickness of the 3D slab of 8 to 10 cm to ensure complete anatomic coverage of the renal arteries, but smaller fields of view may be preferable to improve spatial resolution. A coronal orientation of this 3D slab is used since this ideally remodels the course of the abdominal aorta and the renal arteries and thus allows minimizing the acquisition volume. To further minimize the acquisition time, usually a rectangular field of view is used in the left-to-right direction, but this approach is prone to aliasing from the arms outside the field of view. Usually, this does not substantially degrade the image if the arms are only aliasing into the flanks of the abdomen lateral to the kidney margins. However, in thin individuals, those aliasing artifacts can overlay on the renal arteries themselves, thus requiring the need for a full quadratic field of view. Caution also needs to be taken when parallel acquisition techniques are used, since in that case aliasing artifacts can be propagated into the center of the image, thereby substantially limiting the evaluation of the renal arteries. For 1 mm isotropic spatial resolution, matrix sizes of at least 448 or 512 frequency and phase-encoding steps should be used. Also, acquisition time should be ideally less than 20 seconds, since it is known that even in the case of a perfect breath-holding capacity of the patient, two different physiological processes other than cardiac pulsation result in gradual motion of the vascular bed of the renal arteries. First, there is an involuntary relaxation of the diaphragm over the breath-hold period, resulting in a gradual shift of the retroperitoneum. Second, it has been shown that random involuntary motion is induced by contractions of the diaphragm, which can neither be eliminated by respiratory nor by cardiac gating (10).

In order to understand the challenges for breath-hold high-resolution MRI of the renal arteries, one needs to look into a closer detail of the 3D acquisition: With typical repetition times of 5 milliseconds for fast 3D GRE sequences, the acquisition of a full 448 matrix and an 8-cm thick 3D slab with 1 mm slice thickness would require almost 3 minutes. The recent high performance cardiovascular MR scanners now offer repetition times of 3 milliseconds, which by itself will reduce the acquisition time by about 40% to 108 seconds. In addition, asymmetric k-space sampling is now routinely used on most MR scanners in both phase-encoding directions of approximately 25% each, further reducing the acquisition time to only about 60 seconds. With the use of parallel imaging and an acceleration factor of 2, the acquisition time can be approximately reduced by about half to around 30 seconds. Using a rectangular field of view of about 75%, the acquisition then only lasts 23 seconds. This example highlights the importance of state-of-the-art equipment and new k-space acquisition techniques for renal MRA (Fig. 20-9).

In addition to parallel imaging, other authors have proposed two different strategies for reduction of the number of phase-encoding steps. One approach is to use a spiral echo-planar imaging in the left-to-right phase-encoding direction of the 3D volume with conventional cartesian phase encoding in the anterior-to-posterior direction (11). This approach reduces the acquisition time by approximately 20% to 30% due to the more efficient k-space sampling. However, it is prone to artifacts from nonlinearity of the gradients because the long spiral readout leads to higher sensitivity against B0 inhomogeneities, resulting in image blurring. This artifact can be reduced by unwrapping the phase errors in k-space, which requires knowledge of the spatial distribution of the local off-resonance frequencies or by an algorithm that estimates the offset frequencies from the blurred image itself (12).

Overall, two different approaches for arterial phase imaging of the renal arteries are used:

High Spatial Resolution Single-phase Magnetic Resonance Angiography

With this approach, one single high-resolution data set is acquired during the arterial phase of the contrast media transit for pure imaging of the renal arteries without venous overlay. This approach usually requires bolus timing by a prior injection of a small (1–2 mL) amount of contrast media for determination of the transit time (13). Alternatively, the scan can be initiated after automatic detection of the contrast media bolus arrival (14,15) or real-time visualization of the contrast media bolus arrival (16–18). Two acquisition concepts exist to fulfill the spatial resolution requirements within the given acquisition time. Either an ultrafast sequence with further acceleration by parallel imaging is applied to ensure adequate isotropic spatial resolution within a single breath-hold or an elliptical centric k-space acquisition approach is

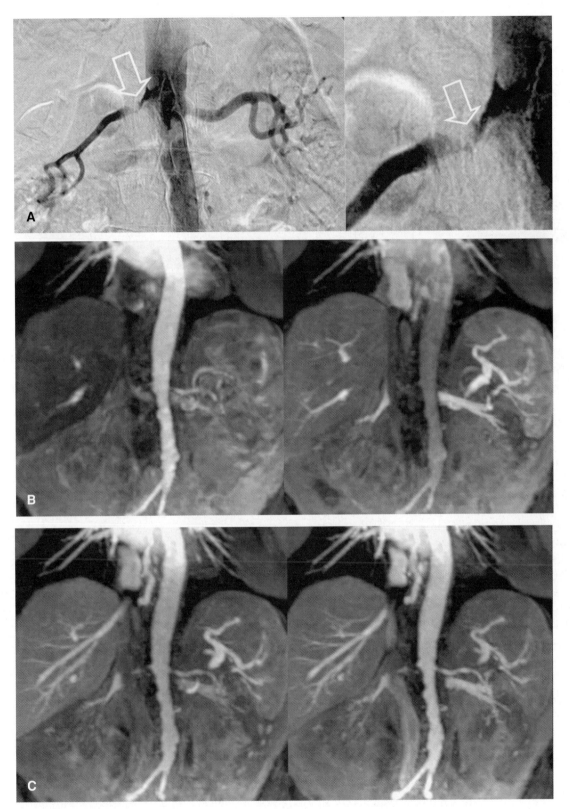

FIGURE 20-9 A: Intra-arterial DSA of a 73-year-old female patient who was suffering from renal hypertension due to her high-grade right-sided RAS (*arrows*). **B:** The magnified view of the stenosis reveals an eccentric narrowing of the renal artery. **C:** The patient then underwent dynamic renal MRA with 2 × 2 mm² in-plane resolution during the first pass of an USPIO contrast agent (SHU 555C). The stenosis can be appreciated on these dynamic images. Since 555C is an intravascular contrast agent, the signal intensity of the vessels remains high even after the first pass. (*Figure 20-9 continues*)

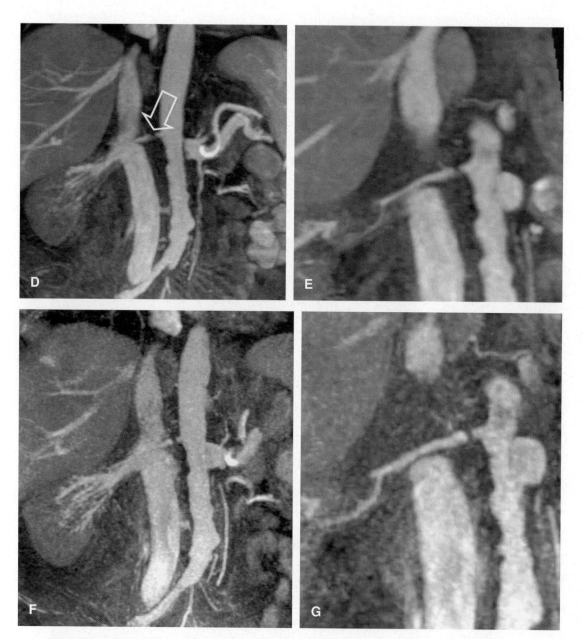

FIGURE 20-9 Continued D: In the high-resolution MRA with an in-plane resolution of 1.3 × 1.3 mm², the stenosis (*arrow*) can be clearly depicted and can be even more appreciated on the magnified view **(E)**. Note that signal is almost exclusively from the vessels, even though this MRA has been acquired during the steady-state phase several minutes after the first injection. Since the contrast agent is cleared from the blood by phagocytosis in the reticuloendothelial system, particularly in liver and spleen, very slowly a second high-resolution MRA with an in-plane resolution of 0.9 × 0.9 mm² was acquired using parallel imaging. **(F, G)**. The contours of these images are better defined, but there is increased image noise due to the application of parallel imaging.

applied. With elliptical centric k-space acquisition, the central portions of k-space are acquired within a very short acquisition time during the beginning of the breath-hold. The acquisition of the high spatial frequency components are carried out during the later phase of the scan (16). Elliptical centric acquisitions commonly use measurement times exceeding one breath-hold; however, due to the rapid acquisition of the central k-space components, motion artifacts are limited even if the patient gradually exhales. On the other hand, very high resolution can be obtained without venous overlay. This approach is commonly used for imaging of the carotids, but there have also been reports on the successful use of this technique for the renal arteries in a larger number of patients (19).

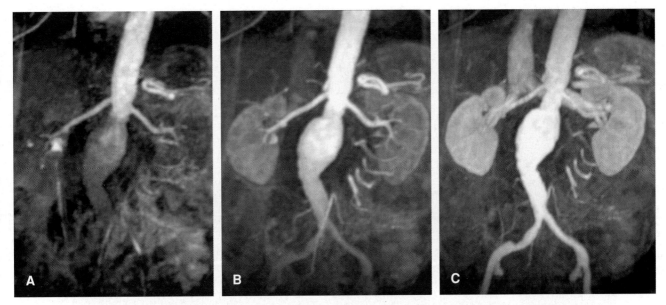

FIGURE 20-10 Coronal MIP views of a multiphasic MRA of a 56-year-old male patient with an abdominal aortic aneurysm. All three phases lasting 6.8 seconds each are acquired in a single breath-hold of 20.4 seconds. **A:** The early arterial phase shows beginning enhancement of the renal arteries. **B:** In the late arterial phase, there is strong arterial contrast of the abdominal vessel without venous overlay of the renal arteries. **C:** In the venous phase, the venous return from both renal arteries can already be appreciated, even though there is still arterial contrast. At this time, the distal end of the aortic aneurysm and the iliac arteries are now completely filled.

Multiphasic Magnetic Resonance Angiography

Multiphasic MRA has been used in different contexts in the literature. Most commonly, the term *multiphasic MRA* refers to a time-resolved approach during the first pass of the contrast media. Multiple 3D Gd-MRA data sets are acquired during one single breath-hold to selectively image the early arterial phase, the late arterial phase, and early venous phase of the contrast media transit (20,21) (Fig. 20-10). This approach has three intrinsic advantages. First, no timing procedure for arrival of the contrast media bolus is required, imaging can directly start after fixed delay, and one of the subsequent data sets will display the contrast media arrival. Second, the short acquisition time of the individual data sets of less than 6 seconds allows better visualization of the segmental and intrarenal segments of the renal arteries before substantial parenchymal enhancement occurs. Third, this approach is less susceptible to involuntary motion of the renal arteries from random diaphragm contractions. Some studies have already shown the improved visualization of the distal renal segments.

On the other hand, spatial resolution is substantially lower due to the short acquisition time of each data set when cartesian k-space sampling is used. With the introduction of undersampled 3D radial imaging (3D-VIPR), time-resolved MRA is possible with isotropic 1 mm spatial resolution but at the cost of lower signal to noise (SNR) and occurrence of substantial streak artifacts at the present time (22).

Thus, time-resolved MRA is a robust technique for depiction of atherosclerotic renal artery occlusive disease, aneurysms (Fig. 20-11), or renal artery dissection; however, caution has to be taken for the evaluation of subtle irregularities of the renal arteries, such as in FMD, neurofibromatosis, or vasculitis.

The other meaning of multiphasic MRA is the acquisition of high-resolution multibreath-hold data sets during the different stages of the contrast media transit, that is, during the arterial phase, the equilibrium phase, and the excretory phase for the acquisition of an MR urography data set (Fig. 20-12).

Three-dimensional Phase Contrast Magnetic Resonance Angiography

This technique was initially developed as a competitor for TOF MR angiography of the renal arteries. While in principle this technique suffers from similar limitations as TOF MRI, such as long measurement times with motion artifacts and limited spatial resolution, it does offer some unique advantages. PC techniques are substantially more sensitive to slow flow, resulting in a better depiction of small distal vessels. The main rationale for the use of this technique, however, is the susceptibility to intravoxel dephasing in areas of accelerated flow and aliasing artifacts at areas of turbulence. While this was initially considered a limitation of the technique, it is now used by some authors

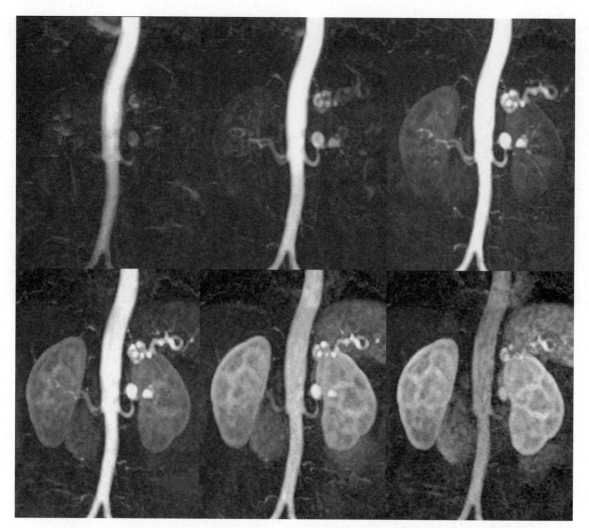

FIGURE 20-11 Time-resolved MRA of the renal arteries in a 52-year-old female patient with hypertension at 3.0 T. The temporal resolution of the single frames is 1.4 seconds. This 3D-MRA was acquired using a TREAT (time-resolved echo-shared angiographic technique) sequence, which combines view sharing with parallel imaging to allow high spatial (1.7 × 1.2 × 5.0 mm³) and a high temporal resolution (1.4 seconds/3D data set). This technique allows detailed analysis of the blood flow dynamics. In this patient with FMD, the dynamic filling process of the renal artery aneurysms can be clearly seen. TREAT also allows assessing the renal perfusion to detect decreased perfusion and delayed perfusion of a single side. (Courtesy of J. Paul Finn, M.D., University of California in Los Angeles.)

as an easy way to detect and grade hemodynamically significant RAS (23) (Fig. 20-13). In order to be sensitive enough for the renal artery flow, the strength and duration of the velocity-encoding gradient (so-called VENC) has to be adapted on a patient-by-patient basis. While in normal individuals a VENC of 50 cm/second is appropriate, the VENC should be set to 40 cm/second in older patients and 20-30 cm/second in patients with compromised renal function.

Qualitative grading of the hemodynamic significance of RAS by means of signal loss on 3D PC MR angiography is done on a four-point scale, with no artifacts or focal tapering of the renal artery for a normal vessel or a mild RAS.

The presence of a focal tapering with some dephasing artifacts marks the presence of a hemodynamically signifi-

cant stenosis greater than 50% in diameter, while a complete focal signal drop-out marks a severe stenosis exceeding 75% in diameter.

Unenhanced Time-of-flight Magnetic Resonance Angiography Techniques

TOF techniques are flow dependent, that is, they require inflow of moving blood into the vascular territory of the renal arteries. As mentioned earlier, standard TOF techniques with two-dimensional (2D) breath-hold multislice methods or 3D free-breathing acquisitions are rarely used in clinical routine due to the adverse effects of motion artifacts and signal voids due to turbulences or in-plane saturation. The introduction of SSFP techniques with navigator

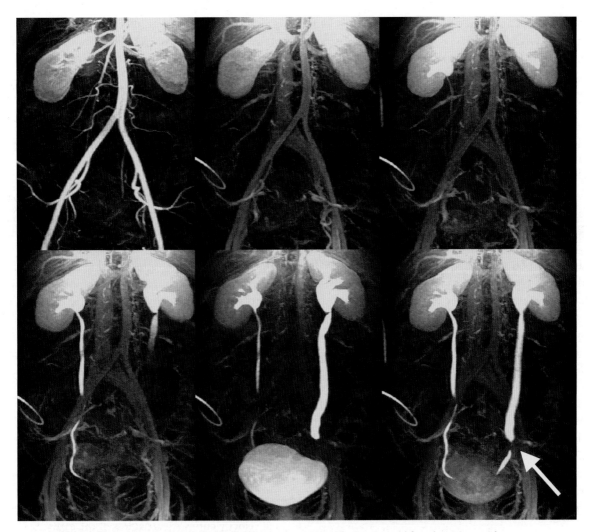

FIGURE 20-12 Coronal MIP view of a multibreath-hold MRA of a 29-year-old female patient with endometriosis-related stenosis of the left ureter. In this multiphasic MRA, the excretion of the kidneys can be well visualized, thereby demonstrating the stenotic segment of the left ureter (*arrow*). There are dilatation of the left ureter and hydronephrosis of the left kidney secondary to the ureteral stenosis.

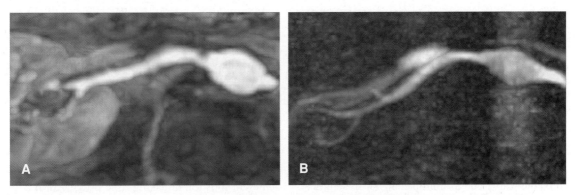

FIGURE 20-13 A: Three-dimensional Gd-MRA of a 62-year-old female patient with a 50% proximal right-sided RAS. **B:** The 3D phase-contrast MRA demonstrates the entire right renal artery without dephasing. Consequently, this stenosis was not considered hemodynamically significant.

correction of respiratory motion has revitalized this completely noninvasive approach.

In one study, these free-breathing renal MRA techniques with SSFP and combined with a slice-selective inversion pulse allowed for selective and high contrast visualization of the renal arteries, including the more distal branches (8). Artifacts from respiratory or cardiac motion were eliminated by cardiac triggering and respiratory gating with a navigator positioned at the diaphragm. Due to the relatively long acquisition times of around 2 minutes, a high in-plane spatial resolution of approximately 1 mm^2 can be achieved with relatively thin slices of 2 mm. Scan orientation for this technique is axial. By using a slice-selective inversion prepulse with an appropriate inversion time (TI), signal of the static tissue can be suppressed depending on the specific relaxation time. On the other hand, inflowing blood, which washes into the imaging volume during the inversion time delay, maintains high signal intensity. Typical inversion times of 300 milliseconds are used. In order to suppress signal from the abdomen as well as from inflowing blood of the inferior vena cava, local presaturation bands should be placed. So far, reliable data only exists in volunteers. Here, the proximal, middle, and distal portion including the intrarenal segmental arteries were well visualized. This technique is still in its early days to estimate its performance in patients with RAS. However, it could hold great potential for patients in whom administration of MR contrast agents is contraindicated, such as in pregnant women with malignant hypertension.

Phase-contrast Magnetic Resonance Flow Measurements

MR cine PC flow measurements were introduced in the late 1990s. Their validity has been shown in comparison studies to invasive US measurements with good correlation between these two modalities (24–26). 2D cine PC flow measurements are based on the principle that spins moving along a gradient experience a phase shift that is proportional to their flow velocity (27). Flow measurements of the renal arteries provide a fast assessment of the hemodynamic significance of a present RAS (5,23,28). These measurements should be performed with cardiac gating using either prospective or retrospective gating. Care needs to be taken to assure that the measurement plane is perpendicular to the vessel axis. This can be easily achieved when the flow measurements are acquired after the 3D Gd-MRA scan using the subvolume maximum-intensity projection (MIP) images of the MRA data set for defining the orientation of the scan plane in multiple angles. In stenosed arteries, the scan plane needs to be positioned at least 1 cm distal or proximal to the stenosis. It is important that the averaged temporal resolution of the sequence is below 30 millisec-

onds in order to reliably display all characteristic components of the velocity curve. For each time frame, a flow-sensitive and a flow-compensated scan are obtained, resulting in a minimum temporal resolution of 2 times repetition time, which is typically in the order of 12 to 15 milliseconds. To acquire a 256×256 matrix for each time frame, a total measurement time of approximately 3 to 4 minutes is required.

Currently, all scanners offer postprocessing software to analyze the series of PC data sets. Regions of interest can be manually drawn along the margins of the vessel cross section. Alternatively, automatic segmentation approaches of the vessel contour can be applied based on fitting a 3D parabolic velocity model to the actual velocity profiles (29). Velocity-time curves are then calculated from the velocity data in each time frame after applying a correction for phase noise and aliasing. Thus, each data point on the curve represents the mean velocity averaged over the vessel area for the individual time frame. It is important for the grading of hemodynamic changes that the cine PC flow curves are scaled to a maximum velocity of 35 to 40 cm/second with the velocity averaged over the vessel area (30). These characteristic changes of the velocity flow profile that correspond to certain degrees of RAS have been invasively validated in the past in animal models and clinically validated in multicenter patient trials (25,26,30). The presence or absence of the three distinct features of the PC flow curve are noted, that is, the "early systolic velocity peak," the subsequent "incision," and the second lower "midsystolic peak." A renal artery without presence of a stenosis is represented by a normal velocity curve. A partial loss of the early systolic peak is an indicator of a hemodynamically nonsignificant low-grade stenosis of 50%. Almost complete loss of the early systolic peak and decrease of the midsystolic peak indicates moderate stenosis of >50%, whereas a featureless flattened flow profile with no systolic velocity components is representative for a high-grade stenosis of >75% (Fig. 20-14).

One disadvantage of standard PC flow measurement techniques using standard GRE techniques is the relatively long scan times of several minutes. This leads to motion artifacts of the PC images with the consequence of overestimation of the vessel area by about 10% to 20%, resulting in about 10% higher mean flow values. Segmented echo-planar imaging cine PC flow measurements are capable of performing cardiac-gated flow measurements in the renal artery with both high temporal and spatial resolutions (31). When eight or more interleaved echo trains are used, a temporal resolution (= repetition time) of below 31 milliseconds can be achieved, thus total imaging time is reduced to a 28-second breath-hold scan for the acquisition of a 256^2 matrix at an RR-interval length of 800 milliseconds. To ensure reliable cardiac gating, an optically decoupled electrocardiogram

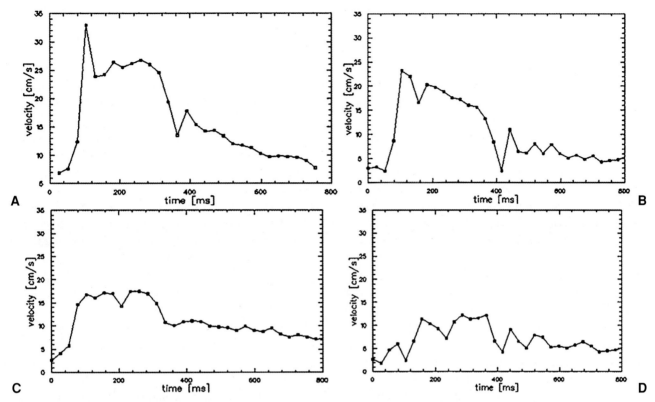

FIGURE 20-14 PC flow measurements of the renal artery. The figure shows the characteristic changes in the flow profile with increasing RAS. **A:** The flow profile of a healthy renal artery with mean early systolic flow velocity peak at approximately 35 cm/second. **B:** Loss of the early systolic peak with otherwise normal flow indicating low-grade RAS (<50%). **C:** With RAS of 50% to 75%, the early systolic peak is absent, and the overall mean flow is becoming impaired. **D:** In the case of a high-grade RAS (>75%), no normal flow pattern can be appreciated. The flow curve appears featureless, and no differentiation of systolic and diastolic flow can be safely achieved.

(ECG) device is preferable, which minimizes the influence of the gradients on the ECG registration. However, one problem of these techniques is the presence of ghosting artifacts from off-resonances around the margins of the vessel.

Measurements of Renal Perfusion

While flow measurements display the flow in the large feeding vessels, perfusion measurements aim at demonstrating the capillary blood flow in the renal parenchyma and, especially, in the highly vascularized renal cortex. The adjunct of renal perfusion measurements to a comprehensive morphologic and functional MR imaging protocol addresses a number of clinical questions. The effects of a chronic RAS with consecutive ischemic nephropathy can be assessed. Renoparenchymal damage independent from the presence of a RAS such as in diabetes, hypertensive nephrosclerosis, or glomerulonephritis can be detected (32,33). Focal disease within the kidney, such as in the presence of segmental RAS or regional ischemic changes in transplants, can be identified and graded by regional assessment of renal perfusion (34).

Currently, there are two main approaches to renal perfusion measurements: arterial spin labeling (ASL) techniques, which use blood as an endogenous contrast agent, and contrast-enhanced techniques, which are based on dynamic imaging of the contrast media transit through the renal parenchyma. ASL techniques are attractive in that they are noninvasive and do not require the administration of contrast agents. Different techniques have been proposed so far in the literature; however, only animal studies or volunteer studies have been performed (35–38).

The main disadvantages that limit broad clinical application are the inherent low SNR and the susceptibility for artifacts. Most ASL techniques such as flow-sensitive alternating inversion recovery (FAIR) measure the signal from arterial blood at a fixed inversion delay after magnetic labeling. As no image information is sampled during this delay, FAIR measurements are inefficient and time consuming. To avoid this problem, a Look-Locker acquisition to sample not one but a series of images after each labeling pulse has been proposed (39). This technique also overcomes the limitation of ASL sequence to yield only a single perfusion-weighted slice without the temporal perfusion information. To increase the SNR and to decrease the susceptibility for artifacts, a True FISP-readout for ASL sequences has been proposed recently (40). In one study of ASL in 46 patients, an overall accuracy of 88% could be achieved to classify kidneys into either healthy or diseased compared with the final clinical diagnosis using a combination of mean arterial blood flow from PC flow measurements and renal perfusion from ASL. While this study was not able to differentiate between primary or secondary parenchymal disease, it showed an extremely high specificity of 99% to exclude any underlying renal disease (32). So, even though these techniques are very promising and possible applications like renal transplant surveillance are in sight, no routine clinical application has been achieved so far.

In contrast to the ASL technique, contrast-enhanced MR perfusion (CE MRP) techniques do not suffer from SNR limitations. The first renal perfusion studies are reported from 1989 (41). Although the technique has evolved since then, CE MRP is not yet widely clinically applied. The basic principle of CE MRP is to administer a bolus contrast agent and to visualize the arrival of the bolus in the renal parenchyma using dynamic imaging of the kidneys with the best temporal resolution possible.

So far, absolute quantification of cortical blood flow is only reliably possible with intravascular contrast agents such as USPIO agents (SHU 555 C, Schering AG, Berlin, Germany; NC 100150, GE Healthcare, Little Chalfont, UK), strongly protein-binding contrast agents (MS-325, Epix Pharmaceuticals, Cambridge, MA, USA), or macromolecular gadolinium complexes (Gadomelitol, Vistarem, Guerbet, Paris, France; Gadomer-17, Schering AG, Berlin, Germany) (42,43). Both T2*-based as well as T1-based perfusion models are applied depending on the relaxation properties of the agent. For the first, double echo T2* sequences should be used to correct for superimposing effects of T1 shortening, while saturation recovery GRE sequences are applied for the latter to ensure a linear relationship between signal intensity and contrast media concentration for a certain range of concentrations. In both cases, the principles of indicator dilution theory can be applied. The regional renal blood volume of the renal cortex can be estimated from the magnitude of the resulting tissue response curve. Assessment of regional renal blood flow in absolute values of mL/100 g of tissue per minute requires the determination of an input function from either the aorta or preferably the renal artery itself (42). The signal of the determined tissue response curve in the cortex of the kidneys needs to be deconvoluted by the signal of the input function in order to calculate the residual function from which the mean transit time can be computed. Regional renal blood flow is calculated from regional renal blood volume divided by the mean transit time. While several of these agents (both gadolinium-chelate–based and

iron-oxide–based) are currently being evaluated in phase 2 and phase 3 trials, none of them have been approved for clinical use yet outside control trials.

With the use of faster MR techniques, semiquantitative assessment of renoparenchymal perfusion with standard extracellular, nonintravascular gadolinium chelates have now become feasible (34). Whereas absolute quantification of renal perfusion is much more difficult due to the rapid excretion of the contrast agent, this type of contrast agent better resembles the sequence of perfusion, filtration, and excretion known from nuclear medicine studies. Recent publications proposed the use of a VIBE sequence for CE MRP with a 2 mL Gd-DTPA bolus and temporal resolution of 2 seconds per image (44). The higher the achievable temporal resolution, the more exact will be the calculation of the perfusion parameters. From these data, signal-intensity versus time (SIVT) curves over user-defined regions of interest (ROI), different parameters can be derived. Since Gd-DTPA behaves at the glomerulus like 99Tc-MAG3, the nuclear medicine marker for renal function, SIVT curves can be analyzed like nuclear medicine studies, which leads to the split renal function (45,46). Fitting the first pass of the SIVT curves with a Gamma variate fit delivers semiquantitative parameters such as mean transit time (MTT), time to maximal signal intensity (Tmax), the maximal upslope steepness (MUS), and the maximal signal intensity (MSI). In order to obtain absolute quantitative perfusion parameters, the renal SIVT curve has to be deconvoluted with the input function that is in the best case the SIVT curve of the renal artery. Due to practicability reasons, the SIVT curve of the aorta is commonly chosen instead. Deconvolution is a complicated mathematical process, which is probably the main obstacle for widespread use of these techniques. It can be easier calculated with intravascular contrast agents that do not leave the vessel bed immediately (33,42,43). For accurate semiquantitative perfusion measurements, sequences with a high linearity between signal intensity and contrast media dose should be applied. The most commonly used type of sequence is a saturation-recovery (SR) Turbo FLASH sequence (47) with a high temporal resolution of 4 slices per second. For the saturation recovery, a series of 90° pulses in a phase angle of 90° is applied, which minimizes inflow-effects and grants good signal linearity. The four slices assure good coverage of the renal parenchyma. The total acquisition time amounts to 5 minutes to cover the first pass as well as the filtration of the contrast agent (Fig. 20-15).

Contrast Medium

Overall, the contrast media administration for 3D Gd-MRA is relatively standardized. Contrast media dose and injection rate mainly depend on the type of contrast media that is used.

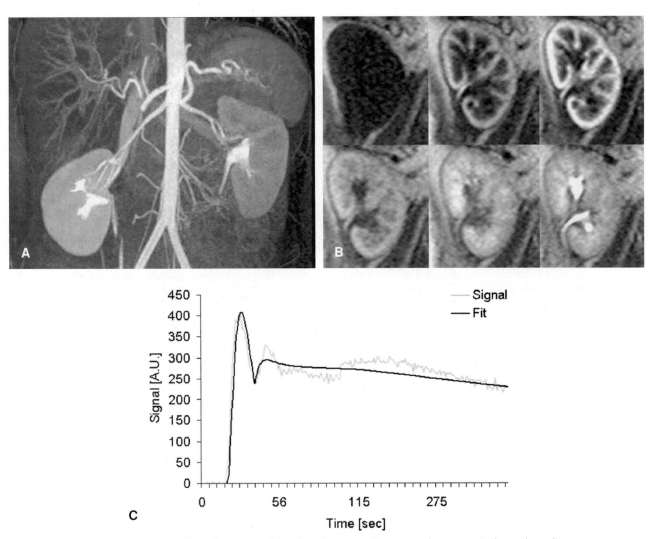

FIGURE 20-15 Renal MRA of a 29-year-old patient demonstrating a normal anatomy. A: The renal vessels can be seen up to the second-order branches. Due to the previous perfusion measurements and the test bolus measurement, there is already excretion of the contrast agent bilaterally. **B:** Exemplary images taken from the renal perfusion measurement in a healthy patient using the SR Turbo FLASH sequence with high temporal resolution. Displayed from **left upper** to **right lower** image: unenhanced scan before the arrival of the contrast agent followed by arrival of the contrast agent in the renal cortex. In the next phase, the renal medulla also is enhanced; the medullar pyramids enhance until the contrast agent is finally excreted. From this perfusion scan, a signal intensity versus time curve **(C)** can be derived from the renal cortex. The figure shows the actually measured points (*signal*) and the gamma variate fit curve (*fit*). The gamma variate fit of a healthy kidney shows a step upslope with a marked first-pass perfusion peak which is followed by another small peak, which represents the recirculation of the contrast agent bolus. The signal from the cortex, then, slowly decays due to filtration and excretion of the contrast agent.

Standard Extracellular Gadolinium Chelates

Standard gadolinium chelates are typically administered at a dose of 0.2 mmol/kg BW with typical injection rates of 1 to 2 mL/second. Some authors also found sufficient image quality with 0.1 mmol/kg BW of standard gadolinium chelates (48). An injection rate of less than 1 mL/second results in a poor bolus profile with consequent poor vessel-to-background contrast. Injection rates exceeding 3 mL/second already cause saturation effects with no further increase in signal intensity but less homogenous contrast throughout the entire acquisition since the bolus travels too rapidly to match the entire 20- second-acquisition of the scan. However, faster acquisition is acceptable with time-resolved approaches, since each of the individual phases only requires a fraction of the bolus passage for optimum contrast enhancement.

Extracellular Nonintravascular Gadolinium Chelates with Special Properties

These agents have similar pharmacokinetics than the previous group; however, they are characterized by higher relaxivity for various reasons. Two of these agents are approved

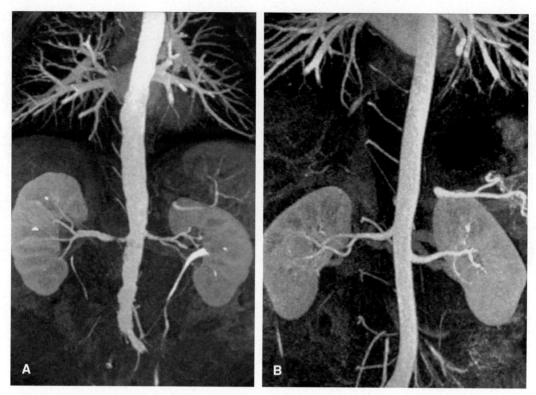

FIGURE 20-16 Comparison of gadobutrol- and Gd-BOPTA-enhanced MRA. A: Three-dimensional MRA of a 47-year-old male with hypertension and right-sided high-grade RAS acquired with 0.15 mmol/kg BW gadobutrol. **B:** MRA of a 32-year-old male patient with hypertension but no renal artery lesion. For this study, 0.15 mmol/kg BW Gd-BOPTA were administered. Both acquisitions had submillimeter spatial resolution and were acquired using parallel imaging techniques. While the former was acquired with an acceleration factor of 2, the latter was acquired with an acceleration factor of 3.

in Europe for CE MRA, namely Gadobutrol (Gadovist, Schering, Germany) and Gadobenate-Dimeglumine (Multihance, Bracco, Italy). While Gadobutrol inherits higher T1-relaxivity due to a double concentration compared with the standard Gadopentetate-Dimeglumine (Magnevist), the higher relaxivity of Multihance is related to a weak protein-binding affinity to albumin (Fig. 20-16).

Many trials have been performed to assess the performance of these agents in terms of dosage and vascular signal intensity. In general, half of the contrast media dose (0.1 mmol/kg BW) is sufficient to equal the results compared with standard gadolinium chelates for CE MRA of the renal arteries (49). At this time, no significant differences between Gadovist and Multihance have been found regarding image quality (49,50). However, injection becomes more difficult, as the smaller contrast media bolus has to be even better synchronized with the MR acquisition to ensure homogenous contrast media plateau during the filling of the center of the k-space. The fraction of protein-bound contrast media of Multihance increases in the equilibrium phase, preserving the arterial plateau phase to a certain extent. Thus, this agent has advantages for long high-resolution 3D acquisitions such as for elliptical centric acquisitions. On the other hand,

Gadobutrol, with its very high relaxivity in the first-pass but short plateau phase, is particularly well suited for fast time-resolved acquisitions. With the advent of parallel acquisition techniques, these agents play a larger role than previously thought. With the use of an acceleration factor of 2, SNR of the acquisition is approximately reduced by a square root of 2. If the acquisition time is kept constant but spatial resolution is doubled, the SNR is again reduced by a square root of 2. Thus, with the use of parallel acquisition techniques and doubling of the spatial resolution at the same time, the SNR of the measurement drops by approximately 50%. In this setting, new gadolinium chelates such as Multihance or Gadovist are important to regain more signal due to their higher relaxivity (49). This, however, seems to require a higher dose than 0.1 mmol/kg BW at the moment to adjust for additional loss of SNR as well as the relatively long scan times of high-resolution MRA.

Intravascular Contrast Agents

The only intravascular contrast agent that is likely to be approved in the near term for CE MRA is MS-325 (Epix Pharmaceuticals, Cambridge, MA, USA). This agent has the advantage that it is both useful for first-pass dynamic CE

MRA and for high-resolution MRA in the steady state. Timing and contrast media injection for the first pass are similar to standard gadolinium chelates with injection rates of about 1 to 2 mL/second. With the advent of motion correction by navigators positioned on the diaphragm, free-breathing 3D CE MRI can now be performed in the steady state with acquisition times of several minutes and a spatial resolution of less than 0.8 mm. One problem for this steady-state high-resolution MRA is artery-vein separation, which is usually possible for the extrarenal arterial vascular tree by means of curved planar reformats. However, intrarenal separation of more distal segmental arteries and veins requires dedicated software that is not yet widely commercially available.

Integration of Renal Artery Injection Protocols into Moving Table Techniques

Frequently, the evaluation of the renal artery is integrated into moving table techniques of the peripheral arteries or into whole-body MRI protocols. For imaging of the renal arteries as part of a peripheral MRI protocol, the injection is usually carried out with biphasic injection protocol with two different injection rates to ensure a bolus travel to the periphery as slow as possible. By this, usually the first half of the dose is injected at 1 mL/second to still achieve a sufficient bolus profile for the renal arteries and then reduced to about 0.5 mL/second to ensure slow but constant flow into the periphery (51). Many other authors now, however, use the so-called hybrid techniques, in which vessel territories prone to venous overlay such as the distal calves and feet are imaged first followed by a moving table technique with imaging of the renal arteries (52). Due to better surface coils and concomitant reduction of the contrast media dose to 0.1 mmol/kg BW, it is no problem to image the renal arteries with good arterial-to-background contrast after previous injection for the calves. This technique is also applied for state-of-the-art whole-body MRI protocols with high spatial resolution in which the carotids and feet are imaged first, followed by a separate injection for the renal arteries and abdomen.

Saline Flush

The administration of contrast agent is always followed by a saline flush of 20 to 30 mL at the same injection rate as the contrast agent. The saline flush guarantees that all of the contrast agent is administered to the patient. Larger amounts of saline can be used for MR urography to enhance the renal excretion. Up to 400 mL of saline can be applied for this indication. Alternatively, 10 mg of furosemide can be intravenously delivered. Administration of contrast agent and saline are best done using an MR compatible injector pump. By this means, a constant flow and a continuous injection without interruption are guaranteed. The constant injection rate provided by the injection pump also allows for good bolus geometry without greater bolus dispersion.

Triphasic Imaging for Parenchymal Enhancement and Magnetic Resonance Urography

Since extracellular contrast agents are freely filtered by the kidneys, excretion of the contrast agent begins virtually after the first pass. To monitor the excretion of the contrast agent, heavily T1-weighted (T1W) sequences such as 3D GRE sequences (vendor acronyms: GRASS, FLASH, FAST) are suitable. Repetitive imaging of the kidneys allows monitoring the arrival of the contrast agent in the kidneys and the excretion of the contrast agent. The time intervals used for imaging depend on the clinical indication. If a dynamic urography is desired, repetitive imaging every 30 to 60 seconds can be performed. By this means, obstruction of the urinary system and their relevance for the urine flow can be obtained. Delayed phase images at least 5 minutes later are necessary to detect excretion, and even later in the kidney with heavily impaired function, which may show considerable delay of excretion.

Postprocessing

Subtraction

Subtraction is a technique that improves vessel-to-background contrast due to elimination of the background signal. This method is routinely used for the peripheral arteries. An important prerequisite for an accurate subtracted data set is that there is no motion occurring between acquisition of the mask and the contrast-enhanced data set. It is known that the depth of inspiration is not absolutely identical between multiple breath-holds. Mask subtraction, therefore, may cause inconsistencies at the margins of the vessel, which are substantial in the case of data sets with a high spatial resolution. This technique should only be reserved for visualization purposes such as MIP display, while exact grading of RAS should be performed on the unsubtracted source images (53).

Three-dimensional Postprocessing

MIP and VR should be reserved for 3D display of complex vascular anatomy. In particular, this approach is helpful to identify accessory renal arteries and renal aneurysms, to resolve the complex courses of transplant arteries and veins, and to identify atypical bypass grafts after surgery. Thick volume MIPs should not be used to grade RAS or to identify renal dissections, since this algorithm only uses the voxel with the highest signal intensity along a certain projection. Thus, other bright structures such as overlaying vessels or aliased fat might erroneously mimic a patent renal artery on a MIP image. VR is a better algorithm, as it allows weighing the contributions from the different signal intensities. Nevertheless, this algorithm is not accurate enough for grading of RAS on MR imaging (54,55). This can be mainly explained by two facts—the typical tortuous course of the renal artery inducing geometric distortions and the eccentricity of atherosclerotic plaques (56).

The renal arteries typically take an oblique course in all three dimensions after originating from the ostium with an initial anterior curve followed by a more cranial and posterior direction. Atherosclerotic changes tend to occur in the proximal segment, predominantly in the anterior or posterior wall, usually resulting in a more oval or irregular shape of the stenosis rather than a round residual lumen (56). Therefore, image reconstruction of the 3D Gd-MRA data sets usually consists of thin, 5 to 10 mm subvolume MIPs based on MPR along the vessel axis. The entire course of the vessel should be displayed in both the axial and coronal view. Due to the isotropic spatial resolution, cross-sectional reformats are then performed perpendicular to the vessel axis in order to assess the reduction of the vessel area at the site of the stenosis or to detect a membrane in case of renal artery dissection.

Image Analysis for Grading of Renal Artery Stenosis

Grading of RAS has to be carried out particularly carefully to obtain accurate and reproducible results. The methods for stenosis grading have evolved over time along with the improvements of spatial resolution.

Image analysis usually includes the grading of the degree of stenosis as well as the assessment of vessel visibility. Before the observer turns to the stenosis grading, he should assess the entire renal artery with respect to its visibility. Vessel visibility is usually scored for the ostium of the renal artery as well as the proximal, distal, hilar, and intrarenal segments. A three-point ordinal scale scoring the visibility as either "not identified," "identified but poorly defined," or "clearly defined with definite evaluation of patency" helps to communicate if this particular vessel segment can at all be evaluated for the presence or absence of a RAS (30).

Absolute measurements of the degree of stenosis can be difficult because of limited spatial resolution. Therefore, a modified grading schema with a five-point ordinal scale has usually been applied grading the stenosis as either "not present," "less than 50%," "equal to or greater than 50%," "greater than 75%" or "occlusion."

Current high spatial resolution 3D data sets allow measurement of the degree of RAS both in the in-plane view

along the vessel axis as well as on the cross-sectional images. Based on the North American Symptomatic Carotid Endarterectomy Trial (NASCET) criteria, the maximal stenosis is then defined as the ratio between the narrowest diameter within the stenosis and the diameter of the nearest normal segment of the main renal artery downstream (1 − [narrowest renal artery diameter/diameter normal distal main renal artery]) × 100%).

In addition, the presence and number of accessory renal arteries should be assessed. Due to the limited spatial resolution of 3D Gd-MRA, stenosis grading is difficult and can usually only be performed on a two-point scale as either "absent/low grade" or "high-grade."

ANATOMY

Normal Anatomy

Normal Arterial Anatomy

Main Renal Arteries

In around 75% of individuals, the renal arteries arise from the aorta immediately below the superior mesenteric artery at the level of the L1-L2 intervertebral disk space, while in the remainder, they may originate anywhere between the lower margins of T12 and L2. Their position is lower in older individuals. Usually, the renal artery ostium is located in the lateral or ventrolateral aspect of the aortic wall, and the renal artery then turns posteriorly in an obtuse angle.

The right renal artery originates closer to the ventral surface in more than 50% of the cases and the left in around 25% of individuals. Location of the orifice in the posterior lateral aortic wall is infrequent and usually involves the left renal artery. The right renal artery passes behind the inferior vena cava, renal vein, duodenum, and pancreatic head.

The left renal artery also lies behind the pancreatic body and renal and splenic veins. In around 60% of individuals, the renal artery divides at the renal hilus, whereas in approximately 15% of the cases an early bifurcation is present (Fig. 20-17).

Intrarenal Branches

It is important to note that the kidney is divided into five vascular segments, which are separately supplied by segmental renal arteries. These segments are called *apical upper*, *middle*, *posterior*, and *lower segments*. The posterior segment comprises the majority of the posterior surface of the kidney, whereas the upper and middle segments are only contributing to the anterior surface. The apical and lower segments have both an anterior and a posterior surface

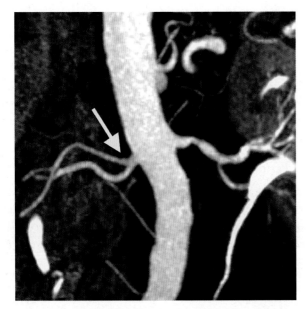

FIGURE 20-17 Coronal MIP view of the abdominal vessels in a 62-year-old male patient with hypertension. There is early (prehilar) branching immediately at the origin of the right renal artery (*arrow*). There is also low-grade stenosis of the left proximal renal artery.

The segmental artery divides into lobar arteries, which further subdivide into two or three interlobar arteries that are located between the renal pyramids. For visualization on MRA or CTA, it is important to note that the proximal interlobar arteries are extraparenchymal and therefore can be seen on time-resolved MRA and CTA. At the corticomedullar junction, a dichotomous branching into arcuate arteries occurs.

The arcuate arteries essentially are end arteries that do not anastomose with each other but subdivide into interlobular arteries, which themselves subdivide and give rise to the afferent glomerular arterioles. Some interlobar arteries penetrate the renal surface as so-called perforating arteries.

On high-resolution CE MRA, usually only the extrarenal segments as well as the anterior and posterior divisions and the proximal aspects of the segmental renal arteries are well seen. The distal segmental arteries are already in close relationship to the renal parenchyma and thus are usually overlaid by enhancement of the latter on single-phase examinations. On time-resolved multiphase MRA, a better visualization of the anterior and posterior divisions as well as the segmental renal arteries has been achieved particularly for the upper and middle segmental artery. The interlobar arteries can be just identified in the proximal parts but cannot be further followed to their subsequent branches due to the small vessel caliber of less than 1 mm in size and the embedding into the renal parenchyma (Fig. 20-18).

component. At the hilus, the renal artery divides into anterior and posterior divisions. Usually, the anterior division supplies the apical, upper, middle, and lower segments and the posterior division supplies the posterior segment. The latter artery courses behind the renal pelvis.

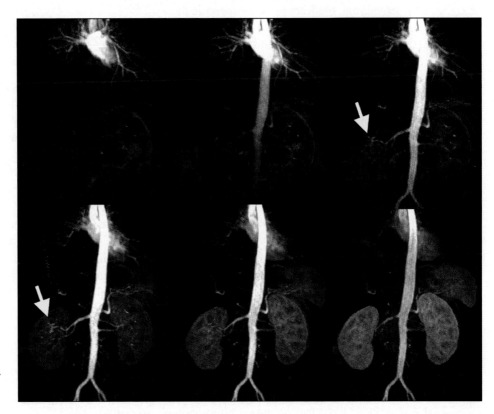

FIGURE 20-18 Coronal MIP view of a TREAT MRA acquired at 3.0 T with a temporal resolution of 1.4 second/3D data set. The high temporal resolution allows to depict the intrarenal branches of the renal arteries (*arrows*). (Courtesy of J. Paul Finn, M.D., University of California in Los Angeles.)

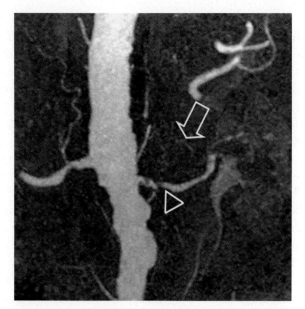

FIGURE 20-19 Coronal MIP view of the MRA of an 82-year-old male patient with chronic occlusion of the left renal artery (*arrowhead*). However, the perfusion of the left kidney is preserved by multiple thin retroperitoneal vessels (one of which is marked by the *arrow*).

Extrarenal Branches

During the extrarenal course, the renal artery gives off several branches, which are only inconsistently seen on CE MRA due to their small caliber. These include the inferior adrenal arteries, which may be solitary or may consist of several arteries. In addition, branches to the perinephric tissues and renal pelvis as well as the proximal ureter arise. Also, the gonadal arteries to the ovaries and testes can arise from the renal arteries.

Capsular Arteries

Capsular arteries usually play no substantial role for the angiographic evaluation of the kidney. However, they can be of high importance in cases of renal artery occlusion or RAS (Fig. 20-19). The three capsular arteries arise from a capsular network that anastomoses freely with perforating arteries and other retroperitoneal arteries, especially lumbar, but also with internal iliac, intercostal, and mesenteric arteries. Thus, these capsular arteries may supply the kidney completely in cases of RAS or occlusion. The capsular arteries either arise from the main renal artery (middle capsular artery) or from other branches such as those of the inferior adrenal artery (superior capsular artery) or the gonadal artery (inferior capsular artery).

Vascular Supply to the Pelvis and Ureters

The renal pelvis is supplied by short branches arising directly from the interlobar and arcuate arteries and occasionally the main renal artery. These branches anastomose with each

other and with ureteral branches, thus forming an important intrarenal collateral pathway. The ureters are supplied by small ureteral branches from the renal artery, directly from the aorta, and from the gonadal arteries. The lower ureter receives blood supply from branches of the common and internal iliac arteries. Longitudinal anastomoses are present along the ureteral wall and provide a collateral pathway.

Perforating Vessels

The perforating vessels are an important collateral pathway to the kidney in the presence of main renal artery obstruction. The perforating arteries may arise from the interlobar, arcuate, or lobar arteries and are accompanied by a vein. As previously mentioned, they anastomose with the capsular arteries and other retroperitoneal arteries.

Normal Venous Anatomy

The intrarenal veins usually accompany the same-named arteries but are usually larger. The arcuate veins join to form the larger vein spot, which do not have a lobar organization, and three to five of those veins form the main renal vein. The right renal vein is 2 to 4 cm in length and joins the inferior vena cava at the same level of the lower third of L1. The left renal vein is 4 to 11 cm in length with a relatively horizontal course in most individuals. It frequently joins the inferior vena cava at a slightly higher lever than the right renal vein.

Asymptomatic Variant Anatomy

Variant Arterial Anatomy

Overall, the renal arteries show a high incidence of variant anatomy (about 40% of the general population), including multiple arteries and early division. Renal arteries can arise anywhere from the proximal abdominal aorta to the iliac arteries, depending on additional variants of the kidney. Thus, imaging must extend from the celiac origin through the bifurcation of the common iliac arteries.

In approximately 60% of individuals, there is a single renal artery, and in the remainder, there are multiple renal arteries. There can be up to four individual arteries for each kidney, which occur with equal frequency on both sides. Multiple arteries are unilateral in about 30% and bilateral in about 12% of individuals. Multiple renal arteries on the same side may occur either as two equivalent-sized renal arteries (approximately 10%), an upper pole renal artery (approximately 7%), a lower pole renal artery (approximately 6%), both upper and lower pole renal arteries (approximately 1%), three renal arteries (approximately 3%), or four or five or more renal arteries (less than 1%).

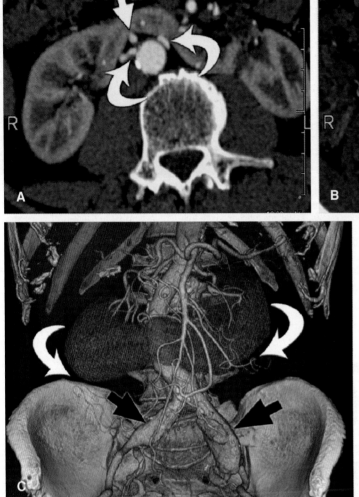

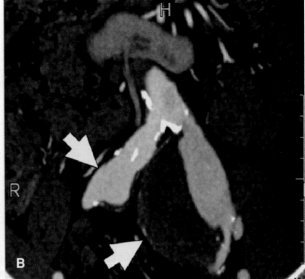

FIGURE 20-20 Horseshoe kidney with bilateral common iliac artery aneurysms. A: Transverse CT section demonstrates a horseshoe kidney with multiple periaortic arterial segments (*curved* and *straight arrows*). **B:** Coronal oblique MPR demonstrates bilateral common iliac artery aneurysms (*arrows*). **C:** Frontal volume rendering demonstrates the relationship between the horseshoe kidney (between *curved arrows*) and the lumina of the common iliac artery aneurysms (*black arrows*). (*Figure 20-20 continues*)

Hilar accessory renal arteries are supplementary vessels that enter the kidney independently at the hilus. Polar accessory renal arteries enter the kidney outside the hilus and typically pierce the renal parenchyma medially to supply the kidney. Accessory renal arteries can originate from virtually any abdominal branch of the aorta. Other than from the aorta, accessory vessels most frequently originate from the common iliac arteries but can also originate from the superior and inferior mesentery, intercostal, lumbar and renal, inferior phrenic, right hepatic, or right colic arteries. It is important to remember that anomalous origins of renal arteries are seen commonly in patients with ectopic or horseshoe kidneys (Fig. 20-20). While the normal course of the right renal artery passes behind the inferior vena cava, 5% of all right renal arteries are dominant crossing the inferior vena cava anteriorly (57).

Detection of Accessory Renal Arteries on Computed Tomographic and Magnetic Resonance Angiography

In respect to accessory renal arteries, several studies exist that report accuracies between 80% and 100%. A recent multicenter trial reported complete agreement between MRA and DSA for the number of accessory renal arteries in only 82% of the cases (median, range 80% to 88% for seven readers) (30). Overestimation of the number of accessory arteries was noted with similar frequency on both MRA and DSA images. Good results have already been reported for the evaluation of kidney donors prior to transplantation in regard to the correct identification of the absolute number and location of supernumerary vessels (58).

Variant Venous Anatomy

Similar to the renal arteries, the renal veins exhibit several anatomical variants (Fig. 20-21). Multiple renal

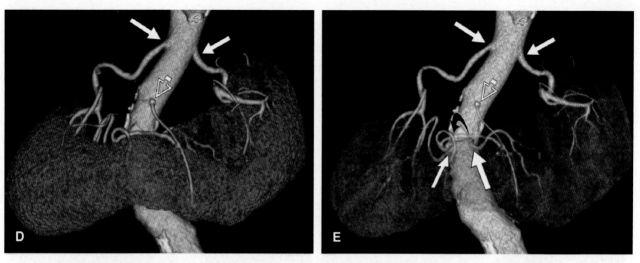

FIGURE 20-20 Continued D: Volume rendering obtained following segmentation of the kidney, renal arteries, and aorta demonstrates two main renal arteries (*white arrows*) and the inferior mesenteric artery arising from the anterior aspect of the aorta with tiny ostial calcification (*open arrow*). **E:** Volume rendering with transfer functions set to diminish renal parenchymal opacity reveals the presence of three additional accessory renal arteries (*additional solid white arrows* and *black curved arrow*) that were not visible in (**D**) due to the opacified horseshoe kidney. This example demonstrates how volume-rendering parameters must be correctly adjusted in order to accurately depict the vascular anatomy. (Figure courtesy of Pietro Sedati and Geoffrey D. Rubin.)

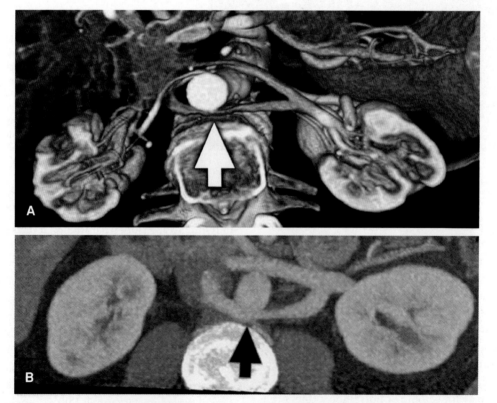

FIGURE 20-21 Circumaortic left renal veins in two different patients. A: Superior volume rendering of a CTA of a potential living renal donor shows a circumaortic left renal vein (*arrow*), the most common renal venous anomaly. **B:** Transverse MIP demonstrates the circumaortic course of the left renal vein in a different patient (*black arrow*) and with separate drainage of the anterior and posterior venous segments into the inferior vena cava. (*Figure 20-21 continues*)

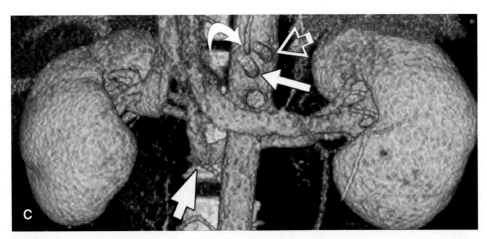

FIGURE 20-21 Continued C: Frontal volume rendering of the same patient as in **(B)** shows the retroaortic course of the left renal vein (*big arrow*) and incidental absence of the celiac trunk, resulting in the common hepatic (*thin arrow*), splenic (*open arrow*), and left gastric (*curved arrow*) arteries arising directly from the aorta. An advantage of volume-rendered CTA when compared with conventional angiography is the ability to display the anatomical relationships between arteries and veins. (Figure courtesy of Pietro Sedati and Geoffrey D. Rubin.)

veins can be found in 10% to 30% of all patients (Fig. 20-22).

The left renal vein, which is three times longer than the right renal vein, contributes most of the variants. Due to its close developmental association with the inferior vena cava, it is prone to congenital abnormalities. In its regular course, the left vein crosses the aorta anteriorly to meet the inferior vena cava. In up to 17% of the cases (59), the left renal vein splits to become a circumaortic renal vein, with one branch crossing the aorta anteriorly and the other branch crossing the aorta posteriorly (60) (Fig. 20-21). In this case, the anterior branch receives the tributaries from the adrenal vein, whereas the gonadal vein and the lumbar vein drain into the posterior branch. Depending on the lumen of the two branches, different patterns for the distribution of the tributaries are possible. Often, the posterior component of a circumaortic left renal has an oblique course, draining into the inferior vena cava several centimeters below the anterior component (Fig. 20-23). In 3.2% of all patients, a purely retroaortic renal vein can be found (61), which can drain in the iliac vein in 0.9%.

Even though most anomalies affect the left renal vein, the right renal vein may also show an aberrant course or an

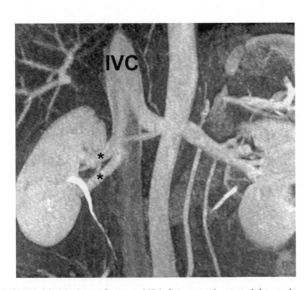

FIGURE 20-22 Coronal venous MRA demonstrating two right renal veins (*) draining into the inferior vena cava (IVC).

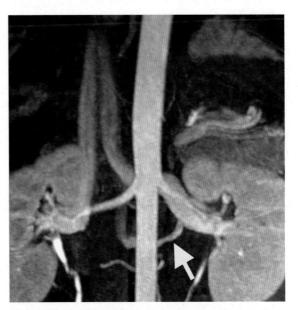

FIGURE 20-23 Variant circumaortic left renal vein with orthotopic main anterior renal vein and inferiorly draining branch (*arrow*). This coronal image depicts the different levels of the renal vein ostia.

anomalous connection with the gonadal vein. Small aberrant veins with connection to the lumbar system or small veins following the ureters down to the gonadal veins may be present on either side. Their presence may be of importance in the case of potential renal transplantation.

The renal veins can be enlarged in several conditions without being symptomatic. Intrarenal tumor-related shunts with high-flow states can lead to increased vessel lumen on the affected side. Due to its tributaries, the left renal vein may be also enlarged in men with varicoceles. Multiparous women often exhibit an enlarged ovary and thus an enlarged left renal vein without being symptomatic. The pathophysiology of this process is not understood. Finally, left renal vein enlargement is observed in patients with splenic vein thrombosis or portal hypertension, resulting in spontaneous splenorenal shunts.

Symptomatic Variant Anatomy

Recent studies have revealed that the presence of accessory renal arteries is not associated with development of hypertension (62) in a single patient. However, if the accessory renal arteries are affected by occlusive disease or renal artery aneurysm, they can become symptomatic and require treatment. Abnormal venous vessels such as retroaortic renal veins or abnormal venous branches can lead to recurrent flank pain, dysuria, and hematuria (63).

Ureteropelvic Junction Obstruction

Aberrant vessels may cause ureteropelvic junction (UPJ) obstruction. Forty-nine percent of all UPJ obstructions in children (57,64) and 29% of all UPJ obstructions in adults can be attributed to crossing vessels. The exact description of the location and number of crossing vessels is important for correct planning of the urologic procedure. In 95% of cases, the crossing vessels are located anteriorly to the UPJ; only in 5% they are found to be posterior. Dominant, precaval right renal arteries, which are found in 5% of all patients, are prone to cause UPJ obstruction when their course is close to the lower pole of the kidney (57) (Fig. 20-24). UPJ obstruction caused by a crossing renal vein is much rarer (Fig. 20-25). Studies comparing DSA as gold standard with CTA found a sensitivity of 100% and a specificity of 96.6% for the detection of crossing vessels with CTA. Studies comparing MRA with DSA have not been published.

In rare cases, huge renal artery aneurysms or arteriovenous malformations may compress the UPJ and lead to obstruction.

Apart from crossing vessels or vessel-related masses, hilar renal masses and retroperitoneal masses can cause UPJ obstruction.

CLINICAL APPLICATIONS

Table 20-1 includes an overview over the most common conditions and diseases encountered when examining the renal vessels.

Role of Parenchymal Cross-sectional Imaging in Addition to Vasculature

With the advances of multidetector technology, both CT and MR now have multiplanar imaging capabilities. For a complete assessment of renal artery disease, evaluation of the renal parenchyma is important and in some cases even mandatory. As discussed later in this chapter, both modalities are well suited for staging and detection of renal cell carcinoma. In addition to intrarenal masses, extrarenal masses such as retroperitoneal fibrosis (Ormond's disease) (65) have to be detected and differentiated from malignant neoplasms (e.g., lymphomas). In the case of large vessel vasculitis, the detection of perivascular soft tissue and especially of vessel wall edema is important to determine the disease activity. In small vessel vasculitis, which can be missed with MRA and CTA, an abnormal patchy enhancement pattern of the parenchyma may be an indirect hint for the radiologist.

The dynamics of contrast enhancement in the kidney is extremely helpful for the establishment of the correct diagnosis both in CT and MR. Regular renal enhancement starts with almost purely cortical enhancement. From the cortex, the contrast agent is filtered into the medulla and finally into the renal pelvis and the ureters. This characteristic enhancement pattern of the kidney is disrupted in some diseases and provides additional information about the disease process. Embolic renal disease (66) and renal infarction lead to focal, wedge-shaped perfusion deficits, while venous stasis or thrombosis leads to hemorrhagic infarction (67), which is easily detected as a hyperdense area in the kidney on CT or as a hyperintense area on T1W MR images. Complete loss of the corticomedullary differentiation (CMD) can be seen with chronic renal failure (68) and acute tubular necrosis (ATN), although loss of CMD is a nonspecific sign (69). In case of infection, such as pyelonephrits or malakoplakia, contrast enhancement of the renal parenchyma is patchy and irregular (70). The kidney often shows an irregular surface and hyperintense signal on T2W images.

Indications for Imaging

Depending on availability of the different imaging methods, the indications for choosing a specific modality may vary. Apart from those previously mentioned, the general condition of the patient and the status of renal function are

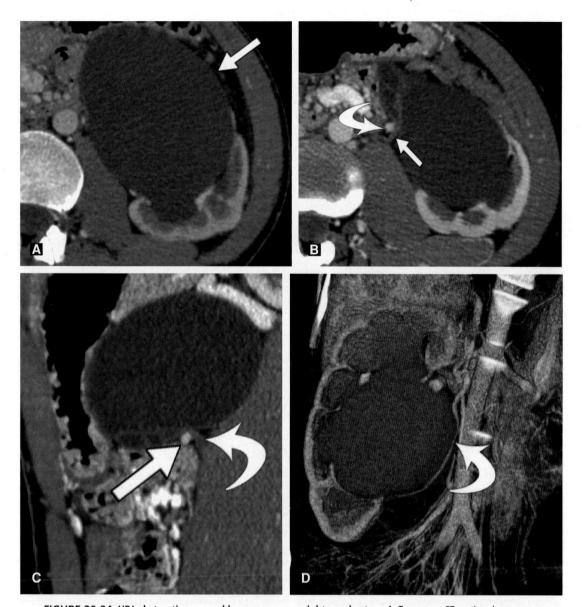

FIGURE 20-24 UPJ obstruction caused by an accessory right renal artery. A: Transverse CT section demonstrates left hydronephrosis and a markedly dilated renal pelvis (*arrow*). **B:** Transverse CT section obtained 2 cm below **(A)**, an artery in close proximity to the UPJ (*curved arrow*), and a band of soft tissue attenuation between the artery and the renal pelvis (*arrow*). **C:** Sagittal MPR demonstrates the presence of severe right-sided hydronephrosis. The ureter is trapped by the crossing artery (*small arrow*) and is normal in caliber distally (*curved arrow*), corresponding to the band of soft tissue seen in **(B)**. **D:** Posterior volume rendering shows the course of the left accessory renal artery, which is responsible for the UPJ obstruction (*curved arrow*). (Figure courtesy of Pietro Sedati and Geoffrey D. Rubin.)

the most important factors for the determination of the best imaging modality.

CT is appropriate for emergency examinations and evaluation of patients with normal renal function or mild dysfunction. If in an emergency situation a patient with impaired renal function is to undergo a CT scan, the patient should be well hydrated before the examination with at least 500 to 1,000 mL of normal saline (71–74). If available, nonionic dimeric isotonic contrast agent may help to avoid contrast-induced nephropathy (75).

Until recently, gadolinium had been considered to be safe in patients with renal dysfunction; however, the recognition of the rare entity of nephrogenic systemic fibrosis (NSF) has substantially limited the use of CE MRA in patients with creatinine clearance of less than 60 mL/minute. Details of NSF can be found in Chapter 5.

The least expensive and most abundant method of screening patients for suspected renal artery diseases is US and Doppler US. However, US is very operator dependent

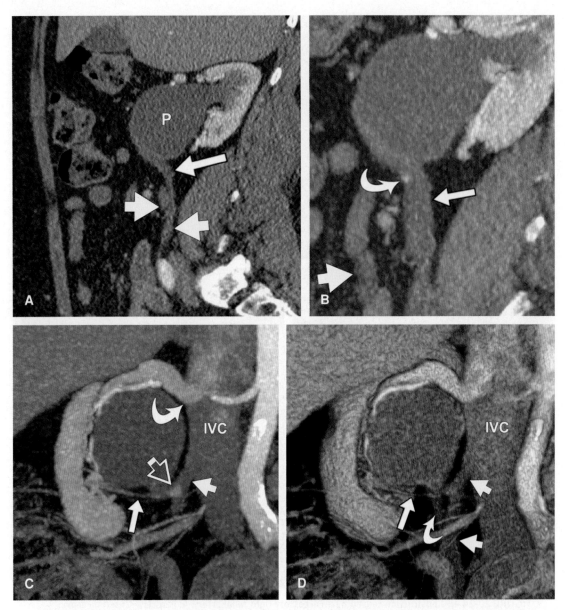

FIGURE 20-25 UPJ obstruction caused by an accessory right renal vein. A: Sagittal MPR through the right kidney demonstrates hydronephrosis with a dilated renal pelvis (*P*), a nondilated ureter (*long arrow*), and an overlapping gonadal vein (*wide arrows*), which mimic the ureter. **B:** Oblique thin-MIP image demonstrates the presence of an enhancing vessel (*curved arrow*) crossing immediately anterior to the ureter (*long arrow*), resulting in mechanical obstruction. The *wide arrow* indicates the adjacent gonadal vein. **C:** Oblique slab MIP demonstrates an accessory renal vein (*long arrow*) crossing the ureter before draining into the gonadal vein (*short solid arrow*) and inferior vena cava (*IVC*). A blush of contrast enhancement is seen in the otherwise unopacified gonadal vein from the accessory renal vein. The dilated renal pelvis displaces the main renal artery and vein (*curved arrow*) superiorly. **D:** Volume rendering illustrates the anterior course of the accessory renal vein (*long arrow*) and the gonadal vein (*short arrows*) relative to the ureter (*curved arrow*). Note how effectively the volume rendering displays these complex anatomical relationships when compared with the MIP (**C**). (Figure courtesy of Pietro Sedati and Geoffrey D. Rubin.)

and may fail because of anatomical constraints in achieving a sufficient acoustic window.

With US, experienced operators can achieve sensitivities of up to 95% for the detection of RAS (81). However, US has high interobserver variability and low sensitivity when performed by inexperienced operators (82,83). With Duplex US, the resistive index (RI) can be calculated from the renal blood flow measurements. The RI was found to be a predictor of a positive postinterventional outcome when RI was <0.8 (84), but other groups found contradictory results with postinterventional improvements in patients with RI >0.8 (85,86). Particularly in obese patients and patients with abdominal bloating, the visibility of the renal vessels can be drastically decreased.

TABLE 20-1

Diseases and Conditions More Commonly Involving the Renal Vasculature

Disease/Condition	Prevalence	Morbidity/Mortality
Multiple renal arteries **Early branching of renal arteries**	Up to 40% of all patients	No morbidity associated, important for renal donor evaluation
Renal vein anomalies	Up to 30% of all patients	No morbidity associated, important for renal donor evaluation
Dominant precaval right renal artery	5% of all patients	Precaval artery can cause ureteropelvic junction obstruction
Renal artery stenosis	4.3% of all patients, prevalence higher with increasing patient age	Hypertension, end-stage renal disease, hemodialysis, cardiac hypertrophy, myocardial infarction
Renal artery aneurysm	Up to 45% of patients with coronary artery disease, peripheral vascular occlusive disease	Hypertension, thrombosis, embolism, rupture
Renal vein thrombosis	1% of all patients	Hypertension, hematuria, loss of renal function
Renal artery dissection	Up to 60% with underlying disease (nephrotic syndrome, clotting disorder)	Hypertension, occlusion of the renal artery
Arteriovenous malformation	Rare disease—suspect after trauma or with fibromuscular dysplasia 0.003% of all patients, prevalence increased after renal trauma	Hypertension, hematuria, right heart failure
Renal artery vasculitis	Rare disease	Hypertension, aneurysms of renal artery, stenoses of renal artery

In patients with nondiagnostic US, CT or MR imaging are the methods of choice for assessment of the renal arteries. Most renal artery pathologies can be safely detected, with the exception of distal FMD and small (<1-2 mm) distal aneurysms in patients with vasculitis, the temporospatial resolution of MRA is often not sufficient. While the superior spatial resolution of CTA may illustrate subtle lesions better than MRA, conventional renal angiography is still required in some cases. Apart from these indications, diagnostic conventional renal angiography is no longer considered as a standard examination. This is mainly due to its invasiveness and cost (76).

Imaging Findings and Pitfalls

Acute thrombembolic occlusion of the renal artery may lead to hematuria and sudden flank pain. The left atrium may be the source of thrombemboli in patients with atrial fibrillation or mitral valve disease. Cholesterol emboli have been reported after cardiac catheter investigation in patients with extensive atherosclerosis in the aortic arc but also without any iatrogenic manipulation. The cholesterol emboli are estimated to account for 5% to 10% of the acute renal failure encountered in patients with clinically significant atherosclerosis (77).

Underlying atherosclerosis in the renal arteries, vasculitis, sickle cell anemia, or trauma may be another reason for thrombus development in the renal arteries. In CT imaging, renal infarction becomes visible by lack of contrast uptake of the entire organ or wedge-shape perfusion defect of the parenchyma. Even in case of complete renal artery occlusion, collateral blood supply by subcapsular vessels may result in a thin rim of enhancing parenchyma (cortical rim sign) (Fig. 20-26).

The assessment of RAS still poses a diagnostic problem. Apart from reviewing also the source images when grading a RAS, there are two additional techniques that one can use. The first technique is to look at the cross-sectional area of the normal renal artery and the stenotic renal artery (Figs. 20-27, 20-28). This technique is most useful in eccentric renal artery stenoses, which may be misinterpreted on a single MIP view and has shown an excellent correlation with the intravascular US. Due to the higher diagnostic accuracy achieved with this technique, also significantly higher interobserver agreements result (78).

A second technique for grading of renal artery stenoses is 3D PC MRA. Due to the long scan time of 4 to 6 minutes, 3D PC MRA yields rather blurry images. However, in PC

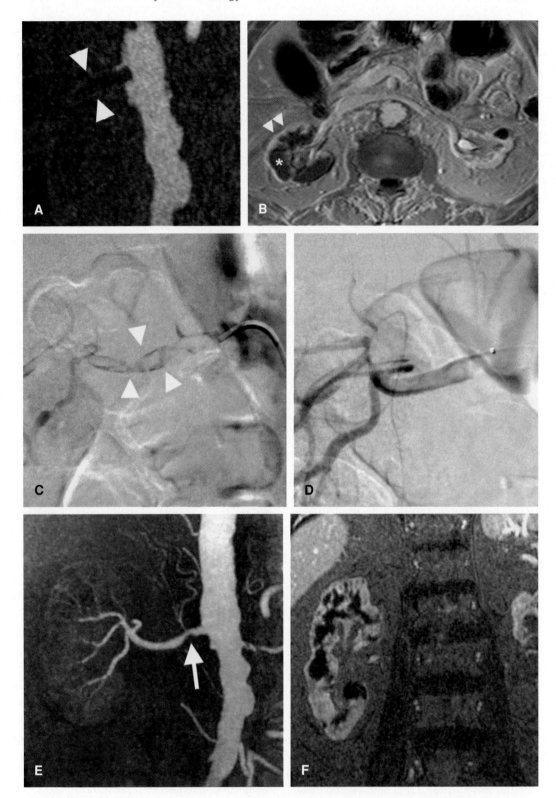

FIGURE 20-26 An 82-year-old male patient with hypertension who presented with deteriorating renal function. A: In the source image of the 3D MRA, a thrombus blocks the right renal artery (*arrowheads*). **B:** In the T1W transverse image postcontrast, the majority of the affected right kidney is not enhancing (∗). Only faint cortical enhancement in some parts of the kidney is visible (*arrowheads*). This is due to blood supply from capsular vessels. **C:** DSA showed complete occlusion of the renal artery with only faint opacification along the vessel wall (*arrowheads*). **D:** Following transcatheter partial thrombectomy, filling of segmental renal arteries to the lower pole is observed. **E:** MRA 3 days after thrombectomy shows patent renal arteries to the periphery. There was only a minor narrowing at the previous site of thrombus (*arrow*). **F:** The coronal MRA images of the late phase show renal enhancement.

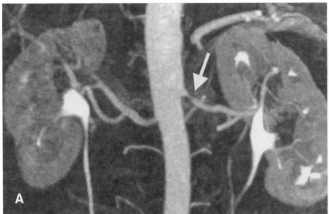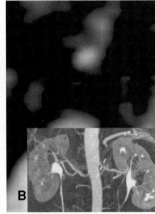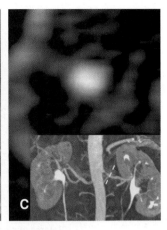

FIGURE 20-27 A: Coronal MIP view of a 56-year-old male patient with left-sided RAS (*arrow*). Note the difference between the **(B)** minimal vessel area in the stenosis and the **(C)** poststenotic cross-sectional diameter of the right renal artery. This stenosis was measured to lead to a 75% reduction of the vessel area and was therefore interventionally treated. Line segments around the left renal artery in the small inset images in B, C show the location of the corresponding MPR.

MRA, spin dephasing occurs with hemodynamically significant stenoses. As discussed previously, this results in a loss of the PC MRA signal and allows detection of hemodynamically significant stenoses (23).

The indications of imaging of the renal arteries with CT and MR are different in most institutions. CT is readily available at most hospitals, easy to use, and fast. Therefore, CT and CTA have their main indication in the emergency diagnostic of abdominal vessel pathologies. In addition, the detection of space-occupying lesions of the retroperitoneum is uncomplicated, and the measurement of the Hounsfield units allows a secure characterization of the lesions.

OCCLUSIVE DISEASES

Renal Artery Stenosis

Atherosclerotic Renal Artery Stenosis

The prevalence of RAS is 4.3% in autopsy studies. RAS is found in up to 22% of patients with infrarenal aortic aneurysm and in up to 45% of patients with peripheral vascular disease (96). Atherosclerosis is the cause of RAS in 90% of patients, while FMD accounts for the remaining 10% of cases (1,90,97,98). Other causes of RAS are listed in Table 20-2.

The prevalence of atherosclerotic RAS increases with age and in patients with hypertension, diabetes mellitus, or coronary artery disease, in whom a prevalence of up to 47% can be reached (97,99–102). If untreated, it leads to

ischemic nephropathy and end-stage renal disease (ESRD) (1). RAS is estimated to account for 10% to 40% of ESRD (103) in patients without identifiably primary renal disease.

To determine the appropriate choice of therapy, the grade, location, configuration, and hemodynamic impact of the RAS have to be described. The most important information about a RAS is the grade of luminal narrowing. While the diameter of stenosis is the most commonly used measurement, recent studies found that the measurement of the area of stenosis yields more reliable results in comparison to intravascular US but also in terms of interreader agreement (78). Particularly for low- to medium-grade stenoses, this technique is much more accurate than the use of the diameter of stenosis and avoids underestimation or overestimation of the stenosis. The measurement of the area of stenosis can also avoid the pitfall of grading the stenosis mistakenly wrong due to the eccentricity of the plaque.

Flow and perfusion measurements can help to determine the hemodynamic significance of a RAS. As for the location of a RAS, two different parts of the renal arteries have to be distinguished, since their treatment differs significantly. Ostial stenoses within the first centimeter of the renal arteries, as in the case of atherosclerotic vessel disease, require stenting for a successful long-term patency. Equally, dissection of the renal artery is primarily treated with stents. Stenoses of the proximal segment of the renal arteries after the initial centimeter are treated by balloon

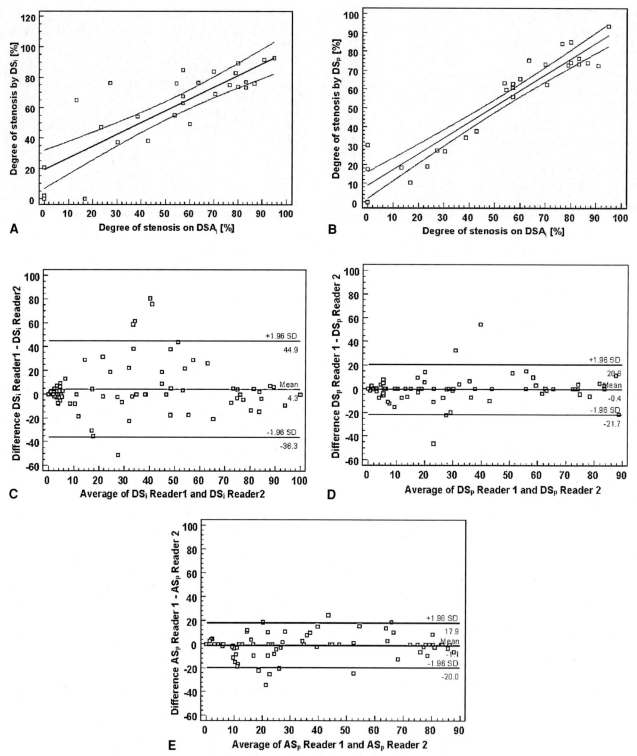

FIGURE 20-28 Correlation of the in-plane and perpendicular diameter stenosis (DSi and DSp) to DSA. A, B: Both DSi and DSp show a linear relationship to DSA; however, the correlation coefficient for DSp is significantly better than for DSi, which in particular can be attributed to the large variation of the results for low values of DSi below 70% to 80%. Comparison of interobserver variability for measurements of the in-plane diameter stenosis (DSi, **C**), perpendicular diameter stenosis (DSp, **D**), and area stenosis (ASp, **E**). For measurements of DSi, interobserver agreement is the worst in the range of 10% to 70% stenosis with the occurrence of both over- and underestimation of the degree of stenosis by up to 80%. This interobserver variability is significantly decreased using measurements of DSp and ASp with the best agreement between the readers for the assessment of the area stenosis. This is particularly evident in the range of low to moderate degrees of stenosis where discrepancies between the readers stay consistently below 25%. (With permission from Schoenberg SO, Rieger J, Weber CH, et al. High-spatial-resolution MR angiography of renal arteries with integrated parallel acquisitions: comparison with digital subtraction angiography and US. *Radiology*. 2005;235:687–698.)

TABLE 20-2

Renal Artery Obstruction

Atherosclerosis

Fibromuscular dysplasia

Congenital coarctation

Neurofibromatosis

Tuberous sclerosis

Takayasu disease

Acute angulation (functional obstruction)

Crossing vessels

Space-occupying lesions (lymph nodes, extrarenal mass, abscess, hematoma, sarcoid, Ormond's disease)

angioplasty with or without stenting. Equally, balloon angioplasty is the treatment of choice in patients with FMD, no matter which part of the renal arteries is affected by the disease.

In addition to these considerations, the size of the kidney plays an important role in assessing the need for intervention. If a cirrhotic kidney without function or heavily impaired function is present, no intervention should be performed. The exact cut-off level for a cirrhotic kidney varies but is thought to be in the range of 7.5-cm length of the long axis of the kidney (1) (Fig. 20-29).

Value of Contrast-enhanced Magnetic Resonance and Computed Tomographic Angiography

Numerous studies have reported RAS sensitivities and specificities of over 90% for 3D Gd-MRA. These studies also demonstrated the superiority of 3D Gd-MRA compared with noncontrast-enhanced TOF techniques (104,105). In contrast, the Dutch multicenter Renal Artery Diagnostic Imaging Study in Hypertension (RADISH) trial reported sensitivities and specificities of 62% and 84% for 3D Gd-MRA and 64% and 92% for CTA when compared with DSA. The average voxel size of the 3D Gd-MRA data sets was about 3 to 6 mm^3; 3D data sets with submillimeter spatial resolution were not acquired in this study. In addition, 3D Gd-MRA was not completed by PC flow measurements for a combined assessment of the degree of RAS. Moreover, CTA technique was similarly insufficient with only one site using MDCT, and no studies performed with <3 mm section thickness. Another limitation of RADISH is the high (38%) prevalence of FMD (106). Data from a multicenter trial on the combined assessment of MRA and flow measurements in comparison to DSA revealed higher accuracies for detection of a high-grade stenosis exceeding 95% (30). In particular, assessing the reduction of the cross-sectional

vessel diameter on orthogonal MPRs appears to effectively reduce misinterpretations (78). Discrepancies in the measured degree of stenosis were reduced from approximately 40% in the coronal plane to only 10% in the orthogonal view (78). Interobserver agreement for the stenosis grading was significantly better by measurements of area of stenosis compared with measurements of diameter of stenosis in-plane.

Due to the still limited spatial resolution of 3D Gd-MRA, data on the accuracy of stenosis grading of small accessory renal arteries are not available. However, the significance of accessory RAS remains controversial. On the one hand, it is known that a high-grade stenosis of an accessory artery can trigger renin release; on the other hand, the necessity for intervention is being questioned due to the small vessel caliber and the resulting risk of occlusion (Fig. 20-30).

Comprehensive Stenosis Grading on Magnetic Resonance

The presence of a significant RAS can be confirmed by adding further morphologic criteria to the diagnostic evaluation of MRA and CTA. The most practical approach is to assess kidney size, cortical thickness, renal parenchyma enhancement, and poststenotic dilatation on the 3D contrast-enhanced data sets. In one study (23), patients with unilateral renal artery occlusive disease benefiting from revascularization revealed a significantly shorter mean ischemic kidney length compared with the contralateral normal kidney as well as a significantly thinner renal cortex. The mean parenchyma enhancement was 15% less on the ischemic side. Poststenotic dilatation >20% was present in 83% of the stenotic arteries. In patients benefiting from revascularization, the mean ischemic kidney length and the mean cortical thickness revealed a significant increase during follow-up after angioplasty.

The addition of PC flow measurements to the standard renal MRA protocol has shown to provide additional diagnostic benefits. First, PC flow measurements by themselves are already sensitive in identifying a high-grade stenosis as compared with DSA, with sensitivities exceeding 90% (28). Second, in combination with 3D Gd-MRA, the overall diagnostic accuracy of MRI for grading of a stenosis increases (30). Third, the add-on of this functional imaging modality to the morphologic stenosis grading significantly reduces interobserver variability between multiple readers and thus increases the consistency of stenosis grading. In addition, the technique helps to identify those lesions with hemodynamic significance, that is, where the autoregulatory capacity is exceeded and loss of renal function is likely to occur (25). In particular, the loss of the early systolic peak

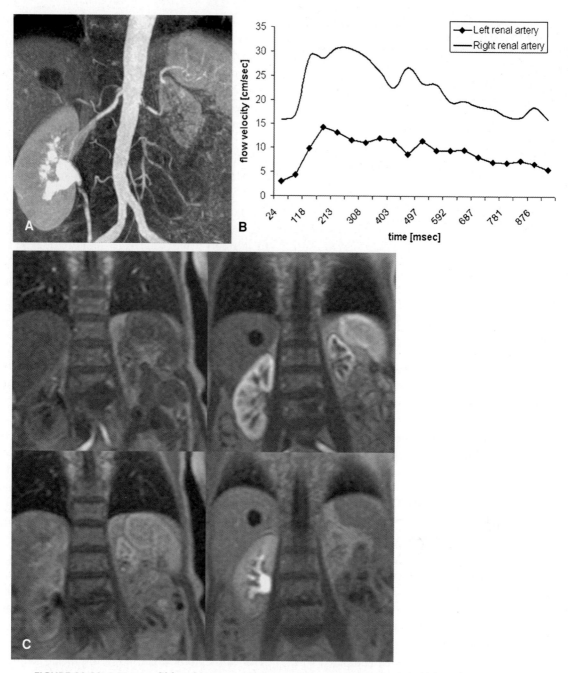

FIGURE 20-29 A 75-year-old female patient with hypertension. The patient revealed a high-grade RAS on the left side with consecutive scarring of the kidney as shown on the MRA **(A)**. In the PC MR flow measurements, a substantially altered flow profile of the affected side with loss of the systolic velocity components becomes visible **(B)**. The dynamic T1W saturation recovery GRE-MR perfusion measurement with a 7-mL bolus of gadolinium revealed decreased first-pass perfusion parameters of the affected left kidney (mean transit time: right 18 seconds, left 29 seconds) but also a complete loss of function of the left kidney with no excretion in the later phases **(C)**. Due to the cirrhosis of and lack of function in the left kidney, the patient was not an appropriate candidate for intervention.

marks the onset of a hemodynamically significant lesion. It is also possible to monitor the success of a surgical or interventional revascularization by quantification of mean flow. One study has shown a significant increase in mean flow after revascularization (28). In addition, the assessment of the velocity flow profile helps to detect early restenosis. It is important to mention that these measurements also can be performed after stent placement, while 3D Gd-MRA is often nondiagnostic due to signal loss at the stenosis site. Care needs to be taken to position the flow measurement plane approximately 1 cm downstream of the stenosis site to avoid phase errors from the metal artifacts (Fig. 20-31).

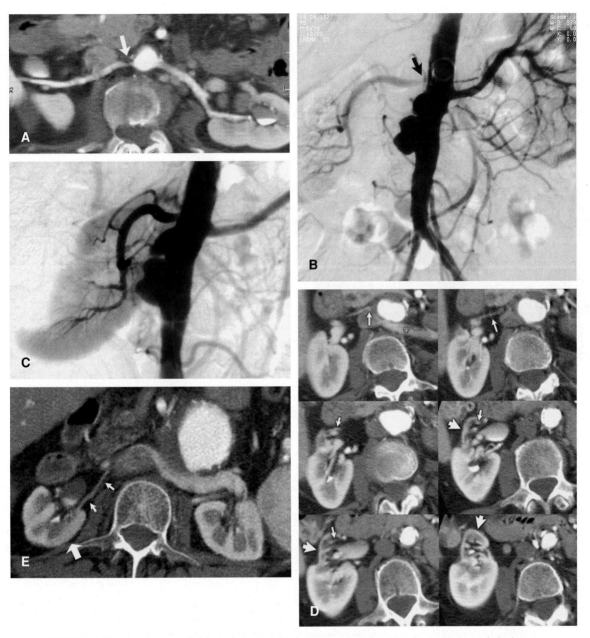

FIGURE 20-30 Accessory renal artery stenoses. A: Curved transverse reformation from a single-row helical CT angiogram performed with 3-mm collimation, 2.0 pitch demonstrates a high-grade stenosis of the proximal right renal artery (*arrow*). **B:** Correlative intra-arterial digital subtraction angiogram (IA-DSA) demonstrates the proximal right RAS (*arrow*), which is partially obscured by an overlying lumbar artery. A small right nephrogram was noted. An infrarenal aortic pseudoaneurysm is demonstrated also. **C:** A 45-degree left anterior oblique IA-DSA obscures the right RAS but demonstrates a defect in the lateral right nephrogram. The cause of this defect was not determined from the IA-DSA study. **D:** Transverse CT reconstructions every 4 mm from cranial to caudal demonstrates a 2- to 3-mm accessory renal artery (*small arrows*) originating from a region of the inferior aspect of the aortic pseudoaneurysm, which is covered with thrombus. The anterior portion of the kidney, supplied by this small accessory renal artery, demonstrates marked atrophy and substantially less cortical enhancement than the superior and posterior portions of the parenchyma, (*wide arrow*), which are supplied by the stenotic main renal artery. Enhancement within the accessory renal artery likely is through hilar collaterals, as the vessel origin is occluded. This vessel was not identified on the IA-DSA study despite a retrospective review of the source images after the CT was performed. Incidentally demonstrated is a retroaortic left renal vein (∗). **E:** Accessory renal artery (*small arrows*) stenosis in a different patient prior to the development of renal atrophy but with reduced opacification in the parenchyma distal to the accessory renal artery (*large arrow*), which is indicative of a hemodynamically significant stenosis. The stenosis at the vessel origin is not shown. This patient also has a retroaortic left renal vein and an abdominal aortic aneurysm. (Figure courtesy of Geoffrey D. Rubin.)

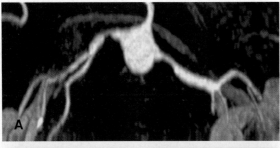
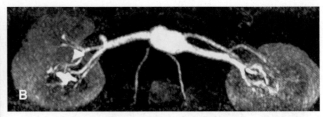
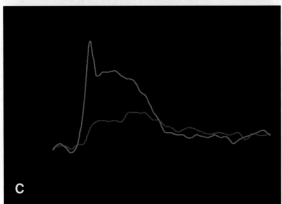

FIGURE 20-31 PC MR flow measurements in patients with and without RAS. A: Transverse MIP of a patient with bilateral RAS. The PC MR flow measurement was positioned on the right renal artery proximal to the bifurcation. **B:** Transverse MIP of a healthy patient without RAS. The PC MR flow measurement was positioned over the left renal artery 1 cm from the ostium. **C:** Plot demonstrating the differences in the flow velocities of the patient in **(A)** (*red line*) and **(B)** (*green line*). The flow of the stenotic renal artery is dramatically decreased; no systolic peak can be marked off any more. (Part **C** reprinted from MR angiography in patients with renal disease. In: Michaely HJ, Schoenberg SO, Rieger JR, et al., eds. *Magnetic Resonance Imaging Clinics of North America.* 2005; 13:131–151. Copyright 2005 with permission from Elsevier.)

Based on the combination of PC flow measurements or 3D PC angiography, a modified grading scheme of RAS can be advised that is less sensitive to errors in the numerical measurement of the morphologic degree of RAS (Table 20-3).

It is important to note that RAS is a progressive disease. More than half of all stenoses progress to high-grade lesions within 3 years (107,108). Due to the high autoregulatory capacity, mean renal artery blood flow will be maintained on a normal level until finally the autoregulatory capacity is exceeded and mean flow suddenly declines, leading to renal failure within a few years (25). Therefore, it is important to follow-up those patients with mild RAS, in which abnormalities in the renal flow profile are already identified.

Renal Perfusion and Renal Artery Stenosis

Further characterization of the functional effects of RAS can be carried out by means of perfusion measurements. Measurements of perfusion using intravascular contrast agents have shown to successfully quantify cortical perfusion with good agreement to invasively determined data (42). Mean cortical perfusion of normal kidney is about 400 mL/100g of tissue/ minute. In cases of high-grade stenosis exceeding 80%, these values can drop to less than 200 mL/100g of tissue/minute. For semiquantitative perfusion measurements with standard gadolinium chelates, significant differences between patients without stenoses or low-intermediate stenoses and those with high-grade stenoses were found for the mean transit time (MTT), the

TABLE 20-3

Modified Grading Scheme of Renal Artery Stenosis Based on Comprehensive Assessment of Morphologic and Hemodynamic Changes

Morphologic Degree of Stenosis	Findings on 3D Gd-MR Angiography	Findings on 2D MR Phase-contrast Flow Measurements	Findings on 3D Phase-contrast MR Angiography
Normal	Normal	Normal flow profile	Normal
Mild	Mild stenosis <50%	Loss of early systolic velocity peak	Normal or mildly stenotic, no intravascular signal loss
Moderate	Stenotic ≥50%	Decrease of midsystolic velocity components	Stenotic, with or without mild intravascular signal loss
Severe	Stenosis >75%	Flattened flow profile with no distinct systolic velocity maximum	Severe intravascular signal loss simulating occlusion

maximum upslope (MUS), and the time to peak (TTP) measurements (34). In patients with RAS MTT/TTP/MUS was 37.2 seconds/25.4 seconds/10.7, while the MTT/TTP/MUS of healthy patients was 21.4 seconds/15.5 seconds/21.3 (34). The different perfusion parameters were also correlated with the patients' serum creatinine levels. Significant correlations were found for MTT and MUS, with moderate correlation coefficients could be found for TTP. Renal perfusion parameters have been found in previous studies to reflect changes in the renal function (109) and to correlate with cardiac risk factors

(110). The importance of renal perfusion is underscored by the fact that patients with impaired renal perfusion parameters have an increased morbidity and mortality.

Another relatively new technique to assess renal perfusion is to use MRA sequences with high temporal resolution (Fig. 20-32). These techniques, TRICKS (GE) or TREAT (Siemens), use view-sharing techniques that undersample the periphery of k-space (111). TREAT also integrates parallel imaging techniques to further increase the temporal resolution (112) and allow detecting decreased perfusion and delayed perfusion of a single side (Fig. 20-33).

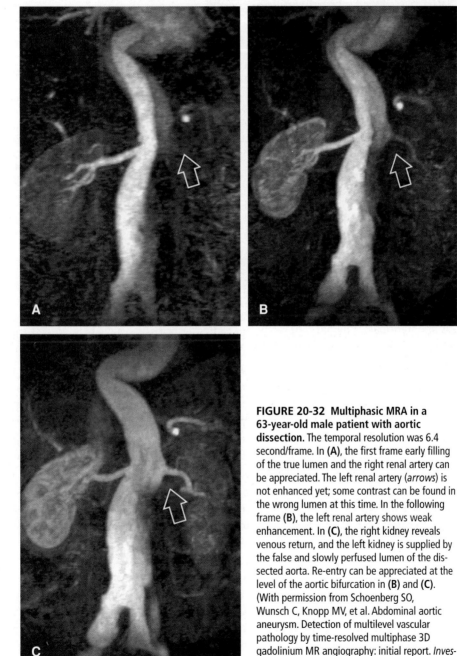

FIGURE 20-32 Multiphasic MRA in a 63-year-old male patient with aortic dissection. The temporal resolution was 6.4 second/frame. In **(A)**, the first frame early filling of the true lumen and the right renal artery can be appreciated. The left renal artery (*arrows*) is not enhanced yet; some contrast can be found in the wrong lumen at this time. In the following frame **(B)**, the left renal artery shows weak enhancement. In **(C)**, the right kidney reveals venous return, and the left kidney is supplied by the false and slowly perfused lumen of the dissected aorta. Re-entry can be appreciated at the level of the aortic bifurcation in **(B)** and **(C)**. (With permission from Schoenberg SO, Wunsch C, Knopp MV, et al. Abdominal aortic aneurysm. Detection of multilevel vascular pathology by time-resolved multiphase 3D gadolinium MR angiography: initial report. *Investigative Radiology* 1999 [Oct];34(10):648–659.)

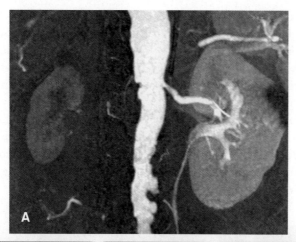

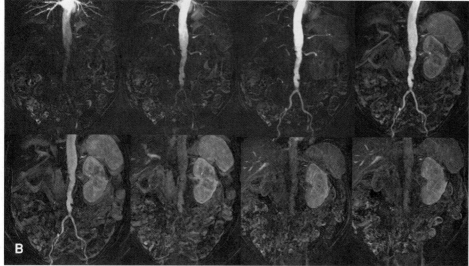

FIGURE 20-33 A: Coronal MIP of a 68-year-old patient with severe atherosclerosis and moderate left RAS. The right kidney shows only weak enhancement; the right renal artery is occluded. **B:** Time-resolved imaging series of the same patient using a TREAT sequence with a temporal resolution of 2 second/3D data set. The left kidney shows regular enhancement, whereas the right kidney demonstrates a delayed and very weak enhancement. This can be explained by remaining right renal perfusion via the capsular arteries. (Courtesy of J. Paul Finn, M.D., University of California in Los Angeles.)

Renal Artery Stenosis and Renoparenchymal Disease

RAS comprises only a small entity in a large complex of overlapping diseases ranging from essential hypertension to primary renoparenchymal disease (1). The high prevalence of coexisting renoparenchymal disease can be considered as an important factor in explaining why a substantial number of patients—around 30%—do not improve after revascularization of RAS (113). Parenchymal disease can result from both primary causes such as diabetes or glomerulonephritis as well as secondary causes resulting from long-standing RAS with the consequence of ischemic kidney disease. Thus far, 3D Gd-MRA has not proven to have greater efficacy in curing renal hypertension or renal insufficiency than US. Due to the relatively high costs of imaging, an aggressive search for RAS by angiographic techniques in patients with hypertension is controversial. Quantitative or semiquantitative perfusion measurements offer an independent measure of parenchymal blood flow in the renal cortex as well as the medulla (32,34,42), allowing an assessment of renal function independent of the presence of RAS (32–34). Abnormalities of these quantitative parameters have been found

in patients with primary parenchymal disease in whom underlying RAS is not present. Thus, these techniques appear to be a promising additional factor to separate renovascular disease from parenchymal causes.

Based on these issues, the determination of which patients with RAS will benefit from an intervention is controversial. While RAS is an important independent factor for 5-year patient survival (114), patients may experience a deterioration in renal function even after a technically successful intervention. Recently, the use of the resistive index in US was reported to be a valuable parameter for the prediction of patient improvement after interventional balloon angioplasty of RAS (82). However, other groups have found contradictory results for the RI as a predictor of successful outcome (83,84). The role for the prediction of outcome after interventional or operative revascularization has not yet been fully established for MR imaging. The potential to differentiate patients with predominantly renovascular or renoparenchymal disease based on a single comprehensive MR exam could represent an important adjunct to the current morphologic evaluation of RAS by 3D Gd-MRA.

Morphologic Assessment Germane to Therapy

An important nuance to RAS imaging that must be assessed when stenting is contemplated in a patient with atherosclerotic occlusive disease is the determination as to whether the lesion is within the renal artery or in the aorta adjacent to the renal artery ostium (Fig. 20-34). When thrombus in the aorta obstructs a renal artery origin, its dilation and stenting can result in a stent that is poorly fixed if it is not sufficiently engaged into the renal artery. Because DSA does not distinguish the true origin of the renal artery relative to the aortic wall in the setting of aortic thrombus, cross-sectional imaging, most effectively using CTA, is important to avoid an unstable stent deployment with the possibility of future migration.

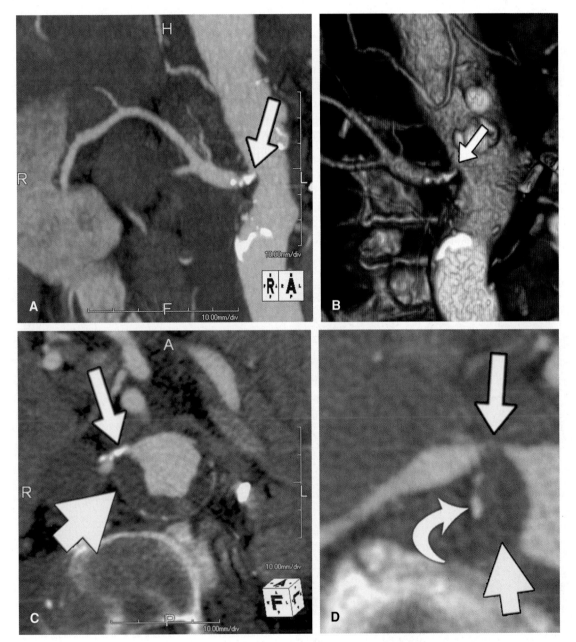

FIGURE 20-34 Aortic thrombus in an aneurysm simulating true RAS. A: MIP and **(B)** volume rendering of a CTA demonstrate apparent right renal arterial osteal stenosis (*arrows*). **C:** Transverse section reveals an abdominal aortic aneurysm with mural thrombus (*wide arrow*). Narrowing of the conduit from the aortic lumen to the renal artery simulates RAS (*narrow arrow*), when in fact this flow-limiting lesion is entirely within the aorta. **D:** A curved planar reformation demonstrates the aortic thrombus (*short arrow*), the high-grade narrowing (*long arrow*), and calcium in the wall of the aortic aneurysm (*curved arrow*) as well as poststenotic dilation in the proximal renal artery. The identification of aortic thrombus causing apparent renal artery stenoses is very important to effective management. Unless a stent deployed to treat this region is anchored at least 1 cm distally in the renal artery, the stent might dislodge and embolize distally down the aorta, as the proximal aortic fixation would be unstable. (Figure courtesy of Pietro Sedati and Geoffrey D. Rubin.)

Fibromuscular Dysplasia

Detection of FMD is of high clinical importance for two reasons. First, these patients are usually young at initial presentation and may require high doses of antihypertensive medications to control blood pressure. Second, FMD responds particularly well to angioplasty, with mean cure rates for blood pressure of about 50% and mean improvement rates of more than 40%. Regarding renal function, similar success rates have been reported with complete cure in about 40% of the cases and improvement in over 55% (118,119). Thus, more than 90% of all patients improve after angioplasty.

FMD can be subdivided into intimal fibroplasia, medial FMD, and adventitial fibroplasia. Whereas the intimal type of FMD is predominately found in infants, the medial type is usually seen in younger women and comprises about 90% of all types of FMD. The etiology of FMD is unknown, but it is considered to be a developmental disease that can be progressive over time.

Involvement of the distal main renal artery as well as the segmental renal arteries is common, whereas the proximal segments are frequently spared. So far, DSA has been the standard of reference for diagnostic evaluation of FMD, since high spatial resolution is mandatory in order to detect and grade the often subtle irregularities. Particular caution has to be taken to rule out FMD at the level of the segmental renal arteries, as modern angioplasty techniques with microcatheters allow dilation of these lesions with favorable outcome. Angiographically, a classic pattern of alternating web-like stenosis with aneurysmal segments is found, accounting for the so-called "string of beads" appearance (Figs. 20-35–20-37). Stenotic segments can be long or short in length. In approximately 40% of cases, the disease is bilateral. In addition, other vascular territories can be affected by FMD, such as the carotid, vertebral, splanchnic, or iliac arteries.

FMD has a varying prevalence in the different studies ranging from 16% to 40% (90,97,120). No large study on the accuracy of 3D Gd-MRA or CTA for the assessment of FMD exists. In most MRA and CTA studies that have reported high accuracies for stenosis grading, either the prevalence of FMD was low or cases with FMD were excluded from the evaluation. The most recent publication reports a sensitivity and specificity for the detection of FMD of 22% and 96% for MRA and of 28% and 99% for CTA, respectively (108). However, as discussed previously,

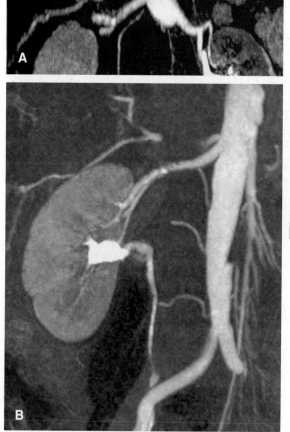

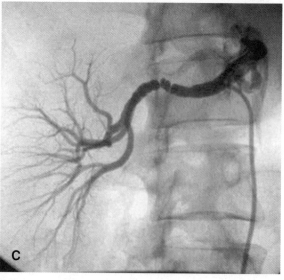

FIGURE 20-35 A–C: FMD in a 35-year-old female patient who presented with severe hypertension. **A:** The transverse MIP of the high-resolution MRA (1 mm³ voxel size) shows subtle vessel wall irregularities at the bifurcation of the renal artery and in the anterior division. **B:** The coronal MIP view confirms the findings. **C:** Patient then underwent conventional angiography, where a good agreement with the MRA was found. After dilatation of the renal artery, the blood pressure dropped drastically to normal values.

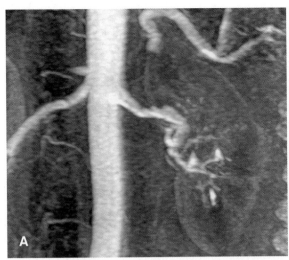 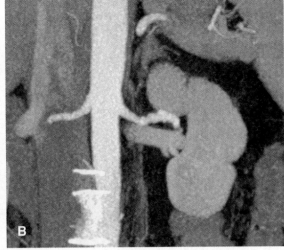

FIGURE 20-36 MRA versus CTA for FMD visualization. A: MRA (Gd-MRA with 2 mm section thickness on a 1.5 T magnetic without parallel imaging) and **(B)** CTA (64 × 0.75 mm) demonstrate the classic string of beads appearance of FMD in the left renal artery. The superior spatial resolution of the CTA when compared with this MRA allows better delineation of the abnormality for a confident diagnosis. (Figure courtesy of Geoffrey D. Rubin.)

there were serious methodologic problems with the MR and CT imaging in this study, resulting in CT techniques that were at least 6 years out of date at the time of its publication in 2004. Therefore, the accuracies of 3D Gd-MRA and CTA are not completely established but are expected to be less than for atherosclerotic stenoses. The challenges for MRA and CTA are subtle irregularities of the renal wall that are not seen due to the limited spatial resolution. Involvement of the distal renal arteries is even more difficult to detect on MRA due to increased motion as well as parenchymal overlay on the segmental renal arteries. While CE MRA has some role in the workup of patients suspected to have FMD, in most practice, the superior spatial resolution and the normal renal function of most patients make CTA the preferred noninvasive examination for diagnosis of FMD. With either technique, severe disease of the main renal arteries can be excluded even with the limited spatial resolution of 1 mm. Also, severe disease of the proximal celiac trunk and superior mesenteric artery can be excluded on the same data sets using sagittal reformats. Finally, patients can be noninvasively screened for significant stenoses of the extracranial and intracranial arteries by the combined use of 3D CE MRA of the carotids and high-resolution 3D TOF MRA at the circle of Willis without putting a young patient at the risk of a catheter angiography (120–122). It is, however, important to note that a negative MRA or a negative CTA of the renal artery does not suffice to exclude distal FMD, and therefore DSA might be required if a strong clinical suspicion is present. Future improvements in spatial resolution of both techniques promise a better depiction of the distal renal arteries.

Rare Causes of Renal Artery Stenosis

While atherosclerosis and FMD account for the vast majority of cases of RAS, some rare conditions may eventually lead to stenotic or occluded renal arteries as well.

Congenital coarctation of the renal arteries usually affects both renal arteries in their ostial segments. Other vascular malformations may also be found in these patients.

In patients with neurofibromatosis, RAS is present in some cases. Fibrous proliferation of the adventitia causes a narrowing of the vessel lumen. These patients should be referred to CTA or MRA as a diagnostic tool, as they are prone to complications during conventional angiography and have only a poor response to angioplasty.

Patients who previously underwent radiation therapy with the renal arteries in the irradiated volume can present with obliterated renal arteries. Depending on the treatment port, either the intrarenal or the extrarenal parts of the renal arteries may be affected.

The detection of renal artery stenoses in all of the above cases is technically feasible using CTA or 3D MRA. Due to the poor soft-tissue contrast of MRA, it is particularly important to obtain morphological sequences of the kidneys to safely cover these uncommon presentations of RAS. Fat-saturated T2W sequences are particularly suited to depict enlarged lymph nodes and to differentiate them from the mesenterial fat tissue. Postcontrast T1W sequences will conveniently show adrenal masses. In CT, no additional acquisitions are necessary, as all information can already be derived from the contrast-enhanced CTA.

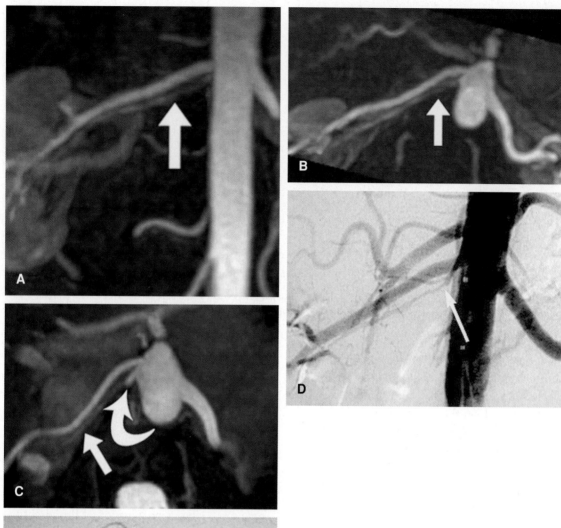

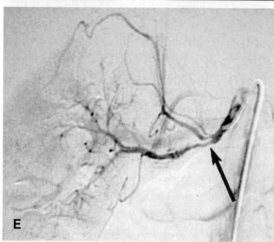

FIGURE 20-37 FMD in an accessory renal artery. A: Coronal and **(B)** transverse MRA demonstrate a thin and irregular accessory renal artery (*arrow*). It is difficult to ascertain if this artery is truly abnormal or normally small and poorly visualized due to limitations in spatial resolution. **C:** Oblique transverse MIP demonstrates a short normal arterial segment (*curved arrow*) proximal to the diseased narrowing of the accessory renal artery (*straight arrow*). This finding allows confident diagnosis of mid and distal accessory renal arterial disease consistent with FMD. It is always important to manipulate the volumetric data to confidently visualize the true origin of aortic branches, as overlap of the renal ostium with the aorta on the MIPs in **(A)** and **(B)** misrepresents the data. **D:** Aortic and **(E)** selective accessory renal arterial injections during DSA confirm medial FMD (*arrows*). (Figure courtesy of Jeffrey Maki.)

Vasculitis

Vasculitis is discussed in detail in Chapter 9. Within the renal arteries, vasculitis can present with stenoses or aneurysms.

In periarteritis nodosa (PAN), the kidneys are involved in 90% of all cases (Fig. 20-38). Hematuria is the main symptom presented in patients. MRA and CTA may rarely show microaneurysms at the bifurcation of the interlobar and arcuate arteries. Conventional subtraction catheter angiography remains the standard diagnostic tool for this study. However, a thinned cortex with a lobulated surface of the kidney at

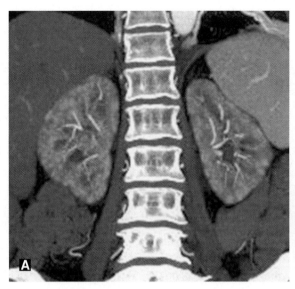
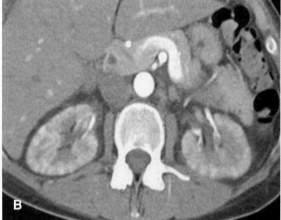

FIGURE 20-38 **A:** Coronal and (**B**) transverse CTA images. The renal arteries appeared normal. The renal cortex demonstrates a patchy, grainy opacification. The patient underwent biopsy, which revealed PAN of the kidneys.

later stages of the disease can be well seen in both CT and MR. Typically, multiple renal infarctions of different ages are seen throughout both kidneys. Using functional MR imaging, lowered perfusion parameters can be appreciated in the affected kidneys. CT may show multiple intrarenal bands of low attenuation, which represent occluded intrarenal arteries.

The autoimmune microvessel disease systemic lupus erythematosus (SLE) has a prevalence of 1 in 2,000 people in the United States. It manifests renal involvement in 50% of all cases. Membranous glomerulonephritis induced by SLE with subsequent nephrotic syndrome is responsible for 30% of all renal vein thromboses, which is a hallmark finding of SLE with renal involvement. Extensive collateral vessels from the renal hilum or the capsular vessels may be seen in cases of renal vein thrombosis. The thrombus can extend into the inferior vena cava. Intrarenal vascular involvement with SLE is less common than with PAN. As with PAN, in SLE, the inflammation of the interlobar arteries causes the formation of microaneurysms. These are rarely seen with MRA and CTA.

Takayasu arteritis (TA) is a granulomatous vasculitis of the large vessels that commonly affects more women than men with a female-to-male ratio of 8:1. While patients of any age may present with TA, 90% of the patients are in their second or third decade of life at initial presentation. Although the disease has a higher prevalence in Asia, it is not uncommon in the United States, where a prevalence of 1 in 1,000 people is estimated. The diagnosis of TA is based on clinical examination as well as on radiologic findings. Since only the major vessels are affected, TA is effectively

assessed with MRA and CTA. These modalities have replaced invasive catheter angiography in TA because they yield more information about the vessel wall involvement beyond the sole grading of stenotic lesions (Fig. 20-39). CTA and MRA may show mural thickening with enhancement after administration of contrast agent (154). These inflammatory changes often precede the development of stenotic lesions. A fat-saturated dark-blood double-inversion recovery T1W technique preferably with EKG-gating allows the best visualization of the vessel wall involvement in

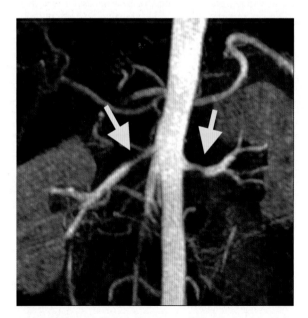

FIGURE 20-39 Coronal MRA of a 24-year-old female patient with long-standing TA. Both renal arteries demonstrate long-extending concentric stenoses (*arrows*).

MR. Additionally, fat-saturated T2W sequences should be acquired to detect vessel wall edema as another sign of active inflammation. Signs of inflammation can be the only diagnostic hint in early stages of the disease when stenoses have not yet developed. Stenotic lesions in TA are caused by inflammatory intimal proliferation and eventually lead to fibrosis of the media and adventitia. They appear as smooth long-extending, symmetric, and focal stenoses. All affected vessels, including the aorta, may finally become completely occluded. Rarely, poststenotic dilatations expand to aneurysms. Serial MRA or CTA is recommended to monitor the course of the disease.

ANEURYSMAL DISEASES

Renal artery aneurysms have a prevalence of 1% (87), with most patients being in their fourth to sixth decade of life (Table 20-4). They account for 22% of all visceral artery aneurysms. The majority of renal artery aneurysms are asymptomatic and are found incidentally with an average size of 2 cm at the initial presentation (Fig. 20-40). Symptomatic renal artery aneurysms may cause nonspecific symptoms such as flank pain, hematuria, and hypertension. Twenty percent of all patients exhibit bilateral renal artery aneurysm; multiple renal artery aneurysms occur in 30%. Approximately 10% to 20% of renal artery aneurysms rupture. Pregnant women are particularly prone to rupture of an aneurysm secondary to the elevated blood flow (88) during pregnancy. The underlying pathophysiology of a renal artery aneurysm is vessel wall damage. This is typically caused by degenerative changes as in atherosclerosis, inflammation as in FMD, or by trauma and iatrogenically.

Atherosclerosis can lead to saccular or fusiform aneurysms in the proximal renal artery and the lobar arteries,

which have a tendency to calcify. Calcified renal artery aneurysms have been reported to have a lower risk of spontaneous rupture, but this observation has recently been questioned (89). Renal artery aneurysms are easily displayed using 3D Gd-MRA and CTA. Three-dimensional postprocessing methods such as VR or shaded surface display (SSD) are necessary to evaluate the anatomical relations of the aneurysm in terms of origin and contact to other vascular structures (Fig. 20-41). Particularly with CT, a circular or incomplete ring of calcification can be demonstrated. Thrombus-containing aneurysms may be responsible for embolic infarcts of the affected kidney.

FMD is the leading cause of renal artery aneurysms. Up to 37% of all patients with FMD develop renal artery aneurysms (90). These saccular or fusiform aneurysms are diagnostically challenging, as they are preferentially located in the lobar and segmental arteries. In medial fibroplasia, the varying gauge of the string of beads of FMD hinders exact determination of aneurysmal extension. Three-dimensional Gd-MRA often fails to demonstrate FMD, especially when present in the segmental renal arteries due to motion artifacts blurring in the image. If multiple aneurysms are present in a patient with FMD-like appearance of the renal arteries, Ehlers-Danlos syndrome should be considered (90,91).

Renal artery aneurysms also arise in the presence of a variety of inflammatory diseases such as PAN, Wegener's granulomatosis, and tuberculosis. These aneurysms typically affect the subsegmental and interlobar arteries and are hardly seen with MRA or CTA. Because of their small diameter, they are also referred to as microaneurysms. Rare pseudoaneurysms of the renal arteries arise from focal infections or from Behçet disease (92). In contrast to true aneurysms, pseudoaneurysms do not involve all wall segments. Postinfectious aneurysms are typically mycotic and are prone to rupture.

Asymptomatic renal artery aneurysms smaller than 2 cm do not warrant intervention but should be followed. Therapy for renal artery aneurysms is indicated in women of childbearing age to prevent rupture of the aneurysm during pregnancy. All symptomatic aneurysms and growing aneurysms require treatment. If the neck of the aneurysm is found to be narrow, transcatheter with coiling can be attempted. If the aneurysm exhibits a broad base, open surgical repair is indicated. The literature reports good success rates for the surgical repair of the renal arteries; however, hypertension is cured or improved in only roughly 60% of patients (93).

Aneurysms of the renal veins are even rarer than renal artery aneurysms. Less than 10 cases have been described in the literature so far (Fig. 3-27). Diagnostically, they are

TABLE 20-4
Renal Artery Aneurysm

Atherosclerosis
Fibromuscular dysplasia
Panarteritis nodosa (microaneurysms)
Neurofibromatosis (microaneurysms)
Lupus erythematosus (microaneurysms)
Wegener's granulomatosis
Syphilis
Tuberculosis
Behçet disease
Ehlers-Danlos syndrome
Infection (mycotic aneurysm)
Trauma

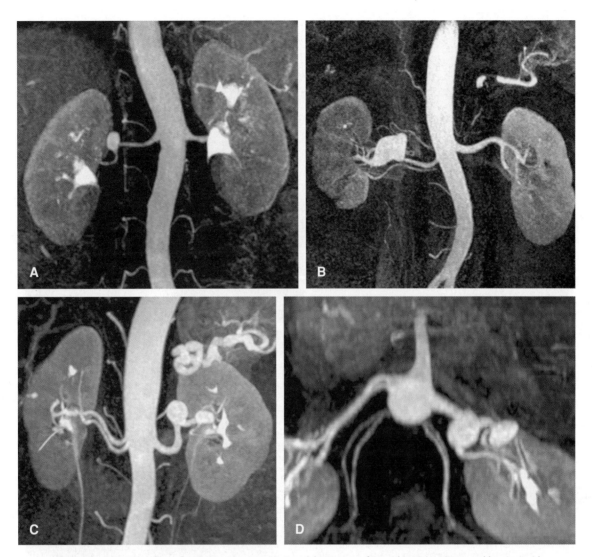

FIGURE 20-40 MRA of renal artery aneurysms. A: Coronal MIP view of a renal MRA in a 52-year-old patient with hypertension. A small (1.5 cm) aneurysm at the branching site of the renal artery can be appreciated. No signs of atherosclerosis and no RAS are found. **B:** Coronal MIP view of a renal MRA in a 68-year-old patient with hypertension. The MRA demonstrates a saccular aneurysm of the left renal artery involving also the lobar arteries. **C, D:** Coronal and transverse MIP view of a renal MRA at 3.0 T of a 38-year-old patient with hypertension and FMD. On the left side, the main renal artery and the branching site as well as the anterior lobar artery show aneurysmatic changes (**C** and **D**). (Courtesy of J. Paul Finn, M.D., University of California in Los Angeles.)

often easy to demark from the surrounding structures. The "layered gadolinium sign" has been described as characteristic for renal vein aneurysms (94).

RENAL ARTERY DISSECTION

Isolated renal artery dissection (RAD) is a rare condition, with approximately 200 cases reported in the literature (Table 20-5). Clinical signs of RAD include progressive renovascular hypertension, decrease of the kidney function, and kidney infarction, if any symptoms occur at all. If the false lumen re-enters the true lumen, the symptoms can

disappear suddenly. RAD typically affects patients in their fourth to sixth decade, with men being four times more often affected than women. Bilateral RAD occurs in 10% to 15% of all patients (127). The most frequent cause of RAD is FMD. In 9% of all patients with FMD, focal RAD can be detected. Other reasons for RAD include atherosclerotic vessel disease, trauma (especially anterior-posterior deceleration), segmental arterial mediolysis, Marfan syndrome, Ehlers-Danlos syndrome, subadventitial angioma, and iatrogenic manipulation. The typical imaging finding in RAD is the appearance of two lumina (Fig. 20-42). Due to its infrequent occurrence, no studies have been published

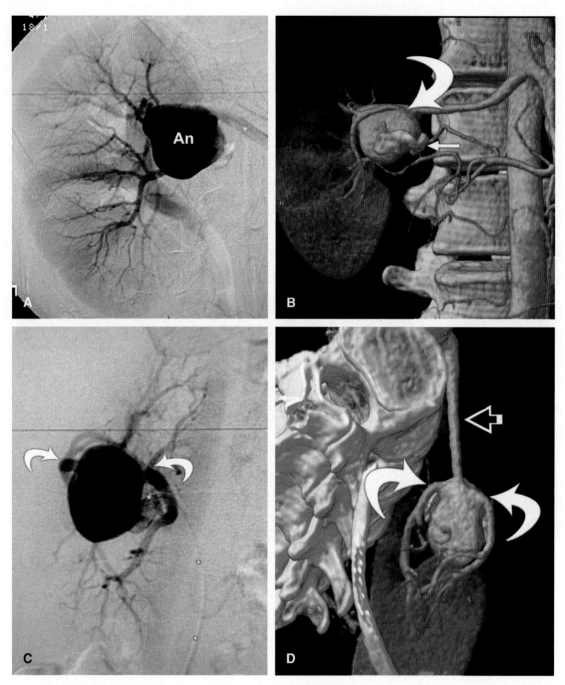

FIGURE 20-41 Right renal artery aneurysm. A: Anteroposterior projection of a selective right renal artery angiogram demonstrates a large aneurysm (*An*) in the renal hilum. The tip of the injection catheter is proximal to the renal artery aneurysm (∗). **B:** Frontal volume rendering from a renal CTA demonstrates a right renal artery aneurysm with peripheral calcification (*small arrow*) and a secondary renal artery branch arising from the superoanterior aspect of the aneurysm (*curved arrow*). **C:** Oblique projection of a selective injection of right renal artery demonstrating the renal artery aneurysm and two efferent renal artery branches supplying the anterior and posterior halves of the kidney, respectively (*curved arrows*). The locations of these arterial origins cannot be ascertained due to overlap with the aneurysm. **D:** Volume rendering best illustrates the relationships between the afferent renal artery (*open arrow*), the renal artery aneurysm, and the two efferent arteries (*curved arrows*). (Figure courtesy of Pietro Sedati and Geoffrey D. Rubin.)

Renal Artery Dissection

Atherosclerosis
Fibromuscular dysplasia
Dissection—aortic aneurysm
Trauma (deceleration)
Marfan syndrome
Ehlers-Danlos syndrome
Iatrogenic
Idiopathic

so far in analyzing the value of MRA or CTA for the detection of RAD.

More commonly, RAD occurs in the presence of aortic dissection (Fig. 20-43). Due to the different blood flow velocities in the false and the true lumen, standard contrast timing techniques may fail or produce artifacts. The MR flow and MR perfusion measurements may show delayed blood flow and contrast agent arrival in the parenchyma. Yet, MR flow measurements may fail if the dissection led to a small residual lumen, whereas MR perfusion measurements are more robust due to the

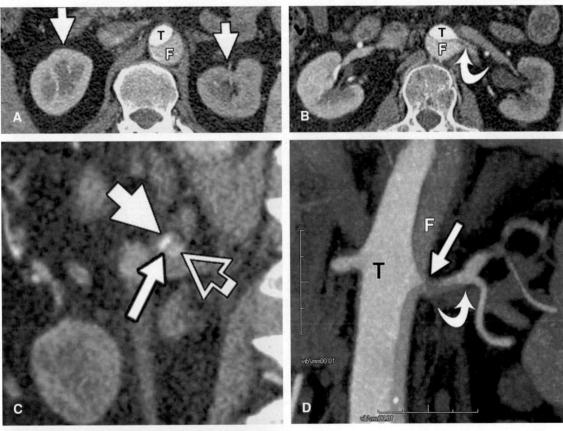

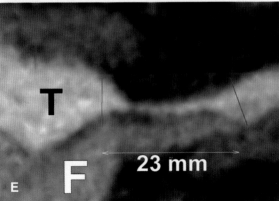

FIGURE 20-42 Type B dissection with flap extending into the right renal artery. A: Axial image demonstrates aortic dissection and differential enhancement of the kidneys (*arrows*). **B:** There is a single left renal artery, which arises from the true lumen. The dissection flap extends into its origin (*arrow*). **C:** MPR perpendicular to the long axis of the renal arteries demonstrates the dissection flap (*thin arrow*), true lumen (*wide arrow*), and the false lumen (*open arrow*). **D:** MIP demonstrates left renal artery true luminal stenosis (*straight arrow*) and the termination of the dissection flap (*curved arrow*). **E:** Curved planar reformation facilitates measurement of the length of the extension of the intimal flap into the left renal artery. (Figure courtesy of Pietro Sedati and Geoffrey D. Rubin.)

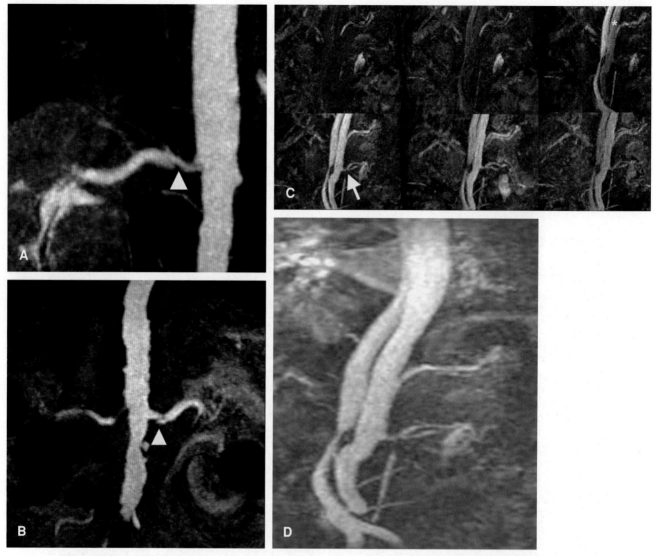

FIGURE 20-43 MR of renal artery dissection. A, B: Focal dissection of the renal artery in patients with atherosclerotic disease (*arrowheads*). Both patients revealed impaired renal artery flow. **C:** Coronal time-resolved renal MRA of a 42-year-old patient with traumatic dissection of the aorta. In the time-resolved multiphasic MRA, the enhancement of the true (first enhancing) and the false (delayed enhancing) lumen of the aorta can be appreciated. This technique proves that the left renal artery (*arrow*) originates from the false lumen (∗). **D:** The coronal MIP view demonstrates a dissection extending into the iliac bifurcation. From this single static image, the origin of the left renal artery cannot clearly be assigned to the true or false lumen.

acquisition of the information along the entire renal cortex. MR flow measurements are, however, a good approach to differentiate between a thrombosed lumen and slow flow, as thrombi may show various signal intensity depending on their age. While even slow flow shows some phase shift in MR flow measurements, thrombus does not. Yet, motion with its related phase-shift artifacts may obscure depiction of the renal arteries. Motion in combination with the small lumen of the distal renal vessels make accurate MR flow measurements in these vessels quite challenging. Another helpful approach is the

use of time-resolved multiphase MRA, which shows the arrival of the contrast agent bolus in the different lumens and thus allows assessing the origin of the renal blood supply (Fig. 20-43).

CTA is a valuable tool for the evaluation of aortic dissection to display the extent of the dissection and the re-entry site. Its superior spatial resolution allows it to characterize intrarenal dissection better than MR methods. While CT cannot quantify renal function like MR, substantial functional information can be gleaned from the pattern of parenchymal enhancement. Whenever variable parenchymal enhancement is observed on CT (or 3D MRA), the key differential consideration is whether delayed enhancement is due to delayed delivery of contrast material that is due to renal arterial supply from an aortic false lumen that has slower flow than the true lumen, or there is a flow limitation within the renal artery resulting in renal ischemia (Fig. 20-44). When the lumen supplying the kidney is clearly visualized from the aorta, through the renal artery osteum and into the mid renal artery, then a stenosis in the lumen may be visible. Alternatively, the intimal flap may collapse against a renal

artery osteum and produce a flow restriction. Another common variant occurs when a renal artery is supplied by both true and false lumen, where fenestrations in the intimal flap within the aorta or within the renal artery result in flow between true and false lumen, equalizing pressure and flow. Complex anatomic relationships such as these are best visualized with CTA due to its superior spatial resolution (Fig. 20-45). When a lumen is thrombosed, the hematoma presents as a high attenuation (>60 H.U.) area in the renal wall with CT. On MR, the detection of renal artery wall hematoma depends on the age of the bleeding

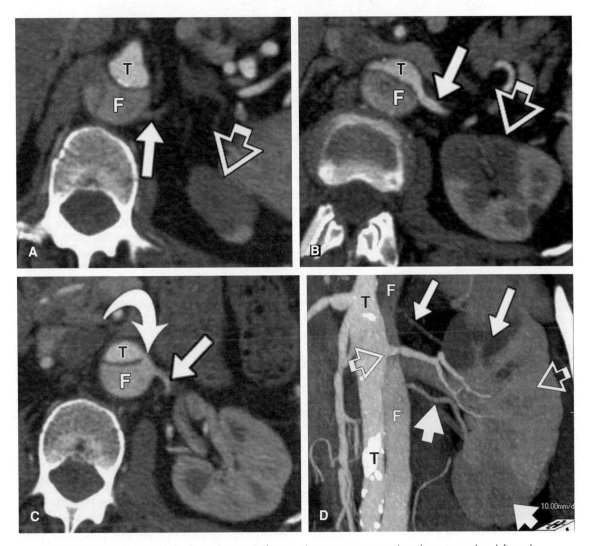

FIGURE 20-44 Type B aortic dissection. A–C: Three contiguous transverse sections demonstrate three left renal arteries. Image **(A)** demonstrates a left renal artery (*straight solid arrow*) arising from the false lumen (*F*), **(B)** demonstrates a second left renal artery (*straight solid arrow*) arising from the true lumen (*T*), and **(C)** shows a third left renal artery (*straight solid arrow*) receiving supply from both true and false lumina with a fenestration near this renal artery's osteum (*curved arrow*) allowing communication between the true and false lumina. There are three different degrees of left renal enhancement due to the differential opacification of the true and false lumina (*white outline arrow* shows relative decreased left renal upper pole enhancement in images **A** and **B**). It is important not to confuse differential renal enhancement due to variable rates of contrast medium delivery through true and false lumina with that of renal ischemia. (*Figure 20-44 continues*)

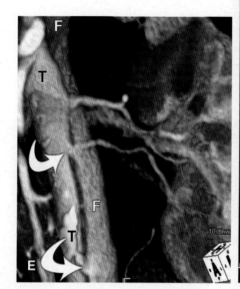
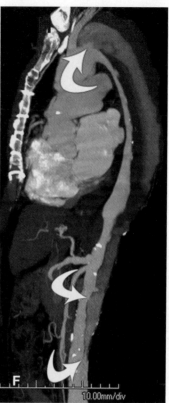

FIGURE 20-44 Continued D, E: Anterior oblique MIP **(D)** and volume-rendered image **(E)** demonstrate the small left upper pole accessory artery arising from the false lumen with corresponding relatively decreased upper pole enhancement (*long arrows*), the main left renal artery arising from the true lumen (*T*) resulting in maximal left renal mid zone enhancement (*open arrow*), and the lower pole accessory artery receiving supply from both true and false lumina resulting in intermediate lower pole enhancement (*short arrow*). Note sites of true-false luminal communication through fenestrations that occur at the sites of exit tears at aortic branches (*curved arrows*). **F:** Sagittal MPR image demonstrates the site of the primary entry tear in the proximal descending aorta (*large curved arrow*) and sites of other fenestrations (*smaller curved arrows*) in the abdominal aorta. The opacification of the false lumen is closely associated with the proximity to fenestrations due to slow flow in the false lumen. (Figure courtesy of Pietro Sedati and Geoffrey D. Rubin.)

and the sequences used. If there is suspicion of renal wall hematoma, dark-blood, fat-saturated T1W images should be acquired if possible with ECG-gating.

VASCULAR COMPRESSION SYNDROMES

While renal artery compression can occur in a wide variety of conditions, its overall prevalence is rare. These conditions include aortic and aortic branch aneurysms, pseudoaneurysms, hematoma, pancreatic pseudocyst, enlarged lymph nodes (123), renal mass (Fig. 20-46), adrenal masses, and retroperitoneal fibrosis.

Median arcuate ligament compression of the renal artery is far less common compared with the prevalence of celiac trunk compression (124). However, recent literature suggests that the prevalence of RAS by compression through the crura of the diaphragm may be underestimated. Particularly, slender patients and patients with aberrant origin of the renal

arteries are prone to develop this compression syndrome. Diagnosis is best made with dynamic MR imaging using SSFP sequences in end-expiration and in-inspiration. A single-phase MRA or CTA may not show the compression. MRA lacks the required soft-tissue contrast to show the crus of the diaphragm.

The differential diagnoses for renal vein compression are very similar to those of the artery involvement. They include (pseudo- and true) aneurysms of the aorta and the renal artery; enlarged lymph nodes (123); retroperitoneal, renal, and adrenal masses; and pancreatic pseudocysts. Because of its close anatomical relation to the aorta and the mesenterial vessels, the left renal vein can be compressed by crossing vessels. This syndrome, also known as "nutcracker" syndrome, is caused by the superior mesenteric artery, which compresses the left renal vein as the vein passes under the proximal part of the SMA (Fig. 20-47). The nutcracker syndrome is a relatively common cause of renal vein

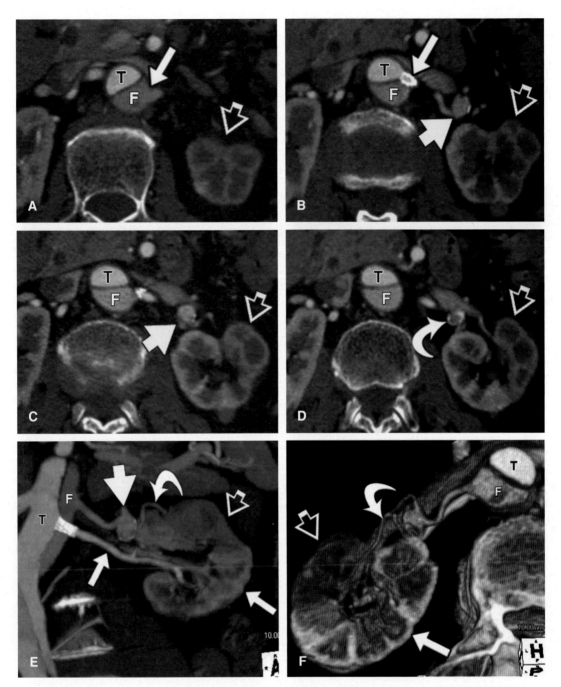

FIGURE 20-45 Type B aortic dissection with false luminal pseudoaneurysm in an accessory renal artery.
A–D: Contiguous, cranial to caudal, transverse CT sections demonstrate true (*T*) and false (*F*) lumina of an abdominal aortic dissection. **A:** An accessory renal artery is supplied by the false lumen (*long arrow*) with cortical thinning and hypoattenuation of the supplied upper polar renal parenchyma (*open arrow*). **B–D:** The main left renal artery originates from the true lumen just inferior to the accessory renal artery. A stent has been placed in the proximal main renal artery to correct a stenosis from the intimal flap at the renal arterial ostium (*long arrow*). A saccular aneurysm of the accessory artery (*wide arrows*) with mural thrombus and calcification (*curved arrow on* **D**) is demonstrated. **E:** Oblique MIP shows differential enhancement of the upper pole (*open arrow*) in distribution of the accessory renal artery arising from the false lumen relative to the lower pole, which is supplied by the stented main renal artery (*long arrows*). The false luminal pseudoaneurysm (*wide arrow*) and one of its efferent arteries (*curved arrow*) are also shown. **F:** Superior volume rendering illustrates the two renal arteries and the differential parenchymal enhancement. (*Figure 20-45 continues*)

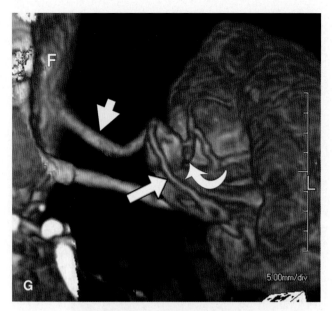

FIGURE 20-45 Continued G: Frontal volume rendering clarifies the complex anatomy of the accessory renal arterial pseudoaneurysm (*wide arrow*), which gives rise to two efferent branches: one to the upper pole (*curved arrow*) and another to the anterior aspect of the lower pole (*long arrow*). (Figure courtesy of Pietro Sedati and Geoffrey D. Rubin.)

compression. The increased intravenous pressure can lead to reflux of blood to the ipsilateral gonadal vein and in chronic stages also to drainage via the contralateral gonadal venous system (125). MRA and CTA show an enlarged left renal vein and prominent gonadal veins, which exhibit early and distinct enhancement. Most of these cases are asymptomatic; however, varicoceles can develop. The left renal vein can also be compressed when it passes behind the aorta to join the inferior vena cava.

RENAL VEIN THROMBOSIS

Renal vein thrombosis (RVT) most commonly affects the left renal vein, probably due to its longer course to the inferior vena cava. The most common reason for RVT is a hypercoaguable state such as dehydration (126), nephrotic syndrome, and clotting factor imbalances (Fig. 20-48). RVT is also quite common with the invasion of renal cell carcinoma into the renal vein; RVT with Wilms' tumor is far less common. RVT also occurs in the post-traumatic state, with pancreatitis (127), secondary to renal vein compression by lymph nodes or abscesses or by continuous spread of

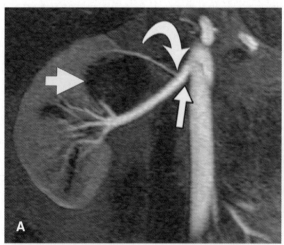

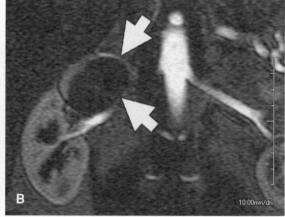

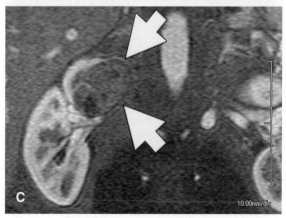

FIGURE 20-46 Renal cell carcinoma displacing arterial branches. A: MIP coronal spoiled gradient echo gadolinium-enhanced MRA demonstrates a single right renal artery (*long arrow*) with prehilar branching (*curved arrow*). These branches are displaced by a low signal mass in the upper pole of the right kidney that is not enhancing (*short arrow*). **B, C:** Coronal source images obtained 20 and 60 seconds following gadolinium injection, respectively, documents the value of delayed images, which establish that the mass enhances and is not a cyst. The arterial branches are not visualized as well as on the MIP (*arrows*). Histopathology revealed a renal cell carcinoma. (Figure courtesy of Pietro Sedati and Geoffrey D. Rubin.)

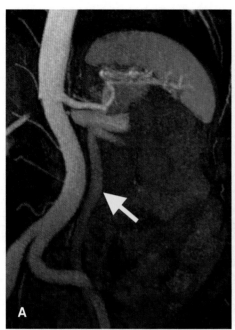
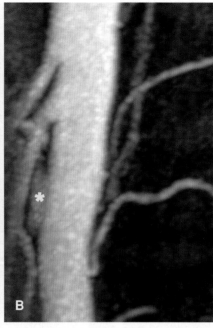

FIGURE 20-47 A: Coronal MIP view of the venous phase of a high spatial resolution MRA demonstrates a dilated gonadal vein on the left side (*arrow*). **B:** In the sagittal MIP view of the same venous phase, a mild compression of the left renal vein (∗) between the superior mesenteric artery and the aorta is shown.

gonadal vein thrombosis into the renal vein. RVT is most common in patients with membranous glomerulonephritis, which occurs in 30% of patients suffering from SLE.

The thrombus may extend into the inferior vena cava up to the right atrium. The classic diagnostic triad of a flank mass, gross hematuria, and thrombocytopenia is only present in 13% of all patients with RVT. Therefore, imaging is often required to establish the diagnosis. If US is not sufficient, MRA or CTA can be used to detect RVT. However, in the setting of decreased renal function, MRA is preferred (Fig. 20-48). Typical radiographic findings of RVT include swelling of the affected kidney in the acute phase and scarring of the kidney with long-standing RVT. MR imaging reveals low signal intensity of the renal parenchyma in both T1W and T2W sequences as well as a compression of the collecting system. The signal intensity loss of the renal cortex in T2W sequences is present from the first day on. Especially in acute RVT, a low signal intensity band at the outer part of the medulla can be seen, which is to represent hemorrhage secondary to the impaired blood drainage. This imaging finding resembles intrarenal changes seen in patients suffering from hemorrhagic fever with renal syndrome. Extensive venous collateral vessels as well as dilatation of the left gonadal vein may be seen in chronic RVT. The collaterals usually arise from the renal hilum around the proximal ureter and of the capsular vessels. The corticomedullary differentiation vanishes from the fifteenth day on T1W images, and the kidney becomes atrophic by 1 month.

The gold standard for diagnosis of RVT, conventional renal venography, is not popular and is hardly used in the clinical routine. MRA and CTA have been shown to be useful and accurate tests for the detection of RVT. With CT, a striated or delayed nephrographic phase may be seen, which is due to the intrarenal stasis of the blood flow. CTA may ease the detection of hemorrhage secondary to the RVT by showing high attenuation signal in the affected kidney. Contrast enhancement of RVT in either CTA or MRA is suspicious for malignant involvement (Fig. 20-49). To detect RVT in the MRA, MPR views of the venous phase are most appropriate. However, no studies comparing conventional venography with MRA or CTA exist to date.

TRAUMA

Renal trauma can be classified into four different grades:

1. Minor renal trauma, including contusion and hematoma of the kidneys
2. Major renal trauma with laceration of the cortex but without urine leak
3. Catastrophic renal trauma with avulsion of the renal vessels
4. Injuries of the UPJ

Renal artery involvement is most common with blunt trauma, which can be prevalent with grades 1 to 4 of the above classification. Therefore, minor trauma does not rule out renal artery involvement. CT is probably the best modality for renal trauma patients due to its short examination times. Depending on the force exerted on the patient during trauma, the degree of renal vessel involvement may vary.

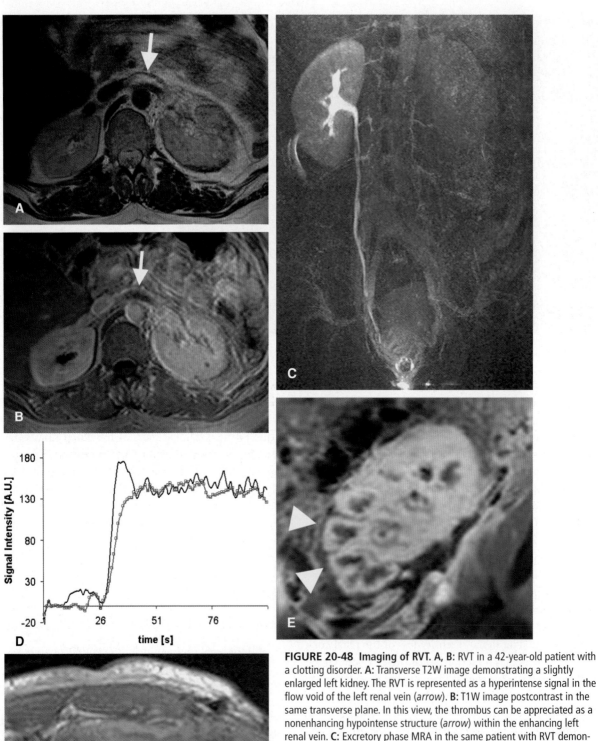

FIGURE 20-48 Imaging of RVT. A, B: RVT in a 42-year-old patient with a clotting disorder. **A:** Transverse T2W image demonstrating a slightly enlarged left kidney. The RVT is represented as a hyperintense signal in the flow void of the left renal vein (*arrow*). **B:** T1W image postcontrast in the same transverse plane. In this view, the thrombus can be appreciated as a nonenhancing hypointense structure (*arrow*) within the enhancing left renal vein. **C:** Excretory phase MRA in the same patient with RVT demonstrates no excretion of the contrast agent in the left kidney. **D:** Signal intensity versus time curve of left renal perfusion. The healthy right kidney (*black curve*) demonstrates a regular pattern with a steep upslope, defined peak, and slow decay of the signal intensity after the peak. The affected side (*red curve*) reveals a delayed and slowed upslope and a lowered, less clearly defined peak. **E:** Postcontrast T1W image of another patient who suffered from venous stasis during renal transplantation. The necrotic areas in the cortex and some of the pyramids are not enhanced (*arrowheads*). In the nonenhanced scan (**F**), there is hyperintensity due to the hemorrhagic infarction of the cortex.

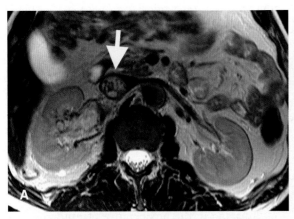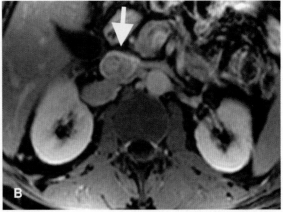

FIGURE 20-49 A: Transverse T2W spin-echo image of a 54-year-old male patient with right-sided renal tumor. With a dark-blood sequence a thrombus is demonstrated in the inferior vena cava (*arrow*). **B:** In the T1W GRE sequence, in transverse orientation there is marked enhancement of the thrombus (*arrow*), suggesting a malignant thrombus that was confirmed histologically after operation.

Deceleration during motor vehicle accidents makes the renal arteries prone for dissection. MRA and CTA may show the dissection flap and intramural hematoma as well as renal infarcts. Renal infarcts present as wedge-shaped hypoattenuating (CT), hypointense (T2W) subcortical areas in the kidney. In the acute phase, the affected kidney may be enlarged due to edema, whereas in the chronic state the kidney shrinks and scars, resulting in an irregular renal surface. Areas of renal infarction do not enhance after contrast administration. A rim sign—marginal cortical perfusion via the perforating arteries in the absence of renal perfusion—may be visible in this case. Renal artery occlusion can occur when the intimal flap occludes the lumen or the lumen thromboses. MRA and CTA then show an abrupt end of the renal artery, and an absent nephrogram can be seen or a rim sign may be visible.

A hallmark finding in renal artery occlusion is the absence of perinephric hematoma, whereas a hematoma may be found solely around the proximal renal artery. If the arterial system of the kidneys communicates with the collecting system, untimely enhancement in the renal pelvis can be seen. If the contrast agent is administered via the superficial femoral vein/external iliac vein, retrograde flow of the contrast agent into the renal vein may be seen in case of renal artery occlusion.

In contrast to the renal arteries, renal vein laceration or secondary RVT is rarely associated with renal pedicle injury. Both renal veins and arteries are involved in the formation of post-traumatic arteriovenous fistulas (AVF). AVFs develop in up to 80% of all patients with penetrating trauma to the kidney, including stab wounds and kidney biopsies. These AVFs rarely impress as space-occupying lesions such as congenital AVMs.

Post-traumatic hypertension by activation of the intrarenal renin-angiotensin system is a potential consequence of post-traumatic AVFs. Other causes for post-traumatic hypertension include intimal flaps of the renal arteries and segmental infarctions of the kidney. Apart from direct vascular injury, indirect impairment of the blood stream to the kidney can cause post-traumatic hypertension due to a subcapsular hematoma with compression of the entire kidney, referred to as a "page kidney" (129,130). CT and MR are both able to demonstrate the subcapsular hematoma. CT may show a crescent-shaped hyerattenuating mass that does not enhance after contrast enhancement. MR will also show a nonenhancing crescent-shaped mass; however, the signal intensities in the different sequences may vary over time. The addition of a T2*W sequence can facilitate the diagnosis.

Overall, a triple-phase CT scan with unenhanced, arterial, and delayed (5 to 10 minute) phase is best for the assessment of renal trauma. This approach allows the detection of hematoma and blood-filled calyces during the nonenhanced phase, depiction of the renal vessels and parenchyma in the arterial phase, and extravasation from the renal collecting system.

VASCULAR IMAGING IN NEOPLASTIC DISEASE

Both MR and CT are well suited for the preoperative assessment of renal cell carcinoma (131–133). Three-dimensional CTA and MRA have been proposed for staging of renal cell carcinoma (134,135). These preoperative examinations are mainly focused on the size and infiltration of the tumor into the adjacent organs and blood vessels. Due to its inherent higher soft tissue contrast, MR is slightly better suited for the detection of tumor extension into the collecting system or perirenal fat.

The preoperative assessment of renal cell carcinoma also has to include the renal arteries and the renal veins. An exact description of the number and size of the arteries feeding the tumor is important to determine the potential for preoperative embolization of the tumor. Preoperative embolization is performed in some institutions to reduce the risk of intraoperative bleeding and the spread of malignant cells. Due to the still-limited spatial resolution of MRA and CTA, tumor vessels as seen in conventional x-ray angiography cannot be seen. To characterize the vascularity of renal tumors, time-resolved MR-techniques have been proposed (139). However, none of these techniques has evolved enough to be a part of clinical routine.

In addition to the renal arteries, renal vein and inferior vena cava involvement must be determined. MR has been reported to be more sensitive than CT in the characterization of renal vein involvement (131,138,146). The tumor thrombus in the renal vein may show as a hypodense structure on CT. Depending on the extent of tumor thrombus, secondary venous stasis in the gonadal, adrenal, or lumbar veins may be seen. With painless swelling of the left scrotum or a dilated left gonadal vein, complete or partial occlusion of the renal vein should be ruled out. Direct extension of tumor thrombus into the gonadal vein can also be seen in some cases. In contrast to RVT of nonmalignant etiology where the thrombus does not enhance, tumor thrombus tends to enhance heterogeneously after the administration of contrast agent. The extension of tumor thrombus into the inferior vena cava drastically changes the surgical approach and may require partial circulatory arrest. Therefore, the entire inferior vena cava, including the right atrium, must be included in the imaging volume. High-resolution, free-breathing T2W sequences are best to exactly assess the level of thrombus extension into the renal vein and the inferior vena cava with MR (Fig. 20-50).

Depending on the vascular supply of the tumor and the patency of draining veins, collateral vessels may be either venous or arterial. While the venous collaterals are located in the renal hilum in most cases, the arterial collaterals typically are at the periphery of the kidney and arise from capsular arteries. Tumor-related shunting and high-flow states can lead to enlargement of the draining vessels (Figs. 20-50, 20-51).

TRANSPLANTATION

Preoperative Planning

Preoperative imaging of potential kidney donors is an increasing indication for renal imaging. Depending on the hospital, CTA or MRA may be preferred for this kind of study (139). Studies comparing MRA with CTA showed comparable inter-reader agreement for both readers as well as similar performance of these modalities compared with conventional angiography for the detection of accessory vessels. MRA has the advantage of avoiding radiation exposure and using non-nephrotoxic contrast agent, but the examination requires a longer period of time and is more expensive than CTA. In addition, CT is able to detect calcifications of the kidney or the ureters. The imaging protocol should include angiography and morphologic imaging of the kidneys to be transplanted and also include a urographic phase for assessment of the proximal ureters.

Imaging in the preoperative planning of renal transplant donors should cover the entire abdominal aorta from the diaphragm to the external iliac arteries in order to detect aberrant renal arterial origins (140). The origin and course of all renal arteries needs to be described in detail for operative planning. Different techniques such as inclusion of an aortic patch with multiple arteries may be considered when there are multiple renal arteries. When reporting on the renal arteries, it is important to look for early branching of the arteries. Early branching is defined by a bifurcation of the renal artery into the segmental arteries within a distance of 2.0 cm or less from the aorta. These patients may not be suitable as renal donors, particularly when early branching is on the right in a retrocaval location.

The renal veins also need to be described in detail. Multiple, duplicated, retroaortic, or bifurcated renal veins as well as anomalies of the gonadal and lumbar vein anastomoses need to be identified. The distance to the orifice of the gonadal vein should be measured and reported. The urographic phase of the examination focuses on the collecting system. Anomalies such as ectasia, duplication of the collecting system, or malrotation of the kidney must be described. The examination has to address the ureters as well. They should be straight and not retracted to facilitate resection. CT is capable of detecting renal or ureteral calculi. MR is only able to demonstrate secondary findings such as hydronephrosis. The parenchyma should be assessed for masses.

In selected instances, preoperative assessment of renal transplant recipients may be indicated. The abdominal aorta and the external and common iliac arteries have to be free of significant disease to provide sufficient blood flow to the kidney allograft. In this setting, CTA may be superior to MRA because it can also display—but also easily overgrade—calcified vessel wall lesions that may be missed with MRA. Since the donor recipients often have been on hemodialysis for longer periods of time, they are prone to venous thromboses. The entire venous system may be involved; however, the upper extremity especially is affected, potentially leading to superior vena cava occlusion

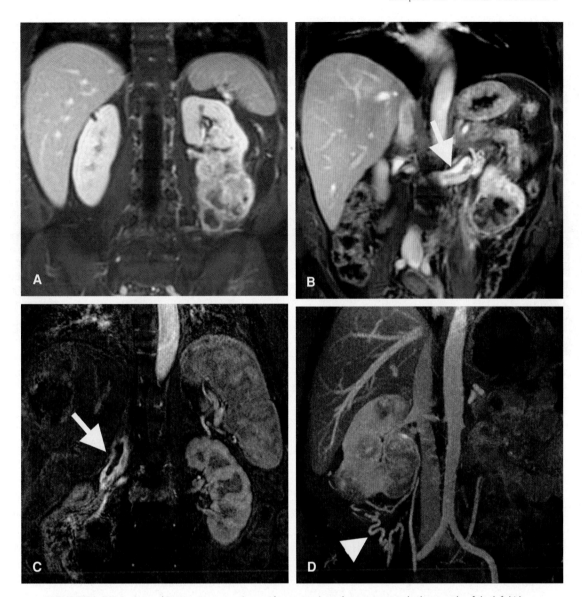

FIGURE 20-50 A: Coronal T1W postcontrast image demonstrating a large tumor at the lower pole of the left kidney. **B:** The same technique reveals thrombus of the left renal vein (*arrow*). Even though the thrombus does not enhance on this image, this thrombus was found to be malignant at operation. **C:** Arterial phase MRA in another patient with renal cell carcinoma on the right. Even though this scan was timed properly for the arterial phase, there is already early venous return on the side of the tumor. The right renal vein and the inferior vena cava reveal tumor thrombus (*arrow*). **D:** Coronal delayed phase MRA scan of a patient with multiple renal cell carcinomas. Note the enlarged capsular vessels inferior of the kidney (*arrowhead*), which hypertrophied to feed the tumor.

and upper extremity stasis. If the inferior vena cava shows thromboses or occlusion, the surgeons may anastomose the renal vein to the mesenteric veins. This is an important piece of information for diagnostic vascular studies posttransplantation to avoid misinterpretation of the findings.

Postoperative Surveillance and Symptomatic Assessment

CT and MR are commonly used in the surveillance of renal transplants (141). While CT offers shorter examination

times and allows easy detection of postoperative complications such as seroma, hematoma, and abscesses, MR may be more suitable for the vascular assessment due to MR contrast agents' lack of nephrotoxicity.

Vascular Assessment

The most common surgical approach for renal transplant vessels is an end to side anastomosis with the external or common iliac artery (Fig. 20-52). In the case of multiple renal arteries, an aortic patch may be used. The transplant renal vein is anastomosed end to side with the recipient's

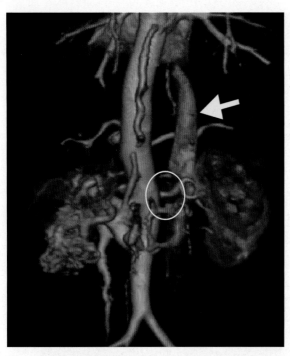

FIGURE 20-51 Posterior-view, volume-rendered MRA of a patient with left-sided renal cell carcinoma. In this patient, the high vascularization of the tumor leads to the development of shunts between the renal vein and the azygous venous system to drain the tumor (*arrow*), while the main renal vein is occluded from tumor (*circle*).

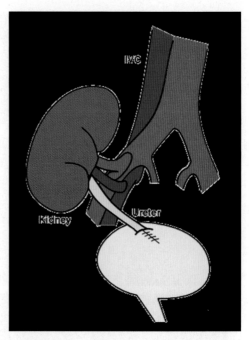

FIGURE 20-52 Scheme of the most common surgical anastomosis of the renal vessels and the ureter in adult patients. The renal artery is anastomosed to the common iliac artery side to side. Sometimes, the external iliac artery is used.

external iliac vein. Normally, the donor's left kidney is used since it provides a longer renal vein. If the right kidney has a sufficiently long renal vein, it can be used as an alternative. If the right renal vein is not long enough, a venous patch may be used to compensate for the shorter right renal vein. There are many variations to this surgical approach, depending on both donor and recipient anatomy (Fig. 20-53).

Owing to its lack of nephrotoxicity, 3D CE MRA has become a standard tool for the evaluation of renal transplants. The recent introduction of iso-osmolar contrast agents for CTA may foster the use of CTA in renal transplant surveillance in the future (75). Currently, there are no studies on this approach. CT offers the additional advantage of being less prone to artifacts if metallic clips were used during the surgical procedure. Most centers, however, do not use metallic clips in renal transplant patients to allow artifactfree MRA.

For renal transplant MRA, a standard 3D CE MRA sequence can be utilized. Due to the pelvic position of the transplant organ and the decreased respiratory motion, longer scan times can be considered to achieve a higher spatial resolution (Fig. 20-54). Prevalences for RAS between 1% and 25% have been reported occurring typically 1 month to 2 years posttransplantation. While proximal RAS at the anastomosis site is mainly a consequence

of the surgical procedure, distal RAS is considered to be a consequence of chronic rejection (142). Therefore, proximal RAS tends to occur in the immediate postoperative period. It is essential to detect possible surgery-induced intimal flap that is causing the RAS high-resolution. MRA has been found to be a highly accurate modality for detection and grading of transplant RAS. Compared with DSA, sensitivities of 100% and specificities ranging from 93% to 97% have been found (143). Since the hemodynamic relevance is characterized by impaired blood flow to the organ, MR flow measurements may be indicated in ambiguous cases. However, they may be hard to position perpendicular to the vessel axis due to the often short and tortuous arterial segment. A possible solution to this dilemma lies in MR-perfusion measurements that can be positioned over the kidney itself and are not restricted by a short transplant renal artery. They allow displaying pathologic perfusion parameters in the affected kidney or even in an affected kidney segment (144). Apart from the transplant renal artery itself, it is also necessary to include the iliac arteries into the field of view. In rare cases, stenoses of the iliac arteries can lead to transplant dysfunction as well (Fig. 20-55).

The etiology of these stenoses includes atherosclerosis and also postsurgical changes. A mild narrowing at the anastomosis site can often be found due to suture or clamp-related injury. If bladder augmentation techniques are used

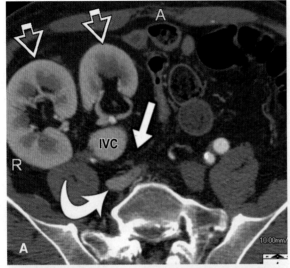

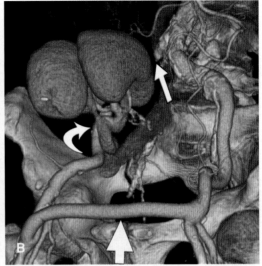

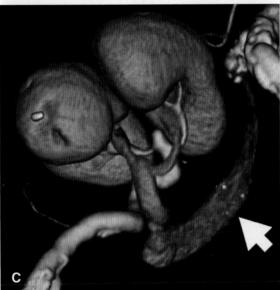

FIGURE 20-53 En-bloc transplant of pediatric kidneys. A: Transverse CT section demonstrates two transplanted kidneys from a pediatric donor (*open arrows*). The transplantation was performed en-bloc with the donor inferior vena cava (*IVC*) and aorta being transplanted together with the renal arteries and veins. The enhancing right common iliac vein (*curved arrow*) receives the drainage from the donor inferior vena cava. The common iliac artery is not seen in its expected location (*straight arrow*). **B:** Volume rendering illustrates the entire graft. The donor aorta is anastamosed to the recipient's external iliac artery (*curved arrow*). The common iliac artery is occluded near its origin (*long arrow*). A femoral to femoral bypass graft carries arterial blood from the left femoral artery to the right to supply the graft. **C:** The donor aorta and renal arteries (*light colored vessels*) and the donor inferior vena cava and renal veins (*dark colored vessels*) are best depicted on the volume rendering. The donor inferior vena cava drains into the recipient's right external iliac vein (*wide arrow*). (Figure courtesy of Pietro Sedati and Geoffrey D. Rubin.)

for surgery, the incidence of RAS is increased. RAS due to kinking of the transplant renal artery may lead to impaired renal blood supply of the allograft, particularly in the early postoperative days (145). Renal allograft torsion with rotation of the vascular pedicle is mainly seen in children with intraperitoneal renal transplant. Rotation of the renal transplant can be detected by changes in graft axis orientation and vascular kinking. Immediate therapy is indicated in these cases to salvage the graft.

Pseudoaneurysms at the anastomosis site are rare, with a prevalence of 1%. They may be asymptomatic or present with renal dysfunction secondary to the compression of the renal vein or artery. They can also occur with infections. Both MRA and CTA can depict pseudoaneurysms. Three-dimensional postprocessing methods such as VR may be necessary to evaluate the anatomical relations of the

pseudoaneurysm in terms of origin and contact to other vascular structures.

Renal artery thrombosis is a very rare and catastrophic early complication in renal transplants. The etiology includes technical errors during operation, hypotension, and atherosclerotic emboli. Renal artery thrombosis presents as absent or delayed and reduced enhancement of the transplant renal artery.

In renal transplants, it is also particularly important to start the venous phase scan immediately after the arterial phase to enable evaluation of the renal vein. RVT in renal transplant patients may arise due to kinking of the renal vein or acute or chronic rejection (146). The imaging findings are the same as with native RVT. Detection of transplant RVT is crucial to prevent loss of the transplant.

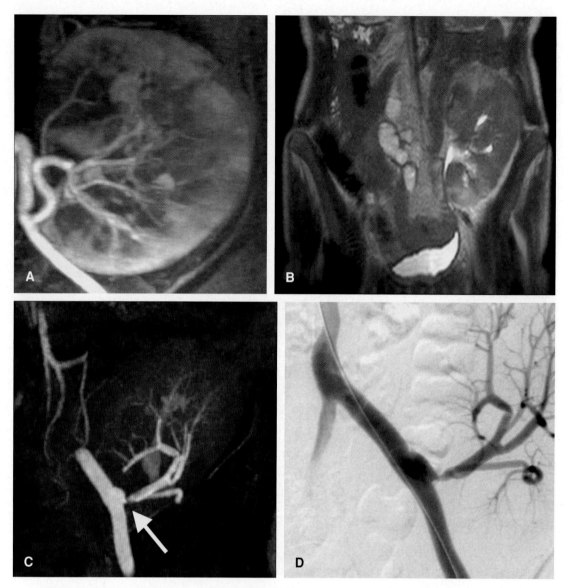

FIGURE 20-54 Complications of renal transplantation in two patients. A: Oblique MIP of the arterial MRA of a renal transplant with increasing serum creatinine level. The MIP shows a normal transplant renal artery but also patchy enhancement of the renal cortex. **B:** The T2W HASTE image of the same patient demonstrates an enlarged transplant kidney with hyperintense patchy renal cortex. This patient underwent biopsy, which revealed malakoplakia, a chronic granulomatous disease of the urinary tract. **C:** Coronal MIP view of a 32-year-old patient with early transplant dysfunction reveals a proximal RAS (*arrow*). Due to the early occurrence of the stenosis, it was regarded as suture-related stenosis. **D:** The conventional angiography confirms the MRA findings. (Parts **C** and **D** reprinted from MR angiography in patients with renal disease. In: Michaely HJ, Schoenberg SO, Rieger JR, et al., eds. *Magnetic Resonance Imaging Clinics of North America.* 2005;13:131–151. Copyright 2005 with permission from Elsevier.)

Parenchymal Assessment

Apart from the variety of vascular processes, renal allograft transplants are prone to a large number of parenchymal diseases and postoperative complications. Early nonvascular complications posttransplantation include acute rejection, ATN, hematoma, abscess, and vascular complications. Late nonvascular complications include chronic rejection, lym-

phocele, malignancies, and opportunistic infections involving the transplanted kidney. Unenhanced CT can be sufficient in the postoperative follow-up. If an abscess is suspected and contrast agent is required, the common precautions for iodine-based contrast agents have to be considered. MRI for parenchymal assessment should include high-resolution T1W and T2W images pre- and postcontrast. To allow

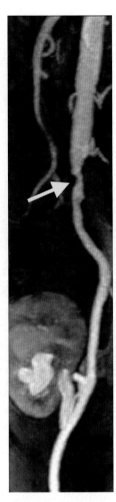

FIGURE 20-55 *A 20-mm oblique sagittal MIP of the arterial phase MRA in a 67-year-old male renal transplant patient. The patient presented with decreasing renal function. The renal arteries were normal, yet the patient revealed a 50% stenosis of the right common iliac artery (*arrow*). Flow measurements proved the hemodynamic significance of the stenosis.*

high resolution and avoid blurring, navigator-based techniques may be used. Time-resolved techniques like perfusion scans or time-resolved MRA sequences add additional information about the parenchymal enhancement pattern. If the acquisition time of the perfusion measurement (using extracellular Gd-chelates) is long enough (usually <4 minutes), excretion of the contrast agent into the calyceal system can be seen. Areas of delayed or lacking excretion are suspicious for parenchymal disease.

If sonography is not diagnostic, unenhanced CT allows fast and easy detection of most complications that arise immediately postsurgery. These include seroma, hematoma, and abscess. While seroma presents as a hypoattenuating mass, hematoma is characterized by high attenuation (40 to 100 Hu). Lymphoceles also appear as hypodense masses but increase in size over time while seromas decrease over time. These conditions do not require therapy in most cases.

Rarely, CT-guided drainage is indicated. Abscesses may arise in the operation field and in the transplanted kidney. They require drainage, which can often be done with CT guidance.

ATN is a reversible disease occurring post-transplantation, probably due to transient hypoxia and closely related to the time of warm ischemia. Since these patients present with increased serum creatinine levels, they are referred to MR in most cases. MR findings of ATN include preserved corticomedullary differentiation in the unenhanced scans with reversal of the typical contrast enhancement pattern after contrast agent administration. The cortex appears hypointense compared with the medulla, where the contrast agent is contained due to the tubular necrosis.

Due to the immunosuppression, malignancies associated with the renal allograft are not uncommon. While renal cell carcinoma and transitional cell carcinoma of the ureter present in the classic way, post-transplantation lymphoproliferative disease (PTLD) is a disease exclusively found in transplant recipients. PTLD arises in the setting of EBV infection and high doses of immunosuppressive drugs. In 75% of the cases, PTLD is found near the allograft and presents as a hypointense lesion in T1W images with weak enhancement. T2W images show hypo- and hyperintense signal behavior of the mass (147). The renal vessels themselves are rarely involved but may be encased (69,148). CT may show a hypoattenuating mass with moderate or no contrast enhancement. Imaging findings may be relatively nonspecific; therefore, PTLD should be considered for every differential diagnosis with unclear findings.

The immunosuppression also exposes patients to a greater risk of infectious disease that often show granulomatous character with the host's decreased immunocompetence. CT and MR show an enlarged allograft with inhomogeneous enhancement after contrast agent administration, as is seen in the case of malakoplakia and reactivated tuberculosis. Nonenhanced T2W images may already display a heterogenous signal intensity of the affected kidney. Even though the diagnosis of chronic rejection is based on biopsy results, imaging may give some clues. In the initial phase, CT and MR may reveal an increased organ size with thickened cortex. As the kidney becomes more fibrotic in the course of the rejection, the cortex thins out. Time-resolved imaging shows decreased and slowed contrast uptake with impaired or lacking excretion of the contrast agent. CT will show a poor nephrogram phase in these kidneys.

STENTS AND POSTOPERATIVE FINDINGS

On MR, postoperative findings of the renal arteries are most often related to stent or clip artifacts. In the case of

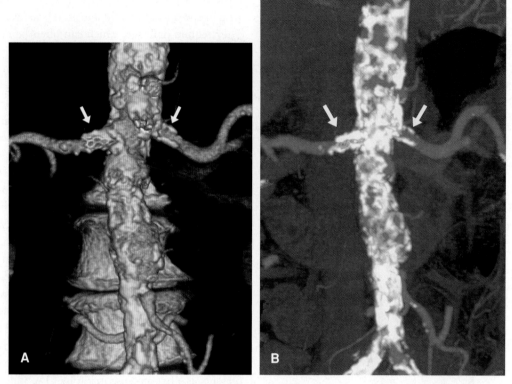

FIGURE 20-56 CTA of bilateral renal stents. A: Volume rendering and **(B)** MIP of a CT angiogram (16 × 1.25 mm) in a patient with extensive aortic calcification. The stents (*arrows*) are more clearly defined on the volume rendering when compared with the MIP due to the improved delineation of the signature stent structure. Overlapping calcification within the proximal renal arteries prevents recognition of the stent structure on the MIP. (*Figure 20-56 continues*)

stents, there is complete loss of signal in a limited stretch of the renal arteries. Newer stents that do not cause local field inhomogeneities and therefore do not lead to a signal loss are currently being developed (149) but are not available clinically. To assess the patency of the stent, MR-flow measurements and MR-perfusion measurements can be used. While a stent artifact most often does not pose a diagnostic challenge, clip artifacts can be misleading. Clips also lead to a local field inhomogeneity and a subsequent signal loss. If they are positioned close to a vessel, their focal signal loss may mimic RAS (150). Again, functional techniques such as flow and perfusion measurements can help to differentiate between artificial and real RAS.

CTA allows for detailed assessment of the position, degree of expansion, and patency of renal artery stents (Fig. 20-56). Special acquisition techniques are not required, but wide windows with relatively high centers are required to minimize blooming of the metal and allow discrimination of the metallic stent and adjacent calcified plaque. Neointimal hyperplasia can result in stenoses forming within stents. It typically appears several months to a year following stent deployment but can develop later.

Abnormal postoperative findings can be classified into acute and chronic complications. The acute complications comprise primarily hematomas, clip-related stenoses, and dissections. Chronically, stenosis can develop at graft anastamoses due to medical hyperplasia.

When examining any patient following renal surgery, close attention has to be paid to the patient's surgical history. In the rare case of inferior vena cava thrombosis, surgeons may anastomose the renal vein to the mesenteric veins. This finding must be differentiated from secondary changes in the draining system, as seen in chronic postoperative renal vein occlusion (Fig. 20-57).

AVMs

Arteriovenous malformations (AVM) are abnormal, direct communications between the arterial and the venous system without connecting capillary vessel bed. Renal AVMs represent a rare disease with a prevalence of 1 in 30,000 patients in autopsy series. They may lead to hypertension and hematuria. Many AVMs do not cause symptoms. Thirty percent of all renal AVMs are congenital; 70% are acquired. Congenital

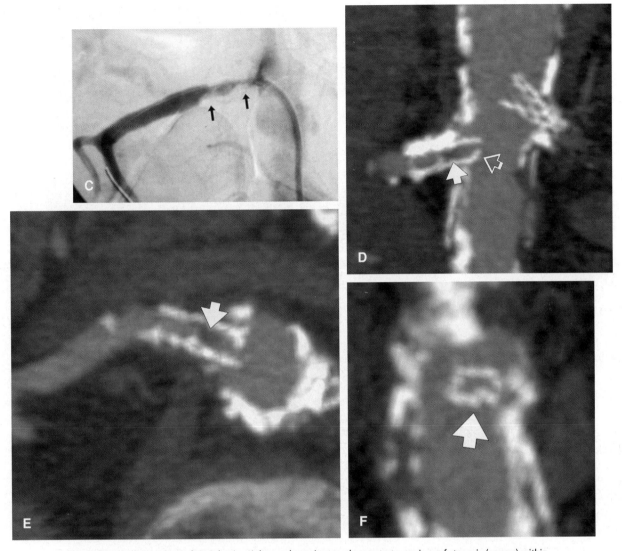

FIGURE 20-56 Continued C: Selective right renal arteriogram demonstrates regions of stenosis (*arrows*) within the stent presumably relating to neointimal hyperplasia. **D:** Coronal and **(E)** transverse MPRs through the central axis of the right stent allow direct visualization of the neointimal hyperplasia as a low attenuation filling defect within the stent (*solid arrow*). Additionally visible is incomplete expansion of the proximal aspect of the stent (*open arrow*). **F:** An axial section perpendicular to the axis of the stent and through its proximal most region confirms the incomplete expansion of the inferior aspect of the proximal stent (*arrow*). (*Figure 20-56 continues*)

AVMs, which are classified as cirsoid, cavernous, or idiopathic, are more common in women than in men. Acquired AVMs that typically arise after renal trauma, including a wide range of different conditions from stab wounds to renal biopsy, are more common in men. Cirsoid AVMs have a dilated corkscrew appearance resembling varicose veins. Depending on the number of involved vessels, cirsoid AVMs may form a renal mass. Since this mass is typically located adjacent to the renal collecting system, hematuria following erosion of the collection system is a common feature with cirsoid AVMs. Cirsoid AVMs most often obtain their

blood supply from segmental and interlobar arteries. Cavernous AVMs are characterized by a single enlarged artery feeding into a cavernous chamber with a single vein draining this chamber. Idiopathic acquired AVMs may arise after erosion of a renal artery aneurysm into the renal vein. They account for only 3% of all AVMs.

Acquired AVMs develop in 80% of all patients with postrenal trauma. In 20% of all cases, a history of renal biopsy can be obtained. Stab wounds and perforating wounds are another common etiologic factor for acquired AVMs. In contrast to congenital AVMs, acquired AVMs are

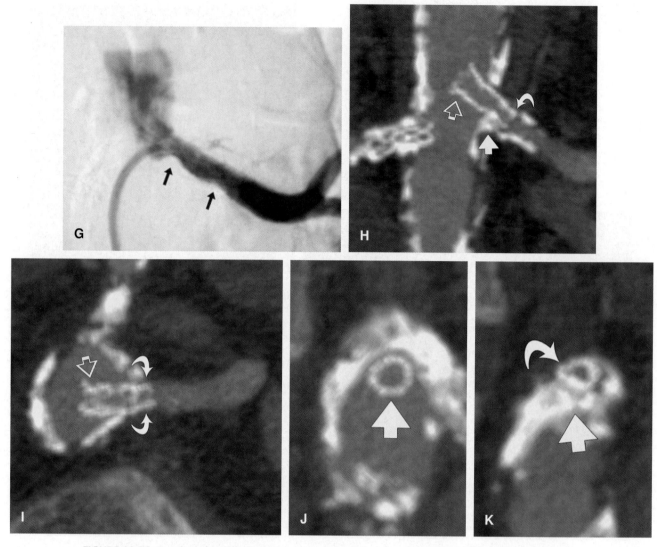

FIGURE 20-56 Continued G: Selective left renal arteriogram demonstrates similar filling defects within the left renal artery, as was seen in (**C**). The presumptive diagnosis of this arteriogram was neointimal hyperplasia as well. **H, I:** Coronal and transverse MPRs through the axis of a left stent demonstrate that the stent is minimally engaged within the renal artery. The majority of the stent is within the aortic lumen (*open arrow*). Approximately 5 mm of the stent is within the renal arterial lumen (*curved arrows*), resulting in an unstable condition with risk of stent dislodgement and embolization distally in the abdominal aorta. Note that the incorrect stent positioning cannot be gleaned from the conventional arteriograms. Examination of the stent lumen fails to demonstrate neointimal hyperplasia. Rather, heavy calcification (*solid arrow*) at the inferior aspect of the renal artery ostium extrinsically impinges on the stent, resulting in incomplete expansion and the appearance of luminal stenosis on the conventional angiogram. The more distal region of narrowing on the angiogram is not within the stent but corresponds to calcified atheroma on the inferior margin of the renal artery distal to the stent. **J:** Axial section perpendicular to the axis of the stent within the aorta demonstrates proper stent expansion (*arrow*). **K:** The distortion of the stent (*curved arrow*) is evident at the renal artery ostium due to compression from the large calcified atheroma on the inferior aspect of the renal artery ostium (*arrow*). This case illustrates a diverse spectrum of key findings that allow substantially greater characterization of stent abnormalities using CT when compared with conventional angiography.

more prone to induce hypertension by the activation of the renin-angiotensin system.

The range of possible imaging findings of AVMs with CT and MR is broad (151). The high flow through the AVM may lead to an early filling of the renal vein and the IVC compared with the other side. The high flow through the kidneys and the fast return of a huge amount of blood can lead to congestive heart failure and cardiomegaly, which is present in 50% of all symptomatic cases. The feeding and draining vessels may exhibit an increased diameter (Fig. 20-58). Cirsoid AVMs in particular tend to appear as a renal mass that shows prominent enhancement to the surrounding renal medulla. Sometimes, the large amount of blood bypassing the cortex leads to a diminished nephrogram and eventually to a cortical atrophy

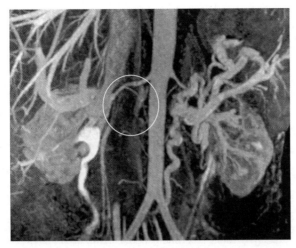

FIGURE 20-57 A 30-mm thin coronal MIP of the venous phase of the MRA in a 68-year-old female presents multiple dilated venous vessels on the patient's left side. No connection between the left kidney and the inferior vena cava can be shown (*circle*). The patient presented with gross hematuria and was thought to suffer from renal AVM. However, it turned out that the patient earlier underwent partial nephrectomy at which the renal veins were erroneously ligated. As a consequence, extensive collateral vessels developed.

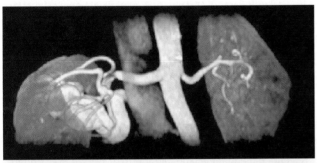

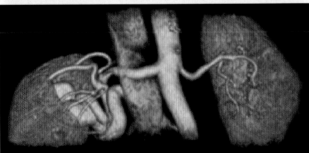

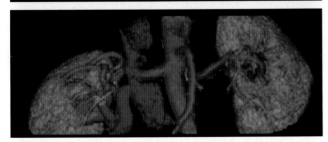

FIGURE 20-58 Renal artery AVM displayed using volume rendering with three different opacity transfer functions. Note the enlarged left renal artery compared with the right due to increased flow as well as the enlarged draining left renal vein.

of parts of the kidneys. Bleeding from the AVMs typically presents as an intraparenchymal lesion.

Embolotherapy is indicated when hematuria, hypertension, or congestive heart failure develops. Arterial embolization is usually the first-line procedure.

REFERENCES

1. Safian RD, Textor SC. Renal-artery stenosis. *N Engl J Med.* 2001;344:431–442.
2. Schoenberg SO, Rieger J, Johannson LO, et al. Diagnosis of renal artery stenosis with magnetic resonance angiography: update 2003. *Nephrol Dial Transplant.* 2003;18: 1252–1256.
3. Schoenberg SO, Rieger J, Nittka M, et al. Renal MR angiography: current debates and developments in imaging of renal artery stenosis. *Semin Ultrasound CT MR.* 2003;24: 255–267.
4. Debatin JF, Spritzer CE, Grist TM, et al. Imaging of the renal arteries: value of MR angiography. *AJR Am J Roentgenol.* 1991;157:981–990.
5. Schoenberg SO, Essig M, Bock M, et al. Comprehensive MR evaluation of renovascular disease in five breath holds. *J Magn Reson Imaging.* 1999;10:347–356.
6. Fleischmann D. Multiple detector-row CT angiography of the renal and mesenteric vessels. *Eur J Radiol.* 2003;45 [Suppl 1]:S79–S87.
7. Goyen M, Debatin JF. Gadopentetate dimeglumine-enhanced three-dimensional MR-angiography: dosing, safety, and efficacy. *J Magn Reson Imaging.* 2004;19:261–273.
8. Spuentrup E, Buecker A, Meyer J, et al. Navigator-gated free-breathing 3D balanced FFE projection renal MRA: comparison with contrast-enhanced breath-hold 3D MRA in a swine model. *Magn Reson Med.* 2002;48:739–743.
9. Wacker FK, Reither K, Ebert W, et al. MR image-guided endovascular procedures with the ultrasmall superparamagnetic iron oxide SH U 555 C as an intravascular contrast agent: study in pigs. *Radiology.* 2003;226:459–464.
10. Vasbinder GBC, Maki JH, Nijenhuis RJ, et al. Motion of the distal renal artery during three-dimensional contrast-enhanced breath-hold MRA. *J Magn Reson Imaging.* 2002;16:685–696.
11. Amann M, Bock M, Floemer F, et al. Three-dimensional spiral MR imaging: application to renal multiphase contrast-enhanced angiography. *Magn Reson Med.* 2002; 48:290–296.
12. Noll DC, Pauly JM, Meyer CH, et al. Deblurring for non-2D Fourier transform magnetic resonance imaging. *Magn Reson Med.* 1992;25:319–333.
13. Hany TF, McKinnon GC, Leung DA, et al. Optimization of contrast timing for breath-hold three-dimensional MR angiography. *J Magn Reson Imaging.* 1997;7:551–556.
14. Foo TK, Saranathan M, Prince MR, et al. Automated detection of bolus arrival and initiation of data acquisition in fast, three-dimensional, gadolinium-enhanced MR angiography. *Radiology.* 1997;203:275–280.
15. Prince MR, Chenevert TL, Foo TK, et al. Contrast-enhanced abdominal MR angiography: optimization of imaging delay time by automating the detection of contrast material arrival in the aorta. *Radiology.* 1997;203:109–114.
16. Wilman AH, Riederer SJ, King BF, et al. Fluoroscopically triggered contrast-enhanced three-dimensional MR angiography with elliptical centric view order: application to the renal arteries. *Radiology.* 1997;205:137–146.
17. Wikstrom J, Johansson L, Karacagil S, et al. The importance of adjusting for differences in proximal and distal contrast bolus arrival times in contrast-enhanced iliac artery magnetic resonance angiography. *Eur Radiol.* 2003; 13:957–963.

18. Butz B, Dorenbeck U, Borisch I, et al. High-resolution contrast-enhanced magnetic resonance angiography of the carotid arteries using fluoroscopic monitoring of contrast arrival: diagnostic accuracy and interobserver variability. *Acta Radiol.* 2004;45:164–170.

19. Riederer SJ, Bernstein MA, Breen JF, et al. Three-dimensional contrast-enhanced MR angiography with real-time fluoroscopic triggering: design specifications and technical reliability in 330 patient studies. *Radiology.* 2000;215:584–593.

20. Schoenberg SO, Knopp MV, Prince MR, et al. Arterial-phase three-dimensional gadolinium magnetic resonance angiography of the renal arteries. Strategies for timing and contrast media injection: original investigation. *Invest Radiol.* 1998;33:506–514.

21. Schoenberg SO, Bock M, Knopp MV, et al. Renal arteries: optimization of three-dimensional gadolinium-enhanced MR angiography with bolus-timing-independent fast multiphase acquisition in a single breath hold. *Radiology.* 1999;211:667–679.

22. Barger AV, Block WF, Toropov Y, et al. Time-resolved contrast-enhanced imaging with isotropic resolution and broad coverage using an undersampled 3D projection trajectory. *Magn Reson Med.* 2002;48:297–305.

23. Prince MR, Schoenberg SO, Ward JS, et al. Hemodynamically significant atherosclerotic renal artery stenosis: MR angiographic features. *Radiology.* 1997;205:128–136.

24. Alfke H, Heverhagen JT, Bandorski D, et al. Prospective comparison of MR phase-contrast velocimetry with intravascular doppler US during infrainguinal artery angioplasty. *J Vasc Interv Radiol.* 2001;12:459–463.

25. Schoenberg SO, Bock M, Kallinowski F, et al. Correlation of hemodynamic impact and morphologic degree of renal artery stenosis in a canine model. *J Am Soc Nephrol.* 2000;11:2190–2198.

26. Schoenberg SO, Just A, Bock M, et al. Noninvasive analysis of renal artery blood flow dynamics with MR cine phase-contrast flow measurements. *Am J Physiol.* 1997;272: H2477–H2484.

27. Bryant DJ, Payne JA, Firmin DN, et al. Measurement of flow with NMR imaging using a gradient pulse and phase difference technique. *J Comput Assist Tomogr.* 1984;8:588–593.

28. Schoenberg SO, Knopp MV, Bock M, et al. Renal artery stenosis: grading of hemodynamic changes with cine phase-contrast MR blood flow measurements. *Radiology.* 1997;203:45–53.

29. Box FM, Spilt A, Van Buchem MA, et al. Automatic model-based contour detection and blood flow quantification in small vessels with velocity encoded magnetic resonance imaging. *Invest Radiol.* 2003;38:567–577.

30. Schoenberg SO, Knopp MV, Londy F, et al. Morphologic and functional magnetic resonance imaging of renal artery stenosis: a multireader tricenter study. *J Am Soc Nephrol.* 2002;13:158–169.

31. Bock M, Schoenberg SO, Schad LR, et al. Interleaved gradient echo planar (IGEPI) and phase contrast CINE-PC flow measurements in the renal artery. *J Magn Reson Imaging.* 1998;8:889–895.

32. Michaely HJ, Schoenberg SO, Ittrich C, et al. Renal disease: value of functional magnetic resonance imaging with flow and perfusion measurements. *Invest Radiol.* 2004; 39:698–705.

33. Schoenberg SO, Aumann S, Just A, et al. Quantification of renal perfusion abnormalities using an intravascular contrast agent (part 2): results in animals and humans with renal artery stenosis. *Magn Reson Med.* 2003;49:288–298.

34. Michaely HJ, Schoenberg SO, Oesingmann N, et al. Functional assessment of renal artery stenosis using dynamic MR perfusion measurements—feasibility study. *Radiology.* 2006;238:586–596.

35. Williams DS, Zhang W, Koretsky AP, et al. Perfusion imaging of the rat kidney with MR. *Radiology.* 1994;190:813–818.

36. Roberts DA, Detre JA, Bolinger L, et al. Renal perfusion in humans: MR imaging with spin tagging of arterial water. *Radiology.* 1995;196:281–286.

37. Wang JJ, Hendrich KS, Jackson EK, et al. Perfusion quantitation in transplanted rat kidney by MRI with arterial spin labeling. *Kidney Int.* 1998;53:1783–1791.

38. Karger N, Biederer J, Lusse S, et al. Quantitation of renal perfusion using arterial spin labeling with FAIR-UFLARE. *Magn Reson Imaging.* 2000;18:641–647.

39. Gunther M, Bock M, Schad LR. Arterial spin labeling in combination with a look-locker sampling strategy: inflow turbo-sampling EPI-FAIR (ITS-FAIR). *Magn Reson Med.* 2001;46:974–984.

40. Martirosian P, Klose U, Mader I, et al. FAIR true-FISP perfusion imaging of the kidneys. *Magn Reson Med.* 2004;51: 353–361.

41. Daly PF, Zimmerman JB, Gillen JS, et al. Rapid MR imaging of renal perfusion: a comparative study of GdDTPA, albumin-(GdDTPA), and magnetite. *Am J Physiol Imaging.* 1989;4:165–174.

42. Aumann S, Schoenberg SO, Just A, et al. Quantification of renal perfusion using an intravascular contrast agent (part 1): results in a canine model. *Magn Reson Med.* 2003;49:276–287.

43. Prasad PV, Cannillo J, Chavez DR, et al. First-pass renal perfusion imaging using MS-325, an albumin-targeted MRI contrast agent. *Invest Radiol.* 1999;34:566–571.

44. Lee VS, Rusinek H, Johnson G, et al. MR renography with low-dose gadopentetate dimeglumine: feasibility. *Radiology.* 2001;221:371–379.

45. Lee VS, Rusinek H, Noz ME, et al. Dynamic three-dimensional MR renography for the measurement of single kidney function: initial experience. *Radiology.* 2003;227: 289–294.

46. Laissy JP, Faraggi M, Lebtahi R, et al. Functional evaluation of normal and ischemic kidney by means of gadolinium-DOTA enhanced TurboFLASH MR imaging: a preliminary comparison with 99Tc-MAG3 dynamic scintigraphy. *Magn Reson Imaging.* 1994;12:413–419.

47. Hawighorst H, Knapstein PG, Weikel W, et al. Cervical carcinoma: comparison of standard and pharmacokinetic MR imaging. *Radiology.* 1996;201:531–539.

48. Lee VS, Rofsky NM, Krinsky GA, et al. Single-dose breath-hold gadolinium-enhanced three-dimensional MR angiography of the renal arteries. *Radiology.* 1999;211:69–78.

49. Herborn CU, Lauenstein TC, Ruehm SG, et al. Intraindividual comparison of gadopentetate dimeglumine, gadobenate dimeglumine, and gadobutrol for pelvic 3D magnetic resonance angiography. *Invest Radiol.* 2003;38:27–33.

50. Essig M, Lodemann KP, LeHuu M, et al. Comparison of MultiHance and Gadovist for cerebral MR perfusion imaging in healthy volunteers. *Radiologe.* 2002;42:909–915.

51. Schoenberg SO, Londy FJ, Licato P, et al. Multiphase-multistep gadolinium-enhanced MR angiography of the abdominal aorta and runoff vessels. *Invest Radiol.* 2001;36: 283–291.

52. Meissner OA, Rieger JR, Weber C, et al. Critical limb ischemia: high-resolution hybrid-MR angiography compared with x-ray angiography for treatment planning. *Radiology.* 2005. In press.

53. Wehrschuetz M, Aschauer M, Portugaller H, et al. Review of source images is necessary for the evaluation of gadolinium-enhanced MR angiography for renal artery stenosis. *Cardiovasc Intervent Radiol.* 2004;27:441–446.

54. Fink C, Hallscheidt PJ, Hosch WP, et al. Preoperative evaluation of living renal donors: value of contrast-enhanced 3D magnetic resonance angiography and comparison of three rendering algorithms. *Eur Radiol.* 2003;13:794–801.

55. Persson A, Dahlstrom N, Engellau L, et al. Volume rendering compared with maximum intensity projection for magnetic resonance angiography measurements of the abdominal aorta. *Acta Radiol.* 2004;45:453–459.

56. Jeremias A, Huegel H, Lee DP, et al. Spatial orientation of atherosclerotic plaque in non-branching coronary artery segments. *Atherosclerosis.* 2000;152:209–215.

57. Yeh BM, Coakley FV, Meng MV, et al. Precaval right renal arteries: prevalence and morphologic associations at spiral CT. *Radiology.* 2004;230:429–433.

58. Winterer JT, Strey C, Wolffram C, et al. Preoperative examination of potential kidney transplantation donors: value of gadolinium-enhanced 3D MR angiography in comparison with DSA and urography. *Rofo Fortschr Geb Rontgenstr Neuen Bildgeb Verfahr*. 2000;172:449–457.

59. Urban BA, Ratner LE, Fishman EK. Three-dimensional volume-rendered CT angiography of the renal arteries and veins: normal anatomy, variants, and clinical applications. *Radiographics*. 2001;21:373–386; questionnaire 549–355.

60. Beckmann CF, Abrams HL. Circumaortic venous ring: incidence and significance. *AJR Am J Roentgenol*. 1979;132: 561–565.

61. Yesildag A, Adanir E, Koroglu M, et al. [Incidence of left renal vein anomalies in routine abdominal CT scans.] *Tani Girisim Radyol*. 2004;10:140–143.

62. Gupta A, Tello R. Accessory renal arteries are not related to hypertension risk: a review of MR angiography data. *AJR Am J Roentgenol*. 2004;182:1521–1524.

63. Fujita K, Munakata A. Left renal haematuria by compression of an unusual vein. *Int Urol Nephrol*. 1991;23:303–306.

64. Rouviere O, Lyonnet D, Berger P, et al. Ureteropelvic junction obstruction: use of helical CT for preoperative assessment—comparison with intraarterial angiography. *Radiology*. 1999;213:668–673.

65. Triantopoulou C, Rizos S, Bourli A, et al. Localized unilateral perirenal fibrosis: CT and MRI appearances. *Eur Radiol*. 2002;12:2743–2746.

66. Kawashima A, Sandler CM, Ernst RD, et al. CT evaluation of renovascular disease. *Radiographics*. 2000;20:1321–1340.

67. Levine E, Grantham JJ, Slusher SL, et al. CT of acquired cystic kidney disease and renal tumors in long-term dialysis patients. *AJR Am J Roentgenol*. 1984;125–131.

68. Semelka RC, Corrigan K, Ascher SM, et al. Renal corticomedullary differentiation: observation in patients with differing serum creatinine levels. *Radiology*. 1994;190:149–152.

69. Hricak H, Terrier F, Demas BE. Renal allografts: evaluation by MR imaging. *Radiology*. 1986;159:435–441.

70. Zimina OG, Rezun S, Armao D, et al. Renal malacoplakia: demonstration by MR imaging. *Magn Reson Imaging*. 2002;20:611–614.

71. Waybill MM, Waybill PN. Contrast media-induced nephrotoxicity: identification of patients at risk and algorithms for prevention. *J Vasc Interv Radiol*. 2001;12:3–9.

72. Erley CM. Nephrotoxicity: focusing on radiocontrast nephropathy. *Nephrol Dial Transplant*. 1999;14[Suppl 4]:13–15.

73. Heyman SN, Rosen S. Dye-induced nephropathy. *Semin Nephrol*. 2003;23:477–485.

74. Murphy SW, Barrett BJ, Parfrey PS. Contrast nephropathy. *J Am Soc Nephrol*. 2000;11:177–182.

75. Aspelin P, Aubry P, Fransson SG, et al. Nephrotoxic effects in high-risk patients undergoing angiography. *N Engl J Med*. 2003;348:491–499.

76. Nelemans PJ, Kessels AG, De Leeuw P, et al. The cost-effectiveness of the diagnosis of renal artery stenosis. *Eur J Radiol*. 1998;27:95–107.

77. Mayo RR, Swartz RD. Redefining the incidence of clinically detectable atheroembolism. *Am J Med*. 1996;100:524–529.

78. Schoenberg SO, Rieger JR, Weber C, et al. MR-angiography of the renal arteries with high spatial resolution using integrated parallel acquisition techniques (iPAT): value of isotropic cross-sectional reformats compared to digital subtraction angiography and intravascular ultrasound. *Radiology*. 2005. In press.

79. Rabbia C, Valpreda S. Duplex scan sonography of renal artery stenosis. *Int Angiol*. 2003;22:101–115.

80. Desberg AL, Paushter DM, Lammert GK, et al. Renal artery stenosis: evaluation with color Doppler flow imaging. *Radiology*. 1990;177:749–753.

81. Berland LL, Koslin DB, Routh WD, et al. Renal artery stenosis: prospective evaluation of diagnosis with color duplex US compared with angiography. Work in progress. *Radiology*. 1990;174:421–423.

82. Radermacher J, Chavan A, Bleck J, et al. Use of Doppler ultrasonography to predict the outcome of therapy for renal-artery stenosis. *N Engl J Med*. 2001;344:410–417.

83. Zeller T, Frank U, Spath M, et al. Color duplex ultrasound imaging of renal arteries and detection of hemodynamically relevant renal artery stenoses. *Ultraschall Med*. 2001;22:116–121.

84. Zeller T, Frank U, Muller C, et al. Duplex ultrasound for follow-up examination after stent-angioplasty of ostial renal artery stenoses. *Ultraschall Med*. 2002;23:315–319.

85. Haustein J, Niendorf HP, Krestin G, et al. Renal tolerance of gadolinium-DTPA/dimeglumine in patients with chronic renal failure. *Invest Radiol*. 1992;27:153–156.

86. Zeltser IS, Liu JB, Bagley DH. The incidence of crossing vessels in patients with normal ureteropelvic junction examined with endoluminal ultrasound. *J Urol*. 2004;172: 2304–2307.

87. Tham G, Ekelund L, Herrlin K, et al. Renal artery aneurysms. Natural history and prognosis. *Ann Surg*. 1983;197:348–352.

88. Cohen JR, Shamash FS. Ruptured renal artery aneurysms during pregnancy. *J Vasc Surg*. 1987;6:51–59.

89. English WP, Pearce JD, Craven TE, et al. Surgical management of renal artery aneurysms. *J Vasc Surg*. 2004;40:53–60.

90. Slovut DP, Olin JW. Fibromuscular dysplasia. *N Engl J Med*. 2004;350:1862–1871.

91. Mattar SG, Kumar AG, Lumsden AB. Vascular complications in Ehlers-Danlos syndrome. *Am Surg*. 1994;60:827–831.

92. Akpolat T, Akkoyunlu M, Akpolat I, et al. Renal Behçet's disease: a cumulative analysis. *Semin Arthritis Rheum*. 2002;31:317–337.

93. Henke PK, Cardneau JD, Welling TH 3rd, et al. Renal artery aneurysms: a 35-year clinical experience with 252 aneurysms in 168 patients. *Ann Surg*. 2001;234:454–462; discussion 462–453.

94. Yoneyama T, Baba Y, Fujiyoshi F, et al. Left renal vein aneurysm: imaging findings. *Abdom Imaging*. 2003;28: 233–235.

95. Sawicki PT, Kaiser S, Heinemann L, et al. Prevalence of renal artery stenosis in diabetes mellitus—an autopsy study. *J Intern Med*. 1991;229:489–492.

96. Missouris CG, Buckenham T, Cappuccio FP, et al. Renal artery stenosis: a common and important problem in patients with peripheral vascular disease. *Am J Med*. 1994;96:10–14.

97. Textor SC. Epidemiology and clinical presentation. *Semin Nephrol*. 2000;20:426–431.

98. Olin JW. Renal artery disease: diagnosis and management. *Mt Sinai J Med*. 2004;71:73–85.

99. Rihal CS, Textor SC, Breen JF, et al. Incidental renal artery stenosis among a prospective cohort of hypertensive patients undergoing coronary angiography. *Mayo Clin Proc*. 2002;77:309–316.

100. Harding MB, Smith LR, Himmelstein SI, et al. Renal artery stenosis: prevalence and associated risk factors in patients undergoing routine cardiac catheterization. *J Am Soc Nephrol*. 1992;2:1608–1616.

101. Olin JW, Melia M, Young JR, et al. Prevalence of atherosclerotic renal artery stenosis in patients with atherosclerosis elsewhere. *Am J Med*. 1990;88:46N–51N.

102. Wachtell K, Ibsen H, Olsen MH, et al. Prevalence of renal artery stenosis in patients with peripheral vascular disease and hypertension. *J Hum Hypertens*. 1996;10:83–85.

103. Scoble JE, Hamilton G. Atherosclerotic renovascular disease. *BMJ*. 1990;300:1670–1671.

104. Vasbinder GB, Nelemans PJ, Kessels AG, et al. Diagnostic tests for renal artery stenosis in patients suspected of having renovascular hypertension: a meta-analysis. *Ann Intern Med*. 2001;135:401–411.

105. Tan KT, van Beek EJ, Brown PW, et al. Magnetic resonance angiography for the diagnosis of renal artery stenosis: a meta-analysis. *Clin Radiol*. 2002;57:617–624.

106. Vasbinder GB, Nelemans PJ, Kessels AG, et al. Accuracy of computed tomographic angiography and magnetic resonance angiography for diagnosing renal artery stenosis. *Ann Intern Med*. 2004;141:674–682; discussion 682.

107. Tollefson DF, Ernst CB. Natural history of atherosclerotic renal artery stenosis associated with aortic disease. *J Vasc Surg*. 1991;14:327–331.

108. Caps MT, Perissinotto C, Zierler RE, et al. Prospective study of atherosclerotic disease progression in the renal artery. *Circulation*. 1998;98:2866–2872.

109. Shariat Razavi I, Stacul F, Cova M, et al. Morpho-functional study of the kidney in patients with kidney disease and liver disease with magnetic resonance. *Radiol Med (Torino)*. 1998;95:72–81.

110. Gandy SJ, Almahri A, Armoogum K, et al. Perfusion parameters of MR renography are associated with cardiovascular disease risk factors and clinical indices of kidney function. Annual conference of the International Society for Magnetic Resonance in Medicine, Kyoto, 2004.

111. Korosec FR, Frayne R, Grist TM, et al. Time-resolved contrast-enhanced 3D MR angiography. *Magn Reson Med*. 1996;36:345–351.

112. Fink C, Ley S, Kroeker R, et al. Time-resolved contrast-enhanced three-dimensional magnetic resonance angiography of the chest: combination of parallel imaging with view sharing (TREAT). *Invest Radiol*. 2005;40:40–48.

113. Isles CG, Robertson S, Hill D. Management of renovascular disease: a review of renal artery stenting in ten studies. *QJM*. 1999;92:159–167.

114. Connolly JO, Higgins RM, Walters HL, et al. Presentation, clinical features and outcome in different patterns of atherosclerotic renovascular disease. *QJM*. 1994;87:413–421.

115. Hillege HL, Girbes AR, de Kam PJ, et al. Renal function, neurohormonal activation, and survival in patients with chronic heart failure. *Circulation*. 2000;102:203–210.

116. Kramer H, Schoenberg SO, Nikolaou K, et al. Cardiovascular screening with parallel imaging and implementation on a whole body MR scanner. *Radiology*. 2005. In press.

117. Ruehm SG, Goyen M, Barkhausen J, et al. Rapid magnetic resonance angiography for detection of atherosclerosis. *Lancet*. 2001;357:1086–1091.

118. Tegtmeyer CJ, Hartwell GD, Selby JB, et al. Results and complications of angioplasty in aortoiliac disease. *Circulation*. 1991;83:153–160.

119. Canzanello VJ, Millan VG, Spiegel JE, et al. Percutaneous transluminal renal angioplasty in management of atherosclerotic renovascular hypertension: results in 100 patients. *Hypertension*. 1989;13:163–172.

120. Begelman SM, Olin JW. Fibromuscular dysplasia. *Curr Opin Rheumatol*. 2000;12:41–47.

121. Michaely HJ, Herrmann KA, Kramer H, et al. The significance of MR angiography for the diagnosis of carotid stenoses. *Radiologe*. 2004;44:975–984.

122. Begelman SM, Olin JW. Nonatherosclerotic arterial disease of the extracranial cerebrovasculature. *Semin Vasc Surg*. 2000;13:153–164.

123. Dion E, Graef C, Haroche J, et al. Imaging of thoracoabdominal involvement in Erdheim-Chester disease. *AJR Am J Roentgenol*. 2004;183:1253–1260.

124. Kopecky KK, Stine SB, Dalsing MC, et al. Median arcuate ligament syndrome with multivessel involvement: diagnosis with spiral CT angiography. *Abdom Imaging*. 1997;22:318–320.

125. Hiromura T, Nishioka T, Nishioka S, et al. Reflux in the left ovarian vein: analysis of MDCT findings in asymptomatic women. *AJR Am J Roentgenol*. 2004;183:1411–1415.

126. Jeong JY, Kim SH, Lee HJ, et al. Atypical low-signal-intensity renal parenchyma: causes and patterns. *Radiographics*. 2002;22:833–846.

127. Ma SK, Kim SW, Kim NH, et al. Renal vein and inferior vena cava thrombosis associated with acute pancreatitis. *Nephron*. 2002;92:475–477.

128. Lacombe M. Isolated spontaneous dissection of the renal artery. *J Vasc Surg*. 2001;33:385–391.

129. Sufrin G. The Page kidney: a correctable form of arterial hypertension. *J Urol*. 1975;113:450–454.

130. Sterns RH, Rabinowitz R, Segal AJ, et al. 'Page kidney'. Hypertension caused by chronic subcapsular hematoma. *Arch Intern Med*. 1985;145:169–171.

131. Ergen FB, Hussain HK, Caoili EM, et al. MRI for preoperative staging of renal cell carcinoma using the 1997 TNM classification: comparison with surgical and pathologic staging. *AJR Am J Roentgenol*. 2004;182:217–225.

132. Catalano C, Fraioli F, Laghi A, et al. High-resolution multidetector CT in the preoperative evaluation of patients with renal cell carcinoma. *AJR Am J Roentgenol*. 2003;180:1271–1277.

133. Hallscheidt PJ, Bock M, Riedasch G, et al. Diagnostic accuracy of staging renal cell carcinomas using multidetector-row computed tomography and magnetic resonance imaging: a prospective study with histopathologic correlation. *J Comput Assist Tomogr*. 2004;28:333–339.

134. Coll DM, Uzzo RG, Herts BR, et al. 3-dimensional volume rendered computerized tomography for preoperative evaluation and intraoperative treatment of patients undergoing nephron sparing surgery. *J Urol*. 1999;161:1097–1102.

135. Friedland GW. Staging of genitourinary cancers. The role of diagnostic imaging. *Cancer*. 1987;60:450–458.

136. Scialpi M, Di Maggio A, Midiri M, et al. Small renal masses: assessment of lesion characterization and vascularity on dynamic contrast-enhanced MR imaging with fat suppression. *AJR Am J Roentgenol*. 2000;175:751–757.

137. Hallscheidt P, Stolte E, Roeren T, et al. The staging of renal-cell carcinomas in MRT and CT—a prospective histologically controlled study. *ROFO*. 1998;168:165–170.

138. Choyke PL, Walther MM, Wagner JR, et al. Renal cancer: preoperative evaluation with dual-phase three-dimensional MR angiography. *Radiology*. 1997;205:767–771.

139. Subramaniam M, Mizzi A, Roditi G. Magnetic resonance angiography in potential live renal donors: a joint radiological and surgical evaluation. *Clin Radiol*. 2004;59:335–341.

140. Pozniak MA, Balison DJ, Lee FT Jr., et al. CT angiography of potential renal transplant donors. *Radiographics*. 1998;18:565–587.

141. Sebastia C, Quiroga S, Boye R, et al. Helical CT in renal transplantation: normal findings and early and late complications. *Radiographics*. 2001;21:1103–1117.

142. Buturovic-Ponikvar J. Renal transplant artery stenosis. *Nephrol Dial Transplant*. 2003;18[Suppl 5]:v74–v77.

143. Chan YL, Leung CB, Yu SC, et al. Comparison of non-breath-hold high resolution gadolinium-enhanced MRA with digital subtraction angiography in the evaluation on allograft renal artery stenosis. *Clin Radiol*. 2001;56:127–132.

144. Michaely HJ, Schoenberg SO, Oesingmann N, et al. Assessment of renal transplants using functional magnetic resonance. MRA workshop, London, ON, 2004;111.

145. Wong-You-Cheong JJ, Grumbach K, Krebs TL, et al. Torsion of intraperitoneal renal transplants: imaging appearances. *AJR Am J Roentgenol*. 1998;171:1355–1359.

146. Yang CW, Lee SH, Choo SW, et al. Early graft dysfunction due to renal vein compression. *Nephron*. 1996;73:480–481.

147. Ali MG, Coakley FV, Hricak H, et al. Complex posttransplantation abnormalities of renal allografts: evaluation with MR imaging. *Radiology*. 1999;211:95–100.

148. Claudon M, Kessler M, Champigneulle J, et al. Lymphoproliferative disorders after renal transplantation: role of medical imaging. *Eur Radiol*. 1998;8:1686–1693.

149. Spuentrup E, Ruebben A, Mahnken A, et al. Artifact-free coronary magnetic resonance angiography and coronary vessel wall imaging in the presence of a new, metallic, coronary magnetic resonance imaging stent. *Circulation*. 2005;111:1019–1026.

150. McCarty M, Gedroyc WM. Surgical clip artefact mimicking arterial stenosis: a problem with magnetic resonance angiography. *Clin Radiol*. 1993;48:232–235.

151. Honda H, Onitsuka H, Naitou S, et al. Renal arteriovenous malformations: CT features. *J Comput Assist Tomogr*. 1991;15:261–264.

Lower Extremities Vasculature

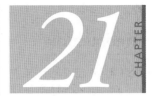

Tim Leiner
Dominik Fleischmann
Neil M. Rofsky

INTRODUCTION

Spectrum and Prevalence of Diseases

Atherosclerotic Peripheral Arterial Occlusive Disease

The vast majority (>80%) of lower extremity arterial disease is due to atherosclerotic peripheral arterial occlusive disease (APAOD). APAOD is a major health care problem in Western society with an estimated prevalence in the general population of 2.5% in persons over 50 years of age. In persons over 70 years of age, the prevalence is estimated at about 7% (1).

Patients who have complaints of APAOD usually present with a history of intermittent *claudication*. This term is derived from the Latin *claudicatio* and means "to limp." Intermittent claudication is caused when blood flow to exercising leg and calf muscles is insufficient compared to metabolic demands. Significant disease in the aortoiliac arteries (Fig. 21-1) typically leads to cramping and pain in buttocks and thighs, while more distally located disease (e.g., tibioperoneal occlusive disease) is often associated with cramping in the foot. Upon cessation of exercise, complaints usually disappear rapidly. The clinical course of intermittent claudication in terms of progression of disease in the symptomatic limb is usually benign since only about a quarter of patients will ever significantly deteriorate (1). With an intervention rate of approximately 5%, only 1% to 3% of all patients with intermittent claudication will ever undergo a major amputation (1).

About 5% or less of patients with intermittent claudication progress to chronic critical ischemia, that is, the oxygen and nutrient supply of the distal lower extremity fall below the level for maintenance of normal cellular processes in resting conditions. Clinically, this is manifested by rest pain and tissue loss (i.e., nonhealing ulcers and gangrene).

The incidence of chronic critical ischemia is estimated to be between 300 and 1,000 per million per year in the general population (1). Because of the severity of com-

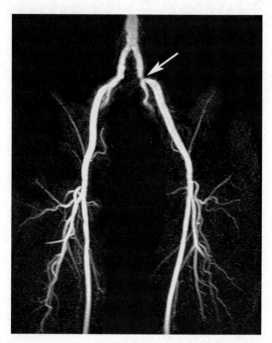

FIGURE 21-1 Proximal stenosis in a claudicant. This MIP image from a 3D gadolinium-enhanced MR angiogram shows a single focal high-grade stenosis in the distal, left common iliac artery (*arrow*) in this patient with left buttock claudication.

plaints, an invasive intervention is attempted in all but the worst cases. Despite advances in endovascular and vascular surgical therapy, however, the rate of major amputation in the general population remains in excess of 0.03% in industrialized countries (2).

The diagnosis of APAOD is made on the basis of the typical history, physical examination (palpation of arterial pulsations), and measurement of the ankle-brachial index (ABI) (1,3). The severity of APAOD is commonly classified according to Fontaine (Table 21-1). More recently, the Society for Vascular Surgery and the International Society for Cardiovascular Surgery introduced a classification, named after Rutherford, that also incorporates hemodynamic and performance criteria (4) (Table 21-2).

TABLE 21-1

Clinical Categories of Peripheral Arterial Occlusive Disease Severity According to Fontaine

Stage	Painfree Walking Distance	Rest Pain	Ulcerations/Gangrene
I	Unlimited	No	No
IIa	>200 m	No	No
IIb	<200 m	No	No
III	0 m	Yes	No
IV	0 m	Yes	Yes

Source: Modified from Becker F. Exploration of arterial function with noninvasive technics. Results in chronic arterial occlusive disease of the lower limbs according to Leriche and Fontaine classification. *Int Angiol.* 1985;4:311–322.

TABLE 21-2

Clinical Categories of Peripheral Arterial Occlusive Disease Severity According to Rutherford

Grade	Category	Clinical Description	Objective Criteria	Treatment Indication
0	0	Asymptomatic, no HSS	Normal treadmill or reactive hyperemia test	Relative
	1	Mild claudication	Completes treadmill test, ankle pressure after >50 mmHg but ≥20 mmHg lower than resting value	Relative
I	2	Moderate claudication	Between categories 1 and 3	Relative
	3	Severe claudication	Cannot complete treadmill test, ankle pressure <50 mmHg after exercise	Relative
II	4	Ischemic rest pain	Resting ankle pressure <40 mmHg; flat or barely pulsatile ankle or metatarsal pulse volume recording; toe pressure <30 mmHg	Absolute
III	5	Minor tissue loss	Resting ankle pressure <60 mmHg; ankle or metatarsal pulse volume recording flat or barely pulsatile; toe pressure <40 mmHg	Absolute
	6	Major tissue loss (above tarso-metatarsal level)	Same as category 5	Absolute

HSS, hemodynamically significant stenosis.

Note: Grades II and III, categories 4, 5, and 6, are embraced by the term *chronic critical ischemia.*

Source: Modified from Rutherford RB, Baker JD, Ernst C, et al. Recommended standards for reports dealing with lower extremity ischemia: revised version. *J Vasc Surg.* 1997;26:517–538.

When a patient presents to the general practitioner or the vascular surgeon with complaints of APAOD, the first-line treatment consists of modification of obvious cardiovascular risk factors such as smoking, hypertension, hypercholesterolemia, and the institution of exercise training (5–7). Generally, options for invasive intervention are considered when complaints become too limiting to pursue ordinary activities.

For patients with intermittent claudication, the decision to intervene is largely dependent on relative criteria (patient and surgeon preference), but for patients with chronic critical ischemia, the need to intervene is more urgent since tissue perfusion does not meet basic metabolic demands, even at rest.

Although only a small minority of patients with APAOD eventually undergo invasive treatment, the estimated annual number of percutaneous and surgical procedures performed for PAOD in the United States alone was over 100,000 in 1986, with sharp increases expected (8), illustrating the large scope of the problem and impact on people's lives.

In contrast to the gradual course of disease perceived with intermittent claudication and chronic critical ischemia is the entity of *acute* limb ischemia. Acute limb ischemia denotes a sudden and rapid decline in limb perfusion, usually producing new or worsening signs and symptoms; often, limb viability is threatened. In patients with APAOD, acute limb ischemia is most often caused by either an embolus or thrombosis. The severity of acute limb ischemia depends on the location and extent of occlusion and the degree to which pre-existing collaterals can be recruited (1).

Other Causes of Peripheral Arterial Disease

Approximately 20% of chronic arterial occlusions are based on diseases other than atherosclerosis that cause luminal narrowing and/or occlusion. The presence, location, and progression of arterial stenoses and occlusions may reflect an underlying systemic disease or may be an expression of regional inflammatory or degenerative processes.

Lower extremity arterial diseases other than APAOD include aneurysmal disease, popliteal entrapment syndrome, cystic adventitial disease, arterial fibrodysplasia, nonspecific aortoarteritis (Takayasu disease), and a host of uncommon vasculitides, the most important of which is thromboangiitis obliterans (Buerger's disease) (9). In addition, congenital connective tissue diseases such as Marfan syndrome, Ehlers-Danlos syndrome, pseudoxanthoma elasticum, homocystinuria, and neurofibromatosis may have peripheral arterial involvement.

Congenital and acquired clotting disorders may also manifest themselves with symptoms of peripheral arterial disease. Rare causes of peripheral arterial disease are primary tumors, radiation therapy, and the iliac syndrome in cyclists. An acute arterial occlusion always necessitates a prompt search for atrial fibrillation, ulcerative endocarditis, and mural thrombi overlying the site of myocardial infarction.

Global View of Unique Aspects and Considerations of Imaging of Coronary Arteries

Given the predominance of APAOD in lower extremity vascular disease, the role of imaging is often one of delineating the anatomy in preparation for an endoluminal (e.g., stent/angioplasty) or surgical (e.g., bypass graft) intervention and to assess whether options for such interventions are feasible. These considerations are well served when information about the number, length, and severity of vascular lesions is accurately detailed (10).

Conventional angiography with the use of iodinated contrast media and, in particular, intra-arterial digital subtraction angiography (IA DSA) has long served as the reference in this regard. However, magnetic resonance angiography (MRA) and computed tomographic angiography (CTA) have emerged as compelling alternatives. The relatively non-invasive nature of these techniques avoids the definable risks associated with catheter-related complications (10,11).

Because both techniques are able to provide an accurate "road map" of the peripheral vasculature, the referring clinician can confidently inform patients that either an angiogram should be performed and percutaneous transluminal angioplasty (PTA) carried out at the same time or, conversely, that the disease is too diffuse and long-segmented or that an occlusive lesion is present that requires a more extensive or complex procedure such as aortofemoral bypass. Some patients, as well as some surgeons, will only be interested in treatment if angioplasty is possible. The use of noninvasive angiography can spare those patients who are not angioplasty candidates and those who do not desire major reconstructive surgery the risks of intra-arterial angiography for diagnostic purposes.

At the other end of the clinical spectrum are patients with chronic critical ischemia. Many of these patients suffer from multilevel disease such as stenoses and obstructions in inflow (aortoiliac) and outflow (femoropopliteal and lower leg) arteries. In patients with chronic critical ischemia, the primary aim is to provide sufficient blood flow to relieve rest pain and heal skin lesions. This can be achieved by PTA and/or arterial reconstructive bypass surgery (12).

The ability to successfully bypass stenoses and obstructions of the lower leg and to perform distal anastomoses of bypass grafts to arteries around the ankle or in the foot has important implications for limb salvage (13). In contradistinction to patients with intermittent claudication, imaging outflow arteries is therefore an *essential* part of the imaging workup and potentially limb-saving in patients with chronic critical ischemia, particularly when it is taken into account that IA DSA is known to fail in visualizing patent crural and foot arteries, which are demonstrated with other modalities (14–16).

The anatomic coverage from the infrarenal aorta down to the pedal arch in the feet in an average patient demands well over 100 cm and encompasses a wide range in the course and caliber of the relevant vessels. The advent of multistation CE MRA imaging protocols and the introduction of multidetector (MD) row CT scanners allows for the routine and successful acquisition of the complete peripheral vascular tree.

What Do Computed Tomography and Magnetic Resonance Bring over Other Imaging and Nonimaging Diagnostic Testing?

In the diagnostic workup of patients with peripheral arterial disease, physical signs and symptoms often guide the clinician toward a diagnosis and suggest the likely disruption of the disease. The battery of available diagnostic tests can often add substantial insights to the disease. Ultimately, an accurate portrayal of the vasculature best guides the treatment management while providing a set of alternatives in the event of complications during the therapeutic intervention.

The available diagnostic tests can be divided into those aimed at a *physiological* assessment of the peripheral circulation and those aimed at providing an anatomical *road map* of the peripheral vasculature, showing the exact location, extent, and severity of the disease process in relation to commonly used anatomical landmarks during interventional radiological and surgical procedures. Table 21-3 provides an overview of these techniques.

Duplex ultrasonography (DU) with color flow is often used to gauge the extent and severity of peripheral arterial disease. This test combines a local anatomical image, obtained in B-mode, with information about the direction, pattern, and magnitude of arterial and venous flow (obtained by Doppler frequency analysis) (17). The severity of stenoses can be derived from peak systolic and end-diastolic velocity measurements, whereby higher peak systolic velocities indicate more severe stenoses (18). Major drawbacks of DU are the long duration of the examination, the operator dependency (19), and the limited ability to ensure that the anatomic coverage is complete. Experienced vascular laboratories with rigorous quality controls are needed for reliable characterization of vascular disease with DU.

Relative to DU, both MD CTA and CE MRA excel in their ability to provide images of the peripheral vascular tree analogous to intra-arterial digital subtraction techniques (20,21). Furthermore, the truly three-dimensional (3D) nature of these data sets allows for evaluations from an infinite number of viewpoints. Another advantage of MD CTA and CE MRA is that examination times are short, and patient tolerance is high. In a recently published study, 41% of patients preferred CE MRA over DU in their workup for suspected peripheral arterial disease, 9% preferred DU, and 50% did not have a preference (22).

Invasive therapy for peripheral arterial disease can be divided into interventional radiological and vascular surgical procedures. The choice of therapy for a range of conditions

TABLE 21-3

Commonly Used Diagnostic Tests for Detection and Grading of Peripheral Arterial Disease

Test	Measures	Interpretation
Ankle-brachial index	Systolic pressure around ankle divided by systolic pressure in arm	When <0.9 peripheral arterial disease is angiographically present in 90% of subjects
Segmental pressure measurements	Arterial pressures in different limb segments (usually with 4 cuffs)	20 mmHg gradient between cuffs indicates significant lesion; allows crude localization of disease
Plethysmography (pulse volume recording)	Visual display of volume changes in limb in response to arterial blood flow	Loss of dicrotic notch on downward part of curve signifies obstruction; in severe disease, waveform may be absent
Doppler wave form analysis	Visual depiction of arterial blood flow pattern using Doppler frequency shift	Increasing levels of stenosis progressively flatten triphasic flow pattern
Duplex ultrasonography	Arterial blood flow pattern and velocity superimposed anatomical (B-mode) image	On localization and determination of disease severity based on peak-systolic and end-diastolic velocity measurements

has been extensively researched in the recently published *Trans-Atlantic Inter-Society Consensus* (TASC) document. In the TASC document, arterial lesions and their preferred treatment are classified according to location, severity, and length (1). The strength and popularity of both MD CTA and CE MRA derive from the fact that both are uniquely suited to guide therapeutic management and arterial access.

IMAGING STRATEGIES

Computed Tomographic Angiography

Lower extremity (peripheral) CTA is a fairly new technique when compared with both ultrasound (US) and MRA. Peripheral CTA became possible only after the introduction of multidetector-row CT technology (MDCT) in 1998, which—for the first time—allowed scanning of the entire lower extremity inflow and runoff vessels in a single CT acquisition and with a single contrast-medium injection at adequate spatial resolution (23). With rapidly developing scanner capabilities and increasing availability of MDCT systems, peripheral CTA gradually entered clinical practice (24–28), and evolved into a robust and reliable modality (29,30). Current state-of-the art 16- through 64-channel CT systems allow the routine acquisition of high-resolution near-isotropic 3D data sets of the peripheral arterial tree (31).

Scanning Technique

Peripheral CT angiograms can be obtained with any MDCT scanner (4-channel and above). No special hardware is required. With a standardized scanning protocol programmed into the scanner, peripheral CTA is a robust technique for elective and emergency situations. When patients are mobile, the study can easily be performed in 10 to 15 minutes of room time. The short acquisition time of

25 to 50 seconds makes it possible to scan acutely ill patients (e.g., in the emergency room setting) as well.

In general, peripheral CTA acquisition parameters follow those of abdominal CTA. Unless automated tube-current modulation is available (which is strongly recommended), a tube voltage of 120 kV and tube amperage of up to 300 mA (depending on the scanner) is used for peripheral CTA, which results in a similar radiation exposure and dose (12.97 mGy, 9.3 mSv) as abdominal CTA (24). Breath holding is required only at the beginning of the CT acquisition through the abdomen and pelvis. Lower amperage (and/or voltage) can and should be used in slim patients. In obese patients, tube voltage and tube current often need to be increased. A medium to small imaging field-of-view (FOV) (using the greater trochanter as a bony landmark) and a medium-soft reconstruction kernel are generally used for image reconstruction.

Scanning Protocol

One (or more) dedicated "peripheral CTA" acquisition and contrast medium injection protocol(s) should be established for each scanner and programmed into the scanner. A full scanning protocol consists of (a) the digital radiograph ("Scout" or "Topogram"); (b) an optional nonenhanced acquisition; (c) one series for a test bolus or bolus triggering; (d) the actual CTA series; and (e) a second, optional ("late phase") CTA acquisition (only initiated on demand) in the event of nonopacification of distal vessels (Fig. 21-2).

Patient Positioning and Scanning Range

The patient is placed feet first and supine on the couch of the scanner. In order to keep the image reconstruction FOV small, and also to avoid off-center stair-step artifacts (32), it is important to carefully align the patient's legs and feet close

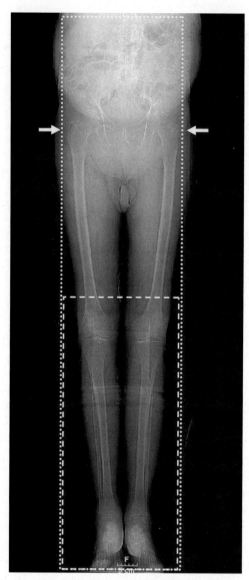

FIGURE 21-2 Digital CT radiograph ("topogram" or "scout view") for prescribing a peripheral CTA. The patient's legs and feet are aligned with the long axis of the scanner. Scanning range (from the T12 vertebral body through the feet) and reconstruction FOV (determined by the greater trochanters [*arrows*]) are indicated by the *dotted line*. A second, optional CTA acquisition is prescribed for the crural/pedal territory (*dashed line*). (Reprinted with permission from Fleischmann D, Hallett RL, Rubin GD. CT angiography of peripheral arterial disease. *J Vasc Interv Radiol.* 2006;17:3–26.)

to the isocenter of the scanner. Tape may be required to hold a patient's knees together. While cushions can be used to stabilize the extremities to the patient's comfort, large cushions under the knees should not be used to keep the FOV small.

Also—as in conventional angiography—excessive plantar-flexion of the feet is avoided to prevent an artifactual stenosis or occlusion of the dorsalis pedis artery ("ballerina sign") (33). The standard anatomic coverage extends from the T12 vertebral body level (to include the renal artery origins) proximally through the patient's feet distally (Fig. 21-2).

The average scan length is between 110 and 130 cm. Smaller scan ranges (e.g., mid-thigh to feet) or a smaller FOV (one leg only) may be selected in specific clinical situations, such as in popliteal arterial entrapment syndrome, or trauma.

In patients with suspected popliteal arterial entrapment syndrome, we use a sling of bedsheet under the patient's forefoot to allow for a provocation maneuver with contraction of the calf muscles against the sheet, which is pulled by the patient during the scan time (Fig. 21-3). Two contrast medium injections (80 mL each) and three CT acquisitions (arterial phase with provocation for the first injection, arterial and venous phases for the second injection, respectively) are given.

Image Acquisition and Reconstruction Parameters

The choice of *acquisition parameters* (detector configuration/pitch) and the corresponding *reconstruction parameters* (section thickness/reconstruction interval) depends largely on the type and model of the scanner. Table 21-4 provides an overview of peripheral CTA acquisition parameters for a wide range of MDCT scanners and reflects our clinical

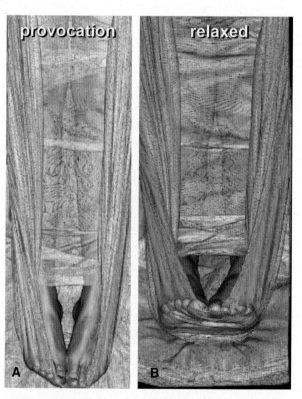

FIGURE 21-3 Provocation maneuver. VR images demonstrate scanning range and provocation maneuver in popliteal arterial entrapment syndrome. A bedsheet is used as a sling under the patient's forefoot. **A:** During the provocation maneuver, the patient extends his or her feet against the resistance of the bedsheet, which is pulled up by the patient at the same time to contract the calf muscles. **B:** Relaxed position.

TABLE 21-4

Multidetector Computed Tomography Acquisition Parameters for Peripheral Computed Tomography—Angiography

	Gantry Rotation Time (seconds)	Detector Configuration (millimeters)[a]	Pitch	Table Increment (millimeters/ 360°)	Table Speed (millimeters/ second)	Scan Time (seconds)	Injection Protocol (Type)
4 Channel MDCT							
GE	0.8	4 × 2.5	1.5	15	19	69	Slow
Sie	0.5	4 × 2.5	1.5	15	30	43	Slow
8-Channel MDCT							
GE	0.5	8 × 1.25	1.35	13.5	27	48	Slow
GE	0.5	8 × 2.50	1.35	27.0	54	24	Fast
16-Channel MDCT							
GE	0.6	16 × 1.25	1.375	35	46	28	Fast
Sie	0.5	16 × 1.5	1.200	33	58	23	Fast
Submillimeter							
GE	0.5	16 × 0.625	1.375	17.5	28	47	Slow
Sie	0.5	16 × 0.750	1.200	18.0	29	45	Slow
64-Channel MDCT							
Sie	0.50	64 × 0.600[b]	~0.8500	17.0	32	40	Slow[c]
Sie	0.33	64 × 0.600[b]	1.1000	21.1	63	20	Fast
GE[d]	0.70	64 × 0.625	0.5625	22.5	32	40	Slow
GE[d]	0.60	64 × 0.625	0.9375	37.5	63	20	Fast

GE, General Electric scanners; Sie, Siemens scanners.

Note: Scan times are shown for a scanning range of 130 cm.

[a]Detector configuration is denoted as number of channels times channel width.

[b]Physical detector configuration is 32 detector rows.

[c]Scan time is fixed to 40 seconds.

[d]64-channel GE scanners have not been used in practice by the authors at the time of writing.

experience with 4-, 16-, and 64-channel Siemens MDCT scanners (Siemens Medical Solutions, Erlangen, Germany), and 4-, 8,- and 16-channel General Electric MDCT scanners (General Electric Healthcare, Milwaukee, WI). Detector configuration is denoted as number of channels times channel width (e.g., 4 × 2.5 mm); section thickness (STh) and reconstruction interval (RI) are expressed as STh/RI (e.g., 3 mm/1.5 mm).

Four-channel Multidetector Computed Tomography

With 4-channel MDCT, the detector configuration is usually set to 4 × 2.5 mm. The corresponding thinnest effective section thickness is approximately 3 mm. With overlapping image reconstruction every 1 to 2 mm, these "standard resolution" data sets are adequate for visualizing the aortoiliac and femoropopliteal vessels and also provide enough detail to assess the patency of crural and pedal arteries if no or only minimal vessel calcification is present. Four-channel MDCT thus provides adequate imaging in patients with intermittent claudication; in acute embolic disease, aneurysms, and anatomic vascular mapping; and also in the setting of trauma.

Such "standard resolution" data sets may not be fully diagnostic, however, when visualization of small arterial branches (crural or pedal) is clinically relevant, such as in patients with critical limb ischemia and predominantly distal disease, notably in the presence of excessive arterial wall calcifications. If higher-resolution imaging is required and if the clinical situation permits a smaller anatomic coverage (e.g., limited to the legs or to popliteal-to-pedal vessels only), exquisite "high-resolution" imaging (Fig. 21-4) can also be achieved with 4-channel systems with 4 × 1 mm or 4 × 1.25 mm detector collimation (24) within acceptable acquisition times.

Eight-channel Multidetector Computed Tomography

A detector configuration of 8 × 1.25 mm permits anatomic coverage of the entire peripheral arterial tree within the same scan time as a 4 × 2.5 mm 4-channel MDCT

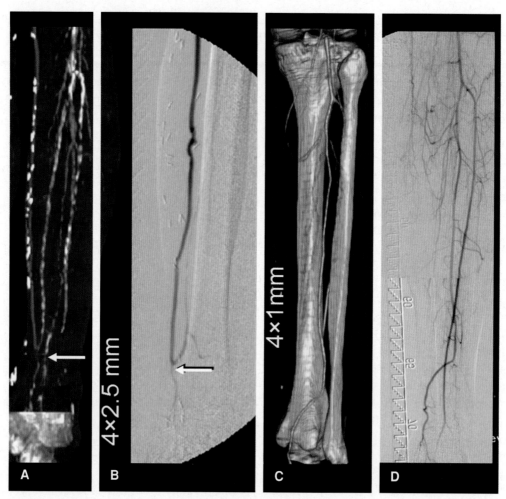

FIGURE 21-4 Comparison of spatial resolution with 4-channel MDCT. A: MIP of the left calf in a patient with femorocriral bypass to the posterior tibial artery was obtained with 4 × 2.5 mm and 3.0 mm/1.0 mm acquisition. Note the blurry appearance of vessel calcifications and the poor visualization of the small arterial branch distal to the anastomosis (*arrow*). **B:** Corresponding DSA with contrast medium injection into the bypass graft. **C:** VR image (posterior view) of another patient's popliteocrural arteries obtained with 4 × 1 mm detector configuration and 1 mm/1 mm section thickness/reconstruction interval. Note the excellent visualization of very small popliocrural vessels. **D:** Corresponding DSA.

acquisition at substantially improved resolution. Images with a nominal section thickness of 1.25 mm, reconstructed at 0.8 mm ("high-resolution"), can routinely be acquired. Crural and even pedal arteries can be reliably identified with these settings. With faster gantry rotation speed (0.5 seconds/360° rotation) and maximum pitch, 8-channel MDCT allows for extended volume coverage—for example, to visualize the entire thoracic, abdominal, and lower extremity arteries within a single acquisition.

Sixteen-channel Multidetector Computed Tomography

When a detector configuration of 16 × 1.25 mm or 16 × 1.5 mm is used, similar "high-resolution" data sets of the peripheral arterial tree can be acquired, if 1.25- to 2-mm thick sections are reconstructed at 0.8- to 1-mm intervals. The acquisition speed with these parameter settings, however, is substantially faster when compared with both 4- and

8-channel systems. In fact, it may be too fast for patients with altered flow dynamics. Sixteen-channel MDCT also allows—for the first time—the routine acquisition of submillimeter "isotropic" data sets of the entire peripheral arterial tree.

With detector configuration settings such as 16 × 0.625 mm or 16 × 0.75, it is possible to reconstruct less than 1-mm thick sections spaced every 0.5 to 0.8 mm. With these settings, the acquisition is "slow," in the range of 40 to 50 seconds, which is comparable to routine 4- (4 × 2.5) and 8- (8 × 1.25) channel system acquisitions. These submillimeter "isotropic" resolution data sets further improve the visualization of small crural or pedal vessels; however, image noise and increased dose and tube-current requirements may be problematic in the abdomen unless automated tube-current modulation is available.

It is important to bear in mind, however, that submillimeter *acquisition* (16 × 0.625 mm, 16 × 0.75 mm) does not necessarily require submillimeter image *reconstruction* (i.e., reconstructing the thinnest possible images). For example, one might routinely choose to reconstruct thicker "high-resolution" (e.g., 1.25 mm) data sets from a submillimeter acquisition. This strategy still allows the user to go back and reconstruct another "isotropic submillimeter" data set at maximum spatial resolution, if clinically necessary.

It is our experience that the reconstruction of a single "high-resolution" (~1.25 to 1.5 mm section thickness) data set obtained with 8- and 16-channel CT and 1-mm section thickness with 64-channel MDCT provides both adequate spatial resolution for the entire peripheral arterial tree while keeping the noise level in the abdomen and pelvis within an acceptable range (Fig. 21-5).

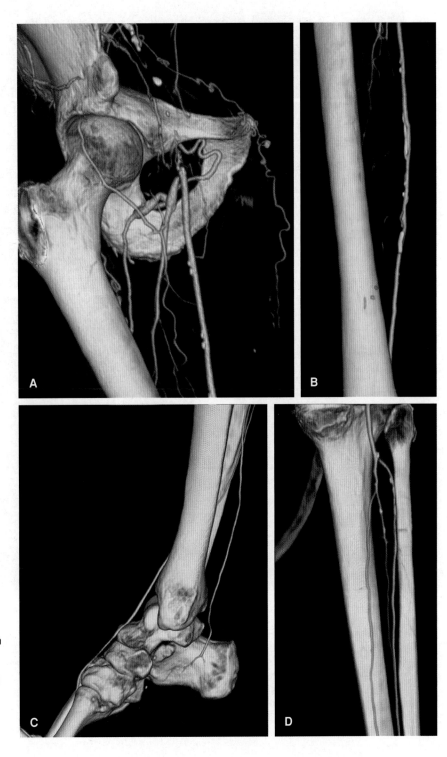

FIGURE 21-5 16-channel MDCT (16 × 1.25 mm, 1.25 mm/0.8 mm) peripheral CT angiogram in a 70-year-old man with right thigh claudication and right iliofemoral artery occlusion demonstrates exquisite detail of small collateral vessels (**A**) as well as femoropopliteal (**B**), pedal (**C**), and crural arteries (**D**). (Reprinted with permission from Fleischmann D, Hallett RL, Rubin GD. CT angiography of peripheral arterial disease. *J Vasc Interv Radiol.* 2006;17:3–26.)

64-channel Multidetector Computed Tomography

Data acquisition with 64-channel MDCT normally ensues on a submillimeter scale (64 × 0.6 mm or 64 × 0.625 mm). Because of peripheral arterial enhancement dynamics, it is important to deliberately "slow down" the acquisition speed with these scanners by selecting a low pitch and refraining

from using the maximum gantry rotation speed, most notably in patients with occlusive disease.

Again, one can use the raw data from the submillimeter acquisition to routinely reconstruct data sets with a section thickness of 1.0 to 1.5 mm ("high-resolution") (Fig. 21-6). "Submillimeter isotropic" images with a section thickness as

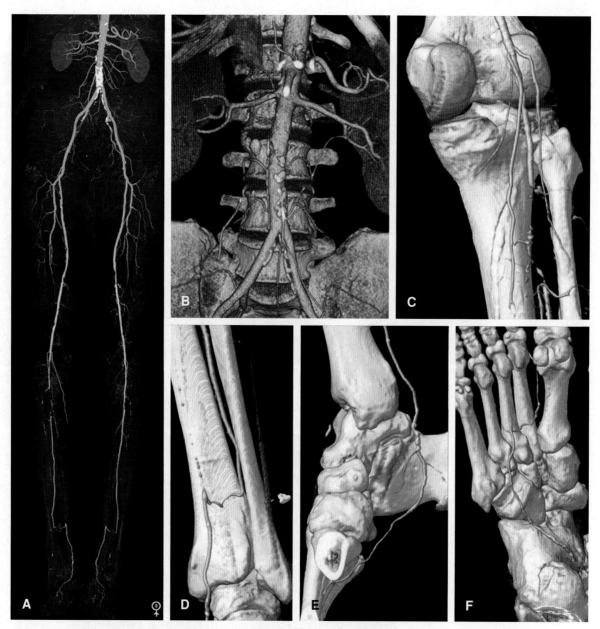

FIGURE 21-6 Sixty-four channel MDCT (64 × 0.6 mm, 1.0 mm/0.7 mm) peripheral CT angiogram in an 83-year-old man with right greater than left calf and foot claudication. Automated tube current modulation (CareDose 4D, Siemens Medical Solutions, Forchheim, Germany) allows submillimeter acquisition and reconstruction with acceptable image noise level in the abdomen and unprecedented spatial resolution down to the plantar arch and metatarsal branches. MIP of the entire data set **(A)**; VR views of the abdomen **(B)**, occlusion of the right popliteal trifurcation with reconstitution of the peroneal artery **(C)**, which reconstitutes the right posterior tibial artery above the ankle via a communicating branch **(D)**, and supplies the foot through the common and lateral plantar arteries **(E)**, which fill the plantar arch **(F)**. (Reprinted with permission from Fleischmann D, Hallett RL, Rubin GD. CT angiography of peripheral arterial disease. *J Vasc Interv Radiol*. 2006;17:3–26.)

small as 0.6 to 1.0 mm spaced every 0.4 to 0.7 mm may be reconstructed from the same acquisition. This maximum spatial resolution may translate into improved visualization and treatment planning of patients with advanced PAOD.

Peripheral CTA data sets are generally large, ranging from 900 to 2,500 images. At Stanford, all images are saved and stored in the Picture Archiving and Communication System (PACS), but this may not be feasible for all institutions. One potential solution to reduce file sizes is to permanently archive 1.5- to 2-mm thick images and to use thinner sections (e.g., submillimeter) only for data viewing and for the generation of permanent high-quality reformatted images.

Contrast Medium Injection Technique

Intravenous iodinated contrast medium is injected into an antecubital vein (20 gauge or larger IV cannula) by using a power injector. The basic principles of contrast medium injection for CTA, such as the relationship of the injection flow rate and the injection duration on arterial enhancement, also apply to peripheral CTA—at least for its aortoiliac portion (34). Peripheral CTA is more complex, however, with respect to synchronizing the enhancement of the entire lower extremity arterial tree with the CT data acquisition speed.

In general, 1.0 to 1.5 g of iodine injected per second (I/s) usually achieves adequate arterial enhancement for an average (75 kg) person. Body weight based adjustments of the injection flow rate and volume are recommended, at least for those subjects with more than 90 kg and those with less than 60 kg of body weight. The injection duration also affects the time course of arterial enhancement. With a continuous IV injection of contrast medium over a prolonged period of time (e.g., 35 seconds), arterial enhancement continuously increases over time (35). This explains why the attenuation values observed in peripheral CT angiograms are usually lowest in the abdominal aorta and peak at the level of the infragenicular popliteal artery (24). In general, biphasic injections result in more uniform enhancement over time, notably with long scan and injection times (>25 to 30 seconds) (32).

Principles of Scan Timing

The time interval between the beginning of the intravenous contrast medium injection and the arrival of the bolus in the aorta—referred to as the contrast medium transit time (t_{CMT})—is very variable between patients with coexisting cardiocirculatory disease and may range from 12 to 40 seconds. Individualizing the scanning delay is thus generally recommended in peripheral CTA. A patient's individual t_{CMT} can be reliably determined with a small test-bolus injection or estimated by using automated bolus-triggering

techniques. The scanning delay may then be chosen to equal the t_{CMT} (the scan is thus initiated as soon as contrast medium arrives in the aorta), or the scanning delay may be chosen at a predefined interval after the t_{CMT}. For example, the notation "t_{CMT} + 5s" means that the scan starts 5 seconds after contrast medium has arrived in the aorta.

Aortopopliteal Bolus Transit Times

The additional challenge in patients with PAOD is related to the well-known fact that arterial stenoses, occlusions, or aneurysms anywhere between the infrarenal abdominal aorta and the pedal arteries may substantially delay downstream vascular opacification (36,37). More specifically, in a group of 20 patients with PAOD, it was found that the transit times of IV-injected contrast medium to travel from the aorta to the popliteal arteries ranged from 4 to 24 seconds (average: 10 seconds), which corresponds to bolus transit speeds as fast as 177 mm/second to as slow as 29 mm/second, respectively (38).

The clinical implication for peripheral CTA is that when a table speed of ~30 mm/second is selected, it is very unlikely (though not impossible) that the data acquisition is faster than the intravascular contrast medium bolus. With increasing acquisition speeds, however, the scanner table may move faster than the intravascular contrast medium column, and the scanner may thus outrun the bolus (Fig. 21-7). Of note, "outrunning-the-bolus" has only been reported in one study, which used a table speed of 37 mm/second (26),

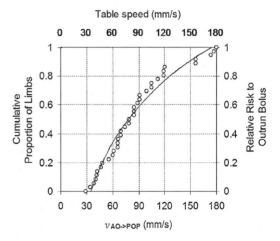

FIGURE 21-7 Plot shows cumulative proportion of limbs as a function of aortopopliteal bolus transit speed (vAO–>POP), with a logarithmic trendline (y = −0.6207Ln(x) + 3.203) fitted to the data (R2 = 0.97). The data can also be interpreted as the relative risk of outrunning the contrast medium bolus as a function of the table speed of the CT scanner, as indicated by the secondary x- and y-axes of the plot, respectively: an increase of the table speed (secondary x-axis) relates to an increased risk of outrunning the contrast medium bolus (secondary y-axis). (Reprinted with permission from Fleischmann D, Hallett RL, Rubin GD. CT angiography of peripheral arterial disease. *J Vasc Interv Radiol*. 2006;17:3–26.)

but it has not been reported in five other published studies on peripheral CTA, all of which used table speeds of 19 to 30 mm/second (24,25,27,28,39).

For the following discussion, it is thus useful to arbitrarily categorize injection strategies for peripheral CTA into those for "slow" acquisitions (≤30 mm/second table speed) and those for "fast" acquisitions (>30 mm/second table speed). Sixty-four-channel MDCT injection strategies will be discussed separately.

Injection Strategies for "Slow" Acquisitions

Detector configuration settings of 4 × 2.5 mm, 8 × 1.25 mm, and 16 × 0.625 mm all translate into an acquisition speed of approximately 30 mm/second. Such a table speed usually translates into a scan time of approximately 40 seconds for the entire peripheral arterial tree. Because the data acquisition follows the bolus from the aorta down to the feet, the injection duration can be chosen approximately 5 seconds shorter than the scan time. For example, for a 40-second acquisition, a 35-second injection duration is sufficient. This would translate into 140 mL of contrast medium if a constant injection rate of 4 mL/second was used. If the beginning of the data acquisition is

timed closely to the contrast arrival time in the aorta (using a test bolus or bolus triggering), biphasic injections achieve more favorable enhancement profiles, with improved aortic enhancement. As an example, our current protocol for a submillimeter acquisition with a Siemens 16-channel scanner is shown in Table 21-5. A similar concept is used for the 64-channel Siemens scanner at our institution as well.

Injection Strategies for "Fast" Acquisitions

Detector configuration settings of 8 × 2.5, 16 × 1.25, or 16 × 1.5 translate into acquisition speeds of 45 to 65 mm/second, which—in some individuals—may be faster than the contrast medium bolus travels through a diseased peripheral arterial tree. In order to prevent the CT acquisition to outrun the bolus, it is necessary to allow the bolus a "head start." This is accomplished by combining a fixed injection duration of 35 seconds to fill the arterial tree and a delay of the start of the CT acquisition relative to the time of contrast medium arrival in the aorta (t_{CMT}). The faster the acquisition, the longer this "diagnostic delay" should be chosen. We use such a strategy with a GE 16-channel scanner with a 16 × 1.25 mm protocol, pitch 1.375, and

TABLE 21-5

Peripheral Computed Tomographic Angiography Injection Protocol for "Slow" Acquisitions

Table speed	≤30 mm/second
Scanning time	≥40 seconds
Examples of acquisition parameters	4 × 2.5 mm 8 × 1.25 mm 16 × 0.75 mm, 16 × 0.625 mm 64 × 0.6 mm, 64 × 0.625 mm (slow pitch and gantry rotation—see Table 21-4)
Injection duration	= scan time − 5 seconds (at least 35 seconds)
Scanning delay	= t_{CMT} (CM arrival in the aorta, as determined by a test bolus or by using automated bolus triggering)
Injection flow rates	Biphasic, 5 to 6 mL/second (1.8 g iodine/second) for 5 seconds 3 to 4 mL/second (1.0 g iodine/second) for remaining (scan time − 10 seconds)
Example	For an acquisition time of 45 seconds, inject 30 mL at 6 mL/second + 115 mL at 3.3 mL/second (300 mg iodine/mL concentration CM) or 25 mL at 4.5 mL/second + 85 mL at 2.5 mL/second (400 mg iodine/mL concentration CM). Total injection duration is 35 seconds (5 + 30). Total CM volume is 145 mL or 110 mL, respectively.

t_{CMT}, contrast medium transit time; CM, contrast medium.
Note: Injection flow rates vary depending on the iodine concentration of the contrast agent used. Iodine injection rate is adequate for a 75-kg individual and should be increased/decreased for subjects >90 kg to <60 kg body weight.

0.6-second gantry rotation period (table speed: 45mm/second). The protocol as well as its generalization to other "fast" acquisitions is shown in Table 21-6. An example of arterial opacification using this approach by using fast scans is shown in Figure 21-5. The limitation of using a very long "diagnostic delay" (>15 seconds between contrast medium arrival and scan initiation) is undesirable opacification of the renal and portal veins and the inferior vena cava.

Injection Strategy for 64-channel Multidetector Computed Tomography

While 32-, 40-, and 64-channel CT systems theoretically allow acquisition speeds of 80 mm/second and more, we deliberately acquire our peripheral CT angiograms at a much slower pace, by prescribing a fixed scan time of 40 seconds for each scan. For a 40-second scan time, we select a gantry rotation of 0.5 seconds and a pitch <1. Automated tube-current modulation is used in this setting to avoid increased radiation dose and also to control image noise (within and across patients). The advantage of always selecting the same 40-second scan time is that it can be combined with fixed (biphasic) injections of 35 seconds duration. The injection flow rates and volumes are then individualized to patient weight, such as shown in Table 21-7. Examples of image quality and opacification are shown in Figure 21-6.

All of the above acquisition and contrast medium injection strategies reduce the risk of outrunning the bolus but do not eliminate it. An example of a patient with extremely delayed flow, most likely caused by decreased cardiac output and altered flow dynamics due to his bilateral iliac and popliteal artery aneurysms, and diffuse arteriomegaly is demonstrated in Figure 21-8. The risk of obtaining nondiagnostic studies is addressed by preprogramming a second CTA acquisition (covering the popliteal and infrapopliteal vasculature) into the scanning protocol. This acquisition is initiated by the CT technologist immediately following the main CTA acquisition only if he or she does not see any contrast medium opacification in the distal vessels.

Other Injection Strategies

The above injection strategies combine individual scan timing (using bolus tracking/test-bolus) in the aorta, with empiric (non-individualized) parameter selection to adjust for a broad range of possible bolus transit speeds down to the feet. Other approaches—using more or less individualization—are also possible. For example, protocols with a fixed, long scanning delay (28s) have been used successfully in the past, notably before automated bolus tracking technique was available on the first 4-channel scanners (28).

TABLE 21-6

Peripheral Computed Tomographic Angiography Injection Protocol for "Fast" Acquisitions in Patients with Peripheral Arterial Occlusive Disease

Table speed	>>30 mm/second
Scanning time	<<40 seconds
Examples of acquisition parameters	8 × 2.5 mm
	16 × 1.25 mm
	16 × 1.5 mm
	64 × 0.6 mm, 64 × 0.625mm (for pitch and rotation—see Table 21-4)
Injection duration	= 35 seconds
Scanning delay	= t_{CMT} + (40 seconds – scanning time)[a]
Injection flow rates	= 1.5 g iodine/second (4 to 5 mL/second)
Examples	Always inject for 35 seconds (e.g., 140 mL at 4 mL/second).
	For a scan time of 30 seconds, start scanning 10 seconds after CM arrived in aorta.
	For a scan time of 25 seconds, start scanning 15 seconds after CM arrived in aorta.
	For a scan time of 20 seconds, start scanning 20 seconds after CM arrived in aorta.

t_{CMT}, contrast medium transit time; CM, contrast medium.
[a]The term *40 seconds – scanning time* is also referred to as the *diagnostic delay*. Iodine injection rate of 1.5 g/second is adequate for a 75-kg individual and should be increased/decreased for subjects >90 kg to <60 kg body weight (20 mg iodine/kg body weight/second). Injection flow rates will vary, depending on iodine concentration of CM.

TABLE 21-7

Integrated 64-Channel Peripheral Computed Tomographic Angiography Acquisition and Injection Protocol

Acquisition	64 × 0.6 mm (number of channels × channel width); 120 kV, automated tube current modulation (250 quality reference mAs)
Pitch, table speed	Variable (depends on volume coverage, usually <1.0). Table is also variable (~30mm/second).
Scan time	FIXED to 40 seconds (in all patients)
Injection duration	FIXED to 35 seconds (in all patients)
Scanning delay	t_{CMT} + 2 seconds (minimum delay with automated bolus triggering, including breath-hold command)
Contrast medium	High concentration (370 mg iodine/mL)
Biphasic injections (body-weight adjusted)	Maximum flow rate for first 5 seconds of injection, continued with 80% of initial flow rate for 30 seconds

Body Weight	Biphasic Injection
<55 kg	20 mL (4.0 mL/second) + 96 mL (3.2 mL/second)
<65 kg	23 mL (4.5 mL/second) + 108 mL (3.6 mL/second)
Average: 75 kg	25 mL (5.0 mL/second) + 120 mL (4.0 mL/second)
>85 kg	28 mL (5.5 mL/second) + 132 mL (4.4 mL/second)
>95 kg	30 mL (6.0 mL/second) + 144 mL (4.8 mL/second)

t_{CMT}, contrast medium transit time.

On the other end of the spectrum are attempts to individualize both the scanning delay and the scanning speed based on both aortic and the popliteal transit times, determined individually with two test boluses (40). All of the above injection protocols can also be used in patients without occlusive disease, but deliberately delaying the scan or slowing down the acquisition is not imperative in this setting. For example, two small injections (60 to 80 mL/second) with short scan times (5 to 6 seconds) for the two arterial acquisitions in popliteal entrapment syndrome are sufficient.

Venous Enhancement

Opacification of deep and superficial veins can be observed in peripheral CTA (24) and is more likely to occur with longer scan times and in patients with active inflammation (e.g., from infected or nonhealing ulcers). Given the rapid arteriovenous transit times observed angiographically in some patients (41), venous opacification cannot be completely avoided. As arterial enhancement is always stronger than venous enhancement when the injection is timed correctly (24), and with adequate anatomic knowledge and postprocessing tools, venous enhancement rarely poses a diagnostic problem.

Visualization and Image Interpretation

Visualization, image interpretation, and effective communication of findings are demanding in peripheral CTA. A powerful medical image postprocessing workstation as well as standardized workflow and visualization protocols are required when peripheral CT angiograms are performed on a regular basis.

Various two-dimensional (2D) and 3D postprocessing techniques are available on today's state-of-the-art workstations. For patients with atherosclerotic disease, a combination of 3D-overview techniques with at least one 2D cross-sectional technique is generally required. The selection of postprocessing techniques not only depends on the type of disease but also on the specific visualization goal: interpretation versus documentation. In the context of interactive exploration of the data sets—usually done by the radiologist interpreting the study during readout—fast navigation and flexible visualization tools are preferred. In the setting of creating standardized sets of static images and measurements for documentation and communication, techniques that allow a protocol-driven generation of predefined views are preferred.

The typical protocol for postprocessing of peripheral CTA in the Stanford 3D laboratory consists of curved

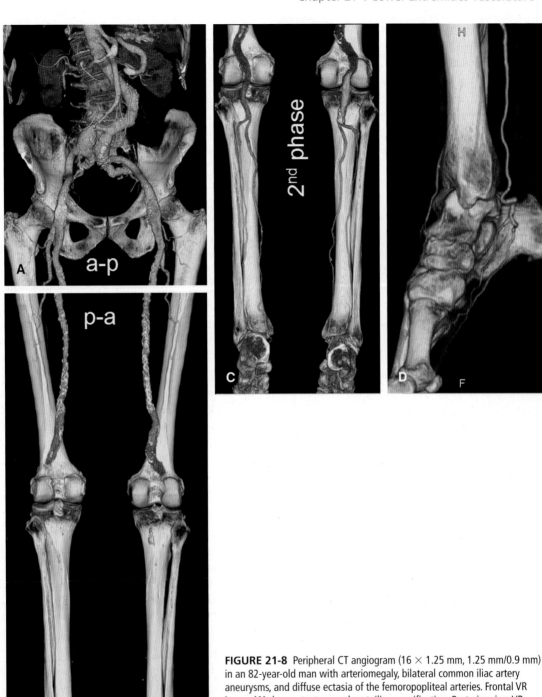

FIGURE 21-8 Peripheral CT angiogram (16 × 1.25 mm, 1.25 mm/0.9 mm) in an 82-year-old man with arteriomegaly, bilateral common iliac artery aneurysms, and diffuse ectasia of the femoropopliteal arteries. Frontal VR image **(A)** demonstrates good aortoiliac opacification. Posterior view VR image **(B)** shows gradually decreasing enhancement of the femoropopliteal arteries bilaterally, with complete lack of enhancement of the popliteal trifurcation and crural arteries. A second phase CTA acquisition was obtained from above the knees down to the feet immediately following the first acquisition. Posterior view of second phase CTA **(C)** shows interval opacification of the bilateral popliteal and crural arteries, down to the feet **(D)**. (Reprinted with permission from Fleischmann D, Hallett RL, Rubin GD. CT angiography of peripheral arterial disease. *J Vasc Interv Radiol.* 2006;17:3–26.)

planar reformations (CPRs); thin-slab maximum-intensity projections (MIPs) through the renal and visceral arteries; bone removal; full-volume MIPs and volume renderings (VRs) of the abdomen, pelvis, and each leg; and filming and archiving of these views. While the creation of such sets of images may be time-consuming even for an experienced technologist, the clinical interpretation is fast and straightforward for the image recipient.

Transverse Source Image Viewing

Reviewing of transverse CT slices is mandatory for the assessment of extravascular abdominal or pelvic pathology. This is facilitated by reconstructing an additional series of contiguous 5-mm thick sections through the abdomen and pelvis. Browsing through the stack of source images is also helpful to gain a first impression on vascular abnormalities, and in select cases—such as in patients with only minimal or no disease, in patients with trauma, or in patients with suspected acute occlusions, source image viewing may be sufficient. Relevant extravascular anatomy, such as the course and position of the medial head of the gastrocnemius muscle in popliteal entrapment syndrome, is readily depicted on the axial images and often inapparent on projection (e.g., MIP) images. Source images may also serve as a reference when 2D- or 3D-reformatted images suggest artifactual lesions. For the majority of cases with vascular disease, however, transverse image viewing is both inefficient and less accurate (27) than viewing reformatted images.

Postprocessing Techniques

Maximum Intensity Projection

Assessment of vascular abnormalities is facilitated when the arterial tree is displayed in an "angiographic" fashion. This can be accomplished with either MIP or VR technique. MIP provides the most "angiographylike" display of the vasculature—particularly when no or only minimal vessel calcifications are present. The disadvantage of MIP is that it requires bone removal from the data set, a time-consuming task. Additionally, inadvertent removal of vessels in close vicinity to bony structures may lead to spurious lesions.

Volume Rendering

Because VR preserves 3D depth information, unlike MIP, bone editing may not be required. Clip planes, volume slabs, and appropriate viewing angles are used to expose the relevant vascular segment. VR is the ideal tool for fast interactive exploration of peripheral CTA data sets. While "snapshot" views obtained during data exploration can be invaluable for communicating a specific finding or detail, VR is somewhat less suited for standardized documentation

of images. In part, this is due to the fact that most PACS workstations do not display the color information on high-resolution grayscale monitors.

The main limitation of both MIP and VR is that vessel calcifications and stents may completely obscure the vascular flow channel (Fig. 21-9). This fundamental limitation precludes its exclusive use in a substantial proportion (approximately 60%) of patients with PAOD (42).

Multiplanar Reformation and Curved Planar Reformation

In the presence of calcified plaque, diffuse vessel wall calcification, or endoluminal stents, cross-sectional views are essential to assess the vascular flow channel (Fig. 21-9). Transverse source images, such as sagittal, coronal, or oblique multiplanar reformations, are useful in an interactive setting, for example in conjunction with VR.

Alternatively, longitudinal cross sections along a predefined vascular centerline, so-called CPRs, can be created (Fig. 21-10). CPRs provide the most comprehensive cross-sectional display of luminal pathology but require either manual or (semi-) automated tracing of the vessel centerlines (43,44). CPR does not require bone editing, but at least two CPRs per vessel segment (e.g., sagittal and coronal views) have to be created in order to fully evaluate eccentric disease.

One problem of (single) CPR images in the context of visualizing the peripheral arterial tree is their limited spatial perception. With bony landmarks out of the curved reconstruction plane, the anatomic context of a vascular lesion may be ambiguous unless clear annotations are present. This limitation has recently been alleviated by an extension of standard CPR to so-called multipath CPR images (43). Multipath CPRs provide simultaneous longitudinal cross-sectional views through the major conducting vessels (Fig. 21-11) without obscuring vessel wall calcifications and stents while maintaining spatial perception (45). This technique is a convenient visualization, documentation, and endovascular treatment-planning tool for peripheral CTA; however, it is not generally available on commercial workstations.

Thin-slab Maximum-intensity Projection, Thin-slab Volume Rendering, and Thick Multi- and Curved Planar Reformation

If applied to subvolumes of the data sets, either by using clip planes, or "slabs" of the volume to focus on a particular area of interest, the resulting images are referred to as *thin-slab MIPs* or *thin-slab VRs*, or *thick MPRs* (or CPRs) (46,47). Interactive real-time variation of the viewing direction, the thickness of the rendered volume, adjustments to

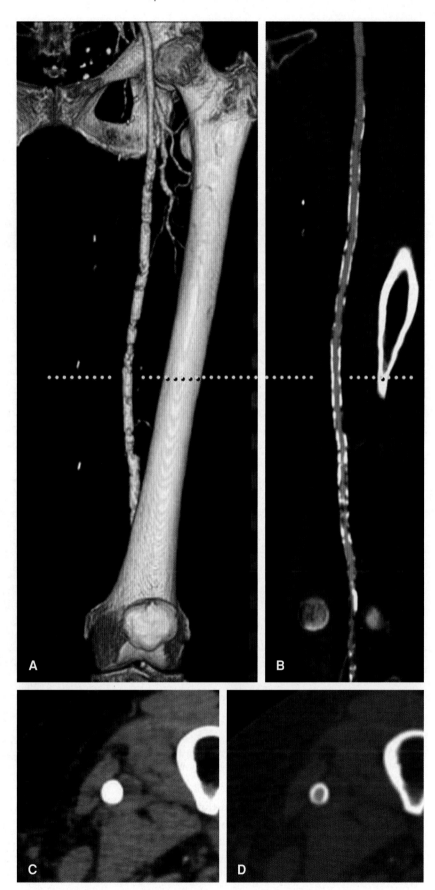

FIGURE 21-9 Peripheral CTA (16 x 1.25 mm, 1.25 mm/0.9 mm) of a 72-year-old woman with a nonhealing left forefoot ulcer. **A:** VR image of the left superficial femoral artery shows excessive vessel wall calcifications, precluding the assessment of the flow channel. Cross-sectional views are required to visualize the vessel lumen. Axial CT images **(B, C)** through mid superficial femoral artery (*dotted line* in **A** and **B**) with viewing window settings (level/width) of 200 HU/600 HU **(B)** does not allow to distinguish between opacified vessel lumen and vessel calcification, which can be distinguished only when an adequately wide window width (300 HU/1200 HU) is used **(C)**. Similar wide window settings are also used for a CPR through the same vessel **(D)**, displaying several areas of wall calcification with and also without stenosis. (Reprinted with permission from Fleischmann D, Hallett RL, Rubin GD. CT angiography of peripheral arterial disease. *J Vasc Interv Radiol.* 2006;17:3–26.)

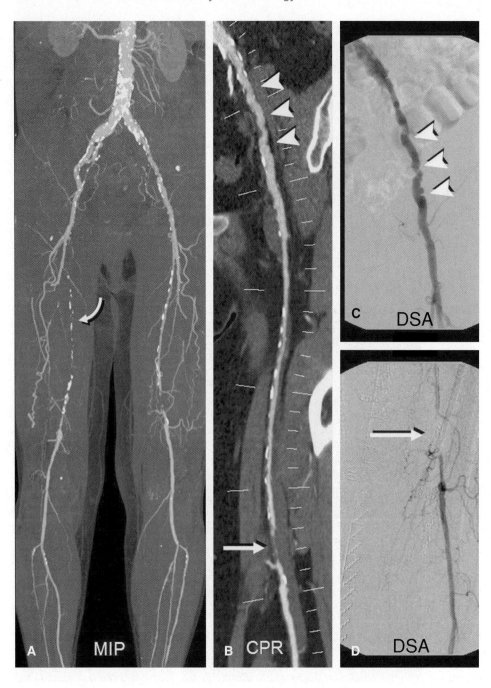

FIGURE 21-10 Peripheral CTA (16 × 0.75 mm, 2.0 mm/1.0 mm) of a 73-year-old woman with intermittent claudication bilaterally. MIP **(A)** shows long right femoropopliteal occlusion (*curved arrow*) and diffuse disease of the left superficial femoral artery with a short distal near-occlusion. CPR **(B)** through left iliofemoral arteries demonstrates multiple mild stenoses of the external iliac artery (*arrowheads*), a diffusely diseased left superficial femoral artery, and short (<3 cm) distal left SFA occlusion (*arrow*). Corresponding selective DSA images of the left external iliac artery **(C)** and the distal left superficial femoral artery **(D)** obtained immediately before PTA/stenting. (Reprinted with permission from Fleischmann D, Hallett RL, Rubin GD. CT angiography of peripheral arterial disease. *J Vasc Interv Radiol.* 2006;17:3–26.)

window-level settings or opacity transfer-functions, and the like is ideal for interactively exploring the data sets.

Automated Techniques for Segmentation and Visualization

While fully automated detection of vessel centerlines, automated segmentation of bony structures, and detection (and subtraction) of vessel wall calcification is highly desirable, no such algorithms have yet been developed. This is not surprising when considering the complex manifestations of vascular disease; the wide range of vessel sizes; the wide overlap in CT density values of opacified blood, plaque, and low-attenuation bone; and the inherently limited spatial resolution and image noise in peripheral CTA data sets. Several software tools for improved and faster editing and for creating centerlines through the arteries have been developed and are available on modern 3D workstations.

Interpretation and Pitfalls

Vascular abnormalities have to be interpreted in the context of a patient's symptoms, stage of disease, and with respect to the available treatment options. For those familiar to reading

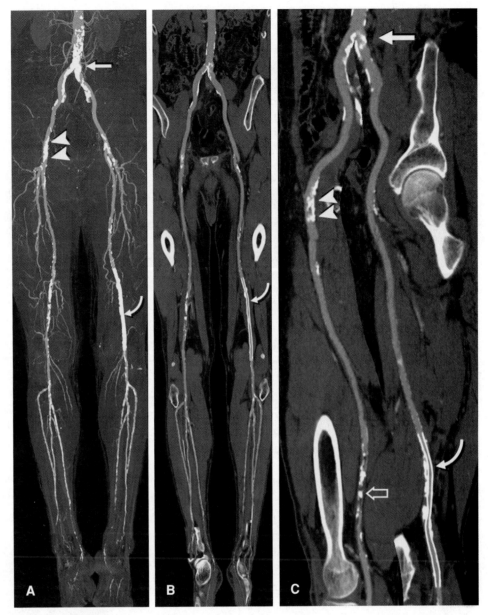

FIGURE 21-11 Peripheral CTA (16 × 0.75 mm, 2.0 mm/1.0 mm) of a diabetic man with bilateral claudication. MIP **(A)** shows arterial calcifications near the aortic bifurcation (*arrow*) as well as in the right (*arrowheads*) and left common femoral arteries, in the right femoropopliteal region, and in the crural vessels. A long stent is seen in the left femoropopliteal segment (*curved arrow*). Frontal view **(B)** and magnified 45° left anterior oblique (LAO) **(C)** multipath CPR images provide simultaneous CPRs through the aorta and bilateral iliac through crural arteries. Note that prominent calcifications cause luminal narrowing in the proximal left common iliac artery (*arrow*) and in the right common femoral artery (*arrowheads*). The left common femoral artery is normal; the long femoropopliteal stent is patent (*curved arrow*). A mixed calcified and noncalcified occlusion of the right distal femoral artery is noted (*open arrow*). (Reprinted with permission from Fleischmann D, Hallett RL, Rubin GD. CT angiography of peripheral arterial disease. *J Vasc Interv Radiol.* 2006;17: 3–26.)

conventional angiograms, the clinical aspect of interpreting a peripheral CTA is usually straightforward. However, visual perception and interpretation of well-known abnormalities in a new and different format (such as VR or CPR images) requires adaptation and familiarity with the specific techniques used.

Probably the most important pitfall related to the interpretation of peripheral CT angiograms is related to using narrow viewing window settings in the presence of arterial wall calcifications or stents. Even at wider-than-normal "CT-angiographic" window settings (Window level/width: 150 Hounsfield units [HU]/600 HU), high-attenuation objects (calcified plaque, stents) appear larger than they really are ("blooming"—due to the point-spread-function of the

scanner), which may lead to an overestimation of a vascular stenosis or suggest a spurious occlusion.

When scrutinizing a calcified lesion or a stented segment by using any of the cross-sectional grayscale images (transverse source images, MPR, or CPR), a viewing window width of at least 1500 HU may be required (Fig. 21-9). Interactive window adjustment on a PACS viewing station or on a 3D workstation are most effective because when printed on film, window settings are usually too narrow.

In the setting of extensive atherosclerotic or media calcification within small crural or pedal arteries, such as those found in diabetic patients and in patients with end-stage renal disease, the lumen may not be resolved regardless of the window/level selection. In these circumstances, other imaging techniques, notably MRI, may be preferable to CTA.

Other interpretation pitfalls result from misinterpretation of editing artifacts (inadvertent vessel removal) in MIP images and pseudostenosis and/or occlusions in CPRs due to inaccurate centerline definition. Most of these artifacts are obvious or easily identified when additional views, complementary viewing modalities, or source images are reviewed.

Magnetic Resonance Angiography

Equipment Considerations

Imaging the lower extremity vasculature demands anatomic coverage of well over 100 cm. As the typical maximum FOV in current commercially available MR scanners is on the order of 40 to 45 cm, the peripheral vascular tree exceeds this by a factor of two to three times. In conventional intra-arterial imaging where the imaging FOV is even smaller, this problem is solved by using a stepping table approach with multiple injections of contrast material or a bolus-chase approach, whereby the bolus of contrast material is filmed and followed down the lower extremity by rapid table translation between several contiguous locations (48). Contrast-enhanced (CE) peripheral MRA essentially uses the same two strategies to image the peripheral vasculature.

When planning a peripheral MRA study, the relative needs for temporal resolution, spatial resolution, and signal-to-noise ratio (SNR) must be balanced. In general, higher main magnetic field strengths, higher maximum gradient amplitudes, and faster gradient systems allow for better imaging protocols to depict peripheral arterial disease. These system attributes are more important for CE MRA, which is currently considered the state-of-the-art for imaging the peripheral vascular tree, than for nonenhanced MRA.

A minimal main magnetic field strength of 1.0 T is needed for peripheral MRA. Systems with powerful gradients offer the greatest efficiency and flexibility.

The use of surface coils increases the SNR and is most important for imaging the tibial vessels, particularly at 1.0 T and 1.5 T. This SNR boost can be invested in temporal or spatial resolution or in combinations of the two. An increase in spatial resolution increases arterial conspicuity and improves disease characterization in small, distal, diseased arteries. An increase in temporal resolution helps to avoid venous enhancement and can display collateral filling patterns to good vantage.

Phased-array surface body- or torso coils can be used to image the lower leg. In addition, dedicated multistation peripheral vascular coils with coverage exceeding 100 cm are widely available (Fig. 21-12). In cases where a protocol

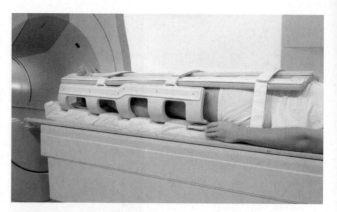

FIGURE 21-12 Lower extremity coil. Commercially available three-station, 12-element phased-array lower extremity coil (Philips Medical Systems; Best, the Netherlands). In each station (aortoiliac, upper legs, and lower legs), there are two anterior and two posterior elements that can be used for signal reception. This coil design also permits parallel imaging. Note that the feet are covered as well, allowing depiction of pedal vasculature with high SNR.

targets a single foot, a head or knee coil can be effective (Fig. 21-13). Several authors have shown that the use of such coils benefits signal-to-noise and anatomical coverage (49–51).

An important technical advance for CE MRA, enabled with the use of localized coils, is parallel imaging (52–54). Parallel imaging speeds up data acquisition by replacing the relatively slow spatial encoding through the use of gradients with a faster spatial encoding that uses coil sensitivity profiles. In theory, acquisition duration can be decreased by a factor R equal to the number of coil elements. However, the acceleration is offset by a reduction in the SNR equal to $\sqrt{R}$.

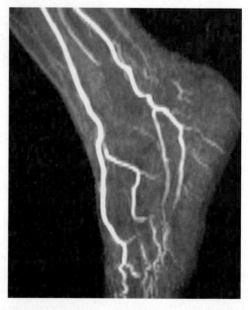

FIGURE 21-13 Pedal vessels obtained by using a head coil. This sagittal MIP, generated from an ECG-triggered 2D TOF sequence, has excellent signal and contrast, demonstrating good-quality pedal vessels.

Different Magnetic Resonance Angiography Techniques for Imaging Peripheral Arterial Disease

Several different MRA techniques have been described to image the peripheral vascular tree. These are (a) phase contrast (PC) MRA, (b) time-of-flight (TOF) or inflow MRA, (c) 3D half-Fourier fast spin echo MRA, (d) balanced steady state free precession (bSSFP) MRA and, (e) CE MRA. The latter technique is currently by far the most widely used, although noncontrast techniques are being re-examined to address recent concerns about nephrogenic systemic fibrosis associated with gadolinium administration. A discussion of this reaction can be found in Chapter 22. A summary of the relative merits and shortcomings of MRA techniques can be found in Table 21-8, and detailed descriptions are found in Chapter 2.

Phase Contrast

In PC MRA, vessel-to-background contrast is generated by displaying the accumulated phase difference in *transverse* magnetization between moving protons in blood and stationary background tissues (55).

In addition to *anatomical* display of the peripheral vasculature, PC MRA provides *physiological* studies with flow quantification. However PC MRA is optimized with a priori knowledge about the maximum blood flow velocity in the vessel of interest, information that is rarely available. If maximum flow exceeds the maximum velocity encoding (VENC) value, aliasing artifacts reduce the signal in the vessel of interest. To avoid this problem, multivelocity encoded PC MRA sequences can be used (56,57). The main advantage of PC MRA is that it is less sensitive to in-plane saturation than TOF MRA.

Steffens et al. (58) compared PC MRA with IA DSA to detect aortoiliac and femoropopliteal APAOD in 115 patients. A sensitivity of 95% and specificity of 90% with near perfect interobserver agreement (kappa value of 0.92) was reported (58). PC MRA is not often used for detection and grading of lower extremity arterial disease because of the success of CE techniques.

Time of Flight

In TOF MRA, vessel-to-background contrast is generated by the inflow of fresh, unsaturated blood to a saturated tissue slice. Saturation of stationary background tissue is achieved when radio frequency (RF) pulses with a repetition time much shorter than tissue T1 values are employed. This results in a relatively low longitudinal magnetization producing relatively lower SI. When inflowing unsaturated blood with its large longitudinal magnetization vector (having not been exposed to the RF pulses) enters the imaging slice, it will be seen as much higher signal intensity. Intravascular protons are also subject to saturation effects, proportional to the time those protons reside in the imaging

---

TABLE 21-8

Advantages and Disadvantages of Different Magnetic Resonance Angiography Techniques for Imaging Peripheral Arterial Occlusive Disease

Technique	Strengths	Weaknesses
PC	Entirely noninvasive Relatively fast	Limited data on clinical utility
TOF	Entirely noninvasive	Overestimation of degree and length of stenoses; other artifacts
	Clinically demonstrated benefit for imaging below-knee lower extremity vasculature	Long duration of examination
Balanced SSFP	Entirely noninvasive	Low SNR at high-resolution imaging No data on clinical utility
3D Half-Fourier FSE	Entirely noninvasive	No data on clinical utility
CE	Extensive data on clinical utility	Possibility of disturbing venous overlay in lower leg station
	Imaging protocols can be tailored to patient and clinical question	Necessity for injection of contrast material; associated cost

PC, phase contrast; TOF, time of flight; SSFP, steady state free precession (see text for explanation); SNR, signal-to-noise ratio; 3D, three dimensional; FSE, fast spin echo; CE, contrast enhanced.

slice. Short repetition time (TR), slow flow, and course of the blood vessel in the imaging slice plane all unfavorably affect vessel-to-background contrast (59).

With slower flow demand, the use of higher TR values allows for the best possible image quality. If protons in arterial blood are subjected to too many successive RF excitations with a short TR, saturation and loss of vessel-to-background contrast will be inevitable. TOF MRA is possible either by imaging successive, independent slices (2D TOF MRA), or by imaging a volume that is later partitioned into separate slices (3D TOF MRA). With 3D TOF MRA, thinner slices can be chosen, but acquisition duration is longer and it is less sensitive to slow flow.

TOF MRA suffers from long imaging times (caused by the use of thin sections, which must be oriented perpendicular to the blood flow) and a number of artifacts inherent to TOF MRA that can overestimate the degree and length of stenoses. Artifacts that may mimic vascular stenosis or occlusion are (a) in-plane saturation (Fig. 21-14), (b) accelerated intravoxel phase dispersion (Fig. 21-15) due to turbulent flow (seen in vicinity of high grade stenoses), (c) signal loss due to saturation bands that eliminate signal from retrograde arterial flow, and (d) slice misalignment due to patient motion between acquisitions of successive slices when 2D TOF techniques are used (Fig. 21-14).

With turbulent flow, as is the case distal to stenoses, the dephasing of spins causes signal loss on MRA images, which can lead to an overestimation of the degree and length of

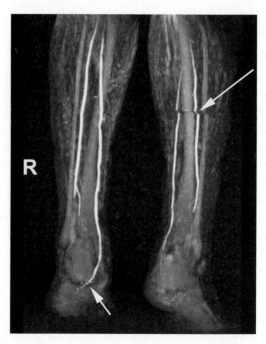

FIGURE 21-14 Slice misalignment artifact (*upper arrow*) due to left lower leg movement during acquisition. The artifact can be differentiated from a stenosis by the typical displacement of the distal arteries with respect to the proximal arteries. Also note gradual extinction of intra-arterial signal in the right foot due to in-plane saturation (*lower arrow*).

stenosis. This artifact is minimized by choosing the shortest echo time (TE) values. For TOF, the shortest TE that can accommodate first-order flow compensation (velocity) is recommended. On the other hand, data from in vitro studies have shown that the magnitude of the signal void artifact

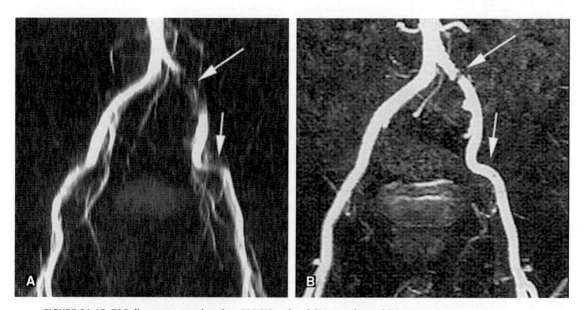

FIGURE 21-15 TOF disease overestimation. TOF **(A)** and gadolinium-enhanced **(B)** MR angiograms in a patient with high-grade left common iliac artery stenosis. Because of intravoxel phase dispersion due to turbulent flow distal to the stenosis the TOF technique is unable to reliably differentiate high-grade stenoses from occlusions (*oblique arrow*). In addition, an in-plane saturation artifact suggests a stenosis in the horizontal part of the left external iliac artery, where in reality there is no stenosis (*vertical arrow*).

directly correlates with the pressure gradient across a stenosis (60).

Saturation bands that selectively image flow from one direction are employed to suppress adjacent venous flow (61,62). Because the signal of *all* blood flowing in a given direction is suppressed, extinction of signal from *retrograde* arterial flow may have undesirable results. For example, in the case of unilateral iliac artery occlusion or superficial femoral occlusion with retrograde flow, the length of disease may be overestimated and eliminate an angioplasty/stent option that may have been appropriate.

Ghosting artifacts result from large variations in blood flow velocity during the cardiac cycle, typically seen in pulsatile vessels. Their occurrence can be prevented by using systolic cardiac synchronization (63) at the expense of acquisition time and possible exacerbation of phase-dispersion artifacts from rapid systolic flow through high-grade stenosis.

TOF MRA was the first technique to show efficacy in MRA of lower extremity occlusive disease (64–66), but selection of optimal imaging parameters is complex (67), and study times are prohibitively long to serve as a routine, comprehensive study of the aorta to the pedal vessels. Despite the disadvantages, TOF MRA has detected run-off vessels in the distal lower leg and foot that were not visualized with conventional x-ray angiographic techniques (15). Furthermore, surgical outcomes for lower extremity bypass grafts based on TOF determined vascular road maps are equivalent to those based on conventional arteriographic road maps (68). At present, the use of nonenhanced TOF MRA is limited to imaging the distal lower leg and foot in patients when CE MRA cannot safely be used or when its image quality is insufficient.

Three-dimensional Half-Fourier Fast Spin Echo

Recently, 3D flow-spoiled, electrocardiogram (ECG)-triggered, half-Fourier fast spin echo imaging has been described for non-CE MRA of the peripheral vasculature (69). With this fresh blood imaging technique in fast-flow vessels, both arteries and veins appear as bright blood when acquired in diastole; however, when acquired in systole, this technique shows black blood arteries and bright blood veins in systole-triggered images (70). Subtraction of systole-triggered images (selective vein) from diastole-triggered images (vein + artery) yields an arterial image.

In peripheral or slow-flow vessels, the technique provides bright blood arteries even in systole, which makes it difficult to separate arteries from veins. Applying the readout direction parallel to the vessel orientation and adding a flow-spoiled gradient pulse in that same direction offer some solutions to this issue (70).

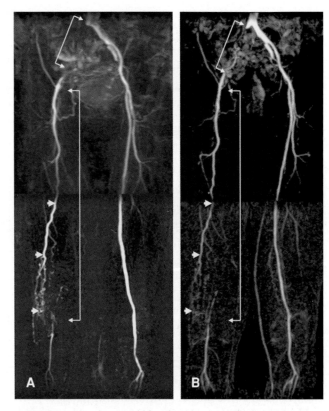

FIGURE 21-16 *A* 69-year-old female with severe intermittent claudication. Both flow-spoiled MRA **(A)** and CE MRA **(B)** demonstrate complete obstructions of the right common iliac artery and the right superficial femoral artery as well as bridging collaterals. (Image courtesy of Joji Urata, MD, Saiseikai Kumamoto Hospital, Kumamoto, Japan.)

Promising results using this technique were reported in healthy volunteers and in preliminary studies in patients (Fig. 21-16). The accuracy of the technique remains to be determined in larger studies.

Balanced Steady State Free Precession

bSSFP can be used for MRI and MRA. A variety of acronyms are used to describe bSSFP pulse sequences; the most used terms are *true fast imaging in steady state free precession* (True-FISP; Siemens Medical Solutions, Erlangen, Germany), *balanced fast field echo* (bFFE; Philips Medical Systems, Best, the Netherlands), and *fast imaging employing steady state excitation* (FIESTA, General Electric, Waukesha, Wisconsin).

These sequences are characterized by a very high SNR and image contrast that is primarily determined by the ratio of T2 to T1. The different T2/T1 ratios of blood and surrounding tissue allow for angiographic, bright blood imaging with bSSFP. Efficient fat saturation is necessary in cases where arteries are surrounded by bright signal fat. Injection of gadolinium chelate contrast media can be helpful to further increase contrast between arteries and surrounding tissue (71).

Balanced SSFP is useful for the quick differentiation of arterial lumen from thrombus in aneurysms and as localizer images to plan subsequent high-resolution CE MRA sequences. More details about bSSFP can be found in recent overviews by Foo et al (71) and Scheffler and Lendhardt (72).

Contrast-enhanced Magnetic Resonance Angiography

Background CE MRA of the peripheral vasculature has evolved into the preferred technique for evaluation of patients with different forms of PAOD in patients for whom its administration is safe. The variety of approaches to peripheral CE MRA allows a tailored strategy to suit the particular clinical question.

A readily available and straightforward approach is the acquisition of three consecutive, identical coronal imaging volumes during injection with a fixed dose (0.2 to 0.3 mmol/kg) or volume (30 to 45 mL) of 0.5 M gadolinium chelate (73–75). This approach is fast and reliable in the vast majority of claudicants. However, image quality of the distal arteries can be contaminated by disturbing venous enhancement for a substantial number of patients (76). Furthermore, the spatial resolution that is usually sufficient for characterizing atherosclerotic aortoiliac lesions is often insufficient for an accurate depiction of the tibial and pedal vessels, particularly when assessing patients with limb-threatening ischemia.

The three-consecutive-station approach does not work well in patients with diabetes mellitus, who are known to primarily have very distal disease (77) and in patients with chronic critical ischemia who have severe stenoses and occlusions from the aorta down to the feet ("multilevel" disease).

As an alternative, tailored prescriptions for each location along with the reordering of the center of k-space can optimize imaging for each station, that is, lower resolution for aortoiliac arteries and higher resolution and more anatomical coverage (to include the pedal arch) for lower leg arteries (78) (Fig. 21-17). Such customization on a per-station basis is the clear preference for performing high-quality peripheral MRA.

The execution of peripheral CE MRA necessitates a compromise between the desire for high spatial resolution and volumetric coverage (requiring long acquisition duration), the desire to avoid disturbing venous enhancement (best achieved with shorter acquisition duration), and the desire for high vessel-to-background contrast. Below, the

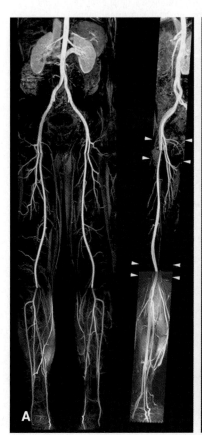 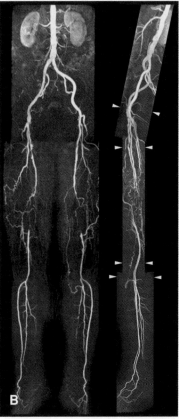

FIGURE 21-17 Tailoring 3D slabs. Coronal and sagittal MIP images of three-station CE MRA examinations 3D moving-bed infusion-tracking peripheral MR angiograms in a 26-year-old healthy male volunteer. The left data set **(A)** was obtained with a fixed-parameter technique (identical imaging parameters for aortoiliac, upper leg, and lower leg arteries); the right data set **(B)** was obtained by using a technique with optimized parameters for each station. Use of flexible parameters permits standard depiction of pedal vasculature **(B)**. On sagittal images, note that volumes for the pelvis and upper and lower legs (containing a different number of partitions) are of different thicknesses (*arrowheads*).

different steps of the peripheral CE MRA examination as well as the practical trade-offs that one is likely to encounter are discussed.

Practical Aspects of Peripheral Contrast-enhanced Magnetic Resonance Imaging

Localizer Scans

Adequate planning of 3D CE MRA volumes ensures optimal image quality in the shortest possible imaging time. Scout scans are usually transverse, thick-slice, low-resolution TOF or, more recently, SSFP acquisitions. Scout views in sagittal or coronal orientation can also be useful. The advantage of using TOF images is that the vascular anatomy can be selectively outlined on MIPs (Fig. 21-18). When the 3D CE MRA volume is planned, transverse source images should *always* be reviewed to ensure that all relevant vascular structures are included in the imaging volume. Failure to do so can result in the exclusion of relevant anatomy from the imaging volume (Fig. 21-19).

Considerations with Regard to Vascular Anatomy

In most patients, peripheral arteries are slightly curved in the anteroposterior direction, and the coverage needed in that dimension is usually less than 10 cm. In the presence of an aortic aneurysm, iliac arterial elongation, collaterals bridging iliac, or superficial femoral arterial obstructions or a femorofemoral crossover bypass graft, the AP coverage needed to depict these vessels may be increased (up to 15 to 20 cm).

In the aortoiliac segment, it is important to keep the acquisition duration to within the capacity of a reasonable breath hold for the individual being studied. By practicing the breath-hold instructions, one can determine a reasonable time frame and avoid confusion during the critical moments of acquisition. In cases where scan duration is incompatible with the breath-holding capabilities of the patient, it is advisable to shorten acquisition duration by increasing slice thickness, by using half-Fourier imaging, or by increasing the parallel imaging factor.

A review of the transverse localizer images ensures that salient structures are included in the 3D CE MRA imaging volume. This is particularly important if a patient has a femorofemoral crossover bypass graft, because these grafts are usually not seen on TOF MIPs due to in-plane saturation artifacts (59).

Other patients who demand special attention are those with (thoraco-) abdominal aortic aneurysms, where flow may be markedly slower compared with patients without

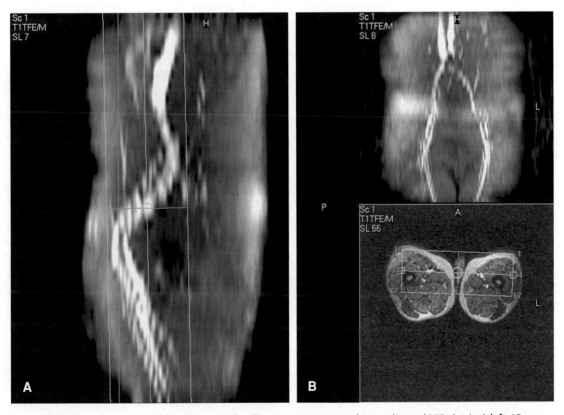

FIGURE 21-18 Low spatial resolution TOF localizer sequence. Image shows orthogonal MIPs (sagittal, **left**; AP, **upper right**; transverse, **lower right**) used to prescribe the 3D CE imaging volume (box enclosed by *thin white line* in **left** and **lower right** panels).

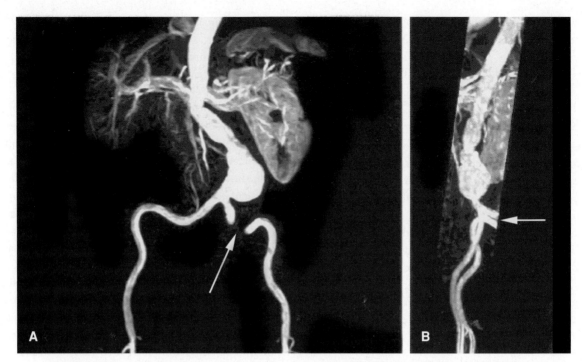

FIGURE 21-19 Exclusion of pelvic arteries from imaging volume. With faulty placement of imaging volume, important vascular anatomy may be excluded. Coronal **(A)** and sagittal **(B)** MIP images of distal aorta and pelvic arteries in a patient with an AAA. On the coronal image, an occlusion in the left common iliac artery cannot be ruled out (arrow in **A**). However, review of the sagittal image shows exclusion of part of the left common iliac artery from the imaging volume (arrow in **B**). This part of the iliac arteries suffered from in-plane saturation in the TOF scan and was not depicted on the sagittal TOF MIP, which led to erroneous planning of the subsequent 3D acquisition. (Modified from Leiner T, Ho KY, Nelemans PJ, et al. Three-dimensional contrast-enhanced moving-bed infusion-tracking [MoBI-track] peripheral MR angiography with flexible choice of imaging parameters for each field of view. *J Magn Reson Imaging*. 2000;11:368–377.)

aneurysms. If insufficient delay time is observed between injection of contrast and imaging, this will result in incomplete enhancement of the aneurysm at the time of imaging (Fig. 21-20). To avoid this problem, either a longer delay between injection and start of acquisition or a multiphasic acquisition should be used (79).

CE MRA is the method of choice for imaging stenoses and occlusions in the aortoiliac (inflow) arteries. The limitations of nonenhanced MRA are particularly evident in this anatomic segment due to the tortuous course of the arteries, pulsatile blood flow, and long imaging times (59,63).

Synchronization of Three-dimensional Contrast-enhanced Magnetic Resonance Angiography Acquisition with Contrast Arrival

A careful synchronization of peak arterial enhancement with the acquisition of the center of k-space is needed in order to obtain a study of diagnostic quality. The time of peak arterial enhancement is a function of many variables, the most important of which are injection rate and volume of contrast media and saline flush (80) as well as cardiac output (81). Because the time of peak arterial enhancement

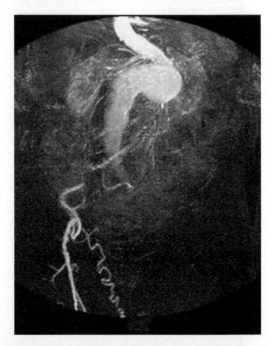

FIGURE 21-20 Incomplete enhancement due to aneurysm. The data acquisition was initiated too early yielding inadequate enhancement of the distal abdominal and iliac vasculature in this patient with thoracoabdominal aortic aneurysm and mimicking occlusions.

can vary substantially between patients, the CE MRA examination needs to be tailored to the individual contrast arrival time. This is important for two main reasons: (a) to prevent ringing artifacts and suboptimal opacification of arteries in the FOV due to starting the acquisition too early (82) and (b) to prevent venous overlay (59).

To determine the delay between the start of injection of contrast medium and the acquisition of central k-space profiles, a 2D TR (1 to 2 seconds per image) test bolus technique can be used (83,84). The optimal scan delay time can be determined by measuring the arrival time in the infrarenal aorta of a small bolus (1 to 3 mL) of contrast medium followed by 25 to 35 mL of saline, injected at the same rate as the full-contrast bolus will be injected later on. A temporal resolution of about 1 to 2 seconds per image should be used.

The scan delay should be chosen to coincide with the frame in which maximum enhancement is observed. Acquisition orientation of the timing bolus in the coronal or sagittal plane provides the exact time at which enhancement commences as well as the rate at which enhancement *progresses* along the 40 to 45 cm of the arterial tree in the FOV (Fig. 21-21). Maki et al. (85) have proposed a further extension of the test-bolus technique by rapidly translating the table to the calf station in order to also determine the bolus arrival time and the time to venous enhancement in the lower leg. Knowledge about the duration between arterial and venous enhancement can then be used to tailor the subsequent 3D CE MRA examination in order to minimize the chance for venous enhancement (85).

More recently, so-called real-time bolus monitoring software packages have been introduced by all major MRI system vendors, and these are now considered by many as the state-of-the-art for peripheral CE MRA (BolusTrak, [Philips Medical Systems, Best, the Netherlands; CareBolus, Siemens Medical Solutions, Erlangen, Germany; and Fluoro Trigger General Electric, Waukesha, WI). Rather than injecting a small amount of contrast material in a separate test-bolus scan, real-time bolus monitoring allows the operator to inject the total volume of contrast material and to proceed with the 3D CE MRA acquisition when the desired signal enhancement in the peripheral arteries has been detected by the scanner or by visual feedback (86–88).

Chapter 5 provides an extensive discussion of the different strategies to appropriately synchronize contrast injection with image acquisition.

Strategies to Optimize Vessel-to-background Contrast

In order to present data in an easily understandable format with the vasculature readily depicted, the signal of background tissues, and fat specifically (because it has the shortest T1), needs to be eliminated.

The most commonly used technique to suppress background signal is subtraction of nonenhanced "mask" images that are identical to the 3D CE MRA volumes (Fig. 21-22). Although subtraction decreases the SNR by a factor of about 1.4 ($\sqrt{2}$ when the number of signals acquired is 1), vessel-to-background contrast improves to the extent that whole-volume MIPs become clinically useful. This has particular benefit when using injection rates below 1.0 mL/second (89). A disadvantage of subtraction is the reliance on coregistration of the mask and CE data sets demanding table repositioning with accuracy on the order of 1 mm or less.

Another way to suppress background tissue is by spectral saturation of signal from protons in fat. Although a fat saturation prepulse can be integrated into the 3D CE MRA sequence, this may take a substantial amount of time, which may force a sacrifice in the achievable spatial resolution for a given acquisition duration. Results of using fat-saturation pulses are mixed, and their use is not universally recommended (90,91).

As discussed previously, a surface coil is mandatory for high-quality imaging of the lower leg arteries, especially in patients with distal disease. Image quality and anatomical coverage is vastly improved when compared with imaging without these coils (49–51).

Strategies to Decrease Venous Enhancement

Venous enhancement is particularly challenging when imaging the lower legs and is quite prevalent in patients with cellulitis (92) and AV communications. Both are often seen in the context of diabetes mellitus (which also comprises a large subgroup of the patients with chronic critical ischemia). The depiction of the lower leg arteries is often paramount in diabetes patients, who are frequent candidates for distal bypass surgery.

Several general acquisition strategies can be used to decrease the chance for disturbing venous enhancement. These are:

(a) increasing acquisition speed
(b) use of a separate acquisition for the lower leg station
(c) use of specialized k-space filling algorithms
(d) use of a TR acquisition strategy
(e) use of infrasystolic venous compression

The most straightforward way of preventing venous enhancement is by shortening acquisition duration first by reducing the TR and TE to the shortest possible values without excessively increasing bandwidth. In addition, partial or fractional echo should be used.

(*text continues on page 950*)

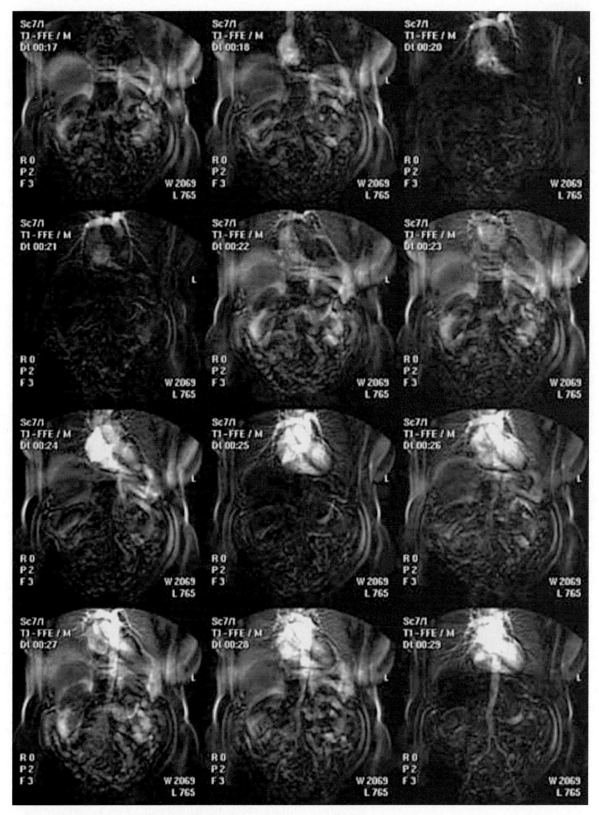

FIGURE 21-21 Bolus monitoring. Individual frames of TR acquisition showing contrast medium arrival and passage through the pulmonary circulation and subsequent enhancement of the systemic circulation (acquisition performed with Philips Medical Systems BolusTrak software). When the injection is started together with the start of image acquisition, the scan delay can be derived from the time displayed in the left upper corner (only frames immediately prior to and after contrast medium arrival are shown).

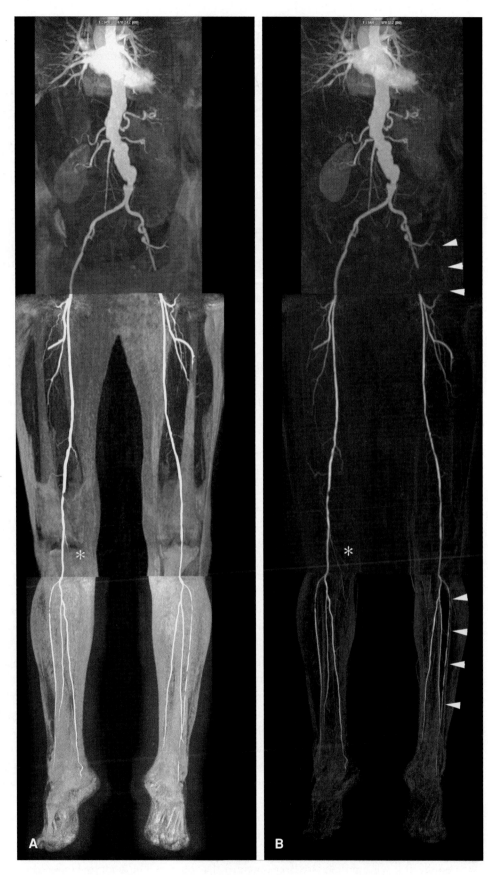

FIGURE 21-22 Subtraction to improve vessel depiction. Multistation CE MRA MIPs of nonsubtracted **(A)** and subtracted **(B)** data sets in a patient with an AAA and occlusion of left external iliac artery. Vessel-to-background contrast is clearly improved when image subtraction of nonenhanced "mask" scans is used. No fat-saturation prepulses were used. Note better visibility of collateral bridging occlusion and lower leg arteries (*arrowheads*).

When the three-consecutive-station approach is used, it is particularly important to image the first two stations (i.e., aortoiliac and upper legs) as fast as reasonably possible. With centrically ordered k-space strategies in the lower station, relatively long (and thus high-resolution) scans can be obtained provided that no or minimal venous enhancement precedes the start of the acquisition.

Multielement (peripheral) surface coils and parallel imaging allow for further increases in acquisition speed (54,93,94). Another way to obtain venousfree images of the lower legs is to switch from a 3D high-resolution acqution to a 2D projectional acquisition, analogous to IA DSA (95). A disadvantage of this latter method is that it is generally limited to a single projection; each unique projection demands a separate injection of contrast medium.

An alternative to the sequential three-station approach is to use a dual-injection protocol in which the lower legs are imaged first and the aortoiliac arteries and upper legs are imaged afterward with a separate acquisition. The rationale for this "hybrid" approach (96) is that it is easier to obtain venousfree, high-resolution 3D images of the lower leg station. The initial acquisition of the lower legs is typically done by using up to 15 to 20 mL 0.5 M Gd-DTPA and can be either mono- or multiphasic. After completing the lower legs, a separate moving table acquisition is performed to image the aortoiliac and upper leg arteries by using the remaining volume of contrast agent (Fig. 21-23).

The greatest benefit of using the hybrid approach can obviously be expected in patients with chronic critical ischemia, patients with arteriovenous fistulas (such as in diabetes mellitus), and patients with cellulitis (95).

Another technique uses separate injections for each imaging station (i.e., three separate acquisitions are performed). Although this approach can be used in the absence of software or hardware needed for rapid table motion, a disadvantage of the multiple injection technique is that the total amount of contrast medium has to be divided into three or more separate injections, each with relatively low doses of contrast medium, while contrast material accumulates with each acquisition. Longer examination times and decreased vessel-to-background contrast may result (97).

Centric k-space filling in general allows for longer acquisition times, facilitating high resolution. These techniques can be used even if the period between arterial and venous enhancement is shorter than the total duration of image acquisition. The underlying principle is to collect central k-space profiles, which primarily determine image contrast, at peak enhancement in the arteries of interest at a time that veins are not or are only minimally enhanced (98,99). The peripheral k-space profiles are later obtained that primarily encode details in the image contributing to high reso-

lution. When centric k-space filling is combined with parallel imaging, the chances of disturbing venous enhancement decrease even further (93,94,100) (Fig. 21-24).

Repetitive centric k-space filling can provide high spatial resolution peripheral MR angiograms with a high temporal frame rate (i.e., "TR" imaging at several seconds per frame). One popular version, *time-resolved imaging of contrast kinetics* (TRICKS), samples the contrast-sensitive central part of k-space more often than the peripheral resolution-sensitive views. After the acquisition is finished, central k-space lines are combined with peripheral lines through a process of temporal interpolation such that a series of TR 3D images of the vasculature are obtained (101). TRICKS can serve as the first acquisition in the tibial station for a hybrid approach to peripheral MRA.

More recently, keyhole *contrast-enhanced timing robust angiography* (CENTRA) was described. With keyhole CENTRA, temporal resolution is increased by repetitive acquisition of the central part of k-space *only*. This information is later combined with a data set containing the peripheral part of k-space, which is acquired as part of the last frame of the TR series (102). Subsequently, these "hybrid k-spaces" can be reconstructed as a series of TR 3D CE-MR angiograms (Fig. 21-25). Temporal resolution can be further increased by combining keyhole imaging with parallel imaging (103).

TR acquisitions such as TRICKS and keyhole CENTRA can obviate timing tests and a separate acquisition of precontrast images for subtraction (104). Hany et al. (105) showed that the use of TRICKS improved small, distal vessel conspicuity and reduced venous overlay in a head-to-head comparison with single injection, three-station peripheral CE MRA protocol.

Although all of these techniques have in common that they are able to reduce venous contamination, the drawback is that they all, to some extent, lead to a reduction in vessel-to-background contrast. For additional details of the techniques mentioned above, we refer the reader to Chapter 2.

Another method to reduce venous contamination is by using mid-femoral (106) or infragenual venous compression with infrasystolic pressures of 50 to 60 mmHg (106,107), with promising results (Fig. 21-26). It remains to be determined if patients with critical ischemia and/or ulcers, in which high-quality lower leg images are most important, can tolerate or benefit from this type of compression.

Combinations of the above techniques can be pursued to further reduce the risk of disturbing venous enhancement.

Resolution Requirements

The work by Hoogeveen et al. (108) and Westenberg et al. (109) has shown that at least three pixels are needed across

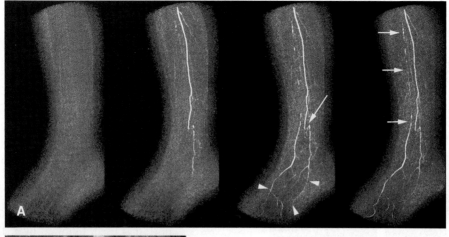

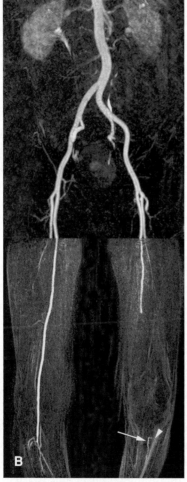

FIGURE 21-23 Hybrid MRA of a 64-year-old male diabetic patient suffering from chronic critical ischemia and with rest pain, imaged with hybrid approach. In (**A**), sequential, sagittal MIPs of 3D CE MRA data set obtained in lower leg station using 15 mL of Gd-DTPA are shown. Image acquisition was started together with the injection and lasted 30 seconds per phase. The acquired resolution of the scans is 1.0 × 1.0 × 1.0 mm³ interpolated to 0.5 × 0.5 × 0.5 mm³. In phase 1, there is no arterial enhancement; in phase 2, there is filling of the fibular artery; in phase 3, the fibular artery has filled the pedal arch (*arrowheads*) through a collateral to the posterior tibial artery (*arrow*). In phase 4, it can be appreciated that the anterior tibial artery is severely diseased (*arrows*) and partially is filled by the pedal arch. In (**B**), a coronal MIP of aortoiliac and upper leg vasculature is shown. There is a complete occlusion of the left superficial femoral artery without significant development of large collaterals. The tibioperoneal trunk (*arrow*) and origin of the anterior tibial artery (*arrowhead*) can clearly be identified.

the lumen of an artery to quantify the degree of stenosis with an error of less than 10%. Thus, higher resolution is needed to accurately characterize stenoses in the distal lower legs or feet as opposed to the larger, proximal iliac arteries. In general, voxel dimensions should be kept as close to isotropic (equal length in all dimensions) as possible to minimize vessel blurring in those projections that introduce lower resolution with more asymmetric voxels. Recom-mended voxel size resolutions are about 4 to 5 mm³ in the aortoiliac arteries, 3 to 4 mm³ in the upper legs, and 1 mm³ or better in the lower legs.

Contrast Media and Injection Protocols

In nearly all of the reported studies on peripheral CE MRA, conventional 0.5 M extracellular contrast agents have been used. The intravascular half-life of commercially

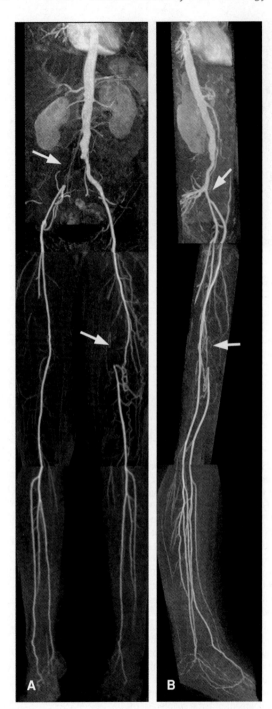

FIGURE 21-24 Centric k-space acquisition with SENSE. A peripheral MR angiogram was obtained in a 59-year-old patient with severe intermittent claudication. Resolution was adapted in each station, and centric k-space filling was used in the upper and lower leg stations. Parallel imaging (SENSE) was used in all stations (aortoiliac: ×2; upper and lower legs: ×3), resulting in acquisition times of 13 seconds, 8 seconds, and 35 seconds for the aortoiliac, upper leg, and lower leg stations, respectively. There are occlusions in the right common iliac artery and left superficial femoral arteries (*arrows*).

approved agents is about 90 seconds (110). Enough contrast must be injected to decrease the T1 of blood to values smaller than those of stationary background tissues. To selectively depict the vasculature, this means that the T1 of blood must be reduced to a value well below that of fat (T1 at 1.5 T = 270 ms).

Typically, between 0.1 and 0.3 mmol/kg of contrast agents is injected (i.e., between 15 and 45 mL for a 75-kg patient), followed by 15 to 30 mL saline injection to flush contrast from injection tubing and veins into the central venous and arterial circulations.

When a TR 2D test-bolus approach is used to image the lower legs and pedal arteries first, usually around 5 to 7 mL of contrast is used, followed by a slightly larger saline flush volume, to make sure that the contrast medium is flushed from tubing and veins into the central circulation. When a hybrid approach is used, the lower legs are usually imaged with 15 to 20 mL of contrast medium and the aortoiliac and upper leg arteries with 20 to 25 mL.

An empirical strategy that works well in clinical practice is to prescribe the contrast injection duration to last for about 40% to 60% of the acquisition duration.

The amount of contrast to be injected as well as injection speed and amount of saline flush depend on variables such as the scan duration and technique used (i.e., single vs. multiple injection). Various single and multiple-phase injection rates and different saline flush volumes have been used successfully.

In general, either a fixed rate of about 1.0 mL/s is used or dual-phase injections with higher initial injection rates of up to 2.0 mL/second for 10 to 20 mL of the contrast medium with a lower rate for the remaining contrast (as low as 0.5 mL/second) (51,111). On older and slower systems, the injection rate is usually kept to well below 1.0 mL/second (73,74).

In a recently published study, Boos and associates (80) found that increasing the amount of contrast injected as well as saline flush volume increases bolus length and improves small vessel conspicuity but does not necessarily result in higher vessel-to-background contrast (80). Conversely, injecting a fixed amount of contrast agent faster leads to a more compact and shorter bolus duration. In another study, Czum et al. (112) demonstrated that by using a dual-phase injection in which the first part of the contrast bolus is injected slowly (0.7 mL/second) and the second part of the injection is faster also improves vessel conspicuity. Sample injection protocols for standard three-sequential-station imaging, a hybrid protocol, and a 2D test bolus protocol are listed in Table 21-9. More details about MR contrast media and administration can be found in Chapter 5.

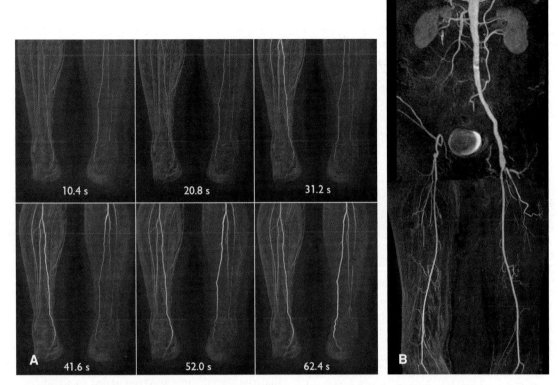

FIGURE 21-25 Keyhole CENTRA. Successive frames of lower leg vasculature **(A)** obtained with TR (10.4 seconds/frame) keyhole CENTRA imaging technique. More proximal, the right common and external iliac arteries are occluded **(B)**. (Image courtesy of Bernd Tombach, MD, Department of Clinical Radiology, Westfalian Wilhelms-University of Muenster, Muenster, Germany.)

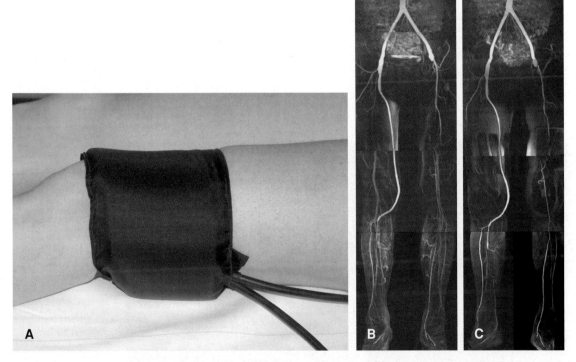

FIGURE 21-26 Venous compression. Supragenual placement of pressure cuff to reduce venous enhancement **(A)**. Intraindividual comparison of three-station CE MRA with **(B)** and without **(C)** venous compression. Use of compression clearly results in less venous enhancement in the lower leg station. (Images **B** and **C** courtesy of Christoph U. Herborn, MD, Department of Radiology, Essen University Hospital, Essen, Germany.)

TABLE 21-9

Suggested Injection Protocols for Commercially Available 0.5 M Gadolinium Chelates

Indication (approach)	Contrast Volume/Injection Rate	Saline Flush Volume/Injection Rate	Comments
Intermittent claudication (three-consecutive station bolus-chase protocol)	15 to 20 mL at 1.0 to 2.0 mL/second 20 to 25 mL at 0.5 to 1.0 mL/second	25 mL at 0.5 to 1.0 mL/second[a]	Dual-phase injection
Chronic critical ischemia	LL: 15 to 20 mL at 2.0 to 3.0 mL/second	25 mL at 2.0 to 3.0 mL/second[a]	Two separate single-phase (hybrid approach)
	Ao/UL: 20 mL at 2.0 to 3.0 mL/second	25 mL at 2.0 to 3.0 mL/second[a]	Injections
Intermittent claudication/ Chronic critical ischemia (2D TR test-bolus approach)	6 mL at 2 mL/second	30 mL at 2.0 mL/second	Lower leg only

LL, lower leg station; Ao/UL, aortoiliac and upper leg stations; 2D, two dimensional; TR, time resolved.
Note: The maximum contrast dose that may be given for all injections together is 0.3 mmol/kg. In this table, a patient body weight of 75 kg was assumed.
[a]Saline is always injected at the same rate as the last phase of the contrast injection.

Novel Contrast Media

Vessel-to-background signal can also be improved by using other contrast agents than the currently used 0.5 M gadolinium chelates. Recently, the first 1.0 M agent (Gadobutrol, Schering AG, Berlin, Germany) has been approved for clinical use in and has a Europeanwide registration for CE MRA.

Gadobutrol is formulated at higher concentration of 1.0 mol/L and about 20% higher relaxivity (T1 relaxivity in blood: 5.2 mM^{-1}s^{-1} at 37°C and 1.5 T), which generates lower blood T1 values compared with other commercially available contrast agents, thus offering an attractive method to increase intravascular signal (113).

In a direct head-to-head comparison between 1.0 M and 0.5 M agents for pelvic MRA, Goyen et al. (114) found that the use of the 1.0 M agent led to significantly higher signal- and contrast-to-noise ratios and better delineation of especially small pelvic arteries (Fig. 21-27). Several other higher relaxivity contrast agents are now in phase II studies or pending approval. An overview of these contrast agents is given by Knopp et al. (115).

Magnetic Resonance Angiography Protocols and Practical Tips

Detailed recommendations for basic imaging parameters can be found in Table 21-10. Since imaging capabilities and

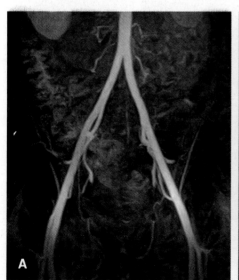 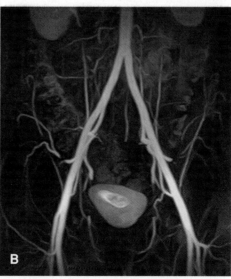

FIGURE 21-27 1.0 M gadolinium contrast agent. Intraindividual comparison of **(A)** 0.5 M (Gd-DTPA) and **(B)** 1.0 M (Gadobutrol; both agents: Schering, Berlin) contrast agents in a healthy volunteer. Note better visibility of branch vessels with use of 1.0 M agent. (Image courtesy of Mathias Goyen, MD, University Medical Center Hamburg-Eppendorf, Hamburg, Germany.)

TABLE 21-10

Recommended Three-dimensional Contrast-enhanced Magnetic Resonance Angiography Sequence Parameters for Three-station Peripheral Contrast-enhanced Magnetic Resonance Angiography

Sequence	Orientation	Coverage	Coil	Repetition Time/Echo Time (milliseconds)	Flip Angle (degrees)	Field-of-view[a] (millimeters)	Matrix	Slice Thickness[b] (millimeters)	Number of Partitions	Bandwidth (kilohertz)	Number of Signals Averaged[c]	Duration (seconds)	Comments
T1w GRE	Coronal	Abdominal aorta to proximal SFA	Body/Surface PA	5/2.5	30 to 40	430 × 300	400 × 200	≤2.5	Tailor to anatomy	40 to 60	0.67	10 to 15	Use parallel imaging when possible
T1w GRE	Coronal	CF to trifurcation	Body/Surface PA	4/1	30 to 40	430 × 350	400 × 256	2.0–2.5	Tailor to anatomy	40 to 60	0.67	7 to 12	Use parallel imaging when possible
T1w GRE	Coronal	P3 to pedal arch	Surface PA	<4/<2	30 to 40	430 × 300	430 × 300	<1.0–1.5	Tailor to anatomy	40 to 60	0.67	30 to 60	Use parallel imaging when possible
T1w SE postcontrast	Transverse	Aneurysm	Body/Surface PA	580/14	90	Tailor to anatomy	Same value as FOV	<5 mm	Tailor to aneurysm	40	1.00	Several minutes	Use parallel imaging when possible

T1w, T1 weighted; GRE, gradient recalled echo; SFA, superficial femoral artery; PA, phased array; CF, common femoral artery; P3, popliteal artery below knee joint; SE, spin echo.

[a]Frequency × Phase.

[b]Noninterpolated, truly acquired slice thickness.

[c]Number below 1 indicates partial or fractional echo.

options vary across vendors, it is advisable to first use the vendor-specified protocols. After gaining experience, customized modifications often evolve as one learns the nuances of a given system. The recommendations below provide a useful framework and should not be regarded as absolute.

It is important to be aware of the patient's ability to undergo the examination and, when needed, to have a low threshold for use of anxiolytic and analgesic agents. Given that the best MRA exams are dependent on pre- and post-contrast data set coregistration, appropriate medications to keep the patient calm and minimize the motion that can result with rest pain can substantially improve the yield of high-quality, diagnostic studies. In addition, baseline instructions to the patient regarding the importance of maintaining a consistent position are beneficial.

Tailored 3D slabs maximize the efficiency of acquisitions. Because of the relatively limited deviation of the main upper leg arteries in the anteroposterior direction, a volume with fewer partitions (hence, decreased scan time) can be used to encompass the femoral-popliteal segment when compared with the aortoiliac vasculature (Fig. 21-28). This is often facilitated by using an oblique coronal acquisition (Fig. 21-28). When the choice for less AP coverage is made, it is possible that collaterals arising from the profunda femoris artery may be (partly) excluded from the imaging volume.

For the below-knee segment, patient preparation involves fixation of feet with Velcro straps or rolled gauze secured with tape. The foot should be no more than 20- to 30-degrees plantar flexion, and 20- to 30-degrees exorotation is the most comfortable position. As for CT and DSA, it is important to avoid extreme plantar flexion, a position that is known to produce pseudostenosis of the dorsalis pedis from tensing of the overlying retinaculum (31). By placing soft foam padding in the popliteal fossa, the calves are suspended, which often results in less potential for venous contamination. In addition, it is useful to apply a tourniquet or blood pressure cuff just above the knee in order to delay venous enhancement (106,116).

Typical imaging parameters for the different approaches discussed previously can be found in Table 21-11. Acquisition durations, as mentioned, were empirically determined from our practices and represent a compromise between the best possible spatial resolution, temporal resolution, and desire to avoid disturbing venous overlay.

When using a 2D thick-slab technique, a temporal resolution of 3 to 5 seconds per phase ensures images free of disturbing venous overlay. The recommended default imaging period is 60 to 90 seconds (approximately 15 to 30 dynamic phases).

When the lower leg is imaged as the last acquisition of a conventional three-station run-off examination, it is safe to limit the duration to no more than 30 seconds. However,

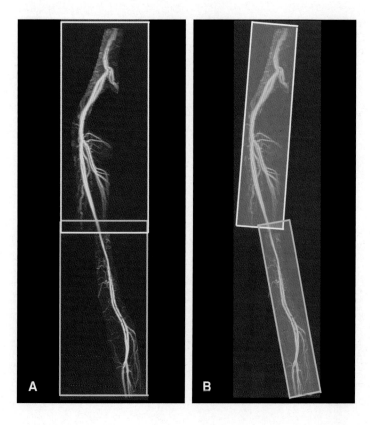

FIGURE 21-28 Tailored slab positioning for efficiency. A: With a fixed-slab approach, the anterior–posterior coverage must be set large enough to accommodate two distinct anatomic paths for the aortoiliac (*white box*) and femoropolitieal (*green box*) segments. **B:** With tailored prescriptions, the segments can be covered independently, with enhanced efficiency. Note the relative requirements of the anatomic coverage: fixed slab > tailored aortoiliac slab > femoropopliteal slab. With equivalent section thickness, scan time diminishes.

TABLE 21-11

Recommended Imaging Parameters for Lower Leg and Pedal Magnetic Resonance Angiography

Sequence	Orientation	Coverage	Coil	Time Repetition/ Echo Time (milliseconds)	Flip Angle (degrees)	Field-of-view[a] (millimeters)	Matrix	Slice Thickness[b] (millimeters)	Number of Partitions	Number of Signals Averaged[c]	Duration (seconds)	Comments
3D CE T1w GRE	Coronal or sagittal	P3 to pedal arch	Body/ Surface PA	<5/<2	30 to 40	430 × 300	Same value as FOV	≤1.0 to 1.5	Tailor to anatomy	0.67	<10, MP <30[d] <45[e]	Use parallel imaging when possible
3D CE T1w GRE	Sagittal	Ankle to pedal arch (single foot only)	Head/ Knee	<5/<2	30 to 40	430 × 300	Same value as FOV	≤1.0	Tailor to anatomy	0.67	<10, MP	Use parallel imaging when possible
2D CE T1w GRE	Sagittal	P3 to pedal arch (single foot only)	Body/ Surface PA	<10/<2	60 to 80	Tailor to anatomy	256	Up to 100	Single thick slice, tailor to anatomy	0.67	3 to 5 (per phase)	
TOF T1w GRE	Transverse	P3 to pedal arch	Surface PA	30/6.9	30 to 40	Tailor to anatomy	256	3.0 to 4.0; 0.0 to 0.5 overlap	Tailor to anatomy	0.67	5 to 10 minutes	Best with flow compensation; set pulse below the slice

3D, three dimensional; CE, contrast enhanced; T1w, T-1 weighted; GRE, gradient recalled echo; P3, popliteal artery below knee joint; PA, phased array; FOV, field-of-view; MP, multiphasic acquisition; 2D, two dimensional; TOF, time of flight.

[a]Frequency × Phase.

[b]Number below 1 indicates partial or fractional echo.

[c]Noninterpolated, truly acquired slice thickness.

[d]When acquired as last station in three-station run-off protocol.

[e]When acquired as dedicated lower leg examination with infrasystolic venous compression.

when elliptical centric sequences in the distal station are combined with methods to reduce venous contamination, longer scan times are often successful.

With infrasystolic venous compression for a dedicated lower-station acquisition, the duration should not exceed 45 seconds. When TRICKS or keyhole CENTRA are used, a temporal resolution of 10 seconds or less per dynamic phase is recommended to demonstrate dynamic features and obtain venous frames. Besides ensuring venous free images, acquisition of multiple phases is also advantageous in case there is a difference in bolus arrival between the two legs. However, in order to improve spatial resolution, a slower frame rate can be obtained with good results in generating at least a single venous free frame (Fig. 21-29).

System-dependent considerations include reconstruction time, available hard disk space on the scanner, and data transfer rates to a postprocessing workstation or PACS; these are usually limiting factors when deciding on parameters. In most cases, it is safe to limit the number of dynamic phases to five; however, the increased computing speeds and capacity on contemporary scanners allow for many more phases to be acquired. Once again, knowing the particular features of one's equipment will provide the most effective protocols.

Magnetic Resonance Angiography Postprocessing Issues

The most commonly used format to display 3D MR angiographic data is the MIP, which is operator independent, free

of intensity thresholding, and fast (117). MIP images can be generated and manipulated in (near) real time, allowing for visualization of 3D CE MRA data sets from any desired angle, which is particularly useful when assessing eccentric stenosis. Review of cross-sectional images, source images and multiplanar thin-section reconstructions should be an integral part of the evaluation.

Because MIP images have a look and feel analogous to IA DSA, particularly when displayed in inverse video mode (Fig. 21-30), they are easily understood by referring clinicians. The MIP algorithm can be especially effective with using thin-slab or (curved) subvolume selections. Whole-volume MIPs can be limited by the superimposition of contrast-enhancing organs or nonessential vascular structures when they have high signal intensities along a particular viewing path.

The easiest and most widely used way of measuring diameter reduction is to simply measure the maximum degree of luminal reduction on MIP images, analogous to how stenoses are measured on IA DSA images. A stenosis is generally considered to be "hemodynamically significant" when reduction of the luminal diameter exceeds 50%. The validity of this approach can be questioned with eccentric stenoses.

A more robust approach is to measure the cross-sectional area, as this is subject to lower interobserver variability (118,119). This is done by first prescribing a center-lumen line on the original partitions and subsequently making

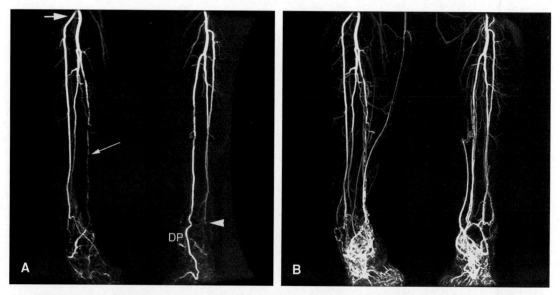

FIGURE 21-29 Hybrid technique with TRICKS and venous compression. A: MIP of 15-second effective temporal resolution TRICKS acquisition allows for high sufficient coverage and spatial resolution, free of disturbing venous contamination. Note the high origin of anterior tibial artery (*short arrow*) and the diffusely diseased posterior tibial artery (*long arrow*) on the right. The posterior tibial artery on the left occludes at the level of the ankle (*arrowhead*) and an excellent left quality dorsalis pedis (*DP*) artery is visualized. **B:** The third of a three-station bolus chase did not fair as well, despite cuff compression. The venous contamination prevents meaningful interpretation.

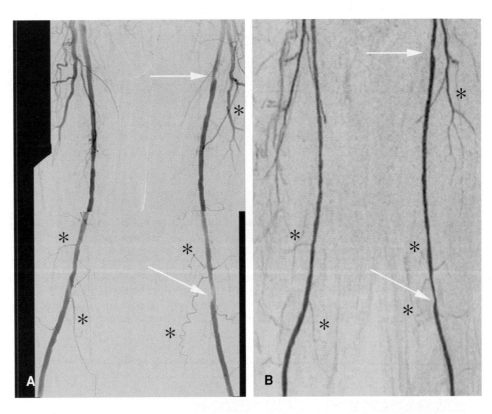

FIGURE 21-30 MIP simulates DSA in superficial femoral arteries in a patient with intermittent claudication. Intra-arterial digital subtraction angiogram **(A)** and MRA MIP displayed in inverse video mode **(B)**. Degree and length of stenosis in the distal left superficial femoral artery are nearly identical with both modalities (*arrows*). Note high-fidelity depiction of small collateral branches (∗).

reformations of the vascular lumen perpendicular to this line (Fig. 21-31).

When determining the stenosis percentage, the vessel boundary should ideally be described in quantitative terms. This can be done by generating a line profile across the vascular lumen and by plotting the range of signal intensities as a function of the position along the line. Commonly used criteria to determine the vascular border are the full width at half maximum (FWHM) or full-width at one-third maximum (109) (Fig. 21-32).

Quantitative analyses of vascular structures can be performed with increasing accuracy and minimal user interaction by using commercially available vessel-tracking software. Postprocessing software packages that find a center-lumen line with minimal user interaction and allow for (semi-)automated extraction of luminal diameter and stenosis percentages are becoming available (Fig. 21-33).

Digital subtraction to increase the contrast between arteries and background tissues is especially useful in the tibial station, as arteries are generally smaller (especially when severely diseased), and hence the amount of gadolinium per voxel and consequently the SNR is lower.

For the larger vessels in the abdominopelvic area and thigh region, subtraction is not absolutely necessary but may improve conspicuity of small branch vessels and collaterals (90,91) (Fig. 21-34). Subtraction is often useful when multiple anatomic segments are studied with repeated injections

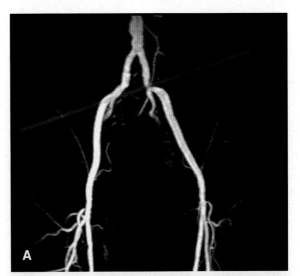

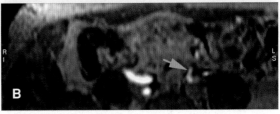

FIGURE 21-31 Oblique reconstruction. A: An MIP from a gadolinium-enhanced MRA in a 57-year-old man with claudication prompts a reconstruction perpendicular to a left common iliac artery stenosis (*orange line*). **B:** An oblique axial slice is generated for review, confirming the high-grade lesion (*arrow*) as compared with the contralateral vessels. The cross-sectional image can be used to assess diameter or area.

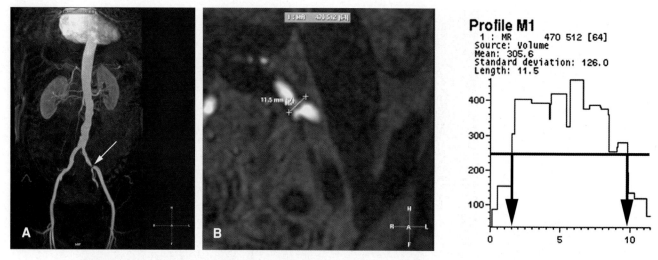

FIGURE 21-32 Full width at half maximum (FWHM) algorithm. Reproducible measurement of residual lumen for determination of stenosis severity using the FWHM algorithm. CE MRA in a 60-year-old female patient shows a moderate to severe stenosis in the left distal common iliac artery (*arrow* in **A**). A line profile drawn on an original partition of the 3D data set (**B**, **left panel**) yields a residual vessel width of 8.25 mm when using the FWHM criterion (**B**, **right panel**).

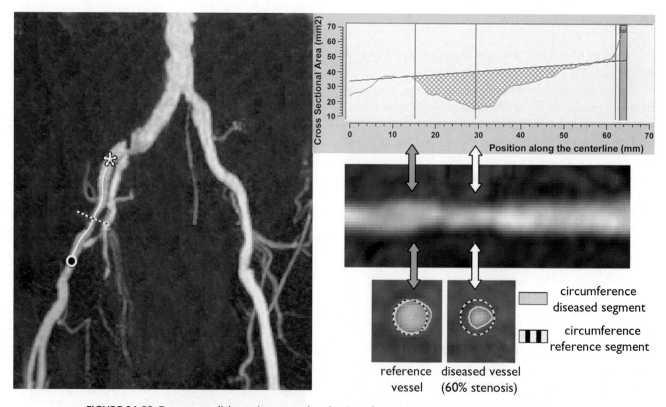

FIGURE 21-33 Two mouse-click, semiautomated evaluation of stenosis severity in a patient with stenoses in right common and external iliac arteries. The *white line* in the **left panel** is the center-lumen line, the *asterisk* and *black and white dot* are the locations of the proximal and distal mouse clicks. The *dotted line* is the site of maximum luminal diameter reduction. The diameter as function of the position along the centerline is displayed in the **upper right panel**. The **middle right panel** shows a curved multiplanar reformation of the part of the vessel between the two mouse-clicks. The **lower panel** shows the closest healthy part of the vessel (**left**) and the part of the vessel with the highest degree of luminal narrowing (**right**). There is a 60% reduction in luminal cross-sectional area at the *dotted line*. (Images obtained with MRA-LKEB software, Leiden University Medical Center, Leiden, the Netherlands.)

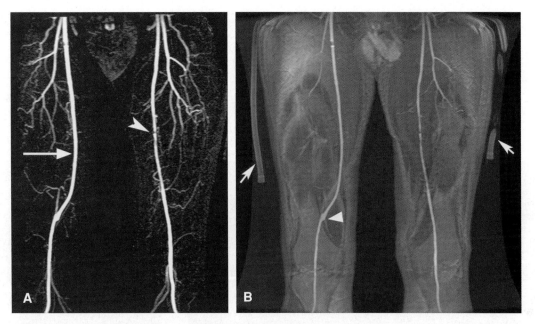

FIGURE 21-34 Considerations for subtraction processing. A: A subtracted MIP image (arterial – pre) of the femoropopliteal segment in this patient being assessed for left claudication emphasizes the excellent detail of the primary vessels and the collateral beds. Note the right femoropopliteal bypass graft (*long arrow*) and a focal high-grade stenosis in the left superficial femoral artery (*arrowhead*). **B:** The nonsubtracted MIP image of the same anatomy has a more limited display of vascular detail but demonstrates osseous and soft tissue features, offering important reference cues to the surgeon and interventionalist. Note the small outpouching of the distal insertion of the femoropopliteal bypass graft (*arrowhead*) in relation to the femoral condyle and the incidentally seen tubing from thigh cuff compression apparatus (*short arrows*).

of contrast medium. In such cases, residual venous enhancement from prior administration may obscure arterial detail in subsequent acquisitions if subtraction is not used (97,120). However, in some cases, a prohibitive arterial signal loss can occur if the mask has residual arterial signal; thus, an assessment of unsubtracted and subtracted data sets should be used to select the best demonstration.

Subtraction of pre- and postcontrast 3D CE MRA data sets can be performed with complex or magnitude image data. The MR raw data, prior to its reconstruction, contains complex values (phase and magnitude information). Complex numbers from the precontrast raw data set can be subtracted from those of the postcontrast data set, and the result can then be reconstructed into the complex subtracted images. Alternatively, subtracted images can be generated by following the magnitude reconstructions of the two data sets and then subtracting their values (117). In practice, the latter is most commonly employed, as it is simple and computationally less intensive.

Complex subtraction has the advantage that it may overcome partial volume effects related to the phase difference between flowing and stationary spins in a voxel. Complex subtraction is especially beneficial for TR thick-slab 2D imaging and to improve conspicuity of small vessels and edges of vessels (117,121).

For therapeutic planning, important cues are provided by the nonvascular tissues. Osseous landmarks are critical for directing the incision site and may influence the selection of graft material by distinguishing suprageniculate from infrageniculate disease (1,120). For example, the readily palpated femoral condyles can serve as a reference point for an incision during a bypass procedure. Landmarks are also important when an iliac-popliteal artery bypass is considered. The anterosuperior iliac spine and pubic tubercle provide the landmarks to plan a suprainguinal retroperitoneal approach.

In this context, it is important to consider that subtraction processing while improving small vessel conspicuity often eliminates the structures surrounding the arteries. As a solution to this limitation, images from the unsubtracted 3D CE MRA data sets can be used to reintroduce relevant landmarks and provide cross referencing to vascular structures (1,120) (Fig. 21-34).

Another very helpful technique for the precise evaluation of vessel morphology is curved multiplanar reformation (cMPR) along the axis of the arterial segment of interest (Fig. 21-35). The technique is particularly useful to obtain views of eccentric stenoses and as a basis to generate views perpendicular to the central axis of the vessel to measure cross-sectional area reduction in stenoses.

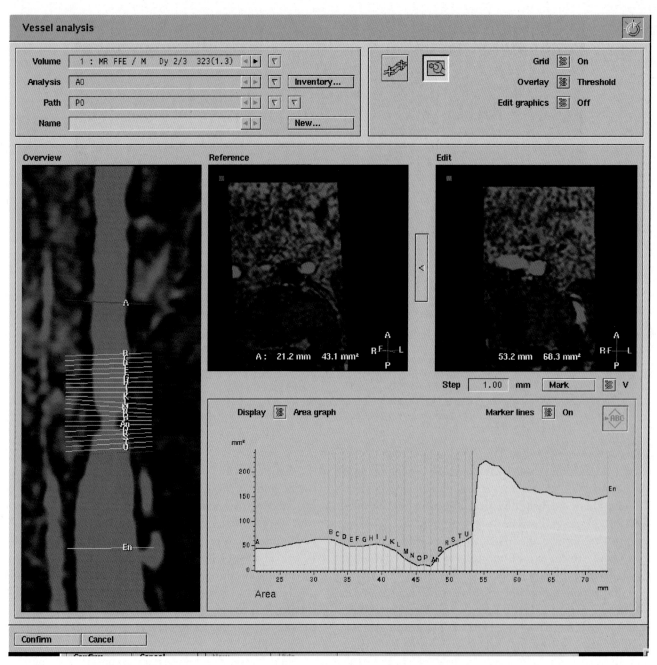

FIGURE 21-35 Curved planar reformation. CPR along vessel axis allows for precise evaluation of vascular morphology with cross-sectional stenosis measurements (generated with Philips Easyvision 4.0 software).

The postprocessing techniques of shaded-surface display (SSD) and VR are less commonly used for MRA. SSD is vulnerable to pseudostenoses and occlusions when the threshold is increased or when SI is low in small artery stenoses. Therefore, SSD is only useful when there is sufficient contrast between the vessel lumen and surrounding tissues. VR employs information about the signal intensity in all voxels. The interested reader is referred to Chapter 6 for detailed information on postprocessing.

The presence of a stenosis or occlusion in a MIP, SSD, or VR should *always* be confirmed by viewing of original, thin-slice partitions of the 3D data set in multiple, orthogonal directions (e.g., coronal, sagittal, and transverse), aided with multiplanar reformations of the arteries preferably perpendicular to the vessel axis. A review of the original partitions can eliminate common interpretative errors such as a pseudostenosis resulting from inadvertent exclusion of relevant vascular anatomy, overprojection of struc-

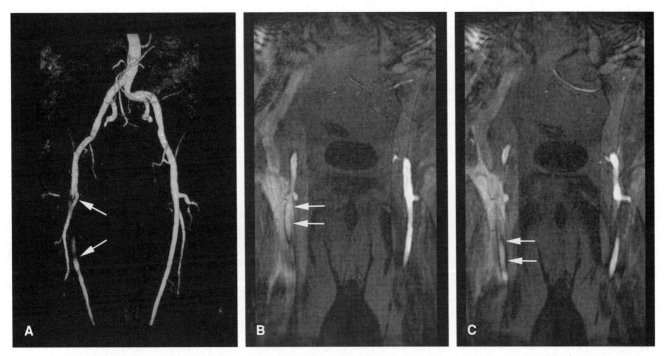

FIGURE 21-36 False stenosis in the right superficial femoral artery on MIP (*arrows* in **A**). Examination of source images reveals wraparound of subcutaneous fat into the superficial femoral artery (aliasing artifact), which is actually widely patent (*arrows* in **B** and **C**). Subtraction of nonenhanced mask partitions from CE partitions resulted in loss of intravascular signal on subtracted images and MIP, where in reality the vessel is nondiseased.

tures with higher signal intensity (e.g., veins, subcutaneous fat, or bone marrow) (Fig. 21-36), or choice of wrong threshold when data is visualized by using SSD or VR.

Source images are necessary for revealing mural thrombus in aneurysms and hence true arterial diameter (Fig. 21-37). It

has been shown that a review of source images in addition to the MIP images significantly increases diagnostic accuracy (122,123).

A summary of sources for MRA pseudo-occlusions is provided in Table 21-12. It should also be noted that the

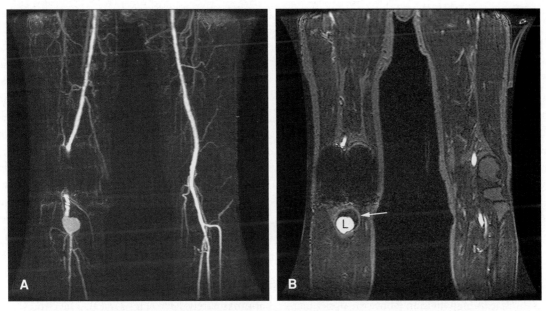

FIGURE 21-37 Source images in aneurysmal disease showing a below-knee popliteal artery aneurysm and metallic prosthesis artifact. A: Frontal MIP image of a patient with a right popliteal artery aneurysm shows that a portion of the above-knee popliteal artery is obscured by the metallic knee prosthesis. **B:** Source image shows the signal void from the prosthesis. Note the enhancing lumen (*L*) and the peripheral thrombus (*arrow*), both comprising the aneurysm.

TABLE 21-12

Causes of Pseudo-occlusion on Contrast-enhanced Magnetic Resonance Imaging

Cause	Typical Imaging Appearance
Mistiming of acquisition in relation to contrast arrival	Loss of intravascular signal in distal part of the imaging volume. Ringing artifact.
Inadvertent exclusion of arterial segments from 3D imaging volume	Abrupt vessel cutoff with distal reconstitution. Can easily be recognized on orthogonal MIP.
Metallic stent	Abrupt vessel cutoff with distal reconstitution. Due to susceptibility artifact. Hyperintense band of signal juxtaposed to signal void.
Surgical clips	Vessel appears stenotic or occluded. Hyperintense band of signal juxtaposed to signal void.
Subtraction artifact	Vessel appears occluded on subtracted source images and MIP. Caused by loss of intravascular signal after subtraction of high-signal intensity, Wrapped-around fat in mask image from 3D CE partitions. Occurs when imaging with a FOV that is smaller than the width of the patient and subcutaneous fat. Arterial segment is patent on original, nonsubtracted partitions.

use of parallel imaging may also lead to errors when phase wrap occurs in the undersampled direction or when reconstruction errors occur.

ANATOMY

Normal Anatomy and Variants

The normal anatomy of the conducting vessels of the lower extremity arterial tree—from the aorta down to the feet—can be divided into an aortoiliac ("inflow") segment and the infrainguinal run-off vessels, which consist of the femoropopliteal segments and the infrapopliteal (crural or tibioperoneal) vessels, which supply the foot. All of the named arteries can be visualized with both MRA and CTA. A typical branching pattern is illustrated in Figure 21-38.

There is a wide variability of normal anatomic arterial branching patterns that do not cause any clinical symptoms. However, some of the normal variants may be clinically significant in the setting of treatment planning. For example, preinterventional knowledge of the level and orientation of the femoral bifurcation may be helpful for arterial access planning, notably if an antegrade puncture is anticipated.

The politeal artery normally divides below the level of the popliteus muscle. A high division (above the upper margin of the popliteus muscle) and take-off of either the anterior or posterior tibial artery is seen in approximately 5%, with formation of either an anterior or posterior tibioper-

oneal trunk (Figs. 21-39, 21-40). In the setting of a high popliteal division, the anterior tibial artery may course anterior to the popliteus muscle (following the phylogenetically older profound popliteal artery [part of the acial artery] of most mammals). The clinical implication of these variants is mainly related to preprocedural planning when selecting a proximal or distal bypass anastomosis.

The variation of crural artery anatomy is best explained by considering the peroneal artery (which is phylogenetically the oldest and most consistently observed branch) as the main vessel and the tibial arteries as its branches. The anterior tibial and the posterior tibial arteries may be hypoplastic or absent. In this case, the peroneal artery usually supplies blood to the respective territories of the dorsalis pedis and common plantar arteries, respectively.

For example, if both the anterior and the posterior tibial arteries are absent, the peroneal artery (*arteria peronea magna*) fills both, the dorsalis pedis artery via its perforating branch and the plantar artery via its communicating branch (Fig. 21-41). The perforating and communicating branches are also not uncommonly seen with normal crural arterial anatomy and may serve as important collaterals. Overall, the peroneal artery is a significant contributor to blood supply of the foot in approximately 12% (Fig. 21-42). The clinical significance is that this situation precludes harvesting of a free fibular flap graft (with its supplying peroneal artery) because it jeopardizes the blood flow to the foot.

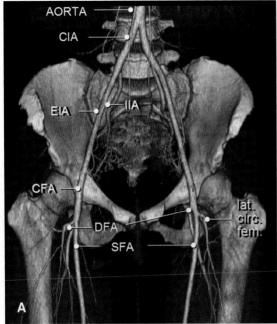

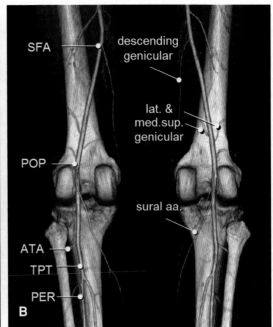

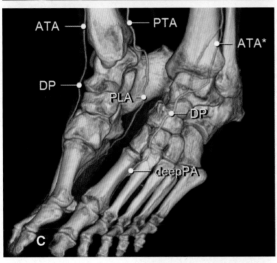

FIGURE 21-38 VR images of the aortoiliofemoral **(A)** territory, the femoropopliteal territory (*posterior view*) **(B)**, and the feet **(C)**. (CIA, common iliac a.; IIA, internal iliac a.; EIA, external iliac a.; CFA, common femoral a.; DFA, deep femoral a.; lat. circ. fem., lateral circumflex femoral a. (normal variant directly off the superficial femoral artery); SFA, superficial femoral a.; POP, popliteal a.; ATA, anterior tibial a.; TPT, tibioperoneal trunk; ATA*, variant anatomy with doubling of the distal anterior tibial artery); PTA, posterior tibial a.; PER, peroneal a.; PLA, lateral plantar a.; DP, dorsalis pedis a.; deep PA, deep plantar a.)

The prevalence of "textbook" arterial anatomy of the foot is only 20% for the dorsalis pedis territory (dorsalis pedis artery, lateral and medial tarsal artery, arcuate artery, deep plantar branch of dorsalis pedis artery that communicates with the deep plantar arch) and 7% for the plantar arch (124). Visualizing the pedal branches becomes relevant in patients with chronic limb-threatening ischemia in whom suitable target vessels for a distal bypass graft are sought. Preoperative imaging with US, MRA, and CTA may be superior to intra-arterial angiography (notably if not done selectively), because these small vessels fill via small collaterals in this setting.

Anatomic Anomalies

The wide variability of anatomic variants and anomalies is explained by the complex embryological development of the leg arteries (124). Figure 21-43 illustrates schematically

how several portions of the original axial artery are progressively replaced by developmentally younger arterial systems. At the level of the hip and thigh, the original axial (sciatic) artery is replaced by the iliofemoral system. The popliteal artery development is particularly complex in primates (see also popliteal vascular entrapment syndrome), but a small portion of the axial artery becomes part of the adult popliteal artery. Another arterial system that develops (commonly seen in monkeys) is the saphenous artery, which becomes the posterior tibial artery in humans. The anterior tibial artery is a new branch, whereas the peroneal artery is again a remnant of the axial (schiatic) artery.

Persistent Sciatic Artery

The sciatic artery is a continuation of the internal iliac artery and normally involutes during fetal development.

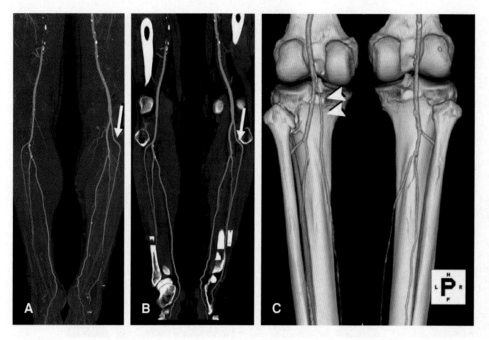

FIGURE 21-39 Two examples of high anterior tibial artery and high posterior tibial artery takeoff. MIP **(A)** and multipath CPR **(B)** of a patient with right superficial femoral artery occlusion shows abnormally high take-off of the anterior tibial artery (*arrow*). VR image (posterior view) **(C)** of a different patient shows high takeoff of the posterior tibial artery (*arrowheads*). The contralateral branching patterns are normal, respectively.

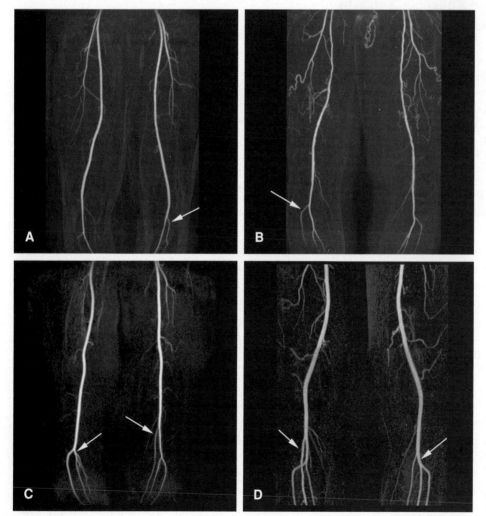

FIGURE 21-40 Common variations in popliteal artery branching pattern. A, B: High origin of left and right anterior tibial arteries, respectively (*arrows;* frequency of 3%). The contralateral legs are classic textbook cases of popliteal artery branching. **C:** Right leg: true trifurcation (*arrow;* frequency of less than 1%); there is a high origin of posterior tibial artery in the left leg (*arrow;* frequency of approximately 1%). **D:** Right leg: high origin of fibular artery (*arrow;* frequency of less than 1%); left leg: short tibioperoneal trunk (*arrow*).

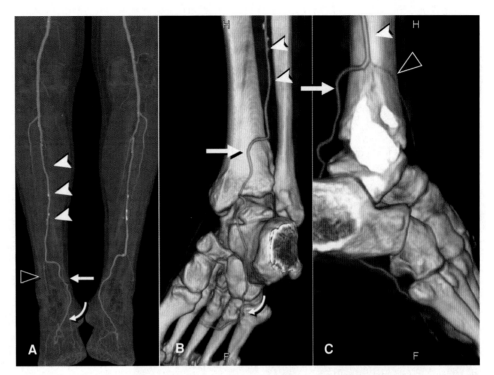

FIGURE 21-41 Bilateral hypoplasia of the anterior and posterior tibial arteries. MIP of the bilateral calves (**A**) and VR images (**B, C**) of the right foot and ankle viewed posteriorly (**B**) and laterally (after removal of the fibula) (**C**) show a single dominant peroneal artery bilaterally (*arrowheads*), which fills the posterior tibial artery (*arrow*) via its communicating branch and the lateral plantar artery (*curved arrow*). A small perforating branch (*open arrowhead*) to the anterior tibial artery/dorsalis pedis artery is also seen.

Persistence of the sciatic artery as the major blood supply to the lower extremity in adults is a rare vascular anomaly—incidence: 0.05% (125)—that may be of clinical significance (Fig. 21-44). Failure to appreciate the persistent sci-atic artery as the major inflow into the lower extremity may lead to inappropriate bypass of apparent occlusive disease of the superficial femoral artery. The persistent sciatic artery is also frequently aneurysmal, which may cause critical limb ischemia resulting from thrombosis or embolization of aneurysm thrombus (126).

FIGURE 21-42 **Variant anatomy**. This patient presented for evaluation of right thigh claudication. The tibial segment of a three-station Gd-MRA bolus-chase study shows bilateral hypoplastic anterior tibial arteries (*arrows*) with the left extending more inferiorly when compared with the right. Both peroneal arteries (*per*) are normal and are seen extending inferiorly to supply the robust dorsalis pedis (*dp*) arteries. The posterior tibial (*pt*) arteries are normal and extend to the feet. Note some venous contamination near the tibial vessel origins.

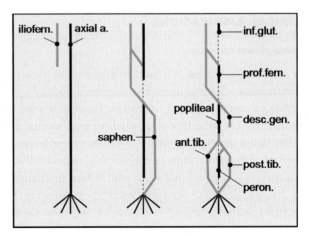

FIGURE 21-43 **Schematic of lower limb arterial development**. The axial (sciatic) artery and its remnant portions are drawn in *black*, newly formed vascular segments are drawn in *gray*. (iliofem., iliofemoral artery; saphen., saphenous artery; inf.glut, inferior gluteal artery; prof.fem., profunda femoris artery; desc.gen., descending genicular artery; ant./post.tib., anterior and posterior tibial arteries; peron., peroneal artery.) (Modified with permission from Lippert H, Pabst R. Arterial variations in man: classification and frequency. München: J.F. Bergmann Verlag; 1985.)

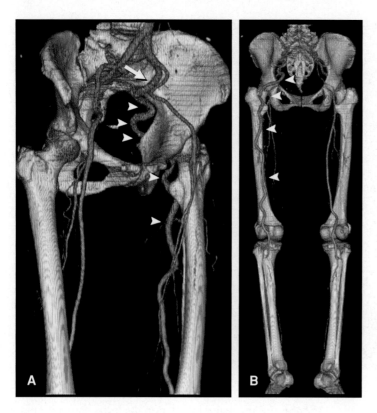

FIGURE 21-44 Persistent sciatic artery. VR right anterior oblique view **(A)** shows large diameter left internal iliac artery (*arrow*), which continues as a persistent sciatic artery (*arrowheads*). Posterior view **(B)** demonstrates the abnormal course of the mildly aneurysmal sciatic artery, which is in continuity with the popliteal artery. (Courtesy of Tamer El-Helw, MD.)

Persistent Saphenous Artery

A persistent saphenous artery, which runs superficially along the great saphenous vein, is an extremely rare variant. The descending genicular artery is a normally present remnant of the saphenous artery (Figs. 21-38, 21-43).

CLINICAL APPLICATIONS

Aneurysmal Diseases

An *aneurysm* is defined as a focal enlargement of an artery to more than 1.5 times its normal diameter. For the aorta, the general cutoff value is 3 cm and for the iliac arteries 1.8 cm. Aneurysms are either *true*, when intima, media, and adventitia are involved, or *false*, if fewer than three layers are involved. False aneurysms are frequently associated with confined rupture of arterial vessel wall, either spontaneous or due to trauma. Morphologically, aneurysms are described as being fusiform or saccular, and they are frequently lined with thrombus. The classification of aneurysms is controversial, as the distinction between diseases previously considered inherited (e.g., Marfan disease) and those considered acquired (e.g., degenerative) is becoming blurred as details are emerging about the genetic mechanisms for many aneurysm types (Table 21-13). The AIDS epidemic has revealed an increasing number of AIDS-related aneurysms (127,128).

The most common aneurysms are of the nonspecific, degenerative type and are predominantly found in the infrarenal abdominal aorta and iliac, femoral, and popliteal arteries. Formerly, this type of aneurysm was known as atherosclerotic, but it is not clear if arterial dilation is a result of atherosclerosis or if aneurysm formation actually results in atherosclerotic changes in the vessel wall (Fig. 21-45). Aneurysmal disease presenting in childhood is most often a complication of umbilical artery catheterization or is caused by Kawasaki or Takayasu diseases (129), and aneurysms caused by heritable connective tissue disorders usually manifest from the second decade onward. These conditions are discussed in more detail in the section on nonatherosclerotic causes of peripheral arterial disease to come.

Abdominal Aortic and Iliac Aneurysms

The topic of abdominal aortic aneurysm (AAA) is covered in Chapter 18. From a technical standpoint, suboptimal depiction of the outflow arteries connected with AAA can be seen with MRA due to slow filling and contrast passage, as was discussed earlier. As a way to minimize this possibility, a dedicated timing scan can be performed to determine the optimal scan delay instead of injecting the entire contrast bolus based on real-time bolus tacking software to start the MRA acquisition.

TABLE 21-13

Etiologic Classification of Arterial Aneurysms

Etiology	Pathologic Change/Mechanism
Primary connective tissue disorders	
Ehlers-Danlos syndrome (mainly types I and IV)	Type V collagen (EDS I) or type III collagen mutations (EDS IV)
Marfan syndrome	Glycine to arginine substitution at residue 239 in fibrillin gene
Miscellaneous	
Focal medial agenesis	Mainly intracranial berry aneurysms, rarely peripheral
Tuberous sclerosis	Thoracic and abdominal aneurysms due to aortic medial defects and hypertension
Turner syndrome	45 XO karyotype (gonadal dysgenesis) with aortic coarctation and infrarenal aneurysms
Menke (kinky hair) syndrome	X-linked syndrome with rapid central nervous and arterial degeneration
Mechanical (hemodynamic)	
Poststenotic	Elevated lateral wall pressures, turbulence, abnormal wall shear stress distal to stenoses, and vibratory forces
Arteriovenous fistula and postamputation related	
Pseudoaneurysms ("false" aneurysms)	
Traumatic	Full-thickness traumatic disruption (e.g., gunshot, stab wound, repeated arterial puncture)
Dissection	Deceleration, compression, and blunt injuries
Pancreatitis related	Periarterial inflammation and digestion of arterial wall
Anastomotic	Any cause of separation between graft and host artery
Arteritis related	
Takayasu disease	Aneurysms in large arteries in up to 30% of patients; possibly autoimmune mediated
Giant cell arteritis	Panarteritis with giant cell infiltration; ascending aorta and axillary branches
Systemic lupus erythematosus visceral branches	
Behçet syndrome	Ascending aorta and sinus of Valsalva
Kawasaki disease	Mucocutaneous lymph node syndrome with coronary artery and peripheral aneurysms
Infectious ("mycotic")	
Bacterial	*Streptococcus, Staphylococcus, Salmonella, Chlamydia pneumoniae*
Fungal	Inoculation of arterial wall after penetrating trauma
Spirochetal	Syphilitic (*Treponema pallidum*)
AIDS	Atypical aneurysms with pristine neighboring vessel segments
Pregnancy related	>50% of aneurysm ruptures in women <40; associated with increased MMP-2 activity
Degenerative	
Nonspecific (previously called *atherosclerotic*)	Complex multifactorial pathogenesis; mainly in aorta, iliac, femoral, and popliteal arteries
Inflammatory variant	Unknown etiology; 5% of AAAs; back pain, weight loss, and ESR elevation
Graft failure	Extremely common in bypass grafts of autologous and prosthetic material

MMP, matrix metalloproteinase; AAA, abdominal aortic aneurysm; ESR, erythrocyte sedimentation rate.

Source: Modified from Glickman BS, Rehm JP, Baxter BT, et al. Arterial aneurysms: etiologic considerations. In: Rutherford RB, ed. *Vascular Surgery*. 5th ed. Philadelphia, PA: WB Saunders; 2000:373–383.

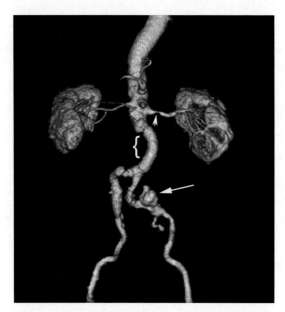

FIGURE 21-45 Aneurysmal disease. This coronal VR image from a gadolinium-enhanced MRA shows diffuse atherosclerotic irregularities, marked vessel tortuosity, a focal left renal artery stenosis (*arrowhead*), and evidence of a tube graft for treatment of an AAA ({). Note the diffuse aneurysmal dilatation of the right common and external iliac arteries and the saccular configuration of a left iliac artery aneurysm (*arrow*).

Alternatively, it is also possible to acquire multiple phases in single or multiple breath holds in order to avoid suboptimal opacification of the arteries distal to the aneurysm. In the presence of a stent graft, the flip angle should be increased to 70 to 90° to improve visualization of the lumen in the stent (also see the section on postinterventional imaging later in this chapter) (130).

In the presence of AAA, there is high coincidence of iliac artery aneurysm, and thus the iliacs should be included in the imaging volume. Isolated iliac artery aneurysms are rare and mostly found in men, and approximately 50% are bilateral. With the widespread use of cross-sectional imaging, more iliac artery aneurysms are now being detected. Invasive treatment is considered when the diameter exceeds 1.8 cm (131,132).

Femoral, Popliteal, and Distal Aneurysms

Aneurysms in the lower extremity are clinically important because of the potential for limb-threatening complications. The association between femoral and popliteal artery aneurysms and AAAs has been well known (133–135). Clinical identification of popliteal or femoral artery aneurysms has been reported to be associated with 62% and 85% incidences of AAAs, respectively (136,137). Therefore, it is mandatory to image the abdominal aorta when a peripheral aneurysm is discovered. Conversely, the incidence of femoral and/or popliteal aneurysms in patients with AAAs is reported to be 12% (133). It should be noted

that most of these lower extremity aneurysms are not detectable on physical examination (138), suggesting that US screening should be considered in AAA patients (especially in male patients, in whom the association is much stronger) (133).

The presence and true size of an aneurysm in peripheral arteries can only be assessed reliably on source images because of intraluminal thrombus in the aneurysm sac. The contrast material only delineates the residual lumen, or collaterals in case of occlusion, and almost always underestimates true luminal diameter.

Peripheral aneurysms are predominantly found in the superficial femoral and popliteal arteries and are of nonspecific, postinterventional, or traumatic origin (Fig. 21-46). Their incidence is rising due to the aging population and widespread use of endovascular and vascular surgical treatment for peripheral arterial disease (139,140).

False aneurysms are now the most frequently encountered type of aneurysm in the femoral artery. Iatrogenic false aneurysms may result from failed hemostasis at the site of arterial puncture and catheter insertion.

Anastomotic aneurysm is another frequently encountered entity and results from failing suture lines at the site of bypass graft insertion onto a native artery (141,142). Infected or mycotic aneurysms are usually the result of IV drug abuse (143). In about half of all cases, peripheral aneurysms are asymptomatic, and they are only discovered in the diagnostic workup of ischemic symptoms such as intermittent claudication, rest pain, or gangrene.

Aneurysms in the common femoral artery are classified as type I, with involvement of only the femoral artery, or type II, when the profunda femoris artery is also involved (144). Isolated aneurysms in the profunda femoris artery are very rare.

Popliteal aneurysms occur slightly more often than aneurysms in the femoral artery. The popliteal artery is considered aneurysmal if its diameter exceeds 0.7 cm (145). Similar to iliac artery aneurysms, popliteal aneurysms are bilateral in about half of all cases; carefully reviewing CT or MRA source images will reveal if this is the case.

Differential diagnostic possibilities such as a Baker cyst (distention of the gastrocnemiosemimembranosus bursa with synovial fluid from the knee), cystic advential disease (multiple loculated cysts in the popliteal artery wall), or other soft tissue tumors can also be investigated in the same imaging session. Aneurysms of the popliteal artery can be complicated by thrombosis, embolization, or rupture. The development of symptoms suggestive of distal embolization by thrombus is an absolute indication for surgical intervention, regardless of the size of the aneurysm (146).

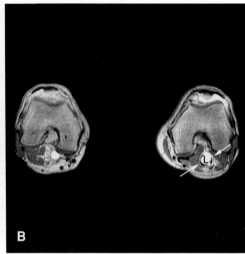

FIGURE 21-46 Aneurysmal lower extremity disease. A: MIP consisting of two out of three stations from a gadolinium-enhanced runoff MRA shows the typical appearance of a tube graft (*T*) for treatment of prior AAA, bilateral common iliac artery aneurysms (left > right), a right common femoral aneurysm, and bilateral superficial femoral artery and popliteal aneurysms. **B:** Axial cross-sectional image at the level of the popliteal artery defines the true diameter (between *arrows*) by demonstrating the vessel lumen (*L*) and peripheral thrombus (thin-rimmed dark material).

Angiographically, embolization presents as occlusion of the lower leg arteries distal to the aneurysm, frequently in combination with severe rest pain. A thrombosed aneurysm presents as an occlusion distal to the superficial femoral artery. Aneurysms in lower leg arteries distal to the popliteal artery are rare and usually are discovered incidentally on the source images (147,148).

The suspected presence of a peripheral arterial aneurysm necessitates bilateral imaging of the entire lower extremity vasculature, from the infrarenal aorta down to the pedal arch, to determine the optimal treatment strategy.

Arteriovenous Malformations

Arteriovenous malformations involving the lower extremity are discussed in Chapter 23.

Atherosclerotic Peripheral Arterial Occlusive Disease

The most common cause of PAOD is atherosclerosis of the infrarenal aorta and lower extremity arteries. Patients with chronic occlusive disease are generally excellent candidates for imaging with CTA and MRA. Acute limb ischemia and other causes of peripheral arterial disease are discussed separately.

Anatomic Framework

The angiographic hallmark of chronic critical ischemia is bilateral, multiple stenoses and occlusions at different levels in the peripheral arterial tree. Patients with diabetes tend to have a distal atherosclerotic occlusive disease distribution and preservation of normal inflow (Fig. 21-47).

It is essential to determine and describe the exact location of a lesion, the length, and the percentage reduction of the luminal diameter. It is also important to describe the morphological *pattern* of occlusive disease.

Vascular surgeons distinguish three distinct patterns of aortoiliac and peripheral occlusive disease (Fig. 21-48). Clinical significance lies in the distinction between types I and II and type III, as this latter group of patients has a much worse prognosis (149,150). For lesions involving the aortic bifurcation and the proximal iliac artery, involvement of the contralateral iliac artery should also be noted, as this will change the preferred interventional treatment strategy. With aortic occlusion (LeRiche syndrome) or unilateral iliac artery occlusion, the site of distal reconstitution should be mentioned, as this will determine the surgical approach.

Aortoiliac Segment

The status of the inflow vasculature, that is, the blood vessels above the inguinal ligament, is crucial for considering therapeutic options. A general rule in vascular surgery is to augment flow by treating the most proximal lesions first because proximal lesions tend to be those that restrict flow to the greatest extent (151–153). It is not uncommon to achieve an improved clinical status by addressing the most proximal disease in cases with multiple, segmental atherosclerotic foci.

The management of aortoiliac lesions has responded to advances in both interventional as well as vascular surgical equipment and techniques. In general, a focal iliac artery stenosis can be treated with angioplasty alone when it is more than 1 cm from both the aortic and iliac artery bifurcations. With more extensive disease, primary stenting is often performed. In an attempt to standardize lesion description and to reconcile this nomenclature with available outcome data, the TransAtlantic Inter-Society Consensus (TASC) Working Group (1) has

defined four different kinds of iliac lesions (Table 21-14, Fig. 21-49).

For category A lesions, there is ample evidence that an endovascular procedure is the treatment of choice. Conversely, for category D lesions, surgery is the treatment of choice. For type B and C lesions, more evidence is needed to make any firm recommendations about the best treatment (1). It is recommended to use TASC nomenclature when reporting the findings of the examination.

The key imaging distinction for the upper leg vasculature is to identify whether there is a relatively short, focal stenosis or high-grade disease over a long segment. This differentiation helps to determine the feasibility for endovascular repair. The most common site of stenoses or occlusions is where the superficial femoral artery courses through the adductor (Hunter) canal.

Femoropopliteal Segment

The TASC working group has developed a morphological classification scheme for the femoropopliteal arteries (Table 21-15, Fig. 21-50). Current best clinical practice is to attempt endovascular treatment in cases where lesion length does not exceed 3 cm. The available evidence indicates that surgery is still the best treatment option when femoropopliteal lesion length exceeds 5 cm.

Newer interventional radiological techniques such as subintimal angioplasty (also known as percutaneous intentional extraluminal recanalization [PIER]), may lead to acceptable patency rates as well, although there is insufficient data available from which to draw firm conclusions at this time (154). In patients with SFA occlusion and concomitant occlusion of the distal popliteal or trifurcation arteries, an isolated popliteal artery segment is considered a suitable target vessel for bypass surgery when there is sufficient collateral outflow to the distal lower leg and foot (155) (Fig. 21-51).

Lower Leg and Pedal Arteries

A depiction of the infragenicular arterial system is critical in patients with chronic critical ischemia (i.e., rest pain and/or tissue loss) and in those with diabetes. For those with intermittent claudication, this is usually not the location of symptomatic lesions nor the target for invasive intervention, except in patients with diabetes mellitus (77).

The main guiding principle behind vascular surgical reconstruction in the lower legs of patients with chronic critical ischemia has evolved from conservative treatment with eventual amputation to restoration of pulsatile flow to the distal lower leg in order to end rest pain and achieve wound healing (156–162). Distal bypass grafting has a much better limb salvage rate than conservative treatment (158,163).

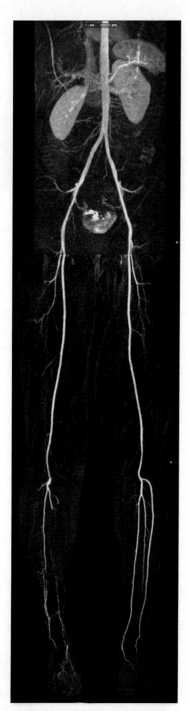

FIGURE 21-47 A 45-year-old female patient with diabetes mellitus type 2. Occlusive disease is confined to the right tibial arteries. The proximal arteries are spared.

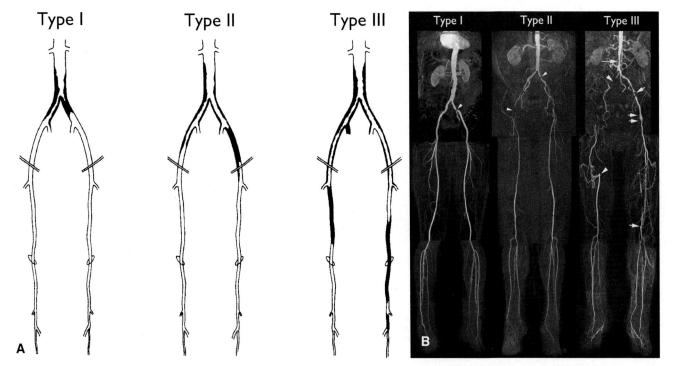

FIGURE 21-48 A: Schematic of different morphological types of peripheral arterial disease. (Reprinted with permission from Brewster DC. Direct reconstruction for aortoiliac occlusive disease. In: Rutherford RB, ed. *Vascular Surgery*. Philadelphia, PA: WB Saunders, 2000:943–972.) **B:** CE MRA appearance of different types of PAOD. Type I: involvement limited to aorta and common iliac arteries; type II: involvement limited to suprainguinal peripheral arteries; type III: central and peripheral arterial occlusive disease (i.e., "multilevel") disease.

Consequently, the vascular surgeon will bypass into the best available outflow vessel, regardless of anatomic level, provided that inflow into the artery and the origin of the graft are uncompromised. The best possible treatment plan is determined with adequate anatomical information about lower leg arteries *and* the pedal arteries in addition to functional information from other tests such as transcutaneous oxygen measurements and targeted high-resolution DU (1,164,165). The status of the vessels that will serve as the outflow from the graft has prognostic information regarding the durability of the graft.

TABLE 21-14

Morphological Stratification of Iliac Lesions According to the TransAtlantic Inter-Society Consensus

Lesion Type	Morphologic Characteristics
TASC type A iliac lesions	Single stenosis <3 cm of CIA or EIA (unilateral or bilateral)
TASC type B iliac lesions	Single stenosis 3 to 10 cm in length, not extending into CFA Total of two stenoses <5 cm long in the CIA and/or EIA, not extending into the CFA
TASC type C iliac lesions	Bilateral 5- to 10-cm long stenoses of CIA and/or EIA, not extending into the CFA Unilateral EIA occlusion not extending into the CFA Unilateral EIA stenosis extending into the CFA Bilateral CIA occlusion
TASC type D iliac lesions	Diffuse, multiple unilateral stenoses involving the CIA, EIA, and CFA (usually >10 cm) Unilateral occlusion, involving both the CIA and EIA Bilateral EIA occlusions Diffuse disease involving the aorta and both iliac arteries Iliac stenoses in a patient with an AAA or other lesion requiring aortic or iliac surgery

TASC, TransAtlantic Inter-Society Consensus; CIA, common iliac artery; EIA, external iliac artery; CFA, common femoral artery; AAA, abdominal aortic aneurysm.
Source: Modified from Dormandy JA, Rutherford RB. Management of peripheral arterial disease (PAD). TASC Working Group. TransAtlantic Inter-Society Consensus (TASC). *J Vasc Surg.* 2000;31:S1–S296.

Type A   **Endovascular Treatment of Choice**

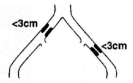

Type B   **Currently, endovascular treatment is more often used but insufficient evidence for recommendation**

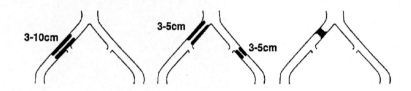

Type C   **Currently surgical treatment is more often used but insufficient evidence for recommendation**

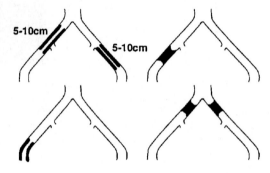

Type D   **Surgical treatment of choice**

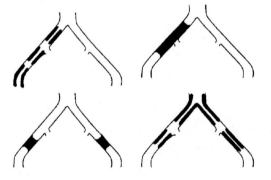

FIGURE 21-49 Aortoiliac TASC lesion types (refer to Table 21-14 for description). (Reprinted with permission from Dormandy JA, Rutherford RB. Management of peripheral arterial disease (PAD). TASC Working Group. TransAtlantic Inter-Society Consensus (TASC). *J Vasc Surg.* 2000;31:S1–S296.)

It is important to recognize variations in the dorsal pedal artery and the medial and lateral plantar branches of the posterior tibial artery, because nonfilling of one of the named segments does not necessarily mean that the vessel is occluded (166). The crucial distinction to report is whether or not the anterior circulation of the foot (most often the dorsalis pedis artery) anastomoses to the posterior circulation (posterior tibial, lateral, and medial plantar arteries) via the deep plantar artery, to constitute the "pedal arch." Occlusion of the entire pedal arch predicts a poor outcome of below-knee bypass grafting (4).

Familiarity with the TASC classification scheme for infrapopliteal lesions can facilitate relevant report generation (Table 21-16).

The STAR Registry report and others have shown distal run-off vessel patency (and diabetes) as the most important lesion characteristic with regard to expected long-term patency (167). Additional improvements in catheter and guide wire design and techniques such as subintimal recanalization (168–171) have expanded the range of lesions that can be adequately treated percutaneously.

TABLE 21-15

Morphological Stratification of Femoropopliteal Lesions According to the TransAtlantic Inter-Society Consensus

Lesion Type	Morphologic Characteristics
TASC type A iliac lesions	Single stenosis <3 cm of CIA or EIA (unilateral or bilateral)
TASC type B iliac lesions	Single stenosis 3 to 10 cm in length, not involving the distal popliteal artery
	Heavily calcified stenoses up to 3 cm in length
	Multiple lesions, each less than 3 cm (stenoses or occlusions)
	Single or multiple lesions in the absence of continuous tibial runoff to improve inflow for distal surgical bypass
TASC type C femoropopliteal lesions	Single stenosis or occlusion longer than 5 cm
	Multiple stenoses or occlusions, each 3 to 5 cm, with or without heavy calcification
TASC type D femoropopliteal lesions	Complete common femoral artery or superficial femoral artery occlusions or complete popliteal and proximal trifurcation occlusions

TASC, TransAtlantic Inter-Society Consensus; CIA, common iliac artery; EIA, external iliac artery.

Source: Modified from Dormandy JA, Rutherford RB. Management of peripheral arterial disease (PAD). TASC Working Group. TransAtlantic Inter-Society Consensus (TASC). *J Vasc Surg.* 2000;31:S1–S296.

Functional Framework: Intermittent Claudication and Critical Limb Ischemia

Patients with lower extremity ischemia can be conveniently divided into two groups from a functional perspective: those with intermittent claudication and those with limb-threatening ischemia. In general, patients with intermittent claudication are considered to have a good prognosis, a benign course, a low rate of amputation, and a limited need for surgical intervention (172,173). In comparison, patients with limb-threatening ischemia are considered to have a much worse prognosis, with a higher rate of amputation if no intervention is performed, particularly in diabetic patients (174).

In the past, the presence of limb-threatening ischemia was the primary indication for pursuing angiographic evaluation as a means to plan surgical revascularization. However, with the expanded diagnostic and therapeutic armamentarium now available, the approach to patients with peripheral vascular disease is changing. The introduction of less invasive alternatives for the diagnosis and treatment of vascular disease has liberalized the indications for pursuing both. A clear shift in this direction can be found when considering those patients with intermittent claudication.

Intermittent Claudication

Intermittent claudication can be thought of as an expression of lower extremity vascular disease that is largely lifestyle limiting. The level of atherosclerotic occlusive disease dictates the symptomatic segment—symptoms typi-

cally occur one level below the segment of disease. Patients with segmental iliac artery stenosis commonly present with buttock and thigh pain from claudication (175). Patients with superficial femoral artery disease usually have calf claudication (one level below the occlusion). Those with profunda femoris artery disease may have isolated thigh claudication; this branch of the common femoral artery provides the main blood supply to the thigh.

It is widely agreed that adverse limb outcomes such as gangrene and amputation are relatively rare among patients with claudication. Amputation rates for this cohort are low—in the range of 1% to 2% per year (1,173). However, claudication is a marker for systemic atherosclerosis, leading to future cardiovascular death and morbidity (176).

When the relatively benign course, from a limb perspective, is considered with the definable risks incurred during and after major reconstructive vascular bypass surgery, conservative treatment is most common for the vast majority of patients with claudication. The risk of surgery is generally not warranted and is usually confined to extreme cases.

In the claudicant group, treatment aims at improving blood supply to the femoral and calf muscles, and it is therefore usually limited to the aortoiliac and femoropopliteal vascular territories. Medical management including exercise regimens, tobacco cessation programs, and drug therapy may improve symptoms (177–179), but patient compliance is often poor. Surgical or endovascular

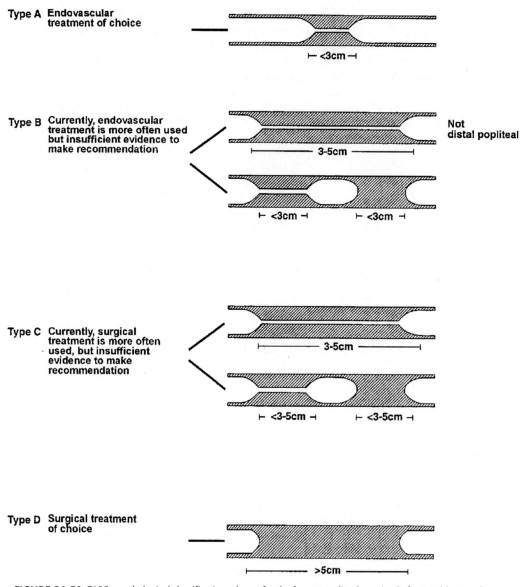

Type A Endovascular treatment of choice

Type B Currently, endovascular treatment is more often used but insufficient evidence to make recommendation

Not distal popliteal

Type C Currently, surgical treatment is more often used, but insufficient evidence to make recommendation

Type D Surgical treatment of choice

FIGURE 21-50 TASC morphological classification scheme for the femoropopliteal arteries (refer to Table 21-15). (Reprinted with permission from Dormandy JA, Rutherford RB. Management of peripheral arterial disease (PAD). TASC Working Group. TransAtlantic Inter-Society Consensus (TASC). *J Vasc Surg*. 2000;31:S1–S296.)

revascularization is then considered. For many patients, angioplasty is more cost-effective than surgical intervention (180).

The original American Heart Association Task Force guidelines (181) and the TASC report (1) have provided guidelines for appropriate treatment. Conventional treatment of aortoiliac lesions and short (<5 cm) femoropopliteal stenoses or occlusions (TASC A or B) typically has been endovascular, whereas longer femoral occlusions (TASC C or D) and occlusions involving the common femoral artery may require surgical revascularization. Factors influencing the method of treatment depend on the lesion morphology (degree of stenosis/occlusion and lesion length) (182); its location; and most importantly, the status of run-off vessels.

IMAGING

CTA and MRA can provide complete delineation of both the femoropopliteal segment and inflow and outflow arteries including lesion number, lengths, stenosis diameter and morphology, adjacent normal arterial caliber, and status of distal run-off vessels (Fig. 21-52). CTA can also demonstrate calcifications. This information guides preprocedure planning with regards to route of access, balloon selection, and expected long-term patency after intervention.

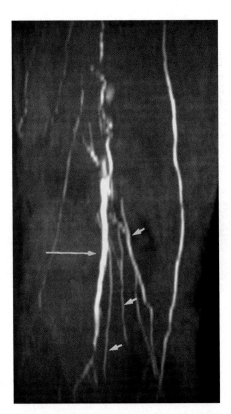

FIGURE 21-51 *A "blind" popliteal segment.* This frontal MIP image from a 2D TOF MR angiogram (TR = triggered; TE = 7 milliseconds; 70° flip angle) shows a popliteal artery (*long arrow*) that is isolated from the circulation. Note the relatively long length of that segment as well as the numerous collateral vessels (*short arrows*). In this case, a bypass to that popliteal segment would be preferred over a longer bypass to an infrageniculate segment. (Reprinted with permission from Adelman MA, Jacobowitz GR. Body MR angiography: a surgeon's perspective. *Magn Reson Imaging Clin North Am.* 1998;6:397–416.)

Eccentric stenoses are better appreciated with CTA and MRA as compared with DSA, and a more accurate determination of diameter reduction is possible in some cases (183). The status of collateral vessels is well assessed on MIP and VR images, and arterial segments distal to long-segment occlusions are well visualized (Figs. 21-10, 21-53).

The calf arteries are not a primary target for endovascular or surgical treatment in the claudicant group but serve as a predictor of expected short- and long-term patency rates after femoropopliteal intervention.

From a financial perspective, preprocedural US or MRA has been shown to be cost-effective relative to catheter angiography (184); it is expected that CTA is also cost-effective in this regard (184,185).

Chronic Limb-threatening Ischemia

Limb-threatening ischemia occurs when the resting blood flow is unable to meet baseline metabolic demands because of arterial occlusive disease. Clinically, this manifests as rest pain (usually affecting the forefoot), ulceration, or gangrene. The pain is typically exacerbated by elevation and alleviated by placing the extremity in a dependent position because gravity increases arterial perfusion.

Gangrene occurs when arterial flow is so poor that areas with the least perfusion undergo spontaneous necrosis. The risk of limb loss is largely determined by the findings at clinical examination in conjunction with the results of noninvasive studies. This information is combined with an assessment of the vascular anatomic structures to determine surgical feasibility.

TABLE 21-16

Morphological Stratification of Infrapopliteal Lesions

Lesion Type	Morphologic Characteristics
TASC type A infrapopliteal lesions	Single stenosis <1 cm in the tibial or peroneal vessels
TASC type B infrapopliteal lesions	Multiple focal stenoses of the tibial or peroneal vessels, each less than 1 cm in length One or two focal stenoses, each less than 1 cm long, at the tibial trifurcation Short tibial or peroneal stenosis in conjunction with femoropopliteal PTA
TASC type C infrapopliteal lesions	Stenoses 1 to 4 cm in length Occlusions 1 to 2 cm in length of the tibial or peroneal vessels Extensive stenoses in the tibial trifurcation
TASC type D infrapopliteal lesions	Tibial or peroneal occlusions longer than 2 cm Diffusely diseased tibial or peroneal vessels

TASC, TransAtlantic Inter-Society Consensus; CIA, common iliac artery; EIA, external iliac artery.
Source: Modified from Dormandy JA, Rutherford RB. Management of peripheral arterial disease (PAD). TASC Working Group. TransAtlantic Inter-Society Consensus (TASC). *J Vasc Surg.* 2000;31:S1–S296.

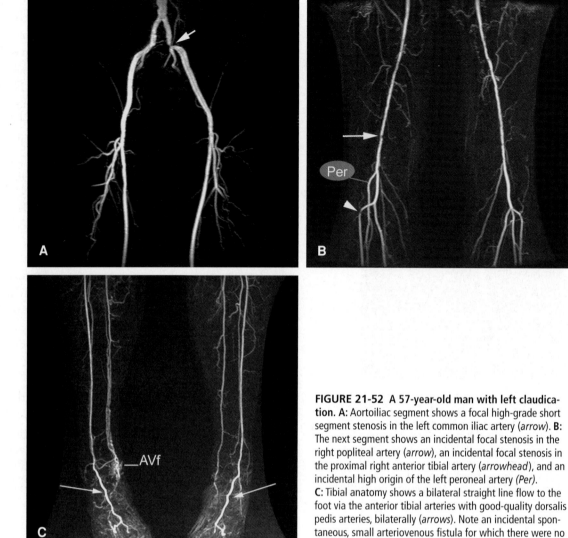

FIGURE 21-52 A 57-year-old man with left claudication. A: Aortoiliac segment shows a focal high-grade short segment stenosis in the left common iliac artery (*arrow*). **B:** The next segment shows an incidental focal stenosis in the right popliteal artery (*arrow*), an incidental focal stenosis in the proximal right anterior tibial artery (*arrowhead*), and an incidental high origin of the left peroneal artery *(Per)*. **C:** Tibial anatomy shows a bilateral straight line flow to the foot via the anterior tibial arteries with good-quality dorsalis pedis arteries, bilaterally (*arrows*). Note an incidental spontaneous, small arteriovenous fistula for which there were no related symptoms or physical findings.

In diabetics, progression of disease is usually much more rapid, and the risk for amputation is much higher (1,186). Diabetics who continue smoking have a dismal prognosis. Amputation rates in this group of patients are up to 40 times higher compared with patients without diabetes (1). Obtaining a full anatomic study from the infrarenal aorta down to the lower leg and pedal arteries is essential in the preinterventional workup of distal peripheral arterial disease.

Although ischemia may be lessened with a proximal procedure, it is crucial to restore pulsatile flow to the level of gangrene in patients with tissue loss. Attempts to achieve such restoration are best pursued when there is arterial continuity to the foot, reiterating the necessity for a complete evaluation down to the pedal arch (187).

A variety of endovascular techniques have shown efficacy in treatment of infrapopliteal lesions (188,189). How-

ever, surgical bypass grafting is the standard approach to revascularization for limb-threatening ischemia. Thus, defining acceptable target vessels for distal bypass with imaging is a crucial component of the vessel analysis in this advanced disease group.

For CTA, utilization of very thin collimation (≤1 mm) and optimization of contrast medium administration will provide improved visualization of these small vessels (Fig. 21-54). The newest generation of 64-channel MDCT machines allows for further increase in spatial resolution and should allow improved visualization of small crural and pedal vessels.

Distal lower extremity MRA is mostly performed by using 3D CE MRA, either as part of a multistation run-off protocol or as a dedicated acquisition. Nonenhanced TOF MRA below the knee has demonstrated efficacy in identifying arteries in the distal lower extremity that could not be

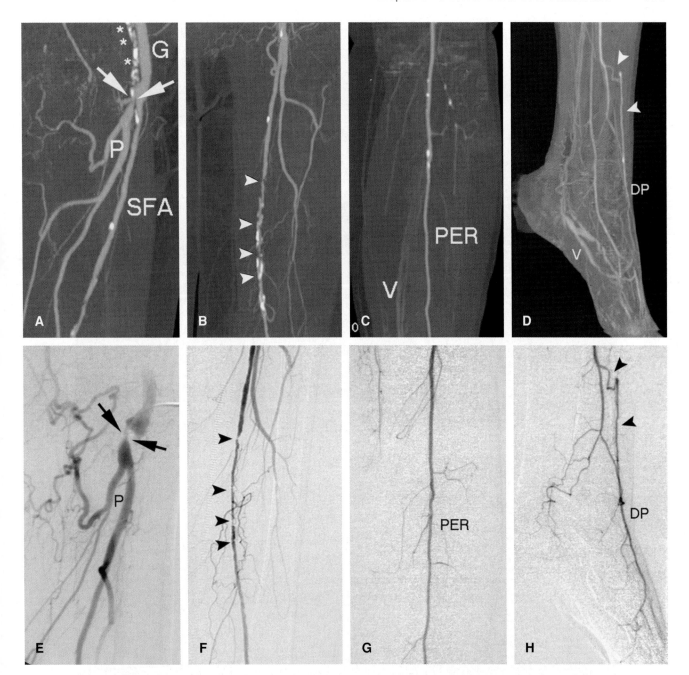

FIGURE 21-53 **Intermittent left leg claudication in a 62-year-old female with a history of tobacco abuse and previous aortobifemoral bypass grafting (ABI was 0.65). A–D: MIP images with bone segmentation. E–H:** DSA images obtained before treatment. **A:** Oblique MIP shows high-grade stenosis (*arrows*) at the origin of the left profunda femoris artery (*P*); a previously placed aortobifemoral graft (*G*) is noted, as is a patent superficial femoral artery (*SFA*). **B:** Coronal MIP of the left thigh demonstrates multifocal moderate to severe stenosis in the SFA (*arrowheads*). The SFA is small in caliber, with soft and calcified plaque present. **C:** Coronal MIP of the calf shows a one-vessel (peroneal, *PER*) runoff to the left foot. Mild venous contamination (*V*) is present. **D:** Sagittal MIP of the left foot shows collateral vessel reconstitution (*arrowheads*) of the dorsalis pedis (*DP*) above the ankle from the peroneal artery. **E:** DSA image from selective catheterization of left profunda femoris artery corroborates the CTA finding of high-grade profunda stenosis (*arrows*). (*P*, profunda femoris artery.) **F:** DSA image of the left SFA shows multiple focal stenoses (*arrowheads*) in the same segment of SFA as demonstrated by CTA. Note the lack of calcium visualization on the subtracted image from DSA. **G:** DSA image of the calf confirms single peroneal vessel runoff. **H:** DSA image of the left foot confirms reconstitution of the dorsalis pedis artery (*DP*) from the peroneal artery (*arrowheads*). (Reprinted with permission from Fleischmann D, Hallett RL, Rubin GD. CT angiography of peripheral arterial disease. *J Vasc Interv Radiol*. 2006;17:3–26.)

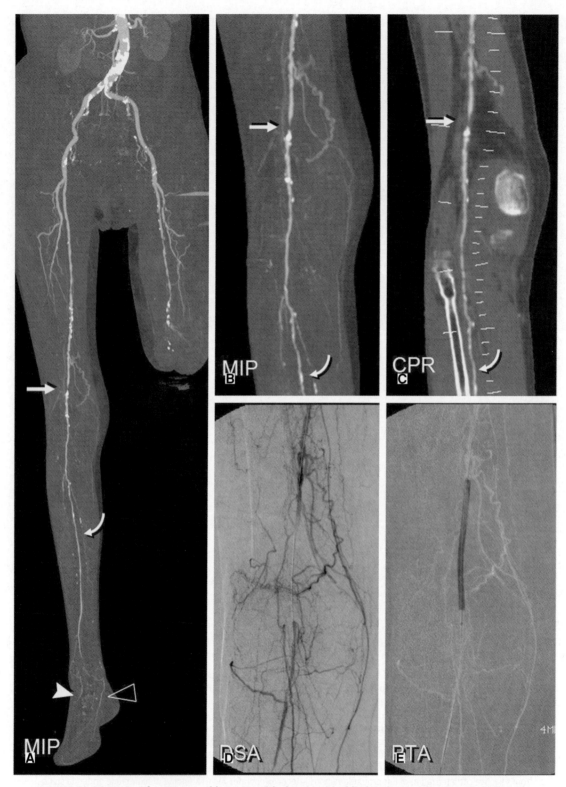

FIGURE 21-54 Image of an 81-year-old woman with chronic critical limb ischemia (Fontaine stage IV) with rest pain of right foot; past medical history is significant for prior above-knee amputation of left lower extremity. A: MIP image of the entire data set demonstrates femoropopliteal artery disease with focal high-grade stenoses and occlusions (*arrow*), and single vessel runoff via the peroneal artery (*curved arrow*), which ends above the ankle. Reconstitution of the dorsalis pedis (*arrowhead*) and the plantar artery (*open arrowhead*) below the ankle. Close-up MIP **(B)** and CPR **(C)** of right popliteal and infrapopliteal segments. Based on CTA images, antegrade access and PTA of the popliteal artery was planned for the next day. **D:** DSA confirms high-grade stenosis (which is occluded by the guide wire) in the diagnostic run. **E:** PTA with 4 mm/8 cm balloon catheter.

visualized with conventional x-ray angiography (so-called *angiographically occult* arteries) (15). While major improvements in 3D CE MRA imaging protocols have largely replaced 2D TOF MRA in most cases, there is a re-emergence of interest in using nonenhanced MRA for patients with severe renal insufficiency. In this regard, the prior documentation of the efficacy of TOF MRA for identifying target vessels for distal bypass (Fig. 21-55) has renewed relevance (15,190).

In the lower leg, subtraction of a nonenhanced mask scan is essential to obtain a high-quality study. In addition, a surface coil is absolutely mandatory at 1.5 T to obtain sufficient SNR, especially when submillimeter resolution is used to interrogate suspected severe distal disease.

Pitfalls

There are several important pitfalls in distal lower extremity and pedal MRA. The most important is disturbing venous enhancement primarily seen in patients with cellulitis and diabetes. A priori identification of these conditions helps to choose the optimal imaging approach (85). In case there is deep venous enhancement in the images, the use of thin-slab MIPs may still allow for a successful evaluation of the data (Figs. 21-56, 21-57).

Exclusion of pedal arterial anatomy can occur when the imaging volume has insufficient AP coverage, and this exclusion is a common mistake. It can be avoided by meticulous review of localizer original partitions.

In patients who have undergone previous orthopedic surgery, the presence of tibial or fibular screws and plates may lead to signal loss due to susceptibility artifacts (Fig. 21-58). Metal clips on bandages may also lead to susceptibility artifacts. A review of the original CE partitions can be clarifying.

Stenosis of the dorsalis pedis artery can artifactually be induced by tight straps and when the foot is imaged by any modality in plantar flexion. The cause of this latter "ballerina sign" artifact is compression of the dorsal pedal artery by the distal part of the retinaculum extensorum (192). Finally, arteries may appear stenotic when poor signal to noise is seen with insufficient contrast enhancement in combination with disproportionately high spatial resolution. Use of an injection rate above 1.0 mL/second as well as a surface coil minimizes this risk.

Diagnostic Accuracy of Magnetic Resonance Angiography for Evaluation of Peripheral Arterial Occlusive Disease

In the early to mid 1990s, several TOF MRA studies with relatively small numbers of patients generated a lot of enthusiasm (66,193–196). However, drawbacks in the acquisition duration—in the order of 1 hour or more—and from image artifacts—overestimation of grade and length of stenoses and occlusions (59,197,198)—have hampered acceptance of TOF MRA techniques as the exclusive approach in routine clinical practice.

As applied to candidates for distal bypass surgery, TOF MRA has shown to be a reasonable alternative to *conventional* DSA and in several instances has been shown to reveal patent arteries that were not seen on conventional arteriograms (15,190). One group has shown that bypasses to these "angiographically occult" arteries have primary patency rates comparable to those of bypasses to arteries that are visualized on conventional arteriograms (68). However, in a recent large trial conducted in over 80 patients with distal peripheral arterial disease, TOF MRA of the pedal arteries yielded relatively high sensitivities of between 75% and 80%; specificities, on the other hand, were poor and ranged between 28% and 39% (199), illustrating the limited role of TOF in current clinical practice to reliably differentiate diseased from healthy vessels.

CE MRA techniques for depiction of the peripheral vascular tree in the lower extremities is widely used in clinical practice. In Table 21-17, the diagnostic accuracies of 3D CE MRA studies of the peripheral arterial tree in comparison to IA DSA are summarized. Sensitivities and specificities are, with few exceptions, very high.

Meta-analysis studies have shown that 3D CE MRA is superior to 2D TOF MRA for the detection and grading of peripheral arterial disease (123,238). One of those studies also demonstrated that a review of source images or multiplanar reformations leads to an almost fivefold increase in the relative diagnostic odds ratio (a measure of the discriminatory power of an examination that represents the odds of a positive examination result among diseased persons relative to the odds of a positive examination result among nondiseased persons) (123).

Diagnostic Accuracy of Computed Tomographic Angiography for Evaluation of Peripheral Arterial Occlusive Disease

Lower extremity CTA (introduced in 1998–1999) is the newest technique for peripheral arterial imaging. Thus, only sparse original data on its accuracy in patients with PAOD are available (Table 21-18) when compared with the body of published data on US or MRA. The majority of published articles on peripheral CTA obtained their results with 4-channel MDCT scanners (24,25,27,28,239,240). These small early series do not allow for clinically meaningful stratification of patients into those with claudication and those with limb-threatening ischemia. Other difficulties in interpreting the results of the published literature are

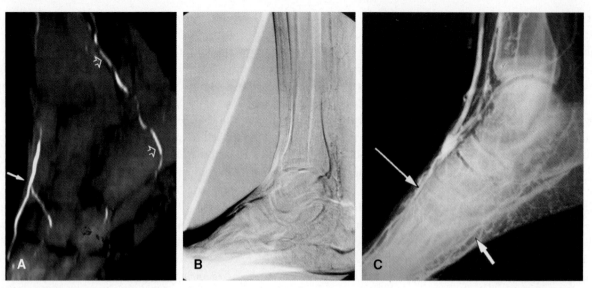

FIGURE 21-55 Occult vessel identified with 2D TOF. Evaluations of the pedal arteries with TOF MRA, conventional DSA, and intraoperative angiography. **A:** Sagittal MIP image from a 2D TOF MR angiogram of the foot (TR = triggered; TE = 7 milliseconds; 70° flip angle) demonstrates an isolated segment of dorsalis pedis artery (*solid arrow*) as well as incomplete posterior tibial artery segments (*open arrows*). **B:** Conventional digital subtraction angiogram obtained prior to MRA does not depict any outflow vessel in the foot because of multiple-level occlusive disease and a limited delivery of contrast medium to the foot. **C:** After depicting the occult pedal artery with MRA, an anterior tibial-dorsalis pedis bypass procedure was performed. This intraoperative angiogram shows outflow through the dorsalis pedis artery (*long arrow*) as well as plantar collateral vessels (*short arrow*). (Reprinted, with permission from Rofsky NM, Adelman MA. MR angiography in the evaluation of atherosclerotic peripheral vascular disease. *Radiology*. 2000;214:325-338.)

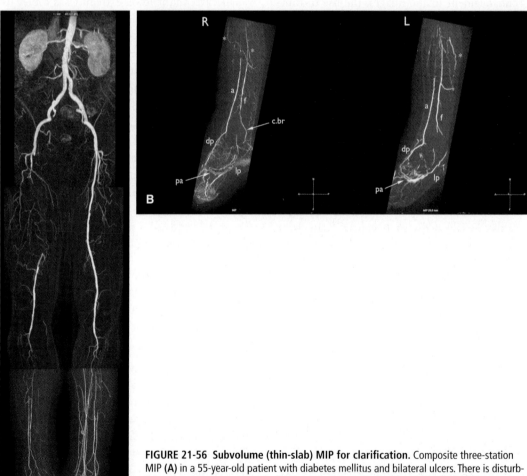

FIGURE 21-56 Subvolume (thin-slab) MIP for clarification. Composite three-station MIP **(A)** in a 55-year-old patient with diabetes mellitus and bilateral ulcers. There is disturbing venous enhancement in the left lower leg. Use of subvolume (thin-slab) MIPs to postprocess the information may improve evaluation **(B)**. The lower leg arteries are filled by collateral branches (∗). (R, right leg; L, left leg; a, anterior tibial artery; f, fibular (peroneal) artery; dp, dorsalis pedis artery; lp, lateral plantar artery; c.br, communicating branch of fibular artery; pa, pedal arch.)

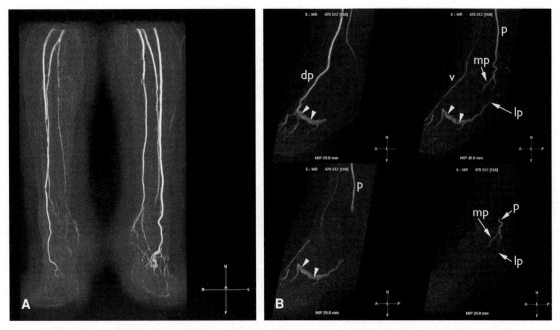

FIGURE 21-57 Improved visualization of pedal vessels. A: Coronal MIP of lower legs, obtained as part of three-consecutive-station CE MRA in a patient with severe intermittent claudication. There is mild venous enhancement in the left foot. **B:** Value of thin-slab sliding MIP reconstructions for delineation of arterial anatomy in the presence of venous enhancement. **Upper left:** A 20-mm subvolume MIP readily demonstrates dorsal pedal artery (*dp*) and pedal arch (*arrowheads*). **Upper right:** A 40-mm subvolume MIP demonstrating lateral plantar artery (*lp*) and continuation of pedal arch. The dorsal pedal vein is also enhanced (*v*). **Lower left:** A 20-mm thin-slab subvolume MIP better demonstrating plantar arch. **Lower right:** selective view of distal posterior tibial artery (*p*), bifurcating into medial plantar (*mp*) and lateral plantar (*lp*) arteries.

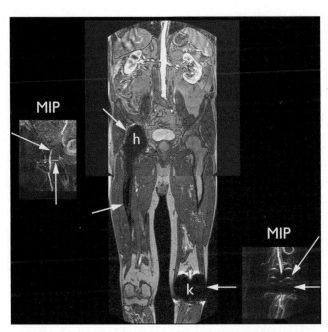

FIGURE 21-58 Susceptibility artifacts can easily be recognized on source images (**middle panel**) as signal voids (h, hip prosthesis; k, knee prosthesis). **Left and right panels** show MIPs of the regions with the hip and knee prostheses. The typical imaging appearance is the presence of a high signal intensity band adjacent to an area of complete signal loss.

the inconsistent thresholds used for grading of "significant" stenoses, variable categorization of anatomic vessel segments, and the use of different visualization and postprocessing tools.

All but one group of authors (240) report good overall sensitivities and specificities for the detection of hemodynamically relevant steno-occlusive lesions with 4-channel MDCT relative to intra-arterial DSA (25,27,28,239) (Table 21-18). In general, both sensitivity and specificity are greater for arterial occlusions than for the detection of stenoses. Accuracies and interobserver agreement are also higher for femoropopliteal and iliac vessels when compared with infrapopliteal arteries when 4-channel CT is used.

In the first study, using submillimeter collimated 16-channel MDCT (30), the overall sensitivities, specificities, and accuracies were all greater than 96%, and there was no evident decrease of performance down to the popliteocrural branches. Pedal arteries have not been specifically analyzed in any published series to date. The presence of vessel calcifications apparently reduces diagnostic performance of MDCT in general (241).

TABLE 21-17

Diagnostic Accuracy of Three-dimensional Gadolinium Chelate–enhanced Magnetic Resonance Angiography of the Peripheral Arteries

Author	Reference	Year	Field Strength	Technique[a]	Number of Patients	Sensitivity (%)[b]	Specificity (%)[b]	Accuracy (%)[b]
Leiner et al.	21	2005	1.5 T	3 CS	295	84	97	94
Binkert et al.	200	2004	1.5 T	Hybrid	30	NR	NR	74.3–87.3
Vavrik	201	2004	1.5 T	3 CS	48	89.5–94.7	93.4–98.1	NR
Bezooijen et al.	93	2004	1.5 T	3 CS	15	89	99	NR
Huber et al.	202	2003	1.5 T	3 CS	20	100	96	NR
Schafer et al.	203	2003	1.5 T	3 CS	30	92–95	97–99	94–99
Wyttenbach et al.	204	2003	1.5 T	3 CS	28	96	93	NR
Hentsch et al.	113	2003	1.0 to 1.5 T	3 CS	203	71–93	87–90	NR
Steffens et al.	205	2003	1.5 T	3 CS	50	99.5	98.8	NR
Nchimi et al.	206	2002	1.5 T	3 CS	49	98	98	92
Cronberg et al.	207	2003	1.5 T	LL only	35	92	64	NR
Klein et al.	208	2003	1.5 T	3 CS	72	59–90	91–96	NR
Morasch et al.	96	2003	1.5 T	Hybrid	60	99	97	98
Pandharipande et al.	209	2002	1.5 T	AoI/FP	20	75–97	94–98	NR
Loewe et al.	210	2002	1.0 T	3 CS	106	96.7	95.8	NR
Swan et al.	104	2002	1.5 T	3 CS TR	69	87–89	90–97	NR
Schoenberg et al.	211	2002	1.5 T	AoI only	41	78–97	75–96	80 to 90
Goyen et al.	212	2002	1.5 T	Total Body	10	95.3	95.2	NR
Khilnani et al.	213	2002	1.5 T	Hybrid	30	91–95% agreement with DSA		
Carriero et al.	214	2002	1.5 T	3 CS	11	94.1	99.2	97.5
Winterer et al.	215	2002	1.5 T	AoI/FP	43	84	60	70
Ruehm et al.	216	2001	1.5 T	Total Body	6	91–94	90–93	NR
Reid et al.	76	2001	1.5 T	3 CS	13	100	NR	NR
Di Cesare et al.	217	2001	1.5 T	AoI/FP	45	97–100	84.8–89.0	NR
Brillet et al.	218	2001	1.5 T	3 CS	15	Kappa 0.75		
Ruehm et al.	91	2001	1.5 T	AoI/FP	23	90	95	NR
Ruehm et al.	75	2000	1.5 T	AoI/FP	61	92.3	99.4	NR
Sueyoshi et al.	219	2000	1.5 T	AoI/FP	13	100	96.5	NR
Huber et al.	220	2000	1.5 T	3 CS	24	100	94–98	NR
Lenhart et al.	221	2000	1.5 T	3 CS	45 (20)	87.5–100.0	96.8–100.0	NR
Lundin et al.	222	2000	1.0 T	3 CS	39	81–94	81–94	NR
Wikström et al.	223	2000	1.5 T	3 CS	30	86	88	NR
Bourlet et al.	224	2000	1.5 T	AoI only	22	96	80	83
Mitsuzaki et al.	225	2000	1.5 T	AoI only	22	91	89	NR
Meaney et al.	74	1999	1.5 T	3 CS	20	81–94	91–97	NR
Link et al.	226	1999	1.5 T	AoI/FP	67	100	83	NR
Oberholzer et al.	227	1999	1.0 T	3 CS	8	89	100	NR
Lenhart et al.	228	1999	1.5 T	3 CS	22 (17)	82–96	87–99	NR
Maspes et al.	229	1999	1.5 T	AoI only	47 (11)	100	87.5	NR
Ho et al.	73	1998	1.5 T	3 CS	28	94	93	NR
Ho et al.	89	1998	1.5 T	AoI only	43	93	98	NR
Yamashita et al.	230	1998	1.5 T	3 FOV	15	96	83	NR
Perrier et al.	231	1998	1.5 T	AoI only	23	92	93	NR
Quinn et al.	232	1997	1.5 T	AoI only	30	100	99	NR
Rofsky et al.	233	1997	1.5 T	2 FOV	15	97	96	97
Poon et al.	234	1997	1.5 T	AoI only	15	100	100	NR
Hany et al.	235	1997	1.5 T	AoI only	39	93–96	96–100	NR
Snidow et al.	236	1996	1.5 T	AoI only	32	100	98	NR
Prince et al.	237	1995	1.5 T	AoI only	43	94	98	NR

3 CS, three-consecutive-station moving table bolus-chase technique; Hybrid, lower legs were imaged with a separate injection of contrast medium prior to imaging aortoiliac and upper leg arteries; NR, not reported; LL, lower legs only; AoI, aortoiliac; FP, femoropopliteal arteries; TR, time-resolved acquisition for lower legs; 3 FOV, three consecutive stations imaged with three separate injections of contrast material; 2 FOV, two consecutive stations imaged with two separate injections of contrast material.

[a]In the case that two different techniques were compared, the best results are reported and number of patients are given for the best technique only.

[b]In the case of multiple readers, the results of the first reader are reported.

TABLE 21-18

Lower Extremity Computed Tomographic Angiography in Comparison to Digital Subtraction Angiography in Patients with Peripheral Arterial Occlusive Disease

Author, Year, Reference	Collimation (M × D)	Section Thickness/ Reconstruction Interval (millimeters)	n	Sensitivity (%)	Specificity (%)	Accuracy (%)
Ofer et al., 2003 (25)						
• >50% stenosis	4.0 × 2.5	3.2/1.6	18	91	92	92
• Occlusion				—	—	—
Martin et al., 2003 (239)						
• >75% stenosis	4 × 5	5.0/2.5	41	92	97	—
• Occlusion				89	98	—
Ota et al., 2004 (27)						
• >50% stenosis (iliac/fem/crur)	4 × 2	2/1	24	99 (97/100/100)	99 (100/96/100)	99 (99/97/100)
• Occlusion				96	98	98
Catalano et al., 2004 (28)						
• >50% steno-occlusion (ao-iliac/fem/pop-crur)	4.0 × 2.5	3/3	50	96 (95/98/96)	93 (90/96/93)	94 (92/97/94)
Portugaller et al., 2004 (39)						
• >50% steno-occlusion (ao-iliac/fem-pop/crur)	4.0 × 2.5	2.5/1.5	50	92 (92/98/90)	83 (95/70/74)	86 (94/88/81)
Edwards et al., 2005 (240)						
• >50% stenosis	4.0 × 2.5	3.2/2.0	44	79 and 72	93 and 93	—
• Occlusion				75 and 71	82 and 81	—
Willmann et al., 2005 (30)						
• >50% steno-occlusion (ao-iliac) (fem) (pop-crur)	16.00 × 0.75	0.75/0.40	39	96 and 97 98 and 97 96 and 97 96 and 97	96 and 97 98 and 98 94 and 96 95 and 96	96 and 97 97 and 98 96 and 96 96 and 96

(M × D), number of channels × channel width in millimeters; fem, femoral; crur, crural; ao-iliac, aorto-iliac; pop-crur, popliteal-through-crural; fem-pop, femoropopliteal.

In a recent study by Ouwendijk et al. (241), diabetes mellitus, cardiac disease, and age were found to be independently predictive for the presence of vessel wall calcifications (all $P < .05$). Regional calcification scores showed that only the effect of age was significantly ($P = .02$) different for the three regions, the effect on the femoropopliteal region being about twice as strong as for the crural region, with the effect on the aortoiliac region between those for the other two regions.

A recent study performed in the Netherlands evaluated the clinical utility, patient outcomes, and costs of peripheral MRA and 16-channel CTA for initial imaging and diagnostic workup of 157 patients with peripheral arterial disease (29). In this randomized prospective study, confidence was slightly greater with CT, patients in the CT group underwent less additional imaging studies, and they had greater improvement of clinical outcomes after treatment, but none of these was statistically significant. However, average diagnostic imaging costs were significantly less with CT ($199 mean unit cost) compared with MRA ($627 mean unit cost).

Utility of Contrast-enhanced Magnetic Resonance Angiography in Comparison to Other Imaging Modalities

Many radiology and vascular surgery departments around the world still routinely use (color-aided) DU as an alternative to diagnostic IA DSA. However, the universal acceptance of DU has been hampered by the need for extensive patient preparation, the relatively high variability between different ultrasonographers (19), and the general lack of a vascular "road map."

In a recent meta-analysis of 31 studies, Visser and Hunink (20) found a significantly higher sensitivity and specificity for CE MRA as compared with DU. These findings have been corroborated by others (21,222,223).

The superior utility of CE MRA when compared with DU is further confirmed from a recent study where treatment plans formulated by three vascular surgeons based on standardized clinical information and the findings from either DU or three-station peripheral CE MRA were compared. In 73 patients, DU provided enough information for treatment planning in a mean of 66% patients versus 92% when CE MRA was used ($P < 0.01$). In addition, treatment plans that were formulated based on CE MRA matched actual treatment in a significantly higher number of patients when compared with DU (242). Patients also tended to prefer CE MRA over DU in their workup (22).

Although it is expected that the diagnostic accuracy of MD CTA will be similar to that of CE MRA, only a few studies have been published to date (25,28,240,243,244).

Acute Limb Ischemia

Acute limb ischemia may occur as the result of embolization or in situ thrombosis of one or more lower extremity arteries or bypass grafts. Acute graft occlusion has become the leading cause of acute lower extremity ischemia in most centers, a by-product of the increased use of bypass grafts for chronic ischemia and their inevitably finite patency (245). Acute ischemia as a complication of acute aortic or iliac dissection is rare but should be considered when there is a history of hypertension accompanied by chest or back pain and in young patients with a marfanoid body habitus.

Emboli originate from the heart in more than 90% of cases. Noncardiac emboli often originate from atherosclerotic disease in the thoracic or abdominal aorta or iliac vessels and aneurysms (246). The etiology of thrombosis is more diverse and includes bypass graft occlusion and thrombotic occlusion of the native artery at the site of an atherosclerotic stenotic lesion and thrombosis within a near normal artery as the result of a hypercoagulable state but also thrombosis as a result of inflammatory diseases (e.g., vasculitis), thrombosis (and distal embolism) of a popliteal artery aneurysm, and popliteal artery entrapment syndrome, dissection, and cystic adventitial disease.

Independent of the etiology, acute limb ischemia classically presents with the "5-P" symptoms: paresthesia, pain, pallor, pulselessness, and paralysis. Particularly in nonembolic acute ischemia, the clinical symptoms may vary substantially, however, and it is often difficult to distinguish embolus from thrombus. The most recent clinical classification specifically separates limbs that are not immediately threatened (Class 2A) and those that are severely threatened to the point where urgent revascularization is necessary for limb salvage (Class 2B) (4) (Table 21-19).

Angiography remains the established gold standard for preprocedural imaging in the setting of acute limb ischemia. Catheter angiography also offers the possibility of thrombolytic or therapy or mechanical thrombectomy at the time of initial angiographic evaluation. Diagnostic information sought by angiography is the exact level and extent of the occlusion and differentiation between embolism and thrombosis (which can become blurred with clot propagation). Documentation of the presence or absence of atherosclerotic disease in other arteries is also important, as is patency of vessels distal to an occluded segment.

TABLE 21-19

Classification and Algorithm for Management of Patients with Acute Limb Ischemia

Class 1	*Viable* (remains so without intervention)	Consider heparin, workup comorbidities, *semielective angiography*	• Observation alone (only class 1) • Percutaneous mechanical thrombectomy • Thrombolytic therapy • Surgical revascularization
Class 2A	*Threatened* (delayed treatment possible)		
Class 2B	*Threatened* (immediate treatment necessary)	Therapeutic heparinization, *urgent angiography*	
Class 3	*Irreversibly ischemic*		Major amputation

Source: Adapted from Rutherford RB, Baker JD, Ernst C, et al. Recommended standards for reports dealing with lower extremity ischemia: revised version. *J Vasc Surg.* 1997;26:517–538.

No formal studies have been carried out to evaluate the accuracy of CE MRA and CTA in the setting of acute limb ischemia, but it is reasonable to consider CE MRA a viable alternative to angiography in patients with class 1 or even class 2 acute ischemia, notably in subjects with decreased renal function. CTA has the potential to completely replace diagnostic angiography in all classes of acute ischemia where vascular imaging is indicated. State-of-the-art MDCTA (16-channel and above) is becoming increasingly available in the emergency setting, and CTA data acquisition is fast, robust, and straightforward. While spatial resolution is below that of arteriography, CTA provides more accurate information on the vessel wall (atheromatous changes as potential embolic source), vessel diameters (partially thrombosed aneurysms), and perivascular abnormalities (cystic adventitial disease). CTA has been used to evaluate both embolism (Fig. 21-59) and thrombosis (Fig. 21-60) with the routine scanning and reconstruction parameters. When using 8- or more channel MDCT, CTA of the chest-abdomen-pelvis and run-off vessels is possible, which allows for assessment of a potential source of atheroembolism. If the scanner allows ECG gating of the chest portion of the acquisition (64-channel MDCT), embolic sources in the left atrium or ventricle may also be detected.

Postinterventional Imaging and Evaluation of Peripheral Arterial Bypass Grafts

As many as 30% of patients develop graft-related complications within the first 2 years after surgery (12). Long-term complications of peripheral arterial bypass grafts include intimal hyperplasia or progression of atherosclerosis, which ultimately may result in graft stenosis and failure (247,248). Timely identification and repair of failing grafts can often avert impending graft failure and improve the secondary bypass graft patency rate (249–252), and it is well known that active postoperative surveillance for restenosis increases mid- and long-term patency rates of peripheral arterial bypass grafts (253).

All grafts benefit from periodic surveillance in search of hemodynamically significant complications and ideally prior to thrombosis. Revision of stenotic lesions can sustain the graft, whereas a revision attempt after graft thrombosis has much worse results. US is the first choice for routine bypass graft surveillance due to its availability, simplicity, and reliability (254,255).

DU surveillance of peripheral bypass grafts for patients treated for critical limb ischemia has led to a reduction of major amputations and consequently to a reduction in costs compared with patients who are not surveyed (256).

CTA and MRA are very convenient problem-solving tools for the workup of patients with nondiagnostic US studies (limited access due to skin lesions, draping, or obesity), when US results are equivocal or when ABI measurements and US give conflicting results (Fig. 21-61). Graft-related complications, including stenosis, aneurysmal changes, and arteriovenous fistulas as well as vascular and extravascular complications can be well demonstrated (Fig. 21-62). CTA and MRA are helpful in the immediate postoperative period, when US is limited due to bandages and wounds (243,257–262) . Despite the high prevalence of metallic clips, MRA diagnostic accuracy has not been adversely affected in most publications (Fig. 21-63), as is detailed in Table 21-20.

Most vascular ligating clips are manufactured of chemically pure titanium. When biodegradable polydioxanone clips are used, no MRA artifacts will be encountered. The proximal and distal anastomoses of the graft should be assessed carefully for the presence of stenoses. Choosing the shortest possible TE value reduces the severity of these artifacts to a minimum. Pseudostenosis from inadvertent exclusion from the coronal imaging volume should always be considered by evaluating the grafts from multiple viewing angles (Fig. 21-64) and by pursuing an adequate patient history.

The chronic and progressive nature of most cases of atherosclerotic peripheral vascular disease will result in many patients who re-present after successful treatment. The history of pre-existing vascular stent grafts, endoprostheses, and vascular surgical ligating clips should be sought when deciding between CTA and MRA for such individuals.

Artifacts from stents, endoprostheses, or clips are much less of a concern when using CTA as compared with MRI/MRA. Because the specific type and the location of a vascular stent are often unknown in a given patient, some institutions triage stent patients toward CTA rather than MRA in order to avoid the diagnostic dilemma of uninterpretable images associated with stent artifacts.

Cross-sectional images, such as CPRs obtained from CTA data sets, allow for adequate assessment of the patency as well as the presence and extent of in-stent stenosis due to intimal hyperplasia or thrombus in large diameter (iliac and femoral) stents (Figs. 21-11, 21-65). CTA has also been used successfully as a research tool to assess the patency of infrapopliteal stents (263).

With MRA, susceptibility artifacts are highly variable in severity but are typically recognized by local or regional distortions or complete signal voids (Fig. 21-66) and may show a rim of high signal if the device edges on source images.

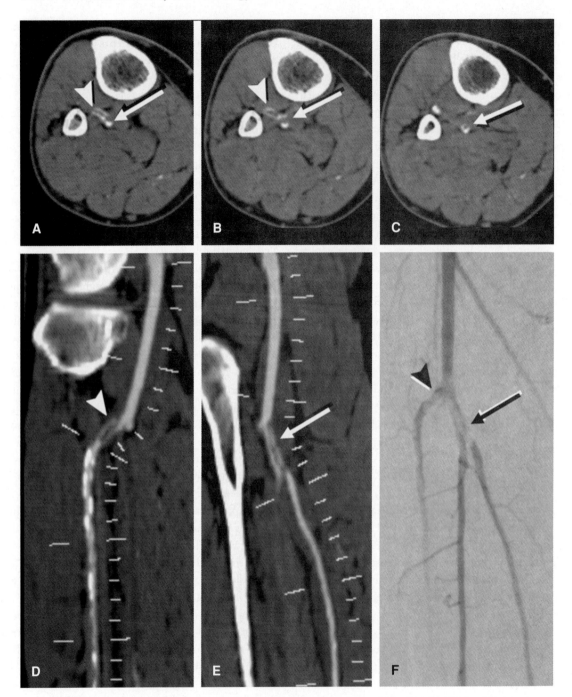

FIGURE 21-59 Acute atheroembolism. Peripheral CT angiogram (4 × 2.5 mm) of a 62-year-old man with abdominal and bilateral common iliac artery aneurysms, complaining of subacute onset of right foot pain. **A–C:** Axial CT images through right proximal calf show embolic filling defects in the anterior tibial artery (*arrowheads*) and the tibioperoneal trunk (*arrows*). **D, E:** Corresponding CPR images from the popliteal artery through the anterior tibial (**D**) and posterior tibial (**E**) arteries display intraluminal filling defects. DSA confirms CTA findings (**F**).

Artifact severity is influenced by the size (especially diameter) and composition of the stent, the size and composition of a ligating clip, the field strength, the TE, the angle to the main magnetic field, and the orientation with respect to the readout gradient (262,264).

Stents made of nitinol suffer least from artifactual signal loss, and stainless steel stents suffer the most. The severity of stent and endograft artifacts is summarized in Table 21-21. In general, an increased angle of the clip or stent orientation with respect to the main magnetic field tends to increase the

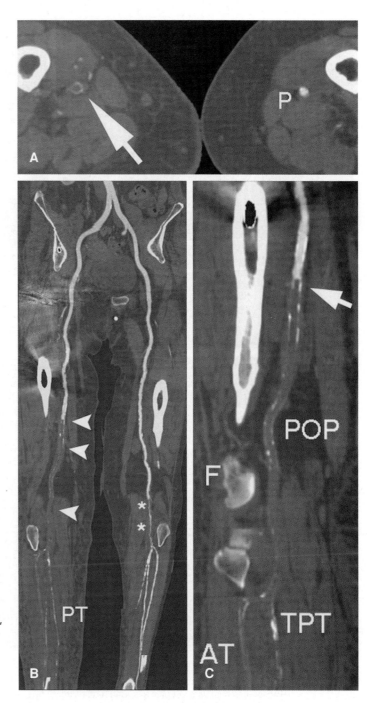

FIGURE 21-60 Acute thrombosis of the femoropopliteal and trifurcation vessels in an 84-year-old woman with an acutely cool right leg; the patient refused angiography. A: Transverse CTA image at the level of the adductor canal shows rounded filling defect in the right popliteal artery (*arrow*). The contralateral left popliteal artery (*P*) is patent at this level. **B:** Large FOV multipath CPR and **(C)** an enlarged image of the popliteal region show extent of right-sided thrombus (*arrowheads*). In addition to the popliteal artery (*POP*), the anterior tibial artery (*AT*), tibioperoneal trunk (*TPT*), and posterior tibial artery (*PT*) are occluded. (*F*, femoral head.) High-grade left popliteal stenosis (∗) is also noted. (Reprinted with permission from Dormandy JA, Rutherford RB. Management of peripheral arterial disease (PAD). TASC Working Group. TransAtlantic Inter-Society Consensus (TASC). *J Vasc Surg*. 2000;31:S1–S296.)

size of the artifactual signal loss. For instance, signal loss in a renal stent will be more severe compared with when the same stent is implanted in an iliac or superficial femoral artery.

Extra-anatomic Bypass Grafts

Extra-anatomic bypass grafts course through a substantially different anatomic pathway than the in situ blood vessels that they replace. The usefulness of autogenous vein grafts as extra-anatomic grafts is limited because of their relatively small diameter and their potential for kinking and shortening when placed beneath an anatomic region that is subject to flexion and mobility (269).

Therefore, prosthetic grafts are usually used and are classified according to their method of construction and basic component. Dacron (DuPont, Wilmington, DE) grafts represent a form of textile or fabric grafts that are constructed by using various methods of knitting or weaving. Nontextile grafts such as expanded polytetrafluoroethylene are the most widely used substrates for extra-anatomic

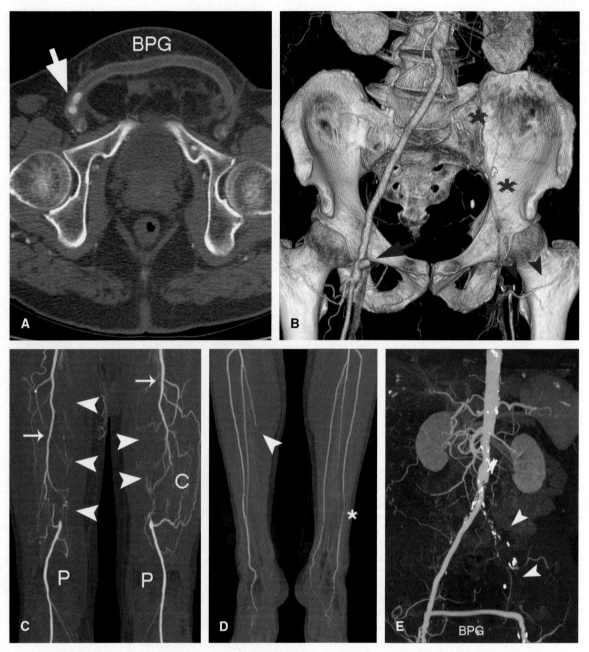

FIGURE 21-61 Utility of peripheral CTA in monitoring bypass graft patency in a 74-year-old male with surgically placed femorofemoral bypass graft for chronic left iliac arterial occlusion. A–D: Initial CTA images. Patient presented with rest pain following recent surgical bypass procedure. Pain and bandages prevented adequate Doppler and physical exam. **A:** Axial CTA image shows lack of contrast opacification of the femorofemoral bypass graft (*BPG*). Only the right common femoral artery is patent (*arrow*). **B:** VR image demonstrates only a short teat of flow at the right bypass graft anastomosis (*arrow*). There is complete occlusion of the left iliac arterial system (*) and reconstitution of the left profunda femoris artery by collaterals to the lateral femoral circumflex artery (*arrowheads*). **C:** MIP at the level of the thighs shows bilateral long-segment SFA occlusions (*arrowheads*), with reconstitution of the popliteal arteries (*P*) via collateral vessels (*C*) from the profunda femoris arteries (*arrows*). **D:** MIP of calf arteries demonstrates three-vessel runoff in the left lower extremity. There is occlusion of the right posterior tibial artery (*arrowhead*) in the mid-calf. Segmentation artifact from automated bone removal is noted (*). **E:** MIP of the abdomen and bilateral groin region 3 days later demonstrates interval surgical revision of the femorofemoral bypass graft (*BPG*), with restored patency. Left iliac occlusion again is noted (*arrowheads*). (Reprinted with permission from Fleischmann D, Hallett RL, Rubin GD. CT angiography of peripheral arterial disease. *J Vasc Interv Radiol.* 2006;17:3–26.)

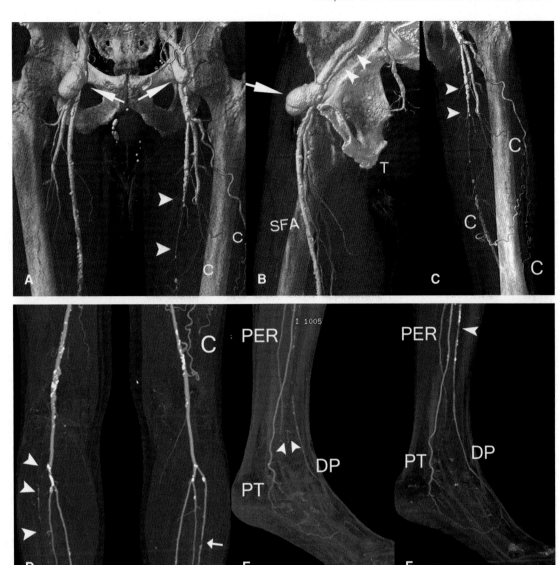

FIGURE 21-62 Perianastomotic pseudoaneurysms with bilateral infrainguinal disease in an 87-year-old man with claudication and history of previous aortobifemoral bypass graft. A: VR image demonstrates bilateral perianastomotic pseudoaneurysms at the distal attachment sites of the aortobifemoral graft and common femoral arteries (*arrows*). There is a long-segment SFA occlusion on the left (*arrowheads*) with collaterals from the profunda femoris artery (*C*). **B:** Thick-slab VR image of right groin (left lateral view) shows the profile of the pseudoaneurysm (*arrow*) as well as the adjacent native external iliac artery (*arrowheads*). The proximal and mid right superficial femoral artery is patent (*SFA*). (*T*, ischial tuberosity.) **C:** VR image of the left thigh demonstrates abundant profunda collateral supply (*C*), which reconstitutes the distal SFA. The length of the occluded segment was approximately 11 cm (*arrowheads*). **D:** MIP of both knees shows occlusion of the right anterior tibial artery at its origin (*arrowheads*). There is a focal significant stenosis in the mid-left anterior tibial artery (*arrow*). Heavy popliteal artery calcific plaque is present bilaterally. **E, F:** MIP of both feet with bone segmentation demonstrates patent posterior tibial arteries (*PT*) at both ankles into the feet. Peroneal arteries (*PER*) are patent to the lower calves. **E:** There is reconstitution of the right dorsalis pedis (*DP*) via peroneal collaterals (*arrowheads*). Left dorsalis pedis is patent. **F:** The focal left anterior tibial stenosis is again identified (*arrowhead*). (Reprinted with permission from Fleischmann D, Hallett RL, Rubin GD. CT angiography of peripheral arterial disease. *J Vasc Interv Radiol.* 2006;17:3–26.)

bypass because they do not require preclotting, are resistant to dilatation, do not leak, and may be less prone to infection than Dacron grafts (269).

Axillobifemoral bypass represents a combination of axillofemoral and femorofemoral grafts and is the most commonly performed extra-anatomic bypass, with 5-year patency rates of 33% to 85% (270). The major indication for axillobifemoral bypass is symptomatic aortoiliac occlusive disease when angioplasty or stenting has failed in patients who are poor candidates for direct aortic grafting.

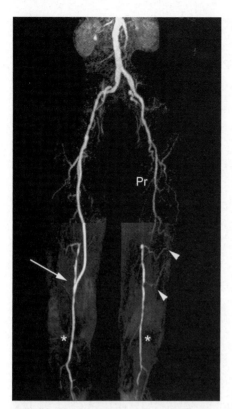

FIGURE 21-63 MRA of a right femoropopliteal bypass graft. Bilateral, long segment superficial femoral artery occlusions are noted with the intact right graft inserting on the superior most aspect of the right popliteal artery (*arrow*). The left extremity shows collaterals (*arrowheads*) from the profundus femoral artery (*Pr*) that reconstitute a diseased distal SFA and popliteal artery. Since the osseous landmarks are absent, the level of the knee joint is indicated for reference (*).

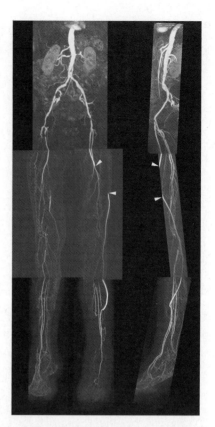

FIGURE 21-64 MRA of femorotibial bypass grafting. Composite three-station coronal (**left panel**) and sagittal (**right panel**) MIPs in 67-year-old male patient with severe intermittent claudication after having undergone bypass femorotibial bypass grafting. On the coronal image, there appears to be an occlusion in the bypass graft. Review of the sagittal image immediately demonstrates that the occlusion is artifactual because of exclusion of the bypass graft from the imaging volume (*arrowheads*).

This bypass is also used in patients with aortic occlusion, multiple failed aortofemoral grafts, infections of the native aorta (Fig. 21-67), or prosthetic grafts and in any situation that precludes an abdominal approach. Axillobifemoral bypass with ligation of both iliac arteries may be used in patients with recurrent peripheral embolization from aortic atheromas. Unilateral axillofemoral bypass is rarely performed because patency rates of the axillobifemoral bypass are superior, possibly the result of better outflow provided by the additional femorofemoral limb (270).

TABLE 21-20

Diagnostic Accuracy of Three-dimensional Contrast-enhanced Magnetic Resonance Angiography for Surveillance of Peripheral Arterial Bypass Grafts

Author	Reference	Year	Field Strength	Technique[a]	Number of Patients	Sensitivity (%)[b]	Specificity (%)[b]	Accuracy (%)[b]
Meissner et al.	262	2004	1.0 T	3 CS	24	NR	NR	100
Loewe et al.	261	2003	1.0 T	3 CS	39	90.0	98.3	89.9
Dorenbeck et al.	260	2002	1.5 T	3 CS	15	100	90	NR
Bertschinger et al.	259	2001	1.5 T	AoI/FP	30	100	100	NR
Loewe et al.	258	2000	1.0 T	3 CS	27	94.7	91.3	NR
Bendib et al.	257	1997	1.5 T	2 FOV	23	91	92	NR

3 CS, three-consecutive-station moving table bolus-chase technique; NR, not reported; AoI, aortoiliac; FP, femoropopliteal arteries; 2 FOV, two consecutive stations imaged with two separate injections of contrast material.
[a]In the case that two different techniques were compared, the best results are reported and number of patients are given for the best technique only.
[b]In the case of multiple readers, the results of the first reader are reported.

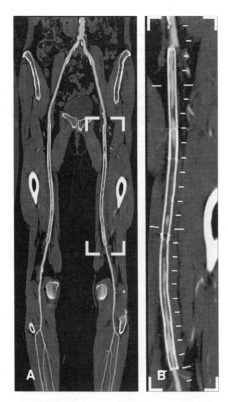

FIGURE 21-65 Stent follow-up with CTA. A: Multipath CPR through the peripheral arterial tree of a patient with prior stent placement in the bilateral superficial femoral arteries. **B:** Close-up view of the left superficial femoral artery demonstrates extensive intimal hyperplasia with multiple high-grade stenoses and occlusion within the stents.

Femorofemoral bypass was widely used for unilateral iliac artery disease, but angioplasty and stenting have resulted in a decrease in the use of this procedure. Femorofemoral bypass can be performed in patients who cannot be revascularized with interventional techniques and

who are poor candidates for direct aortic grafting. It is also used to restore flow to an extremity when one limb of an aortobifemoral graft is occluded and not amenable to thrombectomy or in the setting of acute occlusion from aortic dissection. Five-year patency rates range from 44% to 85%, with the best results obtained when the donor iliac artery and the superficial femoral artery outflow are normal (270).

Thoracic aortofemoral artery bypass is performed in patients with repeated failure of abdominal aortic grafting (Fig. 21-68) or in the hostile abdomen after multiple abdominal surgical procedures in patients who require better inflow than the axillary artery. Patency rates for this bypass at 5 years are approximately 80% (270).

Nonatherosclerotic Causes of Peripheral Arterial Occlusive Disease

Approximately 20% of chronic arterial luminal narrowing or occlusions are caused by conditions other than atherosclerosis. This group of diseases can be divided into systemic vascular diseases with lower extremity involvement or lower extremity diseases with peripheral arterial involvement. Although the spectrum of symptoms is often similar to those seen in APAOD, non-APAOD is usually seen in specific patient groups or at specific anatomic sites or presents with characteristic angiographic features. Obtaining a thorough family history may provide valuable clues with regard to the etiology of the vascular complaints.

Table 21-22 provides an overview of nonatherosclerotic conditions associated with symptoms of peripheral arterial disease. In this section, only conditions involving the lower extremity circulation are discussed. In general, no specific

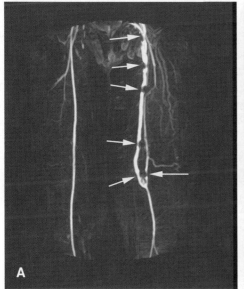
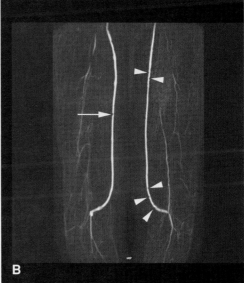

FIGURE 21-66 Signal loss in arterial bypass grafts due to ligating clips. These artifacts are characterized by either complete **(A)** or incomplete **(B)** focal signal loss with an adjacent hyperintense band of signal.

TABLE 21-21

Extent of Artifactual Luminal Narrowing for Different Arterial Stents and Endografts

Graft Type	Manufacturer	Material	Artificial Luminal Narrowing (%) (reference)	Imaging Parameters (FS/PS/TR [milliseconds]/TE [milliseconds])
Noncovered stents				
AVE	Medtronic (Minneapolis, MN)	Stainless steel	30–57 (265)	1.5 T/GRE/4.7/1.9
Cragg Stent	Mintec (Freeport, Bahamas)	Nitinol	16 (266)	1.5T/GRE/6.8/1.4
Easy Wallstent	Schneider (Bülach, Switzerland)	Cobalt alloy	100 (265,266)	1.5 T/GRE/4.7–6.8/ 1.4–1.9
Memotherm iliac	Bard (Karlsruhe, Germany)	Nitinol	4–22 (265)	1.5 T/GRE/4.7/1.9
Palmaz stent	Cordis (Warren, NJ)	Stainless steel	42–100 (265,266)	1.5 T/GRE/4.7–6.8/ 1.4–1.9
Rolling membrane Wallstent	Schneider (Bülach, Switzerland)	Cobalt alloy	32–35 (265)	1.5 T/GRE/4.7/1.9
Sinus iliac	Optimed (Ettlingen, Germany)	Nitinol	9–26 (265)	1.5 T/GRE/4.7/1.9
Smart	Cordis (Warren, NJ)	Nitinol	9–26 (265)	1.5 T/GRE/4.7/1.9
Strecker	Boston Scientific (Natick, MA)	Tantalum	1–19 (265)	1.5 T/GRE/4.7/1.9
Symphony	Boston Scientific (Natick, MA)	Nitinol	8–27 (265)	1.5 T/GRE/4.7/1.9
VascuCoil	Medtronic (Minneapolis, MN)	Nitinol	25–33 (265)	1.5 T/GRE/4.7/1.9
Covered stents				
Corvita stent	Schneider (Bülach, Switzerland)	Cobalt alloy, tantalum core, polycarbonate elastomer	16–33 (266)	1.5 T/GRE/6.8/1.4
Cragg Endopro System 1	Mintec (Freeport, Bahamas)	Nitinol, Dacron cover	0–16 (266)	1.5 T/GRE/6.8/1.4
Hemobahn	Prograft (Palo Alto, CA)	Nitinol, PTFE cover	18–22 (265)	1.5 T/GRE/4.7/1.9
Passager stent	Boston Scientific (Natick, MA)	Nitinol, platinum markers, woven-polyester fabric	1–23 (265,266)	1.5 T/GRE/4.7–6.8/ 1.4–1.9
Endografts				
Ancure	Guidant (Menlo Park, CA)	elgiloy, platinum markers	2–15%[a] (267)	1.5 T/GRE
AneuRx	Medtronic (Santa Rosa, CA)	nitinol, platinum markers	25–34% (267,268)	1.5 T/GRE
Endofit	Endomed (Phoenix, AZ)	nitinol	large artifacts (268)	1.5 T/GRE
Excluder	Gore (Flagstaff, AZ)	nitinol, gold markers	8–15% (267,268)	1.5 T/GRE
Lifepath	Baxter (Morton Grove, IL)	stainless steel	100% (267,268)	1.5 T/GRE
Powerlink	Endologix (Irvine, CA)	stainless steel alloy	large artifacts (268)	1.5 T/GRE
Quantum LP	Cordis (Warren, NJ)	nitinol, tantalum markers	66–71% (267)	1.5 T/GRE
Talent	Medtronic (Santa Rosa, CA)	nitinol	2–7% (267,268)	1.5 T/GRE
Vanguard	Boston Scientific (Natick, MA)	nitinol	little artifacts (268)	1.5 T/GRE
Zenith	Cook (Bloomington, IN)	stainless steel, gold markers	100% (267,268)	1.5 T/GRE

FS, field strength; PS, pulse sequence; TR, repetition time; TE, echo time; GRE, gradient recalled echo.
[a]At attachment site.

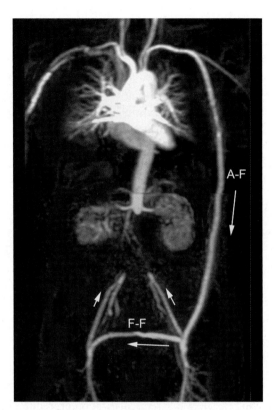

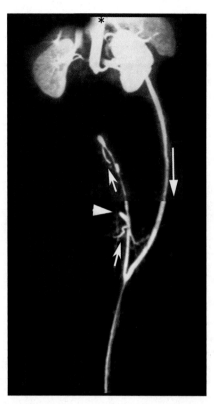

FIGURE 21-67 Extra-anatomic bypass graft in a 46-year-old man who underwent resection of infected native infrarenal aortic aneurysm with placement of left axillobifemoral bypass graft. This spliced MIP from two separate Gd-MRA acquisitions shows a patent axillary limb of left axillobifemoral bypass graft (**A-F**, *descending arrow*). The infrarenal aorta is not seen following ligation and debridement. Discontinuity in the right axillary artery is artifactual and caused by susceptibility effects of concentrated gadolinium during right arm injection. The femorofemoral limb (**F-F**, *left-right arrow*) provides antegrade flow to femoral arteries and fills the iliac arteries (*short arrows*) in a retrograde manner. (Adapted with permission from Krinsky G, Jacobowitz G, Rofsky N. Gadolinium-enhanced MR angiography of extra-anatomic arterial bypass grafts. *AJR Am J Roentgenol.* 1998;170:735–741.)

FIGURE 21-68 Extra-anatomic bypass in a 57-year-old man with history of multiple failed grafts, who underwent resection of infected aortobifemoral graft, ligation of infrarenal aorta, and right leg amputation. This spliced MIP of two consecutive, separate Gd-enhanced MRA acquisitions is comprised of two anatomic segments obtained by using 20 mL of contrast material per segment. Note the extra-anatomic bypass graft (*descending straight arrow*) originating from the descending aorta (*) and anastomosing with the left superficial femoral artery. The native left external iliac, native common iliac, and native common femoral arteries have filled in a retrograde manner (*ascending short arrows*). A small segment of a failed femorofemoral crossover graft (*arrowhead*) can be appreciated.

adaptations of the imaging protocol are necessary when compared with the protocols described previously. Sometimes, there may be a need for associated parenchymal imaging. If necessary, this is mentioned specifically for the condition in question.

Systemic Vascular Diseases with Peripheral Arterial Involvement

Vasculitis

Acute or chronic inflammatory changes of small, medium, and large arteries *or veins* are the hallmarks of vasculitis. In addition to signs and symptoms of peripheral arterial disease, patients with vasculitis frequently also have systemic signs such as fever, malaise, weight loss, and associated rheumatic and cutaneous lesions (271).

Buerger Disease (Thromboangiitis Obliterans)

Buerger disease, or thromboangiitis obliterans (TAO), is a rare segmental inflammatory disease that most commonly affects the small- and medium-sized arteries, veins, and nerves of the arms and legs (272). Buerger disease mainly occurs in young males who have a history of heavy smoking, and the onset of symptoms is almost invariably before the age of 40 to 45 years. The disease should be considered in any young smoking patient with severe peripheral arterial disease. The presence of diabetes mellitus rules out the diagnosis of TAO (273).

Patients may present with claudication of the feet, legs, hands, or arms. As the disease progresses, ischemic pain at rest and ischemic ulcerations on the toes, feet, or fingers may develop. Over 80% of patients present with rest pain and tissue loss.

TABLE 21-22

Nonatherosclerotic Causes of Peripheral Arterial Disease

Conditions associated with vasculitis
Periarteritis nodosa[a]
Hypersensitivity angiitis
   Scleroderma[a]
   Systemic lupus erythematosus[a]
   Serum sickness
   Henoch-Schönlein purpura
   Essential mixed cryoglobulinemia
   Malignancy
Churg-Strauss syndrome
Wegener granulomatosis
Lymphomatoid granulomatosis
Tromboangiitis obliterans (Buerger disease)[a]
Giant cell arteritis
   Temporal arteritis
   Nonspecific aortoarteritis (Takayasu disease)[a]
Miscellaneous vasculitis syndromes
   Relapsing polychondritis[a]
   Behçet disease[a]
   Mucocutaneous lymph node syndrome (Kawasaki syndrome)[a]
   Erythema nodosum
   Hypocomplementemic vasculitis
   Rheumatoid syndromes[a]
Congenital hereditary diseases with arterial involvement
Marfan syndrome[a]
Ehlers-Danlos syndrome[a]
Pseudoxanthoma elasticum[a]
   Homocystinurea[a]
   Neurofibromatosis[a]
   Tuberous sclerosis[a] (Pringle-Bourneville disease)
Congenital nonhereditary diseases with arterial involvement
Cystic adventitial disease[a]
Popliteal artery entrapment syndrome[a]
Persistent sciatic artery[a]
Abdominal aortic hypoplasia[a]
Acquired conditions presenting with symptoms of peripheral arterial disease
Vascular tumors[a]
AIDS-related vasculopathy[a]
Radiation-induced arterial injury[a]
Iliac syndrome in cyclists[a]
Excessive use of ergot alkaloids (ergotism)[a]
Arterial medial fibrodysplasia[a]

[a]Entities involving larger blood vessels.
Source: Based on Rooke TW, Joyce JW. Uncommon arteriopathies. In: Rutherford RB, ed. *Vascular Surgery.* 5th ed. Philadelphia, PA: WB Saunders; 2000:418–434.

Angiographically, TAO is characterized by segmental occlusive lesions (diseased arteries interspersed with normal-appearing arteries) in small- and medium-sized vessels, such as the palmar, plantar, tibial, peroneal, radial, and ulnar arteries and the digital arteries of the fingers and toes. Disease is more severe distally, and proximal arteries are usually normal.

There is a typical pattern of corkscrew collaterals bridging occlusions and no apparent source of emboli. Surgical revascularization is rarely possible for patients with Buerger disease because of the diffuse segmental involvement and distal nature of the disease (Fig. 21-69). Often, no distal target vessel is available for bypass surgery. The only definitive therapy for TAO is complete cessation of smoking.

Takayasu Arteritis

Takayasu arteritis (TA), also known as pulseless disease, is a large vessel vasculitis usually involving the aorta, its main offshoots, and the upper extremities. In up to 15% of cases, the iliac artery and its branches are involved (274).

The successful treatment of TA is limited by both imperfect medical and surgical therapies. Inflammatory aspects of TA are treated with corticosteroids and, in selected patients, other immunosuppressive agents.

Lower extremity revascularization procedures are pursued when extremity ischemia limits routine activities of daily living (275). While revascularization procedures in TA

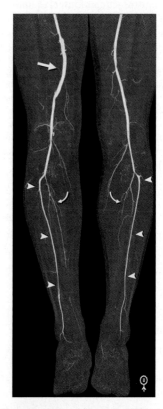

FIGURE 21-69 Thromboangiitis obliterans in a 39-year-old man (64-channel MDCT, 64 × 0.6 mm, 40-seconds scan time). MIP of both thighs and calves shows short, patent femoropopliteal bypass graft (*arrow*) on the right. Note the severely diseased infrageniculate arteries. The anterior tibial arteries are best preserved (*arrowheads*), whereas the peroneal and posterior tibial arteries (*curved arrows*) are occluded bilaterally.

(surgical or percutaneous) are safe and associated with low morbidity and mortality outcomes, as defined by vessel patency, outcomes are influenced by the type of intervention (276). Good short-term outcomes are obtained regardless of the revascularization approach. The best long-term outcomes are achieved by open surgical approaches with bypass grafts as compared with patch angioplasty, endarterectomy, and endovascular revascularization procedures (276,277).

Giant Cell Arteritis

Patients with giant cell arteritis usually suffer from aortic and aortic branch stenoses or temporal arteritis. Large vessel upper extremity involvement is common, but patients may present with symptoms of claudication in the lower extremity. Females are predominantly affected (278).

Giant cell arteritis is characterized angiographically by *symmetric bilateral* stenoses and poststenotic aneurysmal dilatations. Stenoses have a smooth, tapering or "hourglass" aspect. There is usually a rich collateral supply due to the chronic nature of the disease. Ergotism is the main differential diagnosis. With MRI, it may be useful to obtain a delayed T1-weighted postcontrast scan of the vessel in question, as this may provide direct information about inflammatory activity in the vessel wall (279,280).

Periarteritis Nodosa

Periarteritis nodosa is a type of vasculitis that involves the small- and medium-sized arteries of almost all organs. In about 20% of patients, there are characteristic small aneurysms in the visceral, renal, or distal limb vessels. These aneurysms may rupture but regress when patients are treated with steroids (271).

Behçet Disease

Behçet disease is a vasculitis that affects small and large arteries and veins. A major problem is thrombosis, for which lifelong treatment with anticoagulants is necessary. Involvement of all named arteries has been described and consists of arterial thrombosis and saccular aneurysm formation (Fig. 21-70) (281). There is an increased rate of false aneurysm formation at the site of arterial or venous puncture in patients with Behçet disease (282).

Kawasaki Disease

Also known as the mucocutaneous lymph node syndrome, Kawasaki disease is almost exclusively seen in children. Occasionally, aneurysms are found in the upper extremity arteries; the abdominal aorta; and the renal, hepatic and iliac arteries (284). The main clinical problem is aneurysm formation in the coronary arteries, seen in up to 15% of patients (285). Coronary aneurysms can be detected and followed up with coronary MRA (286,287).

AIDS-related Vasculopathy

Infection with HIV and subsequent development of AIDS is known to present with large vessel involvement and aneurysm formation (128,288).

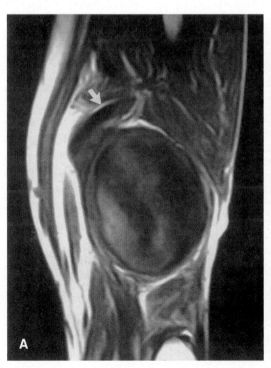
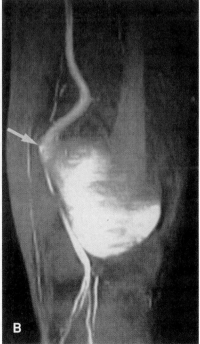

FIGURE 21-70 Popliteal aneurysm in a 30-year-old man with Behçet disease. A: T1-weighted spin echo coronal image of the left knee. Large pseudoaneurysm with central flow void and peripheral thrombus is seen. The popliteal artery (*arrow*) is displaced by the lesion. **B:** 2D-TOF MRA. The neck of the aneurysm (*arrow*) and the displacement of the parent popliteal artery are clearly depicted. (Reprinted with permission from Berkmen T. MR angiography of aneurysms in Behçet disease: a report of four cases. *J Comput Assist Tomogr.* 1998;22:202–206.)

Hereditary Connective Tissue Disorders with Peripheral Arterial Involvement

Marfan Syndrome

Marfan syndrome is caused by an autosomal dominant defect in the cross linking of collagen, and those affected usually come to medical attention when still teenagers (289). About 95% of patients have cardiovascular involvement, mainly aneurysms of the ascending aorta (290). When patients present with symptoms of peripheral arterial disease (291), an active search should be performed for dissections in the descending aorta.

Ehlers-Danlos Syndrome

There are now ten clinical subtypes of Ehlers-Danlos syndrome, an autosomal dominant disease caused by faults in the conversion of procollagen to collagen, leading to diffuse thinning of the arterial media (289,292). In terms of arterial involvement, type IV (arterial-ecchymotic type) is the most important (293). Patients may present with spontaneous arterial rupture, dissections, and arteriovenous fistulas.

Pseudoxanthoma Elasticum

Pseudoxanthoma elasticum is an autosomal recessive disorder that is associated with the accumulation of mineralized and fragmented elastic fibers in the skin, the Bruch membrane in the retina, and in vessel walls (294). Reduction or absence of upper and lower extremity pulses with sparing of the aorta and its branches are characteristic for pseudoxanthoma elasticum. Partially occlusive lower extremity lesions, especially of the femoropopliteal segment, and totally occlusive lesions of the distal upper extremity arteries are common (295).

Other Hereditary Diseases with Peripheral Arterial Involvement

Homocystinuria

Classic homocystinuria is an aminoacidopathy due to cystathionine beta-synthase deficiency (296). Untreated patients with homocystinuria have severe hyperhomocysteinanemia. Pathological sequelae include mental retardation, ectopia lentis, and osteoporosis. However, accelerated atherosclerosis and thrombosis in the arterial and venous systems remain the major cause of morbidity and mortality in untreated patients. If left untreated, half of all patients will have an event before age 30 years. Of note, many patients who present with premature vascular disease have mild hyperhomocysteinanemia (297).

Neurofibromatosis

Neurofibromatosis is an autosomal, dominantly inherited, progressive, generalized dysplasia of mesodermal and neu-roectodermal tissues. Affected patients present in their second and third decades with hypertension and sometimes claudication. The renal arteries are frequently affected as well. Vascular lesions associated with neurofibromatosis are mainly characterized by stenosis, occlusion, aneurysm, pseudoaneurysm, and rupture or fistula formation of small-, medium-, and large-sized arteries (298,299).

Congenital Vascular Diseases Presenting with Symptoms of Peripheral Arterial Occlusive Disease

Congenital Aortic Hypoplasia

Developmental narrowings of the abdominal aorta are rare anomalies and account for fewer than 2% of all aortic coarctations (44,300). Localized segmental narrowings are termed *coarctations*, but when the stenosis extends over a longer distance, the term *hypoplasia* is used (301). No apparent gender predilection has been described, with 46% of affected subjects being male and 54% female (302). The principal clinical features described in reports of children and neonates with this condition are renovascular hypertension resulting from renal artery stenosis and arterial insufficiency of the lower extremities. Due to extensive collateral development, the latter condition is often well tolerated (Fig. 21-71). Physical examination often reveals diminished or absent femoral pulses and an abdominal bruit, generated by turbulent flow in constricted vessels or collateral vessels.

Persistent Sciatic Artery

The sciatic artery is a continuation of the internal iliac artery into the popliteal-tibial arterial axis and provides the major supply to the lower limb bud in early embryologic development (Fig. 21-44). Persistent sciatic artery is a rare congenital anatomical variant in which the primitive artery persists as the legs' major inflow artery. This condition may present with pulsatile mass because of aneurysm formation (303,304). The superficial femoral artery is often hypoplastic or absent. The sciatic artery may be affected by atherosclerosis and cause symptoms of intermittent claudication. Bilateral involvement has been described in up to 50% of cases (305). On physical examination, an apparent paradox is created when the femoral pulse is absent, yet distal pulses are normal, being supplied by the persistent sciatic artery, which enters the leg through the sciatic notch. This is known as the *Cowie sign* (295).

Acquired Conditions Presenting with Symptoms of Peripheral Arterial Disease

Ergotism

Ergotism is a condition characterized by generalized vasoconstriction caused by (excessive) ingestion of

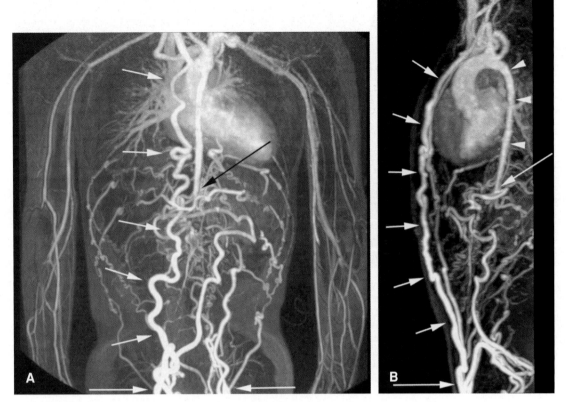

FIGURE 21-71 MRA of congenital aortic hypoplasia in an 8-year-old male. A: Coronal MIP of torso and arms. The descending aorta is hypoplastic and terminates at the level of the kidneys (*black arrow*). The lower extremities receive their blood supply from extensive collaterals in the abdominal wall, such the anastomoses between the right internal thoracic artery and the inferior epigastric artery (*short white arrows* in **A** and **B**) and the lower intercostals and deep circumflex iliac arteries on both sides (*long white arrows* in **A** and **B**). **B:** Sagittal MIP of same imaging volume. (*Arrowheads*, descending aorta; *short white arrows*, anastomosis between the right internal thoracic artery and the inferior epigastric artery; *oblique long white arrow*, termination of descending aorta.)

ergot-containing medications, illicit drugs (lysergic acid diethylamide [LSD]), or foods containing the fungus *Claviceps purpurae*. Ergotamine tartrate and methysergide maleate are prescribed for treatment of migraine headaches and in obstetrics. Dihydroergotamine is used for prevention of deep venous thrombosis (306). The mechanism of action is α-adrenergic blockade mediated vasoconstriction, primarily in the peripheral arteries. Symptoms include intermittent claudication, rest pain, and sometimes tissue loss (306). Angiographic findings are bilateral symmetric vasoconstriction that begins abruptly (305).

External Iliac Artery Endofibrosis (Iliac Syndrome in Cyclists)

Exercise-induced intimal fibrosis affecting mainly the iliac artery is a relatively recently described entity that is a cause of unexplained recurrent lower limb pain in young endurance athletes (307,308). Symptoms often only occur under maximal stress. Approximately one in five top-level cyclists will develop sports-related flow limitations in the iliac arteries (309). There is no relationship with the classical risk factors for atherosclerosis like smoking, hypercholesterolemia, or family predisposition for arterial diseases. The patient's history is paramount for diagnosis (310). Imaging performed in flexion can be helpful (Fig. 21-72).

Vascular Neoplasms

Primary vascular neoplasms of the extremities are rare and are discussed in Chapter 22.

Miscellaneous Conditions

Patients with acute arterial occlusions should be treated for atrial fibrillation, if present, and a careful search must be performed for signs of ulcerative endocarditis as well as

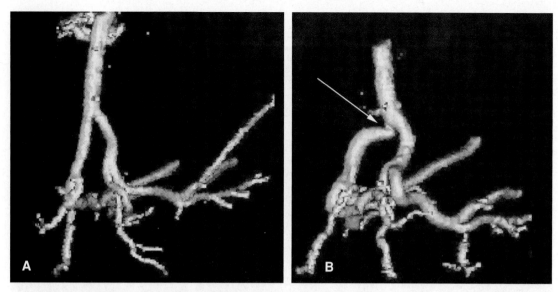

FIGURE 21-72 External iliac artery endofibrosis. Shaded-surface display images of the aortoiliac tree obtained with MRA with flexed hips. Both images are positioned to obtain approximately the same orientation (an oblique posterior view of the arteries with the left artery on the left side). **A:** Reference subject with arteries that run smoothly and straight. **B:** A patient with left-sided iliac artery flow limitations. Note the severe kinking that is visible in the proximal common iliac artery (*arrow*). (Image courtesy of Goof Schep, MD, PhD, Department of Sports Medicine, Maxima Medical Center, Veldhoven, the Netherlands.) (Reprinted with permission from Bender MH, Schep G, de Vries WR, et al. Sports-related flow limitations in the iliac arteries in endurance athletes: aetiology, diagnosis, treatment and future developments. *Sports Med.* 2004;34:427–442.)

mural thrombi overlying the site of myocardial infarction and in aneurysms. Congenital and acquired clotting disorders may also manifest with symptoms of peripheral arterial disease.

Lower Extremity Disease with Peripheral Arterial Involvement

Popliteal Artery Entrapment

The current classification of popliteal arterial entrapment is best explained and understood when based on developmental anatomy of the popliteal fossa (311,312). The mid portion of the popliteal artery (above the upper margin of the popliteus muscle) is a direct remnant of the original axial artery. The definitive distal portion (and "trifurcation") of the popliteal artery is formed by coalescing segments of the newly formed posterior tibial (saphenous) and anterior tibial segments, which are all formed superficially relative to the popliteus muscle.

The original distal popliteal portion of the axial artery runs deep to the popliteus muscle and normally involutes or persists as a small, deep popliteal artery. The development of the "superficial" distal third of the definitive popliteal artery during the 20- to 22-mm stage of the embryo normally takes place after the migration of the

medial head of the gastrocnemius muscle. This muscle mass originates from the posterior aspect of the fibula and lateral tibia, migrates across the popliteal fossa medially, and then finally ascends to the area immediately above the medial femoral condyle.

Types I to III of the popliteal arterial entrapment syndrome represent a continuum of abnormalities where the popliteal artery is "caught" and compressed by the medially migrating medial head of the gastrocnemius muscle (Fig. 21-73). The artery is displaced medially by a fully migrated (I), not fully migrated (II), or a portion (III) of the medial gastrocnemius head, causing narrowing of the popliteal artery, notably with muscle contraction. Type IV is a different developmental abnormality, not related to the gastrocnemius muscle. If the primitive axial artery persists, it lies deep to the popliteus muscle, causing substantial narrowing and arterial damage.

When an entrapment mechanism includes the popliteal artery and vein, this has been termed *type V entrapment* (311). A condition of symptomatic entrapment with stress maneuvers without anatomic abnormality has been termed *type VI* (313). Of note, functional compression with complete interruption of blood flow can also be observed in normal asymptomatic individuals (314).

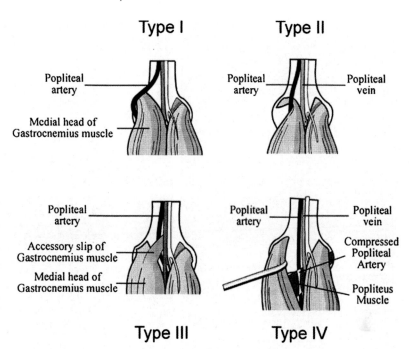

FIGURE 21-73 Types I to IV of popliteal artery entrapment. (Reprinted with permission from Levien LJ, Veller MG. Popliteal artery entrapment syndrome: more common than previously recognized. *J Vasc Surg.* 1999;30:587–598.)

Popliteal entrapment is primarily a disease of young men (male-to-female ratio is 9:1) and presents with calf or foot claudication. It is bilateral in up to 25% of patients (315).

Angiographically, the diagnosis is suggested when there is medial deviation of the proximal popliteal artery (P1 segment) in combination with segmental occlusion or post-stenotic dilatation (145). If no abnormality is seen, additional "stress" views should be obtained during dorsiflexion (with contracted gastrocnemius muscles) (192). The relationship of the popliteal artery to the surrounding soft tissues can be easily demonstrated by reviewing the source images (Fig. 21-74).

CTA and MRA can demonstrate the vessel lumen as well as the surrounding anatomy, facilitating an assessment of the artery–muscle relationship. For MRA, gadolinium-enhanced injections in stress and relaxed maneuvers can be obtained; however, excellent results are readily achieved with flow-sensitive GRE imaging.

Cystic Adventitial Disease

Cystic adventitial disease is due to extrinsic compression of peripheral arteries close to joints by mucoid cysts in the arterial adventitia. In over 85% of cases this concerns the popliteal artery, but the external iliac, common femoral, radial, and ulnar arteries may also be affected (145). The pathogenesis is unknown. Patients are usually males between the ages of 40 and 50 presenting with symptoms of intermittent claudication or popliteal soft tissue mass (316). The diagnosis can be difficult, as APAOD is much more prevalent in this age group (317).

If the cysts are concentric, the arterial lumen will have a smooth "hourglass" shape; if the stenosis is eccentric, the residual lumen will display a "scimitar sign" (Fig. 21-75). When cystic adventitial disease is suspected, MR is the imaging modality of choice, as it can readily demonstrate the arterial stenosis as well as the cysts in addition to other soft tissue and osseous abnormalities. Thus, as an adjunct to the MR angiogram, axial T1- and T2-weighted images should be obtained. On T1-weighted images, cysts have variable signal intensity due to the variable amount of mucoid material. On T2-weighted images, cysts are hyperintense (Fig. 21-76).

In CT, the cystic lesion demonstrates near-water CT attenuation values on transverse source or MPR images. MIP or VR images show the associated luminal narrowing, but the diagnostic information is in the source images (Fig. 21-77).

Radiation-induced Arterial Disease

Radiation therapy is occasionally associated with peripheral arterial disease and may present with intermittent claudication. The affected artery may become fibrotic or stenotic or suffer from accelerated atherosclerosis. Usually, these complications arise several years after therapy (Fig. 21-78). The history provides the most important clue to the diagnosis.

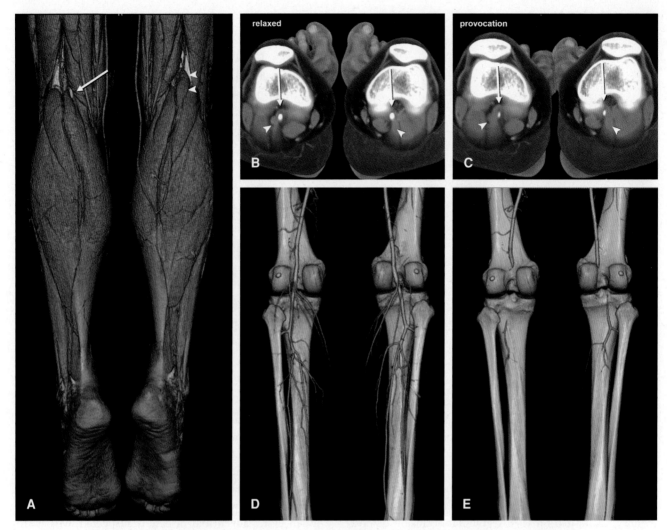

FIGURE 21-74 Bilateral popliteal arterial entrapment syndrome. A: VR posterior view of the calves shows medial course of the left popliteal artery (*arrow*). Note that there is an abnormal accessory slip of the right medial head of the gastrocnemius muscle (*arrowheads*) consistent with type III popliteal arterial entrapment. Grayscale VR images **(B, C)** show that the popliteal artery (*arrows*) runs medial to the medial head of the gastrocnemius muscle (*arrowheads*) bilaterally, with significant narrowing during provocation maneuver **(C)**. Corresponding relaxed and provocation vascular views **(D, E)** show complete obstruction of blood flow during muscle contraction **(E)**.

Trauma

The prevalence of noniatrogenic extremity artery injuries and the different mechanisms of injuries in the civilian population depend on geographic and social factors. In urban environments, for example, arterial injuries most often result from penetrating gunshot or knife wounds (318). The most common causes of blunt injury are motor vehicle accidents and falls. The morbidity of both blunt and penetrating injuries (notably with high-velocity firearms) can be magnified by associated fractures, dislocations, and crush injuries to muscles and nerves (319). The incidence of arterial injury following penetrating (upper and lower) extremity trauma is approximately 10%, in

contrast with 1% following blunt trauma. In contrast, a blunt mechanism accounts for 27% of popliteal artery injuries.

Pathologically, the most common type of arterial injury is a partial laceration or complete transection. Complete transection leads to vessel retraction and thrombosis with subsequent ischemia, whereas partial laceration causes persistent bleeding and/or pseudoaneurysm formation. Both lacerations as well as arterial contusions can be accompanied by intimal flaps, which in turn may or may not lead to vascular obstruction and thrombosis. Concomitant arterial and venous injuries may lead to traumatic arteriovenous fistulas.

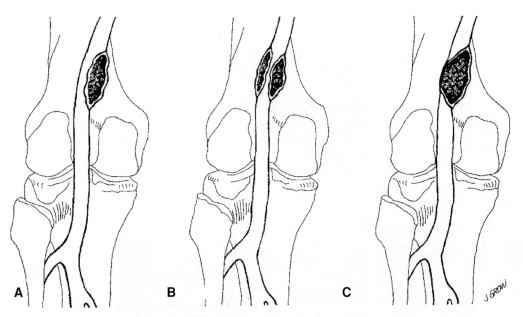

FIGURE 21-75 Adventitial cysts may appear in variable locations on the popliteal artery. The expanding cyst may indent the artery (**A**), the scimitar sign; encircle the artery (**B**), the hourglass sign; or completely occlude the vessel (**C**). (Reprinted with permission from Levien LL, Bergan JJ. Adventitial cystic disease of the popliteal artery. In: Rutherford RB, ed. *Vascular Surgery*. 5th ed. Philadelphia, PA: WB Saunders; 2000:1079.)

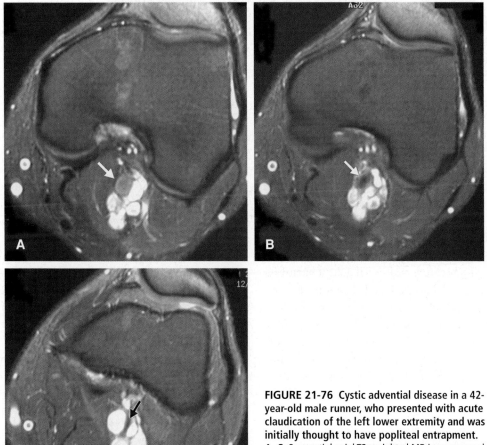

FIGURE 21-76 Cystic advential disease in a 42-year-old male runner, who presented with acute claudication of the left lower extremity and was initially thought to have popliteal entrapment. **A–C:** Sequential axial T2-weighted MR images reveal extensive compression of the popliteal artery by cystic advential disease (*arrow*). (Adapted from Wright LB, Matchett WJ, Cruz CP, et al. Popliteal artery disease: diagnosis and treatment. *Radiographics*. 2004;24: 467–479.)

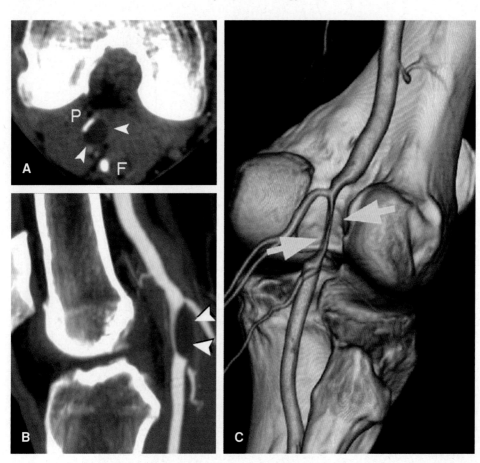

FIGURE 21-77 Adventitial cystic disease in a 55-year-old internist. A: Axial source image from peripheral CTA. There is marked compression of the popliteal artery (*P*) by an ovoid fluid-density lesion (*arrowheads*). Note the predominant transverse compression of the flow lumen. (**F,** fabella.) **B:** Corresponding sagittal thin-slab MIP shows craniocaudal extent of fluid-density lesion in the popliteal arterial wall (*arrowheads*). **C:** VR image viewed obliquely from posteriorly demonstrates severe narrowing of the right popliteal artery (*arrows*). (Reprinted with permission from Fleischmann D, Hallett RL, Rubin GD. CT angiography of peripheral arterial disease. *J Vasc Interv Radiol.* 2006;17: 3–26.)

The most common clinical presentation of traumatic vascular injury is acute ischemia. This holds true for both penetrating and blunt trauma associated with fractures (femoral shaft, proximal tibia) and dislocations (posterior knee dislocations). In general, the clinical signs and symptoms of vascular injury are divided into hard and soft categories, which determine if a patient needs to undergo immediate surgery and/or if imaging is required.

Angiography has been the traditional gold standard for assessing extremity arterial injuries, and the indications for vascular imaging in this setting have been well studied and built into a diagnostic algorithm (320) (Fig. 21-79). With the increasing 24-hour availability of modern MDCT scanners in the emergency setting, however, diagnostic angiography is gradually replaced by CTA. CTA—even with single detector-row scanners—has been shown to be an accurate and useful test in the setting of suspected vascular trauma (321). CT is easily accessible, and exam time is short. Moreover, CTA can be performed in combination with CT of other organ systems (abdomen, chest, etc.) for complete delineation of the distribution and severity of injuries in each individual organ system (322) in the adult and in the pediatric population (322).

Traumatic arterial injuries and the relationship of arterial segments to adjacent fractures and soft tissue injuries are well depicted (Fig. 21-80). CTA reliably depicts hematoma, associated vascular compression, or pseudoaneurysm and can simultaneously show bone fragments. Bullets or other metal artifacts, if present, may limit small portions of the acquired volume.

For initial diagnosis, transverse images are usually sufficient, although multiplanar image reconstruction and viewing may improve rapidity of analysis (Fig. 21-81). The addition of VR images improves depiction of the anatomic relationship between arteries and adjacent bony/soft tissue injuries and foreign bodies. Generation of real-time 3D and/or VR images also promotes rapid communication to, and understanding by, referring clinical services.

Developments in Lower Extremity Magnetic Resonance Angiography

Currently used CE MRA techniques rely on rapid sequential data acquisition during the first arterial passage of intravenously injected extracellular contrast material to depict the peripheral vascular tree. The availability of 3.0 T (Fig. 21-82) and higher field-strength magnets (323) as

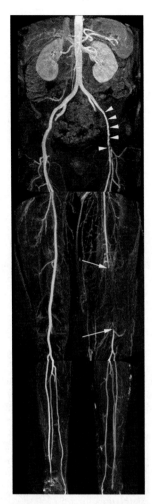

FIGURE 21-78 Radiation-induced peripheral arterial disease. Multistation composite MIP of the lower extremity vasculature demonstrates radiation-induced peripheral arterial disease of left external iliac and common femoral arteries (*arrowheads*). This 66-year-old patient had undergone surgery and radiation therapy for a soft tissue sarcoma 15 years earlier. The patient presented with severe intermittent claudication. The occlusion of the superficial femoral and popliteal arteries (*between arrows*) was due to embolization.

well as further improvements in MRI gradient technology and coil design, and refinements in pulse sequences combined with the use of higher-relaxivity contrast agents (114,115) will also offer significant advantages over current protocols. In the short term, significant advances will come from the application of multiple-station parallel imaging capable coils (94) and coils with much higher numbers of elements (324) that will allow increased acquisition speed and reduce the problem of disturbing venous overlay. Another technical advance that holds considerable promise for the future is *continuously* moving table MRA, which was recently described by Kruger et al. (325) and Sabati et al. (326). The potential advantage of this technique is the ability to track the injected contrast bolus in

real time and to end the acquisition prior to deep venous enhancement.

A different approach to peripheral MRA is the use of contrast agents that remain in the intravascular space for a prolonged period of time, the so-called "blood pool" agents. In the near future, the first generation of blood pool agents is expected to become commercially available (327). Intravascular agents will improve CE MRA on both state-of-the-art as well as older and slower MRI scanners. CE MRA on state-of-the-art systems will benefit from the higher relaxivity of intravascular agents, that is, the loss in vessel-to-background contrast with the use of ultrafast gradient systems, and parallel imaging will be offset because of much faster T1 relaxation in blood. Conversely, CE MRA on older and slower MRI systems will benefit from the longer residence time in the vasculature of these agents. Because of this, synchronization of acquisition with peak arterial enhancement during the first bolus passage will no longer be necessary. However, the problem with data acquisition during the so-called steady-state is simultaneous enhancement of veins. The development of image-processing approaches to artery–vein separation has recently begun, and preliminary results are encouraging (328,329).

The abundance of different MRI techniques and pulse sequences also allows for the extraction of *functional* information in the same imaging session. In a recent study, Zhang et al. (330) demonstrated enhancing soft tissue "spots" at TR 2D projection MRA of the knee, calf, and foot. They found enhancing lesions to be significantly more prevalent in patients with diabetes mellitus. At subsequent follow-up, 13% of patients developed cellulitis or ulceration at the location of the enhancing spot. This finding indicates the ability of CE MRA not only to identify arterial obstructions but also points to a potential role in the prevention of pedal injury and complications.

A combined MRA and magnetic resonance spectroscopy (MRS) approach is also likely to play a prominent role in further understanding the disease process and in the evaluation of novel therapies for severe peripheral arterial disease such as growth-factor augmented collateral vessel development.

In a preliminary study on this subject, Baumgartner and associates (331) demonstrated that a combined protocol, where MRA was used to demonstrate presence of collaterals and MRS of deoxyhemoglobin was used to assess tissue perfusion, was helpful to document therapeutic changes in patients with chronic critical ischemia.

Spectroscopy at 3 T offers improved spectral resolution and the opportunity to assess phosphorus metabolites in a reasonable time period to probe the energetic of the affected muscles. Recent work has suggested links between reduced

(*text continues on page 1008*)

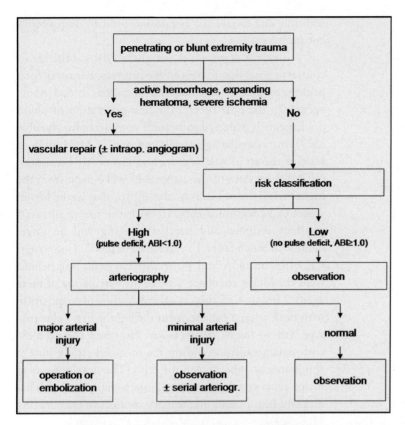

FIGURE 21-79 Diagnostic algorithm for extremity arterial trauma. (ABI, ankle-brachial index.) (Reprinted with permission from Hood DB, Yellin AE, Weaver FA. Vascular trauma. In: Dean R, ed. *Current Vascular Surgical Diagnosis and Treatment*. Norwalk, CT: Appleton & Lange; 1995:405.)

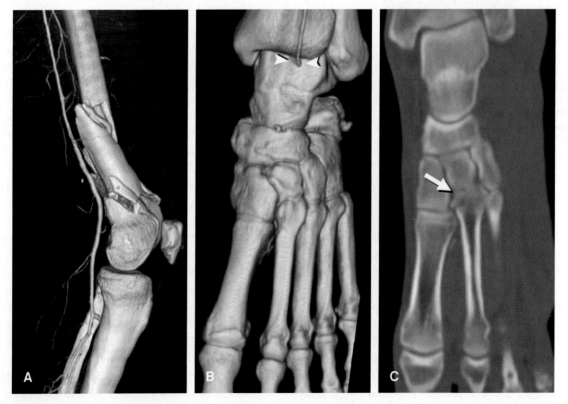

FIGURE 21-80 Peripheral CTA of blunt trauma. This 53-year-old man, who was involved in a motorcycle accident and sustained a left femoral fracture and knee laceration, presented with no palpable dorsalis pedis pulse, but faint Doppler signal was present. **A:** VR view of the left thigh and knee region demonstrates a comminuted distal femoral shaft fracture with mild displacement of the femoropopliteal artery but no evidence of hemorrhage of obstruction. **B:** VR view of the left foot shows abrupt occlusion of the dorsalis pedis artery (*arrowheads*), likely caused by arterial contusion and thrombosis, as suggested by the occult fracture of the base of the second metatarsal bone (*arrow*) in the corresponding reformatted image **(C)**.

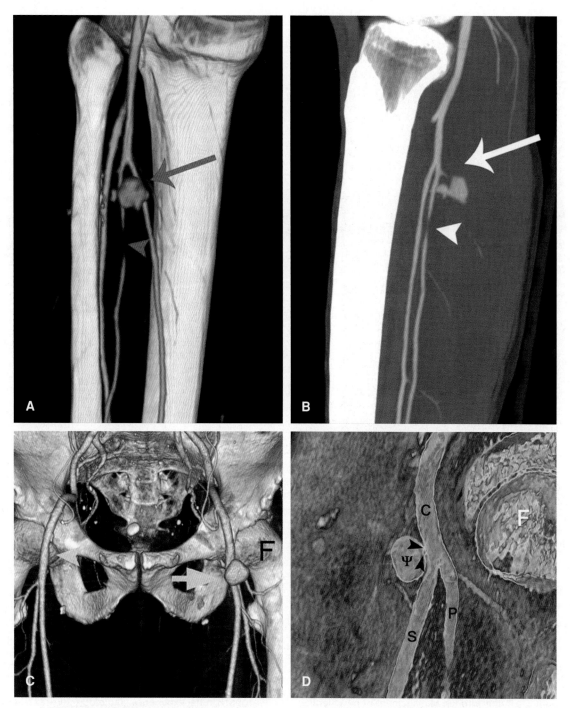

FIGURE 21-81 Peripheral CTA of penetrating trauma. A, B: A 16-year-old male status post gunshot wound to left leg. **A:** Posterior VR image and **(B)** oblique thin-slab MIP of the left calf shows a lobulated pseudoaneurysm arising from the peroneal artery (*arrow*). The immediate distal peroneal artery shows luminal narrowing, most likely spasm (*arrowhead*). The remainder of the trifurcation vessels and adjacent bony structures are intact. **C, D:** A 45-year-old man with groin hematoma after cardiac catheterization. **C:** VR image of the pelvis shows a rounded mass at the left common femoral bifurcation (*arrow*), consistent with pseudoaneurysm. The contralateral right common femoral artery is normal (*arrowhead*). (F, femoral head.) **D:** Sagittal thin-slab VR image with opacity transfer function set to render translucent vessel interior demonstrates a narrow neck (*arrowheads*) of the pseudoaneurysm (ψ), which arises from the common femoral artery (C) immediately proximal to the bifurcation of the superficial femoral (S) and profunda femoris (P) arteries. (F, femoral head.) (Reprinted with permission from Fleischmann D, Hallett RL, Rubin GD. CT angiography of peripheral arterial disease. *J Vasc Interv Radiol*. 2006;17:3–26.)

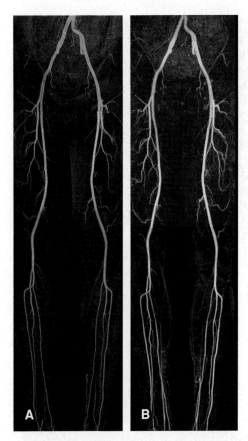

FIGURE 21-82 Peripheral MR angiograms in a 31-year-old healthy volunteer at 1.5 T **(A)** and 3.0 T **(B)**. Both images are coronal, four-station MIP images of the peripheral arteries. Note better visibility of distal arteries at 3.0 T **(B)**. Window and level settings were identical for both data sets. (Reprinted with permission from Leiner T, De Vries M, Hoogeveen R, et al. Contrast-enhanced peripheral MR angiography at 3.0 Tesla: initial experience with a whole-body scanner in healthy volunteers. *J Magn Reson Imaging.* 2003;17:609–614.)

energy reserves observed in the foot muscles of diabetics and impaired microcirculation, suggesting that microcirculation could be a major reason for this difference (332).

REFERENCES

1. Dormandy JA, Rutherford RB. Management of peripheral arterial disease (PAD). TASC Working Group. TransAtlantic Inter-Society Consensus (TASC). *J Vasc Surg.* 2000;31:S1–S296.
2. Dormandy JA, Ray S. The natural history of peripheral arterial disease. In: Tooke JE, Lowe GD, eds. *A Textbook of Vascular Medicine.* London: Arnold; 1996:162–175.
3. Stoffers HE, Kester AD, Kaiser V, et al. Diagnostic value of signs and symptoms associated with peripheral arterial occlusive disease seen in general practice: a multivariable approach. *Med Decis Making.* 1997;17:61–70.
4. Rutherford RB, Baker JD, Ernst C, et al. Recommended standards for reports dealing with lower extremity ischemia: revised version. *J Vasc Surg.* 1997;26:517–538.
5. Beebe HG. Intermittent claudication: effective medical management of a common circulatory problem. *Am J Cardiol.* 2001;87:14D–18D.
6. Regensteiner JG, Gardner A, Hiatt WR. Exercise testing and exercise rehabilitation for patients with peripheral arterial disease: status in 1997. *Vasc Med.* 1997;2:147–155.
7. Gardner AW, Poehlman ET. Exercise rehabilitation programs for the treatment of claudication pain. A meta-analysis. *JAMA.* 1995;274:975–980.
8. Rutkow IM, Ernst CB. An analysis of vascular surgical manpower requirements and vascular surgical rates in the United States. *J Vasc Surg.* 1986;3:74–83.
9. Rudofsky G. Peripheral arterial disease: chronic ischemic syndromes. In: Lanzer P, Topol EJ, eds. *Pan Vascular Medicine.* Berlin: Springer; 2003:1363–1422.
10. Rofsky NM, Adelman MA. MR angiography in the evaluation of atherosclerotic peripheral vascular disease. *Radiology.* 2000;214:325–338.
11. Waugh JR, Sacharias N. Arteriographic complications in the DSA era. *Radiology.* 1992;182:243–246.
12. Dalman RL, Taylor LM Jr. Basic data related to infrainguinal revascularization procedures. *Ann Vasc Surg.* 1990;4:309–312.
13. Kalra M, Gloviczki P, Bower TC, et al. Limb salvage after successful pedal bypass grafting is associated with improved long-term survival. *J Vasc Surg.* 2001;33:6–16.
14. Beard JD, Scott DJ, Evans JM, et al. Pulse-generated runoff: a new method of determining calf vessel patency. *Br J Surg.* 1988;75:361–363.
15. Owen RS, Carpenter JP, Baum RA, et al. Magnetic resonance imaging of angiographically occult runoff vessels in peripheral arterial occlusive disease. *N Engl J Med.* 1992;326:1577–1581.
16. Wilson YG, George JK, Wilkins DC, et al. Duplex assessment of run-off before femorocrural reconstruction. *Br J Surg.* 1997;84:1360–1363.
17. Currie IC, Jones AJ, Wakeley CJ, et al. Non-invasive aortoiliac assessment. *Eur J Vasc Endovasc Surg.* 1995;9:24–28.
18. de Smet AA, Ermers EJ, Kitslaar PJ. Duplex velocity characteristics of aortoiliac stenoses. *J Vasc Surg.* 1996;23:628–636.
19. Ubbink DT, Fidler M, Legemate DA. Interobserver variability in aortoiliac and femoropopliteal duplex scanning. *J Vasc Surg.* 2001;33:540–545.
20. Visser K, Hunink MG. Peripheral arterial disease: gadolinium-enhanced MR angiography versus color-guided duplex US—a meta-analysis. *Radiology.* 2000;216:67–77.
21. Leiner T, Kessels AG, Nelemans PJ, et al. Peripheral arterial disease: comparison of color duplex US and contrast-enhanced MR angiography for diagnosis. *Radiology.* 2005;235:699–708.
22. Visser K, Bosch JL, Leiner T, et al. Patients' preferences for MR angiography and duplex US in the work-up of peripheral arterial disease. *Eur J Vasc Endovasc Surg.* 2003;26:537–543.
23. Rubin GD, Schmidt AJ, Logan LJ, et al. Multidetector-row CT angiography of lower extremity occlusive disease: a new application for CT scanning. *Radiology.* 1999;210:588.
24. Rubin GD, Schmidt AJ, Logan LJ, et al. Multi-detector row CT angiography of lower extremity arterial inflow and runoff: initial experience. *Radiology.* 2001;221:146–158.
25. Ofer A, Nitecki SS, Linn S, et al. Multidetector CT angiography of peripheral vascular disease: a prospective comparison with intraarterial digital subtraction angiography. *AJR Am J Roentgenol.* 2003;180:719–724.
26. Weber OM, Martin AJ, Higgins CB. Whole-heart steady-state free precession coronary artery magnetic resonance angiography. *Magn Reson Med.* 2003;50:1223–1228.
27. Ota H, Takase K, Igarashi K, et al. MDCT compared with digital subtraction angiography for assessment of lower extremity arterial occlusive disease: importance of reviewing cross-sectional images. *AJR Am J Roentgenol.* 2004;182:201–209.
28. Catalano C, Fraioli F, Laghi A, et al. Infrarenal aortic and lower-extremity arterial disease: diagnostic performance of multi-detector row CT angiography. *Radiology.* 2004;231:555–563.

29. Ouwendijk R, de Vries M, Pattynama PM, et al. Imaging peripheral arterial disease: a randomized controlled trial comparing contrast-enhanced MR angiography and multi-detector row CT angiography. *Radiology.* 2005;236: 1094–1103.

30. Willmann JK, Baumert B, Schertler T, et al. Aortoiliac and lower extremity arteries assessed with 16-detector row CT angiography: prospective comparison with digital subtraction angiography. *Radiology.* 2005;236:1083–1093.

31. Fleischmann D, Hallett RL, Rubin GD. CT angiography of peripheral arterial disease. *J Vasc Interv Radiol.* 2006;17: 3–26.

32. Hilfiker PR, Herfkens RJ, Heiss SG, et al. Partial fat-saturated contrast-enhanced three-dimensional MR angiography compared with non-fat-saturated and conventional fat-saturated MR angiography. *Radiology.* 2000;216:298–303.

33. Hartnell GG. Contrast angiography and MR angiography: still not optimum. *J Vasc Interv Radiol.* 1999;10:99–100.

34. Fleischmann D. Use of high-concentration contrast media in multiple-detector-row CT: principles and rationale. *Eur Radiol.* 2003;13[Suppl 5]:M14–M20.

35. Rubin GD, Shiau MC, Schmidt AJ, et al. Computed tomographic angiography: historical perspective and new state-of-the-art using multi detector-row helical computed tomography. *J Comput Assist Tomogr.* 1999;23[Suppl 1]:S83–S90.

36. Bron KM. Femoral arteriography. In: Abrams Herbert L, ed. *Abrams Angiography: Vascular and Interventional Radiology.* Boston: Little Brown; 1983:1835–1875.

37. Versteylen RJ, Lampmann LE. Knee time in femoral arteriography. *AJR Am J Roentgenol* 1989;152:203.

38. Fleischmann D, Rubin GD. Quantification of intravenously administered contrast medium transit through the peripheral arteries: implications for CT angiography. *Radiology.* 2005;236:1076–1082.

39. Portugaller HR, Schoellnast H, Hausegger KA, et al. Multi-slice spiral CT angiography in peripheral arterial occlusive disease: a valuable tool in detecting significant arterial lumen narrowing? *Eur Radiol.* 2004;14:1681–1687.

40. Qanadli SD, Tasu JP, Pelage JP, et al. Cardiovascular imaging. Diagnostic and interventional imaging. *J Radiol.* 1999;80:526–530.

41. Milne EN. The significance of early venous filling during femoral arteriography. *Radiology.* 1967;88:513–518.

42. Roos JE, Fleischmann D, Koechl A, et al. Multipath curved planar reformation of the peripheral arterial tree in CT angiography. *Radiology.* 2007;244:281–290.

43. Kanitsar A, Fleischmann D, Wegenkittl R, et al. CPR: curved planar reformation. In: *IEEE Visualization.* Boston: IEEE Computer Society; 2002:37–44.

44. Terramani TT, Salim A, Hood DB, et al. Hypoplasia of the descending thoracic and abdominal aorta: a report of two cases and review of the literature. *J Vasc Surg.* 2002;36: 844–848.

45. Fleischmann D, Kanitsar A, Lomoschitz E, et al. Multi-path curved planar reformation of the peripheral arterial tree. *Radiology.* 2002;255(P):363.

46. Napel S, Rubin GD, Jeffrey RB Jr. STS-MIP: a new reconstruction technique for CT of the chest. *J Comput Assist Tomogr.* 1993;17:832–838.

47. Raman R, Napel S, Rubin GD. Curved-slab maximum intensity projection: method and evaluation. *Radiology.* 2003;229:255–260.

48. Foley WD, McDaniel D, Milde MW, et al. Digital subtraction angiography of the extremities using table translation. *Radiology.* 1985;157:255–258.

49. Goyen M, Ruehm SG, Barkhausen J, et al. Improved multi-station peripheral MR angiography with a dedicated vascular coil. *J Magn Reson Imaging.* 2001;13:475–480.

50. Fellner FA, Requardt M, Lang W, et al. Peripheral vessels: MR angiography with dedicated phased-array coil with large-field-of-view adapter feasibility study. *Radiology.* 2003;228:284–289.

51. Leiner T, Nijenhuis RJ, Maki JH, et al. Use of a three-station phased array coil to improve peripheral contrast-enhanced magnetic resonance angiography. *J Magn Reson Imaging.* 2004;20:417–425.

52. Pruessmann KP, Weiger M, Scheidegger MB, et al. SENSE: sensitivity encoding for fast MRI. *Magn Reson Med.* 1999;42:952–962.

53. Sodickson DK, Manning WJ. Simultaneous acquisition of spatial harmonics (SMASH): fast imaging with radiofrequency coil arrays. *Magn Reson Med.* 1997;38:591–603.

54. Weiger M, Pruessmann KP, Kassner A, et al. Contrast-enhanced 3D MRA using SENSE. *J Magn Reson Imaging.* 2000;12:671–677.

55. Wedeen VJ, Meuli RA, Edelman RR, et al. Projective imaging of pulsatile flow with magnetic resonance. *Science.* 1985;230:946–948.

56. Swan JS, Grist TM, Weber DM, et al. MR angiography of the pelvis with variable velocity encoding and a phased-array coil. *Radiology.* 1994;190:363–369.

57. Goyen M, Heuser LJ. Improved peripheral MRA using multi-velocity-encoding phase contrast-enhanced MRA techniques. *Acta Radiol.* 2000;41:139–141.

58. Steffens JC, Link J, Muller-Hulsbeck S, et al. Cardiac-gated two-dimensional phase-contrast MR angiography of lower extremity occlusive disease. *AJR Am J Roentgenol.* 1997;169:749–754.

59. Ho KY, Leiner T, de Haan MW, et al. Peripheral MR angiography. *Eur Radiol.* 1999;9:1765–1774.

60. Mustert BR, Williams DM, Prince MR. In vitro model of arterial stenosis: correlation of MR signal dephasing and trans-stenotic pressure gradients. *Magn Reson Imaging.* 1998;16:301–310.

61. Felmlee JP, Ehman RL. Spatial presaturation: a method for suppressing flow artifacts and improving depiction of vascular anatomy in MR imaging. *Radiology.* 1987;164: 559–564.

62. Ehman RL, Felmlee JP. Flow artifact reduction in MRI: a review of the roles of gradient moment nulling and spatial presaturation. *Magn Reson Med.* 1990;14:293–307.

63. Ho KY, de Haan MW, Oei TK, et al. MR angiography of the iliac and upper femoral arteries using four different inflow techniques. *AJR Am J Roentgenol.* 1997;169:45–53.

64. Caputo GR, Higgins CB. Magnetic resonance angiography and measurement of blood flow in the peripheral vessels. *Invest Radiol.* 1992;27[Suppl 2]:S97–S102.

65. Schiebler ML, Listerud J, Baum RA, et al. Magnetic resonance arteriography of the pelvis and lower extremities. *Magn Reson Q.* 1993;9:152–187.

66. Hoch JR, Tullis MJ, Kennell TW, et al. Use of magnetic resonance angiography for the preoperative evaluation of patients with infrainguinal arterial occlusive disease. *J Vasc Surg.* 1996;23:792–800; discussion 801.

67. Owen RS, Baum RA, Carpenter JP, et al. Symptomatic peripheral vascular disease: selection of imaging parameters and clinical evaluation with MR angiography. *Radiology.* 1993;187:627–635.

68. Carpenter JP, Golden MA, Barker CF, et al. The fate of bypass grafts to angiographically occult runoff vessels detected by magnetic resonance angiography. *J Vasc Surg.* 1996;23:483–489.

69. Miyazaki M, Takai H, Sugiura S, et al. Peripheral MR angiography: separation of arteries from veins with flow-spoiled gradient pulses in electrocardiography-triggered three-dimensional half-Fourier fast spin-echo imaging. *Radiology.* 2003;227:890–896.

70. Miyazaki M, Sugiura S, Tateishi F, et al. Non-contrast-enhanced MR angiography using 3D ECG-synchronized half-Fourier fast spin echo. *J Magn Reson Imaging.* 2000;12:776–783.

71. Foo TK, Ho VB, Marcos HB, et al. MR angiography using steady-state free precession. *Magn Reson Med.* 2002;48: 699–706.

72. Scheffler K, Lehnhardt S. Principles and applications of balanced SSFP techniques. *Eur Radiol.* 2003;13:2409–2418.

73. Ho KY, Leiner T, de Haan MW, et al. Peripheral vascular tree stenoses: evaluation with moving-bed infusion-tracking MR angiography. *Radiology*. 1998;206:683–692.

74. Meaney JF, Ridgway JP, Chakraverty S, et al. Stepping-table gadolinium-enhanced digital subtraction MR angiography of the aorta and lower extremity arteries: preliminary experience. *Radiology*. 1999;211:59–67.

75. Ruehm SG, Hany TF, Pfammatter T, et al. Pelvic and lower extremity arterial imaging: diagnostic performance of three-dimensional contrast-enhanced MR angiography. *AJR Am J Roentgenol*. 2000;174:1127–1135.

76. Reid SK, Pagan-Marin HR, Menzoian JO, et al. Contrast-enhanced moving-table MR angiography: prospective comparison to catheter arteriography for treatment planning in peripheral arterial occlusive disease. *J Vasc Interv Radiol*. 2001;12:45–53.

77. Menzoian JO, LaMorte WW, Paniszyn CC, et al. Symptomatology and anatomic patterns of peripheral vascular disease: differing impact of smoking and diabetes. *Ann Vasc Surg*. 1989;3:224–228.

78. Leiner T, Ho KY, Nelemans PJ, et al. Three-dimensional contrast-enhanced moving-bed infusion-tracking (MoBI-track) peripheral MR angiography with flexible choice of imaging parameters for each field of view. *J Magn Reson Imaging*. 2000;11:368–377.

79. Schoenberg SO, Londy FJ, Licato P, et al. Multiphase-multistep gadolinium-enhanced MR angiography of the abdominal aorta and runoff vessels. *Invest Radiol*. 2001;36:283–291.

80. Boos M, Scheffler K, Haselhorst R, et al. Arterial first pass gadolinium-CM dynamics as a function of several intravenous saline flush and Gd volumes. *J Magn Reson Imaging*. 2001;13:568–576.

81. Prince MR. Contrast-enhanced MR angiography: theory and optimization. *Magn Reson Imaging Clin N Am*. 1998;6:257–267.

82. Maki JH, Prince MR, Londy FJ, et al. The effects of time varying intravascular signal intensity and k-space acquisition order on three-dimensional MR angiography image quality. *J Magn Reson Imaging*. 1996;6:642–651.

83. Earls JP, Patel NH, Smith PA, et al. Gadolinium-enhanced three-dimensional MR angiography of the aorta and peripheral arteries: evaluation of a multistation examination using two gadopentetate dimeglumine infusions. *AJR Am J Roentgenol*. 1998;171:599–604.

84. Earls JP, Shaves SC. MR angiography of the thoracic, abdominal, and extremity venous system. *Magn Reson Imaging Clin N Am*. 1998;6:417–435.

85. Maki JH, Wilson GJ, Eubank WB, et al. Predicting venous enhancement in peripheral MRA using a two-station timing bolus. In: *11th Scientific Meeting of the International Society for Magnetic Resonance in Medicine*. Toronto, Ontario: ISMRM; 2003:91.

86. Foo TK, Saranathan M, Prince MR, et al. Automated detection of bolus arrival and initiation of data acquisition in fast, three-dimensional, gadolinium-enhanced MR angiography. *Radiology*. 1997;203:275–280.

87. Luccichenti G, Cademartiri F, Ugolotti U, et al. Magnetic resonance angiography with elliptical ordering and fluoroscopic triggering of the renal arteries. *Radiol Med (Torino)*. 2003;105:42–47.

88. Meaney JF. Magnetic resonance angiography of the peripheral arteries: current status. *Eur Radiol*. 2003;13:836–852.

89. Ho KY, de Haan MW, Kessels AG, et al. Peripheral vascular tree stenoses: detection with subtracted and nonsubtracted MR angiography. *Radiology*. 1998;206:673–681.

90. Leiner T, de Weert TT, Nijenhuis RJ, et al. Need for background suppression in contrast-enhanced peripheral magnetic resonance angiography. *J Magn Reson Imaging*. 2001;14:724–733.

91. Ruehm SG, Nanz D, Baumann A, et al. 3D contrast-enhanced MR angiography of the run-off vessels: value of image subtraction. *J Magn Reson Imaging*. 2001;13:402–411.

92. Wang Y, Chen CZ, Chabra SG, et al. Bolus arterial-venous transit in the lower extremity and venous contamination in bolus chase three-dimensional magnetic resonance angiography. *Invest Radiol*. 2002;37:458–463.

93. Bezooijen R, van den Bosch HC, Tielbeek AV, et al. Peripheral arterial disease: sensitivity-encoded multiposition MR angiography compared with intraarterial angiography and conventional multiposition MR angiography. *Radiology*. 2004;231:263–271.

94. de Vries M, Nijenhuis RJ, Hoogeveen RM, et al. Contrast-enhanced peripheral MR angiography using SENSE in multiple stations: feasibility study. *J Magn Reson Imaging*. 2005;21:37–45.

95. Wang Y, Winchester PA, Khilnani NM, et al. Contrast-enhanced peripheral MR angiography from the abdominal aorta to the pedal arteries: combined dynamic two-dimensional and bolus-chase three-dimensional acquisitions. *Invest Radiol*. 2001;36:170–177.

96. Morasch MD, Collins J, Pereles FS, et al. Lower extremity stepping-table magnetic resonance angiography with multilevel contrast timing and segmented contrast infusion. *J Vasc Surg*. 2003;37:62–71.

97. Westenberg JJ, Wasser MN, van der Geest RJ, et al. Scan optimization of gadolinium contrast-enhanced three-dimensional MRA of peripheral arteries with multiple bolus injections and in vitro validation of stenosis quantification. *Magn Reson Imaging*. 1999;17:47–57.

98. Wilman AH, Riederer SJ. Improved centric phase encoding orders for three-dimensional magnetization-prepared MR angiography. *Magn Reson Med*. 1996;36:384–392.

99. Willinek WA, Gieseke J, Conrad R, et al. Randomly segmented central k-space ordering in high-spatial-resolution contrast-enhanced MR angiography of the supraaortic arteries: initial experience. *Radiology*. 2002;225:583–588.

100. Hu HH, Madhuranthakam AJ, Kruger DG, et al. Improved venous suppression and spatial resolution with SENSE in elliptical centric 3D contrast-enhanced MR angiography. *Magn Reson Med*. 2004;52:761–765.

101. Korosec FR, Frayne R, Grist TM, et al. Time-resolved contrast-enhanced 3D MR angiography. *Magn Reson Med*. 1996;36:345–351.

102. van Vaals JJ, Brummer ME, Dixon WT, et al. "Keyhole" method for accelerating imaging of contrast agent uptake. *J Magn Reson Imaging*. 1993;3:671–675.

103. Hoogeveen RM, von Falkenhausen M, Gieseke J. Fast, dynamic high resolution contrast-enhanced MR angiography with CENTRA keyhole and SENSE. In: *12th Scientific Meeting of the International Society for Magnetic Resonance in Medicine*. Kyoto, Japan: International Society for Magnetic Resonance in Medicine; 2004:9

104. Swan JS, Carroll TJ, Kennell TW, et al. Time-resolved three-dimensional contrast-enhanced MR angiography of the peripheral vessels. *Radiology*. 2002;225:43–52.

105. Hany TF, Carroll TJ, Omary RA, et al. Aorta and runoff vessels: single-injection MR angiography with automated table movement compared with multiinjection time-resolved MR angiography initial results. *Radiology*. 2001;221:266–272.

106. Herborn CU, Ajaj W, Goyen M, et al. Peripheral vasculature: whole-body MR angiography with midfemoral venous compression—initial experience. *Radiology*. 2004;230:872–878.

107. Bilecen D, Jager KA, Aschwanden M, et al. Cuff-compression of the proximal calf to reduce venous contamination in contrast-enhanced stepping-table magnetic resonance angiography. *Acta Radiol*. 2004;45:510–515.

108. Hoogeveen RM, Bakker CJ, Viergever MA. Limits to the accuracy of vessel diameter measurement in MR angiography. *J Magn Reson Imaging*. 1998;8:1228–1235.

109. Westenberg JJ, van der Geest RJ, Wasser MN, et al. Vessel diameter measurements in gadolinium contrast-enhanced three-dimensional MRA of peripheral arteries. *Magn Reson Imaging*. 2000;18:13–22.

110. Schmiedl U, Moseley ME, Ogan MD, et al. Comparison of initial biodistribution patterns of Gd-DTPA and albumin-(Gd-DTPA) using rapid spin echo MR imaging. *J Comput Assist Tomogr*. 1987;11:306–313.

111. Goyen M, Debatin JF, Ruehm SG. Peripheral magnetic resonance angiography. *Top Magn Reson Imaging*. 2001;12:327–335.

112. Czum JM, Ho VB, Hood MN, et al. Bolus-chase peripheral 3D MRA using a dual-rate contrast media injection. *J Magn Reson Imaging*. 2000;12:769–775.

113. Hentsch A, Aschauer MA, Balzer JO, et al. Gadobutrol-enhanced moving-table magnetic resonance angiography in patients with peripheral vascular disease: a prospective, multi-centre blinded comparison with digital subtraction angiography. *Eur Radiol*. 2003;13:2103–2114.

114. Goyen M, Lauenstein TC, Herborn CU, et al. 0.5 M Gd chelate (Magnevist) versus 1.0 M Gd chelate (Gadovist): dose-independent effect on image quality of pelvic three-dimensional MR-angiography. *J Magn Reson Imaging*. 2001;14:602–607.

115. Knopp MV, Tengg-Kobligk H, Floemer F, et al. Contrast agents for MRA: future directions. *J Magn Reson Imaging*. 1999;10:314–316.

116. Bilecen D, Schulte AC, Bongartz G, et al. Infragenual cuff-compression reduces venous contamination in contrast-enhanced MR angiography of the calf. *J Magn Reson Imaging*. 2004;20:347–351.

117. Huang Y, Webster CA, Wright GA. Analysis of subtraction methods in three-dimensional contrast-enhanced peripheral MR angiography. *J Magn Reson Imaging*. 2002;15:541–550.

118. van Bemmel CM, Elgersma OE, Vonken EJ, et al. Evaluation of semiautomated internal carotid artery stenosis quantification from 3-dimensional contrast-enhanced magnetic resonance angiograms. *Invest Radiol*. 2004;39:418–426.

119. de Vries M, de Koning PJ, de Haan MW, et al. Accuracy of semi-automated analysis of 3D contrast-enhanced MR angiography for detection and quantification of aortoiliac stenoses. *Invest Radiol*. 2005;40:495–503.

120. Rofsky NM, Morana G, Adelman MA, et al. Improved gadolinium-enhanced subtraction MR angiography of the femoropopliteal arteries: reintroduction of osseous anatomic landmarks. *AJR Am J Roentgenol*. 1999;173:1009–1011.

121. Wang Y, Johnston DL, Breen JF, et al. Dynamic MR digital subtraction angiography using contrast enhancement, fast data acquisition, and complex subtraction. *Magn Reson Med*. 1996;36:551–556.

122. Hany TF, Schmidt M, Davis CP, et al. Diagnostic impact of four postprocessing techniques in evaluating contrast-enhanced three-dimensional MR angiography. *AJR Am J Roentgenol*. 1998;170:907–912.

123. Nelemans PJ, Leiner T, de Vet HC, et al. Peripheral arterial disease: meta-analysis of the diagnostic performance of MR angiography. *Radiology*. 2000;217:105–114.

124. Lippert H, Pabst R. Arterial variations in man: classification and frequency. München: J.F. Bergmann Verlag; 1985.

125. Mayschak DT, Flye MW. Treatment of the persistent sciatic artery. *Ann Surg*. 1984;199:69–74.

126. Brantley SK, Rigdon EE, Raju S. Persistent sciatic artery: embryology, pathology, and treatment. *J Vasc Surg*. 1993;18:242–248.

127. Nair R, Robbs JV, Chetty R, et al. Occlusive arterial disease in HIV-infected patients: a preliminary report. *Eur J Vasc Endovasc Surg*. 2000;20:353–357.

128. Woolgar JD, Ray R, Maharaj K, et al. Colour Doppler and grey scale ultrasound features of HIV-related vascular aneurysms. *Br J Radiol*. 2002;75:884–888.

129. Roques X, Choussat A, Bourdeaud'hui A, et al. Aneurysms of the abdominal aorta in the neonate and infant. *Ann Vasc Surg*. 1989;3:335–340.

130. Bartels LW, Bakker CJ, Viergever MA. Improved lumen visualization in metallic vascular implants by reducing RF artifacts. *Magn Reson Med*. 2002;47:171–180.

131. Cronenwett JL, Krupski W, Rutherford RB. Abdominal aortic and iliac aneurysms. In: Rutherford RB, ed. *Vascular Surgery*. Philadelphia, PA: WB Saunders; 2000:1246–1280.

132. Brewster DC, Cronenwett JL, Hallett JW Jr., et al. Guidelines for the treatment of abdominal aortic aneurysms. Report of a subcommittee of the Joint Council of the American Association for Vascular Surgery and Society for Vascular Surgery. *J Vasc Surg*. 2003;37:1106–1117.

133. Diwan A, Sarkar R, Stanley JC, et al. Incidence of femoral and popliteal artery aneurysms in patients with abdominal aortic aneurysms. *J Vasc Surg*. 2000;31:863–869.

134. Crawford ES, DeBakey ME. Popliteal artery arteriosclerotic aneurysm. *Circulation*. 1965;32:515–516.

135. Dent TL, Lindenauer SM, Ernst CB, et al. Multiple arteriosclerotic arterial aneurysms. *Arch Surg*. 1972;105:338–344.

136. Graham LM, Zelenock GB, Whitehouse WM Jr., et al. Clinical significance of arteriosclerotic femoral artery aneurysms. *Arch Surg*. 1980;115:502–507.

137. Whitehouse WM Jr., Wakefield TW, Graham LM, et al. Limb-threatening potential of arteriosclerotic popliteal artery aneurysms. *Surgery*. 1983;93:694–699.

138. Bouhoutsos J, Martin P. Popliteal aneurysm: a review of 116 cases. *Br J Surg*. 1974;61:469–475.

139. Levi N, Schroeder TV. Atherosclerotic femoral artery aneurysms: increase in deep femoral aneurysms? *Panminerva Med*. 1996;38:164–166.

140. Lozano F, Sanchez-Fernandez J, Gomez Alonso A. Ruptured aneurysm of the deep femoral artery. Case report and historical review. *J Cardiovasc Surg (Torino)*. 2001;42:821–824.

141. Levi N, Schroeder TV. Anastomotic femoral aneurysms: increase in interval between primary operation and aneurysm formation. *Eur J Vasc Endovasc Surg*. 1996;11:207–209.

142. Khaira HS, Vohra H. True aneurysm in a femoro-popliteal dacron graft—a case report and literature review. *Cardiovasc Surg*. 2002;10:644–646.

143. Levi N, Rordam P, Jensen LP, et al. Femoral pseudoaneurysms in drug addicts. *Eur J Vasc Endovasc Surg*. 1997;13:361–362.

144. Cutler BS, Darling RC. Surgical management of arteriosclerotic femoral aneurysms. *Surgery*. 1973;74:764–773.

145. Wright LB, Matchett WJ, Cruz CP, et al. Popliteal artery disease: diagnosis and treatment. *Radiographics*. 2004;24:467–479.

146. Shortell CK, DeWeese JA, Ouriel K, et al. Popliteal artery aneurysms: a 25-year surgical experience. *J Vasc Surg*. 1991;14:771–776; discussion 776–779.

147. Cappendijk VC, Mouthaan PJ. A true aneurysm of the tibioperoneal trunk. Case report and literature review. *Eur J Vasc Endovasc Surg*. 1999;18:536–537.

148. Monig SP, Walter M, Sorgatz S, et al. True infrapopliteal artery aneurysms: report of two cases and literature review. *J Vasc Surg*. 1996;24:276–278.

149. Hertzer NR. The natural history of peripheral vascular disease. Implications for its management. *Circulation*. 1991;83:I12–I19.

150. Brewster DC. Direct reconstruction for aortoiliac occlusive disease. In: Rutherford RB, ed. *Vascular Surgery*. Philadelphia, PA: WB Saunders; 2000:943–972.

151. Brewster DC, Perler BA, Robison JG, et al. Aortofemoral graft for multilevel occlusive disease. Predictors of success and need for distal bypass. *Arch Surg*. 1982;117:1593–1600.

152. Yao JS. New techniques in objective arterial evaluation. *Arch Surg*. 1973;106:600–604.

153. Sumner DS, Strandness DE Jr. The relationship between calf blood flow and ankle blood pressure in patients with intermittent claudication. *Surgery*. 1969;65:763–771.

154. Spinosa DJ, Leung DA, Matsumoto AH, et al. Percutaneous intentional extraluminal recanalization in patients with chronic critical limb ischemia. *Radiology*. 2004;232:499–507.

155. Samson RH, Showalter DP, Yunis JP. Isolated femoropopliteal bypass graft for limb salvage after failed tibial reconstruction: a viable alternative to amputation. *J Vasc Surg.* 1999;29:409–412.

156. Adelman MA, Jacobowitz GR. Body MR angiography: a surgeon's perspective. *Magn Reson Imaging Clin N Am.* 1998;6:397–416.

157. Hughes K, Domenig CM, Hamdan AD, et al. Bypass to plantar and tarsal arteries: an acceptable approach to limb salvage. *J Vasc Surg.* 2004;40:1149–1157.

158. Aulivola B, Pomposelli FB. Dorsalis pedis, tarsal and plantar artery bypass. *J Cardiovasc Surg (Torino).* 2004;45:203–212.

159. Pomposelli FB, Kansal N, Hamdan AD, et al. A decade of experience with dorsalis pedis artery bypass: analysis of outcome in more than 1000 cases. *J Vasc Surg.* 2003;37:307–315.

160. Pomposelli FB Jr., Marcaccio EJ, Gibbons GW, et al. Dorsalis pedis arterial bypass: durable limb salvage for foot ischemia in patients with diabetes mellitus. *J Vasc Surg.* 1995;21:375–384.

161. Pomposelli FB Jr., Basile P, Campbell DR, et al. Salvaging the ischemic transmetatarsal amputation through distal arterial reconstruction. *J Am Podiatr Med Assoc.* 1993;83:87–90.

162. LoGerfo FW, Gibbons GW, Pomposelli FB Jr., et al. Trends in the care of the diabetic foot. Expanded role of arterial reconstruction. *Arch Surg.* 1992;127:617–620; discussion 620–611.

163. Pomposelli FB Jr., Jepsen SJ, Gibbons GW, et al. A flexible approach to infrapopliteal vein grafts in patients with diabetes mellitus. *Arch Surg.* 1991;126:724–727; discussion 727–729.

164. Holstein PE, Sorensen S. Limb salvage experience in a multidisciplinary diabetic foot unit. *Diabetes Care.* 1999;22[Suppl 2]:B97–B103.

165. Hofmann W, Forstner R, Kofler B, et al. Pedal artery imaging—a comparison of selective digital subtraction angiography, contrast enhanced magnetic resonance angiography and duplex ultrasound. *Eur J Vasc Endovasc Surg.* 2002;24:287–292.

166. Leiner T, Kessels AG, Schurink GW, et al. Comparison of contrast-enhanced magnetic resonance angiography and digital subtraction angiography in patients with chronic critical ischemia and tissue loss. *Invest Radiol.* 2004;39:435–444.

167. Alson MD, Lang EV, Kaufman JA. Pedal arterial imaging. *J Vasc Interv Radiol.* 1997;8:9–18.

168. Clark TW, Groffsky JL, Soulen MC. Predictors of long-term patency after femoropopliteal angioplasty: results from the STAR registry. *J Vasc Interv Radiol.* 2001;12:923–933.

169. Reekers JA, Bolia A. Percutaneous intentional extraluminal (subintimal) recanalization: how to do it yourself. *Eur J Radiol.* 1998;28:192–198.

170. Tisi PV, Mirnezami A, Baker S, et al. Role of subintimal angioplasty in the treatment of chronic lower limb ischaemia. *Eur J Vasc Endovasc Surg.* 2002;24:417–422.

171. Saketkhoo RR, Razavi MK, Padidar A, et al. Percutaneous bypass: subintimal recanalization of peripheral occlusive disease with IVUS guided luminal re-entry. *Tech Vasc Interv Radiol.* 2004;7:23–27.

172. Nadal LL, Cynamon J, Lipsitz EC, et al. Subintimal angioplasty for chronic arterial occlusions. *Tech Vasc Interv Radiol.* 2004;7:16–22.

173. Criqui MH, Fronek A, Klauber MR, et al. The sensitivity, specificity, and predictive value of traditional clinical evaluation of peripheral arterial disease: results from noninvasive testing in a defined population. *Circulation.* 1985;71:516–522.

174. Imparato AM, Kim GE, Davidson T, et al. Intermittent claudication: its natural course. *Surgery.* 1975;78:795–799.

175. Humphrey LL, Palumbo PJ, Butters MA, et al. The contribution of non-insulin-dependent diabetes to lower-extremity amputation in the community. *Arch Intern Med.* 1994;154:885–892.

176. DeBakey ME, Lawrie GM, Glaeser DH. Patterns of atherosclerosis and their surgical significance. *Ann Surg.* 1985;201:115–131.

177. Muluk SC, Muluk VS, Kelley ME, et al. Outcome events in patients with claudication: a 15-year study in 2,777 patients. *J Vasc Surg.* 2001;33:251–257; discussion 257–258.

178. Hiatt WR. Medical treatment of peripheral arterial disease and claudication. *N Engl J Med.* 2001;344:1608–1621.

179. Hiatt WR. Pharmacologic therapy for peripheral arterial disease and claudication. *J Vasc Surg.* 2002;36:1283–1291.

180. Stewart KJ, Hiatt WR, Regensteiner JG, et al. Exercise training for claudication. *N Engl J Med.* 2002;347:1941–1951.

181. de Vries SO, Visser K, de Vries JA, et al. Intermittent claudication: cost-effectiveness of revascularization versus exercise therapy. *Radiology.* 2002;222:25–36.

182. Pentecost MJ, Criqui MH, Dorros G, et al. Guidelines for peripheral percutaneous transluminal angioplasty of the abdominal aorta and lower extremity vessels. A statement for health professionals from a special writing group of the Councils on Cardiovascular Radiology, Arteriosclerosis, Cardio-Thoracic and Vascular Surgery, Clinical Cardiology, Epidemiology and Prevention, the American Heart Association. *Circulation.* 1994;89:511–531.

183. Surowiec SM, Davies MG, Eberly SW, et al. Percutaneous angioplasty and stenting of the superficial femoral artery. *J Vasc Surg.* 2005;41:269–278.

184. Hirai T, Korogi Y, Ono K, et al. Maximum stenosis of extracranial internal carotid artery: effect of luminal morphology on stenosis measurement by using CT angiography and conventional DSA. *Radiology.* 2001;221:802–809.

185. Visser K, de Vries SO, Kitslaar PJ, et al. Cost-effectiveness of diagnostic imaging work-up and treatment for patients with intermittent claudication in the Netherlands. *Eur J Vasc Endovasc Surg.* 2003;25:213–223.

186. Rubin GD, Armerding MD, Dake MD, et al. Cost identification of abdominal aortic aneurysm imaging by using time and motion analyses. *Radiology.* 2000;215:63–70.

187. Nicoloff AD, Taylor LM Jr., Sexton GJ, et al. Relationship between site of initial symptoms and subsequent progression of disease in a prospective study of atherosclerosis progression in patients receiving long-term treatment for symptomatic peripheral arterial disease. *J Vasc Surg.* 2002;35:38–46; discussion 46–37.

188. Dardik H, Ibrahim IM, Sussman B, et al. Morphologic structure of the pedal arch and its relationship to patency of crural vascular reconstruction. *Surg Gynecol Obstet.* 1981;152:645–648.

189. Clair DG, Dayal R, Faries PL, et al. Tibial angioplasty as an alternative strategy in patients with limb-threatening ischemia. *Ann Vasc Surg.* 2005;19:63–68.

190. Dorros G, Jaff MR, Murphy KJ, et al. The acute outcome of tibioperoneal vessel angioplasty in 417 cases with claudication and critical limb ischemia. *Cathet Cardiovasc Diagn.* 1998;45:251–256.

191. Picus D, Hicks ME, Darcy MD, et al. Magnetic resonance imaging of angiographically occult run off vessels in peripheral arterial occlusive disease. *Invest Radiol.* 1993;28:656–658.

192. Kaufman JA. Lower extremity arteries. In: Thrall JA, ed. *Vascular and Interventional Radiology: The Requisites.* Philadelphia, PA: Mosby; 2004:421.

193. Glickerman DJ, Obregon RG, Schmiedl UP, et al. Cardiac-gated MR angiography of the entire lower extremity: a prospective comparison with conventional angiography. *AJR Am J Roentgenol.* 1996;167:445–451.

194. Lewin JS. Time-of-flight magnetic resonance angiography of the aorta and renal arteries. *Invest Radiol.* 1992;27[Suppl 2]:S84–S89.

195. McCauley TR, Monib A, Dickey KW, et al. Peripheral vascular occlusive disease: accuracy and reliability of time-of-flight MR angiography. *Radiology.* 1994;192:351–357.

196. Yucel EK, Kaufman JA, Geller SC, et al. Atherosclerotic occlusive disease of the lower extremity: prospective

evaluation with two-dimensional time-of-flight MR angiography. *Radiology.* 1993;187:637–641.

197. Kaufman JA, McCarter D, Geller SC, et al. Two-dimensional time-of-flight MR angiography of the lower extremities: artifacts and pitfalls. *AJR Am J Roentgenol.* 1998;171: 129–135.

198. Safir J, Purdy D, Zito JL. Cardiac-triggered and segmented two-dimensional MR angiography of peripheral arterial occlusive disease. A pictorial essay. *Clin Imaging.* 1998;22: 134–144.

199. Kreitner KF. Results of four multicenter, phase III, magnetic resonance angiography (MRA) trials with MS-32, a blood-pool contrast agent for the detection of vascular disease in the aortoiliac, renal, and pedal regions. In: *European Congress of Radiology.* Vienna, Austria: European Congress of Radiology, 2004.

200. Binkert CA, Baker PD, Petersen BD, et al. Peripheral vascular disease: blinded study of dedicated calf MR angiography versus standard bolus-chase MR angiography and film hard-copy angiography. *Radiology.* 2004;232:860–866.

201. Vavrik J, Rohrmoser GM, Madani B, et al. Comparison of MR angiography versus digital subtraction angiography as a basis for planning treatment of lower limb occlusive disease. *J Endovasc Ther.* 2004;11:294–301.

202. Huber A, Scheidler J, Wintersperger B, et al. Moving-table MR angiography of the peripheral runoff vessels: comparison of body coil and dedicated phased array coil systems. *AJR Am J Roentgenol.* 2003;180:1365–1373.

203. Schafer FK, Schafer PJ, Jahnke T, et al. [First clinical results in a study of contrast enhanced magnetic resonance angiography with the 1.0 molar gadobutrol in peripheral arterial occlusive disease—comparison to intraarterial DSA.] *Rofo Fortschr Geb Rontgenstr Neuen Bildgeb Verfahr.* 2003;175:556–564.

204. Wyttenbach R, Gianella S, Alerci M, et al. Prospective blinded evaluation of Gd-DOTA- versus Gd-BOPTA-enhanced peripheral MR angiography, as compared with digital subtraction angiography. *Radiology.* 2003;227:261–269.

205. Steffens JC, Schafer FK, Oberscheid B, et al. Bolus-chasing contrast-enhanced 3D MRA of the lower extremity. Comparison with intraarterial DSA. *Acta Radiol.* 2003;44: 185–192.

206. Nchimi A, Brisbois D, Donkers E, et al. [MR aortofemorography versus DSA: prospective evaluation.] *Jbr-Btr.* 2002;85: 246–251.

207. Cronberg CN, Sjoberg S, Albrechtsson U, et al. Peripheral arterial disease. Contrast-enhanced 3D MR angiography of the lower leg and foot compared with conventional angiography. *Acta Radiol.* 2003;44:59–66.

208. Klein WM, Schlejen PM, Eikelboom BC, et al. MR angiography of the lower extremities with a moving-bed infusion-tracking technique. *Cardiovasc Intervent Radiol.* 2003;26: 1–8.

209. Pandharipande PV, Lee VS, Reuss PM, et al. Two-station bolus-chase MR angiography with a stationary table: a simple alternative to automated-table techniques. *AJR Am J Roentgenol.* 2002;179:1583–1589.

210. Loewe C, Schoder M, Rand T, et al. Peripheral vascular occlusive disease: evaluation with contrast-enhanced moving-bed MR angiography versus digital subtraction angiography in 106 patients. *AJR Am J Roentgenol.* 2002;179: 1013–1021.

211. Schoenberg SO, Essig M, Hallscheidt P, et al. Multiphase magnetic resonance angiography of the abdominal and pelvic arteries: results of a bicenter multireader analysis. *Invest Radiol.* 2002;37:20–28.

212. Goyen M, Quick HH, Debatin JF, et al. Whole-body three-dimensional MR angiography with a rolling table platform: initial clinical experience. *Radiology.* 2002;224:270–277.

213. Khilnani NM, Winchester PA, Prince MR, et al. Peripheral vascular disease: combined 3D bolus chase and dynamic 2D MR angiography compared with x-ray angiography for treatment planning. *Radiology.* 2002;224:63–74.

214. Carriero A, Maggialetti A, Pinto D, et al. Contrast-enhanced magnetic resonance angiography MoBI-trak in the study of peripheral vascular disease. *Cardiovasc Intervent Radiol.* 2002;25:42–47.

215. Winterer JT, Schaefer O, Uhrmeister P, et al. Contrast enhanced MR angiography in the assessment of relevant stenoses in occlusive disease of the pelvic and lower limb arteries: diagnostic value of a two-step examination protocol in comparison to conventional DSA. *Eur J Radiol.* 2002;41:153–160.

216. Ruehm SG, Goyen M, Barkhausen J, et al. Rapid magnetic resonance angiography for detection of atherosclerosis. *Lancet.* 2001;357:1086–1091.

217. Di Cesare E, Giordano AV, Santarelli B, et al. [MR-angiography with contrast bolus vs digital angiography in peripheral arterial occlusive disease of the legs.] *Radiol Med (Torino).* 2001;102:55–61.

218. Brillet PY, Tassart M, Bazot M, et al. [Investigation of peripheral vascular bed in critical lower limb ischemia: comparative study between arteriography and magnetic resonance angiography.] *J Mal Vasc.* 2001;26:31–38.

219. Sueyoshi E, Sakamoto I, Matsuoka Y, et al. Symptomatic peripheral vascular tree stenosis. Comparison of subtracted and nonsubtracted 3D contrast-enhanced MR angiography with fat suppression. *Acta Radiol.* 2000;41: 133–138.

220. Huber A, Heuck A, Baur A, et al. Dynamic contrast-enhanced MR angiography from the distal aorta to the ankle joint with a step-by-step technique. *AJR Am J Roentgenol.* 2000;175:1291–1298.

221. Lenhart M, Herold T, Volk M, et al. [Contrast media-enhanced MR angiography of the lower extremity arteries using a dedicated peripheral vascular coil system. First clinical results.] *Rofo Fortschr Geb Rontgenstr Neuen Bildgeb Verfahr.* 2000;172:992–999.

222. Lundin P, Svensson A, Henriksen E, et al. Imaging of aortoiliac arterial disease. Duplex ultrasound and MR angiography versus digital subtraction angiography. *Acta Radiol.* 2000;41:125–132.

223. Wikstrom J, Holmberg A, Johansson L, et al. Gadolinium-enhanced magnetic resonance angiography, digital subtraction angiography and duplex of the iliac arteries compared with intra-arterial pressure gradient measurements. *Eur J Vasc Endovasc Surg.* 2000;19:516–523.

224. Bourlet P, De Fraissinette B, Garcier JM, et al. [Comparative assessment of helical CT-angiography, 2D TOF MR-angiography and 3D gadolinium enhanced MRA in aorto-iliac occlusive disease.] *J Radiol.* 2000;81:1619–1625.

225. Mitsuzaki K, Yamashita Y, Sakaguchi T, et al. Abdomen, pelvis, and extremities: diagnostic accuracy of dynamic contrast-enhanced turbo MR angiography compared with conventional angiography-initial experience. *Radiology.* 2000;216:909–915.

226. Link J, Steffens JC, Brossmann J, et al. Iliofemoral arterial occlusive disease: contrast-enhanced MR angiography for preinterventional evaluation and follow-up after stent placement. *Radiology.* 1999;212:371–377.

227. Oberholzer K, Kreitner KF, Kalden P, et al. [MR angiography of peripheral vessels with automatic tracking table technique at 1.0 in comparison with intra-arterial digital subtraction angiography.] *Rofo Fortschr Geb Rontgenstr Neuen Bildgeb Verfahr.* 1999;171:240–243.

228. Lenhart M, Djavidani B, Volk M, et al. [Contrast medium-enhanced MR angiography of the pelvic and leg vessels with an automated table-feed technique.] *Rofo Fortschr Geb Rontgenstr Neuen Bildgeb Verfahr.* 1999;171: 442–449.

229. Maspes F, Gandini R, Pocek M, et al. [Breath-hold gadolinium enhanced tree-dimensional MR angiography: personal experience in the thoracic-abdominal area.] *Radiol Med (Torino).* 1999;98:275–282.

230. Yamashita Y, Mitsuzaki K, Ogata I, et al. Three-dimensional high-resolution dynamic contrast-enhanced MR angiography

of the pelvis and lower extremities with use of a phased array coil and subtraction: diagnostic accuracy. *J Magn Reson Imaging.* 1998;8:1066–1072.

231. Perrier E, Dubayle P, Boyer B, et al. [Comparison of magnetic resonance angiography with injection of gadolinium and conventional arteriography of the ilio-femoral arteries.] *J Radiol.* 1998;79:1493–1498.

232. Quinn SF, Sheley RC, Szumowski J, et al. Evaluation of the iliac arteries: comparison of two-dimensional time of flight magnetic resonance angiography with cardiac compensated fast gradient recalled echo and contrast-enhanced three-dimensional time of flight magnetic resonance angiography. *J Magn Reson Imaging.* 1997;7:197–203.

233. Rofsky NM, Johnson G, Adelman MA, et al. Peripheral vascular disease evaluated with reduced-dose gadolinium-enhanced MR angiography. *Radiology.*1997;205:163–169.

234. Poon E, Yucel EK, Pagan-Marin H, et al. Iliac artery stenosis measurements: comparison of two-dimensional time-of-flight and three-dimensional dynamic gadolinium-enhanced MR angiography. *AJR Am J Roentgenol.* 1997;169:1139–1144.

235. Hany TF, Debatin JF, Leung DA, et al. Evaluation of the aortoiliac and renal arteries: comparison of breath-hold, contrast-enhanced, three-dimensional MR angiography with conventional catheter angiography. *Radiology.* 1997;204:357–362.

236. Snidow JJ, Johnson MS, Harris VJ, et al. Three-dimensional gadolinium-enhanced MR angiography for aortoiliac inflow assessment plus renal artery screening in a single breath hold. *Radiology.* 1996;198:725–732.

237. Prince MR, Narasimham DL, Stanley JC, et al. Gadolinium-enhanced magnetic resonance angiography of abdominal aortic aneurysms. *J Vasc Surg.* 1995;21:656–669.

238. Koelemay MJ, Lijmer JG, Stoker J, et al. Magnetic resonance angiography for the evaluation of lower extremity arterial disease: a meta-analysis. *JAMA.* 2001;285:1338–1345.

239. Martin ML, Tay KH, Flak B, et al. Multidetector CT angiography of the aortoiliac system and lower extremities: a prospective comparison with digital subtraction angiography. *AJR Am J Roentgenol.* 2003;180:1085–1091.

240. Edwards AJ, Wells IP, Roobottom CA. Multidetector row CT angiography of the lower limb arteries: a prospective comparison of volume-rendered techniques and intra-arterial digital subtraction angiography. *Clin Radiol.* 2005;60: 85–95.

241. Ouwendijk R, Kock MC, van Dijk LC, et al. Vessel wall calcifications at multi-detector row CT angiography in patients with peripheral arterial disease: effect on clinical utility and clinical predictors. *Radiology.* 2006;241:603–608.

242. Leiner T, Tordoir JH, Kessels AG, et al. Comparison of treatment plans for peripheral arterial disease made with multistation contrast medium-enhanced magnetic resonance angiography and duplex ultrasound scanning. *J Vasc Surg.* 2003;37:1255–1262.

243. Willmann JK, Mayer D, Banyai M, et al. Evaluation of peripheral arterial bypass grafts with multi-detector row CT angiography: comparison with duplex US and digital subtraction angiography. *Radiology.* 2003;229:465–474.

244. Willmann JK, Szente-Varga M, Roos JE, et al. Three-dimensional images of extra-anatomic arterial bypass graft using multidetector row spiral computed tomography data with volume rendering. *Circulation.* 2001;104:E154–E155.

245. Ouriel K, Veith FJ, Sasahara AA. A comparison of recombinant urokinase with vascular surgery as initial treatment for acute arterial occlusion of the legs. Thrombolysis or Peripheral Arterial Surgery (TOPAS) Investigators. *N Engl J Med.* 1998;338:1105–1111.

246. Abbott WM, Maloney RD, McCabe CC, et al. Arterial embolism: a 44 year perspective. *Am J Surg.* 1982;143: 460–464.

247. Whittemore A. Current techniques for infrainguinal arterial reconstruction. *Jpn J Surg.* 1990;20:627–634.

248. Nguyen LL, Conte MS, Menard MT, et al. Infrainguinal vein bypass graft revision: factors affecting long-term outcome. *J Vasc Surg.* 2004;40:916–923.

249. Beidle TR, Brom-Ferral R, Letourneau JG. Surveillance of infrainguinal vein grafts with duplex sonography. *AJR Am J Roentgenol.* 1994;162:443–448.

250. Idu MM, Truyen E, Buth J. Surveillance of lower extremity vein grafts. *Eur J Vasc Surg.* 1992;6:456–462.

251. Idu MM, Blankenstein JD, de Gier P, et al. Impact of a color-flow duplex surveillance program on infrainguinal vein graft patency: a five-year experience. *J Vasc Surg.* 1993;17:42–52; discussion 52–43.

252. Idu MM, Buth J, Hop WC, et al. Vein graft surveillance: is graft revision without angiography justified and what criteria should be used? *J Vasc Surg.* 1998;27:399–411; discussion 412–413.

253. Lundell A, Lindblad B, Bergqvist D, et al. Femoropopliteal-crural graft patency is improved by an intensive surveillance program: a prospective randomized study. *J Vasc Surg.* 1995;21:26–33; discussion 33–34.

254. Mills JL, Harris EJ, Taylor LM Jr., et al. The importance of routine surveillance of distal bypass grafts with duplex scanning: a study of 379 reversed vein grafts. *J Vasc Surg.* 1990;12:379–386; discussion 387–379.

255. Moody P, Gould DA, Harris PL. Vein graft surveillance improves patency in femoro-popliteal bypass. *Eur J Vasc Surg.* 1990;4:117–121.

256. Visser K, Idu MM, Buth J, et al. Duplex scan surveillance during the first year after infrainguinal autologous vein bypass grafting surgery: costs and clinical outcomes compared with other surveillance programs. *J Vasc Surg.* 2001;33:123–130.

257. Bendib K, Berthezene Y, Croisille P, et al. Assessment of complicated arterial bypass grafts: value of contrast-enhanced subtraction magnetic resonance angiography. *J Vasc Surg.* 1997;26:1036–1042.

258. Loewe C, Cejna M, Lammer J, et al. Contrast-enhanced magnetic resonance angiography in the evaluation of peripheral bypass grafts. *Eur Radiol.* 2000;10:725–732.

259. Bertschinger K, Cassina PC, Debatin JF, et al. Surveillance of peripheral arterial bypass grafts with three- dimensional MR angiography: comparison with digital subtraction angiography. *AJR Am J Roentgenol.* 2001;176:215–220.

260. Dorenbeck U, Seitz J, Volk M, et al. Evaluation of arterial bypass grafts of the pelvic and lower extremities with gadolinium-enhanced magnetic resonance angiography: comparison with digital subtraction angiography. *Invest Radiol.* 2002;37:60–64.

261. Loewe C, Cejna M, Schoder M, et al. Contrast material-enhanced, moving-table MR angiography versus digital subtraction angiography for surveillance of peripheral arterial bypass grafts. *J Vasc Interv Radiol.* 2003;14: 1129–1137.

262. Meissner OA, Verrel F, Tato F, et al. Magnetic resonance angiography in the follow-up of distal lower-extremity bypass surgery: comparison with duplex ultrasound and digital subtraction angiography. *J Vasc Interv Radiol.* 2004;15:1269–1277.

263. Rand T, Basile A, Cejna M, et al. PTA versus carbofilm-coated stents in infrapopliteal arteries: pilot study. *Cardiovasc Intervent Radiol.* 2006;29:29–38.

264. Weishaupt D, Quick HH, Nanz D, et al. Ligating clips for three-dimensional MR angiography at 1.5 T: in vitro evaluation. *Radiology.* 2000;214:902–907.

265. Lenhart M, Volk M, Manke C, et al. Stent appearance at contrast-enhanced MR angiography: in vitro examination with 14 stents. *Radiology.* 2000;217:173–178.

266. Hilfiker PR, Quick HH, Debatin JF. Plain and covered stent-grafts: in vitro evaluation of characteristics at three-dimensional MR angiography. *Radiology.* 1999;211:693–697.

267. van der Laan MJ, Bartels LW, Bakker CJ, et al. Suitability of 7 aortic stent-graft models for MRI-based surveillance. *J Endovasc Ther.* 2004;11:366–371.

268. Gawenda M, Gossmann A, Kruger K, et al. Comparison of magnetic resonance imaging and computed tomography of 8 aortic stent-graft models. *J Endovasc Ther.* 2004;11:627–634.

269. Brewster DC. Prosthetic grafts. In: Rutherford RB, ed. *Vascular Surgery*. Philadelphia, PA: WB Saunders; 1995:492–521.

270. Krinsky G, Jacobowitz G, Rofsky N. Gadolinium-enhanced MR angiography of extraanatomic arterial bypass grafts. *AJR Am J Roentgenol.* 1998;170:735–741.

271. Fauci AS. The vasculitis syndromes. In: Isselbacher KJ, Braunwald E, Wilson JD, Martin JB, Fauci AS, Kasper DL, eds. *Harrison's Principles of Internal Medicine*. New York: McGraw-Hill; 1994:1670–1679.

272. Olin JW. Thromboangiitis obliterans (Buerger's disease). *N Engl J Med.* 2000;343:864–869.

273. Olin JW, Young JR, Graor RA, et al. The changing clinical spectrum of thromboangiitis obliterans (Buerger's disease). *Circulation.* 1990;82:IV3–IV8.

274. Chung JW, Kim HC, Choi YH, et al. Patterns of aortic involvement in Takayasu arteritis and its clinical implications: evaluation with spiral computed tomography angiography. *J Vasc Surg.* 2007;45:906–914.

275. Kerr GS, Hallahan CW, Giordano J, et al. Takayasu arteritis. *Ann Intern Med.* 1994;120:919–929.

276. Liang P, Tan-Ong M, Hoffman GS. Takayasu's arteritis: vascular interventions and outcomes. *J Rheumatol.* 2004;31:102–106.

277. Fava MP, Foradori GB, Garcia CB, et al. Percutaneous transluminal angioplasty in patients with Takayasu arteritis: five-year experience. *J Vasc Interv Radiol.* 1993;4:649–652.

278. Stanson AW. Imaging findings in extracranial (giant cell) temporal arteritis. *Clin Exp Rheumatol.* 2000;18:S43–S48.

279. Bley TA, Wieben O, Vaith P, et al. Magnetic resonance imaging depicts mural inflammation of the temporal artery in giant cell arteritis. *Arthritis Rheum.* 2004;51: 1062–1063; author reply 1064.

280. Bley TA, Wieben O, Uhl M, et al. High-resolution MRI in giant cell arteritis: imaging of the wall of the superficial temporal artery. *AJR Am J Roentgenol.* 2005;184:283–287.

281. Ko GY, Byun JY, Choi BG, et al. The vascular manifestations of Behcet's disease: angiographic and CT findings. *Br J Radiol.* 2000;73:1270–1274.

282. O'Duffy JD. Vasculitis in Behcet's disease. *Rheum Dis Clin North Am.* 1990;16:423–431.

283. Berkmen T. MR angiography of aneurysms in Behcet disease: a report of four cases. *J Comput Assist Tomogr.* 1998;22:202–206.

284. Bradway MW, Drezner AD. Popliteal aneurysm presenting as acute thrombosis and ischemia in a middle-aged man with a history of Kawasaki disease. *J Vasc Surg.* 1997;26: 884–887.

285. Newburger JW, Burns JC. Kawasaki disease. *Vasc Med.* 1999;4:187–202.

286. Molinari G, Sardanelli F, Zandrino F, et al. Coronary aneurysms and stenosis detected with magnetic resonance coronary angiography in a patient with Kawasaki disease. *Ital Heart J.* 2000;1:368–371.

287. Greil GF, Stuber M, Botnar RM, et al. Coronary magnetic resonance angiography in adolescents and young adults with Kawasaki disease. *Circulation.* 2002;105:908–911.

288. Terada LS, Gu Y, Flores SC. AIDS vasculopathy. *Am J Med Sci.* 2000;320:379–387.

289. Wilcken DE. Overview of inherited metabolic disorders causing cardiovascular disease. *J Inherit Metab Dis.* 2003;26:245–257.

290. Wolff KA, Herold CJ, Tempany CM, et al. Aortic dissection: atypical patterns seen at MR imaging. *Radiology.* 1991;181: 489–495.

291. Crivello MS, Porter DH, Kim D, et al. Isolated external iliac artery aneurysm secondary to cystic medial necrosis. *Cardiovasc Intervent Radiol.* 1986;9:139–141.

292. Germain DP. Clinical and genetic features of vascular Ehlers-Danlos syndrome. *Ann Vasc Surg.* 2002;16:391–397.

293. Germain DP, Herrera-Guzman Y. Vascular Ehlers-Danlos syndrome. *Ann Genet.* 2004;47:1–9.

294. Hu X, Plomp AS, van Soest S, et al. Pseudoxanthoma elasticum: a clinical, histopathological, and molecular update. *Surv Ophthalmol.* 2003;48:424–438.

295. Rooke TW, Joyce JW. Uncommon arteriopathies. In: Rutherford RB, ed. *Vascular Surgery*. Philadelphia, PA: WB Saunders; 2000:418–434.

296. Schwahn B, Rozen R. Polymorphisms in the methylenetetrahydrofolate reductase gene: clinical consequences. *Am J Pharmacogenomics.* 2001;1:189–201.

297. Yap S. Classical homocystinuria: vascular risk and its prevention. *J Inherit Metab Dis.* 2003;26:259–265.

298. Ilgit ET, Vural M, Oguz A, et al. Peripheral arterial involvement in neurofibromatosis type 1—a case report. *Angiology.* 1999;50:955–958.

299. Haust MD. Arterial involvement in genetic diseases. *Am J Cardiovasc Pathol.* 1987;1:231–285.

300. Israel G, Krinsky G, Lee V. The "skinny aorta." *Clin Imaging.* 2002;26:116–121.

301. Boontje AH. Uncommon congenital anomalies of the aorta. *J Cardiovasc Surg (Torino).* 1979;20:33–38.

302. Graham LM, Zelenock GB, Erlandson EE, et al. Abdominal aortic coarctation and segmental hypoplasia. *Surgery.* 1979;86:519–529.

303. Maldini G, Teruya TH, Kamida C, et al. Combined percutaneous endovascular and open surgical approach in the treatment of a persistent sciatic artery aneurysm presenting with acute limb-threatening ischemia—a case report and review of the literature. *Vasc Endovascular Surg.* 2002;36:403–408.

304. de Boer MT, Evans JD, Mayor P, et al. An aneurysm at the back of a thigh: a rare presentation of a congenitally persistent sciatic artery. *Eur J Vasc Endovasc Surg.* 2000;19:99–100.

305. Kadir S. *Diagnostic Angiography*. Philadelphia, PA: WB Saunders; 1986:207–253.

306. Zavaleta EG, Fernandez BB, Grove MK, et al. St. Anthony's fire (ergotamine induced leg ischemia)— a case report and review of the literature. *Angiology.* 2001;52:349–356.

307. Abraham P, Chevalier JM, Leftheriotis G, et al. Lower extremity arterial disease in sports. *Am J Sports Med.* 1997;25:581–584.

308. Abraham P, Bouye P, Quere I, et al. Past, present and future of arterial endofibrosis in athletes: a point of view. *Sports Med.* 2004;34:419–425.

309. Schep G, Bender MH, van de Tempel G, et al. Detection and treatment of claudication due to functional iliac obstruction in top endurance athletes: a prospective study. *Lancet.* 2002;359:466–473.

310. Bender MH, Schep G, de Vries WR, et al. Sports-related flow limitations in the iliac arteries in endurance athletes: aetiology, diagnosis, treatment and future developments. *Sports Med.* 2004;34:427–442.

311. Rich NM, Collins GJ Jr., McDonald PT, et al. Popliteal vascular entrapment. Its increasing interest. *Arch Surg.* 1979;114:1377–1384.

312. Levien LJ, Veller MG. Popliteal artery entrapment syndrome: more common than previously recognized. *J Vasc Surg.* 1999;30:587–598.

313. Rignault DP, Pailler JL, Lunel F. The "functional" popliteal entrapment syndrome. *Int Angiol.* 1985;4:341–343.

314. Chernoff DM, Walker AT, Khorasani R, et al. Asymptomatic functional popliteal artery entrapment: demonstration at MR imaging. *Radiology.* 1995;195:176–180.

315. Andrews RT. Diagnostic angiography of the pelvis and lower extremities. *Semin Interv Radiol.* 2000;17:71–111.

316. Peterson JJ, Kransdorf MJ, Bancroft LW, et al. Imaging characteristics of cystic adventitial disease of the peripheral arteries: presentation as soft-tissue masses. *AJR Am J Roentgenol.* 2003;180:621–625.

317. Cassar K, Engeset J. Cystic adventitial disease: a trap for the unwary. *Eur J Vasc Endovasc Surg.* 2005;29:93–96.

318. Pasch AR, Bishara RA, Lim LT, et al. Optimal limb salvage in penetrating civilian vascular trauma. *J Vasc Surg.* 1986;3:189–195.
319. Mattox KL, Feliciano DV, Burch J, et al. Five thousand seven hundred sixty cardiovascular injuries in 4459 patients. Epidemiologic evolution 1958 to 1987. *Ann Surg.* 1989;209:698–705; discussion 706–697.
320. Hood DB, Yellin AE, Weaver FA. Vascular trauma. In: Dean R, ed. *Current Vascular Surgical Diagnosis and Treatment.* Norwalk, CT: Appleton & Lange; 1995:405.
321. Soto JA, Munera F, Morales C, et al. Focal arterial injuries of the proximal extremities: helical CT arteriography as the initial method of diagnosis. *Radiology.* 2001;218: 188–194.
322. Karcaaltincaba M, Akata D, Aydingoz U, et al. Three-dimensional MDCT angiography of the extremities: clinical applications with emphasis on musculoskeletal uses. *AJR Am J Roentgenol.* 2004;183:113–117.
323. Leiner T, De Vries M, Hoogeveen R, et al. Contrast-enhanced peripheral MR angiography at 3.0 Tesla: initial experience with a whole-body scanner in healthy volunteers. *J Magn Reson Imaging.* 2003;17:609–614.
324. Zhu Y, Hardy CJ, Sodickson DK, et al. Highly parallel volumetric imaging with a 32-element RF coil array. *Magn Reson Med.* 2004;52:869–877.
325. Kruger DG, Riederer SJ, Grimm RC, et al. Continuously moving table data acquisition method for long FOV contrast-enhanced MRA and whole-body MRI. *Magn Reson Med.* 2002;47:224–231.
326. Sabati M, Lauzon ML, Frayne R. Space-time relationship in continuously moving table method for large FOV peripheral contrast-enhanced magnetic resonance angiography. *Phys Med Biol.* 2003;48:2739–2752.
327. Perreault P, Edelman MA, Baum RA, et al. MR angiography with gadofosveset trisodium for peripheral vascular disease: phase II trial. *Radiology.* 2003;229:811–820.
328. van Bemmel CM, Spreeuwers LJ, Viergever MA, et al. Level-set-based artery-vein separation in blood pool agent CE-MR angiograms. *IEEE Trans Med Imaging.* 2003;22:1224–1234.
329. Lei T, Udupa JK, Odhner D, et al. 3DVIEWNIX-AVS: a software package for the separate visualization of arteries and veins in CE-MRA images. *Comput Med Imaging Graph.* 2003;27:351–362.
330. Zhang HL, Kent KC, Bush HL, et al. Soft tissue enhancement on time-resolved peripheral magnetic resonance angiography. *J Magn Reson Imaging.* 2004;19:590–597.
331. Baumgartner I, Thoeny HC, Kummer O, et al. Leg ischemia: assessment with MR angiography and spectroscopy. *Radiology.* 2005;234:833–841.
332. Greenman RL, Panasyuk S, Wang X, et al. Early changes in the skin microcirculation and muscle metabolism of the diabetic foot. *Lancet.* 2005;366:1711–1717.

Upper Extremities Vasculature

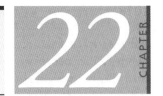

22 CHAPTER

Tim Leiner
Jeffrey C. Hellinger
Neil M. Rofsky

SPECTRUM AND PREVALENCE OF DISEASES

Diagnostic evaluation of suspected upper extremity arterial occlusive disease occurs with less frequency compared to the lower extremity. It accounts for less than 5% of patients presenting with arterial ischemia of an extremity. The abundant collateral networks at the low cervical neck, shoulder, mid arm, elbow and wrist provide robust means to reconstitute distal flow. Furthermore, the upper extremity has less muscle mass and is used less vigorously, as compared to the lower extremity (1).

For these reasons, fewer individuals present with symptomatic disease of the upper versus lower extremity vasculature, and as such, far fewer diagnostic procedures are performed. Another difference between upper and lower extremity vascular disease is highlighted by the fact that surgical and endovascular interventions occur with less frequency in patients presenting with upper extremity ischemia. Many have distal, small vessel disease that is not amenable to repair. In a common vascular practice, upper extremity arterial reconstructions represent only 4% of peripheral arterial reconstructions.

Despite the relative rarity of upper extremity arterial occlusive disease, diagnostic evaluation of the upper extremity vasculature is an important capability for a comprehensive cardiovascular imaging practice. Venous occlusive disease, trauma, hemodialysis access dysfunction, vascular masses, and vascular mapping are other indications for which computed tomographic angiography (CTA) and magnetic resonance imaging (MRI) and angiography (MRA) can play significant diagnostic roles.

With the diverse spectrum of upper extremity vascular disease, a thorough understanding of upper extremity vascular pathology, pathophysiology, and clinical presentation are paramount to implementing imaging strategies and yielding effective interpretations.

The most common cause of upper extremity large vessel arterial occlusive disease is atherosclerosis (2). Arterial occlusive disease of the upper extremity is often caused by nonatherosclerotic disorders such as autoimmune mediated inflammatory and connective tissue disease, trauma, radiation therapy, or thromboembolism.

Arm "claudication" is a typical presentation of most patients with upper extremity arterial disease. These patients typically have exertional pain and fatigue in the arm, forearm, and/or hand, which is relieved with rest. Patients may also present with symptoms from steal phenomena, with Raynaud's phenomenon, with rest pain, or skin and tissue changes such as ulcerations or gangrene. Arterial disease is often associated with an underlying systemic disorder.

Patients with steal syndromes present with upper extremity weakness, dizziness, and sometimes angina. The most common upper extremity steal syndrome is "subclavian steal," with retrograde flow in the vertebral artery to reconstitute the subclavian artery, secondary to ipsilateral proximal subclavian ostial or postostial high-grade stenosis or occlusion.

Another well-known steal phenomenon is coronary steal syndrome, which can be seen when coronary artery bypass grafting is performed with the internal thoracic artery (previously called the internal mammary artery). In the presence of an ipsilateral proximal subclavian artery stenosis or occlusion, flow may reverse in the internal thoracic artery to reconstitute the subclavian artery.

Raynaud's phenomenon, a condition that involves the small- and medium-sized vessels, classically presents in the hand and forearm. It is defined by reversible arterial spasm, which causes a triphasic white-blue-red color response.

For all cases of suspected upper extremity arterial occlusive disease, a prompt and accurate diagnosis is imperative as there is the potential for substantial disability particularly when hand function is adversely affected (2). Gender, age, occupational history, presentation of symptoms, and physical exam are all important to this end (Table 22-1).

Atherosclerotic Arterial Occlusive Disease

The most common locations for upper extremity large vessel involvement include the brachiocephalic and subclavian arteries. However, atherosclerosis can also cause small vessel obstruction by atheromatous embolization or thromboembolism. Patients presenting with symptoms of upper extremity atherosclerotic disease tend to be older compared to those affected by nonatherosclerotic upper extremity arterial occlusive disease (3).

Other Causes of Arterial Disease

The list of nonatherosclerotic conditions affecting the upper extremity vasculature is broad and includes arteritis, compressive syndromes, traumatic injuries, nonatherosclerotic embolization, and a variety of conditions that result from complications of renal insufficiency and surgical interventions (e.g., dialysis access surgery).

The vasculitides can be readily conceptualized based on size of the vessel involved as will be described in the next section. Connective tissue diseases such as Marfan syndrome, Ehlers-Danlos syndrome, pseudoxanthoma elasticum, homocystinurea and neurofibromatosis are well known for their peripheral arterial involvement.

Vascular disease in azotemic patients may involve calciphylaxis, a poorly understood and highly morbid syndrome of vascular calcification and skin lesions (4–7), which can produce medial calcification (also known as Mönckeberg sclerosis) in small- and medium-sized arteries, visible on plain radiographs. These changes are typically found in patients with diabetes mellitus and end-stage renal disease (ESRD) or postrenal transplant. The presence of a distal peripheral pulse helps to distinguish acral calciphylaxis from occlusive disease.

Congenital and acquired clotting disorders may also manifest themselves with symptoms of peripheral arterial disease. Infrequent causes of peripheral arterial disease are fibromuscular dysplasia and primary vascular tumors.

TABLE 22-1

Conditions and Risks for Upper Extremity Arterial Disease

Medical Conditions	Occupational Injury
Atherosclerosis	Vibration syndrome
Thromboembolism	Pneumatic tools
Atheromatous embolization	Grinders
Connective tissue disease	Chain saws
Scleroderma	Electrical shock
CREST syndrome	Thermal injury
Rheumatic arteritis	Hypothenar hammer syndrome
Systemic lupus erythematosus	Mechanical work or auto repair
Polymyositis or dermatomyositis	Lathe operation
Mixed connective tissue disease	Carpentry
Large artery vasculitis	Electrical work
Takayasu disease	Occupational acro-osteolysis—polyvinylchloride
Giant cell arteritis	Athletic activities
Small artery (and vein) vasculitis	Thoracic outlet compression associated with
Thromboangiitis obliterans	Baseball pitching
(Buerger's disease)	Kayaking
Blood dyscrasias	Weightlifting
Cold agglutinins	Rowing
Cryoglobulins and cryofibrinogenemia	Butterfly swimming
Myoproliferative diseases	Golfing
Behçet syndrome	Hand ischemia
Antiphospholipid antibody syndrome	Baseball catching
Thoracic outlet syndrome	Frisbee
Congenital arterial wall defects	Karate
Marfan syndrome	Handball
Pseudoxanthoma elasticum	Pharmacologic history
Ehlers-Danlos syndrome	Drug abuse
Fibromuscular dysplasia	Ergotamine abuse
Iatrogenic injury	Cocaine abuse
Arterial blood gas puncture	Amphetamine abuse
Intra-arterial pressure monitoring	Cannabis use
Cardiac catherization	Drugs
Intra-arterial digital subtraction	β-blockers, vinblastine, bleomycine, cisplatinum
angiography	methylsergide, heavy metals, interferon
Frostbite	(α and β) dopamine overdose
Renal transplantation and related	
azotemic arteriopathy	
Hemodialysis access	
Radiation	
Breast carcinoma	
Hodgkin's disease	
Aneurysms of the upper extremity	

Modified from Greenfield LJ, Rajagopalan S, Olin JW. Upper extremity arterial disease. *Cardiol Clin.* 2002;20(4):623–631.

Disease Classification Based on Vessel Size

Upper extremity vascular disease pathology can be divided based on large, medium, or small vessel involvement. Specific, often mutually exclusive entities can be found within these divisions, particularly when separating diseases that affect the large and small vessels.

Upper extremity large arterial occlusive disease is most often due to atherosclerosis. Claudication symptoms and steal syndromes commonly reflect large vessel involvement.

Nonatherosclerotic conditions that effect the large vessels include subclavian or axillary autoimmune arteritis (Takayasu or giant cell arteritis), thoracic outlet syndrome with resultant intimal damage and subsequent aneurysm formation and distal embolization, radiation arteritis, and penetrating traumatic injury.

Medium- and small-sized arteries and veins are typically involved in thromboangiitis obliterans (TAO), also known as Buerger's or Winiwarter-Buerger disease. Patients with TAO are almost always young (<45 years old); use large amounts of tobacco products (usually, but not limited to, smoking); and characteristically show segmental occlusions in radial, ulnar, palmar, and digital arteries with typical bridging corkscrew collaterals (8).

There are numerous diseases primarily affecting the smaller arteries of the upper extremity (Table 22-1). With inflammatory arteritis, Raynaud's phenomenon is common. Traumatic injury can also involve small and medium vessels. Occupational exposure can lead to vibration or impact-induced small vessel vasospasm in the hand, followed by intimal injury, aneurysm formation, thrombosis, occlusion, and/or distal embolization (Table 22-1). Blunt and penetrating hand trauma can lead to ischemia if the palmar arch is incomplete.

GLOBAL VIEW OF UNIQUE ASPECTS AND CONSIDERATIONS OF IMAGING THIS ORGAN SYSTEM

The upper extremity vascular tree begins at the left ventricular outflow tract, includes the palmar arch and digital arteries, and ends at the entrance of the superior cava into the right atrium. A full upper extremity vascular study, therefore, demands imaging coverage in the order of 70 to 90 cm and also encompasses the inferior part of the cervical region to include the abundant collateral pathways in patients with suspected arterial or venous occlusion. Both MRA and multidetector row CT (MDCT) are capable of imaging over a large field of view with high spatial resolution thereby enabling high-fidelity depiction of the upper extremity vasculature.

Occlusive arterial disease can be evaluated by clinical examination, segmental blood pressure measurements, pulse volume recordings, duplex ultrasonography, and intra-arterial digital subtraction angiography (IA DSA). There is also a firm role for cross-sectional imaging techniques such as MRI and MDCT to provide the necessary preinterventional information about location and severity of vascular disease as well as information about the surrounding tissues. Traditionally, IA DSA had always been reserved for this purpose. However, IA DSA is a procedure that utilizes ionizing radiation and carries a small but definable risk for local and systemic complications due to its invasive nature and the use of nephrotoxic contrast media (9).

Over the past years, MRA and MDCT have emerged as reliable tests for diagnosis and treatment planning. In providing an accurate "roadmap" of upper extremity vasculature to the referring clinician, these techniques aid in the triage of therapeutic options for patients and distinguish disease that is amenable to percutaneous transluminal angioplasty (PTA) from disease that is too diffuse, long-segmented, or complex and thus demands a more extensive interventional procedure or bypass grafting procedure.

At the other end of the clinical spectrum are patients with small vessel disease. Many of these patients suffer from systemic connective tissue disease. In patients with small vessel disease, the primary aim is to provide sufficient blood flow to relieve rest pain and heal skin lesions. This is primarily achieved by medical therapy and not with PTA or arterial reconstructive bypass surgery (2,10).

Noninvasive imaging of distal small vessel disease at the level of the digital arteries is still challenging due to the relatively limited spatial resolution of both MRA and MDCT compared with IA DSA. Continued progress in technology and technique predicts a progressive increased utilization of MRA and MDCT (Fig. 22-1).

The ability to locally administer pharmacological vasodilation by intra-arterial injection of vasodilating agents such as tolazoline represents an important difference between IA DSA and noninvasive imaging. For MRA and MDCT, some degree of vasodilation can be induced by wrapping the hand in warm towels or having the patient hold a warm pack during the examination.

As a practical consideration for any patient presenting with a nontraumatic acute arterial occlusion, a prompt search for atrial fibrillation, ulcerative endocarditis, and mural thrombi overlying the site of myocardial infarction is essential.

WHAT DO COMPUTED TOMOGRAPHY AND MAGNETIC RESONANCE BRING OVER OTHER IMAGING AND NONIMAGING DIAGNOSTIC STRATEGIES?

The cornerstone of the diagnostic workup of patients with upper extremity arterial disease is a thorough physical examination and medical/surgical and occupational history, including any athletic activities in which the patient may be involved. Physical examination should encompass the entire vascular system and not only assessment of peripheral pulsations and local trophic changes. Consequently, one

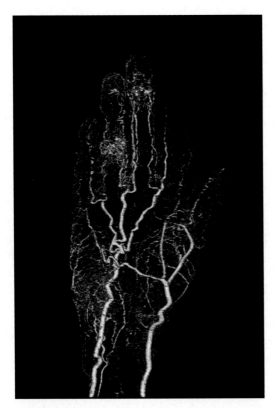

FIGURE 22-1 VR image from a temporally resolved frame of a dynamic CE MRA in a patient with vasospastic disease and degenerative joint changes. The vasculature is well depicted including many of the digital vessels, without the use of pharmacologic vasodilators.

should also search for evidence of systemic hypertension, cardiac murmurs, carotid and abdominal bruits, and signs of subclavian and peripheral arterial aneurysms.

Additional tests can be divided into those aimed at a *physiological* assessment of the peripheral circulation and tests aimed to provide an anatomical *road map* of the peripheral vasculature, showing the exact location, extent, and severity of the disease process, in relation to commonly used anatomical landmarks during interventional radiological and surgical procedures. Table 22-2 shows an overview of these techniques.

One of the most commonly used noninvasive tests to gauge the extent and severity of peripheral arterial disease is color-aided duplex ultrasonography (DU). This test combines a local anatomical image, obtained in B-mode, with information about the direction, pattern, and magnitude of arterial and venous flow (obtained by Doppler frequency analysis) (11).

The severity of stenoses can be derived from peak systolic and end-diastolic velocity measurements, whereby higher peak systolic velocities indicate more severe stenoses (12). A major drawback of DU is the long duration of the examination and the operator dependency (13). It is generally accepted that characterization of location and degree of stenosis requires experienced vascular laboratories with rigorous quality controls.

TABLE 22-2

Commonly Used Diagnostic Tests for Detection and Grading of Upper Extremity Peripheral Arterial Disease

Test	Measures	Interpretation
Segmental arm pressure	Arterial pressures in different arm segments (usually with 2 cuffs), measured in both limbs	>15 mmHg between cuffs or gradient measurements in limbs indicates significant lesion Allows crude localization of disease
Finger pressure digital measurements	Finger blood pressure in proximal phalanges	Normal subjects and patients with vasospastic Raynaud's have blood pressures within 20 mmHg of brachial pressure
Ten-finger arterial wave form analysis	Visual display of volume changes in fingers in response to arterial blood flow	Delayed upstroke and rounded peak baseline bowing away from signifies obstruction; in severe disease waveform may be absent
Digital cold challenge (Nielsen test)	Finger systolic pressure after local ischemic cooling	Decrease in pressure >20% in cooled finger versus control finger testing is indicative of Raynaud's phenomenon
Duplex ultrasonography	Arterial blood flow pattern and velocity	Localization and determination of disease severity based on peak-systolic and end-diastolic velocity measurements

Both MDCT and MRA provide highly detailed images of the peripheral vascular tree analogous to intra-arterial digital subtraction techniques. With truly three-dimensional (3D) data sets, reconstructions can be viewed from an infinite number of perspectives.

In contrast to conventional IA DSA, MDCT and MRA are not limited to depiction of the vascular lumen but also allow uncomplicated visualization of anatomic variants, the vessel wall, and the bony and soft tissues surrounding the vessels.

This capacity is especially important when considering that vascular workups are associated with inflammation, infection, and tumor. Particularly in the evaluation of vasculitides, mural and adjacent soft tissue features provide vital information regarding the status of the disease. Furthermore, the combined attributes of strong soft tissue contrast and the lack of ionizing radiation make MRI ideal for serial follow-up studies when monitoring response to treatment.

As with IA DSA, stress studies can be performed to assess the effect of a change in posture on the vasculature. Both MRA and MDCT are also well suited in the noninvasive follow-up of surgical intervention, including the assessment of the various arterial bypass grafts as well as hemodialysis access sites.

IA DSA has superior in-plane resolution, and based on this feature, it is considered by many as the imaging modality of choice for imaging small vessel disease of the digital arteries. However, the spatial resolution capability of MD CTA and MRA have shown steady improvements.

For example, with state-of-the-art 1.5T and 3.0T MRI imagers and dedicated upper extremity vascular coils, voxel sizes, on the order of 0.7×0.7 mm in plane, on the order of 1.0 mm in the slice direction can be achieved during first arterial passage of contrast medium; with the use of the newest intra-vascular blood-pool contrast agents, this resolution can be improved to 0.4 to 0.5 mm in each direction, resulting in isotropic voxel sizes in the order of 64 to 125 microns.

With the newest MDCT scanners it is routinely possible to achieve isotropic spatial resolutions in the order of 0.4 to 0.5 mm. With such spatial resolution, an assessment of small vascular disease with MRA and CTA is becoming more feasible.

MRA offers physiologic information using phase contrast (PC) techniques. This information regarding flow and velocity offers useful adjuncts to the physiologic road map (14–16). MR spectroscopy can also provide information regarding muscle metabolism (17–23). Finally, MR and to a certain extent CT can also provide information about tissue perfusion. While the impact of the adjunctive tests awaits

further research, such capacities will likely be important as targeted medical and angiogenic therapies emerge in clinical practice.

IMAGING STRATEGIES

Computed Tomographic Angiography

Upper Extremity Computed Tomographic Angiography Technique

Upper extremity computed tomographic angiography (UE CTA) can be performed on all currently available multidetector-row CT scanners (4 to 64 channels) to evaluate a broad spectrum of clinical pathology. Based on the clinical indications, three core protocols are recommended: Aortic Arch with Upper Extremity Runoff, Upper Extremity Runoff, and Upper Extremity Indirect CT Venography (Table 22-3). For each protocol, there are several technical considerations. These include patient preparation, image acquisition, contrast medium administration, image display, and exam transfer and storage.

Patient Preparation

Patient preparation begins by removing all external metallic objects from the patient's chest, neck, and the affected extremity. These objects can limit photon exposure and degrade image quality. The next step is to place an 18- to 22-gauge intravenous (IV) catheter in an upper extremity vein, contralateral to the side of interest. With an ipsilateral venous injection, high density contrast material and related streak artifact in the inflowing veins will render arterial and venous segments nondiagnostic.

As high flow rates are necessary, the antecubital location is the preferred access site. If this location is not possible, other options include the forearm or hand, with the likely need to decrease the contrast medium injection rate. When these secondary sites cannot be accessed, considerations include using a contralateral external jugular vein or a centrally placed venous catheter, which can accommodate power injection.

The final preparation is to position the patient on the CT gantry table. The goal is to isolate the upper extremity in the center of the table. In most cases, patients are positioned supine and head first. The affected extremity is extended above the patient's head and placed isocenter in the gantry, with the palm positioned ventrally and the fingers spread apart (Fig. 22-2). The head is secured in a neutral position, and the contralateral arm is placed at the patient's side.

Pillows, blankets, or both are utilized to support the patient's body and also to raise the height of the upper

TABLE 22-3

Upper Extremity Computed Tomographic Angiography Protocols

Protocol	Coverage	Distance	Application
Aortic Arch with Runoff	Arterial inflow and outflow	700–1,000 mm	Arterial occlusive disease Vasculitis Hemodialysis access Arterial bypass grafts and stents Vascular mapping Vascular masses Trauma
Runoff	Targeted arterial outflow	300–600 mm	Vascular mapping Vascular masses Trauma
Indirect Venogram	Peripheral and central veins Complete Targeted	 700–1,000 mm 400–700 mm	Veno-occlusive disease Vascular mapping Venous stents

extremity so that it is at the same level as the mid axillary line. Tape can be used to secure positioning of the forearm and hand. To ensure that the extremity is as close to the gantry isocenter as possible, patients can either be rotated

into a modified swimmer's position or be placed prone (Fig. 22-3).

If the affected extremity cannot be raised above the patient's head, the exam can be performed with the

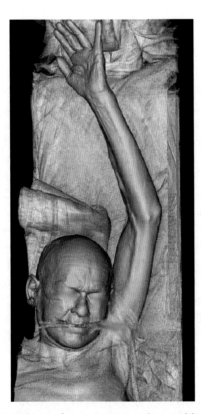

FIGURE 22-2 VR image demonstrates a patient positioned supine for a left upper extremity CTA. The left upper extremity is abducted and hyperextended above the patient's head in the center of the CT gantry table. Bed sheets are folded to support the patient's head and hand. Tape (not depicted) was also utilized to stabilize the forearm and hand.

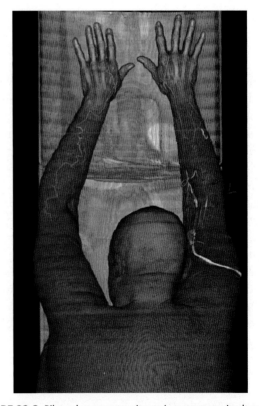

FIGURE 22-3 Bilateral upper extremity angiograms were simultaneously acquired through the patient's forearms and hands. The patient was positioned prone with the forearms and hands as close as possible to the gantry isocenter. The patient's head was supported with a "donut" cushion. Injection was via a right antecubital vein.

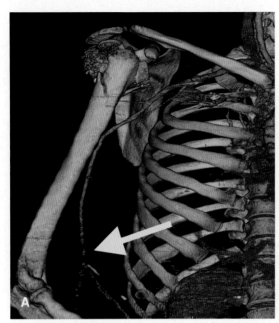
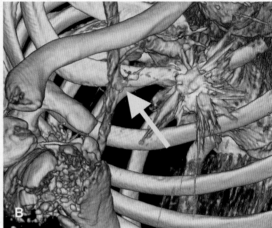

FIGURE 22-4 Right upper extremity 16-channel CTA was performed on a patient who sustained a gunshot injury to the right shoulder, shattering the humeral head. As the patient could not raise the arm, the right arm was placed at the patient's side. Note how the axillary and proximal and mid brachial artery are of diagnostic quality, while the distal brachial artery and proximal radial and ulnar arteries show pseudo-lesions (*arrow*) from noise and spiral artifact (**A**). The study revealed a small traumatic right subclavian pseudoaneurysm (*arrow* in **B**) near retained bullet fragments.

extremity placed alongside the patient's body, with the risk of increased noise and streak artifacts (Fig. 22-4). In this instance, the patient's body should be shifted away from the affected extremity so that the upper extremity can be placed isocenter. To reduce noise in this position, the contralateral upper extremity should be raised out of the field of view. Bilateral exams are acquired by scanning both arms together (targeted runoff for forearm or hand coverage) or by scanning each arm individually (16 to 64 channel scanners).

Functional UE CTA is performed for thoracic outlet syndrome with neutral and challenged CT angiographic acquisitions. In the neutral phase, the affected extremity is placed at the patient's side. In the challenged phase, the arm is raised and the patient's head is turned contralateral, duplicating a combination of Wright (upper extremity abduction with external rotation and the head and chin in neutral position) and Adson's (upper extremity extension with lateral rotation and the head turned toward the affected extremity) provocative maneuvers.

Image Acquisition

Protocol Series Upper extremity CT angiographic protocols can be programmed into the scanners with at least five acquisition series. The first series is a necessary low-dose scout topogram (Fig. 22-5). To prescribe precise coverage and field of view, both anterior-posterior and lateral views are recommended.

The second series is an optional nonenhanced acquisition with 1.25- to 5.0-mm thick images. Coverage may be identical to the planned contrast enhanced acquisition or may target a selected upper extremity region. The primary objective of the optional nonenhanced acquisition is to identify high-density material that may limit CT angiographic image quality and interpretation (i.e., streak artifact) or may be obscured by the contrast medium. These images are essential to confirming the presence and location of calcifications, endovascular stents and stent-grafts, surgical clips, surgical grafts, catheters, bone fragments (i.e., trauma), residual IV contrast, active bleeding, and hematomas.

The third series is a low-dose timing acquisition, which is essential for precise synchronization of the image acquisition with either arterial or venous enhancement or both (see Contrast Medium Administration section, below, for details). The arrival time is determined either real time with bolus tracking software or as a separate timing bolus acquisition.

The fourth series is the CT angiographic acquisition in which the contrast enhanced images are obtained. In adults, a tube voltage of 100 to 120 kV is used along with an

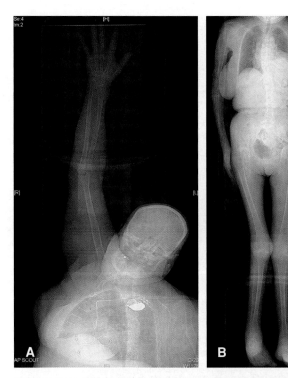

FIGURE 22-5 Coronal topograms for upper extremity CT angiograms performed with the affected extremity isolated above the patient's head (**A**) and with the extremity at the patient's side (**B**). When the extremity is raised above the patient's head, the scan direction is caudadcranial. When placed at the patient's side, the direction is cranialcaudad.

amperage of 275 to 350 mA, unless automated tube current modulation software is utilized. In pediatric applications, 80 to 100 kV is selected as the tube voltage. For patients with a low body mass index, the amperage and tube voltage can be reduced, while for patients of larger body habitus, both may need to be increased. Images are reconstructed with a soft or medium reconstruction kernel.

In the setting of suspected cardiogenic upper extremity thromboembolism, to simplify the diagnostic evaluation, an ancillary consideration is whether retrospective electrocardiogram (ECG) gating through the heart should be combined with the routine non-ECG-gated contrast-enhanced acquisition through the upper extremity vasculature. Breath-holding is required only for the portions of exams that extend through the chest.

The fifth series is an optional delayed post-contrast acquisition. The delayed acquisition is useful in the setting of suspected vasculitis, vascular masses, and hemorrhage. It can also be used to acquire a venous phase after the arterial phase, as in the case of preoperative vascular mapping for hemodialysis creation. A delayed phase can also benefit those instances in which the scan acquisition gets ahead of the contrast medium bolus, a circumstance that is best recognized when the exam is monitored.

Upper Extremity Computed Tomographic Angiogram

Coverage In the Aortic Arch with Upper Extremity Runoff protocol, when the arm is raised, coverage begins at the mid chest to include the aortic arch, and extends in a caudadcranial direction through the fingers, so that the complete inflow and outflow upper extremity vascular tree is evaluated (Fig. 22-6). For an average adult patient, this scan distance may be 700 to 1,000 mm. If the arm is placed at the patient's side, coverage begins at the thoracic inlet and extends through the fingers in a cranialcaudad direction.

In the Upper Extremity Runoff protocol, outflow segments are targeted. Coverage begins at the shoulder or elbow and extends through to the fingers, in a caudadcranial or cranialcaudad direction. The scan distance may range between 300 and 600 mm.

For the Upper Extremity Indirect CT Venogram protocol, central and peripheral veins are evaluated (Fig. 22-7). Scanning the central veins is recommended prior to the peripheral veins, as there is more rapid venous return from the head and neck. The arm may be raised or placed at the patient's side, with the acquisition in either a caudadcranial or cranialcaudad direction, respectively. When the arm is raised, coverage begins at the mid chest to include the cavoatrial junction and progresses cranially. When the arm is at the patient's side, coverage begins at the thoracic inlet and progresses caudally.

Depending on the clinical indications, coverage may extend to either the elbow (400 to 700 mm scan distance) or the hand (700 to 1,000 mm scan distance). For a delayed CT angiographic acquisition, the series may be programmed to cover the entire vascular tree or only the outflow. If the series is needed because contrast did not adequately opacify the forearm and hand arteries on the first acquisition, beginning the delayed scan at the elbow is sufficient.

Acquisition Parameters Table 22-4 lists acquisition (detector configuration, pitch, gantry speed) and reconstruction (slice thickness, reconstruction interval) parameters for complete upper extremity CT angiographic coverage, using 4-, 8-, 16-, and 64-channel multidetector-row CT scanners. Based on the type of multidetector-row CT scanner, selection of these parameters reflects a balance between the desired spatial resolution, the scan distance, and the scan duration. Parameters for 32- and 40-channel scanners can be adapted from 64-channel scanners.

With 4-channel systems, a 4 × 2.5 mm detector configuration is required to scan the complete upper extremity vasculature in a reasonable duration. Then, 2.5-mm

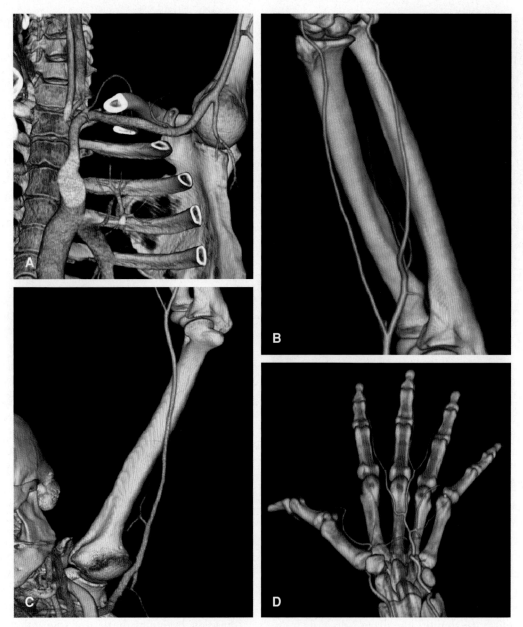

FIGURE 22-6 A left upper extremity CT angiogram was performed using an Aortic Arch with Upper Extremity Runoff protocol. Coverage includes the complete inflow and outflow vascular territories. VR images **(A–D)** are displayed as a four-station angiogram runoff. Note the robust enhancement throughout the vascular tree.

images are reconstructed at 1.0- to 2.0-mm increments, resulting in an effective slice thickness of 3.0 mm. These "standard resolution" acquisitions with up to 1,000 images are adequate to depict the vascular tree to the hand. However, when visualization of the palmar and digital arteries is critical to diagnosis and clinical management, such as in arterial occlusive disease and vasculitis, high-resolution imaging with a 4×1 mm or 4×1.25 mm configuration may be necessary. As the scan duration would be twice as long, the coverage would need to be reduced (i.e., Upper

Extremity Runoff protocol) to minimize venous contamination.

With an 8-channel system, the complete vascular tree is imaged with a high-resolution technique (8×1.25 mm configuration) in duration comparable to 4×2.5 mm acquisitions. Vascular enhancement from the mid chest through the fingers is optimized, while the palmar arch and digital arteries are depicted with reliable detail. This technique also improves visualization of small vessels off the subclavian, axillary, brachial, and proximal radial and ulnar

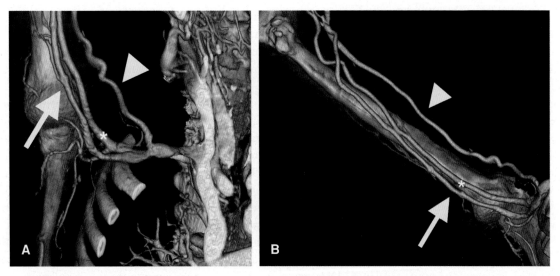

FIGURE 22-7 A right upper extremity venogram was performed with the patient's arm raised. Imaging covered peripheral and central segments. Cephalic (*arrowhead*) and basilic (*arrow*) veins are well depicted (**A**). By using a prolonged injection, the axillary and brachial arteries also show robust enhancement (**B**).

TABLE 22-4

Upper Extremity Computed Tomographic Angiography Acquisition and Reconstruction Parameters

MDCT Scanner	Mode	Detector Configuration (channels × mm)	Pitch	Gantry Rotation Time (sec)	Table Speed (mm/sec)	Scan Time (sec)	Slice Thickness (mm)	RI (mm)	Number of Images
4 Channel									
GE	SR	4 × 2.5	1.5	0.5	30	30	2.5	1.5	600
Phillips	SR	4 × 2.5	1.5	0.5	30	30	2.5	1.5	600
Siemens	SR	4 × 2.5	1.5	0.5	30	30	2.5	1.5	600
Toshiba	SR	4 × 2.0	1.375	0.5	22	41	2	1.0	900
8 Channel									
GE	HR	8 × 1.25	1.35	0.5	27	33	1.25	0.8	1,125
GE	SR	8 × 2.5	1.35	0.5	54	17	2.5	1.5	600
16 Channel									
GE	IR	16 × 0.625	1.375	0.5	28	33	0.625	0.5	1,800
Phillips	IR	16 × 0.75	1.25	0.5	30	30	0.75	0.5	1,800
Siemens	IR	16 × 0.75	1.2	0.5	29	31	0.75	0.5	1,800
Toshiba	IR	16 × 0.5	1.438	0.5	23	39	0.5	0.4	2,250
GE	HR	16 × 1.25	1.375	0.6	46	20	1.25	0.8	1,125
Phillips	HR	16 × 1.5	1.25	0.5	60	15	1.5	0.8	1,125
Siemens	HR	16 × 1.5	1.2	0.5	58	16	1.5	0.8	1,125
Toshiba	HR	16 × 1.0	1.438	0.5	46	20	1.0	0.8	1,125
64 Channel									
GE	IR	64 × 0.625	0.563	0.7	32	28	0.625	0.5	1,800
Siemens	IR	(2) × 32 0.6	0.75	0.5	29	31	0.75	0.5	1,800
GE	HR	32 × 1.25	0.938	0.6	63	14	1.25	0.8	1,125
Siemens	HR	24 × 1.2	1.0	0.5	46	20	1.5	0.8	1,125

SR, standard resolution; HR, high resolution; IR, isotropic resolution; RI, reconstruction interval. Acquisition parameters listed are the detector configuration, pitch, and gantry rotation speed. Reconstruction parameters shown are the slice thickness and reconstruction interval.

Note: Scan times for a distance of 900 mm.

arteries. Data sets are reconstructed every 0.8 mm into images with a nominal section thickness of 1.25 mm, yielding up to 1,250 images. Coverage of the thoracic and abdominal aorta can be combined with an upper extremity CT angiogram using the fastest gantry speed and maximizing the pitch. To minimize venous contamination, increasing the detector width to 2.5 mm (standard resolution) may be necessary.

With 16-channel systems, isotropic resolution and high-resolution modes are utilized. Isotropic exams are acquired with submillimeter collimations (16 × 0.625 mm, 16 × 0.75 mm configurations). These acquisitions further improve visualization of small vessels in the upper extremity vascular tree and are particularly useful for defining anatomic detail in the shoulder, elbow, and hand and for evaluating pediatric upper extremity vasculature. Data sets are generated in a duration similar to 4 × 2.5 mm and 8 × 1.25 mm acquisitions. One of the challenges using this mode is the potential for increased noise and the subsequent need for increasing the amperage, if automated tube current modulation is not utilized. Another challenge is the number of images. Reconstructed at 0.4- to 0.8-mm increments, up to 2,500 images may be generated.

A solution to both the noise and the vast number of slices is to reconstruct images thicker into high-resolution data sets (1.5 mm). Alternatively, the exam can be acquired using a high-resolution mode (16 × 1.25 mm or 16 × 1.5 mm configurations). For most clinical applications with a 16-channel system, the high-resolution mode provides adequate detail to reliably depict the complete upper extremity vasculature.

The table speed with this configuration is often too fast for contrast medium transit in the upper extremity vascular tree. The result is that the acquisition can potentially outrun the bolus, a circumstance that can be largely avoided by slowing the acquisition speed with a lower pitch, by decreasing the gantry rotation speed, or both.

A second solution is to slow the scan by acquiring the study with submillimeter collimation. In this instance, the data set is reconstructed thicker into 1.0- to 1.5-mm thick images. A third solution is to lengthen the delay prior to initiating the scan. These solutions are further addressed in the discussion for contrast medium injection parameters. With a 16-channel system, the increased table speed can be utilized to scan the complete upper extremity vasculature and thoracic and abdominal aorta with a high-resolution technique.

With a 64-channel system, both isotropic (64 × 0.6 mm, 64 × 0.625 mm configurations) and high-resolution (64 × 1.2 mm, 64 × 1.25 mm configurations) modes can also be selected. When using either mode, the table speed is substantially faster than with 16-channel systems. To optimize vascular enhancement through to the digital vessels, it is essential to slow the acquisition speed. Submillimeter collimation, a low pitch, and a slower gantry speed are all options to achieve this goal.

With the submillimeter acquisitions, raw data can be reconstructed into high-resolution data sets (section thickness 1.0 to 1.5 mm, reconstruction interval 0.7 to 0.8 mm), into isotropic resolution data sets (section thickness 0.6 to 0.9 mm, reconstruction interval 0.4 to 0.7 mm) or into both. Automated tube current modulation should be utilized with all isotropic acquisitions to minimize noise and amperage and voltage requirements. Based upon the scan length and duration, an isotropic or a high-resolution technique can be prescribed to image not only through the aorta, but also the lower extremity vasculature.

Contrast Medium Administration

Depending on the degree of noise, arterial enhancement in an upper extremity CT arteriogram should reach at least a minimum of 250 to 300 Hounsfield Units (HU), while venous enhancement for indirect upper extremity venograms should be in the range of 120 to 200 HU. Optimizing this enhancement is dependent on synchronized delivery of contrast medium with an iodine dose of 400 to 600 mg iodine per kilogram (1.3 to 2.0 mL/kg for 300 mg iodine/mL concentration).

For patients who weigh between 60 and 90 kg, the iodine should be delivered at a rate (iodine flux) of 1.0 to 1.5 g iodine per second (3.3 to 5 mL/second for 300 mg iodine/mL concentration). Injection protocols for adult and pediatric upper extremity CT angiograms can achieve these requirements by adjusting the contrast medium concentration (300 to 370 mg iodine per millimeter), injection rate (2.5 to 6 mL/second), injection volume (75 to 150 mL), and/or injection duration based on a patient's body weight, the scan distance, and the speed of the scanner (24).

Strategies for Contrast Medium Administration
Synchronization To account for the variable time for contrast medium to travel from the site of IV injection to the upper extremity vascular tree, it is necessary to determine the transit time using either a test-bolus injection or automatic bolus triggering. For complete upper extremity arterial coverage, either technique can be performed, with the aortic arch serving as the reference level. For targeted upper extremity runoffs, the proximal or distal brachial artery is used as the reference level. In this instance, automated triggering is most practical given the small size (3 to 5 mm) of these arteries.

A test bolus is performed by injecting 15 to 20 cc of contrast at a rate equivalent to that planned for the CT angiogram. Low dose, thick transverse sections are acquired every 2 seconds. A region of interest (ROI) is placed in the reference vessel, generating a time-attenuation curve. The transit time equals the time to the curve's peak, which is then selected as the minimum delay. Automated triggering software is available on all multidetector-row scanners.

During contrast injection, low-dose, single-level sections are acquired. Reference vessel attenuation is monitored in near real time either with a ROI or by visual inspection. The transit time is defined as the time required to reach a predetermined opacification threshold (120 to 150 HU). The scan is then initiated after a short diagnostic delay. In comparison to a test-bolus injection, when utilizing automated triggering, the actual scan delay is longer. This is due to inherent interscan and image reconstruction delays in addition to the diagnostic delay. Depending on the scanner, the minimum scan delay may range between 2 and 8 seconds.

An indirect upper extremity CT venogram can be initiated after determining the arrival time of contrast to the aortic arch. In this instance, the venogram is acquired after an additional 50-second diagnostic delay. If the acquisition proceeds without determining the transit time, the venogram is acquired approximately 70 seconds following the infusion of contrast medium.

Injection Parameters Extrapolating from lower extremity CTA contrast medium principles, upper extremity vascular enhancement is optimized when the table speed does not exceed 30 mm/second (25). For complete inflow and outflow coverage, this translates to scan durations of 25 to 35 seconds (700- to 1,000-mm distance), while for targeted runoff coverage, 10 to 20 seconds (300- to 600-mm distance). Accordingly, upper extremity injection protocols are designed based on slow (≤30 mm/second table speed) and fast (>30 mm/second) acquisitions.

Slow acquisitions occur with 4 × 2.5 mm, 8 × 1.25 mm, or 16 × 0.625 mm configurations. In addition, a 64 × 0.6 mm or 64 × 0.625 mm configuration with a low pitch (≤0.8) and slower gantry speed (≥0.5) produces a table speed around 30 mm/second. When the scan duration is ≥25 seconds with these acquisitions, the injection duration is set to equal the scan duration and a biphasic injection protocol is utilized, rather than a uniphasic injection; the biphasic injection achieves more uniform enhancement for long injection durations (≥25 seconds).

The injection rates and volumes for both phases vary according to the body weight and the contrast medium concentration (Table 22-5). In the first phase, 20% of the total volume is administered at a higher rate (4 to 6 mL/second for 60- to 90-kg patients) over a short duration (i.e., 5 seconds). In the second, the remaining volume is infused at a second, slower injection rate (3 to 5 mL/second for 60- to 90-kg patients) for the duration of the examination. If automated triggering is used, the injection duration is extended to account for the inherent delay with this software.

When the coverage is targeted to the runoff segments and the table speed is ≤30 mm/second, in most acquisitions, the injection duration is also set to equal the scan duration. A uniphasic injection is appropriate for the shorter injection duration (10 to 20 seconds). The injection rate is then derived by determining the patient's appropriate contrast volume for the selected contrast medium concentration and dividing this amount by the injection duration. If the injection rate exceeds the tolerable limit for the accessed vein, the iodine concentration, the injection duration, or both should be increased. If the injection duration is increased, the diagnostic delay should be increased by the same amount.

Fast acquisitions occur with 8 × 2.5 mm, 16 × 1.25 mm, and 16 × 1.5 mm configurations. With a 64-channel system, a collimation greater than 1.0 (32 × 1.25 mm, 24 × 1.2 mm configurations), a high pitch (>1.0), and a fast gantry speed (≤6.0) will routinely result in fast acquisitions. These scan parameters translate into table speeds of 45 to 65 mm/second. For an Aortic Arch with Upper Extremity Runoff protocol, if the injection duration is set to equal the scan duration, an insufficient iodine dose may be delivered and the scan acquisition may be too fast for the required transit time through the upper extremity vascular tree.

The key strategy to prevent the acquisition from "outrunning" the contrast bolus is to use a fixed biphasic injection of 30 to 35 seconds and increase the scan delay such that the scan and injection durations end simultaneously (Table 22-6). For an Upper Extremity Runoff protocol, a fixed 15- to 20-second uniphasic injection is selected, and the scan delay is similarly increased. To attain the required iodine dose, the injection rate and concentration are varied according to the body weight. One cautionary note with this approach is that if the delay is too long (>15 seconds), unwarranted venous opacification in the inflow and outflow regions may result. In this instance, the table speed should be slowed down.

Saline Flush Saline flush is administered with a dual-chamber injector immediately following the contrast medium infusion. For UE CTA, the saline injection improves contrast utilization and reduces perivenous streaks artifacts. A volume of 30 to 40 mL injected at a rate equal to the contrast medium injection rate is sufficient. If a biphasic contrast medium protocol is utilized, the saline injection rate defaults to the second injection rate.

TABLE 22-5

Injection Protocols for Upper Extremity Computed Tomographic Angiography with Multidetector Computed Tomography Table Speed ≤30 mm/second

Weight (kg)	Scan Delay (s)	Iodine Dose‡ (g)	Iodine Flux (g) @ (g/s)		Volume (mL)	Biphasic Injection (mL) @ (mL/s)		Volume (mL)	Biphasic Injection (mL) @ (mL/s)		Volume (mL)	Biphasic Injection (mL) @ (mL/s)	
51–60	t_{CMT}+2–8*	27.5	5.5 @ 1.1	22.0 @ 1.0	92	18 @ 3.7	73 @ 3.2	79	16 @ 3.1	63 @ 2.7	74	15 @ 3.0	59 @ 2.6
61–70	t_{CMT}+2–8*	32.5	6.5 @ 1.3	26.0 @ 1.1	108	22 @ 4.3	87 @ 3.8	93	19 @ 3.7	74 @ 3.2	88	18 @ 3.5	70 @ 3.1
71–80	t_{CMT}+2–8*	37.5	7.5 @ 1.5	30.0 @ 1.3	125	25 @ 5.0	100 @ 4.3	107	21 @ 4.3	86 @ 3.7	101	20 @ 4.1	81 @ 3.5
81–90	t_{CMT}+2–8*	42.5	8.5 @ 1.7	34.0 @ 1.5	142	28 @ 5.7	113 @ 4.9	121	24 @ 4.9	97 @ 4.2	115	23 @ 4.6	92 @ 4.0
91–100	t_{CMT}+2–8*	47.5	9.5 @ 1.9	38.0 @ 1.7	158	32 @ 6.3	127 @ 5.5	136	27 @ 5.4	109 @ 4.7	128	26 @ 5.1	103 @ 4.5
101–110	t_{CMT}+2–8*	52.5	11.0 @ 2.1	42.0 @ 1.8	175	35 @ 7.0	140 @ 6.1	150	30 @ 6.0	120 @ 5.2	142	28 @ 5.7	114 @ 4.9
111–120	t_{CMT}+2–8*	57.5	12.0 @ 2.3	46.0 @ 2.0	192	38 @ 7.7	153 @ 6.7	164	33 @ 6.6	131 @ 5.7	155	31 @ 6.2	124 @ 5.4

CM, contrast medium; t_{CMT}, contrast medium transit time; ‡, average.

*When automated triggering is used, the overall scan delay and injection duration are increased by a value equivalent to the inherent delay (i.e., 1–8 sec). The iodine dose (500 mg I/kg) and flux are optimized by adjusting the injection rate and volume.

TABLE 22-6

Injection Protocols for Upper Extremity CTA with MDCT Table Speed >30 mm/sec

Scan Time (s)	Scan Delay (s)	Iodine Dose (g)	Iodine Flux @ (g/s)	300 mg I/mL CM Volume (mL)	Biphasic Injection (mL)	@	(mL/s)	350 mg I/mL CM Volume (mL)	Biphasic Injection (mL)	@	(mL/s)	370 mg I/mL CM Volume (mL)	Biphasic Injection (mL)	@	(mL/s)
30	t_{CMT}	35	7 @ 1.4	117	23	@	4.7	100	20	@	4.0	95	19	@	3.8
			28 @ 1.1		93	@	3.7		80	@	3.2		76	@	3.0
24	$t_{CMT}+6$*	35	7 @ 1.4	117	23	@	4.7	100	20	@	4.0	95	19	@	3.8
			28 @ 1.1		93	@	3.7		80	@	3.2		76	@	3.0
20	$t_{CMT}+10$*	35	7 @ 1.4	117	23	@	4.7	100	20	@	4.0	95	19	@	3.8
			28 @ 1.1		93	@	3.7		80	@	3.2		76	@	3.0
16	$t_{CMT}+14$*	35	7 @ 1.4	117	23	@	4.7	100	20	@	4.0	95	19	@	3.8
			28 @ 1.1		93	@	3.7		80	@	3.2		76	@	3.0
12	$t_{CMT}+16$*	35	7 @ 1.4	117	23	@	4.7	100	20	@	4.0	95	19	@	3.8
			28 @ 1.1		93	@	3.7		80	@	3.2		76	@	3.0

CM, contrast medium; t_{CMT}, contrast medium transit time.

*A diagnostic delay is added to the beginning of the scan duration so that the delivery of contrast medium and the scan acquisition end together. If automated triggering is used, the diagnostic delay will be reduced by an amount equal to the inherent delay (2 to 8 seconds). Higher concentration contrast medium affords reduced injection rates and volumes. Saline flush is always used.

Note: Injection parameters are for an Aortic Arch with Upper Extremity Runoff CT angiogram performed on a 70-kg patient with a scan distance of 900 mm and table speeds >30 mm. The scan times are <25 seconds. A biphasic protocol with a total injection duration of 30 seconds is required to achieve robust enhancement. Contrast medium transit time is established with automated triggering or bolus timing.

TABLE 22-7

Visualization Techniques

	Display	Principle Use	Advantages	Disadvantages
MIP	2D	• Angiographic overview	• "Slice" through dataset in transverse, coronal, sagittal, and oblique projections • Depict small caliber UE vessels • Depict poorly enhancing vessels • Communicate findings	• Vessel, bone, visceral overlap • Limited stent lumen evaluation • Limited by heavy calcium
VR	3D	• Angiographic overview	• "Slice" through dataset in transverse, coronal, sagittal, and oblique projections • Structural overview • Spatial perception • Communicate findings	• Opacity-transfer function dependent
MPR	2D	• Vessel Analysis • Structure • Flow lumen • Vessel wall	• "Slice" through dataset in transverse, coronal, sagittal, and oblique projections • Accurate display of stenoses, occlusions, calcification, stents	• Limited spatial perception
CPR	2D	• Vessel Analysis • Flow lumen • Vessel wall	• Complete longitudinal vessel cross sectional display • Accurate display of stenoses, occlusions, calcification, stents	• Operator dependent

MIP, maximum intensity projection; VR, volume rendering; MPR, multiplanar reformation; CPR, curved planar reformation; 2D, two dimensional; 3D, three dimensional.

Image Display

Interpretation and communication of upper extremity CT angiogram findings require efficient and effective image display. Two-dimensional (2D) and 3D visualization techniques are a fundamental alternative to transverse source image review and necessitate use of an advanced postprocessing workstation. Each technique has advantages and disadvantages (Table 22-7). These impact whether a technique is used for vessel overview or analysis. The quality of all postprocessed images is directly dependent on the resolution of the CT data set and the degree of contrast enhancement. A thorough treatment of the general topic can be found in Chapter 6.

Visualization Techniques Four principle visualization techniques for displaying the upper extremity vasculature are standard on currently available workstations: maximum intensity projection (MIP), volume rendering (VR), multiplanar reformations (MPR), and curved planar reformations (CPR). Their interactive use is the basis for real time interpretation. Generation of protocol-driven static postprocessed images accommodates review of the transverse source images, coronal reformations, sagittal reformations, and oblique reformations on PACS or a workstation. With all techniques, it is important to use flexible angiographic window and level settings. This includes a wide window setting to account for vascular calcification, high-contrast attenuation, or both.

Vessel Tree Overview MIP and VR provide robust angiographic displays of the upper extremity vasculature. Either can be used to rapidly formulate a structural overview and determine the location of vascular abnormalities. MIP collapses the brightest pixels of the volumetric acquisition into 2D displays, while VR applies user defined color, opacity, and light transfer functions to generate 3D displays.

For CTA, VR offers a comprehensive means to display the upper extremity vasculature and relationships with extravascular structures (Fig. 22-8). Both MIP and VR are dependent on prerendering editing to remove bone and other anatomical structures that may obscure visualization of upper extremity vasculature.

Alternatively, variable sliding thin slabs or cut planes can be utilized with interactive rotation, magnification, window and level settings, and VR transfer. Thin slabs are also employed when targeting upper extremity vascular segments for more focused angiographic evaluation.

MPRs with coronal, sagittal, and oblique projections provide limited overview of the upper extremity vascular

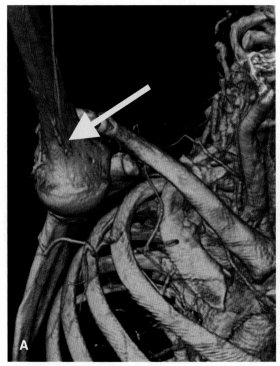 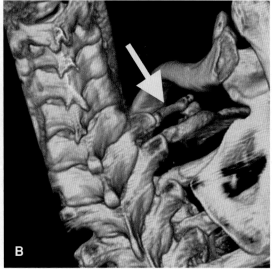

FIGURE 22-8 Cervical rib associated with arterial occlusion. A patient with right upper extremity claudication underwent 16-channel CTA. VR images demonstrated subclavian artery occlusion with reconstitution at the brachial profunda origin (*arrow* in **A**). Review of the source images localized the occlusion to be at level of the anterior scalene muscle. Further review of the skeletal system using VR demonstrated a cervical rib (*arrow* in **B**)

segments. MPR application requires stepping through each image. As vessels curve in and out of the planes, standard MPRs cannot display an entire upper extremity vascular segment in one image.

The solution lies in the generation of longitudinal cross-sectional 2D CPR static or rotational displays by drawing a center line through the vessel lumen on the axial, coronal, or sagittal images. This is performed manually or with automated vessel tracking software. Still, only targeted segments will be displayed. An alternative means to improve the spatial perception of MPR is to apply a thick slab (thick MPR).

Vessel Analysis MPR and CPR techniques are more suited for detailed interrogation of upper extremity vascular segments. Analysis of transverse MPR cross sections, orthogonal longitudinal CPR cross sections, or both is performed through each suspected region of abnormality. These techniques are fundamental for assessing calcified atheromatous plaque, noncalcified plaque, vessel wall thickening, lumen patency, and stent patency. MIP and VR techniques are limited in this evaluation, particularly with diffuse vessel wall calcification. Orthogonal (coronal and sagittal) CPR views are necessary, as eccentric lesions may not be accurately depicted on one view alone.

Source Images Reviewing the axial source images serves two important needs. One is to assess the extravascular anatomy, which may include the chest, neck, head, upper arm, forearm, and hand, depending on the coverage. This review is required not only to detect incidental pathology, but also to evaluate relevant extravascular structures, such as the presence of a cervical rib and the course and size of the anterior scalene muscle in the case of suspected thoracic outlet syndrome.

The second objective of axial source image review is to verify image quality and confirm vascular disease when artifacts are suspected on the 2D and 3D images. Review of the axial source images is facilitated by generating 3- to 5-mm thick reconstructions. Alternatively, the coronal and sagittal reformations can be used.

Magnetic Resonance Angiography

Equipment Considerations

The typical maximum field of view (FOV) in current commercially available imagers is on the order of 40 to 45 cm. This means that the upper extremity vascular tree exceeds the maximum FOV of the MR imager by two times. With contrast-enhanced (CE) MRA, a stepping table strategy with multiple injection can be used when both the proximal and distal upper extremity vessels need to be depicted, similar to the approach often used with IA DSA (26).

When the user divides the typical total dose (0.2 to 0.3 mmol/kg) of extracellular contrast agents into two injections (i.e., one for each FOV), the arterial signal intensity sufficiently exceeds that of the venous signal, with each injection timed appropriately.

When designing an MR imaging protocol, the clinician always has to weigh the relative need for temporal resolution, spatial resolution, and signal-to-noise ratio (SNR).

In general, higher main magnetic field strengths, ($\geq$1.5T), higher maximum gradient amplitudes, and faster gradient systems allow for better imaging protocols for the depiction of peripheral arterial disease. These system attributes are particularly important for CE MRA.

For upper extremity MRA, an absolute requirement is the use of surface coils in order to increase SNR. SNR is the currency enabling high temporal and spatial resolution. The extent of spatial resolution relates to arterial conspicuity, and when sufficient, disease characterization in small, distal, diseased arteries can be maximized.

Alternatively, an increase in SNR can be used to increase acquisition speed in order to avoid venous enhancement or provide temporal information regarding arrival times of contrast in vessels of interest. The use of phased-array surface body- or torso-coils are important for imaging the upper extremity and hand (Fig. 22-9). In addition, some MRI vendors now offer dedicated multi-station peripheral vascular coils with full body coverage.

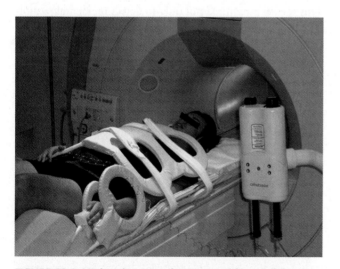

FIGURE 22-9 MR imaging setup demonstrated for parallel imaging accelerated MR angiography of the left upper extremity on a Philips Intera 1.5T MR system. The left hemithorax and upper extremity are covered by the four-element synergy body coil (upper and lower anterior and posterior elements). The forearm and hand are covered by the two-element Flex-M coil.

An important technical advance that has shown to be beneficial for CE MRA in general is parallel imaging (26–29). Parallel imaging is used to speed up data acquisition. In theory, with parallel imaging the acquisition duration can be decreased by a factor R equal to the number of coil elements. However, the SNR is reduced by a factor equal to $\sqrt{R}$.

Magnetic Resonance Angiography Techniques for Imaging Peripheral Arterial Disease

Several different MRA techniques have been described to image the upper extremity vascular tree. These are: (a) TOF or inflow MRA; (b) PC MRA; and (c) CE MRA. A summary of the relative merits and shortcomings of these techniques can be found in Chapter 2. Newer techniques such as 3D half-Fourier fast spin echo MRA and balanced steady state free precession (bSSFP) MRA are potentially promising techniques but have not been applied to upper extremity imaging and will therefore not be discussed in this chapter.

Time-of-flight Magnetic Resonance Angiography

In TOF MRA, vessel-to-background contrast is generated by the inflow of fresh, unsaturated blood in a saturated tissue. Saturation bands are essential to achieve a selective display of arterial or venous structures (30–32).

Saturation bands are essential to achieve a selective display of arterial or venous structures, as the flow in these systems is, for the most part, in opposite directions. Such an approach can have an undesirable effect in suppressing retrograde flow in a vessel, distal to a high grade stenotic or obstructive lesion.

TOF MRA suffers from the long imaging times, an inconsistent orientation through the tortuous path of the upper extremity vasculature, and inherent artifacts that result in overestimation of the degree and length of stenoses (Fig. 22-10).

Most published TOF upper extremity studies have focused on the assessment of dialysis access fistulae, and tend to suffer from overestimation (30–35). Thus, in clinical practice, TOF is typically restricted to those patients who cannot receive contrast media or for cases benefiting from a quick and limited assessment of flow direction (e.g., subclavian steal syndrome).

Phase-contrast Magnetic Resonance Angiography

In addition to anatomical display of the peripheral vasculature, PC MRA allows for physiological studies because flow can be quantified in a noninvasive manner.

Although anatomic PC MRA is less sensitive to in-plane saturation than TOF MRA, PC MRA is not often

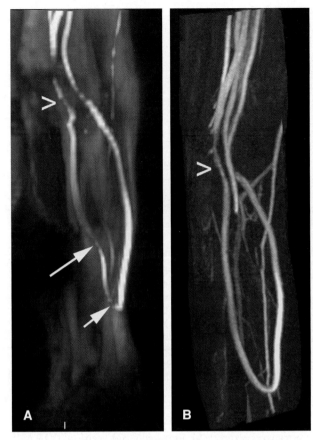

FIGURE 22-10 Coronal maximum intensity projections of TOF **(A)** and corresponding CE MR **(B)** angiograms in patient with a flow-declined hemodialysis access loop graft. The TOF study suggests high-grade stenoses in three parts of the loop graft (*arrows* and > in **A**). The corresponding CE MRA study confirms mild to moderate luminal narrowing in the draining vein just proximal to the anastomosis (> in **B**). Suggested luminal narrowing in **(A)** is due to in-plane saturation (*short arrow*) and suboptimal nonperpendicular orientation of the vessel in relation to the imaging slice plane.

used for detection and grading of upper extremity arterial stenoses because of the reliance on CE techniques (see below).

PC MRA is mainly used to assess the direction of flow in the cervical arteries in cases of suspected subclavian steal syndrome. The technique has also been used in a limited number of studies investigating the feasibility of MRA to assess hemodialysis access fistulae (36).

Contrast-enhanced Magnetic Resonance Angiography

Background CE MRA of the upper extremity vasculature is the preferred MRA technique for evaluation of patients with different forms of upper extremity arterial disease.

Because of the general propensity of upper extremity arterial disease to affect either the more centrally located large- and medium-sized vessels or more distally located

forearm and hand arteries, the most common approach is to acquire a single FOV, focusing on either region. The dose of contrast medium used is usually between 0.2 and 0.3 mmol/kg, or between 30 and 45 mL for a 75 kg patient (37–40).

As stated previously, when imaging both the central vasculature as well as that of the forearm and hand, contrast medium administration can be split into two separate injections, with the first injection used to image the distal, smaller vessels. It is paramount with this approach that examination parameters are optimized for spatial resolution and coil selection relevant to the individual acquisitions.

Practical Aspects of Upper Extremity Contrast-enhanced Magnetic Resonance Angiography

Localizer Scans The CE MRA portion of the upper extremity MRA examination can usually be completed within several minutes. However, adequate planning of the high spatial resolution 3D CE MRA volumes is essential to ensure optimal image quality in the shortest possible imaging time. The exact spatial location of the 3D CE MRA imaging volumes that cover the upper extremity vascular tree is prescribed on 'scout' or 'localizer' images.

Scout scans are usually generated from transverse, thick slice, low-resolution TOF scans (Fig. 22-11), or more recently, steady state free precession (SSFP) acquisitions (Fig. 22-12). Scout views in sagittal or coronal orientation are also useful, and are easily obtained in less than a minute. The use of low-resolution TOF acquisitions to supply the scout images can show a cursory view of the vascular anatomy with MIPs, especially of the brachial and forearm arteries.

When the 3D CE MRA volume is planned, transverse source images should always be reviewed to ensure that all relevant vascular structures are included in the imaging volume. Failure to do so can result in the exclusion of relevant anatomy from the imaging volume (see below). Sample localizer protocols are listed in Tables 22-8 and 22-9.

In addition to using localizer images to prescribe the 3D CE MRA imaging volume, standard T1- and T2-weighted images and fat-saturated T2 images can be used to check that coverage is sufficient and includes all of the region of interest that needs to be visualized. These images are typically available in cases requiring both soft tissue analysis and vascular assessment (e.g., surgical planning for extremity tumors).

Considerations with Regards to Vascular Anatomy In most patients, coverage needed in the anteroposterior direction is usually less than 10 cm. In the presence of an aortic root aneurysm or collaterals bridging subclavian artery obstructions or bypass grafts

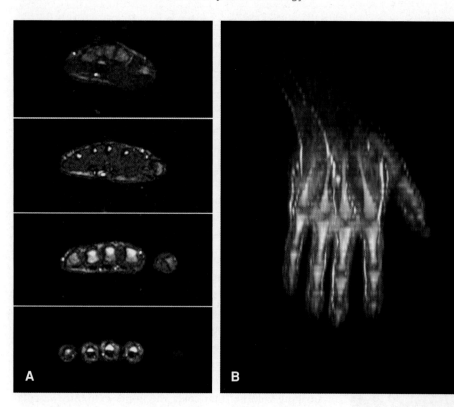

FIGURE 22-11 TOF localizer scans of the hand. In **panel A**, four transverse source images are shown. Vascular structures appear as bright "dots" in the soft tissues of the hand with bright to intermediate signal intensity. **Panel B** shows the resulting MIP of all slices. Total acquisition time for this localizer sequence was about 1 minute.

(e.g., subclavian-to-subclavian, subclavian-to-carotid), the AP coverage needed to depict these vessels may be increased (up to 15 to 20 cm). The 3D CE MRA imaging volume should be positioned based on the localizer images to ensure that the relevant structures are not excluded. When there is any doubt as to the presence of collaterals, a test bolus injection with a small amount of contrast medium can be used to answer this question.

It is also important to realize that bypass grafts coursing in a transverse direction are usually not seen on TOF MIPs generated from axial acquisitions, as these are vulnerable to in-plane saturation (41). Other patients who demand special attention are those with large thoracic aortic aneurysms where contrast media may pool, risking incomplete enhancement of the aneurysm and the distal vessels at the time of imaging. To avoid this problem, either a longer delay between injection

TABLE 22-8

Sample Time of Flight Localizer Imaging Protocol

Parameter	Value
Sequence	Gradient recalled echo
TR/TE (ms)	11/6.9
Flip angle (°)	50
FOV (mm)	450 × 450
Orientation	Transverse
Matrix	256 × 128
Slice thickness (mm)	5.0
Slices	30
Slice gap (mm)	10
Duration	45 s (total duration for 3 stations: 135 s)

TR, repetition time; TE, echo time; FOV, field of view.

TABLE 22-9

Sample bSSFP Localizer Imaging Protocol

Parameter	Value
Sequence	bSSFP (TrueFISP, bFFE or bTFE, FIESTA)*
TR/TE (ms)	6.0/3.0
Flip angle (°)	90
FOV (mm)	450 × 450
Orientation	Coronal
Matrix	256 × 256
Slice thickness (mm)	8.0
Slices	25
Slice gap (mm)	0
Duration	40 s (total duration for three stations: 120 s)

TR, repetition time; TE, echo time; FOV, field of view.
*See text for explanation of abbreviations.

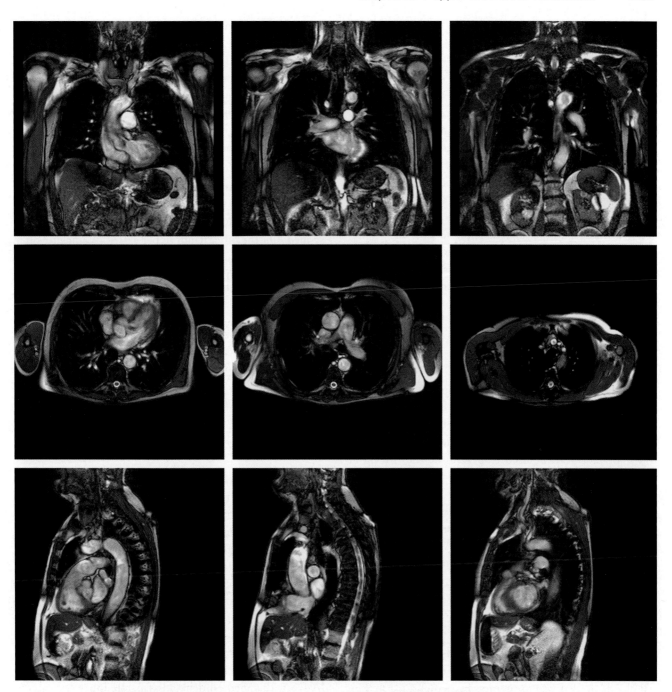

FIGURE 22-12 SSFP localizer sequence for imaging of the thorax and proximal upper extremity. SSFP sequences provide a rapid overview in multiple orientations of relevant anatomy such as the aortic arch and branch vessels in this patient. Coronal **(upper row)**, transverse **(middle row)**, and sagittal **(lower row)** images are acquired in less than 1 second per image, enabling large volume coverage in a single breath-hold.

and start of acquisition, or a multiphasic acquisition should be used (40, 42). A test bolus may be of value to establish when all the arteries in the area of interest are opacified (see below).

Synchronization of Three-dimensional Contrast-enhanced Magnetic Resonance Angiography Acquisition with Contrast Arrival Careful synchronization of peak arterial enhancement with acquisition of the center of

k-space is essential to obtain a study of diagnostic quality. The time of peak arterial enhancement is a function of many variables, the most important of which are injection rate and volume, amount and rate of saline flush (43), and cardiac output (44). Because the time of peak arterial enhancement can vary substantially between patients, the CE MRA examination needs to be tailored to the individual contrast arrival time.

This is important for two main reasons: (a) to prevent ringing artifacts and suboptimal opacification of arteries in the FOV due to starting the acquisition too early (45), and (b) to prevent disturbing venous overlay (41).

To determine the delay between the start of injection of contrast medium and the acquisition of central k-space profiles, a 2D time-resolved test bolus technique can be used. The optimal scan delay time can be determined by measuring the arrival time in the arterial bed of interest of a small bolus (1 to 3 mL) of contrast medium followed by 25 to 35 mL of saline, injected at the same rate as the full contrast bolus will be injected later on (46). A temporal resolution of about 1 to 2 seconds per image should be used.

The scan delay should be chosen to coincide with the frame in which maximum enhancement is observed. Acquisition orientation of the timing bolus scan should be in the coronal or sagittal plane, as this will not only provide the exact time at which enhancement commences, but also the rate at which enhancement progresses along the 40 to 45 cm of the arterial tree in the FOV.

For patients in whom two acquisitions are planned, such as forearm imaging followed by upper arm and central imaging, timing information from one station can be used to determine the optimal scan delay for the second acquisition. For example, enhancement of the distal brachial artery can be used to determine the timing of opacification of the forearm arteries as well as the upper arm arteries.

With real time bolus monitoring (see Chapter 5), the operator is able to inject the total volume of contrast material and proceed with the 3D CE MRA acquisition when the desired signal enhancement in the arterial bed of interest has been detected by the scanner, or by visual feedback (47–49). For an extensive discussion of the different strategies to appropriately synchronize contrast injection with image acquisition, please refer to Chapter 5.

Strategies to Optimize Vessel-to-background Contrast Because the T1 of fat is close to that of CE arterial blood, another way to suppress background tissue is by spectral saturation of signal from protons in fat. Although a fat saturation prepulse can be integrated into the 3D CE MRA sequence, this may impact scan time, and decrease the achievable spatial resolution in a given acquisition duration.

Another vulnerability with fat suppression, particularly in the proximal vessels emanating from the aortic arch, is the inadvertent loss of vascular signal from a poorly shimmed field. In this case, water suppression may result in the unintended suppression of the gadolinium signal (Fig. 22-13) (50). Thus, the use of fat-saturation pulses for upper extremity MRA is not universally recommended (51,52).

Another useful technique to maximize vessel to background is the use of subtraction of a precontrast data set from a postcontrast data set, which will be described in detail in a later section of this chapter.

The use of a surface coil is essential for high spatial and temporal resolution imaging, especially in patients with distal disease. Image quality and anatomical coverage is vastly improved when compared with imaging without these coils (53–55).

Optimization Strategies Venous enhancement may contaminate high spatial resolution arterial imaging when acquisition speeds that are too long or too slow are prescribed. On the other hand, upper extremity imaging often entails venous imaging as well, especially in patients undergoing a preoperative imaging workup prior to creation of dialysis access. Below, several general acquisition strategies that can be used to optimize upper extremity CE MRA are discussed. These are:

1. Increasing acquisition speed
2. Use of a separate acquisition for the forearm and hand
3. Use of specialized k-space filling algorithms
4. Use of a time-resolved acquisition strategy
5. Use of infrasystolic venous compression
6. Use of suprasystolic arterial compression

The most straightforward way of ensuring a selective arterial phase is by shortening acquisition duration. This should be done, first of all, by lowering repetition time (TR) and echo time (TE) to the shortest possible value, without excessively increasing bandwidth. In addition, partial or fractional echo should be used. With the introduction of multielement (peripheral) surface coils and parallel imaging, acquisition speed can be increased further (28,56,57).

Venous free imaging is readily obtained by employing a 2D projectional acquisition, where through plane resolution is entirely sacrificed, analogous to IA DSA (58). Like IA DSA, this method demands separate injections of contrast medium for each projection, and therefore this approach is infrequently used in the upper extremity.

In cases where the entire upper extremity needs to be imaged, it is unusual to use a "moving table" approach, as is common for the lower extremity. To avoid the limitations of imaging two stations in rapid succession, we recommend use of a dual-injection protocol in which the forearm and hand are imaged first, and the thoracic and proximal upper extremity are imaged afterward in a separate acquisition.

The rationale for this "hybrid" approach is that it is easier to obtain high-resolution 3D images of the small distal

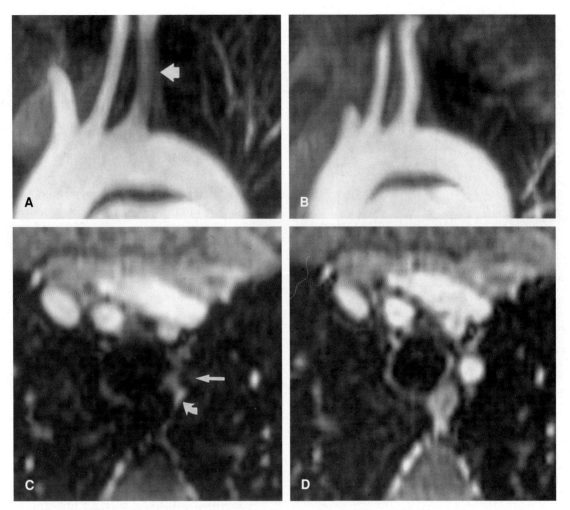

FIGURE 22-13 Images obtained in a 47-year-old man with progressive left upper extremity pain and weakness. 3D MR angiography was performed to exclude a left subclavian artery stenosis or thrombosis. **A:** MIP image from a fat-saturated 3D MR angiographic examination (6.0/1.2, 20° flip angle) shows moderate loss of signal intensity within the proximal segment of the left subclavian artery (*arrow*). **B:** The patient returned 6 days later for repeat imaging. An identical 3D MR angiographic examination was performed, except that fat suppression was not used. Corresponding MIP image shows a normal left subclavian artery. **C:** Delayed fat-saturated 2D GRE MR image (150/2.1, 90° flip angle) shows a signal void (*straight arrow*) within the left subclavian artery. Adjacent mediastinal fat (*curved arrow*) is not saturated. **D:** Corresponding 2D GRE MR image obtained with otherwise identical imaging parameters, except that no fat-saturation pulse was used, shows normal intravascular signal intensity within the left subclavian artery. Partial signal intensity loss in the surrounding fat is secondary to opposed-phase effects. (Reprinted with permission from Siegelman ES, Charafeddine R, Stolpen AH, et al. Suppression of intravascular signal on fat-saturated contrast-enhanced thoracic MR arteriograms. *Radiology*. 2000;217(1):115–118.)

arteries free of disturbing venous enhancement. The initial acquisition of the forearm and hand is typically done using up to 15 to 20 mL 0.5 M Gd-DTPA with a monophasic injection. Because synchronization of central k-space lines is optimized with regard to contrast enhancement in the forearm arteries, venous enhancement is virtually eliminated. After imaging of the distal upper extremity is completed, a second acquisition is performed to image the aorta, arch vessels, and brachial artery using the remaining volume of contrast agent (Fig. 22-14).

A disadvantage of the multiple injection technique is that the total amount of contrast medium has to be divided into two or more separate injections of much less contrast medium. This may lead to longer examination times and a decrease in vessel-to-background contrast compared with a single, double to triple dose injection.

Over the past few years, all major MR vendors have implemented dedicated centric k-space filling algorithms (see Chapter 2). Centric k-space filling avoids venous contamination and accounts for the common situation in which the time between arterial and venous enhancement is shorter than the duration of the high spatial resolution 3D CE MRA acquisition.

Greater flexibility is available when centric k-space filling is combined with parallel imaging; the chances of

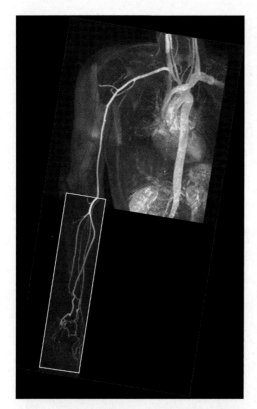

FIGURE 22-14 Composite MIP of hybrid dual-injection approach for imaging the upper extremity. First, the distal upper extremity arteries (enclosed by box) were imaged during injection of 17 mL of gadolinium-DTPA. Subsequently, the proximal upper extremity and aortic arch vessels were imaged during a second injection with the same amount of contrast material. Note lack of venous enhancement in the proximal station.

disturbing venous enhancement decrease even further (56,57,59).

Repetitive centric k-space filling techniques obtain high spatial resolution peripheral MR angiograms with high temporal frame rate (i.e., time-resolved imaging at several seconds per frame). Korosec et al. (60) first described this concept as time-resolved imaging of contrast kinetics (TRICKS). Refinements to the TRICKS technique allow for further increases in acquisition speed (61–63).

A technique similar to TRICKS is keyhole contrast-enhanced timing robust angiography (CENTRA). With keyhole CENTRA, temporal resolution is increased by repetitive acquisition of the central part of k-space only. This information is later combined with a data set containing the peripheral part of k-space, which is acquired as part of the last frame of the time-resolved series (64). Subsequently, these hybrid k-spaces can be reconstructed as a series of time-resolved 3D CE MR angiograms (Fig. 22-15). Temporal resolution can be further increased by combining keyhole imaging with parallel imaging (65). Other seg-

mented k-space acquisition schemes have been described as well (66).

Time-resolved acquisitions obviate the need for test bolus injections (67). Although there are no published data on the benefits of TRICKS or keyhole CENTRA for imaging upper extremity vessels, Hany et al. (68) found that the use of TRICKS improved small, distal vessel conspicuity and reduced venous overlay in a head-to-head comparison with single injection, three-station lower extremity CE MRA.

A technique to optimize upper extremity venous imaging is the use of infrasystolic venous compression proximal to the cubital fossa with pressures of 50 to 60 mmHg (69). In contrast to the lower extremities, venous compression is more often used to induce venous dilatation and improve visualization of these structures. Knowledge about maximum venous diameter is important for vascular surgeons to determine the type of arteriovenous fistula (AVF) that will be created in patients with ESRD requiring dialysis access (see the section on Dialysis Access Fistulas).

The use of suprasystolic arterial compression, also known as timed arterial compression (TAC), employs a blood pressure cuff wrapped around the upper arm and inflated to 200 mmHg to arrest all blood flow at a predetermined scan delay. The exact delay time is determined with a serial 2D MR technique (BolusTrak; Philips), with a small test bolus of contrast medium, followed by saline flush.

Compared with their standard first-pass MRA technique with an acquisition time of 23 seconds and voxel size of $1.17 \times 0.59 \times 0.7$ mm^3 (483 microns), use of TAC MRA permitted a four-fold increase in spatial resolution, to a voxel size of $0.59 \times 0.29 \times 0.7$ mm^3 (120 microns) (70). The improved spatial resolution permitted full diagnostic assessment of the palmar metacarpal, common metacarpal, common palmar, and proper digital arteries, in addition to radial, ulnar, and palmar arch arteries, which could also be evaluated with the standard approach (Fig. 22-16).

Resolution Requirements To accurately describe degree and length of peripheral arterial occlusive disease (PAOD), it is paramount that the resolution of the 3D data set needs to meet minimal standards. For instance, it is known from the work by Hoogeveen et al. (71) and Westenberg et al. (72) that at least three pixels are needed across the lumen of an artery to quantify the degree of stenosis with an error of less than 10%. When this constraint is kept in mind, the greater spatial resolution demands to accurately quantify stenoses in the distal forearm or hand arteries as opposed to the aortic arch vessels become obvious.

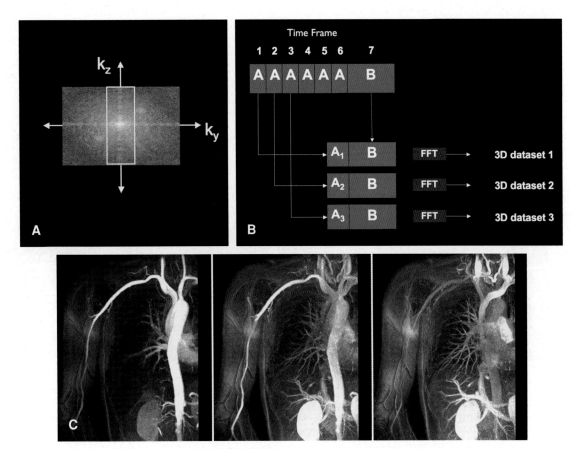

FIGURE 22-15 Keyhole CENTRA acquisition scheme. With this technique, temporal resolution is increased by acquiring the center of k-space (white box in **A**) multiple consecutive times (green boxes in **B**). The peripheral part of the k-space is acquired after the last center is acquired. After the acquisition has been completed, all k-space centers are combined with the peripheral part and reconstructed to a series of 3D volumes. In **(C)**, an example is shown of a keyhole CENTRA acquisition of the aortic arch and proximal upper extremity vessels. In this acquisition, the central part was set to 25% of the entire k-space, yielding a temporal resolution of about 6 seconds. Total acquisition time for this sequence was 6 + 6 + 18 = 30 seconds.

Voxel dimensions should be kept as close to isotropic as possible so that vessel blurring is minimized when viewing projections that differ from the plane of acquisition. Recommended voxel sizes are about 3 to 4 mm³ or less in the thoracic and proximal upper extremity arteries, 1 to 2 mm³ or less in the forearm, and 1 mm³ or better in the hand. Resolution of 500 microns or below are recommended.

Contrast Media and Injection Protocols

The IV cannula should always be placed in the upper extremity contralateral to the side of interest because the presence of undiluted contrast medium in a vein close to the artery of interest may cause artifactual signal loss (also see the section on Magnetic Resonance Angiography Postprocessing Issues).

Most of the reported studies on upper extremity CE MRA used conventional 0.5 M extracellular contrast agents. Typically, between 0.1 and 0.3 mmol/kg of contrast agent is injected (i.e., between 15 and 45 mL for a 75-kg patient), followed by a 15 to 30 mL saline injection to flush contrast from injection tubing and veins into the central venous and arterial circulations.

With conventional 0.5 M extracellular contrast agents, typically, a dose between 0.1 and 0.3 mmol/kg typically is injected (i.e., between 15 and 45 mL for a 75-kg patient), followed by a 15 to 30 mL saline injection to flush contrast from injection tubing and veins into the central venous and arterial circulations.

Currently, there is no single preferred injection protocol for upper extremity CE MRA, although an empirical strategy that works well in clinical practice is that the contrast injection duration should be about 40% to 60% of the acquisition duration. The rationale for this strategy is twofold.

First, due to contrast dilution at the leading and trailing edges of the bolus, as well as variable transit times

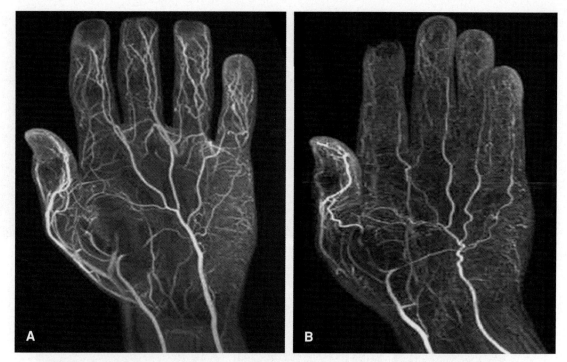

FIGURE 22-16 Example of the effect of TAC on CE MRA of the hand. Images acquired at ultra-high spatial resolution of 0.59 × 0.29 × 0.7 mm³ normally suffer from substantial venous enhancement in the first pass due to long acquisition times **(panel A)**. Application of suprasystolic TAC enables acquisition of images largely free of venous enhancement at spatial resolutions close to intra-arterial DSA. (Images are courtesy of Professor Klaus Wentz, M.D., Ph.D., of RODIAC Diagnostic Centers, Kilchberg, Switzerland.)

through different portions of the pulmonary circulation, contrast bolus length will increase in the body (usually with about 5 to 7 seconds) (73). Second, contrast that is injected after about half of the typical scan duration (in the order of 10 to 20 seconds) will not arrive in the arterial bed of interest before k-space lines contributing to contrast enhancement in the image are acquired (in cases where centric k-space filling is used).

The amount of contrast to be injected as well as injection speed and amount of saline flush are dependent on other variables such as scan duration and technique used (i.e., single vs. multiple injection). Different authors have used various single- and multiple-phase injection rates and different saline flush volumes.

In general, a fixed rate of about 2.0 to 3.0 mL/second is used (55, 74). On older and slower systems, the injection rate is usually set to between 1.0 and 3.0 mL/second (75,76).

In a recently published study focusing on abdominal aortic CE MRA, Boos et al. (43) found that increasing the amount of contrast injected as well as saline flush volume increases bolus length and improves small vessel conspicuity, but does not necessarily result in higher vessel-to-background contrast. A sample injection protocol for upper extremity CE MRA is listed in Table 22-10. More details regarding nuances of contrast administration can be found in Chapter 5.

Novel Contrast Media Vessel to background signal can also be improved by using other contrast agents than the currently used 0.5 M gadolinium chelates. Recently, the first 1.0 M agent (gadobutrol [Gadovist]; Schering AG, Berlin, Germany) has been approved for clinical use and has a European-wide registration for CE MRA. Gadobutrol is formulated at higher concentration of 1.0 mol/L and about 20% higher relaxivity (T1 relaxivity in blood: 5.2 mM^{-1}s^{-1} at 37°C and 1.5 T). These properties generate lower blood T1 values compared with other commercially available contrast agents, thus offering an attractive method to increase intravascular signal (77).

In a direct head-to-head comparison between 1.0 M and 0.5 M agents for pelvic MRA, Goyen et al. found that the use of the 1.0 M agent led to significantly higher signal- and contrast-to-noise ratios and better delineation of especially small pelvic arteries (78). There have been no specific studies investigating the utility of higher relaxivity contrast agents for the upper extremity.

Higher relaxivity compared to extracellular agents is achievable with certain agents (79,80). Gadofosveset (Vasovist [formerly known as MS-325]; Schering AG, Berlin, Germany) is a higher relaxivity agent available for use in Europe. With these agents a lower dose can achieve the same vessel-to-background contrast as ECF agents, or, conversely, the imaging of smaller vessels benefits from the higher SNR (Fig. 22-17).

TABLE 22-10

Suggested Injection Protocol for Commercially Available 0.5 M Gadolinium Chelates

Indication (approach)	Contrast Volume/ Injection Rate	Saline Flush Volume/ Injection Rate	Comments
3D CE MRA	35 mL at 3.0 mL/s	25 mL at 3.0 mL/s*	Use multiphase approach whenever possible
2D time-resolved test bolus approach	2–3 mL at 3.0 mL/s	30 mL at 3.0 mL/s	Can be used to detect subclavian steal phenomenon

3D, three dimensional; CE MRA, contrast-enhanced magnetic resonance angiography; 2D, two dimensional.
*Saline is always injected at the same rate as the last phase of the contrast injection.
Note: The maximum contrast dose that may be given for all injections together is 0.3 mmol/kg. In this table, a patient body weight of 75 kg was assumed.

Magnetic Resonance Angiography Postprocessing Issues

Although the same postprocessing techniques can be used for displaying CTA and MRA datasets, there are specific nuances to maximize the MRA results.

Subtraction Imaging

The T1 decrease in peripheral arterial blood due to injection of 0.1 to 0.3 mmol/kg 0.5 M gadolinium chelate contrast medium is generally insufficient to selectively enhance arteries and suppress background tissue on ray-casting algorithms such as whole-volume MIP, especially in cases of small distally located and diseased arteries. Therefore, the signal of background tissues, and fat specifically (because it has the shortest T1), need to be eliminated in order to present data to clinicians in an easily understandable format.

The most commonly used technique to suppress background signal is subtraction of nonenhanced "mask" images that are identical to the 3D CE MRA volumes. Although subtraction decreases the SNR by a factor of about 1.4 ($\sqrt{2}$ when the number of signals acquired is 1), vessel-to-background contrast improves to the extent that whole-volume MIPs become clinically useful, especially when using injection rates below 1.0 mL/second (Fig. 22-18) (75). A disadvantage of using mask scans is that patients may move in between acquisition of the mask and CE parts of the scan, which can lead to subtraction misregistration artifacts.

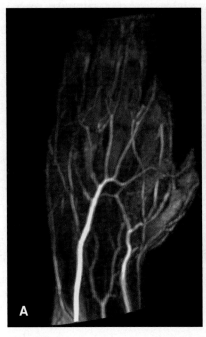 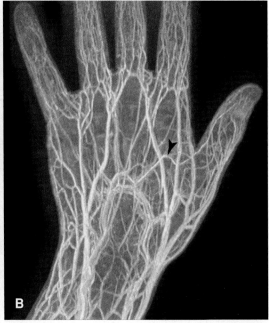

FIGURE 22-17 Whole-volume MIPs of first-pass (**panel A**) and steady state (**panel B**) acquisitions using 0.03 mmol/kg gadofosveset. The first-pass image clearly shows the superficial and deep palmar arches. Because of the limited spatial resolution (1.0 × 1.0 × 1.0 mm³), it is difficult, however, to evaluate the digital arteries. The steady state acquisition was acquired at 0.4 × 0.4 × 0.4 mm³ resolution (64 microns). The improved spatial resolution is clearly reflected in the much higher level of detail, such as the depiction of the princeps pollicis artery and its branches into the thumb (*arrowhead* in **B**). Note that MIP is not the preferred evaluation of steady state images because of the concomitant venous enhancement.

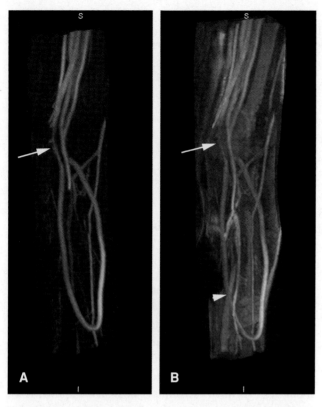

FIGURE 22-18 Effect of image subtraction on vessel conspicuity in a patient with flow-declined arteriovenous loop graft in the antecubital fossa. Whole-volume MIP of subtracted images **(panel A)** shows a moderately severe stenosis in the vein draining the loop graft (*arrow*). In contrast, the MIP of the nonsubtracted images **(panel B)** shows a severe stenosis bordering on occlusion (*arrow*). This overestimation is due to overprojection of subcutaneous fat with signal intensity similar to that in the vessel. Note a similar phenomenon in the ascending part of the graft where it crosses bone marrow in the ulna (*arrowhead*).

Subtraction is especially useful in the smaller arteries of the forearm and hand (51,52).

While subtraction improves small vessel conspicuity, it has the disadvantage that the tissues surrounding the arteries are often lost (81). Therefore, the use of VR nonsubtracted 3D CE MRA data sets can be very useful for cross-referencing vascular structures to important anatomical landmarks used for therapeutic purposes.

Osseous anatomy of the extremity as well as the exact position of veins on the skin surface in relation to underlying muscular and bony structures is particularly important for referring vascular surgeons (Fig. 22-19), especially if CE MRA is used as the sole preoperative imaging modality (81).

For the larger vessels in the thorax and proximal upper extremity, subtraction is not absolutely necessary, but may be useful to improve conspicuity of small branch vessels and collaterals.

Subtraction can also be a useful technique when multiple anatomic segments are studied with repeated injections of contrast medium. In such cases, residual venous enhancement from prior administration may obscure arterial detail in subsequent acquisitions if subtraction is not used (81,82).

Image Rendering Options

On almost all of today's commercially available postprocessing workstations, MIP images can be generated and manipulated in (near) real time. This makes it possible to view 3D CE MRA data sets from any desired angle, and is particularly useful when assessing eccentric stenoses.

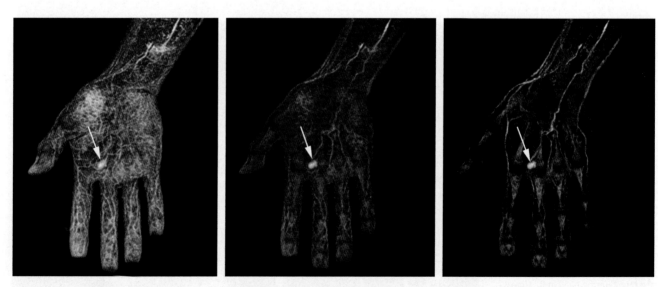

FIGURE 22-19 Color VRs at different thresholds in a patient with an aneurysm of the third common palmar digital artery at the level of the third metacarpal head. The images show the relation of the aneurysm to surrounding soft tissues and metacarpal bones.

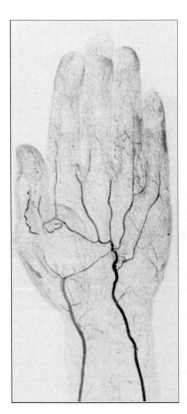

FIGURE 22-20 Example of MIP of MRA of the hand acquired at ultra-high spatial resolution of 0.59 × 0.29 × 0.7 mm³, displayed in inverse video mode. (Image courtesy of Professor Klaus Wentz, M.D., Ph.D., of RODIAC Diagnostic Centers, Kilchberg, Switzerland.)

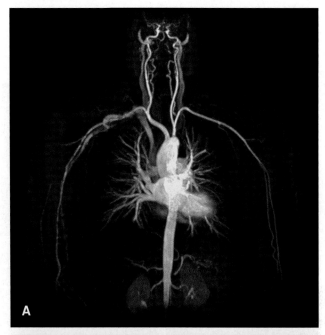

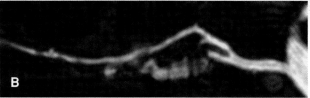

FIGURE 22-21 Principle of cMPR. Whereas arteries can be hard to differentiate from surrounding structures such as veins in simple MIPs (right subclavian artery in **panel A**), cMPR—in effect, a thin-slab MIP of a curved surface—allows for selective visualization of the artery **(panel B)**. This tool is particularly useful where the artery is in close proximity to structures with similar signal intensity such as contrast-filled veins.

A review of cross-sectional images remains an integral part of the evaluation. Because MIP images have a look and feel analogous to IA DSA, particularly when displayed in inverse video mode (Fig. 22-20), they are easily understood by referring clinicians.

The MIP algorithm works best when using thin-slab or (curved) subvolume selections. In whole-volume MIPs, contrast-enhancing organs or other vascular structures may superimpose over smaller arteries when they have higher signal intensities along a particular viewing path.

Another very helpful technique for the precise evaluation of vessel morphology is curved multiplanar reformation (cMPR) along the axis of the arterial segment of interest (Fig. 22-21).

Other commonly used postprocessing techniques are shaded surface display (SSD) and volume rendering (VR). With SSD, all information in voxels with signal intensity below a predefined threshold is discarded. SSD is mainly useful for the depiction of complex anatomic relationships between large vessels. SSD is vulnerable to pseudostenoses and pseudo-occlusions, and its use should be reserved for circumstances where sufficient contrast between the vessel lumen and surrounding tissues exists.

With VR, the information about the signal intensity in all voxels is retained. Color scales are commonly used in VR to code ranges of signal intensities in order to better differentiate the vasculature from various surrounding tissues (Fig. 22-22).

It must be stressed, however, that the presence of a stenosis or occlusion in a MIP, SSD, or VR must always be confirmed by viewing of original, thin-slice partitions of the 3D data set in multiple, orthogonal directions (e.g., coronal, sagittal, and transverse), aided with MPRs of the arteries, preferably perpendicular to the vessel axis.

Artifactual stenosis in the subclavian artery can result from undiluted contrast medium in the ipsilateral subclavian vein during infusion. The high venous gadolinium concentration often yields susceptibility artifacts, in turn leading to signal loss in the adjacent subclavian artery, mimicking stenosis. Acquisition of a second phase, immediately after the first, will almost always reveal the true status of the subclavian artery as dilution and washout of the

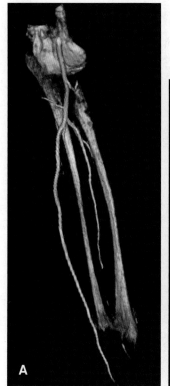

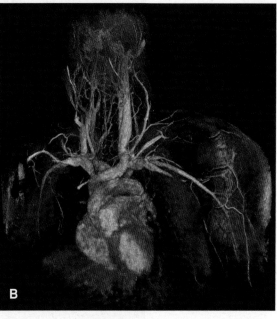

FIGURE 22-22 Examples of color VRs of the antecubital fossa and distal upper extremity arteries **(A)** and the central thoracic and cervical arteries and veins **(B)**. VR is a particularly powerful technique to show the vessels in relation to each other and surrounding anatomical structures. Display of MR angiographic data sets with VR can greatly aid the vascular surgeon in planning the exact approach to a certain vessel in relation to overlying bony and soft tissue landmarks.

contrast medium ameliorates the susceptibility artifacts (Fig. 22-23).

For aneurysms, the source image review is needed to determine the true arterial diameter of an aneurysm since mural thrombus can be readily appreciated, yielding improved diagnostic accuracy (83,84).

ANATOMY

Arterial System

The upper extremity vascular tree begins at the aortic arch and extends through to the digital arteries. It is composed of a main conduit that gradually tapers to the level of the elbow, at which point it branches into three main forearm arteries. These three arteries course to the hand and supply an intricate network in the palm and fingers.

Clinically, the main arteries can be separated into inflow and outflow segments. Inflow arteries include the aortic arch, brachiocephalic artery, and right and left subclavian arteries, while the outflow arteries include the axillary, brachial, radial, ulnar, and interosseous arteries. The proximal upper extremity vasculature is demonstrated schematically in Figure 22-24 with detailed text to follow.

Beginning at the subclavian artery, second order branches arise from the main arteries, often with considerable variabil-

ity. In the setting of arterial occlusive disease, the second order branches form important collateral pathways at the shoulder, upper arm, or elbow to ensure arterial flow to the hand.

Within the hand, a parallel, interconnected system of volar and dorsal arteries also is designed to optimize hand perfusion. This duplicated anatomy forms the basis for examining hand perfusion with a capillary refill test and an Allen's test (86).

Inflow

With conventional left aortic arch anatomy, the brachiocephalic artery arises as the first artery off the aortic arch and gives origin to the right subclavian artery at the level of the right sternoclavicular joint. The left subclavian artery arises directly from the aortic arch just distal to the left common carotid artery, at the level of the fourth thoracic vertebrae. The subclavian arteries are divided into three segments, each of which can exhibit pathology specific to the individual segment.

The first subclavian artery segment courses vertically and laterally from the ostium, toward the ipsilateral medial border of the scalenus anterior muscle. This segment gives origin to the vertebral artery, internal mammary artery, and thyrocervical trunk. These branches arise in close proximity to each other, near the medial border of the scalenus anterior. On the left, the costocervical trunk also arises from this segment.

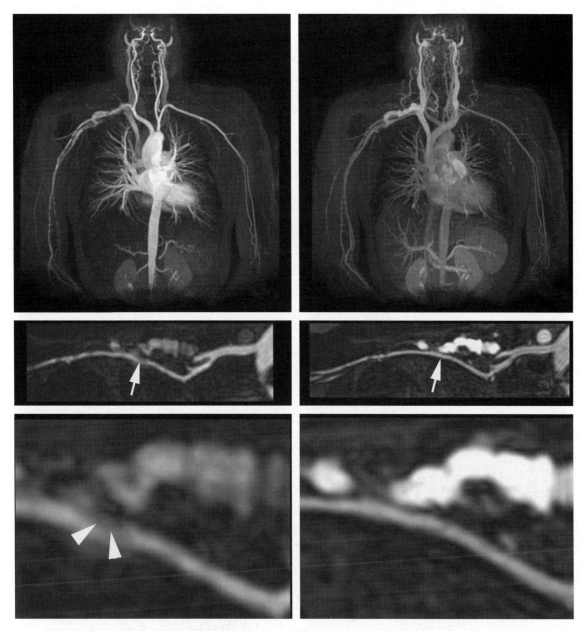

FIGURE 22-23 Whole-volume MRA MIP of the central thoracic and upper extremity vessels. The **upper two panels** show whole-volume MIPs of the first and second dynamic phases. The **middle two panels** are cMPRs showing mild luminal narrowing in the left, arterial phase image (*left arrow*). Zoomed views of the area with the arrows in the middle two panels more clearly show intra-arterial signal loss due to susceptibility artifacts emanating from the right subclavian vein (*arrowheads* in **lower left panel**). The second, mixed arterial and venous phase shows no abnormalities in the subclavian artery (*right arrow*).

The thyrocervical trunk gives rise to three main branches, the inferior thyroid artery, the suprascapular artery, and the superficial cervical artery. The inferior thyroid artery supplies the infero-posterior thyroid gland and parathyroid glands. It anastomoses with the ipsilateral superior thyroid.

The suprascapular artery supplies the superior shoulder musculature, including the supraspinatous, infraspinatus, and the subscapular fossa. In addition, the suprascapular artery supplies flow to the acromioclavicular and glenohumeral joints. The suprascapular artery forms anastomoses with the dorsal scapular, thoracoacromial, subscapular, and circumflex scapular arteries.

The superficial cervical artery supplies the trapezius and surrounding muscles. It anastomoses with the descending branch of the occipital artery.

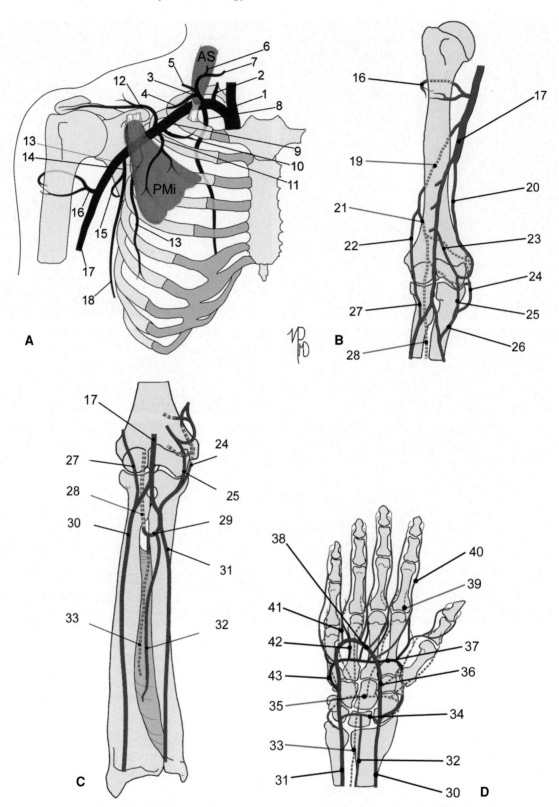

FIGURE 22-24 Schematic drawing of normal upper extremity arterial anatomy. Illustrated by Nancy Prendergast, M.D. (Adapted from Kadir S. Arterial anatomy of the upper extremities. In: *Atlas of Normal and Variant Angiographic Anatomy.* Philadelphia: WB Saunders; 1991:63–91.) (Figure 22-24 continues)

1. Subclavian artery
2. Vertebral artery
3. Thyrocervical trunk
4. Subscapular artery
5. Superficial cervical artery
6. Ascending cervical artery
7. Inferior thyroid artery
8. Internal thoracic (mammary) artery
9. Axillary artery
10. Superior thoracic artery
11. Pectoral branch off thoracoacromial
12. Acromial branch off thoracoacromial
13. Lateral thoracic
14. Subscapular
15. Circumflex scapular
16. Circumflex humeral
17. Brachial
18. Thoracodorsal
19. Profunda brachial
20. Superior ulnar collateral
21. Middle collateral
22. Radial collateral

23. Inferior ulnar collateral
24. Posterior branch of ulnar recurrent
25. Anterior branch of ulnar recurrent
26. Ulnar recurrent
27. Radial recurrent
28. Interosseous recurrent
29. Common interosseous
30. Radial
31. Ulnar
32. Anterior interosseous
33. Posterior interosseous
34. Palmar carpal branch
35. Dorsal carpal branch forming the dorsal carpal rete
36. Superficial palmar branch of radial artery
37. Deep palmar arch
38. Superficial palmar arch
39. Dorsal metacarpal arteries
40. Proper palmar digital arteries
41. Common palmar digital arteries
42. Palmar metacarpal
43. Deep palmar branch of ulnar artery

FIGURE 22-24 (Continued)

In nearly 30% of cases, the thyrocervical branches may arise independently. In approximately 16%, the trunk may arise with one independent branch. In nearly 50%, the superficial cervical artery may arise together with the dorsal scapular artery (deep cervical artery). In this instance, the common arterial segment, which supplies the superficial cervical and dorsal scapular arteries, is termed the transverse cervical artery. The second segment of the subclavian artery is a short, horizontal portion that is posterior to the scalenus anterior muscle. On the right, the main branch is the costocervical trunk. On the left, more commonly, as mentioned, this branch arises from the first segment. Major subdivisions of the costocervical trunk include the superior intercostal artery and deep cervical artery, to supply the posterior intercostal spaces and posterior neck musculature, respectively. In approximately 10% of cases, the trunk is absent, and the divisions arise directly from the subclavian artery.

The third segment courses downward from the lateral border of the scalene anterior muscle to the outer margin of the first rib, at which point it becomes the axillary artery. The dorsal scapular artery commonly arises from this segment, supplying muscles at the medial border of the scapula. Alternatively, it may arise from the second segment or from the transverse cervical artery. The dorsal scapular anastomoses with the suprascapular and circumflex scapular arteries.

Outflow

In the axilla, the axillary artery extends from the lateral margin of the first rib to the inferior margin of the teres major, at which point it becomes the brachial artery. It is divided into three portions, based on its relation to the pectoralis minor. Each segment usually has at least one branch vessel; however, considerable variation exists. The first segment lies proximal to the pectoralis minor. The superior thoracic artery arises from this segment to supply the first three intercostal spaces by communicating with the intercostal arteries. Less commonly, the superior thoracic artery may be absent or may arise from the thoracodorsal artery.

The second segment lies posterior to the pectoralis minor. The thoracoacromial and lateral thoracic arteries arise from this segment. The thoracoacromial gives origin to pectoral, acromial, clavicular, and deltoid branches. The lateral thoracic artery supplies the lateral chest wall, providing branches to the pectoralis, serratus anterior, and subscapularis muscles. The lateral thoracic may share a common origin with the thoracoacromial or the subscapular.

The third axillary arterial segment is lateral to the pectoralis minor. Its major branches are the subscapular and humeral circumflex arteries. The subscapular artery divides after a short length into the circumflex scapular and the thoracodorsal arteries. The humeral circumflex artery divides into anterior and posterior humeral circumflex arteries. In approximately 10%, the humeral circumflex and subscapular arteries arise from a common origin.

In the upper arm, the brachial artery extends from the lateral border of the teres major to the antecubital fossa, where it divides into radial and ulnar arteries. Major branches of the brachial artery are the brachial profunda, superior ulnar collateral, inferior ulnar collateral, nutrient, and muscular arteries. Distally, the brachial profunda divides into the radial collateral and middle collateral arteries. These arteries anastomose with the radial recurrent and interosseous recurrent arteries along the anterior and posterior aspects of the lateral epicondyle, respectively.

The superior ulnar collateral and the inferior ulnar collateral arteries also form anastomotic networks around the elbow. The superior ulnar collateral communicates with the posterior ulnar recurrent artery and the inferior ulnar collateral communicates with the anterior ulnar recurrent artery at the posterior and anterior aspects of the medial epicondyle, respectively.

The inferior ulnar collateral also gives off a branch posterior to the medial epicondyle, which communicates with the superior ulnar collateral and posterior ulnar recurrent arteries. Less commonly, a branch off the superior ulnar collateral may course anterior to the medial epicondyle to communicate with the anterior ulnar recurrent artery.

In the forearm, the radial, ulnar, and interosseous arteries are the major runoff vessels to the hand (Fig. 22-24). Just below the elbow, the brachial artery branches into radial and ulnar arteries. The radial artery courses superficial in the lateral forearm, medial to the brachioradialis, surrounded by skin and fasciae anteriorly. At the radial styloid, the radial artery bifurcates into superficial and deep branches.

The ulnar artery courses in the medial forearm, anterior to the flexor digitorum profundus muscle. Proximally, the ulnar has a deep course surrounded by the pronator teres, flexor digitorum superficialis, flexor carpi radialis, and palmaris longus. Distally, however, it is superficial, surrounded by integument and fasciae.

The ulnar artery crosses into the wrist superficial to the flexor retinaculum and lateral to the pisiform. Immediately distal to the pisiform, the ulnar artery divides into a larger superficial branch and a smaller deep branch.

Regarding the interosseous arteries, a common interosseous artery arises off the proximal ulnar artery and divides into volar and dorsal interosseous branches. These course in the respective interosseous membranes to the wrist. As discussed previously, the radial, interosseous, anterior ulnar and posterior ulnar recurrent arteries are vital for collateral flow around the elbow.

Aberrant anatomy for the radial and ulnar arteries includes anomalous high origin off the axillary or brachial arteries. This occurs more frequently with radial arteries (14% to 17%) as compared with ulnar arteries (2% to 3%). A variant of this is a persistent superficial brachial artery.

Arterial Anatomy of the Hand

In the hand, the arterial anatomy is distinguished by a four arch system. Two are in the carpus, while two are in the palm. The carpal arch system has volar and dorsal compo-

nents. Single volar or dorsal carpal branches off the radial and ulna anastomose to form the respective carpal arches. The volar interosseous artery drains into both the volar and dorsal carpal arches, while the dorsal interosseous artery only anastomoses with the dorsal carpal arch.

The radial and ulnar arteries communicate to form superficial and deep palmar arches (Fig. 22-24). The deep arch is formed by the anastomosis of the radial and ulnar artery deep branches. The deep branch of the radial artery crosses dorsally in the anatomical snuff box over the scaphoid and trapezium, deep to the abductor pollicis longus and extensor pollicis longus and brevis. The deep branch then courses between the first dorsal interosseous muscles to enter the palm. The radial artery continues along the bases of the metacarpals, until the fifth metacarpal, at which point the radial artery anastomoses with the deep branch off the ulnar artery.

The superficial palmar arch is located approximately 1 cm distal to the deep arch. It is formed primarily from the superficial palmar branch off the ulnar artery, which crosses the palm anterior to the flexor retinaculum. A complete "true" superficial arch is formed when the radial artery superficial branch anastomoses with the ulnar superficial branch. However, this may occur in only one third of cases. More commonly, the superficial arch is completed by the ulnar artery through anastomoses at the digital level or by anastomosis with an artery off the deep arch (i.e., radialis indices).

Regarding the metacarpal and digital arteries, the superficial palmar arch supplies three common palmar digital arteries, and the deep arch supplies three metacarpal arteries. These branches join in the interosseous space and then divide into proper palmar digital arteries, which supply the adjacent digits—ulnar side of the second finger, both sides of the third and fourth fingers, and the radial side of the fifth finger. The ulnar side of the fifth finger is supplied directly by a proper digital artery from the superficial arch, while the thumb and radial side of the second finger are supplied directly from the deep palmar arch.

For the thumb, the princeps pollicis ascends from the deep arch to the base of the thumb and divides into two branches that supply the radial and ulnar sides of the thumb. For the radial side of the second finger, the radialis indices commonly arises from the deep arch. However, the radialis indices may arise from the princeps pollicis. In addition, the radialis indices often has an anastomosis with the superficial arch.

The dorsal carpal arch also plays a role in digital perfusion to all four fingers. The dorsal arch gives origin to three dorsal metacarpal arteries. These course in the second

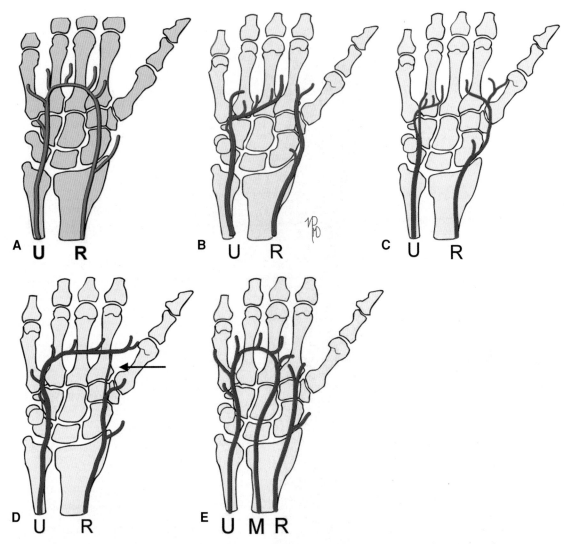

FIGURE 22-25 Common variants of the arterial anatomy in the hands. A: Classic radioulnar arch. **B, C:** Examples of incomplete deep palmar arch. **D:** Complete superficial palmar arch in which ulnar artery is the main contributor that anastomoses with small branch (*arrow*) of the deep arch in the first digital interspace. **E:** Mediano-ulnar arch. (U, ulnar artery; R, radial artery; M, median artery. Illustrated by Nancy Prendergast, M.D. Adapted with permission from Kadir S. Arterial anatomy of the upper extremities. In: *Atlas of Normal and Variant Angiographic Anatomy*. Philadelphia: WB Saunders; 1991:63-91.)

through fourth dorsal interosseous spaces and divide into paired dorsal digital arteries that extend to the tufts of the fingers. At the distal phalyngeal tufts, the dorsal digital arteries anastomose with palmar digital arteries from the superficial arch.

Communication between the dorsal and palmar systems also occurs by way of proximal and distal perforating arteries between the dorsal metacarpal arteries and the deep and superficial palmar arches, respectively.

The complex and rich vascular network of the vascular anatomy found in the hand is highly variable. In the previ-

ous discussion the classic anatomy was emphasized. Some examples of common variants are found in the series of diagrams shown in Fig. 22-25.

Venous System

The upper extremity venous system consists of superficial and deep veins. The superficial veins lie within the superficial fascia, while the deep veins accompany the upper extremity arteries (venae comitans). Valves are present in both the superficial and deep veins, with a greater frequency in the deep system (Fig. 22-26).

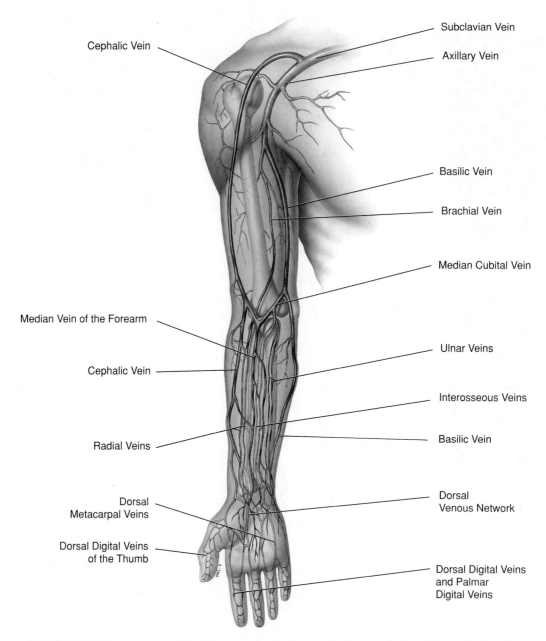

FIGURE 22-26 Venous anatomy of the right upper extremity. (Reprinted with permission from Uflacker R. *Atlas of Vascular Anatomy: An Angiographic Approach.* 2nd ed. Philadelphia: Lippincott Williams & Wilkins; 2007.)

In the hand, forearm, and upper arm, the superficial system is the principal venous drainage, and as a result, overall caliber for these peripheral veins is larger than in the deep system. The smaller deep veins are further distinguished in that they accompany the arteries in pairs. The peripheral superficial and deep venous systems communicate at multiple levels via venous networks and perforating venous connections.

Within the axillae and thorax, major venous drainage occurs only into a deep system as single veins that accom-pany the adjacent artery. The inlet to these intrathoracic central veins is defined by the costoclavicular space.

Superficial Veins of the Upper Extremity

Beginning at the fingers and extending through the upper arm, the superficial system consists of the dorsal digital veins, dorsal metacarpal veins, dorsal venous plexus, palmar digital veins, palmar venous plexus, median cubital vein, median antecubital vein, cephalic vein, and the basilic vein.

In the hand, dorsal digital veins for the ulnar aspect of the index finger, radial aspect of the fifth finger, and both sides of the third and fourth fingers drain into three dorsal metacarpal veins. These in turn drain into the dorsal venous plexus.

On the radial side of the hand, this plexus is joined by dorsal veins from the thumb and the dorsal vein of the radial aspect of the index finger to form the cephalic vein. On the ulnar side of the hand, the dorsal vein from the ulnar aspect of the fifth finger joins the plexus. The ulnar portion of the plexus then drains into the basilic vein.

The proper palmar digital veins communicate with the dorsal digital veins through intercapitular veins at the metacarpal heads. One route of drainage for the proper palmar digital veins is into the palmar venous plexus over the thenar and hypothenar eminences. This plexus drains into the median antecubital vein.

In the forearm, the cephalic, basilic, median cubital, and median antecubital veins can have variable anatomy. In general, the cephalic and basilic veins course on the radial and ulnar aspects, respectively. Either or both may be dominant. The cephalic vein crosses the ventrolateral antecubital fossa between the brachioradialis and the biceps brachii muscles, while the basilic vein crosses the ventromedial antecubital fossa, between the biceps brachii and pronator teres.

The median cubital vein directly connects the cephalic and basilic veins in the antecubital fossa. These veins may also be connected by a dorsal oblique vein in the forearm. An accessory cephalic vein may be present, joining the cephalic vein below the elbow. This accessory cephalic vein may arise from a dorsal forearm venous plexus or may arise from the cephalic vein above the wrist.

The median antecubital vein courses along the ventromedial forearm. It ends either in the basilic or the median cubital veins. Alternatively, the median antecubital, as with the median cubital vein, may divide into one branch that drains into the basilic (median basilica vein) and the other into the cephalic (median cephalic) vein.

In the upper arm, the basilic and cephalic veins are medial and lateral to the biceps brachii, respectively. The basilic vein ascends initially within the superficial fascia, but then perforates the deep fascia at the mid arm level. The vein then courses on the medial aspect of the brachial artery until the inferior margin of the teres major muscle. At this level, the basilic vein joins the brachial vein to form the axillary vein.

The cephalic vein ascends within superficial fascia entering the infraclavicular fossa posterior to the pectoralis major. The vein then crosses into the clavipectoral fossa with ultimate drainage into the superior aspect of the axillary vein, below the clavicle.

Deep Veins of the Upper Extremity

Peripherally, upper extremity deep veins include the superficial palmar venous arches, deep palmar venous arches, radial veins, ulnar veins, interosseous veins, brachial veins, and the axillary vein. Centrally, the deep veins consist of the subclavian and brachiocephalic veins.

In the hand, in addition to proper palmar digital veins draining into the superficial palmar venous plexus, the proper palmar digital veins also drain into the common palmar digital and palmar metacarpal veins. The common palmar digital veins converge into the superficial palmar venous arches, while the palmar metacarpal veins form the deep palmar venous arches. Palmar metacarpal veins also communicate to the dorsal metacarpal veins via perforating veins. Both pairs of the venous arches parallel the respective arterial arches.

The superficial palmar arches drain into the ulnar veins, and the deep palmar arches drain into the radial veins. Branches from the deep palmar arches and the proximal ulnar and radial veins coalesce to form a carpal venous plexus, which drains into the volar and dorsal interosseous veins.

In the forearm, the radial, ulnar, and interosseous paired veins ascend on either side of their respective companion arteries. Proximal to the elbow, the interosseous veins drain into the ulnar veins, and the ulnar vein gives off a draining branch to the median cubital vein. At the elbow, the radial and ulnar veins coalesce to form the paired brachial veins.

In the upper arm, the paired brachial veins ascend on either side of the brachial artery, receiving small venous branch tributaries. At the level of the teres major, the brachial veins coalesce with the basilic vein to form the axillary vein. The medial brachial vein may join the basilic vein prior to this junction. The axillary vein courses as a single structure to the level of the first rib, medial and inferior to the axillary artery. In addition to the cephalic vein, the axillary vein receives venous tributaries corresponding to the axillary arterial branches.

In the thorax, the subclavian vein extends from the outer margin of the first rib to the level of the clavicular head, where it joins with the internal jugular vein to form the brachiocephalic vein. The subclavian vein lies superior and posterior to the subclavian artery and courses posterior to the scalenus anterior. Important tributaries include the external jugular, anterior jugular, and dorsal scapular veins. The thoracic duct drains into the left subclavian vein at the confluence with the left internal jugular vein, and the right lymphatic duct drains into the right subclavian vein at the confluence with the right internal jugular vein.

The right and left brachiocephalic veins join together to form the superior vena cava, which then drains into the right atrium. The right brachiocephalic vein has a short vertical course and lies anterior and to the right of the brachiocephalic artery. The left brachiocephalic vein has a longer, horizontal course, and lies anterior to the brachiocephalic, left common carotid, and left subclavian arteries. Common tributaries include the vertebral, internal mammary, inferior thyroid, and supreme intercostal veins (85,87,88).

CLINICAL APPLICATIONS

Arterial Occlusive Disease

Arterial occlusive disease of proximal upper extremity vessels may be due to atherosclerosis, embolism, inflammatory arteritis, previous radiation therapy, or other iatrogenic causes and trauma. In addition, there are a host of uncommon causes that may manifest themselves with lesions in the upper extremity arterial bed. A prior review of a series with 136 patients requiring operative correction showed atherosclerosis to be the most common cause of occlusive disease in the brachiocephalic artery (89).

In that series, subclavian artery atherosclerosis was associated with distal ischemia; thrombosis of the subclavian artery was due to compression by cervical ribs, arteritis, and the use of this vessel for creation of a Blalock-Taussig operation (subclavian to pulmonary arterial anastomosis).

Axillary and brachial artery lesions were principally caused by trauma (mainly by gunshot wounds, laceration, or blunt trauma). Atherosclerosis, embolism, and radiation injury were also seen in some patients.

The causes of injury to the radial, ulnar, and more distal arteries were trauma, intra-arterial cannulas for measuring blood pressure, and various small vessel diseases (89).

Patients with chronic occlusive disease are generally excellent candidates for imaging with MDCT or MRA. Patients with acute ischemia, on the other hand, present an emergency situation; the decision to obtain an imaging test is based on clinical grounds and the presumed etiology of the occlusion.

In patients with a suspected embolus or thrombosis, immediate endoluminal evaluation/treatment or surgical exploration is indicated. Despite the excellent capabilities of MDCT and MRA, there is, however, a paucity of literature on upper extremity imaging with cross-sectional modalities other than duplex ultrasonography.

Because of the abundant collateral pathways, lesions of the brachiocephalic vessels often do not present with upper extremity claudication, in contrast to occlusive lesions in the proximal arteries supplying the lower extremities.

Although some patients may present with arm claudication, cerebral symptoms resulting from perfusion changes (i.e., subclavian steal syndrome) and embolization of thrombi generated at the site of ulcerated lesions are actually the most important reasons for referral.

The subclavian steal syndrome occurs when use of the upper extremity increases its demand for blood and the arm "steals" it from the cerebral circulation through the ipsilateral vertebral or brachiocephalic artery. It is important to realize that not all patients with an angiographic steal phenomenon are symptomatic. In fact, only about one third of all patients with angiographically proven steal syndromes suffer from characteristic complaints (90–92).

MRA offers a comprehensive assessment combining a depiction of the arterial stenosis and the ability to depict reversed flow in the vertebral artery (Fig. 22-27).

A recent review by Azakie et al. (3) of 94 cases of symptomatic atherosclerotic occlusive disease of the brachiocephalic artery found that 85 of 94 patients (88%) presented with symptoms of cerebral hypoperfusion (n = 52; 55%) combined with transient ischemic attack (n = 40; 43%) or stroke (n = 5; 5%). Right upper extremity claudication and digital embolization were the presenting symptoms in only 26 of 94 patients (28%).

Exact delineation of the site of occlusive disease is important from a therapeutic point of view, as many vascular surgeons prefer extrathoracic procedures to intrathoracic endarterectomy or bypass procedures, except in the management of complex occlusive disease of two or more major vessels.

The options for repairing brachiocephalic lesions are percutaneous transluminal angioplasty (PTA), and stenting, when needed, or surgical procedures such as endarterectomy, aortobrachiocephalic (or carotid or subclavian) bypass grafting through a median sternotomy, and axilloaxillary bypass.

Left subclavian lesions can be repaired by PTA, by carotid-subclavian bypass, or subclavian-carotid reimplantation. On the right side, PTA, subclavian endarterectomy and carotid-subclavian bypass are possible alternatives.

Common carotid occlusion can be repaired by endarterectomy on the right side, but subclavian to carotid bypass is usually a simpler procedure. Multiple lesions of the arch vessels can be repaired with PTA or bypass grafts from the aortic arch.

In general, PTA and surgery for aortic arch branch vessel disease have good long-term success rates, with better results being reported for surgery. Reported long-term primary patency rates for PTA in two recent, large series

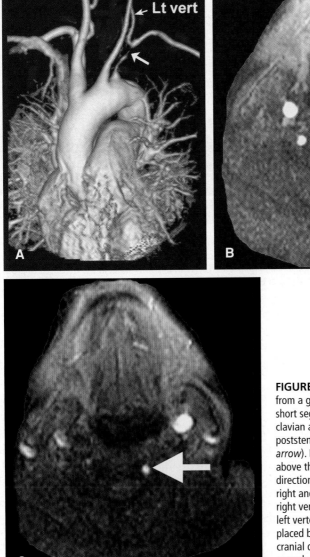

FIGURE 22-27 Subclavian steal. A: VR image from a gadolinium-MRA study shows a stenosis and short segment occlusion of the prevertebral left subclavian artery (*large white arrow*) and flow in the poststenotic segment of the left vertebral artery (*short arrow*). **B:** 2D TOF with a saturation band placed above the slice suppresses flow in a cranial-caudad direction, resulting in selective demonstration of the right and left common carotid arteries and only the right vertebral artery; note the absence of flow in the left vertebral artery. **C:** 2D TOF with a saturation band placed below the slice suppresses flow in the caudad-cranial direction, and shows flow in the veins and retrograde flow in the left vertebral artery (*arrow*), identifying subclavian steal physiology.

were 72% (n = 38) (93), and 93% (n = 89) (94). In the 94 surgical cases studied by Azakie et al. (3), postoperative survival rate was 96% at 1 year, 85% at 5 years, and 67% at 10 years. Freedom from recurrence requiring operation was 100% at 1 year, 99% at 5 years, and 97% at 10 years (3).

The choice for either PTA or surgery should be made on an individual basis, weighing the additional risks of surgery versus the lower long-term patency of PTA. At present, PTA will often be attempted first. Both techniques carry similar small risks for stroke (3,93,94).

Atherosclerotic Upper Extremity Occlusive Disease

Aortic Arch and Branch Vessels

Symptomatic atherosclerotic occlusive disease of the upper extremity is uncommon. Morphologically, atherosclerotic lesions can be distinguished from other causes by their eccentricity and irregularity, and not uncommonly by the presence of ulceration. Conversely, lesions associated with vasculitis tend to result in smooth, concentric narrowing over a longer trajectory, and rare causes of peripheral arterial

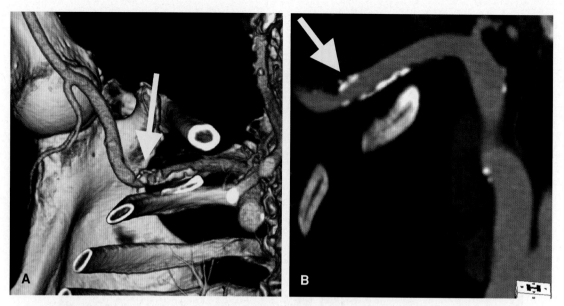

FIGURE 22-28 CTA was performed in a patient with right upper extremity claudication. A VR image **(A)** reveals a short segment atherosclerotic lesion at the distal subclavian artery (*arrow*). A rotating curved planar reformation shows that the majority of the lesion results in no hemodynamic significance **(B)**. With the arm raised, at the transition to the axillary artery, luminal narrowing approaches 50% (*arrow* in **B**).

disease such as fibromuscular dysplasia or ergotamine use are characterized angiographically by a characteristic "string of beads" appearance.

Atherosclerotic lesions are most commonly found in the brachiocephalic artery, followed by the subclavian artery (Fig. 22-28) Lesions involving the subclavian artery are three times more common on the left than on the right (95). Stenoses and occlusions in the brachiocephalic and other arch vessels are found in relatively young patients with mean ages ranging between 50 and 61 years (91,96). No consistent gender predilection exists with conflicting results that favor females (3) or males (91).

Factors associated with atherosclerotic disease of the aortic arch vessels are the general risk factors for developing atherosclerotic occlusive disease, the most important being smoking and hypertension. A key consideration for management options is the presence of concomitant carotid artery and coronary artery disease. In the large series mentioned previously, the prevalence of concomitant coronary artery disease ranged from 26% to 65% (3,91,96).

For aortic arch and major branch vessels, PC acquisitions to determine the direction of flow in the carotid and vertebral arteries can be combined with a high spatial resolution CE MRA luminogram to depict the location and severity of any stenotic lesions.

Because of the high frequency of neurologic symptoms, it is advisable to image the carotid arteries in the same session. Several examples of atherosclerotic disease of the aortic arch vessels are shown (Figs. 22-29 to 22-31). (A sample imaging protocol is listed in Table 22-11.)

The true frequency of atherosclerotic lesions in these vessels is unknown since the abundant collateral networks at both the shoulder and elbow levels substantially contribute to the masking of symptoms. Special groups of patients are those who underwent aortic arch and arch vessel surgery and those with ESRD (see below). It is well known that the latter group of patients suffer from accelerated atherosclerosis (97,98) and may require distal upper extremity bypass surgery (99).

Forearm and Hand Arteries

Except for patients with ESRD, atherosclerosis is rarely the cause of symptomatic ischemia due to lesions in the forearm and hand arteries. Patients with dialysis access shunts also have a relatively high frequency of arterial lesions supplying the access. This is discussed in more detail in the section on Imaging of Dialysis Access below. (Sample imaging protocols are listed in Tables 22-12 and 22-13).

Embolic Disease of the Upper Extremity

Embolism to the upper extremity vasculature is one manifestation of arterial disease, and this condition results in a clinical presentation of acute ischemia. When an embolism lodges distally in the digits, it can present as the "blue-finger syndrome" (100).

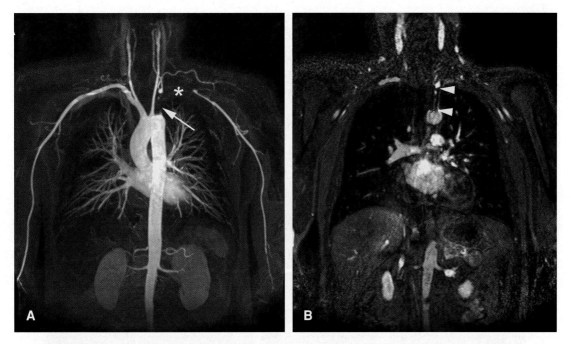

FIGURE 22-29 A 70-year-old male patient with recurrent complaints of left upper extremity claudication. There are two occlusions in the proximal left subclavian artery (*arrow* and *asterisk* in **A**). The latter occlusion is relatively well collateralized via the thyrocervical trunk. Close inspection of the source images reveals that the more proximal occlusion is in fact due to a susceptibility artifact due to the presence of a stent (between *arrowheads* in **B**). In this case, it would be advisable to rule out in-stent restenosis with CTA.

In a series of 36 patients with acute ischemia of the upper limb, 17 (47.2%) had embolic occlusion, 9 (25%) had iatrogenic thrombosis in the brachial artery, and 10 (27.8%) had primary arterial thrombosis (101).

Emboli to the upper limb account for 15% to 20% of all peripheral emboli and typically originate from the heart (70% of cases) secondary to conditions such as cardiac arrhythmias (most commonly atrial fibrillation), ventricular aneurysms, myocardial infarction, blood dyscrasias, paradoxical emboli, and bacterial endocarditis (39,102–104).

Acute ischemia of the arm may also be caused by emboli arising from the heart, from subclavian or axillary aneurysms, or as the result of trauma, the latter from penetrating, blunt, or iatrogenic events. The broad range of etiologies for thromboembolism is outlined in Chapter 9. Some special circumstances related to upper limb emboli are listed in Table 22-14.

A special consideration is the possibility of thromboembolism from upstream aneurysmal disease. This can be seen after trauma as a consequence of chronic thoracic outlet compression, in which the presence of a cervical rib is quite common (105–107). Beyond the point of compression, the subclavian artery often shows poststenotic dilatation with aneurysm formation containing thrombus, which can serve as a source of distal thromboembolism (Fig. 22-32).

Additional points of compression include the pectoralis minor tendon where it attaches to the coracoid process in the axilla and the head of the humerus, which can stretch and damage the axillary artery in extreme rotations typical of throwing athletes (113). Digital arterial embolism can result from the ulnar artery aneurysms that can be associated with the hypothenar hammer syndrome.

Patients presenting with digital ischemia have a broad differential diagnosis, and a key step in the evaluation is to ascertain whether there is disease in the proximal vessels. Upstream findings prompt the likelihood that the digital features are distal manifestations of that proximal disease.

When upstream vessels are normal, the workup can proceed toward distinguishing between arterial obstruction and vasospasm. Predisposing clinical circumstances (e.g., atrial fibrillation, recent myocardial infarction, penetrating trauma) can often suggest the etiology, but noninvasive tests can help to establish the suspected diagnosis of embolism and to guide the level for incision or catheter placement. Duplex sonography can be an important strategy in this regard.

Imaging Findings

The classic finding at angiography is a complete occlusion producing the classic "meniscus sign," a filling defect or abrupt vessel cutoff. Although abrupt arterial occlusion

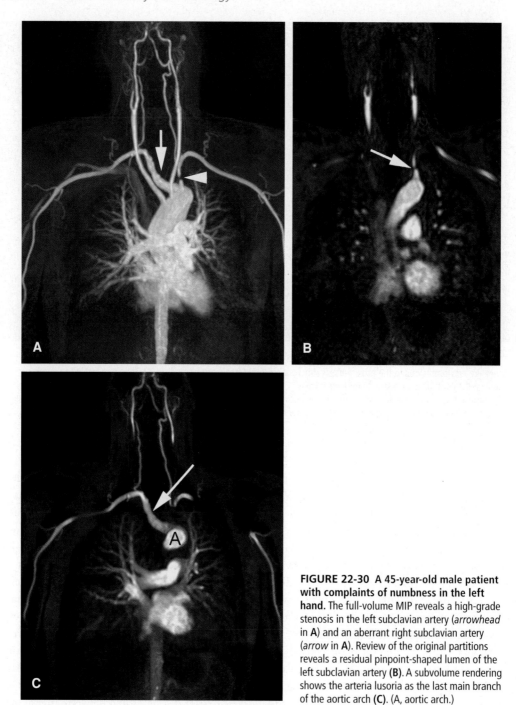

FIGURE 22-30 A 45-year-old male patient with complaints of numbness in the left hand. The full-volume MIP reveals a high-grade stenosis in the left subclavian artery (*arrowhead* in **A**) and an aberrant right subclavian artery (*arrow* in **A**). Review of the original partitions reveals a residual pinpoint-shaped lumen of the left subclavian artery (**B**). A subvolume rendering shows the arteria lusoria as the last main branch of the aortic arch (**C**). (A, aortic arch.)

suggests embolic disease, only discrete intraluminal filling defects allow reliable distinction of embolism from other occlusive etiologies (Fig. 22-33).

Larger emboli will occlude the larger proximal vessels, with the brachial artery bifurcation being the most common site in the upper extremity (Fig. 22-33) (114). Microemboli to the arteries of the hand typically produce segmental occlusions of the common and proper digital arteries with abrupt termination of blood flow. With

dynamic acquisitions, soft tissue perfusion details can provide adjunctive information. CE MRA is a simple way to monitor patients following thrombolysis and is sensitive in the detection of collateral vessel filling (Fig. 22-34) (39).

Treatment Considerations

The treatment options for acute peripheral arterial occlusion caused by thrombosis or embolism include thrombolytic therapy; surgical embolectomy/thrombectomy; and

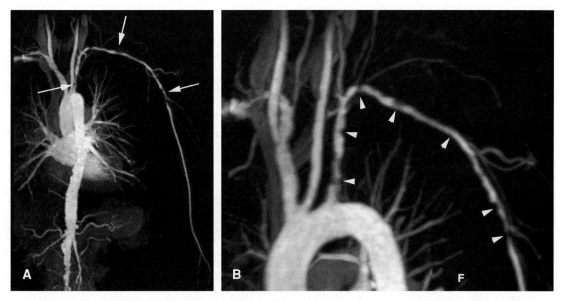

FIGURE 22-31 A 65-year-old male patient with known atherosclerosis. The whole-volume MIP **(A)** shows multiple irregular stenoses in the left subclavian artery of moderate- to high-grade severity (*arrows*). This is confirmed on the zoomed left anterior oblique projection (*arrowheads* in **B**).

more recently, rheolytic therapy (115). With rheolytic therapy, water jet technology creates a low-pressure zone at the catheter tip and a subsequent vacuum effect that draws in vessel thrombus to allow for its removal. Regardless of the approach, the objective is to preserve limb and life by restoration of blood flow.

The presence of significant atherosclerotic subclavian artery stenosis can be addressed by balloon angioplasty and stent implantation. The use of the stent is thought to prevent embolic events (2).

The Vasculitides

Inflammation of the walls of vessels, called vasculitis, can affect vessels of any type in virtually any organ (see Chapter 10 for in depth information). The upper extremity is a frequent site of many forms of vasculitis. In contrast to atherosclerotic occlusive disease, patients have constitutional signs and symptoms such as fever, myalgias, arthralgias, and malaise, in addition to local manifestations of downstream ischemia (Fig. 22-35). Vasculitides are associated with laboratory abnormalities such as elevated erythrocyte sedimentation rate, antineutrophilic cytoplasmic antibodies (ANCA), and antiendothelial cell antibodies (116,117).

Angiographically, vasculitis is suggested by the presence of smooth stenoses over a longer trajectory compared with atherosclerotic occlusive disease. One of the most important features supporting the diagnosis is vessel wall thickening and enhancement, which can readily be appreciated by cross-sectional imaging. The imaging protocol in suspected

vasculitis should therefore include delayed, postcontrast imaging and with MR, sequences geared toward optimally demonstrating the soft tissues will provide added value.

Large Artery Vasculitis in the Upper Extremity

Takayasu Arteritis

Takayasu arteritis is an inflammatory condition of the arterial wall affecting the aorta, aortic branches to the head and upper extremity, and the renal arteries (118). The absence of upper-extremity arterial pulses was a feature of the disease present in the intial description by Mikto Takayasu in 1908 (118–121).

The estimated incidence of Takayasu arteritis in the United States is 2.6 cases per 1,000,000 population per year (120,122), but the disease is more often observed in patients of Asian origin. Females are much more often affected than men (about eight to nine times more often), with most patients being in the second and third decades of life.

The clinical manifestations of Takayasu arteritis are usually divided into early and late phases, with a classic triphasic pattern of expression. Nonspecific systemic features such as low-grade fever, malaise, weight loss, and fatigue characterize the early or prepulseless phase.

This is followed by a vascular inflammatory phase and a late quiescent and occlusive phase (38,123). Characteristic features in the late phase include diminished or absent pulsations, hence the alternative name "pulselessness" disease,

TABLE 22-11

Recommended Magnetic Resonance Sequence Parameters for Aortic Arch and Proximal Upper Extremity Magnetic Resonance Angiography

Sequence	Orientation	Coverage	TR/TE (ms)	FA (degrees)	FOV (mm)	Matrix	Slice Thickness* (mm)	No. of Partitions	BW (kHz)	NSA	Duration (s)	Comments
bSSFP	Coronal	Aortic arch to distal brachial artery	6.0/3.0	90	430 × 430	400 × 256	5–10	30–60	500–700	1	30–60 s	
2D PCA	Transverse	Neck/carotid and vertrebral arteries	20/5	15	260 × 260	256 × 256	10	1 1	200–500	2 2	30–60 s	To detect subclavian steal. Set VENC to 120 cm/s
2D timing	Coronal	Aortic arch to distal brachial artery	4.0/1.5	30–40	430 × 430	256 × 256	80–100	1	500–700	0.67	>60	
3D GRE	Coronal	Aortic arch to distal brachial artery	<4.0/<2.0	30–40	430 × 300	430 × 300	1.0–2.0	Tailor to anatomy	200–500	0.67	40–50 (≥2 dyn)	Use parallel imaging
T1w postcontrast	Transverse	Location of suspected vasculitis	580/14	90	385 × 270	385 × 270	3.0	Tailor to anatomy	200–500	1	Several minutes	Use parallel imaging

TR, repetition time; TE, echo time; FA, flip angle; FOV, field of view (frequency × phase); BW, bandwidth; NSA, number of signals averaged (number below 1 indicates partial or fractional echo); bSSFP, balanced steady state free precession; 2D PCA, two-dimensional phase-contrast angiography; 3D GRE, three-dimensional gradient refocused echo; VENC, velocity encoding; dyn, dynamic scans.

*Noninterpolated, truly acquired slice thickness.

TABLE 22-12

Recommended Magnetic Resonance Sequence Parameters for Magnetic Resonance Angiography of the Forearm and Hand

Sequence	Orientation	Coverage	TR/TE (ms)	FA (degrees)	FOV (mm)	Matrix	Slice Thickness* (mm)	No. of Partitions	BW (kHz)	NSA	Duration (s)	Comments
bSSFP	Coronal	Distal brachial artery to digits	6.0/3.0	90	430 × 430	400 × 256	5–10	30–60	500–700	1	30–60	
2D timing	Coronal	Distal brachial artery to digits	4.0/1.5	30–40	430 × 430	256 × 256	40–60	1	500–700	0.67	>60	
3D GRE	Coronal	Distal brachial artery to digits	<4.0/ <2.0	30–40	430 × 300	430 × 300	1.0	Tailor to anatomy	200–500	0.67	40–50 (≥2 dyn)	Use parallel imaging
T1w post-contrast	Transverse	Location of suspected vasculitis	580/14	90	385 × 270	385 × 270	3.0	Tailor to anatomy	200–500	1	Several minutes	Use parallel imaging

TR, repetition time; TE, echo time; FA, flip angle; FOV, field of view (frequency × phase); BW, bandwidth; NSA, number of signals averaged (number below 1 indicates partial or fractional echo); bSSFP, balanced steady state free precession; 2D, two dimensional; 3D GRE, three-dimensional gradient refocused echo; dyn, dynamic scans.

*Noninterpolated, truly acquired slice thickness.

TABLE 22-13

Recommended Magnetic Resonance Sequence Parameters for Magnetic Resonance Angiography of the Hand and Digits

Sequence	Orientation	Coverage	TR/TE (ms)	FA (degrees)	FOV (mm)	Matrix	Slice Thickness* (mm)	No of Partitions	BW (kHz)	NSA	Duration (s)	Comments
bSSFP	Coronal	Wrist and hand	6.0/3.0	90	430 × 430	400 × 256	5	30–60	500–700	1	30–60 s	
2D timing	Coronal	Wrist and hand	4.0/1.5	30–40	220 × 150	256 × 256	40–60	1	500–700	0.67	>60	
3D GRE	Coronal	Wrist and hand	<5.0/ <2.0	30–40	220 × 150	220 × 150	≤1.0	Tailor to anatomy	200–500	0.67	40–50 (≥2 dyn)	Use parallel imaging
T1w post-contrast	Transverse	Location of suspected abnormality	580/14	90	150 × 75	300 × 150	1.0	Tailor to anatomy	200–500	1	Several minutes	Use parallel imaging
T1-weighted steady state	Coronal	Wrist and hand	<5.0/ <2.0	20	220 × 150	368 × 248	≤0.6		200		About 5 minutes	In combination with blood pool or agent TAC only

TR, repetition time; TE, echo time; FA, flip angle; FOV, field of view (frequency × phase); BW, bandwidth; NSA, number of signals averaged (number below 1 indicates partial or fractional echo); bSSFP, balanced steady state free precession; 2D, two dimensional; 3D GRE, three-dimensional gradient refocused echo; dyn, dynamic scans; TAC, timed arterial compression (see text).

*Noninterpolated, truly acquired slice thickness.

TABLE 22-14

Unique Etiologies of Upper Limb Thromboembolism

Thoracic outlet compression [105–107]
Brachial artery fibromuscular dysplasia [108,109]
Hypothenar hammer syndrome [110]
Occluded axillary-femoral bypass grafts [111,112]
Radial artery catheterization injury [40]

and stenoses in virtually any limb- or organ-supplying artery (120,124).

Excellent regional collateral circulation and the lack of specificity of early symptoms often results in a delayed diagnosis. Because of the varied presentation several diagnostic criteria have been proposed, as discussed in Chapter 10.

Imaging findings in Takayasu arteritis include segmental or long and diffuse stenosis, occlusion, dilatation, and aneurysm formation (Figs. 22-36, 22-37). Because of the chronic nature of the disease, patients are often evaluated serially at 3- to 6-month intervals. In this light, and considering the young age of many patients, MRI can be considered as the preferred imaging modality.

The diffuse nature of this disease demands broad anatomic coverage that should include the entire aorta; the brachiocephalic vessels; and the celiac, renal, and mesen-

teric arteries (Figs. 22-38, 22-39). In the presence of suggestive symptoms, the pulmonary and coronary circulation should be interrogated as well.

Giant Cell Arteritis

Polymyalgia rheumatica and giant cell arteritis (GCA) are closely related conditions that affect persons of middle age and older and often occur together. These conditions are considered by many to be different phases of the same disease (125). The incidence of polymyalgia rheumatica and GCA increases after the age of 50 years and peaks between 70 and 80 years of age.

Polymyalgia rheumatica is an inflammatory condition of unknown cause characterized by aching and morning stiffness in the cervical region and shoulder and pelvic girdles. It is an immune mediated synovitis that usually responds rapidly to low doses of corticosteroids and has a favorable prognosis.

GCA is an immune-mediated vasculitis of the large- and medium-sized arteries. Clinical manifestations may be nonspecific and variable, including features attributable to systemic inflammation and local complications of vascular injury. GCA most commonly affects the temporal arteries (125,126) but involvement of the extracranial arteries is increasingly being recognized (127).

Extracranial GCA may affect the aorta or branches of the aortic arch, particularly the subclavian, axillary, and

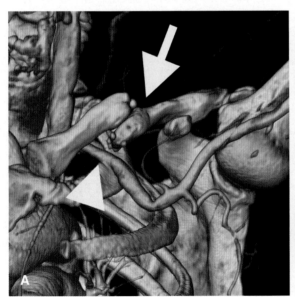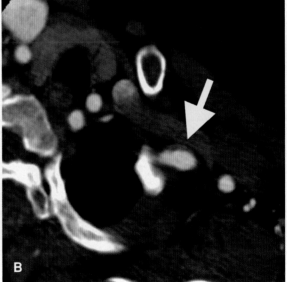

FIGURE 22-32 16-channel left UE CTA was performed to evaluate a patient with recurrent arterial thromboembolism. Six hours following surgical thrombectomy, the patient again had a cool hand. VR images reveal a mid clavicle nonunion fracture (*arrow* in **A**) with compression on the subclavian-axillary artery segment at the costoclavicular space (*arrowhead* in **A**) consistent with cervicoaxillary compression syndrome—costoclavicular subtype. Compression resulted in a focal axillary artery pseudoaneurysm with mural thrombus (*arrow* in **B**) and recurrent downstream arterial embolization.

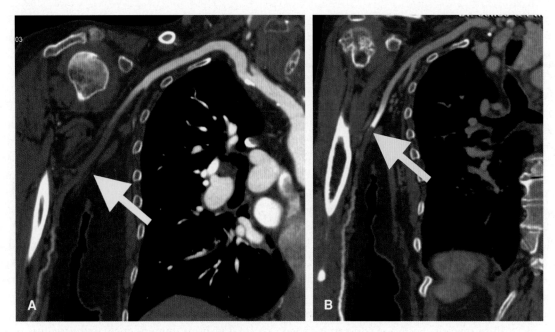

FIGURE 22-33 Upper extremity embolic disease. Two consecutive passes of the left upper extremity with a 16-slice MDCT show an abrupt cutoff of the brachial artery opacification. **A:** The first pass shows the proximal vasculature with high-quality enhancement and less density in the brachial just distal to the embolus (*arrow*). **B:** Note the increased density of contrast immediately upstream to a well-defined embolus (*arrow*) visualized on the second pass. (Courtesy of Dr. Ruben Sebben, Dr. Jones, and Partners Medical Imaging, Adelaide, Australia.)

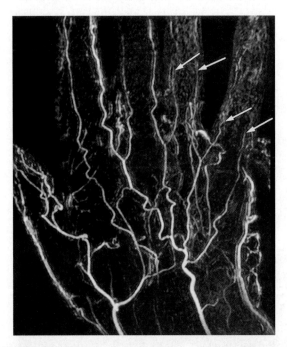

FIGURE 22-34 Microemboli. A 53-year-old man with sudden onset of ischemia in the left fourth and fifth digits. CE MR angiogram obtained to monitor patient response following urokinase injection shows abrupt termination of the proper digital vessels of the fourth and fifth digits (*arrows*). (Adapted with permission from Connell DA, Koulouris G, Thorn DA, et al. Contrast-enhanced MR angiography of the hand. *Radiographics.* 2002;22:583–599.)

brachial arteries (128–131). In rare cases, the lower extremity may be involved (132). Upper extremity arterial stenosis is seen as a manifestation of GCA in 4% to 15% of cases, but based on sonography and positron emission tomography data, the disease may be present yet remain undetected (133–135).

When the branches of the aortic arch, particularly the subclavian and axillary arteries, become narrowed, patients often complain of arm claudication (135). Pulses in the neck or arms may be decreased or absent.

The diagnosis of extracranial GCA is established using clinical and serological criteria as well as typical angiographic and sonographic findings (136). At MR, areas of inflammation are characterized by hyperenhancement (Figs. 22-40, 22-41) (137–141).

The histopathological and radiographic findings of GCA may sometimes be indistinguishable from those observed in Takayasu arteritis or isolated angiitis of the central nervous system. The age at onset and the distribution of lesions will facilitate the differentiation.

A high rate of negative findings in the temporal artery biopsy specimens is fairly typical of the extracranial GCA patient population, suggesting compartmentalization of the vasculitis (130). While an elevated erythrocyte sedimentation rate is often seen in GCA and is part of the diagnostic

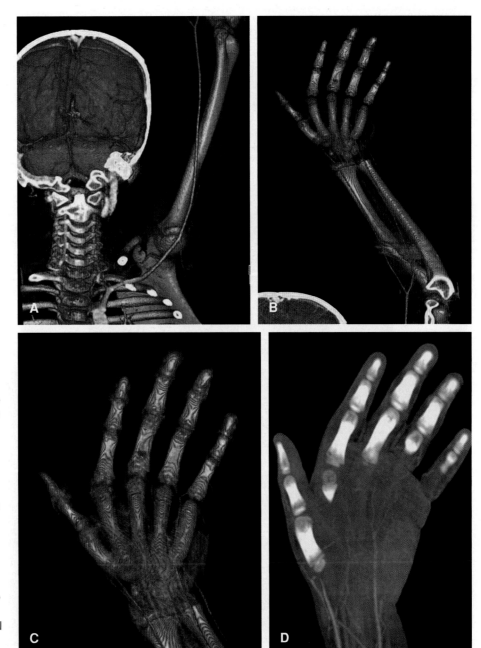

FIGURE 22-35 A 7-year-old boy presented with subacute ischemia in the left third through fourth fingers. Clinically, based on elevated inflammatory markers, small vessel vasculitis was suspected. CTA was performed to exclude proximal outflow disease in the subclavian through brachial segments. The child was positioned supine with the arm raised. Coverage extended through to the fingers. Images confirmed normal proximal outflow segments (**A,** VR image) with diminished enhancement in the radial, ulnar, and interosseous arteries (**B,** VR image). Palmar and digital arteries in the hand (**C,** VR image; **D,** MIP image) were poorly enhanced. The patient was treated for 4 weeks with oral steroid and vasodilator medications. (*Figure 22-35 Continues*)

criteria established by the American College of Rheumatology, up to 22.5% of patients with GCA have a normal erythrocyte sedimentation rate before treatment (143).

The C-reactive protein level has been found to be a more sensitive indicator of disease activity than the erythrocyte sedimentation rate both at diagnosis and during relapse (144). The excellent soft tissue contrast and lack of ionizing radiation make MRI ideal for serial follow-up studies being used to monitor response to treatment (Fig. 22-40) (142,145).

Thromboangiitis Obliterans (Buerger's Disease)

The conventional angiographic features of Buerger's disease involve the small- and medium-sized vessels, such as the palmar, plantar, tibial, peroneal, radial, and ulnar arteries and the digital arteries of the fingers and toes. Arteriographic findings may be suggestive but are not pathognomonic (8). The presence of diabetes mellitus rules out the diagnosis of thromboangiitis obliterans.

Findings include segmental occlusive lesions (diseased arteries interspersed with normal-appearing arteries), more

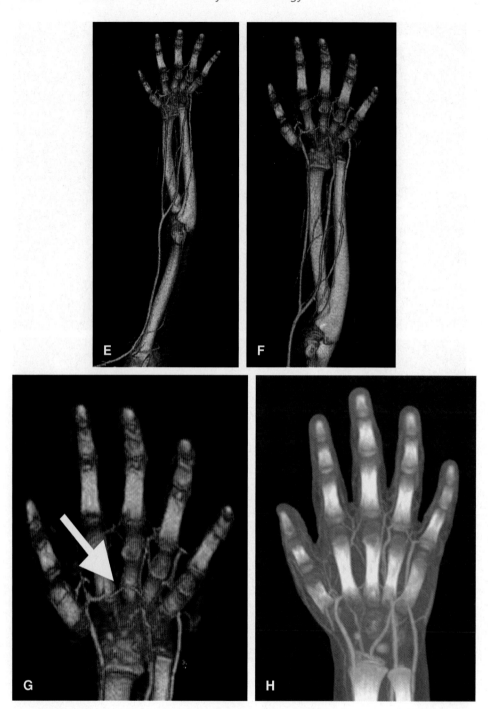

FIGURE 22-35 (Continued)
Follow-up CTA was performed with the extremity at the patient's side—a secondary goal of this exam was to evaluate the thoracic and abdominal aorta. Imaging revealed stable caliber and enhancement in the proximal outflow. **(E)** with now robust enhancement and caliber in the radial, ulnar, interosseous, palmar, and common digital arteries **(F)**. The deep arch was intact (*arrow* in **G**). Paired digital arteries were well enhanced to nearly the proximal interphalangeal joint spaces **(H)**.

severe disease distally with normal proximal arteries and no evidence of atherosclerosis; collateralization around areas of occlusion (corkscrew collaterals), and no apparent source of emboli (146,147).

In a retrospective analysis of 825 patients with thromboangiitis obliterans (TAO), there were 42 patients (5.1%) with upper extremity arterial involvement only, 616 (74.7%) with lower extremity involvement only, and 167 (20.2%) with both (148). The most frequently affected arteries were the anterior (41.4%) or posterior (40.4%) tibial arteries in the lower extremities, and the ulnar artery (11.5%) in the upper extremities. There were no significant differences in the distribution of arterial involvement between men and women or between the right and left sides. In total, approximately 25% of the patients had upper extremity involvement.

In another study of 85 patients with TAO, 16 (19.1%) patients had no arm complaints (degree I ischemia).

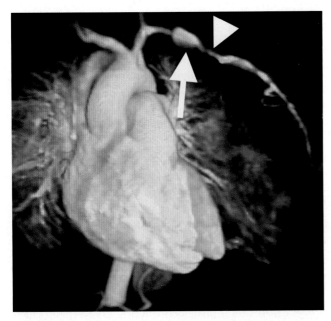

FIGURE 22-36 Female patient with Takayasu arteritis. This VR image from a CE MRA of the left subclavian artery demonstrates diffuse involvement, including both aneurysmal dilatations (*arrow*) and stenotic disease (*arrowhead*).

Thirty-eight (45.2%) patients complained of numbness and paresthesia, chiefly of the tips of the fingers on both hands. Six (7.1%) persons complained of pains in the hands at physical exercise. Ulcers and necroses of the fingers were present in 24 (28.6%) patients (149). There are not many reports of MRA or CTA of TAO.

The only proven strategy to prevent progression of the disease and avoid its serious complications, including the need for amputation, is the complete discontinuation of cigarette smoking or other use of tobacco in any form (8). Sympathectomy can improve distal flow (150).

The diffuse segmental involvement and distal nature of the disease together with the lack of sufficient distal target vessels that typifies the condition usually makes surgical revascularization impossible. In those individuals with severe ischemia and an identifiable distal target vessel, bypass surgery with the use of an autologous vein can be considered (150).

FIGURE 22-37 43-year-old female patient with known Takayasu disease presenting with severe recurrent complaints of fever and malaise. The patient had undergone previous bypass surgery for left subclavian artery occlusion, connecting the left common carotid artery with the axillary artery. Coronal whole-volume MIP (**A**) shows the bypass bridging the occluded left subclavian artery (*asterisks*). Note occlusion of both carotid arteries (*arrows*). Left anterior oblique projection (**B**) confirms right carotid occlusion (*arrow*). Note that there are three vessels originating from the aortic arch, the third being a variant left vertebral artery branching directly off the aortic arch. There is mild luminal narrowing present in this artery (*arrowhead*). Right anterior oblique projection (**C**) confirms left common carotid occlusion with retrograde filling of the carotid bulb via the circle of Willis (*arrow*). Coronal source image (**D**) confirms luminal narrowing in the vertebral artery as seen in (**B**). Note smooth segmental narrowing typical for arteritides.

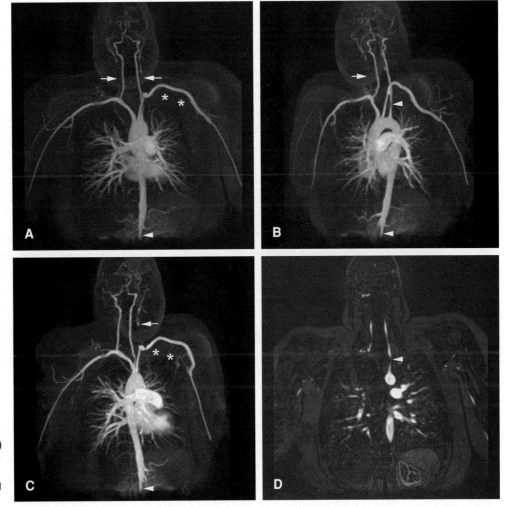

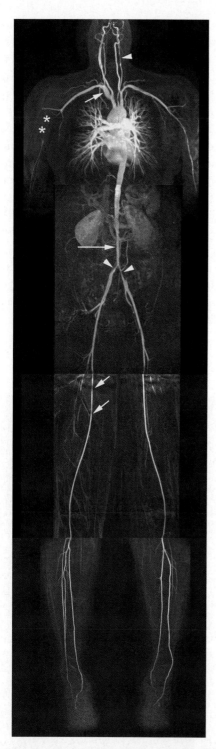

FIGURE 22-38 29-year-old female patient with known Takayasu disease. The patient was evaluated for recurrent right upper extremity claudication. In addition, the patient reported complaints of bilateral lower extremity claudication. Merged MIP of total-body MRA acquisition shows multiple smooth segmental stenoses in the central artery in the left vertebral artery (originating directly from the aortic arch; *upper two arrowheads*), the infrarenal aorta (*long horizontal arrow*), both common iliac arteries (*lower arrowheads*), and the right superficial femoral artery (*oblique short arrows*). In addition, there is aneurysmal dilatation of the proximal right subclavian artery (*upper oblique arrow*) and an occluded axillary artery (*).

Small Artery Vasculitis in the Upper Extremity

The small vessel vasculitis diseases demonstrate an obliterative fibrosis that causes digital ischemia and gangrene. Rheumatoid arthritis, Sjögren's syndrome, Wegener's granulomatosis, and microscopic polyarteritis nodosa can display a small vessel arteritis in the upper extremities.

Raynaud's Phenomenon

Raynaud's phenomenon is defined as a reversible spasm of the small- and medium-sized arteries resulting in a characteristic triphasic white-blue-red color response: (a) cessation of digital artery flow producing well-demarcated finger pallor, followed by (b) vasorelaxation and return of arterial flow and subsequent postcapillary venule constriction resulting in desaturated blood, producing cyanosis, followed by (c) postischemic hyperemia, replacing cyanosis with rubor (2,151,152).

A distinction is made between primary Raynaud's phenomenon (formerly Raynaud's disease), if there is no underlying illness, and secondary Raynaud's phenomenon (formerly Raynaud's syndrome), if there is an associated disorder detected on assessment. The classification of Raynaud's is, however, subject to continuous discussion in the literature. Some authors do not make the distinction between primary and secondary Raynaud's because patients who at first only appear to suffer from primary Raynaud's may develop an associated disorder after many years of follow-up.

In primary Raynaud's phenomenon, patients have an abnormally strong vasospastic response to cold or emotional stimuli with anatomically normal arteries. Primary Raynaud's typically occurs in young women, is bilateral and not associated with ischemic ulcerations, has a benign course, and requires only symptomatic treatment.

Secondary Raynaud's is suggested by the following findings: an age of onset of more than 30 years; episodes that are intense, painful, asymmetric, or associated with skin lesions; clinical features suggestive of a connective tissue disease (e.g., arthritis and abnormal lung function); specific autoantibodies; and evidence of microvascular disease on microscopy of nail fold capillaries (152–154).

Raynaud's complex of symptoms is very common. Various survey studies that have been conducted in the general population in several different countries found the prevalence to range from several percent up to 30%. In these studies, between 70% and 90% of all reported patients were women. In a large U.S. registry of 1,137 patients presenting with Raynaud's, 356 (31.3%) suffered from pure vasospasm with no associated disease, 391 patients (34.4%) had associated connective tissue disease, and 389 patients (34.3%) suffered from other underlying diseases (155).

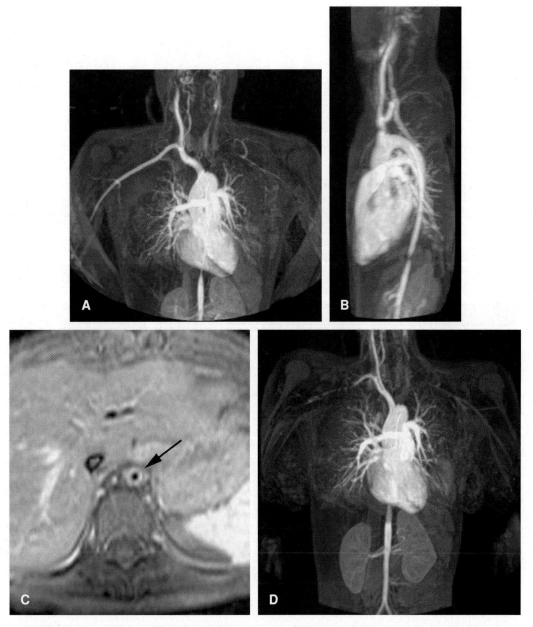

FIGURE 22-39 A 19-year-old female with known history of Takayasu arteritis. A, B: MIP reconstructions from 3D GRE gadolinium-enhanced MRA demonstrates complete occlusion of the left common carotid artery and left subclavian artery at their origins, with partial reconstitution of the left subclavian artery via collaterals, which then occludes at the level of the brachial artery. Left vertebral artery is occluded. Note narrowing of distal thoracic aorta. **C:** Axial T1 TSE postgadolinium image shows narrowing, wall thickening, and wall enhancement involving the stenotic segment in the distal thoracic aorta (*arrow*). **D:** MIP reconstruction performed 2 years later demonstrates progressive disease with multifocal narrowing and irregularity of the right subclavian artery, with occlusion of the brachial artery. (Courtesy of Avneesh Gupta, M.D., Boston University Medical Center.)

Small vessel involvement is characteristic of connective tissue disorders such as scleroderma, CREST syndrome (Calcinosis cutis, Raynaud's syndrome, Esophageal motility disorder, Sclerodactyly, and Telangiectasia), rheumatoid arthritis, mixed connective tissue disease, systemic lupus erythematosus, polymyositis, and dermatomyositis (156–158). It is seen in more than 90% of patients with scleroderma.

Angiographic findings in Raynaud's patients and for those with vasospastic disorders, in general, tend to be descriptive and are not specific. The findings are characterized by narrowing and tapering of the proper digital vessels

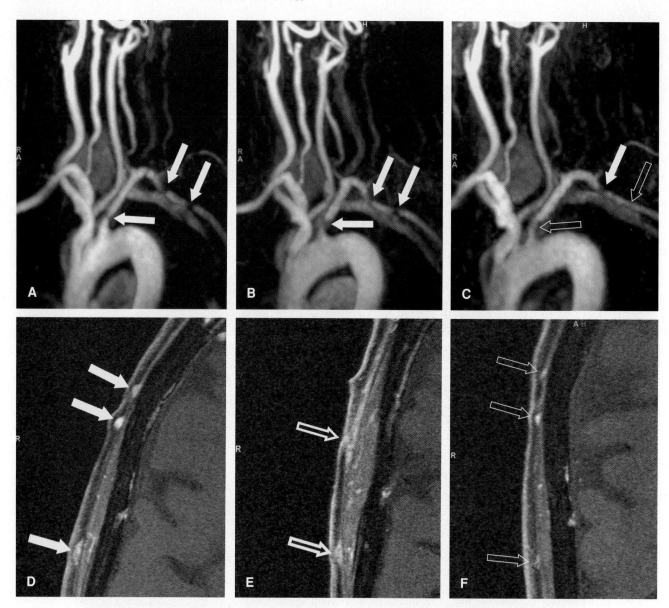

FIGURE 22-40 MR angiography of the aortic arch and the supra-aortic arteries reveals three sequential stenoses of the left subclavian artery (*arrows* in **A**) that are still present after 2 weeks of corticosteroid treatment (*arrows* in **B**). Follow-up after 2-1/2 months of continued steroid medication revealed a substantial improvement (*open arrows* in **C**), while one stenosis (*solid arrow* in **C**) remained. Enlarged high-resolution MR images of the left superficial temporal artery in cross section (*arrows* in **D**) depict mural inflammatory enhancement that had decreased after 2 weeks of steroid medication (*open arrows* in **E**) and had almost entirely vanished after 2-1/2 months (*light arrows* in **F**). (Courtesy of Thorsten Bley, M.D., Department of Diagnostic Radiology, University of Freiburg, Freiburg, Germany. Reprinted with permission from Bley TA, Ness T, Warnatz K, et al. Influence of corticosteroid treatment on MRI findings in giant cell arteritis. *Clin Rheumatol.* 2007. Sep;26(9):1541–1543.)

(Fig. 22-42). Capillary congestion in the fingertips has been described (39).

Angiography is not considered necessary to establish the diagnosis, because cold water testing or other provocative maneuvers are usually diagnostic. MRA and CTA have greater value for cases in which more proximal obstruction is suspected.

Cervicoaxillary Compression (Thoracic Outlet) Syndromes

Neurovascular shoulder compression encompasses a group of related anatomical disorders affecting the brachial plexus and subclavian and axillary arteries and veins. Compression occurs at either the interscalene triangle, costoclavicular space, or retropectoralis minor space, with the interscalene

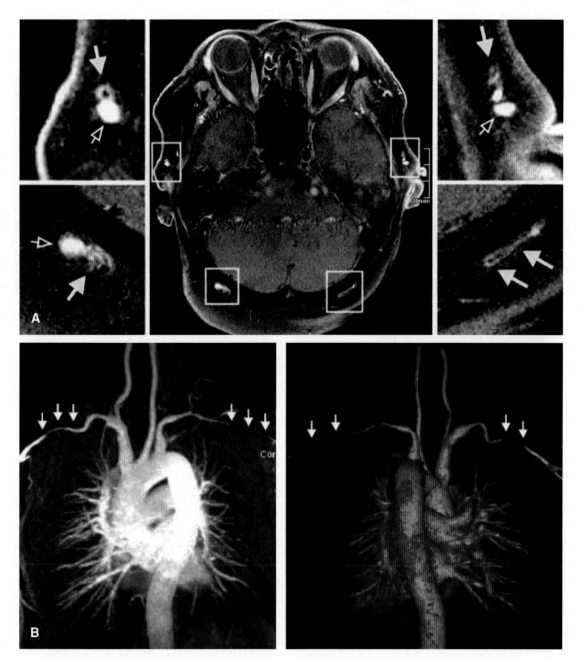

FIGURE 22-41 A 67-year-old female patient with histologically proven GCA and associated inflammatory signal changes in the superficial cranial arteries **(top)** and stenoses in the supraaortic vessels **(bottom)**. High-resolution T1-weighted head images **(A)**. Mural inflammatory signal enhancement in superficial cranial arteries can clearly be identified and is shown for the magnified occipital and temporal arteries. Signal enhancement due to the accumulation of contrast agent and circumferential luminal thickening can be appreciated for all four arteries (*solid white arrows*). Note the flow void in the arterial system due to higher velocity (outflow effects) if compared with venous signal (*open white arrows*). CE MRA **(B)**. MIP **(left panel)** and 3-D VR **(right panel)** based on CE MRA of the thoracic aorta. Multisegmental stenoses in the left and right subclavian arteries are clearly visible (*solid white arrows*). (Courtesy of Thorsten Bley, M.D., Department of Diagnostic Radiology, University of Freiburg, Freiburg, Germany. Reprinted with permission from Bley TA, Ness T, Warnatz K, et al. Influence of corticosteroid treatment on MRI findings in giant cell arteritis. *Clin Rheumatol.* 2007. Sep;26(9):1541–1543.)

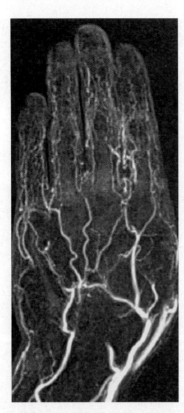

FIGURE 22-42 Single-dose Gd-BOPTA MR angiography of the hand in a 37-year-old female patient with Raynaud's syndrome demonstrates tapering and attenuation of the digital vessels. (Reprinted with permission from Winterer JT, Scheffler K, Paul G, et al. Optimization of contrast-enhanced MR angiography of the hands with a timing bolus and elliptically reordered 3D pulse sequence. *J Comput Assist Tomogr.* 2000;24:903–908.)

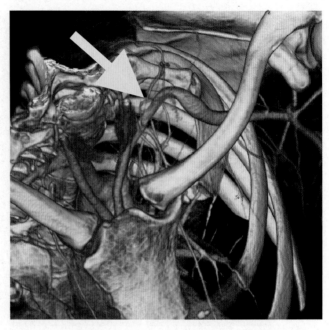

FIGURE 22-43 CTA was performed in a patient with left upper extremity claudication, fatigue, and parasthesias. Note the focal narrowing just proximal to the costoclavicular space (*arrow*). This corresponds to compression by the anterior scalene muscle. Findings are consistent with cervicoaxillary compression syndrome—thoracic outlet subtype.

triangle being the most common level. Fibrous bands, anomalous muscles, cervical ribs, or acquired bone derangements are potential causes. Traditionally, this disorder has been termed the thoracic outlet syndrome.

As the thoracic outlet is anatomically defined by the interscalene space, cervicoaxillary compression syndrome (CAS) has been proposed to more precisely characterize patients. Compression can then be categorized into thoracic outlet (Fig. 22-43), costoclavicular, and pectoralis minor subtypes (160).

Presenting symptoms will vary based on the level and degree of compression as well as the particular anatomic structures compressed in the area of the thoracic outlet (161). Clinically, patients can be divided into neurogenic, vascular, mixed (neurogenic and vascular), and nonspecific subtypes. Symptoms with neurogenic CAS include upper extremity muscle atrophy, sensory deficients, paresthesias, and less likely pain. Symptoms are most commonly caused by either neurologic or arterial impingement. Subclavian artery occlusion, stenosis, and aneurysm formation may occur with or without peripheral emboli.

Arterial CAS patients may experience claudication with fatigue, numbness, pallor, pulselessness, and coolness. Downstream embolization can occur both chronically and acutely. Venous CAS is distinguished by upper extremity heaviness, edema, skin discoloration, fatigability, heaviness, thrombosis, and venous collaterals (162).

Nonspecific CAS is the most common, but more challenging clinical presentation. Pain is more frequent, whereas neurologic and vascular symptoms are more variable (163).

Evaluation begins with provocative maneuvers during physical examination, typically hyperabduction with external rotation. Cervical radiographs are often obtained to exclude a cervical rib. Nerve conduction studies and electromyography are often obtained to investigate affected nerve and muscle territories. Provocative duplex sonography with or without digital plesmyography can efficiently screen the vasculature directly. CTA and MRI MRA provide the most in-depth evaluations. The imaging goals are to define the cervicoaxillary muscle, bone, and soft tissue anatomy, while dynamically assessing the arteries and veins in neutral and provocative positions.

Image Acquisition for Cervicoaxillary Compression Syndrome

With CTA, images are first acquired with the patient in a neutral position. The affected extremity is placed at the patient's side, while the contralateral upper arm is raised to minimize noise. Neutral images only need to be acquired through the shoulder. Upper extremity positions are then reversed with the affected arm now hyperextended, abducted above the patient's head. Imaging covers the entire inflow and outflow anatomy. Volume rendering technique provides a robust means to display the cervicoaxillary vasculature, collateral pathways, and nonvascular anatomy.

With MRI, high-resolution T1-weighted and T2-weighted fast spin echo images are obtained to delineate the anatomy and detect underlying causes of compression. TOF sagittal images are then acquired with the patient's arms alongside his or her body. Arms are repositioned with the affected arm in hyperabduction and external rotation.

A saturation band can be applied medial to the imaging slice when evaluating the subclavian vein or lateral to the imaging slice when evaluating the subclavian artery. This allows for MIP reconstruction of the vessel of interest without overlapping signal from the other vessel. Since no IV contrast is required, a potential advantage of TOF imaging is the possibility to repeat these acquisitions with different stress maneuvers without suffering from venous contamination. Among the limitations of TOF imaging are intraluminal filling defects related to turbulent or pulsatile flow, in-plane saturation effects, lengthy acquisitions, and need for multiple acquisitions for vessels with tortuous anatomy in which a single acquisition perpendicular to the vessel of interest is not feasible (Fig. 22-44). MIP reconstructions of

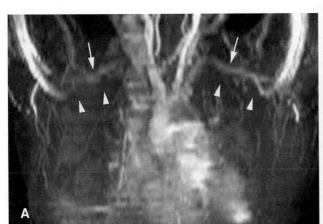
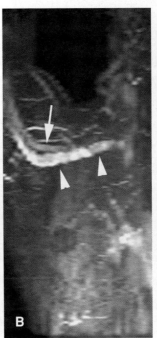
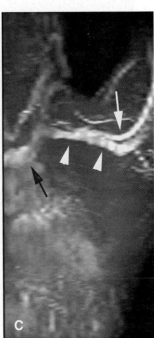
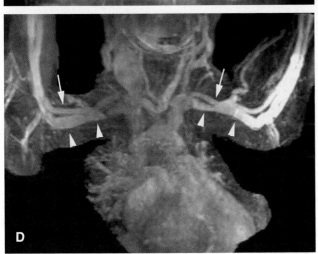

FIGURE 22-44 A: Coronal MIP reconstruction of a 2D TOF acquisition in the axial plane without a saturation band shows strong flow-related signal in the vertically oriented vessels (i.e., carotid, jugular, axillary, and brachial vessels). No flow is visualized in the region of the subclavian veins (*white arrowheads*). Based on this acquisition, differentiation between thrombosis and in-plane saturation is challenging. There is also decreased flow-related signal in the subclavian arteries (*white arrows*), which indicates the presence of in-plane saturation. Due to faster transit time of arterial blood through the imaging plane, the in-plane saturation effects are reduced compared with those of slow-flowing veins. **B, C:** Coronal MIP reconstructions from a sagittal 2D TOF acquisition of the right **(B)** and left **(C)** upper extremities. With the vessels now perpendicular to the imaging plane, there is strong flow-related signal in the subclavian veins (*white arrowheads*) and arteries (*white arrows*) bilaterally. Note that in this imaging plane, the portions of the veins with a more vertical orientation such as the distal left brachiocephalic vein (*black arrow*) and the axillary vein, show progressively lower signal due to in-plane saturation. **D:** Coronal MIP reconstruction from a gadolinium-enhanced 3D fat-saturated T1-weighted gradient-echo acquisition during the delayed venous phase shows normal enhancement of both subclavian veins (*white arrowheads*), which are widely patent. There is also normal enhancement of the subclavian arteries (*white arrows*).

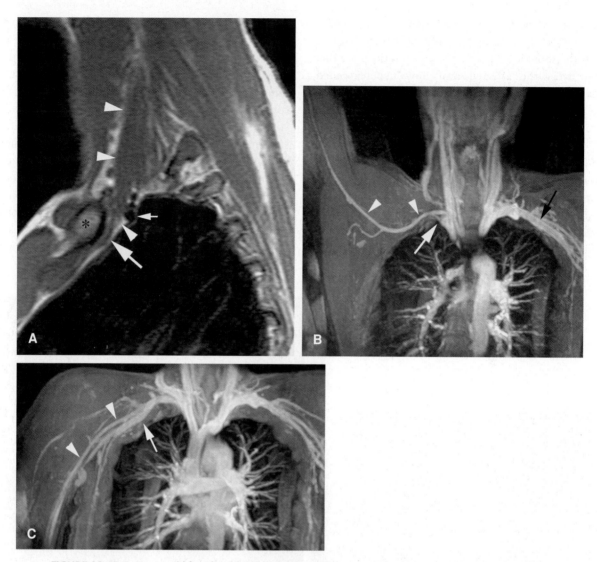

FIGURE 22-45 A 40-year-old female with right recurrent upper extremity edema. Patient had prior thrombosis of her right subclavian vein treated with fibrinolysis and angioplasty and then attempted rib dissection at a different
hospital. **A:** Right sagittal T1-weighted fast spin echo image shows a flat configuration of the right subclavian vein
(*large arrow*), which is compressed between the clavicle (∗) anteriorly and the anterior scalene muscle (*arrowheads*)
posteriorly. The subclavian artery (*small arrow*) is identified just above and slightly posterior to the vein. **B:** Coronal MIP
reconstruction of a 3D fat-saturated T1-weighted gradient-echo acquisition during the delayed venous phase performed with the right upper extremity in the abducted position shows lack of filling of the subclavian vein along its
entire course, with an abrupt cut-off (*white arrow*) at the level of the thoracic outlet. The left subclavian vein (*black
arrow*) and both internal jugular veins are widely patent. Note normal enhancement in the right subclavian artery
(*white arrowheads*). **C:** Coronal MIP reconstruction from a repeated acquisition with the same technique as **(B)** after a
second injection of gadolinium with both arms in neutral position shows normal venous patency bilaterally. The subclavian vein (*white arrow*) is clearly visible and symmetrical in appearance to the contralateral side. The right subclavian
artery (*white arrowheads*) is also normal in appearance. These findings confirm the presence of right subclavian vein
occlusion at the thoracic outlet only during abduction.

the TOF images of the subclavian vessels before and after
stress maneuvers provide an overview of the presence of
extrinsic compression of these vessels at the thoracic outlet.
Cardiac gating may help to reduce pulsatility artifacts.

A rapid determination of patency in the major veins of the
chest can be achieved with sparsely sampled TOF MR imaging. This is a useful initial evaluation preempting premature

termination of the study by the patient or when IV access is
compromised. In the thorax, the authors acquire three to five
TOF slices in a sagittal orientation, which allow for a rapid
assessment of brachiocephalic and subclavian vein patency.

A gadolinium-enhanced MRA MRV examination is also
feasible and is performed in neutral and challenged positions
(Fig. 22-45). Acquisitions during the arterial and delayed

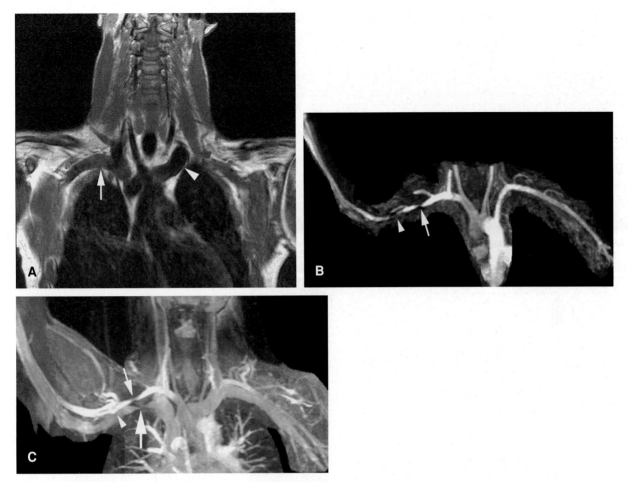

FIGURE 22-46 An 18-year-old male with coldness and numbness in his right hand when holding his arm over his head. A: Coronal T1-weighted fast spin echo image shows normal flow voids in the left brachiocephalic vein (*white arrowhead*) and right subclavian vein (*white arrow*). **B:** Coronal MIP reconstruction of a 3D fat-saturated T1-weighted gradient-echo acquisition during the arterial phase obtained with the right arm abducted shows two apparent areas of narrowing in the right subclavian artery. The patient's IV access was in the right antecubital fossa. Arterial phase images in the extremity that receives the gadolinium injection, as concentrated gadolinium in the adjacent vein. **C:** Coronal MIP reconstruction of the subsequent acquisition during the delay phase using the same sequence as in **(B)** shows resolution of the more distal stenosis (*white arrowhead*), which confirms its artifactual nature due to T2* effects of the flowing gadolinium in the adjacent vein. A persistent stenosis in the proximal right subclavian artery (*small white arrow*) and vein (*large white arrow*) are seen at the level of the thoracic outlet.

venous phases provide excellent delineation of the arterial and venous anatomy of the entire chest, and ideally, the volume coverage should extend to the hand. Compared to TOF imaging, this technique provides superior vessel coverage, is less prone to artifacts, and provides anatomic information from which the underlying cause for the thoracic outlet syndrome can be inferred (164). Gadolinium-enhanced MR imaging is well suited to demonstrate the presence of stenosis, obstruction, thrombosis, or aneurysm formation.

The presence of a focal stenosis in the subclavian artery during the first acquisition of the dynamic examination must be interpreted with caution as the injected concentrated gadolinium in the adjacent subclavian vein can cause arterial pseudostenosis/occlusion secondary to blooming

artifact due to T2* effects. In this situation, evaluation of the artery during the delayed venous phase typically reveals no abnormality in this vessel. Absence of abnormal findings in the subclavian vein and artery does not exclude this condition and imaging must be acquired during stress maneuvers (Fig. 22-46).

The use of blood pool agents facilitates a high quality arterial and venous study (Fig. 22-47), although the prolonged half-life of this class of agent can limit a pure angiographic rendering in both rest and abducted positions.

Focal narrowing along the course of the proximal upper vasculature, particularly at the point where the subclavian artery is adjacent to the anterior scalene muscle, is highly suggestive of the anatomy associated with CAS.

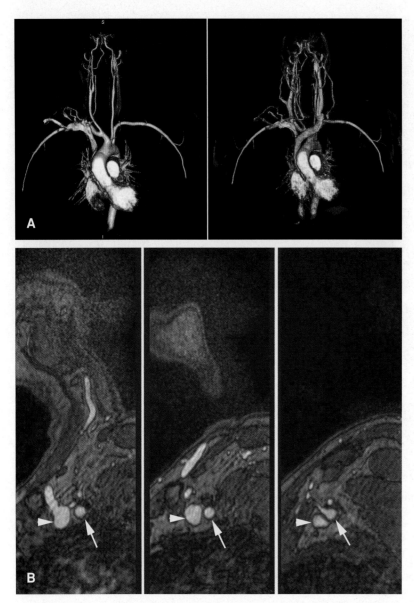

FIGURE 22-47 A 64-year-old patient with left upper extremity claudication and absence of radial pulse. The referring surgeon suspected thoracic outlet syndrome. Multiple-phase dynamic CE MRA during injection of 0.03 mmol/kg of the blood pool agent contrast medium Vasovist reveals normal left subclavian artery without evidence of damage **(A)**. Sagittal reconstructions of high spatial resolution (0.75 × 0.75 × 0.75 mm³) steady state acquisition **(B)** allows for evaluation of both the subclavian artery (*oblique arrows*) and vein (*arrowheads*). There is no evidence of aneurysmal widening or thrombus formation, thus refuting the diagnosis of thoracic outlet syndrome.

However, the appropriate clinical context is vital when interpreting CTA and MRA studies in patients suspected of thoracic outlet syndrome. Elevation of the upper extremity may falsely confer an impression of the disorder, since focal narrowing can be seen in asymptomatic individuals (Fig. 22-48).

Venous compression at the prescalene space is observed on MR imaging after postural maneuvers in 63% of patients with symptoms related to thoracic outlet compression versus 47% of healthy volunteers (162). In addition, an increased thickening of the subclavius muscle was noted in the symptomatic population (162).

Trauma

Vascular injuries of the upper extremity represent approximately 30% to 50% of all peripheral vascular injuries. The majority of injuries are to the brachial artery, and most injuries are due to penetrating trauma (165,166) (Fig. 22-49). Blunt injuries account for between 6% and 10% of upper extremity vascular trauma and are often associated with musculoskeletal injuries and neural injuries (167). The functional impact of the traumatic event is often related to concomitant injury to peripheral nerves. However, timely restoration of blood flow is essential to optimize outcome.

Physical examination and limited Doppler ultrasonography are the mainstays of diagnosis (168,169). Arteriography is generally reserved when multiple sites of injury are known or suspected or if any question remains after physical examination and noninvasive studies (168). More recently, CTA in patients with traumatic extremity injuries

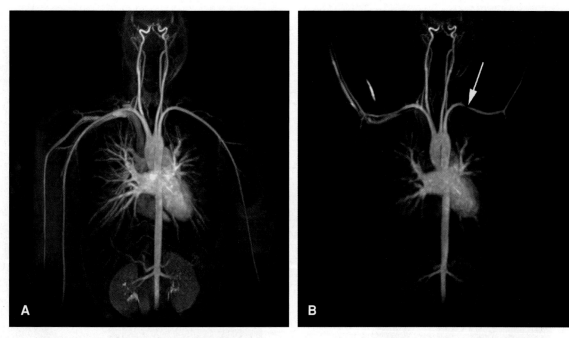

FIGURE 22-48 Physiological subclavian artery narrowing in an asymptomatic individual. **A:** When the arms are placed next to the torso, the artery is completely normal in appearance. **B:** When elevating the arms in the abducted position, there is subtle, focal narrowing of the subclavian artery (*arrow* in **B**). The clinical context is critical since this phenomenon can be seen when the arms are elevated in normal individuals.

is an alternative to conventional angiography (170,171). MRA may also be used for this assessment (172), but availability and concerns for metallic orthopedic hardware limits widespread utilization in evaluating trauma patients.

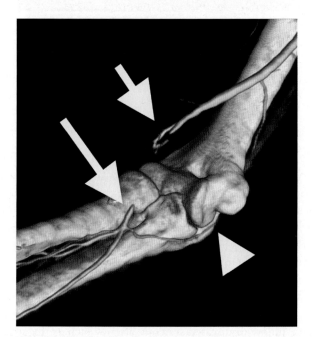

FIGURE 22-49 A penetrating laceration to the right forearm was investigated with 8-channel CTA. The distal brachial (*short arrow*) and proximal radial (*long arrow*) arteries are occluded. Reconstitution primarily occurs via the ulnar collateral network (*arrowhead*).

Anticoagulation with heparin should be given if not otherwise contraindicated. Revascularization should be completed within the critical ischemic time: 4 hours for proximal injuries and 12 hours for distal injuries. Surgical revascularization methods include resection and primary repair or resection with an interposition graft. Various endovascular techniques, including the placement of embolization coils, intravascular stents, and the use of stented grafts, have been used in the setting of traumatic upper extremity injuries (173,174). The sequence of repair of multiple injuries to the extremity usually begins with arterial revascularization followed by skeletal stabilization and nerve and tendon repair.

Venous injuries to the arm rarely require repair. Injuries to more central veins such as the brachial and axillary veins may be treated with ligation since the extensive collateral venous network typically provides sufficient venous return.

Orthopedic Injuries

Vascular injuries may accompany skeletal fractures, with a reported incidence of these combined injuries between 0.3% and 6.4% (175–177) (Fig. 22-50). Vascular repair generally precedes the orthopedic fixation, since the ischemic component typically dominates the clinical outcome. The associations between orthopedic injuries and arterial injuries are as follows: supracondylar fracture of the humerus—brachial artery; clavicular/first rib fracture—

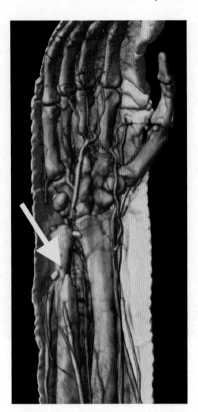

FIGURE 22-50 Physical exam on a patient who sustained blunt trauma to the distal forearm was remarkable for an absent palpable ulnar artery. CTA revealed an occluded ulnar artery at the level of a distal ulnar fracture (*arrow*). The radial artery supplied inflow to the hand, with retrograde flow across the deep arch to reconstitute the ulnar artery near the hamate hook.

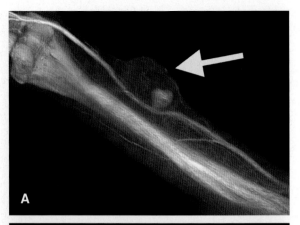

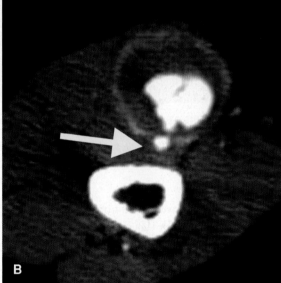

FIGURE 22-51 Two days after attempting to place arterial line catheter, 8-channnel CTA was obtained to investigate a pulsatile mass. VR (**A**) and axial source (**B**) images demonstrate a focal distal brachial pseudoaneurysm with a focal neck (*arrow* in **B**).

subclavian artery; shoulder dislocation—axillary artery; and elbow dislocation—brachial artery.

Intra-arterial Injections

Inadvertent intra-arterial injections of medications not intended for intra-arterial use and unintended arterial injections of illicit drugs can cause acute arterial occlusion, distal thromboembolism, mycotic aneurysm, and chronic ischemia. The causative agent may induce an intense inflammatory response with endothelial injury and possibly thrombosis. Brachial artery injuries and mycotic aneurysms are common, and surgical ligation is a common treatment option for the latter.

Catheterizations

Iatrogenic injuries to the upper extremity vasculature are not common and may follow arterial or venous punctures. Arterial complications include dissection, aneurysm, pseudoaneurysm and arterial-venous fistulae (178–180) (Fig. 22-51). The increased use of radial artery catheterizations seems to have rare complications with a recent report citing only three major vascular complications of 500 cases (181).

Postoperative Assessments

Surgical revascularization is relatively uncommon for the upper extremity. Proximal disease, particularly when associated with the subclavian steal syndrome, may be approached with endovascular therapy, a carotid-subclavian bypass, or an axillary-axillary bypass. From the surgical perspective, axillary-axillary bypass is not often used because it requires a long segment of prosthetic graft material to be passed underneath the skin overlying the sternum and it offers no real advantage over carotid-subclavian bypass.

The subclavian artery is a common conduit to provide inflow to diseased systemic arteries such as the aorta (Figs. 22-52, 22-53). Subclavian-carotid artery bypass is performed for symptomatic common carotid artery occlusive disease when the external or internal carotid artery is a

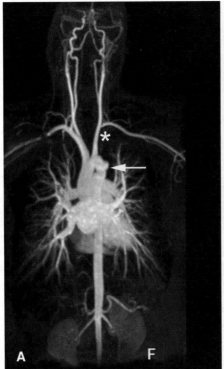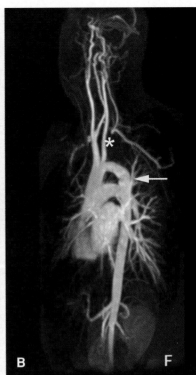

FIGURE 22-52 Routine postoperative follow-up examination of a 20-year-old patient having undergone surgical repair for aortic coarctation. The patient did not report any symptoms. Coronal **(A)** and left anterior oblique **(B)** whole-volume MIPs show luminal irregularities in the proximal descending aorta at the site of surgical repair (*arrows*). The proximal left subclavian artery (∗) has been sacrificed to patch the aorta (subclavian flap angioplasty).

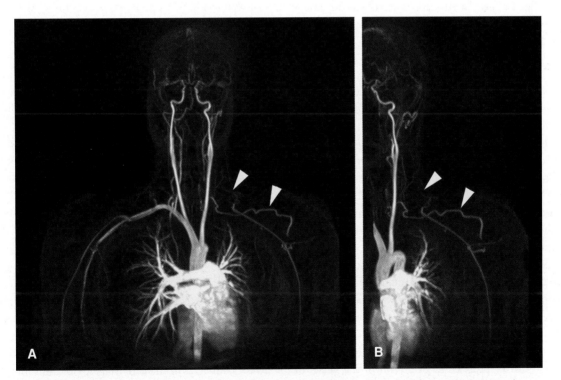

FIGURE 22-53 A 17-year-old female patient who complained of weakness in the left arm. The patient underwent surgical repair for an aortic coarctation at the age of 7 years. High-resolution MRA shows missing left subclavian artery **(A)** because it was used in a subclavian patch angioplasty procedure to repair the coarctation. Collateral branches arising from the costocervical trunk (*medial arrowhead*) and the thyrocervical trunk (*lateral arrowhead*) reconstitute the axillary artery. A left anterior oblique view **(B)** better shows the origin of the collaterals.

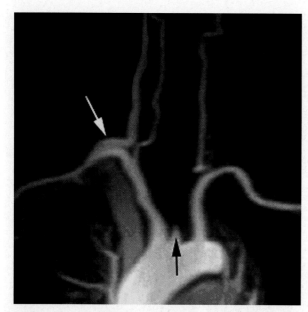

FIGURE 22-54 Subclavian-carotid bypass graft. This MIP image demonstrates a right subclavian-carotid bypass graft (*white arrow*) to restore adequate cerebral blood flow in a 44-year-old woman with Takayasu arteritis and bilateral common carotid artery occlusions. Note the proximal occlusion of the left common carotid artery (*black arrow*).

suitable outflow vessel and the ipsilateral subclavian artery is normal (Fig. 22-54). In addition, the subclavian artery can serve as a conduit to direct blood to the lungs in cyanotic heart disease (Fig. 22-55).

Radiation Arteritis

Arterial occlusive disease and neuromuscular disorders are uncommon delayed complications of local radiation therapy for underlying malignancies (182). Radiation-induced brachial plexopathy, the most common iatrogenic neuromuscular complication after treatment of breast cancer, may be difficult to distinguish from plexopathy due to recurrent neoplasm. Vascular injury due to radiation is a rare sequela of radiation therapy, in general, and subclavian or axillary arteriopathy is also an uncommon sequela of radiation therapy to the axilla (183).

The disorder shows histologic changes that include fibrosis of the internal elastic membrane, injury to the vasa vasorum and ischemic necrosis of the vessel wall, periarterial fibrosis, and hyalinization and thickening of the vessel wall with fibrin deposition (184,185). Such changes may lead to a reduction in vessel diameter due to vessel wall thickening and may progress to occlusion of the vessel or predispose to thrombus formation, ulceration, and distal embolization.

The onset of symptoms ranges from 1 to 42 years after radiation therapy and often follows a latency period of more than 10 years (185). These symptoms most commonly include skin changes and reduced mobility of the arm. With arterial damage, symptoms include pain, claudication, or numbness, and these may be accompanied by ischemic signs such as peripheral cyanosis or ulceration.

The angiographic appearance of radiation-induced subclavian or axillary arteriopathy may mimic primary atherosclerotic disease with focal occlusion or stenosis with or without ulceration (Fig. 22-56). The areas most commonly affected are the mid to distal subclavian artery or the subclavian-axillary junction. Radiation-induced arteriopathy may appear as a vasculits. Little published data exist regarding the CT and MR appearances of radiation-induced arteriopathy. In one study focusing on MR of the cerebral vasculature, wall thickening and prominent ring enhancement of the wall were seen in large cerebral arteries (186). Based on study patients with radiation treatment to the head and neck with MR, Becker at al. showed that radiation arteriopathy may manifest as occlusion, subocclusive sclerotic or atheromatous plaque, localized mural thrombus, aneurysm, or, rarely, spontaneous rupture (187).

Radiation arteritis should be distinguished from other vascular diseases, such as large-vessel vasculitis characterized by long, tapered smooth stenosis, and from thoracic outlet syndrome due to external compression of the subclavian artery.

OCCUPATIONAL AND ENVIRONMENTAL CONDITIONS

Occupational vascular disorders account for substantial morbidity and medical costs and include injuries caused by work accidents and those caused by cumulative trauma due to vibration, the performance of repetitive motions (Fig. 22-57), exposure to polyvinylchloride, electrical burns, and athletic injuries.

This section will focus on the latter four categories of disorders. Gross vascular trauma is covered in the preceding section.

Vibration-induced White Finger

Vibration-induced white finger (VWF) is a hand-arm vibration syndrome that occurs in up to 50% of workers who use handheld vibration tools such as pneumatic tools, hammers, chain saws, and grinders, operating at a frequency of 20 to 1,000 Hz. In the early stages, vibration injury may be manifested as numbness and tingling in one or more exposed fingers.

Later, a Raynaud-like phenomenon is seen with blanching of the fingertips on exposure to cold, followed by

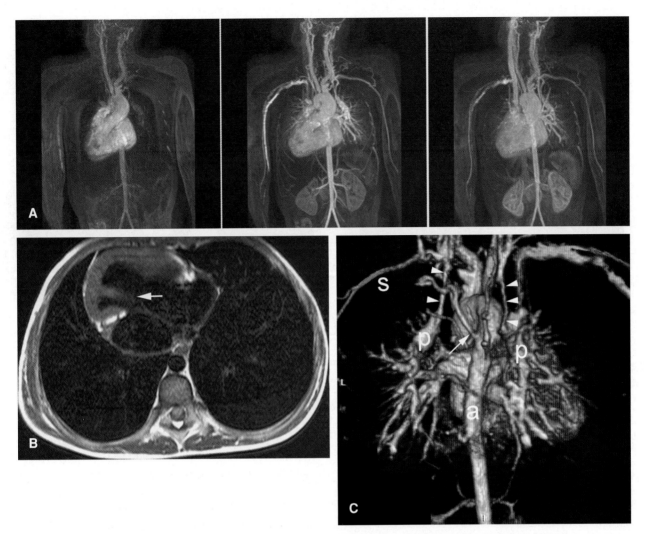

FIGURE 22-55 An 8-year-old patient with double-inlet left ventricle, rudimentary right ventricle, severely hypoplastic right atrioventricular valve, atrial septal defect, and atresia of the pulmonary trunk and bifurcation and dextrocardia. The patient had undergone a Raskind atrioseptostomia and had received bilateral modified Blalock-Taussig (BT) shunts as a neonate. The patient complained of shortness of breath and underwent CE MRA to determine the status of the BT shunts. Multiphase dynamic CE MRA (**A**) clearly demonstrates the dextrocardia and a stenosis at the origin of the brachiocephalic trunk (**A**). Note the delayed opacification of the pulmonary circulation, which is seen only after opacification of the systemic circulation. ECG-triggered black blood T1-weighted MRI demonstrates the rudimentary right ventricle and the large ventricular septal defect (*arrow* in **B**). VR in the posteroanterior projection (**C**) clearly shows the diffusely narrowed BT shunts (*arrowheads*). Note major aortopulmonary collateral (*arrow*). (s, subclavian artery; p, pulmonary artery; a, descending aorta.)

reactive hyperemia. Episodes may last up to 1 hour. Continued exposure to vibration may induce cyanosis in the affected fingers. Tissue loss, however, is rare, with only about 1% of the cases progressing to ulceration and gangrene (188).

The exact mechanism of injury is unknown, but vibration-induced local platelet adhesion at sites of intimal damage and impaired vasodilatation due to peripheral nerve damage are thought to play important roles (189). The diagnosis is made from the history of using vibrating tools

and from the Raynaud's symptoms. Symptoms of peripheral ischemia may be accompanied by other vegetative symptoms such as hearing loss, reduced heart rate variation, and shorter systolic time intervals (190). The first-line investigation to detect digital artery occlusion is systolic pressure measurements of the affected fingers with transcutaneous Doppler ultrasound, followed by MRA and/or CTA. In advanced disease, conventional x-ray arteriography is considered because of the superior capabilities to depict small hand vessels.

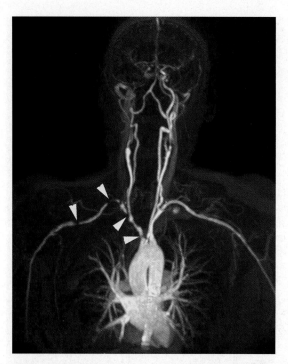

FIGURE 22-56 Radiation-induced arteritis in a 64-year-old female patient who had undergone amputation of the right breast for breast cancer with subsequent radiotherapy two decades earlier. The patient consulted a neurologist because of 12 transient episodes of blurry vision and one episode of ataxia over the past 3 months as well as right upper extremity weakness. Whole-volume MIP reveals multiple high-grade lesions in the brachiocephalic trunk and right subclavian artery (*arrowheads*) as well as high-grade stenoses in the right common and internal carotid arteries, and the left internal carotid artery (*arrows*). There was a subclavian steal phenomenon in the right vertebral artery (not shown).

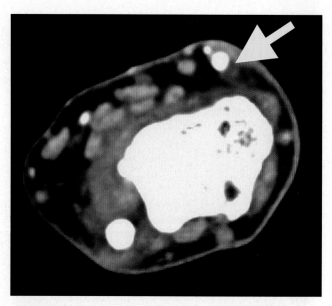

FIGURE 22-57 A right upper extremity CT angiogram was performed in a patient who felt a focal pulsatile mass near the radio-carpal articulation. The patient was a carpenter and regularly placed direct forces on this region. Cross-sectional imaging reveals a focal thrombosed radial pseudoaneurysm (*arrow*).

Typical arteriographic findings include multiple segmental occlusions sometimes bridged by corkscrew collaterals. In severe cases, entire digital arteries can be occluded, often accompanied by an incomplete palmar arch. Therapy consists of calcium antagonists and discontinuation of use of vibrating tools.

Hypothenar Hammer (Hand) Syndrome

Finger ischemia caused by embolic occlusion of digital arteries originating from the palmar ulnar artery in a person repetitively striking objects with the heel of the hand, causing trauma to the hypothenar eminence, has been termed hypothenar hammer syndrome (HHS). Other names for this disorder include hypothenar hand syndrome, post-traumatic digital ischemia, and pneumatic tool disease. Injury to the distal ulnar artery at the level of the hamate bone is characteristic with digital ischemia typically sparing the thumb (Fig. 22-58).

The ulnar artery appears to be most vulnerable in the distal portion of Guyon's canal, which is bounded medially by the pisiform and the hook of the hamate and dorsally by the transverse carpal ligament; in this area, the protective capabilities of palmaris brevis muscle are least effective. The type of arterial abnormality often depends on the nature of the damage to the vessel. Intimal damage favors thrombotic occlusion, whereas injury to the media favors palmar aneurysms (191,192) (Fig. 22-59). Indeed, thrombosis and aneurysm are common features seen angiographically with HHS (193).

Diverse occupations or avocations, such as carpenter, mechanic, mountain biker, and stapler in which the palm is exposed to repetitive trauma, presumably lead to ulnar artery injury and HHS. Degeneration or thrombosis of the palmar ulnar artery is believed to be a consequence of the repetitive trauma. Symptomatic finger ischemia can result from embolization to digital arteries from the abnormal palmar ulnar artery segment.

However, it is worthy of noting that while repetitive occupational hand trauma is common, HHS is an infrequent condition. It is possible that a large cohort of people with ulnar artery pathology exists in an asymptomatic form and thus escapes medical attention. Another explanation is that predisposing factors give rise to HHS (194) prompting recent investigations to assess such potential predisposing factors (194,195).

Ferris et al. found a noteworthy incidence of bilateral palmar ulnar artery disease with segmental occlusion, or a

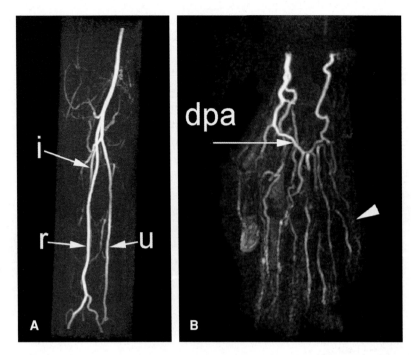

FIGURE 22-58 A 37-year-old construction worker suspected of having hypothenar hammer syndrome. CE MRA of the forearm **(A)** reveals normal radial (*r*), ulnar (*u*), and interosseous artery (*i*). Dedicated imaging of the hand **(B)** reveals an occluded superficial palmar arch but patent deep palmar arch (*dpa*). There is scarce vascular supply to the fourth and fifth fingers (*arrowhead*). These findings are typical of the hypothenar hammer syndrome.

typical corkscrew appearance and variable areas of ectasia. In that study, the corkscrew angiographic pattern, characteristic of fibromuscular dysplasia (FMD), was supported by histologic results of resected segments. Thus, evidence suggests that preexisting FMD of the palmar ulnar artery in these patients makes the artery more prone to form

intraluminal thrombus from repetitive striking of the palm (195).

Patients often present clinically with Raynaud's phenomenon (numbness, paresthesias, coldness, and blanching of more digits) of the dominant hand (196).

Angiographic assessment is useful for defining the type of lesion—spasm, aneurysm, or occlusion—and predisposing features such as the aforementioned corkscrew appearance suggesting FMD. Relatively few reports of diagnosis with CT and MRA exist (37,197,198).

Treatment is often supportive, with surgical intervention reserved for occluded palmar ulnar arteries in the presence of significant ischemic symptoms.

Surgical intervention consists of excision of the abnormal palmar ulnar artery segment and interposition grafting. Such grafting may harvest a forearm vein, the distal saphenous vein, or an epigastric artery. Surgery may be indicated for patent ulnar arteries with typical elongation and corkscrew deformity, with or without symptoms of finger ischemia, to eliminate onset or recurrence of digital artery embolism, although this is not universally accepted (195).

Acro-osteolysis

Acro-osteolysis (AO) is a clinical syndrome resulting from occupational exposure to vinyl chloride. The syndrome has three main components: (a) Raynaud's phenomenon of the fingers and sometimes the toes, (b) skin changes resembling scleroderma on the back of the hands or distal third of the flexor side of the forearm, and (c) evidence of bone resorption

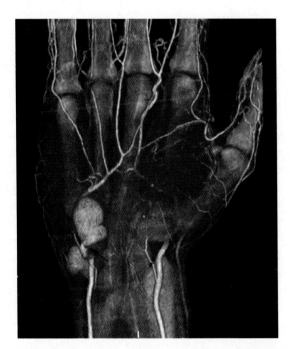

FIGURE 22-59 Hypothenar hammer syndrome. CTA depicts a distal ulnar artery aneurysm arising at the junction with the palmar arch. (Courtesy of Dr. Ruben Sebben, Dr. Jones, and Partners Medical Imaging, Adelaide, Australia.)

in the terminal phalanges of the fingers, radial and ulnar styloid processes, sacroiliac joints, and lower poles of the patellas.

Bone resorption is detected by the presence of band-like translucencies. In advanced cases, complete destruction of the tuft of the phalanx and partial or complete occlusion of the digital arteries may occur. Patients exposed to vinyl choride are also at increased risk of developing angiosarcoma of the liver, often decades after start of exposure. Of note, vinyl chloride particles have been detected in livers of patients undergoing hemodialysis and are thought to be due to microscopic fragments of dialysis tubing within blood pumps necessary for hemodialysis (199).

The angiographic findings in AO include multiple arterial stenoses and occlusions of the digital arteries with non-specific hypervascularity adjacent to the areas of bony resorption (200). The reason for the hypervascularity is not clear but may be due to stasis of contrast medium in digital pulp arteries secondary to shortening and retraction of the fingers (188).

Electrical Injuries

Almost any part of the body can be injured by electrical current. The extent of injury to any given tissue depends on many factors, including tissue type and the amount and duration of the electrical current. After nerve tissue, blood vessels are most susceptible to electrical injury (201). Currents of less than 1,000 V cause injuries limited to the immediate underlying skin and soft tissues. High voltage (>1,000 V) usually causes extensive damage (188).

Because of its grasping function, the hand and arm are often involved. In addition, cardiac and respiratory arrest can be induced, even without intermediate tissue damage.

It is extremely important to realize that high voltage injuries—especially lightning strikes—may cause vasospasm so severe that the entire extremity can appear cyanotic, cold, and pulseless. However, this may resolve spontaneously and completely within hours (202). Therefore, early amputation should never be performed.

Long-term vascular injuries include extensive occlusion of the forearm and digital arteries. In addition, damage to the arterial media may lead to aneurysm formation weeks to months after injury. In a study of 28 patients with electrical injuries, 8 arteriograms were normal; 6 arteriograms showed changes to the small arteries; and in 38 extremities, the main arteries were injured. In the latter group, there were 24 total occlusions, narrow and irregular lumens in 10 cases, and occlusions with distal refilling in 4 cases. Changes in the main arteries were most often seen near major joints where the internal body resistance and the density of current are higher (203).

Thermal Vascular Injury

Burns

Serial examination of burn wounds can be very useful, since the depth of injury is often underestimated on initial examination. Furthermore, devitalized tissue may appear viable for some time after injury, and often, some degree of progressive microvascular thrombosis around the periphery of wounds is seen. Consequently, the wound appearance changes over the days following injury. Angiography is often not necessary to establish the site and extent of vascular injury. In individual cases, it can be desirable to visualize arterial involvement—for instance, in cases of eschars exerting traction on underlying viable tissues.

Frostbite

Frostbite represents a spectrum of injury ranging from irreversible cellular destruction to reversible changes seen after rewarming. These changes include increases in tissue edema, circulatory stasis, and progressive thrombosis leading to further tissue necrosis. As is the case with burn injury, it can be desirable to visualize arterial involvement in cases of eschars exerting traction on underlying viable tissues. Escharotomy is a commonly performed procedure in cases of vascular compromise.

Athletic Vascular Injury

Arterial insufficiency is often low on the list of differential diagnoses when assessing young athletes, and is often missed or delayed for this reason. Arterial pathology often masquerades as neuromuscular injury, yet it is firmly established that (professional) athletes who engage in strenuous physical activity may develop upper extremity ischemia due to arterial injury (204).

Arterial injury in athletes may present with symptoms of acute arterial or venous occlusion due to thrombosis or embolus, or sometimes even with arterial rupture. Injury to distal arteries is often manifested by Raynaud's phenomenon.

Athletes who engage in overextended shoulder motion such as baseball pitchers, volleyball players, butterfly swimmers, weightlifters, and oarsmen can present with symptoms of thoracic outlet compression. The specific vascular changes associated with thoracic outlet compression are discussed in more detail in the previous section on Cervicoaxillary Compression (Thoracic Outlet) Syndrome.

Effort thrombosis (Paget-von Schrötter syndrome) is a condition that deserves mention in this context. Effort thrombosis describes spontaneous thrombosis of the upper extremity after repetitive motion/exercise, usually in the dominant upper extremity (81,205). This entity is most common in young males and is associated with pulmonary embolism in up to 30% of cases (206). There is an anatomic predisposition in 75% of the cases, including cervical ribs, exostoses, fibrous bands, and muscular hypertrophy (anterior scalene/subclavius muscles) (81). MRI allows for the diagnosis of venous thrombosis and identification of the associated anatomic predisposition (207).

Injuries to the distal forearm and digital arteries may result in HHS, and this is typically seen in baseball catchers, volleyball and handball players, practitioners of karate, mountain bikers and touring cyclists, cricketers, and Frisbee players. The athlete may complain of Raynaud-like symptoms, hypothenar pain, and a tender palpable mass, which may be present in cases of aneurysm formation. In severe cases, patients may present with rest pain and finger ulceration (113,188,208).

The first-line diagnostic investigations consist of Allen's test and Doppler flow studies of the digital arteries. Angiographic findings include nonspecific palmar arch and digital artery occlusion.

Surgical repair of arterial occlusion is rarely indicated in nonacute cases, but if there is an aneurysm, it should be excised (208).

DIALYSIS ACCESS FISTULAS

ESRD, a permanent and often nonreversible decline in renal function, is an increasingly important medical problem, ultimately requiring hemodialysis in the vast majority of patients. The incidence and prevalence of ERSD as well as the number of patients requiring hemodialysis have sharply risen over the past few years. In 2004, an estimated 1.22 million patients were on hemodialysis worldwide, representing a 20% increase over 2001 (209–211).

A well functioning vascular access is the cornerstone of hemodialysis treatment in ESRD patients and can be achieved by either insertion of a central venous catheter or by surgical creation of an AVF or graft.

The fistula is created by the anastomoses of antecubital veins with either brachial or radial arteries. Alternatively, a graft can be constructed that connects an artery to a vein (Fig. 22-60).

The access of first choice is the autogenous AVF because it has better long-term performance and patency rates when compared to arteriovenous grafts (AVG) and central venous catheters (CVC). Furthermore, AVFs have

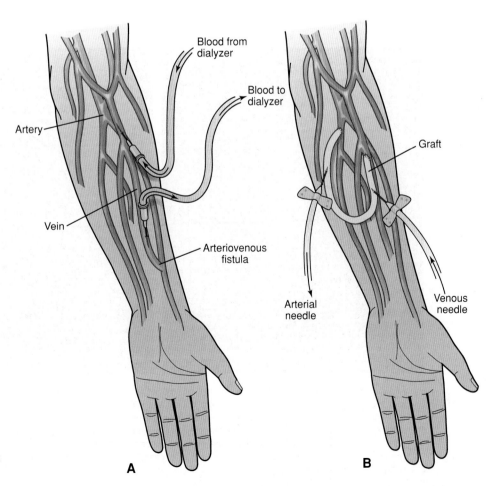

FIGURE 22-60 Schematic diagrams of arteriovenous dialysis access. A: The AVF results from the anastomosis of the patient's own veins and arteries. **B:** Connection of a forearm artery with a vein can be facilitated by a prosthetic graft.

Blood from dialyzer

Blood to dialyzer

Artery

Vein

Arteriovenous fistula

Graft

Arterial needle

Venous needle

A

B

lower vascular access-related morbidity, mortality, and health care costs compared with AVG and CVC (199–214). In contrast, prosthetic vascular grafts require about five times more therapeutic interventions compared with AVF to keep the access functioning (37,212–214).

To avoid vascular access–related complications as much as possible, the Dialysis Outcome Quality Initiative (K-DOQI) and Good Nephrological Practice guidelines advocate an all AVF policy, that is, at least 70% of all newly created accesses should consist of autogenous AVF (215,216). However, the major drawback of AVF creation is the relatively high frequency of early thrombosis—up to 10% of all newly created AVFs thrombose within the first week after creation—and nonmaturation.

Nonmaturation is defined as an AVF being inadequate for hemodialysis due to insufficient flow-volume or insufficient venous distension. The most important causes of nonmaturation are thought to be flow-limiting stenoses in the arteries proximal to the arteriovenous anastomosis and poor venous outflow due to small caliber vessels or preexisting stenoses or occlusions (Fig. 22-61) (217–221).

Furthermore, the presence of large-caliber side branches may also jeopardize AVF maturation due to a dis-

advantageous flow distribution (222,223). Different studies have reported AVF nonmaturation rates within the first months after creation from 5% up to 54% (220,224–230) (Fig. 22-62).

To increase the number of mature and functional AVFs, adequate history taking, physical examination, and preoperative assessment of upper extremity vessels are an absolute necessity (215,216,225).

Increasingly, arterial and venous diameters as well as the presence and location of preexisting atherosclerotic occlusive disease and venous stenoses, occlusions, and side branches are used to guide the choice of fistula type and location. Consequently, interest has risen in preoperative imaging of upper extremity vessels. The goal of preoperative imaging is assessment of vessel caliber and identification of sites where arteries and veins are of suboptimal quality for access purposes.

Imaging Prior to Dialysis Access Fistulae Creation

Both CTA and MRA can be used to assess the arterial and venous structures relevant to the creation of access fistulae. Concerns regarding the use of contrast media punctuate the dialog when considering alternatives.

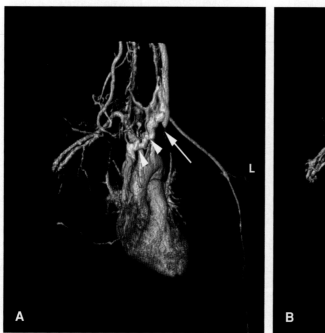
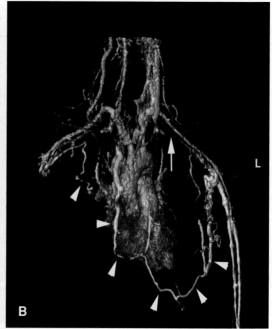

FIGURE 22-61 Color VRs of central veins in a 66-year-old patient with terminal renal failure awaiting dialysis access fistula creation. The patient had a history of multiple jugular venous catheters on both sides. The examination was performed to assess central venous patency. Early venous phase imaging **(A)** reveals multiple irregularities in the brachiocephalic vein (*arrowheads*) and tapering of the distal left internal jugular vein (*arrow*). The late venous phase **(B)** shows an occluded left subclavian vein (*arrow*) bridged by an extensive collateral venous network in the chest wall functioning as the primary conduit for return of venous blood coming from the left upper extremity to the superior vena cava (*arrowheads*).

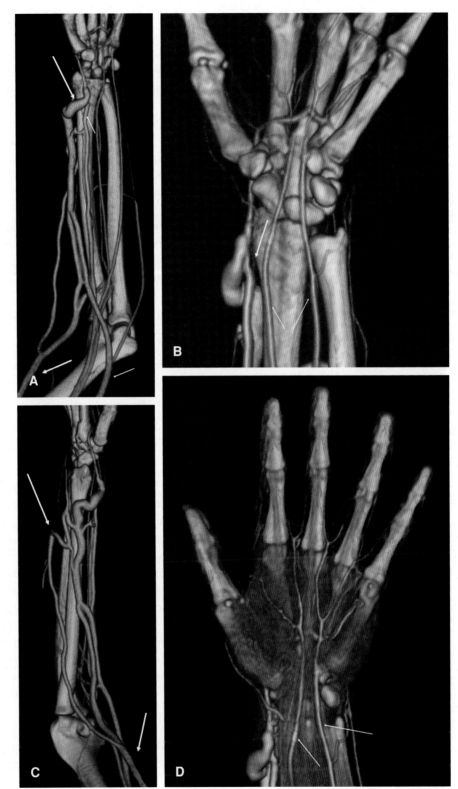

FIGURE 22-62 64-channel MD CTA was performed to evaluate a left upper extremity Brescia-Cimino fistula **(A)**. The fistula was created 6 months prior. However, it did not completely mature. As this case demonstrates, lack of hemodialysis maturation can result from arterial inflow stenosis and competing collateral outflow veins. Part **(A)** shows the radial artery (*narrow short arrow*) to cephalic vein (*wide long arrow*) anastomosis overlying the distal radius. Outflow drainage in the upper arm is through both cephalic (*wide short arrow*) and basilic (*narrow long arrow*) veins. Interrogation of the anastomosis reveals moderate inflow stenosis (*wide arrow* in **B**). Part **(C)** demonstrates that a portion of the immediate outflow drains away from the forearm cephalic vein and into a competing venous network (*long arrow*). The network ultimately drains into the more central cephalic vein system (*short arrow*). As noted in parts **(B)** and **(D)**, the fistula is likely high flow, resulting in degree of "steal phenomenon." The princeps pollicus and radialis indices are poorly opacified. The volar interosseous artery (*short arrow*) is enlarged and along with the ulnar artery (*long arrow*), provides the dominant supply to the palm and digits.

Prior to the CE era, non-CE TOF MR venography of the upper extremity already showed better correlation with surgical findings (kappa 0.78) compared with conventional x-ray venography (kappa 0.56) in patients undergoing preoperative evaluation (231). However, TOF MRA is prone to artifacts, and stenoses can be overestimated (49).

CE MRA protocols enable image acquisition with higher spatial (submillimeter voxel-size) and temporal resolutions (<20 seconds per dynamic scan) with good to excellent image quality (70,232). In CE MRA, arterial and venous images are acquired in the coronal or sagittal plane during injection of contrast media. For arterial imaging, 0.2 to 0.3 mmol/kg 0.5 M extracellular gadolinium chelate contrast medium has been injected in a contralateral antecubital or dorsal hand vein. For venous imaging, diluted (1:15) contrast media is injected in an ipsilateral dorsal hand vein.

At the time of this writing, new concerns regarding the safety of Gd-enhanced MRA in patients with ESRD (see the end of this section) may result in a revival of noncontrast techniques for this and other applications.

Because intrathoracic vessels are prone to movement during respiration, patients should hold their breath for about 15 to 20 seconds, depending on the temporal and spatial resolutions and other technical factors related to system performance. Contrast medium is injected at speeds up to 3.0 mL/second, followed by 25 mL of saline flush.

Spatial resolution in recent reports is typically in the order of $1.0 \times 1.0 \times 1.2$ mm^3 (craniocaudal/frequency direction $\times$ left-right/phase-encoding directions $\times$ anteroposterior/slice direction). Using this approach for imaging, upper extremity arteries and veins can be visualized with high accuracy (232). However, because the average upper extremity length of an adult is about 70 to 80 cm, depicting the entire upper extremity requires imaging of at least two FOV because of the limited MR-bore length.

The use of 1- to 2-mL test dose of contrast medium prior to the CE acquisition, or the use of real time bolus monitoring software, facilitates a selective demonstration of the arterial segments.

Arterial Assessment

In addition to careful attention to timing of the acquisition with respect to the contrast media injection, as stated in the technical section of this chapter, Wentz et al. (70) reported good results using CE MRA for imaging digital arteries with timed arterial compression. With that approach to stop arterial flow, longer scan times of a smaller FOV facilitate increased spatial resolution without venous enhancement. Planken et al. reported a multiphasic approach using multiple dynamic scans that resulted in

good to excellent subjective image quality images (232,233).

Venous Assessment

Reported CE MR venography techniques use either direct injection of diluted contrast media (1:15 to 1:25 mL of gadolinium chelate in saline solution) in the ipsilateral extremity during image acquisition or contralateral IV injection of nondiluted contrast media, and acquisition during delayed venous enhancement after initial arterial first pass (234–237). Both techniques have their strengths and weaknesses.

Direct venography yields better vessel opacification with lower contrast dose as compared with the contralateral injection approach. However, direct injection without use of a proximal cuff may lead to selective enhancement of veins.

This is in contradistinction to the contralateral injection or indirect approach that will result in opacification of all veins, albeit with lower vessel to background contrast. On the other hand, timing considerations are more challenging with the contralateral injection approach.

To increase vessel-to-background contrast, subtraction techniques can be applied, although misregistration artifacts, particularly in central venous imaging, may result (235,238–240). Furthermore, there is a risk for early enhancement of central veins in the first pass (i.e., SVC), and in that circumstance, subtraction may obscure the demonstration of these vessels.

CE MR venography using delayed venous enhancement techniques showed poor performance for detection of central venous stenosis and occlusions (sensitivity and specificity 50% and 80%, respectively) (241,242). Shankar et al. (243) have demonstrated that noncontrast MR venography, is more accurate for assessment of central venous patency prior to central venous catheter insertion compared with duplex ultrasonography with a sensitivity and specificity of 71% and 89% for detection of central venous stenosis and occlusions (243).

For venous mapping prior to surgery, direct CE MR venography offers a low-dose option; it is easy to perform, well tolerated, and highly accurate for detection of venous stenosis and obstructions in the upper extremity and central veins (Figs. 22-63 and 22-64) (234–237,244,245). Furthermore, direct CE MR venography diameter measurements are more accurate compared with duplex ultrasonography when using surgical measurements as a standard of reference (246).

Only sparse data exist regarding the clinical value of preoperative cross-sectional imaging. Future studies using up-to-date equipment and scan protocols should better determine its clinical impact.

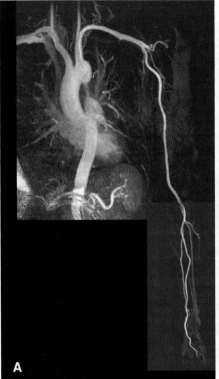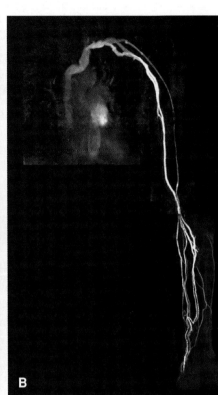

FIGURE 22-63 Composite MIPs of combined arteriography **(A)** and direct venography **(B)** in a patient awaiting dialysis access construction. The arteriogram was obtained by injection of contast medium in the contralateral antecubital vein. Distal arteries were depicted in the first acquisition using 15 mL gadolinium-DTPA. A second injection of 15 mL was used to depict the proximal arterial tree. Proximal and distal veins were depicted by direct injection of 50 and 50 mL 1/15 diluted gadolinium-DTPA in a hand vein. To avoid selective opacification of draining veins, an MR-compatible blood pressure cuff was placed above the elbow and inflated to 60 mmHg.

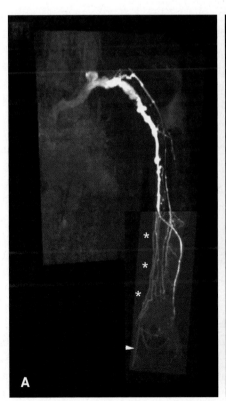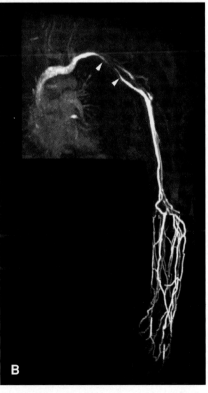

FIGURE 22-64 Two-station composite MIPs of direct venograms of the left upper extremity in two different patients awaiting dialysis access construction. In **(A)**, an example is shown of preferential drainage via the cephalic and median cubital veins. Note suboptimal filling of the basilic vein (*asterisks*) and IV cannula (*arrowhead*). In **(B)**, an example is shown of a segmental smooth filiform stenosis of the left subvclavian vein (*arrowheads*). This is the same patient as in Figure 22-37. The same protocol was used as described in the previous figure.

Use of Gadolinium Contrast Agents in Patients with End-stage Renal Disease

The most widely used gadolinium chelates for CE MRA purposes are gadopentate dimeglumine (Magnevist, Schering, Berlin, Germany), gadodiamide (Omniscan, GE Health, Oslo, Norway), and gadoteridol (ProHance, Bracco Diagnostics, Milan, Italy). The total incidence of adverse events related to gadolinium use for CE MRA appears to be less than 5%. The incidence of any single adverse event is approximately 1% or lower.

By far, the most common events are nausea, headache, and emesis (247). When used intravenously, no detectable nephrotoxicity has been reported, and the rates of adverse events are extremely low (248–250).

Recently, concerns have arisen regarding the accumulation of free gadolinium in patients with renal failure (247). During the last decade, approximately 230 cases of nephrogenic systemic fibrosis (NSF), previously known as nephrogenic fibrosing dermopathy, have been reported worldwide (251).

The reported clinical signs and symptoms of NSF are subacute progressive swelling of extremities followed by more proximal involvement and severe skin induration, pain, muscle restlessness, and loss of skin flexibility. NSF can lead to serious physical disability and wheelchair requirement (251). The incidence of NSF seems to be low, and the pathophysiology is unknown (251). To date, the use of gadolinium in the form of gadodiamide (Omniscan) has the strongest association with NSF (251).

An international NSF registry at Yale University (New Haven, CT) maintains records on patients with NSF worldwide. At the time of this writing, the site had records of 215 patients (252). More than 95% of all NSF patients surveyed (approximately 100 at the time of this writing) had been exposed to a gadolinium chelate within 2 to 3 months prior to disease onset. The majority of the patients were being maintained with dialysis.

After contemplating the risk/benefit ratio and carefully considering the alternative diagnostic options prevention of dehydration, strategies such as using the lowest effective dose of contrast media possible and consideration of prompt dialysis after contrast media injection have been suggested to address the potential complications of this disorder (252).

Imaging Dialysis Access Fistulae

AVFs for hemodialysis vascular access have a high risk of thrombosis due to stenoses that jeopardize flow and patency (253) (Fig. 22-65). Prompt detection and treatment of these stenoses can prevent thrombosis and subsequent loss of access and additional surgery (215).

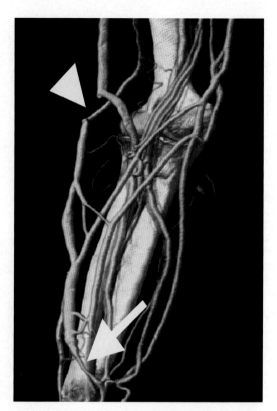

FIGURE 22-65 CT angiography was performed to evaluate a dysfunctioning Brescia-Cimino AVF. While the anastomosis is patent, a high-grade short segment stenosis is present in the immediate venous outflow (*long arrow*). In addition, there is focal occlusion of the cephalic vein at the antecubital fossa (*short arrow*).

Flow-limiting stenoses can be found anywhere along the vascular tree from the left ventricle to the right atrium.

Although most lesions are found close to the arteriovenous anastomosis, patients with ESRD are known to suffer from accelerated atherosclerosis leading to stenoses in the arteries supplying the upper extremity.

For instance, Duijm et al. found 19 relevant stenoses in the arteries supplying the access in 14 of 101 patients (14%) with a dysfunctional vascular access (254). Many ESRD patients also have a history of subclavian or jugular venous cathethers, the presence of which may cause severe stenoses in the superior vena cava.

In current clinical practice, stenosis detection and grading in AVF and the venous outflow segments are performed using Duplex ultrasonography and digital subtraction angiography (DSA). Duplex ultrasonography is highly reliable to detect stenoses in close proximity to the arteriovenous anastomosis, but it remains difficult to evaluate subclavian and intrathoracic vascular structures.

At DSA, the arterial part of the AVF is visualized according to the method of Staple, using a proximal cuff to interrupt flow in order to achieve retrograde filling of the arterial part of the AVF (255). Analysis of DSA images acquired with this method can be difficult due to vessel overlap, especially at the level of the anastomosis.

Due to temporary flow interruption, the hemodynamic situation is altered, which may lead to overestimation of vessel diameter at DSA. A further drawback that limits the value of DSA for diagnostic purposes is incomplete retrograde filling, resulting in failure to visualize the arterial part of the AVF and feeding artery in most patients (30,256). Both CE MRA and MDCT do not suffer from these drawbacks and are capable of highly accurate depiction of stenoses in AVF, as well as the supplying arteries and draining veins (31).

Both CT and MRI can provide information regarding the degree of vascular impairment (30,31,233,256–258). This capacity helps to stratify patients into those who can have PTA (single or multiple stenoses) versus those who require an operative procedure (occlusion). The results of one study suggest that conventional angiography can be reserved for candidates for percutaneous intervention (31).

The main advantage of using noninvasive techniques in the evaluation of flow-limited AVF is that prior to an intervention, all relevant lesions in the inflow trajectory (starting at the left ventricle) and the outflow trajectory (ending in the right atrium) can be identified, thus allowing for a faster, more targeted DSA-guided procedure. MRA also provides an opportunity to measure flow rates using PC velocity mapping in the same session that the vascular anatomy is visualized.

The option for MRA versus MD CTA requires careful consideration. Vascular clips may create artifacts with either and can be more severe with one or the other depending on the constituent materials of the clip. Another important consideration when imaging those patients with AVF-related complications is when individuals find it difficult to hold their upper extremities absolutely still—even mild quivering may lead to image degradation (257).

The new safety concerns when using Gd-chelates in ESRD patients, as stated previously, need to be weighed against the known risks of using iodinated contrast media. Use of iodinated contrast media may lead to temporary or permanent deterioration of residual renal function in up to 20% of the cases (259).

Further deterioration of renal function should be avoided because loss of residual renal function is associated with higher morbidity and mortality rates (260,261). Another risk with the use of iodinated contrast media is the chance that renal function recovery will be lost, even after initiation of hemodialysis therapy. Residual kidney functions such as secretion of organic acids and various endocrine functions cannot be provided by dialysis and should therefore be preserved as long as possible (260).

MAGNETIC RESONANCY ANGIOGRAPHY IMAGE PROTOCOL AND RESULTS

The MR imaging protocol consists of the standard building blocks of a localizer and subsequent 3D high spatial resolution CE MRA. Some authors have advocated using PC velocity mapping in addition to the anatomical evaluation (256,262). Because of the extremely high flow rates in the AVF, a time-resolved sequence employing TRICKS or keyhole CENTRA is recommended for this region (Fig. 22-66).

Dynamic phases should not exceed 10 seconds each. Voxel size should be in the order of $1.0 \times 1.0 \times 1.0$ mm^3. The high-flow kinetics are also the reason that, in contrast to the lower extremities, moving table approaches have not been used for upper extremity imaging in case the access is located in the forearm.

Almost all studies in patients with AVF have used an approach with separate injections and acquisitions for the

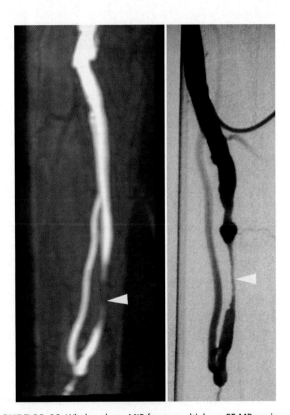

FIGURE 22-66 Whole-volume MIP from a multiphase CE MR angiogram of assessing a radiocephalic AVF obtained in the left arm of a 61-year-old male patient. A high-grade stenosis seen on CE MRA (*arrowhead* in **left panel**) with the corresponding DSA (*arrowhead* in **right panel**). The window settings have been changed to show that the CE MRA shows a residual lumen at the site of stenosis. (Reprinted with permission from Planken RN, Tordoir JH, Dammers R, et al. Stenosis detection in forearm hemodialysis arteriovenous fistulae by multiphase contrast-enhanced magnetic resonance angiography: preliminary experience. *J Magn Reson Imaging*. 2003; 17(1):54–64.)

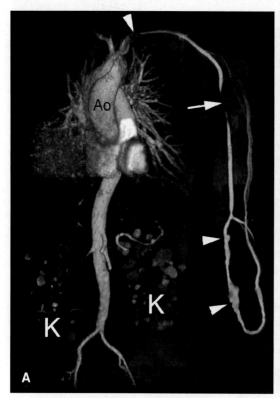
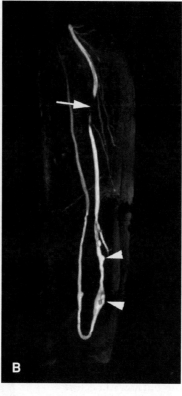

FIGURE 22-67 A 67-year-old patient with polycystic kidney disease and flow-declined hemodialysis access fistula in the left forearm **(A)**. There are high-grade stenoses in the subclavian (*top arrowhead*) and brachial artery supplying the shunt (*arrow*). In addition, there are multiple aneurysmal dilations in the loop graft (*lower arrowheads* in **A**). Note enhancement of residual kidney parenchyma. Zoomed subvolume MIP of the left forearm and antecubital region **(B)** more clearly shows high-grade stenosis (*arrow*) and aneurysms (*arrowheads*). (K, kidney.)

distal upper extremity containing the AVF (always imaged first) and proximal upper extremity. A double to triple contrast dose (0.2 to 0.3 mmol/kg or between 30 and 45 mL for a 75-kg person) of a standard extracellular agent has been used to obtain diagnostic images of excellent quality (Fig. 22-67).

Again, a careful risk-to-benefit assessment of such a high-dose strategy and a consideration of the alternatives needs to be pursued in patients with substantial renal insufficiency. Given that both gadolinium chelates and iodinated contrast are readily dialyzed, the use of CTA should be stongly considered in patients with chronic ESRD when there is no significant native renal function, in order to avoid the potential risk of NSF.

With the need to separately image the proximal and distal upper extremity vascular territories, the total amount of contrast medium is usually divided into two separate injections with half the total dose each. In cases where the access is located in the upper arm, it is almost always possible to depict it in a single FOV, with a single injection of contrast medium (Figs. 22-68, 22-69). Combinations of noncontrast and CE approaches will likely emerge to address the potential concerns regarding NSF.

Published studies on MRA of flow-compromised AVF have all found high sensitivities for the detection of flow-limiting lesions. In one of the earliest papers on CE MRA of access shunts, Planken et al. (233) found a sensitivity of 100% and positive predictive value of 70% on patient level for the detection of flow-limiting stenoses of >50% luminal reduction, in 15 patients with flow-declined AVF. Specificity was low (10%), however, at the 50% cut-off level.

The reasons for the poor specificity were low spatial resolution (voxel size of 3.1 mm^3) and the presence of a lot of borderline stenoses on DSA. However, because of the potentially deleterious consequences of missing a stenosis, a high sensitivity is much more important. More recent, larger studies have found very high sensitivity and specificity, both close to 100%, mainly because of the improved spatial resolution (263,264).

COMPUTED TOMOGRAPHIC ANGIOGRAPHY IMAGE PROTOCOL AND RESULTS

A successful protocol reported by Neyman et al. (265) using a 64-slice system is presented. A craniocaudal acquisition is obtained using 0.6-mm collimation, 0.37-second rotation speed, 0.75-mm slice thickness, and 0.5-mm reconstruction interval. An arterial acquisition is obtained after a 20- to 25-second delay following initiation of contrast injection, using 100 to 120 mL IV contrast infused at

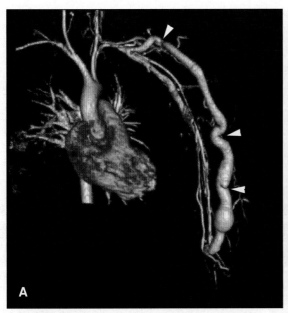
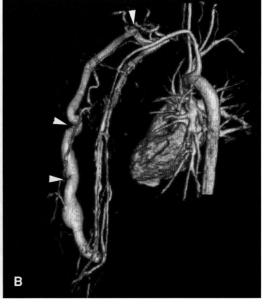

FIGURE 22-68 Anteroposterior **(A)** and posteroanterior **(B)** color VRs of the arterial phase in a 53-year-old patient with a flow-declined radiocephalic hemodialysis access shunt in the left upper extremity. Note severe kinking and dilatation at multiple sites in the venous outflow part of the access (*arrowheads*).

4 mL/second, and is followed by a venous phase acquisition. Using this protocol, imaging of the fistula and downstream complications such as digital infection can be visualized (Fig. 22-70).

An analysis of 14 patients having both MD CTA and DSA studies revealed no significant difference in the detection and grading of stenoses at the anastomosis sites, graft loops, and draining veins of failing hemodialysis AVFs (Fig. 22-71) (257). The 3D capability of MD CTA is able to depict vascular lesions with unique perspectives, helping to select patients for PTA or surgical procedures (Fig. 22-72).

MD CTA can characterize stenoses, graft and stent neointimal hyperplasia, and puncture site pseudoaneurysms.

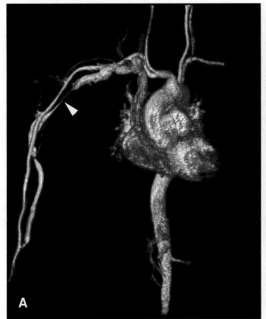
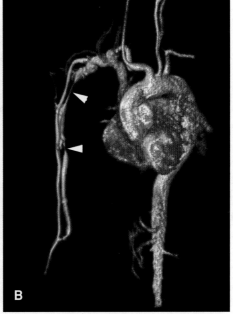

FIGURE 22-69 Coronal **(A)** and left anterior oblique **(B)** color VR of failing brachiobasilic hemodialysis access shunt in the right upper extremity in a 65-year-old patient. There are high-grade short distal and segmental proximal venous stenoses. CE MRA can depict both the arterial inflow and venous outflow trajectory with high fidelity.

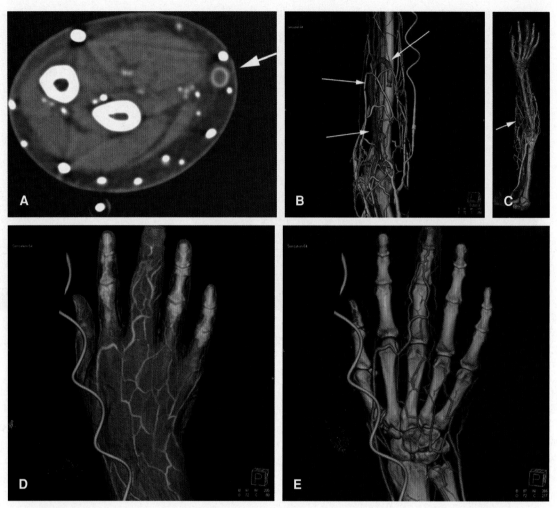

FIGURE 22-70 A 31-year-old woman with ESRD on hemodialysis, with a right arm dialysis graft, presented with low-grade fever and right finger swelling. **A:** Axial CE multislice CT of the right arm shows thrombosed graft (*arrow*). **B:** Coronal oblique color-coded VR from the same CT data set shows the entire graft (*arrow*) in red, owing to lower density relative to bone and arteries. **C:** Coronal color-coded VR of the right arm and hand from the same CT data set shows arteries (*white structures*) from the shoulder to the hand without stairstep or motion artifact. The graft (*arrow*) is displayed in red due to the relatively lower density of the graft material. The index finger has increased vascularity due to infection. **D:** Posterior color-coded VR of the hand with parameters selected to display skin and soft tissues shows soft tissue swelling and increased vascularity of the index finger due to infection. White tubing from the IV catheter line is seen coursing along the side of the hand. **E:** Posterior color-coded VR with parameters selected to display bone and vasculature depicts the small vessels causing increased perfusion of the infected digit. (Reprinted with permission from Neyman EG, Johnson PT, Fishman EK. Hemodialysis fistula occlusion: demonstration with 64-slice CT angiography. *J Comput Assist Tomogr.* 2006;30:157–159.)

RECONSTRUCTIVE SURGERY CONSIDERATIONS

Surgical wound reconstruction progresses in complexity from direct wound closure to skin grafting to local tissue transfer ("flap") and ultimately to free tissue transfer ("free flap") (266). For these procedures, vascular integrity is an important determinant of successful short- and long-term outcomes. In many instances, tissue perfusion and arterial and venous patency can be assessed preoperatively by physical examination. Depending on the complexity of the wound, the complexity of the planned surgical reconstruc-tion, and the presence of underlying vascular disease, imaging may be necessary (Fig. 22-73).

With upper extremity applications, vascular imaging is most commonly utilized prior to tissue transfer reconstructions, whether the upper extremity is to be the donor or recipient site. In many instances, reconstruction follows tumor resections or traumatic injuries.

Accurate preoperative diagnostic mapping is essential not only to ensure flap viability but also to prevent hand ischemia. The primary objectives are (a) to assess the patency and caliber of the target arteries and veins; (b) to assess the

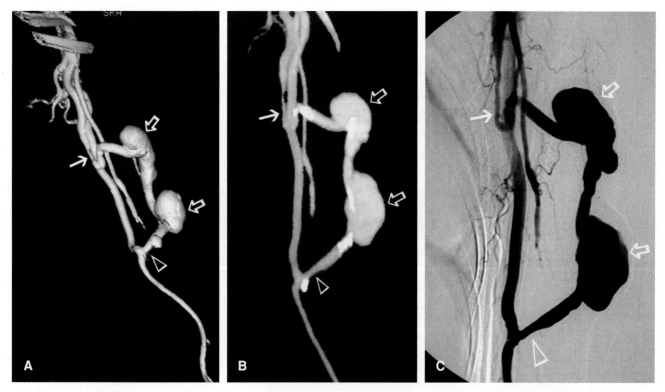

FIGURE 22-71 A 56-year-old woman with insufficient flow of brachiobasilic graft AVF. MD CTA images in 3D shaded-surface **(A)** and 2D MIP **(B)** displays show proximal grade 1 stenosis (*arrowhead*), two lobulated aneurysms (*open arrows*) of graft, and grade 3 stenosis of draining vein (*solid arrow*). DSA image **(C)** obtained 2 days later shows similar findings. (Reprinted with permission from Ko, et al. *AJR*. 2005;185:1268–1274.)

patency of and communication between the deep and superficial and palmar arches; and (c) to screen for normal variant origins, atherosclerotic disease, perivascular fibrosis, radiation arteritis, and other vascular abnormalities.

In select instances, duplex ultrasound with digital plethysmography provides a cost-effective means to map out the upper extremity arteries and veins. It has a limited role when the upper extremity arterial inflow and central veins require evaluation. CT and MR provide more comprehensive evaluations. In addition to intrathoracic assessment, these modalities also have the advantage of evaluating fasciomusculocutaneous and osseous structures. Selecting the optimum CT or MR protocol depends on whether the upper extremity will be used as a donor or recipient site. MRI may be contraindicated if orthopedic hardware is present at the region of interest.

Regarding the use of the upper extremity as a donor, radial and ulnar composite free flaps are often utilized for head and neck reconstructions (267–269). Forearm fasciocutaneous, musculocutaneous, osseofasciocutaneous, and osseomusculocutaneous flaps are potential considerations. As the radial and ulnar artery may arise aberrantly from as high as the axillary artery, CT and MR scan coverage should

begin at the subclavian artery. Imaging extends to the digital arteries. Head and neck recipient territories can be screened by using a wide FOV.

Regarding recipient reconstructions in the upper extremity, pedicle or free flaps may be used for the chest wall, upper arm, forearm, or hand. Common muscle donor sites include the latissimus dorsi, rectus abdominis (transverse rectus abdominis musculocutaneous, TRAM), serratus anterior, and gracilis muscles, while common fascial and fasciocutaneous sites include radial forearm, lateral arm, scapular, and temporoparietal fascial flaps (266,270).

Bone defects can be reconstructed using fibula free flaps and small fibular grafts (270). If fingers require reconstruction, toes can be transferred at the time of wound reconstruction (270).

Depending on the level of reconstruction, vascular anastomosis may be to the thoracodorsal, internal mammary, brachial, radial, ulnar, or palmar arch vessels. In distinction to donor evaluations, CTA and MRA coverage for upper extremity recipient evaluations can be more targeted.

For example, when the recipient vessels are either the thoracodorsal or internal mammary artery, as with TRAM breast reconstructions, CT and MRI coverage includes the

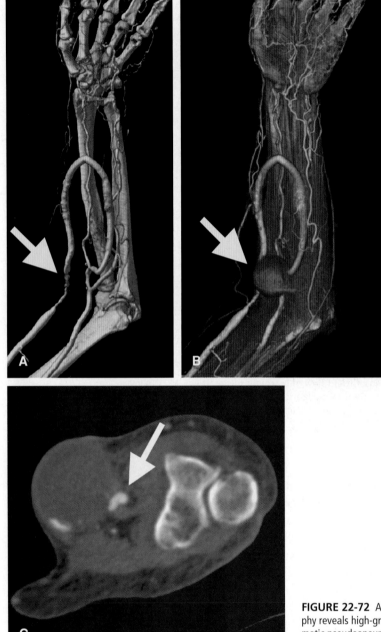

FIGURE 22-72 A right forearm loop graft imaged with 64-channel CT angiography reveals high-grade outflow stenosis (*arrow* in **A**) with a thombosed anastomotic pseudoaneurysm (*arrow* in **B**), which compresses the arterial inflow (*arrow* in **C**). The graft was successfully revised surgically.

complete inflow territory and only the outflow territory through to the mid to distal brachial artery. For wounds in the upper arm, forearm, or hand, in the absence of underlying vascular disease, targeted *runoff* coverage is recommended, beginning one vascular segment above the wound and extending through to the fingers.

Venous Occlusive Disease

Upper extremity venous occlusive disease occurs less frequently as compared with the lower extremity. It is reported to occur in

0.15% to 0.2% of hospitalized patients. Of documented cases with acute to subacute venous thrombosis, upper extremity involvement can account for up to 18% (228,271). Over the past recent decades, the incidence of upper extremity venous thrombosis has increased paralleling the increased used of central venous catheters and transvenous pacemaker wires (228).

Deep veins are most commonly involved, in particular the subclavian vein followed by the axillary vein (228). Less commonly, thrombus is located in the brachial veins and forearm deep veins either alone or synchronously. Infrequently,

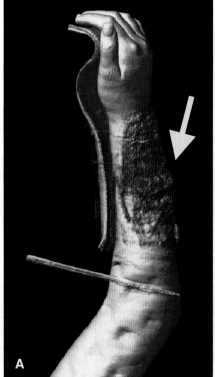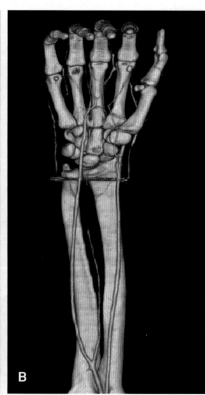

A

B

FIGURE 22-73 Prior to free-flap reconstruction of a dorsal forearm degloving injury (*arrow* in **A**), CT angiography was performed. Patent radial, ulnar, and interosseous arteries are demonstrated, along with an intact palmar arch and digital arteries (**B**).

central thrombus may extend into the brachiocephalic vein, the superior vena cava, or both. Internal jugular thrombus may be found in nearly 50% of patients with upper extremity venous thrombosis (228).

Etiologies for upper extremity venous occlusive disease are characterized as either primary or secondary. Primary thrombosis occurs spontaneously or with effort in the setting of intrinsic thrombophilia, musculoskeletal shoulder compression, or both. Important causes of thrombophilia include mutations of factor V Leiden and prothrombin and deficiencies of antithrombin, protein C, and protein S (272).

In a review of 115 patients with upper extremity deep venous thrombosis, Martinelli et al. (272) showed that hyperhomocysteinemia and strenuous upper extremity muscular activity do not directly increase the risk for thrombosis. This group also observed that in female patients with thrombophilia, the use of oral contraceptives further increased the risk for upper extremity thrombosis by approximately twofold (272).

Secondary thrombosis occurs as a result of extrinsic factors that increase the inherent thrombotic state. Extrinsic factors may be the cause in at least 70% of upper extremity venous thrombosis cases (228). The most common factors are IV devices and malignancy.

IV devices include permanent and temporary central venous catheters as well as transvenous pacemaker wires. As mentioned previously, it is the use of these devices that has led to the increased incidence of upper extremity venous thrombosis. In distinction to lower extremity venous occlusive disease, oral contraceptives, surgery, pregnancy, puerperium, and prolonged immobilization alone do not increase the risk for upper extremity venous occlusive disease (272).

Patients with upper extremity venous occlusive disease may present with arm and forearm enlargement, pain, heaviness, and skin discoloration. Physical exam is most notable for edema. Additional findings include erythema and prominent ipsilateral veins with or without a palpable cord. With complete venous outflow obstruction, arterial inflow may be compromised as well, leading to arterial ischemia with or without gangrene.

Onset of symptoms is usually slow and progressive, rather than acute. Such is the case with chronic shoulder compression, which leads to progressive venous remodeling and narrowing.

Prompt recognition of upper extremity venous thrombosis is essential. Mortality can be as high as 30% with pulmonary embolism occurring in 5% to 9% (225,228). Diagnostic evaluation focuses on four principal areas. The first is confirming the presence of thrombus and estimating its burden. The second is determining whether thrombus is occlusive or nonocclusive. The third is assessing the end-organ sequelae, including upper extremity edema and pulmonary embolism. The fourth is identifying primary and secondary risk factors.

Treatment most commonly consists of anticoagulation. Additional treatment options include pharmacologic and mechanical thrombectomy. When possible, risk factors should be removed. This often entails removal of a central venous catheter. In the setting of thoracic compression, surgical decompression is the treatment of choice. With the appropriate treatment, the recurrence rate for upper extremity deep venous thrombosis is less than 2%. Even with appropriate treatment, thrombophilia can increase the recurrence rate by nearly threefold (272).

Duplex ultrasonography is the first-line modality to evaluate suspected upper extremity venous thrombosis. Advantages

include that it does not use radiation or contrast medium, it can be performed at the bedside, and it provides dynamic functional information. Functional evaluation includes caliber assessment in neutral and challenged positions as well as flow and waveform assessment during inspiration and expiration. Duplex is useful when thrombus is located in the outflow veins or in the peripheral aspect of the subclavian vein.

Duplex sonography is operator dependent and has a limited role in central vein evaluation, including the brachiocephalic vein and the superior vena cava. Duplex is also limited when there is a poor acoustic window. In these instances, CT and MR venography are excellent alternatives (239) (Fig. 22-74). Both are also excellent modalities to more frequently provide alternative diagnoses (Fig. 22-75).

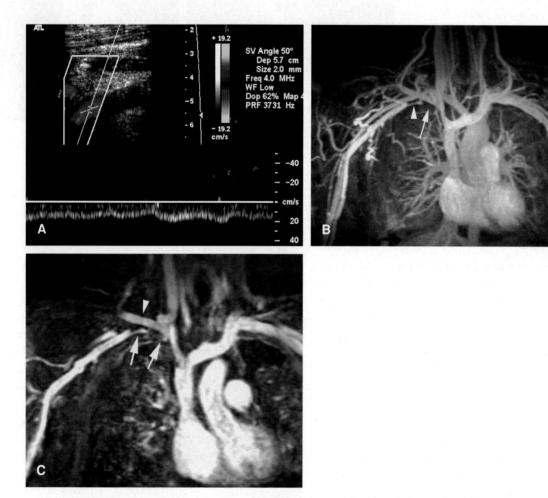

FIGURE 22-74 A 23-year-old male with Hodgkin's lymphoma and prior catheters in the right upper extremity thrombus now presenting with edema in the right arm. A: Doppler ultrasound of the right subclavian vein in a patient with right upper extremity swelling shows normal wall-to-wall color flow and normal respiratory variability of the waveform on spectral evaluation. Due to its location, not all portions of the subclavian vein are accessible to Doppler ultrasound evaluation. The patient went on to receive MRI due to high clinical suspicion for thrombosis. **B:** Coronal MIP reconstruction from the delay venous phase 3D fat-saturated T1-weighted gradient-echo acquisition shows lack of enhancement of the distal right subclavian vein (*arrow* and *arrowhead*), indicating occlusion. This is better depicted in **(C)**, a coronal MIP reconstruction from a subtracted (delay venous phase—precontrast) 3D fat-saturated T1-weighted gradient-echo acquisition. Note the large venous collateral (*arrowhead*) seen, which is consistent with chronic occlusion.

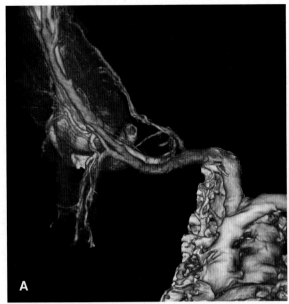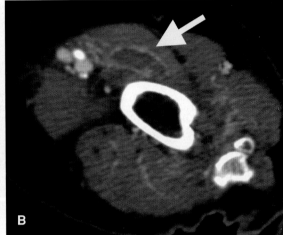

FIGURE 22-75 A right upper extremity venogram performed on a 16-channel multidetector-row scanner in a patient with erythema, warmth, and swelling reveals patent peripheral and central veins, excluding deep venous thrombosis (**A**). Review of source images, however, demonstrates an intramuscular abscess (*arrow* in **B**), associated with stranding and consistent with myositis.

Indirect upper extremity multidetector-row CT venography provides a comprehensive evaluation of the complete upper extremity venous system and imaged nonvascular structures. Using a single bolus of contrast medium, information is gathered very rapidly. As previously discussed, coverage extends from the mid chest through to the fingers or elbow. Breath-holding is required only through the chest.

Key principles to achieving robust image quality for volumetric imaging include dosing iodine strictly according to body weight, timing the acquisition to either the late arterial or equilibrium phase, and using a section thickness not greater than 2.0 mm. Timing is optimized by using a diagnostic delay of approximately 50 to 60 seconds after the arrival of contrast medium in the aortic arch.

To attain both arterial and venous enhancement, the injection rate is decreased so that the injection duration is approximately one half to three quarters of the diagnostic delay. A saline infusion is also used to minimize streak artifact. Functional venous imaging with neutral and challenged positioning is readily achieved with two separate injections and acquisitions.

A standard MRI and MRV protocol should include high-resolution T1-weighted and T2-weighted fast spin echo sequences, a 2D gradient-recalled echo sequence (ideally oriented perpendicular to the flow direction), and an option for a 3D coronal gradient echo gadolinium-enhanced multiphase MRA MRV. The T1- and T2-weighted sequences are obtained to evaluate nonvascular anatomy as well as to characterize thrombus.

As with indirect CTV, assessment of nonvascular anatomy should evaluate the shoulder, muscles, ligaments, and soft tissues. The 2D gradient-echo sequences are utilized to specifically assess for intraluminal filling defects. Often, these sequences are sufficient to confirm or exclude the presence of upper extremity venous thrombus.

TOF sequences are vulnerable to flow artifacts in-plane saturation effects, particularly when a single acquisition plane is prescribed for vascular anatomy that is tortuous and varying in its orientation. Multiple properly oriented TOF acquisitions are possible, but this is a bit cumbersome, results in long exam times, and can be difficult to assemble as a continuous, large FOV. 2D GRE sequences are particularly useful when gadolinium cannot be administered.

An alternative to 2D gradient sequences for bright blood imaging is an axial, static steady state free precession sequence, although this approach may obscure thromboses containing short T1 components (273).

With the coronal Gd-enhanced MRA MRV, high-resolution images are obtained through the upper extremity and chest, first in the arterial phase and then with at least two subsequent acquisitions in the early and late venous phases. An additional option is a delayed fat-saturated spoiled gradient recalled acquisition.

Timing for the arterial phase is either to the arch or the mid upper arm, depending on the field of coverage and positioning. As with CT, imaging can be performed during neutral and stress positioning when compression symptoms are suspected.

VASCULAR MASSES: ANEURYSMS, CONGENITAL LESIONS, TUMORS, AND TUMORLIKE CONDITIONS

Upper extremity vascular masses form a broad category that includes aneurysmal disease, congenital lesions, tumors, and tumorlike conditions. Clinical history, presentation, and physical findings are all essential for selecting the imaging strategy, further diagnostic assessment, and subsequent treatment planning.

Imaging strategies include combinations of radiography, ultrasound, Tc-99m red blood cell (RBC) scintigraphy, CT, and MRI. Conventional radiographs are useful to localize a mass and also to screen for bone erosion, phleboliths, and other soft tissue calcifications. Ultrasound provides an efficient means to confirm a vascular mass and to evaluate the degree of vascular and solid components. Tc-99m RBC scintigraphy evaluates the flow and degree of vascularity as well as the extent of the mass.

CT and MRI offer the most comprehensive evaluations. The location, size, extent, and composition of the mass are characterized; inflow, outflow, and downstream vascular territories are surveyed; and local osseous and soft tissue structures are assessed. By providing comprehensive evaluations, both CT and MRI are also the most useful to plan treatment strategies. CT and MRI techniques are tailored to the location and the type of vascular mass. Following surgical or endovascular interventions, ultrasound, CT, and MRI can be used to monitor disease and assess for postoperative complications.

Aneurysmal Disease

Upper extremity aneurysms are rare. The majority are arterial; however, venous aneurysms can also occur. A true aneurysm is designated when the vessel wall contains intact intima, media, and adventitia. A false or pseudoaneurysm is designated when the endothelial lining and other vessel wall components are disrupted and the enlarged contour is maintained by the adjacent soft tissues, a fibrous capsule, or both.

Upper extremity arterial aneurysms may be isolated or multiple and may occur anywhere from the subclavian artery through to the digital arteries and, depending on the etiology, may be accompanied by arterial aneurysms elsewhere (Fig. 22-76).

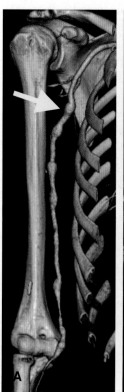 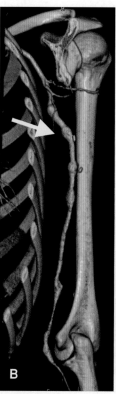 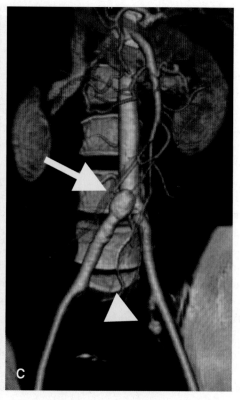

FIGURE 22-76 CT angiography was performed through the bilateral upper extremities and thoracic and abdominal aorta by placing the upper extremities at the patient's side and scanning from the thoracic inlet through to the fingertips and pelvis. Multiple tandem aneurysms are present in both brachial arteries (*arrows* in **A** and **B**). In addition, aneurysms are present at the proximal right common and left internal iliac arteries (*arrow* and *arrowhead* in **C**, respectively).

Etiologies include atherosclerotic degeneration, connective tissue disorders (i.e., Marfan syndrome, Ehlers-Danlos), vascular dysplasia (FMD, tuberous sclerosis), medium artery arteritis (i.e., GCA, Takayasu arteritis), inflammatory disorders (i.e., Kawasaki disease), trauma (true and false aneurysms), and infection (mycotic) (274). In pediatric patients, when none of these causes are identified and vessel wall degeneration is not suspect, the etiology is presumed to be congenital (274).

Patients usually present with a slow-growing, pulsatile mass. It is not uncommon that the aneurysm is asymptomatic. Alternatively, pain, paresthesias, extremity weakness, swelling, or a combination thereof may occur secondary to extrinsic mass compression on adjacent soft tissues, veins, and nerves. Mural thrombus often lines the inside of the aneurysm. This can lead to distal embolization and digital ischemia. Depending on the aneurysm size, rupture can occur. Treatment options include aneurysmectomy alone, aneurysmectomy with primary repair, and aneurysmectomy with end-to-end anastomosis or interposition graft repair. In select cases, endovascular repair, with an appropriately sized stent graft, is a consideration.

Upper extremity venous aneurysms are single, solitary venous dilatations without intervening components of varicose veins, arteriovenous malformations, or pseudoaneurysms. Concurrent varicose veins and arteriovenous malformations, however, may present in the venous distribution.

These result in elevated venous pressures, potentiating aneurysm growth. Venous aneurysms may be congenital in origin or degenerative (i.e., trauma, infection) (275). Patients most commonly present with an asymptomatic palpable mass. Less commonly, the venous aneurysm elicits pain and causes edema. Potential complications include thrombophlebitis and thromboembolism, the latter of which may lead to pulmonary embolism. Rupture rarely occurs. Surgical treatment options are similar to arterial aneurysms: aneurysmectomy alone, aneurysmectomy with primary repair, and aneurysmectomy with end-to-end anastomosis or interposition graft repair.

Upper extremity aneurysms are often assessed with duplex ultrasound followed by CT or MRI. Duplex ultrasound is a fast and efficient modality to confirm a suspected aneurysm and to distinguish the aneurysm from a vascular malformation, vascular tumor, or a solid tumor. It is also useful to determine whether the aneurysm is arterial or venous. CT and MR angiograms can help to identify additional aneurysms in the ipsilateral upper extremity, in other vascular territories, or both.

With all evaluations, aneurysm location, size, neck morphology, and thrombus composition are defined.

Aneurysms should be distinguished as true or false, and active extravasation should be excluded.

For CT angiographic evaluation of arterial aneurysms, either an Aortic Arch and Runoff protocol or the Runoff protocol can be utilized. Coverage extends to the digits to assess for downstream embolization. To optimize arterial enhancement to the digits, the table speed should be <30 mm/second.

Depending on the aneurysm size and if the aneurysm is in the subclavian, axillary, or brachial region, as contrast may stagnate in an aneurysm, the reference level for either a timing bolus or automated triggering may need to be chosen distal to the aneurysm. CT venograms are obtained either as a delayed acquisition following the arterial phase or as a dedicated single acquisition using an appropriate diagnostic delay. Coverage extends to the chest to assess the thromboembolism burden and exclude a pulmonary embolism.

MR acquisitions include standard high resolution T1-weighted and T2-weighted fast spin echo sequences as well as 3D MRA with delayed venograms. Initially, a steady state free precision sequence can be rapidly acquired to screen the upper extremity and plan the examination. The T1- and T2-weighted sequences, with or without fat saturation, are obtained to characterize the aneurysm and nonvascular structures.

The multiphase angiogram-venogram affords a dynamic evaluation, which is key to assessing relative flow and excluding concurrent arteriovenous malformations. Coverage and timing considerations are similar to those for CTA. Multiphase acquisitions are also of benefit should the first pass acquisition not coincide precisely with arterial enhancement (Fig. 22-77).

Congenital Lesions

Upper extremity congenital vascular masses arise from errors in fetal angiogenesis. They are divided into tumors and vascular malformations based upon clinical history, biologic features, and histologic findings (276,277). Chapter 23 is devoted to pediatric vascular anomalies and includes a comprehensive discussion of congenital lesions related to the vascular system.

MRI and MRA have been considered the modality of choice to evaluate and similarly classify these lesions. (278,279). However, CTA also offers a robust means to display and characterize congenital vascular masses. Treatment includes pharmacologic, percutaneous, endovascular, and surgical options (279).

Vascular Tumors

The main congenital vascular tumor is infantile hemangioma. Others include congenital hemangiomas (involuting

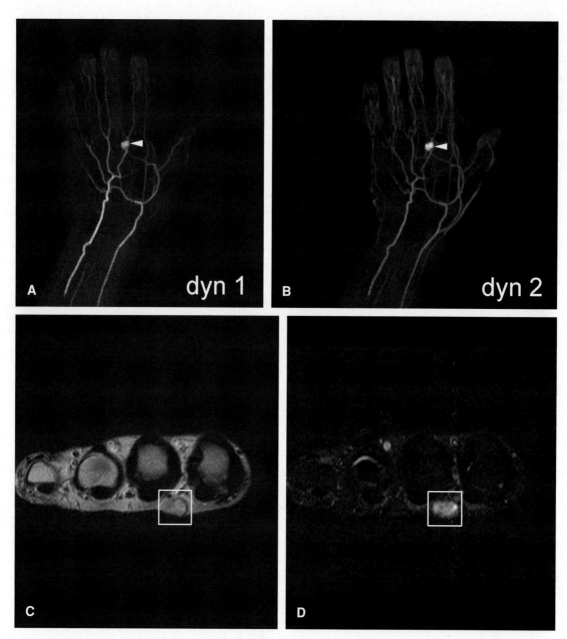

FIGURE 22-77 A 28-year-old male patient presenting with pulsatile mass on the volar aspect between second and third fingers. Whole-volume MIPs clearly demonstrate a multilobulated aneurysm of the third common palmar digital artery at the level of the third metacarpal head **(A)**. Cross-sectional T1-weighted **(C)** and fat-saturated T2-weighted **(D)** images delineate the aneurysm (enclosed in white box) in relation to the other soft tissues in the hand and show the superficial location. (Dyn 1 and 2, first and second dynamic phases.)

and noninvoluting), angioblastomas (tuft angioma), and kaposiform hemangioendotheliomas. Congenital hemangiomas are variants of infantile hemangiomas. Angioblastomas and kaposiform hemangioendotheliomas more commonly develop during early childhood and are discussed in the Tumor subsection of this chapter.

Seven percent of infantile hemangiomas occur in the upper extremity (280). These lesions are benign endothelial tumors that manifest in the neonatal period, arising in

superficial or deep soft tissues or both. Up to 40% are present at birth, while the majority develop during the first month of life (280,281).

Hemangiomas have an approximate three to one female-male predominance and more commonly develop in light-skinned children and those who are premature (281).

Infantile hemangiomas are characterized by two growth phases: proliferation and involution. Congenital hemangiomas are distinguished in that they are fully developed at birth and either involute rapidly or remain at the same size. Although the time course for proliferation and involution varies among patients with infantile hemangiomas, generalizations can be made.

During the first 5 to 6 months, infantile hemangiomas rapidly proliferate, out of proportion to the child's growth (277,280). Over the next 5 to 6 months, tumoral growth rate slows, becoming proportionate to the child's growth (282,283). The mass stabilizes and reaches a maximum size by 10 to 12 months. Tumors may be bright red to blue in color depending on their location in the superficial or deep soft tissues. Lesions are firm and do not change in size or shape with arm elevation (282). As the tumor proliferates, potential complications may occur, including ulceration, pain, bleeding, infection, and high-output cardiac failure (281).

Involution begins over the next 6 months and continues slowly during the subsequent few years. Tumor color changes to dull red and then to gray-yellow, and the tumor texture becomes soft.

While the majority of lesions completely resolve, it is not uncommon to have residual sequelae, including atrophied wrinkled skin, scars, hypopigmentation, telangectasias, and a small fibrofatty mass. Lesions that involute after six years of age are more likely to leave residual sequelae (280). The natural history allows for a conservative approach to most upper extremity hemangiomas. The exceptions are large masses and any that limit upper extremity function.

Diagnostic imaging is not usually required to make the initial diagnosis. However, imaging is useful to establish the extent of soft tissue involvement, exclude differential lesions (angioblastoma, kaposiform hemangioendothelioma, and infantile fibrosarcoma), and also exclude coexistent visceral and intracranial congenital vascular lesions.

Imaging assists in monitoring lesion changes, planning treatment, and assessing response to treatment. Imaging characteristics reflect the tumor's biologic activity at the time of imaging.

In the proliferative phase, radiographs are usually normal. Duplex ultrasound reveals a hypervascular mass of variable echotexture. On MRI, hemangiomas show iso- to hypointense signal relative to muscle on T1-weighted sequences and hyperintense signal on T2-weighted images. Flow voids are present on spin echo images. On CT, the mass is usually isodense to muscle. MRA and CTA demonstrate homogenous enhancement with feeding and draining vasculature.

In the involuting phase, findings on ultrasound, MRI, and CT highlight the fibrofatty infiltration. Duplex, MRA, and CTA all show reduced vascularity.

Vascular Malformations

Approximately 20% of vascular malformations occur in the upper extremity (280). These lesions are composed of endothelial-lined vessels without intervening parenchyma.

All vascular malformations are present at birth but may not come to clinical attention until childhood, adolescence, or early adulthood. Growth is proportionate to the patient unless stimulated by hormonal changes, trauma, infection, or other stressors (276,279,280). Lesions never involute.

Most vascular malformations occur sporadically with equal gender distribution (280). Cases of autosomal dominant inheritance have been described (284,285).

Vascular malformations are classified according to physiologic flow and tissue composition. Low-flow anomalies include venous, lymphatic, capillary, and mixed tissue types. High-flow malformations include arteriovenous malformations and AVFs.

Low-flow anomalies account for the majority of upper extremity vascular malformations, reaching nearly 90% of clinical presentations (279). Among the low-flow anomalies, venous malformations (46%) are most common, followed by lymphatic (17%), capillary (12%), or mixed (12%) (279). Imaging characteristics for each vascular malformation reflect the specific tissue.

Venous Malformations

Venous malformations are composed of dilated venous spaces. Phleboliths and in-situ thrombus are common as a result of slow flow and stasis. Venous malformations present as a nonpulsatile soft, blue mass that decompresses with arm elevation (279). Alternatively, if identified early, it may present as a blue plaque.

Depending on the size and extent, upper extremity pain, swelling, and paresthesias are frequent complaints, and decreased upper extremity function may occur. (279). Function is improved with compression garments (279).

Radiographs and noncontrast CTs are useful to detect the phleboliths. Ultrasound reveals serpiginous hypoechoic, compressible vascular spaces. On MRI, slow-flow malformations are characterized by T1-hypointense and T2-hyperintense signal. Short inversion time inversion recovery (STIR) sequences are often recommended for determining the extent of a malformation and are often supplemented by dynamic Gd-enhanced studies (78,286) (Fig. 22-78). Phleboliths can be recognized with MR as punctuate foci of hypointense signal T1- and T2-weighted imaging but may be difficult to detect. MRA and CTA both demonstrate homogenous enhancement, unless thrombus is present.

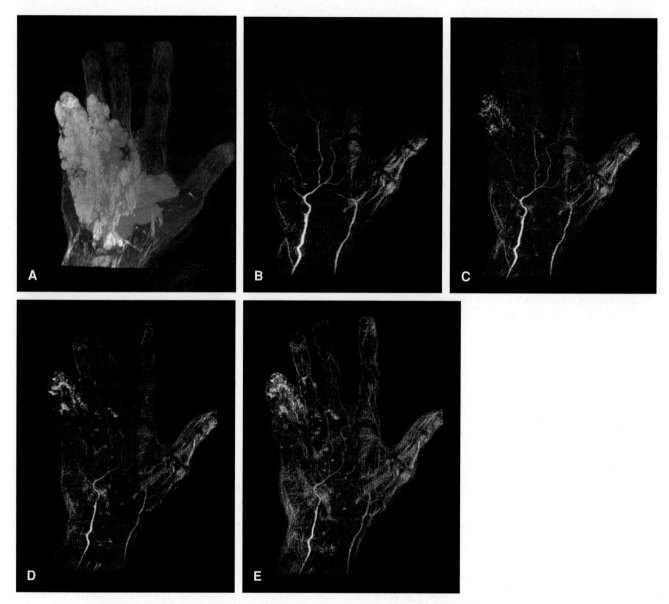

FIGURE 22-78 Slow-flow vascular malformation demonstrated with MR. A: Coronal STIR sequence reconstructed as a thin-slab MIP shows lobulated high-signal extensively throughout the hand, involving the shortened fifth digit, the proximal fourth and third digits, and palmar soft tissues. **B–E:** Serial, coronal VR images obtained during the dynamic acquisition of a gadolinium-ehanced 3D study show progressive enhancement of the affected digital and palmar soft tissues as well as the underlying vascular anatomy. Lack of early draining veins refutes the presence of an AVF.

Lymphatic Malformations

Lymphatic malformations develop as a result of errors in lymphatic channel segmentation with lymphatic channel obstruction. Cystic spaces result, and an increasing size of the malformation reflects fluid accumulation in these spaces. The cysts are susceptible to infection and hemorrhage.

These malformations are found primarily in the neck, axillae, and chest. Rarely will they occur in the upper arm, forearm, or hand (287). Patients with an upper extremity lymphatic malformation may present with a progressively

enlarging, palpable nonpulsatile mass, which is slightly firm and does not decompress on arm elevation (279). The mass may be painful and is often associated with swelling (279,287).

Large anomalies can lead to cutaneous eruptions and dimpling (279). Functional impairment can occur, depending on the extent of upper extremity involvement and bulk size of the lesion (279). Ultrasound is remarkable for a multiloculated cystic mass. Cysts may be anechoic, hypoechoic, or hyperechoic, reflective of the variable fluid composition

(287). On MRI, macrocysts show intermediate to high T1 and hyperintense T2 signal. MRA and CTA are remarkable for enhancement only in the septae between the cystic spaces.

Capillary Malformations

Capillary malformations ("port wine stains") are composed of dilated capillary and venules in the upper dermis. At birth, they present as geographic pink cutaneous discolorations. As they grow, malformations may become red to purple.

Upper extremity capillary malformations can involve the ipsilateral chest wall (279). Imaging is not usually required to reach a diagnosis but may be useful when demonstrating extent of the malformation is of interest. Additionally, MRI MRA or CTA may be useful to evaluate for coexistent disease, including additional vascular malformations.

Arteriovenous Malformation

Arteriovenous malformations are direct communications between arteries and veins without intervening capillaries. Blood shunts rapidly from the arterial system across the connection(s) and into the venous system, resulting in enlargement of feeding arteries and draining veins. Arteriovenous malformations may involve the hand, forearm, upper arm, or the whole upper extremity.

Classification schemes are based on the caliber and number of inflow arteries, the number and complexity of macro- and microfistulous connections, the caliber and number of outflow veins, and the clinical presentation (142,279,288,289).

An arteriovenous malformation typically presents as a warm, red mass with or without pain, pulsatility, thrill, or a bruit. There is no alteration in the mass size or contour with positional changes. Pain may be with exertion, at rest, or both. If presenting at birth, swelling with or without red discoloration may be the only sign (279). Depending on the complexity of the malformation, increased warmth, extremity heaviness, hyperhydrosis, hyperostosis, distal ischemia, ulceration, bleeding, and congestive heart failure may occur.

Duplex ultrasound can readily diagnose an upper extremity arteriovenous malformation. MRI MRA or CTA is usually required to more thoroughly evaluate the extent of the malformation and plan appropriate treatment (Fig. 22-79). On duplex ultrasound, the lesion has hypoechoic tubular structures with pulsatile high velocity flow. There is decreased arterial inflow resistance and arterialization of the venous outflow.

MRI is remarkable for a tangle of multiple tubular T1- and T2-weighted spin echo signal voids in the absence of an

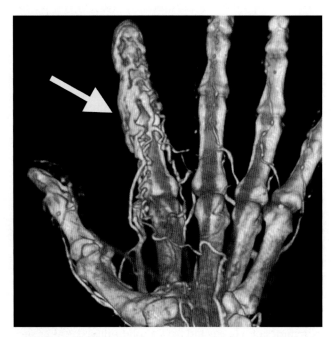

FIGURE 22-79 64-channel CT angiography was obtained prior to surgical resection of an index finger arteriovenous malformation. The VR image confirms an extensive arteriovenous malformation (*arrow*) supplied by both radial and ulnar arteries. No direct palmar arch communication was identified between the radial and ulnar systems.

intervening mass. These structures are hyperintense on fat-suppressed T2-weighted fast spin echo and STIR sequences. PC-MRI can quantitate flow and velocity through the malformation and demonstrate directionality and characterize the inflow arteries, the macro and microfistulous communications, and draining outflow veins. Recognition of the early draining vein is essential to the diagnosis.

Tumors

Upper extremity vascular tumors include benign and malignant growths. They may arise from endothelial cells, pericytes, or vessel smooth muscle cells. Presentation varies from skin discolorations to large palpable masses.

Large tumors may cause extrinsic mass effect on soft tissues, nerves, and veins, resulting in upper extremity pain, paresthesias, edema, varicosities, or a combination thereof. Definitive treatment for most requires surgical resection. Adjunct therapies for malignant tumors include chemotherapy and radiotherapy.

Pretreatment, diagnostic imaging goals are to (a) define the tumor, its extent, and its vascular supply and (b) exclude local invasion and distant metastasis. Posttreatment, depending on the time course and tissue type, the imaging objectives are to assess for residual disease, recurrent disease (local and distant), and any known metastasis.

Tumor appearances on CTA and MRI/MRA reflect the degree of vascular and solid tissue components as well as the presence of necrosis and hemorrhage.

Benign

Angioleiomyoma

Angioleiomyomas are well-encapsulated, well-circumscribed benign tumors that arise from smooth muscle cells in the tunica media of superficial and deep soft tissue veins. Less commonly, they may also arise in arteries. Histologically, angioleiomyomas are divided into three subtypes: solid, venous, and cavernous (290). Degenerative changes can occur leading to dystrophic calcification, thrombus formation, myxoid changes, and stromal hyalinization (291).

Angioleiomyomas most commonly present as small (<2 cm), slow-growing, painful nodules during the fourth to sixth decades of life (290). Most occur in the lower extremities of women and have a solid subtype. Other sites include the upper extremity, head, and upper trunk.

In distinction to lower extremity angioleiomyomas, upper extremity angioleiomyomas are more prevalent in men and demonstrate a cavernous subtype (290). Frequent upper extremity locations include the hand, wrist, and forearm. When the hand is involved (10% to 17% overall) (292,293), tumors are typically localized to the volar surface and do not arise beyond the distal interphalangeal joints (294). In the absence of pain, tumors in the hand can reach larger sizes (295,296).

The differential diagnosis for these benign nodular subcutaneous masses includes hemangiomas, ganglions, fibromas, schwannomas, lipomas, and giant tendon sheath tumors (297,291). A foreign body granuloma or inclusion cyst are additional considerations (291).

Imaging features vary based on the tissue subtype and the degree of degeneration. Radiographs and noncontrast CTs may demonstrate phleboliths. Duplex ultrasound shows a well-defined hypoechoic mass, with increased vascularity (298). Tc-99m RBC scintigraphy reveals increased flow on first-pass perfusion and increased activity on early and delayed blood pool images, localized to the mass (299).

On MRI, angioleiomyomas are characterized by T1 signal intensity, which is isointense to slightly hyperintense to that of muscle; regions of hyperintense and hypointense T2 signal intensity correspond to smooth muscle and fibrous tissue, respectively. Tubular signal voids on T2-weighted images correspond to intratumoral vascular channels and a T2 hypointense rim corresponds to the fibrous capsule (295–297,300).

With MRA and CTA, the mass demonstrates prominent enhancement with reported homogenous and heterogenous patterns (295–297,300). Both MRA and CTA are useful to define the vascular supply (296,300).

Angioblastoma (Tufted Angioma)

Angioblastomas are rare, benign subcutaneous proliferations of capillary "tufts," distinguished by "cannon ball" arrangements. These tumors typically present in early childhood (the majority less than 5 years of age) as red macules, papules, or both, along the midline axis of the body, involving the neck, shoulders, and upper torso. Proximal upper extremities may also be involved.

Diagnosis is usually achieved by biopsy, and in most instances, diagnostic imaging is not required. However, MRI MRA (301) or CTA can be obtained to evaluate the extent of soft tissue infiltration.

This is particularly important in the setting of Kasabach-Merritt syndrome.

This syndrome consists of a thrombocytopenic consumptive coagulopathy in an infant presenting with a reddish or purple mass in association with local and distant ecchymoses. The coagulopathy and thrombocytopenia can lead to a rapid increase in size of the mass.

Specimens typically reveal a kaposiform hemangioendothelioma but may show features of angioblastoma, or a mixture of the two tissue types. Histologically, angioblastomas overlap with the more agressive kaposiform hemangioendothelioma, and it has been questioned if the angioblastoma is a precursor (302).

Glomus Tumors

Glomus tumors are rare, benign hamartomas derived from glomus bodies (303,304). Glomus bodies function as specialized intradermal arteriovenous thermoregulatory structures. They are located throughout the body, but are most concentrated in the digits, palms, and soles of the feet (304).

Blood flow through this shunt, and in essence temperature to the skin, is controlled by contractile, epithelioid glomus cells along with neuroreticulum and smooth muscle fibers in the surrounding capsule (304). Glomus tumors are composed of the normal cell makeup and are distinguished by the presence of proliferating epithelioid (glomus) cells and connective tissue surrounding vascular channels (303).

Histologically, tumors are categorized into three types based on the predominance of either hyalinized connective tissue (type I, myxoid), glomus cells (type II, solid), or vascular spaces (type III, angiomatous) (303,305).

Clinically, glomus tumors can be categorized as solitary or multiple. The majority of cases are solitary. These can arise wherever there are glomus bodies, but most commonly arise in the extremities, typically within the digit and subungual region (303,304).

Glomus tumors account for 1.0% to 4.5% of upper extremity tumors (306). Fifty percent to 80% of upper extremity glomus tumors occur in the hand, and among hand lesions, 63% to 77% are subungual (48,303,304). When arising in the digit, solitary tumors are more commonly found in females. Extradigital lesions have a male predominance (303,304,306).

Patients classically present in the third to fifth decade with a triad of pain insensitivity, cold intolerance, and point tenderness. Lesions appear as red to purple plaques or nodules, are ovoid or round in shape, and measure less than 1 cm in size (range up to 3 cm) (303,304). Subungual lesions often cause nail deformities. Histologically, either myxoid, solid, or vascular tissue may predominate (303,304).

In distinction to solitary glomus tumors, multiple glomus tumors have been shown to have autosomal dominant inheritance (307). They typically are located extradigital, occur at a younger age with a male predominance, and elicit no symptoms. Lesions present as red to blue plaques or nodules. Histologically, vascular spaces comprise the majority of the tumor (303,305).

Diagnostic assessment begins by using targeted clinical tests: Love's pin test, Hildreth's tourniquet pin test, cold insensitivity test, and transillumination (308,309).

The cold insensitivity and Hildreth's pin tests are most accurate, with reported sensitivities of 100% and 71% to 92% and specificities of 100% and 91% to 100%, respectively. Love's test achieves 100% sensitivity but 0% specificity, while transillumination has a reported sensitivity of 23% to 38% and a specificity of 90% (308,309).

In many instances, these clinical tests are sufficient to reach a diagnosis, localize the tumor, and plan an operative approach. However, in approximately 30% of cases, depending on the size and depth of the lesion, physical examination does not localize the lesion with enough accuracy to confidently plan an operative approach (48).

Diagnostic imaging can be performed, as preoperative localization is essential to achieving complete surgical excision and minimizing postoperative scarring as well as avoiding postoperative nail deformity (48,310). With each modality, interpretation should be made in context to the clinical presentation, as the image findings are often nonspecific.

Screening may begin with radiography and ultrasound. Radiographs are useful for suspected subungual tumors, as long-standing lesions can result in cortical erosion. However, erosive changes may only be seen in up to 60% of cases (311).

Duplex ultrasound reveals a hypoechoic, hypervascular mass and can depict tumors as small as 3 mm (48,311). False negative results can occur, particularly with less than 3 mm or flattened lesions (311). In this situation, repeating duplex sonography or obtaining an MRI MRA is recommended (48).

MRI is useful for patients with obscure symptoms and negative or equivocal radiographs, ultrasound, or both. It is also advocated to assess recurrent glomus tumors, which are typically due to incomplete tumor excision. Glomus tumors demonstrate T1 hypointensity and T2 hyperintensity. In approximately one third of recurrent lesions, tumors have isointense to hypointense T2 signal character (312). MRA should routinely be combined with MRI to increase the study yield (Fig. 22-80) (312,313).

On MRA, tumors show mild to moderate enhancement in the arterial phase with progressive homogenous enhancement on the delayed phase. A similar enhancement pattern is seen with CTA, based on extradigital applications (314).

Intramuscular Hemangioma

Intramuscular hemangiomas are rare, benign skeletal muscle tumors. These tumors are distinct from infantile hemangiomas and congenital hemangiomas. Intramuscular hemangiomas typically present in adolescence or early

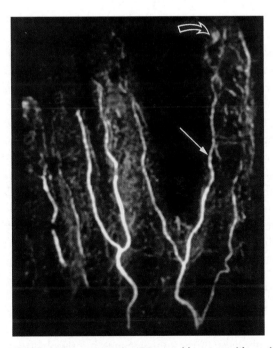

FIGURE 22-80 Glomus tumor in a 37-year-old woman with a painful focus in the pulp of the right second digit. CE MRA shows the proper digital vessels, with the ulnar artery to the second digit (*straight arrow*) coursing toward a small enhancing lesion in the fingertip (*curved arrow*). A glomus tumor was confirmed at surgery. (Reprinted with permission from Connell DA, Koulouris G, Thorn DA, Potter HG, et al. Contrast-enhanced MR angiography of the hand. *Radiographics.* 2002;22:583-599.)

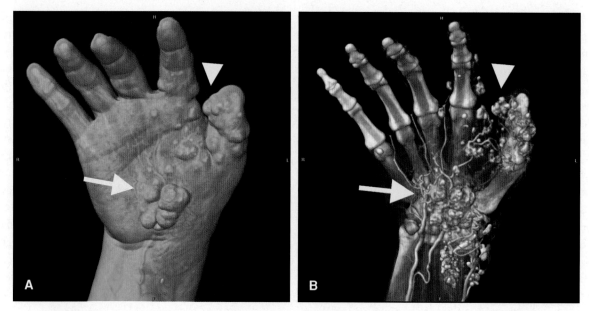

FIGURE 22-81 CT angiography was performed to map out the extent of an infiltrative intramuscular hemangioma. As shown in skin **(A)** and vascular **(B)** VR images, the hemangioma is supplied predominantly by the ulnar artery and has two epicenters—one in the palm (*arrow*) and the other in the thenar eminence (*arrowhead*). Multiple phleboliths are present.

adulthood as an enlarging firm, painful mass without skin discoloration, as the tumor infiltrates through the muscle and does not involute (Fig. 22-81).

Histologically, they are composed of vascular channels intermixed with variable nonvascular elements, including smooth muscle, fibrous septae, myxoid stroma, thrombus, and hemosiderin. Diagnostic imaging reflects this heterogeneity, and diagnosis in many instances relies on tissue specimen.

Radiographs and noncontrast CT will demonstrate phleboliths. Ultrasound may demonstrate a soft tissue mass with increased vascularity. MRI reveals a mass often with tubular signal voids, and the STIR sequence is a reliable technique for demonstrating the extent of the lesion. More commonly, the mass shows intermediate to high T1 and hyperintense T2 spin echo signal intensity with the latter having a serpentine pattern. CE MRA and, presumably, CTA reveal serpentine enhancement in the mass (315).

Intermediate-Grade

Hemangioendotheliomas Hemangioendotheliomas are rare tumors arising from endothelial cells. They typically grow in the subcutaneous and deep soft tissues, but are also found in muscle, bone, lung, liver, and spleen.

Histologically, these tumors are defined by proliferation of capillary or venous channels surrounded by endothelial cells intermixed with sheets of epithelial cells, spindle cells, lymphocytes, or a combination of these cells.

Traditionally, these tumors have been considered of intermediate grade between hemangiomas and hemangiosarcomas. However, various histological subtypes exist, and each can be categorized as either benign (grade I; infantile hemangioendothelioma, spindle cell hemangioendothelioma, kaposiform hemangioendothelioma, intravascular papillary hemangioendothelioma); intermediate (grade II; retiform hemangioendothelioma, polymorphous hemangioendothelioma, composite hemangioendothelioma, endovascular papillary angioendothelioma); or malignant (grade III; epithelioid hemangioendothelioma) based on the degree of vascular channel development, cellular atypia, and mitotic figures (316).

Imaging features for hemangioendotheliomas in the upper extremity are often nonspecific. Depending on the subtype and the tissue and bone involvement, radiographs and noncontrast CT may demonstrate phleboliths with a soft tissue or an expansile osteolytic mass. On MRI, lesions have heterogenous character, with low to intermediate T1 and intermediate to high T2 signal intensity. CTA and MRA show hypervascular masses with homogenous enhancement. Vascular channels are not typically depicted (317).

Malignant

Angiosarcomas Angiosarcomas are aggressive tumors composed of endothelial cells lining vascular channels. Most commonly, they arise in the skin or soft tissues, in particular the extremities (282). Other sites include the breast, liver, spleen, and heart. In the extremities, cutaneous are more common than soft tissue hemangiosarcomas.

Tumors vary from well to poor differentiation, reflective of the degree of vascular channel formation, cellular atypia, and mitotic figures. Local invasion and distant metastasis are common.

Risk factors for upper extremity angiosarcomas may include chronic lymphedema (318), localized radiation (319,320), and foreign bodies (286,321). Among these, chronic lymphedema is the most prevalent factor.

Angiosarcomas arising in the setting of long-standing lymphedema is known as Stewart-Treves syndrome (318). It was originally described in postmastectomy patients, but can occur with any congenital or acquired abnormality (i.e., trauma, surgery, radiation), which results in lymphatic dilatation and stasis. Upper extremity immobility with long-term dependent positioning could also place a patient at higher risk (322).

Upper extremity angiosarcomas may present as regional bruising, defined plaque(s), nodule(s), or a mass depending on whether it arises in the skin or soft tissues. Raised margins, ulceration, necrosis, and intratumoral hemorrhage are common.

Patients are frequently asymptomatic, leading to delayed presentations. With larger size masses, compression symptoms may be present. Diagnosis is ultimately made by tissue biopsy; endothelial cell origin is confirmed by detection of Factor VIII antigen and CD31 and CD34 markers.

Radiographs, ultrasound, CT, and MRI all play important roles in evaluating these patients. Radiographs and ultrasound serve as first-line modalities for screening. Both radiographs and noncontrast CT can evaluate calcification, bone destruction, and the tumor matrix.

On CT, without contrast, tumors typically have a nonspecific attenuation that is isodense to muscle. However, they may be hyperdense (323).

On MRI, tissue characteristics are also nonspecific. Angiosarcomas demonstrate isointense T1- and hyperintense T2-weighted signal intensities. Foci of hypointense T1 and T2 signal typically reflects regions of hemorrhage. Signal voids may also reflect the vascular channels.

Following contrast medium delivery, upper extremity CTA and MRA will show marked tumor enhancement, with an outline of feeding vessels. Vascular channels may be depicted.

Hemangiopericytomas Hemangiopericytomas are rare vascular tumors that can grow throughout the body, including the upper extremity. They are derived from pericytes, which are found in capillaries, deep to the endothelial basement membrane. These cells provide a contractile function, regulating capillary size and blood flow.

Hemangiopericytomas are divided into infantile and adult subtypes. Infantile hemangiopericytomas account for approximately 10% of cases and are defined as those presenting at less than one year of age (324,325).

The infantile type has a 2:1 male-to-female ratio and most commonly is found in the superficial soft tissues. This is distinct from the adult type, which occurs equally among genders and is found typically in deeper structures (326).

Both types most often manifest as slow growing, firm, and painless masses. Because of the lack of direct innervation, it is not uncommon that patients do not present until the masses reach considerable size. Upper extremity hemangiopericytomas of 9 × 10 × 15 cm (327) and 9 × 6.6 × 5 cm (328) have been reported in infants and adults, respectively.

Histologically, both infantile and adult hemangiopericytomas demonstrate proliferating spindle and ovoid tumor cells surrounding endothelial-lined vascular spaces. The tumor and endothelial cells are separated by a basement membrane.

A silver stain is necessary to identify reticulin sheaths that surround the tumor cells, thereby distinguishing the hemangiopericytoma from hemangioendotheliomas and other vascular and nonvascular soft tissue tumors that may also have vascular channels with spindle cells (325,328). Tumor cells in both types have variable degrees of cellular atypia and mitotic activity.

The histology of hemangiopericytomas, however, does not always predict the clinical course. Whereas up to approximately 50% of adult cases may metastasize, infantile hemagiopericytomas have a more benign clinical course and rarely spread (75,318).

Regarding diagnostic imaging for hemangiopericytomas, radiographs and CT may show speckled calcifications (329). On MRI, lesions typically have intermediate T1 and hyperintense T2 signal intensity.

Both CTA and MRA demonstrate hypervascular masses with vascular cystic spaces interspersed with solid tissue. Depending on the size, variable degrees of necrosis and hemorrhage may be present. Feeding arteries and draining veins are readily depicted. The feeding arteries typically form a common trunk that then enters the mass and arborizes in a radial fashion within and around the tumor (330).

Kaposi's Sarcoma Kaposi's sarcoma is a rare, cutaneous vascular tumor that is frequently aggressive—both local and distant. Four clinical forms are recognized: *classic* (European endemic), *lyangiopaphic* (African endemic), *transplant* associated, and AIDS associated (epidemic) (331).

The classic form typically occurs in the distal extremities. Upper extremity involvement is less common. When

Kaposi's sarcoma is diagnosed in the upper extremity, an immunosuppressed state (transplant or AIDS associated) should be questioned.

Depending on the clinical setting and tumor behavior, patients may present with multiple red to purple macules, plaques, nodules, or a combination of these lesions. Mucosal surfaces, lymph nodes, and viscera may be involved (331,332).

Histologically, tumors are composed of proliferating capillary vascular channels surrounded by atypical endothelial cells and a stroma of spindle cells with an inflammatory infiltrate (333). Diagnosis is confirmed with biopsy. CTA or MRI MRA is not usually required, unless local invasion, metastasis, or internal organs require evaluation.

Tumorlike Conditions

Pyogenic Granuloma

Pyogenic granulomas are hyperplastic lobular capillary hemangiomas that typically develop rapidly in response to traumatic soft tissue injury. Lesions are commonly red, pedunculated masses with friable surfaces that bleed easily. Lesions may also be sessile. Diagnosis is made clinically; noninvasive vascular imaging is not required. The differential diagnosis includes Kaposi's sarcoma, squamous cell carcinoma, and amelanotic melanoma. Treatment options include surgical excision, laser ablation, electrocautery, and silver nitrate cautery (334).

Bacillary Angiomatosis

Bacillary angiomatosis is a cutaneous capillary proliferative process. It is caused by Bartonella gram-negative bacilli (*B. quintana, B. henselae*), most commonly in immunocompromised patients. It can also occur in immunocompetent hosts. Clinically, bacillary angiomatosis manifests as single or multiple angiomatous papules or nodules.

Diagnosis is confirmed with tissue cultures, stains, and if necessary, electron microscopy. Noninvasive vascular imaging is not required. The differential diagnosis includes Kaposi's sarcoma, pyogenic granulomas, histiocytoid hemangioma, and lobular capillary hemangioma. Treatment is with antibiotics (erythromycin) (335).

ACKNOWLEDGMENT

Dr. Leiner would like to express his gratefulness to Dr. R. Nils Planken, M.D., Ph.D, for help with preparation of the illustrations.

REFERENCES

1. Kaufman JA. Upper-extremity arteries. In: Kaufman JA, Lee MJ, eds. *Vascular and Interventional Radiology: The Requisites.* Philadelphia: Mosby, 2004:142–162.
2. Greenfield LJ, Rajagopalan S, Olin JW. Upper extremity arterial disease. *Cardiol Clin.* 2002;20:623–631.
3. Azakie A, McElhinney DB, Higashima R, et al. Innominate artery reconstruction: over 3 decades of experience. *Ann Surg.* 1998;228:402–410.
4. Angelis M, Wong LL, Myers SA, et al. Calciphylaxis in patients on hemodialysis: a prevalence study. *Surgery.* 1997;122:1083–1089; discussion 1089–1090.
5. Hafner J, Keusch G, Wahl C, et al. Calciphylaxis: a syndrome of skin necrosis and acral gangrene in chronic renal failure. *Vasa.* 1998;27:137–143.
6. Wilmer WA, Magro CM. Calciphylaxis: emerging concepts in prevention, diagnosis, and treatment. *Semin Dial.* 2002;15:172–186.
7. Worth RL. Calciphylaxis: pathogenesis and therapy. *J Cutan Med Surg.* 1998;2:245–248.
8. Olin JW. Thromboangiitis obliterans (Buerger's disease). *N Engl J Med.* 2000;343:864–869.
9. Waugh JR, Sacharias N. Arteriographic complications in the DSA era. *Radiology* 1992;182:243–246.
10. Johnston KW. Upper extremity ischemia. In: Rutherford RB, ed. *Vascular Surgery.* Philadelphia: WB Saunders; 2000:1111–1115.
11. Currie IC, Jones AJ, Wakeley CJ, et al. Noninvasive aortoiliac assessment. *Eur J Vasc Endovasc Surg.* 1995;9:24–28.
12. de Smet AA, Ermers EJ, Kitslaar PJ. Duplex velocity characteristics of aortoiliac stenoses. *J Vasc Surg.* 1996;23:628–636.
13. Ubbink DT, Fidler M, Legemate DA. Interobserver variability in aortoiliac and femoropopliteal duplex scanning. *J Vasc Surg.* 2001;33:540–545.
14. Chai P, Mohiaddin R. How we perform cardiovascular magnetic resonance flow assessment using phase-contrast velocity mapping. *J Cardiovasc Magn Reson.* 2005;7:705–716.
15. Gatehouse PD, Keegan J, Crowe LA, et al. Applications of phase-contrast flow and velocity imaging in cardiovascular MRI. *Eur Radiol.* 2005;15:2172–2184.
16. Ringgaard S, Oyre SA, Pedersen EM. Arterial MR imaging phase-contrast flow measurement: improvements with varying velocity sensitivity during cardiac cycle. *Radiology.* 2004;232:289–294.
17. Stueckle CA, Claeys L, Haegele K, et al. Diagnostic value of proton MR spectroscopy in peripheral arterial occlusive disease: a prospective evaluation. *AJR Am J Roentgenol.* 2006;187:1322–1326.
18. Morikawa S, Inubushi T, Kito K, et al. Imaging of phospho-energetic state and intracellular pH in human calf muscles after exercise by 31P NMR spectroscopy. *Magn Reson Imaging.* 1994;12:1121–1126.
19. Itoh M, Iio M, Kawai M, et al. 31P-NMR spectroscopy of myopathies: clinical application of whole-body MR. *Radiat Med.* 1986;4:41–45.
20. Bottomley PA, Lee Y, Weiss RG. Total creatine in muscle: imaging and quantification with proton MR spectroscopy. *Radiology.* 1997;204:403–410.
21. Constantinides CD, Gillen JS, Boada FE, et al. Human skeletal muscle: sodium MR imaging and quantification-potential applications in exercise and disease. *Radiology.* 2000;216: 559–568.
22. Nirkko AC, Rosler KM, Slotboom J. Muscle metabolites: functional MR spectroscopy during exercise imposed by tetanic electrical nerve stimulation. *Radiology.* 2006;241:235–242.
23. Williams DM, Fencil L, Chenevert TL. Peripheral arterial occlusive disease: P-31 MR spectroscopy of calf muscle. *Radiology.* 1990;175:381–385.
24. Fleischmann D. High-concentration contrast media in MDCT angiography: principles and rationale. *Eur Radiol.* 2003;13 Suppl 3:N39–N43.
25. Fleischmann D, Rubin GD. Quantification of intravenously administered contrast medium transit through the peripheral arteries: implications for CT angiography. *Radiology.* 2005;236:1076–1082.
26. Pruessmann KP, Weiger M, Scheidegger MB, et al. SENSE: sensitivity encoding for fast MRI. *Magn Reson Med.* 1999;42:952–962.

27. Sodickson DK, Manning WJ. Simultaneous acquisition of spatial harmonics (SMASH): fast imaging with radiofrequency coil arrays. *Magn Reson Med*. 1997;38:591–603.

28. Weiger M, Pruessmann KP, Kassner A, et al. Contrast-enhanced 3D MRA using SENSE. *J Magn Reson Imaging*. 2000;12:671–677.

29. Niendorf T, Sodickson DK. Parallel imaging in cardiovascular MRI: methods and applications. *NMR Biomed*. 2006;19: 325–341.

30. Bos C, Smits JH, Zijlstra JJ, et al. MRA of hemodialysis access grafts and fistulae using selective contrast injection and flow interruption. *Magn Reson Med*. 2001;45:557–561.

31. Cavagna E, D'Andrea P, Schiavon F, et al. Failing hemodialysis arteriovenous fistula and percutaneous treatment: imaging with CT, MRI and digital subtraction angiography. *Cardiovasc Intervent Radiol*. 2000;23:262–265.

32. Gehl HB, Bohndorf K, Gladziwa U, et al. Imaging of hemodialysis fistulas: limitations of MR angiography. *J Comput Assist Tomogr*. 1991;15:271–275.

33. Konermann M, Sanner B, Laufer U, et al. Magnetic resonance angiography as a technique for the visualization of hemodialysis shunts. *Nephron*. 1996;73:73–78.

34. Laissy JP, Menegazzo D, Debray MP, et al. Failing arteriovenous hemodialysis fistulas: assessment with magnetic resonance angiography. *Invest Radiol*. 1999;34:218–224.

35. van Erkel AR, Pattynama PM. Receiver operating characteristic (ROC) analysis: basic principles and applications in radiology. *Eur J Radiol*. 1998;27:88–94.

36. Oudenhoven LF, Pattynama PM, de Roos A, et al. Magnetic resonance, a new method for measuring blood flow in hemodialysis fistulae. *Kidney Int*. 1994;45:884–889.

37. Winterer JT, Ghanem N, Roth M, et al. Diagnosis of the hypothenar hammer syndrome by high-resolution contrast-enhanced MR angiography. *Eur Radiol*. 2002;12:2457–2462.

38. Nastri MV, Baptista LP, Baroni RH, et al. Gadolinium-enhanced three-dimensional MR angiography of Takayasu arteritis. *Radiographics*. 2004;24:773–786.

39. Connell DA, Koulouris G, Thorn DA, et al. Contrast-enhanced MR angiography of the hand. *Radiographics*. 2002;22:583–599.

40. Lee VS, Lee HM, Rofsky NM. Magnetic resonance angiography of the hand. A review. *Invest Radiol*. 1998;33:687–698.

41. Ho KY, Leiner T, de Haan MW, et al. Peripheral MR angiography. *Eur Radiol*. 1999;9:1765–1774.

42. Schoenberg SO, Londy FJ, Licato P, et al. Multiphase-multistep gadolinium-enhanced MR angiography of the abdominal aorta and runoff vessels. *Invest Radiol*. 2001;36: 283–291.

43. Boos M, Scheffler K, Haselhorst R, et al. Arterial first pass gadolinium-CM dynamics as a function of several intravenous saline flush and Gd volumes. *J Magn Reson Imaging*. 2001;13:568–576.

44. Prince MR. Contrast-enhanced MR angiography: theory and optimization. *Magn Reson Imaging Clin North Am*. 1998;6:257–267.

45. Maki JH, Prince MR, Londy FJ, et al. The effects of time varying intravascular signal intensity and k-space acquisition order on three-dimensional MR angiography image quality. *J Magn Reson Imaging*. 1996;6:642–651.

46. Earls JP, Rofsky NM, DeCorato DR, et al. Breath-hold single-dose gadolinium-enhanced three-dimensional MR aortography: usefulness of a timing examination and MR power injector. *Radiology*. 1996;201:705–710.

47. Foo TK, Saranathan M, Prince MR, et al. Automated detection of bolus arrival and initiation of data acquisition in fast, three-dimensional, gadolinium-enhanced MR angiography. *Radiology*. 1997;203:275–280.

48. Luccichenti G, Cademartiri F, Ugolotti U, et al. Magnetic resonance angiography with elliptical ordering and fluoroscopic triggering of the renal arteries. *Radiol Med (Torino)*. 2003;105:42–47.

49. Meaney JF. Magnetic resonance angiography of the peripheral arteries: current status. *Eur Radiol*. 2003;13:836–852.

50. Siegelman ES, Charafeddine R, Stolpen AH, et al. Suppression of intravascular signal on fat-saturated contrast-enhanced thoracic MR arteriograms. *Radiology* 2000;217:115–118.

51. Leiner T, de Weert TT, Nijenhuis RJ, et al. Need for background suppression in contrast-enhanced peripheral magnetic resonance angiography. *J Magn Reson Imaging*. 2001;14:724–733.

52. Ruehm SG, Nanz D, Baumann A, et al. 3D contrast-enhanced MR angiography of the run-off vessels: value of image subtraction. *J Magn Reson Imaging* 2001;13:402–411.

53. Fellner FA, Requardt M, Lang W, et al. Peripheral vessels: MR angiography with dedicated phased-array coil with large-field-of-view adapter feasibility study. *Radiology* 2003;228:284–289.

54. Goyen M, Ruehm SG, Barkhausen J, et al. Improved multi-station peripheral MR angiography with a dedicated vascular coil. *J Magn Reson Imaging*. 2001;13:475–480.

55. Leiner T, Nijenhuis RJ, Maki JH, et al. Use of a three-station phased array coil to improve peripheral contrast-enhanced magnetic resonance angiography. *J Magn Reson Imaging*. 2004;20:417–425.

56. Bezooijen R, van den Bosch HC, Tielbeek AV, et al. Peripheral arterial disease: sensitivity-encoded multiposition MR angiography compared with intraarterial angiography and conventional multiposition MR angiography. *Radiology* 2004;231:263–271.

57. de Vries M, Nijenhuis RJ, Hoogeveen RM, et al. Contrast-enhanced peripheral MR angiography using SENSE in multiple stations: feasibility study. *J Magn Reson Imaging*. 2005;21:37–45.

58. Wang Y, Winchester PA, Khilnani NM, et al. Contrast-enhanced peripheral MR angiography from the abdominal aorta to the pedal arteries: combined dynamic two-dimensional and bolus-chase three-dimensional acquisitions. *Invest Radiol* 2001;36:170–177.

59. Hu HH, Madhuranthakam AJ, Kruger DG, et al. Improved venous suppression and spatial resolution with SENSE in elliptical centric 3D contrast-enhanced MR angiography. *Magn Reson Med*. 2004;52:761–765.

60. Korosec FR, Frayne R, Grist TM, et al. Time-resolved contrast-enhanced 3D MR angiography. *Magn Reson Med*. 1996;36:345–351.

61. Barger AV, Block WF, Toropov Y, et al. Time-resolved contrast-enhanced imaging with isotropic resolution and broad coverage using an undersampled 3D projection trajectory. *Magn Reson Med*. 2002;48:297–305.

62. Peters DC, Korosec FR, Grist TM, et al. Undersampled projection reconstruction applied to MR angiography. *Magn Reson Med*. 2000;43:91–101.

63. Vigen KK, Peters DC, Grist TM, et al. Undersampled projection-reconstruction imaging for time-resolved contrast-enhanced imaging. *Magn Reson Med*. 2000;43: 170–176.

64. van Vaals JJ, Brummer ME, Dixon WT, et al. "Keyhole" method for accelerating imaging of contrast agent uptake. *J Magn Reson Imaging*. 1993;3:671–675.

65. Hoogeveen RM, von Falkenhausen M, Gieseke J. Fast, dynamic high resolution contrast-enhanced MR angiography with CENTRA keyhole and SENSE. In: 12th Scientific Meeting of the International Society for Magnetic Resonance in Medicine. Kyoto, Japan: International Society for Magnetic Resonance in Medicine; 2004.

66. Foo TK, Ho VB, Hood MN, et al. High-spatial-resolution multistation MR imaging of lower-extremity peripheral vasculature with segmented volume acquisition: feasibility study. *Radiology*. 2001;219:835–841.

67. Swan JS, Carroll TJ, Kennell TW, et al. Time-resolved three-dimensional contrast-enhanced MR angiography of the peripheral vessels. *Radiology*. 2002;225(1):43–52.

68. Hany TF, Carroll TJ, Omary RA, et al. Aorta and runoff vessels: single-injection MR angiography with automated table movement compared with multiinjection time-resolved MR angiography initial results. *Radiology*. 2001;221:266–272.

69. Planken RN, Keuter XH, Hoeks AP, et al. Diameter measurements of the forearm cephalic vein prior to vascular access creation in end-stage renal disease patients: graduated pressure cuff versus tourniquet vessel dilatation. *Nephrol Dial Transplant.* 2006;21:802–806.

70. Wentz KU, Frohlich JM, von Weymarn C, et al. High-resolution magnetic resonance angiography of hands with timed arterial compression (tac MRA). *Lancet.* 2003;361:49–50.

71. Hoogeveen RM, Bakker CJ, Viergever MA. Limits to the accuracy of vessel diameter measurement in MR angiography. *J Magn Reson Imaging.* 1998;8:1228–1235.

72. Westenberg JJ, van der Geest RJ, Wasser MN, et al. Vessel diameter measurements in gadolinium contrast-enhanced three-dimensional MRA of peripheral arteries. *Magn Reson Imaging.* 2000;18:13–22.

73. Prince MR, Grist TM, Debatin JF. *3D Contrast MR Angiography.* Berlin: Springer; 2003.

74. Goyen M, Debatin JF, Ruehm SG. Peripheral magnetic resonance angiography. *Top Magn Reson Imaging.* 2001;12:327–335.

75. Hoey SA, Letts RM, Jimenez C. Infantile hemangiopericytoma of the musculoskeletal system: case report and literature review. *J Pediatr Orthop.* 1998;18:359–362.

76. Meaney JF, Ridgway JP, Chakraverty S, et al. Stepping-table gadolinium-enhanced digital subtraction MR angiography of the aorta and lower extremity arteries: preliminary experience. *Radiology.* 1999;211:59–67.

77. Hentsch A, Aschauer MA, Balzer JO, et al. Gadobutrol-enhanced moving-table magnetic resonance angiography in patients with peripheral vascular disease: a prospective, multi-centre blinded comparison with digital subtraction angiography. *Eur Radiol.* 2003;13:2103–2114.

78. Goyen M, Lauenstein TC, Herborn CU, et al. 0.5 M Gd chelate (Magnevist) versus 1.0 M Gd chelate (Gadovist): dose-independent effect on image quality of pelvic three-dimensional MR-angiography. *J Magn Reson Imaging.* 2001;14:602–607.

79. Knopp MV, Tengg-Kobligk H, Floemer F, et al. Contrast agents for MRA: future directions. *J Magn Reson Imaging.* 1999;10:314–316.

80. Caravan P, Cloutier NJ, Greenfield MT, et al. The interaction of MS-325 with human serum albumin and its effect on proton relaxation rates. *J Am Chem Soc.* 2002;124:3152–3162.

81. Rofsky NM, Morana G, Adelman MA, et al. Improved gadolinium-enhanced subtraction MR angiography of the femoropopliteal arteries: reintroduction of osseous anatomic landmarks. *AJR Am J Roentgenol.* 1999;173:1009–1011.

82. Westenberg JJ, Wasser MN, van der Geest RJ, et al. Scan optimization of gadolinium contrast-enhanced three-dimensional MRA of peripheral arteries with multiple bolus injections and in vitro validation of stenosis quantification. *Magn Reson Imaging.* 1999;17:47–57.

83. Hany TF, Schmidt M, Davis CP, et al. Diagnostic impact of four postprocessing techniques in evaluating contrast-enhanced three-dimensional MR angiography. *AJR Am J Roentgenol.* 1998;170:907–912.

84. Nelemans PJ, Leiner T, de Vet HC, et al. Peripheral arterial disease: meta-analysis of the diagnostic performance of MR angiography. *Radiology.* 2000;217:105–114.

85. Kadir S. Arterial anatomy of the upper extremities. In: Atlas of normal and variant angiographic anatomy. Philadelpphia: WB Saunders; 1991:63–91.

86. Fuhrman TM, Pippin WD, Talmage LA, et al. Evaluation of collateral circulation of the hand. *J Clin Monit* 1992;8:28–32.

87. Kadir S. Arteriography of the upper extremity. In: *Diagnostic Angiography.* Philadelphia: WB Saunders; 1986:207–253.

88. Whitehouse WM, Erlandson EE. Upper extremity revascularization. In: Rutherford RB, ed. *Vascular Surgery.* Philadelphia: WB Saunders; 2000:1162–1170.

89. Holleman JH, Hardy JD, Williamson JW, et al. Arterial surgery for arm ischemia. A survey of 136 patients. *Ann Surg.* 1980;191:728–736.

90. Cherry KJ, Jr., McCullough JL, Hallett JW, Jr, et al. Technical principles of direct innominate artery revascularization: a comparison of endarterectomy and bypass grafts. *J Vasc Surg.* 1989;9:718–723; discussion 723–724.

91. Kieffer E, Sabatier J, Koskas F, et al. Atherosclerotic innominate artery occlusive disease: early and long-term results of surgical reconstruction. *J Vasc Surg.* 1995;21:326–336; discussion 336–337.

92. Reul GJ, Jacobs MJ, Gregoric ID, et al. Innominate artery occlusive disease: surgical approach and long-term results. *J Vasc Surg.* 1991;14:405–412.

93. Korner M, Baumgartner I, Do DD, et al. PTA of the subclavian and innominate arteries: long-term results. *Vasa.* 1999;28:117–122.

94. Huttl K, Nemes B, Simonffy A, et al. Angioplasty of the innominate artery in 89 patients: experience over 19 years. *Cardiovasc Intervent Radiol.* 2002;25:109–114.

95. Hass WK, Fields WS, North RR, et al. Joint study of extracranial arterial occlusion. II. Arteriography, techniques, sites, and complications. *JAMA.* 1968;203:961–968.

96. Berguer R, Morasch MD, Kline RA. Transthoracic repair of innominate and common carotid artery disease: immediate and long-term outcome for 100 consecutive surgical reconstructions. *J Vasc Surg.* 1998;27:34–41; discussion 42.

97. Dikow R, Zeier M, Ritz E. Pathophysiology of cardiovascular disease and renal failure. *Cardiol Clin.* 2005;23:311–317.

98. Guerin AP, Marchais SJ, Metivier F, et al. Arterial structural and functional alterations in uraemia. *Eur J Clin Invest.* 2005;35 Suppl 3:85–88.

99. Nehler MR, Dalman RL, Harris EJ, et al. Upper extremity arterial bypass distal to the wrist. *J Vasc Surg.* 1992;16:633–640; discussion 640–642.

100. Gaines PA, Swarbrick MJ, Lopez AJ, et al. The endovascular management of blue finger syndrome. *Eur J Vasc Endovasc Surg.* 1999;17:106–110.

101. James EC, Khuri NT, Fedde CW, et al. Upper limb ischemia resulting from arterial thromboembolism. *Am J Surg.* 1979;137:739–744.

102. Banis JC, Jr., Rich N, Whelan TJ, Jr. Ischemia of the upper extremity due to noncardiac emboli. *Am J Surg.* 1977;134:131–139.

103. Widlus DM, Venbrux AC, Benenati JF, et al. Fibrinolytic therapy for upper-extremity arterial occlusions. *Radiology.* 1990;175:393–399.

104. Travis JA, Fuller SB, Ligush J Jr, et al. Diagnosis and treatment of paradoxical embolus. *J Vasc Surg.* 2001;34:860–865.

105. Haimovici H. Arterial thromboembolism of the upper extremity associated with the thoracic outlet syndrome. *J Cardiovasc Surg (Torino).* 1982;23:214–220.

106. Scher LA, Veith FJ, Samson RH, et al. Vascular complications of thoracic outlet syndrome. *J Vasc Surg.* 1986;3:565–568.

107. Hood DB, Kuehne J, Yellin AE, et al. Vascular complications of thoracic outlet syndrome. *Am Surg.* 1997;63:913–917.

108. Cheu HW, Mills JL. Digital artery embolization as a result of fibromuscular dysplasia of the brachial artery. *J Vasc Surg.* 1991;14:225–228.

109. Haueisen H, Stierli P, Roeren T. [Fibromuscular dysplasia of the brachial artery—2 case reports and review of the literature.]. *ROFO.* 1999;170:119–122.

110. Lorelli DR, Shepard AD. Hypothenar hammer syndrome: an uncommon and correctable cause of digital ischemia. *J Cardiovasc Surg (Torino)* 2002;43:83–85.

111. McLafferty RB, Taylor LM, Jr., Moneta GL, et al. Upper extremity thromboembolism caused by occlusion of axillofemoral grafts. *Am J Surg.* 1995;169:492–495.

112. Mawatari K, Muto Y, Funahashi S, et al. The potential risk for upper extremity thromboembolism in patients with occluded axillofemoral bypass grafts: two case reports. *Vasc Surg.* 2001;35:67–71.

113. Yao JS. Upper extremity ischemia in athletes. *Semin Vasc Surg.* 1998;11:96–105.

114. Champion HR, Gill W. Arterial embolus to the upper limb. *Br J Surg.* 1973;60:505–508.

115. Puma JA, Haq SA, Sacchi TJ. Acute upper extremity arterial occlusion: a novel role for the use of rheolytic thrombectomy and intravascular ultrasound. *Catheter Cardiovasc Interv.* 2005;66:291–296.
116. Falk RJ, Jennette JC. ANCA small-vessel vasculitis. *J Am Soc Nephrol.* 1997;8:314–322.
117. Jennette JC, Falk RJ. Small-vessel vasculitis. *N Engl J Med.* 1997;337:1512–1523.
118. Numano F, Okawara M, Inomata H, et al. Takayasu's arteritis. *Lancet.* 2000;356:1023–1025.
119. Takayasu M. A case with peculiar changes of the retinal central vessels. *Acta Soc Ophthalmol Jpn.* 1908;12:554–555.
120. Johnston SL, Lock RJ, Gompels MM. Takayasu arteritis: a review. *J Clin Pathol.* 2002;55:481–486.
121. Sheikhzadeh A, Tettenborn I, Noohi F, et al. Occlusive thromboaortopathy (Takayasu disease): clinical and angiographic features and a brief review of literature. *Angiology* 2002;53:29–40.
122. Hall S, Barr W, Lie JT, et al. Takayasu arteritis. A study of 32 North American patients. *Medicine (Baltimore).* 1985;64:89–99.
123. Aluquin VP, Albano SA, Chan F, et al. Magnetic resonance imaging in the diagnosis and follow up of Takayasu's arteritis in children. *Ann Rheum Dis.* 2002;61:526–529.
124. Sharma BK, Jain S, Suri S, et al. Diagnostic criteria for Takayasu arteritis. *Int J Cardiol.* 1996;54 (suppl):S141–S147.
125. Salvarani C, Cantini F, Boiardi L, et al. Polymyalgia rheumatica and giant-cell arteritis. *N Engl J Med.* 2002;347:261–271.
126. Levine SM, Hellmann DB. Giant cell arteritis. *Curr Opin Rheumatol* 2002;14:3–10.
127. Weyand CM, Goronzy JJ. Giant-cell arteritis and polymyalgia rheumatica. *Ann Intern Med* 2003;139:505–515.
128. Stanson AW. Imaging findings in extracranial (giant cell) temporal arteritis. *Clin Exp Rheumatol.* 2000;18:S43–S48.
129. Lambert M, Weber A, Boland B, et al. Large vessel vasculitis without temporal artery involvement: isolated form of giant cell arteritis? *Clin Rheumatol.* 1996;15:174–180.
130. Brack A, Martinez–Taboada V, Stanson A, et al. Disease pattern in cranial and large-vessel giant cell arteritis. *Arthritis Rheum.* 1999;42:311–317.
131. Walz-Leblanc BA, Ameli FM, Keystone EC. Giant cell arteritis presenting as limb claudication. Report and review of the literature. *J Rheumatol.* 1991;18:470–472.
132. Bley TA, Warnatz K, Wieben O, et al. High-resolution MRI in giant cell arteritis with multiple inflammatory stenoses in both calves. *Rheumatology (Oxford).* 2005;44:954–955.
133. Schmidt WA, Natusch A, Moller DE, et al. Involvement of peripheral arteries in giant cell arteritis: a color Doppler sonography study. *Clin Exp Rheumatol.* 2002;20:309–318.
134. Blockmans D, Stroobants S, Maes A, et al. Positron emission tomography in giant cell arteritis and polymyalgia rheumatica: evidence for inflammation of the aortic arch. *Am J Med.* 2000;108:246–249.
135. Klein RG, Hunder GG, Stanson AW, Sheps SG. Large artery involvement in giant cell (temporal) arteritis. Ann Intern Med 1975;83:806–812.
136. Both M, Aries PM, Muller-Hulsbeck S, et al. Balloon angioplasty of arteries of the upper extremities in patients with extracranial giant-cell arteritis. *Ann Rheum Dis.* 2006;65:1124–1130.
137. Bley TA, Uhl M, Venhoff N, et al. 3-T MRI reveals cranial and thoracic inflammatory changes in giant cell arteritis. *Clin Rheumatol.* 2007;26:448–450.
138. Bley TA, Weiben O, Uhl M, et al. Assessment of the cranial involvement pattern of giant cell arteritis with 3T magnetic resonance imaging. *Arthritis Rheum.* 2005;52:2470–2477.
139. Bley TA, Wieben O, Uhl M, et al. Integrated head-thoracic vascular MRI at 3 T: assessment of cranial, cervical and thoracic involvement of giant cell arteritis. *Magma.* 2005;18:193–200.
140. Bley TA, Wieben O, Uhl M, et al. High-resolution MRI in giant cell arteritis: imaging of the wall of the superficial temporal artery. *AJR Am J Roentgenol.* 2005;184:283–287.
141. Bley TA, Wieben O, Vaith P, et al. Magnetic resonance imaging depicts mural inflammation of the temporal artery in giant cell arteritis. *Arthritis Rheum.* 2004;51:1062–1063; author reply 1064.
142. Bley TA, Ness T, Warnatz K, et al. Influence of corticosteroid treatment on MRI findings in giant cell arteritis. *Clin Rheumatol.* 2007;26:1541–1543.
143. Salvarani C, Hunder GG. Giant cell arteritis with low erythrocyte sedimentation rate: frequency of occurence in a population-based study. *Arthritis Rheum.* 2001;45:140–145.
144. Hayreh SS, Podhajsky PA, Raman R, et al. Giant cell arteritis: validity and reliability of various diagnostic criteria. *Am J Ophthalmol.* 1997;123:285–296.
145. Bley TA, Markl M, Wieben O. Inflammatory hyperenhancement persists in delayed high-resolution MRI in giant cell arteritis. *AJR Am J Roentgenol.* 2006;186:1197–1198.
146. Lambeth JT, Yong NK. Arteriographic findings in thromboangiitis obliterans with emphasis on femoropopliteal involvement. *Am J Roentgenol Radium Ther Nucl Med.* 1970;109:553–562.
147. Buchon R, Jacob J, Vicens JL, et al. [Arteriographic aspects of Buerger's disease. Apropos of 18 cases]. *Ann Radiol (Paris).* 1989;32:391–398.
148. Sasaki S, Sakuma M, Kunihara T, et al. Distribution of arterial involvement in thromboangiitis obliterans (Buerger's disease): results of a study conducted by the Intractable Vasculitis Syndromes Research Group in Japan. *Surg Today.* 2000;30:600–605.
149. Pokrovskii AV, Kuntsevich GI, Dan VN, et al. Diagnosis of occlusive lesions of upper extremity arteries in patients with thromboangiitis obliterans. *Angiol Sosud Khir.* 2003;9:86–94.
150. Bozkurt AK, Besirli K, Koksal C, et al. Surgical treatment of Buerger's disease. Vascular 2004;12:192–197.
151. Block JA, Sequeira W. Raynaud's phenomenon. *Lancet.* 2001;357:2042–2048.
152. Wigley FM. Clinical practice. Raynaud's phenomenon. *N Engl J Med.* 2002;347:1001–1008.
153. Kallenberg CG. Early detection of connective tissue disease in patients with Raynaud's phenomenon. *Rheum Dis Clin North Am.* 1990;16:11–30.
154. Kallenberg CG, Wouda AA, Hoet MH, et al. Development of connective tissue disease in patients presenting with Raynaud's phenomenon: a six year follow up with emphasis on the predictive value of antinuclear antibodies as detected by immunoblotting. *Ann Rheum Dis.* 1988;47:634–641.
155. Porter JM, Edwards JM. Occlusive and vasospastic diseases involving distal upper extremity arteries—Raynaud's syndrome. In: Rutherford RB, ed. *Vascular Surgery.* Philadelphia: WB Saunders; 2000:1170–1183.
156. McLafferty RB, Edwards JM, Taylor LM Jr, et al. Diagnosis and long-term clinical outcome in patients diagnosed with hand ischemia. *J Vasc Surg.* 1995;22:361–367; discussion 367–369.
157. Mills JL, Friedman EI, Taylor LM Jr., et al. Upper extremity ischemia caused by small artery disease. *Ann Surg.* 1987;206:521–528.
158. Seibold JR. Critical tissue ischaemia in scleroderma: a note of caution. *Ann Rheum Dis.* 1994;53:289–290.
159. Winterer JT, Scheffler K, Paul G, et al. Optimization of contrast-enhanced MR angiography of the hands with a timing bolus and elliptically reordered 3D pulse sequence. *J Comput Assist Tomogr.* 2000;24:903–908.
160. Ranney D. Thoracic outlet: an anatomical redefinition that makes clinical sense. *Clin Anat.* 1996;9:50–52.
161. Urschel HC, Patel A. Thoracic Outlet Syndromes. *Curr Treat Options Cardiovasc Med.* 2003;5:163–168.
162. Demondion X, Bacqueville E, Paul C, et al. Thoracic outlet: assessment with MR imaging in asymptomatic and symptomatic populations. *Radiology.* 2003;227:461–468.
163. Huang JH, Zager EL. Thoracic outlet syndrome. *Neurosurgery.* 2004;55:897–902; discussion 902–893.

164. Charon JP, Milne W, Sheppard DG, et al. Evaluation of MR angiographic technique in the assessment of thoracic outlet syndrome. *Clin Radiol.* 2004;59:588–595.

165. Andreev A, Kavrakov T, Karakolev J, et al. Management of acute arterial trauma of the upper extremity. *Eur J Vasc Surg.* 1992;6:593–598.

166. Dennis JW, Frykberg ER, Crump JM, et al. New perspectives on the management of penetrating trauma in proximity to major limb arteries. *J Vasc Surg.* 1990;11:84–92; discussion 92–93.

167. Fitridge RA, Raptis S, Miller JH, et al. Upper extremity arterial injuries: experience at the Royal Adelaide Hospital, 1969 to 1991. *J Vasc Surg.* 1994;20:941–946.

168. Schwartz M, Weaver F, Yellin A, et al. The utility of color flow Doppler examination in penetrating extremity arterial trauma. *Am Surg.* 1993;59:375–378.

169. Meissner M, Paun M, Johansen K. Duplex scanning for arterial trauma. *Am J Surg.* 1991;161:552–555.

170. Soto JA, Munera F, Morales C, et al. Focal arterial injuries of the proximal extremities: helical CT arteriography as the initial method of diagnosis. *Radiology.* 2001;218:188–194.

171. Rieger M, Mallouhi A, Tauscher T, Lutz M, Jaschke WR. Traumatic arterial injuries of the extremities: initial evaluation with MDCT angiography. *AJR Am J Roentgenol.* 2006;186:656–664.

172. Yaquinto JJ, Harms SE, Siemers PT, et al. Arterial injury from penetrating trauma: evaluation with single-acquisition fat-suppressed MR imaging. *AJR Am J Roentgenol.* 1992;158:631–633.

173. Castelli P, Caronno R, Piffaretti G, et al. Endovascular repair of traumatic injuries of the subclavian and axillary arteries. *Injury.* 2005;36:778–782.

174. Ohki T, Veith FJ, Kraas C, et al. Endovascular therapy for upper extremity injury. *Semin Vasc Surg* 1998;11:106–115

175. Atteberry LR, Dennis JW, Russo-Alesi F, et al. Changing patterns of arterial injuries associated with fractures and dislocations. *J Am Coll Surg.* 1996;183:377–383.

176. Cone JB. Vascular injury associated with fracture-dislocations of the lower extremity. *Clin Orthop Relat Res.* 1989;243:30–35.

177. Frykberg ER, Dennis JW, Bishop K, Laneve L, Alexander RH. The reliability of physical examination in the evaluation of penetrating extremity trauma for vascular injury: results at one year. *J Trauma.* 1991;31:502–511.

178. Coskunfirat OK, Ozgentas HE. True aneurysm of the radial artery after iatrogenic injury and successful reconstruction with an interposition vein graft. *J Reconstr Microsurg.* 2003;19:143–146.

179. Noguchi M, Hazama S, Tsukasaki S, et al. Iatrogenic pseudoaneurysm in a hemodialysis patient: the hidden hazard of a high radial artery origin. *Heart Vessels.* 2004;19:98–100.

180. Dogan OF, Demircin M, Ucar I, et al. Iatrogenic brachial and femoral artery complications following venipuncture in children. *Heart Surg Forum.* 2006;9:E675–E680.

181. Hildick-Smith DJ, Walsh JT, Lowe MD, et al. Transradial coronary angiography in patients with contraindications to the femoral approach: an analysis of 500 cases. *Catheter Cardiovasc Interv.* 2004;61:60–66.

182. Rubin DI, Schomberg PJ, Shepherd RF, et al. Arteritis and brachial plexus neuropathy as delayed complications of radiation therapy. *Mayo Clin Proc.* 2001;76:849–852.

183. Andros G, Schneider PA, Harris RW, et al. Management of arterial occlusive disease following radiation therapy. *Cardiovasc Surg.* 1996;4:135–142.

184. Budin JA, Casarella WJ, Harisiadis L. Subclavian artery occlusion following radiotherapy for carcinoma of the breast. *Radiology.* 1976;118:169–173.

185. Hashmonai M, Elami A, Kuten A, et al. Subclavian artery occlusion after radiotherapy for carcinoma of the breast. *Cancer.* 1988;61:2015–2018.

186. Aoki S, Hayashi N, Abe O, et al. Radiation-induced arteritis: thickened wall with prominent enhancement on cranial MR images report of five cases and comparison with 18 cases of Moyamoya disease. *Radiology.* 2002;223:683–688.

187. Becker M, Schroth G, Zbaren P, et al. Long-term changes induced by high-dose irradiation of the head and neck region: imaging findings. *Radiographics.* 1997;17:5–26.

188. Yao JS. Occupational vascular problems. In: Rutherford RB, ed. *Vascular Surgery.* Philadelphia: WB Saunders; 2000: 1232–1240.

189. Stoyneva Z, Lyapina M, Tzvetkov D, et al. Current pathophysiological views on vibration-induced Raynaud's phenomenon. *Cardiovasc Res.* 2003;57:615–624.

190. Aleksic M, Heckenkamp J, Gawenda M, et al. Occupation-related vascular disorders of the upper extremity-two case reports. *Angiology.* 2006;57:107–114.

191. Kleinert HE, Volianitis GJ. Thrombosis of the Palmar Arterial Arch and Its Tributaries: Etiology and Newer Concepts in Treatment. *J Trauma.* 1965;83:447–457.

192. Kleinert HE, Burget GC, Morgan JA, et al. Aneurysms of the hand. *Arch Surg.* 1973;106:554–557.

193. Vayssairat M, Debure C, Cormier JM, et al. Hypothenar hammer syndrome: seventeen cases with long-term follow-up. *J Vasc Surg.* 1987;5:838–843.

194. Hammond DC, Matloub HS, Yousif NJ, et al. The corkscrew sign in hypothenar hammer syndrome. *J Hand Surg [Br].* 1993;18:767–769.

195. Ferris BL, Taylor LM, Jr, Oyama K, et al. Hypothenar hammer syndrome: proposed etiology. *J Vasc Surg.* 2000;31:104–113.

196. Pineda CJ, Weisman MH, Bookstein JJ, et al. Hypothenar hammer syndrome. Form of reversible Raynaud's phenomenon. *Am J Med.* 1985;79:561–570.

197. Coulier B, Goffin D, Malbecq S, et al. Colour duplex sonographic and multislice spiral CT angiographic diagnosis of ulnar artery aneurysm in hypothenar hammer syndrome. *Jbr-Btr.* 2003;86:211–214.

198. Drape JL, Feydy A, Guerini H, et al. Vascular lesions of the hand. *Eur J Radiol.* 2005;56:331–343.

199. Vale JA, Proudfoot AT, Meredith TJ. Poisoning from hydrocarbons and chlorofluorocarbons and volatile substance abuse. In: Weatherall DJ, Ledingham JGG, Warrell DA, eds. *Oxford Textbook of Medicine.* Oxford: Oxford University Press; 1996:1083–1093.

200. Falappa P, Magnavita N, Bergamaschi A, et al. Angiographic study of digital arteries in workers exposed to vinyl chloride. *Br J Ind Med.* 1982;39:169–172.

201. Fish R. Electric shock, Part I: Physics and pathophysiology. *J Emerg Med.* 1993;11:309–312.

202. Cooper MA. Lightning injuries: prognostic signs for death. *Ann Emerg Med.* 1980;9:134–138.

203. Vedung S, Arturson G, Wadin K, et al. Angiographic findings and need for amputation in high tension electrical injuries. *Scand J Plast Reconstr Surg Hand Surg.* 1990;24:225–231.

204. McCarthy WJ, Yao JS, Schafer MF, et al. Upper extremity arterial injury in athletes. *J Vasc Surg.* 1989;9:317–327.

205. Urschel HC, Jr., Razzuk MA. Neurovascular compression in the thoracic outlet: changing management over 50 years. *Ann Surg.* 1998;228:609–617.

206. Prandoni P, Polistena P, Bernardi E, et al. Upper-extremity deep vein thrombosis. Risk factors, diagnosis, and complications. *Arch Intern Med.* 1997;157:57–62.

207. Pedrosa I, Aschkenasi C, Hamdan A, et al. Effort-induced thrombosis: diagnosis with three-dimensional MR venography. *Emerg Radiol.* 2002;9:326–328.

208. Mosley JG. Arterial problems in athletes. *Br J Surg.* 2003;90:1461–1469.

209. Moeller S, Gioberge S, Brown G. ESRD patients in 2001: global overview of patients, treatment modalities and development trends. *Nephrol Dial Transplant.* 2002;17:2071–2076.

210. Grassmann A, Gioberge S, Moeller S, et al. ESRD patients in 2004: global overview of patient numbers, treatment modalities and associated trends. *Nephrol Dial Transplant.* 2005;20:2587–2593.

211. Meichelboeck W. ESRD 2005—A Worldwide Overview—Facts, Figures and Trends. In: Mickley V, ed. *4th International Congress of the Vascular Access Society (VAS).* Berlin, Germany: Karger, 2005:227–261.

212. Kherlakian GM, Roedersheimer LR, Arbaugh JJ, et al. Comparison of autogenous fistula versus expanded polytetra-fluoroethylene graft fistula for angioaccess in hemodialysis. *Am J Surg.* 1986;152:238–243.

213. Leapman SB, Boyle M, Pescovitz MD, et al. The arteriovenous fistula for hemodialysis access: gold standard or archaic relic? *Am Surg.* 1996;62:652–656; discussion 656–657.

214. Staramos DN, Lazarides MK, Tzilalis VD, et al. Patency of autologous and prosthetic arteriovenous fistulas in elderly patients. *Eur J Surg.* 2000;166:777–781.

215. III. NKF-K/DOQI Clinical Practice Guidelines for Vascular Access: update 2000. *Am J Kidney Dis.* 2001;37:S137–181.

216. Tordoir JH, Mickley V. European guidelines for vascular access: clinical algorithms on vascular access for haemodialysis. *Edtna Erca J.* 2003;29:131–136.

217. Konner K, Hulbert-Shearon TE, Roys EC, et al. Tailoring the initial vascular access for dialysis patients. *Kidney Int.* 2002;62:329–338.

218. Malovrh M. Noninvasive evaluation of vessels by duplex sonography prior to construction of arteriovenous fistulas for haemodialysis. *Nephrol Dial Transplant.* 1998;13:125–129.

219. Malovrh M. Native arteriovenous fistula: preoperative evaluation. *Am J Kidney Dis.* 2002;39:1218–1225.

220. Mihmanli I, Besirli K, Kurugoglu S, et al. Cephalic vein and hemodialysis fistula: surgeon's observation versus color Doppler ultrasonographic findings. *J Ultrasound Med.* 2001;20:217–222.

221. Zeebregts C, van den Dungen J, Bolt A, et al. Factors predictive of failure of Brescia-Cimino arteriovenous fistulas. *Eur J Surg.* 2002;168:29–36.

222. Beathard GA, Arnold P, Jackson J, et al. Aggressive treatment of early fistula failure. *Kidney Int.* 2003;64:1487–1494.

223. Turmel-Rodrigues L, Mouton A, Birmele B, et al. Salvage of immature forearm fistulas for haemodialysis by interventional radiology. *Nephrol Dial Transplant.* 2001;16:2365–2371.

224. Allon M, Robbin ML. Increasing arteriovenous fistulas in hemodialysis patients: problems and solutions. *Kidney Int.* 2002;62:1109–1124.

225. Hingorani A, Ascher E, Markevich N, et al. Risk factors for mortality in patients with upper extremity and internal jugular deep venous thrombosis. *J Vasc Surg.* 2005;41:476–478.

226. Huber TS, Ozaki CK, Flynn TC, et al. Prospective validation of an algorithm to maximize native arteriovenous fistulae for chronic hemodialysis access. *J Vasc Surg.* 2002;36:452–459.

227. Miller PE, Tolwani A, Luscy CP, et al. Predictors of adequacy of arteriovenous fistulas in hemodialysis patients. *Kidney Int.* 1999;56:275–280.

228. Mustafa S, Stein PD, Patel KC, et al. Upper extremity deep venous thrombosis. *Chest.* 2003;123:1953–1956.

229. Robbin ML, Gallichio MH, Deierhoi MH, et al. US vascular mapping before hemodialysis access placement. *Radiology.* 2000;217:83–88.

230. Tordoir JH, Rooyens P, Dammers R, et al. Prospective evaluation of failure modes in autogenous radiocephalic wrist access for haemodialysis. *Nephrol Dial Transplant.* 2003;18:378–383.

231. Menegazzo D, Laissy JP, Durrbach A, et al. Hemodialysis access fistula creation: preoperative assessment with MR venography and comparison with conventional venography. *Radiology.* 1998;209:723–728.

232. Planken RN, Tordoir JH, Duijm LE, et al. Current techniques for assessment of upper extremity vasculature prior to hemodialysis vascular access creation. *Eur Radiol.* 2007; In Press.

233. Planken RN, Tordoir JH, Dammers R, et al. Stenosis detection in forearm hemodialysis arteriovenous fistulae by multiphase contrast-enhanced magnetic resonance angiography: preliminary experience. *J Magn Reson Imaging.* 2003;17:54–64.

234. Li W, David V, Kaplan R, et al. Three-dimensional low dose gadolinium-enhanced peripheral MR venography. *J Magn Reson Imaging.* 1998;8:630–633.

235. Shinde TS, Lee VS, Rofsky NM, et al. Three-dimensional gadolinium-enhanced MR venographic evaluation of patency of central veins in the thorax: initial experience. *Radiology.* 1999;213:555–560.

236. Ruehm SG, Zimny K, Debatin JF. Direct contrast-enhanced 3D MR venography. *Eur Radiol.* 2001;11:102–112.

237. Ruehm SG. MR venography. *Eur Radiol.* 2003;13:229–230.

238. Lebowitz JA, Rofsky NM, Krinsky GA, et al. Gadolinium-enhanced body MR venography with subtraction technique. *AJR Am J Roentgenol.* 1997;169:755–758.

239. Kroencke TJ, Taupitz M, Arnold R, et al. Three-dimensional gadolinium-enhanced magnetic resonance venography in suspected thrombo-occlusive disease of the central chest veins. *Chest.* 2001;120:1570–1576.

240. Oxtoby JW, Widjaja E, Gibson KM, et al. 3D gadolinium-enhanced MRI venography: evaluation of central chest veins and impact on patient management. *Clin Radiol.* 2001;56:887–894.

241. Haire WD, Lynch TG, Lund GB, et al. Limitations of magnetic resonance imaging and ultrasound-directed (duplex) scanning in the diagnosis of subclavian vein thrombosis. *J Vasc Surg.* 1991;13:391–397.

242. Baarslag HJ, Van Beek EJ, Reekers JA. Magnetic resonance venography in consecutive patients with suspected deep vein thrombosis of the upper extremity: initial experience. *Acta Radiol.* 2004;45:38–43.

243. Shankar KR, Abernethy LJ, Das KS, et al. Magnetic resonance venography in assessing venous patency after multiple venous catheters. *J Pediatr Surg.* 2002;37:175–179.

244. Thornton MJ, Ryan R, Varghese JC, et al. A three-dimensional gadolinium-enhanced MR venography technique for imaging central veins. *AJR Am J Roentgenol.* 1999;173:999–1003.

245. Goyen M, Barkhausen J, Kuehl H, et al. [Contrast-enhanced 3D MR venography of central thoracic veins: preliminary experience]. *Rofo Fortschr Geb Rontgenstr Neuen Bildgeb Verfahr.* 2001;173:356–361.

246. Planken RN, Tordoir JH, Duijm LE, et al. Magnetic resonance angiographic assessment of upper extremity vessels prior to vascular access surgery: feasibility and accuracy. *Eur Radiol.* In press.

247. Shellock FG, Kanal E. Safety of magnetic resonance imaging contrast agents. *J Magn Reson Imaging.* 1999;10:477–484.

248. Cochran ST, Bomyea K, Sayre JW. Trends in adverse events after IV administration of contrast media. *AJR Am J Roentgenol.* 2001;176:1385–1388.

249. Prince MR, Arnoldus C, Frisoli JK. Nephrotoxicity of high-dose gadolinium compared with iodinated contrast. *J Magn Reson Imaging.* 1996;6:162–166.

250. Tombach B, Bremer C, Reimer P, et al. Renal tolerance of a neutral gadolinium chelate (gadobutrol) in patients with chronic renal failure: results of a randomized study. *Radiology.* 2001;218:651–657.

251. Marckmann P, Skov L, Rossen K, et al. Nephrogenic systemic fibrosis: suspected causative role of gadodiamide used for contrast-enhanced magnetic resonance imaging. *J Am Soc Nephrol.* 2006;17:2359–2362.

252. Kuo PH, Kanal E, Abu-Alfa AK, et al. Gadolinium-based MR Contrast Agents and Nephrogenic Systemic Fibrosis. *Radiology.* 2007;242:647–649.

253. Murphy GJ, White SA, Nicholson ML. Vascular access for haemodialysis. *Br J Surg.* 2000;87:1300–1315.

254. Duijm LE, Liem YS, van der Rijt RH, et al. Inflow stenoses in dysfunctional hemodialysis access fistulae and grafts. *Am J Kidney Dis.* 2006;48:98–105.

255. Staple TW. Retrograde venography of subcutaneous arteriovenous fistulas created surgically for hemodialysis. *Radiology*. 1973;106:223–224.

256. Waldman GJ, Pattynama PM, Chang PC, et al. Magnetic resonance angiography of dialysis access shunts: initial results. *Magn Reson Imaging*. 1996;14:197–200.

257. Ko SF, Huang CC, Ng SH, et al. MDCT angiography for evaluation of the complete vascular tree of hemodialysis fistulas. *AJR Am J Roentgenol*. 2005;185:1268–1274.

258. Lin YP, Wu MH, Ng YY, et al. Spiral computed tomographic angiography-a new technique for evaluation of vascular access in hemodialysis patients. *Am J Nephrol*. 1998;18:117–122.

259. Geoffroy O, Tassart M, Le Blanche AF, et al. Upper extremity digital subtraction venography with gadoterate meglumine before fistula creation for hemodialysis. *Kidney Int*. 2001;59:1491–1497.

260. Jansen MA, Hart AA, Korevaar JC, et al. Predictors of the rate of decline of residual renal function in incident dialysis patients. *Kidney Int*. 2002;62:1046–1053.

261. Merkus MP, Jager KJ, Dekker FW, et al. Predictors of poor outcome in chronic dialysis patients: The Netherlands Cooperative Study on the Adequacy of Dialysis. The NECOSAD Study Group. *Am J Kidney Dis*. 2000;35:69–79.

262. Misra S, Woodrum DA, Homburger J, et al. Assessment of wall shear stress changes in arteries and veins of arteriovenous polytetrafluoroethylene grafts using magnetic resonance imaging. *Cardiovasc Intervent Radiol*. 2006;29:624–629.

263. Doelman C, Duijm LE, Liem YS, et al. Stenosis detection in failing hemodialysis access fistulas and grafts: comparison of color Doppler ultrasonography, contrast-enhanced magnetic resonance angiography, and digital subtraction angiography. *J Vasc Surg*. 2005;42:739–746.

264. Froger CL, Duijm LE, Liem YS, et al. Stenosis detection with MR angiography and digital subtraction angiography in dysfunctional hemodialysis access fistulas and grafts. *Radiology*. 2005;234:284–291.

265. Neyman EG, Johnson PT, Fishman EK. Hemodialysis fistula occlusion: demonstration with 64-slice CT angiography. *J Comput Assist Tomogr*. 2006;30:157–159.

266. Willcox TM, Smith AA. Upper limb free flap reconstruction after tumor resection. *Semin Surg Oncol*. 2000;19:246–254.

267. Chepeha DB, Moyer JS, Bradford CR, et al. Osseocutaneous radial forearm free tissue transfer for repair of complex midfacial defects. *Arch Otolaryngol Head Neck Surg*. 2005;131:513–517.

268. Chepeha DB, Wang SJ, Marentette LJ, et al. Radial forearm free tissue transfer reduces complications in salvage skull base surgery. *Otolaryngol Head Neck Surg*. 2004;131:958–963.

269. Wax MK, Rosenthal EL, Winslow CP, et al. The ulnar fasciocutaneous free flap in head and neck reconstruction. *Laryngoscope*. 2002;112:2155–2160.

270. Pederson WC. Upper extremity microsurgery. *Plast Reconstr Surg*. 2001;107:1524–1537; discussion 1538–1529, 1540–1523.

271. Kroger K, Schelo C, Gocke C, et al. Colour Doppler sonographic diagnosis of upper limb venous thromboses. *Clin Sci (Lond)*. 1998;94:657–661.

272. Martinelli I, Battaglioli T, Bucciarelli P, et al. Risk factors and recurrence rate of primary deep vein thrombosis of the upper extremities. *Circulation*. 2004;110:566–570.

273. Pedrosa I, Morrin M, Oleaga L, et al. Is true FISP imaging reliable in the evaluation of venous thrombosis? *AJR Am J Roentgenol*. 2005;185:1632–1640.

274. Fann JI, Wyatt J, Frazier RL, et al. Symptomatic brachial artery aneurysm in a child. *J Pediatr Surg*. 1994;29:1521–1523.

275. Ranero-Juarez GA, Sanchez-Gomez RH, Loza-Jalil SE, et al. Venous aneurysms of the extremities. Report of 4 cases and review of literature. *Angiology*. 2005;56:475–481.

276. Mulliken JB, Glowacki J. Hemangiomas and vascular malformations in infants and children: a classification based on endothelial characteristics. *Plast Reconstr Surg*. 1982;69:412–422.

277. Bruckner AL, Frieden IJ. Hemangiomas of infancy. *J Am Acad Dermatol*. 2003;48:477–493; quiz 494–476.

278. Meyer JS, Hoffer FA, Barnes PD, et al. Biological classification of soft-tissue vascular anomalies: MR correlation. *AJR Am J Roentgenol*. 1991;157:559–564.

279. Upton J, Coombs CJ, Mulliken JB, et al. Vascular malformations of the upper limb: a review of 270 patients. *J Hand Surg [Am]*. 1999;24:1019–1035.

280. Finn MC, Glowacki J, Mulliken JB. Congenital vascular lesions: clinical application of a new classification. *J Pediatr Surg*. 1983;18:894–900.

281. Chiller KG, Passaro D, Frieden IJ. Hemangiomas of infancy: clinical characteristics, morphologic subtypes, and their relationship to race, ethnicity, and sex. *Arch Dermatol*. 2002;138:1567–1576.

282. McClinton MA. Tumors and aneurysms of the upper extremity. *Hand Clin*. 1993;9:151–169.

283. Smolinski KN, Yan AC. Hemangiomas of infancy: clinical and biological characteristics. *Clin Pediatr*. 2005;44:747–766.

284. Boon LM, Mulliken JB, Vikkula M, et al. Assignment of a locus for dominantly inherited venous malformations to chromosome 9p. *Hum Mol Genet*. 1994;3:1583–1587.

285. Breugem CC, Alders M, Salieb-Beugelaar GB, et al. A locus for hereditary capillary malformations mapped on chromosome 5q. *Hum Genet*. 2002;110:343–347.

286. Ben-Izhak O, Kerner H, Brenner B, et al. Angiosarcoma of the colon developing in a capsule of a foreign body. Report of a case with associated hemorrhagic diathesis. *Am J Clin Pathol*. 1992;97:416–420.

287. Rossi G, Iannicelli E, Almberger M, et al. Cystic lymphangioma of the upper extremity: US and MRI correlation (2004:11b). *Eur Radiol*. 2005;15:400–402.

288. Hill RA, Pho RW, Kumar VP. Resection of vascular malformations. *J Hand Surg [Br]*. 1993;18:17–21.

289. Al-Qattan MM, Murray KA, El-Shayeb A. Arteriovenous vascular malformations confined to the hand: an algorithm of management based on a new classification. *J Hand Surg [Br]*. 2006;31:266–273.

290. Hachisuga T, Hashimoto H, Enjoji M. Angioleiomyoma. A clinicopathologic reappraisal of 562 cases. *Cancer*. 1984;54:126–130.

291. Ramesh P, Annapureddy SR, Khan F, et al. Angioleiomyoma: a clinical, pathological and radiological review. *Int J Clin Pract*. 2004;58:587–591.

292. Calle SC, Eaton RG, Littler JW. Vascular leiomyomas in the hand. *J Hand Surg [Am]*. 1994;19:281–286.

293. Kataoka M, Yano H, Fukunaga T, et al. Giant vascular leiomyoma in the hand. *Scand J Plast Reconstr Surg Hand Surg*. 1997;31:91–93.

294. Uchida M, Kojima T, Hirase Y, et al. Clinical characteristics of vascular leiomyoma of the upper extremity: report of 11 cases. *Br J Plast Surg*. 1992;45:547–549.

295. Moritomo H, Murase T, Ebara R, et al. Massive vascular leiomyoma of the hand. *Scand J Plast Reconstr Surg Hand Surg*. 2003;37:125–127.

296. Nagata S, Nishimura H, Uchida M, et al. Giant angioleiomyoma in extremity: report of two cases. *Magn Reson Med Sci*. 2006;5:113–118.

297. Hwang JW, Ahn JM, Kang HS, et al. Vascular leiomyoma of an extremity: MR imaging-pathology correlation. *AJR Am J Roentgenol*. 1998;171:981–985.

298. Gomez-Dermit V, Gallardo E, Landeras R, et al. Subcutaneous angioleiomyomas: gray-scale and color Doppler sonographic appearances. *J Clin Ultrasound*. 2006;34:50–54.

299. Lim ST, Kim MW, Sohn MH. Tc-99m RBC perfusion and blood-pool scintigraphy in the evaluation of vascular leiomyoma of the hand. *Ann Nucl Med*. 2002;16:293–296.

300. Yagi K, Hamada Y, Yasui N. A leiomyoma arising from the deep palmar arterial arch. *J Hand Surg [Br]*. 2006;31:680–682.

301. Herron MD, Coffin CM, Vanderhooft SL. Tufted angiomas: variability of the clinical morphology. *Pediatr Dermatol.* 2002;19:394–401.
302. Enjolras O, Wassef M, Mazoyer E, et al. Infants with Kasabach-Merritt syndrome do not have "true" hemangiomas. *J Pediatr.* 1997;130:631–640.
303. Tsuneyoshi M, Enjoji M. Glomus tumor: a clinicopathologic and electron microscopic study. *Cancer.* 1982;50:1601–1607.
304. Heys SD, Brittenden J, Atkinson P, et al. Glomus tumour: an analysis of 43 patients and review of the literature. *Br J Surg.* 1992;79:345–347.
305. Looi KP, Teh M, Pho RW. An unusual case of multiple recurrence of a glomangioma. *J Hand Surg [Br].* 1999;24:387–389.
306. Schiefer TK, Parker WL, Anakwenze OA, et al. Extradigital glomus tumors: a 20-year experience. *Mayo Clin Proc.* 2006;81:1337–1344.
307. Brouillard P, Boon LM, Mulliken JB, et al. Mutations in a novel factor, glomulin, are responsible for glomuvenous malformations ("glomangiomas"). *Am J Hum Genet.* 2002;70:866–874.
308. Bhaskaranand K, Navadgi BC. Glomus tumour of the hand. *J Hand Surg [Br].* 2002;27:229–231.
309. Giele H. Hildreth's test is a reliable clinical sign for the diagnosis of glomus tumours. *J Hand Surg [Br].* 2002;27:157–158.
310. Takata H, Ikuta Y, Ishida O, Kimori K. Treatment of subungual glomus tumour. *Hand Surg.* 2001;6:25–27.
311. Fornage BD. Glomus tumors in the fingers: diagnosis with US. *Radiology.* 1988;167:183–185.
312. Theumann NH, Goettmann S, Le Viet D, et al. Recurrent glomus tumors of fingertips: MR imaging evaluation. *Radiology.* 2002;223:143–151.
313. Al-Qattan MM, Al-Namla A, Al-Thunayan A, et al. Magnetic resonance imaging in the diagnosis of glomus tumours of the hand. *J Hand Surg [Br].* 2005;30:535–540.
314. Kim JK, Won JH, Cho YK, et al. Glomus tumor of the stomach: CT findings. *Abdom Imaging.* 2001;26:303–305.
315. Memis A, Arkun R, Ustun EE, et al. Magnetic resonance imaging of intramuscular haemangiomas with emphasis on contrast enhancement patterns. *Clin Radiol.* 1996;51:198–204.
316. Ibarra RA, Kesava P, Hallet KK, et al. Hemangioendothelioma of the temporal bone with radiologic findings resembling hemangioma. *AJNR Am J Neuroradiol.* 2001;22:755–758.
317. Bruegel M, Waldt S, Weirich G, et al. Multifocal epithelioid hemangioendothelioma of the phalanges of the hand. *Skeletal Radiol.* 2006;35:787–792.
318. Roy P, Clark MA, Thomas JM. Stewart-Treves syndrome-treatment and outcome in six patients from a single centre. *Eur J Surg Oncol.* 2004;30:982–986.
319. Westenberg AH, Wiggers T, Henzen-Logmans SC, et al. Post-irradiation angiosarcoma of the greater omentum. *Eur J Surg Oncol.* 1989;15:175–178.
320. Monroe AT, Feigenberg SJ, Mendenhall NP. Angiosarcoma after breast-conserving therapy. *Cancer.* 2003;97:1832–1840.
321. Jennings TA, Peterson L, Axiotis CA, et al. Angiosarcoma associated with foreign body material. A report of three cases. *Cancer.* 1988;62:2436–2444.
322. Sinclair SA, Sviland L, Natarajan S. Angiosarcoma arising in a chronically lymphoedematous leg. *Br J Dermatol.* 1998;138:692–694.
323. Sugita R, Takezawa M, Itinohasama R. Primary angiosarcoma of the chest wall: CT and MR findings. *Radiat Med.* 2002;20:101–103.
324. Kauffman SL SA. Haemangiopericytoma in children. *Cancer.* 1960;13:695–710.
325. Enzinger FM, Smith BH. Hemangiopericytoma. An analysis of 106 cases. *Hum Pathol.* 1976;7:61–82.
326. O'Hara M. A clinico-pathological study of infantile hemangiopericytoma. *Pathol Res Prac.* 1989;185:114–115.
327. Jenkins JJ, 3rd. Congenital malignant hemangiopericytoma. *Pediatr Pathol.* 1987;7:119–122.
328. Kasdan ML, Stallings SP. Malignant hemangiopericytoma of the forearm. *Plast Reconstr Surg.* 1993;91:533–536.
329. Alpern MB, Thorsen MK, Kellman GM, et al. CT appearance of hemangiopericytoma. *J Comput Assist Tomogr.* 1986;10:264–267.
330. Kato N, Kato S, Ueno H. Hemangiopericytoma: characteristic features observed by magnetic resonance imaging and angiography. *J Dermatol.* 1990;17:701–706.
331. Babal P, Pec J. Kaposi's sarcoma - still an enigma. *J Eur Acad Dermatol Venereol.* 2003;17:377–380.
332. Cottoni F, Masala MV, Piras P, et al. Mucosal involvement in classic Kaposi's sarcoma. *Br J Dermatol.* 2003;148:1273–1274.
333. Leu HJ, Odermatt B. Multicentric angiosarcoma (Kaposi's sarcoma). Light and electron microscopic and immunohistological findings of idiopathic cases in Europe and Africa and of cases associated with AIDS. *Virchows Arch A Pathol Anat Histopathol* 1985;408:29–41.
334. Walsh JJt, Eady JL. Vascular tumors. *Hand Clin.* 2004;20:261–268, v–vi.
335. Amsbaugh S, Huiras E, Wang NS, et al. Bacillary angiomatosis associated with pseudoepitheliomatous hyperplasia. *Am J Dermatopathol.* 2006;28:32–35.

Pediatric Techniques and Vascular Anomalies

CHAPTER 23

Orhan Konez
Katharine L. Hopkins
Patricia E. Burrows

BACKGROUND AND IMPORTANCE

Pediatric vascular anomalies (commonly referred to as *birthmarks* or *vascular birthmarks*) are a heterogeneous group of lesions for which numerous classification systems have been proposed. The most commonly used classification system, based on endothelial characteristics of different lesions, is derived from work of Mulliken and Glowacki (1). It divides pediatric vascular anomalies into two categories (Table 23-1). Vascular tumors—including hemangiomas and hemangioendotheliomas—are proliferative endothelial cell neoplasms. Most hemangiomas tumors develop during infancy, proliferate rapidly, stabilize for a period of time,

and then slowly regress (2). In contrast, vascular malformations are developmental anomalies of vasculogenesis and angiogenesis, composed of dysplastic vessels. They generally are present at birth, grow in proportion to the body during childhood, and do not involute. Vascular malformations are classified further according to flow characteristics—high or low—and predominant channel involvement—arteriovenous (AVM), capillary (CM), venous (VM), lymphatic (LM), or combined (2,3).

Morbidity associated with pediatric vascular anomalies is variable and is influenced by lesion type, size, location, and behavior. Mass effect may cause compression of vital structures, airway compromise, or visual impairment. Other

TABLE 23-1

Classification of Vascular Anomalies

I. Hemangiomas and Congenital Vascular Tumors	Infantile hemangioma Rapidly involuting congenital hemangioma (RICH) Noninvoluting congenital hemangioma (NICH) Intramuscular hemangioma Kaposiform hemangioendothelioma (KHE)
II. Vascular Malformations A. High flow	Arteriovenous malformation (AVM) Arteriovenous fistula (AVF)
B. Low flow	Venous malformation (VM) Lymphatic malformation (LM) Lymphatic-venous Malformation (LVM) Capillary malformation (CM) (port-wine stain)
C. Combined i. High flow	Parkes-Weber syndrome (CAVM or CLAVM with limb overgrowth)
ii. Low flow	Klippel-Trenaunay syndrome (CLVM with limb overgrowth) Maffucci syndrome (VM-like lesions with enchondromatosis) Proteus syndrome, Banayan Riley Rubalcava syndrome

Note: High- or low-flow grouping solely based on the flow dynamics within the lesion. If there is a rapid arteriovenous shunt, the lesion is considered high flow, if not, it is considered a low-flow anomaly.

Source: Mullikan JB, Glowacki J. Hemangiomas and vascular malformations in infants and children: a classification based on endothelial characteristics. *Plast Reconstr Surg.* 1982;69:412–420.

local complications such as ulceration, infection, hemorrhage, and ischemia may occur (4,5). Systemic effects, which may be life threatening, include high-output congestive heart failure, anemia, consumptive coagulopathy, and altered drug pharmacokinetics (2,4,6). In some children, diffuse vascular malformations are associated with inhibition or acceleration of bone growth, soft tissue hypertrophy, ectopic adipose tissue, and limb gigantism (7,8). Vascular lesions may also cause considerable disfigurement—either temporary or permanent—with secondary effects on self-image and psychosocial development. Many of the pediatric vascular anomalies occur as part of syndromes. Familial forms are less common than sporadic ones. Characteristics of individual lesions as well as frequently associated syndromes will be discussed in detail in this chapter.

In total, pediatric vascular anomalies are quite common. Hemangioma is diagnosed in 10% to 12% of infants and children and is the most frequently encountered pediatric soft tissue neoplasm (3,4,8). Venous malformations, many of which are silent, are estimated to occur in up to 50% of the general population (9). Since some lesions result in greater morbidity and require more aggressive therapy than others, accurate diagnosis has important implications with respect to treatment and prognosis (2,4).

IMAGING STRATEGIES

Overview

Many pediatric vascular anomalies can be correctly diagnosed based on clinical presentation and physical examination alone; others require diagnostic imaging. The characteristic imaging features are summarized in Table 23-2. Sonography is often the first imaging study performed. Grayscale sonography, spectral analysis, and color Doppler ultrasound all have value in characterizing vascular lesions (5,10). The advantages of ultrasound are that it uses no ionizing radiation; requires no sedation or contrast administration; and is noninvasive, relatively inexpensive, and readily available. Disadvantages of ultrasound include limited soft tissue differentiation, poor echo transmission through air and bone, and operator dependence. Radiologists and sonographers who are inexperienced with respect to the sonographic evaluation of vascular anomalies may have difficulty differentiating the lesions.

Magnetic resonance imaging (MRI) and computed tomography (CT) complement sonography and, particularly when lesions are large or complex, provide additional information about soft tissue content and extent (3,10). Because of their excellent spatial resolution and

TABLE 23-2

Imaging Findings in Pediatric Vascular Anomalies

Lesion	Subset	Ultrasound	Magnetic Resonance Imaging				Computed Tomography	Angiography
			GRE	T1WI	T2WI	CE T1WI		
Vascular Tumors								
Hemangioma	Proliferating	STM with HFV; low RI	HFV in and around STM	STM; iso- or hypointense to muscle; flow voids	High signal, lobulated STM; flow voids	STM with uniform, intense enhancement	STM with uniform, dense enhancement; dilated vessels	Dilated feeding arteries and veins; capillary stain
	Involuting	As above	As above					As above
	Involuted	Echogenic avascular STM	No HFV	Variable fat content High signal (fat)	Variable fat content Decreased signal (fat)	No enhancement	Variable fat content Fat density; no enhancement	Avascular
Kaposiform hemangioendothelioma		Diffuse infiltrating STM with HVF	Mildly dilated vessels in and around STM	Diffuse STM; STT and skin thickening	Diffuse increased signal; subcutaneous stranding	Diffuse enhancement	Diffuse, enhancing STM; subcutaneous stranding	Hypervascular; diffuse capillary stain
Vascular Malformations								
Arteriovenous malformation		HFV with low RI; AV shunt; +/− STT	HVF throughout	STT; flow voids	Variable increased signal; flow voids	Diffuse enhancement	Enhancing vessels and STT	Dilated feeding arteries; nidus; early opacification of draining veins
Capillary malformation		Not seen						
Venous malformation		Heterogeneous STM; low velocity flow; compressible	No HFV; signal voids due to phleboliths	Signal isointense to muscle; +/− high signal thrombi	Septated, high-signal STM; signal voids due to phleboliths	Diffuse or heterogeneous enhancement	STM with variable enhancement; lamellated calcifications (phleboliths)	Contrast puddling on venous phase; sinusoidal spaces and varices on direct injection
Lymphatic malformation	Macrocystic	Cystic STM; +/− vessels in septae	No HFV	Low signal, septated STM	High-signal STM with fluid/fluid levels	Rim or no enhancement	STM; low attenuation; no or rim enhancement	Avascular STM; dilated or anomalous veins
	Microcystic	Echogenic STT; avascular	No HFV	STT; hypo- or isointense to muscle	Diffuse increased signal; subcutaneous stranding	No enhancement	Diffuse STT; nonenhancing subcutaneous stranding	Avascular STM or capillary staining

GRE, gradient recalled echo; T1WI, T1-weighted image; T2WI, T2-weighted image; CE T1WI, contrast-enhanced T1-weighted image; STM, soft tissue mass; HVF, high-flow vessels; STT, soft tissue thickening; AV, arteriovenous.
Source: Modified from Burrows PE, Laor T, Paltiel H, et al. Diagnostic imaging in the evaluation of vascular birthmarks. *Dermatol Clin.* 1998;16:455–488.

three-dimensional (3D) display capabilities, MRI and CT are superior techniques for defining positional relationships with respect to deep organs and vital structures. Magnetic resonance angiography (MRA) and computed tomographic angiography (CTA) may also be used to delineate feeding arteries and draining veins prior to interventional or surgical treatment (11,12). In patients with vascular syndromes, information may be gained from these modalities regarding associated anomalies as well. In many cases, invasive arteriography is only necessary for purposes of embolization (3).

Magnetic Resonance Imaging and Magnetic Resonance Angiography

MRI is the noninvasive imaging modality of choice for diagnosing and characterizing pediatric vascular anomalies (3,8,10). In comparison to ultrasound, MRI provides superior soft tissue differentiation and better defines positional relationships. In comparison to CT, MRI has three important advantages. It allows assessment of flow dynamics for distinguishing low-flow from high-flow lesions. It provides superior soft tissue characterization, and it uses no ionizing radiation.

Noninvasive MRA is being used with increasing frequency to map out feeding arteries and draining veins in vascular lesions that require sclerotherapy, transcatheter embolization, or surgical resection. MR angiograms rival conventional catheter angiograms in quality and are relatively noninvasive. They are performed at the same time as standard diagnostic MRI, are typically achieved without additional sedation, and, in contrast to CTA and conventional angiography, do not use ionizing radiation. 3D contrast-enhanced (CE) MRA can be repeated multiple times during arterial and venous phases of enhancement, providing time-resolved images without cumulative radiation exposure. Accordingly, MRA has a distinct safety advantage over other angiographic techniques for pediatric imaging (13). In addition, it has greater sensitivity than CTA and conventional angiography for low-flow vascular malformations.

During assessment of pediatric vascular anomalies, particularly those associated with specific syndromes, MRI and MRA are valuable tools for defining related abnormalities. For example, in patients with low-flow vascular malformations of an extremity, magnetic resonance venography (MRV) may be used to search for concomitant abnormalities of the superficial and deep venous systems (Klippel-Trenaunay syndrome [KTS]) (3). Similarly, in patients with suspected PHACES (anomalies of the *P*osterior fossa, facial *H*emangiomas, cervical and cerebral *A*rteries, *C*ardiovascular system, *E*ye and ear, and *S*ternum) syndrome, MRI and MRA provide information about facial hemangiomas as well as anomalies of the posterior fossa, heart, aorta, and head and neck arteries (14).

The primary disadvantages of MRI and MRA are that they may be lengthy, noisy, and potentially frightening examinations for children. Special measures must be taken to reduce motion and eliminate anxiety during scanning. Technical parameters must also be modified to accommodate pediatric patients. Rapid scanning techniques should be used whenever possible.

Equipment

MRI scanners have undergone considerable development over the past decade. Improved gradient performance has reduced scan time, making vascular and soft tissue imaging much easier to perform in infants and children. Although techniques reported in this chapter are optimized for 1.5 T MRI scanners, the U.S. Food and Drug Administration (FDA) has recently approved use of field strengths up to 4 T for clinical imaging. To date, experience with high-field-strength MRI in children is limited, but benefits are likely to include improved signal-to-noise ratio (SNR), increased spatial and contrast resolution, better delineation of small vascular and soft tissue abnormalities, reduced scan duration, and lower contrast doses (15–17). In order to maximize application of these benefits to the pediatric population, concomitant advances in support equipment will be necessary. At this time, commercial MRI-compatible pulse oximeters and power injectors are available for high-field-strengths magnets, while MRI-compatible anesthesia infusion pumps and ventilators are only marketed for use in field strengths up to 1.5 T.

Sedation

The vast majority of children younger than 6 years of age require sedation for MRI. On occasion, even older children may benefit from sedation, particularly if they are developmentally delayed or if imaging protocols are long in duration. Sedation is more often needed for MRI than for CT due to longer scan duration, noisier image acquisition, and more intimidating gantry configuration (18).

To avoid complications of sedation, such as aspiration, respiratory arrest, hypoxic-ischemic brain injury, and death, safeguards must be implemented (18,19). Both the American Academy of Pediatrics and the American Society of Anesthesiologists have published guidelines recommending development and implementation of a structured sedation program by every institution at which pediatric sedation is performed (20,21). While prescribing sedation according to such guidelines is relatively safe and effective, sedating children without a structured policy may have disastrous consequences for the patient (19,22–26). Each institutional sedation program should address variables that influence the safety and efficacy of pediatric sedation, including education and availability of personnel, patient screening, preparation and monitoring practices, sedative prescription, and complication preparedness. Only experienced persons who are capable of providing pediatric life support should administer sedation. Pediatric resuscitation equipment must be immediately available, and patients should be carefully chosen, prepared, and monitored (18).

Because patient visibility is limited in the MRI scanner, continuous electronic monitoring of sedated children is particularly important during scanning. MRI-compatible pulse oximeters with pediatric probes should be used with appropriate precautions to prevent thermal injury. MRI-compatible electrocardiographic equipment, blood pressure monitoring devices, and ventilators are commercially available as well and may be used when clinically indicated.

Certain patients with vascular anomalies—including those with mass lesions adjacent to the airway and those with systemic hemodynamic compromise—require special consideration when undergoing sedation for imaging procedures. Because endotracheal intubation, assisted ventilation, and pharmacologic support may be necessary, sedation is best performed in such cases by an anesthesiologist or other specialist experienced in advanced pediatric airway and circulatory management. Whenever possible, unstable respiratory or hemodynamic status should be corrected before the patient is transported to the imaging department.

A number of different sedatives are effective for pediatric imaging. Oral chloral hydrate (50 to 100 mg/kg; maximum dose 200 mg) is the most commonly used sedative in infants under 18 months of age. In children 18 months of age or older, intravenous sodium pentobarbital is the most widely used agent (2 to 6 mg/kg titrated slowly to effect; maximum dose 200 mg in children weighing <55 kg or 300 mg in children weighing >55 kg). A detailed review of safe sedation practices and available sedatives can be found in recent review articles (18,27).

Respiratory Motion

Short repetition time (TR) and echo time (TE) sequences that can be completed during a single breath hold negate the adverse effects of respiratory motion on MR image quality and are useful when imaging cooperative patients who have lesions in the chest or upper abdomen. When imaging uncooperative or sedated children who are unable to hold their breath, other techniques must be implemented to compensate for respiratory motion. The most commonly used technique is signal averaging, by which each phase-encoding step is repeated a number of times. The phase-

encoding data are averaged, improving the SNR and reducing motion artifact. The disadvantage of this technique is that imaging time increases in direct proportion to the number of signals averaged (28).

Respiratory gating techniques have also been developed to reduce respiratory motion artifact. Respiratory gating synchronizes signal readout to occur at a consistent phase of the respiratory cycle, usually end-expiration, when motion is at a minimum. In patients with regular respiratory rates, images with sharper anatomic detail and reduced ghosting artifact are produced, but imaging time is increased because data acquisition is limited to a portion of the respiratory cycle. This technique is used predominantly with T2-weighted fast spin echo (FSE) sequences and is not compatible with T1-weighted imaging (29).

With respiratory ordered phase encoding (ROPE), phase-encoding steps are reordered according to the respiratory cycle, based on the patient's breathing pattern at the beginning of the examination. Without increasing imaging time, ROPE minimizes ghosting artifact but does not eliminate image blurring (28,30). It is incompatible with FSE sequences due to the phase-ordering requirements of those sequences (31).

Clinical Protocols

Sequences commonly used for evaluating pediatric vascular anomalies are listed in Table 23-3. MRI protocols commonly begin with a bright blood gradient recalled echo (GRE) sequence to detect high-flow vessels. Presence of high-flow vessels distinguishes AVMs and hemangiomas from other pediatric vascular anomalies. For characterizing soft tissue content and defining lesion extent, T1-weighted spin echo (SE) sequences (with and without intravenous contrast) and T2-weighted FSE sequences are used. Both T1-weighted CE SE and T2-weighted FSE sequences are performed with frequency-selective fat saturation to increase conspicuity of lesions relative to fat.

When imaging hepatic hemangiomas and hemangioendotheliomas, dynamic CE MRI scanning is desirable for demonstrating characteristic early peripheral puddling of contrast and delayed central enhancement. Rapid T1-weighted gradient-echo images are obtained either throughout the lesion or at a single location at 20- to 60-second intervals for up to 10 minutes (32,33).

Because pediatric vascular anomalies may be larger than is apparent on physical examination, imaging should begin with a large field of view (FOV). Once the boundaries of a vascular lesion have been defined, application of a narrow FOV will increase spatial resolution. Reducing slice thickness also improves spatial resolution. Thicknesses of 3 to 6 mm are commonly used in infants and children.

TABLE 23-3

Magnetic Resonance Imaging and Magnetic Resonance Angiography of Pediatric Vascular Anomalies

Favored Sequences	Alternatives
Bright blood GRE	
T1-weighted SE	
T2-weighted FSE with fat saturation	Short tau inversion recovery (STIR)
Time-resolved contrast-enhanced 3D spoiled gradient recalled echo (SPGR) MR DSA	TOF angiography, 2D or 3D; PC angiography, 2D or 3D
OR	
Dynamic CE T1-weighted SPGR (for hepatic vascular tumors only)	
CE T1-weighted SE with fat saturation	

Reducing slice thickness has the disadvantage of prolonging scan duration, which may result indirectly in patients awakening or moving before completion of all desired sequences. Accordingly, the need for increased spatial resolution should be carefully weighed and, if possible, counterbalanced by use of rapid imaging sequences and streamlined imaging protocols.

The acquisition matrix (referring to the number of frequency-encoding steps × phase-encoding steps) has a direct relationship on both spatial resolution and scan duration. A 256 × 192 matrix is used for most SE sequences. When imaging small body parts or when using a large FOV, increased matrix size (up to 512 × 384) may be necessary to preserve resolution (28).

Although reducing FOV, reducing slice thickness, and increasing the acquisition matrix will improve spatial resolution in pediatric MRI, it also reduces the SNR. In order to maintain an adequate SNR, surface coils must be used. Very few surface coils have been designed specifically for imaging children. Therefore, creative use of surface coils designed for adults is necessary. Infants can be placed in standard adult head surface coils to image any body part. Older children are scanned with adult extremity, torso, or other surface coils. The smallest available surface coil that will cover the region of interest should be used. Especially when patients are sedated and unable to communicate, meticulous attention must be paid to manufacturer-recommended safety precautions in order to prevent serious thermal injuries.

When formulating MRI protocols, radiologists should keep in mind that scanning might be terminated prematurely if children awaken from sedation or are unable to be still. Imaging sequences that are critical to diagnosis should always be performed first, with additional sequences added only as time permits. A combination of sequences in at least two planes is used to maximize diagnostic yield in the available scan time. Familiarity with associated anomalies and characteristic patterns of disease distribution is required to ensure that a comprehensive diagnostic scan is completed.

MRA of pediatric vascular anomalies and associated syndromes may be performed in a number of ways. The most commonly used methods are time of flight (TOF), phase contrast (PC), and CE 3D MRA. With TOF angiography, contrast is achieved by subjecting stationary tissue to repeated radio frequency (RF) pulses until spins become saturated and give off relatively little signal. In comparison, fully magnetized spins entering the imaging volume, such as those in flowing blood, give off a large signal (34). Both two-dimensional (2D) and 3D TOF acquisitions are possible.

In 2D TOF, contiguous cross-sectional GRE images are generated in a plane perpendicular to the vessels of interest, usually the axial plane. By application of a spatial presaturation band proximal or distal to the imaging volume, either arterial or venous signal can be suppressed. Use of thin slices (on the order of 2 mm) reduces saturation of blood as it flows through the imaging plane. Flip angle and TR also affect the degree to which in-plane flow is saturated. Low flip angles (30 to 60 degrees) favor signal from slow-flowing blood, whereas high flip angles (60 to 90 degrees) favor signal from fast-flowing blood. At the same time, as the flip angle increases, unwanted signal from stationary tissue decreases. A flip angle of 60 degrees is often chosen in compromise (34). A long TR (>40 milliseconds) reduces saturation of in-plane flow but lengthens imaging time. A short TE reduces intravoxel dephasing, the phenomenon by which spins with different phases in the same voxel interfere with one another, resulting in signal loss (34).

Two-dimensional TOF MRA is degraded by presence of short T1 intravascular thrombus, which may mimic or obscure flowing blood. Due to in-plane saturation effects, the technique is potentially insensitive to slowly flowing blood and to vessels coursing parallel to the imaging plane. In addition to intravoxel dephasing, 2D TOF MRA is susceptible to ghosting artifacts from respiration and pulsatile flow (34).

For 3D TOF MRA, an RF pulse is applied to the entire imaging volume, rather than to individual slices, with every TR. The data are then segmented into individual slices by Fourier transformation. Because SNR depends on data from the entire imaging volume rather than from individual slices, SNR is greater for 3D than for 2D TOF. Three-dimensional imaging also permits smaller voxel dimensions, yielding isotropic spatial resolution and reduced intravoxel dephasing. The major disadvantage of 3D TOF imaging is that blood becomes progressively saturated as it flows through the larger imaging volume, resulting in signal variance along the length of a vessel. To diminish this effect, flip angle is reduced to 30 to 40 degrees and, in some cases, is varied as a function of depth in the volume. Choosing a TE such that fat and water are out of phase (e.g., 2.3 or 6.8 milliseconds at 1.5 T) helps to suppress background signal in the setting of a smaller flip angle. TR is lengthened to increase T1 recovery (34).

In PC angiography, contrast is achieved by manipulating the phases of spinning protons such that those in flowing blood are different than those in stationary tissues. The result is that signal intensity is proportional to flow velocity. Unlike TOF angiography, PC techniques can be used to quantify velocity and flow, to determine direction of flow, and to differentiate flowing blood from thrombus. PC angiography has excellent background suppression and can be sensitized to slow flow. Like TOF, it can be acquired in either 2D or 3D modes (34).

Two-dimensional PC imaging is performed in thick slabs rather than thin slices and requires a very short scan time. It is susceptible to intravoxel dephasing, and, unlike TOF techniques, does not provide cross-sectional source data perpendicular to the vessels of interest. Nor does it allow reprojection of angiographic images from any angle (34).

When performing PC angiography, one must specify a velocity-encoding value (Venc). PC images have the greatest sensitivity to blood flowing at velocities close to the Venc (34). When imaging pediatric vascular anomalies, it is sometimes useful to repeat rapid 2D PC acquisitions with different Venc values. Images performed with a low Venc (10 to 20 cm/second) are relatively sensitive to slow-flow and draining veins, whereas images performed with a high Venc (100 cm/second) better demonstrate high-flow lesions and feeding arteries (34).

The acquisition principles for 3D PC angiography are similar to those for 3D TOF. Data for the entire imaging volume are acquired with every TR and then segmented into individual slices by Fourier transformation. Three-dimensional PC imaging takes longer to perform than either 2D PC or 3D TOF imaging. Advantages include sensitivity to slow flow, high SNR, and good background suppression. Three-dimensional PC imaging has better spatial resolution and less susceptibility to intravoxel dephasing than 2D PC imaging. It is more susceptible to dephasing than 3D TOF. Postprocessing allows angular reprojection of angiographic images (34).

CE MRA has become the noninvasive angiographic method of choice for imaging many vascular anomalies. A T1-shortening agent is injected intravenously, and rapid 3D T1-weighted spoiled gradient echo (SPGR) imaging is performed during enhancement of the target vasculature. Gradient echo pulse sequences allow rapid data acquisition. Spoiling of residual magnetization after each echo improves T1 contrast and suppresses background signal. Because CE MRA does not rely on flow and phase-shift effects for intravascular contrast, motion and flow artifacts associated with TOF and PC imaging are not encountered (13).

Data for 3D CE MRA are collected over the entire scan time, resulting in excellent SNR. Isotropic spatial resolution can be achieved with submillimeter section thicknesses. Generally, a TE close to 2.3 milliseconds is used. This TE improves background suppression at 1.5 T, since signals from fat and water are out of phase. In addition, it minimizes the effects of dephasing and T2* signal decay. To reduce scan time, TR is shortened as much as possible, preferably without broadening bandwidth above 32 kHz. Narrower bandwidths improve SNR. Flip angles of 45 to 60 degrees are favored for arterial phase imaging, high-contrast doses, and long TRs, while flip angles of 30 to 45 degrees are reserved for venous phase imaging, lower contrast doses, and ultrashort TRs (<5 milliseconds) (13).

With 3D CE MRA, large FOV imaging can be performed in the plane of the vessels of interest, reducing both the number of slices and the amount of time necessary to image a large vascular territory. Partial Fourier imaging reduces scan time further by decreasing the number of phase-encoding steps without diminishing image resolution (13). On MRI scanners with high-performance gradients, imaging can be completed in seconds and, in patients who are old enough to cooperate, within a single breath hold.

Although many techniques have been described for CE MRA, time-resolved 3D MR digital subtraction angiography

(DSA) is best suited for evaluating pediatric vascular anomalies. With time-resolved 3D MR DSA, very rapid scanning allows acquisition of complete data sets before arrival of contrast in the target vessels as well as during arterial, parenchymal, and venous phases of enhancement. Digital subtraction is then performed to separate the vascular phases and improve the contrast-to-noise ratio (13). Patterns of contrast enhancement can be evaluated in addition to relative rates of enhancement in feeding arteries and draining veins.

A major benefit of time-resolved 3D MR DSA techniques in pediatric imaging is that precise bolus timing is unnecessary. Contrast is injected rapidly, usually at a rate of 2 to 3 mL/second, and serial acquisitions of less than or equal to 10-second duration are performed in rapid succession. At least one acquisition will certainly coincide with the arterial phase of enhancement, and at least one will coincide with the venous phase of enhancement. Accordingly, there is no need for use of bolus-tracking techniques or test injections to determine contrast arrival time in the target vasculature (13).

For optimal isolation of arterial and venous phases in children with rapid recirculation times, temporal resolution must be maximized. Most high-performance MRI scanners are now capable of completing a 3D MRA acquisition in 6 to 10 seconds. Data processing techniques have been developed to improve temporal resolution further. 3D TRICKS (3D time-resolved imaging on contrast kinetics) is one such method. It uses frequent central k-space sampling, zero-filling, and temporal interpolation of data to generate 3D images as frequently as every 2 seconds (13).

For targeted 3D CE MRV of an extremity, direct venography has also been described (35). Peripheral intravenous access is secured in the affected extremity, and contrast is injected directly into the venous system during imaging. A relatively high-contrast dose is used (0.3 mmol gadolinium chelate/kg), diluted at least 10:1 with normal saline to prevent signal loss from T2 shortening and to allow prolonged injection. 3D SPGR imaging is begun soon after initiation of contrast injection and repeated several times until the venous system is completely filled. Digital subtraction of a precontrast scan improves results. This technique is superior to indirect CE MRV in terms of contrast-to-noise ratios (35).

Intravenous Contrast

When administered intravenously, gadolinium chelates shorten T1 relaxation times, resulting in positive contrast enhancement (increased signal intensity) on T1-weighted pulse sequences. After injection, they distribute predominantly in the blood pool and extracellular fluid compartments of the body, where they remain until they are excreted by the kidneys. Redistribution from the blood pool to the extracellular fluid space is completed in approximately 11 minutes (13). Biologic half-lives of the contrast agents are between 1 and 2 hours (36).

With respect to MRI of pediatric vascular anomalies, intravenous contrast agents help to distinguish lymphatic malformations—which enhance only peripherally or not at all—from enhancing hemangiomas and venous malformations. For standard CE MRI at 1.5 T, gadolinium chelates are generally injected at a dose of 0.1 mmol/kg. At 3 T, the contrast dose may be halved (0.05 mmol/kg) because of increases in SNR and contrast resolution. For CE MRA, doses of 0.2 to 0.3 mmol/kg are used (35,37).

Intravenous contrast may be injected either manually or with an MRI-compatible power injector. In comparison to manual injection, power injection provides more uniform delivery of contrast material with no delay between injection of the contrast agent and saline flush (37). Power injection is used predominantly for CE MRA and is not necessary for standard CE MRI. It must be used with caution in infants and children who are sedated or unable to communicate, particularly when injection is performed through intravenous catheters located in hands, wrists, or feet. Regardless of the mode of injection, intravenous positioning of the catheter with both free blood return and unrestricted saline injection should be confirmed prior to contrast administration.

Contrast injection is most often performed through 20 to 24 gauge peripheral intravenous catheters. Either manual or power injection can be performed via this route. Alternatively, contrast may be injected by hand through central venous catheters or peripherally inserted central catheters (PICCs). Power injection of gadolinium contrast agents through central lines and PICCs has not been studied rigorously in children.

Risks associated with extravasation are lower for gadolinium chelates than for iodinated CT contrast agents because of the lower osmolality and lower volumes of contrast used for MRI (13,38). Nonetheless, animal models demonstrate that extravascular gadolinium chelate extravasation may lead to soft tissue inflammation and necrosis. Soft tissue damage is greatest with gadopentetate dimeglumine (Magnevist) and least with gadoteridol (ProHance) and gadodiamide (Omniscan). These latter agents are lower in osmolality (39).

When possible, injection sites are monitored visually so that contrast extravasation can be recognized and stopped immediately. Visual inspection is most important when patients are nonverbal or sedated and are unable to report injection site pain. Monitoring the injection site is generally not problematic for standard CE MRI, because the patient may be removed from the bore of the magnet prior to contrast injection and then repositioned in time to begin scanning. Although scanning is usually begun within 1 minute of contrast injection, precise bolus timing for standard CE MRI sequences is unnecessary.

For dynamic CE MRI or CE MRA, the patient must be positioned within the magnet bore to allow initiation of scanning during or immediately after contrast injection. Contrast is generally injected through a length of tubing, and the injection site may not be visible from outside the magnet bore. In this setting, power injection of the contrast agent and saline flush must be performed with caution.

Contrast injection should always be followed by an intravenous saline flush. The volume of gadolinium agents used in pediatric MRI is very small, and a large percentage may remain in the intravenous catheter tubing after injection. A saline flush clears contrast from the tubing. It prevents artifactual signal loss due to intravenous pooling of concentrated gadolinium (40). In addition, it reduces the risk of secondary venous thrombosis (13). Intravenous access should be maintained for at least 10 minutes following contrast injection so that intravenous fluids and medications can be administered, if needed, for allergic reaction. Serious allergic reactions are rare (36).

Computed Tomography and Computed Tomographic Angiography

Although MRI is preferred for assessing pediatric vascular anomalies, CE CT may replace or complement MRI in some cases. While MRI takes 20 minutes or more to perform, CT can be completed in less than a minute and provides a rapid alternative to MRI in children with unstable cardiovascular status or respiratory compromise. It is useful in patients who have contraindications to sedation or MRI. In addition, it has a role in imaging patients with embolization coils or surgical clips in whom MRI is degraded by magnetic susceptibility artifact.

In the setting of pediatric vascular anomalies, the primary roles of CT are to characterize soft tissue content; to define positional relationships; and, in some cases, to delineate osseous involvement. CE CT is preferable to MRI in imaging vascular anomalies of the neck, bowel, and lungs. Although CT is better than MRI for demonstrating phleboliths in venous malformations, plain radiographs reveal phleboliths at a lower radiation dose to the patient (3).

High-resolution CTA has become feasible in recent years with introduction of helical and multislice CT scanners.

Large vascular territories can now be imaged within seconds, minimizing the detrimental effect of motion on image quality. CTA has better spatial resolution than MRA but uses ionizing radiation. Radiation exposure is cumulative, and doses are particularly high when multiphasic scans are performed to resolve arterial and venous phases of enhancement. At this time, concerns regarding the potential for carcinogenesis in infants and children limit the use of multiphasic CTA in the pediatric population. It should be used only when imperative for diagnosis and when MRA is contraindicated.

Examples of specific imaging protocols are included in Table 23-4. When performing CT and CTA in children, unique technical considerations arise, stemming from the wide spectrum of patient sizes, hemodynamic states, and maturity levels encountered.

Equipment

Since 1990, CT technology has been rapidly and continually improving. Multislice scanners, collecting several channels of data simultaneously, provide a speed advantage over older single-slice helical and incremental models. Subsecond

TABLE 23-4

Sample Computed Tomography and Computed Tomographic Angiography Protocols for Evaluation of Pediatric Vascular Anomalies

CT parameter:	Multidetector CT		
Detector rows:	4 to 16		
Collimator thickness (mm):	1.0 to 2.5		
Pitch:	1		
Slice thickness (mm):	5 and 1.0 to 2.5		
Reconstruction interval (mm):	5 and 0.5 to 1.3		
kVp:	80 to 120		
mAs:			
<10 kg	Chest 40; A/P 60		
11 to 20 kg	Chest 50; A/P 70		
21 to 30 kg	Chest 60; A/P 80		
31 to 40 kg	Chest 70; A/P 100		
41 to 50 kg	Chest 90; A/P 130		
51 to 70 kg	Chest 120; A/P 150		
>70 kg	Chest 140+; A/P 170+		
Gantry rotation interval (seconds):	1.0	1.0	0.5
IV contrast dose (mL/kg):	1 to 3 (300 mg iodine/mL)		
Injection rate: (mL/seconds):			
24 gauge IV	1.2 to 2.0		
22 gauge IV	1.2 to 2.5		
20 gauge IV	2.0 to 3.0		
Scan delay:	Determined by bolus tracking		
IV, intravenous.			

gantry rotation times also increase scan speed. Radiologists can use increased speed to shorten scan duration (scanning quickly through a region of interest without reducing collimation) or to increase *z*-axis resolution (scanning for a given period of time with thinner collimation). When imaging pediatric vascular anomalies, increased speed translates into reduced patient motion, improved 2D and 3D image quality, and greater latitude with respect to scan timing and contrast injection.

Image processing workstations, particularly those with intuitive user interfaces, automated operations, and ultrafast performance characteristics, facilitate rapid creation of multiplanar and 3D images, thereby improving scan interpretation, treatment planning, and communication of results. Picture archival and communications systems (PACS) also ease handling of the massive amounts of data that result from high-resolution vascular CT and CTA.

Sedation

To eliminate misregistration artifact in CT, patients must remain motionless during image acquisition. Neonates and infants under 12 months of age, when fed and swaddled, may sleep through a CT examination. Older children sometimes require sedation, although its use has diminished considerably in recent years with the use of faster helical and multislice CT scanners (41–43). Pappas et al. (43) reported a sedation rate of only 3.3% in children younger than 7 years of age who were undergoing multislice body CT (43). In practice, strict age restrictions for sedation are not useful. Rather, the decision to give sedation or not should be adapted to the needs of the individual child (18). The same sedation safety precautions should be used for CT as for MRI.

Respiratory Motion

Misregistration due to respiratory motion may diminish the diagnostic value of CT directed to the chest or abdomen. This is particularly true when target lesions are small relative to respiratory excursion and when respiratory rates are rapid, as is often the case in children. Whenever possible, respiratory motion should be minimized during image acquisition. Cooperative children over 5 to 7 years of age are able to suspend respiration voluntarily for periods of up to 30 seconds, providing a satisfactory window in which to complete data acquisition (44). A practice session before scanning allows appraisal of each child's breath holding skills and increases the likelihood that he or she will follow instructions correctly during imaging.

In children under 5 to 7 years of age who are too young to hold their breath voluntarily, images obtained during quiet respiration may be diagnostic. Ventilation can be suspended briefly in children who are intubated and paralyzed under general anesthesia. Alternatively, a 15- to 25-second respiratory pause (Hering-Breuer reflex) may be induced in children who are sedated but not intubated by using positive pressure ventilation applied through a face mask apparatus (45). This latter technique, known as *controlled ventilation*, is noninvasive and well tolerated by both infants and children. It has been applied primarily to high-resolution CT scanning of the chest but is also applicable to other pediatric CT protocols. Two operators perform the maneuver, one controlling the face mask device and the second applying gentle cricoid pressure to minimize air passage down the esophagus. Through the face mask, positive pressure (25 cm water) is applied to augment the patient's spontaneous inspiratory efforts. Additional breaths are delivered to induce hypocarbia and apnea. For a given patient, the number of additional breaths required to induce apnea as well as the duration of the respiratory pause are reproducible and can be determined by a "trial run" before CT scanning. Once apnea is achieved, maintenance of positive pressure lengthens its duration and allows chest imaging during full lung inflation (45).

Radiation Dose, mA, kVp, and Pitch

Children are more sensitive than adults to radiation and have a higher risk of experiencing the carcinogenic and genetic effects (46). In addition, because x-ray beam attenuation decreases as body mass decreases, CT imparts a higher effective radiation dose to children than to adults (47). Based on models assuming a linear extrapolation of risks from intermediate to low doses, Brenner et al. (48) have estimated that the lifetime cancer mortality risk attributable to radiation exposure at the age of 1 year is 0.18% for abdominal CT and 0.07% for head CT (48). Although the veracity of these risk estimates is debated, radiologists widely agree that patient radiation exposure should be kept as low as is reasonably achievable (ALARA) (49,50). To this end, care should be taken to avoid unnecessary scans, to implement radiation-reducing technology, and to choose age-appropriate scan parameters. When feasible, CT should be replaced by other diagnostic imaging modalities that do not use ionizing radiation, such as ultrasound and MRI. It is also important that radiologists and technologists be educated about specific parameters that affect radiation dose and take an active role in minimizing exposure to each patient.

The first parameter to consider is tube current, often expressed as a function of time (milliamperes-seconds or mAs). mAs determines the quantity of x-rays to which the patient is exposed and is directly related to radiation dose. The number of x-rays required to create a diagnostic image decreases as patient size decreases, because small patients attenuate the x-ray beam less than large patients. Therefore, pediatric CT can and should be performed with a lower mAs than adult CT (49). A number of strategies have been proposed to tailor mAs to patient size. The most commonly used strategies involve mAs gradation according to patient weight, height, or cross-sectional dimensions (49,51,52). Specific recommendations regarding mAs are included in Table 23-4.

The potential disadvantage of decreasing mAs is increased image noise. Noise is inversely related to the number of x-rays that reach the CT detectors. While reducing mAs in a given patient increases image noise, this effect is balanced as patient size decreases by a reduction in x-ray beam attenuation (49). Accordingly, mAs can be reduced in smaller patients without degradation of image quality, assuming no change in section thickness. If section thickness is reduced to improve spatial resolution in small patients, there will be a concomitant increase in image noise. Section thickness, mAs, and noise must be balanced to achieve diagnostic image quality while minimizing radiation dose.

Several authors suggest that CT tube potential can also be reduced in small patients without significant degradation of image quality (47,53–55). Tube potential determines x-ray beam energy and is exponentially related to radiation dose (46,52). Most CT examinations are performed with a tube potential of 120 peak kilovoltage (kVp) (56). Theoretically, lowering tube potential to 80 kVp would improve bone, iodine, and soft tissue contrast in small patients while reducing radiation dose as much as 65% (47,54,57). Because of the complex relationship between tube potential, image noise, tissue contrast, and patient size, additional study into modulation of this parameter is needed.

Pitch is a third parameter that can be adjusted to reduce radiation dose in helical CT. Increasing pitch reduces redundant tissue exposure and shortens the time during which the x-ray beam is turned on. Few comparisons of pitch and radiation exposure have been made in children. Vade et al. (58) reported a 33% reduction, and Donnelly et al. (49) reported a 28% reduction in radiation dose using a pitch of 1.5 as compared to 1.0 on single-slice helical scanners. To maintain constant image noise levels, some multislice CT scanners automatically increase tube current (mA) in proportion to increases in pitch (59). On these scanners, the benefits of increasing pitch are negated unless mA is manually reduced. The potential disadvantage of increasing pitch is broadening of the section sensitivity profile with loss of z-axis resolution. Reducing collimation and using an overlapping image reconstruction interval minimizes this effect (60). Helical CT and CTA in children

are most often performed with a pitch of 1.5 (56). When subsecond gantry rotation intervals are used, a pitch close to 1.0 is advised.

In comparison to single-slice CT, multislice CT geometry changes radiation dose in several ways (61,62). Septa between detectors in the z-axis direction absorb radiation that consequently contributes to patient dose but not to image data. This effect increases as the number of detector rows increases. Radiation dose is also increased by broadening of the x-ray beam in the z-axis direction, such that edges of the beam create a penumbra beyond the margins of the active detector elements. While ensuring uniform x-ray exposure to each detector element, broadening of the x-ray beam further reduces radiation dose efficiency (61). At the same time, dose efficiency is somewhat increased because beam collimation is relatively large with respect to focal spot size (high umbra:penumbra ratio) (62).

Growing concern regarding CT's potential for carcinogenesis has led CT manufacturers to implement both hardware and software modifications that reduce radiation dose (51,54,63,64). Positive changes include implementation of solid-state detectors, improved anode ratings, focal spot tracking, and soft-beam x-ray filtration (50,52,65). Commercial CT scanners now allow preprogramming of pediatric-specific tube current settings for a number of standard imaging protocols (63,64). Real-time current modulation has also been developed, tailoring mA in response to changes in patient geometry and x-ray absorption during data acquisition (52,66). In addition, commercial CT consoles are now required to display the volume CT dose index ($CTDI_{vol}$) (52). $CTDI_{vol}$ estimates the average radiation dose in a scan volume with reference to a standardized CT phantom. Some CT scanners also display the dose length product [$DLP = CTDI_{vol}$ (milligrays) $\times$ Scan length (cm)]. Access to these dose descriptors at the time of scan planning enables radiologists and technologists to predict and actively reduce radiation exposure on a case-by-case basis (46).

Additional patient protection is achieved by shielding radiosensitive organs (lenses, thyroid gland, breasts, and gonads) during CT scanning. Organs both inside and outside of the scan volume may be shielded (52). Fricke et al. (67) reported a 29% reduction in breast radiation dose with bismuth in-plane shielding during multislice CT of the chest. Similarly, Hopper et al. (68) reported a 40% to 50% reduction in radiation dose to the lenses with bismuth-coated latex eye shielding during CT of the head. Both groups claimed no loss of diagnostic information. Beaconsfield et al. (69) demonstrated a 45% reduction in thyroid radiation and a 76% reduction in breast radiation with lead shielding of these organs during CT of the head. Hidajat et al. (70) showed a 95% reduction in absorbed testicular dose with use of a testis shield during abdominal CT.

Additional Scan Parameters

Several additional scan parameters must be selected when planning CT scans of pediatric vascular anomalies. These include collimator thickness, section thickness, reconstruction interval, FOV, and z-axis coverage.

Collimator thickness is chosen before scanning is initiated. For conventional and single-slice helical CT, collimator thickness is equivalent to nominal section thickness. Values in the range of 3 to 5 mm would be appropriate for imaging pediatric vascular anomalies. Thinner collimation is generally avoided when imaging children with conventional or single-slice CT scanners, because an increase in mA is required to keep quantum noise levels constant. Consequently, CT angiograms, 3D reconstructions, and multiplanar reformations created on these scanners are of lower quality than those created on multislice CT scanners.

On multislice CT scanners, collimator thickness defines the minimum section thickness that can be achieved after scanning is completed. Values in the range of 1.0 to 2.5 mm would be appropriate for imaging pediatric vascular anomalies, as long as mAs is not increased concurrently. By a process known as z-filtering, section thickness can then be manipulated retrospectively. Sections of 3 to 5 mm with noise levels comparable to those achieved on conventional or single-slice scanners are created for axial image interpretation. Sections of 1.0 to 2.5 mm can also be generated to serve as superior source images for CTA, 3D reconstruction, and multiplanar reformation. Accordingly, the advantages of high-resolution, thin-collimation imaging can be achieved without penalty in terms of quantum noise or radiation dose. Choosing a reconstruction interval that is 33% to 50% smaller than the section thickness reduces partial volume averaging effects and also improves the quality of postprocessed images (44).

FOV should closely approximate the diameter of the anatomic region of interest. Because pixel size is directly proportional to FOV, decreasing FOV improves spatial resolution and reduces partial volume averaging effects (55). To prevent unnecessary radiation exposure, scan coverage in the z-axis direction must be closely confined to the anatomic region of interest. When determining FOV and z-axis coverage, radiologists should be aware that pediatric vascular anomalies may be larger than is apparent on physical examination, may be multifocal, and may be associated with other anomalies. FOV and z-axis coverage should accommodate potential patterns of disease distribution.

Frontal and/or lateral digital scout radiographs, used to determine FOV and z-axis coverage, are performed with a low tube current (30 to 40 mA). Precontrast axial CT scans are generally avoided unless imperative for diagnosis. The same is true of multiphase scans, which may double or triple radiation dose. If multiphase imaging is required, whether to evaluate arterial and venous anatomy or to assess contrast enhancement patterns over time, then it should be performed with a low mA and, when possible, at a single scan location.

Intravenous Contrast

Optimum contrast enhancement of pediatric vascular anomalies depends on predictable and uniform delivery of contrast material to the target organs and vessels. Injection techniques applied to infants and children are different than those used in adults. Smaller patients require smaller contrast doses; smaller intravenous catheters mandate reduced injection rates and altered scan delays. Because children come in a wide range of sizes, contrast enhancement techniques are scaled to the individual patient.

Use of low-osmolality nonionic intravenous contrast is preferred in pediatric CT, despite its increased cost (71). In comparison to ionic contrast media, the nonionic agents have fewer minor side effects such as unpleasant taste, nausea, vomiting, flushing, and injection site discomfort (72). Although not life-threatening, these side effects may lead to patient motion during image acquisition (72,73). Indeed, reduced patient motion and improved scan quality have been demonstrated with use of nonionic contrast agents in both children and adults (72,74).

Contrast doses ranging from 1 to 3 mL/kg are used for pediatric CT and CTA, with a dose of 2 mL/kg used most frequently (300 mg iodine/mL, total dose not to exceed 5 mL/kg) (56,60). To reduce perivenous artifact resulting from concentrated iodine, contrast may be diluted 3:1 with normal saline (44,75). Although both manual injection and power injection are used for pediatric CT and CTA, power injection provides more uniform and predictable enhancement. Its use is gaining acceptance but is not universal due to concerns regarding the potential for catheter rupture, contrast extravasation, and soft tissue injury (44,56,76). Infants and young children are thought to be at higher risk of contrast extravasation and its sequelae because they are unable to communicate effectively. The risk of extravasation increases when tourniquets are not released prior to injection, when multiple attempts have been made to gain intravenous access, and when injection is made through catheters that have been indwelling for more than 20 hours (77). Morbidity also increases when extravasation occurs in the dorsum of the wrist, hand, or foot or in a limb with preexisting vascular or lymphatic compromise (77). In children with vascular anomalies in an extremity, contrast injection in the affected limb should performed with caution or, when possible, avoided entirely.

There is no correlation between injection rate and complication rate (78). If safety measures are followed, actual complication rates associated with contrast injection are low (<0.3%) (76). It is imperative that stable intravenous positioning of the catheter be verified prior to contrast administration. Both free return of venous blood and unrestricted injection of a saline flush should be demonstrated. In addition, injection sites should be monitored carefully during contrast administration to allow immediate recognition and cessation of contrast extravasation. Recently, extravasation detection accessories (EDAs) have become available on commercial power injectors. EDAs work by detecting changes in soft tissue impedance that occur with contrast extravasation. If such changes are detected, further contrast infusion is halted automatically. Although the sensitivity of EDAs in detecting clinically relevant extravasation in adult patients approaches 100%, their use in children has not been reported (77,79). If extravasation occurs, management includes elevation of the affected limb, application of a cold compress, and observation for compartment syndrome.

Contrast administration for pediatric CT and CTA is most often performed through 20 to 24 gauge peripheral intravenous catheters (56). Butterfly needles may be unsuitable for power injection because of their relative instability, higher risk of extravasation, and potential inadequacy should intravenous fluid or medication be required on an emergent basis (76,80). There is very little information available on the safety of contrast injection through central lines in children. In a retrospective review of power injection through pediatric central lines, Kaste and Young (76) reported a complication rate of 0.35% (catheter rupture in one of 283 injections). The injection rates studied (0.3 to 0.8 mL/second) were lower than those used by other authors for pediatric body CT (55,73).

Information about the feasibility of injecting contrast through PICCs is also limited. PICC manufacturers currently recommend only gravity infusion or use of standard infusion pumps, and there is considerable uncertainty as to whether rapid bolus injection of contrast material through PICCs is safe and efficacious (81). Maximum tolerated flow rates are dependent on catheter diameter (direct relationship) as well as on catheter length and contrast viscosity (indirect relationship). In vitro analysis of 35-cm and 45-cm silicone PICCs showed inadequate peak contrast flow rates through 3 French (F) catheters (<0.7 mL/second) and marginally adequate flow rates through 4F single-lumen and 6F dual-lumen catheters (0.9 to 1.6 mL/second). In contrast, 5F single-lumen and 7F dual-lumen PICCs tolerated flow

rates above those typically used for pediatric CT (>3 mL/second) (81). Comprehensive in vivo analysis of contrast injection through PICCs has yet to be performed.

Viscosity should be reduced by warming contrast according to the manufacturer's instructions prior to injection. Injection rates used in infants and children vary considerably. Particularly for CTA, they are tailored to deliver the entire volume of contrast within a period of time that is equal to or less than the duration of image acquisition (55). With power injectors, the following injection rates have been recommended: 1.2 to 2.0 mL/second through 24-gauge peripheral catheters, 1.2 to 2.5 mL/second through 22-gauge peripheral catheters, and 2.0 to 3.0 mL/second through 20-gauge peripheral catheters (44,55). Manual contrast injection rates generally range from 1.0 to 2.0 mL/second (44). Although contrast injection rates used for pediatric CT are lower than those used in adults, they provide adequate vascular enhancement in the range of 150 to 200 Hounsfield units (HU) (44).

It is important in pediatric CT that contrast injection be followed by a normal saline flush. Contrast volumes used in infants and children are so small that a large percentage may remain within the intravenous catheter tubing following injection. A saline flush ensures that the entire contrast dose is delivered to the patient and reduces intravenous contrast stasis. The saline volume should be adequate to fill the intravenous catheter tubing and move the contrast bolus toward the heart. Intravenous access should be maintained for at least 10 minutes following contrast injection in case intravenous fluid resuscitation or medication are required for treatment of an allergic reaction.

Scan Delay

Scan timing is complicated in pediatric CT by variability in patient size, hemodynamic status, contrast volume, and contrast administration techniques. For standard CT imaging, scan delays are often determined empirically based on contrast volume, lesion location, and estimated contrast circulation time. Short empiric delays are appropriate for scanning central lesions in infants and toddlers with small contrast volumes and rapid circulation times. In addition, they are used when contrast is injected through a central venous catheter. Longer scan delays are required when contrast is injected slowly or through a peripheral intravenous catheter, when the target lesion is peripheral in location, or when patient size approaches that of an adult.

Empiric scan delays vary, not only from patient to patient but from scanner to scanner. For conventional (step-and-shoot) pediatric body CT, it was common practice to begin scanning after intravenous injection of approximately half of the contrast bolus. Longer scan delays are necessary for helical body CT because scan speed may exceed the rate of contrast circulation. For single-slice helical CT, scanning is begun after completion of the contrast bolus—with a 0- to 10-second delay for neck and chest CT and with a 10- to 20-second delay for abdominopelvic CT. For multislice helical CT, scanning of the neck and chest is initiated 10 to 15 seconds after completion of the contrast bolus, while scanning of the abdomen and pelvis is initiated 20 to 30 seconds after completion of the contrast bolus.

Empiric scan delays are inherently inexact and may be hampered by individual variations in enhancement rate. Commercial automated bolus-tracking methods provide an alternative means of determining scan delay and have been associated with improved contrast enhancement (60,82). Following initiation of contrast injection, serial single-level CT images are generated of a region of interest. Enhancement in the region of interest is tracked graphically, and scanning is begun once a desired degree of enhancement is achieved (e.g., >45 HU in the liver or >100 HU in the aorta). Bolus tracking is the preferred technique for determining scan delay in CTA, when precise bolus timing is necessary. For CT arteriography, scanning should coincide with peak arterial enhancement. For scanning in the venous phase, delayed images are necessary. The primary disadvantage of bolus tracking is a small increase in radiation dose to the patient. Radiation dose can be minimized during bolus tracking by lowering tube current (24 to 40mA) and increasing interscan delay (3 to 6 seconds) (44,60,82).

The use of a test injection is another method that has been described for determining scan delay. Several milliliters of contrast are injected intravenously in a "trial run" prior to completion of the diagnostic CT scan. As with bolus tracking, passage of contrast through a target region of interest is monitored by using serial single-level CT images, and time to peak enhancement is determined graphically. Although test injections have been applied successfully in adult CT (83), they are sometimes problematic in pediatric CT and are performed infrequently. Timing is difficult to reproduce, particularly when manual contrast injection is used. In infants and small children, test injections consume a large percentage of the maximum allowable contrast dose, sparing little contrast for the diagnostic scan. In addition, test injections increase radiation exposure, lengthen scan duration, and risk awakening sedated or sleeping patients (44).

Postprocessing Options

The postprocessing options that are most beneficial with respect to evaluating pediatric vascular anomalies are multiplanar reformation (MPR), curved planar reformation (CPR), volume rendering (VR), and maximum intensity projection (MIP). In most cases, postprocessing can be accomplished easily and rapidly, either at the CT or MRI console or at an independent workstation (44,55).

MPR creates 2D tomographic images in orthogonal or oblique planes. It is used to delineate the extent of vascular masses and malformations as well as to define complex spatial relationships. Curved structures that course in and out of the plane—such as vessels—may be better displayed with CPR. Like MPR, CPR results in 2D tomograms; however, the CPR display plane curves along points that are manually positioned within the structure of interest.

VR involves assignment of a color scale opacity level to each voxel in a data set in proportion to tissue signal or attenuation values. Grayscale lighting effects are applied simultaneously, reflecting signal or attenuation gradients between neighboring voxels. This technique is most helpful for depicting complex 3D spatial relationships.

MIPs provide an angiographic effect. Imaginary rays are cast through a volume of data, and the maximum signal intensity or attenuation value encountered is projected onto a 2D image. A number of different projection angles may be used to view the anatomy of interest from different perspectives or to rotate it around an axis. With this technique, images similar to those achieved with conventional angiography are generated. Even blood vessels that do not lie in a single plane can be demonstrated in their entirety. MIP reconstruction is much simpler with 3D CE MRA than with CTA, because MRA signal emanates only from CE vessels and not from surrounding tissues. With CTA, high-attenuation CE vessels may be masked by other highly attenuative structures such as bone. Accordingly, these structures must be edited from the image (13). The minimum intensity projection (MinIP) is a variation of the MIP technique that is useful for showing mass effect upon the airways.

Reconstruction quality depends heavily on quality of the source data. Volumetric data acquisitions with isotropic voxel dimensions and a small FOV provide the best foundation for multiplanar and 3D reconstructions. In this setting, resolution is nearly identical in all three orthogonal planes, and reconstructed images share the same resolution as the original axial sections. For CT reconstructions, a 33% to 50% overlapping reconstruction interval reduces stair-step artifact, while a soft reconstruction algorithm minimizes noise in both source images and processed images (44).

VASCULAR ANOMALIES: DISEASE CONDITIONS AND CLINICAL APPLICATIONS OF MAGNETIC RESONANCE AND COMPUTED TOMOGRAPHY

Vascular anomalies consist of vascular tumors (hemangiomas, endotheliomas, and angiosarcomas) and various forms of low- and high-flow vascular malformations. The basic difference between the two groups is that vascular tumors demonstrate endothelial cell proliferation, whereas vascular malformations have relatively normal endothelial cell turnover (Table 23-1) (1). The diagnostic approach to these complex conditions requires a solid understanding of the nature of these conditions. Assessment of flow dynamics and extent of the anomaly is necessary for the differential diagnosis as well as for therapeutic decision making. In simple terms, high-flow anomaly means that there is a rapid shunt from the arterial system to the venous system, whereas fluid movement is slow in low-flow anomalies. This differentiation is important not only for diagnosis but also to determine the treatment modality. For example, low-flow anomalies (venous malformations, lymphatic malformations, etc.) are associated with swelling, pain, and consump-

tion coagulopathy and generally respond to sclerotherapy (sclerosant solution injection with direct puncture of the malformation), whereas high-flow anomalies evolve over time and carry much more significant risks (e.g., cardiac volume overload, tissue ischemia, and significant bleeding). Also, treatment is more complex, usually involving embolization using a transcatheter approach.

Imaging Workup and Findings

Most vascular anomalies can be diagnosed clinically. Of those requiring imaging for diagnosis, MRI is adequate in most patients. The vascular anomalies protocol typically include T1-weighted SE images; T2-weighted fat-saturated SE or inversion recovery images; gradient echo imaging without saturation band; and, finally, postcontrast fat-saturated

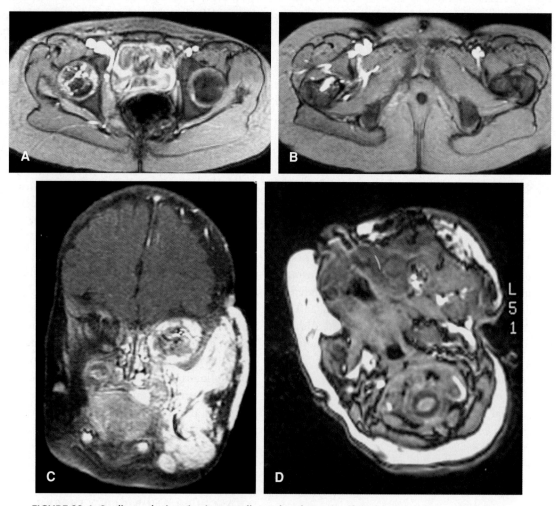

FIGURE 23-1 Gradient echo imaging is generally used to determine if the lesion is a low- or high-flow anomaly. A, B: Arteriovenous malformation. **C, D:** Infantile hemangioma. **E–G:** Noninvoluting hemangioma. **H, I:** Venous malformation. **J, K:** Lymphatic malformation. Axial gradient echo images **(A, B)** obtained through the inguinal area in a patient with AVM show hyperintensities in the proximal femur and surrounding soft tissues representing the nidus. Please note that the femoral vasculature on the right appears significantly larger than the left. Enlargement of the main artery and draining vein in the diseased body area is a strong indicator of a hemodynamically significant arteriovenous shunt. **(C)** and **(D)** show a large infantile hemangioma in the left face extending into the left orbit. A postcontrast coronal T1-weighted image **(C)** demonstrates signal voids representing arterial feeders. An axial gradient echo image **(D)** demonstrates high signals in these vessels. (*Figure 23-1 continues*)

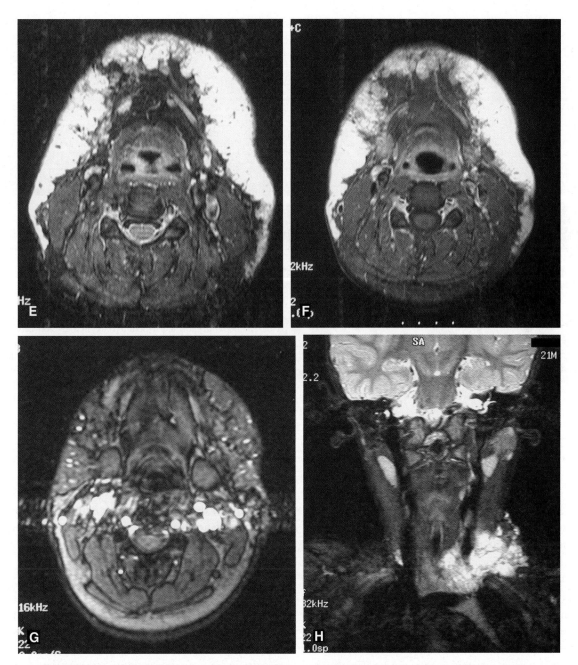

FIGURE 23-1 (Continued) (E) is a T2-weighted image of a noninvoluting hemangioma in the mandibular area. The lesion demonstrates a high T2 signal. **(F)** is a postgadolinium T1-weighted image of the same tumor lesion demonstrating intense contrast enhancement. An axial gradient echo image **(G)** of the same tumor demonstrates multiple, small hyperintensities in the tumor representing small arterial feeders. A large venous malformation in the left lower neck is seen on the T2-weighted coronal image **(H)** as a hyperintense and irregular but sharply marginated vascular lesion. (*Figure 23-1 continues*)

T1-weighted images (Table 23-3). For a complete workup, CE MRA can be added to this protocol. If this sequence is needed, it should be performed after the gradient echo sequence, before obtaining postcontrast T1-weighted images so that the whole scan can be completed with one contrast injection. The interpretation scheme of MRI for a possible vascular anomaly can be summarized as follows

(84): if the anomaly shows evidence of high-flow vascular channels (hyperintensities on gradient echo and signal voids on SE), diagnostic considerations are limited to AVM, arteriovenous fistula (AVF), and hemangioma or other vascular tumor (Fig. 23-1). The most important feature distinguishing hemangiomas from AVMs or AVFs is the presence of a tumoral mass lesion, which can be

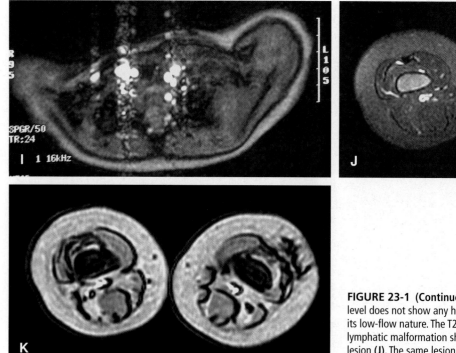

FIGURE 23-1 (Continued) Gradient echo image **(I)** at the same level does not show any hyperintensities in the lesion, confirming its low-flow nature. The T2-weighted axial image in a patient with lymphatic malformation shows a sharply marginated, hyperintense lesion **(J)**. The same lesion does not demonstrate any hyperintensity on the axial gradient echo image **(K)** due to its low-flow nature.

appreciated on MRI by T2-hyperintense solid tissue showing intense contrast enhancement. If the anomaly does not show high-flow signal characteristics, the differential includes low-flow anomalies such as venous malformation, lymphatic malformation, or lymphatic-venous malformation (capillary malformation is not in this list, as these malformations are superficial and do not require imaging for diagnosis). If the low-flow anomaly shows no contrast enhancement or a minimal degree of peripheral contrast enhancement ("rings and archs"), a lymphatic malformation should be considered foremost in the differential (Fig. 23-2). If the anomaly shows noticeable patchy areas of contrast enhancement within the fluid spaces, a venous malformation should be suspected. To simplify, hemangiomas consist of solid tissue with high-flow supplying and draining channels, and vascular malformations consist of channels only. Another obvious difference is that hemangiomas present in the first few months of age, and most involute by age 9 years, so a patient presenting beyond the age of 9 years generally does not have a hemangioma.

Some patients with vascular anomalies benefit from dedicated vascular imaging (either conventional angiography or noninvasive angiography such as MRA or CTA) to confirm the anticipated diagnosis and to tailor the interventional treatment approach. For example, given a low-flow anomaly, an arteriogram would show no arterial feeders

(confirming the diagnosis), and it may outline the venous drainage channels of the malformation, which in turn help the interventionalist to make an appropriate plan for sclerotherapy. If the malformation is a high-flow anomaly, the arterial feeder or feeders are demonstrated beforehand, possibly helping plan subsequent transcatheter embolization or surgical intervention.

Some type of flow-sensitive sequence should be included in MRI evaluation of patients with vascular anomalies. Standard GRE sequences are useful because they demonstrate the relationship of fast-flow vessels to the mass lesion, in cross section. CE MRA, when applied optimally, results in high-quality vascular images that compare well with standard invasive angiography. Dynamic MRA, in which a series of images is obtained over time, is useful in predicting the type of channel abnormality present and may provide information not seen on conventional angiography. For example, opacification of the abnormal channels in venous malformations is quite poor in the delayed phases of conventional arteriograms, whereas they are usually fully opacified during CE MRA (Fig. 23-3).

The development of multidetector CT scanners has greatly improved the practicality of CTA. When imaging with 4-row CT scanners, the relatively long acquisition resulting from the slow table speed typically results in difficulties separating the arterial and venous components of

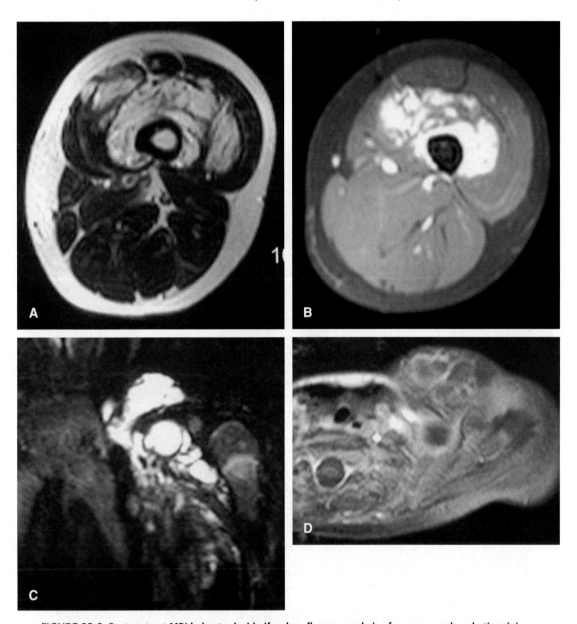

FIGURE 23-2 Postcontrast MRI helps to decide if a slow-flow anomaly is of a venous or lymphatic origin. A, B: Venous malformation. **C, D:** Lymphatic malformation. An axial T2-weighted SE image **(A)** shows a relatively large hyperintense lesion wrapping the femur anteriorly, involving multiple muscle groups. This lesion demonstrates significant contrast enhancement on the postcontrast axial T1-weighted image **(B)**. VMs typically demonstrate significant contrast enhancement. LMs, on the other hand, demonstrate minimal peripheral or no contrast enhancement, while VMs and LMs both demonstrate significant high T2 signal. A macrocystic LM in the left shoulder area, demonstrating multiloculated cystic spaces on a T2-weighted coronal SE image **(C)** and a mild degree of peripheral rim enhancement on a postcontrast axial T1-weighted SE image **(D)**.

AVMs (Fig. 23-4). With 16- to 64-row scanners, it is possible to scan the entire body in less than 30 seconds and an extremity in less than 10 seconds, resulting in improved characterization of AVMs (Fig. 23-5). With this speed, the images are usually not degraded by motion or breathing (it can be completed in a single breath hold). The major limitation of the technique remains the undesired (particularly in children) radiation exposure, although the absorbed dose

using CTA has proven to be less than that for conventional arteriography (85).

In the following sections, the different types of vascular anomalies are detailed with their definitions, histopathological features, prevalence, location, imaging strategies, and imaging findings as well as therapeutic approaches. Vascular imaging techniques including the indications and applications of MRA and CTA, and therapeutic techniques

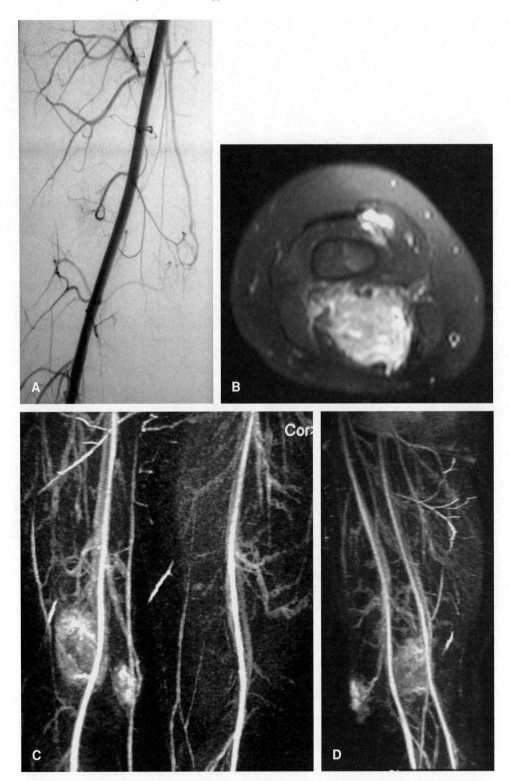

FIGURE 23-3 Small venous malformation near the patella. A catheter-based conventional arteriogram shows no arterial feeders or opacification of the lesion **(A)**. However, in this patient, one of the small popliteal muscular branches had been reportedly catheterized and incorrectly embolized with absolute alcohol. An axial fat-saturated T2-weighted SE image **(B)** obtained after alcohol embolization demonstrates two hyperintense areas, a larger one in the popliteal area and a smaller one near the patella. The larger lesion in the popliteal region represents muscle necrosis due to alcohol embolization. The smaller lesion is the original VM. Unfortunately, attempting arterial embolizations in low-flow anomalies is a common form of mismanagement. CE MRA **(C, D)** demonstrates the VM with a draining vein into the femoral vein. The muscle necrosis area also shows significant contrast enhancement due to edema and necrosis-related muscular inflammation. The femoral artery and vein in the other leg appear unremarkable. (*Figure 23-3 continues*)

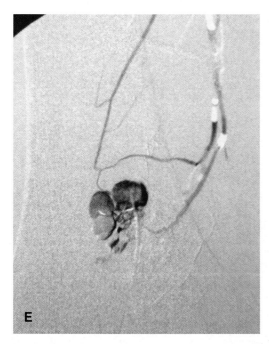

E

FIGURE 23-3 (Continued) Direct percutaneous puncture of the malformation was performed in an attempt to perform sclerotherapy **(E)**, which showed a cloverleaf-shaped malformation with small draining veins.

including transcatheter embolization and sclerotherapy based on disease entity imaging and pathological characteristics are stressed in these sections.

HEMANGIOMAS AND VASCULAR TUMORS

Pediatric hemangiomas and vascular tumors include the following: infantile, rapidly involuting congenital hemangiomas (RICHs), noninvoluting congenital hemangiomas (NICHs), those that are intramuscular, and kaposiform hemangioendothelioma (KHE).

Definition, Clinical Presentation, and Histopathology

Infantile hemangiomas are benign neoplasms of infancy composed of proliferating endothelial cells (84,86). They are the most common tumors of early childhood, with an estimated prevalence of 1% to 3% of all neonates and 10% of infants by 1 year of age (90–93). There is marked female preponderance (up to 6.6:1) (94,95). Twenty percent of patients may suffer from more than one lesion. Prematurity is a well-known risk factor, particularly in those neonates who fall below 1,500 grams in weight (96). Also, they are more common in infants whose mothers have undergone chorionic villus sampling (97). It is estimated that 10% of patients have a history of affected family members. Rare families do show an autosomal dominant

inheritance pattern for hemangiomas (98). Histologically, these tumors are characterized by lobulated masses of capillaries lined by plump endothelial cells with thick basement membranes (86,87). Cellular markers of endothelial cell proliferation are present, and vascular growth factors (e.g., vascular endothelial growth factor [VEGF] and basic fibroblast growth factor [bFGF]) are often increased systemically. Histopathological features of hemangiomas in the involution phase include dilatation of the vascular lumina, flattening of endothelial cells, and the presence of fibrofatty tissue. GLUT-1 (glucose transporter 1) is present in the endothelial cells at all phases. Programmed cell death (apoptosis) is believed to be the mechanism of hemangioma involution.

Infantile hemangiomas have a distinctive life cycle, characterized by proliferating and involuting phases. Most appear within a few weeks after birth and undergo rapid initial proliferation, with a subsequent plateau at age 9 to 10 months, and then much slower involution, which may last until 5 to 10 years of age. Typical proliferating phase cutaneous hemangiomas are bright red, flat, or raised skin lesions with or without prominent adjacent superficial veins. Deep hemangiomas may have normal overlying skin or may show a subtle bluish discoloration. On palpation, infantile hemangiomas are generally firm and rubbery to the touch. In the involuting phase, hemangiomas become softer and paler. While the hemangioma involutes completely, the lesion may leave a wrinkled crepe paper–like appearance on the skin due to the loss of cutaneous collagen and elastin, and residual fibrofatty tissue may give the impression of a persistent mass. Ulceration in the proliferating phase results in scarring.

Although any area of the body may be affected, approximately 60% occur on the head and neck, followed by the trunk (25%) and extremities (15%) (99). The exact prevalence of visceral hemangiomas is unknown, as most of these lesions (typically liver hemangiomas) are found incidentally. However, symptomatic visceral hemangiomas are reported to be in 11.4% of patients (94). Hemangiomas can develop in almost any internal organ. Visceral hemangiomas are most common in the presence of five or more cutaneous lesions, and the involvement of three or more organs constitutes *disseminated hemangiomatosis*. Central nervous system (CNS) involvement is uncommon. In most cases, intracranial hemangiomas occur on dural or pial surfaces, either in contiguity with orbital lesions or in patients with disseminated hemangiomatosis. Hemangiomas in the beard area of the face have a high association with airway obstruction.

Hepatic hemangiomas can be entirely asymptomatic, but they often lead to hepatomegaly; high-output congestive

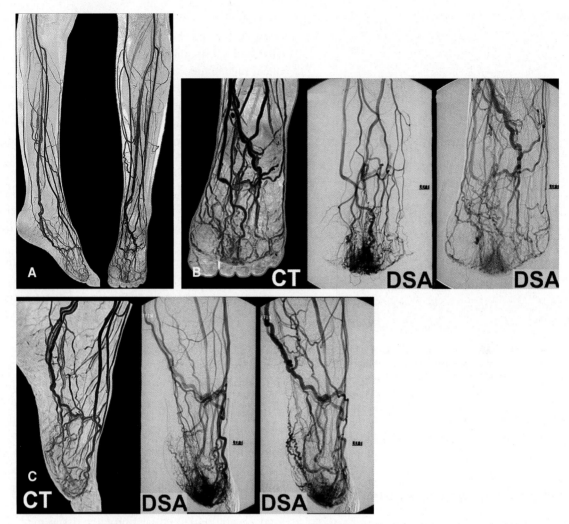

FIGURE 23-4 Four-row CTA of forefoot AVM. A: MIPs with inverted grayscale demonstrate the scan range from the distal popliteal artery through the tip of the foot. A 4 × 1.0 mm acquisition with 1.5 pitch and 0.5 second rotation time resulted in a 40-second-long acquisition. This scan was performed from cranial to caudal, and because of the prolonged duration resulting from the 4-row acquisition, extensive venous opacification is observed, most notably distally during the later phases of the scan. Differential flow in the superficial and deep venous systems is evident as the saphenous vein demonstrates greater opacification proximally than do the posterior tibial and popliteal veins. **B:** Frontal and **(C)** lateral views of the foot demonstrate from **left to right**, CTA, arterial-phase DSA, and venous-phase DSA. DSA was performed with a selective injection in the popliteal artery. The two DSA views were obtained 5 seconds apart and document the rapidity of arteriovenous shunting through this lesion. While the DSA acquisition allows separation of arterial and venous structures, the slower acquisition of the CTA does not allow this separation. Moreover, the higher spatial resolution of the DSA acquisition is evident in the demonstration of smaller vessels. (Courtesy of Geoffrey D. Rubin, MD.)

heart failure; anemia; and, occasionally, thrombocytopenia. Massive involvement with hemangioma, especially in the liver, has been associated with severe hypothyroidism, due to the production of 3-iodinine-dehydrogenase by the endothelial cells.

Although they are considered to be postnatal benign neoplasms, infantile hemangiomas can be associated with adjacent somatic developmental anomalies. The most common include cleft sternum and midline abdominal raphe, PHACES syndrome, spinal dysraphia (100), and anogenital anomalies. The PHACES syndrome was initially named by Frieden et al. (14). This syndrome consists of plaquelike (usually) facial hemangioma, posterior fossa anomalies (cystic), cerebral arterial abnormalities, aortic coarctation and arch anomalies, eye anomalies, and/or sternal clefting. Cerebrovascular anomalies include absence or hypoplasia of carotid or vertebral trunks, persistent embryonic vessels such as persistent trigeminal artery, occlusion or stenosis of intracranial arteries, and aneurysms. Occlusion resulting in cerebral infarction can occur postnatally. Cerebral dysgenesis

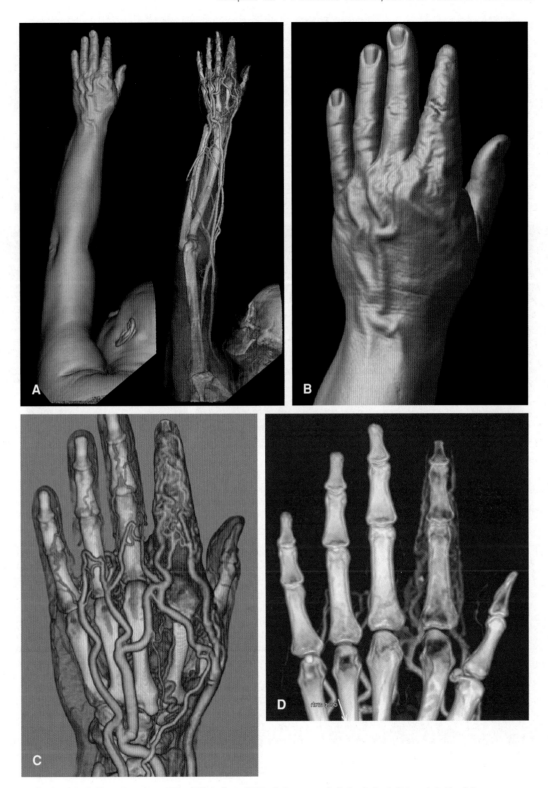

FIGURE 23-5 Sixty-four-row CTA of high-flow AVM of the second digit of the left hand. A: The full scan range is illustrated in these two VRs with opacity transfer functions selected to demonstrate both the skin **(left)** and underlying vascular and musculoskeletal structures **(right)**. The proper positioning for upper extremity CTA is demonstrated. The arm being injected is not shown but is held in anatomic position at the patient's side. **B:** VR with opacity transfer function to show surface anatomy accentuated by a high degree of specular reflection illustrates distended veins on the dorsum of the left hand as well as a shortened and swollen second digit without a fingernail. **C:** Alteration of the opacity transfer function illustrates the opacification of both arterial and venous channels with the nidus of the AVM involving the entirety of the second digit. **D:** Two-cm thick ray-sum projection illustrates demineralization throughout the phalanges of the involved second digit as well as acro-osteolysis of the second digit. (*Figure 23-5 continues*)

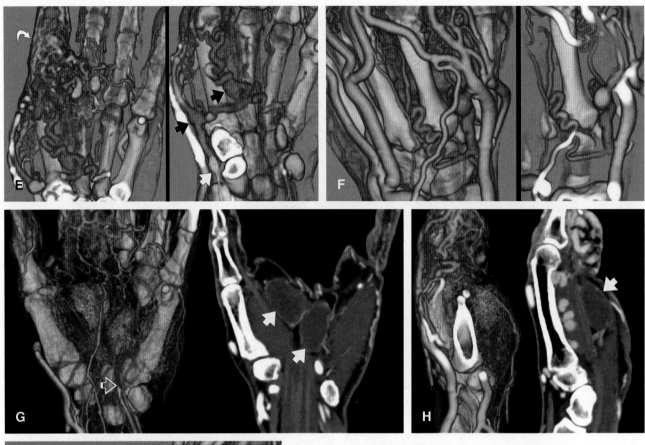

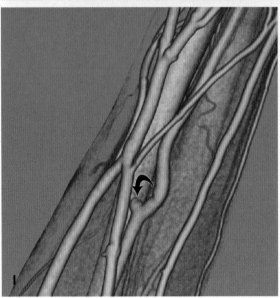

FIGURE 23-5 (Continued) E: Two-cm thick-slab VR images of the palmar aspect of the hand demonstrates the enlarged radial artery (*wide white arrow*) with distal aneurysms of enlarged tributary branches (*black arrows*) supplying the nidus of the AVM (*curved white arrow*). The close proximity of the tortuous vascular channels in the hand necessitates the use of thin-slab VRs to help separate the overlapping structures. **F:** A VR of the dorsum of the hand **(left)** illustrates the complex vascular channels. Arteries are separable from veins based upon their color due to the use of a sharp color transition applied to the opacity transfer function. Because the arteries are slightly less enhancing during this distal phase of the scan, they appear to be reddish orange, while the venous channels are lighter in color. The creation of a thin-slab **(right)** allows better visualization of the tortuous and aneurysmal arterial branches present on both sides of the base of the second metacarpal. The assessment of unenhancing structures is key to a complete assessment of this complex lesion. Frontal/coronal **(G)** and lateral/sagittal **(H)** VRs and MPRs illustrate large, thrombosed aneurysms (*blue structures* on VRs and *solid arrows* on MPRs), corresponding to the distal ulnar artery and lateral aspect of the deep palmar arch. The point of ulnar arterial occlusion is indicated with the *open white arrow*. **(I)** The aberrant flow conditions resulting from this AVM can result in aneurysm formation in proximal vessels. An 8-mm aneurysm has developed off the radial artery in the mid-forearm (*curved black arrow*). Careful scrutiny of the entire vascular system from axilla to tips of the fingers is required to completely characterize the abnormality. (Courtesy of Geoffrey D. Rubin, MD.)

and intracranial hemangioma have been added recently to the list of associations.

RICHs, in contrast, are fully grown at birth and regress relatively rapidly thereafter, often completing involution by 12 to 18 months of age. Typically, the masses are warm and occasionally have bruits or even a palpable thrill. Many are extremely

vascular and subsequently misdiagnosed as AVMs. Superficial lesions often have a blue-purple telangiectatic appearance surrounded by a pale halo. Their histopathology includes the presence of large thin-walled vascular channels, vascular thrombi, calcifications, hemosiderin, and cystlike vascular aneurysms (88). They do not stain positively for GLUT-1.

NICHs are also fully formed at birth but do not involute spontaneously. They are generally seen as tumorlike soft tissue masses that vary in size, from a few centimeters to 10 to 15 cm, and generally are soft to palpation and not painful, but most have a palpable warmth with a component of fast arterial flow. Like RICHs, they often have a telangiectatic appearance with a paler halo. NICHs, in contrast to infantile hemangiomas and RICHs, persist indefinitely (101). Histopathological features include lobular collections of small, thin-walled vasculature with a large central vessel. Interlobular areas contain predominantly dilated, often dysplastic veins, and arteries are increased in number. These lesions also lack positive staining for GLUT-1.

Intramuscular hemangiomas are uncommon distinct entities consisting of focal masses of capillaries in a fibrous stroma interspersed between striated muscle bundles in a pseudo-infiltrative fashion that mimics malignancy. They are GLUT-1 negative and do not involute. Unfortunately, in much existing literature, the term *intramuscular hemangioma* is used to describe venous malformations.

The exact prevalence of RICH, NICH, and intramuscular hemangiomas are unknown, but these are significantly less common than infantile hemangiomas.

KHEs are uncommon, usually diffuse tumors that are most commonly located in the trunk, extremities, and retroperitoneum (102). They are commonly associated with Kasabach-Merritt phenomenon (KMP) (severe coagulopathy due to platelet trapping resulting in spontaneous hemorrhage) but can also, less commonly, be seen with normal platelet counts. KHEs may be present at birth or may develop within the first few months after birth. An ill-defined purpuric mass with scattered bruising and petechiae is a common presentation. KMP is characterized by severe coagulopathy (usually with platelet counts below 25,000) secondary to platelet trapping, resulting in spontaneous hemorrhage (103). KHEs are histopathologically distinct from the common hemangiomas of infancy (89). The lesions involute slowly but sometimes start involution much later than infantile hemangiomas and do not regress completely. Residua of KHEs are common and include cutaneous red stains; telangiectatic streaks; and firm, irregular subcutaneous masses (104). These residue differ markedly from involuted common infantile hemangioma. Spindle-shaped endothelial cells, diminished pericytes and mast cells, and microthrombi and hemosiderin deposits are histopathological features of KHEs. The lesions are GLUT-1 negative.

Indications for Imaging

Imaging is not indicated in the majority of infantile hemangiomas, as they are easily diagnosed by most experienced physicians. For confirmation of a suspected hemangioma,

ultrasound is usually preferred as an initial imaging tool because of its portability, low cost, and lack of requirement for sedation. MRI is the ideal imaging modality to confirm diagnosis and evaluate lesion extent and associated anomalies in atypical patients as well as in those being considered for active therapy. There is little role for CT except to image hemangiomas of the bowel.

Infantile hemangiomas are quite consistent in their MRI appearance. In the early phases (proliferating and plateau phases), the tumor is a focal and lobulated homogeneous mass that is isointense to muscle on T1-weighted images and hyperintense on T2-weighted images (84). Typical infantile hemangioma is a rounded, sharply marginated mass lesion or less commonly an infiltrative but well-defined mass lesion. Postcontrast T1-weighted images typically show intense and homogeneous enhancement (Fig. 23-6). High-flow vessels, the largest of which are draining veins, are present typically within and around the tumor and appear as signal voids on SE sequences and high-signal foci on short TE gradient echo sequences (84). During the involuting phase, the vascularity and contrast enhancement of the tumor are less conspicuous, and progressive fibrofatty replacement can be seen. If CT is performed at this stage, increased fatty tissue is easily recognized with some residual vessels (Fig. 23-7). Calcifications in the tumoral mass are not features of infantile hemangioma but may be seen in RICHs (105). Also, if the tumor is located adjacent to a bone, smoothly marginated cortical erosions can be seen (10). With these imaging findings in association with appropriate age and clinical behavior, most hemangiomas can be diagnosed with high certainty and require no biopsy. If there is any deviation from this characteristic appearance, biopsy is recommended.

Hepatic hemangiomas, also called *hemangioendotheliomas*, have some unique imaging features (Fig. 23-8). Their angioarchitecture is variable, ranging from simple hypervascular nodules supplied by hepatic arteries and portal veins to direct arteriovenous, arterioportal and portovenous fistulas, sometimes with bizarre venous varices or other anomalies. In multifocal hemangiomas, the tumor nodules resemble infantile hemangiomas, appearing as homogenous, centripetally enhancing T2-hyperintense spheres with flow voids. Large flow voids within the nodules typically represent portovenous fistulas. Focal hepatic hemangiomas may have extremely high flow or slow flow, the latter with centripetal sinusoidal channels. They may also have areas of nonenhancement centrally. Recently presented evidence suggests that these focal lesions are a form of RICH.

While MRI findings in NICH are identical to those in infantile hemangioma, those in RICH may be sufficiently different to lead to misdiagnosis. While RICH consists of a

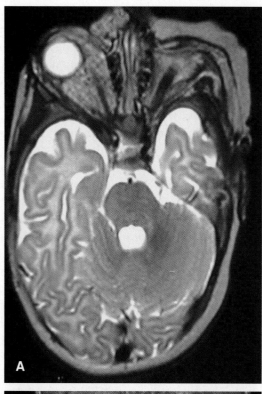

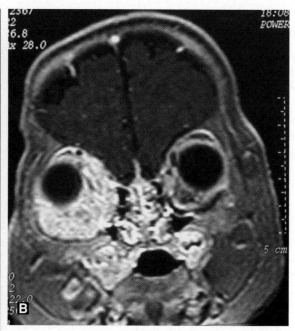

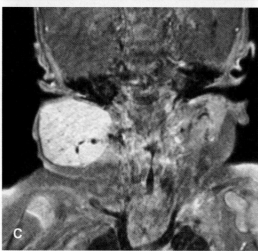

FIGURE 23-6 Infantile hemangioma. An axial T2-weighted SE image **(A)** through the orbits shows a large mass lesion in the right orbit displacing the intraorbital structures. Small pinpoint signal voids represent small arteries. The mass demonstrates significant, relatively homogeneous contrast enhancement on the postcontrast scan **(B)**, consistent with infantile hemangioma. A postcontrast T1-weighted SE image **(C)** from another patient with a large neck mass demonstrates a rounded, sharply marginated, homogeneously enhancing mass with small signal voids (due to arterial flow) within the periphery and around the mass. This appearance is characteristic for infantile hemangiomas in the proliferating phase. With typical MR findings that support the clinical diagnosis, no tissue sampling is needed for diagnosis in most infantile hemangioma patients.

focal mass and high-flow feeding and draining vessels, the vessels may predominate, leading to diagnosis of AVM. Alternatively, the mass lesion appears heterogeneous due to the presence of arterial aneurysms and thrombi and parenchymal infarcts, suggesting the diagnosis of malignancy such as congenital fibrosarcoma. MRA is useful in these patients in order to delineate the vascular architecture of the lesion in case of subsequent resection or embolization (88) (Fig. 23-9).

The imaging findings of intramuscular hemangiomas are similar to infantile hemangiomas, except the margins may appear less smooth. These masses usually require surgi-

cal excision or transcatheter embolization, so the investigation of the lesion's vascular architecture can be quite useful (Fig. 23-10). CT does not allow direct visualization of the hemangiomas as effectively as MRI. Phleboliths are common and readily visible on CT. CT can also provide a preoperative map of the arteries around the intramuscular hemangiomas (Fig. 23-11).

Generally speaking, MRA is not essential for the diagnosis of infantile hemangioma. MRA may be quite valuable if there are any concerns regarding associated arterial anomalies, such as is seen in PHACES syndrome, and in patients with high output cardiac failure, in whom

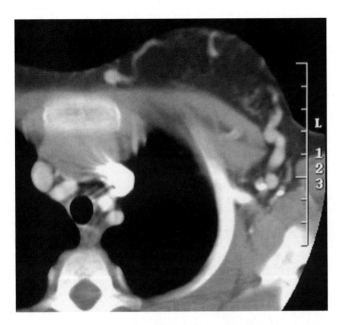

FIGURE 23-7 Infantile hemangioma (involuted). A postcontrast CT scan through the upper chest shows prominent vasculature with increased fatty tissue, but no or minimal residual mass lesion. This appearance is typical at the late-involution phase of infantile hemangiomas.

embolization may be necessary. The field of imaging should cover larger areas in this clinical setting (e.g., MRA of the chest, head, and neck in a patient with a large facial hemangioma). MRA images can be constructed by using the already acquired gradient echo images (utilizing the TOF MRA technique), but the diagnostic value of this technique is limited in these patients since the technique suffers due to artifacts and signal loss due to tortuous vasculature and complex flow directions of the tumor vasculature. When flow-dependent MRA techniques (TOF or PC) are used for MRA, neovasculature can be demonstrated (Fig. 23-12). However, vascular signal losses are common, and the scan time for completing these techniques for a relatively large area imposes a major limitation. PC MRA may particularly be useful for assessment of the venous drainage pattern of the mass lesion as well as the intracranial sinuses and venous architecture of the head and neck. Therefore, in patients with large facial hemangiomas where PHACES syndrome is considered, this technique

(*text continues on page 1147*)

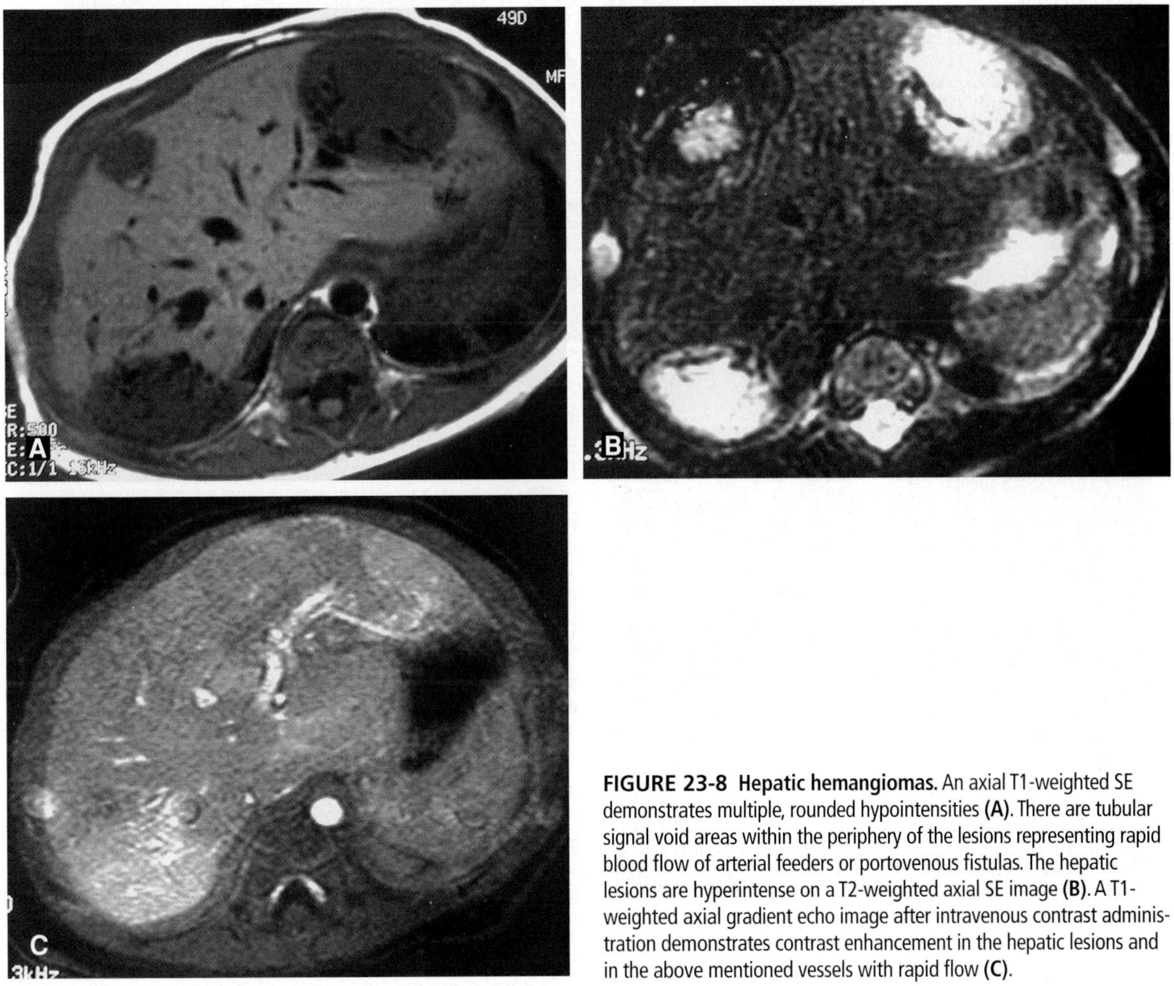

FIGURE 23-8 Hepatic hemangiomas. An axial T1-weighted SE demonstrates multiple, rounded hypointensities **(A)**. There are tubular signal void areas within the periphery of the lesions representing rapid blood flow of arterial feeders or portovenous fistulas. The hepatic lesions are hyperintense on a T2-weighted axial SE image **(B)**. A T1-weighted axial gradient echo image after intravenous contrast administration demonstrates contrast enhancement in the hepatic lesions and in the above mentioned vessels with rapid flow **(C)**.

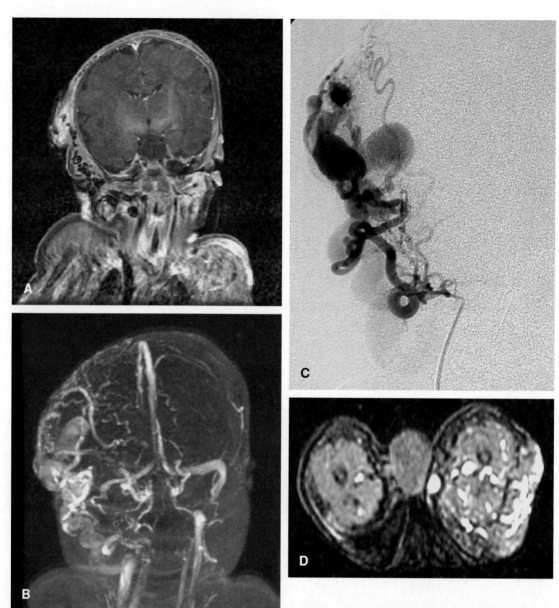

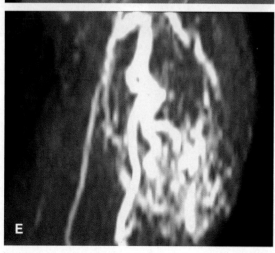

FIGURE 23-9 Rapidly involuting congenital hemangioma. A–C: RICH in the temporofrontal region. **D, E:** Large RICH in the left thigh. A coronal, postcontrast T1-weighted image **(A)** shows a tumoral mass in the extracranial temporofrontal area that demonstrates heterogeneous contrast enhancement and multiple, tubular signal voids representing abnormal vasculature in the area. TOF MRA without any saturation band demonstrates the abnormal arteries feeding the tumor and large draining veins **(B)**. The appearance of the lesion on catheter-based conventional arteriogram with iodinated contrast injection in the temporal artery **(C)** correlates well with the MRA. The large, round vascular spaces represent arterial aneurysms and venous ectasis, which are not seen in infantile hemangiomas and result in some of the heterogeneity as seen in the SE imaging study of these lesions. In a different patient with RICH located in the thigh, an axial gradient echo image **(D)** shows multiple flow-related hyperintensities representing arterial feeders of the tumor. Lateral **(E)** TOF MRA images confirm the hypervascularity of this congenital tumor.

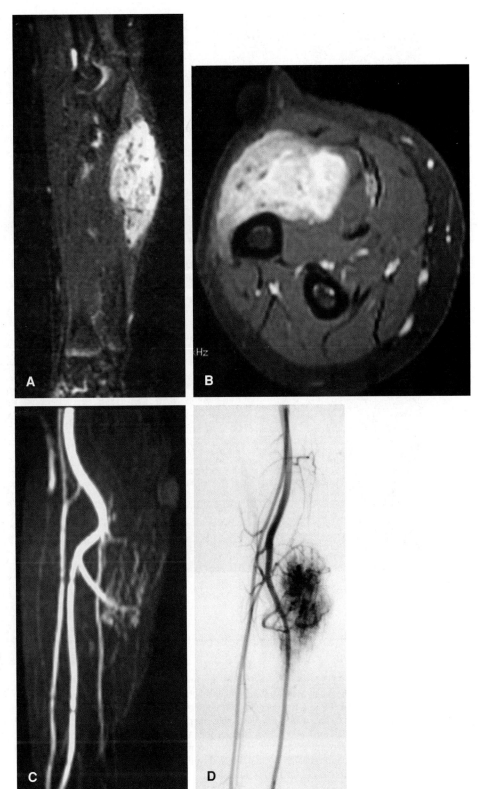

FIGURE 23-10 Intramuscular hemangioma. A sagittal T2-weighted inversion recovery image of the forearm (**A**) shows a well-marginated hyperintense lesion with small flow-related signal voids in the tumor, representing small intralesional arteries. The lesion enhances intensely as seen on an axial postcontrast T1-weighted image (**B**). Small signal void areas in the lesion represent small intratumoral arteries. CE MRA (**C**) reveals arterial feeds, as well as intralesional small arteries, but no arteriovenous shunting. Catheter-based conventional arteriogram (**D**) shows multiple arterial feeders from the distal brachial and ulnar arteries with tiny, irregular intralesional vasculature resulting in intense heterogeneous contrast accumulation in the lesion. Note that there is a high origin of the radial artery (anatomic variant).

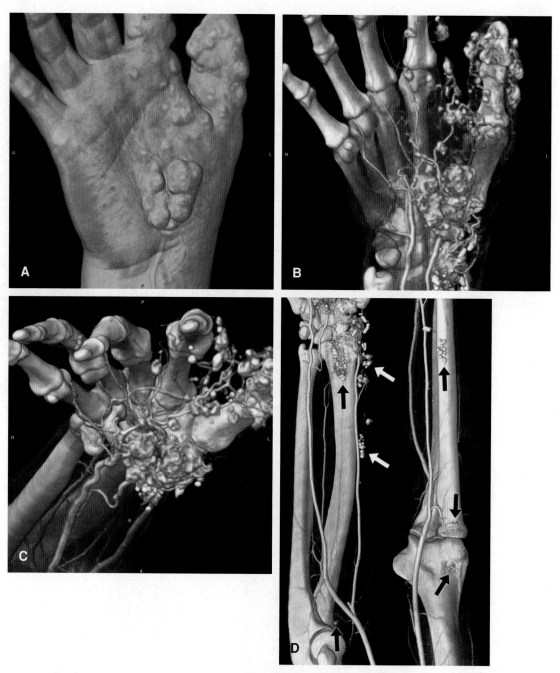

FIGURE 23-11 CTA of upper extremity intramuscular hemangiomata. A: VR of the right hand illustrates the superficial deformities associated with multiple hemangiomata. **B:** Alteration of the opacity transfer function to render the skin and soft tissues transparent allows visualization of the underlying hemangiomata, which are readily visualized due to extensive phleboliths as well as some enhancement of the soft tissue masses themselves. **C:** Interactive rotation of the VR at the workstation allows creation of nonstandard views and depiction of the complex spatial relationships between feeding arteries, draining veins, and soft tissue masses. **D:** Although the largest hemangiomata are in the hand, numerous phleboliths (*arrows*) can be seen throughout the forearm and proximal to the volar aspect of the capitellum. (Courtesy of Geoffrey D. Rubin, MD.)

should be used. The TOF MRA technique has the advantage of relatively rapid scanning and better demonstration of fast-flow vasculature in and around the lesion through the axial source images. CE MRA is the most popular technique, however, mainly because it is quick with minimal or no confusion related to complex flow dynamics of the lesion or the area of interest. The main disadvantage of the technique is the opacification of the arteries and veins at the same time due to rapid cervicofacial arteriovenous circulation, particularly in the head and neck, where most hemangiomas are located.

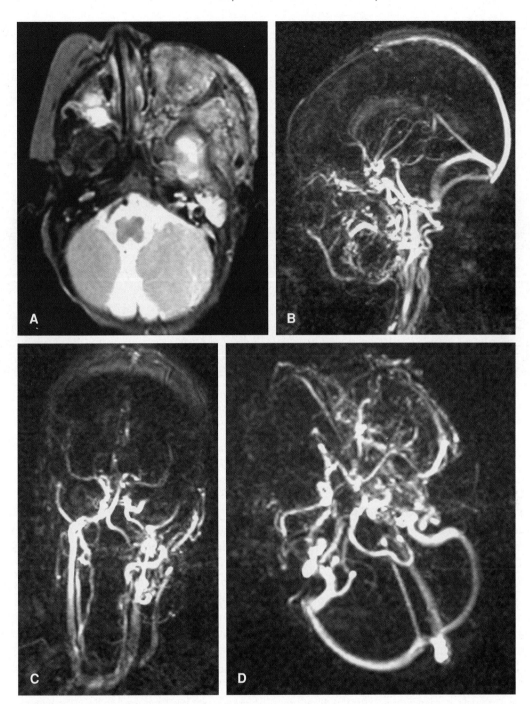

FIGURE 23-12 Infantile hemangioma. An axial T2-weighted SE image **(A)** shows an extensive left facial lesion, which is slightly hyperintense and heterogeneous. PC MRA of the head **(B–D)** reveals significantly increased hypervascularity in and around the lesion, which is typical for infantile hemangioma. (*Figure 23-12 continues*)

With the availability of 16 or greater channel CT scanners, CTA postprocessing may become an ideal imaging tool in some of these patients, particularly if associated vascular abnormalities are suspected (e.g., PHACES syndrome) primarily because the study can be performed with minimal sedation or no sedation at all. On the other hand, radiation exposure in infants and children remains a major

concern, and there is limited data available at the current time.

Imaging features of KHE are generally easy to distinguish from those of infantile hemangiomas (Fig. 23-13). KHE usually demonstrates ill-defined margins and inhomogeneous intensity and enhancement patterns. Unlike a common hemangioma, KHE characteristically involves multiple

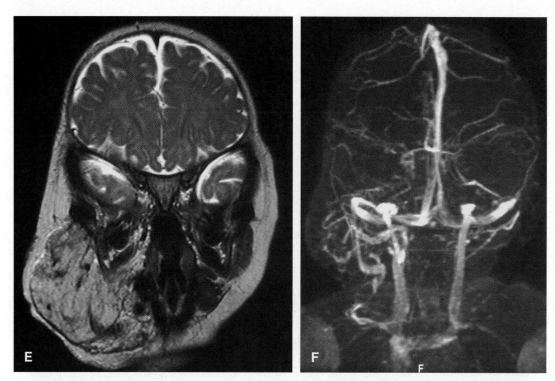

FIGURE 23-12 (Continued) A coronal T2-weighted SE image **(E)** from a different patient with infantile hemangioma demonstrates similar T2 signal characteristics with arterial signal voids in and around the lesion. Due to questionable hydrocephalus in this patient, PC MRV **(F)** was performed to rule out any extrinsic compression of the jugular venous return. MRV clearly demonstrates widely patent internal jugular veins in addition to confirming patency of the intracranial sinuses. The tumor has multiple, relatively large draining veins. In large head and neck infantile hemangiomas, MR angiography of the head and neck and chest is quite useful in ruling out vascular abnormalities that may be related to PHACES syndrome.

tissue planes with cutaneous thickening, subcutaneous stranding, and edema. Additionally, signal voids within the tumoral mass (due to hemosiderin deposition) can also be noted in some cases. Hypervascularity is a dominant feature of some KHE, although superficial feeding and draining vessels are less frequent and less conspicuous than with an infantile hemangioma. Destructive changes in the adjacent bones are common in KHE, whereas this is a rare occurrence in hemangiomas. Since some of these tumors require transcatheter embolization, obtaining MRA or CTA is of considerably more value in these tumors than in infantile hemangiomas. Similar imaging features can be seen in lymphangioendothelioma, which is much less common.

The differential diagnostic considerations of vascular masses presenting in early infancy include sarcomas, particularly congenital or infantile fibrosarcoma (106); rhabdomyosarcoma; and teratoma. In general, hemangiomas are characterized by discrete margins and homogeneous contrast enhancement, whereas sarcomas tend to be heterogenous (106,107). KHE without KMT may be confused with sarcomas. Any mass lacking the characteristic imaging and clinical features of hemangioma should be biopsied.

Treatment

Whether hemangiomas need to be treated or not is a subject of controversy because most hemangiomas eventually involute. Approximately 50% of hemangiomas involute in patients by the age of 5 years, 70% involute by age 7 years, and 90% involute by age 9 years (93,108). Some patients with involuted infantile hemangiomas require corrective surgery for residual telangiectasia, epidermal atrophy, and/or excessive fibrofatty tissue. However, there are a few instances in which a consensus exists among physicians who commonly treat or follow these patients. The term *endangering hemangiomas* has been used to describe hemangiomas whose location or hemodynamic effects threaten the life or function of the infant. These instances include periorbital hemangioma (causing a threat to vision); visceral hemangiomas (liver, gastrointestinal, brain, etc.); hemangiomas with high output cardiac failure; hemangiomas with significant or persistent ulcerations; and, finally, airway hemangiomas (109).

Pharmacological intervention is the first line of treatment; the most commonly used agent is corticosteroids. Treatment should be initiated during the proliferating phase of the tumor; it may be ineffective in later stages. The generally recommended steroid dosage (prednisone) ranges from 2

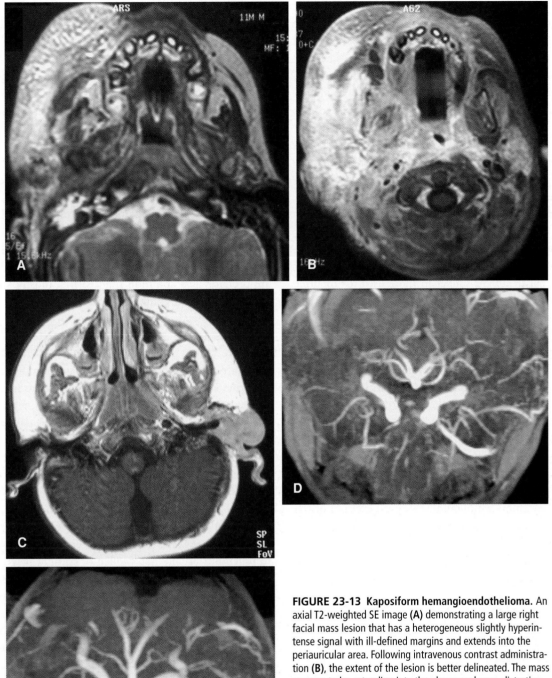

FIGURE 23-13 Kaposiform hemangioendothelioma. An axial T2-weighted SE image **(A)** demonstrating a large right facial mass lesion that has a heterogeneous slightly hyperintense signal with ill-defined margins and extends into the periauricular area. Following intravenous contrast administration **(B)**, the extent of the lesion is better delineated. The mass appears to be extending into the pharyngeal area, distorting the airway as well as the carotid sheath structures on the right. The contrast-enhancement pattern of this tumor is intense but somewhat heterogeneous. A postcontrast axial T1-weighted image **(C)** from another patient with KHE demonstrates a more focal mass in the periauricular area with homogeneous intense contrast enhancement. TOF MRA **(D, E)** demonstrates arterial feeders of this tumor.

to 3 mg/kg/day. If steroids are ineffective, vincristine can be tried. Interferon alpha is effective but is rarely used because of a high incidence of spastic diplegia. Intratumoral steroid injections can be used in small focal lesions, such as hemangiomas involving the nose or eyelids. A flash lamp pulsed dye laser can be used in selected cases to promote healing of ulcerations or fading of cutaneous lesions. Early resection is indicated in "endangering" hemangiomas that do not respond quickly to pharmacotherapy. Embolization is reserved for treatment of cardiac failure refractory to pharmacotherapy or severe bleeding. RICHs and hepatic hemangiomas are the most frequently embolized lesions.

In the treatment of RICHs, it is important to avoid misdiagnosis of AVMs. While most of these involute rapidly without treatment, symptomatic ones (e.g., high-output cardiac failure) are managed with pharmacological and/or interventional treatment similar to those used for infantile hemangiomas. Both noninvoluting and intramuscular hemangiomas are unlike infantile or congenital hemangiomas and require surgical treatment. Arterial embolization prior to surgical excision is sometimes indicated (110).

KHE associated with extremely low platelet counts and sometimes markedly decreased fibrinogen levels (KMT) (89,111) also are managed like infantile hemangiomas, using angiogenesis inhibitors. Additional treatment options include radiation, antiplatelet aggregating agents, cytotoxic drugs, and antifibrinolytic agents (112–120). KHE has a mortality rate of approximately 24% related to the coagulopathy or to complications of local tumor infiltration (89). Transcatheter embolization and/or surgical excision of the tumoral mass can be performed in selected cases. Particles (PVA or embospheres) are the most commonly used embolic agents. Platelet transfusions should be avoided, as these result in tumor growth.

HIGH-FLOW MALFORMATIONS

Definition, Clinical Presentation, and Histopathology

High-flow malformations include both AVMs and AVFs. AVMs are vascular anomalies that are characterized by abnormal communications resulting in shunting between veins and arteries. Classically, the arteries and veins are connected by a plexiform network of tortuous and dysplastic vessels referred to as a nidus. Many AVMs, however, lack a discrete nidus, consisting either of a large number of direct AVFs, or a diffuse collection of fine channels, possibly arteriolovenular shunts. Histologic demonstration of the arteriovenous shunts is difficult without laborious sectioning and special techniques. Histopathological sections show beds of capillaries, venules, and arterioles within a densely fibrous or fibromyxomatous background, intermixed with numerous larger caliber

arteries and thick-walled veins (121). Adventitial fibrosis and irregular intimal fibrosis in the veins (due to high flow and pressure) and dilated lymphatics can be commonly demonstrated (121). AVMs are congenital malformations but usually are not obvious at birth. Osler-Weber-Rendu syndrome (hereditary hemorrhagic telangiectasia) is an autosomal dominant disease characterized by mucocutaneous telangiectasias and AVMs in multiple organ systems. An AVF is a simple connection between an artery and a vein that can be congenital or secondary to a penetrating injury (Fig. 23-14).

High-flow vascular malformations are much less common than those with low flow. Most commonly, AVMs involve the brain or head and neck, followed by the lower extremities and trunk (122). AVMs are congenital lesions, but most are first noted in the second or third decades of life (123). There is no gender predominance (123). AVFs are probably less common than AVMs, mostly located in the head and neck, pulmonary circulation, or liver.

The clinical manifestations of AVM are variable, depending upon extent and flow characteristics. While extensive lesions with direct shunting present in infancy with cardiac volume overload, most are asymptomatic initially and evolve over time. Progressively increasing shunting results in vascular dilation, swelling, venous hypertension, and tissue ischemia. Progression may be accelerated after certain triggers such as trauma or the hormonal changes of puberty or pregnancy as well as after iatrogenic trauma including biopsy, proximal ligation, subtotal excision, or proximal embolization. Common symptoms of AVM include pain, swelling, hemorrhage, and heart failure. Kohout et al. (124) describe the Schobinger staging of AVMs. In stage 1, the stage of quiescence, the lesion is warm to touch but usually not swollen or painful. Stage 2 represents the stage of expansion, characterized by swelling, prominent veins, and pulsatility. Stage 3, destruction, results from tissue ischemia related to venous hypertension and arterial steal and involves increasing pain and ulceration. Stage 4, decompensation, is uncommon and includes the features of stage 3 plus high-output cardiac failure. Findings on clinical examination include the presence of a pulsatile mass, redness, increased temperature, pulsations, bruits, and thrills. Soft tissue and bone overgrowth, frequently with an overlying cutaneous capillary malformation, are typically present. Diffuse enlargement or overgrowth of the involved extremity is common in lesions involving the entire limb, often referred to as Parkes Weber syndrome (PWS).

AVMs involving the lungs, gastrointestinal system, and brain are features of hereditary hemorrhagic telangiectasia (HHT). Pulmonary AVMs or AVFs usually cause cyanosis, clubbing, and polycythemia as well as cerebral infarcts and abscesses (due to loss of the normal filtering function of the pulmonary vasculature). Approximately 15% to 20% of

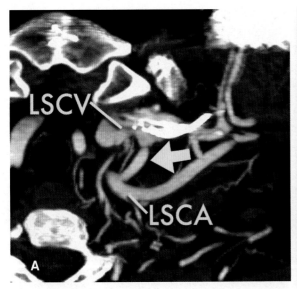
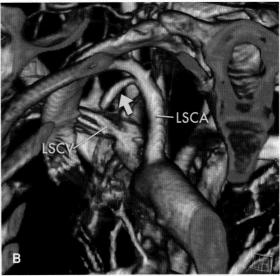

FIGURE 23-14 Arteriovenous fistula. Ultrasonographic examination of the subclavian veins to rule out subclavian thrombosis revealed no evidence of thrombosis, but an arteriovenous communication between the subclavian artery and vein in a young patient with pacer wires placed via the left subclavian vein. Etiology for this AVF is most likely a vascular trauma during the pacer placement. CTA **(A, B)** revealed an abnormal connecting vascular channel (*straight arrows*) between the subclavian artery and vein. With the currently available multidetector scanners, CTA offers a rapid angiographic imaging with high resolution but requires careful timing to image vascular anomalies, particularly in the head and neck due to rapid arteriovenous circulation.

patients with HHT have pulmonary AVMs, and approximately half of these patients are asymptomatic. Gastrointestinal bleeding and cardiac overload are seen in abdominal AVM. Patients may present with abdominal pain due to ischemic insult to the gut or thrombosis of the dilated venous channels of the alimentary system AVMs. Spinal AVMs are usually separated into four groups based on their location (paraspinal, epidural, dural, and intradural) (125). Spinal AVMs are associated with chronic or acute myelopathy or subarachnoid hemorrhage. AVFs can involve any organ system and may be symptomatic early in life due to high-output cardiac failure. Diagnosis often results from detection of a bruit or pulsatile mass in an asymptomatic patient (3).

Imaging Evaluation and Findings

Although the gold standard for diagnosing high-flow malformations is conventional arteriography, the high-flow nature of the malformation can be confirmed easily with a Doppler examination (Fig. 23-15). Characteristic Doppler findings include high-flow, low-resistance arteries and arterial waveforms in the draining veins (126). Spectral analysis reveals high venous peak velocity and a low resistive index. A low resistive index is also commonly found in hemangiomas; therefore, a high venous peak velocity appears to be the most reliable indicator to distinguish AVMs from other vascular anomalies (126).

MRI with MRA is the most comprehensive modality for the assessment of these lesions (Figs. 23-16, 23-17). CTA has advantages of rapid imaging and higher image res-

olution (Figs. 23-18, 23-19). Conventional angiography usually is reserved for patients requiring invasive treatment.

The characteristic MRI appearance of an AVM is that of an ill-defined soft tissue abnormality with enlarged vascular channels associated with dilated feeding and draining vessels and without a discrete mass. The area of the "nidus" appears heterogeneous. The high-flow vessels of the AVM appear as linear or punctuate signal voids on SE imaging with corresponding bright signal intensity on flow-enhanced gradient echo sequences. Skin thickening and increased fat deposition may be seen (10). A masslike appearance can be seen in some AVMs, which usually occurs secondary to edema particularly if an AVM nidus is in a closed space such as in a muscle sheath. In these cases, it may be difficult to differentiate AVMs from other soft tissue mass lesions on the basis of MRI alone. AVMs can involve bone, producing lytic bone expansion, lacy or hyperostotic changes, or cortical thinning. Direct bone involvement is indicated by the presence of high-flow intraosseous channels. CT also shows the lytic and sclerotic changes.

MRA findings depend upon the size of the communicating channels (Fig. 23-20). In stage 1 AVMs, including those in many patients with PWS, diffuse enlargement of arteries and veins may be the only finding. Early opacification of the venous channels is a hallmark of AVM and results in simultaneous visualization of arteries and veins in the region of the interest on CE MRA. In order to decrease venous contamination, the scan time should be kept at a minimum, and multiple phases should be acquired. A method called *time-resolved imaging of contrast kinetics* (TRICKS) can be used to solve the

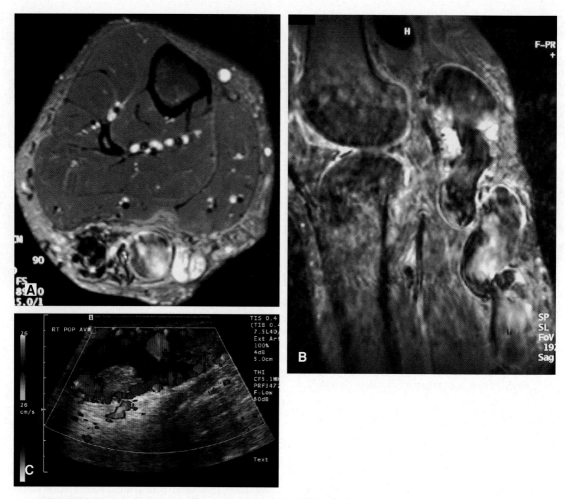

FIGURE 23-15 Arteriovenous malformation. (A) Axial and **(B)** sagittal postcontrast T1-weighted images demonstrate large, irregular vasculature in the posterior upper calf/popliteal region, which demonstrates heterogeneous intensities due to irregular, fast blood flow. Image artifacts are due to the pulsatile nature of this lesion. A color Doppler image **(C)** demonstrates typical multidirectional flow in the lesion. (*Figure 23-15 continues*)

timing problems or venous contamination (127). Source images may provide useful anatomic information prior to treatment (128). Steel coils used for embolization cause severe signal loss and image distortion. Platinum coils usually result in minimal distortion.

TOF technique can be used to demonstrate the arterial feeders, although the vasculature in the nidus makes a mixed signal due to multidirectional flow (Fig. 23-14). A similar mixed signal can also be seen in the draining veins due to arterialized multidirectional disoriented draining veins. PC MRA has very limited use in AVMs. Compared with CE MRA, TOF and PC MRA techniques are more susceptible to artifactual signal loss associated with the saturation of slow-flowing blood. Overall, it has been reported that flow-based MRA techniques can distinguish high-flow anomalies (e.g., AVM) from low-flow malformations (e.g., VM), but these MRA techniques add little practical information to the diagnostic process (11).

In infancy, AVMs may be confused with hemangiomas. Since infantile hemangiomas usually present with dilated arterial feeders and draining veins, the main imaging feature distinguishing an AVM from an infantile hemangioma is the lack of a mass lesion in AVMs. However, as mentioned previously, some AVMs in closed spaces demonstrate a masslike signal abnormality on MRI. One example of this is lingual AVMs (129). In lingual AVMs, the presence of ill-defined margins in AVMs versus lobulation in hemangiomas may be the only distinguishing imaging features (129). Clinical history and examination as well as age must be taken into account.

Treatment

AVMs generally permeate the involved tissues and are difficult to cure. Because of the morbidity associated with treatment as well as the low probability of achieving a cure in most types of AVM, treatment is not recommended in asymptomatic patients. Embolization (closing off the nidus

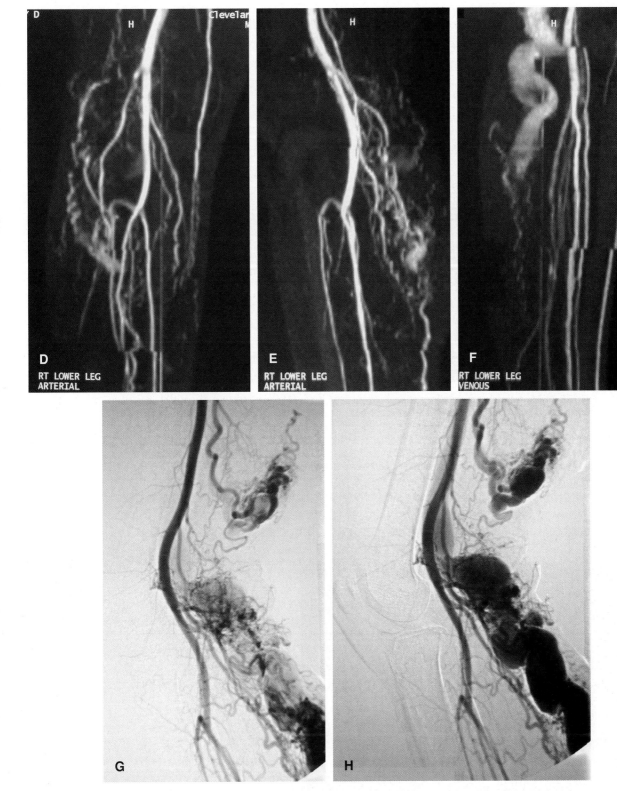

FIGURE 23-15 (Continued) TOF MRA images **(D, E)** obtained with suppression of the venous flow demonstrate arterial feeders of the malformation and the nidus. Draining veins are not seen. TOF MRV **(F)** obtained with arterial flow saturation demonstrates a large, varicoid draining vein of the AVM. The deep extremity veins appear patent. Conventional catheter-based arteriograms in early arterial phase **(G)** and delayed arterial phase **(H)** show a typical, large AVM lesion with large draining veins, correlating well with the MRA and MRV findings.

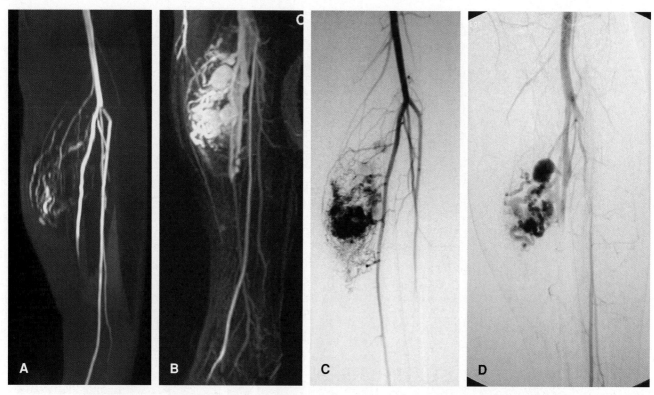

FIGURE 23-16 Arteriovenous malformation. A 2D TOF MRA image **(A)** of the left calf shows normal trifurcation of the popliteal artery and an AVM with small arterial feeders from the popliteal artery as well as from the posterior tibial artery. However, the size of the lesion is better delineated by CE MRA **(B)**. On the other hand, rapid flow into the draining veins is the limiting factor to assess the arterial feeders in CE MRA due to obscuration of small feeders by large draining veins. Arterial- **(C)** and venous- **(D)** phase images of a conventional catheter-based arteriogram clearly demonstrate the arterial feeders and draining veins and correlate well with the MRAs.

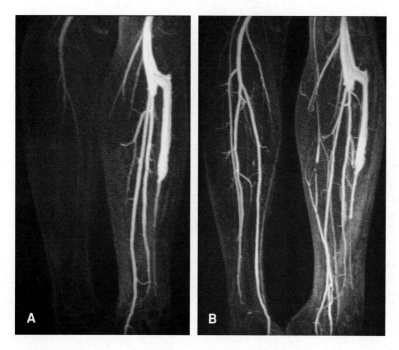

FIGURE 23-17 Arteriovenous fistula. A young female patient presented for a diagnostic workup for possible vascular lesion in the left calf. A CE MRA **(A)** shows rapid opacification of the run-off arteries and the posterior tibial vein in the left leg. There is relatively slow flow in the right run-off arteries. Tibial arteries in the right leg appear normal in the second phase of the CE scan **(B)**. (*Figure 23-17 continues*)

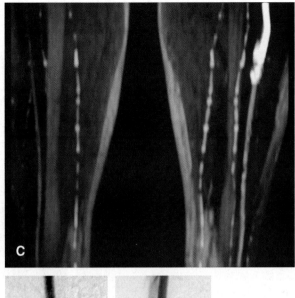

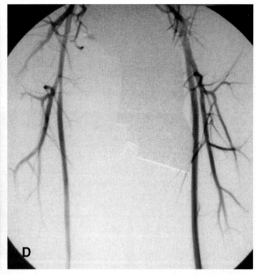

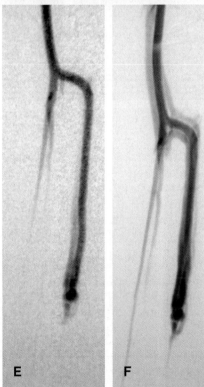

FIGURE 23-17 (Continued) TOF MRV **(C)** demonstrates the deep veins as well as the arteriovenous communication level and enlargement of the posterior tibial vein above this level. A catheter-based conventional pelvic arteriogram **(D)** demonstrates enlarged iliac and femoral arteries on the left due to an arteriovenous shunt in the left leg. The early arterial phase of the selective left leg arteriogram **(E)** clearly demonstrates the level of arteriovenous communication. In order to obtain a detailed assessment of high-flow anomalies, an arteriogram should be performed with high rates of image acquisition and short injection times. A slightly delayed phase of conventional arteriogram clearly outlines the venous drainage of the AVF **(F)**.

of the AVM with various materials and substances) is generally effective in AVMs to stabilize the malformation, but the method of treatment should be selected based on the stage of the malformation (Fig. 23-21). In stage I, embolization is not feasible, as there is not enough shunting (130). In stages III and IV, embolization is the treatment of choice, if the vascular anatomy is appropriate. In some patients with focal lesions, surgical excision is feasible, with preoperative embolization to decrease blood loss during resection.

Embolization usually is performed using a supraselective transcatheter approach, often supplemented by percutaneous

injection of the nidus. The percutaneous approach may be the only option when the nidus cannot be reached with catheters due to difficult anatomy or closure of the arterial feeders by previous surgical ligation or coil embolization. In general, ligation or coil embolization of the arterial feeders usually results in recruiting several small arterial feeders and also makes the AVM worse in some patients; therefore, embolization or surgical ligation of the arterial feeders should be avoided.

Permanent embolization agents, including absolute alcohol and NBCA (n-butyl-2-cyanoacrylate), are most

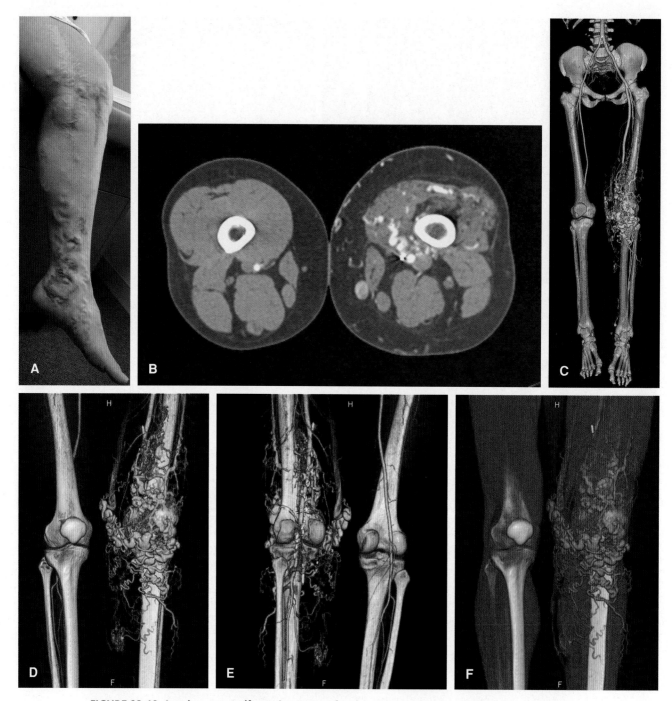

FIGURE 23-18 Arteriovenous malformation. A young female patient presents with a history of long-standing high-flow vascular anomaly around the knee with multiple failed surgical attempts **(A)**. MRA is not favored due to multiple metallic surgical clips that would cause significant image distortion. An axial source image **(B)** from CTA just above the knee shows an enlarged circumference of the leg; atrophic muscles; and multiple, various-sized enhancing vessels. There is a tiny metal density/artifact seen from a metallic surgical clip. Source images of CTA are valuable in terms of evaluating the underlying soft tissues. CTA can cover large portions of the body **(C)** in a short period of time (commonly less than 30 seconds) to investigate additional potential vascular abnormalities. With the currently available image-processing techniques, the area of interest can be further assessed in multiple projections and window settings to optimize the visualization of the diseased vessels **(D–F)**.

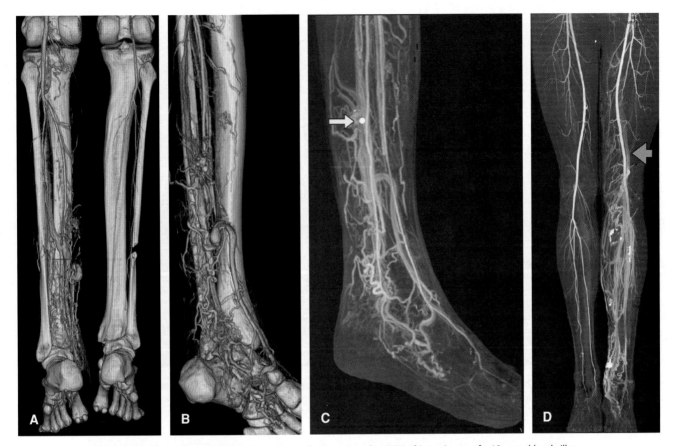

FIGURE 23-19 Leg-length discrepancy due to lower extremity AVM. This tragic case of a 19-year-old male illustrates the impact of AVMs on limb growth and the potentially clinically occult nature of early AVMs. **A:** Posterior VR of a CTA illustrates an extensive AVM in the left lower leg. An examination of the position of the calcanei relative to the tibial plateaus illustrates that the left lower leg is longer than the right. An osteotomy in the right fibula as well as curvature of the proximal tibia are sequela of prior right leg-lengthening Iliazarov procedure. The procedure had been performed at age 14 to equalize the lower leg lengths prior to the diagnosis of the left lower leg AVM. While the procedure had been successful at the time, continued growth of the left lower leg has resulted in the current limb-length discrepancy. **B:** The complex interrelationships of arterial and venous channels are evident on the VR; however, arterial and venous channels are difficult to distinguish. **C:** Arteriovenous differentiation is easier on the MIP, where the inflowing arteries are brighter than the draining veins. The relative spatial relationships evident on the VR are not visible, however. A phlebolith (*arrow*) is evident in a venous channel. **D:** MIP of the bilateral lower extremities provides comparative visualization of the arterial system. Venous opacification, while extensive in the left leg, has not occurred in the right leg. The degree of opacification in the left leg is greatest in the calf with early filling of the distal superficial femoral vein (*arrow*). (Courtesy of Geoffrey D. Rubin, MD.)

effective in primary treatment of AVM. The use of these agents requires expert catheter skills and experience. Devastating complications are possible. Most AVMs require several sessions generally 2 months apart with regular follow-up. Particulate embolic agents (embospheres, PVAs) are more appropriate for preoperative embolization.

The goal of embolization is to ablate the nidus but not the feeding arteries. Similarly, ligation of the arterial feeders should not be performed. Unlike AVMs, AVFs usually are curable by embolization or ligation (131).

LOW-FLOW MALFORMATIONS

Low-flow malformations include those that are venous (cavernous hemangiomas), lymphatic, lymphatic-venous (LVM), and capillary (port-wine stains).

Definition, Clinical Features, and Histopathology

Venous Malformations

VMs are the most common symptomatic type of vascular malformation. Forty percent of VMs are located in the head and neck, 40% in the extremities, and the remaining 20% on the trunk (9). Most VMs are spongy, masslike lesions that are composed of abnormal veins (veins with a relative lack of smooth muscle cells in their walls), although many also involve identifiable conducting veins. Morphologic types include focal sequestered VM; multifocal sequestered lesions; and diffuse, nonsequestered lesions composed of varicose channels and venous lakes. The latter communicate freely with the venous circulation. Multifocal VMs are often familial. VMs are commonly (and erroneously) referred to as *hemangiomas* or *cavernous hemangiomas*.

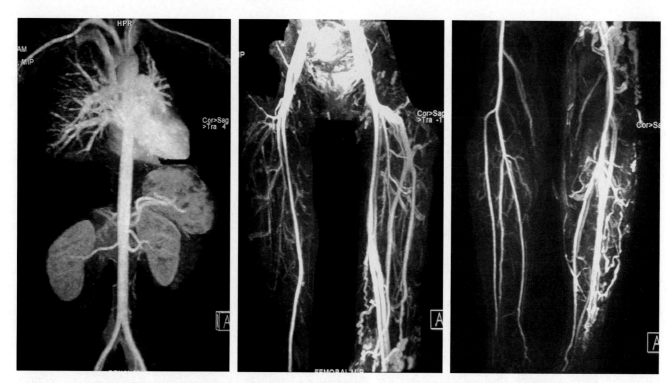

FIGURE 23-20 Arteriovenous malformation. CE MRA of the aorta and lower extremities demonstrates an extensive AVM in the left leg. The left iliac and femoral arteries appear larger than the right. This is a common finding in high-flow anomalies due to the significant arteriovenous shunt in the diseased extremity. There are multifocal niduses resulting in early opacification of the left leg veins.

In general, low-flow vascular malformations enlarge proportionately with the growth of the child. Enlargement is secondary to channel dilation, often caused by intralesional thrombosis in VM. The characteristic physical findings in VMs include a soft and easily compressible soft tissue mass (or swelling) that is associated with bluish skin discoloration. Engorgement with dependency, activity, venous compression, or maneuvers that increase venous pressure is typical. Thrombosis and thrombophlebitis may occur (9). Although VMs are considered benign entities, those in critical locations can result in significant morbidity. Examples include cervicofacial VMs that compress or intrinsically involve the airway, sometimes requiring tracheostomy; orbital VMs, resulting in progressive loss of vision; diffuse facial/calvarial VMs associated with sinus pericranii (abnormal communication between intracranial and extracranial circulations); and developmental intracranial venous anomalies. Diffuse extremity VMs may be associated with a limb-length discrepancy, with the affected limb being shorter than the normal one as well as consumption coagulopathy. Intraosseous VMs can cause structural weakening of the osseous shaft and pathologic fractures. Involvement of a joint by VM may result in hemosiderin-arthropathy due to repeated intra-articular bleeding, which is most commonly encountered in the knee. VMs of the gastrointestinal tract most commonly cause chronic bleeding and anemia, and they may be part of blue rubber bleb nevus syndrome (BRBNS). Lesions that involve the foregut can be associated with portal venous anomalies (absence of the portal vein, portal hypertension, etc).

BRBNS is a hereditary condition in which patients continuously develop focal VM over their lifetimes. The cutaneous lesions are blue and dome shaped and vary in size from one millimeter to several centimeters. They can be pedunculated. Most patients have multiple muscular and gastrointestinal lesions. The latter are associated with bleeding, often leading to blood transfusions and resections as well as intussusception and bowel obstruction.

Glomuvenous malformation (GVM) (or glomangioma) is a rare familial (autosomal dominant) form of venous malformation. It presents with multiple small nodular superficial venous malformations that are often tender. GVM differs from typical VMs because of the presence of numerous glomus cells (immature smooth muscle cells) that line the ectatic vascular channels (132).

Lymphatic and Lymphatic-venous Malformations

LMs consist of masses of endothelial-lined, thin-walled channels that contain lymphatic fluid. LMs were formerly

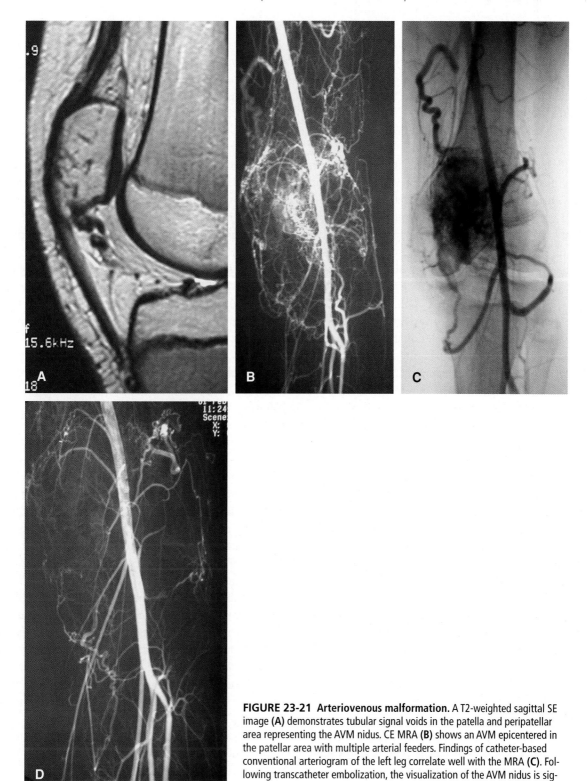

FIGURE 23-21 Arteriovenous malformation. A T2-weighted sagittal SE image **(A)** demonstrates tubular signal voids in the patella and peripatellar area representing the AVM nidus. CE MRA **(B)** shows an AVM epicentered in the patellar area with multiple arterial feeders. Findings of catheter-based conventional arteriogram of the left leg correlate well with the MRA **(C)**. Following transcatheter embolization, the visualization of the AVM nidus is significantly diminished **(D)**.

termed *lymphangiomas, cavernous lymphangiomas,* or *cystic hygromas.* They are usually classified as microcystic, macrocystic, or mixed and diffuse or focal. Microcystic LMs are characterized with no visible cystic lesions on MRI, while macrocystic LMs are characterized with easily noticeable cystic spaces on MRI. MRI of mixed LM demonstrates cystic- and solid-appearing sections in the malformation. The term *cystic hygroma* was previously used to describe the macrocystic LM that contains a small number of large cysts.

LVMs are a combination of LMs and anomalous venous channels. True combinations of spongy VM and LM are uncommon, although after surgery for LM, venous blood can circulate in the recurrent LM. The venous anomalies associated with LM include dilated venous channels and persistent embryonic veins.

The incidence of LMs is similar in males and females. The most common location is the head and neck, followed by the axilla, extremities, and trunk. The majority of lesions are noticed before 2 years of age but presentation later in life is not uncommon (1). LMs may be associated with a number of genetic syndromes including Turner syndrome and trisomy 13, 18, and 21 (1).

LMs most commonly occur in the cervicofacial region (approximately 75%), but they can involve any structure except the brain. Most diffuse LMs are apparent in infancy. They grow proportionately with the child's growth but characteristically enlarge transiently with systemic viral infections or acutely due to intralesional hemorrhage or infection. The overlying skin can be normal, or it may have tiny characteristic vesicles, often commingled with a capillary stain. LMs of the floor of the mouth and tongue are usually characterized by vesicles, swelling, and bleeding, typically with overgrowth of the mandibular body. LMs of the orbit typically cause proptosis (sudden proptosis is usually due to intralesional bleeding), which may require surgical or interventional decompression to preserve vision. Mediastinal LMs often accompany cervical and/or axillary lesions and may be associated with airway obstruction or chylothorax. Some LMs are characterized by chylous reflux and leakage as well as swelling. Diffuse LMs involving a limb can cause diffuse or localized swelling with soft tissue and skeletal overgrowth. Pelvic LMs can be associated with bladder outlet obstruction, constipation, or recurrent sepsis. Disappearing bone disease (Gorham-Stout syndrome) is a rare disease entity that is considered multifocal LM with progressive osteolysis and is often associated with fatal chylous effusions.

Capillary Malformations

Capillary malformations (CM) are seen most commonly in the skin, where they are referred to as *port-wine stains*. They often co-exist with deep vascular malformations, especially AVM and LM, and with subcutaneous fatty overgrowth. CM is present in 0.4% of newborns (133). CM is seen most commonly on the face, followed by neck, trunk, and extremities (134).

Imaging Strategies and Findings

Imaging should be tailored to the clinical need. In the presence of typical clinical findings, imaging may not be necessary. To identify high-flow components, Doppler ultrasound may be sufficient. To determine the extent as well as the nature of a lesion, MRI is best. Plain radiographs are useful mainly to determine the presence of osseous or thoracic complications. In VMs, radiography may show round, lamellated calcifications (phleboliths) in the soft tissues with or without a soft tissue mass or prominence. Osseous involvement can be appreciated as focal areas of cortical thinning with increased trabeculae (10). LMs can also be associated with cortical thinning with increased trabeculae, hyperostosis, or focal lytic lesions. LMs rarely are associated with progressive osteolysis; this condition has been termed *Gorham-Stout syndrome* (also known as disappearing bone disease) (135,136).

MRI serves in these conditions not only to confirm the diagnosis but also to plan therapy (e.g., surgery vs. sclerotherapy). Most VMs, LMs, and LVMs are hyperintense on T2-weighted images and are isointense or hypointense compared with muscle on T1-weighted images. They usually are septated and sharply marginated but frequently involve more than one tissue plane. For planning sclerotherapy, it is useful to be able to determine the size of the channels or cysts. Round signal voids representing thrombi or phleboliths are commonly seen in VMs but usually are not present in LMs. Fluid-fluid levels are common in LMs, especially after a history of intralesional hemorrhage. In LMs with multiple macrocysts, the individual cysts may have different signal intensity if bleeding has occurred in one cyst and not another. Small fluid levels can be seen in VMs, especially those containing large channels (3). Signal voids due to high flow on SE sequences or flow-related hyperintensities on gradient echo sequences are not features of these malformations. Contrast-enhancement patterns are the most reliable means of distinguishing VM from LM. Patchy or inhomogeneous enhancement of the channel lumen is a feature of VMs, while dilated conducting veins in LVM may enhance more densely and homogeneously. LMs generally show enhancement of the rims but not the contents of the cysts. Other nonenhancing cystic malformations, including brachial cleft, foregut duplication, and thyroglossal duct cysts, may be difficult to distinguish from LM.

LM can be multifocal, involving multiple sites in the same patient. Multifocal LM typically involves multiple bones, including the spine, as well as soft tissues, including the spleen. Chylous effusions occur most frequently in this type of lesion. In the presence of severe bone loss, this condition has been termed *Gorham* or *Gorham-Stout syndrome* (137). LVMs have elements of LM and associated abnormalities of major conducting veins (e.g., persistent embryonic veins, abnormal dilation of normal veins, and absence or maldevelopment of deep venous system). Often, delineation of the venous anatomy is necessary before attempting any surgical or percutaneous intervention.

The angioarchitecture of VM is variable. While there is no generally accepted classification, they include focal, multifocal, and diffuse forms. Focal lesions may be intramuscular, cutaneous, or mucosal and usually consist of collections of abnormal interconnecting channels or spaces that are "sequestered" or drain through fairly small channels to normal adjacent conducting veins. They are quite easily treated by sclerosant injection. Lesions demonstrating small arterial feeders with intense and rapid opacification and prominent draining veins may be classified as capillary-venous malformation, and these lesions are commonly confused with AVMs on noninvasive angiographic studies (Figs. 23-22, 23-23). Diffuse VMs involve multiple tissue layers, usually including muscle, subcutaneous fat, skin, and sometimes bone. In diffuse lesions, the malformed veins are not sequestered but communicate directly with the main conducting veins, which frequently are abnormal as well. Diffuse VMs are difficult to treat effectively, as injected sclerosant can directly enter the circulation, potentially causing deep venous thrombosis, pulmonary embolism, or systemic effects of ethanol. Some patients with diffuse venous malformations have focal eccentric varices, which can exert considerable mass effect on adjacent structures. Unlike in LMs or LVMs, the deep veins are generally present but may be dilated or malformed. Diffuse cervicofacial VMs have a high incidence of developmental venous anomalies of the brain and of calvarial VM with sinus pericranii.

Multifocal VMs are most commonly seen in the familial forms of VM, including the following:

1. *Blue rubber bleb nevus syndrome.* The musculoskeletal lesions have a typical appearance on MRI, looking like multifocal clusters of fluid-filled cavities. Gastrointestinal lesions are serosal or mucosal. Pedunculated or polypoid mucosal lesions can result in intussusception. They are seen frequently in the liver, where they are generally asymptomatic but result in the presence of phleboliths.
2. *Mucocutaneous familial venous malformations.* In this form, patients present in a very similar fashion to BRBNS but do not have gastrointestinal involvement.
3. *Mucocutaneous and cerebral venous malformations.* In this familial condition, patients have progressive development of CNS "cavernous malformations," generally referred to as inhomogeneous, enhancing focal lesions with hemosiderin. Some lesions are tiny and are picked up most reliably with gradient imaging.
4. *Glomuvenous malformations.* Although GVMs differ from common VMs clinically and histologically, imaging features are very similar. GVMs usually appear as

focal, nodular superficial lesions. On direct contrast venography, the focal lesion is seen as a lobulated space, generally communicating directly with a small cutaneous vein. MRI may show similar features, with tiny veins appearing to connect to the nodules.

While SE imaging is optimal to demonstrate the extent of the VM, CE is useful to assess the flow pattern (Figs. 23-24–23-26). If the gadolinium is injected through the involved body part (e.g., via a foot vein for a leg VM), the opacification of the venous system in the involved area is optimal, since the veins but not the arteries are opacified in the early phases. This approach should be used particularly in extremity low-flow anomalies with possible association with a maldeveloped deep venous system (e.g., Klippel-Trenauney Syndrome). Other MRA techniques (TOF and PC) have limited use in this malformation, but the source images of TOF are typically used to rule out high-flow vessels in these malformations (e.g., ruling out AVM).

While CT is a good imaging modality to demonstrate osseous changes in these low-flow anomalies, poor tissue contrast limits the delineation of the soft tissue lesion (Figs. 23-27, 23-28). Also, although contrast enhancement of VMs is conspicuous on MRI, opacification of the venous channels of VMs with iodinated contrast is quite poor because the contrast material usually reaches the VM after the scan is completed (CT scan time is very short) and the sensitivity of iodinated contrast on CT is significantly less than that of gadolinium compounds on MRI. Because of the lesser enhancement capabilities of iodinated contrast on CT, CTA also suffers from similar problems and has a limited role in the evaluation of these malformations (138). On the other hand, CT is quite sensitive to demonstrate phleboliths.

Conventional arteriography is not appropriate in most patients with low-flow malformations but may be necessary when other studies are indeterminate or when associated anomalies such as sinus pericranii or small AVFs are suspected. Selective arteriography may demonstrate puddling of contrast material within the sinusoidal spaces and abnormal veins of the VM; however, a direct intralesional injection of contrast material is a better examination in order to opacify the lesion and to show its extent, the interconnecting channels, and the venous drainage pattern. Multiple percutaneous access sites may be necessary to opacify the various portions of the malformation.

CM (port-wine stain) is a common form of vascular anomaly that usually does not require imaging. The value of MRI in CM is to rule out a possible underlying vascular anomaly. Patients with CM distribution of the first branch of the trigeminal nerve (V1) should be evaluated for the possibility of Sturge-Weber syndrome (139).

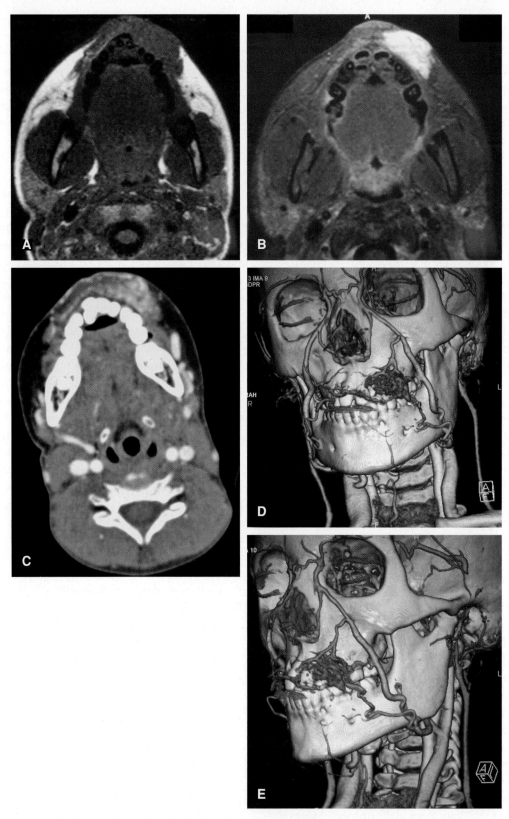

FIGURE 23-22 Capillary venous malformation in a young boy, who presented with an obvious vascular anomaly in the upper lip area. Pre- and postcontrast MRI shows a homogeneously enhancing, sharply marginated lesion in the left lip area **(A, B)**. This appearance is strongly suggestive of a VM. A source CT image from CTA demonstrates heterogeneous enhancement of the lesion **(C)**. On CTA **(D, E)**, the vascular malformation and the draining vein (draining into the facial vein) are seen clearly. The facial artery is seen extending into the region, but it is unclear if there are arterial feeders to this lesion from the facial artery (due to obscuration by the intense enhancement of the lesion). The timing of the scanning after the intravenous contrast injection plays a major role to evaluate vascular lesions accurately, particularly in children and in the head and neck due to rapid arteriovenous circulation. (*Figure 23-22 continues*)

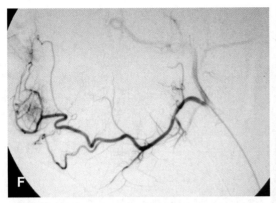
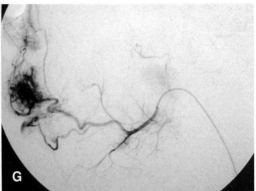

FIGURE 23-22 (Continued) A catheter-based conventional arteriogram (contrast injection in the facial artery) shows tiny arterial feeders into the malformation **(F)**. A slightly delayed angiographic image **(G)** shows intense enhancement of the malformation. Opacification of the draining veins is delayed, confirming the fact that this lesion is not an AVM.

Treatment

VMs are managed conservatively with graded compression stockings and aspirin (to decrease clotting). Since most low-flow malformations involve one or multiple muscle groups (and bones in some cases), a surgical approach is not feasible in the majority of patients. Sclerotherapy (direct injection of sclerosant agent into the lesion under various imaging guidance techniques) is the first-line therapeutic approach. Currently, the most commonly used sclerosant agent is absolute ethanol. Other less commonly used sclerosants include ethanolamine oleate (Ethamolin) and sodium tetradecyl sulfate. Some small, focal lesions are amenable to resection.

LMs and LVMs are also treated either by sclerotherapy or resection. Both techniques are most effective in macrocystic LM. It is quite difficult to treat microcystic LMs. Most CMs do not cause health problems; patients seek medical help due to concern for a suspected underlying condition or, more commonly, for cosmetic reasons. Pulsed dye laser is the standard treatment (140).

OVERGROWTH SYNDROMES WITH VASCULAR ANOMALIES

Definition, Clinical Features, and Histopathology

The overgrowth syndromes associated with vascular anomalies include Klippel-Trenaunay, Sturge-Weber, Parkes Weber, Proteus, Banayan Riley Rubalcava (BRR), and Mafucci.

Klippel-Trenaunay Syndrome

The medical community at times has used the terms *Klippel-Trenaunay syndrome* and *Klippel-Trenaunay-Weber syndrome* interchangeably. The consensus today is that KTS is characterized by low-flow vascular anomalies, while PWS is characterized by high-flow vascular anomalies. KTS is a rare, sporadic, slow-flow combined vascular anomaly (capillary-lymphatic-venous malformation [CLVM])

that is characterized by a triad of capillary malformations (port-wine stain), varicose veins (VM), and bony and/or soft tissue hypertrophy. A lymphatic component is present, evidenced either by lymphedema or by lymphatic vesicles, usually intermingled with the capillary malformation in the lateral or anterior aspect of the thigh and knee. Venous abnormalities in the involved extremity are common. KTS can be inherited in a multifactorial way and a range of vascular malformations can be observed in family members (141). Some cases of KTS are caused by a mutation in or gain-of-function translocation involving the VG5Q gene (142).

While most patients with KTS have increased length of the affected limb, the syndrome may rarely be associated with hypotrophy. The symptoms and findings associated with the disorder may vary in range and severity from case to case. Anomalous lateral veins, which are typically on the lateral aspect of the thigh, become prominent because of absent or incompetent valves and deep venous anomalies. The lateral venous anomaly is known as the marginal vein of Servelle. Thrombophlebitis (53%) and thromboembolic episodes (11%) are the main complications, which require careful surveillance (143). Other anomalies associated with KTS include syndactyly, macrodactyly, polydactyly, and hip dysplasia (144). A small percentage of KTS patients have been reported to have cerebral and cerebellar hemihypertrophy (145) or Sturge-Weber syndrome (146). However, this does not warrant a cerebral MRI if there are no supporting clinical findings.

Sturge-Weber Syndrome

Sturge-Weber syndrome is a neurocutaneous disorder characterized with capillary or venular malformation of the leptomeninges (typically in the parieto-occipital region) and skin of the face. Facial CMs of the Sturge-Weber syndrome are typically located in the distribution of the first division

(*text continues on page 1166*)

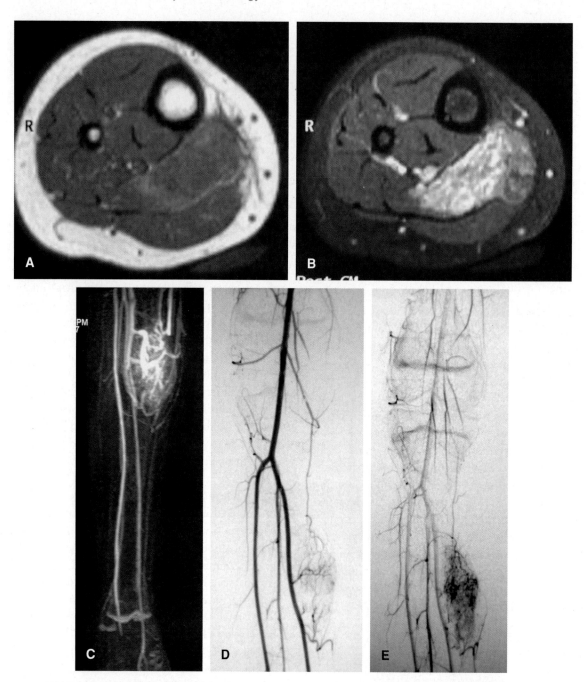

FIGURE 23-23 Capillary venous malformation in a young girl, who presented with a painful vascular malformation in the calf. Pre- and postgadolinium axial T1-weighted images **(A, B)** show intense heterogeneous contrast enhancement of the malformation located in the posterior upper calf involving the soleus muscle. A CE MRA **(C)** shows a significantly hypervascular lesion with opacification of both run-off arteries and draining veins. Due to prominent contrast accumulation in the lesion, it is difficult to evaluate whether there are arterial feeders that can be catheterized for embolotherapy. A catheter-based conventional arteriogram shows multiple, tiny arterial feeders from the posterior tibial artery **(D)**. A slightly delayed phase of the conventional arteriography **(E)** shows heterogeneous opacification of the malformation without rapid opacification of the draining veins.

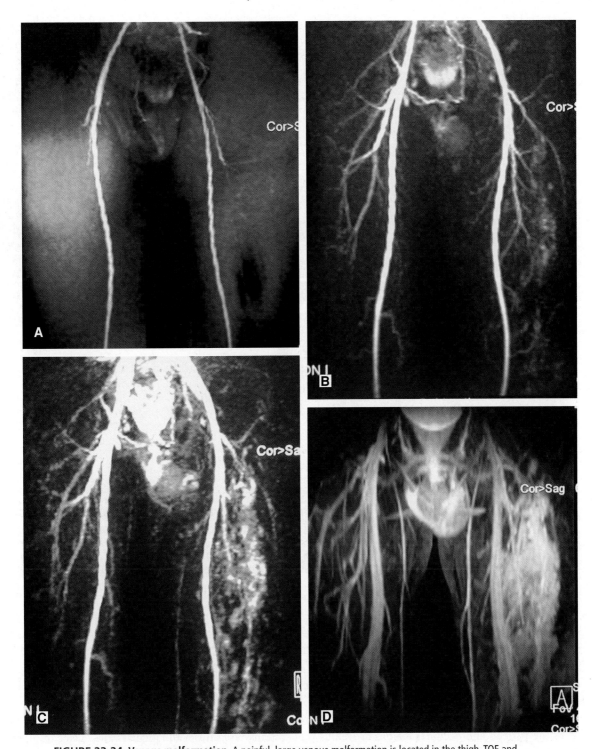

FIGURE 23-24 Venous malformation. A painful, large venous malformation is located in the thigh. TOF and postcontrast MRA were performed. TOF MRA demonstrated no detectable arterial flow within the malformation **(A)**. The external iliac, superficial, and deep femoral arteries appear normal and symmetric. A multiphase CE MRA **(B–D)** demonstrates progressive contrast accumulation in the malformation. Without the TOF technique, it would be difficult to rule out high-flow anomalies.

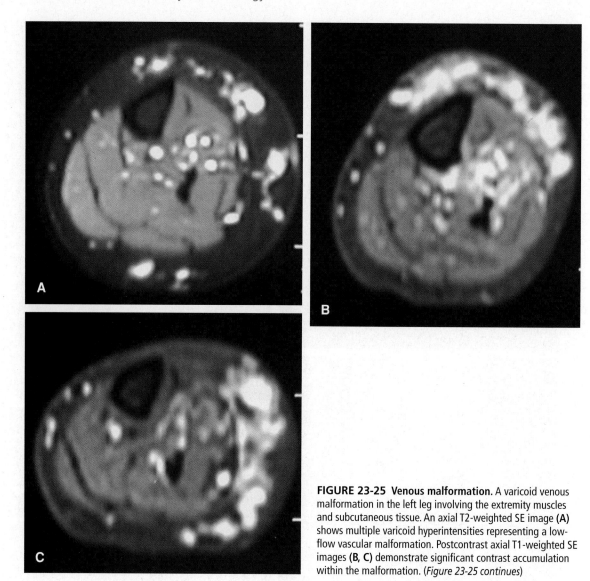

FIGURE 23-25 Venous malformation. A varicoid venous malformation in the left leg involving the extremity muscles and subcutaneous tissue. An axial T2-weighted SE image **(A)** shows multiple varicoid hyperintensities representing a low-flow vascular malformation. Postcontrast axial T1-weighted SE images **(B, C)** demonstrate significant contrast accumulation within the malformation. (*Figure 23-25 continues*)

of the trigeminal nerve (139). Only 8% of patients with CM have Sturge-Weber syndrome. Buphthalmos and ocular choroidal vascular malformations are common.

The neurological manifestations of Sturge-Weber syndrome vary, depending on the location of the leptomeningeal malformations, which most commonly are located in the parietal and occipital regions as well as the secondary effects of these vascular malformations. Patients with Sturge-Weber syndrome may develop seizures, hemiparesis, developmental delay, and glaucoma. The characteristic "tram-track" pattern of dystrophic calcification that can be identified on skull radiographs and CT is due to ischemic atrophy and thus may be a late finding (147). The earliest intracranial findings are the presence of pial enhancement and enlargement of the choroid plexus. CE MRI is felt to be more sensitive than CT. Other findings

include a prominent deep collateral venous system, cortical atrophy and later calcification, and thickening of the calvarium (Fig. 23-29). Patients have progressive overgrowth of the facial soft tissues and bone on the affected side. The globe can be enlarged and misshapen (buphthalmos). In severe cases, MRA/MRV can also reveal reduced flow in the transverse sinuses and jugular veins, a lack of superficial cortical veins, and reduced flow signal from the middle cerebral artery (148).

Parkes Weber Syndrome

PWS is a diffuse high-flow malformation that involves the entire extremity (usually a lower limb) with limb overgrowth. A cutaneous capillary malformation is present, and some patients also have a lymphatic component. PWS usually presents with cutaneous warmth and a bruit or thrill on

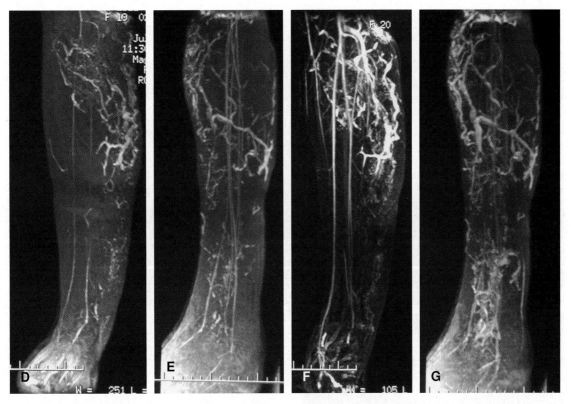

FIGURE 23-25 (Continued) Frontal **(D)** and lateral views **(E)** of an early phase of CE MRA show relatively rapid opacification of the malformation. The enhancement of the malformation is progressive with relatively rapid opacification of the draining anterior tibial vein, as seen in the second phase of the CE MRA **(F, G)**.

clinical examination. Dilated veins; lengthening of the affected limb; and hypertrophy in girth owing to muscle overgrowth, increased fat, and lymphedema are typical. Asymptomatic cardiac volume overload is frequent. Usually, patients demonstrate progressive worsening with pain and ulceration as the high-flow lesion evolves.

Proteus Syndrome

Proteus syndrome is a highly variable complex disease that appears to affect patients in a mosaic manner (149) and is commonly associated with high- and low-flow vascular anomalies. Patients have verrucous nevus, lipomas and/or lipomatosis, macrocephaly, asymmetric limbs with partial gigantism of the hands and feet, and cerebriform plantar thickening (150). The vascular anomalies in this entity include various forms, including fast-flow malformations such as AVMs and low-flow malformations such as LMs and/or VMs. Ocular manifestations in Proteus syndrome include strabismus, nystagmus, high myopia, and retinal pigmentary abnormalities (151). Many of the associated lesions are absent at birth and develop progressively. CNS manifestations of this syndrome include hemimegalencephaly, subependymal calcified nodules, and periventricular cysts (152). Common complications of Proteus syn-

drome include progressive skeletal deformities, invasive lipomas and malignant tumors, and deep venous thrombosis with pulmonary embolism (153).

Banayan Riley Rubalcava Syndrome

BRR syndrome is another uncommon overgrowth syndrome, associated with macrocephaly, lipomas and other tumors, ectodermal dysplasia, and vascular malformations. Sixty percent of patients have PTEN mutation, and there is overlap with Cowden syndrome. While low-flow vascular malformations are the most commonly reported, patients may present with multiple high-flow malformations (Fig. 23-30).

Maffucci Syndrome

Maffucci syndrome is a rare congenital anomaly combining bony exostoses and enchondromas with soft tissue low-flow malformations that are similar to VMs. Lesions contain spindle-cell hemangioendotheliomas, a reactive vascular proliferation within a pre-existing vascular malformation. There is no recognized genetic basis. The vascular malformations of Maffucci syndrome are blue or purple, soft, compressible, and occasionally tender. These vascular lesions exhibit clinical, radiologic, and pathologic features

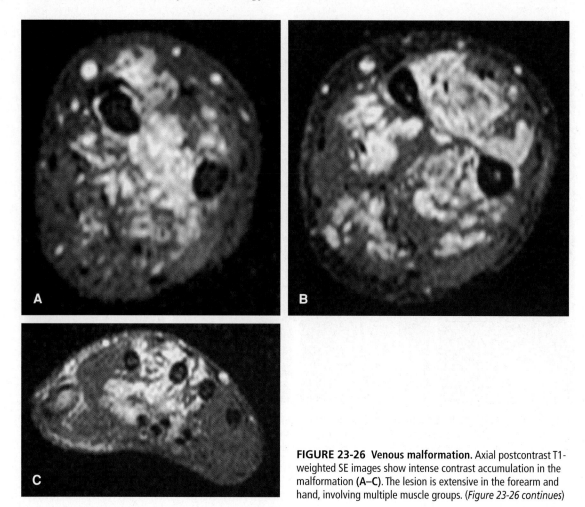

FIGURE 23-26 Venous malformation. Axial postcontrast T1-weighted SE images show intense contrast accumulation in the malformation **(A–C)**. The lesion is extensive in the forearm and hand, involving multiple muscle groups. (*Figure 23-26 continues*)

of VMs. The patients with Maffucci syndrome are usually symptomatic because of a growth disturbance of the affected bones, and the vascular malformations may be painful. Osseous lesions usually appear in children, while the vascular lesions manifest in older patients. Bony and vascular lesions may be unilateral or bilateral. Malignant transformation, most commonly chondrosarcoma, occurs in 20% to 30% of patients.

Epidermal Nevus Syndrome

Epidermal nevus syndrome is a rare, multisystem congenital disease that is characterized by epidermal nevi as well as skeletal, neurologic, ocular, urogenital, and vascular abnormalities. The disease affects boys and girls equally and presents between birth and 14 years of age. Affected individuals may live 40 years. Although the exact cause of epidermal nevus syndrome is not known, an autosomal dominant pattern of inheritance is observed in approximately two thirds of cases.

The spectrum of vascular findings in epidermal nevus syndrome include arterial aneurysms and coarctations, AVMs, and patent ductus arteriosus (Fig. 23-31).

Imaging Strategies and Findings

Plain radiography to evaluate leg-length discrepancy and MRI are the mainstay of imaging the overgrowth syndromes that involve the limbs. KTS can be recognized by prenatal ultrasound examination (154). Currently, conventional leg venography is the gold standard in the evaluation of the deep venous system and the superficial varicoid veins. The use of ascending and descending phlebography, tourniquets, and dependency of the limb optimize this assessment (86). However, conventional leg venography is a relatively invasive diagnostic test that also has several limitations, which are particularly important in children. These limitations include a difficulty of opacifying the deep venous system due to the flow of contrast through incompetent perforators into capacious superficial channels, contrast

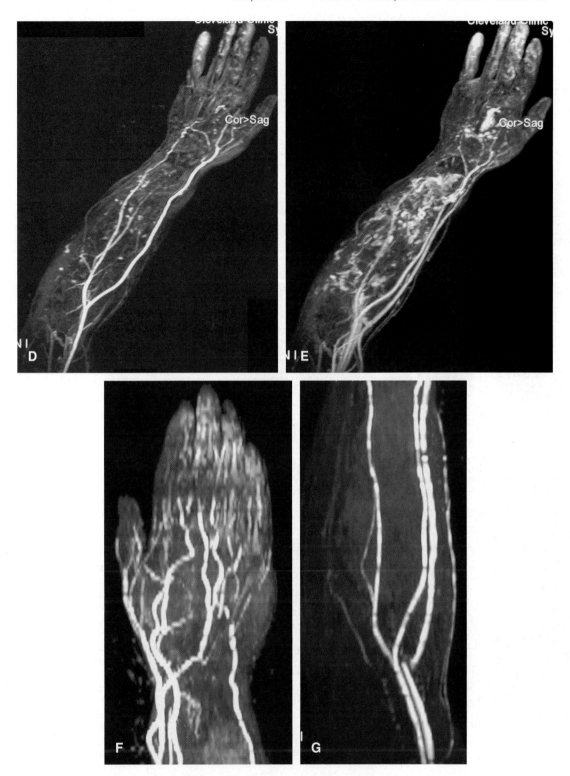

FIGURE 23-26 (Continued) CE MRA early **(D)** and slightly delayed **(E)** phases demonstrate progressive opacification of the malformation and draining veins. TOF MRV of the hand and forearm demonstrates normal extremity veins without visualization of the malformation. TOF MRV **(F–G)** is a useful technique to confirm the patency of the deep veins in the extremities but an unreliable technique to assess the flow dynamics of low-flow anomalies.

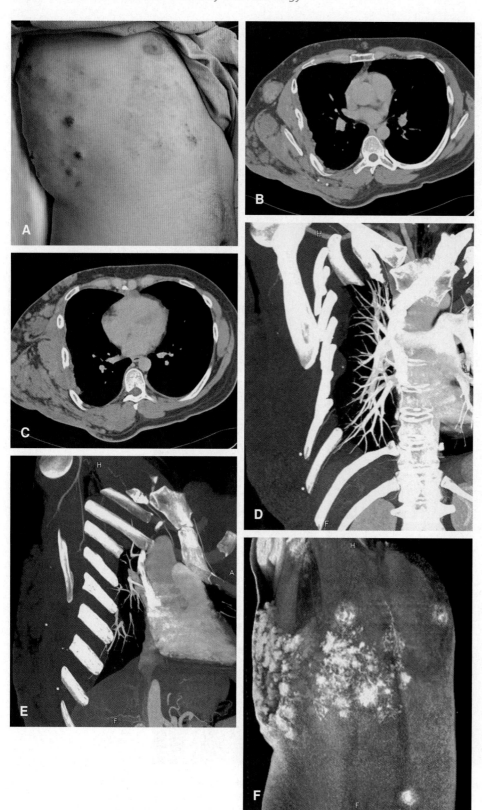

FIGURE 23-27 Large venous malformation in the chest wall. A young male patient presents with an extensive, deformative venous malformation in the chest wall (**A**). Source images of CTA (**B, C**) demonstrate a large soft tissue density malformation with barely detectable contrast enhancement. The chest wall appears significantly deformed. CTA (**D, E**) demonstrates normal nearby arteries (subscapular and subcostal) but no abnormal arterial flow in the malformation. There is a large, heterogeneous soft tissue abnormality and small phleboliths. A small phlebolith is also seen in the intrathoracic component of the malformation. With the narrow window setting, irregular areas of contrast enhancement are seen throughout the malformation (**F**). Overall, the sensitivity of the CTA in detecting low-flow anomalies is lower than in MR.

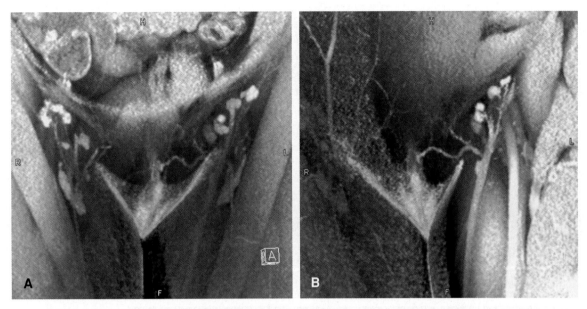

FIGURE 23-28 Vulvar venous malformation. A young female presents with a small vascular malformation in the left vulva. Due to an incorrect diagnosis of this lesion as a high-flow anomaly, CTA was suggested. CTA did not show any arterial feeder to the area, but with an appropriate window setting, a small asymmetric draining vein was noted (draining into the femoral vein), consistent with a small vulvar venous malformation **(A, B)**. The draining vein is easily noticeable in this case due to the fatty background, which is an advantage in demonstration of the vascular opacification in CTA.

limitations in children, and lack of appropriate peripheral venous access.

MRI is important to assess the deep lymphatic, venous, and adipose components in the affected limb, since the presence of each is highly variable (Figs. 23-32, 23-33). For example, limb "overgrowth" in KTS can be due to fat, LM, VM, or combinations of the three. The distribution of the abnormal tissue is important; those patients with involvement mainly of the subcutaneous tissue are amenable to surgical debulking, while those with muscular involvement likely are not. Extension of LM into the pelvis through the ischiorectal fossa is common and is associated with an increased incidence of sepsis. Pelvic macrocysts can obstruct the rectum and the urinary system. MRA and MRV can be performed by CE MRA with multiple phases that also allows the complete evaluation of the deep and superficial veins in the diseased extremity. At the same time, AVF or AVM (PWS) can be ruled out. If the contrast material is injected via a peripheral vein of the diseased extremity, excellent imaging of the venous system can be obtained without any arterial contamination as long as the timing of the scan is set appropriately. However, this approach would cause a "venous contamination" in the diseased extremity, which would then result in poor differentiation between KTS and PWS. Therefore, this approach (injecting IV contrast via the involved extremity) should be selected to image the

venous system in the diseased extremity if PWS or other high-flow anomalies are not suspected.

MRV has been proved to be as effective as contrast venography in the evaluation of the deep venous system in patients with KTS (155) (Figs. 23-32, 23-33). Another advantage of MRV is that the entire extremity can be assessed for additional varicosities, whereas the varicosities are not fully opacified by either leg venography or direct intralesional contrast injections. By obtaining MRV in multiple phases, physiologic information on how the normal and abnormal venous channels fill in the diseased extremity can be obtained (this is usually impractical in conventional venography, as tourniquets are used to redirect the contrast material from the varicoid veins into the deep venous system). In general, image-degrading artifacts due to breathing are usually not a problem. In addition to using the MIP images with varying degrees of rotation, source images should be used to identify the deep and superficial and varicoid venous channels separately and to evaluate the deep venous system fully. If the TOF MRA technique is being used for extremity venography, then 2D imaging is more suitable than 3D imaging because a larger FOV is possible without the risk of proton saturation within the volume of interest, particularly if the flow is slow (156). When 2D TOF venography is performed without gadolinium, the deep veins may erroneously appear to be absent due to slow flow. It is important to correlate the MRV images with

(text continues on page 1175)

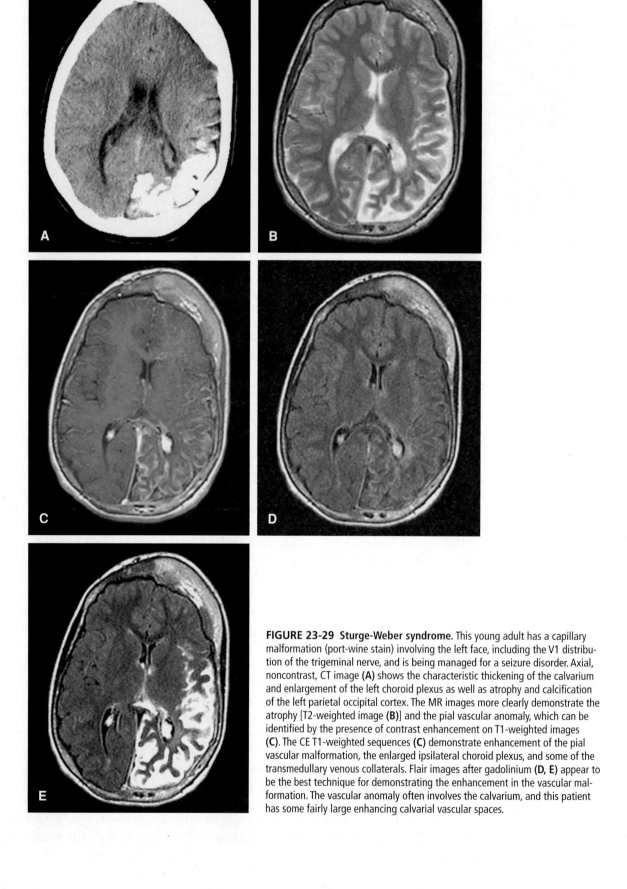

FIGURE 23-29 Sturge-Weber syndrome. This young adult has a capillary malformation (port-wine stain) involving the left face, including the V1 distribution of the trigeminal nerve, and is being managed for a seizure disorder. Axial, noncontrast, CT image **(A)** shows the characteristic thickening of the calvarium and enlargement of the left choroid plexus as well as atrophy and calcification of the left parietal occipital cortex. The MR images more clearly demonstrate the atrophy [T2-weighted image **(B)**] and the pial vascular anomaly, which can be identified by the presence of contrast enhancement on T1-weighted images **(C)**. The CE T1-weighted sequences **(C)** demonstrate enhancement of the pial vascular malformation, the enlarged ipsilateral choroid plexus, and some of the transmedullary venous collaterals. Flair images after gadolinium **(D, E)** appear to be the best technique for demonstrating the enhancement in the vascular malformation. The vascular anomaly often involves the calvarium, and this patient has some fairly large enhancing calvarial vascular spaces.

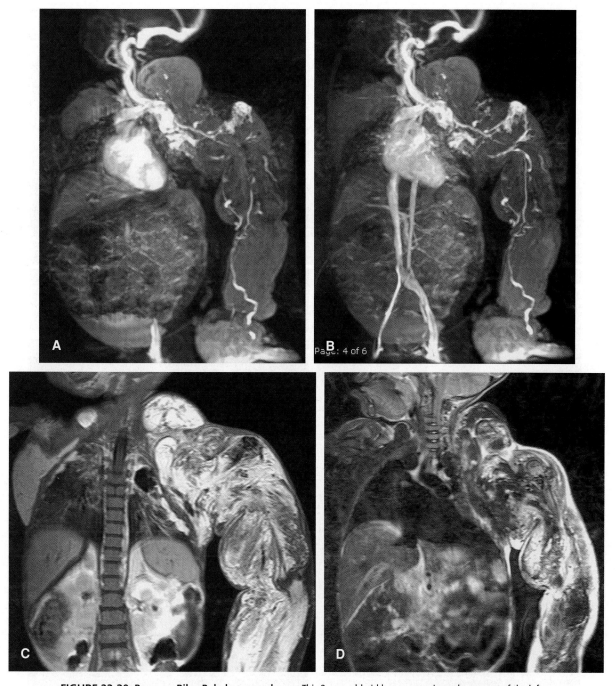

FIGURE 23-30 Banayan Riley Rubalcava syndrome. This 2-year-old girl has progressive enlargement of the left neck and upper extremity, with a continuous murmur in the left shoulder area. CE MR angiogram **(A, B)** shows dilation of the left internal jugular and innominate veins, with AVMs in the left shoulder and axilla as well as anomalous veins in the forearm. There is also enlargement of the left iliac vessels secondary to the presence of additional AVMs in the left lower extremity. On the SE imaging, however, the T1-weighted images **(C)** show extensive ectopic lipomatous tissue throughout the left chest wall, neck, and left upper extremity, accounting for much of the limb overgrowth. There is a similar fatty mass in the right axilla. The T2-weighted imaging **(D)** also shows low-flow vascular malformations indicated by T2 hyperintense areas in the affected soft tissues.

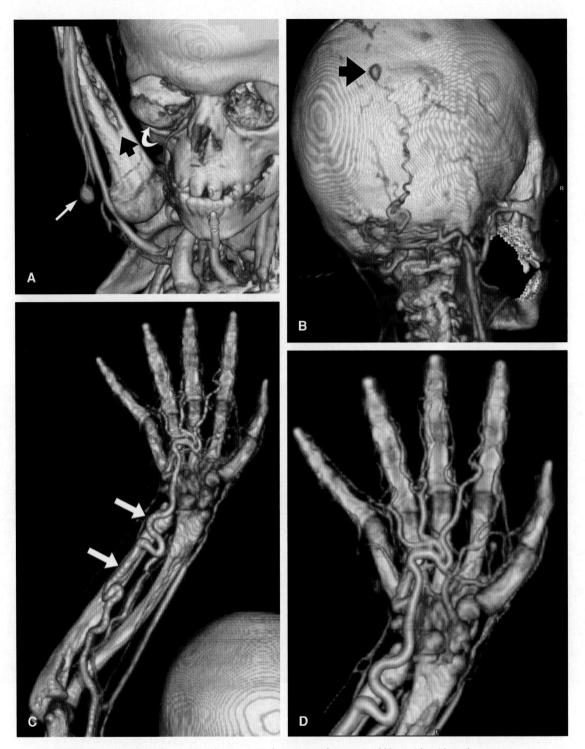

FIGURE 23-31 Epidermal nevus syndrome. A: VR from a CTA of an 8-year-old boy with epidermal nevus syndrome who developed multiple aneurysms and arterial malformations of the right side of his body. An aneurysm of the circumflex humoral artery (*straight white arrow*) is present. The humoral shaft is eroded by bony hemangioma (*black arrow*). His malformed right globe has been replaced with a prosthetic eye (*curved white arrow*). **B:** Posterior oblique VR of the same CTA reveals a saccular aneurysm of an enlarged branch of the occipital artery (*arrow*). **C:** Frontal VR of the right forearm and hand reveals an enlarged and tortuous ulnar artery (*arrows*) due to an AVM in the right hand **(D)**. (Images courtesy of Frandics P. Chan, MD, PhD, and Geoffrey D. Rubin, MD.)

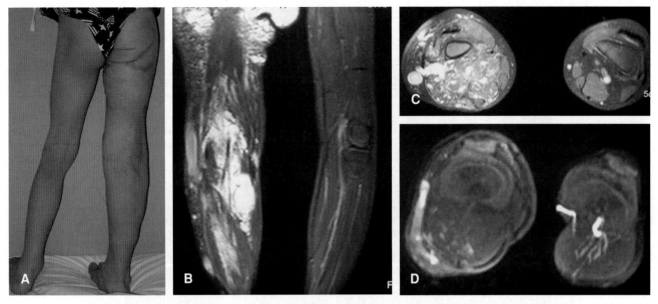

FIGURE 23-32 Klippel-Trenaunay syndrome. A young male patient presents with KTS involving the right leg **(A)**. The right leg is enlarged with patches of skin discoloration and varicoid venous enlargements. T2-weighted SE images **(B, C)** show scattered abnormal high signals throughout the leg, consistent with capillary LVM. The MRV **(D)** does not demonstrate the malformation but does reveal varicosities of the primitive marginal vein.

those from T2-weighted, IR, or postgadolinium sequences in order to clearly identify the deep veins.

CTA can also be an effective means of assessing KTS, particularly in patients where biphasic acquisitions are required to capture arterial and venous phases of enhancement (Fig. 23-34). The appropriate delay for maximal venous opacification is age dependent but ranges from 60 to 180 seconds following acquisition of the arterial phase. When timing is uncertain, monitoring sections can be acquired over the superficial femoral vein as a guide to trigger the venous-phase acquisition.

Most patients with PWS have generalized enlargement of the arteries and veins as well as true hypertrophy of the muscles of the affected limb. T2-weighted and postgadolinium sequences often show patchy increased signal in some of the muscles. They may, in addition, have focal arteriovenous shunts, increased subcutaneous fat, and lymphedema (Fig. 23-35). They do not have lymphatic cysts. In addition to MRA, CTA can be useful to evaluate the arterial tree and abnormal feeding arteries (Fig. 23-36).

Patients with Proteus and BRR syndromes may have either high- or low-flow anomalies or a combination of the two. In addition, they usually have extensive deposits of ectopic fat. Common locations for this fat include the peritoneum, the paraspinal muscles, and the limbs.

Treatment

Venous insufficiency resulting in chronic pain usually improves with support garments. The key to successful therapy of KTS is precise documentation of the venous anatomy and function. If a KTS patient has a patent and adequate deep venous system, abnormal varicoid veins (usually painful) and/or slow-flow malformations can be treated by sclerotherapy or surgical excision. However, it should be noted that symptomatic improvement may not be accomplished in a significant number of patients despite surgical resection of varicose veins or several procedures may be required (143). The goal of surgery is to improve function, reduce bleeding from cutaneous lymphatic vesicles, and reduce the frequency of infection. Episiodesis is the most common operation, carried out at the appropriate age to eliminate the leg-length discrepancy. Debulking of the limb is performed in patients with extensive subcutaneous LM, sometimes with stripping or ligation of the symptomatic superficial veins, including lateral embryonic veins. If the deep venous system is hypoplastic or absent, intervention on an abnormal superficial or collateral system is contraindicated (it may lead to more varicosities and edema) (155). Partial pedal amputation is sometimes performed to allow the child to wear shoes and ambulate. There currently is no effective treatment for patients with PWS unless they have focal arteriovenous shunts that can be embolized.

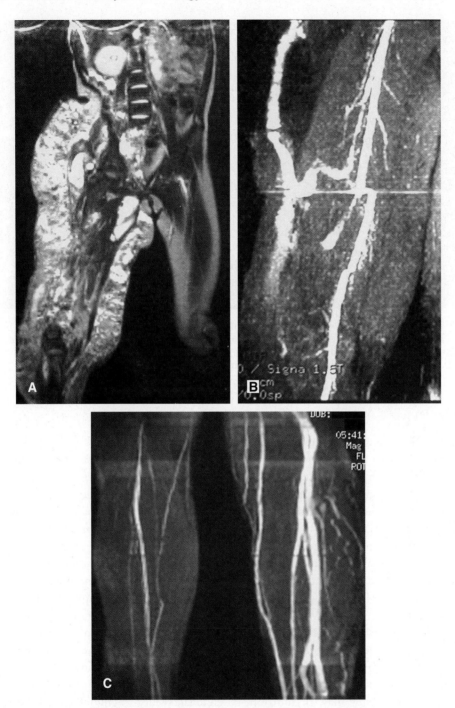

FIGURE 23-33 Klippel-Trenaunay syndrome. A coronal T2-weighted SE image **(A)** demonstrates extensive, heterogeneous hyperintense soft tissue involving the right leg and extends into the pelvis. The soft tissue abnormality represents capillary LVM. TOF MRV **(B)** demonstrates patent deep veins and a large marginal vein in the lateral thigh extending superiorly and also connecting to the deep venous system at the mid-thigh level. Nonvisualization of the deep veins with large veins draining into a large marginal vein is seen on TOF MRV images in a different patient with KTS **(C)**.

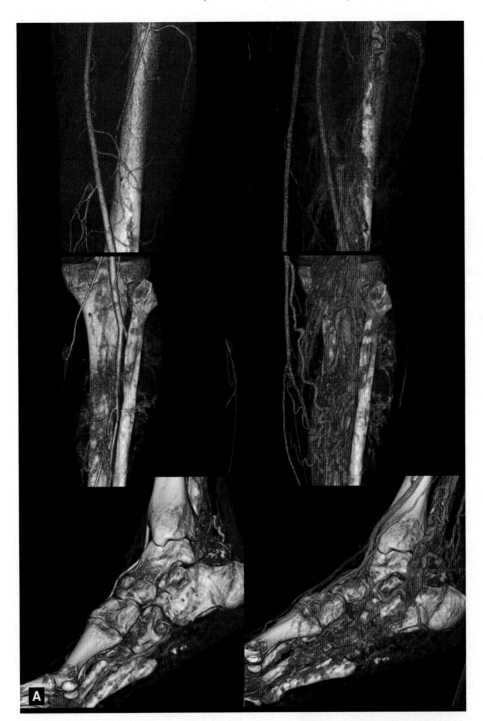

FIGURE 23-34 Klippel-Trenaunay syndrome CTA. A: Arterial **(left column)** and venous **(right column)** phases of a dual-phase CT angiogram displayed by using VR of the right lower extremity. A plethora of arterial branches from the superficial femoral artery and crural arteries are demonstrated on the arterial phase; however, the vessels are not enlarged. Within the calf, localized regions of increased opacification in a clustered nodular appearance can be observed around these arterial branches, but early venous filling, as would be seen in an AVM, is not observed. On the venous phase, enlarged and tortuous venous channels dominate the calf, posterior ankle, and dorsum of the foot with the lesser degree of involvement in the thigh. (*Figure 23-34 continues*)

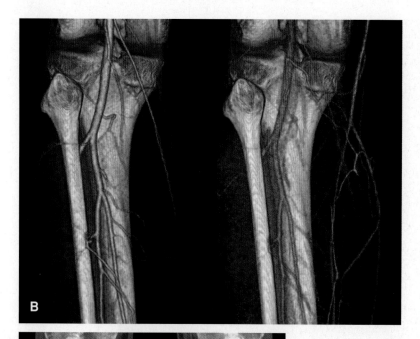

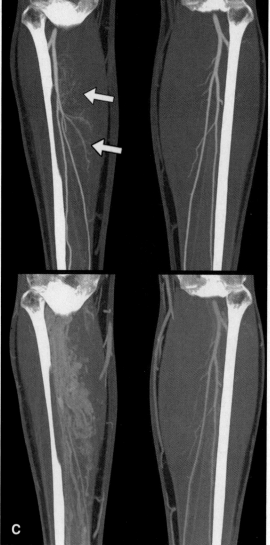

FIGURE 23-34 (Continued) (B) Arterial **(left)** and venous **(right)** phases of the normal proximal left calf are shown for comparison. **(C)** MIP through the two calves in the arterial **(upper row)** and venous **(lower row)** phases allow the clearest visualization of the early opacification of the capillary–venous malformations, which have a cotton wool–type appearance, at the ends of arterial branches (*arrows*). The majority of the malformation and abnormal venous channels are only visible on the delayed phase. (*Figure 23-34 continues*)

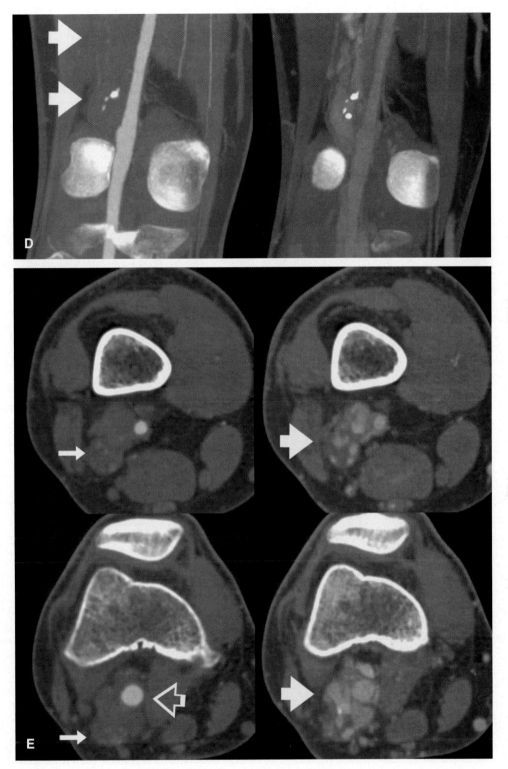

FIGURE 23-34 (Continued) (D) Arterial **(left)** and venous **(right)** thin-slab MIPs demonstrate an aneurysm of the popliteal artery, which is an atypical feature in KTS. *Arrows* indicate a soft tissue mass on the arterial phase that is observed to completely opacify on the venous phase corresponding to dilated venous channels. Calcification within the mass corresponds to a phlebolith. **E:** Selected transverse sections in the arterial **(left column)** and venous **(right column)** phases illustrate the popliteal artery aneurysm (*open arrow*) as well as the minimal venous opacification upon arterial phase imaging (*small arrow*) when compared with venous phase images (*large arrows*). (Courtesy of Geoffrey D. Rubin, MD.)

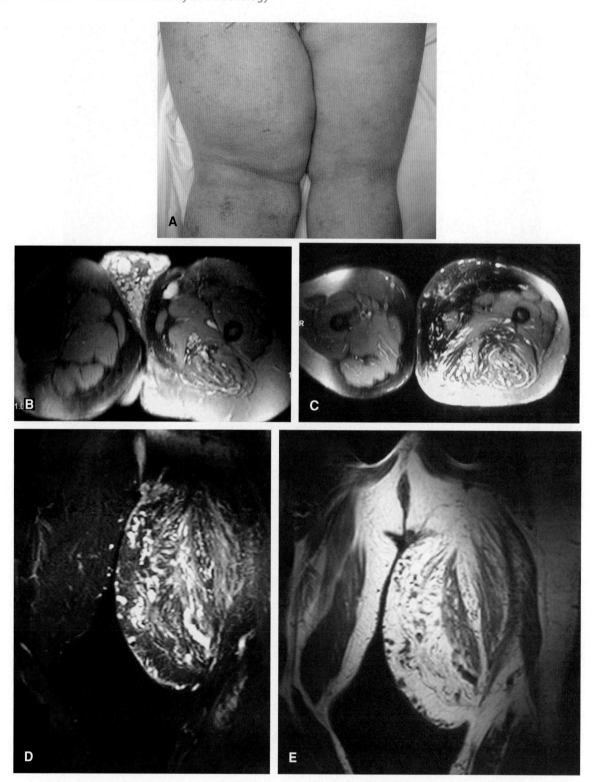

FIGURE 23-35 Combined vascular malformation (multifocal AVM) with fatty overgrowth. A photo **(A)** shows a significantly enlarged left leg with small subcutaneous varicosities. T2-weighted axial SE **(B, C)** and coronal inversion recovery **(D)** images demonstrate multiple regions of hyperintensity in the subcutaneous tissue and also involving multiple muscle groups and the scrotum. The abnormalities appear hypointense on the T1-weighted coronal SE image **(E)**. (*Figure 23-35 continues*)

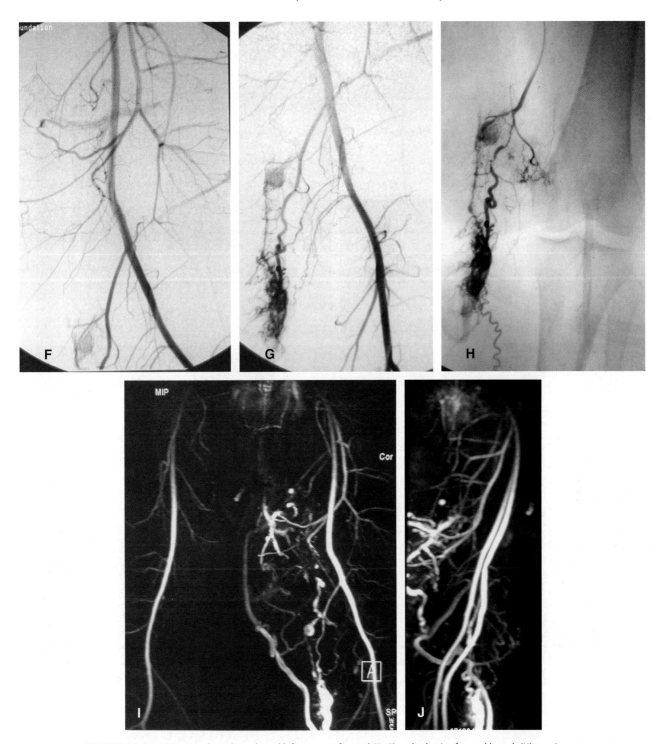

FIGURE 23-35 (Continued) Catheter-based left common femoral **(F, G)** and selective femoral branch **(H)** arteriograms show multiple, direct arteriovenous connections. CE MRA in frontal and lateral projections **(I, J)** demonstrate abnormal arteriovenous connections. There is an enlarged left femoral artery with early opacification of the greater saphenous vein.

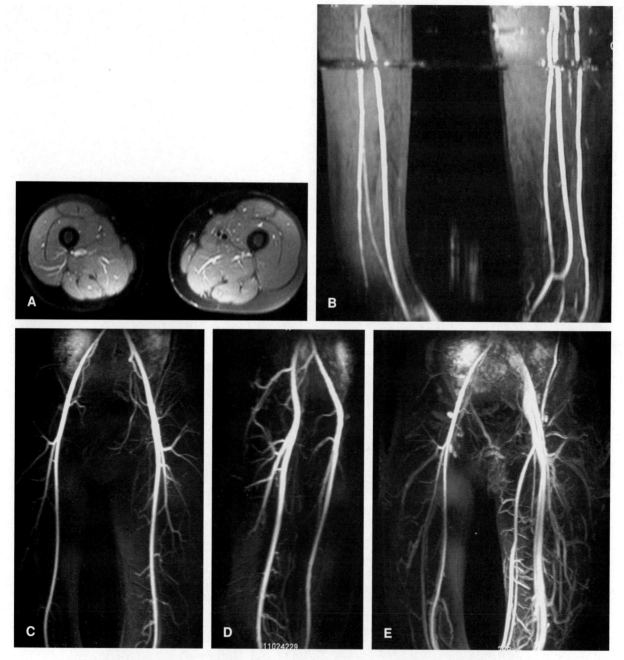

FIGURE 23-36 Parkes Weber syndrome. A young boy presents with a vascular anomaly in the left leg associated with mild patchy skin discoloration over the leg and the same side of the trunk. Initial assessment of the malformation was made by MRI and MRA. An axial T2-weighted image **(A)** shows an increased left leg circumference with increased vascularity but no obvious solitary abnormality. TOF MRA also shows increased vascularity in the left leg, but the image is degraded by motion artifacts **(B)**. Multiphase CE MRA of the legs **(C–E)** demonstrates an enlarged left femoral artery **(C, D)** and its branches (compared with the right) and early opacification of the deep veins **(E)**. (*Figure 23-36 continues*)

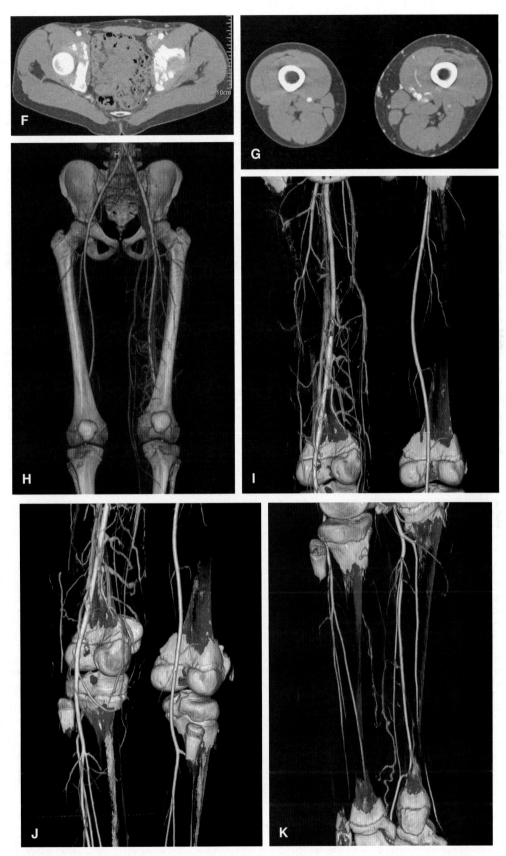

FIGURE 23-36 (Continued) Source CT images from CTA (**F, G**) show similar findings to that of the axial T2-weighted images (**A**). The circumference of the left leg is significantly larger than the right. The left common femoral artery and vein are larger than the right. There is an early opacification of the left common femoral vein on the cross-sectional CT images. CTA (**H–K**) clearly demonstrates arteriovenous connections in the entire leg with early opacification of the extremity veins.

SUMMARY

In conclusion, although vascular anomalies may seem complex to the unfamiliar imager, most can be diagnosed accurately by using a well-planned imaging protocol designed to determine extent, tissue characteristics, enhancement pattern, and flow characteristics and considering basic clinical information such as the age of the patient and evolution of the lesion. The use of correct terminology based on the biologic classification is mandatory, as the application of appropriate therapy depends upon it.

REFERENCES

1. Mulliken JB, Glowacki J. Hemangiomas and vascular malformations in infants and children: a classification based on endothelial characteristics. *Plast Reconstr Surg*. 1982;69:412–420.
2. Jackson IT, Carreno R, Potparic Z, et al. Hemangiomas, vascular malformations, and lymphovenous malformations: classification and methods of treatment. *Plast Reconstr Surg*. 1993;91:1216–1230.
3. Burrows PE, Laor T, Paltiel H, et al. Diagnostic imaging in the evaluation of vascular birthmarks. *Dermatol Clin*. 1998;16:455–488.
4. Silverman RA. Hemangiomas and vascular malformations. *Pediatr Clin North Am*. 1991;38:811–834.
5. Dubois J, Garel L. Imaging and therapeutic approach of hemangiomas and vascular malformations in the pediatric age group. *Pediatr Radiol*. 1999;29:879–893.
6. Boon LM, Burrows PE, Paltiel HJ, et al. Hepatic vascular anomalies in infancy: a twenty-seven-year experience. *J Pediatr*. 1996;129:346–354.
7. Rogalski R, Hensinger R, Loder R. Vascular abnormalities of the extremities: clinical findings and management. *J Pediatr Orthop*. 1993;13:9–14.
8. Murphey MD, Fairbairn KJ, Parman LM, et al. Musculoskeletal angiomatous lesions: radiologic-pathologic correlation. *Radiographics*. 1995;15:893–917.
9. Enzinger FM, Weiss SW. Benign tumors and tumor-like lesions of blood vessels. In: Enzinger FM, ed. *Soft Tissue Tumors*. St. Louis: CV Mosby Co.; 1988:489–532.
10. Robertson R, Robson CD, Barnes PD, et al. Head and neck vascular anomalies of childhood. *Neuroimaging Clin North Am*. 1999;9:115–132.
11. Dobson MJ, Hartley RW, Ashleigh R, et al. MR angiography and MR imaging of symptomatic vascular malformations. *Clin Radiol*. 1997;52:595–602.
12. Fasulakis S, Adronikou S. Comparison of MRE angiography and conventional angiography in the investigation of intracranial arteriovenous malformations and aneurysms in children. *Pediatr Radiol*. 2003;33:378–384.
13. Prince MR, Grist TM, Debatin JF. Basic Concepts. In: *3D Contrast MR Angiography*. 1st ed. Berlin: Springer-Verlag; 1999:3–39.
14. Frieden IJ, Reese V, Cohen D. PHACE syndrome. The association of posterior fossa brain malformations, hemangiomas, arterial anomalies, coarctation of the aorta and cardiac defects, and eye abnormalities. *Arch Dermatol*. 1996;132:307–311.
15. Reichenbach JR, Barth M, Haacke EM, et al. High-resolution MR venography at 3.0 Tesla. *J Comput Assist Tomogr*. 2000;26:949–957.
16. Campeau NG, Huston J 3rd, Bernstein MA, et al. Magnetic resonance angiography at 3.0 Tesla: initial clinical experience. *Top Magn Reson Imaging*. 2001;12:183–204.
17. Takahashi M, Uematsu H, Hatabu H. MR imaging at high magnetic fields. *Eur J Radiol*. 2003;46:45–52.
18. Hopkins KL, Davis PC, Sanders DL, et al. Sedation for pediatric imaging studies. *Neuroimaging Clin North Am*. 1999;9:1–10.
19. Cote CJ. Sedation for the pediatric patient: a review. *Pediatr Clin North Am*. 1994;41:31–58.
20. American Academy of Pediatrics, Committee on Drugs. Guidelines for monitoring and management of pediatric patients during and after sedation for diagnostic and therapeutic procedures. *Pediatrics*. 1992;89:1110–1115.
21. American Society of Anesthesiologists Task Force on Sedation and Analgesia by Non-Anesthesiologists. Practice guidelines for sedation and analgesia by non-anesthesiologists. *Anesthesiology*. 1996;84:459–471.
22. Cote CJ. Monitoring guidelines: do they make a difference? [commentary]. *AJR Am J Roentgenol*. 1995;165:910–912.
23. Hollman GA, Elderbrook MK, VanDenLangenberg B. Results of a pediatric sedation program on head MRI scan success rates and procedure duration times. *Clin Pediatr*. 1995;34:300–305.
24. Vade A, Sukhani R, Dolenga M, et al. Chloral hydrate sedation of children undergoing CT and MR imaging: Safety as judged by American Academy of Pediatrics guidelines. *AJR Am J Roentgenol*. 1995;165:905–909.
25. Egelhoff JC, Ball WS, Koch BL, et al. Safety and efficacy of sedation in children using a structured sedation program. *AJR Am J Roentgenol*. 1997;168:1259–1262.
26. Cote CJ, Notterman DA, Karl HW, et al. Adverse sedation events in pediatrics: a critical incident analysis of contributing factors. *Pediatrics*. 2000;105:805–814.
27. Krauss B, Green SM. Sedation and analgesia for procedures in children. *N Engl J Med*. 2000;342:938–945.
28. Rawson JV, Siegel MJ. Techniques and strategies in pediatric body MR imaging. *Magn Reson Imaging Clin N Am*. 1996;4:589–598.
29. Barish MA, Jara H. Motion artifact control in body MR imaging. *Magn Reson Imaging Clin N Am*. 1999;7:289–301.
30. Bailes DR, Gilderdale DJ, Bydder GM, et al. Respiratory ordered phase encoding (ROPE), a method for reducing respiratory motion artifacts in magnetic resonance imaging. *J Comput Assist Tomogr*. 1985;9:835–838.
31. Paley MR, Ros PR. MR imaging of the liver—a practical approach. *Magn Reson Imaging Clin N Am*. 1997;5:415–429.
32. Semelka RC, Sofka CM. Hepatic hemangioma. *Magn Reson Imaging Clin N Am*. 1997;5:241–253.
33. Mortele KJ, Mergo PJ, Urrutia M, et al. Dynamic gadolinium-enhanced MR findings in infantile hepatic hemangioendothelioma. *J Comput Assist Tomogr*. 1998;22:714–717.
34. Korosec FR, Mistretta CA. MR angiography: basic principles and theory. *Magn Reson Imaging Clin N Am*. 1998;6:223–256.
35. Prince MR, Grist TM, Debatin JF. 3D contrast MR venography. In: *3D Contrast MR Angiography*. 1st ed. Berlin: Springer-Verlag; 1999:163–171.
36. Runge VM, Nelson KL. Contrast agents. In: Stark DD, Bradley WG, eds. Magnetic Resonance Imaging. 3rd ed. Vol. 1. St. Louis: Mosby; 1999:257–275.
37. Mitzuzaki K, Yamashita Y, Ogata I, et al. Optimal protocol for injection of contrast material at MR angiography: study of healthy volunteers. *Radiology*. 1999;213:913–918.
38. Bellin M-F, Jakobsen JA, Tomassin I, et al. Contrast medium extravasation injury: guidelines for prevention and management. *Eur Radiol*. 2002;12:2807–2812.
39. Runge VM, Dickey KM, Williams NM, et al. Local tissue toxicity in response to extravascular extravasation of magnetic resonance contrast media. *Invest Radiol*. 2002;37:393–398.

40. Krinsky G, Rofsky NM. MR angiography of the aortic arch vessels and upper extremities. *Magn Reson Imaging Clin N Am.* 1998;6:269–292.
41. White KS. Reduced need for sedation in patients undergoing helical CT of the chest and abdomen. *Pediatr Radiol.* 1995;25:344–346.
42. Kaste SC, Young CW, Holmes TP, et al. Effect of helical CT on the frequency of sedation in pediatric patients. *AJR Am J Roentgenol.* 1997;168:1001–1003.
43. Pappas JN, Donnelly LF, Frush DP. Reduced frequency of sedation of young children with multisection helical CT. *Radiology.* 2000;215:897–899.
44. Cohen RA, Frush DP, Donnelly LF. Data acquisition for pediatric CT angiography: problems and solutions. *Pediatr Radiol.* 2000;30:813–822.
45. Long FR, Castile RG. Technique and clinical applications of full-inflation and end-exhalation controlled-ventilation chest CT in infants and young children. *Pediatr Radiol.* 2001;31:413–422.
46. Frush DP, Donnelly LF, Rosen NS. Computed tomography and radiation risks: what pediatric health care providers should know. *Pediatrics.* 2003;112:951–957.
47. Ware DE, Huda W, Mergo PJ, et al. Radiation effective doses to patients undergoing abdominal CT examinations. *Radiology.* 1999;210:645–650.
48. Brenner DJ, Elliston CD, Hall EJ, et al. Estimated risks of radiation-induced fatal cancer from pediatric CT. *AJR Am J Roentgenol.* 2001;176:289–296.
49. Donnelly LF, Emery KH, Brody AS, et al. Minimizing radiation dose for pediatric body applications for single-detector helical CT. *AJR Am J Roentgenol.* 2001;176:303–306.
50. Linton OW, Mettler FA. National conference on dose reduction in CT, with emphasis on pediatric patients. *AJR Am J Roentgenol.* 2003;181:321–329.
51. Fox SH, Toth T. Dose reduction on GE CT scanners. *Pediatr Radiol.* 2002;32:718–723.
52. Kalra MK, Maher MM, Toth TL, et al. Strategies for CT radiation dose optimization. *Radiology.* 2004;230:619–628.
53. Lieberman K, Huda W, Chang J, et al. How should x-ray techniques be modified for pediatric patients in head CT [abstract]? *Radiology.* 2002;225(P):593.
54. Suess C, Chen X. Dose optimization in pediatric CT: current technology and future innovations. *Pediatr Radiol.* 2002;32:729–734.
55. Seigel MJ. Multiplanar and three-dimensional multi-detector row CT of thoracic vessels and airways in the pediatric population. *Radiology.* 2003;229:641–650.
56. Hollingsworth C, Frush DP, Cross M, et al. Helical CT of the body: a survey of techniques used for pediatric patients. *AJR Am J Roentgenol.* 2003;180:401–406.
57. Paterson A, Frush DP, Donnelly LF. Helical CT of the body: are settings adjusted for pediatric patients? *AJR Am J Roentgenol.* 2001;176:297–301.
58. Vade A, Demos TC, Olson MC, et al. Evaluation of image quality using 1:1 pitch and 1.5:1 pitch helical CT in children: a comparison study. *Pediatr Radiol.* 1996;26:891–893.
59. Mahesh M, Scatarige JC, Cooper J, et al. Dose and pitch relationship for a particular multislice CT scanner. *AJR Am J Roentgenol.* 2001;177:1273–1275.
60. Frush DP, Donnelly LF. Helical CT in children: technical considerations and body applications. *Radiology.* 1998;209:37–48.
61. Thornton FJ, Paulson EK, Yoshizumi TT. Single versus multidetector row CT: comparison of radiation doses and dose profiles. *Acad Radiol.* 2003;10:379–385.
62. Rydberg J, Buckwalter KA, Caldemeyer KS, et al. Multisection CT: scanning techniques and clinical applications. *Radiographics.* 2000;20:1787–1806.
63. Morgan HT. Dose reduction for CT pediatric imaging. *Pediatr Radiol.* 2002;32:724–728.
64. Westerman BR. Radiation dose for Toshiba CT scanners. *Pediatr Radiol.* 2002;32:735–737.
65. Dixon AK, Dendy P. Spiral CT: how much does radiation dose matter? *Lancet.* 1998;352:1082–1083.
66. Kalender WA, Wolf H, Suess C, et al. Dose reduction in CT by anatomically adapted tube current modulation: experimental results and first patient studies. *Radiology.* 1997;205P:471.
67. Fricke BL, Donnelly LF, Frush DP, et al. In-plane bismuth breast shields for pediatric CT: effects on radiation dose and image quality using experimental and clinical data. *AJR Am J Roentgenol.* 2003;180:407–411.
68. Hopper KD, Neuman JD, King SH, et al. Radioprotection to the eye during CT scanning. *AJNR Am J Neuroradiol.* 2001;22:1194–1198.
69. Beaconsfield T, Nicholson R, Thornton A, et al. Would thyroid and breast shielding be beneficial in CT of the head? *Eur Radiol.* 1998;8:664–667.
70. Hidajat N, Schroder RJ, Vogl T, et al. The efficacy of lead shielding in patient dosage reduction in computed tomography. *Rofo Fortschr Geb Rontgenstr Neuen Bildgeb Verfahr.* 1996;165:462–465.
71. Cohen MD, Smith JA. Intravenous use of ionic and nonionic contrast agents in children. *Radiology.* 1994;191:793–794.
72. Cohen MD, Herman E, Herron D, et al. Comparison of intravenous contrast agents for CT studies in children. *Acta Radiologica.* 1992;33:592–595.
73. Cohan RH, Ellis JH, Garner WL. Extravasation of radiographic contrast material: recognition, prevention, and treatment. *Radiology.* 1996;200:593–604.
74. Stockberger SM, Kickling JA, Liang Y, et al. Spiral CT with ionic and nonionic contrast material: evaluation of patient motion and scan quality. *Radiology.* 1998;206:631–636.
75. Rubin GD, Lane MJ, Bloch DA, et al. Optimization of thoracic spiral CT: effects of iodinated contrast medium concentration. *Radiology.* 1996;201:785–791.
76. Kaste SC, Young CW. Safe use of power injectors with central and peripheral venous access devices for pediatric CT. *Pediatr Radiol.* 1996;26:499–501.
77. Birnbaum BA, Nelson RC, Chezmar JL, et al. Extravasation detection accessory: clinical evaluation in 500 patients. *Radiology.* 1999;212:431–438.
78. Jacobs JE, Birnbaum BA, Langlotz CP. Contrast media reactions and extravasation: relationship to intravenous injection rates. *Radiology.* 1998;209:411–416.
79. Powell CC, Li J, Rodino L, et al. A new device to limit extravasation during contrast-enhanced CT. *AJR Am J Roentgenol.* 2000;174:315–318.
80. Gothlin J. The comparative frequency of extravasal injection at phlebography with steel and plastic cannulas. *Clin Radiol.* 1972;23:183–184.
81. Williamson EE, McKinney JM. Assessing the adequacy of peripherally inserted central catheters for power injection of intravenous contrast agents for CT. *J Comput Assist Tomogr.* 2001;25:932–937.
82. Frush DP, Spencer EB, Donnelly LF, et al. Optimizing contrast-enhanced abdominal CT in infants and children using bolus-tracking. *AJR Am J Roentgenol.* 1999;172:1007–1013.
83. Ruben GD, Dake MD, Semba CP. Current status of three-dimensional spiral CT scanning for imaging the vasculature. *Radiol Clin North Am.* 1995;33:51–70.
84. Konez O, Burrows PE. Magnetic resonance of vascular anomalies. *Magn Reson Imaging Clin N Am.* 2002;10:363–388.
85. Rubin GD, Walker PJ, Dake MD, et al. Three-dimensional spiral computed tomographic angiography: an alternative imaging modality for the abdominal aorta and its branches. *J Vasc Surg.* 1993;18(4):656–664.
86. Mulliken JB, Young AE, eds. *Vascular Birthmarks: Hemangiomas and Malformations.* Philadelphia: WB Saunders; 1988.
87. Vikkula M, Boon LM, Mulliken JB, et al. Molecular basis of vascular anomalies. *Trends Cardiovasc Med.* 1998;8,281–292.

88. Konez O, Burrows PE, Mulliken JB, et al. Angiographic features of rapidly involuting congenital hemangioma (RICH). *Pediatr Radiol.* 2003;33:15–19.

89. Sarkar M, Mulliken JB, Kozakewich HP, et al. Thrombocytopenic coagulopathy (Kasabach-Merritt phenomenon) is associated with Kaposiform hemangioendothelioma and not with common infantile hemangioma. *Plast Reconstr Surg.* 1997;100:1377–1386.

90. Pratt AG. Birthmarks in infants. *Arch Dermatol.* 1967;67:302–305.

91. Jacobs AH, Walton RG. The incidence of birthmarks in the neonate. *Pediatrics.* 1976;58:218–222.

92. Holmdahl K. Cutaneous hemangiomas in premature and mature infants. *Acta Paediatr.* 1955;44(4):370–379.

93. Jacobs AH. Strawberry hemangiomas: the natural history of the untreated lesion. *Calif Med.* 1957;86(1):8–10.

94. Enjolras O, Gelbert F. Superficial hemangiomas: associations and management. *Pediatr Dermatol.* 1997;14(3):173–179.

95. Blei F, Walter J, Orlow SJ, et al. Familial segregation of hemangiomas and vascular malformations as an autosomal dominant trait. *Arch Dermatol.* 1998;134:718–722.

96. Amir J, Metzker A, Krikler R, et al. Strawberry hemangioma in preterm infants. *Pediatr Dermatol.* 1993;1:58–68.

97. Burton BK, Schulz CJ, Angle B, et al. An increased incidence of haemangiomas in infants born following chorionic villus sapling (CVS). *Prenat Diagn.* 1995;15:209–214.

98. Berg JN, Walter JW, Thisanagayam U, et al. Evidence for loss of heterozygosity of 5q in sporadic haemangiomas: are somatic mutations involved in haemangioma formation? *J Clin Pathol.* 2001;54:249–252.

99. Esterly NB. Cutaneous hemangiomas, vascular stains and malformations, and associated syndromes. *Curr Probl Pediatr.* 1996;26(1):3–39.

100. Albright AL, Gartner JC, Wiener ES. Lumbar cutaneous hemangiomas as indicators of tethered spinal cords. *Pediatrics.* 1989;83:977–980.

101. Enjolras O, Mulliken JB, Boon LM, et al. Noninvoluting congenital hemangioma: a rare cutaneous vascular anomaly. *Plast Reconstr Surg.* 2001;107:1647–1654.

102. Zukerberg LR, Nickoloff BJ, Weiss SW. Kaposiform hemangioendothelioma of infancy and childhood. An aggressive neoplasm associated with Kasabach-Merritt syndrome and lymphangiomatosis. *Am J Surg Pathol.* 1993;17:321–328.

103. Kasabach HH, Merritt KK. Capillary hemangioma with extensive purpura: report of a case. *Am J Dis Child.* 1940;59:1063–1070.

104. Enjolras O, Mulliken JB, Wassef M, et al. Residual lesions after Kasabach-Merritt phenomenon in 41 patients. *J Am Acad Dermatol.* 2000;42:225–235.

105. Konez O, Burrows PE, Kozakewich HPW, et al. Non-invasive imaging features of rapidly involuting congenital hemangioma. Scientific abstract. *ARRS.* 2003.

106. Boon LM, Fishman SJ, Lund DP, et al. Congenital fibrosarcoma masquerading as congenital hemangioma: report of two cases. *J Pediatr Surg.* 1995;30(9):1378–1381.

107. Hayward PG, Orgill DP, Mulliken JB, et al. Congenital fibrosarcoma masquerading as lymphatic malformation: report of two cases. *J Pediatr Surg.* 1995;30(1):84–88.

108. Bowers RE, Graham EA, Tomlinson KM. The natural history of the strawberry nevus. *Arch Dermatol.* 1960;82:667–680.

109. Frieden IJ, ed. Management of hemangiomas. Special symposium notes. *Pediatr Dermatol.* 1997;14(1):57–83.

110. Cohen AJ, Youkey JR, Clagett GP, et al. Intramuscular hemangioma. *JAMA.* 1983;249:2680–2682.

111. Mulliken JB, Fishman SJ, Burrows PE. Vascular anomalies. *Curr Probl Surg.* 2000;37(8):519–684.

112. Evans J, Batchelor ADR, Stark G, et al. Haemangioma with coagulopathy: sustained response to prednisone. *Arch Dis Child.* 1975;50(10):809–812.

113. Sadan N, Horowitz I, Choc L, et al. Giant hemangioma with thrombocytopenia and osteolysis successfully treated with prednisone. *J Pediatr Orthop.* 1989;9(4):472–475.

114. Miller JG, Orton CI. Long-term of a case of Kasabach-Merritt syndrome successfully treated with radiotherapy and corticosteroids. *Br J Plast Surg.* 1992;45(7):559–561.

115. de Prost Y, Teillac D, Bodemer C, et al. Successful treatment of Kasabach-Merritt syndrome with pentoxifylline. *J Am Acad Dermatol.* 1991;25(5 Pt 1):854–855.

116. Perez-Payrols J, Pardo-Masferrer J, Gomez-Bellvert C. Treatment of life threatening infantile hemangiomas with vincristine (letter). *N Engl J Med.* 1995;333:69.

117. Bell AJ, Chisholm M, Hickton M. Reversal of coagulopathy in Kasabach-Merritt syndrome with tranexamic acid. *Scand J Haematol.* 1986;37(3):248–252.

118. Shulkin BL, Argenta LC, Cho KJ, et al. Kasabach-Merritt syndrome: treatment with epsilon-aminocaproic acid and assessment with indium 111 platelet scintigraphy. *J Pediatr.* 1990;117(5):746–749.

119. Hu B, Lachman R, Phillips J, et al. Kasabach-Merritt syndrome-associated Kaposiform hemangioendothelioma successfully treated with cyclophosphomide, vincristine, and actinomycin D. *J Pediatr Hematol Oncol.* 1998;20(6):567–569.

120. Haisley-Royster C, Enjolras O, Frieden IJ, et al. Kasabach-Merritt phenomenon: a retrospective study of treatment with vincristine. *J Pediatr Hematol Oncol.* 2002;24(6):459–462.

121. North P, Kozakewich H. Vascular malformations and tumors in children. Society for Pediatric Pathology workshop notes. Vancouver, BC, 2004.

122. Enzinger FM, Weiss SW. Hemangioendothelioma: vascular tumors of intermediate malignancy. In: Enzinger FM, ed. *Soft Tissue Tumors.* St. Louis, MO: CV Mosby Co.; 1988:533–544.

123. Enjolras O, Logeart I, Gelbert F, et al. Arteriovenous malformations: a study of 200 cases. *Ann Dermatol Venereol.* 2000;127(1):17–22.

124. Kohout MP, Hansen M, Pribaz JJ, et al. Arteriovenous malformations of the head and neck: natural history and management. *Plast Reconstr Surg.* 1998;102:643–654.

125. Rodesch G, Lasjaunias P. Spinal cord arteriovenous shunts: from imaging to management. *Eur J Radiol.* 2003;46:221–232.

126. Paltiel HJ, Burrows PE, Kozakewich HPW, et al. Soft-tissue vascular anomalies: utility of US for diagnosis. *Radiology.* 2000;214:747–754.

127. Korosec FR, Frayne R, Grist TM, et al. Time-resolved contrast-enhanced 3D MR angiography. *Magn Reson Med.* 1996;36(3):345–351.

128. Hirai T, Korogi Y, Ikushima I, et al. Usefulness of source images from three-dimensional time-of-flight MR angiography after treatment of cavernous dural arteriovenous fistulas. *Radiat Med.* 2003;21(5):205–209.

129. Khong P-L, Burrows PE, Kozakewich HP, Mulliken JB. Fast-flow lingual vascular anomalies in the young patient: is imaging diagnostic? *Pediatr Radiol.* 2003;33:118–122.

130. Holt PD, Burrows PE. Interventional radiology in the treatment of vascular lesions. *Facial Plast Surg Clin N Am.* 2001;9(4):585–599.

131. Burrows PE, Fellows KE. Techniques for management of pediatric vascular anomalies. In: Cope C, ed. Current techniques in interventional radiology. 2nd ed. Philadelphia: Current Science; 1995:11–27.

132. Boon LM, Mulliken JB, Vikkula M, et al. Assignment of a locus for dominantly inherited venous malformations to chromosome 9. *Hum Mol Genet.* 1994;3:1583–1587.

133. Tsai FJ, Tsai CH. Birthmarks and congenital skin lesions in Chinese newborns. *J Formos Med Assoc.* 1993;92(9):838–841.

134. Mills CM, Lanigan SW, Hughes J, et al. Demographic study of port wine stain patients attending a laser clinic: family history, prevalence of naevus anaemicus and results of prior treatment. *Clin Exp Dermatol.* 1997;22(4):166–168.

135. Gorham LW, Stout AP. Massive osteolysis (acute spontaneous absorption of bone, phantom bone, disappearing bone): its relations to hemangiomatosis. *J Bone Joint Surg.* 1955;37:986–1004.

136. Konez O, Vyas PK, Goyal M. Disseminated lymphangiomatosis presenting with massive chylothorax. *Pediatr Radiol.* 2000;30(1):35–37.

137. Hsu TS, Cooper LT, Maus TP, et al. Cutaneous and gastrointestinal tract hemangiomas associated with disappearing bones: Gorham syndrome. *Int J Dermatol.* 2001;40(11):726–728.

138. Konez O, Burrows PE. Evaluation of patients with vascular anomalies using multidetector CT angiography with volumetric three dimensional rendering. Abstract presentation. ISSVA, Wellington, New Zealand, 2004.

139. Bioxeda P, de Misa RF, Arrazola JM, et al. Facial angioma and the Sturge-Weber syndrome: a study of 121 cases. *Med Clin (Barc).* 1993;29:101(1):1–4.

140. Labreze-Leaute C, Boralevi F, Pedespan JM, et al. Pulsed dye laser for Sturge-Weber syndrome. *Arch Dis Child.* 2002;87(5):434–435.

141. Aelvoet GE, Jorens PG, Roelen LM. Genetic aspects of the Klippel-Trenaunay syndrome. *Br J Dermatol.* 1992;126(6):603–607.

142. Tian X-L, Kadaba R, You S-A, et al. Identification of an angiogenic factor that when mutated causes susceptibility of Klippel-Trenaunay syndrome. *Nature.* 2004;427:640–645.

143. Samuel M, Spitz L. Klippel-Trenaunay syndrome: Clinical features, complications and management in children. *Brit J Surg.* 1995;82:757–761.

144. Jacob AG, Driscoll DJ, Shaughnessy WJ, et al. Klippel-Trenaunay syndrome: spectrum and management. *Mayo Clin Proc.* 1998;73:28–36.

145. Torregrosa A, Marti-Bonmati L, Higueras V, et al. Klippel-Trenaunay syndrome: prevalence of brain hemihypertrophy with MR imaging. Abstract presentation. ECR 1999.

146. Williams DW III, Elster AD. Cranial CT and MR in the Klippel-Trenaunay-Weber syndrome. *AJNR Am J Neuroradiol.* 1992;13:291–294.

147. Yock DH Jr. *Magnetic Resonance Imaging of CNS Disease.* 2nd ed. St. Louis: Mosby; 1995:552.

148. Vogl TJ, Stemmler J, Bergman C, et al. MR and MR angiography of Sturge-Weber syndrome. *AJNR Am J Neuroradiol.* 1993;14(2):417–425.

149. Biesecker LG, Happle R, Mulliken JB, et al. Proteus syndrome: diagnostic criteria, differential diagnosis, and patient evaluation. *Am J Med Genet.* 1999;84(5):389–395.

150. Bilkay U, Tokat C, Ozek C, et al. Proteus syndrome. *Scand J Plast Reconstr Surg Hand Surg.* 2003;37(5):307–310.

151. De Becker I, Gajda DJ, Gilbert-Barness E, et al. Ocular manifestations in Proteus syndrome. *Am J Med Genet.* 2000;92(5):350–352.

152. Dietrich RB, Glidden DE, Roth GM, et al. The Proteus syndrome: CNS manifestations. *AJNR Am J Neuroradiol.* 1998;19(5):987–990.

153. Biesecker LG. The multifaceted challenges of Proteus syndrome. *JAMA.* 2001;285(17):2240–2243.

154. Christenson L, Yankowitz J, Robinson R. Prenatal diagnosis of Klippel-Trenaunay-Weber syndrome as a cause for in utero heart failure and severe post-natal sequelae. *Prenatal Diag.* 1997;17:1176–1180.

155. Laor T, Burrows PE, Hoffer FA. Magnetic resonance venography of congenital vascular malformations of the extremities. *Pediatr Radiol.* 1996;26:371–380.

156. Wallner B, Edelmann RR, Kim D. Magnetic resonance angiography. In: Kim D, Orron DE, eds. *Peripheral Vascular Imaging and Intervention.* St. Louis: Mosby–Year Book; 1992:201–203.

Venous System

Ivan Pedrosa
Eric Zeikus
Douglas E. Green
Marc V. Gosselin

INTRODUCTION

Methods available for imaging the venous system are plentiful, including conventional, direct venography, grayscale and Doppler ultrasound (US), contrast-enhanced (CE) computed tomography (CT), and both noncontrast and CE magnetic resonance imaging (MRI). With the current imaging technologies, the venous system anatomy and pathology can be readily and reliably demonstrated.

Relatively noninvasive assessments of the venous system can be achieved over large fields-of-view (FOVs) with CT and MR. The cross-sectional evaluations available from both modalities provide excellent soft tissue detail and high levels of contrast between the veins and adjacent structures; this offers a depiction of venous anatomy, an ability to delineate masses affecting the veins, a demonstration of intraluminal pathology, and the capacity to reveal communications with other structures.

This chapter will review the anatomy, anomalies, and pathology of the systemic veins and the expanding role for both multidetector CT (MDCT) and MRI in venous evaluations. Clinical applications are discussed in detail, emphasizing detection of central venous thrombosis, thrombus characterization, definition of venous anatomy pre-central venous catheterization, and primary neoplasms of the veins as well as pitfalls in interpretation.

Spectrum and Prevalence of Diseases

Delineation of venous patency and anatomy is required in various clinical scenarios. Venous thrombosis is a common medical condition and can cause venous thromboembolism, which accounts for up to 250,000 hospitalizations and approximately 50,000 deaths per year in the United States (1). Its incidence is increased among elderly patients, those with reduced mobility (e.g., postsurgical states), pregnancy and postpartum states, oral contraceptives, hormone replacement therapy, and malignancy, as well as among patients with underlying hematological disturbances, coagulopathies, or prolonged medical illness (2). Incidence is also increased in patients with extrinsic venous compression, long-term indwelling catheters for hemodialysis, chemotherapy, and hyperalimentation (3).

Localized venous thrombosis may influence surgical management in patients with renal and hepatic tumors. Imaging studies are indicated not only to confirm the presence or absence of thrombus but also to evaluate for an underlying cause, the extent and chronicity of thrombus, and to characterize the thrombus as bland or tumoral. This information can directly impact the patient's prognosis and the suitability for surgical resection as well as the optimal surgical approach.

Venous occlusion has become a frequent problem in patients with long-term indwelling catheters. In these patients, defining the venous anatomy and patency is critical in order to achieve venous catheterization. In addition, due to a myriad of congenital variants, evaluation of venous anatomy is essential for central venous line placement in patients with anomalously coursing catheters seen on chest radiography. Evaluation of inferior vena cava (IVC) and renal venous anatomy may be critical in patients with anatomic variants receiving an IVC filter.

EMBRYOLOGY, ANATOMY, AND CONGENITAL ANATOMIC VARIANTS

Embryologic Development and Anatomy

Thoracic Veins: Upper Extremity and Intrathoracic Systemic Veins (Superior Vena Cava and Azygous System)

The internal and external jugular veins drain the face, neck, and head. They extend to drain into the brachiocephalic veins bilaterally. About 2.5 cm superior to this end point, there are a pair of valves in the internal jugular system. The vertebral vein drains in the brachiocephalic vein and also has a pair of valves near its orifice (4).

The subclavian vein arises at the outer edge of the first rib and represents the continuation of the axillary vein. It unites with the jugular vein in the region behind the sternoclavicular joint, forming the brachiocephalic vein. The right brachiocephalic vein is shorter and courses in a straighter and more vertical plane behind the sternum. The left brachiocephalic typically courses anterior to the brachiocephalic arteries. It unites with the contralateral brachiocephalic vein to form the superior vena cava (SVC) (4,5).

The tributaries of the brachiocephalic veins include the thymic, internal thoracic, inferior thyroid, intercostal, and pericardiophrenic veins. The internal thoracic veins extend along the medial aspect of the sternum and receive blood from the anterior intercostals and abdominal veins, such as the inferior epigastric veins. The right internal thoracic vein opening lies near the origin of the SVC, and thus, catheters can occasionally extend into the vein (4,5).

The pericardiophrenic vein drains the pericardium, pleural, and diaphragmatic regions and interconnects with the inferior phrenic vein, which drains into the IVC. This vein courses along the mediastinum with the phrenic nerve. This allows another central collateral pathway to bypass any central venous obstructions.

Azygous and Hemiazygous Systems

The azygous vein represents a collection of different venous systems draining the posterior chest wall and lumbar spinal region. It originates as a continuation from the right lumbar vein, and as it ascends, it receives the numerous posterior intercostal veins before coursing anterior over the right main bronchus into the SVC. There are between one and four valves, usually incomplete, located throughout the azygous and hemiazygous system. Usually, a valve is present within the azygous arch and can occasionally be seen on CT when there is reflux of contrast material (6).

The hemiazygous venous system is similar to the azygous system, receiving similar drainage but predominantly from the left intercostal veins. The two systems have numerous interconnections between them along the posterior ascending vertebral portion. It empties into the azygous vein at about the fifth vertebral body level.

The intercostal veins are divided three regions: supreme, superior, and standard intercostals. In each intercostal space are one posterior and two anterior intercostal veins.

The supreme intercostal veins (first intercostal space) drain into the brachiocephalic vein. The superior intercostal veins receive the drainage from the second through fourth intercostal veins, with the left also receiving flow from the hemiazygous vein. The right superior intercostal vein empties into the posterior superior aspect of the arch of the azygous vein. The left superior intercostal vein drains into the left brachiocephalic vein and also receives flow from the hemiazygous vein. The next eight posterior intercostal vessels drain directly into the azygous-hemiazygous system. The anterior veins drain into the internal mammary and musculophrenic venous systems (5).

A comprehensive understanding of the embryology that underlies the multiplicity of possible congenital variants is beyond the scope of this text, but some valuable references are provided to the interested reader (7–10). In general, redundant development and the variance in the selective regression of multiple separate venous systems results in either a conventional configuration of the central veins or alternative configurations. Given the complex sequence of appearance and regression of multiple vessels, there are many possible anatomical variants.

Congenital Variants

Superior Vena Cava/Azygous System Anomalies

Most variants of the SVC and azygous systems are asymptomatic unless they are associated with congenital heart disease.

Persistent Left Superior Vena Cava

A persistent left SVC can be seen with (double SVC) or without (left SVC) a right SVC. Up to 67% of patients with persistent left SVC have a bilateral or double SVC due to patency of the right and left anterior cardinal veins (11). Prevalence in the general population is 0.3%, while it reaches over 11% in patients with congenital heart disease (12). The right brachiocephalic trunk empties normally into the right atrium.

The left brachiocephalic trunk can flow into the coronary sinus, and with this pattern, patients can be asymptomatic (13). The left trunk can also empty into the left atrium or into the left superior pulmonary vein, both of which cause mixing of deoxygenated and oxygenated blood, causing profound hypoxemia and erythrocytosis (14,15). In addition, 50% to 70% of patients with this form are at risk of paradoxical embolism because of accompanying lesions (atrial septal defect, unroofed coronary sinus, or direct communication of the vein to the left atrium) (11).

In the absence of a right SVC, the left SVC usually empties into the coronary sinus, which in turn empties into the right atrium (Fig. 24-1). It derives from persistence of the left anterior cardinal vein instead of the right anterior cardinal vein. Individuals with the anomaly are asymptomatic. Incidence is 0.3% to 0.5% of the general population and 3% to 5% of patients with congenital heart disease.

A double or persistent left SVC draining into the coronary sinus should be considered as a potential cause of a dilated coronary sinus detected on transesophageal echocardiograms (13).

Anomalous Pulmonary Venous Drainage

Typically, four pulmonary veins drain into the left atrium; however, anatomic variants are common. In a study on 201 patients undergoing chest CT for pulmonary embolism, pulmonary stenosis, or aortic injury, conventional anatomy with two atrial ostia for the right upper and lower lobe

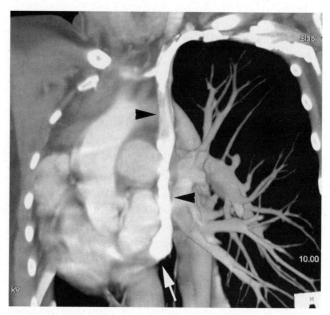

FIGURE 24-1 Left SVC. VR reconstruction of a CE CT of a patient with a persistent left-sided SVC (*black arrowheads*). Note its course, emptying into the coronary sinus (*white arrow*).

veins, with the middle lobe vein joining the upper lobe vein, was present in 68% of patients (16). Anatomic variants were noted on the right lung in the rest of patients with independent drainage of the middle lobe vein (or veins) directly into the left atrium (26% of patients) (16). In the same study, variability in the left lung was less common, with 86% of patients having two ostia for the left upper and lower lobe veins (16). A common trunk for these two veins was the most common anatomic variant (14%) (16).

Anomalous pulmonary venous drainage (APVD) is a spectrum of pulmonary venous anomalies that result from failure of connection between the primitive pulmonary splanchnic plexus and the common pulmonary vein derived from the atrium (10). APVD has been classified into four groups depending on the level of the drainage of the anomalous vein: supracardiac, cardiac, infradiaphragmatic, and mixed (10). Pulmonary venous blood drains directly into the right side of the heart or systemic veins, causing an extracardiac left-to-right shunt (10). APVD can be total, when all pulmonary veins drain anomalously, or partial, when one or more of the pulmonary veins drain normally within the left atrium (Figs. 24-2, 24-3). For survival, total APVD requires the presence of a right-to-left shunt via a cardiac septal defect or patent ductus arteriosus (10). A more detailed discussion of APVD can be found in Chapter 16.

Hypogenetic lung (Scimitar) syndrome is the result of an abnormal development of the lung, occurring almost

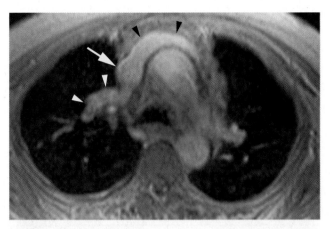

FIGURE 24-2 Partial anomalous pulmonary venous return—right upper pulmonary vein. Axial 2D magnetization-prepared T1-weighted gradient echo image during the delayed venous phase shows the left bra-chiocephalic vein (*black arrowheads*) joining with the SVC (*white arrow*). The right upper pulmonary vein (*white arrowheads*) is identified draining into the SVC, indicating partial anomalous pulmonary venous return. The rest of the pulmonary veins (not shown) drained normally into the left atrium.

always on the right. A small lung is associated, with a small or absent pulmonary artery and systemic arterial supply as well as anomalous venous return (10). The anomalous pulmonary venous return usually drains into the IVC below the right hemidiaphragm, although it may drain in the

suprahepatic portion of the IVC (Fig. 24-4), hepatic vein, portal vein, azygous vein, coronary sinus, or right atrium (10). Other anomalies can be present, including anomalies of the right bronchial tree, which is commonly a mirror image of the left, and diverticula (10). Other cardiovascular anomalies are also frequent (10).

Absence of the Azygous Vein

This very rare asymptomatic anomaly occurs as the result of embryologic developmental failure of the cranial aspect of the right supracardinal veins. The azygous vein receives nearly all the venous drainage from the right intercostal veins. In agenesis of the azygous vein, the hemiazygous vein plays an important role in the hemodynamics, draining almost all of the right and left intercostal veins. This condition increases the venous flow into the left superior intercostal vein (17).

Inferior Vena Cava Anomalies

Many of the IVC system anomalies can occur as isolated entities or in combination.

Double Inferior Vena Cava

This derives from the persistence of both supracardinal veins. Prevalence is 0.2% to 0.3%. The left infrarenal IVC

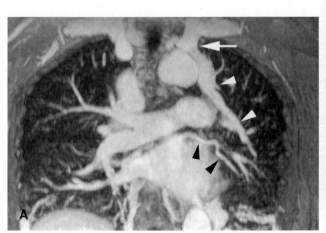
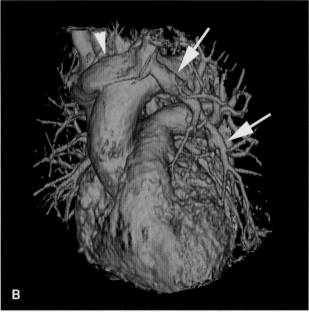

FIGURE 24-3 Partial anomalous pulmonary venous return—left upper pulmonary vein. A: Coronal thick-slab MIP reconstruction of a 3D fat-saturated T1-weighted gradient echo acquisition obtained during the delayed venous phase shows an aberrant left upper lobe pulmonary vein (*white arrowheads*) draining into the left subclavian vein (*white arrow*). Note a tiny vestigial left superior pulmonary vein (*black arrowheads*) draining into the left atrium. The right and inferior left pulmonary veins (not shown) drained normally into the left atrium. **B:** VR reconstruction of the same acquisition as **(A)** better displays the relationship of the aberrant left pulmonary vein (*white arrows*) draining into the left brachiocephalic vein (*white arrowhead*) in this case of partial anomalous pulmonary venous return.

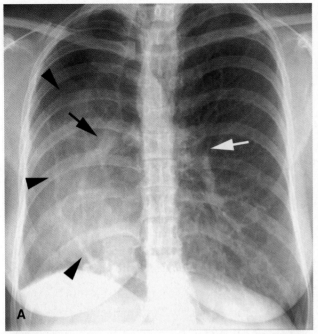

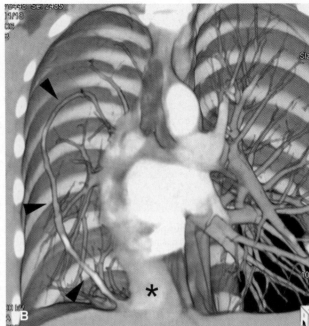

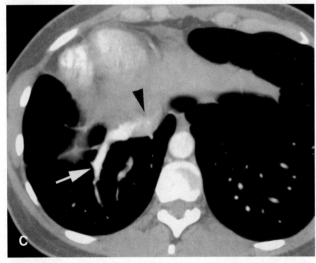

FIGURE 24-4 Scimitar syndrome. A: Anteroposterior chest radiograph showing a curvilinear opacity in the right lung base (*black arrowheads*). Note the small-sized right lung with rightward tracheal deviation and mediastinal shift. The right pulmonary artery (*black arrow*) is also small compared with the left pulmonary artery (*white arrow*). **B:** 3D VR reconstruction from a CT angiogram in the same patient confirms the presence of an aberrant (scimitar) pulmonary vein (*black arrowheads*) in the right lung draining into the inferior vena cava (*). **C:** Axial CE CT image (same acquisition as **B**) better demonstrates the aberrant (scimitar) vein (*white arrow*) emptying into the suprahepatic IVC (*black arrowhead*).

typically joins with the left renal vein, and the right infrarenal IVC has a conventional configuration (Figs. 24-5, 24-6).

Left Inferior Vena Cava

This derives from regression of the right supracardinal vein with persistence of the left supracardinal vein. The left IVC typically joins with the left renal vein, which merges with the right renal vein to form a normally positioned right-sided suprarenal IVC. Prevalence is 0.2% to 0.5%.

Double Right Inferior Vena Cava

This is a very uncommon variant, with two cases reported in the literature. The anomaly occurs by persistence of the infrarenal portions of both the supracardinal and subcardinal

veins. The ureter must course laterally with respect of the two veins to rule out a persistent right posterior cardinal vein.

Azygous Continuation of the Inferior Vena Cava

Also known as absence of the hepatic segment of the IVC with azygous continuation, this condition occurs following anastomotic failure between the right vitelline vein and the right subcardinal vein, with resulting atrophy of the right subcardinal vein. Blood is thus diverted through the subcardinal-supracardinal anastomosis into the supracardinal system. The azygous vein is derived from thoracic segments of the supracardinal vein and drains normally into the SVC.

Azygous continuation of an anomalous IVC is seen in 0.6% of patients with congenital heart disease and has

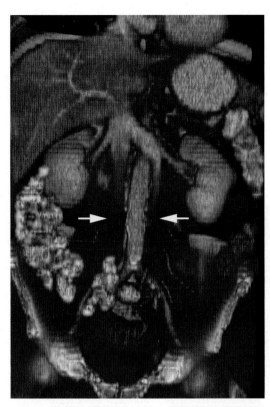

FIGURE 24-5 Double IVC demonstrated with CT. Coronal *volume rendering* reconstruction from a CE MDCT examination of the abdomen and pelvis shows an IVC (*white arrows*) at each side of the aorta. The left IVC drains into the left renal vein. (Courtesy of Alejandro Zuluaga.)

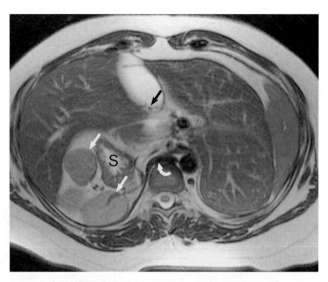

FIGURE 24-7 Polysplenia. Axial T2-weighted FSE image shows a midline liver and a gallbladder, which contains a few small gallstones (*black arrow*). Multiple right-sided splenules (*white arrows*) are seen. Note lack of visualization of the IVC in this patient with azygous continuation, which is visualized as a retrocrural flow void (*curved arrow*). The stomach (*S*) is on the right.

been associated with the polysplenia/asplenia syndrome. It is a common cause of dilatation of the azygous vein. The IVC is usually interrupted at the level of the intrahepatic IVC, and blood returning from the abdomen and legs is routed through the azygous and hemiazygous veins (Fig. 24-7).

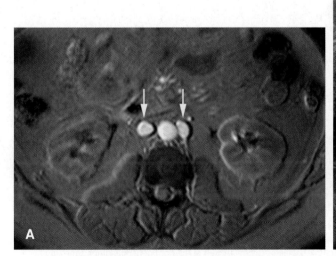

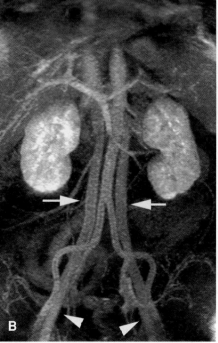

FIGURE 24-6 Double IVC demonstrated with MR. A: Axial TOF image shows two large patent vessels (*white arrows*) at each side of the aorta. **B:** Coronal MIP reconstruction from a 3D T1-weighted gradient echo sequence obtained during the delayed phase confirms the enhancement of the duplicated IVC (*white arrows*). Note continuation of each IVC with each ipsilateral iliac and femoral (*white arrowheads*) veins. (Courtesy of Stanford University Cardiovascular Imaging.)

Occasionally, the hemiazygous vein may be the main collateral pathway from the abdomen to the chest (Fig. 24-8). The hepatic veins drain into the hepatic segment of the IVC, which drains directly into the right atrium (8).

The IVC passes posterior to the diaphragmatic crura to anastomose with the azygous vein. Conventional renal venous anatomy is preserved, except that both right and left gonadal veins drain into the ipsilateral renal vein.

Left Infrarenal Inferior Vena Cava with Hemiazygous Continuation

This results from a persistence of the left supracardinal vein, with regression of the right supracardinal vein. The left supracardinal vein eventually becomes the hemiazygous vein in the thorax, which empties via the normal pathway. The right and left renal veins and suprarenal IVC are of conventional configuration.

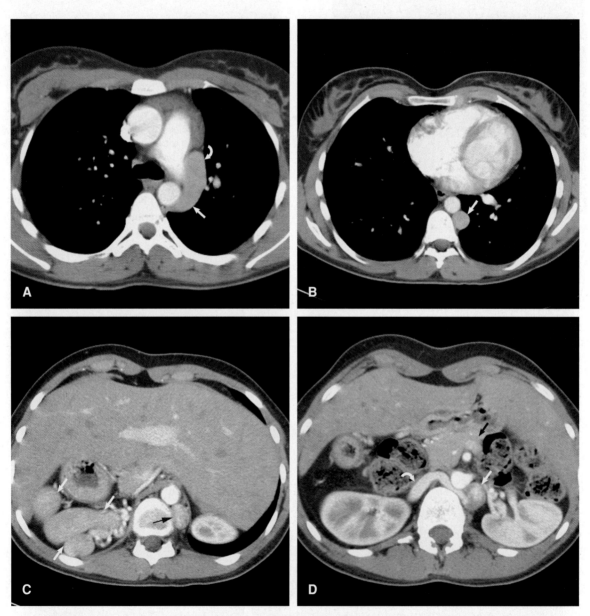

FIGURE 24-8 Polysplenia with hemiazygous continuation. Axial CE CT images of the chest in a patient with polysplenia shows an enlarged hemiazygous vein (*white arrows* in **A** and **B**). **C:** Axial CT image at the level of the upper abdomen shows a midline liver anteriorly and multiple splenules (*white arrows*) in the right upper quadrant. The enlarged hemiazygous vein (*black arrow*) is seen again. **D:** Axial CT image inferior to **C** shows communication between the azygous vein (*white arrow*) and the IVC (*curved arrow*), crossing the midline behind the aorta. A truncated tail of the pancreas and absence of the uncinate process is seen. There is an abnormal relationship of the superior mesenteric vessels (*black arrow*) indicating intestinal malrotation. Overall, these findings are all hallmark imaging findings of polysplenia.

Absence of the Infrarenal Inferior Vena Cava

The venous drainage of the lower extremities occurs via multiple collaterals in the lumbar, sacral, and inferior epigastric systems. It is thought by many not to be a true congenital anomaly but instead caused by in utero thrombosis of the infrarenal IVC.

Renal Vein Anomalies

Retroaortic Left Renal Vein

A persistence of the dorsal arch of the renal collar, with regression of the intersubcardinal anastomosis, gives rise to a retroaortic left renal vein. The prevalence is 2.1%. A single left renal vein passes posterior to the aorta (Fig. 24-9).

Circumaortic Left Renal Vein

Circumaortic left renal vein occurs from persistence of the dorsal limb of the embryonic left renal vein and the dorsal arch of the renal collar. Prevalence has been reported as high as 8.7%. The superior vein receives the left adrenal vein and courses anterior to the aorta. The inferior left renal vein receives the gonadal vein and courses posterior to the aorta.

Double Inferior Vena Cava with Retroaortic Right Renal Vein and Hemiazygous Continuation of the Inferior Vena Cava

This anomaly is the result of failure of anastomosis of the right subcardinal vein to the vitelline vein, with persistence of the left supracardinal system. The right renal vein and infrarenal right supracardinal vein meet and pass posterior to the aorta to meet the left supracardinal vein, the cranial aspects of which become the hemiazygous vein, which empties via the conventional pathway via a rudimentary azygous vein. There is persistence of the dorsal right renal collar and atrophy of the ventral collar. There are multiple additional variations on where the hemiazygous vein can empty, including the coronary vein or via the accessory hemiazygous vein into the left brachiocephalic vein.

Double Inferior Vena Cava with Retroaortic Left Renal Vein and Azygous Continuation of the Inferior Vena Cava

This occurs due to persistence of both supracardinal veins and the dorsal arch of the left renal collar, with regression of the ventral arch of the left renal collar. The anastomosis of the right subcardinal vein to the vitelline vein also fails. The left supracardinal vein empties into the left renal vein, which then empties into the right supracardinal system, the cranial aspect of which becomes the azygous vein. The azygous vein then drains normally into the SVC. This can reportedly be diagnosed with US by visualizing the renal artery crossing abnormally anterior to the IVC.

Retrocaval Ureter

This rare anomaly is also referred to as circumcaval ureter. With the exception of one case described in the literature, it always occurs on the right. The anomaly is due to failure of the right supracardinal venous system to develop, so the infrarenal segment of the IVC is formed by persistence of the right posterior cardinal vein, which anatomically lies ventrolateral to the embryonic kidney. Thus, the developing ureter will be located dorsal to the infrarenal IVC. Patients with this anomaly may develop partial right ureteral obstruction or recurrent urinary tract infections. Treatment is via surgical relocation of the ureter.

Double Inferior Vena Cava with Left Retrocaval Ureter

There are only three reported cases of this extremely rare anomaly. The embryologic development is similar to a double IVC, except that the left IVC is formed not from persistence of the left supracardinal vein but by persistence of the left subcardinal vein. The subcardinal vein lies ventral to the developing left kidney.

Periureteral Venous Ring

This anomaly is caused by persistence of the infrarenal anastomosis between the right posterior cardinal vein and right supracardinal vein adjacent to the right ureter. The anomaly is rare, with approximately 20 reported cases, and it can cause unilateral renal obstruction.

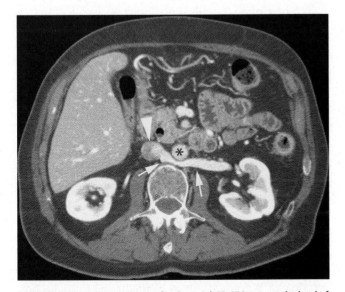

FIGURE 24-9 Retroaortic renal vein. Axial CE CT image at the level of the upper abdomen shows a retroaortic left renal vein (*white arrows*) as it crosses behind the aorta (∗) to join the IVC (*white arrowhead*).

Complex Anomalies

Double Superior Vena Cava and Inferior Vena Cava

This is an uncommon anomaly that is rarely reported in the literature. It occurs from persistence of the left anterior cardinal vein, the left supracardinal vein, and the left subcardinal vein. The abdominal venous systems are thus bilaterally symmetrical. The left SVC and IVC both empty into the left atrium, however, and cause cyanotic heart disease.

Left Superior Vena Cava and Inferior Vena Cava

This occurs from persistence of the left anterior cardinal vein in the thorax and the supracardinal vein in the abdomen. There is failure of the anastomosis between the right subcardinal vein and the vitelline vein, and the left supracardinal vein persists above the level of the left renal vein and continues on into the thorax as the hemiazygous vein, which anastomoses with the left SVC formed from the left anterior cardinal vein. This empties into the coronary sinus and into the right atrium.

Azygous Continuation of the Inferior Vena Cava with Left Superior Vena Cava

This occurs from failure of anastomosis of the right vitelline vein with the right subcardinal vein in conjunction with persistence of the right supracardinal vein and left anterior cardinal vein. The left SVC empties into the coronary sinus and then into the right atrium.

Left Inferior Vena Cava with Hemiazygous Continuation and Double Superior Vena Cava

This occurs exactly as left SVC and IVC except for persistence of the thoracic portions of both anterior cardinal veins.

Double Inferior Vena Cava with Azygous Continuation

This occurs from persistence of both abdominal supracardinal systems and the intersupracardinal anastomosis at the level of the diaphragm. There is atrophy of the left abdominal supracardinal system above the anastomosis and persistence of the right with continuity with the azygous. The blood from the left lower abdomen empties into the right supracardinal system via the intersupracardinal anastomosis, which then empties via the azygous vein into the SVC. There is agenesis of the suprarenal IVC with both renal veins draining via the supracardinal system. The hepatic veins drain conventionally into the right atrium.

Double Inferior Vena Cava with Azygous and Hemiazygous Continuation

This occurs exactly as double IVC with azygous continuation except that the intersupracardinal anastomosis regresses. The hemiazygous follows conventional drainage through the azygous into the SVC.

Absence of the Suprarenal Inferior Vena Cava with Azygous and Hemiazygous Continuation

This occurs from regression of the right vitelline vein and both suprarenal subcardinal veins. Below the renal veins, both supracardinal and subcardinal veins persist, along with the supracardinal-subcardinal anastomosis. Blood flows via the ipsilateral supracardinal systems into the azygous and hemiazygous veins, which drain conventionally into the SVC. There has been only one reported case of this anomaly.

Absent Superior Vena Cava with Azygous Drainage into the Inferior Vena Cava

This occurs from regression of both anterior cardinal veins. Drainage of the thorax is from the supracardinal system, which flows retrograde via the azygous and hemiazygous veins and anastomoses with the IVC at the level of the renal hilum. There is one case report of this anomaly.

Double Inferior Vena Cava with Hemiazygous Continuation of the Left Inferior Vena Cava

This is similar to double IVC except that the left renal vein empties into the left IVC, and the suprarenal supracardinal vein persists and continues into the thorax as the hemiazygous, which drains conventionally into the azygous vein. The right IVC is otherwise conventional.

TECHNICAL CONSIDERATIONS

Computed Tomography

Computed tomographic venography (CTV) has several intrinsic advantages over conventional venography. CT has superior contrast resolution, allowing the use of less concentrated contrast material. Less concentrated contrast material reduces the incidence of phlebitis (18). Venous structures poorly opacified by conventional venography are well visualized with CT (19). CT can also depict important extraluminal pathology.

CTV can be performed with either direct or indirect opacification. In direct venography, contrast is injected into an upstream vein and then imaged as during the first pass of media through the vein of interest. With indirect venography, veins are imaged after contrast has passed through the arterial system. Indirect venography has two important advantages that can offset the generally diminished contrast enhancement relative to direct techniques: (a) concurrent imaging of pulmonary or systemic arteries can be performed, and (b) direct injection into the peripheral veins of the hand or foot is averted.

The advantages in volume coverage speed performance enjoyed by the MDCT scanner are not as essential in venous imaging. Most venous pathology can be diagnosed with anisotropic data sets, and the enhancement of venous structures follows a broader trajectory than their companion arteries. The greater tube heating tolerances of modern, direct cooled tubes with MDCT facilitates combined arterial and indirect venous examinations.

CT evaluation after metallic stent placement in the venous system represents an important capability. MDCT imaging allows for accurate evaluation of the intrastent lumen (Fig. 24-10), while MRI suffers from susceptibility effects cause by certain metallic stents. CT is the examination of choice in patients with venous stents in whom there is clinical concern for occlusion or stenosis and no contraindication for iodinated contrast.

Magnetic Resonance

Magnetic resonance venography (MRV) can be performed without (nonenhanced) and with (enhanced) the intravenous administration of contrast media. Nonenhanced techniques include flow-dependent or flow-independent sequences. CE MRV is usually performed with three-dimensional (3D) gradient echo sequences, although a two-dimensional (2D) approach with sequential acquisition can be useful in patients with limited breath-hold capacity.

Breath-hold imaging should be attempted in cooperative patients when imaging veins in the chest; abdomen; and to a lesser extent, the pelvis. Breathing artifacts degrade image quality and impair visualization of blood vessels. Additional artifacts secondary to physiologic motion can arise from cardiac pulsations and bowel peristalsis. Nonenhanced fast imaging and single-shot pulse sequences minimize

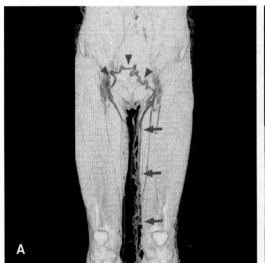
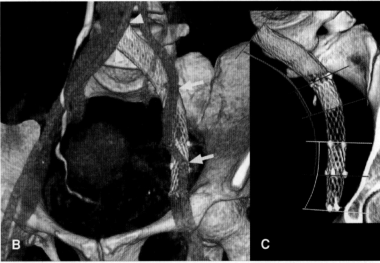
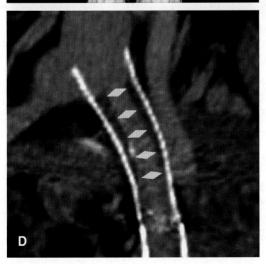

FIGURE 24-10 Neointimal hyperplasia after stenting. Neointimal hyperplasia 2½ years after common and external iliac vein stenting. CT scan from a 40-year-old female with a history of chronic DVT, 2½ years after left common and external iliac venous stenting to treat May-Thurner syndrome. **A:** VR shows extensive superficial varicosities (*arrows*) along the medial aspect of the left thigh draining into the right deep venous system through a network of superficial epigastric veins (*arrowheads*). **B:** VR of the pelvis shows three stents extending from the proximal common iliac vein to the distal external iliac vein. Note that the right common iliac artery (*arrowheads*) and the left common and external iliac arteries (*arrows*) cross over these stented segments. Although unusual, in this case, both the right and the left common iliac arteries resulted in compression of the left common iliac vein to cause the May-Thurner syndrome. **C:** VR shows the metallic structure as well as the overlap of the three stents (extent of stents demonstrated with different colors). **D:** Magnified curved planar reformations shows the longitudinal cross section of the stents. In the segment marked by *yellow diamonds,* there are linear areas of low density paralleling the stent wall, which result in luminal narrowing. Findings indicate moderate neointimal hyperplasia in the proximal stent. (Courtesy of Stanford University Cardiovascular Imaging.)

these artifacts and can facilitate the evaluation of central veins in the chest, abdomen, and pelvis.

In general, suspended respiration is most reproducible during end-expiration. This is an essential consideration for subtraction postprocessing (see subtraction technique). End-expiratory breath holding is maximized by a brief coaching session prior to the exam, informing the patient about the importance of avoiding extremes in respiratory efforts. A nasal cannula to administer oxygen can greatly increase the individual's breath-hold ability (20). MRI at end-inspiration with or without oxygen supplementation can further improve a patient's respiratory capacity. A temporary suspension of the respirator in ventilated patients generally yields high-quality, motionfree images. Finally, if these strategies fail, rapid, motion-insensitive MR sequences are frequently used as a nonbreath-hold protocol.

Nonenhanced Techniques

Flow-independent Sequences

Spin Echo Imaging With traditional T1- and T2-weighted spin echo (SE) sequences, moving blood appears homogeneously hypointense or black as the excited spins exit the imaged slice. This exit phenomenon yields no signal and is commonly termed as *flow void* (21). With flow void, intraluminal thrombus is appreciated as signal residing within a vessel lumen. Thrombus signal intensity depends on age of the thrombus but does not necessarily follow the same predictable time-dependent appearance as intracranial hemorrhage. Slow flow in a patent vessel can also demonstrate increased signal (21). Conventional T1- and T2-weighted SE sequences are not recommended as a first-line strategy for chest and abdominal MRV, as these require long acquisition times.

Fast Spin Echo Imaging Fast spin echo (FSE) sequences (or turbo SE sequences) can be used to decrease long acquisition times associated with conventional SE sequences. For FSE sequences, multiple 180-degree refocusing pulses are applied after each 90-degree pulse, and the subsequent echoes are used to fill in the lines of k-space sequentially (22). With multiple phase-encoded steps performed per repetition time (TR), the speed of sequence acquisition is reduced proportional to the echo train length.

It is possible to use FSE to exploit the long T2 characteristics of blood and provide bright signal within blood vessels, independent from the direction or velocity of the flow (23). The T2 of blood depends on its oxygenation level and thus varies from 60 milliseconds in venous blood (oxygenation between 60% and 75%) to 220 milliseconds for arterial blood (24).

The T2 of venous blood is substantially longer than that of the other tissues on FSE acquisitions with long tau (time

between 180° refocusing pulses) (25). A short echo time (TE) (<100 milliseconds) and a longer inter-TE can augment the signal difference between venous and arterial blood (25). At 1.5 T, a TE of 50 milliseconds provided maximum contrast-to-noise in the calf veins using a fat-saturated FSE sequence (23) although a TE >60 milliseconds can offer adequate suppression of the muscle (25). Fat-saturation techniques further improve suppression of the background signal, allowing for improved depiction of the veins, particularly when maximum intensity projection (MIP) algorithms are used.

The FSE MR venographic method can produce high-quality MR venograms in small extremity veins (e.g., calf and forearm) and is especially sensitive for depicting small branch veins (23).

In clinical practice, FSE sequences may have some value in cases where intravenous contrast is not recommended and other nonenhanced techniques provide inconclusive results. Improved visualization of small vessels in the calf by using FSE sequences has been described compared with time-of-flight (TOF) imaging (23).

Short tau inversion recovery (STIR) sequences can be effective in demonstrating slowly flowing blood as bright signal and can facilitate the depiction of vascular malformations (26,27).

Single-shot Turbo Spin Echo Imaging In single-shot FSE imaging, all lines of k-space for a given slice are filled by multiple 180-degree refocusing pulses applied after a single excitation pulse (22). The "effective TE" in single-shot imaging represents the time between the excitation pulse and the particular TE of the echo train in which the central k-space line is acquired. Low-frequency lines in the center of k-space are typically sampled earlier in the echo train to provide adequate T2-weighted contrast and optimal signal-to-noise ratio (SNR). However, there is inherent blurring of single-shot images due to signal decay during the acquisition of the long echo train.

Half-Fourier techniques are commonly applied in conjunction with single-shot FSE sequences to further decrease acquisition time. These techniques rely on the inherent symmetry of k-space. By acquiring approximately 60% of the data to fill the k-space in half-Fourier techniques, such as half-Fourier single-shot turbo spin echo (HASTE, Siemens, Erlanger, Germany) or single-shot fast spin echo (SSFSE, General Electric Healthcare, Waukesha, WI), the remainder of the k-space can be mathematically calculated based on its symmetry. Since single-shot echo train imaging can be performed either with or without half-Fourier reconstruction, the acronym *HASTE*, which clearly connotes the use of half-Fourier reconstruction, will be used for the remainder of this chapter.

HASTE allows for very fast T2-weighted imaging, with most slices taking less than 1,000 milliseconds to acquire.

The quality of single-shot imaging is related to gradient performance. As a specific absorption rate (SAR)–intensive sequence, the number of slices obtainable in a multislice sequence can be constrained and compensated for with reduced flip angle (FA)–refocusing pulses.

Multislice acquisitions are acquired in a sequential manner, with each slice completely acquired before it proceeds to the acquisition of the next slice. This sequence provides a motion-insensitive strategy for imaging patients with limited or no breath-hold capacity. If the patient can cooperate, however, breath holding is still recommended to preserve sequential display of the anatomy.

HASTE images, like conventional T1- and T2-weighted SE images, characteristically demonstrate a flow void within the vessels as the excited protons exit the imaging slice. Slow flow may allow the blood protons to spend enough time within the imaging slice to provide intravascular signal. Since HASTE acquisitions are T2 weighted and the T2 of blood is relatively long, vessels with slow flow may demonstrate very bright signal in these images. For more uniform suppression of blood signal, so-called *double inversion* strategies can be effective (28,29).

Bright signal from slow flow should not be confused with thrombus, the latter typically demonstrating intermediate gray signal intensity on HASTE sequences (Fig. 24-11). While this may be a source confusion, in the authors' experience, the negative predictive value of HASTE imaging when intravascular flow voids are present is excellent.

The inherent T2 contrast and short acquisition times make this sequence an excellent approach for an initial survey of the body as well as dynamic acquisitions during Valsalva maneuvers. Dynamic HASTE imaging is a widely available technique that provides a rapid screening for venous thrombosis without the need for intravenous administration of contrast.

Dynamic single-shot FSE images are acquired perpendicular to the vessel of interest by using the following parameters: TR 800 milliseconds; TE 62; FA 120; 192 × 256 matrix; slice thickness = 6 mm. Images are obtained during end expiration at a relaxed status and following a sequence command. The patient is instructed to perform a series of seven gradually increasing and then decreasing Valsalva maneuvers (relax, mild push, moderate push, extreme push, moderate push, mild push, relax). These seven images can then be displayed as a single acquisition in a movie loop that facilitates visualization of changes in signal intensity and vessel size.

The Valsalva maneuver increases the intrathoracic pressure with a subsequent decrease in the venous return to the heart. Valsalva also decreases blood velocity and causes enlargement of peripheral veins. With gradually increasing Valsalva effort, normal veins become gradually larger, reflecting vessel distensibility, and increased signal intensity of the blood can appear as a result of slow flow and temporary pooling (Fig. 24-12). The demonstration of both increased signal intensity within the vessel lumen and expansion of vessel caliber in response to a Valsalva maneuver has excellent negative predictive value to exclude venous thrombosis (unpublished data). Thrombosed veins demonstrate intermediate gray signal intensity before and after Valsalva maneuvers on these images without apparent signal intensity change or vessel enlargement (Fig. 24-13).

Steady-state Free Precession Imaging Steady-state free precession (SSFP) imaging is a coherent steady-state technique in which a fully balanced gradient waveform is used to recycle transverse magnetization to preserve signal intensity in species with a long T2 (30). Examples of these techniques among different manufacturers include true fast imaging with steady-state precession (true FISP, Siemens, Erlanger, Germany), fast imaging employing steady state acquisition (FIESTA, GE Healthcare, Waukesha, WI), or balanced fast field echo (balanced FFE, Philips, Bothell, WA). The transverse magnetization is maintained in the steady state from one TR to the next by rewinding the gradient waveforms on all axes (30). The gradients are perfectly balanced, and the total gradient area is zero at the end of each cycle (30).

Image contrast depends on the T2/T1 ratio and is nearly independent of blood flow (31). The high T2/T1 ratio of blood yields high signal intensity on true FISP images without intravenous contrast material (30). The

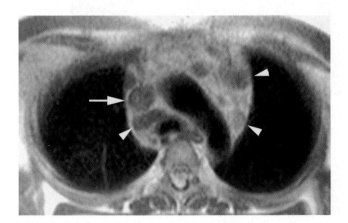

FIGURE 24-11 Acute SVC thrombosis on HASTE. Axial HASTE image through the level of the aortic arch in a 22-year-old female with history of Hodgkin lymphoma now referred for new face and neck swelling shows a normal flow void in the aortic arch. Multiple enlarged mediastinal lymph nodes are also present (*white arrowheads*). There is loss of the normal flow void in the SVC (*white arrow*), which shows intermediate signal intensity, indicating thrombus. Note the similarity of signal intensity to that of adjacent lymph nodes. Postcontrast images (not shown) confirmed the presence of occlusive thrombus in the SVC.

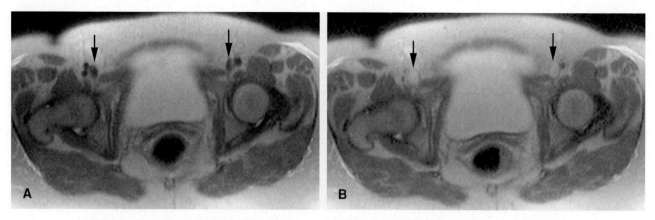

FIGURE 24-12 Dynamic Valsalva HASTE imaging—normal signal intensity patterns. Imaging was performed for a 25-year-old woman with acute onset of shortness of breath 3 days after vaginal delivery. **A:** Axial HASTE images at the level of the inguinal region obtained at rest shows normal flow voids in the femoral veins (*arrows*). **B:** Axial HASTE images obtained at the same level as image (**A**) during maximum Valsalva effort demonstrates increased size and signal intensity in the femoral veins, findings that virtually exclude the diagnosis of venous thrombosis in this location.

rapid nature of this sequence provides diminished sensitivity to motion.

SSFP images obtained perpendicular to the vessel or vessels of interest are usually the most useful. Multislice acquisitions are acquired in a sequential manner, with each image acquired in approximately 1 second or less. This imaging approach is insensitive to respiratory artifacts and

allows for a rapid evaluation of the entire chest, abdomen, or pelvis in a single breath hold. Short TRs and very short TEs are recommended to decrease artifacts related to T2* decay and off-resonance effects.

SSFP imaging has been proposed as an alternative to gadolinium-enhanced magnetic resonance angiography (MRA) for rapid assessment of patients with suspected

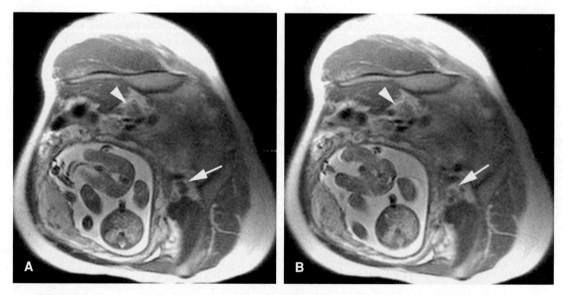

FIGURE 24-13 Dynamic Valsalva HASTE imaging of left iliac deep vein thrombosis in a 42-year-old pregnant woman (20 weeks gestational age) with acute left lower extremity swelling. TOF imaging (not shown) in the supine position failed to show flow in the left iliac vein. The patient was placed in the right lateral decubitus in an attempt to decompress the left iliac vein. **A:** Axial HASTE image at the level of the upper pelvis obtained at rest shows normal flow void in the right iliac vein (*arrow*). The left iliac vein (*arrowhead*) is enlarged and shows intermediate signal intensity. **B:** Axial HASTE image obtained during maximum Valsalva maneuver. The right iliac vein (*white arrow*) increases in size and signal intensity, confirming the presence of normal flow. The appearance of the left iliac vein (*white arrowhead*) remains unchanged, which is consistent with venous thrombosis. Follow-up gadolinium-enhanced MR after delivery following anticoagulation therapy showed a narrowed recanalized left iliac vein.

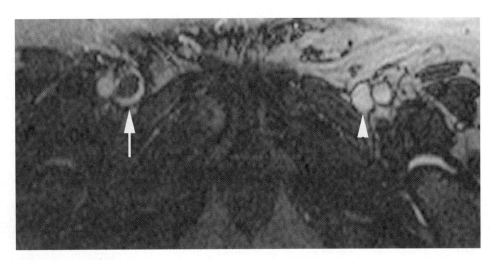

FIGURE 24-14 SSFP imaging of right common femoral deep vein thrombosis. Axial SSFP through the common femoral vessels in a patient with prior renal transplant and right lower extremity edema shows a round hypointense filling defect (*white arrow*) within the right common femoral vein. Note the difference in caliber compared with the normal left common femoral vein (*white arrowhead*), which demonstrates uniform normal high signal. High signal blood surrounds the filling defect in the right common femoral vein, indicating an acute partially occlusive thrombus.

acute aortic dissection (32) and comprehensive evaluation of the entire hepatic vasculature in potential liver donors (33). It allows for thrombus to be visualized as intravascular filling defects with low signal intensity compared with the surrounding hyperintense blood (Fig. 24-14) and has been recently proposed as a noninvasive, fast approach for detection of venous thrombus in the veins of the abdomen, pelvis, and lower extremities (34).

Pulsatility artifacts in SSFP images (30) may cause heterogeneous signal intensity that can be misinterpreted as

thrombus (35). These artifacts are more common at the level of the confluence of veins or in areas where the veins change abruptly in direction. Furthermore, venous thrombus can be missed on these images in patients scanned in the subacute stage (1 to 3 weeks after onset of symptoms) (35) (Fig. 24-15). This is presumably related to the thrombus having T2/T1 characteristics similar to that of the blood pool. Increased signal intensity on T1- and T2-weighted images of carotid thrombi induced in swine has been described with the relative increase in SI significantly

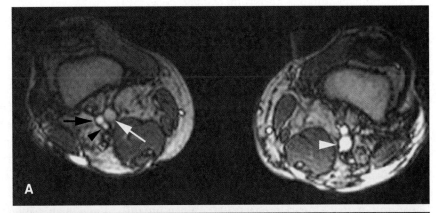

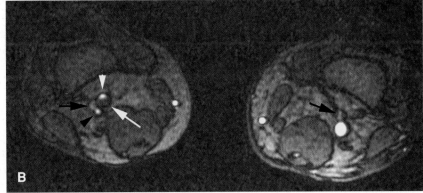

FIGURE 24-15 Popliteal thrombus missed with true FISP imaging. A: Axial true FISP image at the level of the popliteal fossa in a patient with suspected right-sided venous thrombosis shows slightly heterogeneous high signal intensity in the right popliteal vein (*white arrow*). Incidentally, a duplicated deep venous system is appreciated with an accessory right popliteal vein (*black arrowhead*). Laterally, the right popliteal artery (*black arrow*) is noted. A single left popliteal vein (*white arrowhead*) is seen. **B:** Axial TOF image acquired at the same level as **(A)**, with a saturation band above the imaging slice to eliminate the inflowing signal from arterial spins. A nonocclusive thrombus (*white arrow*) is visualized in the right popliteal vein, which demonstrates flow anteriorly (*white arrowhead*). Normal flow is seen in the accessory right popliteal vein (*black arrowhead*) as well as the left popliteal vein. Note the lack of signal in the popliteal arteries (*black arrows*) due to the use of a superior saturation band.

higher on T2-weighted images than that on the T1-weighted images occurring during the first 3 weeks (36). This phenomenon may account for increased signal intensity within the thrombus and false-negative results of SSFP imaging in patients who are imaged in the subacute stage (35). Nevertheless, SSFP imaging can be valuable in patients without intravenous access and suspected venous thrombosis in whom gadolinium-enhanced techniques are not feasible. This is particularly true in those patients with limited breath-hold capability due to the relatively motion-insensitive nature of this sequence compared with other unenhanced techniques (e.g., TOF, phase contrast [PC]). In a recent study, SSFP had a sensitivity of 66% and a specificity of 77% for the diagnosis of venous thrombosis when compared with gadolinium-enhanced T1 gradient echo images (35).

A potential advantage of SSFP imaging is the possibility to obtain cine acquisitions with the use of cardiac triggering (30). Cardiac triggering may reduce pulsatile artifacts and thus improve the homogeneity of the signal within vessels. To the authors' knowledge, the impact of cardiac triggering in the diagnostic accuracy of MRV with SSFP sequences has not yet been explored. However, in their experience, this approach is particularly valuable in the evaluation of the SVC and segments of the IVC close to the right atrium. Cardiac triggering virtually eliminates pulsation artifact in these vessels and allows for continued display of intraluminal thrombus during the cardiac cycle (37) (Fig. 24-16). Extreme degrees of motion of venous thrombus within the SVC and IVC may correlate with higher risk for thromboembolic events.

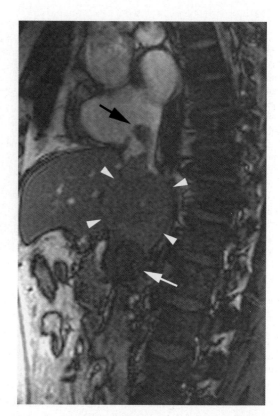

FIGURE 24-16 True FISP imaging of IVC thrombus extending into the right atrium. Sagittal FISP through the IVC shows expansion of the intrahepatic segment of the cava (*white arrowheads*), with complete loss of normal bright blood signal within the IVC, indicating complete thrombosis. Slightly lower signal intensity is seen in the infrahepatic IVC (*white arrow*), which corresponds to a previously placed IVC filter. A fragment of thrombus that extends into the right atrium (*black arrow*) is only attached to the larger IVC thrombus by a thin stalk and is at risk for detachment and embolization.

Flow-dependent Sequences ("Bright Blood" Magnetic Resonance Venography)

Time-of-flight Imaging A major accomplishment for MR imaging was the realization that TOF properties could be exploited for MR vascular imaging (38–41). TRs shorter than the longitudinal relaxation time (T1) of the stationary spins within the imaging slice lead to decreased signal from partial saturation effects (41). When unsaturated blood spins (not excited by the spatially selected radio frequency pulses) move from outside the slice into the imaging slice, they produce a much stronger signal than the partially saturated signal of the stationary spin within the imaging slice (41). This produces the "entry slice phenomenon" or "inflow enhancement," in which signal intensity within the vessels is strong while signal in the stationary tissue is weak. For details on TOF imaging techniques, please refer to Chapter 2.

TOF optimization to depict slow flow within veins includes prescription of the imaging slices perpendicular to the vessel of interest and the use of thin sections (3 to 5 mm). A determination of vessel patency over a large FOV with TOF can be time-consuming. Fewer slices with inter-slice spacing reduce the total acquisition time. A demonstration of bright intraluminal signal in those slices will establish vessel patency. However, the relatively limited sampling could result in undetected, small partial thrombosis and in an inability to render a meaningful MIP reconstruction. This sparsely sampled TOF approach can be effective before gadolinium-enhanced MRV is performed for assessment of vessel patency and the direction of flow within the vein of interest.

Increased signal intensity caused by the entry-slice phenomenon is not directional. Systemic arteries and veins, when adjacent to each other, tend to run in opposite directions, but both appear bright on the slice imaged with TOF. A saturation band is used to selectively eliminate the signal from the flowing spins entering the slice from a chosen direction (42). For uniform suppression, the saturation

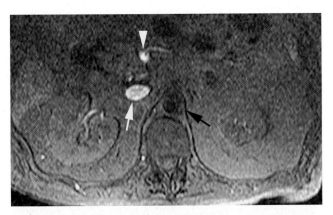

FIGURE 24-17 Saturation band showing portal venous flow direction. A saturation band may be applied either above or below the imaging slice to suppress signal from spins moving into the imaging slice from above or below, respectively. Appropriate usage of saturation bands allows for evaluation of flow direction. In normal circumstances, blood flow in the portal vein is in a caudal-cranial direction and parallels flow in the IVC. In this image with a saturation band above the imaging slice, flow-related signal is only seen in the caudad to craniad direction, within both the IVC (*white arrow*) and portal vein (*white arrowhead*). This indicates both portal vein patency as well as appropriate hepatopetal flow direction. Note that signal intensity within the aorta (*black arrow*) is suppressed by the saturation band.

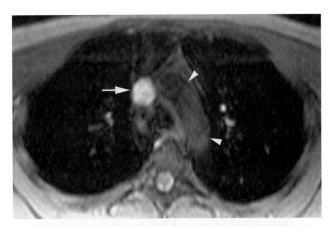

FIGURE 24-18 Normal TOF imaging of the great vessels with an inferior saturation band. Axial TOF image of the chest acquired with an inferior saturation band shows normal craniocaudal flow in the SVC (*white arrow*). Flow in the aortic arch (*white arrowheads*) entering the slice inferiorly has been saturated by the inferior saturation band.

FAs (<20°) can lead to decreased suppression of the background signal as well as a poor SNR. Very high FAs (>45°) can cause saturation of the slower venous blood signal. A MIP algorithm applied to TOF images can generate venogram-like images, displaying the venous anatomy (and

band is applied in a consistent, close proximity to the slice, referred to as a *traveling saturation band*.

MRV is performed by saturating the signal from the arterial spins. Placement of the saturation band, either above or below the imaging slice, depends on the anatomic location of the slice as it relates to the heart. Below the heart, the aortic signal is suppressed by placing the saturation band above the slice. In so doing, bright signal is selectively displayed within those vessels that have blood entering from below the slice (i.e., IVC, portal vein) (Fig. 24-17). This approach can be used for determination of both the vessel patency and its flow direction.

Above the heart, axial venographic TOF images are acquired with a saturation band applied below the imaging slice in order to eliminate the signal from arterial spins (Fig. 24-18). For the subclavian veins, sagittal images are needed for a perpendicular orientation with respect to the vessel orientation (Fig. 24-19). In order to suppress the arterial signal, the saturation band located medial to the imaging slice (left to the slice for the right hemithorax and right to the slice for the left hemithorax) will provide MRV TOF images of the subclavian veins.

Typical MR acquisition parameters for TOF imaging are TR = 25 to 30 milliseconds; TE = 6 to 10 milliseconds; FA = 30 to 45°; thickness 3 to 5 mm; matrix 128 × 256, and application of flow compensation gradients. Low

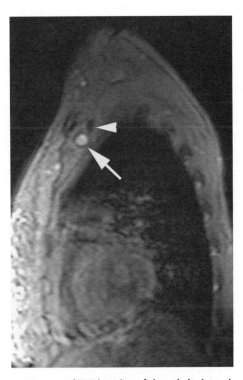

FIGURE 24-19 Normal TOF imaging of the subclavian vein with a medial saturation band. Sagittal TOF image at the level of the left mid clavicular line obtained with a saturation band positioned medial to the slice shows homogeneous high signal intensity in the left subclavian vein (*white arrow*), while the signal in the subclavian artery (*white arrowhead*) has been saturated.

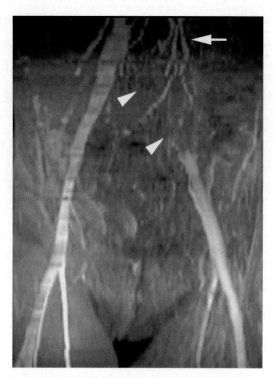

FIGURE 24-20 TOF imaging of left iliac venous thrombosis. MIP reconstruction of an axial multislice TOF acquisition of the pelvis shows lack of signal intensity in the left iliac vein (*white arrowheads*) due to thrombosis. Multiple smaller collateral veins (*white arrow*) are identified in the region.

the extent of occlusion) in a familiar and readily accepted manner (Fig. 24-20).

With TOF, venous thrombosis will appear as a hypointense filling defect within the hyperintense column of flowing blood (43–46). MR using 2D TOF has demonstrated good correlation with conventional venography in the diagnosis of venous thrombosis (44,47–49). Reported sensitivity and specificity are also high compared with duplex sonography (49). Pitfalls can result from in-plane saturation of the intraluminal signal simulating venous thrombus, particularly when blood is not flowing orthogonal to the imaging slice. Turbulent flow can manifest as an area of low signal intensity, seen often near venous confluences, also mimicking a filling defect. Subacute clot can demonstrate high signal intensity similar to that of the flowing blood, blending imperceptive with the normal blood signal (50). Thrombus that is not completely occlusive, especially small areas of clot adhering to the vessel wall, can be difficult to visualize by TOF (45).

Phase Contrast Imaging PC is another technique that exploits the moving nature of blood to create an image. Spins moving in the presence of a magnetic field gradient

accumulate additional phase shift (51–53). The amount of shift is directly proportional to the velocity of the spins and the strength of the gradient (52).

Flow-induced phase shifts arise only from the component of motion along the gradient direction. Thus, three orthogonal gradient directions must be employed in evaluating multidirectional flow (53). The strength of the gradient must also be carefully matched to the velocity of the blood being imaged.

Thus, it is desirable to know the velocity of the blood to be imaged before performing the imaging. Ideally, velocity-encoding values should be chosen to exceed the maximum expected velocity by about 25% (25). For PC imaging of the venous system, a velocity-encoding value of approximately 20 cm/second is typically used (25). Phase contrast venography (PCV) is rarely used in the body.

Contrast-enhanced Magnetic Resonance Venography

Three-dimensional T1-weighted gradient echo sequences allow for assessment of larger anatomic areas, with excellent spatial resolution during a single breath hold, and largely eliminate the artifacts from flow turbulence and in-plane saturation that typify noncontrast MRV techniques (45,54). The 3D sequences are acquired during and after intravenous administration of gadolinium contrast media. CE MRV relies on the T1-shortening effect of intravenous gadolinium preparations on blood, yielding high signal intensity.

CE MRV can be done either directly or indirectly. Direct MRV consists of injection of dilute contrast in the distal aspect of the affected extremity, with subsequent image acquisition. Indirect MRV relies on circulation of injected concentrated contrast media, with subsequent imaging at calculated vascular phases (arterial, venous, delay).

Contrast Agents Conventional gadolinium contrast agents, distributed in the extravascular, extracellular fluid (ECF), offer excellent signal to noise during a delayed, equilibrium phase and yield intense homogeneous venous enhancement even after administration of a single dose of gadolinium. The relative safety and efficacy of gadolinium venography makes it an excellent choice for patients with certain degrees of renal insufficiency or an allergy to iodinated contrast media (55–57). Gadolinium venography has been useful to identify venous access for patients with renal failure (58). Recent concerns associating severe renal insufficiency, gadolinium contrast administration, and nephrogenic systemic fibrosis will need to be considered when balancing the risk:benefit ratio for gadolinium venography in this patient population (59–61).

Blood pool agents (e.g., MS-325, NC100150) offer prolonged and strong venous enhancement (62,63)

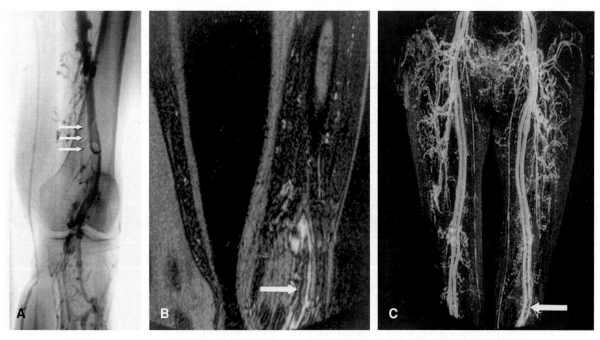

FIGURE 24-21 Superficial femoral vein thrombus with blood pool MR contrast media (Clariscan). Thrombus in the superficial femoral vein (*arrows*) with exact agreement between conventional venography (**A**) and MRV (**B, C**). The MIP image does not show the full extent of the disease (**C**). Despite motion degradation, the study was rated diagnostic. (With permission from Aschauer M, Deutschmann HA, Stollberger R, et al. Value of a blood pool contrast agent in MR venography of the lower extremities and pelvis: preliminary results in 12 patients. *Magn Reson Med.* 2003;50:993–1002.)

(Fig. 24-21). This capacity can significantly improve diagnostic conspicuity and contrast in iliocaval venous opacification compared with extracellular contrast media–enhanced MRV (63). The prolonged half-life may offer additional convenience with the possibility of contrast material administration preceding transfer of the patient to the imaging suite.

Indirect Magnetic Resonance Venography
Three-dimensional T1-weighted gradient echo sequences cover a large area of anatomy in a single vascular phase. Twenty- to twenty-five-second acquisitions provide sufficient anatomic coverage during end expiration breath holds, when needed. Subsequent vascular contrast phases can then be obtained, while allowing the patient time to breathe in the interim. With reproducible breath-holding, subtraction technique can be used to maximize target to background contrast and to generate a venogram (64).

After a timing run and calculation of an appropriate delay time, the authors perform indirect MRV by using a 3D fat-saturated T1-weighted gradient echo sequence (TR = 4.2, TE = 1.7, FA = 25, 160 × 256 matrix, slice thickness 1.5 to 2.5 interpolated, slab thickness 80 to 160 mm). Fat saturation should be avoided in the chest and neck, where inadvertent water suppression could eliminate the gadolinium signal (65). Contrast administration consists of a double dose (0.2 mmol/kg body weight) of gadopentetate dimeglumine (Magnevist, Berlex Laboratories, Wayne, NJ) through intra-

venous access in an antecubital vein. When upper extremity thrombosis is in question, the contralateral arm is injected.

With conventional extracellular-gadolinium agents, a biphasic administration yields good-quality enhancement of the blood pool. The total dose of gadolinium is administered as follows: 0.1 mmol/kg body weight at 2 cc/second immediately followed by 0.1 mmol/kg body weight at 0.8 cc/second, in a single injection. An additional 20 cc of saline flush is injected at 0.8 cc/second. Evaluation of the visceral veins, including the portal and renal veins, is typically performed with a single dose of gadolinium (0.1 mmol/kg body weight at 2 cc/second) with excellent results.

Bolus injection timing is essential when a selective venous study is desired. First, a "vein-free" arterial phase is captured by using a timing examination with administration of 1 cc of gadopentetate dimeglumine at a rate of 2 cc/second through a peripheral intravenous line in an antecubital vein, as previously described by Earls and associates (66). This approach ensures acquisition of the central region of the k-space during the middle of the administered bolus, thus guaranteeing appropriate arterial enhancement throughout that entire 3D data set. The delay time (Td), or the time between injection initiation and the scan start time, can be effectively calculated with the following equation:

$$Td = Tc + Ti/2 - Ts/2$$

where Tc is the circulation time, Ti is the injection time for the first component of the injection (administered at 2 cc/second), and Ts is the scan acquisition time. Tc is the time between injection initiation and the peak arterial enhancement in the anatomic region of interest (ROI), and it is estimated by the timing run.

For example, if the contrast arrives to the abdominal aorta 20 seconds after initiation of the injection of 1 cc of gadolinium at 2 cc/second, then Tc equals 20. If the patient's weight is 80 kg, a double dose (0.2 mmol/kg body weight) will be 80 × 0.4 = 32 cc. A single dose (16 cc) is given intravenously at 2cc/second followed by a second dose (16 cc) at 0.8 cc/second in a single injection. The injection time for the first component of the injection given at 2 cc/second is 16/2 = 8 seconds. For an acquisition time of 24 seconds, the time delay for starting the acquisition would be:

$$\mathbf{Td} = 20 + 8/2 - 24/2 = 20 + 4 - 12 = \mathbf{12\ seconds}$$

In this example, acquisition of the first 3D data set (arterial phase) should be timed so that the acquisition is initiated 12 seconds into the gadolinium administration. Breathing instructions are typically given before starting the acquisition. Hyperventilation prior to the breath-hold procedure improves the patient's performance. In the authors' experience, two cycles of the command "breath in, breath out" take approximately 6 seconds and yield good results. Therefore, in the theoretical patient, two sets of breathing instructions would be started 6 seconds after the initiation of the contrast injection, and the acquisition would be started immediately after completing the breathing instructions (12 seconds after initiation of the injection of contrast).

After the "venous-free" acquisition is obtained during the arterial phase, two additional acquisitions are obtained at 40 seconds and 90 seconds delay after the arterial peak. Typically, delayed blood pool acquisitions are used for making the diagnosis.

The arterial (A) acquisition can be used as a mask that is subtracted from the delayed blood pool phase, the latter containing both arteries and veins (AV) (64). MIP reconstructions of the subtraction result, AV − A, resemble conventional venography images (64) (Fig. 24-22).

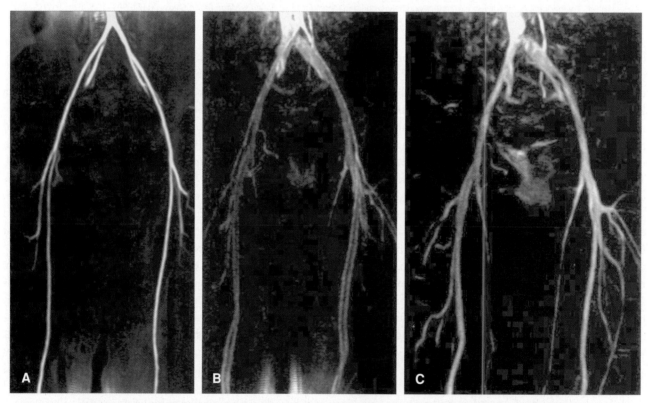

FIGURE 24-22 Indirect MRV with subtraction display in a 49-year-old woman. This woman with clinically suspected iliac deep venous thrombosis represents source data lacking appreciable flow-related enhancement. **A:** MIP MR image from arterial phase gadolinium-enhanced 3D MR acquisition (5/2;FA, 50) shows normal aortoiliac system. **B:** MIP MR image from blood pool phase gadolinium-enhanced 3D MR acquisition (5/2; FA, 50) shows normal aortoiliac veins and arteries. **C:** MIP MR image from subtraction venogram (blood pool phase minus arterial phase) shows normal venous anatomy. (Adapted with permission from Lebowitz JA, Rofsky NM, Krinsky GA, et al. Gadolinium-enhanced body MR venography with subtraction technique. *AJR Am J Roentgenol*. 1997;169:755–758.)

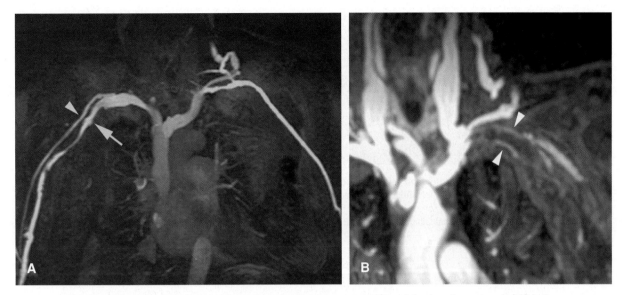

FIGURE 24-23 Direct MRV. A: MIP reconstruction of a 3D fat-saturated T1-weighted gradient echo acquisition during the simultaneous administration of diluted gadolinium (1:20) through distal veins of both arms shows the normal right cephalic (*white arrowhead*) and subclavian (*white arrow*) veins. A single vessel is seen on the **left**, which corresponds to a mildly enlarged cephalic vein. Similar to conventional venography, patent veins are readily seen with direct venography, while thrombosed veins are not seen. **B:** Thick-slab MIP reconstruction of a 3D fat-saturated T1-weighted gradient echo acquisition obtained during the delayed venous phase after **(A)** coned in on the proximal left subclavian vein. There is occlusive thrombus (*white arrowheads*) in the left subclavian vein. Note the enhancement of its wall, indicating subacute (likely less than 2 weeks) thrombosis. Direct MRV can be followed by delayed acquisition indirect venography, which allows for exquisite visualization of thrombosed vessels.

Three-dimensional T1-weighted gradient echo sequences provide accurate reconstructions in any plane, facilitating the evaluation of tortuous veins and veins that are oriented parallel to the acquisition plane.

Direct Venography Direct gadolinium-enhanced MRV (67) uses a very low concentration of gadolinium chelate to avoid first-pass susceptibility effects that can obscure key information. Diluted gadolinium contrast media (3 cc in 60 cc of saline for a 1:20 solution) is injected directly through peripheral intravenous access in the affected extremity. Bilateral intravenous access may be needed in both upper extremities for the assessment of the SVC in order to minimize mixing artifacts from nonopacified blood entering the SVC from the contralateral extremity. A tourniquet in the lower extremities helps to prevent enhancement of the superficial venous system (67).

A 3D fat-saturated T1-weighted gradient echo sequence as described earlier is used when direct MRV is performed during the administration of the contrast media. The acquisition can be started 7 to 10 seconds after the initiation of contrast media delivery. Multiple acquisitions may be obtained over time to improve visualization of small veins and veins with slow flow enhancing in a delayed fashion.

This technique improves visualization of patent veins compared with indirect MR techniques. In addition, lack of arterial enhancement facilitates the interpretation of these examinations as well as multiplanar and volumetric reconstructions (i.e., MIP, volume rendering [VR]). The diagnosis of venous thrombosis is made based on the nonvisualization of a particular venous segment. However, similar to conventional venography, early acquisitions during the administration of contrast may fail to demonstrate venous pathology or can be difficult to interpret. Delayed imaging after the direct MR examination is completed may yield images similar to those of the indirect MR technique. These are useful for the visualization of venous pathology, including occluded veins (Fig. 24-23).

THROMBUS STAGING

The ability to accurately age a thrombus (thrombus staging) has implications for patient management. Patients presenting within 3 days, 1 to 2 weeks, and 3 to 4 weeks after the first appearance of the symptoms have complete or partial resolution of the thrombotic occlusion after fibrinolytic therapy in approximately 95%, 82%, and 69% of the cases, respectively (68). Conversely, patients with clinical symptoms for 5 to 8 weeks prior to initiating this therapy have a

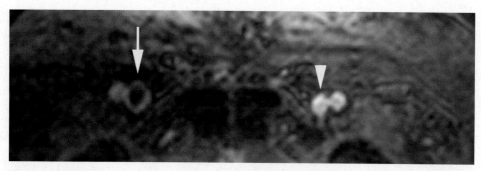

FIGURE 24-24 MRV of acute deep vein thrombosis. Axial reconstruction from a coronal 3D fat-saturated T1-weighted gradient echo acquisition during the delayed venous phase in a patient with right lower extremity swelling. There is expansion of the right common femoral vein (*white arrow*) compared with the left (*white arrowhead*). A centrally located intraluminal filling defect and wall enhancement are also present, indicating acute thrombosis.

low incidence of recanalization (68). Furthermore, the onset of clinical symptoms can be insidious or misinterpreted as secondary to other diseases or conditions, causing a delay in diagnosis. Thus, the decision to proceed with fibrinolytic therapy can be controversial and would ideally be based on a capacity to identify and date a thrombus.

Acute venous thrombosis typically presents as a centrally located filling defect that causes expansion of the affected vein (69) (Fig. 24-24). The thrombus can be completely or partially occlusive. In vivo, acute venous thrombosis is associated with an inflammatory response within the vein wall and perivenous tissues apparently mediated by proinflammatory cytokines and adhesion molecules (69). A vein that is chronically occluded will decrease in caliber (45). Not uncommonly, chronically occluded veins are undetectable by imaging studies as they become a thin fibrotic remnant.

Collateral vessels are a secondary sign that is also indicative of subacute to chronic occlusion (Fig. 24-25). Over time, the thrombus will reorganize. Recanalization occurs from the center of the thrombus out to the periphery, and flow will initially be re-established through the center of the thrombus. With organization, the remaining thrombus is adherent to the periphery of the vessel wall. Chronically thrombosed veins will not change caliber with a physiologic maneuver such as a Valsalva maneuver.

US examinations can suggest the age of the thrombus based on its echogenicity and location within the lumen. An increase in echogenicity is expected as organization of the venous thrombus occurs, although this can vary among patients (70). US elastography has been proposed as a valuable tool to stage venous thrombi based on the fact that thrombus elasticity decreases with age due to the organization process (71).

With CT, venous thrombosis is diagnosed when a complete, partial, or juxtamural filling defect representing a clot is seen in an opacified vein. Indirect signs can include perivenous soft tissue infiltration suggestive of edema and dense mural enhancement (72). The accuracy of CT in distinguishing between acute and chronic thrombus is not known. Acute thrombus can be identified on a noncontrast CT as a hyperdense mass within the lumen of a vein. Chronic thrombus may be calcified; other features include clot recanalization, small unopacified retracted veins, and multiple venous collaterals (73).

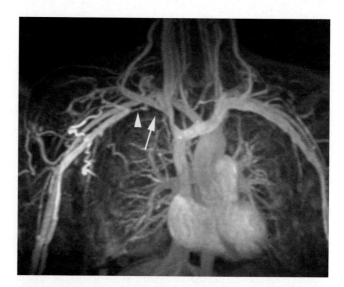

FIGURE 24-25 Chronic thrombosis. MIP reconstruction from a coronal subtracted (delay phase minus precontrast) 3D fat-saturated T1-weighted gradient echo acquisition in a patient with Hodgkin disease and right arm swelling. There is complete thrombosis of the right subclavian vein (*white arrow*) just before the anastomosis with the internal jugular vein. A thin sliver of central enhancement (*white arrowhead*) is identified in the more distal subclavian vein, indicating partial recanalization. Note the extensive collateral vessels in the right upper chest/back compared with the asymptomatic left side.

MR imaging can provide valuable information regarding the age of the venous thrombus, but appearances can vary with the imaging strategy.

The MR appearance of arterial thrombus relative to its age has been described in a swine model (36). The signal characteristics of arterial thrombi as well as the changes detected over time are associated with different oxygenation states of the hemoglobin, changes in intracellular and matrix content of proteins, and the hydration of the cellular components (36).

Oxyhemoglobin, a diamagnetic compound present within acute thrombus (a few hours after induction), does not cause shortening of the T1 or T2 relaxation times. This may explain the intermediate signal intensity on T1 and increased signal intensity on T2 of acute thrombus (36).

One week after thrombus induction, an increase in signal intensity on T1- and T2-weighted images was noted within thrombi. The presence of methemoglobin with short T1 relaxation time is responsible for the increased signal intensity on T1-weighted images (36). Increased signal intensity on T2-weighted images is due to increased water content of lysed red blood cells (36).

The relative increase in signal intensity was significantly higher on T2-weighted images than that on the T1-weighted images, and the strongest statistical significance occurred during the first 3 weeks. The signal intensity decreased in chronic thrombus (6 weeks after induction), demonstrating intermediate signal intensity both on T1- and T2-weighted images (36).

In vitro relaxation time measurements of venous thrombus show marked reduction in T1- and T2-weighted images during the acute phase, which can help in differentiating clot from stagnant flow (74). As the clot ages, there is further shortening of its T1 and, to a lesser extent, of its T2 (74). However, the in vitro assessment may not apply to the behavior in the more complex and dynamic conditions found in vivo.

When clot organization occurs, usually 5 days after induction, it incorporates to the vessel wall and thus makes its visualization challenging (74). An organized clot may be visible only as an area of wall thickening with no difference in signal intensity than that of the vessel wall (74). The appearance of thrombus within a vein changes over time.

Partially occlusive thrombus is visible as a filling defect surrounded by flow at the periphery of the vein, which can be visualized on TOF imaging as well as on T1 postcontrast GRE sequences as a peripheral rim of high signal intensity (45). Occlusive thrombus fills the vein lumen entirely, and no flow is present.

On MRI, the perivenous inflammatory response seen with acute venous thrombosis is characterized by increased signal intensity on T2-weighted images within the vein wall and perivenous tissues, presumably due to edema (45). Signal intensity of the actual acute thrombus material on T1 GRE or SE sequences is usually isointense to the vein wall; partial or complete loss of the normal intraluminal flow void may also be appreciated.

Signal intensity of venous thrombi increases over time (75) (Fig. 24-26). In addition, acute thrombosis is associated with enhancement of the vessel wall on gadolinium-enhanced T1-weighted images (69). Wall enhancement occurs at the level of adhesion of the thrombus to the vein wall (69) (Fig. 24-27).

Increased signal intensity in the surrounding tissues can be explained by extravasation of gadolinium from the vessel wall in areas of capillary leak caused by the strong inflammatory response initiated by acute deep vein thrombosis (45,69). Increased signal intensity decreases over time as the thrombus is incorporated into the vein wall and inflammation resolves, usually over the course of 14 days (69). This decrease in signal intensity over time could be used to chronologically differentiate acute from subacute thrombosis.

Signal intensity of the subacute to chronic thrombus is variable, with the thrombus usually appearing heterogeneous on most sequences. Subacute thrombus can appear as high signal intensity on T1 GRE sequences, TOF sequences (50), and true FISP sequences (35) (Fig. 24-28). With SSFP imaging, the bright signal of clot can blend with the bright signal of the blood pool and may go undetected (35).

With CE T1 GRE sequences, reorganized thrombus can appear as zones of increased signal intensity in the periphery of the vein (69). Chronic thrombus usually demonstrates very low signal intensity on T1- and T2-weighted sequences.

THROMBUS CHARACTERIZATION

An important consideration in clinical practice is differentiation of bland versus tumor thrombus. While bland thrombus is typically treated with anticoagulation or fibrinolytic therapy, tumor thrombus should be managed in the context of the primary neoplasm.

Bland Thrombus

The term *bland thrombus* is generally applied to any filling defect within a vessel that is not comprised of malignant cells. The key finding for bland thrombus on an imaging examination is the lack of enhancement after administration of contrast.

Given that CT is routinely performed after contrast administration, determination of thrombus enhancement

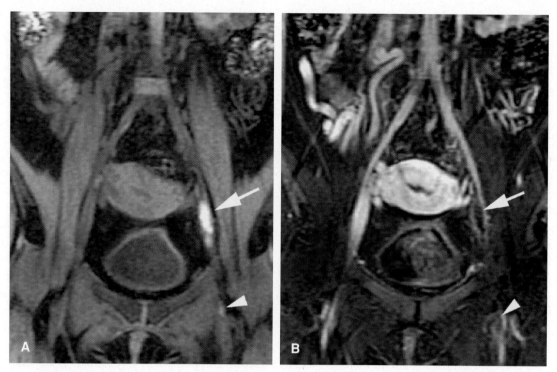

FIGURE 24-26 Bright thrombus on T1-weighted imaging. A: Unenhanced coronal 3D fat-saturated T1-weighted gradient echo in a patient with a previous history of left lower extremity DVT shows an ovoid area of high signal within the left external iliac vein (*white arrow*), indicating subacute thrombus. A smaller focus of high signal (*white arrowhead*) is identified more distally in the left common femoral vein. **B:** Coronal subtracted (contrast enhanced during the delayed venous phase minus the unenhanced phase) confirms the presence of venous thrombus in the external iliac (*white arrow*) and common femoral (*white arrowhead*) veins as nonenhancing filling defects corresponding to the areas of high signal intensity on **(A)**.

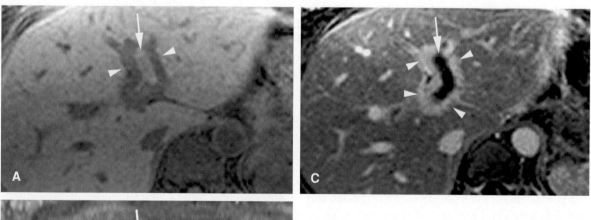

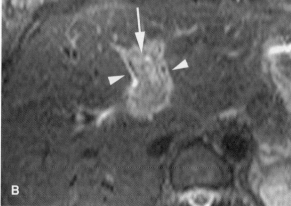

FIGURE 24-27 Venous wall edema and enhancement in acute deep vein thrombosis in a 48-year-old male with abdominal pain. A: Axial unenhanced 3D fat-saturated T1-weighted gradient echo image through the level of the left portal vein shows a tubular area of high signal intensity (*white arrow*) representing thrombus in the left portal vein, surrounded by low signal intensity (*white arrowheads*). **B:** Axial STIR gradient echo image through the same level as **(A)** shows heterogeneous hyperintense thrombus (*white arrow*) in the left portal vein surrounded by high signal intensity edema (*white arrowheads*), which corresponds to the area of low signal intensity on **(A)**. **C:** Subtraction (portal venous phase minus precontrast) 3D fat-saturated T1-weighted gradient echo image shows avid enhancement of the left portal vein wall (*white arrowheads*). Nonenhancing thrombus within the left portal vein (*white arrow*) is now more apparent.

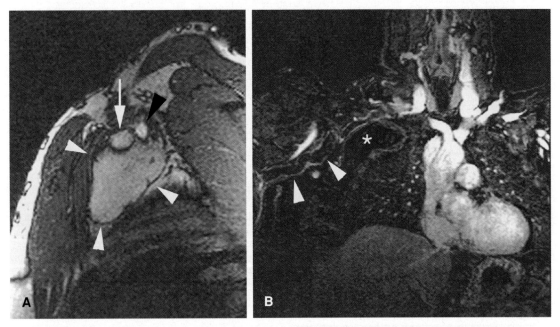

FIGURE 24-28 Bright thrombus on true FISP imaging in a 53-year-old man with right upper extremity edema.
A: Sagittal FISP image through the right subclavian vessels shows the right subclavian vein (*white arrow*) and artery (*black arrowhead*). Just beneath these vessels is a mass (*white arrowheads*), which demonstrated signal intensity similar to that of fat on all sequences (not shown) and represented a lipoma. The signal in the subclavian vein is slightly less but very similar to that in the artery. Subacute thrombus can demonstrate intermediate to high signal intensity on FISP images and thus may be missed. **B:** Curved reconstruction along the right subclavian vein from a coronal subtracted (delay phase minus precontrast) 3D fat-saturated T1-weighted gradient echo acquisition in the same patient shows no enhancement of the mass (*). Extensive nonenhancing filling defect in the right subclavian vein (*white arrowheads*) is present, indicating complete thrombosis.

may require that the patient returns for imaging without contrast. In that scenario, it is important to use the same scanner and to keep all other parameters constant. Theoretically, delayed images obtained following contrast administration might show de-enhancement, as has been seen in renal masses (76) to facilitate characterization. However, to the best of the authors' knowledge, this approach has not been validated for thrombus.

On MR, the presence or absence of thrombus contrast enhancement can be readily assessed by using subtraction techniques (post–pre-contrast) in cooperative patients when anatomic co-registration is satisfactory. Bland thrombus typically appears as a black intraluminal filling defect on subtraction imaging during the delay venous phase (Fig. 24-29). In less cooperative patients, measurement of signal intensity in the thrombi with ROIs before and after gadolinium administration should be pursued.

Tumor Thrombus

Determination of tumor thrombus can impact both an indication for surgery and the surgical approach. Tumor thrombus, compared with bland thrombus, is composed of a cohesive mass of malignant cells that have invaded the blood vessel. Tumor thrombus must have a vascular supply to support the neoplastic tissue. Demonstration of thrombus enhancement after contrast administration is the most valuable finding to predict tumor thrombus. However, intense enhancement has been described in chronic organized bland thrombus within the heart 10 to 20 minutes after administration of gadolinium (77).

Occasionally, benign neoplastic thrombus can be seen, and, therefore, tumor thrombus is not always equivalent to malignant thrombus. Benign intravascular tumors including spindle cell tumors, lipomas, and intravascular papillary endothelial hyperplasia (Masson tumor) can be seen as enhancing intraluminal filling defects on MRI. Most frequently, however, enhancing intraluminal masses represent local venous invasion of malignant neoplasms (e.g., hepatocellular carcinoma, renal cell carcinoma [RCC]); less frequently, primary venous sarcomas are responsible for the presence of enhancing intravenous masses.

Differentiation of benign from malignant portal vein thrombosis in patients with cirrhosis has been described

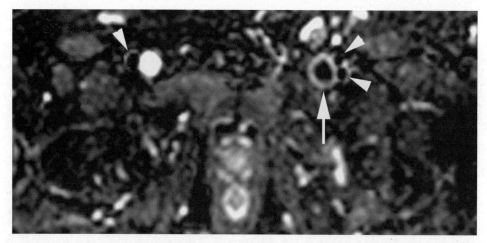

FIGURE 24-29 Bland thrombus in a 51-year-old male with a history of extragonadal germ cell tumor and renal cell carcinoma, now presenting with left lower extremity edema. Axial reformatted subtraction (delay phase minus arterial phase) 3D fat-saturated T1-weighted gradient echo image shows expansion of the left common femoral vein, which contains a central thrombus (*white arrow*). Note the difference in caliber of the left common femoral vein compared with the right. Also note signal void in the common femoral artery on the right (*white arrowhead*) as well as the superficial and deep femoral arteries on the left (*white arrowheads*) on this subtracted image (acquired by subtracting the arterial phase from the venous phase).

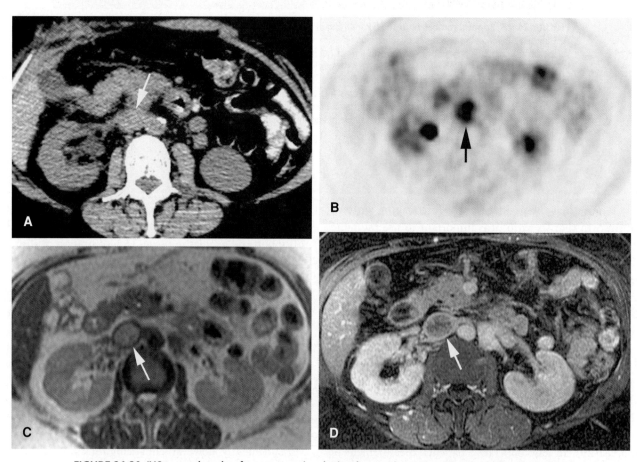

FIGURE 24-30 IVC tumor thrombus from metastatic colonic adenocarcinoma in a 57-year-old female. A: Axial noncontrast CT image from a CT/PET examination at the level of the lower pole of the left kidney shows expansion of the IVC (*white arrow*). **B:** Axial reconstructed PET image with CT attenuation correction from the same fluorodeoxyglucose (FDG)-PET scan as that in **(A)** at a similar level shows avid focal FDG uptake in the IVC (*black arrow*), which is well above that of blood pool in the adjacent aorta, indicating tumor in the IVC. **C:** Axial HASTE image through the same level as **(A)** also demonstrates expansion of the IVC (*white arrow*), with heterogeneous hyperintense thrombus in its lumen. Note the loss of the normal flow void in the IVC compared with the normal flow void in the adjacent aorta. **D:** Axial subtraction (venous phase minus precontrast) 3D fat-saturated T1-weighted gradient echo image through the same level as **(C)** confirms enhancement within the thrombus (*white arrow*), indicating tumor thrombus. The circumferential rim of high signal could indicate either enhancement of the IVC wall or blood flowing around the tumor thrombus.

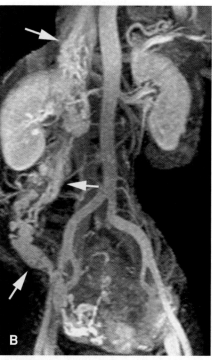

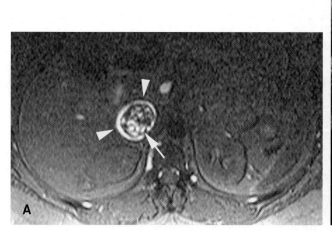

FIGURE 24-31 TOF imaging of invasive leiomyomatosis. A: Axial TOF image with a saturation band above the imaging slice in a patient with bilateral lower extremity edema shows expansion of the intrahepatic segment of the IVC, which contains a heterogeneous filling defect (*white arrow*). Flow-related signal surrounds the filling defect nearly circumferentially (*white arrowheads*). Note the presence of flow-related signal within the thrombus itself, indicating vascular flow within the tumor thrombus. **B:** Coronal MIP reconstruction from a subtracted (arterial minus precontrast phase) 3D fat-saturated T1-weighted gradient echo sequence shows extensive vascularization (*arrows*) extending from the pelvis to the right gonadal vein and IVC, which represents dilated blood vessels within invasive leiomyomatosis.

using US (78) and CT (79). Doppler US can identify vascularity within the thrombus, although it can suffer from limited visualization of deep central veins within the chest and abdomen, particularly in patients with a large body habitus. Determination of subtle thrombus enhancement on CT can be difficult. Furthermore, pseudoenhancement related to beam hardening after contrast administration can mimic thrombus enhancement.

The excellent inherent soft tissue contrast and sensitivity for detection of small amounts of gadolinium suits MR as a robust imaging technique for thrombus characterization (Fig. 24-30). It is important to realize, however, that the demonstration of enhancement may be elusive in rare cases with extremely hypovascular neoplasms.

Although variable, signal intensity of tumor thrombus is frequently increased on T2-weighted images and can be similar to the primary neoplasm. Caution must be exercised in diagnosing tumor thrombus on noncontrast MRV sequences. Slow venous flow can demonstrate increased signal intensity on T2-weighted SE and FSE images, which can mimic venous thrombi (80).

Similarly, turbulent flow and/or pulsatile flow can cause intraluminal filling defects, which can be misinterpreted as venous thrombi on flow-dependent MR strategies (e.g., TOF imaging). This is especially true at the confluence of veins with rapid flow (e.g., confluence of renal veins and IVC or jugular veins with subclavian veins) and at locations where veins change dramatically in orientation (e.g., common femoral to external iliac veins). Although noncontrast MRV cannot discriminate accurately between bland and tumor thrombus based on its signal characteristics, flow within thrombus can be detected occasionally with these techniques (Fig. 24-31). The location and context of the filling defect, such as in the portal vein or hepatic veins in the presence of a hepatic mass or within the renal vein in the presence of a renal mass, can suggest the diagnosis.

Bland and tumor thrombus can coexist in the same patient. Bland thrombus can develop secondary to slow flow caused by occlusive tumor thrombus and, therefore, is frequently located "upstream" to the tumor thrombus. On subtracted 3D T1 GRE postcontrast images, bland thrombus

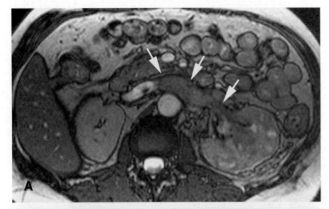

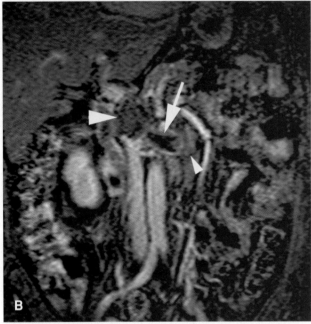

FIGURE 24-32 Renal mass with both bland and tumor thrombus as shown in MR images of a patient presenting for staging. A: Axial true FISP image through the left renal vein shows diffuse heterogeneous signal intensity in the left kidney, representing the patient's known infiltrating mass. There is expansion of the left renal vein (*white arrows*), which contains intermediate signal intensity. Note normal high blood pool signal intensity in the IVC and aorta. **B:** Coronal subtracted (venous phase minus precontrast) 3D fat-saturated T1-weighted gradient echo image shows expansion of the left renal vein, which contains a heterogeneous enhancing filling defect (*small white arrowhead*) consistent with tumor thrombus. The distal left renal vein just proximal to its confluence with the IVC is filled by a nonenhancing thrombus (*white arrow*). A rhomboid area of low signal intensity in the IVC (*large white arrowhead*) represents an IVC filter. At surgery and pathology, tumor thrombus was found in the left renal vein extending from the left kidney to the level of the IVC filter. The presence of enhancement in the thrombus allows for accurate characterization as tumor thrombus, while lack of enhancement does not exclude tumor thrombus.

is visualized as a homogeneous nonenhancing (black) filling defect immediately adjacent to the enhancing (variable intermediate-to-bright signal intensity) tumor thrombus (Fig. 24-32).

CLINICAL APPLICATIONS

Jugular Veins

Evaluation of the jugular veins is usually part of a comprehensive evaluation of the central veins in the neck and chest. This is frequently performed in the context of patients with a prior history of indwelling catheters before repeated central venous catheterization is attempted. Patients with malignancies are at risk for jugular vein thrombosis as well (81). Evaluation of jugular venous outflow is also essential in evaluating intracranial venous patency in diseases such as cerebral sinus thrombosis. The craniocaudad direction and relatively straight course of the jugular veins is favorable for TOF MRI. However, intraluminal filling defects related to turbulent flow are not uncommon. CE MRV is usually performed because it provides not only excellent evaluation of the jugular veins but also an outstanding assessment of the rest of the central veins in the chest, including collateral circulation (Figs. 24-25, 24-39, 24-41).

The appearance of jugular vein occlusion varies from a distended vessel with a centrally located filling defect (acute/subacute thrombosis) (Fig. 24-33) to nonvisualization of the vessel (chronic occlusion). Jugular vein wall edema as well as edema in the adjacent soft tissues of the neck is common in acute thrombosis. The presence of collateral veins suggests chronic thrombosis to some degree. Central venous catheters can be visualized as linear filling defect within the patent vein. Visualization of the catheter within the thrombosed segment of the vein or in chronically occluded nonvisualized vessels is virtually impossible.

Extrinsic compression of the jugular veins can be seen secondary to enlarged lymph nodes (e.g., lymphoma). Head and neck squamous cell neoplasms often cause vascular compromise. Tumors that arise in the parotid or submandibular glands can also cause jugular occlusion from direct spread. Jugular vein thrombosis can present as a soft tissue mass in patients with malignancies (82). Neck irradiation can cause narrowing and occlusion of the jugular veins.

Traumatic injury and subsequent thrombosis of the jugular vein can occur. While arterial injuries are the main concern in the presence of a seat belt sign in the neck after motor vehicle accidents (83), internal jugular vein thrombosis may also occur (Fig. 24-34). Bilateral traumatic internal jugular vein thrombosis may occur after trauma and can cause significant elevation of the intracranial pressure (84). Penetrating trauma to the neck may result in arteriovenous fistulas (AVFs) between the carotid and jugular venous system (Fig. 24-35).

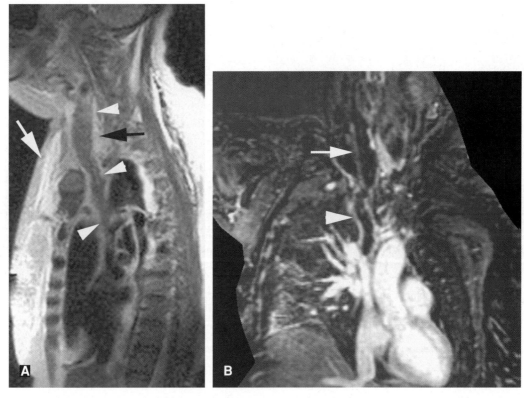

FIGURE 24-33 Acute internal jugular venous thrombosis. A: Sagittal HASTE image through the right neck and chest shows loss of the normal flow void within the right internal jugular and right brachiocephalic veins (*white arrowheads*), which are expanded and filled with intermediate signal intensity material, indicating thrombus. Note the increased signal intensity in the wall of the internal jugular vein (*black arrow*) and subcutaneous tissues (*white arrow*), indicating edema. **B:** Curved coronal reconstruction from a subtracted (delayed postcontrast minus precontrast) 3D fat-saturated T1-weighted gradient echo acquisition confirms the presence of thrombus as a nonenhancing filling defect expanding the right internal jugular vein (*white arrow*) and brachiocephalic vein (*white arrowhead*).

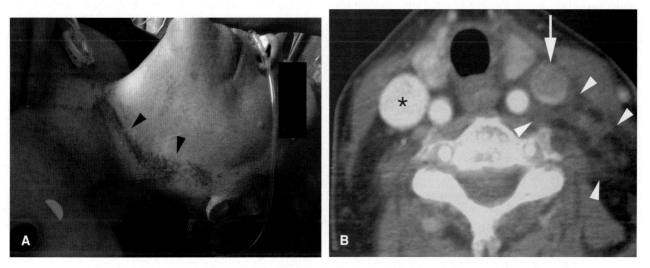

FIGURE 24-34 Traumatic internal jugular thrombosis due to seat belt injury. A: Photograph of a patient with traumatic thrombosis of the left internal jugular vein after a motor vehicle accident. A linear bandlike area of ecchymosis is present over the left lateral aspect of the neck (*black arrowheads*) in the expected distribution of the shoulder portion of a seat belt. **B:** Axial CE CT scan through the neck shows extensive fat stranding in the lateral left neck (*white arrowheads*). Normal enhancement is seen in the right internal jugular vein (*). A filling defect of intermediate density is present in the left internal jugular vein (*white arrow*), indicating an acute thrombus. A crescentic area of increased density surrounds the filling defect, indicating flow around the acute thrombus. Findings are consistent with acute internal jugular vein thrombosis secondary to seat belt injury.

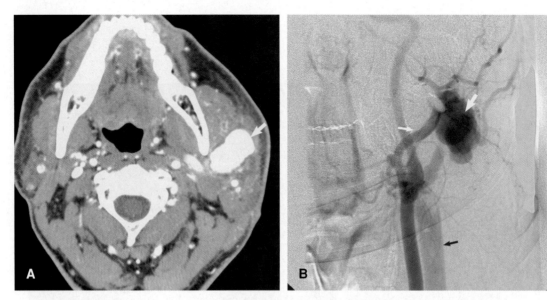

FIGURE 24-35 Traumatic arteriovenous fistula (AVF) from gunshot wound. A: CE CT in a patient with a gunshot wound to the left neck shows a large collection (*white arrow*) that enhances to the same degree as the arteries in the same image, which is consistent with a pseudoaneurysm. **B:** Selective catheter angiogram in the left common carotid artery confirms the presence of a lobulated pseudoaneurysm (*large white arrow*), which is fed by the internal maxillary (*small white arrow*). Early venous return in an enlarged internal jugular vein (*black arrow*) is diagnostic of an AVF.

Retropharyngeal infection that spreads into the carotid space can also cause septic thrombophlebitis in the jugular veins (85). Lemierre syndrome or postanginal septicemia (necrobacillosis) is caused by an acute oropharyngeal infection with secondary septic thrombophlebitis of the internal jugular vein (86). Fusobacterium species, micro-organisms normally present in the oral cavity, are responsible for most cases of this condition.

The infected jugular vein can serve as a source for distant metastatic emboli. In the preantibiotic era, this condition often had a fulminant course with a mortality rate of 90% (87). While oropharyngeal infections are the primary site of infection in most cases, the interval between this infection and the presence of septicemia can be as long as 1 week (86). For this reason, the clinical symptoms related to the oropharyngeal infection are not infrequently cleared at the time the patient develops symptoms related to septicemia. Therefore, this condition can be confused with other conditions, including bacterial endocarditis with septic emboli or poststreptococcal glomerulonephritis (86). However, in Lemierre syndrome (Fig. 24-36), a sore throat is still the most common symptom during the primary infection (88).

The lungs are the most common location of metastatic infection and are involved in approximately 82% to 95% of cases (87,88). The classic radiologic appearance of the pulmonary involvement is similar to that of other septic emboli with multiple peripheral, round, and wedge-shaped opacities that progress rapidly to cavitation. However, cavitation may not be obvious at the time of the initial presentation and is not specific for septic emboli (87). MRI can demonstrate extensive edema in the soft tissues of the neck with associated jugular vein thrombosis. Intense vein enhancement is seen and occasionally, enhancing cavitated lesions secondary to pulmonary septic emboli can be demonstrated.

Upper Extremities

Evaluation of patients with suspected venous pathology in the upper extremities requires not only an accurate depiction of pathology within the veins of the affected extremity but also a comprehensive assessment of the central veins in the chest (subclavian and brachycephalic veins and SVC).

CTV is best performed with indirect technique by using a single bolus of contrast, a section thickness of not greater than 2.0 mm and a delay of approximately 60 seconds after arrival of contrast medium in the aortic arch. Chapter 22 provides further details.

Due to the complex 3D anatomy of the upper extremity and central veins in the chest, TOF and other flow-sensitive techniques are not ideal for the MR evaluation of these vessels. With TOF, multiple acquisitions in different planes are required for complete assessment of these vessels to avoid in-plane saturation effects. For example, the SVC is

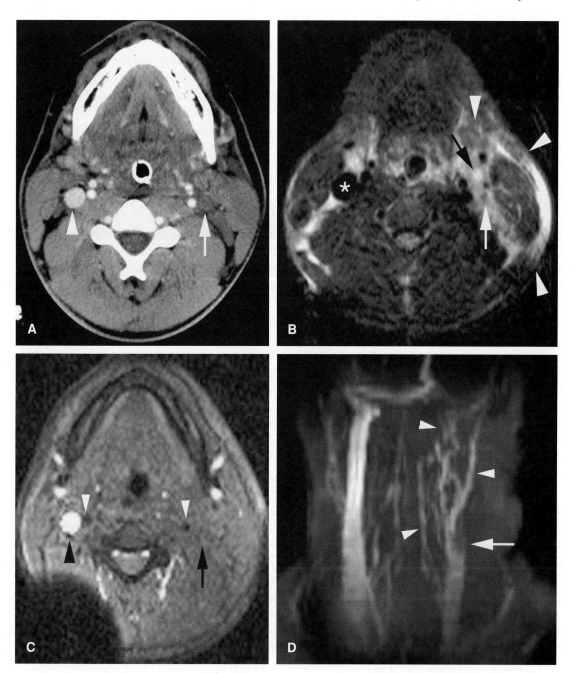

FIGURE 24-36 Lemierre syndrome in an 18-year-old male with sepsis, neck pain, and difficulty breathing 6 days after dental procedure. A: Axial CE CT scan shows no enhancement in the left internal jugular vein (*white arrow*) compared with the normal enhancing right internal jugular vein (*white arrowhead*). Multiple lymph nodes are identified in the left neck. **B:** Axial STIR image in the same patient reveals extensive edema surrounding the left sternocleidomastoid muscle (*white arrowheads*). A flow void is present in the patent right internal jugular vein (∗). Intermediate signal intensity thrombus (*white arrow*) fills the left internal jugular vein. Central increased signal intensity within an adjacent lymph node (*black arrow*) is consistent with necrosis. **C:** Axial TOF with an inferior saturation band shows no flow-related signal within the left internal jugular vein (*black arrow*). Normal flow signal is present in the right internal jugular vein (*black arrowhead*). Note the signal void in the internal carotid arteries (*white arrowheads*) bilaterally due to the use of a superior saturation band. **D:** Coronal MIP reconstruction from the same TOF imaging acquisition as **(C)** better illustrates lack of flow-related signal in the distal left internal jugular vein. A meniscus-shaped filling defect (*white arrow*) in the mid left internal jugular is consistent with thrombus. Multiple collateral vessels (*white arrowheads*) are present.

best imaged on straight axial images, while the brachiocephalic and subclavian veins are best assessed in the sagittal plane. Distally toward the axillary and brachial veins, oblique axial or even straight axial images are needed to acquire the images perpendicular to these vessels. The overall acquisition time for a complete evaluation of the chest and upper extremity veins by using TOF imaging is impractical in clinical practice, and it should be reserved only for those patients in whom gadolinium or iodinated contrast administration is not possible.

A rapid determination of patency in the major veins of the chest can be achieved with sparsely sampled TOF MRI. This is a useful initial evaluation pre-empting a premature termination of the study by the patient or when intravenous access is compromised. In the thorax, the authors acquire three to five TOF slices in a sagittal orientation, which allow for a rapid assessment of brachiocephalic and subclavian vein patency. A saturation band medial to the imaging slice can be used to selectively saturate the inflowing spins within the artery. Similarly, a limited number of slices in the axial plane provided a rapid assessment of the patency of the SVC. This approach does not exclude the presence of nonocclusive thrombus but allows for rapid determination of patency in the major veins of the chest.

A comprehensive evaluation of the entire chest and proximal upper extremities is best accomplished by using a 3D T1-weighted gradient echo sequence in a single breath hold. A properly timed 3D examination during the bolus of gadolinium provides images during the arterial and venous phases. Multiplanar and MIP reconstructions provide accurate delineation of the anatomy and permit interrogation of the veins of interest in different orthogonal planes, facilitating the detection of intraluminal filling defects.

Thrombosis in the upper extremity can be either primary or secondary. Primary thrombosis of the subclavian and/or axillary veins is called *effort thrombosis* or *Paget–von Schrötter syndrome*. However, secondary thrombosis is much more common with the current frequent use of central lines.

Effort thrombosis describes spontaneous thrombosis of the upper extremity after repetitive motion/exercise, usually in the dominant upper extremity (89,90). This entity is most common in young males and is associated with pulmonary embolism in up to 30% of cases (91). There is an anatomic predisposition in 75% of cases including cervical ribs, exostoses, fibrous bands, muscular hypertrophy (anterior scalene/subclavius muscles) (90). MRI allows for the diagnosis of venous thrombosis and

identification of the associated anatomic predisposition (92) (Fig. 24-37).

Thoracic outlet syndrome is a controversial entity in which the symptoms depend on the particular anatomic structure that is compressed in the area of the thoracic outlet (93). The relevant structures include the subclavian artery and vein, brachial plexus, and sympathetic nerves. Occasionally, multiple symptoms may result from compression of a combination of these anatomic structures. Symptoms are most commonly caused by either neurologic or arterial impingement. Pain, numbness and tingling, or heaviness in the effected limb are common complaints. Subclavian artery occlusion, stenosis, and aneurysm formation may occur with or without peripheral emboli (93). Symptoms can develop due to venous compression and/or occlusion, including edema, cyanosis, fatigability, heaviness, and thrombosis (94). Further details, along with the imaging findings, are described in Chapter 22.

Secondary thrombosis of the subclavian vein occurs in 33% to 60% of patients with central catheters and pacemakers and approximately 60% to 70% of patients with upper extremity DVT have central catheters (81,95). Patients with longer catheter dwell time were more likely to develop central vein abnormalities (96). Other causes include trauma, tumors, intravenous drug abuse (IVDA), infection, and hypercoagulable states (97,98). Subclavian vein thrombosis is clinically evident in only 3% of cases. There is associated pulmonary embolism in 36% of cases (99).

Evaluation of the central veins in the chest may be warranted in patients with an edematous upper extremity with a normal Doppler evaluation. Doppler US is still the diagnostic modality of choice to evaluate the subclavian and more distal upper extremity veins, due to its availability and accuracy. However, the sonographic evaluation of the brachiocephalic veins and SVC is not possible with Doppler US. MRI offers excellent visualization of these vessels, and detection of thrombosis of the brachial veins and IVC with MR is comparable to conventional venography (100) (Fig. 24-38).

An evaluation of the upper extremity veins is often warranted in patients with malfunctioning hemodialysis grafts or fistulas and is described in detail in Chapter 22.

Central Vein Access

Patients with end-stage renal disease as well as oncologic/hematologic patients are good candidates for noninvasive vascular imaging of the central veins of the body, especially following multiple failed attempts of central venous catheterization. With increased 3D capabilities and thin-section imaging, effective venous mapping

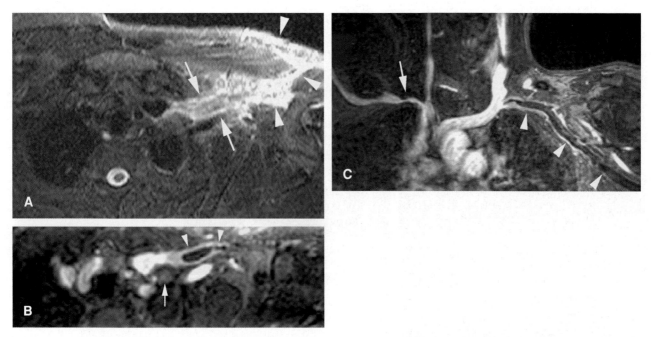

FIGURE 24-37 Paget–von Schrötter syndrome. Effort-induced thrombosis of the subclavian vein (Paget–von Schrötter syndrome) in a 44-year-old left-handed male with left arm swelling and pain. **A:** Axial STIR image shows expansion of the left subclavian vein with high signal intensity thrombus (*white arrows*) in its lumen. Note extensive high signal from edema in the vessel wall and surrounding soft tissues (*white arrowheads*) caused by acute thrombus. **B:** Axial reformatted image from a coronal 3D fat-saturated T1-weighted gradient echo acquisition shows a low signal intensity filling defect in the left subclavian vein (*white arrowheads*), with associated intense enhancement of its wall. The left subclavian artery is seen immediately posterior to the thrombosed left subclavian vein. A hypertrophied left anterior scalene muscle (*white arrow*) is seen causing extrinsic compression upon the left subclavian vein at the transition point between the patent and thrombosed lumen. Hypertrophy of the anterior scalene muscle is one of the anatomic variants that predispose to effort-induced thrombosis. **C:** CE coronal 3D fat-saturated T1-weighted gradient echo image during the venous phase confirms extensive thrombosis of the left subclavian and axillary veins (*white arrowheads*). Intense wall enhancement in these vessels is consistent with acute thrombosis. Note mild narrowing of the right subclavian vein (*white arrow*) with the patient's arm abducted, which illustrates the anatomic predisposition of this patient to develop this condition. (With permission from Pedrosa I, Aschkenasi C, Hamdan A, et al. Effort-induced thrombosis: diagnosis with three-dimensional MR venography. *Emerg Radiol.* 2002;9:326–328.)

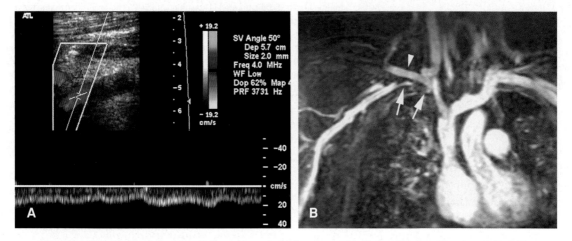

FIGURE 24-38 Right subclavian vein thrombus not visible sonographically in a 23-year-old male with Hodgkin lymphoma and prior catheters in the right upper extremity, now presenting with edema in the right arm. A: Doppler US of the right subclavian vein shows normal wall-to-wall color flow and normal respiratory variability of the waveform on spectral evaluation. Due to its location, not all portions of the subclavian vein are accessible to Doppler US evaluation. The patient went on to receive MRI due to high clinical suspicion for thrombosis. **B:** Coronal MIP reconstruction from a coronal subtracted (delay venous phase minus precontrast) 3D fat-saturated T1-weighted gradient echo acquisition shows lack of enhancement of the distal right subclavian vein (*white arrows*), indicating occlusion. A large venous collateral (*white arrowhead*) is seen, which is consistent with chronic occlusion.

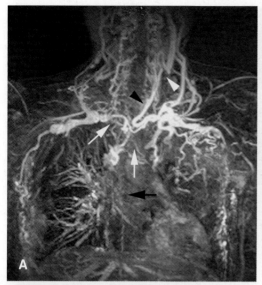

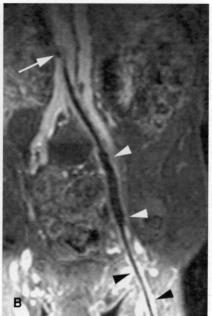

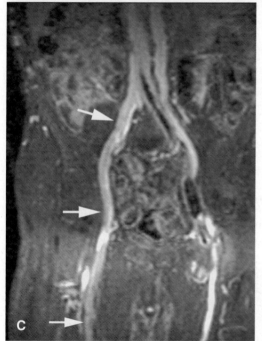

**FIGURE 24-39 Venous road map in a 51-year-old man with chronic renal insuffi-
ciency and multiple previous central venous catheters.** The patient needs venous access
for hemodialysis, although multiple attempts to gain access in the thorax were unsuccessful.
MRI was requested to establish the status of the central venous system. **A:** 3D MIP reconstruction from a coronal subtracted (delay phase minus arterial phase) acquisition in the chest shows
occlusion of the lower left internal jugular vein (*white arrowhead*), which is bypassed via the
external jugular vein (*black arrowhead*). Both right and left brachiocephalic veins (*white
arrows*) are occluded. The right internal jugular vein and both axillary veins are also occluded.
Note extensive collateral vessels over the chest, neck, and back. The SVC (*black arrow*) is not
visualized as it enhanced during the arterial phase, which was used as the mask for this subtraction. Careful review of the source unsubtracted images showed a patent SVC (not shown).
Given the lack of upper extremity access, MR evaluation of the abdomen and pelvis was subsequently performed during the same session, which revealed a patent venous system. Based on
these findings, the decision was made to insert a left femoral catheter. **B:** The patient underwent
MR imaging 4 months later for evaluation of left lower extremity edema. Coronal curved reformation from a 3D fat-saturated T1-weighted gradient echo acquisition during the delayed
venous phase shows the left iliac system with a long tubular filling defect, representing the
patient's existing catheter (*black arrowheads*). Note that the filling defect enlarges in the external iliac vein, representing pericatheter thrombosis (*white arrowheads*). A small, rounded filling
defect at the catheter tip (*white arrow*) likely represents a fibrin cap. **C:** Coronal curved reformation from the same acquisition as **(B)** shows the patent right venous system (*white arrows*)
from the common femoral vein to the IVC.

can be performed prior to patients receiving chemotherapy, hyperalimentation, or hemodialysis (58,101)
(Fig. 24-39). An evaluation of central lines and detection of thrombus along their course or at their tip is
also possible.

The ability for gadolinium-enhanced MRV to provide a road map of the venous system to select a candidate
vein for catheterization was demonstrated by Shinde et al.
(58). In that study, an appropriate vessel could be identified for successful placement of a catheter, indwelling
venous access device, or arteriovenous (AV) hemodialysis
graft in nine patients in whom placement location was

selected based on the information obtained from MR
venograms (58).

Thoracic Collateral Flow

Hyperdense contrast is an expected appearance in the central systemic veins that drain toward the heart. When seen
in other systemic thoracic veins, it indicates diversion of
contrast into collateral routes, driven by higher central pressures caused by obstruction or cardiac abnormalities.
Dilated collaterals often require some time to develop.
Therefore, the obstruction to flow is usually chronic and
not related to the acute narrowing seen when the arm is

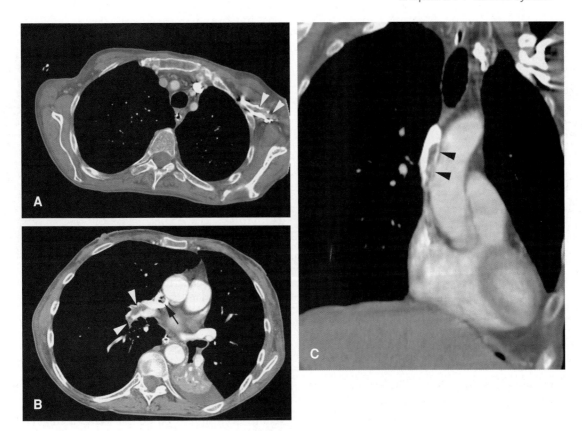

FIGURE 24-40 Left subclavian thrombosis with pulmonary embolus. A: CE CT image at the level of the upper thorax demonstrates left subclavian thrombosis (*white arrowheads*). **B:** Axial CT image at an inferior level shows nonocclusive SVC thrombosis (*black arrow*) with concurrent right pulmonary emboli present (*white arrowheads*). **C:** Coronal reformation better demonstrates the extent of SVC thrombosis (*black arrowheads*).

elevated above the patient's head during the actual CT examination. Significant dilatation of collateral routes does suggest the presence of developing SVC syndrome. In cases of SVC obstruction, collateral pathways from systemic veins may divert blood along the ligamentum teres and into the left portal vein (102). This results in focal enhancement of segment IV (103,104).

Perhaps the most common cause of hyperdense opacification to dilated collateral routes is obstruction to a portion of the central vein. Potential etiologies of obstruction can be grouped into intrinsic and extrinsic venous abnormalities. Intrinsic venous etiologies of stenosis or occlusion include prior indwelling catheter, pacemaker leads, prior trauma, radiation therapy, and thrombosis (hypercoagulable state and effort-induced thrombosis) (Fig. 24-40). The increased use of indwelling catheters has made a relatively significant contribution to the overall incidence of venous stenosis and occlusion (101,105).

Extrinsic compression of the venous system may occur from thoracic outlet syndromes (aberrant scalene muscle insertion, cervical ribs, and healing first rib or clavicular

fractures), fibrosing mediastinitis and neoplasm, especially small cell carcinoma and lymphoma (Fig. 24-41). Occasionally, constrictive pericardial disease may contribute to SVC obstruction. Cardiac etiologies, such as right heart failure, intracardiac masses, or valvular disease, may distend the collaterals and induce IVC reflux of hyperdense contrast but tend not to have well-developed routes, as there is no focal obstruction to bypass.

The opacification of selected thoracic venous routes serves as an indicator of the site of obstruction and the likely direction of venous flow. A general rule of thumb is that the thoracic collateral routes shift inferiorly as the venous obstruction occurs more centrally. The major routes available are divided into the superior venous system, posterior system, and anterolateral system. These routes of diverted blood flow interconnect to form an encompassing thoracic venous loop (106).

The superior venous network involves the anterior jugular venous system, which acts to connect the subclavian, external jugular, and internal jugular veins bilaterally. Often seen with these collaterals are a number of

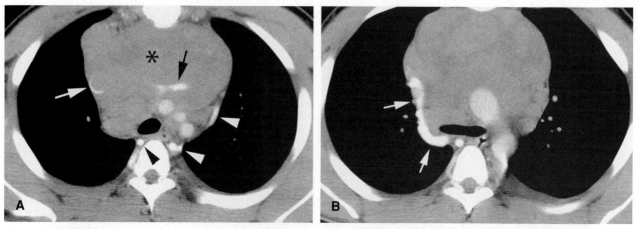

FIGURE 24-41 SVC narrowing secondary to lymphoma. A: CE CT image at the level of the mid thorax demonstrates a large mediastinal mass (∗), which represents lymphoma. The mass severely compresses and invades the suprazygous SVC lumen (*white arrow*) and encases the left brachiocephalic vein (*black arrow*). Collateral flow via the posterior intercostals (*white arrowheads*) into the hemiazygous system is seen. The azygous vein (*black arrowhead*) is also densely opacified with intravenous contrast. **B:** Collateral flow via the posterior intercostals also feeds the azygous vein (*white arrows*), which demonstrates antegrade flow into the infrazygous SVC, bypassing the more proximal obstruction.

parascapular venous network vessels. The venous plexus around the shoulder is likely a more specific indicator of subclavian or brachiocephalic obstruction (107) (Fig. 24-42). The anterior jugular venous system includes the transverse arch between the clavicles and the horizontal vein located behind each clavicle. These will enlarge and demonstrate hyperdense opacification when there is an obstruction to the subclavian or brachiocephalic veins. The

internal jugular veins, which drain the brain, face, and neck regions, are often asymmetric in size. Internal jugular venous occlusion often demonstrates a collateral venous opacification of the superior venous network (Fig. 24-43).

The posterior system predominantly revolves around the azygous and hemiazygous network, which interconnects with the lumbar, paraspinal, and intercostal venous systems. This route of collateral flow can be seen with SVC or distal

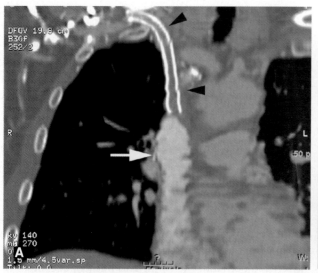
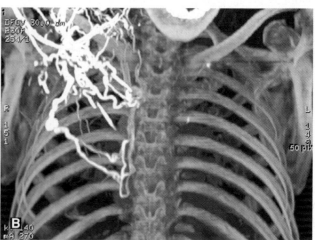

FIGURE 24-42 Thrombosed right brachiocephalic vein stent in a patient with a previously placed stent in the right brachycephalic/subclavian vein, now presenting with right upper extremity edema. A: Coronal reformation from axial CT shows lack of intraluminal enhancement in a right brachiocephalic stent (*black arrowheads*). The SVC (*white arrow*) is widely patent and received the contrast through the azygous vein (not shown). Irregularity along the medial SVC wall is due to cardiac pulsation and should not be mistaken for thrombus. **B:** MIP reconstruction from the same acquisition as in **(A)** better displays the extensive collateral network in the right anterior chest wall and shoulder.

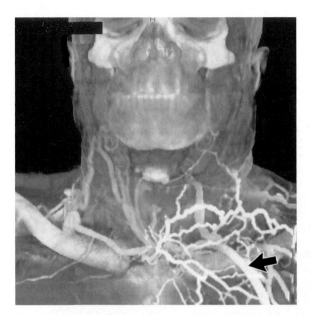

FIGURE 24-43 Anterior neck venous collaterals. Anterior VR CT image shows collateral vessels of the anterior neck and chest wall that developed in a patient with jugular vein thrombosis (not shown). These collateral vessels drain through the external jugular, left subclavian, transthoracic, and intercostal channels to the left brachiocephalic vein. (*Arrow*, central venous catheter.) (With permission from Lawler LP, Corl FM, Fishman EK. Multi-detector row and volume-rendered CT of the normal and accessory flow pathways of the thoracic systemic and pulmonary veins. *Radiographics*. 2002;22[Spec No]:S45–S60.)

brachiocephalic obstruction (106,108). Some opacification can occur in normal individuals if the infusion rate of contrast is high enough. However, a concurrent increase in size of the azygous and hemiazygous diameter should support a collateral route from a central obstruction (107).

The level of the central venous obstruction will determine the direction of flow within the azygous and hemiazygous system. When there is supra-azygous central venous obstruction, the anterograde collateral flow is usually routed within the paraspinal and intercostal veins, which serve as a conduit to the azygous-hemiazygous system. The collateral flow empties into the SVC caudal to the obstruction. This anterograde flow of contrast is confirmed when there is an abrupt transition within the azygous vein between opacified and unopacified blood (Fig. 24-44). When the obstruction is located caudal to the azygous vein (infra-azygous), there is retrograde flow extending to the lumbar, pericardial, and diaphragmatic collateral network. The contrast column is continuous within the azygous and hemiazygous veins, confirming the direction as retrograde (108) (Fig. 24-45). The anterolateral system is represented by interconnections of anterior intercostal, internal mammary, and long thoracic veins. This network serves as a conduit for bypassing SVC obstructions, delivering hyperdense contrast to the IVC via pericardiophrenic, musculophrenic, lumbar, and hepatic veins (Fig. 24-46). Though this system of collaterals is not the preferred route for SVC obstructions, it does usually demonstrate significant opacification when there is concomitant SVC and azygous obstruction (108).

Superior Vena Cava and Brachiocephalic Veins

With the exception of evaluation of pulsed Doppler waveforms for loss of respiratory variability and transmitted cardiac pulsations, sonography is limited in its evaluation of the brachiocephalic veins and SVC. The deep anatomic

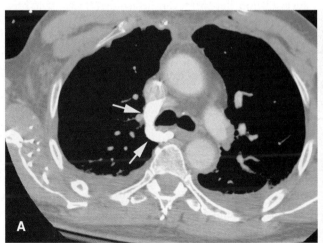
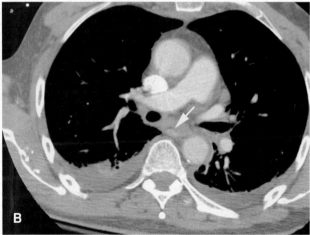

FIGURE 24-44 Antegrade flow within the azygous vein. Two images of a CE thoracic CT examination that demonstrates an abrupt transition between the more cranial contrast-opacified azygous arch (*arrows* in **A**) and the more caudal non-opacified azygous vein (*arrow* in **B**). Intense enhancement of the azygous arch supports forward flow to the infrazygous SVC, bypassing a suprazygous SVC obstruction or brachiocephalic stenosis.

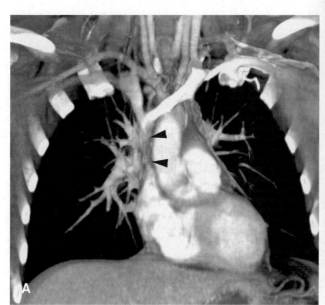
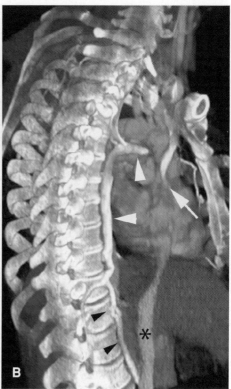

FIGURE 24-45 Retrograde flow within the azygous vein. A: Coronal MIP reconstruction from a CE CT examination shows severe intrinsic stenosis of the infra-azygous SVC (*black arrowheads*). **B:** Sagittal MIP reconstruction from the same examination as that in (**A**) confirms narrowing of the infra-azygous SVC (*white arrow*). A continuous column of contrast within the azygous vein (*white arrowheads*) extends below the diaphragm (*black arrowheads*) and drains into the IVC (∗), which is faintly enhancing. These findings indicate retrograde flow within the azygous vein, which bypasses the infra-azygous SVC narrowing.

location of these structures and the osseous structures of the chest wall (i.e., clavicles, sternum, and ribs) limit the sonographic evaluation of these vascular structures with a transthoracic approach. Due to venous mixing artifact and beam-hardening artifact from dense iodinated contrast flowing through the SVC, CE CT is also limited in SVC assessment. Inflow of unenhanced blood from the contralateral upper extremity and from the jugular veins on CE CT typically causes heterogeneous enhancement with an appearance of filling defects within the SVC and brachiocephalic veins, which is difficult to differentiate from thrombus.

MRV does not have those shortcomings and thus is a good choice for SVC evaluation. Full assessment of the central thoracic venous structures with MR is best performed with multiple complementary sequences. Fast dark blood techniques (i.e., double inversion half-Fourier turbo SE) provide a rapid assessment of these veins in a single breath hold, although differentiation between slow flow and thrombus may not be possible based on the increased intra-

luminal signal intensity. TOF techniques are useful for a rapid screening of patency in these vessels. Three to five thin slices (3-mm thickness) can be acquired in a single breath hold. To maximize the inflow phenomenon, the acquisition is prescribed perpendicular to the vessel of interest—axial for the SVC and sagittal for the brachiocephalic veins.

TOF imaging has been shown accurate in the evaluation of the thoracic veins, with excellent correlation of findings at MR and conventional venography (111). TOF imaging carries with it relatively long examination times and artifact vulnerability, as described previously.

Dynamic gadolinium-enhanced 3D GRE sequences provide a detailed assessment of these vessels in a much shorter time. Direct MRV is feasible by acquiring 3D data sets during the first pass after gadolinium administration. As mentioned earlier, gadolinium contrast is typically diluted to avoid T2* effects and subsequent decreased signal intensity within the injected vein. Bilateral evaluation of the upper extremity veins (brachiocephalic, subclavian, axillary veins) as well as the SVC requires simultaneous

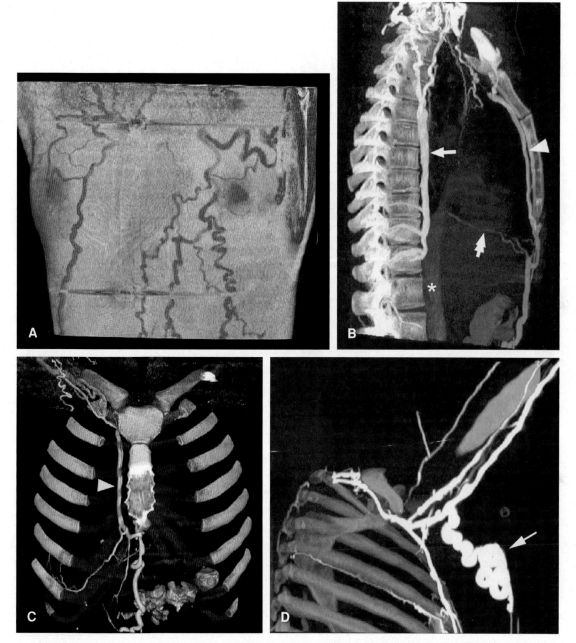

FIGURE 24-46 SVC occlusion on CT in a 26-year-old female with history of facial swelling. A: VR following right-side contrast medium injection demonstrates extensive filling of the subcutaneous venous network of the antero-lateral chest wall due to compromised thoracic venous inflow in this patient with thrombotic occlusion of the brachio-cephalic veins and SVC. **B:** Right lateral thick-slab MIP image shows the collateralization of inflow into the right azy-gous (*arrow*) and internal mammary veins (*arrowhead*). Note the small phrenic veins (*double arrow*), which are fed by the internal mammary vein and drain into the IVC (*). **C:** A VR demonstrates the dilated internal mammary vein (*arrow*) draining into dilated and tortuous inferior epigastric veins. **D:** Sagittal oblique thin-slab MIP image following a left-side injection demonstrates inflow of intravenous contrast material over the left basilic, brachial, and cephalic veins with a major outflow over a dilated and tortuous lateral thoracic vein (*arrow*). A rare collateral pathway involves a systemic-to-pulmonary venous communication via vessels developed in pleural adhesions. This very uncommon pathway can potentially lead to right-to-left shunting in the setting of SVC obstruction. (From Wilson ES. Systemic to pulmonary venous communication in the superior vena caval syndrome. *AJR Am J Roentgenol.* 1976;127:247–249; and Stock-berger SM, West KW, Cohen MD. Right-to-left shunt from systemic venous to pulmonary venous system developing after SVC obstruction. *J Comput Assist Tomogr.* 1995;19:312–315.)

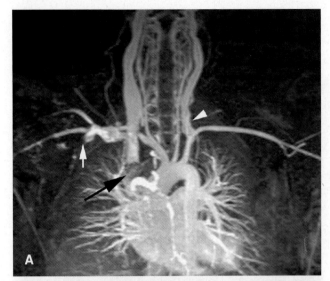

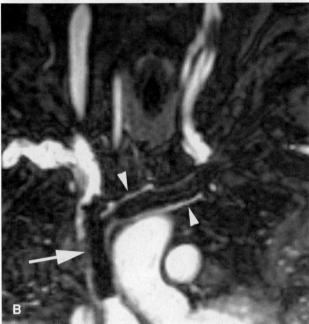

FIGURE 24-47 Acute thrombosis of the SVC and left brachiocephalic vein. A: Coronal MIP reconstruction from a subtracted (venous phase minus precontrast) 3D fat-saturated T1-weighted gradient echo acquisition shows lack of enhancement of the SVC (*black arrow*) and left brachiocephalic vein. The right internal jugular and brachiocephalic veins are patent. The right subclavian is occluded (*white arrow*) in its middle third. The left internal jugular vein is patent (*white arrowhead*). **B:** Coronal oblique reconstruction from the same acquisition as that in **(A)** better demonstrates expansion of the lumen of the SVC (*white arrow*) and left brachiocephalic vein (*arrowheads*) by acute thrombus.

administration of gadolinium through separate intravenous access sites in the right and left upper extremities. Indirect MRV allows for evaluation of the thoracic veins during the equilibrium phase (Fig. 24-47). A sensitivity of 100% has been reported for the detection of venous

thrombosis in the thoracic veins when using gadolinium-enhanced indirect MRV (54,100,112).

SVC syndrome is a clinical diagnosis with symptoms of dyspnea; facial, tongue, neck, or arm swelling; hoarseness; stridor; nasal congestion; headaches; syncope; and lethargy. Symptoms are the result of chronic obstruction of venous outflow from the head and upper extremities due to SVC obstruction below the azygous-SVC confluence. It is most commonly seen as a complication of thoracic malignancy in the Western world, with lung cancer the most common etiology (113,114). Worldwide, SVC syndrome is also commonly caused by histoplasmosis, which causes idiopathic fibrosing mediastinitis (115). The area of SVC narrowing is easily seen on MRV, and often, the cause of the narrowing is also delineated (Fig. 24-48). Other causes include central catheters, pacemakers, mediastinal fibrosis, and aortic aneurysms (Fig. 24-49). Multiple collateral vascular pathways are also usually present and are seen best on 3D reformatted images. The progression of collateral vessels is also a clue suggesting progression of SVC narrowing. Stenosis and/or occlusion of the brachiocephalic veins is a common event in patients with long-standing indwelling catheters (Fig. 24-50).

The patency and caliber of the SVC and its relation to adjacent structures can be evaluated in patients with lymphoma and other anterior or superior mediastinal masses such as thymomas, germ cell neoplasms, goiter or thyroid neoplasms, and mesothelioma. Septic thrombophlebitis of the SVC can be seen as a rare complication of hemorrhagic mediastinitis resulting from inhalational anthrax.

Anomalously coursing venous catheters on x-ray are also well evaluated with CTV and MRV. Positioning within a persistent left or double SVC can be documented. A fibrin plug on the tip of a catheter is often visualized as a rounded or amorphous area of low signal intensity at the catheter tip, which is larger than the catheter tubing. Occasionally, a fibrin sheath around the tip of the catheter can be large enough to compromise the lumen of the SVC and cause symptoms (Fig. 24-51).

Normally with CT studies, the contralateral systemic veins are the last to enhance while imaging the lung apices, even with a contrast delay of up to or greater than 50 seconds. Therefore, on routine multidetector thoracic CT or pulmonary computed tomographic angiography (CTA) exams, prompt opacification of the contralateral systemic veins with the artery should alert the radiologist to the presence of a peripheral AVF. This may be in the arm, the neck, or potentially the head, either iatrogenic or traumatic. When the contralateral subclavian vein demonstrates early temporal enhancement (equal to arterial), then an upper extremity AVF is likely present, usually secondary to a dialysis fistula

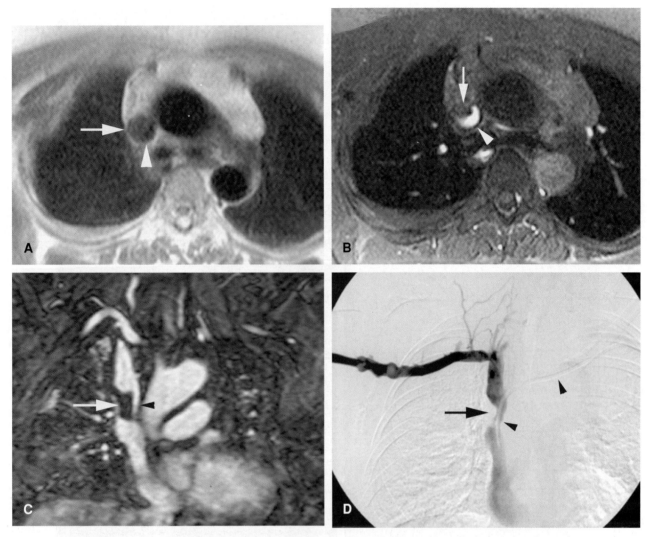

FIGURE 24-48 Partially occlusive SVC thrombus in a 46-year-old woman with breast carcinoma and facial edema. A: Axial dark blood HASTE image shows loss of the normal flow void in right lateral aspect of the SVC, which is filled with intermediate signal intensity material (*white arrow*). An area of lower signal intensity medially (*white arrowhead*) represents a normal flow void, indicating that the thrombus is only partially occlusive. **B:** Axial TOF image obtained with an inferior saturation band at the same level as that in **(A)** confirms the lack of wall-to-wall flow-related signal in the SVC. A crescentic area of high signal (*white arrowhead*) indicates flow around the partially occlusive thrombus (*white arrow*), which appears as a filling defect. **C:** Coronal 3D fat-saturated T1-weighted gradient echo acquisition during the delayed venous phase after administration of gadolinium in the same patient shows a signal void in the SVC (*white arrow*), indicating thrombus that is partially occlusive as enhanced blood flows past the thrombus medially (*black arrowhead*). **D:** Conventional direct venogram image confirms the presence of a nonocclusive thrombus (*black arrow*) in the SVC. Note the ghost artifact from a hemodialysis catheter (*black arrowheads*) in the left subclavian vein extending into the SVC.

(Fig. 24-52). This is a subtle finding but well described in the lower extremities and IVC on abdominal and pelvic CT exams.

Pulmonary Veins

Gadolinium-enhanced MR imaging provides a detailed examination of the pulmonary vasculature and possible collateral pathways in the chest in a single breath hold, without using ionizing radiation or iodinated contrast (116). There is excellent correlation between the MR findings and those at cardiac catheterization, echocardiogram, and intraoperative findings (116). MR provides additional information regarding the anatomy of the pulmonary veins (number and size) and presence of stenosis or aneurysmal dilatation as well as presence of additional vascular anomalies (116).

An increased interest in the assessment of the anatomic configuration and size of the pulmonary veins is the result of new therapies for the treatment of atrial fibrillation

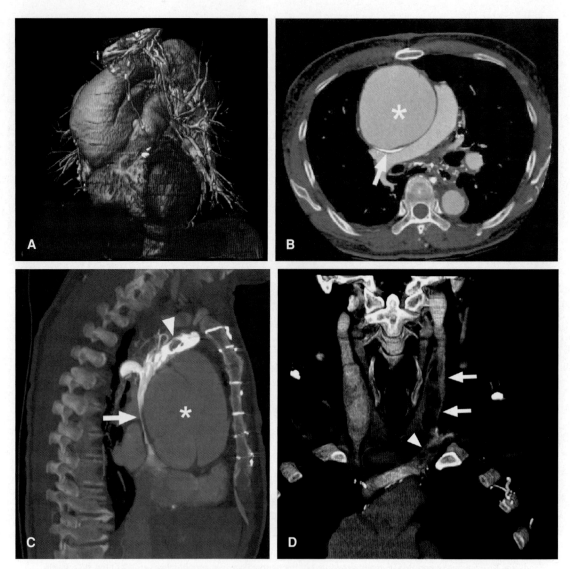

FIGURE 24-49 SVC narrowing from ascending aortic aneurysm in a 50-year-old patient with type A aortic dissection and ascending aortic aneurysm, presenting with progressive facial swelling. VR **(A)** demonstrates a large aneurysm of the ascending aorta. Transverse section **(B)** and right lateral thin-slab MIP **(C)** demonstrates severe compression of the SVC (*arrow*) and the right pulmonary artery by the marked dilatation of the ascending aorta (∗). A filling defect (*arrowheads*) in the left brachiocephalic vein represents thrombus formed in situ due to sluggish venous inflow from the downstream extrinsic obstruction. A VR **(D)** shows the extent of the venous thrombus in the left brachiocephalic vein (*arrowhead*) into the left internal jugular vein (*arrow, thrombus material black*). (Courtesy of Stanford University Cardiovascular Imaging.)

with radio frequency ablation (117). This is discussed in Chapter 16.

Pulmonary venous thrombosis can occur in patients with intrathoracic malignancies, particularly lung cancer (Fig. 24-53), and can affect surgical approach. Thrombus in the pulmonary veins can be the source for systemic embolism, including that in patients with stroke or distal extremity arterial occlusion (118). Thrombosis can also occur following surgery, particularly partial or complete pneumonectomy (Fig. 24-54). Preoperative recognition of

this condition is important because systemic tumor emboli can occur during the resection of the intravenous component of the tumor, which can lead to a life-threatening complication (119). Extension of the tumor thrombus into the left atrium may require a different surgical approach. Pulmonary venous thrombus can be recognized with CT (120), transesophageal echo (121), and positron emission tomography (PET). PET imaging can demonstrate direct extension of the tumor into the left atrium and confirm the tumoral nature of the thrombus (122).

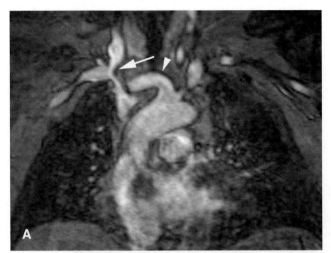

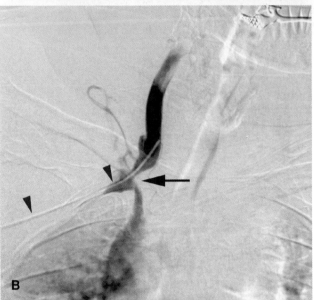

FIGURE 24-50 Narrowed brachicephalic vein from prior indwelling venous catheters in a 53-year-old male with right upper extremity and facial edema as well as end-stage renal disease, renal transplant, and multiple prior central venous catheterizations. A: Coronal 3D fat-saturated T1-weighted gradient echo acquisition demonstrates narrowing at the confluence of the right brachicephalic and internal jugular veins (*white arrow*). The right subclavian artery is denoted by the *white arrowhead*. **B:** Conventional direct venogram of the chest after positioning of the catheter (*arrowheads*) in the right internal jugular vein through the subclavian vein confirms the presence of a focal narrowing (*arrow*) at the confluence of the right internal jugular, subclavian, and brachicephalic veins.

Three-dimensional gadolinium-enhanced MRI provides excellent evaluation of the pulmonary veins in patients with lung cancer (123).

Primary neoplasms of the pulmonary veins are rare. Most primary tumors are sarcomas, although those originating in the pulmonary arteries are much more common than those with origin in the pulmonary veins

(124). Pulmonary vein leiomyosarcoma is the most common primary neoplasm originating in the pulmonary vein. Pulmonary vein leiomyosarcomas are more common in women and often extend into the left atrium at the time of diagnosis (125). Prognosis is poor, although complete surgical excision can provide long-term survival (125).

Inferior Vena Cava

While the exact number of patients who develop IVC thrombosis is unknown because of the variations in clinical presentation, approximately 4% to 15% of cases with lower extremity deep venous thrombosis may have cranial extension of the thrombus into the IVC (126). With an estimated 165,000 to 493,000 cases of DVT per year in the United States based on population-based studies, an extrapolated 6,600 to 74,000 cases of IVC thrombosis are expected (126). In addition, IVC thrombosis occurs in patients with certain intra-abdominal malignancies, particularly RCC (127). CT and MR play an important role not only in the diagnosis of IVC thrombosis but also in determining its extension. Medical and surgical management is frequently decided based on this information.

CT imaging at the late arterial phase is helpful in the detection of neovascularity and tumoral enhancement. The IVC is subject to flow artifacts that can make detection of thrombus difficult. Scanning at more delayed phases can reduce the artifact. However, enhancement can also be diminished. In the lower extremities, as discussed later, Szapiro et al. found that peak enhancement ranged from 93 H.U. to 137 H.U. and occurred from 93 to 147 seconds following injection, depending on the vein. However, qualitative assessment favored scanning at 210 seconds because opacification was more homogeneous (128). Presumably, this pattern holds for the IVC.

MR imaging offers an evaluation of the IVC with noncontrast (i.e., black blood sequences, bright blood sequences) and gadolinium-enhanced approaches. Similar to other anatomic locations, gadolinium-enhanced MRI provides a faster evaluation because assessment of a large anatomic area, including IVC and iliac veins, is frequently needed.

Dark blood imaging of the entire abdomen and pelvis in two separate breath holds is feasible with HASTE. Cardiac gating is used, either by applying cardiac leads to the chest wall or a peripheral detector of the pulse pressure wave. This ensures homogeneous intraluminal dark signal in the patent veins. IVC thrombus is readily seen as intraluminal filling defects with heterogeneous intermediate-to-high signal intensity. Bright blood images acquired

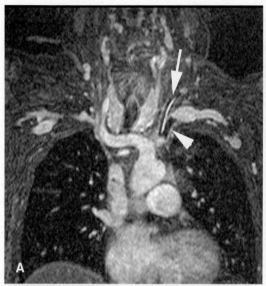

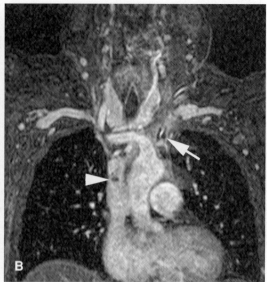

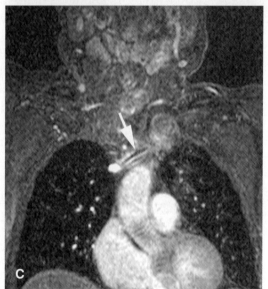

FIGURE 24-51 Malfunctioning port secondary to a fibrin sheath. A: Coronal subtracted (delayed postcontrast minus precontrast) image of the chest in a patient with a malfunctioning chemotherapy port shows a nonenhancing intraluminal filling defect (*arrowhead*) attached to the catheter (*arrow*) as it enters in the left subclavian/brachio-cephalic vein. **B:** Coronal subtracted image from same acquisition as that in **(A)** at a slightly more anterior location shows inferior extension of the nonenhancing filling defect (*arrow*), which surrounds the catheter. A roundlike-appearing filling defect (*arrowhead*) is noted distally surrounding the very tip of the catheter, which was located in the upper SVC. **C:** Coronal subtracted image from the same acquisition at a slightly more anterior location than that in **(B)** shows circumferential low signal filling defect surrounding the catheter (*white arrow*) as it courses through the brachio-cephalic vein. These findings are consistent with a fibrin sheath.

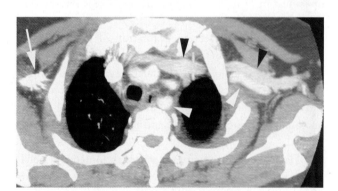

FIGURE 24-52 Early subclavian vein opacification by arteriovenous fistula. CT image at the level of the upper chest obtained 20 seconds after administration of a bolus of contrast through a right antecubital vein shows early opacification of the left subclavian vein (*black arrowheads*), which is similar in density to the subclavian artery (*white arrowheads*). Dense right-sided contrast (*white arrow*) is being injected. This is diagnostic for a left arm arterial-venous direct connection, which in this case was a dialysis fistula.

with TOF sequences offer an excellent evaluation of the IVC and iliac veins at the expense of long acquisition times. Turbulent flow, however, can cause foci of decreased signal that can simulate thrombi. Cardiac gating and decreased slice thickness (3 to 4 mm) can partially reduce this problem.

A coronal acquisition using a 3D fat-saturated T1-weighted spoiled gradient echo sequence allows for imaging of the venous anatomy in the abdomen and pelvis, including the entire IVC from the diaphragm to the level of the external iliac veins. A double dose of gadolinium administered with a biphasic injection produces excellent signal in the veins during the delayed acquisitions (approximately 2 minutes after injection). A venous-only data set is generated by subtraction technique (venous-arterial), as discussed previously.

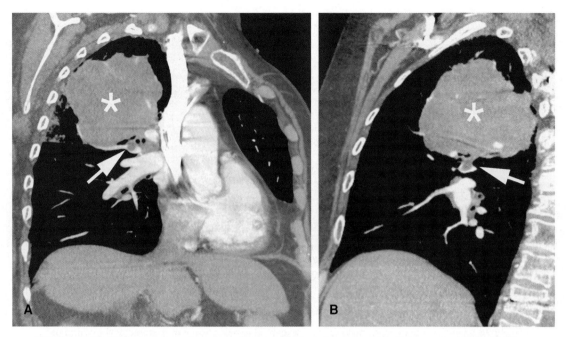

FIGURE 24-53 Right superior pulmonary vein thrombus from lung cancer. A: Oblique coronal thick-slab MIP image of the chest showing a large right upper lobe lung mass (∗). There is a filling defect in the right upper pulmonary vein (*white arrow*), indicating thrombus. **B:** Sagittal multiplanar reformatted image redemonstrating the large right upper lobe mass (∗). The filling defect in the right superior pulmonary vein (*white arrow*) is contiguous with the mass and appears to be the same density, which is higher than expected for bland thrombus. The constellation of findings likely indicates tumor thrombus.

The IVC can be divided into the suprahepatic, intra/infrahepatic, and infrarenal segments. The suprahepatic segment is a short segment that extends from the right atrium to the hepatic veins. The intra/infrahepatic IVC extends from the hepatic veins to the renal veins. The segment that extends from the renal veins to iliac bifurcation can be characterized as infrarenal IVC. While this classification does not correspond to anatomic differences in the IVC per se, it has some clinical implications, as thrombosis of the IVC in these different anatomic locations typically relates to different causes.

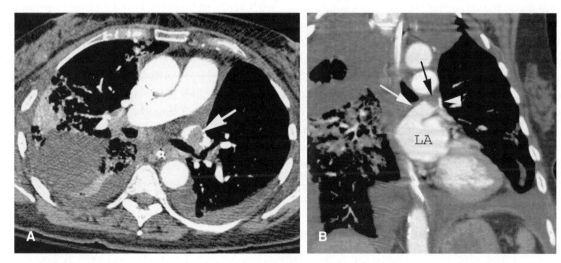

FIGURE 24-54 Left superior pulmonary vein thrombosis following partial pneumonectomy in a 56-year-old male 3 days after left upper lobectomy for lung carcinoma. A: Axial CE CT image through the left superior pulmonary vein demonstrates a centrally located filling defect (*white arrow*), representing thrombus. The right-sided pleural effusion and pulmonary consolidation is due to pneumonia. **B:** Oblique coronal reformation from the same acquisition as that in **(A)** better demonstrates location of the thrombus (*black arrow*) in the left upper pulmonary vein (*white arrow*) next to the surgical clip (*white arrowhead*). (LA, left atrium.)

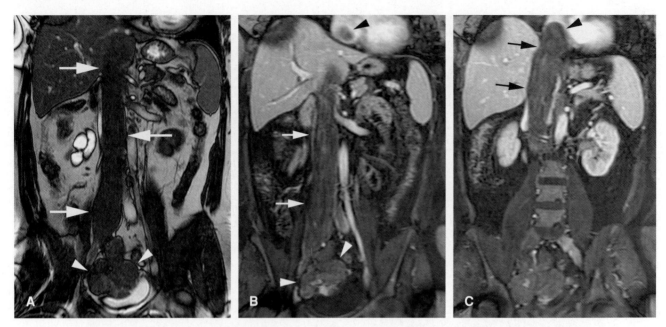

FIGURE 24-55 Intravenous leiomyomatosis in a 44-year-old female with prior hysterectomy for fibroids and prior episode of cardiac arrest secondary to pulmonary embolism. Patient has a known thrombus in the IVC, which was refractory to anticoagulation therapy. **A:** Coronal FISP image showing expansion of the IVC (*white arrows*), which demonstrates uniformly low signal intensity instead of the normal high signal intensity demonstrated by vascular structures. The low signal intensity indicates thrombus within the IVC. Although the uterus had been removed, multiple round low signal intensity pelvic masses are present, which have the similar signal intensity to that of the IVC thrombus (*white arrowheads*). **B:** Coronal fat-saturated 3D T1-weighted spoiled gradient echo (SPGR) image acquired during the delayed venous phase through the same level as that in **(A)** shows vague areas of increased signal intensity (*white arrows*) within the IVC thrombus, which were not seen on the precontrast acquisition (not shown) and therefore indicate enhancement. Similarly, a low-level enhancement is noted in the fibroids (*white arrowheads*). The thrombus in the IVC was contiguous with the enhancing fibroids via the internal iliac veins. Note the filling defect in the right atrium (*black arrowhead*). **C:** Coronal fat-saturated 3D T1-weighted SPGR image from the same acquisition as that in **(C)** at a slightly more posterior location better shows the tumor thrombus expanding the intrahepatic IVC (*black arrows*) and extending into the right atrium (*black arrowhead*). The subtle areas of increased signal intensity were not seen on the precontrast images (not shown) and therefore represent enhancement. Enhancement within thrombus is diagnostic of tumor thrombus, and this constellation of findings indicates intravenous leiomyomatosis.

Thrombosis of the infrarenal IVC is most commonly caused by extension of pelvic deep venous thrombosis but can also be due to extrinsic compression, hypercoagulable state, pregnancy, congenital anomalies (such as webs or interruption), neoplasms, cranial extension of right gonadal vein thrombosis, trauma/hematoma, or vascular stasis. Pelvic neoplasms can grow into the IVC through extensive venous collaterals or directly along the right gonadal vein. The latter is more common with ovarian neoplasms and intravenous uterine leiomyomatosis (Fig. 24-55). Occasionally, tumor thrombus in the renal vein in patients with RCC can extend inferiorly into the infrarenal IVC. The IVC is involved in 4% to 15% of patients with RCC (129). More commonly, patients with IVC extension of renal vein tumor thrombus have bland thrombus in the infrarenal IVC caused by the venous stasis secondary to the obstruction. Frequently, patients may present with symptoms secondary to lower extremity DVT, and the renal tumor is discovered during the imaging workup. Similarly, patients may present

with acute pulmonary embolism after embolization of fragments of the IVC thrombus into the pulmonary circulation.

Thrombosis of the infra- and intrahepatic segments of the IVC can be caused by cranial extension of infrarenal IVC thrombosis. This IVC segment is the most commonly involved by tumor thrombus extending from the renal veins. While RCC is most frequently the neoplasm that causes infrahepatic IVC thrombosis, other renal tumors (i.e., angiomyolipoma, transitional and squamous cell carcinoma) (130,131), and primary retroperitoneal tumors (e.g., retroperitoneal sarcomas, adrenal cortical carcinoma) may rarely extend into the IVC. Other causes include trauma, extrinsic compression (i.e., hepatic neoplasms, retroperitoneal masses and lymphadenopathy, aortic aneurysm), iatrogenic (i.e., surgery, insertion of central venous catheters, IVC filters), and hypercoagulable states (Fig. 24-56).

IVC thrombosis is present in 4% to 15% of patients with RCC (129). The reported accuracy in the detection of

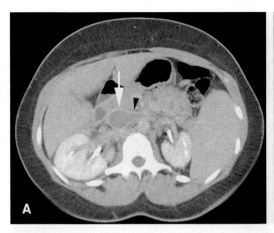 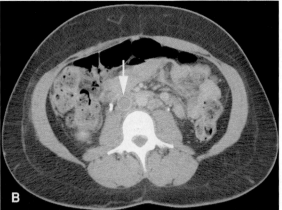

FIGURE 24-56 Spontaneous IVC thrombosis from essential thrombocytopenia in a 37-year-old female with no previous medical history and progressive bilateral lower extremity edema. There is extensive occlusive thrombus within the IVC (*arrow*) extending into the left renal vein (*arrowhead*). The thrombus further extends into the iliac veins (not shown). The patient was diagnosed shortly afterward with essential thrombocytopenia.

tumor extension within the renal vein and IVC for MR is superior to that of CT, although this is based on data prior to the multidetector era (132). Extension of tumor thrombus into the IVC is not a contraindication for surgical resection of the primary renal tumor. Patients with RCC and venous thrombus extending into the IVC without metastatic disease elsewhere have survival rates as high as 68% at 5 years after resection of the renal neoplasm (129).

Thrombosis of the suprahepatic IVC can be due to any of the above entities, along with cardiac causes (atrial myxoma or thrombosis). Distinction between congenital and chronic traumatic occlusion of the suprahepatic IVC may not be possible (Fig. 24-57). Primary hepatocellular carcinoma can grow along the hepatic veins into the suprahepatic IVC and right atrium (Fig. 24-58). Prognosis in these circumstances is poor, and patients usually undergo chemotherapy (133). Improvement in functional status and lower extremity edema has been reported in patients with IVC thrombosis and intracardiac extension of hepatocellular carcinoma after endovascular SVC-to-IVC transatrial stent placement, with and without percutaneous portocaval shunt (134). However, partial hepatectomy with segmental resection of the inferior vena cava has been reported in selected cases (135). Presurgical diagnosis of tumor thrombus extension into the right atrium in patients with renal cell and hepatocellular carcinoma is mandatory, as cardiopulmonary bypass is typically needed during the surgical resection (129,136,137).

Flattening of the IVC may be an indicator of hypovolemia in a trauma patient. Jeffrey and Federle (138)

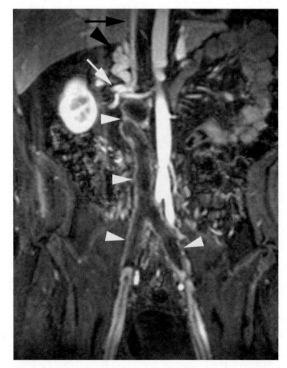

FIGURE 24-57 IVC thrombosis due to post-traumatic narrowing. Coronal curved reconstruction from a coronal 3D fat-saturated T1-weighted gradient echo acquisition during the portal venous phase in a patient with bilateral lower extremity edema shows extensive thrombus filling the infrarenal IVC and extending into both common iliac veins (*white arrowheads*). The right renal vein (*white arrow*) empties into a markedly narrowed suprarenal IVC (*black arrow*). Retroperitoneal collaterals (*black arrowhead*) are noted adjacent to the suprarenal IVC. The patient had a history of remote trauma due to a motor vehicle accident during which there may have been injury to the IVC, thus explaining the imaging findings. Expansion by thrombus of the infrarenal IVC and iliac veins is consistent with acute thrombosis.

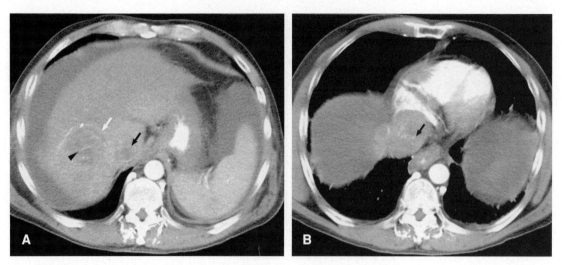

FIGURE 24-58 IVC tumor thrombus from HCC. A: Axial CE CT image in a patient with HCC shows a round area of heterogeneous enhancement (*white arrow*) in the right lobe of the liver, which contains arterial neovascularity (*black arrowhead*). Heterogeneous hypoenhancement in the IVC is suggestive of tumor thrombus (*black arrow*). **B:** Axial image slightly superior to **(A)** confirms invasion of the IVC by the tumor, with extension into the right atrium. Note the arterial neovascularization of the tumor mass (*black arrow*).

described an IVC flattened on at least three contiguous 1-cm slices as a sign of impending cardiovascular collapse in trauma patients. Mirvis et al. (139) studied 13 trauma patients who had been hypotensive in the field or on admission with diffuse small bowel abnormalities (shock bowel). Ten of these patients were found to have a flattened cava (an anteroposterior diameter at the level of the renal veins of 9 mm or less).

The significance of a flattened cava in patients without trauma is uncertain. A retrospective study of 500 nearly consecutive abdominal CT scans in patients without a history of trauma found a flattened cava in 70 (14%). (A flattened cava was defined to have a ratio of maximal transverse diameter to maximal anteroposterior diameter of at least 3:1 at one or more of four predefined levels.) Of those 70 patients, 21 had definite evidence of hypovolemia or hypotension, and three had possible evidence of hypovolemia or hypotension. This left 46 (66%) of patients with no evidence of hypovolemia or hypotension (140).

CT can demonstrate contained rupture of the IVC. Signs include retroperitoneal hematoma surrounding the IVC, irregular vessel contour, and extravasation (141). Injury of the retrohepatic IVC is associated with a poor outcome (142). The surrounding liver can tamponade bleeding, and the patient may, therefore, be hemodynamically stable. Before repairing a retrohepatic caval injury, the surgeon may opt for preoperative caval balloon tamponade to reduce the risk of exsanguination.

Fat can herniate into the caval lumen through a mural laceration (143). Fat can also be seen in the cava, following embolization from a major bone fracture. Occasionally, a fat collection can appear to be within the lumen of the IVC because of a partial volume artifact at the level of the diaphragm (Fig. 24-59). Multiplanar reformations can be helpful in evaluating this finding (144).

Aneurysms of the IVC have been rarely described, with approximately 16 cases reported in the literature. The cause is unknown, although there may be a relation to anomalous connections in the embryologic venous system. IVC aneurysms may be associated with other congenital anomalies. Acquired aneurysms after trauma have also been described. Saccular aneurysms are more common, while the fusiform type has also been described. Thrombosis, pain, rupture, and lower extremity swelling may be present. There is an increased risk for pulmonary embolism in the presence of thrombus. Contrast layering in the dependent portion of the IVC, the so called *layered contrast sign*, on MRA has been reported. Surgical intervention is recommended due to a high incidence of symptoms in isolated aneurysm of the infrarenal IVC (Fig. 24-60) and in those cases with associated agenesis of the IVC above or below the hepatic veins (145).

Hepatic Veins

The hepatic venous outflow occurs through the right, middle, and left hepatic veins in most individuals. At autopsy, a single right, median, and the left hepatic veins are found in 98.3%, 88.3%, and 76.3% of the cases, respectively (146).

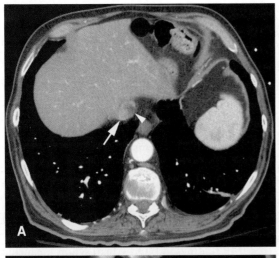

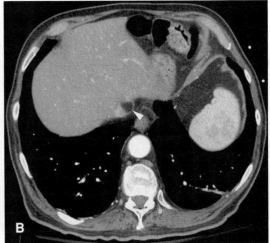

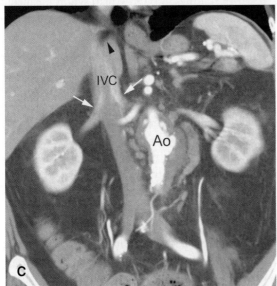

FIGURE 24-59 IVC pseudothrombus in a 62-year-old man with a mycotic abdominal aortic aneurysm being evaluated with CTA. A: Axial CE CT image obtained during the arterial phase at the level of the right hemidiaphragm shows an irregularly shaped low density filling defect (*white arrowhead*) within the IVC (*white arrow*). **B:** Axial CE CT image from same acquisition as that in (**A**) at a slightly more inferior location better demonstrates the fat attenuation of the filling defect (*white arrowhead*) within the IVC and the continuation of the filling defect with the intra-abdominal fat. This confirms that the filling defect in (**A**) represents partial volume effect from intra-abdominal fat. **C:** Coronal reformatted image from the same acquisition as that in (**A**) better demonstrates the extension of intra-abdominal fat (*black arrowhead*) next to the IVC at the level of the diaphragm, which simulates an intraluminal filling defect in the IVC. The infrahepatic IVC is partially opacified by dense contrast from the renal veins (*white arrows*). Note the irregular mycotic aortic aneurysm (*Ao*).

Accessory hepatic veins for the segments V and VIII of the liver occur in 43% and 49%, respectively (146). The incidence of short hepatic veins in segments 6 and 7 is 38% (146). Identification of accessory or replaced hepatic veins is critical when planning a hepatectomy for split transplantation from living liver donors (146). MDCT and gadolinium-enhanced MR images provide excellent evaluation of the hepatic venous anatomy for this purpose (33). CT is particularly helpful in the evaluation of patients with hepatic trauma. The presence of a major hepatic venous injury in the setting of liver trauma correlates with an increased risk for delay bleeding (147) (Fig. 24-61).

Enlargement of the hepatic veins is common in patients with elevated right heart filling pressures. In patients with right-sided heart failure, intravenously administered contrast media may reflux into the azygous and hemiazygous system and into the hepatic veins (Fig. 24-62).

Retrograde opacification of the IVC or hepatic veins on CT is a specific but insensitive sign of increased right-sided heart pressures (148). However, while this finding is useful when low injection rates are used (= or <3 mL/second), its reliability decreases with the use of high injection rates (>3 mL/second) (148).

Obstruction of hepatic venous outflow or Budd-Chiari syndrome may occur secondary to the obstruction of the hepatic veins or the IVC. Idiopathic, congenital (webs or interruption of the IVC), IVC and/or hepatic vein thrombosis due to hypercoagulable states, tumors, inflammatory and autoimmune diseases (Behçet disease, phlebitis, etc.), trauma, and veno-occlusive disease after liver transplant are among the different causes of this condition.

In acute stages, the liver on CT is enlarged and diffusely hypodense. These findings are attributed to hepatic congestion (149). Thrombosis of the hepatic veins may be

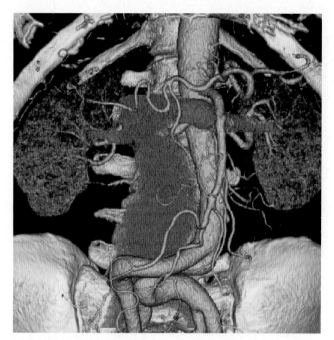

FIGURE 24-60 IVC aneurysm. Coronal VR reconstructions showing aneurysmal dilatation of the infrarenal IVC (*blue*). The suprarenal IVC was widely patent upon review of the source images (not shown). Note the marked tortuosity of the iliac arteries (*yellow*).

directly visualized as a hypodense clot surrounded by an enhancing vessel wall. Normal or increased enhancement of the caudate lobe is seen, as it has a separate drainage to the IVC. Subcapsular enhancement may also be noted, as these areas are drained by capsular veins (150). Patchy,

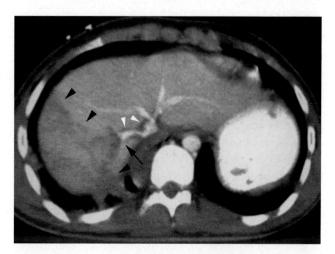

FIGURE 24-61 Traumatic hepatic venous injury. Axial CE CT image at the level of the upper abdomen in a patient after a motor vehicle accident shows heterogeneous enhancement of the posterior right lobe of the liver (*black arrowheads*), which is consistent with a hepatic contusion. The hepatic contusion extended inferiorly along the entire right lobe, and frank laceration was present in the inferior aspect of the liver (not shown). Note an abrupt cut-off (*black arrow*) in the right hepatic vein, representing a traumatic injury of this vessel. Low-attenuation (*white arrowheads*) tracking along the right hepatic vein and surrounding the intrahepatic IVC represents blood.

heterogeneous enhancement is noted in the rest of the liver, as would be expected with diminished perfusion.

In chronic stages, the hepatic veins may not be visualized. Intrahepatic venous collateral pathways may be present. The caudate lobe and left lobe may be enlarged, while the rest of the liver atrophies. The liver contour is irregular, and regenerating nodules may enhance during the arterial phase, potentially leading to an erroneous diagnosis of hepatocellular carcinoma (HCC). Unlike HCC, though, regenerating nodules in Budd-Chiari syndrome are small (0.5 cm to 4.0 cm), multiple, and homogeneous (151). Extrahepatic findings are due to secondary portal hypertension (HTN) and include ascites, splenomegaly, and varices.

MR findings in Budd-Chiari syndrome include hepatic vein thrombosis, hepatic vein occlusion and narrowing, and IVC thrombosis or narrowing (152). Patency of the central hepatic veins does not exclude Budd-Chiari syndrome. Obstruction at the level of the small- or intermediate-sized veins may occur with normal central hepatic veins (152–154). Intrahepatic collaterals are typically seen as "comma-shaped" enhancing vessels (152,155).

The caudate lobe of the liver is typically preserved in this condition as it drains, separately from the rest of the liver, directly into the IVC and not through the hepatic veins. Peripheral areas of heterogeneous high signal intensity on T2-weighted images and decreased signal intensity on T1-weighted images with normal signal intensity in the caudate lobe has been described in the acute presentation of the Budd-Chiari syndrome (156). At pathology, this finding correlates with hepatic ischemia, congestion, and hemorrhage (156). Ascites is common due to acute liver failure. The caudate lobe demonstrates increased enhancement during the arterial phase on dynamic postgadolinium images and persists during the delayed venous phase (156) (Fig. 24-63).

With time, peripheral atrophy of the liver may occur with either greater or lesser enhancement than the normal liver on dynamic gadolinium-enhanced images. This occurs as a result of the combination of decreased portal perfusion and dilatation of hepatic sinusoids (152). The caudate lobe, preserved due to its independent venous drainage, hypertrophies to compensate for the atrophy in the rest of the liver. In chronic stages of Budd-Chiari syndrome, maintained parenchymal ischemia can lead to nodular regenerative hyperplasia. Regenerative nodules in patients with chronic Budd-Chiari syndrome are typically multiple (>10), small (<4 cm in diameter), and display homogeneous high signal intensity on T1- and T2-weighted images (157). Decreased signal intensity on T2-weighted images has also been described in these nodules (152,158). There is

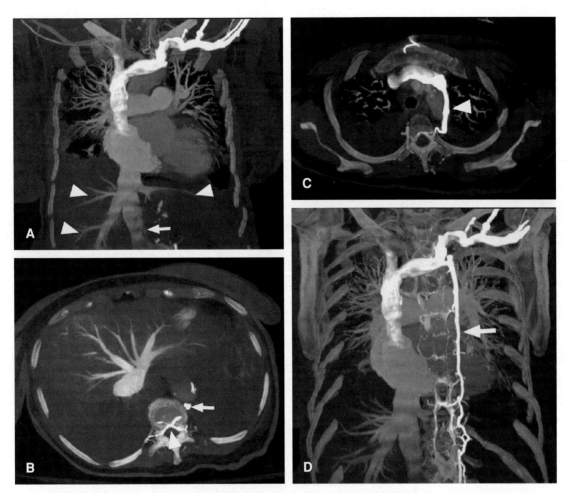

FIGURE 24-62 Hepatic venous reflux in a 74-year-old-female referred for probable pulmonary embolism demonstrates sequelae of elevated right heart filling pressures. Coronal slab MIP **(A)** demonstrates undiluted contrast material inflow in the left subclavian vein, the left brachiocephalic vein, and SVC. Note the transit of contrast material through the right atrium into the intrahepatic segment of the IVC (*white arrow*) as well as hepatic veins (*white arrowheads*). Once the contrast material enters the right atrium, it is diluted by unopacified blood and is thus less attenuative. Axial thin-slab MIP **(B)** demonstrates filling of all three hepatic veins, indicating relatively high right ventricular filling pressures that overcome the higher hydrostatic pressures required to fill the anteriorly located left and middle hepatic venous branches in this supine patient. Note the intense opacification of the hemiazygous vein (*white arrow*) and transvertebral veins (*white arrowhead*). Elevated right atrial pressures result in backflow of contrast material into the azygous arch (not shown) and into the left superior intercostal vein (*white arrowhead* in **C**), which drains into the hemiazygous system (*white arrow* in **D**). The greater degree of opacification present in these veins indicates that the contrast material has not been diluted by unopacified blood and thus has not entered the heart, indicating retrograde flow in the hemiazygous vein. The lesser degree of opacification in the azygous arch indicates admixture with unopacified blood entering from right intercostal veins. (Courtesy of Stanford University Cardiovascular Imaging.)

increased incidence of HCC in chronic Budd-Chiari, with reported incidence of 6% (159).

Veno-occlusive disease (VOD) is a variant of hepatic venous outflow obstruction that typically affects patients undergoing bone marrow transplantation. A nonthrombotic occlusion of the terminal hepatic venules and small sublobular veins results from fibrous obliteration of these vessels in 5% of patients after bone marrow transplantation (152). This condition typically occurs within 3 weeks of marrow infusion (152). Imaging studies are frequently used to exclude other causes for

acute liver failure, as the imaging findings in VOD are not specific. MR imaging may be used when differentiation between extremely slow flow and thrombus is not possible on US. Other findings hepatomegaly with compression of the hepatic veins, ascitis, and gallbladder wall edema are not specific (152).

Preoperative imaging is used to evaluate the vascular architecture in living transplant donors and recipients and in patients with liver neoplasms who are candidates for resection. In a study of 107 donor and recipient candidates, at least one surgically important vascular variant was seen in 70

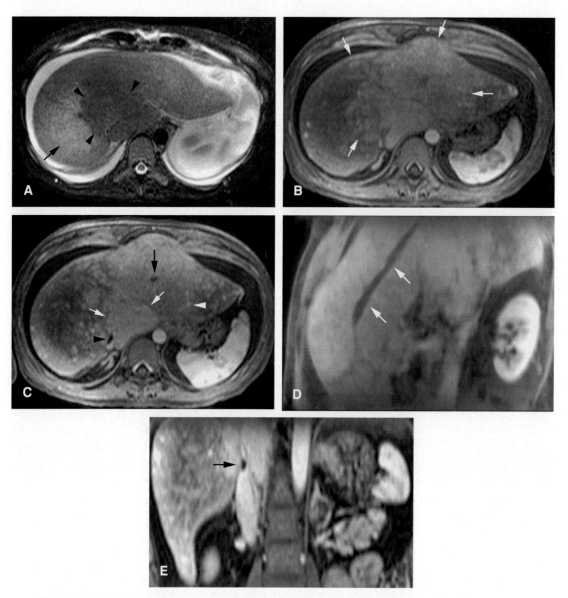

FIGURE 24-63 Budd-Chiari syndrome in a 26-year-old woman with right upper quadrant pain. US showed ascites and multiple hypoechoic lesions within the liver. **A:** Axial STIR image shows heterogeneous high signal intensity throughout the liver, particularly within the right lobe (*black arrow*). Note enlargement of the caudate lobe, which is typical of Budd-Chiari syndrome (*black arrowheads*). **B:** Axial CE 3D fat-saturated GRE (VIBE) image during the portal venous phase shows markedly decreased enhancement of the liver, with areas of heterogeneous patchy enhancement (*white arrows*). **C:** Axial CE 3D fat-saturated GRE (VIBE) image obtained during the equilibrium phase confirms the thrombosis of the left hepatic vein (*black arrow*). A filling defect is visualized within the IVC (*black arrowhead*), consistent with intraluminal thrombus. Note the normal enhancement of caudate lobe (*white arrows*) related to its independent venous drainage. Also note the curvilinear, comma-shaped areas of high signal intensity (*white arrowhead*), indicating intrahepatic collaterals. **D:** Sagittal reconstruction of the CE VIBE acquisition during the equilibrium phase better demonstrates thrombosis of the left hepatic vein (*white arrows*). **E:** Coronal reconstruction of the CE VIBE acquisition during the equilibrium phase demonstrates marked narrowing of the intrahepatic segment of the IVC with intraluminal thrombus (*black arrow*). (Adapted with permission from Morrin MM, Pedrosa I, Rofsky NM. Magnetic resonance imaging for disorders of liver vasculature. *Top Magn Reson Imaging.* 2002;13:177–190.)

patients (65%) (160). Of the total of 129 variants, 52 (40%) involved hepatic veins, and 26 (20%) involved portal veins. In a study of 42 patients with hepatic neoplasms who were candidates for resection, 11 (26%) had hepatic vein anomalies, and 7 (17%) had portal vein anomalies (161).

The most common hepatic vein anomaly is an accessory inferior right hepatic vein (Fig. 24-64). This anomaly is more important in donors than in recipients. If the cross-sectional diameter is greater than 5 mm, the accessory inferior right hepatic vein must be reanastomosed to

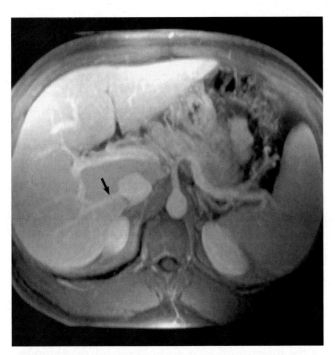

FIGURE 24-64 Accessory right hepatic vein. MIP of an axial 3D fat-saturated T1-weighted gradient echo acquisition during the delayed venous phase after administration of gadolinium demonstrates an inferior accessory hepatic vein (*black arrow*) that is draining segment VI.

the recipient's cava to avert graft congestion due to inadequate drainage. The branch draining the right superior anterior segment (segment VIII) may drain into the middle hepatic vein. In harvesting the right lobe, the surgical plane courses about 1 cm to the right of the middle hepatic vein. Segment VIII, then, loses its venous drainage, resulting again in graft congestion unless its draining vein is reanastomosed in the recipient.

Renal Veins

Most individuals have a single renal vein for each kidney, although variations in the number and location of the renal veins can occur. The left renal vein is typically longer (5.9 +/− 1.5 cm) than the right (2.4 +/− 0.7 cm) (162), as it has to cross the midline to drain into the normally right-sided IVC. Both renal veins are normally similar in caliber, with an average diameter of approximately 1.2 cm (162). An additional renal vein is much more common on the right side (26%) than on the left (2.6%) (163). A second additional vein on the right side is found in approximately 5% of the postmortem examinations (163). Valves are not present within renal veins (164).

Variations in the morphology of the left renal vein are common. A renal collar or circumaortic vein is present when the left renal vein divides into two separate components, with each one of them crossing the midline anterior and posterior to the abdominal aorta, respectively. Each component drains independently into the IVC, with the retroaortic component being typically inferior to the one anterior to the aorta. This anatomic variation is present in approximately 0.3% of autopsy studies (165). A single retroaortic renal vein is found in approximately 5% of postmortem examinations (165).

The presence of a retroaortic or circumaortic renal vein should be recognized on imaging studies, as it may have significant implications in specific clinical circumstances, including IVC filter placement, spermatic vein embolization, adrenal or renal venous sampling (166), retroperitoneal surgical approach to abdominal aortic aneurysms (167,168), or renal surgery (169). Failure to recognize the dorsal component of the renal vein during retroperitoneal surgery may lead to life-threatening hemorrhage or nephrectomy (170). A retroaortic component of the renal vein is readily visible on CT and MR imaging studies, and for MR, particularly on gadolinium-enhanced images. The renal veins show intense enhancement during the late arterial phase of CE examinations (171); a delayed venous phase is not necessary for visualization of the renal vein anatomy. However, a delayed venous acquisition may be important to determine the presence of tumor enhancement within the renal vein.

Laparoscopic living donor nephrectomy is a less invasive alternative to open surgery. As the operative FOV is quite limited, preoperative information about venous anatomy is useful to select an appropriate kidney for transplant and to plan the surgery. Renal vein anomalies, as described above, should be noted. It is important to note large lumbar veins draining into the renal vein as well as the location of the left adrenal vein (172).

Renal vein thrombosis may be secondary to glomerulonephritis, sepsis, lupus nephritis, diabetic nephropathy, amyloidosis, sarcoidosis, sickle cell anemia, malignancy, dehydration, and trauma (173). With CT and MR, filling defects in the renal vein implicate thrombosis. Secondary signs of renal vein thrombosis, including a delayed cortical nephrogram and global parenchymal enlargement, are well demonstrated.

With CT, the renal veins are well seen during the early corticomedullary phase of enhancement, the recommended for renal vein evaluation. In the acute state, renal vein thrombosis is seen as a hypoattenuating filling defect within an enlarged renal vein. Over time, thrombus may contract, and extensive collateral vessels may develop.

MR imaging in patients with renal vein thrombosis can demonstrate renal swelling, indistinct corticomedullary differentiation on T1-weighted images, and decreased signal intensity of the renal cortex and medulla on T1- and T2-weighted images (173). Obliteration of the fat in the renal sinus, compression of the renal collecting system, marked attenuation of the renal veins, multiple perirenal venous collaterals, and dilatation of the gonadal vein are ancillary findings that can be found in these patients (174). A band of low signal intensity in the outer part of the medulla is typically present, although this finding can also be noted in patients with hemorrhagic fever with renal syndrome (HFRS) (173). Decreased signal intensity in the outer medulla is better appreciated on T2-weighted images in these patients (173). This finding is likely a consequence of the outer medulla's sensitivity to ischemia (175). Congestion and hemorrhage of the outer medulla at pathology account for the MR imaging findings both in patients with HFRS and renal vein thrombosis (173).

Patients with renal cell neoplasms have an increased risk for tumor invasion of the renal vein. Although this is much more common in patients with RCC, other primary malignant tumors of the kidney, including transitional cell carcinoma and tumors of the adrenal gland, can present with renal vein invasion (176,177). Rarely, benign neoplasms like angiomyolipoma (AML) can demonstrate aggressive local behavior and extend into the renal vein or even the IVC.

2D TOF images can be used as a fast screening protocol for evaluation of the renal veins, particularly in patients with left renal masses. A saturation band medial to the imaging slice can be applied to eliminate signals within the arteries. In a single breath hold, three to five sagittal slices provide a fast assessment of the patency of the renal veins. Gadolinium-enhanced 3D T1-weighted gradient echo acquisitions provide excellent delineation of the renal veins as well as the presence or absence of thrombus. Subtraction images during the delayed venous phase are particularly helpful in the characterization of the thrombus. Enhancing thrombus should be considered tumoral; lack of enhancement is suggestive of bland thrombus, although it does not exclude tumor thrombus entirely.

The presence or absence of left renal vein thrombosis and its extent when present is critical information for planning the surgical approach. The superior mesenteric artery (SMA) is used as an anatomic landmark for the midline. If the thrombus in the left renal vein is proximal to the SMA, a left flank approach is used (Fig. 24-65). This approach allows for retraction of the tumor thrombus in its entirety in the majority of cases (Fig. 24-66). If the thrombus extends beyond the SMA, a midline incision is preferred because tumor thrombus located in the left renal vein to the right of the SMA is typically unreachable from a left flank incision (Fig. 24-67).

Renal vein thrombosis is a serious postoperative complication of kidney transplantation that leads to graft loss in

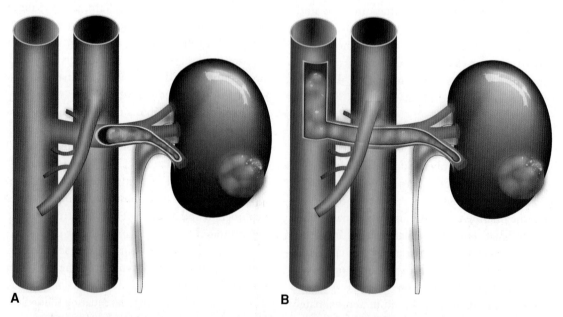

A   **B**

FIGURE 24-65 Implications of tumor thrombus in the left renal vein. A: Schematic representation of the left renal vein system showing tumor thrombus within the left renal vein (*black arrow*), which does not cross the midline, which is denoted by the SMA. This type of venous extension is usually amenable to a standard flank incision. **B:** In this same schematic illustration, the tumor thrombus (*black arrows*) now extends past the level of the SMA and extends into the IVC. A midline incision is usually required to access the thrombus in the right hemiabdomen and perform a left nephrectomy during a single surgical procedure.

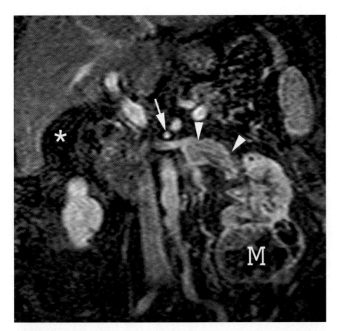

FIGURE 24-66 Left renal vein tumor thrombus extending to the SMA in a 68-year-old man with gross hematuria and renal mass and suggestion of renal vein thrombus on prior CT (not shown). Coronal subtracted (venous phase minus precontrast) 3D fat-saturated T1-weighted gradient echo image at the same level shows heterogeneous enhancement in the renal mass (*M*) in the lower pole of the left kidney. As this is a subtraction image, the nonenhancing gallbladder contents (*∗*) become black and serve as an internal control for enhancement. High signal within the left renal venous thrombus (*white arrowheads*) represents enhancement, and thus it can be characterized as tumor thrombus. The tumor thrombus in the left renal vein does not extend beyond the SMA (*white arrow*). A standard left intercostal flank approach was used at surgery, which allowed for resection of both the renal mass and the venous thrombus.

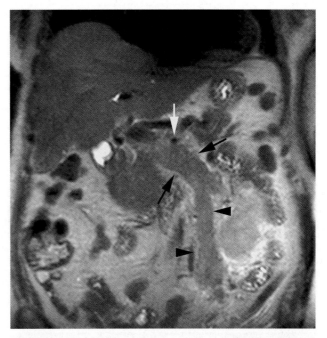

FIGURE 24-67 Left renal vein tumor thrombus extending beyond the SMA. Coronal HASTE in a patient with an infiltrating left renal mass shows expansion of the left renal vein (*black arrows*) and left gonadal vein (*black arrowheads*), which are filled with intermediate signal intensity thrombus. The SMA (*white arrow*) is visualized as a normal flow void.

almost all cases (178,179). Retransplantation and history of peritoneal dialysis are the stronger risk factors for renal vein thrombosis in transplant recipients (178). This complication occurs in approximately 0.5% to 4.0% of patients, with some series reporting incidences as high as 10% (180), and typically presents early after surgery, between the second and seventh postoperative day (180). Lack of collateral veins increases the risk for infarct and rupture of the transplanted kidney. Acute/hyperacute rejection and surgical technical errors have been associated with renal vein thrombosis, although a cause is not found in the majority of cases. Extrinsic compression, excessive length of the vein, and increased motility of the graft are some of the causes associated with the surgical technique.

Other causes include thrombophilic disorders and immunosuppressive medication (181). Reversal diastolic flow, lack of normal venous wave form, and diffuse enlargement of the kidney secondary to edema can be appreciated on duplex US in transplanted patients with renal vein thrombosis (182). Occasionally, kinking of a long tortuous

vein can cause occlusion without thrombosis presenting with acute pain in the area of the transplant and findings at US similar to those of renal vein thrombosis (181). Most patients with clinical suspicion for allograft vein thrombosis are taken to the operating room without delay based on the appropriate US findings and clinical presentation. In patients with an unclear diagnosis, further imaging can confirm the presence of thrombus within the renal vein. MR and CT imaging provide a comprehensive evaluation of the ileofemoral system, which allow for depiction of thrombus not only in the renal vein but also in the rest of the pelvic veins (Fig. 24-68). Renal AVFs can be evaluated with CT and MR imaging, which are particularly useful in visualization of the feeding arterial feeder and draining vein (Fig. 24-69). Further information on the renal vessels can be found in Chapter 20.

Portomesenteric System

The portomesenteric system includes the veins that drain the blood from the abdominal gastrointestinal tract (with the exception of the lower part of the rectum) and those from the spleen, pancreas, and gallbladder. All of these veins convey the blood to the liver by the portal vein. The main portal vein is approximately 8 cm in length and is formed by the confluence of the splenic and SMVs. The diameter

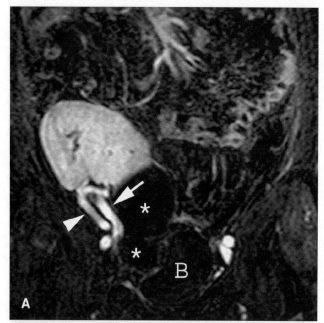

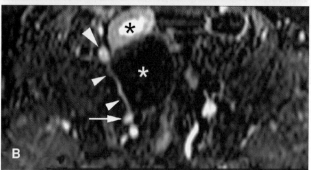

FIGURE 24-68 Compression of external iliac vein by a pelvic lymphocele, causing impairment in function of renal transplant and right lower extremity edema in a 58-year-old female with right cadaveric renal transplant 2 months prior to this visit, with continuous increase in creatinine levels and now complaining of right thigh swelling and pain. **A:** Coronal subtracted (venous phase minus precontrast) 3D fat-saturated T1-weighted gradient echo image showing the patent renal artery (*arrowhead*) and vein (*arrow*) of the renal transplant in the right lower quadrant. A lobulated fluid collection (*) is identified, below and medial to the transplanted kidney and adjacent to the urinary bladder (*B*). **B:** Axial reconstruction from the coronal acquisition better demonstrates the relation of the fluid collection (*white* *) located posterior to the renal transplant (*black* *) and the iliac vessels. Note marked extrinsic compression and narrowing of the mid external iliac vein (*small arrowheads*). The proximal (*arrow*) and distal (*large arrowhead*) portions of the external iliac vein are normal in caliber. The fluid collection was percutaneously drained and represented a lymphocele. Creatinine levels returned to baseline, and her symptoms in the right lower extremity resolved shortly after the drainage.

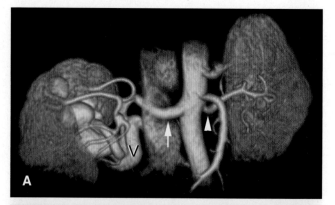

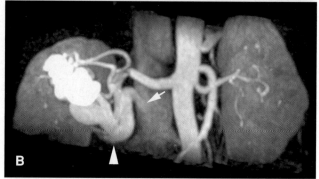

FIGURE 24-69 Renal AVF. **A:** Coronal VR image from an axial fat-saturated 3D T1-weighted SPGR shows single right (*white arrow*) and left (*white arrowhead*) renal arteries. Note massive dilated vessels in the right renal hilum compared with the left and early filling of the dilated right renal vein (*V*) during the arterial phase. **B:** Coronal MIP presentation better demonstrates the markedly dilated right renal vein (*white arrowhead*) as it drains into the IVC (*arrow*). Note the lack of opacification of the left renal vein, indicating early filling of the right renal vein.

of the portal vein may vary significantly in healthy volunteers, depending on their sex, age, respiration, posture, and meals (183). Reported upper limits for the portal, splenic, and superior mesenteric vein diameters are 16, 12, and 11 mm, respectively, as determined for volunteers in the fasting state, supine decubitus position, and deep inspiration (183).

The portal vein bifurcates into a right and left portal vein in 89% of healthy individuals evaluated for liver donation (184). The right portal vein bifurcates into an anterior and a posterior branch. The cystic vein enters into the right portal vein before the latter enters into the right lobe of the liver. The left portal vein divides into a superior and an inferior branch. Anatomic variants of the portal vein include trifurcation (origin of the left portal vein at the bifurcation of the right portal vein into anterior and posterior branches) and anomalies in configuration of the right portal vein (origin of the left portal vein from the right anterior portal vein branch or early origin of the right posterior portal vein) in 4% and 6% of individuals, respectively (184). Recognition of portal vein anatomic variants may be important in patients undergoing hepatic surgery. Lee et al. (184) found a higher association of biliary anomalies in patients with portal vein anomalies (58%) than in patients with hepatic arterial anomalies (30%). Tributaries of the portomesenteric system include the short gastric veins, gastroepiploic vein, coronary vein, pancreatic veins, and the inferior mesenteric vein.

Cross-sectional imaging, particularly with CT, can demonstrate important ancillary findings of vascular disease such as bowel wall thickening, pneumatosis, and portomesenteric venous gas. In the setting of bowel ischemia, pneumatosis intestinalis and portomesenteric venous gas strongly suggest the presence of transmural infarction (185,186). CT allows the detection of smaller amounts of portomesenteric venous gas than does plain film.

Pneumatosis and portomesenteric venous gas may also be seen in a variety of nonischemic diseases. Therefore, clinical correlation is needed before surgery is recommended (187). The differential diagnosis includes iatrogenic and idiopathic causes, trauma, inflammation, infection, neoplasm, and obstruction. Portomesenteric venous gas without pneumatosis can be seen with mesenteric abscess, portal pyelophlebitis, sepsis, and trauma as well as after gastrointestinal surgery or liver transplant.

Portal Vein

An assessment of portal vein patency is a common indication for imaging. CE CTA and CE MRA are both established techniques for this purpose (188). Venous thrombosis is seen as persistent, well-defined intraluminal filling defects with central low attenuation or low signal for CTA and MRA, respectively (Fig. 24-70). MRA techniques are less sensitive for detection of calcification and often have difficulty visualizing vessels with metallic stents.

TOF MRA can assess for portal vein patency as well as direction of flow. With a saturation band placed superior to the slice, a bright portal vein confirms its patency, and flow paralleling the IVC flow confirms a hepatopetal direction (Fig. 24-17). If no signal is seen within the portal vein, then the flow is reversed (hepatofugal) or the vein is occluded. The ambiguity in the latter circumstance can be solved by examining the portal vein on the postcontrast images. If normal enhancement of the portal vein is noted on dynamic postcontrast images, then reverse flow (hepatofugal flow) in the portal vein is likely (Fig. 24-71). Alternatively, repeating the TOF acquisition with the saturation band below the imaging slice can help to make this diagnosis. If the flow is reversed (hepatofugal), the portal vein becomes bright (matching the aorta) and the IVC becomes black.

Thrombosis of the portal vein can occur secondary to intra-abdominal infection, hypercoagulable state, trauma,

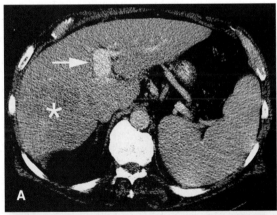
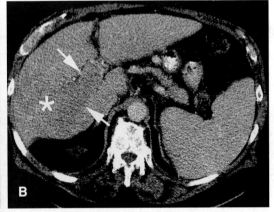
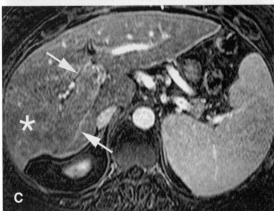

FIGURE 24-70 CT and MR imaging of portal vein tumor thrombus. A: Axial CT image through the level of the left portal vein shows a large, heterogeneously enhancing mass (∗) infiltrating the majority of the right lobe. The left portal vein (*arrow*) is widely patent. **B:** Axial CT image at a slightly more inferior level than that in **(A)** again shows the large mass (∗) and lack of visualization of the right portal vein (*arrows*). **C:** Axial subtracted (portal venous phase minus precontrast) image through the same level as that in **(B)** also shows the mass (∗). The right portal vein (*arrows*) is expanded and filled with enhancing tumor thrombus.

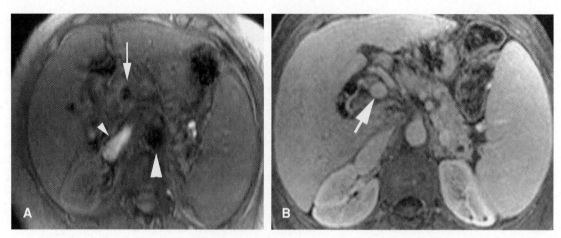

FIGURE 24-71 Hepatofugal flow with TOF MRI. A: Oblique axial TOF image through the hepatic hilum shows normal flow-related signal in the IVC (*small white arrowhead*). An expected flow void is present in the aorta (*large white arrowhead*), as the image was acquired with a saturation band above the imaging slice. No flow-related signal is present in the main portal vein (*white arrow*). This could indicate either thrombosis or reversed flow. **B:** Axial CE fat-saturated 3D T1-weighted SPGR image through a similar level during the delayed venous phase shows normal wall-to-wall enhancement in the main portal vein (*arrow*), ruling out portal vein thrombosis. Thus, the lack of signal in the portal vein in **(A)** indicates flow in the same direction as the aorta, which is reversed, or hepatofugal, flow.

postoperative state, neoplasm, congenital causes, pregnancy, and oral contraceptives (189). HCC is the most common neoplasm causing portal vein tumor thrombus (Fig. 24-72). Reduced portal blood flow can also occur secondary to hepatic parenchymal disease and abdominal sepsis (infectious or ascending thrombophlebitis). Portal vein thrombosis is idiopathic in approximately 8% to 15% of cases (189). Patients can present with abdominal pain, especially when thrombus extends to the SMV (189).

Differentiation between recent and chronic portal vein thrombosis may have clinical implications (190). Recanalization of the portal vein is common in patients with recent thrombosis who are treated with early anticoagulation therapy (190). This therapy, however, tends to fail in patients with chronic portal vein thrombosis; recanalization in this group of patients is uncommon (190). Clinical and imaging findings that suggest recent thrombosis include recent abdominal pain, no evidence of chronic portal HTN

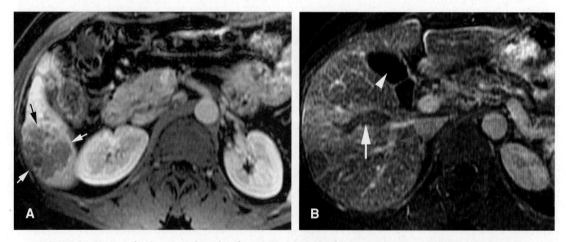

FIGURE 24-72 Portal vein tumor thrombus from HCC. A: Axial 3D fat-saturated T1-weighted gradient echo image obtained during the portal venous phase in a patient with hepatitis C cirrhosis shows a round heterogeneously hypoenhancing mass in segment VI of the liver (*arrows*), consistent with HCC. **B:** Axial subtracted (portal venous phase minus precontrast) 3D fat-saturated T1-weighted fat-saturated gradient echo image shows hypoenhancing thrombus (*arrow*) in the anterior branch of the right portal vein. Note the lack of enhancement in the gallbladder (*white arrowhead*), which serves as an internal control. The posterior branch of the right portal vein (*red arrowhead*) shows normal enhancement.

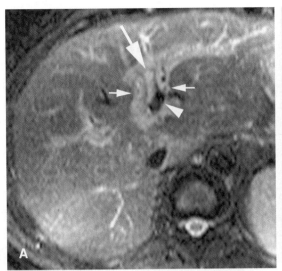 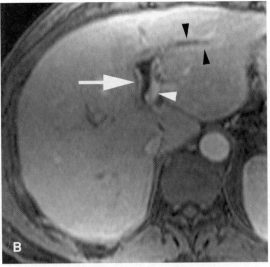

FIGURE 24-73 Portal venous thrombus secondary to infection (pyelophlebitis) in a 59-year-old man with fever, chills, and right upper quadrant pain for 4 weeks. A: Axial STIR image through the left **(A)** and right **(B)** portal veins shows increased intraluminal signal intensity (*large white arrow*) and, in the setting of subacute thrombosis, increased signal intensity surrounding the left portal vein (*small white arrows*) is consistent with edema. A small area of normal flow void is seen within a more proximal segment of the left portal vein (*white arrowhead*). **B:** Axial 3D fat-saturated T1-weighted fat-saturated gradient echo image acquired during the portal venous phase through the left portal vein shows filling of the intrahepatic portal veins (*arrow*) by nonenhancing thrombus. Wall enhancement of the central and more peripheral (*black arrowheads*) left portal veins is consistent with subacute thrombus. A small portion of the patent, enhancing left (*white arrowhead*) portal vein is again demonstrated.

(gastrointestinal bleed, ascites, collateral portosystemic circulation, or splenomegaly), and lack of portal cavernous transformation cross-sectional imaging (190).

In the authors' experience, recent thrombus demonstrates high signal intensity on T2-weighted images. However, this finding is not specific, as tumor thrombus can also show increased signal intensity. CE MR images can help to differentiate tumor from acute bland thrombus. Tumor thrombus shows enhancement after contrast administration, which is better appreciated on subtraction imaging. Acute bland thrombus does not enhance, although enhancement in the wall of the portal vein is common. High signal intensity of the thrombus on T2-weighted images and increased enhancement after administration of gadolinium in the wall of the portal vein during the acute/subacute stages is probably related to inflammation (Fig. 24-73). These findings have been described as a sign of acute/subacute thrombosis in other anatomic locations (69).

Segmental portal vein occlusion may result in wedge-shaped areas of increased signal intensity on T2-weighted images and decreased signal intensity on T1-weighted images (191). Increased enhancement during the arterial phase on CTA or dynamic gadolinium-enhanced MR images is the result of compensatory increased arterial blood flow for the affected segment (192,193). Typically, enhancement of the affected hepatic segment during the portal and delayed venous phases becomes homogeneous (192). Chronic occlusion of a segmental branch of the portal vein may lead to focal fatty sparing (193).

Mixing of enhanced and unenhanced blood at the portosplenic confluence can be a source of confusion. Blood in the splenic vein enhances with intravenous contrast earlier than in the SMV; at the portosplenic confluence, this mixing creates a heterogeneous appearance that can be confused with a filling defect. CE images during the equilibrium phase should equilibrate the heterogeneity of mixing.

Portal hypertension is defined as a portal venous pressure of greater than 10 mmHg. Collagen deposition in the spaces of Disse, and intrahepatic endogenous vasoconstrictors and mesenteric vasodilators are proposed to be responsible for increased blood flow and pressure in the portal venous system (194). Regardless, the end result is the development and enlargement of portosystemic collateral vessels.

With a progressive increase in portal venous pressure, flow in the portal vein changes from the normal flow toward the liver (hepatopetal) to flow away from the liver (hepatofugal). Reversal flow is secondary to intrahepatic arterioportal communication through the vasa vasorum (arterioles) supplying the wall of the portal veins and direct shunting of blood from the hepatic arteries through the capillary system and into the portal vein (195). The hepatic

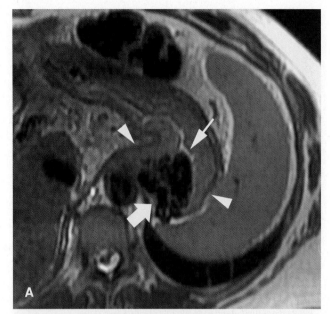

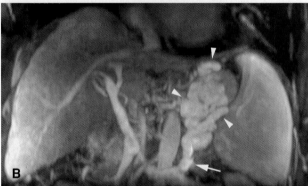

FIGURE 24-74 Gastric varices. A: Axial T1-weighted in-phase gradient echo image in a patient with nonalcoholic steatohepatitis (NASH) and long-standing portal HTN shows large flow voids (*thick arrow*) in the wall (*arrowheads*) of the gastric fundus. Note the intraluminal extension (*thin arrow*) of the varices. **B:** Coronal reformation of an axial 3D fat-saturated T1-weighted gradient echo acquisition during the delayed venous phase better displays the extensive gastric varices (*arrowheads*) and their communication (*arrow*) with the splenic vein.

apparent gastroesophageal varices at endoscopy; an episode of life-threatening hemorrhage occurs in 30% of them (196). The risk of bleeding has been associated with the size of the gastroesophageal varices as well as the Child class, although it seems independent from the portal venous pressure (197). Gastroesophageal varices follow the course of the left gastric vein extending from the superior aspect of the portal venous confluence cranially along the lesser curvature of the stomach toward the gastroesophageal junction draining within the veins of the lower esophageal plexus (194).

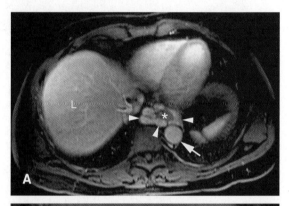

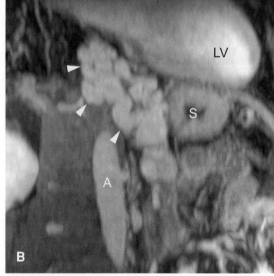

FIGURE 24-75 Esophageal varices in a 52-year-old man with hepatitis C cirrhosis who presented for transplant evaluation. A: Axial 3D fat-saturated T1-weighted SPGR image obtained during the portal venous phase through the lower thorax shows the dome of the liver (*L*) and the descending aorta (*white arrow*). Multiple tubular enhancing structures (*white arrowheads*) are present around the esophagus (***), indicating paraesophageal varices. **B:** Oblique coronal reformatted image from an axial 3D fat-saturated T1-weighted SPGR acquisition during delayed venous phase shows the aorta (*A*) and the stomach (*S*) below the left ventricle (*LV*). This image better demonstrates the tubular nature of the large paraesophageal varices (*white arrowheads*).

arterial inflow overwhelms the portal venous inflow, as the hepatic arterial pressure (similar to the systemic arterial pressure) exceeds the portal venous pressure (5 to 10 mmHg) (194).

Patients with diffuse liver disease and portal HTN develop large portosystemic collateral vessels. Common varices include the left gastric vein, short gastric veins (Fig. 24-74), paraumbilical veins, and splenic vein. Gastroesophageal varices, predominantly supplied by the left gastric vein (coronary vein), are the most clinically relevant venous collaterals in patients with portal HTN (Fig. 24-75). Up to 30% of patients with portal HTN have

A recalized paraumbilical vein can be seen in patients with portal HTN along the anterior aspect of the falciform ligament, the ligamentum teres (corresponding to the atrophied umbilical vein). The paraumbilical vein originates from the left portal vein and typically ends at the level of the umbilicus (Fig. 24-76). Most commonly, venous flow from the paraumbilical varix drains into the systemic circulation via one of the two inferior epigastric veins (194). Alternatively, a cephalic course of the paraumbilical vein communicates via the substernal veins or internal mammary veins with the intercostal and azygous veins (194). A herniated paraumbilical vein at the level of the umbilicus may be misinterpreted on physical examination as a hernia (194). Enlarged veins in the anterior abdominal wall, the so-called *caput medusae*, may be present in patients with advance portal HTN.

Spontaneous retroperitoneal shunts can also be found, including splenorenal, iliolumbar, intercostal, and phrenic vein shunts (194). The estimated incidence of spontaneous splenorenal and gastrorenal anastomoses in patients with portal hypertension is around 16% (198). Large spontaneous spleno- and/or gastrorenal shunt might prevent development of large esophageal varices (199). However, the risk for variceal bleeding and chronic hepatic encephalopathy is not affected by the presence of these shunts (199). Splenorenal shunts occur when venous varices off the splenic vein communicate directly with the left renal vein.

CE MDCT and gadolinium-enhanced MR images with multiplanar and 3D reconstructions are particularly helpful in understanding the anatomy in these complex vascular networks. An enlarged left renal vein is typically present (Fig. 24-77). MRI is superior to US in demonstrating spontaneous splenorenal shunts (200). Frequently, venous collaterals off the splenic vein are very convoluted and extend cephalically or caudally for a great distance before they eventually communicate with the left renal vein (194). Rarely, spontaneous communication between the mesenteric circulation and the IVC, a mesocaval shunt, may occur (Fig. 24-78).

Anastomosis between distal branches of the inferior mesenteric vein and inferior hemorrhoidal veins are normally encountered at the level of the rectum. Patients with portal HTN may develop important hemorrhoidal bleeding from enlarged varices in the rectal wall. Venous flow in collaterals originating in the inferior mesenteric vein may also return to the systemic circulation through the gonadal veins (194).

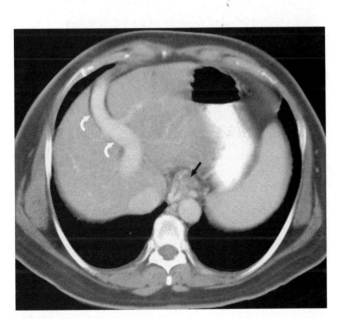

FIGURE 24-76 Recanalized paraumbilical vein. Axial CE CT image at the level of the upper abdomen in a patient with cirrhosis shows a recanalized paraumbilical vein (*curved arrows*). Note the presence of gastroesophageal varices (*black arrow*).

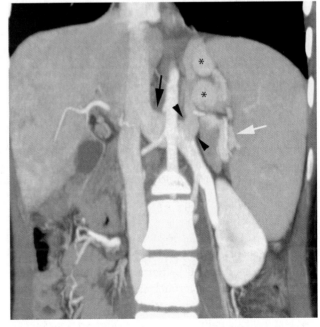

FIGURE 24-77 Splenorenal shunt. Coronal VR reconstruction from a CE MDCT examination shows large varices in the splenic hilum (∗) arising from the splenic vein (*white arrow*) and draining (*black arrowheads*) into the enlarged renal vein (*black arrow*).

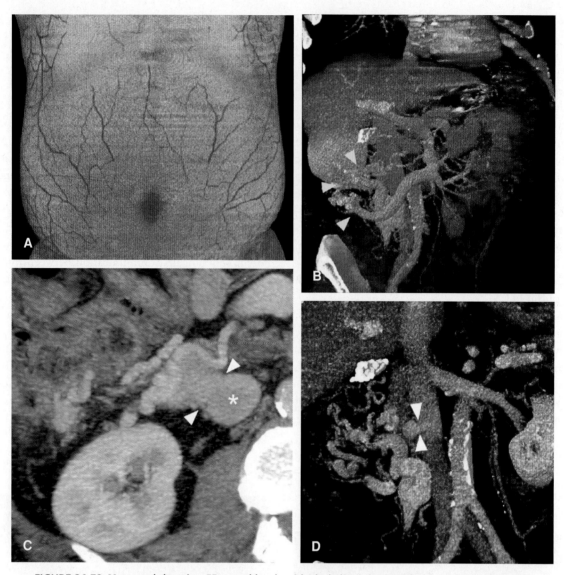

FIGURE 24-78 Mesocaval shunt in a 55-year-old male with alcoholic cirrhosis with spontaneous mesocaval shunt. A: VR demonstrates the extensive subcutaneous venous network (caput medusae) formed due to diverted splanchnic venous flow in this patient with portal HTN. **B:** VR demonstrates multiple venous collaterals (*arrowheads*) originating from SMV, forming a spontaneous mesocaval shunt at the level of the infrahepatic IVC. **C:** Transverse image as well as a **(D)** demonstrate the area (*arrowheads*) where the venous collaterals drain into the IVC (*). The high spatial resolution of CT enables visualization of the 1- to 2-mm collateral veins forming the shunt but, unlike MR, cannot document the direction of flow in the portal vein, which by inference from the well-developed venous collaterals is likely to be hepatofugal. (Courtesy of Stanford University Cardiovascular Imaging.)

Extrahepatic aneurysms of the portal vein are uncommon and can be caused by portal HTN, diffuse hepatic disease, or congenital or abnormal weakness of the portal vein wall (201–203). Although most cases are asymptomatic and incidentally discovered by cross-sectional imaging examinations, these patients may present with mild abdominal pain (201). Occasionally, patients present with symptoms related to complications like jaundice or gastrointestinal bleeding (204,205). Complications of portal vein aneurysm include thrombosis with or without complete occlusion of the portal vein, rupture, portal-systemic shunt, and mass effects on adjacent viscera (201,204,205). Obstructive jaundice and gastric outlet obstruction may be secondary to mass effect on the common bile duct and duodenum, respectively, by large extrahepatic portal vein aneurysms (201). Life-threatening severe portal HTN may occur after acute thrombosis of the portal vein aneurysm (201).

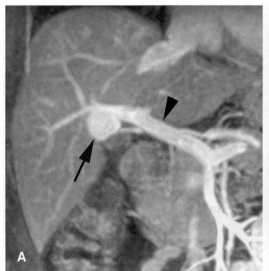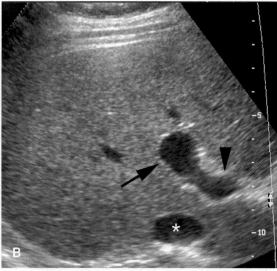

FIGURE 24-79 Portal vein aneurysm. A: Coronal MIP reconstruction from an axial 3D fat-saturated T1-weighted gradient echo acquisition during portal venous phase in a patient evaluated for unrelated symptoms shows the main portal vein (*black arrowhead*) and an aneurysmal segment adjacent to the porta hepatis (*black arrow*) enhancing to the same degree as portal venous blood on all phases of the acquisition. **B:** Transverse US image in the same patient confirmed a focal area of aneurysmal dilatation of the portal vein (*black arrow*) compared with the normal caliber main portal vein (*black arrowhead*). The IVC is denoted by (*).

Portal vein aneurysms can be demonstrated in utero by US (202). Fusiform and saccular configurations may be seen in these aneurysms (205,206). A diameter greater than 20 mm is considered as diagnostic of extrahepatic portal vein aneurysm (201). US can accurately measure the size of the portal vein. Thrombus and flow within the aneurysm can be readily detected with color and pulse Doppler US. CT and MR imaging can be used to confirm the diagnosis and to provide a more comprehensive evaluation of the portomesenteric system prior to surgical correction (Fig. 24-79).

Superior Mesenteric Vein

The SMV drains the blood from the small intestine and cecum as well as from the ascending and transverse portions of the colon. The SMV is formed at the level of the right lower quadrant by the union of the veins that return blood from the terminal, the ileum, the cecum, and vermiform appendix. From this location, the SMV ascends between the two layers of the mesentery on the right side and immediately adjacent to the SMA. Patients with intestinal malrotation demonstrate the SMV either in front or on the left side of the SMA (207) (Fig. 24-80). Patients with underlying intestinal malrotation are at risk for midgut volvulus (Fig. 24-81). Tributaries of the SMV include the ileocolic, right colic, middle colic, right gastroepiploic, and pancreaticoduodenal veins. In the upper abdomen, the SMV con-

fluences with the splenic vein to form the portal vein just behind the neck of the pancreas.

The diagnosis of mesenteric venous thrombosis is often difficult to make clinically and accounts for 10% to 15% of all cases of mesenteric ischemia (208,209). Risk factors include intra-abdominal infection (Fig. 24-82), portal HTN, pancreatitis (Fig. 24-83), visceral malignancy, perforated viscus, prior abdominal surgery, hypercoagulable states, women taking oral contraceptives, and smoking (188). In up to 50% of patients, no underlying cause is found (210). MD CTA or gadolinium-enhanced MRV should be the diagnostic imaging modalities of choice when there is high clinical suspicion (188). The inherent high-resolution of MDCT reconstructions may be helpful in patients with mesenteric venous stenosis (Fig. 24-84). SMV stenosis can also be seen in patients with sclerosing mesenteritis (Fig. 24-85).

TOF may also demonstrate a filling defect or complete obstruction of the SMV, although these images are prone to false positives from turbulent flow.

Nonocclusive thrombus is appreciated on CE images as a filling defect in the lumen of the vessel, whereas occlusive thrombus is seen as lack of enhancement within the SMV (Fig. 24-86). Sensitivity, specificity, and accuracy of MR for the detection of thrombosis in the portal venous system are 100%, 98%, and 99%, respectively (211), and CT will establish the diagnosis in upward of 90% of patients (212).

(*text continues on page 1251*)

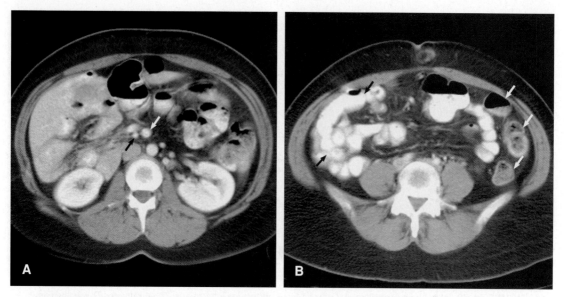

FIGURE 24-80 Intestinal malrotation. A: Axial CE MDCT image in a patient with intestinal malrotation shows an inverted relationship between the SMV (*white arrow*) and the SMA (*black arrow*). Normally, the SMA, the smaller vessel of the two, lies to the left side (as oriented to the patient) of the SMV. **B:** Axial CT image at a slightly lower level than that in (**A**) shows the small bowel in the right hemiabdomen (*black arrows*) and the colon in the left hemiabdomen (*white arrows*).

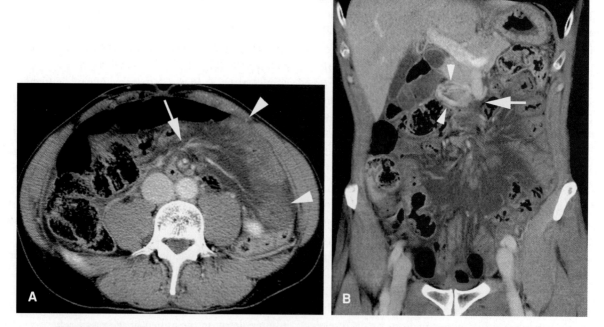

FIGURE 24-81 Midgut volvulus. A: Axial CE CT image during the portal venous phase through the level of the mid abdomen reveals bowel wall thickening and mesenteric edema (*white arrowheads*) around several jejunal loops. Note the abnormal configuration of the mesenteric vasculature with a swirled appearance and confluence of the vessels toward the mesenteric root (*white arrow*). **B:** Coronal reformatted image of the same acquisition as that in (**A**) confirms the swirled configuration of the mesenteric vessels in the mid abdomen (*white arrowheads*). There is an abrupt cutoff of the SMV (*white arrow*), indicating obstruction due to rotation around the vascular axis. At surgery, a midgut volvulus with associated bowel ischemia was found.

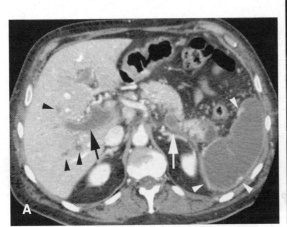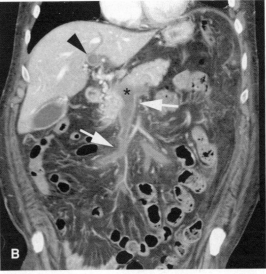

FIGURE 24-82 Extensive portomesenteric thrombosis from Enterococcal sepsis in a 55-year-old male with abdominal pain. A: Axial CT image shows extensive thrombus and wall enhancement within the right portal vein (*black arrow*), multiple additional peripheral right portal venous branches (*black arrowheads*), and the splenic vein (*white arrow*). Small peripheral areas of splenic perfusion are present in the almost completely infarcted spleen (*white arrowheads*). **B:** Coronal reformatted image demonstrates the extensive thrombosis along the portosplenic confluence (∗) and the SMV and its branches (*white arrows*). The thrombosed main portal vein (*black arrowhead*) is partially visualized.

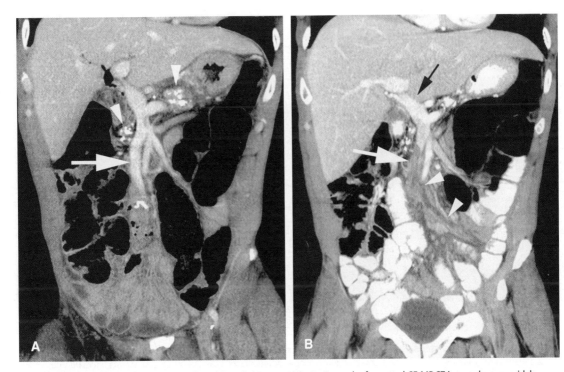

FIGURE 24-83 SMV thrombosis from chronic pancreatitis. A: Coronal reformatted CE MDCT image shows a widely patent SMV (*white arrow*). Note the calcifications in the head and tail of the pancreas (*white arrowheads*), indicating chronic pancreatitis. **B:** Coronal reformatted image of CE MDCT scan obtained 2 weeks following the scan in (**A**), after the patient presented with acute pain, demonstrates new thrombus in the SMV (*white arrow*) and its branches (*white arrowheads*). The main portal vein is patent (*black arrow*).

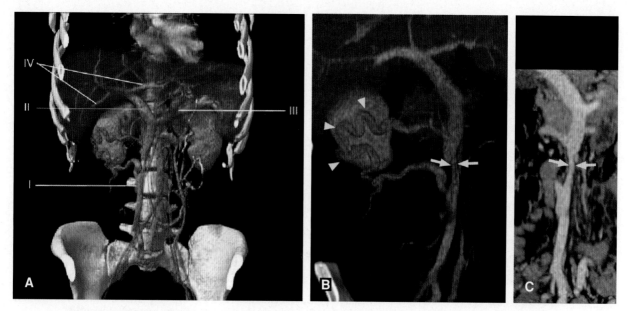

FIGURE 24-84 Idiopathic SMV stenosis in a 27-year-old female with history of gastric bypass with abdominal pain. A: VR demonstrates the normal mesenteric venous return. (I, SMV; II, portal vein; III, splenic vein; IV, left and right hepatic veins.) **B, C:** A tight focal stenosis (*arrows*) of the SMV is present, with formation of an intramesenteric collateral pathway (*arrowheads*) anterior to the right kidney. Coronal reformation reveals no extrinsic mass causing the focal stenosis.

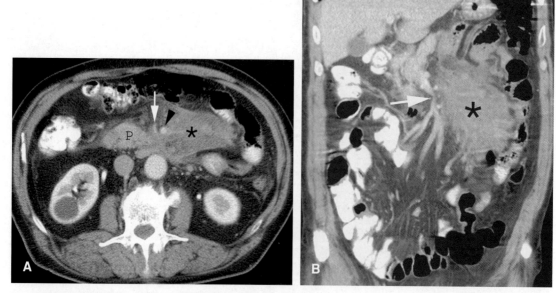

FIGURE 24-85 SMV stenosis from sclerosing mesenteritis. A: Axial CE CT image through the mid abdomen in a patient with sclerosing mesenteritis shows a low-density mesenteric-based mass (∗) and the pancreatic head (*P*). The SMV (*white arrow*) is appropriately located to the right of the SMA (*arrowhead*) but is distorted and tethered, increasing the anteroposterior dimension. Note the high-density internal contrast, indicating that the vessel remains patent. **B:** Coronal reformatted image from the same acquisition better demonstrates the focal waistlike area of narrowing of the SMV (*white arrow*). Note the dilated venous branches leading up to the stenotic segment. The extent of the large mass (∗) is better appreciated on the reformatted image.

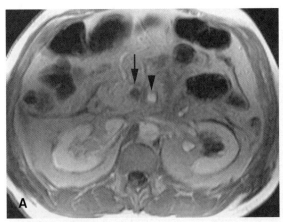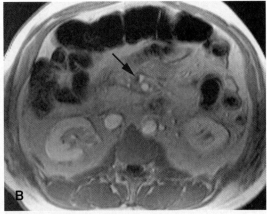

FIGURE 24-86 Partially occlusive SMV thrombus. A: Axial 2D magnetization-prepared T1-weighted gradient echo image acquired during the delayed venous phase through the mid abdomen shows a lack of enhancement in the SMV (*black arrow*) due to thrombosis. Note normal enhancement within the SMA (*black arrowhead*). **B:** Axial image from the same acquisition as that in (**A**) at a slightly lower level shows inferior extension of the SMV thrombus (*arrow*). The thrombus here is partially occlusive, as normal enhancement is present within the left side of the vessel.

Conventional angiography for the diagnosis of venous thrombosis in the portomesenteric system has been virtually replaced with CTV and MRV (211,212). Its use may be limited to patients with a history of thrombophilia in whom small-vessel mesenteric venous thrombosis is suspected and has not been seen with other imaging (212).

The presence of a filling defect with expansion of the lumen of the SMV suggests acute thrombosis. Bowel wall thickening and mesenteric edema in the presence of acute SMV thrombosis are of concern with bowel ischemia. The presence of bowel wall pneumatosis with/without air in the mesenteric veins is concerning for transmural infarction. These indirect findings may also be appreciated in the bowel on MR examinations in patients with mesenteric ischemia. SMV thrombosis is associated with bowel wall thickening and mesenteric congestion on MR (213). Occasionally, the so-called *target sign* described on CT can be appreciated on MR images with alternating layers of low and high signal in the thickened wall. Postcontrast images can show lack of enhancement of the bowel wall in the ischemic segments (214).

Physiologic derangements associated with small bowel ischemia can be evaluated with MRI by using alternative MR sequences. MR oximetry using a T2-weighted multi-echo sequence can detect differences in oxygen desaturation between the IVC and SMV after acute segmental mesenteric ischemia in a porcine model (215). After obtaining the blood sample required for calibration, the T2 values can be used as a marker of oxygen saturation (215). Differences in T2 values between the IVC and SMV suggest acute mesenteric ischemia (215).

A similar approach has also been validated in dogs with nonocclusive mesenteric ischemia due to hemorrhagic shock (216). PC imaging can be used for determination of flow velocity in the SMA and SMV before and after a meal challenge (217,218). Flow in the SMV can be used as an accurate predictor of flow in the SMA (218). Fasting and postprandial flow determinations with PC imaging in the SMV of healthy volunteers and patients without chronic mesenteric ischemia show a substantial postprandial flow augmentation (217). Patients with chronic mesenteric ischemia have significantly less postprandial augmentation compared with healthy volunteers (217). Real-time interactive MRI can demonstrate segmental hypomotility of the small intestine in patients with ischemia (188,219).

Splenic Vein

The splenic vein extends from the splenic hilum in the left upper quadrant to the right immediately adjacent to the upper and back part of the pancreas, inferior to the splenic artery. The splenic vein ends behind the neck of the pancreas at the level of its confluence with the SMV to form the portal vein. The splenic vein is typically large in caliber and has a smooth course, which differs from the very tortuous configuration that typifies the splenic artery.

Splenic vein thrombosis is frequently associated with pancreatic pathology (e.g., pancreatitis, carcinoma). Although some authors have suggested an increased risk of gastric variceal bleeding in patients with splenic vein thrombosis secondary to pancreatitis, the incidence of this complication is only 4% (220). Other causes of splenic

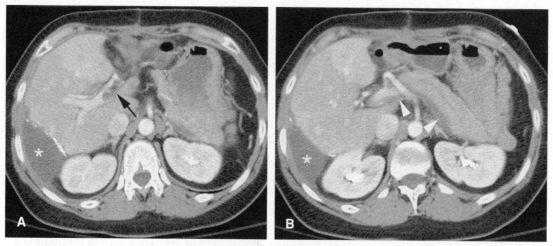

FIGURE 24-87 Splenic vein thrombosis after abdominal surgery. A: Axial CE CT image through the mid abdomen in a patient with recent partial right hepatectomy shows postoperative fluid (∗) adjacent to the suture margin in the surgical bed. A filling defect in the main portal vein (*black arrow*) is consistent with thrombus. **B:** Axial CE CT image inferior to (**A**) shows inferior extension of the thrombus along the extrahepatic portal vein and complete filling of the splenic vein by occlusive thrombus (*white arrowheads*). The postoperative fluid collection (∗) is noted again.

vein thrombosis overlap with those of portal vein and SMV thrombosis, including hypercoagulable states, trauma, abdominal surgery (Fig. 24-87), and infection.

Although the true incidence of splenic vein thrombosis after splenectomy is unknown (not every patient is imaged after surgery), this complication occurs in at least 7% of these patients (221). Most patients respond to anticoagulant therapy, although in some instances, thrombus may extend to the portal vein and eventually cause cavernous transformation of this vessel (221).

CE MDCT and gadolinium-enhanced MRI can demonstrate splenic vein thrombosis and the collateral venous pathways. Patients with obstruction of the splenic vein typically show dilatation of the gastroepiploic vein along the greater curvature of the stomach. The gastroepiploic vein drains the blood from the spleen into the portomesenteric system, ending either directly in the anterior aspect of the SMV or joining first to the middle colic vein (with blood return from the transverse colon) to form the gastrocolic trunk, which then unites the SMV (Fig. 24-88).

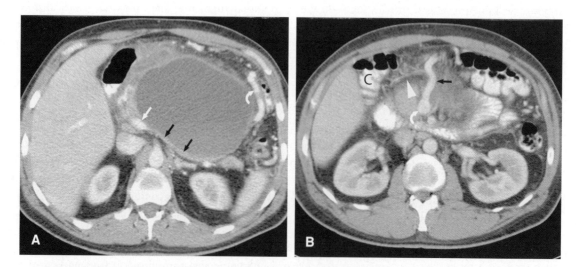

FIGURE 24-88 Splenic vein thrombosis from pancreatitis with a pseudocyst. A: Axial CE MDCT image shows the portal vein (*white arrow*) and lack of enhancement in the expected location of the splenic vein (*black arrows*), which is consistent with occlusion. An enlarged gastroepiploic vein (*curved arrow*) is seen lateral to the large pseudocyst. **B:** Axial MDCT image at a lower level than B shows the enlarged gastroepiploic vein as it joins the middle colic vein (*white arrowhead*) to form the gastroepiploic trunk (*black arrow*), which drains into the SMV (*curved arrow*). This is the most common collateral pathway for drainage of the spleen in patients with splenic vein occlusion. The hepatic flexure portion of the colon is indicated (*C*).

Enlargement of the gastroepiploic vein anterior to the stomach should always increase the suspicion of splenic vein occlusion/stenosis. Due to the convoluted configuration of the gastroepiploic vein, its course is better displayed by using 3D and multiplanar reconstructions (Fig. 24-89).

Pelvic, Gonadal, and Iliac Veins

Most cases of venous thrombosis of the pelvic veins are secondary to cephalad extension of thrombus from the femoropopliteal system (222). Isolated thrombus in pelvic veins is much less common, although it is more frequent in the postpartum period (222). Less than 10% of patients with DVT will have isolated ileofemoral disease (223). This circumstance tends to occur in certain well-recognized clinical situations, including the puerperium. During this period, deep vein thrombosis typically occurs in the ileofemoral region, with over 90% of cases involving the left leg, likely secondary to compression of the left common iliac vein by the right iliac artery and the gravid uterus (224).

Patients with pelvic malignancies are also at risk to develop primary thrombosis of pelvic veins. A significant increased risk for pulmonary embolism exists with pelvic vein thrombosis (222). Other causes include trauma, prior surgery (Fig. 24-90), infection, and hypercoagulable states.

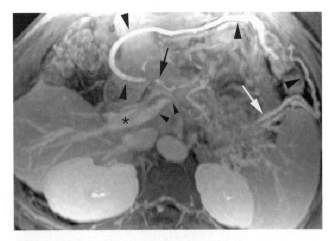

FIGURE 24-89 Collateral splenic venous drainage—the gastrocolic trunk. Axial thick-slab MIP reconstruction from a 3D fat-saturated T1-weighted gradient echo acquisition during the portal venous phase shows the portal vein (*), which tapers at the level of the portosplenic confluence (*small black arrowheads*). The splenic vein is not visualized due to occlusion by the patient's known pancreatic carcinoma. A large gastroepiploic vein (*white arrow*) is seen arising from the splenic hilum and extending along the greater curvature of the stomach (*large arrowheads*). This is the most common collateral pathway for venous drainage of the spleen in patients with splenic vein occlusion. The gastroepiploic vein may drain directly into the SMV/portal vein, as in this patient (*black arrow*), or after joining the middle colic vein to form the gastrocolic trunk.

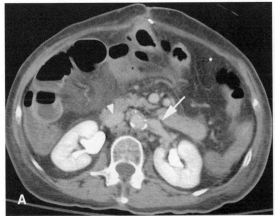

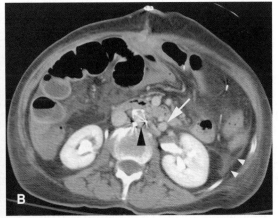

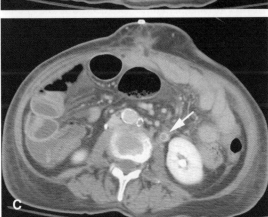

FIGURE 24-90 Gonadal vein thrombosis following abdominal surgery. A: Axial CE CT image obtained during the delayed venous phase at the level of the left renal vein in a patient with recent repair of an abdominal aortic aneurysm. The confluence of the left gonadal vein and left renal vein (*white arrow*) enhances to the same degree as the IVC (*arrowhead*) at this level. **B:** Axial CE CT image slightly inferior to (**A**) shows postoperative clips about the aorta (*black arrowhead*) and anterior skin staples. The left gonadal vein (*white arrow*) is patent, demonstrating the same contrast density as the IVC. Note inflammatory changes in the left lateroconal fascia (*white arrowheads*) after surgical retroperitoneal approach to the abdominal aneurysm. **C:** Axial CE CT image inferior to (**B**) now demonstrates a round filling defect in the left gonadal vein (*white arrow*).

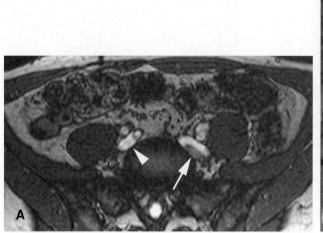
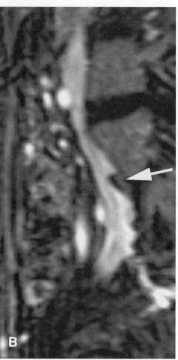

FIGURE 24-91 Partially occlusive right common femoral vein thrombus in a 43-year-old male with a history of Crohn disease status post ileectomy and multiple pulmonary embolisms with negative bilateral Doppler US of the lower extremities. A: Axial true FISP image through the common iliac vessels shows normal uniform high signal in the right common iliac vein (*white arrowhead*). There is an oval intermediate signal intensity filling defect in the posterior aspect of the left common iliac vein (*white arrow*). **B:** Oblique sagittal reformatted image from a 3D fat-saturated T1-weighted gradient echo image through the left iliac system obtained during the delayed postgadolium-enhanced venous phase in the same patient confirms the presence of a partially occlusive thrombus, seen as a low signal intensity filling defect (*white arrow*), in the left common iliac vein.

Considering the radiation sensitivity of the pelvic reproductive organs, MR should be a first-line study in younger patients. MR is helpful for the assessment of the pelvic veins in patients with suspected extension of thrombus from the lower extremities. MR is superior to Doppler US in the evaluation of the iliac and deep pelvic veins and in the objective assessment of the extent of deep vein thrombosis. Doppler US examination of the lower extremities is negative in up to 20% to 50% of patients with proven pulmonary embolism (225). Thrombosis of deep pelvic veins accounts for the source of pulmonary embolism in a substantial number of these patients. MRV using TOF images can detect thrombus in the pelvic veins in up to 30% of these patients (225) (Fig. 24-91).

Three-dimensional gadolinium-enhanced MR images provide exquisite detail of the iliofemoral system. Subtraction postprocessing can render 3D venograms without arterial signal (Fig. 24-92) (54). Reported sensitivity for the diagnosis of iliac and femoral vein thrombosis using gadolinium-enhanced MRV is 100% when compared with conventional venography (54).

May-Thurner syndrome is an anatomic variant in which the left iliac vein is compressed between the anterior aspect of the spine and the overlying (typically right) iliac artery. While this circumstance is frequently present in asymptomatic patients, it has been associated with the development of symptomatic acute venous thrombosis of the left iliac vein (226). The diagnosis of left lower extremity DVT is typically made by US, although the evaluation of the proximal extent of the thrombus and the relationship between the iliac artery and vein is usually not possible with this technique. Thrombolysis and/or thrombus aspiration followed by stent placement in the iliac vein are technically and clinically (resolution of the symptoms) successful in 96% and 95% of patients, respectively (227). However, early and late complications of this strategy have been reported, including upward stent migration into the right ventricle (227,228).

Compression of the iliac veins by pelvic masses is also a cause of lower extremity edema and, potentially, venous thrombosis. MRV can help to distinguish between two different situations—extrinsic compression and venous

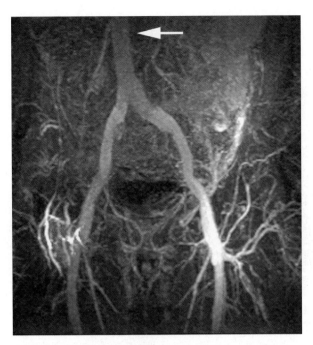

FIGURE 24-92 Normal pelvic MRV. Coronal MIP reconstruction from a subtracted 3D fat-saturated T1-weighted gradient echo acquisition shows normal pelvic venous anatomy to the level of the mid IVC (*arrow*). Subtraction of an acquisition timed during the arterial phase from one acquired during the delayed blood pool phase allows for a selective demonstration of venous structures.

thrombosis—whereas the former is typically treated by reducing the size of the compressing mass (i.e., surgery, radiotherapy, chemotherapy) or by intravascular stenting, the latter requires anticoagulation or fibrinolysis therapy (Fig. 24-93).

There is an increased risk for venous thromboembolism during pregnancy and even higher risk during puerperium (2). Women under the age of 40 years have a 10-fold increased frequency of pulmonary embolism compared with men of the same age (229). Up to 50% of these cases are related to pregnancy in the female group, and many others are related to oral contraceptives (229). The incidence of venous thrombosis in pregnancy is approximately 0.13 to 0.70 per 1,000 women (230,231). The risk for venous thrombosis is even higher during the puerperium, with an incidence of 2.3 to 6.1 per 1,000 women who have this condition (2). Tobacco smoking, history of prior superficial vein thrombosis, and postpartum hemorrhage compound the risk (232). The clinical diagnosis may be challenging, because lower extremity symptoms are typically absent unless there is also involvement of the external and common iliac veins (222).

Septic thrombophlebitis of the gonadal veins most often is seen in the postpartum state and is associated with

endometritis. Postpartum ovarian vein thrombophlebitis should be suspected in patients with persistent fever (233). The incidence of septic pulmonary embolism without treatment in these patients is 40% (2). Ovarian vein thrombosis is less common during pregnancy; 80% to 90% of the cases occur in the right side (234). Abdominal pain related to ovarian vein thrombosis may be difficult to differentiate clinically from appendicitis or ovarian torsion (234). US assessment of the gonadal veins may be limited due to the deep location of these vessels; presence of bowel gas; and in the puerperium, an enlarged uterus.

Both gonadal veins are visualized by US in approximately 78% of parturient women (235). One of the two gonadal veins is not visible in 17%, while none of them is visible in 4% of these patients (235). CT may render false-positive results due to poor opacification of these vessels. Kubik-Huch et al. (236) found gonadal vein thrombosis in 9 out of 27 patients with puerperal fever. The sensitivity, specificity, and accuracy for this diagnosis was 55.6%, 41.2%, and 46.2% for US and 77.8%, 62.5%, and 68.0% for CT (Fig. 24-94). MRI rendered conclusive results in all evaluated patients, resulting in a sensitivity and specificity of 100% (236). MR should be considered the modality of choice for its diagnosis in those patients with inconclusive US findings. TOF images can accurately detect gonadal vein thrombosis without the need for intravenous contrast administration (234). Gadolinium-enhanced MR images can confirm this diagnosis (Fig. 24-95).

MRI evaluates the pelvic veins without using ionizing radiation and without a strict need for intravenous contrast, benefiting patients who are pregnant, of young age, or with a history of contrast allergy. The predominantly vertical course of the gonadal veins favors the use of axial TOF images. When there is extrinsic compression of the iliac vessels by the gravid uterus, thin sections can optimize sensitivity to detecting the resultant slow flow. A lateral decubitus position with the affected side up may help decompress the vessel of interest, allowing for improved detection of slow flow. Dynamic single-shot acquisitions during Valsalva maneuvers (see Magnetic Resonance in the Technical Considerations section) can rule out the presence of thrombus when the vein of interest distends and increases in signal intensity with increasing efforts. Persistent intermediate signal intensity within a distended vessel without change in appearance during the Valsalva maneuvers on single-shot images is consistent with thrombus (Fig. 24-96).

Enlargement of the right gonadal vein during pregnancy is common, particularly during the second and third trimester. It seems to be more common than dilatation of this vein on the left side. This finding has been described previously at laparotomy in pregnant patients with right-sided

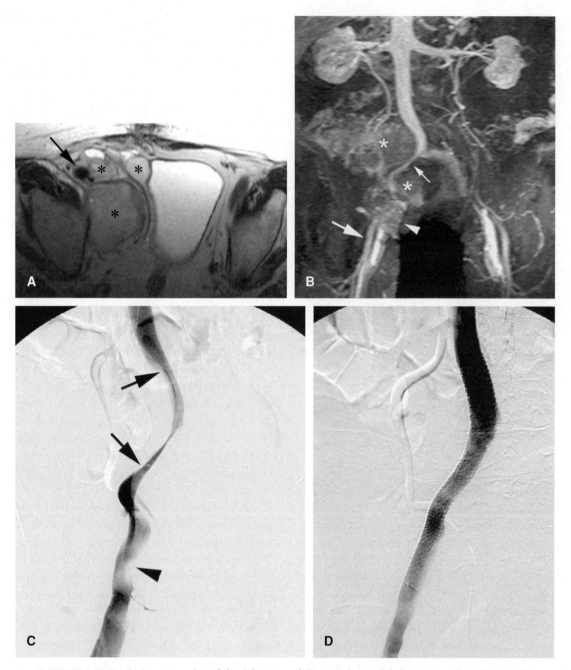

FIGURE 24-93 Extrinsic compression of the right external iliac vein by a pelvic liposarcoma in a 78-year-old patient with recurrent liposarcoma in the pelvis and severe right lower extremity edema. **A:** Axial T2-weighted HASTE image at the level of the lower pelvis shows multiple masses (*), some of which surround the external iliac vessels (*arrow*). **B:** Coronal MIP reconstruction from a subtracted (delayed phase minus arterial phase) acquisition shows extrinsic compression and attenuation of the common iliac vein (*small arrow*) by the heterogeneously enhancing masses (*) in the right pelvis. A portion of the mass extends inferiorly (*white arrowhead*) and obscures the right external iliac vein on this MIP reconstruction, although it was thought to be patent after reviewing the source images. The right common femoral vein (*large arrow*) is widely patent. Based on these findings, the patient was referred for conventional venography instead of receiving treatment with anticoagulation therapy. **C:** Conventional direct iliac venogram in the same patient confirms the presence of extrinsic compression with a smooth impression along the lateral aspect of the common iliac vein (*black arrows*) as well as an additional impression from the more inferior aspect of the mass (*black arrowhead*). No thrombosis was noted. **D:** Conventional direct iliac venogram followed angioplasty and stenting, which relieved the narrowing. The patient's right leg edema subsequently subsided.

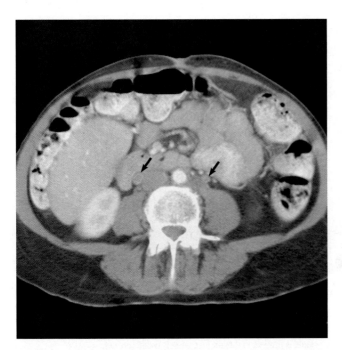

FIGURE 24-94 Bilateral gonadal vein thrombosis following pelvic surgery. Axial CE MDCT image in a patient with recent gynecologic surgery and bilateral ovarian vein thrombophlebitis shows low-attenuation filling defects in both the right and left ovarian veins (*black arrows*).

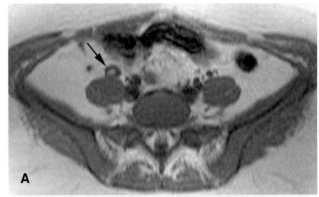

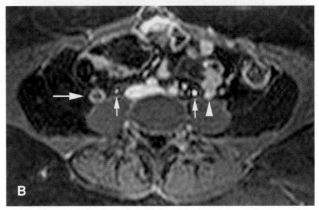

FIGURE 24-95 Unilateral gonadal vein thrombus in a 40-year-old female with prior history of thyroid lymphoma and question of right gonadal vein thrombosis in follow-up CT (not shown). A: Axial T1 GRE image through the mid pelvis shows expansion of the right gonadal vein (*black arrow*), which contains a hyperintense filling defect. **B:** Axial delay phase 3D fat-saturated T1-weighted gradient echo image through the same level shows normal enhancement of the left gonadal vein (*white arrowhead*). There is a hypointense filling defect in the right gonadal vein (*white arrow*), indicating thrombus. Note the high signal intensity in the ureters (*small arrows*) bilaterally from excreted gadolinium. Above the sacral promontory, the ureters are located medial to the gonadal vein and are often useful landmarks for finding the gonadal veins.

abdominal pain and suspected acute appendicitis (237). The ureter can be extrinsically compressed and even obstructed by the right gonadal vein, as has been demonstrated with intravenous urography and retrograde ureteral pyelography in pregnant women with right-sided abdominal pain (238). This has been proposed as the cause for right-sided abdominal pain, the so-called *right ovarian vein syndrome*, in pregnant patients (238,239) (Fig. 24-97). However, it is unclear if this is the only mechanism responsible for the abdominal pain, as a significant number of patients with this finding have no evidence of right hydronephrosis (240). In the authors' experience, enlargement of the right gonadal vein per se may be the cause of the abdominal pain in some of these patients. Rarely, spontaneous rupture of a dilated right ovarian vein causing life-threatening hemorrhage may occur (239,241).

Clinically, pelvic congestion syndrome is a diagnosis of exclusion, with manifestations of chronic pelvic pain. The condition is often exacerbated by prolonged standing, intercourse, or pregnancy, or during menses. The major symptoms are low abdominal pain, dyspareunia or postcoital ache, gluteal or thigh varices, and emotional disturbances (242). Other causes of pelvic pain, including endometriosis, need to be excluded. The pathogenesis is similar to that of

venous varicosities of the lower extremities. Up to 83% of patients have extrinsic compression of the left renal vein between the aorta and the SMA, the so-called *nutcracker phenomenon* (242). Increased pressure in the left renal vein causes congestion and retrograde flow in the left ovarian vein and subsequent development of pelvic varicosities (Figs. 24-98, 24-99). However, the clinical scenario is critical because passive reflux from the left renal vein to the left gonadal vein can occur in asymptomatic women (243).

Bilateral surgical ligation of the gonadal veins, including the use of a laparoscopic transperitoneal para-aortic approach, can help to reduce pelvic congestion syndrome symptoms (244). Transcatheter embolization of the gonadal veins has been proposed as well (242,245). An initial clinical success rate has been reported in 86% of these patients, with a long-term benefit in 75% (242). Transcatheter

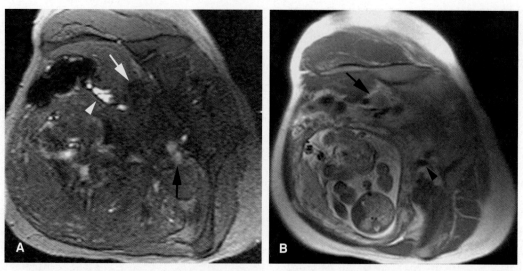

FIGURE 24-96 Left external iliac vein deep vein thrombosis in a 42-year-old pregnant woman with twin pregnancy and left leg swelling after a plane flight. A: Axial TOF image at the level of the iliac bifurcation. The image was acquired with the patient in the right lateral decubitus position to alleviate pressure on the left venous system and with a superior saturation band, nulling signal in the arteries. The normal right internal and external iliac arteries are present as areas of high signal intensity (*black arrow*). No normal flow-related signal is present in the left iliac vessels (*white arrow*), indicating thrombosis. Pelvic collateral veins are present (*white arrowhead*). **B:** Axial HASTE in the same patient shows expansion of the left external iliac vein (*black arrow*), which contains intermediate signal intensity, representing thrombus. Compare with the contralateral normal right external iliac vein (*black arrowhead*), which demonstrates a normal flow void.

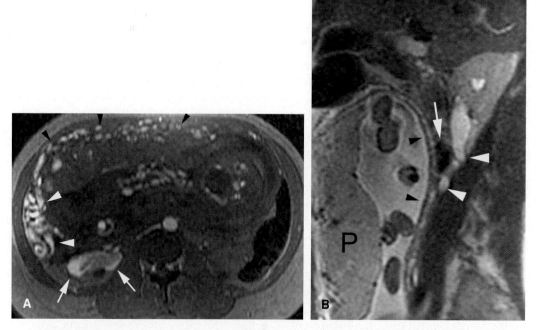

FIGURE 24-97 Gonadal vein varix in a 23-year-old pregnant female, at 32 weeks gestational age, with right upper quadrant pain. A: Axial TOF without a saturation band shows multiple uterine vessels (*black arrowheads*) within the anterior myometrium of the gravid uterus. The appendix was normal (not shown). Multiple dilated veins (*white arrowheads*) are present on the right side of the uterus, which connected to a larger dilated vessel (*white arrows*) that drained superiorly into the IVC, representing a right ovarian vein varix. **B:** Sagittal HASTE in the same patient shows the placenta (*P*) of the gravid uterus. The ovoid area of low signal (*white arrow*) located posterior to the myometrial wall (*black arrowheads*) represents a flow void in the right gonadal vein varix. Note the dilated right renal collecting system and ureter (*white arrowheads*) posterior to the varix. A dilated right ovarian vein, causing right renal obstruction, has been proposed as a cause of acute right lower quadrant pain in pregnant patients.

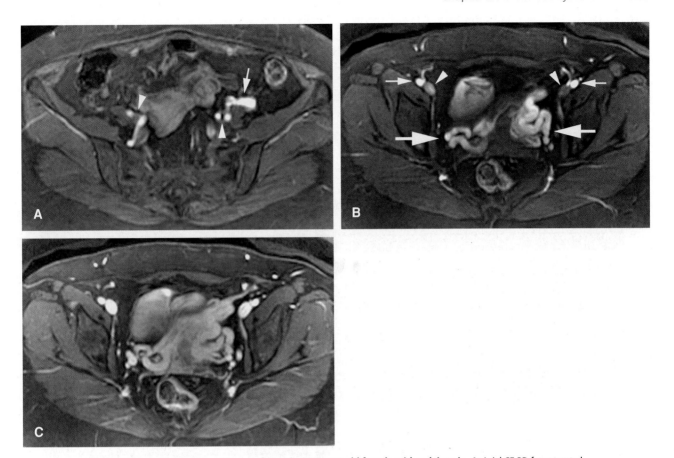

FIGURE 24-98 Pelvic congestion syndrome in a 56-year-old female with pelvic pain. A: Axial CE 3D fat-saturated T1-weighted gradient echo image obtained during the arterial phase through the pelvis shows normal enhancement in the internal and external iliac arteries (*white arrowheads*) without opacification of the iliac veins. Additional tortuous vessels are present on the left (*white arrow*), which connect superiorly with the left gonadal vein (not shown). Note that these vessels demonstrate early arterial enhancement, indicating reflux of enhanced blood from the left renal vein. The fact that blood has refluxed from the left renal vein indicates increased venous pressure. **B:** Axial CE 3D fat-saturated T1-weighted gradient echo image slightly inferior to **(A)** obtained 40 seconds after the arterial peak shows the enhancing external iliac arteries (*small white arrows*) and unopacified veins (*white arrowheads*). There are multiple enhancing collateral veins (*large white arrows*) bilaterally. **C:** Axial CE 3D fat-saturated T1-weighted gradient echo image at the same level as that in **(B)** obtained 90 seconds after the arterial peak shows more complete filling of the asymmetrically enlarged left pelvic collateral veins. There is now wall-to-wall enhancement in the external iliac veins bilaterally. When seen in conjunction with the clinical symptoms of chronic pelvic pain, demonstration of retrograde flow in dilated pelvic veins from the gonadal vein is consistent with pelvic congestion syndrome.

embolization reduces the pain intensity, number of pain attacks, and emotional disturbances (242).

Sonographic findings of pelvic congestion syndrome include left ovarian vein with reversed caudal flow, the presence of varicocele, dilated arcuate veins crossing the uterine myometrium, polycystic changes of the ovary, and variable duplex waveform during the Valsalva maneuver (246). CTV and MRV can demonstrate not only the normal appearance of the ovarian veins in healthy women but also passive reflux from the left renal vein to the left gonadal vein even in asymptomatic women (243,247). As an isolated finding, reflux in the gonadal veins is unlikely to be associated with pelvic congestion syndrome (247). For this reason, this diagnosis should only be made when appropriate clinical history

accompanies the imaging findings (243). Pelvic varices have a characteristic appearance on contrast CT and MR examinations, with tortuous and dilated parauterine and ovarian veins best seen on delayed postcontrast images (248).

The nutcracker syndrome should be considered in women with symptoms of pelvic venous congestion and hematuria (249). Compression of the left renal vein can be readily appreciated on MRI or CT and confirmed by retrograde cine-video-angiography with determination of the renocaval gradients (249). Internal and external renal stenting as well as gonadocaval bypass are effective treatments in patients with nutcracker syndrome (249).

Intravenous leiomyomatosis is a rare condition in which the female pelvic veins are invaded by benign proliferating

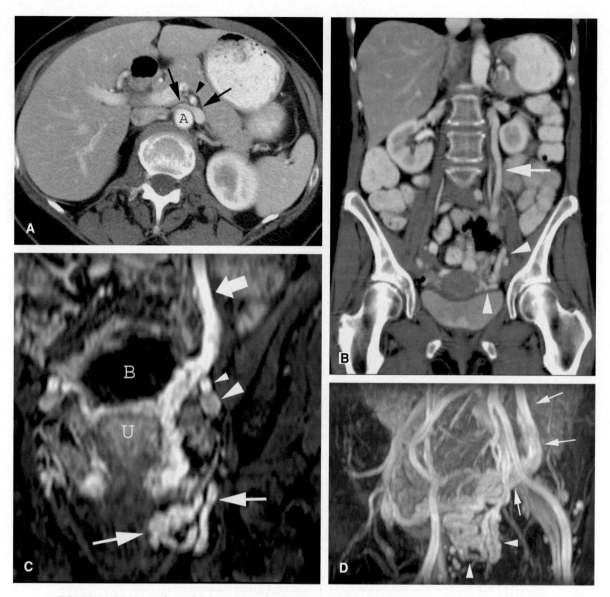

FIGURE 24-99 Nutcracker pelvis in a 60-year-old female with left pelvic pain. A: Axial CE CT image through the mid abdomen obtained during the portal venous phase shows the left renal vein (*black arrows*) being narrowed as it courses between the aorta (*A*) and the SMA (*black arrowhead*). **B:** Coronal reconstructed CT image from same acquisition as that in **(A)** shows a dilated left ovarian vein (*white arrow*), which connected in different images (not shown) with asymmetrically enlarged left pelvic veins (*white arrowheads*). The dilatation of the left gonadal vein is the result of increased venous pressure from the narrowed left renal vein as it courses between the aorta and SMA, the so-called *nutcracker phenomenon*. **C:** Coronal reformatted thin-slab MIP from an axial 3D fat-saturated T1-weighted SPGR acquisition during the late arterial phase in the same patient at the level of the bladder (*B*) and uterus (*U*). Note the differential enhancement between the left external iliac artery (*small arrowhead*) and vein (*large arrowhead*) due to the timing of the acquisition. The left gonadal vein (*thick white arrow*) is dilated and enhances avidly, which confirms retrograde flow from the renal vein. This reconstruction again suggests the connection of the left gonadal vein with the enlarged left uterine veins (*thin white arrow*), which also show early enhancement. **D:** 3D VR oblique reconstruction from same acquisition as that in **(C)** shows the dilated left ovarian vein (*white arrows*) anastomosing with the dilated left uterine veins (*white arrowheads*).

smooth muscle cells (250,251). The smooth muscle cells originate most commonly from uterine leiomyomas but can also rarely arise from the tunica media of the pelvic venous wall itself (251). Up to 25% of cases arise from veins other than the pelvic veins (250,252–254). The proliferating smooth muscle cells can extend throughout the pelvic veins and into the IVC, right atrium, and right ventricle (250).

CE MRI will show enhancing thrombus within the myometrial and pelvic veins, commonly in conjunction with uterine leiomyomas. Prominent vessels may also be obvious on TOF images (Fig. 24-31). IVC involvement (Fig. 24-55) and cranial extension into the heart and right atrium, if present, are important to document. Approximately 30 cases with intracardiac extension of intravenous leiomyomatosis have been reported (250).

The diagnosis should be considered in a females with an intracardiac mass and either a history of uterine fibroids or hysterectomy (251). Occasionally, extension into the pulmonary artery (255) or even pulmonary parenchymal deposits (256) can be found. MR imaging can also be helpful in those patients with large uterine fibroids in whom US findings are equivocal—for example, differentiation of intravenous leiomyomatosis from malignant degeneration of uterine fibroids.

Lower Extremities

Direct spiral CTV of the lower extremities was described in 1994 (257). With this approach, a 22-gauge angiocatheter is placed in the dorsal vein of each foot. Tourniquets placed around each ankle direct flow into the deep veins. Forty milliliters of nonionic contrast with an iodine concentration of 300 mg iodine/mL is diluted with 200 mL saline and then simultaneously injected at 4 mL/second into both legs via a Y-adapter. After a 35-second delay, a 100-cm vol-

ume from the ankles to the IVC is scanned. Immediately following the study, 100 mL of saline is injected into both cannulas to flush contrast material from the veins. The 1994 report used a single-slice helical scanner with a scan duration of 50 seconds. These injection parameters may need to be changed if using a multidetector scanner.

Advantages of this technique over conventional venography include the reduction in contrast material concentration and volume. As Bettmann et al. (18) found a substantially decreased rate of phlebitis when the concentration of contrast was reduced from 60% to 45%, it is reasonable to expect a further decrease when using a 20% concentration. The quality of venous opacification is improved, particularly in the deep femoral veins, pelvic veins, and the IVC. This can lead to the detection of thrombi in these locations that would be missed by conventional venography (19).

Direct CTV has been shown to have high sensitivity and specificity (100% and 92%) when compared with conventional venography (19).

CTV can be performed following a CT pulmonary angiogram (Fig. 24-100) (258). Indirect CTV is attractive for several reasons. It may be offered at a low cost, as it involves no additional contrast administration and only limited extra scanning time, although this assertion has been challenged (259). Direct injection into foot veins is

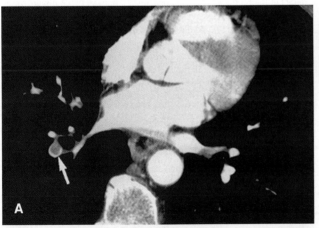
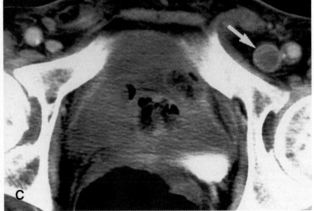
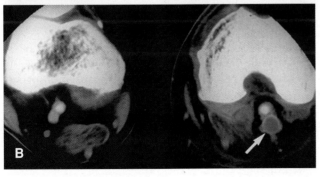

FIGURE 24-100 Transverse CE CT venogram and pulmonary angiogram obtained from a 71-year-old man with pulmonary embolism and deep vein thrombosis. **A:** CT scan obtained at the level of the lower chest shows an embolus in a right lower lobe pulmonary artery (*arrow*). **B:** Venous phase CT scan obtained at the level of the knee shows deep vein thrombosis as a nonenhancing filling defect that expands the left popliteal vein (*arrow*). **C:** CT scan obtained at the inguinal level shows thrombus in the left common femoral vein (*arrow*). (With permission from Loud PA, Katz DS, Bruce DA, et al. Deep venous thrombosis with suspected pulmonary embolism: detection with combined CT venography and pulmonary angiography. *Radiology.* 2001;219:498–502.)

averted. CT might provide a reproducible baseline for follow-up, guide the placement of caval filters, and potentially salvage suboptimal examinations of the chest (260).

Scan timing is not as critical as with CT arteriography, as venous enhancement rises slowly then has a gradual decline (262). Szapiro et al. (128) found that peak enhancement ranged from 93 H to 137 H and occurred from 93 to 147 seconds following injection, depending on the vein. However, qualitative assessment favored scanning at 210 seconds because opacification was more homogeneous (128). Five or 10-mm thick sections were obtained at 4 cm intervals from the diaphragm to the ankles. It was believed but not validated that the increased yield of deep vein thrombosis that might be obtained by contiguous scanning would not justify the increased radiation dose (roughly double) (260). However, recent work suggests that the intervening gaps cause unnecessary false-negative results (optimized image reconstruction for detection of deep venous thrombosis at MD CTV (263). The use of elastic stockings decreases filling of superficial veins, directing blood into the deep veins and increasing their enhancement by 30% to 34% (264).

Findings are more subtle than with direct CTV, as enhancement is less intense. Pitfalls are numerous (265). The most common is an apparent filling defect secondary to inhomogeneous venous opacification (Fig. 24-101). Suboptimal opacification may cause a false-negative examination. Beam-hardening artifacts from orthopedic hardware can obscure visualization of a segment of vein or cause spurious filling defects.

The sensitivity of indirect CTV ranges from 71% to 100%. The specificity ranges from 93% to 100% (259,261,266–269). Of particular interest is the frequency of positive indirect CT venograms in the absence of pulmonary embolism, as these patients should be anticoagulated. Estimates of the frequency of this occurrence range from 2% (270) to 4% (260). Recently, it has been shown that even with the improved sensitivity of MDCT for direct detection of pulmonary embolism, the addition of indirect CTV in this setting increased the diagnosis of venous thromboembolism in 27.4% of patients (271).

The definitive role of indirect CTV requires further investigation. An important concern is the gonadal radiation dose, which is several orders of magnitude higher than with pulmonary CTA alone (272). For scanning younger patients, the radiation dose delivered to the gonads and pelvis has to be accounted for in a decision process that considers CTV. Additionally, there is a financial impact. Peterson and associates (259) found that CTV cost $46.88 more than US, while charges differed by $602.00 (259). Finally, the technique ultimately needs to be validated with outcome data.

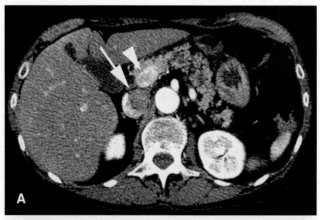

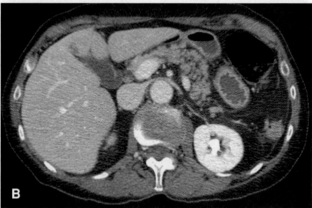

FIGURE 24-101 Mixing artifacts on CT. A: Axial CE CT image obtained during the late arterial phase through the main portal vein shows a large filling defect in the IVC (*white arrow*) and a more subtle, potential filling defect in the portal vein (*white arrowhead*). **B:** Axial CE CT image obtained during the delay venous phase shows normal enhancement in the portal vein and IVC, confirming that both filling defects were caused by mixing of enhanced and unenhanced blood. The confluence of the renal veins and IVC and the portal vein with the splenic vein are common location for mixing artifacts during the late arterial phase. These are the result of mixing early enhancing venous return from the kidneys and the spleen, with unenhanced blood from the infrarenal IVC and SMV, respectively.

Below the inguinal ligament, Doppler US is the preferred modality to evaluate venous patency due to its lower cost and availability. The reported sensitivity and specificity of US to detect venous thrombus in the lower extremity exceed 95% and 98%, respectively (223). Both TOF and gadolinium-enhanced MRV can be performed to evaluate veins as distal as the calf with sensitivity and specificity ranging from 92% to 100% and 94% to 100% compared with both contrast venography and Doppler US (44,54,273). MR evaluation may be necessary in patients where US imaging is inconclusive or if it is limited by hematoma, obesity, or other surgical changes.

Approximately 10% to 20% of patients with clinically suspected DVT will have thrombosis isolated to the veins of the calf (274). Proximal extension of DVT from the calf occurs in at least 20% to 30% of patients with calf vein DVT, which leads to a higher risk of developing clinically important pulmonary embolic events (223). Reported sensitivity and specificity of US for the diagnosis of isolated calf vein thrombosis are very variable, with reported sensitivities as low as 13% (223,275). Moderate discrepancy among US, MRV, and conventional venography examination has also been reported in the diagnosis of calf DVT (276). In patients with a high clinical suspicion, a second modality may be useful if the initial study is negative (276). Gadolinium-enhanced MRV with a dedicated peripheral vascular coil can display the lower extremity veins from the IVC to the tibial veins with image quality comparable to that of the conventional venography examinations (273).

Direct thrombus visualization in the lower extremities is achievable with a T1-weighted magnetization-prepared 3D gradient echo sequence without the need for intravenous contrast administration (277). A water-only excitation radio frequency pulse helps to abolish the fat signal, and the effective inversion time is selected to nullify the blood signal (277). In a prospective blinded study using conventional venography as the gold standard, the sensitivity and specificity of this method for the diagnosis of lower extremity deep vein thrombosis were over 92% and 90%, respectively (277). The sensitivities for isolated calf, femoropopliteal, and ileofemoral deep vein thrombosis were approximately 83% to 92%, 97%, and 100%, respectively (277).

Approximately 50% of patients with previous lower extremity DVT show complete resolution 12 to 24 months after the acute event (223). Valvular insufficiency and venous reflux is not uncommon after DVT. Because saturation bands are typically applied above the imaging slice with TOF imaging in order to eliminate flow signal from the arteries, venous flow may be partially or completely saturated in patients with a history of deep vein thrombosis and venous reflux in the lower extremity veins. CE MRV can be helpful to recognize this situation by demonstrating normal enhancement of the veins on images acquired during the delayed venous phase.

Primary Venous Neoplasms

Primary venous neoplasms are rare entities that consist of leiomyosarcomas, epithelioid hemangioendotheliomas, and vascular leiomyomas. Neoplasms most commonly arise from the large, central veins, and it is more common for a smooth muscle neoplasm to arise from venous walls than from arteries. Most are malignant, and of the three, leiomyosarcoma is the most common. Data is limited, based mostly on small series and case reports.

Leiomyosarcoma is the most common primary venous neoplasm of the vena cava and the second most common

primary adult tumor of retroperitoneal origin (278). It can arise from any vein, but occurs most commonly in the mid-abdominal IVC. As of 1996, there were 218 reported cases of primary leiomyosarcoma of the IVC (279). There is a 5:1 female-to-male predominance, and age at diagnosis is most common in the fifth to seventh decades (280–283).

Three different growth patterns have been reported for retroperitoneal leiomyosarcomas: (a) completely extraluminal (62% of cases), (b) completely intraluminal (5% of cases), and (c) combination intra- and extraluminal (33% of cases)(278). Clinical symptoms are due to venous thrombosis or symptoms from metastasis. Venous leiomyosarcomas spread via expansion and extension up or down the involved vein. Depending on the grade, direct invasion of adjacent structures is possible.

In a series of 25 patients from Memorial Sloan-Kettering Cancer Center, metastatic spread occurred locally (33% of cases), to the liver (29%), and to the lungs (5%) (284). Depending on the portion of the IVC where the leiomyosarcoma arises, there can be obstruction of the hepatic veins with resultant Budd-Chiari syndrome, obstruction of the renal veins, and obstruction of the infrarenal IVC, causing IVC syndrome. Appearance at MRI is that of a heterogeneous signal-intensity soft-tissue retroperitoneal mass, with or without central necrosis. It is common to visualize collateral vessels. Tumors arising from peripheral veins (i.e., extremities) may have similar appearance (Fig. 24-102).

The tumors are usually of high grade but are predominantly slow growing, allowing formation of collateral vessels (285). Due to slow growth and nonspecific clinical symptoms, stage is often advanced at the time of diagnosis, and life expectancy is poor. Size is often greater than 10 cm at the time of diagnosis. Treatment is by wide surgical excision followed by ligation, primary repair and/or patching, or synthetic grafting. Survival is poor, with an average of 3.5 years of survival time (285).

Epithelioid hemangioendotheliomas are extremely rare entities, with 33 cases reported in English-language literature as of 2000 (286). From the limited data, most occur in the lower extremity veins, commonly in the femoral vein (286), but case reports describe SVC involvement (287). There is no male-to-female predominance, and age at diagnosis is variable (286).

The spectrum of individual tumor behavior is varied, but most are slow growing. Approximately 30% of cases develop metastases, most commonly to regional lymph nodes and to the lungs (286). Survival is relatively good, even in the presence of metastatic disease, with a less than 20% mortality rate at 3 to 5 years (286). Imaging studies show a soft tissue mass associated with the vein, which can demonstrate calcification (287).

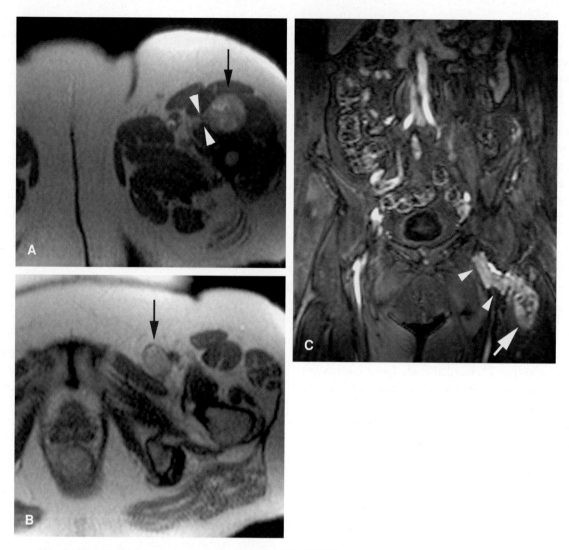

FIGURE 24-102 Thigh leiomyosarcoma. A: Axial T2-weighted HASTE sequence through the proximal thigh shows a heterogenous hyperintense mass (*arrow*) with predominantly well-defined contours. However, a small ill-defined area and outpouching of the mass is seen in its medial aspect (*arrowheads*). **B:** Axial image from the same acquisition as that in **(A)** at a slightly superior level shows intraluminal extension of the mass (*arrow*) in the common femoral vein. **C:** Coronal section from a 3D fat-saturated T1-weighted gradient echo acquisition during the arterial phase shows avid heterogeneous enhancement of the mass (*arrow*). Enhancing tumor thrombus (*arrowheads*) is seen along the common femoral vein. After surgical resection of the mass and the thrombus, histopathologic analysis confirmed leiomyosarcoma with intravascular extension.

Vascular leiomyomas, or angioleiomyomas, are rare, benign tumors that are composed of smooth muscle and vascular endothelium (288–291). Approximately 800 cases have been reported in the English literature (288). Vascular leiomyomas have been postulated to lie in a spectrum of vascular smooth muscle proliferation ranging from hemangiomas to solid leiomyomas (292), while other authors believe that they are hamartomas (291,292). They can occur anywhere in the body, but approximately 89% occur in the extremities (291). Several classification systems have been proposed, dividing vascular leiomyomas into capillary/solid (67%), venous (23%), and cavernous (11%) subtypes (291).

Approximately 60% of vascular leiomyomas present as painful cutaneous masses (289,291). One feature reported as being distinct to vascular leiomyomas is increased lesion size with physical activity, especially if the lesion is in the hand (289). Preoperative diagnosis is rarely correct unless there is a high degree of suspicion (288,289). Surgical excision is curative. Radiographic literature is sparse, and other literature simply reports that vascular leiomyomas appear as a mass on CT (Fig. 24-103), US, and MRI, which can demonstrate calcification (288–290).

Intravascular papillary endothelial hyperplasia (Masson tumor) (IPEH) is characterized by an exuberant endothelial proliferation within the lumen of medium-sized veins (294). This entity, first described by Masson in 1923 as a neoplasm-inducing endothelial proliferation, is now considered to be a reactive vascular proliferation following traumatic vascular stasis (294). The head, neck, fingers, and trunk are more common locations, with some of these lesions rarely reported in the abdomen (294).

Microscopically, tuftlike or papillary proliferation of endothelial cells are present and almost always intimately associated with a thrombus (294). Angiosarcoma is the primary differential diagnosis that must be excluded before the diagnosis of IPEH is made. The following features have been reported in IPEH: (a) well circumscribed or encapsulated, (b) proliferative process limited completely to the intravascular spaces, (c) lack of extreme nuclear atypia and frequent mitotic figures, (d) papillae composed of fibrohyalinized tissue of two or more endothelial cell layers without any covering, (e) lack of true endothelial lining, (f) pseudochannels without irregular and anastomosing blood vessels in the stroma, and (g) lack of necrosis (294).

The diagnosis is typically made after surgical resection of the lesion because the imaging findings in IPEH are not specific. A masslike proliferation adjacent to or within the lumen of a vessel can be seen on cross-sectional imaging examinations (Fig. 24-104). Prior history of major trauma in the anatomic area of the lesion may suggest the diagnosis, but surgical resection is still needed.

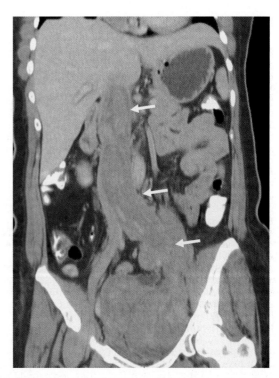

FIGURE 24-103 Vascular leiomyoma in a 49-year-old woman with abdominal discomfort for 1 month. Coronal reformation image shows tumor extension from the left common iliac vein to the IVC (*arrows*). (With permission from Chen BB, Chen CA, Liu KL. Leiomyomatosis with extension to the left gluteal muscle, inferior vena cava, and right atrium. *AJR Am J Roentgenol.* 2006;187:W546–W547.)

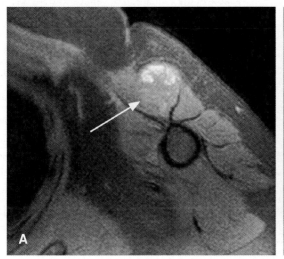
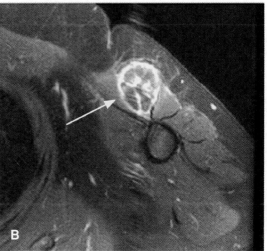

FIGURE 24-104 Intravascular papillary endothelial hyperplasia (Masson tumor) in a 68-year-old woman with a mixed form of IPEH combined with intramuscular hemangioma, cavernous type. A: Fat-suppressed T1-weighted axial image (TR, 533 milliseconds; TE, 9 milliseconds) clearly depicts hyperintense regions associated with thrombi. **B:** Same sequence after gadolinium administration shows enhancement at the periphery and the septalike structure of the mass. (Adapted with permission from Lee SH, Suh JS, Lim BI, et al. Intravascular papillary endothelial hyperplasia of the extremities: MR imaging findings with pathologic correlation. *Eur Radiol.* 2004;14:822–826.)

REFERENCES

1. Kniffin WD Jr, Baron JA, Barrett J, et al. The epidemiology of diagnosed pulmonary embolism and deep venous thrombosis in the elderly. *Arch Intern Med.* 1994;154: 861–866.
2. Kim V, Spandorfer J. Epidemiology of venous thromboembolic disease. *Emerg Med Clin North Am.* 2001;19:839–859.
3. Bernardi E, Piccioli A, Marchiori A, et al. Upper extremity deep vein thrombosis: risk factors, diagnosis, and management. *Semin Vasc Med.* 2001;1:105–110.
4. Godwin JD, Chen JT. Thoracic venous anatomy. *AJR Am J Roentgenol.* 1986;147:674–684.
5. Lawler LP, Corl FM, Fishman EK. Multi-detector row and volume-rendered CT of the normal and accessory flow pathways of the thoracic systemic and pulmonary veins. *Radiographics.* 2002;22[Spec No]:S45–S60.
6. Yeh BM, Coakley FV, Sanchez HC, et al. Azygos arch valves: prevalence and appearance at contrast-enhanced CT. *Radiology.* 2004;230:111–115.
7. Abdulla R, Blew GA, Holterman MJ. Cardiovascular embryology. *Pediatr Cardiol.* 2004;25:191–200.
8. Bass JE, Redwine MD, Kramer LA, et al. Spectrum of congenital anomalies of the inferior vena cava: cross-sectional imaging findings. *Radiographics.* 2000;20:639–652.
9. Minniti S, Visentini S, Procacci C. Congenital anomalies of the venae cavae: embryological origin, imaging features and report of three new variants. *Eur Radiol.* 2002;12: 2040–2055.
10. Zylak CJ, Eyler WR, Spizarny DL, et al. Developmental lung anomalies in the adult: radiologic-pathologic correlation. *Radiographics.* 2002;22[Spec No]:S25–S43.
11. Tak T, Crouch E, Drake GB. Persistent left superior vena cava: incidence, significance and clinical correlates. *Int J Cardiol.* 2002;82:91–93.
12. Gris P, Wilmet B, Benchillal A, et al. [Persistent left superior vena cava. Apropos of 2 cases.] *Rev Pneumol Clin.* 1995;51: 33–35.
13. Gonzalez-Juanatey C, Testa A, Vidan J, et al. Persistent left superior vena cava draining into the coronary sinus: report of 10 cases and literature review. *Clin Cardiol.* 2004;27: 515–518.
14. Metzler B, Hillebrand H, Eulenbruch HP, et al. [Persistent left superior vena cava with right-left shunt into the left atrium.] *Dtsch Med Wochenschr.* 2002;127:83–86.
15. Mornex JF, Brune J, Termet H, et al. [An unusual cause of hypoxia: anastomosis of the right superior vena cava into the left auricle. Surgical correction.] *Rev Fr Mal Respir.* 1983;11:149–155.
16. Marom EM, Herndon JE, Kim YH, et al. Variations in pulmonary venous drainage to the left atrium: implications for radiofrequency ablation. *Radiology.* 2004;230:824–829.
17. Arslan G, Ozkaynak C, Cubuk M, et al. Absence of the azygous vein associated with double superior vena cava—a case report. *Angiology.* 1999;50:81–84.
18. Bettmann MA, Paulin S. Leg phlebography: the incidence, nature and modification of undesirable side effects. *Radiology.* 1977;122:101–104.
19. Baldt MM, Zontsich T, Stumpflen A, et al. Deep venous thrombosis of the lower extremity: efficacy of spiral CT venography compared with conventional venography in diagnosis. *Radiology.* 1996;200:423–428.
20. Marks B, Mitchell DG, Simelaro JP. Breath-holding in healthy and pulmonary-compromised populations: effects of hyperventilation and oxygen inspiration. *J Magn Reson Imaging.* 1997;7:595–597.
21. Miller SW, Holmvang G. Differentiation of slow flow from thrombus in thoracic magnetic resonance imaging, emphasizing phase images. *J Thorac Imaging.* 1993;8: 98–107.
22. Mugler JP 3rd. Overview of MR imaging pulse sequences. *Magn Reson Imaging Clin N Am.* 1999;7:661–697.
23. Bluemke DA, Wolf RL, Tani I, et al. Extremity veins: evaluation with fast-spin-echo MR venography. *Radiology.* 1997;204:562–565.
24. Wright GA, Hu BS, Macovski A. 1991 I.I. Rabi Award. Estimating oxygen saturation of blood in vivo with MR imaging at 1.5 T. *J Magn Reson Imaging.* 1991;1: 275–283.
25. Vogt FM, Herborn CU, Goyen M. MR venography. *Magn Reson Imaging Clin N Am.* 2005;13:vi, 113–129.
26. Saks AM, Paterson FC, Irvine AT, et al. Improved MR venography: use of fast short inversion time inversion-recovery technique in evaluation of venous angiomas. *Radiology.* 1995;194:908–911.
27. Herborn CU, Goyen M, Lauenstein TC, et al. Comprehensive time-resolved MRI of peripheral vascular malformations. *AJR Am J Roentgenol.* 2003;181:729–735.
28. Stemerman DH, Krinsky GA, Lee VS, et al. Thoracic aorta: rapid black-blood MR imaging with half-Fourier rapid acquisition with relaxation enhancement with or without electrocardiographic triggering. *Radiology.* 1999;213: 185–191.
29. Simonetti OP, Finn JP, White RD, et al. "Black blood" T2-weighted inversion-recovery MR imaging of the heart. *Radiology.* 1996;199:49–57.
30. Carr JC, Simonetti O, Bundy J, et al. Cine MR angiography of the heart with segmented true fast imaging with steady-state precession. *Radiology.* 2001;219:828–834.
31. Plein S, Bloomer TN, Ridgway JP, et al. Steady-state free precession magnetic resonance imaging of the heart: comparison with segmented k-space gradient-echo imaging. *J Magn Reson Imaging.* 2001;14:230–236.
32. Pereles FS, McCarthy RM, Baskaran V, et al. Thoracic aortic dissection and aneurysm: evaluation with nonenhanced true FISP MR angiography in less than 4 minutes. *Radiology.* 2002;223:270–274.
33. Carr JC, Nemcek AA Jr, Abecassis M, et al. Preoperative evaluation of the entire hepatic vasculature in living liver donors with use of contrast-enhanced MR angiography and true fast imaging with steady-state precession. *J Vasc Interv Radiol.* 2003;14:441–449.
34. Spuentrup E, Buecker A, Stuber M, et al. MR-venography using high resolution True-FISP. *Rofo.* 2001;173:686–690.
35. Pedrosa I, Morrin M, Oleaga L, et al. Is true FISP imaging reliable in the evaluation of venous thrombosis? *AJR Am J Roentgenol.* 2005;185:1632–1640.
36. Corti R, Osende JI, Fayad ZA, et al. In vivo noninvasive detection and age definition of arterial thrombus by MRI. *J Am Coll Cardiol.* 2002;39:1366–1373.
37. Seelos KC, Funari M, Higgins CB. Detection of aortic arch thrombus using MR imaging. *J Comput Assist Tomogr.* 1991;15:244–247.
38. Dumoulin CL, Hart HR Jr. Magnetic resonance angiography in the head and neck. *Acta Radiol Suppl.* 1986;369:17–20.
39. Keller PJ, Drayer BP, Fram EK, et al. MR angiography with two-dimensional acquisition and three-dimensional display. Work in progress. *Radiology.* 1989;173:527–532.
40. Gao JH, Holland SK, Gore JC. Nuclear magnetic resonance signal from flowing nuclei in rapid imaging using gradient echoes. *Med Phys.* 1988;15:809–814.
41. Laub GA. Time-of-flight method of MR angiography. *Magn Reson Imaging Clin N Am.* 1995;3:391–398.
42. Felmlee JP, Ehman RL. Spatial presaturation: a method for suppressing flow artifacts and improving depiction of vascular anatomy in MR imaging. *Radiology.* 1987;164: 559–564.
43. Edelman RR, Wentz KU, Mattle H, et al. Projection arteriography and venography: initial clinical results with MR. *Radiology.* 1989;172:351–357.
44. Carpenter JP, Holland GA, Baum RA, et al. Magnetic resonance venography for the detection of deep venous thrombosis: comparison with contrast venography and duplex Doppler ultrasonography. *J Vasc Surg.* 1993;18: 734–741.

45. Polak JF, Fox LA. MR assessment of the extremity veins. *Semin Ultrasound CT MR.* 1999;20:36–46.
46. Spritzer CE, Sostman HD, Wilkes DC, et al. Deep venous thrombosis: experience with gradient-echo MR imaging in 66 patients. *Radiology.* 1990;177:235–241.
47. Spritzer CE, Norconk JJ Jr., Sostman HD, et al. Detection of deep venous thrombosis by magnetic resonance imaging. *Chest.* 1993;104:54–60.
48. Dupas B, el Kouri D, Curtet C, et al. Angiomagnetic resonance imaging of iliofemorocaval venous thrombosis. *Lancet.* 1995;346:17–19.
49. Laissy JP, Cinqualbre A, Loshkajian A, et al. Assessment of deep venous thrombosis in the lower limbs and pelvis: MR venography versus duplex Doppler sonography. *AJR Am J Roentgenol.* 1996;167:971–975.
50. Insko EK, Siegelman ES, Stolpen AH. Subacute clot mimicking flow in a thrombosed arterial bypass graft on two-dimensional time-of-flight and three-dimensional contrast-enhanced MRA. *J Magn Reson Imaging.* 2000;11:192–194.
51. Dumoulin CL, Souza SP, Walker MF, et al. Three-dimensional phase contrast angiography. *Magn Reson Med.* 1989;9:139–149.
52. Pelc NJ, Bernstein MA, Shimakawa A, et al. Encoding strategies for three-direction phase-contrast MR imaging of flow. *J Magn Reson Imaging.* 1991;1:405–413.
53. Rofsky NM. MR angiography of the hand and wrist. *Magn Reson Imaging Clin N Am.* 1995;3:345–359.
54. Fraser DG, Moody AR, Davidson IR, et al. Deep venous thrombosis: diagnosis by using venous enhanced subtracted peak arterial MR venography versus conventional venography. *Radiology.* 2003;226:812–820.
55. Rofsky NM, Weinreb JC, Bosniak MA, et al. Renal lesion characterization with gadolinium-enhanced MR imaging: efficacy and safety in patients with renal insufficiency. *Radiology.* 1991;180:85–89.
56. Haustein J, Niendorf HP, Krestin G, et al. Renal tolerance of gadolinium-DTPA/dimeglumine in patients with chronic renal failure. *Invest Radiol.* 1992;27:153–156.
57. Prince MR, Arnoldus C, Frisoli JK. Nephrotoxicity of high-dose gadolinium compared with iodinated contrast. *J Magn Reson Imaging.* 1996;6:162–166.
58. Shinde TS, Lee VS, Rofsky NM, et al. Three-dimensional gadolinium-enhanced MR venographic evaluation of patency of central veins in the thorax: initial experience. *Radiology.* 1999;213:555–560.
59. Marckmann P, Skov L, Rossen K, et al. Nephrogenic systemic fibrosis: suspected causative role of gadodiamide used for contrast-enhanced magnetic resonance imaging. *J Am Soc Nephrol.* 2006;17:2359–2362.
60. Grobner T. Gadolinium—a specific trigger for the development of nephrogenic fibrosing dermopathy and nephrogenic systemic fibrosis? *Nephrol Dial Transplant.* 2006;21:1104–1108.
61. Kuo PH, Kanal E, Abu-Alfa AK, et al. Gadolinium-based MR contrast agents and nephrogenic systemic fibrosis. *Radiology.* 2007;242(3):647–649.
62. Aschauer M, Deutschmann HA, Stollberger R, et al. Value of a blood pool contrast agent in MR venography of the lower extremities and pelvis: preliminary results in 12 patients. *Magn Reson Med.* 2003;50:993–1002.
63. Sharafuddin MJ, Stolpen AH, Dang YM, et al. Comparison of MS-325- and gadodiamide-enhanced MR venography of iliocaval veins. *J Vasc Interv Radiol.* 2002;13:1021–1027.
64. Lebowitz JA, Rofsky NM, Krinsky GA, et al. Gadolinium-enhanced body MR venography with subtraction technique. *AJR Am J Roentgenol.* 1997;169:755–758.
65. Siegelman ES, Charafeddine R, Stolpen AH, et al. Suppression of intravascular signal on fat-saturated contrast-enhanced thoracic MR arteriograms. *Radiology.* 2000;217:115–118.
66. Earls JP, Rofsky NM, DeCorato DR, et al. Breath-hold single-dose gadolinium-enhanced three-dimensional MR aortography: usefulness of a timing examination and MR power injector. *Radiology.* 1996;201:705–710.
67. Li W, David V, Kaplan R, et al. Three-dimensional low dose gadolinium-enhanced peripheral MR venography. *J Magn Reson Imaging.* 1998;8:630–633.
68. Theiss W, Wirtzfeld A, Fink U, et al. The success rate of fibrinolytic therapy in fresh and old thrombosis of the iliac and femoral veins. *Angiology.* 1983;34:61–69.
69. Froehlich JB, Prince MR, Greenfield LJ, et al. "Bull's-eye" sign on gadolinium-enhanced magnetic resonance venography determines thrombus presence and age: a preliminary study. *J Vasc Surg.* 1997;26:809–816.
70. O'Shaughnessy AM, Fitzgerald DE. Determining the stage of organisation and natural history of venous thrombosis using computer analysis. *Int Angiol.* 2000;19:220–227.
71. Geier B, Barbera L, Muth-Werthmann D, et al. Ultrasound elastography for the age determination of venous thrombi. Evaluation in an animal model of venous thrombosis. *Thromb Haemost.* 2005;93:368–374.
72. Zerhouni EA, Barth KH, Siegelman SS. Demonstration of venous thrombosis by computed tomography. *AJR Am J Roentgenol.* 1980;134:753–758.
73. Ghaye B, Szapiro D, Willems V, et al. Pitfalls in CT venography of lower limbs and abdominal veins. *AJR Am J Roentgenol.* 2002;178:1465–1471.
74. Rapoport S, Sostman HD, Pope C, et al. Venous clots: evaluation with MR imaging. *Radiology.* 1987;162:527–530.
75. Spritzer CE, Trotter P, Sostman HD. Deep venous thrombosis: gradient-recalled-echo MR imaging changes over time—experience in 10 patients. *Radiology.* 1998;208:631–639.
76. Macari M, Bosniak MA. Delayed CT to evaluate renal masses incidentally discovered at contrast-enhanced CT: demonstration of vascularity with deenhancement. *Radiology.* 1999;213:674–680.
77. Barkhausen J, Hunold P, Eggebrecht H, et al. Detection and characterization of intracardiac thrombi on MR imaging. *AJR Am J Roentgenol.* 2002;179:1539–1544.
78. Dodd GD 3rd, Memel DS, Baron RL, et al. Portal vein thrombosis in patients with cirrhosis: does sonographic detection of intrathrombus flow allow differentiation of benign and malignant thrombus? *AJR Am J Roentgenol.* 1995;165:573–577.
79. Tublin ME, Dodd GD 3rd, Baron RL. Benign and malignant portal vein thrombosis: differentiation by CT characteristics. *AJR Am J Roentgenol.* 1997;168:719–723.
80. Matsuo M, Kanematsu M, Nishigaki Y, et al. Pseudothrombosis with T2-weighted fast spin-echo MR images caused by static portal venous flow in severe cirrhosis. *J Magn Reson Imaging.* 2002;15:199–202.
81. Hingorani A, Ascher E, Markevich N, et al. Risk factors for mortality in patients with upper extremity and internal jugular deep venous thrombosis. *J Vasc Surg.* 2005;41:476–478.
82. Mamede RC, Resende e Almeida KO, de Mello-Filho FV. Neck mass due to thrombosis of the jugular vein in patients with cancer. *Otolaryngol Head Neck Surg.* 2004;131:968–972.
83. Rozycki GS, Tremblay L, Feliciano DV, et al. A prospective study for the detection of vascular injury in adult and pediatric patients with cervicothoracic seat belt signs. *J Trauma.* 2002;52:618–623; discussion 623–614.
84. Duke BJ, Ryu RK, Brega KE, et al. Traumatic bilateral jugular vein thrombosis: case report and review of the literature. *Neurosurgery.* 1997;41:680–683.
85. Gidley PW, Ghorayeb BY, Stiernberg CM. Contemporary management of deep neck space infections. *Otolaryngol Head Neck Surg.* 1997;116:16–22.
86. Golpe R, Marin B, Alonso M. Lemierre's syndrome (necrobacillosis). *Postgrad Med J.* 1999;75:141–144.
87. Screaton NJ, Ravenel JG, Lehner PJ, et al. Lemierre syndrome: forgotten but not extinct—report of four cases. *Radiology.* 1999;213:369–374.

88. Chirinos JA, Lichtstein DM, Garcia J, et al. The evolution of Lemierre syndrome: report of 2 cases and review of the literature. *Medicine (Baltimore)*. 2002;81:458–465.

89. Urschel HC Jr, Razzuk MA. Neurovascular compression in the thoracic outlet: changing management over 50 years. *Ann Surg*. 1998;228:609–617.

90. Adelman MA, Stone DH, Riles TS, et al. A multidisciplinary approach to the treatment of Paget-Schroetter syndrome. *Ann Vasc Surg*. 1997;11:149–154.

91. Prandoni P, Polistena P, Bernardi E, et al. Upper-extremity deep vein thrombosis. Risk factors, diagnosis, and complications. *Arch Intern Med*. 1997;157:57–62.

92. Pedrosa I, Aschkenasi C, Hamdan A, et al. Effort-induced thrombosis: diagnosis with three-dimensional MR venography. *Emerg Radiol*. 2002;9:326–328.

93. Urschel HC, Patel A. Thoracic outlet syndromes. *Curr Treat Options Cardiovasc Med*. 2003;5:163–168.

94. Demondion X, Bacqueville E, Paul C, et al. Thoracic outlet: assessment with MR imaging in asymptomatic and symptomatic populations. *Radiology*. 2003;227:461–468.

95. Marinella MA, Kathula SK, Markert RJ. Spectrum of upper-extremity deep venous thrombosis in a community teaching hospital. *Heart Lung*. 2000;29:113–117.

96. Gonsalves CF, Eschelman DJ, Sullivan KL, et al. Incidence of central vein stenosis and occlusion following upper extremity PICC and port placement. *Cardiovasc Intervent Radiol*. 2003;26:123–127.

97. Martinelli I, Battaglioli T, Bucciarelli P, et al. Risk factors and recurrence rate of primary deep vein thrombosis of the upper extremities. *Circulation*. 2004;110:566–570.

98. Joffe HV, Kucher N, Tapson VF, et al. Upper-extremity deep vein thrombosis: a prospective registry of 592 patients. *Circulation*. 2004;110:1605–1611.

99. Prandoni P, Bernardi E. Upper extremity deep vein thrombosis. *Curr Opin Pulm Med*. 1999;5:222–226.

100. Kroencke TJ, Taupitz M, Arnold R, et al. Three-dimensional gadolinium-enhanced magnetic resonance venography in suspected thrombo-occlusive disease of the central chest veins. *Chest*. 2001;120:1570–1576.

101. Butty S, Hagspiel KD, Leung DA, et al. Body MR venography. *Radiol Clin North Am*. 2002;40:899–919.

102. Yedlicka JW, Schultz K, Moncada R, et al. CT findings in superior vena cava obstruction. *Semin Roentgenol*. 1989;24:84–90.

103. Ishikawa T, Clark RA, Tokuda M, et al. Focal contrast enhancement on hepatic CT in superior vena caval and brachiocephalic vein obstruction. *AJR Am J Roentgenol*. 1983;140:337–338.

104. Maldjian PD, Obolevich AT, Cho KC. Focal enhancement of the liver on CT: a sign of SVC obstruction. *J Comput Assist Tomogr*. 1995;19:316–318.

105. White CS. MR imaging of thoracic veins. *Magn Reson Imaging Clin N Am*. 2000;8:17–32.

106. Chasen M, Charnsangavej C. Venous chest anatomy: clinical implications. In: *RSNA Categorical Course in Diagnostic Radiology: Chest Radiology* ; 1992.

107. Engel IA, Auh YH, Rubenstein WA, et al. CT diagnosis of mediastinal and thoracic inlet venous obstruction. *AJR Am J Roentgenol*. 1983;141:521–526.

108. Gosselin MV, Rubin GD. Altered intravascular contrast material flow dynamics: clues for refining thoracic CT diagnosis. *AJR Am J Roentgenol*. 1997;169:1597–1603.

109. Wilson ES. Systemic to pulmonary venous communication in the superior vena caval syndrome. *AJR Am J Roentgenol*. 1976;127:247–249.

110. Stockberger SM, West KW, Cohen MD. Right-to-left shunt from systemic venous to pulmonary venous system developing after SVC obstruction. *J Comput Assist Tomogr*. 1995;19:312–315.

111. Hartnell GG, Hughes LA, Longmaid HE, et al. Body magnetic resonance angiography and its effect on the use of alternative imaging—experience in 1026 patients. *Br J Radiol*. 1995;68:963–969.

112. Thornton MJ, Ryan R, Varghese JC, et al. A three-dimensional gadolinium-enhanced MR venography technique for imaging central veins. *AJR Am J Roentgenol*. 1999;173:999–1003.

113. Escalante CP. Causes and management of superior vena cava syndrome. *Oncology* (Williston Park). 1993;7:61–68; discussion 71–72, 75–77.

114. Parish JM, Marschke RF Jr, Dines DE, et al. Etiologic considerations in superior vena cava syndrome. *Mayo Clin Proc*. 1981;56:407–413.

115. Urschel HC Jr, Razzuk MA, Netto GJ, et al. Sclerosing mediastinitis: improved management with histoplasmosis titer and ketoconazole. *Ann Thorac Surg*. 1990;50:215–221.

116. Prasad SK, Soukias N, Hornung T, et al. Role of magnetic resonance angiography in the diagnosis of major aortopulmonary collateral arteries and partial anomalous pulmonary venous drainage. *Circulation*. 2004;109:207–214.

117. Haissaguerre M, Jais P, Shah DC, et al. Spontaneous initiation of atrial fibrillation by ectopic beats originating in the pulmonary veins. *N Engl J Med*. 1998;339:659–666.

118. Gandhi AK, Pearson AC, Orsinelli DA. Tumor invasion of the pulmonary veins: a unique source of systemic embolism detected by transesophageal echocardiography. *J Am Soc Echocardiogr*. 1995;8:97–99.

119. Mansour KA, Malone CE, Craver JM. Left atrial tumor embolization during pulmonary resection: review of literature and report of two cases. *Ann Thorac Surg*. 1988;46:455–456.

120. Dore R, Alerci M, D'Andrea F, et al. Intracardiac extension of lung cancer via pulmonary veins: CT diagnosis. *J Comput Assist Tomogr*. 1988;12:565–568.

121. Tassan S, Chabert JP, Tassigny C, et al. [Peripheral embolic arterial accident due to pulmonary vein thrombosis revealing bronchial carcinoma.] *Ann Cardiol Angeiol (Paris)*. 1998;47:11–13.

122. Pitman AG, Solomon B, Padmanabhan R, et al. Intravenous extension of lung carcinoma to the left atrium: demonstration by positron emission tomography with CT correlation. *Br J Radiol*. 2000;73:206–208.

123. Takahashi K, Furuse M, Hanaoka H, et al. Pulmonary vein and left atrial invasion by lung cancer: assessment by breath-hold gadolinium-enhanced three-dimensional MR angiography. *J Comput Assist Tomogr*. 2000;24:557–561.

124. Yi ES. Tumors of the pulmonary vasculature. *Cardiol Clin*. 2004;22:vi–vii, 431–440.

125. Oliai BR, Tazelaar HD, Lloyd RV, et al. Leiomyosarcoma of the pulmonary veins. *Am J Surg Pathol*. 1999;23:1082–1088.

126. Geehan D. Inferior Vena Caval Thrombosis. http// www.emedicine.com/MED/topic2718.htm, accessed March, 2007.

127. Sosa RE, Muecke EC, Vaughan ED Jr, et al. Renal cell carcinoma extending into the inferior vena cava: the prognostic significance of the level of vena caval involvement. *J Urol*. 1984;132:1097–1100.

128. Szapiro D, Ghaye B, Willems V, et al. Evaluation of CT time-density curves of lower-limb veins. *Invest Radiol*. 2001;36:164–169.

129. Vaidya A, Ciancio G, Soloway M. Surgical techniques for treating a renal neoplasm invading the inferior vena cava. *J Urol*. 2003;169:435–444.

130. Rubio-Briones J, Palou Redorta J, Salvador Bayarri J, et al. Incidentally detected renal angiomyolipoma with tumour thrombus into the inferior vena cava. *Scand J Urol Nephrol*. 1997;31:189–191.

131. Oh SJ, Lim DJ, Cho JY, et al. Squamous cell carcinoma of the renal pelvis with invasion of the infradiaphragmatic inferior vena cava. *Br J Urol*. 1998;82:918–919.

132. Semelka RC, Shoenut JP, Magro CM, et al. Renal cancer staging: comparison of contrast-enhanced CT and gadolinium-enhanced fat-suppressed spin-echo and gradient-echo MR imaging. *J Magn Reson Imaging*. 1993;3:597–602.

133. Chang JY, Ka WS, Chao TY, et al. Hepatocellular carcinoma with intra-atrial tumor thrombi. A report of three cases

responsive to thalidomide treatment and literature review. *Oncology*. 2004;67:320–326.

134. Wallace MJ. Transatrial stent placement for treatment of inferior vena cava obstruction secondary to extension of intracardiac tumor thrombus from hepatocellular carcinoma. *J Vasc Interv Radiol*. 2003;14:1339–1343.

135. Sarmiento JM, Bower TC, Cherry KJ, et al. Is combined partial hepatectomy with segmental resection of inferior vena cava justified for malignancy? *Arch Surg*. 2003;138:624–630; discussion 630–631.

136. Belis JA, Pae WE Jr, Rohner TJ Jr, et al. Cardiovascular evaluation before circulatory arrest for removal of vena caval extension of renal carcinoma. *J Urol*. 1989;141:1302–1307.

137. Yogita S, Tashiro S, Harada M, et al. Hepatocellular carcinoma with extension into the right atrium: report of a successful liver resection by hepatic vascular exclusion using cardiopulmonary bypass. *J Med Invest*. 2000;47:155–160.

138. Jeffrey RB Jr, Federle MP. The collapsed inferior vena cava: CT evidence of hypovolemia. *AJR Am J Roentgenol*. 1988;150:431–432.

139. Mirvis SE, Shanmuganathan K, Erb R. Diffuse small-bowel ischemia in hypotensive adults after blunt trauma (shock bowel): CT findings and clinical significance. *AJR Am J Roentgenol*. 1994;163:1375–1379.

140. Eisenstat RS, Whitford AC, Lane MJ, et al. The "flat cava" sign revisited: what is its significance in patients without trauma? *AJR Am J Roentgenol*. 2002;178:21–25.

141. Hewett JJ, Freed KS, Sheafor DH, et al. The spectrum of abdominal venous CT findings in blunt trauma. *AJR Am J Roentgenol*. 2001;176:955–958.

142. Milliken J. IVC injuries. *J Trauma*. 1983;23:207–212.

143. Sheafor DH, Foti TM, Vaslef SN, et al. Fat in the inferior vena cava associated with caval injury. *AJR Am J Roentgenol*. 1998;171:181–182.

144. Han BK, Im JG, Jung JW, et al. Pericaval fat collection that mimics thrombosis of the inferior vena cava: demonstration with use of multi-directional reformation CT. *Radiology*. 1997;203:105–108.

145. Gradman WS, Steinberg F. Aneurysm of the inferior vena cava: case report and review of the literature. *Ann Vasc Surg*. 1993;7:347–353.

146. Chaib E, Ribeiro MA Jr, Saad WA, et al. The main hepatic anatomic variations for the purpose of split-liver transplantation. *Transplant Proc*. 2005;37:1063–1066.

147. Poletti PA, Mirvis SE, Shanmuganathan K, et al. CT criteria for management of blunt liver trauma: correlation with angiographic and surgical findings. *Radiology*. 2000;216:418–427.

148. Yeh BM, Kurzman P, Foster E, et al. Clinical relevance of retrograde inferior vena cava or hepatic vein opacification during contrast-enhanced CT. *AJR Am J Roentgenol*. 2004;183:1227–1232.

149. Mathieu D, Vasile N, Menu Y, et al. Budd-Chiari syndrome: dynamic CT. *Radiology*. 1987;165:409–413.

150. Erden A, Erden I, Karayalcin S, et al. Budd-Chiari syndrome: evaluation with multiphase contrast-enhanced three-dimensional MR angiography. *AJR Am J Roentgenol*. 2002;179:1287–1292.

151. Brancatelli G, Federle MP, Grazioli L, et al. Benign regenerative nodules in Budd-Chiari syndrome and other vascular disorders of the liver: radiologic-pathologic and clinical correlation. *Radiographics*. 2002;22:847–862.

152. Morrin MM, Pedrosa I, Rofsky NM. Magnetic resonance imaging for disorders of liver vasculature. *Top Magn Reson Imaging*. 2002;13:177–190.

153. Hommeyer SC, Teefey SA, Jacobson AF, et al. Venocclusive disease of the liver: prospective study of US evaluation. *Radiology*. 1992;184:683–686.

154. van den Bosch MA, van Hoe L. MR imaging findings in two patients with hepatic veno-occlusive disease following bone marrow transplantation. *Eur Radiol*. 2000;10:1290–1293.

155. Stark DD, Hahn PF, Trey C, et al. MRI of the Budd-Chiari syndrome. *AJR Am J Roentgenol*. 1986;146:1141–1148.

156. Noone TC, Semelka RC, Siegelman ES, et al. Budd-Chiari syndrome: spectrum of appearances of acute, subacute, and chronic disease with magnetic resonance imaging. *J Magn Reson Imaging*. 2000;11:44–50.

157. Vilgrain V, Lewin M, Vons C, et al. Hepatic nodules in Budd-Chiari syndrome: imaging features. *Radiology*. 1999;210:443–450.

158. Rha SE, Lee MG, Lee YS, et al. Nodular regenerative hyperplasia of the liver in Budd-Chiari syndrome: CT and MR features. *Abdom Imaging*. 2000;25:255–258.

159. Kashyap AS, Kashyap S. Hepatocellular carcinoma. *Lancet*. 1999;354:253.

160. Erbay N, Raptopoulos V, Pomfret EA, et al. Living donor liver transplantation in adults: vascular variants important in surgical planning for donors and recipients. *AJR Am J Roentgenol*. 2003;181:109–114.

161. Sahani D, Saini S, Pena C, et al. Using multidetector CT for preoperative vascular evaluation of liver neoplasms: technique and results. *AJR Am J Roentgenol*. 2002;179:53–59.

162. Satyapal KS, Rambiritch V, Pillai G. Morphometric analysis of the renal veins. *Anat Rec*. 1995;241:268–272.

163. Satyapal KS, Rambiritch V, Pillai G. Additional renal veins: incidence and morphometry. *Clin Anat*. 1995;8:51–55.

164. Satyapal KS, Kalideen JM. Absence of renal vein valves in humans and baboons. *Ann Anat*. 1996;178:481–484.

165. Satyapal KS, Kalideen JM, Haffejee AA, et al. Left renal vein variations. *Surg Radiol Anat*. 1999;21:77–81.

166. Trigaux JP, Vandroogenbroek S, De Wispelaere JF, et al. Congenital anomalies of the inferior vena cava and left renal vein: evaluation with spiral CT. *J Vasc Interv Radiol*. 1998;9:339–345.

167. Baldridge ED Jr, Canos AJ. Venous anomalies encountered in aortoiliac surgery. *Arch Surg*. 1987;122:1184–1188.

168. Aljabri B, MacDonald PS, Satin R, et al. Incidence of major venous and renal anomalies relevant to aortoiliac surgery as demonstrated by computed tomography. *Ann Vasc Surg*. 2001;15:615–618.

169. Lin CH, Steinberg AP, Ramani AP, et al. Laparoscopic live donor nephrectomy in the presence of circumaortic or retroaortic left renal vein. *J Urol*. 2004;171:44–46.

170. Mitty HA. Circumaortic renal collar. A potentially hazardous anomaly of the left renal vein. *Am J Roentgenol Radium Ther Nucl Med*. 1975;125:307–310.

171. Kawamoto S, Lawler LP, Fishman EK. Evaluation of the renal venous system on late arterial and venous phase images with MDCT angiography in potential living laparoscopic renal donors. *AJR Am J Roentgenol*. 2005;184:539–545.

172. Scatarige JC, Horton KM, Ratner LE, et al. Left adrenal vein localization by 3D real-time volume-rendering CTA before laparoscopic nephrectomy in living renal donors. *Abdom Imaging*. 2001;26:553–556.

173. Jeong JY, Kim SH, Lee HJ, et al. Atypical low-signal-intensity renal parenchyma: causes and patterns. *Radiographics*. 2002;22:833–846.

174. Tempany CM, Morton RA, Marshall FF. MRI of the renal veins: assessment of nonneoplastic venous thrombosis. *J Comput Assist Tomogr*. 1992;16:929–934.

175. Brezis M, Rosen S, Silva P, et al. Renal ischemia: a new perspective. *Kidney Int*. 1984;26:375–383.

176. Geiger J, Fong Q, Fay R. Transitional cell carcinoma of renal pelvis with invasion of renal vein and thrombosis of subhepatic inferior vena cava. *Urology*. 1986;28:52–54.

177. Gollub MJ, Bosniak MA, Schlossberg P, et al. Extension of a secondary adrenal neoplasm into the inferior vena cava. *Abdom Imaging*. 1994;19:359–360.

178. Ojo AO, Hanson JA, Wolfe RA, et al. Dialysis modality and the risk of allograft thrombosis in adult renal transplant recipients. *Kidney Int*. 1999;55:1952–1960.

179. Galmes I, Burgos FJ, Borrego J, et al. [Vascular complications in renal transplantation.] *Actas Urol Esp*. 1995;19:8–14.

180. Giustacchini P, Pisanti F, Citterio F, et al. Renal vein thrombosis after renal transplantation: an important cause of graft loss. *Transplant Proc.* 2002;34:2126–2127.

181. Voiculescu A, Pfeiffer T, Brause M, et al. Acute pain over the kidney graft and Duplex-sonographic findings mimicking complete renal transplant vein thrombosis. *Nephrol Dial Transplant.* 2002;17:2268–2269.

182. Grenier N, Douws C, Morel D, et al. Detection of vascular complications in renal allografts with color Doppler flow imaging. *Radiology.* 1991;178:217–223.

183. Goyal AK, Pokharna DS, Sharma SK. Ultrasonic measurements of portal vasculature in diagnosis of portal hypertension. A controversial subject reviewed. *J Ultrasound Med.* 1990;9:45–48.

184. Lee VS, Morgan GR, Lin JC, et al. Liver transplant donor candidates: associations between vascular and biliary anatomic variants. *Liver Transpl.* 2004;10:1049–1054.

185. Kernagis LY, Levine MS, Jacobs JE. Pneumatosis intestinalis in patients with ischemia: correlation of CT findings with viability of the bowel. *AJR Am J Roentgenol.* 2003;180:733–736.

186. Wiesner W, Mortele KJ, Glickman JN, et al. Pneumatosis intestinalis and portomesenteric venous gas in intestinal ischemia: correlation of CT findings with severity of ischemia and clinical outcome. *AJR Am J Roentgenol.* 2001;177:1319–1323.

187. Iannitti DA, Gregg SC, Mayo-Smith WW, et al. Portal venous gas detected by computed tomography: is surgery imperative? *Dig Surg.* 2003;20:306–315.

188. Bradbury MS, Kavanagh PV, Bechtold RE, et al. Mesenteric venous thrombosis: diagnosis and noninvasive imaging. *Radiographics.* 2002;22:527–541.

189. Sobhonslidsuk A, Reddy KR. Portal vein thrombosis: a concise review. *Am J Gastroenterol.* 2002;97:535–541.

190. Condat B, Pessione F, Helene Denninger M, et al. Recent portal or mesenteric venous thrombosis: increased recognition and frequent recanalization on anticoagulant therapy. *Hepatology.* 2000;32:466–470.

191. Itai Y, Ohtomo K, Kokubo T, et al. Segmental intensity differences in the liver on MR images: a sign of intrahepatic portal flow stoppage. *Radiology.* 1988;167:17–19.

192. Schlund JF, Semelka RC, Kettritz U, et al. Transient increased segmental hepatic enhancement distal to portal vein obstruction on dynamic gadolinium-enhanced gradient echo MR images. *J Magn Reson Imaging.* 1995;5:375–377.

193. Yu JS, Rofsky NM. Magnetic resonance imaging of arterioportal shunts in the liver. *Top Magn Reson Imaging.* 2002;13:165–176.

194. Henseler KP, Pozniak MA, Lee FT Jr, et al. Three-dimensional CT angiography of spontaneous portosystemic shunts. *Radiographics.* 2001;21:691–704.

195. Bookstein JJ, Cho KJ, Davis GB, et al. Arterioportal communications: observations and hypotheses concerning transsinusoidal and transvasal types. *Radiology.* 1982;142:581–590.

196. Collini FJ, Brener B. Portal hypertension. *Surg Gynecol Obstet.* 1990;170:177–192.

197. Lebrec D, De Fleury P, Rueff B, et al. Portal hypertension, size of esophageal varices, and risk of gastrointestinal bleeding in alcoholic cirrhosis. *Gastroenterology.* 1980;79:1139–1144.

198. Wind P, Alves A, Chevallier JM, et al. Anatomy of spontaneous splenorenal and gastrorenal venous anastomoses. Review of the literature. *Surg Radiol Anat.* 1998;20:129–134.

199. Ohnishi K, Sato S, Saito M, et al. Clinical and portal hemodynamic features in cirrhotic patients having a large spontaneous splenorenal and/or gastrorenal shunt. *Am J Gastroenterol.* 1986;81:450–455.

200. Naik KS, Ward J, Irving HC, et al. Comparison of dynamic contrast enhanced MRI and Doppler ultrasound in the preoperative assessment of the portal venous system. *Br J Radiol.* 1997;70:43–49.

201. Jin B, Sun Y, Li YQ, et al. Extrahepatic portal vein aneurysm: two case reports of surgical intervention. *World J Gastroenterol.* 2005;11:2206–2209.

202. Gallagher DM, Leiman S, Hux CH. In utero diagnosis of a portal vein aneurysm. *J Clin Ultrasound.* 1993;21:147–151.

203. Glazer S, Gaspar MR, Esposito V, et al. Extrahepatic portal vein aneurysm: report of a case treated by thrombectomy and aneurysmorrhaphy. *Ann Vasc Surg.* 1992;6:338–343.

204. Thomas TV. Aneurysm of the portal vein: report of two cases, one resulting in thrombosis and spontaneous rupture. *Surgery.* 1967;61:550–555.

205. Brock PA, Jordan PH Jr, et al. Portal vein aneurysm: a rare but important vascular condition. *Surgery.* 1997;121:105–108.

206. Ohnami Y, Ishida H, Konno K, et al. Portal vein aneurysm: report of six cases and review of the literature. *Abdom Imaging.* 1997;22:281–286.

207. Berrocal T, Lamas M, Gutieerrez J, et al. Congenital anomalies of the small intestine, colon, and rectum. *Radiographics.* 1999;19:1219–1236.

208. Rhee RY, Gloviczki P. Mesenteric venous thrombosis. *Surg Clin North Am.* 1997;77:327–338.

209. Rhee RY, Gloviczki P, Mendonca CT, et al. Mesenteric venous thrombosis: still a lethal disease in the 1990s. *J Vasc Surg.* 1994;20:688–697.

210. Deron J, Russell A. Mesenteric venous thrombosis. http://www.emedicine.com/med/topic2753.htm, accessed December, 2006.

211. Kreft B, Strunk H, Flacke S, et al. Detection of thrombosis in the portal venous system: comparison of contrast-enhanced MR angiography with intraarterial digital subtraction angiography. *Radiology.* 2000;216:86–92.

212. Kumar S, Sarr MG, Kamath PS. Mesenteric venous thrombosis. *N Engl J Med.* 2001;345:1683–1688.

213. Warshauer DM, Lee JK, Mauro MA, et al. Superior mesenteric vein thrombosis with radiologically occult cause: a retrospective study of 43 cases. *AJR Am J Roentgenol.* 2001;177:837–841.

214. Klein HM, Klosterhalfen B, Kinzel S, et al. CT and MRI of experimentally induced mesenteric ischemia in a porcine model. *J Comput Assist Tomogr.* 1996;20:254–261.

215. Chan FP, Li KC, Heiss SG, et al. A comprehensive approach using MR imaging to diagnose acute segmental mesenteric ischemia in a porcine model. *AJR Am J Roentgenol.* 1999;173:523–529.

216. Li KC, Pelc LR, Puvvala S, Wright GA. Mesenteric ischemia due to hemorrhagic shock: MR imaging diagnosis and monitoring in a canine model. *Radiology.* 1998;206:219–225.

217. Burkart DJ, Johnson CD, Reading CC, et al. MR measurements of mesenteric venous flow: prospective evaluation in healthy volunteers and patients with suspected chronic mesenteric ischemia. *Radiology.* 1995;194:801–806.

218. Burkart DJ, Johnson CD, Ehman RL. Correlation of arterial and venous blood flow in the mesenteric system based on MR findings. 1993 ARRS Executive Council Award. *AJR Am J Roentgenol.* 1993;161:1279–1282.

219. Holsinger AE, Wright RC, Riederer SJ, et al. Real-time interactive magnetic resonance imaging. *Magn Reson Med.* 1990;14:547–553.

220. Heider TR, Azeem S, Galanko JA, et al. The natural history of pancreatitis-induced splenic vein thrombosis. *Ann Surg.* 2004;239:876–880; discussion 880–882.

221. Petit P, Bret P, Atri M, et al. Splenic vein thrombosis after splenectomy: frequency and role of imaging. *Radiology.* 1994;190:65–68.

222. Volturo GA, Repeta RJ Jr. Non-lower extremity deep vein thrombosis. *Emerg Med Clin North Am.* 2001;19:vi, 877–893.

223. Fraser JD, Anderson DR. Deep venous thrombosis: recent advances and optimal investigation with US. *Radiology.* 1999;211:9–24.

224. Ginsberg JS, Brill-Edwards P, Burrows RF, et al. Venous thrombosis during pregnancy: leg and trimester of presentation. *Thromb Haemost.* 1992;67:519–520.

225. Stern JB, Abehsera M, Grenet D, et al. Detection of pelvic vein thrombosis by magnetic resonance angiography in patients with acute pulmonary embolism and normal lower limb compression ultrasonography. *Chest.* 2002;122:115–121.

226. Kibbe MR, Ujiki M, Goodwin AL, et al. Iliac vein compression in an asymptomatic patient population. *J Vasc Surg.* 2004;39:937–943.

227. Kwak HS, Han YM, Lee YS, et al. Stents in common iliac vein obstruction with acute ipsilateral deep venous thrombosis: early and late results. *J Vasc Interv Radiol.* 2005;16:815–822.

228. Mullens W, De Keyser J, Van Dorpe A, et al. Migration of two venous stents into the right ventricle in a patient with May-Thurner syndrome. *Int J Cardiol.* 2006;110:114–115.

229. Coon WW. Epidemiology of venous thromboembolism. *Ann Surg.* 1977;186:149–164.

230. Treffers PE, Huidekoper BL, Weenink GH, et al. Epidemiological observations of thrombo-embolic disease during pregnancy and in the puerperium, in 56,022 women. *Int J Gynaecol Obstet.* 1983;21:327–331.

231. Kierkegaard A. Incidence and diagnosis of deep vein thrombosis associated with pregnancy. *Acta Obstet Gynecol Scand.* 1983;62:239–243.

232. Danilenko-Dixon DR, Heit JA, Silverstein MD, et al. Risk factors for deep vein thrombosis and pulmonary embolism during pregnancy or post partum: a population-based, case-control study. *Am J Obstet Gynecol.* 2001;184:104–110.

233. Quarello E, Desbriere R, Hartung O, et al. [Postpartum ovarian vein thrombophlebitis: report of 5 cases and review of the literature.] *J Gynecol Obstet Biol Reprod (Paris).* 2004;33:430–440.

234. Nagayama M, Watanabe Y, Okumura A, et al. Fast MR imaging in obstetrics. *Radiographics.* 2002;22:563–580; discussion 580–582.

235. Smith MD, Felker RE, Emerson DS, et al. Sonographic visualization of ovarian veins during the puerperium: an assessment of efficacy. *Am J Obstet Gynecol.* 2002;186:893–895.

236. Kubik-Huch RA, Hebisch G, Huch R, et al. Role of duplex color Doppler ultrasound, computed tomography, and MR angiography in the diagnosis of septic puerperal ovarian vein thrombosis. *Abdom Imaging.* 1999;24:85–91.

237. Ameur A, Lezrek M, Boumdin H, et al. [Right ovarian vein syndrome: report of a case and review of the literature.] *Ann Urol (Paris).* 2002;36:368–371.

238. Arvis G. [Right ovarian vein syndrome.] *Ann Urol (Paris).* 1985;19:65–66.

239. Renuka T, Dhaliwal LK, Gupta I. Hemorrhage from ruptured utero-ovarian veins during pregnancy. *Int J Gynaecol Obstet.* 1998;60:167–168.

240. Pedrosa I, Levine D, Eyvazzadeh AD, et al. MR imaging evaluation of acute appendicitis in pregnancy. *Radiology.* 2006;238:891–899.

241. Foley MR, Sonek JD, Lavender LM, et al. Spontaneous rupture of uteroovarian veins in pregnancy: two case reports. *Am J Obstet Gynecol.* 1987;156:962–964.

242. d'Archambeau O, Maes M, De Schepper AM. The pelvic congestion syndrome: role of the "nutcracker phenomenon" and results of endovascular treatment. *JBR-BTR.* 2004;87:1–8.

243. Nascimento AB, Mitchell DG, Holland G. Ovarian veins: magnetic resonance imaging findings in an asymptomatic population. *J Magn Reson Imaging.* 2002;15:551–556.

244. Gargiulo T, Mais V, Brokaj L, et al. Bilateral laparoscopic transperitoneal ligation of ovarian veins for treatment of pelvic congestion syndrome. *J Am Assoc Gynecol Laparosc.* 2003;10:501–504.

245. Venbrux AC, Chang AH, Kim HS, et al. Pelvic congestion syndrome (pelvic venous incompetence): impact of ovarian and internal iliac vein embolotherapy on menstrual cycle and chronic pelvic pain. *J Vasc Interv Radiol.* 2002;13:171–178.

246. Park SJ, Lim JW, Ko YT, et al. Diagnosis of pelvic congestion syndrome using transabdominal and transvaginal sonography. *Am J Roentgenol.* 2004;182:683–688.

247. Rozenblit AM, Ricci ZJ, Tuvia J, et al. Incompetent and dilated ovarian veins: a common CT finding in asymptomatic parous women. *AJR Am J Roentgenol.* 2001;176:119–122.

248. Coakley FV, Varghese SL, Hricak H. CT and MRI of pelvic varices in women. *J Comput Assist Tomogr.* 1999;23:429–434.

249. Scultetus AH, Villavicencio JL, Gillespie DL. The nutcracker syndrome: its role in the pelvic venous disorders. *J Vasc Surg.* 2001;34:812–819.

250. Grella L, Arnold TE, Kvilekval KH, et al. Intravenous leiomyomatosis. *J Vasc Surg.* 1994;20:987–994.

251. Kaszar-Seibert DJ, Gauvin GP, Rogoff PA, et al. Intracardiac extension of intravenous leiomyomatosis. *Radiology.* 1988;168:409–410.

252. Dunlap HJ, Udjus K. Atypical leiomyoma arising in an hepatic vein with extension into the inferior vena cava and right atrium. Report of a case in a child. *Pediatr Radiol.* 1990;20:202–203.

253. Jurayj MN, Midell AI, Bederman S, et al. Primary leiomyosarcomas of the inferior vena cava. Report of a case and review of the literature. *Cancer.* 1970;26:1349–1353.

254. Wray RC Jr, Dawkins H. Primary smooth muscle tumors of the inferior vena cava. *Ann Surg.* 1971;174:1009–1018.

255. Akatsuka N, Tokunaga K, Isshiki T, et al. Intravenous leiomyomatosis of the uterus with continuous extension into the pulmonary artery. *Jpn Heart J.* 1984;25:651–659.

256. Nishizawa J, Matsumoto M, Sugita T, et al. Intravenous leiomyomatosis extending into the right ventricle associated with pulmonary metastasis and extensive arteriovenous fistula. *J Am Coll Surg.* 2004;198:842–843.

257. Stehling MK, Rosen MP, Weintraub J, et al. Spiral CT venography of the lower extremity. *AJR Am J Roentgenol.* 1994;163:451–453.

258. Loud PA, Klippenstein DL. Lower extremity deep venous thrombosis in cancer patients: correlation of presenting symptoms with venous sonographic findings. *J Ultrasound Med.* 1998;17:693–696; quiz 697–698.

259. Peterson DA, Kazerooni EA, Wakefield TW, et al. Computed tomographic venography is specific but not sensitive for diagnosis of acute lower-extremity deep venous thrombosis in patients with suspected pulmonary embolus. *J Vasc Surg.* 2001;34:798–804.

260. Katz DS, Loud PA, Bruce D, et al. Combined CT venography and pulmonary angiography: a comprehensive review. *Radiographics.* 2002;22[Spec No]:S3–S19; discussion S20–S24.

261. Loud PA, Katz DS, Bruce DA, et al. Deep venous thrombosis with suspected pulmonary embolism: detection with combined CT venography and pulmonary angiography. *Radiology.* 2001;219:498–502.

262. Yankelevitz DF, Gamsu G, Shah A, et al. Optimization of combined CT pulmonary angiography with lower extremity CT venography. *AJR Am J Roentgenol.* 2000;174:67–69.

263. Das M, Muhlenbruch G, Mahnken AH, et al. Optimized image reconstruction for detection of deep venous thrombosis at multidetector-row CT venography. *Eur Radiol.* 2006;16(2):269–275. Epub 2005 Aug 2.

264. Abdelmoumene Y, Chevallier P, Barghouth G, et al. Technical innovation. Optimization of multidetector CT venography performed with elastic stockings on patients' lower extremities: a preliminary study of nonthrombosed veins. *AJR Am J Roentgenol.* 2003;180:1093–1094.

265. Garg K, Mao J. Deep venous thrombosis: spectrum of findings and pitfalls in interpretation on CT venography. *AJR Am J Roentgenol.* 2001;177:319–323.

266. Cham MD, Yankelevitz DF, Shaham D, et al. Deep venous thrombosis: detection by using indirect CT venography. The Pulmonary Angiography-Indirect CT Venography Cooperative Group. *Radiology.* 2000;216:744–751.

267. Coche EE, Hamoir XL, Hammer FD, et al. Using dual-detector helical CT angiography to detect deep venous thrombosis in patients with suspicion of pulmonary embolism: diagnostic value and additional findings. *AJR Am J Roentgenol.* 2001;176:1035–1039.

268. Duwe KM, Shiau M, Budorick NE, et al. Evaluation of the lower extremity veins in patients with suspected pulmonary embolism: a retrospective comparison of helical CT venography and sonography. 2000 ARRS Executive Council Award I. American Roentgen Ray Society. *AJR Am J Roentgenol.* 2000;175:1525–1531.

269. Garg K, Kemp JL, Wojcik D, et al. Thromboembolic disease: comparison of combined CT pulmonary angiography and venography with bilateral leg sonography in 70 patients. *AJR Am J Roentgenol.* 2000;175:997–1001.

270. Richman PB, Wood J, Kasper DM, et al. Contribution of indirect computed tomography venography to computed tomography angiography of the chest for the diagnosis of thromboembolic disease in two United States emergency departments. *J Thromb Haemost.* 2003;1:652–657.

271. Ghaye B, Nchimi A, Noukoua CT, et al. Does multi-detector row CT pulmonary angiography reduce the incremental value of indirect CT venography compared with single-detector row CT pulmonary angiography? *Radiology.* 2006;240:256–262.

272. Rademaker J, Griesshaber V, Hidajat N, et al. Combined CT pulmonary angiography and venography for diagnosis of pulmonary embolism and deep vein thrombosis: radiation dose. *J Thorac Imaging.* 2001;16:297–299.

273. Ruehm SG, Wiesner W, Debatin JF. Pelvic and lower extremity veins: contrast-enhanced three-dimensional MR venography with a dedicated vascular coil-initial experience. *Radiology.* 2000;215:421–427.

274. Cogo A, Lensing AW, Wells P, et al. Noninvasive objective tests for the diagnosis of clinically suspected deep-vein thrombosis. *Haemostasis.* 1995;25:27–39.

275. Eskandari MK, Sugimoto H, Richardson T, et al. Is color-flow duplex a good diagnostic test for detection of isolated calf vein thrombosis in high-risk patients? *Angiology.* 2000;51:705–710.

276. Sica GT, Pugach ME, Koniaris LS, et al. Isolated calf vein thrombosis: comparison of MR venography and conventional venography after initial sonography in symptomatic patients. *Acad Radiol.* 2001;8:856–863.

277. Fraser DG, Moody AR, Morgan PS, et al. Diagnosis of lower-limb deep venous thrombosis: a prospective blinded study of magnetic resonance direct thrombus imaging. *Ann Intern Med.* 2002;136:89–98.

278. Hartman DS, Hayes WS, Choyke PL, et al. From the archives of the AFIP. Leiomyosarcoma of the retroperitoneum and inferior vena cava: radiologic-pathologic correlation. *Radiographics.* 1992;12:1203–1220.

279. Mingoli A, Cavallaro A, Sapienza P, et al. International registry of inferior vena cava leiomyosarcoma: analysis of a world series on 218 patients. *Anticancer Res.* 1996;16:3201–3205.

280. Redla S, Kantor R. Case of the month. A lump in the abdomen. *Br J Radiol.* 1999;72:517–518.

281. Singh-Panghaal S, Karcnik TJ, Wachsberg RH, et al. Inferior vena caval leiomyosarcoma: diagnosis and biopsy with color Doppler sonography. *J Clin Ultrasound.* 1997;25:275–278.

282. Bailey RV, Stribling J, Weitzner S, et al. Leiomyosarcoma of the inferior vena cava: report of a case and review of the literature. Ann Surg. 1976;184:169–173.

283. Coughlin JR, Andrews S. Growth of a leiomyosarcoma of the inferior vena cava. *Can Assoc Radiol J.* 1992;43:221–224.

284. Hollenbeck ST, Grobmyer SR, Kent KC, et al. Surgical treatment and outcomes of patients with primary inferior vena cava leiomyosarcoma. *J Am Coll Surg.* 2003;197:575–579.

285. Dzsinich C, Gloviczki P, van Heerden JA, et al. Primary venous leiomyosarcoma: a rare but lethal disease. *J Vasc Surg.* 1992;15:595–603.

286. Charette S, Nehler MR, Whitehill TA, et al. Epithelioid hemangioendothelioma of the common femoral vein: case report and review of the literature. *J Vasc Surg.* 2001;33:1100–1103.

287. Ferretti GR, Chiles C, Woodruff RD, et al. Epithelioid hemangioendothelioma of the superior vena cava: computed tomography demonstration and review of the literature. *J Thorac Imaging.* 1998;13:45–48.

288. Wang CP, Chang YL, Sheen TS. Vascular leiomyoma of the head and neck. *Laryngoscope.* 2004;114:661–665.

289. Ramesh P, Annapureddy SR, Khan F, et al. Angioleiomyoma: a clinical, pathological and radiological review. *Int J Clin Pract.* 2004;58:587–591.

290. Kugimoto Y, Asami A, Shigematsu M, et al. Giant vascular leiomyoma with extensive calcification in the forearm. *J Orthop Sci.* 2004;9:310–313.

291. Hachisuga T, Hashimoto H, Enjoji M. Angioleiomyoma. A clinicopathologic reappraisal of 562 cases. *Cancer.* 1984;54:126–130.

292. Duhig JT, Ayer JP. Vascular leiomyoma. A study of sixtyone cases. *Arch Pathol.* 1959;68:424–430.

293. Chen BB, Chen CA, Liu KL. Leiomyomatosis with extension to the left gluteal muscle, inferior vena cava, and right atrium. *AJR Am J Roentgenol.* 2006;187:W546–W547.

294. Hong SG, Cho HM, Chin HM, et al. Intravascular papillary endothelial hyperplasia (Masson's hemangioma) of the liver: a new hepatic lesion. *J Korean Med Sci.* 2004;19:305–308.

295. Lee SH, Suh JS, Lim BI, et al. Intravascular papillary endothelial hyperplasia of the extremities: MR imaging findings with pathologic correlation. *Eur Radiol.* 2004;14:822–826.

Index

Note: Page numbers followed by *f* indicate figures; page numbers followed by *t* indicate tables.